Herb, Nutrier

and Drug Interactions

Clinical Implications and Therapeutic Strategies

Herb, Nutrient, and Drug Interactions

Clinical Implications and Therapeutic Strategies

Mitchell Bebel Stargrove, ND, LAc

Private Practice, A WellSpring of Natural Health, Inc., Beaverton, Oregon
President, MedicineWorks.com/Health Resources Unlimited, Inc., Beaverton, Oregon
Founder, Editor-in-Chief, IBIS: Integrative BodyMind Information System
Adjunct Professor, Oregon College of Oriental Medicine, Portland, Oregon
Guest Lecturer, National College of Natural Medicine, Portland, Oregon

Jonathan Treasure, MA, MNIMH, RH (AHG)

Medical Herbalist, Centre for Natural Healing, Ashland, Oregon

Dwight L. McKee, MD

Diplomate, American Boards of Internal Medicine, Medical Oncology, and Hematology
Board Certified in Integrative and Holistic Medicine
Certified Nutrition Specialist, Private Practice, Aptos, California
Scientific Director, Life Plus International, Batesville, Arkansas; Cambridgeshire, England

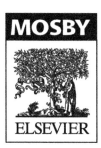

MOSBY

ELSEVIER

11830 Westline Industrial Drive
St. Louis, Missouri 63146

HERB, NUTRIENT, AND DRUG INTERACTIONS:
CLINICAL IMPLICATIONS AND THERAPEUTIC STRATEGIES   ISBN: 978-0-323-02964-3
Copyright © 2008 by Mitchell Bebel Stargrove and Lori Beth Stargrove

---

Notice

Knowledge and best practice in this field are constantly changing. As new research and experience broaden our knowledge, changes in practice, treatment and drug therapy may become necessary or appropriate. Readers are advised to check the most current information provided (i) on procedures featured or (ii) by the manufacturer of each product to be administered, to verify the recommended dose or formula, the method and duration of administration, and contraindications. It is the responsibility of the practitioner, relying on his or her own experience and knowledge of the patient, to make diagnoses, to determine dosages and the best treatment for each individual patient, and to take all appropriate safety precautions. To the fullest extent of the law, neither the Publisher nor the Authors assume any liability for any injury and/or damage to persons or property arising out of or related to any use of the material contained in this book.

The Publisher

Library of Congress Control Number 2007933790

Vice President and Publisher: Linda Duncan
Senior Editor: Kellie White
Senior Developmental Editor: Jennifer Watrous
Publishing Services Manager: Patricia Tannian
Senior Project Manager: Anne Altepeter
Interior Designer: Paula Catalano
Cover Designer: Paula Catalano

Support Team and Reviewers

PROJECT FACILITATOR

Lori Beth Stargrove, ND

Private Practice, President, A WellSpring of Natural Health, Inc., Beaverton, Oregon

TECHNICAL ASSISTANCE, ICON DESIGN, AND DATABASE MANAGEMENT

Raphael B. Stargrove

WebWeaver Design

CONTRIBUTORS

Kimberly Ann Brown, MSAOM, LAc

Research Coordinator, Helfgott Research Institute, Portland, Oregon

Gonzalo Flores, MAcOM, LAc

Private Practice, Groundspring Healing Center, Portland, Oregon

REVIEWERS

Ruth Bar Shalom, ND, LAc

Private Practice, Holistic Medical Center, Santa Cruz, California

Timothy C. Birdsall, ND, FABNO

Vice President, Integrative Medicine, Cancer Treatment Centers of America, Zion, Illinois

Carlo Calabrese, ND, MPH

Senior Investigator, Helfgott Research Institute, Portland, Oregon
Research Professor, National College of Natural Medicine, Portland, Oregon

Hyla Cass, MD

Assistant Clinical Professor of Psychiatry, UCLA School of Medicine, Los Angeles, California
Private Practice, Pacific Palisades, California

Subhuti Dharmananda, PhD

Director, Institute for Traditional Medicine, Portland, Oregon

Michael F. Holick, PhD, MD

Professor of Medicine, Physiology, and Biophysics and Director of the General Clinical Research Center, Boston University Medical Center, Boston, Massachusetts

Alena M. Langsjoen, MS

Laboratory Director, Coenzyme Q10 Laboratory, Inc., Tyler, Texas

Peter H. Langsjoen, MD, FACC

Private Practice in Cardiology
Research in Biomedical and Clinical Aspects of Coenzyme Q10, Tyler, Texas
Affiliated with East Texas Medical Center Hospital and Mother Francis Health System Hospital, Tyler, Texas

Rick Marinelli, ND, MAcOM, LAc

Private Practice, Natural Medicine Clinic, Portland, Oregon
Clinical Professor, National College of Natural Medicine, Portland, Oregon
Doctoral Faculty, Oregon College of Oriental Medicine, Portland, Oregon

Russell B. Marz, ND, LAc

Private Practice, Tabor Hill Clinic, Portland, Oregon
Associate Professor of Nutrition, National College of Natural Medicine, Portland, Oregon
President, Omnivite Nutrition, Inc., Portland, Oregon

Lewis Mehl-Madrona, MD, PhD

Professor, Integrative Psychiatry, University of Arizona, Department of Medicine, Program in Integrative Medicine, Tucson, Arizona; University of Saskatchewan College of Medicine, Saskatoon, Saskatchewan

William A. Mitchell, ND

Co-Founder; Clinical Professor, Advanced Integrated Therapeutics, Bastyr University, Kenmore, Washington
Private Practice, Seattle, Washington

Shauna Rey, ND

Staff Naturopathic Physician, Midwestern Regional Medical Center, Cancer Treatment Centers of America, Zion, Illinois

Peggy M. Rollo, ND, LAc

Private Practice, Portland, Oregon

Kia Sanford, MS, CN

Private Practice, Ashland, Oregon

Lori Beth Stargrove, ND

Private Practice, A WellSpring of Natural Health, Inc., Beaverton, Oregon

Maret G. Traber, PhD

Professor of Nutrition; Principal Investigator, Linus Pauling Institute, Oregon State University, Corvallis, Oregon

Don West, RPh

Lloyd Center Pharmacy, Portland, Oregon

To those who have inspired us,
who have welcomed us,
who have taught, and supported us,
in our challenges, growth, shortcomings, and successes;

Those with whom we share our lives and work,
with whom we play, create, grow, and endure,
as we evolve together,
in our understanding, appreciation, and respect for one another;

Those who come to us, who trust and challenge us,
who ask difficult questions and want honest responses,
who honor us with the challenge and privilege of serving them
in their healing and self-discovery;

That we may care for each and all, including ourselves,
just a little bit better,
working together in a sincere effort
toward healing, truth, and peace
in every interaction.

Acknowledgments

Reviewers:

Ruth Bar Shalom, ND, LAc
Timothy C. Birdsall, ND
Carlo Calabrese, ND, MPH
Hyla Cass, MD
Subhuti Dharmananda, PhD
Michael F. Holick, PhD, MD
Alena M. Langsjoen, MS
Peter H. Langsjoen, MD, FACC
Rick Marinelli, ND, MAcOM, LAc
Russell B. Marz, ND, LAc

Lewis Mehl-Madrona, MD, PhD
William A. Mitchell, ND
Shauna Rey, ND
Peggy M. Rollo, ND, LAc
Kia Sanford, MS, CN
Lori Beth Stargrove, ND
Maret G. Traber, PhD
Don West, RPh

Special gratitude and appreciation for inspiration, participation, support, and patient perseverance to:

Lori Beth Stargrove, ND
Jillellen McKee, DO
Joanne Chase
The Bebel and Kopacz, Isenberg, and Sternheim families
Raphael B. Stargrove
Tara R. Stargrove
Sage S. Stargrove
Richard W. Bebel
Mary A. Bebel
Norbert Isenberg, PhD
Edith Isenberg, RN
Stephanie Sandstrom
Owen Treasure
Kellie White
Jennifer Watrous
Anne Altepeter
Roger L. McWilliams
Inta Ozols
Linda Duncan
Sara Snyder
Larry Park
Claire de la Mer
Marilyn Wasson
Kelley Schaefer-Levi
Jacob S. Gill
Tatiana Lifshitz
David Weitzer, LMT
Janice Weitzer, LMT
Satya Ambrose, ND, LAc
Duncan Soule, MD
David Young, DC
Grant Dawson, DC
John Bastyr, ND
William Turska, ND
Robert Broadwell, ND, LAc
William A. Mitchell, ND

Joseph E. Pizzorno, Jr, ND
Jared L. Zeff, ND, LAc
Tieraona Low Dog, MD
Wayne Jonas, MD
David S. Riley, MD
Pamela Snider, ND
John Weeks
Robert Stern, DC, CFE
Bruce Canvasser, ND
Heiner Freuhauf, PhD, LAc
Clyde Jensen, PhD
Eric F. Stephens, DAOM, LAc
David M. Eisenberg, MD
Robert Scholten, MSLIS
Ted J. Kaptchuk, OMD
Steve Austin, ND
Timothy C. Birdsall, ND
Alan R. Gaby, MD
Jonathan V. Wright, MD
Christopher A. Foley, MD
Melvin R. Werbach, MD
Bruce N. Ames, PhD
Candace B. Pert, PhD
Micheal R. Ruff, PhD
Leland Kaiser, PhD
Mildred S. Seeling, MD, MPH, FACN
Gonzalo Flores, MAcOM, LAc
John K. Chen, PhD, PharmD, OMD, LAc
Jerry Cott, PhD
Iris Bell, MD, PhD
Jackie Wootton, MEd
Joseph J. Jacobs, MD, MBA
Subhuti Dharmananda, PhD
Ethan Depweg, MAcOM, LAc
Peter Eschwey, MAcOM, LAc
Sheila Barnhart

Nicki Scully
Mark Hallert
Terry L. Neal
Parvinder S. Kohli
James A. Spake, MEd, LMT
Prof. Wang Qingyu
Sri Dadaji Mahendranath
Dr. T.H. Trismegistus

Prof. D. Mahalakshmi
Prof. Ganapati
Our patients
Our teachers and mentors
National College of Natural Medicine
Oregon College of Oriental Medicine
The healing environs of the Pacific Northwest

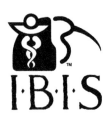

Foreword

Dietary supplements are among the most commonly used complementary and alternative medical therapies in the United States, with sales reportedly exceeding $20 billion in 2005. Newspapers, magazines, and the mass media feed our curiosity for new supplements and ways to manage our health on a daily basis. New dietary supplement formulations flood the shelves of pharmacies, health food stores, retail chains, and Internet outlets. Consumers want to know what works and are willing to pay for products that may make them feel better. However, consumers are also growing frustrated with inconsistencies in product quality and perceived lack of regulatory oversight. Surveys indicate that health care professionals are both interested in learning about, and concerned over the widespread use of, dietary supplements. This is not surprising given the contradictory scientific data and provocative titles in medical journals linking supplements with dangerous adverse events and lack of efficacy. Although many supplements are safely used by the public, there is little question that the complex chemistry of botanicals and multi-ingredient formulations may have profound effects, both beneficial and harmful, on our human physiology.

Dietary supplements marketed in the United States before passage of the Dietary Supplements Health Education Act (DSHEA) in 1994 are not required to demonstrate safety or efficacy, an a priori belief that since these products were already in the marketplace, one could assume a certain level of safety. The assumption that these products are safe and free from adverse effects may lead to excessive dosing, concomitant use with prescription and over-the-counter (OTC) medications, and failure to disclose supplement use to health care providers. According to a large, federally sponsored survey, approximately 28 million Americans are taking dietary supplements with their prescription medications, and 69% of them have not told their primary care provider. As a physician who is also an herbalist, I find that patients generally feel comfortable talking to me about their use of supplements and alternative therapies. Yet, even with my training, I constantly brush up against the edge of my knowledge and experience when a patient asks if taking ginkgo, ginseng, saw palmetto, hawthorn, coenzyme Q10, magnesium, L-carnitine, multivitamin, and a Chinese herbal formulation called *xin li shu kang wan* will interact in any way with his quinapril, amiodarone, clopidrogel bisulfate, simvastatin, and esomeprazole! A difficult question for anyone to answer, but even more for those without any formal training in natural products and limited to the typical 12- to 15-minute patient encounter. As was shown with St. John's wort, however, herb-drug interactions can occur and can be very serious.

It would be easy to assume that if adverse events and interactions with drugs were really a problem, it would be glaringly apparent given the number of people using these products. However, as Chair of the United States Pharmacopeia Dietary Supplements Information Expert Committee, I can attest to the difficulty in determining and establishing safety for many of the dietary supplement ingredients in the marketplace. Many botanicals and nutritional supplements lack detailed pharmacokinetic and pharmacodynamic data. The adverse event reporting systems that are currently in place for drugs are woefully inadequate for monitoring dietary supplement products, given the vast number of complex and unique formulations in the marketplace and the variety of names used on the label (i.e., Latin binomial, common,

foreign language). This makes it almost impossible to enter, retrieve, or analyze information from electronic databases when an adverse event is suspected. Unlike prescription and OTC medications, it can be difficult to ascertain if the adverse event was caused by the ingredient(s) declared on the label, or actually resulted from the accidental or intentional adulteration, substitution, or contamination of the product with a toxic botanical, heavy metal, or pharmaceutical agent. Accurate identification of the dietary supplement is essential for determining causality; however, the point of contact for most serious adverse events is generally a physician who has neither the training nor the funds for collecting, submitting, and paying a laboratory with expertise in analyzing complex botanical or supplement products. This further complicates evaluation of adverse event reports in the medical literature, because product identity is seldom verified. In most cases, the evidence for causality is based primarily on the fact that the supplement cannot be excluded, rather than clear evidence of toxicity. And yet, in the absence of better pharmacological data and an optimal adverse event reporting system, case reports remain a necessary, if problematic, mechanism for monitoring safety.

With the primary emphasis on adverse interactions, the topic of beneficial interactions has received little attention. It is well recognized that statin medications deplete coenzyme Q10 in the body. Preliminary evidence suggests that administering 50 to 100 mg per day of the supplement may reduce the myopathies that are reported by about 20% of patients using this class of lipid-lowering medications. A growing body of evidence supports the administration of glutamine during chemotherapy to prevent neuropathy, whereas selenium was shown to reduce the nephrotoxicity associated with cisplatin. Low serum folate levels decrease the effectiveness of antidepressant medications. An integrative approach would utilize therapies that reduce or mitigate the adverse effects of medications deemed necessary for the patient whenever possible.

It is within this climate that I enthusiastically welcome this book, a collaboration written by experienced clinicians within the fields of conventional, integrative, and natural medicine for health professionals who wish to counsel their patients effectively on the safe and beneficial use of dietary supplements. As the title suggests, this book addresses herb-drug interactions, nutrient-drug interactions, and drug-induced nutrient depletions in a clinically oriented, integrative manner. The authors demonstrate an appropriate balance between recommendation and risk based on the overall strength of the scientific evidence and their own clinical experience. The text is well referenced, balanced, and objective, and the use of icons and summary tables allows the clinician to quickly identify areas of potential risk, as well as potential benefit. This book is a major contribution to the field of integrative medicine and an invaluable resource to practitioner and researcher alike.

Tieraona Low Dog, MD
Director of Education, Program in Integrative Medicine
Clinical Assistant Professor, Department of Medicine
University of Arizona College of Medicine
Chair, United States Pharmacopeia Dietary Supplements
Information Expert Panel

We are in the midst of a critical historic juncture in the evolution of medicine. Three major currents are influencing the practice of medicine, the science underlying its methodology, and the relationship between caregiver and patient. First, a significant proportion of patients are exercising greater levels of self-education and self-care, requesting greater opportunity for informed decision making and often demanding a realignment of the usual power relationships in conventional medicine. Second, the emergence of personalized medicine, particularly but not only in the form of genomics, pharmacogenomics, and nutrigenomics, offers the promise of tailoring efficacy while decreasing adverse effects in a manner that offers a modern scientific approach to individualization of care beyond generic pathology and lowest-common-denominator generalizations. Third, the now well-established recognition of medical pluralism mandates greater communication and collaboration between health care providers of various medical traditions from diverse cultures and philosophies, methodologies and therapeutics. Together, these factors give a profoundly transdisciplinary impetus to the development of enhanced clinical strategies synthesizing the science of medicine and the art of healing in a process-oriented approach to the individual patient.

Within the context of these converging influences, the issues arising from the potential interactions between conventional drug therapies and herbal and nutritional therapies present both a challenge and an opportunity. The challenge involves unanticipated adverse drug reactions (ADRs). The opportunity involves the potential for enhancing the depth and breadth of the mainstream medical model, ultimately improving the success of clinical outcomes. After more than two decades of complementary and "alternative" medicine ("CAM") and subsequent optimistic portents of an era of "integrative medicine," the average practitioner surveying the medical landscape for substantive changes in the clinical care model usually sees only glimmers of vision, moments of inspiration, and select ideal cases. Such aspirations may be suitable for some, but most clinicians would be content simply with effective tools for understanding other disciplines, how their patients are using them, and the implications when mixing pharmaceutical medicines and other modalities. Nevertheless, our patients are using a diverse array of medical approaches, and we all are entering a world of transdisciplinary care and personalized medicine, complexity models of physiology, and unprecedented access to information. In this context, the discovery of new synergies and unparalleled collegial collaboration offer the promise of enhanced patient empowerment and novel clinical strategies. Ultimately, we must always keep in mind that our first and only loyalty can be to our patients and their health, even if it forces us to grapple with the unfamiliar and acknowledge the unconventional.

PURPOSE AND FUNCTION

The present work derives from the clinical needs of practicing health care professionals who have been compiling, analyzing, and publishing assessments on interactions for two decades. Interactions between drugs and nutrients first became a subject of review and education in 1988 during the development of the *Integrative BodyMind Information System (IBIS)* database.

On publication of that reference tool, clinicians increasingly requested deeper coverage of interactions issues involving nutrients and herbs, in response to widespread and growing use of such products by their patients and clinicians' desire to integrate such agents into their therapeutic repertoire. In 1997, exhortations from physicians and educators precipitated a dedicated focus on interactions issues in a clinical context and catalyzed development of the *Interactions* software database, subsequently published in 2000. That reference work essentially functioned as the first edition of the research and writing that has evolved into the present publication. Through that experience and several years of input and feedback from health care professionals and educators around the world, as well as inquiries from an online reporting and resource website, the models, methods, and tools applied in the creation of this publication were developed and refined. In particular, a year of intensive investigation, dialogue, and debate produced the pioneering system of interaction characterization, literature evaluation, and clinical probability applied in reviewing, compiling, and assessing the relevant scientific and medical literature. Thus, the current volume represents the indirect outcome of almost 20 years of work and 10 years of direct efforts.

Interactions between pharmaceutical drugs and "natural" products such as nutrients and herbs constitute an area of immediate concern and growing awareness wherever patients are receiving health care and members of the public are engaged in self-care through use of these substances. Many patients naively assume that nutrient and herbal products are "natural" and that this somehow implies they are "safe." More disturbing is the acknowledged fact that many patients often withhold disclosure of nutrient and herbal intake or use of nonconventional care from their conventional health care providers. This combination suggests the need for deep inquiry and analysis into the doctor-patient relationship and the coordination of medical care. In the meantime, however, clinicians need a guide to working with patients using nutrients and herbs and guidelines for crafting their interventions to coordinate these elements. This book is most directly intended to serve this need among health care professionals, educators, and students throughout the whole range of medical professions. The depth of coverage, the emphasis on research, and the focus on practical implications address the needs of this professional audience. Secondarily, this information will be of benefit to individuals in other professions, ranging from librarians to retail staff, faced with questions from the general public regarding these issues.

An overview of the presently available literature reveals the predominance of two types of print and electronic publications covering this subject matter: those intended for the professional market and those intended for a consumer/patient audience. The same data may also be disseminated differently for use by both audiences. In both cases, most publications can fairly be characterized as lacking in depth and incomplete or overreaching in conclusions.

The professional literature tends to assume that patients using nutrients and herbs ("dietary supplements") are doing so without supervision of health care professionals trained and experienced in the therapeutic application of nutritional and botanical therapies. Lack of disclosure by patients also tends to be the case, and greater awareness, frank discussion, and informed decision making in these areas are necessary for effective clinical management as well as patients' perception of respect for their choices. Similarly, especially in complex and chronic conditions, the use of multiple providers from several different health care disciplines is increasingly common. Professionals in all disciplines can increase clinical efficacy and patient safety through open dialogue and collegial (peer-to-peer) collaboration. However, interactions literature is often prepared by health care professionals without training or experience in nutritional and botanical therapies. Therefore, the advantages of purposefully combining, strategically sequencing, or deliberately avoiding such interventions are usually not addressed in a comprehensive and practical way. In addition, the interactions reference texts and guides developed for consumers are limited in depth, often avoid critical issues, and sometimes prey on readers' fears by exaggeration and headline hyperbole. Furthermore, the commercial context of their use frequently presents an apparent conflict of interest, especially when provided as aids in product selection in a retail setting. Similarly, these guides are presented as online educational tools appended to broader coverage of "alternative medicine" within the context of medical, pharmaceutical, or insurance websites. Either situation implies significant constraints as to thoroughness, rigor, and efficacy because caution is justifiably the operative premise. The issue of apparent conflict of interest and possible bias must always be considered in a setting funded and presented by commercial interests, both for what is said and what is avoided. Inherently, the scope, thoroughness, and standards of evidence tend to be different for consumer education (or promotional) publications than for professional publications because of the vast divergence in educational level, operational needs, and responsibility. Overall, the literature available to most of the general public, whether magazines, books, friends and family, or the Internet, tends to avoid recommendation of these agents at therapeutic doses or in a manner that might be construed as treating diagnosed conditions.

By contrast, in this book we explore many methods of using nutritional and herbal interventions not only as "dietary supplements" but also as components of comprehensive, transdisciplinary therapeutic strategies. This approach diverges fundamentally from typical drug interactions databases marketed for physicians, especially those for handheld devices, that list telegraphic warnings (often unsubstantiated) about "supplements" without context or qualification. Where concomitant administration of nutrients and herbs might harm a patient or significantly interfere with predictable effects of conventional medications, the priority of ensuring patient safety is established throughout the text by providing cautions and suggesting modifications based on scientific literature and clinical experience.

METHODOLOGY AND STRUCTURE

The methodology applied in developing this publication involved two steps. First, input was gathered from among the authors and other clinicians, as well as pharmacists and educators, as to potential interactions they were seeing in clinical practice and of substantive clinical relevance, particularly potential risk or observed therapeutic value. Second, available reference works on interactions, including drug-drug interactions literature, were reviewed for scope, depth, methodology, and presentation. This method ensures that we incorporated the best of all approaches, building on those from our own

experience, and avoiding or countering those methods and characteristics that lead to poorly founded, overreaching, or misleading conclusions. Ultimately, the team that produced this book was determined to make realistic assessment of clinical relevance and evidence quality its foundation. Only a product that would meet the standards of what we would feel confident using in our own practices would be acceptable for publication. Thus, the research and editorial team consists of practicing health care professionals trained in therapeutic nutrition, botanical medicine, pharmacology, and pharmacognosy with experience on a daily basis in general family practice and specialty care, with an emphasis on internal medicine, oncology, and hematology. This text is therefore itself a result of collaboration among practicing experts from different modalities that is emblematic of the transdisciplinary collaboration that ultimately is required to understand and manage drug-nutrient and drug-herb interactions. This fact alone distinguishes this text from other publications that claim to cover the topics but present one-sided, theoretical, or partial approaches that necessarily lack the transdisciplinary insight and clinical relevance of this collaboration. Perhaps most importantly, our authors are deeply enmeshed in collaborative care on a daily basis, bringing together health care professionals from multiple disciplines and combining therapies from multiple modalities.

In areas where the available resources appeared to be limited, immature, or flawed, the authors systematically addressed three primary needs. First, the lack of a multidisciplinary approach inherent in the existing literature leads to the common tendency, for example, to assert potential interactions imputed from assumed pharmacological theory, without any corroboration from clinical experience with the interacting agents. Other than research into certain well-known drug-induced nutrient depletion patterns, direct clinical trials of adequate power are nearly absent from literature pertaining to drug-herb and drug-nutrient interactions. Overall, the primary source evidence tends to be delayed and reactive, fragmented, or tangential to other research objectives, or simply unapparent to those not trained and experienced in these fields. Consequently, many interactions supported by readily available evidence are simply not described in most texts. Also, many interactions based on substandard or preliminary evidence are given more weight than they deserve. In such cases, contextualization and "debunking" of the putative or alleged interactions often result from the necessary "reality check." This problem also derives from overreliance on secondary literature (e.g., reviews, meta-analyses) and derivative material in topical publications. Second, no previously available text, including our first effort, incorporates sufficient detail to assess effectively the quality of the original data; the strengths and limitations of the study design, size, and duration; or the characteristics or even the dose, form, or other critical particulars of the agents involved. Third, *clinical relevance* and *therapeutic implications* need to be the primary goal of analysis of all interactions.

In light of these many factors, this text relies primarily on evidence from clinical trials whenever possible, using reasonable extrapolations from human research as secondary evidence and relegating animal studies or in vitro experiments to a supportive role. Published case reports are assessed based on the strength of their relevance, detail, and quality. Extrapolations can be reasonable or not. Our in-depth examination of the published literature revealed that the available secondary and derivative literature contains at worst an abundance of confusion and at best a lack of clarity on decisive facts, such as proper identification of a nutrient or herb and the plant part used, naturally occurring nutrients or whole herbs versus synthetic forms or extracts, doses outside the range of those considered safe and clinically effective, diverse modes of administration, and distinctive or even divergent characteristics of subject populations. In particular, the repeated citation of a poor-quality case report, irrelevant finding, or flawed research in multiple publications suggests superficial recycling of citations by secondary authors without full text review of original sources or critical analysis of conclusions. The pervasive interchanging as equivalents of *Ephedra* (the plant) and ephedrine (a pharmaceutical alkaloid) provides a stark illustration of this problem and its reverberations, despite the presumed good intentions of those making the assertions. In contrast, this text notes if studies use forms of an agent that experienced practitioners would shun, or doses too high for safety or too low for therapeutic efficacy. Perhaps most important is the recognition that uninformed administration of agents, or combinations of agents, in a manner wholly detached from the logic, methodology, or standards and guidelines of appropriate clinical practice and historical context from which they are derived, does not constitute an "adverse event" or "interaction."

A significant gap often exists between the research literature and clinical practice in regard to the origins and form of many agents studied in the scientific literature. Not all nutrients or botanically derived preparations can accurately be described as "natural" medicines; many do not appear in nature and are more accurately placed in the province of "pharmaceutical preparations" rather than herbs or nutrients as traditionally understood or historically practiced. Thus, a gradient can be articulated spanning pharmaceutical nutrients (e.g., dl-alpha-tocopherol, i.e., racemic synthetic vitamin E), isolated preparations of naturally occurring nutrient and botanical constituents, foods and herbs in whole or minimally modified forms (with inherent diversity and variability of constituents), and nutrients and herbs in combinations or formulae (with even greater complexity). Often the isolated constituents and synthetic preparations or mixed isomers used in research studies contrast sharply with the forms (whether naturally occurring or crafted in accordance with traditional methodologies) typically used by practitioners trained and experienced in nutritional and botanical therapeutics. Moreover, the issues affecting interactions analysis are confounded by the recurrent paradox observed in innumerable papers on broader topics in which authors voice contradictory assumptions and conclusions; first, that whole-food sources are safer and more effective than, and generally preferable to, nutrients (or herbal) constituents in pill or tablet form, but second, that foods, herbs, nonstandardized extracts or isolates, or multicomponent formulae do not fit the methodology of study designs oriented to assessing single-agent pharmaceutical interventions. The resulting statements that naturally occurring and synthetic forms are equivalent, and recurrent findings that food (or herbal) sources provide benefits not found in synthetic supplemental or extracted forms, at least not in those specific forms studied, suggest that naturally occurring forms, identical in origin, to food (or plant) sources may be the missing link. Further, authors of research papers, and even more so those who read abstracts or press releases and then write articles on these papers for the professional and lay press, often fail to discriminate between studies using naturally occurring forms, dosage levels, and modes of administration typical in experienced clinical practice and studies using isolates or synthetic variants. Consequently, ill-founded extrapolations and unsubstantiated conclusions and warnings often result that diverge from the actual research findings and even more so from real-world clinical implications. In general, it might be stated that foods are a common preference among practitioners

emphasizing nutritional therapies in their clinical practice. However, the therapeutic efficacy of food sources can be limited by several critical factors, including difficulty in achieving necessary dose thresholds of specific nutrients or constituents on a consistent basis because of volume of food sources required, low rates of compliance in the regular consumption of such required doses of necessary food items, and, in more recent decades, declining nutrient quality of commercially available foods.

Similarly, just as there is a large divergence between primary literature and the secondary literature of reviews and meta-analyses, an even greater separation exists between primary sources and editorial news coverage in both professional publications and popular press, as well as in educational materials and tools available to the typical patient/consumer. In particular, three primary limitations appear on analysis. First, the nature of study populations is often not defined, particularly with reference to critical distinctions between healthy subjects and those with diagnosed conditions. The related factors, such as genetic risk and pharmacogenomic variability, gender and age, health status, and socioeconomic vulnerabilities, are only considered on rare occasions. Second, critical factors in study design, such as cohort size, dose, form, duration of administration, and other potentially confounding influences, can significantly alter outcomes and the interpretation of findings. In many cases, these variables would be significant enough to create major divergences in assessing conclusions because characteristics of a given study could plausibly alter effects, but such characteristics were not mentioned or factored into the analysis and conclusions. Third, certain health care professionals, most notably naturopathic physicians and herbalists of the Euro-American, Chinese–East Asian, and Ayurvedic traditions, employ botanical formulations and nutritional therapeutics as a primary clinical intervention. Whether in these settings or in multidisciplinary integrative approaches, the use of multiple agents within a therapeutic strategy is typical practice, and especially in herbal medicine, single agents are rarely expected to provide the properties, potency, or personalization that a compound formula provides. Such treatment strategies are very difficult to assess adequately using research models or methodologies that assume single-agent interventions, which are uncommon in patients with chronic diseases and complex cases.

The methodology applied in this text emphasizes that supplementation of nutrients (and rarely, nutritive use of herbs) in healthy populations is distinct from unsupervised, concomitant use of nutrient support in individuals concurrently taking prescription drugs (especially those with known nutrient-depleting effects) and from purposeful coadministration of nutrients or herbs with conventional drugs within the context of clinical management by health care professionals applying integrative principles. Therefore, the organization of these interactions monographs involves a spectrum of categories, including "avoidance," "benefit," and "management."

By incorporating summary tables as well as in-depth analysis of each interaction analysis, our text provides a useful combination of brevity and thoroughness by presenting an accurate overview as well as answering needs for deeper access to substance and detail. We refer to this publication as a "comprehensive" reference work because our goal is to articulate the subject in a broad and practical manner, not merely to catalogue available data without reference to origins, therapeutic context, patterns of usage, and clinical implications. In response to feedback from users of the previous software publications and in pursuit of strategic design goals, the current text not only increases the breadth and depth of the topics under consideration, but more importantly also applies a systematic method of analysis and presentation aimed at enhancing the clinical utility of the reviewed information and subsequent analysis. The structure and presentation of each monograph are designed to enable rapid review through summary analysis and coded characterizations of the character, significance, and evidence quality of each substantiated interaction, while also providing greater depth with a thorough review of evidence, mechanisms, and evolution of the scientific literature on the subject.

Each monograph provides basic information on physiology and function of the given nutrient or herbal agent, followed by a summary of established interactions and a review of clinically relevant data that contextualizes the discussion of interactions with specific drugs, including known or potential therapeutic uses and historical/ethnomedicine precedent, deficiency symptoms, dietary sources, nutrient preparations, typical therapeutic and supplemental dosing, laboratory assessment, and safety profile, with nutrient adverse effects, contraindications, and precautions and warnings. The Strategic Considerations section of each monograph discusses the broader clinical role of the particular agent, emphasizing implications of interactions, and further assesses the clinical relevance of the available data, patterns of interactions, and contentious or unresolved issues; this section also presents broad clinical reviews for substances for which substantive interactions evidence is lacking. Each review of a particular interaction dyad is divided into those with substantive evidence, primarily focusing on clinical trials and qualified case reports, and those relying on preliminary, speculative, and/or questionable data. Within each interaction pair, the pharmaceutical agent, and/or drug class, is introduced by generic name(s) and a summary characterization regarding type(s) of interaction(s) involved, quality of the evidence base, and estimated probability of clinical relevance, followed by subsections presenting mechanism(s) of action, evidence and practical clinical implications, suggestions, and cautions.

Presenting the development of evidence chronologically and thematically places emphasis on critical factors such as study design, number and characteristics of subjects, study duration, form, and dosage. Data from in vitro experiments and animal research are primarily used to examine possible mechanisms of action and to elucidate or qualify evidence from human research. In general, the standards applied in evaluating the strength of evidence are less demanding than those appropriate to evaluation of clinical trial relevance. Furthermore, patient safety is emphasized as the highest value, with a focus on optimizing outcomes while minimizing adverse effects. Overall, given the emerging state of interactions literature, the threshold of inclusion applied in weighing the available evidence is often of a lower standard than ideal, and conclusions are often qualified as such, with the oft-repeated recommendation that "further research through well-designed and adequately powered clinical trials is warranted." Specific citations are appended to each monograph, and a separate file listing Reference Literature underpinning the overview presentations for each nutrient monograph is available.

The *default bias* often displayed in the medical literature assumes that interactions involving herbs and nutrients result in adverse effects. Not only are such outcomes merely one of several possible effects, but such reports are also often of substandard quality in the professional literature and are typically caricatured and misrepresented in the popular press. In assessing the quality of evidence, we have appreciated the taxonomy articulated by Fugh-Berman and Ernst (2001) for the review and assessment of report reliability in the area of herb-drug interactions. As noted in their meta-analysis, the data used in making claims of interactions are frequently inadequate and unreliable. Thus, these authors concluded that more than two thirds of published reports reviewed were "unevaluable" and graded only 13% as "well-documented." They also noted that, in contrast to most drugs that contain a single pharmacological agent, most herbal products in use, and thus likely to be involved in possible interactions, tend to contain a variety of pharmacologically active constituents. The typical use of multiple herbs within a formulation further complicates the possibilities of ascribing causal relationships.

The literature of nutrient-drug interactions is typically not much better in quality than that of herb-drug interactions, with the possible exception of research into drug-induced nutrient depletions. Generally, the research cited is limited by several factors: inadequate patient history; presence of concurrent conditions or pathologies; involvement of one or more medications (particularly those with known interactions or adverse effects); lack of adequate recording of such comedications; failure to adequately describe, assay, or otherwise document alleged interactors; incomplete chronology or consideration of time relation of intake among substances; and incomplete consideration of alternative explanations for adverse effects. The need for improvements in the methodology, gathering, and analysis of reports and research of interactions involving herbs and nutrients will benefit all concerned and enable distinctions among harmful, beneficial, and bimodal interactions and clarify the frequency, intensity, and risk parameters influencing such events. Our conscious intention in assessing data is to tilt toward safety and emphasize conservative, nontoxic interventions. The development of this text has also emphasized avoidance of unreasonable and poorly founded extrapolations, especially speculative construction of "backwards interactions" based on tenuous assumptions. For example, asserting that because an herb may relieve symptoms assumed to derive from estrogen deficiency, the herb inherently will adversely interact with agents intended to elevate estrogen levels; or when a nutrient or herbal preparation demonstrates a beneficial effect on glycemic control, it is somehow interpreted as adversely "interacting" with hypoglycemic medications. In fact, however, such effects often represent a therapeutic synergy worth investigating.

Awareness of narrow therapeutic index, titration in response to gradual introduction or withdrawal of any agent, and individualized assessment and evolving interventions stand as the recurrent issues and key operative watchwords in safe and effective implementation of interactions in a clinical setting. Overall, developing methods for approaching potential interactions can help health care professionals avoid inherently dangerous situations; minimize, neutralize, or counter risks and potential adverse effects or impaired therapeutic responses; and engineer increased therapeutic potency through additive, synergistic, or strategic combinations.

Many of the limitations in the scientific literature relating to interactions reflect and parallel those in the broader study of herbal and nutritional therapies in general. The scientific literature available to those attempting to assess the probability and clinical significance of interactions among various agents is inherently incomplete and inclined to be reactive. Whether in the area of drug-drug interactions or those involving nutrients or herbs, the instances of purposeful research into adverse interactions are rare. Case reports and circumstantial findings tend to dominate the literature and are of highly variable quality, with the clear majority qualifying as incomplete and unreliable. Further, although the scientific study of combined drug and nutrient therapies is emerging, and study of drug-induced nutrient depletions is occasionally commanding attention (again, usually in reaction to accumulating reports of adverse outcomes), the literature investigating drug-herb interactions is in a highly preliminary, and often woeful, state. Again, unqualified case reports tend to dominate the headlines, and only recently have experienced practitioners of herbal medicine become involved in designing clinical trials or evaluating case reports. Notably, most discussions of herbs in the conventional literature involve single herbs, and if being used for treatment, then only using a generic, pathology-focused treatment model, when in fact experienced health care professionals almost always prescribe herbs in formulae that are modified to match peculiar individual patient characteristics and that evolve over time in response to changes in the patient's condition. Similarly, the dosages, clinical indications, prescribing methodology, preparation methods, and even plant parts used in most published trials often reflect little on the professional practice of herbal medicine. In other words, the two groups are usually talking about different things, and the designs of most studies have limited relevance to clinical practice of European, American, or East Asian schools of herbal medicine. Thus, we see a surge in discussion of the use of St. John's wort for depression, when a poll of professional herbal prescribers before such papers would have revealed no consistent use of the plant for that condition as a broad psychiatric diagnostic category; perhaps for melancholy and head injuries, but not "depression." Even more disturbing are studies using parts of plants never used or rarely used by herbalists or in doses at grossly different levels of potency than typical in clinical practice. Similar issues arise when looking at studies of vitamins, minerals, or other nutrients where single-agent interventions using forms usually avoided by professional prescribers, and often at doses considered ineffectual, produce insignificant outcomes. "Well, what would you expect; that's why we don't do it that way," is the usual response from experienced botanical/nutritional practitioners. The major consequences of such ill-conceived research are wasted money and resources and lost opportunities at evolving scientific knowledge and collegial collaboration.

The secondary literature discussing interactions involving herbs and nutrients amplifies and distorts the problems with the primary source material. Again, "news" tends to be hyperbolic and inflammatory and information delayed, reactive, and overrun with incestuous overuse of poorly qualified and superficially analyzed or incomplete reviews of the primary literature; consequently the conclusions are often poorly founded and hasty, of questionable clinical relevance, and misleading in their therapeutic implications. "The devil is in the details," and more often than not, no one bothered to look into the details. Although not nearly as "glamorous" and headline producing as adverse events and dangerous interactions, the areas of drug-induced nutrient depletions and integrative interventions combining drugs, nutrients, and/or herbs represent the bulk of substantive interactions material. Beyond simply correcting problematic interactions resulting from ignorance and lack of communication, these potential avenues of purposeful interactions management also constitute the most promising opportunities for the development of scientific knowledge capable of delivering the clinical interventions most likely to result in successful outcomes. Again, we see the necessity of distinguishing between supplemental use of nutrients, especially vitamins and minerals, on a broad level for undifferentiated populations and the clinical application of botanical and nutritional agents as therapeutic interventions in their own right or as part of multicomponent strategies. The quantity and quality

of clinical trials focusing on, or at least taking note of, interactions will grow as researchers in conventional medicine become more conversant with nutrient and herbal therapies and engage practitioners experienced in such modalities in study design. All these observations emphasize the need to develop tools to facilitate submission of clinical data with complete and pertinent details to high-quality case reports of herb-drug-nutrient interactions, with the active cooperation of all parties involved. High-quality case reports can form the basis for meaningful clinical research and allow the emergence of informed and clinically relevant pharmacovigilance.

Grappling with drug-drug interactions is well known for its difficulties, and the emerging field of drug-nutrient and drug-herb interactions introduces many other complications, as mentioned. Because interactions involving drugs are commonplace and can be dangerous, those involving nutrients and herbs need not seem particularly unusual. Most notoriously, as one noted PharmD commented in conversation: "We just assume that warfarin interacts with everything." Drug-drug interactions are known for variability based on dose, timing, gender, hepatic function, and other drug clearance parameters. Reliably predicting interactions involving more than two agents, of any type, inherently invokes greater uncertainty, and any declarations other than probability are best viewed with skepticism. As a result, throughout the interactions literature, including that covering drug-drug interactions, there is often an implicit understanding that such interactions are strictly pharmacodynamic or pharmacokinetic and thus completely within the province of pharmacology. On close examination, however, such assumptions often unravel as it becomes apparent that interactions operate at many levels, and that firm distinctions are elusive and assurances of a complete mechanism of action may be hasty. Interestingly, many combinations described as interactions are not really *interactions* in the narrow technical definition. Although some may be "interactions" in some broader definition, a large proportion of adverse events derive from situations more accurately described as "contraindications" or "inappropriate prescriptions" (e.g., excessive additive effects; contrary actions; effective but inappropriately sequenced interventions; patients too young, compromised, or otherwise inappropriate for a certain agent[s] at the given dose).

Within the interactions literature, scant attention has been paid to the methodology by which interactions are analyzed. Borgert and associates (2005) noted in this connection that the "commonest approach was the no method approach." In general, there is insufficient quantitative dose-response data in herb and nutrient interaction studies to meet rigorous criteria for the accurate demonstration of supra-additive and subadditive effects of different dose levels for a given pair of agents.

THE INTERACTIONS UNIVERSE

The evaluation schema and detailed definitions and standards used in this text are provided in the following Interactions Evaluation Guide. The primary emphasis of this taxonomy is to establish an operational characterization of each interaction pair based on clinical priorities. In summary, the type and clinical significance of each known or potential interaction are parsed according to several variables: pharmacokinetic, pharmacodynamic, or clinical/strategic; adverse, beneficial, or bimodal (bidirectional); prevention or reduction of adverse effects; compensatory or protective response to probable depletions; negligible, cautionary, or avoidance levels of probable effects; and suitability for self-care or necessity of professional management. The levels of probability of clinically significant interaction are graded as "1. Certain," "2. Probable," "3. Possible," "4. Plausible," "5. Improbable," or "6. Unknown." In a parallel assessment, the available and reviewed evidence is evaluated according to strength and quality: "Consensus," "Emerging," "Preliminary," "Mixed," or "Inadequate." The overall position of each interaction pair within this taxonomy is clearly data dependent, and when the available data suggested ambiguity or conflict, a final assignation was established by review and agreement of the entire editorial team.

In this text, all interactions are considered as potentially operating on several levels within the genomic variability and physiology of individual patients, their behavior and local environment, the clinical strategy and therapeutic relationship(s), and among practitioners. These multiple levels may be represented as a set of concentric circles (see figure).

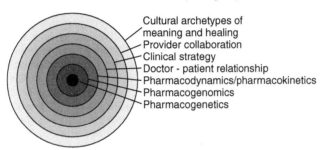

Cultural archetypes of meaning and healing
Provider collaboration
Clinical strategy
Doctor - patient relationship
Pharmacodynamics/pharmacokinetics
Pharmacogenomics
Pharmacogenetics

Interactions Universe

Within this "interactions universe," multiple interventions are more often the rule than the exception, and interactions may be influenced by several different levels; as always, these effects may vary based on patient characteristics and the timing relationship between different interventions. Some interactions may be significantly affected by pharmacogenomic variability, with those involving warfarin, statin drugs, or folic acid being prime examples. In other cases, by shifting the perspective to clinical strategy, what may appear superficially as an interaction may simply be a clinical contraindication; that is, the therapeutic intent of one agent is antagonistic to the other agent, and these would generally be avoided in combination. More subtly, concomitant use of two agents may be characterized as "divergent" or "distracting," in which the action of a secondary or adjuvant therapy could theoretically reduce the action of the primary agent and thereby reduce overall therapeutic efficacy. A similar interaction pattern might be described as "dissonant" when two interventions are potentially appropriate but often can be incompatible in their action or mode of administration. Likewise, from a strategic perspective, some agents in pairs or in clusters, particularly when applied in a logical sequence, may act in a "consonant" manner. Thus, two agents given simultaneously may provide minimal benefit but administered sequentially may enhance therapeutic outcomes through strategic synergy. Two examples of such patterns are seen in the relationship between antibiotics and probiotic flora and, in a more complex form, between chemotherapy and antioxidants. Further, as recognition of herbs and nutrients as therapeutic agents, rather than mere supplements, grows, so does the need for expanding study of interactions between and among herbs and nutrients. Classical herbal traditions all have guidelines regarding synergies and contraindications for coadministration; such a methodology is inherent to formula building. However, research is only coming into the light in regard to such phenomena as the potential adverse effects on healthy intestinal bacterial flora from herbs with direct antibacterial activity, as opposed to indirect immune-enhancing

activity. Once again, we see the need to place all substances with known or potential pharmacological activity on a level playing field using objective research design and integrative clinical approaches.

The complexities of these various influences on drug activity are rarely discussed in the literature with regard to resultant "interactions" and possible clinical implications. For example, clinicians of many modalities might recommend exercise, but how often do they consider the potential impact of exercise on drug metabolism? Might not a sudden increase in physical activity significantly change clearance of certain drugs as much as or more than many common nutrients or herbs? Similarly, in an era when every patient (except those on warfarin) is advised to "eat more fruits and vegetables," how can we calculate the impact of a significant change in dietary habits, especially for the better? Do we want to discourage patient initiative and motivation? Here, for example, one might consider the use of pomegranate juice in the patient with a family history of prostate cancer, or high intake of vegetables in someone with a family history of vascular disease. The recent finding that pomegranate juice, like grapefruit juice, inhibits the 3A4 isotype of cytochrome P450 enzymes involved in the metabolism of many pharmaceuticals, adds another level of complexity to prescribing and pharmacovigilance. Further, when the recommendation of dietary fiber and healthy oils is almost universal, doesn't every clinician need to advise patients about the known pharmacokinetic effects on drug metabolism of increasing fiber (which can bind many medications) or of eating more fish or olive oil, with the unknown implications of the effects of lipids on simultaneously consumed drugs? In considering these possibilities, we realize the limitations of scientific knowledge and clinical experience regarding pharmacokinetics of dietary intake, which does not even take into account the wide, pharmacogenomically determined variability among patients in the activity of hepatic enzymes and other systems of detoxification.

CLINICAL IMPLICATIONS

The questions raised here and throughout this text challenge the attentive reader to reconsider drug activity within the full context of therapeutic strategy and patient outcomes. Simply put, is it a higher priority to manage therapies for the sake of the patients or for the stability of their drug levels? Ultimately, the question arises: when do we counsel patients to avoid healthy behavior on the basis of the possible risk of disrupting predictable drug levels? Even with such cautions and qualifications, can we be certain this is really obtainable? How does such an approach address interindividual biochemical and metabolic variability? These issues have been discussed in nutrition therapeutics for decades (e.g., Roger Williams, PhD, discoverer of pantothenic acid and father of the concept of "metabolic individuality") and are foundational to the methodology of many of the so-called alternative medical traditions. For example, after emphasizing to patients the importance of the modern mantra of "eat right and exercise," how do we accept the paradox of telling "warfarinized" patients with cardiovascular disease to refrain from eating green vegetables, while also asserting repeatedly that food sources of nutrients are inherently superior to pharmaceutical supplemental sources?

Most experienced health care professionals understand that many "disruptive" behaviors (in terms of medication levels) are not really "problematic" in an absolute sense, and that simply refraining from such behaviors is not the answer. In fact, the patient who abruptly stops using a nutrient or herb, drops something from the diet, or radically changes habits out of fear and ill-informed warnings is actually at greater risk from sudden changes. Carried to its extreme, might we not recommend to patients that they sit on the couch and eat only nonnutritive food so as best to maintain stable drug levels? Do we want our patients to imitate the in vitro experiments that we so often caution ourselves not to extrapolate so freely into human physiology? Thus, for example, with patients receiving oral anticoagulants, it would be more desirable, both from a health perspective and in terms of building patient rapport, if we could work with them on increasing healthy foods in their diet, teaching them to maintain a stable intake of dietary vitamin K, while monitoring their INR and titrating it with the appropriate warfarin dosage to maintain the desired clinical effect.

In reviewing the broad literature relevant to interactions between drugs and natural products, four key factors seem paramount and decisive to safety and efficacy: doctor-patient communication and trust; therapeutic index and rapidity of response; monitoring, feedback, and titration; and the urgent need for high-quality research and well-documented case reports together with communication and collaboration. Moreover, the overview of all the findings involving such interactions strongly suggests that other than a minority of clearly dangerous and contraindicated combinations of agents, most interactions are therapeutically advantageous when managed properly, and some portion are between these two polarities, where they pose clinically significant risks only when frank discussion and full disclosure are lacking and corrective measures are not implemented. In some cases, nutritional and herbal therapies may impair activity of a drug by promoting healthy physiological functions (our primary goal) and thereby increase metabolism of stressful or toxic substances, including many drugs. Thus, in these circumstances, the issue is not necessarily incompatibility, but rather lack of coordination and inappropriate timing, such as separation of bile sequestrant intake from the ingestion of fat-soluble nutrients, which tend to be depleted by such a drug, or separating intake of an immune-supportive nutrient such as zinc from antibiotics when the two might chelate when ingested simultaneously.

Although some observations and recommendations in this text may appear unfamiliar to some medical practitioners, the material used is inherently conservative, and the clinical suggestions are designed to be both pragmatic and clinically oriented, with an emphasis on objectivity and evidence, safety and efficacy. Apart from research into certain well-known drug-induced nutrient depletion patterns, direct clinical trials of adequate power are nearly absent from literature pertaining to drug-herb and drug-nutrient interactions. The scant number of reports of well-qualified and clinically significant adverse events suggests that dangers may be less than some have anticipated or declared, especially given the widespread use of herbs and nutrients and the overlap with medication intake. Moreover, research directed at the potential value of the anecdotal evidence available in qualified case reports strongly suggests that these could be a resource of premier value, given the complexities of interactions and the metabolic idiosyncrasies of patients.

Drug-induced nutrient depletion patterns constitute a significant proportion of drug-nutrient interactions. In these situations, awareness of interference with physiological functions of key nutrients or simple decline in available nutrient levels contributes directly or indirectly to known adverse drug effects and offers simple and safe interventions for reducing adverse effects, increasing patient comfort and compliance, and improving therapeutic efficacy and clinical outcomes. Research in this area was largely established in professional discourse by Daphne A. Roe, MD, who focused on such phenomena, particularly in geriatric patients, more than three decades ago. Growing awareness of nutrient use by patients and interest in nutritional therapies within conventional medicine suggest that this body of scientific literature will expand in coming years.

In essence, the issue of interactions presents physicians and other health care professionals with the challenge of working as allies, treating all interventions as options to be evaluated as tactics with a potential to enhance the therapeutic strategy. Thus, we may come to reframe the term "alternative medicine" not as "unconventional" or "competing" but rather as a range of options within a comprehensive repertoire to be considered in light of the patients' risks, needs, and history, as well as their preferences and values, motivation and compliance. Furthermore, effective clinical practice requires more flexible approaches, given the limitations of predictive models, especially when we question whether any model can accurately comprehend and predict the outcomes if more than two factors interact in a patient whose natal pharmacogenomic individuality has been modified by a lifetime's layers of stressors, trauma, and supports. These complexities suggest the need for an evolving and customized response in providing medical care, especially when treating chronic disease, in which some generic elements of treatment intertwine with some highly individualized aspects, and all components shift through phases of the clinical strategy and are crafted to optimize multiple interventions. The nature of the therapeutic relationship and its central role in such a setting emphasize the primacy of establishing and maintaining trust and frank open communication, the ability to be supportive and challenging, especially regarding diet and other lifestyle factors, and the need to be nonjudgmental, flexible, and responsive.

These issues point to patient self-care and utilization of multiple health care professionals from different modalities or specializations as central but often-ignored factors in the clinical reality of drug-herb and drug-nutrient interactions. In discussions of diverse approaches to health care and medicine, two distinct but often-related issues often become confused and inappropriately intermingled.

First, patients are using a wide range of medical treatments, ingesting unsupervised and untested permutations of substance combinations, and experimenting with both ancient and novel techniques and behaviors for enhancing wellness and treating disease. Since the early 1990s, conventional medicine has become increasingly aware of the patterns of utilization of health care services provided by health care professionals other than medical physicians (MDs), as well as use of nonconventional therapies by MDs. Likewise, the emerging educational, legal, and professional infrastructures of accredited educational institutions, professional associations, and licensing laws reveal the continued growth of naturopathic physicians, chiropractors, acupuncturists, massage therapists, medical herbalists, and others. Providing safe and effective clinical care in this environment requires knowledge, mutual respect, communication, and collaboration among health care providers working with individual patients, recognizing, affirming, and utilizing their choices, instincts, experiences, and intuitions. These issues become even more complex when patients have ready access to previously unavailable medical information and demand a partnership based on informed decision making. Professionals may have difficulty accepting that each patient, especially patients with chronic disease, holds this final responsibility and control and that health care providers are simply participants in this critical aspect of the patient's life and personal evolution.

Demographic data indicate that higher educational and income levels are associated with the use of natural medicine and alternative therapies. Whether acting from healthy initiative or desperation, these patients deserve respect in their health care choices and support in obtaining coherent medical care. Self-care is a strong tradition within American, English, and other cultures. Whether Culpepper or the Thomsonian and Hygienic movements, individuals, families, and communities have long fought for their right to continue their traditions of care that predate professional medicine. Although potentially challenging to our authority as educated health care professionals (and to the time constraints of daily practice), education and initiative, informed decision making, and self-empowerment can be our greatest allies in promoting health, preventing illness, and treating disease, with proper timing and strategic coordination. Here, must we not defer to the obvious necessity and professional duty to build trust based on honesty and full disclosure? Enabling frank discussions can provide the most reliable means of respecting patients' choices and satisfying their needs within a context of communication and mutual respect, collaboration and coordination among an integrative team of health care professionals.

This brings us to the second broad and often-unstated issue deeply involved in adverse events and interactions involving patients utilizing the services of multiple health care providers. Short of learning many types of medicine directly, clinicians of every type, whether conventional MDs, practitioners of natural medicine traditions, or practitioners from indigenous medical traditions, can benefit from cultivating collegial alliances with professionals from the diverse health care traditions that their patients utilize, as a means of developing practical familiarity and experience in cross-referrals. Each of these schools of medicine possesses its own respective models, techniques, and tools, and each derives from unique circumstances of history, demographics, and culture. Although simply the result of a lack of opportunity in some cases, ignorance of other health care systems often results from indefensible reliance on ill-founded rumors and inherited prejudices. Rarely does an MD really know the particulars of the chiropractic profession, or vice versa. Likewise, many practitioners of nutritional therapies have little substantive training in herbal medicine, and vice versa, to say nothing of the huge differences among European phytotherapy, American botanical medicine, and Chinese herbal tradition. Unfortunately, besides the notable exception of numerous pharmacists, our patients sometimes have a broader view of the numerous medical options in their repertoire than their health care providers, and that knowledge base is often far wider than deep. None of these parochial attitudes and behaviors serves the interest of our patients or respects their choices and values. Our responsibility as health care professionals is to serve our patients' needs, have access to information regarding the substances they choose to ingest and the procedures they find beneficial, and build collaborative relationships with providers experienced in those approaches, regardless of whether we agree with or support those choices. Ultimately, is any other option professionally ethical, clinically responsible, or therapeutically effective?

Reports of adverse events or interactions involving nutritional therapies or botanical agents almost universally derive from situations of patient self-medication, usually without disclosure or coordinated planning by the health care providers, and often involve faulty preparation, adulteration, contamination, or other departures from typical responses to known interventions. In contrast, substantive reports of adverse events or interactions regarding nutritional therapies or botanical agents prescribed, administered, and supervised by health care professionals trained and experienced in the respective therapies are virtually nonexistent. The few exceptions typically represent interventions considered within the standards of care but subsequently determined to be inappropriate to specific patient populations or in particular dosages or preparations. Thus, MDs, naturopathic physicians, and qualified herbalists have rarely been involved in situations of adverse reactions or interactions with prescribed nutritional or herbal treatments; in fact, they usually are enthusiastic advocates of scientific research through well-designed trials that might ensure safety, clarify indications, and enhance efficacy.

Based on our education, training, and clinical experience and strongly influenced by the process of compiling and analyzing the material in this text, we offer the following final thoughts. First, the issue of interactions involves not only avoiding unnecessary risks, but also recognizing unforeseen opportunities. The greater promise in integrative medicine lies not in the use of naturally occurring agents, such as an herb, food, or nutrient, to treat standard diagnoses in place of pharmaceutical agents, nor in the benefits of expanding the clinical repertoire of conventional medicine, but in rendering its medicines more effective, especially in combination with innovations in pharmacogenomics, systems physiology, and new research methodologies. More profoundly, the very movement of engaging with transdisciplinary approaches and their underlying models offers all practitioners and providers, conventional or otherwise, an inseparable corollary to the restructuring of their practice, the potential for transformation and expansion of their own consciousness, and an openness to a greater vision of the mysterious and miraculous in medicine.

Mitchell Bebel Stargrove, ND, LAc
Jonathan Treasure MA, MNIMH, RH(AHG)
Dwight L. McKee, MD

Bibliography

Adams KM, Lindell KC, Kohlmeier M, Zeisel SH. Status of nutrition education in medical schools. Am J Clin Nutr 2006;83(4):941S-944S.

Aiken LH. Achieving an interdisciplinary workforce in health care. N Engl J Med 2003;348:164-166.

Anonymous. Complementary and alternative medicine: what people 50 and over are using and discussing with their physicians. National Center for Complementary and Alternative Medicine. Accessed January 2007. http://nccam.nih.gov/timetotalk/.

Armstrong SC, Cozza KL, Sandson NB. Six patterns of drug-drug interactions. Psychosomatics 2003;44(3):255-258.

Aronson JK. Unity from diversity: the evidential use of anecdotal reports of adverse drug reactions and interactions. J Eval Clin Pract 2005;11(2):195-208.

Aronson JK, Hauben M. Anecdotes that provide definitive evidence. BMJ, 2006;16;333(7581):1267-1269 (review).

Astin JA, Pelletier KR, Marie A, Haskell WL. Complementary and alternative medicine use among elderly persons: one-year analysis of a Blue Shield Medicare supplement. J Gerontol A Biol Sci Med Sci 2000;55(1):M4-M9.

Berman B, Bausell R, Lee W-L. Use and referral patterns for 22 complementary and alternative medical therapies by members of the American College of Rheumatology: results of a national survey. Arch Intern Med 2002;162(7):766-770.

Borgert CJ, Borgert SA, Findley KC. Synergism, antagonism, or additivity of dietary supplements: application of theory to case studies. Thromb Res 2005;117(1-2):123-132.

Casagrande SS, Wang Y, Anderson C, Gary TL. Have Americans increased their fruit and vegetable intake? The trends between 1988 and 2002. Am J Prev Med 2007;32(4):257-263.

Cherkin DC, Deyo RA, Sherman KJ et al. Characteristics of visits to licensed acupuncturists, chiropractors, massage therapists, and naturopathic physicians. J Am Board Fam Pract 2002;15(6):463-472.

Davis DR, Epp MD, Riordan HD. Changes in USDA food composition data for 43 garden crops, 1950 to 1999. J Am Coll Nutr 2004;23:669-682.

Druss BG, Marcus SC, Olfson M et al. Trends in care by nonphysician clinicians in the United States. N Engl J Med 2003;348(2):130-137.

Druss BG, Rosenheck RA. Association between use of unconventional therapies and conventional medical services. JAMA 1999;282(7):651-656.

Eisenberg DM, Kessler RC, Foster C et al. Unconventional medicine in the United States: prevalence costs, and patterns of use. N Engl J Med 1993; 328(4):246-252.

Eisenberg DM, Kessler RC, Van Rompay MI et al. Perceptions about complementary therapies relative to conventional therapies among adults who use both: results from a national survey. Ann Intern Med 2001;135(5):344-351.

Fugh-Berman A, Ernst E. Herb-drug interactions: review and assessment of report reliability. Br J Clin Pharmacol 2001;52(5):587-595.

Ginsburg GS, Konstance RP, Allsbrook JS, Schulman KA. Implications of pharmacogenomics for drug development and clinical practice. Arch Intern Med 2005;165(20):2331-2336 (review).

Goldstein M, Brown ER, Ballard-Barbash R et al. The use of complementary and alternative medicine among California adults with and without cancer. eCAM 2005;2:557-565.

Grinnell F, Bishop JP, McCullough LB. Bioethical pluralism and complementarity. Perspect Biol Med 2002;45(3):338-349 (review).

Harnack LJ, Rydell SA, Stang J. Prevalence of use of herbal products by adults in the Minneapolis/St Paul, Minn, metropolitan area. Mayo Clin Proc 2001;76(7):688-694.

Hidaka M, Okumura M, Fujita K et al. Effects of pomegranate juice on human cytochrome P450 3A (CYP3A) and carbamazepine pharmacokinetics in rats. Drug Metab Dispos 2005;33(5):644-648.

Howard N, Tsourounis C, Kapusnik-Uner J. Dietary supplement survey of pharmacists: personal and professional practices. J Altern Complement Med 2001;7(6):667-680.

Jadad AR, Moore RA, Carroll D et al. Assessing the quality of reports of randomized clinical trials: is blinding necessary? Control Clin Trials 1996;17(1):1-12.

Kaptchuk TJ. The double-blind, randomized, placebo-controlled trial: gold standard or golden calf? J Clin Epidemiol 2001;54(6):541-549.

Kaptchuk TJ, Eisenberg DM. Varieties of healing. 1. Medical pluralism in the United States. Ann Intern Med 2001;135:189-195.

Kessler RC, Davis RB, Foster DF et al. Long-term trends in the use of complementary and alternative medical therapies in the United States. Ann Intern Med 2001;135(4):262-268.

Lafferty WE, Bellas A, Corage Baden A et al. The use of complementary and alternative medical providers by insured cancer patients in Washington State. Cancer 2004;100(7):1522-1530.

Laine C, Goodman SN, Griswold ME, Sox HC. Reproducible research: moving toward research the public can really trust. Ann Intern Med 2007;146(6): 450-453.

Leung JM, Dzankic S, Manku K, Yuan S. The prevalence and predictors of the use of alternative medicine in presurgical patients in five California hospitals. Anesth Analg 2001;93(4):1062-1068.

Mann HJ. Drug-associated disease: cytochrome P450 interactions. Crit Care Clin 2006;22(2):329-345, vii (review).

Millen AE, Dodd KW, Subar AF. Use of vitamin, mineral, nonvitamin, and non-mineral supplements in the United States: the 1987, 1992, and 2000 National Health Interview Survey results. J Am Diet Assoc 2004;104(6):942-950.

Pal D, Mitra AK. MDR- and CYP3A4-mediated drug-herbal interactions. Life Sci 2006;78(18):2131-2145 (review).

Paramore LC. Use of alternative therapies: estimates from the 1994 Robert Wood Johnson Foundation National Access to Care Survey. J Pain Symptom Manage 1997;13(2):83-89.

Pelletier KR, Marie A, Krasner M, Haskell WL. Current trends in the integration and reimbursement of complementary and alternative medicine by managed care, insurance carriers, and hospital providers. Am J Health Promot 1997;12(2):112-122 (review).

Roe D. Drug-Induced Nutritional Deficiencies, AVI Publishing, Westport, Conn, 1976.

Rothwell PM. External validity of randomised controlled trials: "to whom do the results of this trial apply?" Lancet 2005;365(9453):82-93.

Rothwell PM. Treating individuals. 2. Subgroup analysis in randomised controlled trials: importance, indications, and interpretation. Lancet 2005; 365(9454):176-186.

Rothwell PM, Mehta Z, Howard SC et al. Treating individuals. 3. From subgroups to individuals: general principles and the example of carotid endarterectomy. Lancet 2005;365(9455):256-265.

Stamford BA. Curing health and medical coverage. Am Journalism Rev 2000;56-59.

Tang C, Lin JH, Lu AY. Metabolism-based drug-drug interactions: what determines individual variability in cytochrome P450 induction? Drug Metab Dispos 2005;33(5):603-613 (review).

Treasure J. MEDLINE and the mainstream manufacture of misinformation. Herbal Hypotheses 2;2006. http://www.herbological.com/downloads.html.

Treasure J. Warding off evil in the 21st century: St. John's wort as a xenosensory activator. Herbal Hypotheses 1;2005. http://www.herbological.com/downloads.html.

Votova K, Wister AV. Self-care dimensions of complementary and alternative medicine use among older adults. Gerontology 2007;53(1):21-27.

You, the reader, are invited to send additions, corrections, citations, and other input and feedback to Interactions2@MedicineWorks.com, and to join the interactions forum at http://interactions.medicineworks.com/forum/.

Interactions Evaluation Guide

INTERACTION PROBABILITY GUIDE

I. Probability of Clinically Significant Interaction

Interactions are by definition probable events. As with any statistical variable, meaningful prediction must be based on knowledge of the numerator and denominator.

Probabilities assigned to the interactions in the text are based on the following criteria of combined likelihood and clinical relevance.

1. Certain

Interaction occurrence is definite. Available research and clinical experience both indicate that purposeful coadministration is likely to provide increased therapeutic effect in beneficial interactions. With adverse interaction, concomitant use is definitely to be avoided, even when under the active care of an appropriately trained and experienced health care professional. In most cases, however, it is inadvisable to make sudden changes in usage if the individual's medical condition has been stable.

2. Probable

There is relatively high probability of this interaction occurring, all other factors being equal. Conservative practice implies considering these interactions operationally as definite, unless there are compelling reasons to the contrary. Available evidence or clinical experience indicates that purposeful coadministration may enhance therapeutic intervention. With adverse interaction, concomitant use is generally to be avoided, except when under the active care of an appropriately trained and experienced health care professional. In most cases, however, it is inadvisable to make sudden changes in usage if the individual's medical condition has been stable.

3. Possible

There is variable probability of this interaction occurring, depending on specific circumstances. Operationally, the probability of the interaction may be relatively low for most individuals; however, interindividual and intraindividual variation in probable occurrence of the interaction is likely, depending on multifactorial circumstances, including atypical dosages, certain preexisting medical conditions altering pharmacokinetic or pharmacodynamic parameters, particular risk associated with life stage susceptibilities, and pharmacogenomic and biochemical variability.

4. Plausible

Interaction of plausible, but not proven, likelihood. Although the mechanism and rationale of this interaction appear reasonable based on current knowledge, the available evidence is inadequate to support a conclusive judgment as to the likelihood of its occurrence or the variables influencing the character of such an interaction. However, potential clinical significance of the interaction may warrant careful consideration within integrative therapeutic strategies. This may be based on currently accepted clinical practices among appropriately qualified professionals in botanical and nutritional therapeutics, despite lack of currently available published evidential support.

5. Improbable

This interaction is unlikely to occur in most individuals, all other factors being equal. When taken at commonly used dosages for appropriate medical conditions as prescribed by health care professional(s) trained and experienced in botanical and/or nutritional therapeutics, the probability of clinically significant interaction occurring appears to be minimal.

6. Unknown

Data are contradictory, inconclusive, or insufficient to assign probability status.

INTERACTION TYPE AND CLINICAL SIGNIFICANCE GUIDE

II. Type and Clinical Significance of Interaction

Generally applicable principles:

- If the individual's prior medical condition has been stable, *any* changes to the therapeutic regimen involving addition or withdrawal of nutrients, botanicals, or pharmaceuticals should not be made abruptly. Transitions in protocols are de facto potential foci for interaction instability that may, if ignored, significantly affect intended therapeutic outcomes.
- Individuals vary in response to any pharmacological agent because of individual biochemical or pharmacogenomic variability, as well as health status and medical conditions.
- Professional management implies supervision by collaborating health care professionals with appropriate training in nutritional and/or botanical therapeutics within an integrative medical framework.

✗ Potential or Theoretical Adverse Interaction of Uncertain Severity

Interaction is theoretically possible based on known pharmacological characteristics of each substance. Inadequate information is currently available to determine clinical significance of potential risk. Pending conclusive research, close supervision and regular monitoring by a health care professional are warranted for any concomitant use.

✗✗ Minimal to Mild Adverse Interaction—Vigilance Necessary

Interaction represents a low to moderate risk, but potential severity warrants supervision of patient during concomitant use. Concomitant use is therapeutically feasible within the context of multidisciplinary collaboration, along with supervision and monitoring by health care professional(s) trained in conventional pharmacology and experienced with clinical herbal medicine and/or therapeutic nutrition.

✗✗✗ Potentially Harmful or Serious Adverse Interaction—Avoid

Interaction represents a significant to severe risk of adverse effect and should be avoided. Concomitant use should be deliberately avoided outside the context of close supervision and regular monitoring, including laboratory monitoring wherever feasible, by health care professional(s) trained in conventional pharmacology and experienced with clinical herbal medicine and/or therapeutic nutrition.

◇ Impaired Drug Absorption and Bioavailability, Negligible Effect

Interaction is adverse but of minimal clinical significance. Nonetheless, modification of dosage, timing, or mode of administration may reduce potential for adverse effects of interaction.

◇◇ Impaired Drug Absorption and Bioavailability, Precautions Appropriate

Interaction is of mild to moderate severity. Modification of dosage, timing, or mode of administration will reduce adverse effects of interaction.

◇◇◇ Impaired Drug Absorption and Bioavailability, Avoidance Appropriate

Interaction has clinically significant adverse effects. Concomitant use should be avoided, especially outside the context of close supervision and regular monitoring by health care professional(s) trained in conventional pharmacology and experienced with clinical herbal medicine and/or therapeutic nutrition. Modification of dosage, timing, or mode of administration may contribute to minimizing severity in cases in which benefit of concurrent administration outweighs risks.

◇ Adverse Drug Effect on Herbal Therapeutics, Strategic Concern

Interaction in which drug may interfere with therapeutic effect of herbal prescription because of the drug's pharmacological properties. Alterations in drug dosage, timing, or other factors may prevent, ameliorate, or compensate for adverse effects of or interference with herbal therapeutics and optimize therapeutic effect, with appropriate clinical management within an integrative therapeutic strategy, without compromising therapeutic efficacy of either intervention.

◇ Adverse Drug Effect on Nutritional Therapeutics, Strategic Concern

Interaction in which drug may interfere with therapeutic effect of nutrient prescription because of the drug's pharmacological properties. Alterations in drug dosage, timing, or other factors may prevent, ameliorate, or compensate for adverse effects of or interference with nutritional therapeutics and optimize therapeutic effect, with appropriate clinical management within an integrative therapeutic strategy, without compromising therapeutic efficacy of either intervention.

◇≈≈ Drug-Induced Adverse Effect on Nutrient Function, Coadministration Therapeutic, with Professional Management

Interaction in which standard-practice use of pharmaceutical agent will usually interfere with normal physiological nutrient function because of predicted drug action. Appropriate coadministration of nutrient, with appropriate clinical management within an integrative therapeutic strategy, will counter adverse metabolic effects of drug on nutrient and may optimize therapeutic effect without compromising therapeutic efficacy of pharmaceutical intervention.

◇≈≈ Drug-Induced Adverse Effect on Nutrient Function, Supplementation Therapeutic, Not Requiring Professional Management

Interaction in which standard-practice use of pharmaceutical agent will usually interfere with normal physiological nutrient function because of drug action. Appropriate concomitant supplementation with (or coadministration of) nutrient will counter adverse metabolic effects of drug on nutrient and may optimize therapeutic effect without compromising therapeutic efficacy of pharmaceutical intervention. Clinical management is usually not required.

◇◇ Drug-Induced Effect on Nutrient Function, Supplementation Contraindicated, Professional Management Appropriate

Interaction in which prescription pharmaceutical agent intentionally interferes with normal physiological nutrient function through predicted drug action. Nutrient dietary intake is typically restricted and supplementation or administration contraindicated to optimize therapeutic effect and avoid compromising therapeutic efficacy of pharmaceutical intervention.

⊕✗ Bimodal or Variable Interaction, with Professional Management

Interaction is inherently neither beneficial nor adverse, unless ignored. Based on known pharmacological characteristics of each substance (or reasonable extrapolations therefrom), interaction is theoretically possible. Depending on the specific clinical contextualization (patient, population, diagnosis, setting) and practitioner training and experience, the interaction may be deliberately utilized by an appropriately trained and experienced health care professional for increasing clinical efficacy with appropriate clinical management within an integrative therapeutic strategy. Although clinically significant in certain circumstances, this interaction may be of only minor significance in other contexts.

Note: In situations in which "Bimodal" is assigned to an interaction dyad in the text, the possible variations are also listed.

⊕ Potential or Theoretical Beneficial or Supportive Interaction, with Professional Management

Beneficial interaction is theoretically possible based on known pharmacological data. However, inadequate substantive data exist currently to determine clinical significance of potential benefit. Coordinated use with appropriate clinical management within an integrative therapeutic strategy may theoretically increase therapeutic efficacy. Pending conclusive research, concomitant use may warrant close supervision and regular monitoring by a health care professional.

⊕⊕ Beneficial or Supportive Interaction, with Professional Management

Interaction in which intentional therapeutic use of nutrient or botanical preparation concomitantly with drug therapy can provide additive or synergistic effect and increase therapeutic efficacy for most individuals when taken at appropriate dosages with professional supervision and monitoring as needed. Some individuals may derive greater benefit because of medical conditions or individual pharmacogenomic and biochemical variability. Coadministration can be therapeutically efficacious within the context of multidisciplinary collaboration and supervision by health care professional(s) trained in conventional pharmacology and experienced with clinical herbal medicine and/or therapeutic nutrition.

⊕⊕⊕ Beneficial or Supportive Interaction, Not Requiring Professional Management

Interaction in which concurrent administration can generally be considered safe for patient self-care. Based on available evidence, it is improbable that the therapeutic benefit of additive or synergistic interaction or nutritive support has the potential to induce an undesired and possibly adverse additive or interference effect, although discussion and communication with prescribing physician are advised.

≈≈ Drug-Induced Nutrient Depletion, Supplementation Therapeutic, with Professional Management

Interaction in which appropriate use of nutrient, given clinical management within an integrative therapeutic strategy, can prevent or counter nutrient depletion caused by drug without compromising therapeutic efficacy for most individuals when taken at commonly used dosages. Concomitant use therapeutically efficacious within the context of multidisciplinary collaboration and supervision by health care professional(s) trained in conventional pharmacology and experienced with clinical therapeutic nutrition.

≈≈≈ Drug-Induced Nutrient Depletion, Supplementation Therapeutic, Not Requiring Professional Management

Interaction in which simultaneous use can generally be considered safe for patient self-care. Based on examined evidence, appropriate therapeutic use of nutrient adjunctively with drug therapy likely to provide correct drug-induced nutrient depletion pattern and improve therapeutic outcomes for most individuals, without interfering with drug efficacy, when taken at appropriate dosages. Based on available evidence, it is improbable that the therapeutic benefit of additive or synergistic interaction or nutritive support has the potential to induce an undesired and possibly adverse additive or interference effect, although discussion and communication with prescribing physician are advised.

≈◇◇ Drug-Induced Nutrient Depletion, Supplementation Contraindicated, Professional Management Appropriate

Interaction in which prescription medication intentionally interferes with normal physiological nutrient metabolism and may produce nutrient depletion pattern through predicted drug action. Nutrient dietary intake is typically restricted and supplementation (or coadministration) contraindicated to optimize therapeutic effect and avoid compromising therapeutic efficacy of pharmaceutical intervention. Concomitant use is generally contraindicated for most individuals. In some unusual circumstances, nutrient might be prescribed under appropriate parameters of dosage, timing, and duration, with clinical management and monitoring within the context of multidisciplinary collaboration and supervision by health care professional(s) trained in conventional pharmacology and experienced with therapeutic nutrition.

☼ Prevention or Reduction of Drug Adverse Effect

Interaction in which intentional coadministration of nutrient or herb concurrently with drug therapy within an integrative therapeutic strategy can prevent, reduce, or counter adverse drug effects without compromising therapeutic efficacy for most individuals when taken at appropriate dosages, under professional guidance.

☼ Prevention or Reduction of Herb or Nutrient Adverse Effect

Interaction in which appropriate use of medication is intended to prevent, reduce, or counter adverse nutrient or herb effects in conditions characterized by nutrient overload, exogenous toxicity, and metabolic derangement, without inducing

clinically significant nutrient deficiency pattern or obstructing the role of herbal prescription for appropriate individuals when taken at therapeutic dosages. Concomitant use is contraindicated unless specifically determined as therapeutically efficacious within the context of multidisciplinary collaboration and supervision by health care professional(s) trained in conventional pharmacology and experienced with therapeutic nutrition.

? Interaction Possible but Uncertain Occurrence and Unclear Implications

Interaction is of uncertain character, significance, and predictability of occurrence, reflective of inconsistent and/or inadequate evidence. Prudence dictates avoiding concomitant use while assuming neither risk nor benefit until more data become available. Pending further clinical research findings, it is prudent to avoid concomitant use outside the context of close supervision and regular monitoring by health care professional(s) trained in conventional pharmacology and experienced with clinical herbal medicine and/or therapeutic nutrition.

STRENGTH AND CHARACTER OF SOURCE EVIDENCE GUIDE

III. Strength and Quality of Source Evidence

The source material for each topic is evaluated using the following composite indicators to offer an assessment of the overall character of the literature reviewed for that nutrient-drug or herb-drug pair.

● Consensus

Interaction demonstrated by a converging consensus of clinical experience, research literature, and known pharmacology, including significant findings from published clinical or preclinical human studies of strong design, size, and relevance; well-documented and consistent case reports; and established pharmacokinetic and pharmacodynamic data.

◉ Emerging

Interaction supported by emerging pattern of clinical experience, research literature, and known pharmacology, including human studies of adequate design, size, and relevance; limited but consistent, well-documented case reports; unpublished papers and presentations; and probable pharmacokinetics or pharmacodynamics.

○ Preliminary

Interaction suggested by preliminary data, involving fragmentary or partial evidence; reports derived from anecdotal clinical experience, preliminary research literature, or general pharmacological principles; research findings based on animal or in vitro experimental studies; or human studies characterized by inadequate design, size, and significance; limited or incomplete case reports; or extrapolations from pharmacokinetic or pharmacodynamic data.

▽ Mixed

Interaction proposed on the basis of partial, contradictory, or otherwise inconclusive evidence, including from single sources; unsubstantiated or incomplete case reports; inappropriate or methodologically flawed studies; or nonsignificant data.

□ Inadequate

Interaction proposed using obsolete, discredited, speculative, or otherwise inadequate or inappropriate evidence from derivative or secondary sources, including conjecture or unjustified extrapolation, inappropriate or flawed methodology, or studies of questionable relevance.

Contents

SECTION III: CROSS-INDEXES

INDEX, 891

Monograph references are located on the CD at the back of the book.

They can also be found at medicineworks.com

Aloe

Botanical Name: *Aloe vera* (L.) Burm.
Pharmacopoeial Name: Aloe vera gel.
Synonym: *Aloe barbadensis* (Mill.).
Common Names: Aloe gel, aloe vera gel.

Summary

Drug/Class Interaction Type	Mechanism and Significance	Management
Chemotherapy and radiotherapy associated with mucositis ⊕/☼	Aloe gel may ameliorate chemotherapy-induced oral and gastrointestinal mucositis.	Use prophylactically and symptomatically during chemotherapy with agents known to induce mucositis.
Wound care, surgery ⊕/⊕	Aloe gel incorporated into conventional dressings improves healing in wound care settings.	Commercial hydrogel dressings available.

HERB DESCRIPTION

Family

Aloaceae (formerly in Liliaceae).

Related Species

Aloe ferox Mill., *A. africana* Mill., *A. spicata* Baker., *A. perryi* Baker.; the *Aloe* genus has more than 300 species. *Aloe vera* has been widely hybridized in commerce, and cultivars are the primary source of the gel.

Habitat and Cultivation

Native to Africa, widespread in cultivation throughout subtropical regions in North and South America, West Indies, and East Asia; the cactuslike aloe is also a popular houseplant.

Parts Used

Aloe gel is a mucilaginous, colorless liquid derived from the central parenchymatous cells of the fresh leaves of aloe.

Note: Aloe gel and aloe latex are completely distinct remedies. The anthraquinone-containing dried juice, a yellow-orange latex, or sap exuded from the outer or pericycle (vascular bundles) area of the leaf, is often known as "Cape aloe" or "Curacao aloe." Some traditional cultures have used the root as a medicine, but this is not a current Western usage. Aloe latex can be considered with the Rhamnacae species such as cascara (*Rhamnus purshiana* DC), the buckthorns (*R. frangula* L. and *R. cathartica* L.), as well as senna leaf and fruits (*Cassia senna* L.) and rhubarb root (*Rheum palmatum* L.). All these species contain closely related anthraquinone glycosides that dominate their pharmacology, particularly the pronounced laxative and purgative activity associated with these herbs.

Common Forms

100% Fresh gel and freeze-dried concentrates, typically 4.5:1 concentrate, equivalent to 11.25 mg/mL of acemannan.
Standardized Extracts: Preparations based on acemannan (acetylated mannose polysaccharide) obtained by hydroethanolic extraction from the inner leaf gel. Multiple proprietary products are available, including Carrysyn (73% acemannan, Carrington Laboratories).

Note: "Aloe juice" is not a pharmacopoeial term; it describes varied products sold commercially that contain diluted gel. These products may contain only small amounts of the active gel constituents and may incorporate added thickeners such as pectins and starch. These juice products are usually anthraquinone free.

HERB IN CLINICAL PRACTICE

Overview

Aloe vera gel, the clear, colorless mucilage from the central parenchyma of the leaf, is primarily known for promoting topical healing of burns, wounds, incisions, frostbite, ulcers, and related inflammatory problems. The gel is also widely incorporated into natural cosmetic and skin care products. Modern research interest has focused on identifying the active polysaccharide components of the gel and investigating their potential immunomodulatory properties as biological response modifiers.[1] Internal applications are also of interest, such as for inflammatory bowel disease, and a positive trial in active ulcerative colitis patients is available.[2,3]

Proprietary aloe extracts based on hydrogel are available in professional and consumer markets. These are either stabilized by means of rapid pasteurization or freeze-dried as a soluble powder; both forms contain standardized amounts of the main active polysaccharide (acemannan). Professional products are available in a variety of applications for wound care, burn treatment, diabetic care, general first-aid dressings, and management of radiation and chemotherapy adverse effects. Limited clinical evidence supports these applications, although promotion of wound healing appears to be better supported by the available data than burn treatment.

In the United States, popular dietary supplement products combining freeze-dried acemannan with other ingredients are "network marketed" as "glyconutritionals." These are promoted as nonspecific immunostimulants, often with wide-ranging therapeutic claims, including for the treatment of cancer and human immunodeficiency virus (HIV). Evidence for such claims is not substantial at this time and is partly extrapolated from non–peer-reviewed data supplied to the U.S. Patent Office based on in vitro or uncontrolled animal studies using parenteral routes of administration.[4]

1

Aloe gel and its derivative products are not officially approved for internal medical use, although some proprietary topical hydrogel products have been approved by the U.S. Food and Drug Administration (FDA). The botanical literature emphasizes the anthraquinone herb rather than the gel. The World Health Organization (WHO) monograph series includes both remedies separately, but this is the exception.[5] Comprehensive literature reviews relating to recent immunological research on the gel are unavailable, although there are surveys of the data up to the late 1990s.[6] The available clinical trial evidence on aloe gel extracts was systematically reviewed in 1999 by Vogler and Ernst.[7]

Historical/Ethnomedicine Precedent

Aloe leaf has been in recorded use for centuries, with documentation by Dioscorides, Pliny, and Galen, as well as in traditional Ayurvedic and Chinese medicine. The gel was allegedly used by Cleopatra for cosmetic skin enhancement, but Europeans became more familiar with uses of the gel from African tribes and subsequently planted specimens of *Aloe* spp. throughout their colonies, which became rapidly naturalized in subtropical zones. Aloe spread in the United States, especially Florida, where it was used by the Seminole people for healing burns and stings. The gel remains in widespread popular folk use; currently it is often kept as a houseplant, with a leaf cut to obtain fresh gel as treatment for sunburn, thermal burns, insect bite, and other first-aid needs.

Known or Potential Therapeutic Uses

External/Topical: Treatment of abscesses, burns, surgical incisions, wounds, ulcers (oral, leg), dermatitis, and psoriasis. Internal: Antiviral (HIV/herpes simplex virus [HSV]), dysglycemia, inflammatory bowel disease, immunomodulation, peptic ulcer preventive, ulcerative colitis.

Key Constituents

The gel is more than 97% water by weight. The solid matter is approximately 65% carbohydrate, predominantly in the form of a long-chained, polydispersed, beta-(1,4)-acetylated mannan (acemannan).[8,9] Sterols, organic acids (especially oxalate), and various amino acids make up the remainder. Novel dihydrocoumarins have recently been described.[10] Naturally occurring enzymes are present in the fresh gel, and pasteurization is necessary to stabilize the gel to prevent enzymatic degradation.

Therapeutic Dosing Range

Fresh Juice Concentrate: 25 mL up to four times daily.
Standardized Extracts: 500 to 800 mg-equivalent acemannan daily.

INTERACTIONS REVIEW
Strategic Considerations

The WHO monograph on aloe gel does not ascribe any interactions involving the herb.[5] The anthraquinone-containing *Aloe* latex is not considered here, but the reader should refer to the Cascara monograph for some interactions typical of the anthraquinone-containing botanicals.

In the setting of externally applied medications, aloe interactions are limited to various combination preparations, using the hydrogel as a vehicle with related materials (e.g., algal gums, synthetic hydrogels) or as an ingredient of creams and ointments in combination with anti-inflammatory agents.

The topical effects of the gel are thought to be the result of several mechanisms.[11,12] Anti-inflammatory effects have been established experimentally in the treatment of adjuvant arthritis, paw edema, frostbite, and diabetic ulceration in animal models,[11,13-15] as well as in human mucosal $CaCO_2$ cells in vitro.[2] The mechanisms involved are probably multifactorial and include inhibition of prostaglandin synthesis, antioxidant quenching of free radicals, and bradykinin inhibition, as well as promotion of connective tissue development, inhibition of collagenase (and metalloproteinase) activity, and stimulation of cell-mediated immunity.[14,16-21] Research at Carrington Laboratories has established that the pectins present in aloe vera gel are efficient stabilizers of peptides, which constitute a large class of tissue growth factors and immunomodulators, and may explain some of the observed activities of the plant gel (by increasing the half-life of peptide cytokines and growth factors).[22]

Since the 1930s, when aloe gel was first investigated for the topical treatment of "roentgen dermatitis," there have been persistent attempts to establish its efficacy for topical treatment of ultraviolet B (UVB) and x-ray radiation burns, although with consistently mixed results.[23] Recent animal tests have been positive,[24] but the only randomized controlled clinical trial available failed to show any benefit of the gel against placebo on chest wall and breast irradiation in 108 breast cancer patients.[25] Another oncological use is in chemotherapy-induced mucositis, although only oral (aphthous stomatitis) treatment has received substantial evidential support, and a proprietary aloe hydrogel product has been FDA approved for aphthous ulcer treatment.[26]

Internal use of the gel has been examined in relation to potential antiviral and immunostimulating effects for HIV patients, as well as for glycemic regulation in diabetic patients. Neither of these indications is well supported, nor are they in current general use clinically by practitioners of natural or botanical medicine. Suggestions of potential synergistic interactions with antivirals and antidiabetic agents are discussed later (see Theoretical, Speculative, and Preliminary Interactions Research). A recent United Kingdom trial established positive support for the use of aloe gel internally for ulcerative colitis.[2,3] Wide variation in commercial and proprietary processing methods, leading to products with differing activities, may underlie much of the conflicting results in clinical trials in various applications of "stabilized" *Aloe vera* products. The only relatively uniform activity would be from fresh gel obtained from freshly harvested aloe leaves, which are, however, logistically difficult to use in studies.

One recent, small, crossover-design human trial found a significant effect of aloe on the pharmacokinetics of vitamin C and vitamin E absorption. When single doses of the vitamins were consumed orally with 2 oz of aloe gel or whole-leaf extract, absorption of both the water-soluble and fat-soluble vitamins were significantly slowed, leading to longer half-life in plasma. The authors suggested that aloe could be used to complement the absorption of these nutrients.[27]

Data on the effects of aloe gel on drug-metabolizing enzymes and transporters are not available.

HERB-DRUG INTERACTIONS

Chemotherapy and Radiotherapy Associated with Mucositis, Including Bleomycin, Fluorouracil/5-FU, and Methotrexate

Including Bleomycin (Blenoxane), cisplatin (cis-diaminedichloroplatinum, CDDP; Platinol, Platinol-AQ), cyclophosphamide (Cytoxan, Endoxana, Neosar, Procytox), docetaxel (Taxotere), doxorubicin (Adriamycin, Rubex), etoposide (Eposin, Etophos, VePesid, VP-16), fluorouracil (5-FU; Adrucil, Efudex, Efudix, Fluoroplex), gemcitabine (Gemzar), irinotecan (camptothecin-11, CPT-11; Campto, Camptosar), methotrexate (Folex, Maxtrex, Rheumatrex), paclitaxel (Paxene, Taxol).

Interaction Type and Significance

⊕   **Potential or Theoretical Beneficial or Supportive Interaction, with Professional Management**

☼   **Prevention or Reduction of Drug Adverse Effect**

Probability:
4. Plausible

Evidence Base:
✗☐ Inadequate

Effect and Mechanism of Action
Inflammation of the oral mucosa (mucositis) induced by chemotherapeutic agents or ionizing radiation may be reduced by topical application of aloe vera gel.

The interaction is unsupported by published direct evidence but is based on established pharmacology and empirical clinical practice.

Research
Mucositis can be a dose-limiting toxicity of certain chemotherapies (notably 5-FU) and not only compromises normal physiological function, but also can present a portal to systemic infection complications in granulocytopenic patients following secondary infection.[28] An acemannan-containing product has been licensed by the FDA for aphthous stomatitis, although clinical trial evidence for the efficacy of aloe in this setting is equivocal.[26,29] There is also some experimental evidence for the efficacy of aloe gel as a cytoprotective agent for gastrointestinal (GI) mucosa, in addition to moderate gastric acid inhibition activity.[2,30-32] Radiation oncology has also investigated aloe gel as a topical preventive against adverse effects and one trial tested the effects of aloe gel in head and neck radiotherapy for prevention of oral mucositis; although a positive effect was noted, it was not statistically significant.[33] Preclinical and clinical studies on radiation-induced dermatitis and mucositis prevention by aloe gel have been conducted but, to date, have failed to demonstrate convincing benefits of aloe in symptom reduction.[23,34-36]

Finally, aloe gel has been shown in vitro to exhibit hematopoietic activity, which lends additional, if indirect, support to its use in combination with conventional cancer treatments.[37]

Integrative Therapeutics, Clinical Concerns, and Adaptations
Topical oral wash ("swish and swallow") formulations containing aloe gel, often combined with agents such as glutamine and licorice extracts, have been employed empirically by practitioners using botanical/nutritional approaches to reduce chemotherapy-induced mucositis and stomatitis and are associated with anecdotal reports of symptom reduction. The antiviral and antifungal effects of aloe gel, along with its putative immunostimulatory and hematopoietic effects, lend additional circumstantial support to aloe gel as a choice of remedial agent for oral mucositis in this setting. Although the indirect GI mucositis also caused by chemotherapeutic drugs is, to some extent, a different issue clinically from oral mucositis, the same general approach with aloe gel has been used for prophylaxis of this GI toxicity. Further data and clinical trials are required to establish whether the anecdotal combination treatment is efficacious.

Surgery and Other Wound Care

Evidence: Polyethylene oxide sheet dressing (Vigilon).
Extrapolated, based on similar properties: Hydrogel dressings.

Interaction Type and Significance
⊕/⊕   **Beneficial or Supportive Interaction, with Professional Management**

Probability:
2. Probable

Evidence Base:
▽ Mixed

Effect and Mechanism of Action
Addition of aloe vera gel to polyethylene oxide hydrogel dressings may improve abrasive wound healing in the context of professional wound management. The extent and significance of the benefit of combining aloe gel with conventional dressings are unknown.

Research
Polyethylene oxide is a cross-linked hydrogel containing 96% water that is supported on a low-density mesh of polyethylene sheet for dressing wounds with limited epidermal involvement, such as dermabrasions, minor burns, and pressure ulcers. One clinician-researcher reported that the addition of aloe vera gel to this dressing format increased dermabrasion wound-healing rates.[38,39] Another surgical report from an obstetrical practice, however, suggested that application of aloe vera gel actually delayed the healing of surgical wounds, with complications of healing in 21 women.[40] A small trial compared the effects of an aloe vera hydrogel to a non–aloe-containing hydrogel in the healing rates of pressure ulcers and found no significant differences between the preparations.[41] Oral surgical aloe hydrogel products have shown some efficacy on molar extraction sites.[42]

Integrative Therapeutics, Clinical Concerns, and Adaptations
Despite the general evidence for promotion of wound healing by aloe vera gel, further studies are needed before recommending its use in any situation other than uncomplicated, superficial wounds. Evidence from specialized wound care settings remains inconclusive, and although skilled wound care management is available in these contexts, the use of aloe vera gel for intensive wound care requires professional monitoring.

THEORETICAL, SPECULATIVE, AND PRELIMINARY INTERACTIONS RESEARCH, INCLUDING OVERSTATED INTERACTIONS CLAIMS

Antivirals: Acyclovir and Related Purine Nucleoside Analog Antivirals; Zidovudine/AZT and Related Reverse-Transcriptase Inhibitor (Nucleoside Analogs and Nonnucleosides) Antiretroviral Agents

Evidence: Acyclovir (Zovirax), zidovudine (azidothymidine, AZT, ZDV, zidothymidine; Retrovir).
Extrapolated, based on similar properties: Zidovudine combination drugs: abacavir (ziager), zidovudine, and lamivudine

(Combivir); abacavir (ziager), lamivudine, and zidovudine (Trizivir); didanosine (ddI, dideoxyinosine; Videx), dideoxycytidine (ddC, zalcitabine; Hivid), lamivudine (3TC, Epivir), stavudine (D4T, Zerit), tenofovir (Viread).

A preliminary in vitro study examined the potential synergistic effects of acemannan with both azidothymidine (AZT) and acyclovir on human U1 cells infected with HSV-1 and HIV-1. The investigators found a synergistic antiviral effect in which suboptimal drug doses, when combined with acemannan, produced significant antiviral effects. The authors suggest this should be further investigated as a possibly beneficial clinical interaction for HIV/AIDS patients because the mechanisms of the drug and herb were considered to be mutually exclusive.[43] Only one subsequent trial has investigated the effect of the combination in HIV patients and found no effect of acemannan on CD4 count decline compared with the control groups, which included coadministration with AZT over 48 weeks of treatment.[44]

Glyburide and Related Sulfonylurea Hypoglycemics

Evidence: Glyburide (glibenclamide; Diabeta, Glynase, Glynase Prestab, Micronase, Pres Tab).
Extrapolated, based on similar properties: Acetohexamide (Dymelor), chlorpropamide (Diabinese), glimepiride (Amaryl), glipizide (Glucotrol, Glucotrol XL), tolazamide (Tolinase), tolbutamide (Orinase, Tol-Tab); combination drugs: glipizide and metformin (Metaglip), glyburide and metformin (Glucovance).

Aloe has been attributed with mild antidiabetic activity and is often listed as such in surveys of hypoglycemic medicinal plants.[45,46] Vogler and Ernst's review[7] concluded that aloe may be useful as an adjunctive treatment in diabetes, but the studies were limited in number and methodologically poor, and their conclusion is controversial. The possible use of different plant parts (i.e., latex, gel) further confounds interpretation. A human trial with glyburide comedication has not been replicated,[47] although its findings have been cited as evidence of an aloe gel–glyburide interaction.[48] One negative human study failed to show hypoglycemic effect of the juice, and an animal study demonstrated an actual hyperglycemic action of the gel.[49,50] Animal studies suggest that antioxidant activity may exert indirect antidiabetic effects.[51,52] The use of aloe in any form for glycemic control of type 1 or type 2 human diabetes is not common current clinical practice, at least not in Western botanical medicine. This is therefore a speculative interaction postulated by reverse extrapolation from a nonestablished pharmacological effect.

Hydrocortisone and Related Topical Corticosteroids

Evidence: Hydrocortisone 17-butyrate, acetate, probutate, or valerate (hydrocortisone topical; Acticort 100, Aeroseb-HC, Ala-Cort, Ala-Scalp HP, Allercort, Alphaderm, Bactine, Beta-HC, Caldecort Anti-Itch, Cetacort, Cort-Dome, Cortaid,

Cortef, Cortifair, Cortizone, Cortone, Cortril, Delacort, Dermacort, Dermarest, DriCort, DermiCort, Dermtex HC, Epifoam, Gly-Cort, Hi-Cor, Hydro-Tex, Hytone, LactiCare-HC, Lanacort, Lemoderm, Locoid, MyCort, Nutracort, Pandel, Penecort, Pentacort, Proctocort, Rederm, S-T Cort, Synacort, Texacort, Westcort).
Extrapolated, based on similar properties: Alclometasone (Aclovate, Modrasone), amcinonide (Cyclocort), beclomethasone, betamethasone dipropionate/valerate (betamethasone topical; Alphatrex, Beta-Val, Betaderm, Betanate, Betatrex, Diprolene AF, Diprolene, Diprosone, Luxiq, Maxivate, Teladar, Uticort, Valisone), clobetasol (clobetasol topical; Cormax, Dermoval, Dermotyl, Dermovate, Dermoxin, Eumosone, Lobate, Olux, Temovate, Temovate E, Topifort), clobetasone (Eumovate), clocortolone (clocortolone pivalate topical; Cloderm), desonide (DesOwen, Tridesilon), desoximetasone (Topicort, Topicort LP), desoxymethasone, dexamethasone (Aeroseb-Dex, Decaderm, Decadron, Decaspray), diflorasone (Apexicon, Florone, Maxiflor, Psorcon), diflucortolone (Nerisona, Nerisone), fluocinolone (Derma-Smoothe/FS, Fluonid, Synalar, Synemol), fluocinonide (Fluonex, Lidex, Lidex-E, Lonide, Vanos), fludroxycortide (flurandrenolone), fluocortolone (Ultralan), flurandrenolide (Cordran, Drenison), fluticasone (Cutivate), halobetasol (Ultravate), halcinonide (Halog), mometasone (Elocon, mometasone topical), triamcinolone, (Aristocort, Triderm, Kenalog, Flutex, Kenonel, triamcinolone topical); triamcinolone and nystatin (Mycolog II).

A single animal study used rodent paw models of inflammation to compare the effect of topical hydrocortisone acetate alone and in combination with aloe hydrogel. The combination was found to be more efficacious than the synthetic steroid alone at reducing edema and inflammation in this model.[53] This combination is frequently reported as a (beneficial) interaction; however, the combination does not appear to be used at all in practice and, although theoretically plausible, remains clinically undemonstrated at present and appears to be overstated.

Sevoflurane

Sevoflurane
A single perioperative incident of excessive bleeding was attributed to preoperative aloe consumption.[54] In fact, the anesthetic sevoflurane is a potent inhibitor of platelet aggregation, and the procedure was biopsy of a hemangioma. In this case it seems unlikely that the excessive hemorrhage could be reliably attributed to aloe consumption. Isoflurane is suggested as a preferred anesthetic to sevoflurane in situations with high risk of perioperative bleeds.[55] No other reports of aloe and bleeding or enhanced anticoagulation have been made.

The 55 citations for this monograph are located under Aloe on the CD at the back of the book.

Astragalus

Botanical Name: *Astragalus membranaceus* (Fisch.) Bunge.
Pharmacopoeial Name: Radix astragali.
Common Names: Astragalus, milk vetch root, Huang-Qi.

Summary

Drug/Class Interaction Type	Mechanism and Significance	Management
Acyclovir Purine nucleoside analog antivirals ⊕	Astragalus promotes T helper cell type 1 (Th1) immunity. Possible additive antiviral activity, against herpes simplex virus type 1 (HSV-1). Experimental support only; interaction not established clinically.	Consider coadministration during drug therapy for HSV family viruses.
Aldesleukin Recombinant interleukin-2 (rIL-2) ⊕/☼	Astragalus may synergistically increase effects of rIL-2. Experimental evidence only; interaction not clinically established.	Theoretically, coadministration may enhance therapeutic outcome of IL-2 treatment.
Cyclophosphamide Myelosuppressive chemotherapy ☼/⊕⊕/⊕ ✗	Astragalus promotes myelopoiesis; may protect white blood cell (WBC) counts during chemotherapy with cyclophosphamide, platinum agents, or other myelosuppressive chemotherapies. In nonmalignant disease applications, theoretically an adverse interaction.	Coadminister and continue after myelosuppressive chemotherapy until WBC count normalized; used with related herbs in formula.
Interferon alpha (IFN-α) ☼/⊕	Astragalus increases endogenous IFN; can be used to support IFN therapy or potentiate drug, allowing reduced drug dose and increased tolerability. Empirical clinical support; no trial evidence.	Consider coadministration in chronic viral conditions treated with IFN.
Thrombolytics ⊕	Astragalus increases fibrinolytic capacity by promoting tissue-type plasminogen activator (tPA). Astragalus may additively support fibrinolytic drug therapies. Interaction not clinically established.	Consider use in hyperviscosity or high-risk thrombotic patients with appropriate drugs.

HERB DESCRIPTION

Family

Fabaceae.

Related Species

Astragalus membranaceus var. *mongholicus* (Bunge).

Habitat and Cultivation

Perennial member of the legume family, native to Northern China, Mongolia, and Siberia and now under organic cultivation in the United States. The genus contains more than 400 species. Wild "locoweeds" (various *Astragalus* spp.) are a common livestock forage food. Gum tragacanth is derived from a related species, *A. gummifer.*

Parts Used

Radix (root).

Common Forms

Dried Sliced Root: Often soaked, then pressed or flattened; variant preparation may be honey-roasted in Chinese medicine.
Powdered Root: For decoction, liquid extracts and tablets.
Tincture and Fluid Extracts: 60% to 70% ethanol; usually include a water-extraction phase for polysaccharides, then preserved in ethanol.
Standardized Extracts: Several preparations are available. There is no consensus on marker compounds for standardization at this time; individual manufacturers' preparations may vary.

HERB IN CLINICAL PRACTICE

Overview

Astragalus has been used for more than 2000 years in Chinese medicine and is one of several important materia medica imports into Western botanical medicine. The herb is primarily used in Western herbalism as an immunomodulating agent and for cardiovascular disease. Interest in the herb as an adjunct to chemotherapy in oncological settings is increasing, but a recent Cochrane review found limited evidence of value for astragalus decoctions in improving adverse effects of chemotherapy in colorectal cancer patients.[1] Another, more recent meta-analysis reviewed trials in which astragalus was combined with platinum agents in non–small cell lung cancer; evidence showed that the combination may provide increased effectiveness in terms of tumor response, reduced toxicity of the chemotherapy, survival time, or performance status.[2]

Most available scientific literature is published in Chinese and has not been directly accessed for this survey. Much of the experimental data on astragalus are based on isolated polysaccharide fractions, either in vitro or by intraperitoneal administration in vivo. Extrapolation from this data to human oral consumption of powdered crude herb or liquid extracts may not be appropriate, particularly with regard to dosage. Chinese clinical trials usually use the herb in combination formulae with other herbs, such as ginseng, dang gui, poria, and rhemannia, because this is the typical manner of clinical administration. The available data have been used to discuss the interactions later.

Astragalus, as with other East Asian herbs incorporated into the Western materia medica relatively recently, is not monographed by the German Commission E, European Scientific

Cooperative on Phytotherapy (ESCOP), or World Health Organization (WHO). Astragalus does have an *American Herbal Pharmacopoeia* monograph,[3] and the literature has been reviewed by McKenna et al.[4] and Wagner et al.[5] Bensky et al.[6] provide an authoritative review, and Chen and Chen[7] relate traditional Chinese uses to conventional pharmacology.

Historical/Ethnomedicine Precedent

Chinese uses include spleen *(Pi) qi* tonification, lung *(Fei) qi* tonification, and "securing the exterior"; promoting pus discharge and growth of new tissue and providing immune support. These features may contribute to a number of different biomedical pathological conditions. Astragalus is traditionally used in Chinese medicine in combination formulae for a wide range of conditions, from the common cold to chronic renal failure.[7]

Known or Potential Therapeutic Uses

Cardioprotection (anti-ischemic, fibrinolytic, antioxidant); immunostimulation (reversal of leukopenia, myelosuppression); general prophylaxis of infection, stress, hypertension, certain viral infections (coxsackieviruses B2 and B3, parainfluenza type 1, viral myocarditis, Japanese endocarditis, HSV-1), nephritis, nephropathy, oxidative stress psoriasis, prostatic hypertrophy, and Takayasu arteritis.

Key Constituents

Polysaccharides (astragalans or astragologlucans); triterpene saponins (astragolides I-VII); isoflavones and other flavonoids; amino acids, minerals, essential oils, and phytosterols.

Therapeutic Dosing Range

Dried Root: 10 to 15 g daily; by decoction, maximum 120 g in Chinese medicine.
Hydroethanolic Extracts: 10 to 20 mL daily (based on 1:1 equivalent).

INTERACTIONS REVIEW
Strategic Considerations

Astragalus is used in Western botanical medicine as a tonic, adaptogenic, immunomodulating herb with negligible toxicity. It is myeloprotective, with added cardioprotective, hepatoprotective, and antioxidant properties, which make it a potentially useful adjunct in contexts involving immunosuppression, whether through disease processes, such as human immunodeficiency virus (HIV) and chronic fatigue immune dysfunction syndrome (CFIDS), or drug induced, such as myelosuppressive chemotherapies for the treatment of malignancies and immunosuppression in allograft patients. Recent research on the cardiac properties of the herb may help expand the Western use of astragalus beyond the narrow confines of "immunomodulation."[9,10]

Astragalus use with pharmaceutical immunosuppression (i.e., allograft patients) may be theoretically problematic, but there are no reports of adverse interactions arising from its use in this context. Combination with immunosuppressants may be regarded as contraindicated in practice. Several interactions described later are based on pharmacodynamic effects of the herb on immune parameters. These interactions are not generally supported by published clinical trials; however, strategic coadministration of the herb in some of the therapeutic contexts described is anecdotally established practice among some practitioners of botanical and integrative medicine.

Effects on Drug Metabolism and Bioavailability

There is currently no evidence of interactions resulting from the effects of astragalus on drug-metabolizing systems. A rodent study examining the hepatoprotective effects of astragalus saponins against acetaminophen-induced toxicity found a significant increase in hepatic cytochrome P450 (CYP) levels after astragalus administration.[11] Although studies are lacking, clinically significant pharmacokinetic interactions have not been reported to date.

HERB-DRUG INTERACTIONS

Acyclovir and Related Purine Nucleoside Analog Antivirals

Evidence: Acyclovir (Zovirax).
Extrapolated, based on similar properties: Purine nucleoside analog antivirals; famciclovir (Famvir), ganciclovir (Cytovene), valciclovir (Valcivir, Valcyclovir, Valtrex).

Interaction Type and Significance

⊕ **Potential or Theoretical Beneficial or Supportive Interaction, with Professional Management**

Probability:	Evidence Base:
4. Plausible	○ **Preliminary**

Effect and Mechanism of Action
A synergistic pharmacodynamic interaction increases the antiviral efficacy of the drug. Astragalus has established activity against a number of viruses in experimental and in vivo environments. Mechanisms remain to be clarified, but in general, T helper cell type 1 (Th1) cytokines and cell-mediated immune responses are enhanced by astragalus extracts.

Research
Zuo et al.[12] demonstrated a potentiation of acyclovir against herpes simplex virus type 1 (HSV-1)–infected mice when combined with astragalus that was greater than the effects of either agent alone, when measured by reduced mortality and extended survival time.

Integrative Therapeutics, Clinical Concerns, and Adaptations
Coadministration or pretreatment with astragalus may be useful as a possible adjunct to pharmaceutical antiviral therapies, based on limited available evidence. The interaction remains to be confirmed by clinical studies.

Aldesleukin (IL-2)

Interleukin-2 (IL-2), recombinant interleukin-2 (rIL-2); Proleukin.

Interaction Type and Significance

⊕ **Potential or Theoretical Beneficial or Supportive Interaction, with Professional Management**
☼ **Prevention or Reduction of Drug Adverse Effect**

Probability:	Evidence Base:
3. Possible	○ **Preliminary**

Effect and Mechanism of Action

The coadministration of astragalus and rIL-2 may produce a synergistic pharmacodynamic interaction. Astragalus extracts enhance several aspects of Th1-mediated immunity. Interleukin-2 immunotherapy is used to enhance cell-mediated immunity. Astragalus appears to potentiate IL-2 synergistically, which is one plausible mechanism of its ability to increase Th1 (cell-mediated) over Th2 immune activity.

Research

Co-incubation of lymphokine-activated killer (LAK) cells with astragalus F3 (fractionated extract) polysaccharide (55 µg/mL) achieved the same "tumor cell kill" when combined with 100 units/mL of IL-2, as did untreated LAK combined with 1000 units/mL of IL-2, suggesting a tenfold potentiation.[13] In a related study by the same group using LAK cells from patients with acquired immunodeficiency syndrome (AIDS), measured activity against melanoma cell lines increased tenfold when IL-2 was combined with astragalus F3, allowing a 50% reduction in effector/target cell ratio.[14,15] Similar results of tenfold potentiation with the F3 fraction and IL-2 with murine renal cell carcinoma have been reported.[16]

Integrative Therapeutics, Clinical Concerns, and Adaptations

Patients undergoing low-dose cytokine therapy using IL-2 may benefit from concurrent use of astragalus extracts or combinations, allowing a lower dose of IL-2 to be used and thus reducing potential adverse effects of the immunotherapy. Astragalus tends to favor Th1 over Th2 through additional mechanisms and may be considered a useful synergist in this therapeutic context. Direct clinical evidence for the interaction is not available.

Cyclophosphamide and Related Myelosuppressive Chemotherapy, Especially Alkylating Agents

Evidence: Cyclophosphamide (Cytoxan, Endoxana, Neosar, Procytox).

Extrapolated, based on similar properties: Busulfan (Myleran), carboplatin (Paraplatin), chlorambucil (Leukeran), cisplatin (*cis*-diaminedichloroplatinum, CDDP; Platinol, Platinol-AQ), dacarbazine (DIC, DTIC, DTIC-Dome, imidazole carboxamide), ifosfamide (Ifex, Mitoxana), mechlorethamine (Mustargen, nitrogen mustard), melphalan (Alkeran), oxaliplatin (Eloxatin), phenylalanine mustard (Melphalan), pipobroman (Vercyte), streptozocin (Zanosar), temozolomide (Temodar), thiotepa (Thioplex), uracil mustard (uramustine).

Interaction Type and Significance

☼ **Prevention or Reduction of Drug Adverse Effect**
⊕⊕ **Beneficial or Supportive Interaction, with Professional Management**
⊕/✗ **Bimodal or Variable Interaction, with Professional Management**

Probability:
2. Probable

Evidence Base:
◉ **Emerging**

Effect and Mechanism of Action

Astragalus reduces the effects of cyclophosphamide-induced suppression of cell-mediated immunity, increasing white blood cell (WBC) counts in chemotherapy-induced leukopenia and neutropenia, and is lymphoproliferative at splenic and bone marrow levels. In the context of cyclophosphamide treatment of nonmalignant disease, the interaction is theoretically

adverse, although properly speaking, this is a "contraindicated" combination.

Research

Several studies using cells from human cancer and healthy control patients in graft-versus-host (GVH) reaction models suggest that astragalus polysaccharide extracts promote cell-mediated immunity and reverse cyclophosphamide-induced immunosuppression.[13,17,18] Water extracts increase phagocytosis in carbon clearance tests, stimulate splenic lymphocyte proliferation, and increase tumor necrosis factor alpha (TNF-α) and interleukin-6 (IL-6) production by macrophages.[19] Proliferative effects on bone marrow stem cells and peripheral WBCs was observed after intraperitoneal (IP) administration of astragalus in mice.[20] Rodent macrophages were activated by astragalus polysaccharide in vitro, partly through nuclear factor kappa B (NF-κB) activation.[21] Clinical trials with intravenous (IV) astragalus polysaccharide coadministered with chemotherapy have been reported in the Chinese literature with positive results on outcome, versus chemotherapy alone, in terms of survival as well as quality-of-life measures.[22,23]

Clinical Implications and Adaptations

The astragalus-cyclophosphamide interaction has been classified as adverse by some authorities, presumably in the context of cyclophosphamide used in autoimmune disease treatment rather than cancer therapy.[24] Astragalus extracts may be incorporated into integrative protocols designed to support patients undergoing any myelosuppressive chemotherapies. Combination formulae are typically used in these applications, and experimental evidence indicates that such combinations may be more efficacious than the single herb against cyclophosphamide immunotoxicity.[25] Lymphopenia also occurs frequently in cancer patients, before, during, and after chemotherapeutic interventions, and correlates with decreased immunocompetence. To the degree that astragalus and other botanicals can support lymphocyte counts in such patients, these agents may be of clinical benefit, although controlled trials are required to demonstrate efficacy.

Interferon Alpha (IFN-α)

Interferon Alpha (IFN-α): Alferon N, Intron A, Roferon-A.

Interaction Type and Significance

☼ **Prevention or Reduction of Drug Adverse Effect**
⊕ **Potential or Theoretical Beneficial or Supportive Interaction, with Professional Management**

Probability:
4. Plausible

Evidence Base:
○ **Preliminary**

Effect and Mechanism of Action

Astragalus increases endogenous interferon (IFN) production by leukocytes and thus may potentiate the effects of therapeutic recombinant interferon (rIFN) administration. It is not established whether this is an additive or synergistic effect. Preliminary clinical support is available.

Research

An experimental study compared administration of a combination of recombinant IFN-2α with astragalus in a cell culture model of HSV-1–infected diploid human cells. The combination exhibited greater antiviral activity than the rIFN alone.[26] In a human trial, healthy volunteers were given 8 g/day of astragalus. After 2-week and 2-month periods of administration, blood levels of IFN were significantly elevated compared with controls.[27] The effect of IFN in treatment of 235 patients with chronic viral cervicitis was potentiated by astragalus, the combination being more effective as topical treatment than either IFN or astragalus alone. Interferon and astragalus combinations were superior to either agent alone against the human cold in a human trial using topical nasal spray application. Duration of symptoms was reduced significantly.

Integrative Therapeutics, Clinical Concerns, and Adaptations

Astragalus is known to have antiviral activity and to increase cell-mediated immunity. It is not clear to what extent augmentation of IFN levels underlies these effects; coordinated use of astragalus extracts may potentiate or synergize with IFN treatments (e.g., for viral hepatitis).

Thrombolytic Agents

Parenteral alteplase, recombinant (Activase); anistreplase (Eminase); reteplase, recombinant (Retavase); streptokinase (Streptase); urokinase (Abbokinase, Abbokinase Open-Cath).

Interaction Type and Significance

⊕ **Potential or Theoretical Beneficial or Supportive Interaction, with Professional Management**

Probability: Evidence Base:
4. Plausible   ○ Preliminary

Effect and Mechanism of Action

Astragalus extracts increase fibrinolysis and improve rheological characteristics of whole blood. Coadministration with various forms of antithrombotic therapy may be supportive, although clinical evidence is unavailable.

Research

Astragaloside IV fractionated extracts increased fibrinolytic potential of human umbilical vein endothelial cells in culture. The effect was mediated by upregulation of tissue-type plasminogen activator (tPA) expression and downregulation of plasminogen activator inhibitor (PA-I).[28] Increased PA-I activity relative to tPA and urokinase-type plasminogen activator (uPA) activity strongly correlates with cardiovascular morbidity and mortality. Reduced fibrinolytic capacity is a major cardiovascular disease risk in younger men. PA-I type 1 (PAI-1) is a risk factor for recurrence of myocardial infarction (MI), and high PAI-1 levels predict a first MI in middle-aged men and women.[29-31]

Integrative Therapeutics, Clinical Concerns, and Adaptations

Astragalus extracts may be supportive of strategies aimed at prophylaxis and treatment of thrombosis in at-risk populations. There are no reports that astragalus extracts adversely interfere with normal hemostasis or interact adversely

with typical anticoagulant drugs, which generally do not act through tPA. Combination with natural fibrinolytic agents such as Wobenzyme, nattokinase, and lumbrokinase may be appropriate in integrative protocols targeting hypercoagulable states.

THEORETICAL, SPECULATIVE, AND PRELIMINARY INTERACTIONS RESEARCH, INCLUDING OVERSTATED INTERACTIONS CLAIMS

Aminoglycoside Antibiotics

Amikacin (Amikin), gentamicin (G-mycin, Garamycin, Jenamicin), kanamycin (Kantrex), neomycin (Mycifradin, Myciguent, Neo-Fradin, NeoTab, Nivemycin), netilmicin (Netromycin), paromomycin (monomycin; Humatin), streptomycin, tobramycin (AKTob, Nebcin, TOBI, TOBI Solution, TobraDex, Tobrex).

A combination of astragalus and *Lu Han Cao* (Herba Pyrolae) was injected into guinea pigs subsequently administered intraperitoneal (IP) aminoglycosides, and the combination was found to prevent toxicity and nephrotoxicity.[32] Chen and Chen[7] overstate this as an interaction. Because the formula included another herb ingredient and parenteral administration, it should not be extrapolated to astragalus alone in oral administration without further supporting data.

Oral Hypoglycemic Agents and Insulin

Buformin (Andromaco Gliporal, Buformina), chlorpropamide (Diabinese), glimepiride (Amaryl), glipizide (Glucotrol; Glucotrol XL), glyburide (Glibenclamide; Diabeta, Glynase, Glynase Prestab, Micronase, Pres Tab), insulin (animal-source insulin: Iletin; human analog insulin: Humanlog; human insulin: Humulin, Novolin, NovoRapid, Oralin), metformin (Dianben, Glucophage, Glucophage XR); combination drugs: glipizide and metformin (Metaglip), glyburide and metformin (Glucovance); tolazamide (Tolinase), phenformin (Debeone, Fenformin), tolbutamide (Orinase, Tol-Tab).

A traditional Chinese use of astragalus combinations includes effects that would be recognized in modern pharmacology as lowering blood glucose.[7] There is also some experimental support for this theoretical interaction using streptozocin-induced rodent models of diabetes. It has been suggested that this implies a potential adverse interaction with oral hypoglycemics, a speculation that has no foundation, and if anything is contrary to the known effects and uses of the herb in this context. Data even suggest that insulin sensitivity may be increased by the herb.[33] Astragalus is also potentially beneficial in preventing diabetic cardiomyopathy.[34]

The 34 citations for this monograph are listed under Astragalus on the CD at the back of the book.

Bilberry

Botanical Name: *Vaccinium myrtillus* L.
Pharmacopoeial Names: Myrtilli folium, Myrtilli fructus.
Common Names: Blueberry, bilberry, whortleberry, huckleberry.

HERB DESCRIPTION

Family

Ericaceae.

Related Species

There is considerable bioregional diversity of wild blue-fruited *Vaccinium* spp., whose berries are very similar nutritionally and medicinally to the official species, *V. myrtillus* L. (e.g., in the U.S. Pacific Northwest alone, *V. ovatum* Pursh., *V uliginosum* L., *V. occidentale* Gray., *V ovalifolium* Smith., *V deliciosum* Smith., *V. membranaceum*, Dougl.). Horticultural cultivars are also common.

Parts Used

Fruit (berries); the leaf, a separate remedy, has been used in traditional herbal medicine but currently is not widely used.

Common Forms

Leaf: Dried leaf (infusion), dried-leaf hydroethanolic extract.
Berry (Fruit): Dried whole fruit; hydroethanolic tincture and liquid extracts; standardized extract (Myrtocyan, Tegens, MirtoSelect) in capsule form containing 25% anthocyanidins, with 36% anthocyanosides.

INTERACTIONS REVIEW

Strategic Considerations

Bilberry is currently best known for the properties of the anthocyanidin (Greek *antos,* "flower," and *kyanos,* "blue") and proanthocyanidin content of the fruit (berries). Anthocyanidins and proanthocyanidins are naturally occurring polyphenolic flavonoids widely present in berries and other fruit, also responsible for the blue-red pigmentation in many flowers and fruits. The chemistry and biological activities of the anthocyanidins and anthocyanins (aglycones and glycosides, respectively) have been extensively studied; the representative compound is cyanidin and its glycosides.[1,2]

Although the phytomedical literature on bilberry is dominated by the pharmacology of the anthocyanins and proanthocyanins and their glycosides, these are present at a level of only 0.1% to 0.25% in the fresh fruit. The catechin (tannin) content of the fruit, however, is actually an order of magnitude higher, 5% to 10%. This implies that standardized extracts that are widely used in commerce represent a highly concentrated product, and the safe therapeutic dose range is wide, from 120 to 480 mg standardized extract per day (equivalent to upper dose of ~500.0 g fresh, or ~100.00 g dry, berry/day). At these dose levels, bilberry concentrated extracts can be considered as a "phytonutriceutical" product, better classified with other concentrated flavonoid supplements, such as quercitin, rutin, and the oligomeric proanthocyanidins (OPCs). Resveratrol and the related compound pterostilbene may also be present in significant quantities in the concentrated extracts. Pterostilbene appears to have hypocholesterolemic properties mediated by its binding affinity to the peroxisome proliferator activated receptor (PPAR) and shares some of the chemopreventive and antioxidant characteristics of resveratrol.[3,4]

The German literature describes use of 10% dried bilberry fruit decoction as a safe supportive treatment of nonspecific diarrhea, including pediatric cases, and for topical inflammations of the mouth and throat, including oral candidiasis.[5-8] These uses are not widespread in North American clinical practice and are unlikely to invoke interactions with pharmaceutical agents.

The concentrated extracts, enriched in anthocyanins, have a range of pharmacological actions, including antioxidant, chemoprotective, vasoprotective, antiulcer, anti-inflammatory and antiatherogenic, antiaggregatory, and ophthalmic effects. Clinical evidence supports their use in peripheral vascular disorders (e.g., venous insufficiency, capillary fragility) and in ophthalmic disorders. Recent reviews of these data include the therapeutic monograph from the European Scientific Cooperative on Phytotherapy (ESCOP)[9] and a survey by McKenna et al.[10] Data relating to berry and fruit polyphenols and cancer chemoprevention has been reviewed by Prior and Joseph.[11] Experimental data demonstrating direct anticancer effects of anthocyanins is emerging.[12] In clinical practice, concentrated bilberry extracts are most likely to be used for disorders of microcirculation, and the specific advantage of the anthocyanins is their affinity for ophthalmic neurovasculature; conditions such as optic neuritis of multiple sclerosis, macular degeneration, glaucoma, and diabetic retinopathy are often the key prescribing indications.

Interactions between standardized bilberry extracts and pharmaceutical drugs have received minimal study. A single study reported a reduction in platinum compound toxicity without compromise to antitumor efficacy in an Ehrlich tumor rodent model using oral anthocyanins at 300 mg/kg coadministered with cisplatin.[13] No English translation of this report has been published, and the platinum interaction has not been confirmed by other studies or clinical reports and is not reviewed further here.

Pharmacokinetic data suggest that human intestinal flora are essential for hydrolysis of the glycoside form to the anthocyanin and proanthocyanin aglycones.[14-16] This suggests that iatrogenic reduction in microflora populations induced by antibiotics may reduce the bioavailability of the bilberry polyphenols, although evidence for this is not available.

Effects on Drug Metabolism and Bioavailability

Effects of bilberry extracts, or anthocyanins and proanthocyanins, on drug metabolism have not been well studied. Chemopreventive effects of fruits and berries have been examined in a few studies examining the mechanism of these effects, including possible inhibition of cytochrome P450 (CYP) 1A1 and 2E1 xenobiotic (aryl hydrocarbon carcinogen)–metabolizing enzymes.[17-20] The data are inconclusive but suggest low or minimal effects on these enzymes. Resveratrol, present in small amounts in bilberries, may inhibit CYP1B1, but this is not a significant drug-metabolizing cytochrome in humans although it is overexpressed in hormone-dependent tumor tissue.[21] Recent experimental evidence suggests that bilberry extracts

9

potently inhibit organic anion-transporting polypeptide B (OATP-B), which is an intestinal transporter responsible for mediating absorption of several drugs.[22] The flavonoid fraction of bilberry seems likely to be the active inhibitory component, but the in vivo significance of this inhibition remains to be established. Pharmacokinetic interactions between bilberry extracts or ingredients have not been reported.

HERB-DRUG INTERACTIONS

Antiplatelet Thromboprophylactics

Acetylsalicylic acid (acetosal, acetyl salicylic acid, ASA, salicylsalicylic acid; Arthritis Foundation Pain Reliever, Ascriptin, Aspergum, Asprimox, Bayer Aspirin, Bayer Buffered Aspirin, Bayer Low Adult Strength, Bufferin, Buffex, Cama Arthritis Pain Reliever, Easprin, Ecotrin, Ecotrin Low Adult Strength, Empirin, Extra Strength Adprin-B, Extra Strength Bayer Enteric 500 Aspirin, Extra Strength Bayer Plus, Halfprin 81, Heartline, Regular Strength Bayer Enteric 500 Aspirin, St Joseph Adult Chewable Aspirin, ZORprin); combination drugs: ASA and caffeine (Anacin), ASA, caffeine, and propoxyphene (Darvon Compound), ASA and carisoprodol (Soma Compound), ASA, codeine, and carisoprodol (Soma Compound with Codeine), ASA and codeine (Empirin with Codeine), ASA, codeine, butalbital, and caffeine (Fiorinal); cilostazol (Pletal), clopidogrel (Plavix), dipyridamole (Permole, Persantine), ticlopidine (Ticlid); combination drug: ASA and extended-release dipyridamole (Aggrenox, Asasantin)

Interaction Type and Significance

✗ **Potential or Theoretical Adverse Interaction of Uncertain Severity**

Probability:	Evidence Base:
5. Improbable	☐ Inadequate

Effect and Mechanism of Action

Aspirin (ASA) is a well-documented antiplatelet agent acting through inhibition of cyclooxygenase production of thromboxane A_2 (TXA_2). Ticlopidine interacts with glycoprotein IIb/IIIa to inhibit adenosine diphosphate (ADP)–induced fibrinogen binding to activated platelets and has been used for prevention of thrombosis when aspirin is poorly tolerated. Because of reports of hematological adverse effects associated with ticlopidine, clopidogrel is currently the preferred antiplatelet agent in such cases. As with ticlopidine, clopidogrel (Plavix) is an irreversible antiplatelet drug operating via ADP receptor antagonism. The potential interaction is therefore an additive pharmacodynamic increase in antiplatelet activity. Such an additive effect may theoretically increase the likelihood of bleeding disorders related to disturbances of primary hemostasis.

Research

Preliminary in vitro evidence suggested that concentrated anthocyanidins can inhibit platelet aggregation, probably by a decrease in cyclic adenosine monophosphate (cAMP) or an inhibition of TXA_2 formation at the platelet level.[23,24] A later study examined the effect of standardized bilberry extract in 30 healthy adults for 30 and 60 days, at an oral dose of 160 mg three times daily (tid). The subjects were divided into three groups: extract alone, extract combined with vitamin C (1000 mg tid), or vitamin C alone. Platelet aggregation was studied in vitro in relation to ADP- and collagen-induced stimulation. The bilberry extract/vitamin C group had a higher level of inhibition of aggregation than either the bilberry or the vitamin C group. Aggregation returned to baseline 120 days after treatment discontinuation.[25]

Integrative Therapeutics, Clinical Concerns, and Adaptations

If thromboprophylaxis is being affected by use of aspirin, there is at least a theoretical benefit in using bilberry extracts, not only to enhance the antiplatelet effects, but also because bilberry anthocyanidins have been shown (in rodent models) to be inhibitory of experimental chemically induced gastric ulceration, and to promote ulcer healing.[26,27] However, combining deglycyrrhizinated licorice (DGL) with aspirin in such cases may be a more cost-effective and reliable way of reducing the nonsteroidal anti-inflammatory drug (NSAID)–induced mucosal irritation and bleeding. Patients taking chronic high doses of concentrated bilberry extracts in combination with pharmaceutical antiplatelet agents should be advised to report any symptoms of peripheral bleeding such as epistaxis or susceptibility to bruising, but the effect of dietary intake is likely negligible. This hypothetical interaction is probably of marginal clinical significance.

THEORETICAL, SPECULATIVE, AND PRELIMINARY INTERACTIONS RESEARCH, INCLUDING OVERSTATED INTERACTIONS CLAIMS

Oral Hypoglycemic Agents and Insulin

Buformin (Andromaco Gliporal, Buformina), chlorpropamide (Diabinese), glimepiride (Amaryl), glipizide (Glucotrol; Glucotrol XL), glyburide (Glibenclamide; Diabeta, Glynase, Glynase Prestab, Micronase, Pres Tab), insulin (animal-source insulin: Iletin; human analog insulin: Humanlog; human insulin: Humulin, Novolin, NovoRapid, Oralin), metformin (Dianben, Glucophage, Glucophage XR); combination drugs: glipizide and metformin (Metaglip), glyburide and metformin (Glucovance); tolazamide (Tolinase), phenformin (Debeone, Fenformin), tolbutamide (Orinase, Tol-Tab).

Traditionally, bilberry leaf was used as an antidiabetic tea before the ready availability of insulin for management of blood sugar levels. This use was emphasized in German phytotherapy and is discussed at length by Wichtl.[6] However, as pointed out by Weiss,[5] bilberry leaf, in common with other herbal infusions touted as antidiabetic teas, does not afford a clinically significant degree of glycemic control, and bilberry leaf infusions are not in general use by diabetic patients. Bilberry leaf is "unapproved," according to the Commission E monograph, because of lack of evidence for the antidiabetic function. One study of a rodent model of streptozotocin-induced (STZ) diabetes suggested that a short-term drop in blood glucose was seen compared with nondiabetic control animals after acute oral doses of bilberry leaf at a rate of 3.0 g/kg for 4 days (equivalent to cumulative human dose of ~840 g dried leaf).[28] Extrapolations from this study that infer interactions with insulin or hypoglycemic agents are unwarranted, given the excessive dose used and the lack of clinical use of the leaf in modern Western botanical medicine.

Warfarin and Related Oral Vitamin K Antagonist Anticoagulants

Anisindione (Miradon), dicumarol, ethyl biscoumacetate (Tromexan), nicoumalone (acenocoumarol; Acitrom, Sintrom), phenindione (Dindevan), phenprocoumon (Jarsin, Marcumar), warfarin (Coumadin, Marevan, Warfilone).

Some secondary sources have speculated that, because of the in vitro antiplatelet actions previously discussed, interactions may occur between concentrated bilberry extracts and warfarin or related "vitamin K antagonist" oral anticoagulants, as well as antiplatelet drugs.[29-31] Although some foods (e.g., avocado) have been reported to interact with warfarin, without a direct effect on vitamin K, the mechanisms of these interactions remain unclear. Combining antiplatelet and anticoagulant medications can result in increased risk of bleeding in certain individuals, so it remains a theoretical possibility that chronic coadministration of very high doses of bilberry extract with warfarin could result in an increased risk of bleeding. However, this remains a speculative extrapolation, without supportive data.

The 31 citations for this monograph are located under Bilberry on the CD at the back of the book.

Black Cohosh

Botanical Name: *Cimicifuga racemosa* (L.) Nutt.
Pharmacopoeial Name: Rhizoma cimicifugae racemosae.
Synonym: *Actea racemosa* L.
Common Names: Black cohosh, black snakeroot, macrotys (historical).

SUMMARY

Drug/Class Interaction Type	Mechanism and Significance	Management
Androgen blockade LHRH antagonists Antiandrogens ☼/⊕	Black cohosh reduces drug-induced vasomotor adverse effects. Established effect in women, but only anecdotal support for the interaction in men.	Coadminister with professional management and monitoring.
Hormone replacement therapy (HRT) Estrogens/progestins ☼/⊕⊕	Black cohosh supports reduced HRT doses, or tapered withdrawal by reducing symptoms associated with climacteric.	Consider adoption, especially for HRT withdrawal.
Tamoxifen, Raloxifene (SERMS) ⊕⊕/☼	Black cohosh reduces drug-induced climacteric symptoms, may synergize with SERM antitumor effects in estrogen receptor—positive cancer.	Consider coadministering with professional management.

LHRH, Luteinizing hormone—releasing hormone; *SERMs*, selective estrogen response modulators.

HERB DESCRIPTION

Family
Ranunculaceae.

Related Species

None; blue cohosh (*Caulophyllum thalactroides* L.) is a different species botanically and medicinally. Asian varieties sold as *sheng ma* may be derived from *Actea foetida* or *Actea dahrica* and are not interchangeable.

Habitat and Cultivation

Native to eastern North America; 95% of black cohosh is wildcrafted, and the impact of annual harvests of 600,000 to 700,000 pounds (1998) on the viability of wild populations is a cause for concern.

Parts Used

Rhizome and roots.

Common Forms

Dried: Powdered rhizome and root.
Tincture: 1:3 to 1:10 60% alcohol-dried.
Fluid Extract: 1:1 60% to 90% alcohol-dried.
Standardized Extracts: Commercial extracts standardized to 2.5% triterpene glycosides are available. Clinical trials have largely been based on Remifemin, a proprietary isopropanolic formulation available as liquid and tablet form equivalent to a 1:1 g/mL fluid extract, or BNO 1055, an ethanolic extract sold as Klimadynon/Menafem. (See constituents discussed later for labeling of 27-deoxyactein marker compound.)

Note: Herbal practitioners may use fresh herb material, but this is not common in commerce.

HERB IN CLINICAL PRACTICE

Overview
Modern use of black cohosh is dominated by its perception as a remedy for various symptoms associated with menopause. In 1989 the German Commission E approved its use for dysmenorrhea, premenstrual discomfort, and neurovegetative ailments associated with menopause. Increasing concern about the adverse effects of conventional hormone replacement therapy (HRT), coupled with clinical trial support for menopausal applications and promotion of standardized European isopropanolic preparations of black cohosh, has led to a narrowing of focus on the herb as a gynecological remedy, especially for menopausal issues. Therapeutic monographs of the herb include those by the British Herbal Medical Association (BHMA),[1] German Commission E,[2] and more recently by the World Health Organization (WHO),[3] *American Herbal Pharmacopoeia*,[4] and European Scientific Cooperative on Phytotherapy (ESCOP).[5]

Contrary to initial research assumptions of its "estrogenic" properties, recent studies on black cohosh suggest that it is in fact antiestrogenic. Lacking any phytoestrogenic isoflavone constituents, newer data have demonstrated dopaminergic and serotonergic receptor binding. Ongoing developments in estrogen receptor molecular biology continue to add to the complex emerging picture. The traditionally known affinities of black cohosh for the nervous and musculoskeletal systems, its cardiovascular effects, and the broad scope of its gynecological indications (which extend far beyond the specific issue of climacteric symptoms) increasingly appear to have an underlying basis in the neuroendocrine pharmacology of the herb, although this awaits full elucidation.

Historical/Ethnomedicine Precedent

Black cohosh was used by Native Americans for general malaise, various gynecological conditions, kidney ailments, malaria, rheumatism, sore throat, and snakebite.[6] The early colonists also used the herb, reputedly for menorrhea, uterine disorders, nervous disorders, lumbago, snakebite, and various infectious conditions, including malaria.[7] *Cimicifuga* was a primary remedy for the Eclectic physicians, who termed it "macrotys." The Eclectics used different forms of the herb, including fresh and dried extracts and a "resinoid" concentrate. This was employed for a wide range of neuromuscular, gynecological, and obstetrical conditions, including neuralgia, headache, rheumatism, false labor, labor, postpartum pain, "partus preparator" (to encourage natural contractions during labor), mastitis, atony of the uterus, and amenorrhea, as well as for a variety of nervous system disorders, including chorea, convulsions, delirium tremens, nervous excitability, spasmodic cough, and pertussis. Interestingly, Eclectic use included male urogenital conditions such as orchalgia and spermatorrhea as well as infections such as smallpox.[8-10] Grieve includes the indication of St. Vitus' dance (Sydenham's chorea) in children.[11] Boericke[12] emphasized depression as a key mental indication for *Cimicifuga* as a homeopathic medicine.

Known or Potential Therapeutic Uses

Antirheumatic, antispasmodic, uterine tonic; treatment of climacteric symptoms and ovarian insufficiency, especially associated with iatrogenically induced menopause; mild depression, especially associated with cyclical or climacteric changes; fibromyalgia.

Key Constituents

Triterpene glycosides: More than 20 identified, including 23-epi-26 deoxyactein, which is often incorrectly labeled as "27-deoxyactein" on commercial standardized product labels.[13]

Flavonoids: Early reports of the presence of the phytoestrogenic isoflavones formononetin and biochanin A have not been substantiated by recent analytical data and are not present in the standardized isopropanolic extract Remifenin.[14,15]

Aromatic acids: Hydroxycinnamic acid esters of fukiic and piscidic acid; fukinolic and cimicifugic acids, along with ferulic isoferulic and caffeic acids.

Novel polyphenolics have recently been described.[16]

Other components include up to 20% resin ("cimicifugin").[17]

Therapeutic Dosing Range

From 0.2 to 4.0 mL/day (1:1 equivalent) hydroethanolic extracts.

Recent clinical trials using isopropanolic extracts average a modest daily dose of 40 to 80 mg-equivalent dried herb.

INTERACTIONS REVIEW
Strategic Considerations

Black cohosh therapeutic monographs typically do not identify any drug interactions.[2,3,5] The herb appears to be relatively safe and is well tolerated with minimal toxicity at therapeutic doses.

A recent comprehensive safety review by Low Dog et al.[18] analyzed uncontrolled reports, postmarketing surveillance, and human clinical trials of more than 2800 patients involving black cohosh. The trials demonstrated a low incidence (5.4%) of adverse events, of which 97% were minor, and none resulted in discontinuation of therapy. No severe events were attributable to the herb. The authors concluded that black cohosh was safe when used for menopausal symptoms and is a safe alternative for women in whom estrogen therapy is contraindicated.[18] However, both this and other safety reviews[19] mainly examined isopropanolic extracts as used in clinical trials, and the data do not necessarily apply to traditional preparations, which are often used at higher doses. According to the manufacturers of Remifemin, animal tests suggest that higher equivalent doses, up to 500 times the 40-mg oral dose of isopropanolic preparations, are well tolerated over 6 months.

Despite the apparently benign toxicity of the herb according to clinical trial data, there have been persistent anecdotal reports of hepatotoxicity linked to black cohosh consumption. A recent National Institutes of Health (NIH) workshop discussed such reports and concluded that at present, hepatoxicity has not been conclusively demonstrated, although vigilance, including liver function monitoring, may be appropriate when higher doses are used.[20,21]

The absence of published interactions data and reports requires integrative practitioners to make the best possible assessments about potential interactions in light of the known pharmacology of the herb. Given increasing concerns about the risks of breast cancer associated with female HRT, arguably one of the more common clinical settings for use of the herb is the coadministration of black cohosh with HRT. Related concerns are potential interactions between black cohosh and drugs used for other aspects of menopause, such as the bisphosphonates for osteoporosis.

Hormone-dependent malignancies are another important area where drug-herb interactions must be considered. Premenopausal patients with reproductive malignancies are likely to experience more severe menopausal symptoms, especially vasomotor effects, as a result of chemotherapy-induced menopause than are postmenopausal patients.[22,23] The use of HRT in either population is contraindicated because of the proliferative activity of estrogens and the increased risk of renewed tumorigenesis.[24,25] The possible efficacy of black cohosh for symptom relief in these populations has not been the subject of systematic long-term studies, although some data are available; nevertheless, anecdotally the use of black cohosh is widespread in this setting.[26] The potential interaction between adjunctive tamoxifen and black cohosh in this population has been subject of small number of preclinical and clinical investigations.[27-30] (See SERMs later.)

Related adjuvant endocrine pharmacotherapies, such as aromatase inhibitors, including the more selective third-generation drugs, are restricted in use to postmenopausal patients.[24] Black cohosh does not contain the isoflavones with known in vitro aromatase inhibition (e.g., red clover, soy) and has no known aromatase inhibitory activity. Currently, no data relate coadministration of black cohosh with aromatase inhibitors.

Women for whom estrogen therapy is contraindicated and those with a history of estrogen-dependent malignancies should avoid black cohosh, according to some sources.[31] Recent studies on the pharmacology and clinical effects of black cohosh have been reviewed by Borrelli et al.[32,33] The current consensus is that the herb is primarily antiestrogenic, with receptor-binding tests negative for alpha or beta estrogen receptor (ER), and that it lacks estrogenic effects on uterine tissue.[34-40] Despite the predominant evidence for nonestrogenicity, as evidenced by assays on immortal ER-positive lines such as the MCF7 (breast) and Ishihara (endometrial) cell lines, data on cell proliferation are conflicting, with a few studies suggesting proliferation at low doses, although not at higher doses.[41-44] In contrast, a recent poster report suggested that MMT-neu transgenic rats (in which mammary tumors develop through spontaneous activation of the HER-2/neu oncogene), when treated with equivalent oral doses of isopropanolic black cohosh, show increased metastatic progression to the lung at necropsy.[45] However, the black cohosh–treated animals did not differ from controls in latency or incidence of mammary tumor formation. Publicity about this poster report suggesting that black cohosh is unsafe for breast cancer patients would appear premature given that the weight of emerging evidence is against proliferative effects of the herb.[46] Further evidence is needed to establish safety definitively, and use of black cohosh in oncological settings should be restricted to health care professionals with appropriate clinical expertise in the use of botanicals in reproductive malignancies.

Evidence that both serotonergic and dopaminergic pathways may be involved in the mediation of some of the clinical effects of black cohosh on menopausal symptom reduction is gathering weight from initial experimental studies on serotonin receptor binding of the extract.[47] Borrelli et al.[33] hypothesized that serotonin may account for the apparent low-dose estrogenic effects, and this hypothesis has also been adopted by experienced researchers in the field such as Jarry et al.[48] Significantly, recent clinical evidence exists for the effectiveness of selective serotonin reuptake inhibitors (SSRIs; e.g., paroxetine, venlafaxine, fluoxetine) in reducing hot flashes in breast cancer patients.[49-51] Circumstantial support for this theory is also found in ER research which suggests possible activation effect of ER transcription by serotonin.[52]

The ER itself is an intensive focus of ongoing study, and the complexities of coactivation factors and pharmacogenomic variation within the alpha and beta receptor subtypes continue to expand the picture.[53-55] The complexity of ER biology may account for some of the earlier contradictory research findings; for instance, the biphasic nature of dose-response curves exhibited by estrogens and phytoestrogens has been studied as an example of the general phenomenon of *hormesis* (biphasic or U-shaped dose response curves), adding a further explanatory dimension to the multifactorial mechanisms involved.[56,57]

In clinical practice, combination prescriptions of herbs are often employed, but these are rarely studied in trials. An exception is a recent positive trial of the paired combination of St. John's wort (*Hypericum perforatum*) and black cohosh for climacteric symptoms.[58] The study indirectly lends further support to the thesis that menopausal symptoms are caused by neurotransmitter imbalances, given the known pharmacology of St. John's wort, which is devoid of phytoestogenic effects. (See St. John's Wort monograph.)

Overall, the pharmacodynamics of black cohosh are complex and not fully understood. The focus on menopause may have detracted from wider considerations; for example, black cohosh compounds are chemoprotective against menadione-induced deoxyribonucleic acid (DNA) damage.[59] The model of black cohosh emerging from current research in many ways is more coincident with the traditional picture of the remedy as a neuroendocrine rather than a hormonal agent.

Effects on Drug Metabolism and Bioavailability

Pharmacokinetic interactions between black cohosh and prescription drugs have not been recorded to date. Preliminary clinical data suggest a potential for interactions with drugs metabolized by cytochrome P450 2D6 (CYP2D6), following a probe drug study with desobriquin on 12 healthy volunteers by Gurley et al.[60] This study failed to find any effect of black cohosh extracts on CYP1A2, CYP2E1, and CYP3A4, despite significant inhibition of CYP2D6. The preparation was a commercial black cohosh extract standardized to 0.2% triterpene glycosides administered at 1090 mg orally twice daily for 28 days. An in vitro study tested separate black cohosh triterpene compounds for inhibitory activity against recombinant CYP3A4 oxidation of nifedipine. Separate isolated triterpenes demonstrated moderate IC_{50} (median inhibitory concentration) effects, but the whole extract demonstrated a notable inhibition, with IC_{50} of 0.027 mg/mL. The authors suggested potential for interactions with 3A4-metabolized drugs; however, this conflicts with the available clinical evidence from Gurley's group, who established that black cohosh extracts had no effect in vivo on the 3A4 substrate midazolam.[61]

Drugs metabolized by CYP2D6 include important tricyclic antidepressants, SSRIs, antipsychotics, stimulants (e.g., risperidone), analgesics, and tamoxifen. CYP2D6 is a narrow-band (high-affinity) low-throughput cytochrome, and many of the drugs metabolized by 2D6 can also be oxidized by 3A4. Polymorphisms of 2D6 are well known, and "poor metabolizers" have been shown to exhibit higher adverse effect levels with several drugs that are 2D6 substrates. Genotyping of patients for whom for prescription of 2D6 substrate drugs is indicated has been proposed as advisable.[62] Coadministration of black cohosh with drugs that are substrates of 2D6 should be avoided, or related drugs that are not 2D6 substrates should be selected, but interactions with 3A4 substrates are unlikely.

Modulation of drug transporters by black cohosh has received little study. Gurley et al.[63] found no effect of the herb (40 mg/day for 14 days) on digoxin pharmacokinetics, suggesting a negligible action on P-glycoprotein (P-gp). An experimental model of the human organic anion-transporting polypeptide B (OATP-B) revealed a moderate inhibitory effect on estrone-3-sulfate uptake after black cohosh addition; however, the number of known OATP-B substrates in humans is limited at present, although it does include DHEA-S and estrone.[64]

HERB-DRUG INTERACTIONS

Androgen Blockade Chemotherapies

Chemotherapy, antiandrogens: Bicalutamide (Casodex), cyproterone (Androcur, Cyprohexal, Cyprostat, Cyproteron, Procur, Cyprone, Ciproterona, Cyproteronum, Neoproxil, Siterone), flutamide (Chimax, Drogenil, Euflex), nilutamide (Anandron, Nilandron).

Chemotherapy, estrogens: Diethylstilbestrol (DES; Stilphostrol).

Chemotherapy, luteinizing hormone–releasing hormone (LHRH) agonists: Goserelin (Zoladex), leuprolide (Eligard, Lupron, Lupron Depot, Viadur), triptorelin (De-capeptyl Trelstar, Trelstar LA).

Chemotherapy, gonadotropin-releasing hormone (GnRH) receptor antagonists/LHRH antagonists: Abererelix, etrorelix (Cetrotide), ganirelix (Antagon).

5α-Reductase inhibitors: Dutasteride (Avidart, Avodart, Avolve, Duagen, Dutas, Dutagen, Duprost), finasteride (Propecia, Proscar).

Steroid/androgen synthesis blockade: Ketoconazole (Nizoral).

Interaction Type and Significance
☼ **Prevention or Reduction of Drug Adverse Effect**
⊕ **Potential or Theoretical Beneficial or Supportive Interaction, with Professional Management**

Probability:
4. Plausible

Evidence Base:
☐ Inadequate

Effect and Mechanism of Action
Androgen deprivation combining one or more endocrine agents (or orchiectomy) in prostate cancer patients leads to well-documented adverse effects of hot flashes and loss of libido in more than 50% of patients. Black cohosh extracts may reduce vasomotor symptoms in patients with androgen deprivation.

Research
To date, research into the effects of black cohosh on vasomotor symptoms has been in women undergoing menopause, whether the natural climacteric or chemically or surgically induced. (See later discussion of interactions with HRT and SERMs.)

Reports
Currently, there are no published reports on the use of black cohosh for adverse effects of androgen blockade, although a recent general review of the subject by Moyad[65] highlights the pressing need for research on this topic.

Integrative Therapeutics, Clinical Concerns, and Adaptations
Although the clinical efficacy of black cohosh in reducing hot flashes is not always consistent, interest in the use of the herb remains high among menopausal women and is a focus of ongoing research. On the other hand, information regarding use of lifestyle and integrative strategies or alternative therapies for andropausal symptoms is scarce. The spectrum of clinical and laboratory abnormalities associated with androgen deprivation therapy has been characterized as "androgen deprivation syndrome" (ADS) by prostate oncologist Strum, who suggests that ADS is an accelerated and exaggerated form of male menopause (andropause) involving a spectrum of possible symptoms, including mental and emotional changes and bone and joint pain.[66] The traditional indications of black cohosh for depression and rheumatic conditions, as well as its effects on vasomotor symptoms, suggest that its consideration is appropriate in the context of integrative oncological management of prostate cancer patients experiencing ADS, and clinical investigation is warranted.

Hormone Replacement Therapy (HRT): Estrogen-Containing and Synthetic Estrogen and Progesterone Analog Medications

HRT, estrogens: chlorotrianisene (Tace); conjugated equine estrogens (Premarin); conjugated synthetic estrogens (Cenestin); dienestrol (Ortho Dienestrol); esterified estrogens (Estratab, Menest, Neo-Estrone); estradiol, topical/transdermal/ring (Alora Transdermal, Climara Transdermal, Estrace, Estradot, Estring FemPatch, Vivelle-Dot, Vivelle Transdermal); estradiol cypionate (Dep-Gynogen, Depo-Estradiol, Depogen, Dura-Estrin, Estra-D, Estro-Cyp, Estroject-LA, Estronol-LA); estradiol hemihydrate (Estreva, Vagifem); estradiol valerate (Delestrogen, Estra-L 40, Gynogen L.A. 20, Progynova, Valergen 20); estrone (Aquest, Estragyn 5, Estro-A, Estrone '5', Kestrone-5); estropipate (Ogen, Ortho-Est); ethinyl estradiol (Estinyl, Gynodiol, Lynoral).

HRT, estrogen/progestin combinations: Conjugated equine estrogens and medroxyprogesterone (Premelle cycle 5, Prempro); conjugated equine estrogens and norgestrel (Prempak-C); estradiol and dydrogesterone (Femoston); estradiol and norethindrone, patch (CombiPatch); estradiol and norethindrone/norethisterone, oral (Activella, Climagest, Climesse, FemHRT, Trisequens); estradiol valerate and cyproterone acetate (Climens); estradiol valerate and norgestrel (Progyluton); estradiol and norgestimate (Ortho-Prefest).

HRT, estrogen/testosterone combinations: Esterified estrogens and methyltestosterone (Estratest, Estratest HS). (See also Estrogen Replacement Therapy [ERT] later.)

Interaction Type and Significance
☼ **Prevention or Reduction of Drug Adverse Effect**
⊕⊕ **Beneficial or Supportive Interaction, with Professional Management**

Probability:
1. Certain

Evidence Base:
◉ Emerging

Effect and Mechanism of Action
Black cohosh extracts have been demonstrated to reduce several menopausal discomforts, especially vasomotor symptoms such as hot flashes and night sweats, through nonestrogenic mechanisms for which female HRT is also prescribed. Coadministration can be used to assist drug withdrawal, to reduce drug dosage or form of drug administration, or to decrease exposure to undesirable levels of exogenous estrogen.

Research
There is no research directly analyzing the effects of combining HRT and black cohosh, and the majority of clinical trials preclude use of HRT as an inclusion criterion, comparing the effects of black cohosh alone to placebo. Coadministration data are generally confined to survey information (see Reports), although two German open-label trials that included coadministration groups (Petho 1987, Warnecke 1985) were cited in McKenna et al.[67] but were unavailable for review; apparently these trials did not demonstrate significant interactions or adverse effects.

Reports
Recent survey data on menopausal women in Western countries reveal extensive use of dietary, botanical, and nutritional supplements for menopausal complaints.[68-71] Significant proportions of survey participants admitted to concurrent use of HRT with herbal therapies for menopause, ranging from 16% in the San Francisco Bay area survey by Kam et al.[69] to 46% in the Seattle area survey by Newton et al.[70] (n = 886). Black cohosh was the third most popular supplement used (after soy extracts and ginkgo). Almost all participants believed the natural therapies used were beneficial.

Integrative Therapeutics, Clinical Concerns, and Adaptations
Changing perceptions of menopause (which is increasingly seen as a normal life cycle transition for which "natural" and folk remedies are more appropriate than mainstream medical interventions), coupled with increasing concern about the risks of breast cancer associated with female HRT, has led to widespread self-prescribed use of black cohosh (among other agents) as a "replacement" for HRT.[72] Practitioners familiar with botanical therapies use black cohosh in formulations to assist tapered withdrawal from HRT. It is also used to facilitate transition from combination regimens of conjugated estrogens

and synthetic progestins to lower doses of "safer" bioidentical HRT protocols using estriol and natural progesterone, or Bi-est or Tri-est compounded hormonal formulations (i.e., estrone, estradiol, and estriol compounded formulations). Black cohosh is rarely used alone in this context, but rather is used as one ingredient of formulae addressing the specific pattern of the individual case. Use of laboratory test data of urinary 2α-/16α-hydroxyestrone ratio as a screening test is advisable to determine incorporation of related interventions affecting estrogen metabolism in postmenopausal women; the 2α-substituted estrogen metabolites have much less tumor-promoting activity than those with 16α-substituted structure. Typical associated complementary interventions include the dietary consumption of brassicaceous vegetables, use of soy isoflavones and indole-3-carbinol supplements, and lifestyle factors such as physical exercise and weight reduction, all of which favor the shift from the 16α-hydroxylation to the 2α-hydroxylation pathway.

Selective Estrogen Response Modulators (SERMs)

Raloxifene (Evista), tamoxifen (Nolvadex), toremifene (Fureston).

Interaction Type and Significance

☼ **Prevention or Reduction of Drug Adverse Effect**
⊕⊕ **Beneficial or Supportive Interaction, with Professional Management**

Probability:	Evidence Base:
4. Plausible	○ Preliminary

Effect and Mechanism of Action

Black cohosh extracts reduce vasomotor adverse effects associated with SERMs and may synergize with the antiproliferative effects of these agents in the adjuvant setting for ER-positive breast cancers.

Research

The mechanism of this interaction is not currently understood, although the reduction of hot flashes is unlikely to be directly mediated through ER effects. Preliminary evidence for enhancement of the antiproliferative effects of tamoxifen by black cohosh in MCF-7 (estrogen-dependent breast cancer) cells was demonstrated by Bodinet and Freudenstein,[27] who found significant inhibition of proliferation by the extract alone and a synergistic increase when combined with tamoxifen. Nisslein and Freudenstein[30,73] found similar synergistic effects with tamoxifen for both mammary and endometrial cancer lines in rodent models; in the endometrial model the effects did not result in increased tumor growth or metastasis, either with black cohosh alone or with the black cohosh–tamoxifen combination.

Two trials have examined the effects of black cohosh on tamoxifen-induced hot flashes. Jacobson et al.[29] used isopropanolic black cohosh extracts at 40 mg for 60 days in placebo/tamoxifen, black cohosh/tamoxifen, black cohosh/no tamoxifen, and placebo/no tamoxifen groups. They studied incidence and severity of hot flashes and sampled changes in follicle-stimulating hormone (FSH) and luteinizing hormone (LH) levels before and after treatment. The decline in hot flashes was 27% over baseline, but differences between the black cohosh and placebo groups were only significant in the degree of reduction of sweating. This contrasts with a more recent study by Hernadez Munoz and Pluchino,[28] who compared the use of tamoxifen alone (20 mg/day) to the same dose combined with 20 mg of ethanolic standardized black cohosh extract daily, administered for 12 months in 136 breast cancer survivors age 32 to 52 years. Almost half the intervention group were free from hot flashes, and the incidence of severe hot flashes was 24% in the intervention group and 73.9% in the usual-care (tamoxifen-only) group. Pockaj et al.[74] conducted a survey of black cohosh use among menopausal women with hot flashes, 13 of whom had a history of breast cancer or were taking tamoxifen or raloxifene, and found that a significant number had reduced symptoms and that no adverse effects of the herb were noted.

Integrative Therapeutics, Clinical Concerns, and Adaptations

Endocrine therapy with tamoxifen remains a standard adjuvant approach in ER-positive breast cancer for both premenopausal and postmenopausal women, despite issues of tumor flare, development of drug resistance, and a range of adverse effects. Adverse effects of tamoxifen include hot flashes, vaginal bleeding and discharge, and a range of central nervous system (CNS) symptoms, such as mood changes, irritability, and depression. In addition, tamoxifen increases the risk of endometrial cancer and blood clots because of its estrogen-like activity, although it also lowers blood lipid levels and enhances bone density for the same reason.

Practitioners experienced in the use of botanical medicines in integrative cancer care settings may consider black cohosh (along with the isoflavone and lignan phytoestrogens) as potential supportive agents for reduction of hot flashes induced by tamoxifen. Furthermore, the experimental data suggest a potential improvement in anticancer efficacy for the combination. Large-scale clinical trials of these agents (vs. placebo) in combination with endocrine therapies are needed to evaluate fully the potential effects of such combination therapies. (See also Androgen Blockade Chemotherapies earlier.)

THEORETICAL, SPECULATIVE, AND PRELIMINARY INTERACTIONS RESEARCH, INCLUDING OVERSTATED INTERACTIONS CLAIMS

Estrogen Replacement Therapy (ERT)

Warnings about black cohosh causing "estrogen excess" with ERT have been made by Miller.[75] This suggestion is not only speculative, but also in conflict with the known pharmacology of the herb. (See previous sections on HRT with estrogens and estrogen/progestin combinations.)

Iron

It has been suggested that black cohosh extracts may deplete iron from supplemental sources because of the tannin content of the herb.[76] Black cohosh rhizome and roots are not excessively tannin rich, and circumstantial evidence for the interaction is absent, so this interaction can be regarded as wholly speculative.

The 76 citations for this monograph are located under Black Cohosh on the CD at the back of the book.

Cascara

Botanical Name: *Rhamnus purshiana* DC.
Pharmacopoeial Name: Cortex rhamni purshianae.
Synonym: *Frangula purshiana* (DC) A. Gray ex J.C. Cooper.
Common Names: Cascara, cascara sagrada.

HERB DESCRIPTION

Family

Rhamnaceae.

Related Species

Alder buckthorn, *Rhamnus frangula* L. (syn. *Frangula alnus*, Miller.), buckthorn, *Rhamnus catharticus* L.

Parts Used

Dried bark (aged at least 1 year, stored in dark).

Common Forms

Dried bark: Powdered or cut for decoction.
Fluid Extract: 1:1 25% alcohol.[1]
Other liquid and solid preparations.

INTERACTIONS REVIEW

Strategic Considerations

Cascara bark is a major representative of the anthraquinone-containing herbs that are principally used for short-term relief of constipation. The anthraquinone-containing laxative group of botanicals traditionally includes related Rhamnaceae species such as the buckthorns (*Rhamnus frangula* L. and *R. catharticus* L.), senna leaf and fruits (*Cassia senna* L.), rhubarb root (*Rheum palmatum* L.), and aloe latex (*Aloe ferox*, Miller). The different crude drugs in this group have a large medical and commercial application as stimulant laxatives for the preparation of patients for radiological or colonoscopic procedures, softening of stool before anorectal surgical procedures, and treatment of constipation linked to drug-induced or lifestyle causes. In traditional botanical medicine, cascara and its relatives have long been used for short-term treatment of constipation, with a more recent history of folk use in herbal cancer treatments (e.g., the Hoxsey formula).

The widespread availability of both over-the-counter (OTC) and dietary supplement preparations containing stimulant laxatives has emphasized the problem of adverse effects from laxative abuse, with public education through cautionary product labeling suggesting restrictions for duration of use and contraindications for consumers.[2] Most of the professional literature echoes this concern. Cascara bark was approved for constipation by the German Commission E[3] and is the subject of monographs by the British Herbal Medical Association (BHMA),[1] World Health Organization (WHO),[4] and most comprehensively by the European Scientific Cooperative on Phytotherapy (ESCOP).[5]

A distinction should be made between appropriate therapeutic use of cascara and related botanicals and the uncontrolled, self-prescribed consumption of these agents by certain individuals. These latter, for psychological reasons, either consider normal bowel movement frequency to be unhealthy or compulsively exhibit behaviors classified in the eating disorder group of diagnoses (i.e., bulimia, anorexia, binge eating) and use purgation (and/or vomiting) as a self-imposed means of eliminating ingested food. Although such abuse exists, preoccupation with the purgative aspects of these herbs and their anthraquinone constituents is only one concern to integrative practitioners. A broader consideration of the activity of these botanicals in light of recent research suggests therapeutic applications in other fields, such as cancer chemotherapy.

Recent findings have revealed that the earlier concept of all stimulant laxatives acting through gut motility mechanisms is oversimplistic. Multiple mechanisms are involved, including almost every aspect of active and passive electrolyte transport, such as sodium/potassium-adenosinetriphosphatase (Na^+, K^+-ATPase), cyclic nucleotides, protein kinase C, calcium (Ca^{++}) dependence, autocoids or neurotransmitter release, increased mucosal permeability, and histological damage.[6-11] Furthermore, it has become clear that significant differences exist between the mechanism of action of the different agents; for example, senna does not stimulate platelet-activating factor (PAF) or inducible nitric oxide synthase (iNOS), as occurs with cascara.[6,8]

In the field of cancer biology, hydroxyanthraquinone agents such as emodin, once considered to be potentially carcinogenic, have more recently been studied for a variety of antiproliferative effects, mediated by inhibition of both nuclear factor kappa B (NF-κB) and tyrosine kinase.[12,13] These results have particular impact on HER-2/neu overexpression, as discussed later in the context of cascara's possible therapeutic combination with herceptin. Parenthetically, it should be noted that a significant number of conventional chemotherapeutic agents, notably doxorubicin, idarubicin, epirubicin, and mitoxantrone, are all anthraquinone derivatives. Interestingly, drug resistance to these agents may be reduced by plant-based polyphenols, including aloe-emodin, probably by inhibition of NF-κB.[14] Experimental studies with whole-herb extracts are rare, and most available data derive from studies using isolated anthraquinone ingredients such as emodin and aloe-emodin, and extrapolations to whole-plant effects must be qualified.

Pharmacokinetic interactions involving modification of drug absorption resulting from decreased transit times induced by cascara administration should not be overlooked. Stockley[15] reports only one such interaction between quinidine and a senna preparation in which quinidine AUC (area under curve) levels were reduced to 25% of baseline 12 hours after administration of a dose of Liquedepur. This is in contrast to the German Commission E, who proposed potential for interactions between all laxative herbs and antiarrhythmic drugs because of electrolyte disturbances (hypokalemia) rather than drug depletion from reduced bioavailability. The onset of enhanced bowel motility and the formation of soft or semisolid stool after administration of anthraquinone laxatives are known to lag 6 to 8 hours after ingestion, a result of the bowel flora hydrolysis of anthrone conjugates into the active aglycone drug form.[16] The extended delay should be taken into account if pharmaceuticals with a therapeutically narrow range are already being administered to the patient before cascara administration. As always, clinical context and goals of coadministration are relevant for evaluating the significance of a potential interaction, and the cautions persistently repeated in relation to these drugs in the botanical literature (possible hypokalemia) are only discussed here in the section Theoretical, Speculative, and Preliminary Interactions Research.

Effects on Drug Metabolism and Bioavailability

Some evidence suggests that the naturally occurring anthraquinones such as emodin and chrysophanol are substrates that may undergo bioactivation into carcinogenic (mutagenic/genotoxic) intermediates through cytochrome P450 1A1 and 1A2.[17] However, in vitro data suggest that they may inhibit the same enzymes.[18,19] Extrahepatic cytochromes, such as CYP1B1 (which is often overexpressed in certain reproductive malignancies), have been experimentally induced by emodin in a human lung cancer cell line.[20] Similar experimental models also suggest inhibitory effects on phase 2 enzymes, including glutathione-S-transferase P1 and N-acetyltransferase.[21,22] These effects may be due to inhibition or downregulation of transcription factors NF-κB and activating protein 1 (AP-1).[22,23] At present, the pharmacokinetic effects of anthraquinone herbs on drug metabolism are not well characterized, but the possibility of clinically significant effects cannot be ruled out.

HERB-DRUG INTERACTIONS

Trastuzumab

Trastuzumab (Herceptin).

Interaction Type and Significance
⊕ **Potential or Theoretical Beneficial or Supportive Interaction, with Professional Management**

Probability:	Evidence Base:
4. Plausible	☐ Inadequate

Effect and Mechanism of Action
Anthraquinone constituents of cascara, especially emodin, inhibit proliferation of HER-2/neu–overexpressing cancer cells and may additively interact with the monoclonal antibody, which also inhibits proliferation of HER-2/neu–overexpressing malignancy.

Research
Emodin, an anthraquinone constituent (and metabolite) of cascara, has been demonstrated to have antiproliferative effects, including induction of differentiation and apoptosis, through different mechanisms in several cancer cell lines, including breast, cervical, non–small cell lung cancer (NSCLC), and hepatoma, through a variety of mechanisms.[24-29] As a known inhibitor of the HER-2 tyrosine kinase domain,[30] emodin is particularly effective against HER-2/neu–overexpressing cells, and the continuing work by Zhang et al.[12,31] suggests that several beneficial interactions may occur between emodin and chemotherapy for HER-2/neu–overexpressing malignancies.

The HER-2 proto-oncogene is structurally related to the epidermal growth factor receptor. HER-2/neu is a p185 protein tyrosine kinase receptor and is a major target of antiproliferative drugs. Trastuzumab (Herceptin) is a successful first-generation monoclonal antibody drug that targets the HER-2/neu receptor. Currently, trastuzumab is licensed only for treatment of HER-2/neu–overexpressing metastatic breast cancer in patients with prior chemotherapy failure.[32,33] Gefitinib (Iressa, AstraZeneca) has been approved for treatment of NSCLC in patients who have failed treatment with traditional chemotherapeutic agents.[34] Currently, no studies have directly examined the interaction of trastuzumab and emodin. However, emodin has been shown in vitro to reduce drug resistance of HER-2/neu–overexpressing NSCLC cells to cisplatin, doxorubicin, and etoposide, as well as with paclitaxel in HER-2/neu–positive breast cancer cells.[25,31]

Integrative Therapeutics, Clinical Concerns, and Adaptations
At this time, use of natural tyrosine kinase inhibitors, such as curcumin from turmeric or emodin from cascara and related anthraquinone-containing herbs, is tentatively beginning to be explored in integrative oncological protocols. In practice, effective daily doses to achieve cytotoxicity from emodin have been calculated to be between 160 and 180 mg.[35] An issue with these doses is the possibility of mutagenicity from emodin itself. Despite in vitro tests that suggest mutagenicity, however, this factor has been considered a minimal risk factor in humans.[36-38]

The controversial Hoxsey anticancer formula incorporated several anthraquinone-containing herbs, including those with high levels of emodin. Anecdotally, the strongest support for Hoxsey formula came from breast and some skin cancers, several of which are now known to overexpress HER-2/neu.[39]

In China, other herbs containing emodin have been used in cancer therapy, notably *Polygonum cuspidatum*.[35] Practitioners of integrative oncology use the herb in this setting in botanical formulae for prevention of cancer recurrence, following conventional treatments. It should also be considered as a remedy for opiate-induced constipation in opiate-dependent cancer patients, in whom it might also synergize with certain chemotherapies.

THEORETICAL, SPECULATIVE, AND PRELIMINARY INTERACTIONS RESEARCH, INCLUDING OVERSTATED INTERACTIONS CLAIMS

Digoxin and Related Cardiac Glycosides and Antiarrhythmic Drugs

Amiodarone (Cordarone, Pacerone), deslanoside (cedilanin-D), digitoxin (Cystodigin), digoxin (purgoxin; Digitek, Lanoxin, Lanoxicaps), disopyramide (Norpace), dofetilide (Tikosyn), flecainide (Tambocor), ibutilide (Corvert), ouabain (g-strophanthin), procainamide (Procan-SR, Pronestyl), quinidine (Quinaglute, Quinidex, Quinora), sotalol (Betapace, Betapace AF, Sorine).

Potential electrolyte and acid-base disturbances resulting from chronic diarrhea caused by inappropriately prolonged use (or abuse) of cascara extracts was considered by the German Commission E. In their 1984 monograph on cascara, the Commission included a warning about the possibility of adverse interactions with cardiac glycosides, as well as other antiarrhythmic drugs, caused by hypokalemia. This was extended to a possible additive adverse interaction with known potassium-depleting drugs, such as thiazide diuretics and corticosteroids, as well as licorice root.[3] Over time, through force of repetition, this has now become a consensus interactions concern associated with all the stimulant laxative botanicals.

There are no actual clinical reports of this speculative interaction occurring. Therapeutic context should be acknowledged before general warnings about interactions are given. Laxative abuse is a possible context to consider.

Estimates of the incidence of laxative abuse are scarce. A review of 73 published studies suggested an incidence of approximately 4.0% in the general population, but 14% among bulimic patients.[40] The diagnosis of bulimia predominantly affects females and is rare in older populations likely to be taking antiarrhythmic medication. Also, hypokalemia is a rarely reported adverse effect of laxative use, although decades ago the issue was sporadically noted.[41] A single case report from the psychiatric literature does suggest that two severe episodes of torsades de pointes in a mentally ill woman were the result of electrolyte disturbance from the stimulant laxative bisacodyl.[42] No antiarrhythmics were being used by this patient; however, a preclinical study that examined the effect of coadministered bisacodyl on digoxin serum levels found a significant reduction in serum cardiac glycoside levels compared with controls, which the authors considered a result of absorption losses caused by the laxative.[43]

Beyond the situation of overt or covert laxative abuse, the dangers of a hypokalemia-induced interaction seem remote. *Stockley's Drug Interactions*[15] does not report drug-induced hypokalemia cases from any cause, including stimulant laxatives interacting with cardiac glycosides. As suggested by at least one commentator, these adverse effects are overstated and unlikely to be the basis of a clinically relevant interaction.[44,45] Unless a patient is borderline hypokalemic from potassium-wasting diuretic therapy without potassium supplementation, diarrhea-induced hypokalemia would require at least five voluminous liquid stools per day for several days, which is an improbable consequence of normal therapeutic administration of cascara.

The 45 citations for this monograph are located under Cascara on the CD at the back of the book.

Cayenne

Botanical Name: *Capsicum annuum* L. *var annuum*.
Pharmacopoeial Names: Capsici fructus, capsici fructus acer.
Common Names: Cayenne, chili pepper, red pepper, hot pepper.
Note: Conventionally, "chili" or "cayenne" refers to the hottest varieties, "paprika" to intermediate varieties, and "sweet" or "bell" pepper to the mild, nonpungent types. None are "true peppers" of the Piperaceae, such as black pepper, *Piper nigrum* L.

SUMMARY

Drug/Class Interaction Type	Mechanism and Significance	Management
Acetylsalicylic acid, nonsteroidal anti-inflammatory drugs (NSAIDs), and other ulcerogenic agents ☼/?	Cayenne is ulceroprotective; interaction little used in practice. Superior alternative botanical agents available.	Coadministration unnecessary; use more effective agents.
Enalapril Angiotensin-converting enzyme (ACE) inhibitors ✗	Cayenne may exacerbate ACE inhibitor—induced cough during early coadministration; isolated report.	Monitor, avoid, or reduce drug and herb dose, if feasible.
NSAIDs, oral corticosteroids, antiarthritic medications ⊕⊕⊕	Topical administration may improve symptom relief from anti-inflammatories or enable lower drug doses.	Consider adopting in chronic arthritis patients with escalating medication requirements.

HERB DESCRIPTION

Family

Solanaceae.

Related Species

Capsicum annuum L. *var frutescens, Capsicum annuum* L. *var longum, Capsicum annuum* L. *var glabriusculum,* (Dunal) Heiser and Pickersgill *Capsicum minimum* (Roxb). Typically, pungent varieties are classed as *C. annuum* and its varieties, whereas the nonpungent peppers are classed as *C. frutescens.*

Habitat and Cultivation

Native to Central America; naturalized to tropical and subtropical zones globally; now cultivated worldwide.

Parts Used

Dried ripe fruit.

Common Forms

Dried: Powdered fruit.
Oleoresin: Crude extract.
Tincture: Typically, 1:10 to 1:20, 60% to 90% ethanol.
Topical: Cream and ointments containing 0.02% to 0.05% capsaicinoids.

HERB IN CLINICAL PRACTICE

Overview

The widespread use of cayenne as a dietary ingredient contrasts with a relative lack of information about the clinical pharmacology of the whole herb. The crude herb extract, capsicum "oleoresin," contains more than 100 different volatile components (many of which are not yet fully characterized) and must be distinguished from isolated capsaicin, which unlike the oleoresin, has been subject to considerable pharmacological research.

Activity of capsaicin and its congeners is responsible for several of the traditional therapeutic effects of cayenne, especially the topical treatment of painful peripheral disorders. Capsaicin has been used extensively in neuro-pharmacological research, and its vanillyl moiety lent its name to the *vanilloid receptor* (VR). The VR is a chemically and thermally gated cation channel that is opened by heat and closed by capsaicin. Capsaicin activation causes the release of various neuropeptides at the VR, including substance P, which mediates pain sensation in afferent peripheral nocioceptive pathways, with recent evidence suggesting additional mechanisms of central noradrenergic activation through the locus coeruleus.[1] The VR is distributed widely in sensory afferent innervation of joints, muscles, and the integumentary, respiratory, digestive, and urogenital systems, as well as in the mucous membranes of the oral cavity and the cornea.[2]

Apart from its irritant effects (well known to police departments), internal use of capsaicin isolate has also been limited by some controversy over the potential mutagenic and tumorigenic toxicities of the compound.[3] Another naturally occurring vanillyl compound, resinferatoxin (RTX), derived from *Euphorbia resinefera,* has been used as a more potent capsaicin analog, therapeutically investigated as an intravesical treatment for incontinence, and is preferred to capsaicin because of a better adverse effects and toxicity profile.[4] Capsaicin itself has been synthesized, and synthetic analogs such as nonivamide (pellargonic acid vanillamide) are also available, sometimes employed as adulterants in capsicum samples.

Therapeutic use of isolated capsaicin and the oleoresin for external use is approved in the United States and several European Union (EU) countries as an ingredient in topical over-the-counter (OTC) preparations for analgesia in various neuralgic and myalgic conditions, with strengths typically

0.02% to 0.05% for creams and ointments. The German Commission E approved capsicum ("Paprika" monograph) for external use only and suggested limits to duration of administration (2 days), which appear to be conservative.[5] Literature reviews of the herb are sparse, except for a recent survey by McKenna et al.[6]

Historical/Ethnomedicine Precedent

Cayenne has been used for thousands of years by Native American and Meso-American peoples (*chili* is the Mayan term for cayenne) and was introduced to Europe following Spanish exploration of the Americas in the fifteenth century CE. Besides its near-universal use as a pungent spice additive to the human diet, cayenne is used in the major systems of traditional medicine, including Ayurveda, Chinese, Kampo, Korean, and African.

Generally, cayenne has been used topically as a rubefacient and counterirritant for arthritis and myalgias and as an analgesic for neuralgias and rheumatic pain. Internally, it has been used as a heating and stimulating remedy for colds and respiratory conditions, colic, and dyspepsia and as a digestive and circulatory stimulant. In Western botanical medicine, cayenne was associated with the popular folk medicine doctrines of Samuel Thomson in the United States in the mid-nineteenth century. "Thomsonian medicine" was based on a primitive energetic system that used cayenne in life-threatening illness "to raise vital heat." Thomsonian medicine later became refined and incorporated into the "Physiomedicalist school" of botanical medicine, which placed less emphasis on "heroic" therapeutic strategies of high doses of cayenne and other stimulants. In traditional Western botanical medicine, cayenne is primarily used internally as a stimulating cardiovascular and digestive tonic and topically as an analgesic.

Known or Potential Therapeutic Uses

External: Arthritis, chilblains, cluster headaches, myalgias, fibromyalgia and rheumatic pains, neuralgias and neuropathies (including diabetic neuropathy, postherpetic neuropathy, shingles, postsurgical neuropathic pain), osteoarthritis, pruritus, psoriasis, rhinopathy.
Internal: Atony of gastrointestinal (GI) tract, chemoprevention, diaphoretic and antipyretic in feverish conditions, noninflammatory flatulent dyspepsia, peripheral circulatory insufficiency, peptic ulcer prophylaxis.

Key Constituents

Pungent "capsaicinoid" principles, 0.5% to 1.5%, consisting principally of capsaicin (8-methyl-6-noneoyl-vanillylamide) and related vanillyl derivatives, dihydrocapsaicin, nordihydrocapsaicin, homohydrocapsaicin, and homocapsaicin.

Cayenne also contains several carotenoids, including carotene, lutein, and zeaxanthin; high levels of vitamins C and A; flavonoids; and steroidal alkaloid glycosides.

Therapeutic Dosing Range

Powdered Dried Herb (cayenne pepper): 30 to 250 mg, two or three times daily.
Tincture: 0.25 to 1.0 mL three times daily; 1:1 equivalent.
Topical: 0.025% capsaicinoid cream applied up to four times daily.

INTERACTIONS REVIEW
Strategic Considerations

The German Commission E monograph for cayenne lists no known interactions, and interactions reports for cayenne are rare.[5] The reason in part may be the rather narrow mainstream patterns of use as a topical analgesic. Synergistic interactions with coadministered analgesic and anti-inflammatory drugs are theoretically possible in this context, and some supportive data on this are available. However, topical herb-drug combinations are not widely employed in current clinical practice (see later discussion of antiarthritic medications). The dose of capsaicinoids in OTC topical preparations varies from 0.02% to 0.05%, applied up to four times daily to the affected area. Therapeutic context is itself apparently a determinant of capsaicin activity; animal experiments suggest that the analgesic effects of the compound are heightened in inflammatory states compared with noninflammatory controls.[7]

Internal prescription of cayenne by practitioners of botanical medicine usually follows traditional prescribing principles; thus cayenne is often incorporated in rather small quantities as an adjunctive ingredient of polypharmacy prescriptions to confer qualities of stimulation, warmth, and dispersion to the principal formula ingredients. The *British Herbal Pharmacopoeia* recommended dose for internal consumption is 30 to 120 mg, thrice daily. Assuming a "high" capsaicin content of approximately 1% capsaicinoids, this would deliver a daily amount of less than 5.0 mg capsaicinoids daily.[8] This is somewhat less than the typical human chronic dietary consumption levels in cultures where cayenne is a principal dietary spice, estimated at approximately 0.5 to 1.0 mg/kg.[2] In this context, interactions that have been extrapolated on the basis of experimental and animal data, involving relatively high levels of isolated capsaicin administered parenterally, are not directly applicable to clinical practice. (See Theoretical, Speculative, and Preliminary Interactions Research.)

Effects on Drug Metabolism and Bioavailability

The effects of dietary levels of cayenne intake on GI motility and secretion theoretically may lead to pharmacokinetic effects on drug absorption through direct actions on gut permeability, gastric acid levels, and intestinal transit times. Early reports suggested that cayenne increases gastric acid secretion, but recent studies do not confirm this.[9] An experimental study with a human ileocarcinoma cell line demonstrated increased cell permeability (tight junction gap increase) on administration of cayenne, although the opposite effect was observed with other spices (e.g., black pepper).[10] Animal evidence is inconclusive, although an ulceroprotective effect has been demonstrated in several studies, possibly related to increased mucous secretion and anti-inflammatory effects.[11-14]

In humans, hot pepper sauce (e.g., Tabasco) appears to slow gastric emptying, but overall orocecal time is unchanged, indicating increased intestinal transit.[15] This corresponds with the empirical observation that diarrhea can result from hot spicy food ingested by individuals who do not consume it regularly. Other evidence suggests a general metabolic stimulation; resting metabolic rate increases after cayenne spice ingestion in a meal, and the simultaneous increases in oxygen uptake, lipolysis, and carbohydrate metabolism may be associated with a degree of beta-adrenergic stimulation.[16,17] Gender differences in these effects have also been recorded.[18,19] Currently, dietary cayenne studies suggest that absorption of drugs ingested with cayenne-spiced food may be enhanced, regardless of the drug's characteristics. The degree to which this effect may be clinically significant is variable and unpredictable. Furthermore, some experimental data appear to conflict with this general conclusion; in rats, for example, cayenne coadministration appears to reduce the oral bioavailability of aspirin.[20]

Pharmacokinetic effects of capsaicin on drug-metabolizing enzymes have been an area of research interest, partly because of apparently conflicting data on carcinogenicity of the compound from epidemiological and experimental studies. Capsaicin itself is a substrate of hepatic CYP450 2E1, a cytochrome that shares with 1A1 and 1A2 the role of metabolism of potentially carcinogenic aromatic hydrocarbons.[21] Other pathways for capsaicin metabolism have been investigated, including aliphatic hydroxylation.[22] Capsaicin has been reported to be a tumor promoter, carcinogen, and potential mutagen.[23] At the same time, it has also been found to have antigenotoxic, antimutagenic, and anticancer effects.[24,25] More recently, capsaicin has also been found to inhibit nuclear factor kappa B (NF-κB) and to have proapoptotic effects, which support a multimechanism basis for its chemopreventive properties.[26-28]

Capsaicin and dihydrocapsaicin directly inhibit CYP2E1, which has been suggested as a mechanism of its anticarcinogenic effects.[25,29-33] The primary drug substrates of 2E1 include the halogenated aliphatic anesthetics (enflurane, halothane, isoflurane, methoxyflurane, sevoflurane), as well as acetaminophen and ethanol. Ethanol, smoking, obesity, and diabetes all induce 2E1, which is unusual among the CYP450 enzymes in being subject to so many environmental influences. However, capsaicin can also undergo bioactivation.[23,24] The formation of reactive intermediates from capsaicin may also be a result of pan-P450 metabolism of capsaicin, according to a recent study by Reilly et al.,[34] who report that this is an essential part of detoxification of capsaicin rather than bioactivation because the intermediates can be "trapped" by addition of glutathione (GSH), suggesting that they are normally conjugated harmlessly. Overall, current data seem to indicate that capsaicin either can be metabolized as a straightforward detoxification or can be bioactivated, generating intermediates that may have direct or indirect toxicity through pan-P450 enzyme inhibition or covalent adduct formation with hepatic microsomal deoxyribonucleic acid (DNA), depending on the circumstances. Animal experiments suggesting prolongation of pentobarbital- and phenobarbital-induced sleeping times may support the pan-P450 inhibition by reactive intermediates (these agents are multi-P450 substrates, and pharmacokinetic-increased levels would require pan-P450 inhibition).[35]

Preliminary experimental evidence also suggests that capsaicin inhibits P-glycoprotein (P-gp). Drug resistance to vinblastine in a P-gp–overexpressing, multidrug-resistant carcinoma cell line (KB-C2) was significantly inhibited in vitro by capsaicin at 50 μmol.[36] Further data on the effects of capsaicin on drug resistance are needed before clinical extrapolations can be made.

Knowledge of the impact of chronic capsaicin or cayenne ingestion combined with pharmaceuticals on this complex system is clearly incomplete. However, obvious pharmacokinetic interactions resulting from CYP2E1 inhibition have not been reported, with the possibly relevant exception of theophylline (see later).

HERB-DRUG INTERACTIONS

Acetylsalicylic Acid, Nonsteroidal Anti-Inflammatory Drugs (NSAIDs), and Other Ulcerogenic Agents

Evidence: Acetylsalicylic acid (acetosal, acetyl salicylic acid, ASA, salicylsalicylic acid; Arthritis Foundation Pain Reliever, Ascriptin, Aspergum, Asprimox, Bayer Aspirin, Bayer Buffered Aspirin, Bayer Low Adult Strength, Bufferin, Buffex, Cama Arthritis Pain Reliever, Easprin, Ecotrin, Ecotrin Low Adult Strength, Empirin, Extra Strength Adprin-B, Extra Strength Bayer Enteric 500 Aspirin, Extra Strength Bayer Plus, Halfprin 81, Heartline, Regular Strength Bayer Enteric 500 Aspirin, St. Joseph Adult Chewable Aspirin, ZORprin); combination drugs: ASA and caffeine (Anacin), ASA, caffeine, and propoxyphene (Darvon Compound), ASA and carisoprodol (Soma Compound), ASA, codeine, and carisoprodol (Soma Compound with Codeine), ASA and codeine (Empirin with Codeine), ASA, codeine, butalbital, and caffeine (Fiorinal), ASA and extended-release dipyridamole (Aggrenox, Asasantin).

Extrapolated, based on similar properties: Nonsteroidal anti-inflammatory drugs (NSAIDs):

COX-1 inhibitors: Diclofenac (Cataflam, Voltaren), combination drug: diclofenac and misoprostol (Arthrotec), diflunisal (Dolobid), etodolac (Lodine), fenoprofen (Dalfon), furbiprofen (Ansaid), ibuprofen (Advil, Excedrin IB, Motrin, Motrin IB, Nuprin, Pedia Care Fever Drops, Provel, Rufen), combination drug: hydrocodone and ibuprofen (Reprexain, Vicoprofen), indomethacin (indometacin; Indocin, Indocin-SR), ketoprofen (Orudis, Oruvail), ketorolac (Acular ophthalmic, Toradol), meclofenamate (Meclomen), mefenamic acid (Ponstel), meloxicam (Mobic), nabumetone (Relafen), naproxen (Aleve, Anaprox, Naprosyn), oxaprozin (Daypro), piroxicam (Feldene), salsalate (salicylic acid; Amigesic, Disalcid, Marthritic, Mono Gesic, Salflex, Salsitab), sulindac (Clinoril), tolmetin (Tolectin).

COX-2 inhibitors: Celecoxib (Celebrex).

Interaction Type and Significance

☼ **Prevention or Reduction of Drug Adverse Effect**

? **Interaction Possible but Uncertain Occurrence and Unclear Implications**

Probability:	Evidence Base:
3. Possible	○ **Preliminary**

Effect and Mechanism of Action

Internal administration of cayenne may be protective against drug-induced mucosal ulceration by NSAIDs and related agents. The interaction is likely, but arguably of minimal clinical importance.

Research

Animal studies have provided inconclusive data on the effect of capsaicin on gastric mucosa, either alone or in combination with ulcerogenic agents.[11,13,14,37,38] Early studies suggested that cayenne might increase gastric acid secretion.[9] In more recent human studies, Myers et al.[39] found that red pepper (and black pepper) increased gastric cell exfoliation but had no effect on gastric secretion. Meanwhile, one rodent study found a protective effect against aspirin-induced ulceration in rats.[11] This effect was confirmed in humans in a small preclinical study by Yeoh et al.,[40] who found that 20 g cayenne per day coadministered with 600 mg aspirin daily led to a significant protective effect against gastric ulceration assessed endoscopically.[40] A study comparing 103 peptic ulcer patients with matched controls examined chili consumption and found that higher chili consumption was significantly associated with lower ulcer incidence.[41] Another study of 84 healthy volunteers found that capsaicin administered in low doses intragastrically was protective against ethanol- and indomethacin-induced mucosal damage when coadministered, but not when the capsaicin was given for 2 weeks before drug administration.[42]

Integrative Therapeutics, Clinical Concerns, and Adaptations

Although this interaction appears to be reasonably established by experimental evidence, the clinical significance is arguably rather low. Internal administration of cayenne at medicinal doses daily to counter aspirin adverse effects seems a relatively unfavorable strategy, given the availability of other herbal agents that are ulceroprotective, anti-inflammatory, and also lack any irritant properties. (See monographs for Aloe and Licorice.)

Enalapril and Related Angiotensin-Converting Enzyme (ACE) Inhibitors

Evidence: Enalapril (Vasotec)
Extrapolated, based on similar properties: Benazepril (Lotensin), combination drug: benazepril and amlodipine (Lotrel), captopril (Capoten), combination drug: captopril and hydrochlorothiazide (Acezide, Capto-Co, Captozide, Co-Zidocapt), cilazapril (Inhibace), combination drug: enalapril and felodipine (Lexxel), combination drug: enalapril and hydrochlorothiazide (Vaseretic), fosinopril (Monopril), lisinopril (Prinivil, Zestril), combination drug: lisinopril and hydrochlorothiazide (Prinzide, Zestoretic), moexipril (Univasc), perindopril (Aceon), quinapril (Accupril), ramipril (Altace), trandolapril (Mavik).

Interaction Type and Significance

✗ Potential or Theoretical Adverse Interaction of Uncertain Severity

Probability:	Evidence Base:
2. Probable	⦿ **Emerging**

Effect and Mechanism of Action

Cough is a known adverse effect associated with ACE inhibitors. Coadministration with cayenne can exacerbate cough symptoms, probably through more than one mechanism. The clinical significance is minimal.

Research

A form of "sensory hyperreactivity" cough induced by capsaicin alone has been described.[43-45] This may be mediated by VRs in the bronchial tree.[46] Vagal afferents that also include vanilloid pathways (C fibers) can be stimulated by capsaicin; however, experimentally this does not appear to cause a cough reflex but induces apnea (in primates).[47] Capsaicin inhalation has also been used to identify a subset of asthmatic patients with chemical sensitivity to inhaled irritants in a controlled manner, providing a degree of exposure management control in sensitive individuals.[48]

The mechanism of ACE inhibitor–induced cough is believed to be related to elevations in bradykinin (ACE is a kininase).[49] Yeo et al.[50,51] conducted a series of small investigations into ACE inhibitor–induced cough and capsaicin with normal and hypertensive patients using enalapril. Skin (delayed-type hypersensitivity, DTH) testing revealed that enalapril cough was associated with bradykinin, not substance P, reactivity. The drug-induced cough lessened over 28 days, and its sensitivity to capsaicin exacerbation also decreased. Adjusting the dose of enalapril downward (5 vs. 20 mg/day) reduced the frequency and severity of cough, but it did not appear to alter consistently the effect of capsaicin on the cough, leading the authors to conclude that there was a wide range of dose-dependent variation in response to capsaicin.[50,51]

Reports

An isolated report is available, with poor documentation standards (i.e., concurrent medications not listed). A 53-year-old woman had been taking an (unidentified) ACE inhibitor for several years without adverse effects, but experienced cough symptoms every time she applied a capsaicin-containing cream (0.075% capsaicin).[52]

Clinical Implications and Adaptations

Differential diagnosis of cough includes possible ACE inhibitor–induced cough. This is reversible on cessation of the drug and will likely diminish over a 28-day period of drug administration. Exacerbation by capsaicin is possible in some individuals, but the interaction is probably of minimal significance. Management strategies are empirical, with cessation or reduction of the herb or drug.

Nonsteroidal Anti-Inflammatory Drugs (NSAIDs), Analgesics, Oral Corticosteroids, and Other Antiarthritic Medications

Nonsteroidal anti-inflammatory drugs (NSAIDs):
   COX-1 inhibitors: Diclofenac (Voltaren, Cataflam), combination drug: diclofenac and misoprostol (Arthrotec), diflunisal (Dolobid), etodolac (Lodine), fenoprofen (Dalfon), furbiprofen (Ansaid), ibuprofen (Advil, Excedrin IB, Motrin, Motrin IB, Nuprin, Pedia Care Fever Drops, Provel, Rufen), combination drug: hydrocodone and ibuprofen (Reprexain, Vicoprofen), indomethacin (indometacin; Indocin, Indocin-SR), ketoprofen (Orudis, Oruvail), ketorolac (Acular ophthalmic, Toradol), meclofenamate (Meclomen), mefenamic acid (Ponstel), meloxicam (Mobic), nabumetone (Relafen), naproxen (Aleve, Anaprox, Naprosyn), oxaprozin (Daypro), piroxicam (Feldene), salsalate (salicylic acid; Amigesic, Disalcid, Marthritic, Mono Gesic, Salflex, Salsitab), sulindac (Clinoril), tolmetin (Tolectin).
   COX-2 inhibitors: Celecoxib (Celebrex).
Acetylsalicylic acid: acetosal, acetyl salicylic acid, ASA, salicylsalicylic acid; Arthritis Foundation Pain Reliever, Ascriptin, Aspergum, Asprimox, Bayer Aspirin, Bayer Buffered Aspirin, Bayer Low Adult Strength, Bufferin, Buffex, Cama Arthritis Pain Reliever, Easprin, Ecotrin, Ecotrin Low Adult Strength, Empirin, Extra Strength Adprin-B, Extra Strength Bayer Enteric 500 Aspirin, Extra Strength Bayer Plus, Halfprin 81, Heartline, Regular Strength Bayer Enteric 500 Aspirin, St. Joseph Adult Chewable Aspirin, ZORprin; combination drugs: ASA and caffeine (Anacin), ASA, caffeine, and propoxyphene (Darvon Compound), ASA and carisoprodol (Soma Compound), ASA, codeine, and carisoprodol (Soma Compound with Codeine), ASA and codeine (Empirin with Codeine), ASA, codeine, butalbital, and caffeine (Fiorinal), ASA and extended-release dipyridamole (Aggrenox, Asasantin).
Corticosteroids, oral: Betamethasone (Celestone), cortisone (Cortone), dexamethasone (Decadron), fludrocortisone (Florinef), hydrocortisone (Cortef), methylprednisolone (Medrol), prednisolone (Delta-Cortef, Orapred, Pediapred, Prelone),

prednisone (Deltasone, Liquid Pred, Meticorten, Orasone), triamcinolone (Aristocort).

Interaction Type and Significance

⊕⊕⊕ **Beneficial or Supportive Interaction, Not Requiring Professional Management**

Probability:	Evidence Base:
1. Certain	◉ Emerging

Effect and Mechanism of Action

Topical capsaicin preparations, when coadministered with antiarthritic medications, can result in increased symptom relief because of substance P modulation by capsaicin. The interaction may be used to reduce the dose of pharmaceuticals to lessen potential drug adverse effects. The interaction is not widely exploited but may be of considerable significance to chronic arthritis patients.

Research

Five controlled clinical trials conducted to date support the use of topical capsaicin preparations for symptom relief in both osteoarthritis (OA) and rheumatoid arthritis (RA). The preparation used most frequently in the trials was Zostrix (GenDerm), containing 0.025% capsaicin administered topically to affected areas four times daily.[53-55] The mechanisms of pain reduction lie in the ability of capsaicin to modulate substance P–mediated nociceptive pathways (see previous discussion).[53,56,57] The effects are similar to the pain relief mechanisms in other conditions and are not primarily antiinflammatory.[58] The trial conducted by Deal et al.[59] involved both OA (70) and RA (31) patients, who were allowed to continue taking their antiarthritis medications, including NSAIDs, corticosteroids, and analgesics. Analgesic effects of capsaicin are more pronounced in inflammatory states than in normal controls, according to one animal study.[7]

Integrative Therapeutics, Clinical Concerns, and Adaptations

This is a straightforward example of an additive (or possibly synergistic) and beneficial interaction caused by convergent clinical effects operating through different mechanisms (inflammation and nociception) for drug and herb, respectively. The interaction is apparently benign and noncontroversial and could be recommended to patients interested in either increased levels of symptom relief other than that offered by pharmaceuticals or decreased dose levels of pharmaceuticals to reduce adverse effects.

THEORETICAL, SPECULATIVE, AND PRELIMINARY INTERACTIONS RESEARCH, INCLUDING OVERSTATED INTERACTIONS CLAIMS

Antacids

Aluminum carbonate gel (Basajel), aluminum hydroxide (Alternagel, Amphojel); combination drugs: aluminum hydroxide, magnesium carbonate, alginic acid, and sodium bicarbonate (Gaviscon Extra Strength Tablets, Gaviscon Regular Strength Liquid, Gaviscon Extra Strength Liquid); aluminum hydroxide, magnesium hydroxide, and simethicone (Advanced Formula Di-Gel Tablets, co-magaldrox, Di-Gel, Gelusil, Maalox, Maalox Plus, Mylanta, Wingel); aluminum hydroxide, magnesium trisilicate, alginic acid, and sodium bicarbonate (Alenic Alka, Gaviscon Regular Strength Tablets); calcium carbonate (Titralac, Tums); magnesium hydroxide (Phillips' Milk of Magnesia MOM); combination drugs: magnesium

hydroxide and calcium carbonate (Calcium Rich Rolaids); magnesium hydroxide, aluminum hydroxide, calcium carbonate, and simethicone (Tempo Tablets); magnesium trisilicate and aluminum hydroxide (Adcomag trisil, Foamicon); magnesium trisilicate, alginic acid, and sodium bicarbonate (Alenic Alka, Gaviscon Regular Strength Tablets); combination drug: sodium bicarbonate, aspirin, and citric acid (Alka-Seltzer).

Mills and Bone[60] suggest a possible adverse interaction between antacid medications and cayenne resulting from gastroirritant and hypersecretory effects of the herb. Reports of such interactions are lacking, and most data suggest gastroprotective effects follow internal cayenne consumption, with increased mucus and blood flow rather than hyperacidity at the gastric mucosa. Clinically, it is common practice to advise patients with acid-related ulcers to avoid spicy food, and internal administration of stimulants such as cayenne is unusual in GI-sensitive individuals. On balance, this suggested interaction appears entirely speculative.

Anticoagulant and Antiplatelet Medications

Anticoagulants, oral vitamin K antagonists: Anisindione (Miradon), dicumarol, ethyl biscoumacetate (Tromexan), nicoumalone (acenocoumarol; Acitrom, Sintrom), phenindione (Dindevan), phenprocoumon (Jarsin, Marcumar), warfarin (Coumadin, Marevan, Warfilone).
Anticoagulants, heparin, unfractionated (UFH): Heparin (Calciparine, Hepalean, Heparin Leo, Minihep Calcium, Minihep, Monoparin Calcium, Monoparin, Multiparin, Pump-Hep, Unihep, Uniparin Calcium, Uniparin Forte).
Anticoagulants, heparinoids: Danaparoid (Orgaran), fondaparinux (Arixtra).
Anticoagulants, low-molecular-weight heparins: Ardeparin (Normiflo), dalteparin (Fragmin), enoxaparin (Lovenox), tinzaparin (Innohep).
Anticoagulants, thrombin inhibitors, hirudins: desirudin (Iprivask, Revasc), lepirudin (Refludan).
Antiplatelet thromboprophylactics: Acetylsalicylic acid (acetosal, acetyl salicylic acid, ASA, salicylsalicylic acid; Arthritis Foundation Pain Reliever, Ascriptin, Aspergum, Asprimox, Bayer Aspirin, Bayer Buffered Aspirin, Bayer Low Adult Strength, Bufferin, Buffex, Cama Arthritis Pain Reliever, Easprin, Ecotrin, Ecotrin Low Adult Strength, Empirin, Extra Strength Adprin-B, Extra Strength Bayer Enteric 500 Aspirin, Extra Strength Bayer Plus, Halfprin 81, Heartline, Regular Strength Bayer Enteric 500 Aspirin, St. Joseph Adult Chewable Aspirin, ZORprin); combination drugs: ASA and caffeine (Anacin), ASA, caffeine, and propoxyphene (Darvon Compound), ASA and carisoprodol (Soma Compound), ASA, codeine, and carisoprodol (Soma Compound with Codeine), ASA and codeine (Empirin with Codeine), ASA, codeine, butalbital, and caffeine (Fiorinal); cilostazol (Pletal), clopidogrel (Plavix), dipyridamole (Persantine), ticlopidine (Ticlid); combination drug: ASA and extended-release dipyridamole (Aggrenox, Asasantin).
Blood viscosity reducing agents: Pentoxifylline (Pentoxil, Trental).

Isolated capsaicin has definitively been demonstrated to have some antiplatelet effects in vitro and in animal experiments. The mechanism of these effects is not understood and their relevance to human hemostasis unclear. Some experimental evidence suggests antiplatelet activity of capsaicin may be related to cell membrane fluidization.[61, 62]

Another study has demonstrated a nitric oxide (NO)–releasing effect that is modulated by capsaicin-sensitive afferent neurons, which may implicate the vanilloid pathway.[63] Capsaicin has effects on at least three stimuli of platelet activation: platelet-activating factor (PAF), collagen, and thromboxane.[64,65] At present, the levels of capsaicin (IC_{50} for collagen-induced in vitro effect was 87 μg/mL), and prolongation of tail bleed times in mice required a dose of 25 mg/kg capsaicin.[66] These levels are more than an order of magnitude higher than typical human doses from therapeutic topical or chronic dietary administration. Some epidemiological data, however, suggest that dietary use of cayenne may be related to lower incidence of thromboses in chronic cayenne consumers. A study comparing 88 Thai subjects to 55 Caucasian Americans found higher fibrinolytic parameters in the latter than in the Thai (cayenne user) group.[67] Finally, traditional herbalist Dr. Christopher[68] recommended cayenne as a hemostatic to stop external bleeding and promote wound healing, and Felter and Lloyd[69] suggest it can also be taken internally as an antihemorrhagic, especially for postpartum bleeding. At present, clinically significant interactions with antiplatelet, fibrinolytic, or anticoagulant medications are unreported and appear improbable.

Cisplatin

Evidence: Cisplatin (*cis*-diaminedichloroplatinum, CDDP; Platinol, Platinol-AQ).
Extrapolated, based on similar properties: Carboplatin (Paraplatin), oxaliplatin (Eloxatin).

One study using a rodent model demonstrated some reduction in cisplatin-induced nephrotoxicity in animals after single-dose cisplatin when coadministered with intragastric capsaicin.[70] The authors suggested that this was caused by antioxidant mechanisms, because renal glutathione and superoxide dismutase levels rose with the capsaicin treatment. High doses of capsaicin (10 mg/kg) were used, and the applicability of these data to human oncology settings is difficult to establish until more studies are performed.

Monoamine Oxidase (MAO) Inhibitors

MAO-A inhibitors: Isocarboxazid (Marplan), moclobemide (Aurorix, Manerix), phenelzine (Nardil), procarbazine (Matulane), tranylcypromine (Parnate).

MAO-B inhibitors: Selegiline, deprenyl, L-deprenil, L-deprenyl; (Atapryl, Carbex, Eldepryl, Jumex, Movergan, Selpak); pargyline (Eutonyl), rasagiline (Azilect).

Newell et al.[71] suggest a potential adverse interaction between MAO inhibitors and capsaicin, presumably based on extrapolations of "sympathomimetic-like" effects associated with acute cayenne ingestion, such as transient increases in resting metabolic rate. Capsaicin is not an adrenomimetic agent and lacks any direct sympathetic activity; this extrapolation appears to be an overextension of the known pharmacology and is unsupported by clinical reports.

Theophylline/Aminophylline

Theophylline/aminophylline (Phyllocontin, Slo-Bid, Slo-Phyllin, Theo-24, Theo-Bid, Theocron, Theo-Dur, Theolair, Truphylline, Uni-Dur, Uniphyl), combination drug: ephedrine, guaifenesin, and theophylline (Primatene Dual Action).

Two studies by the same investigator examined the kinetics of theophylline and cayenne (dried fruit orally) coadministration. Single-dose coadministration demonstrated an increase in clearance of the drug. However, cayenne pretreatment for 1 week led to decreased levels of the theophylline metabolite 1-methyluric acid (1-MU), suggesting a potential increase in theophylline levels from inhibition of theophylline metabolism.[72,73] Slight increases in theophylline levels are associated with increased adverse effects, which could indicate a potential interaction; however, the effects in humans are unknown and reports unavailable. The author's speculation that xanthine oxidase inhibition is affected by cayenne may or may not be correct. Theophylline is primarily metabolized by CYP1A; however, a secondary pathway of theophylline metabolism by 2E1 exists, and this P450 enzyme is inhibited by capsaicin.[74]

The 74 citations for this monograph are located under Cayenne on the CD at the back of the book.

Dang Gui

Botanical Name: *Angelica sinensis* (Oliv.) Diels.
Pharmacopoeial Name: Angelicae radix.
Synonym: *Angelica polymorpha* Maxim. *var sinensis* Oliv.
Common Names: Dang gui, dong quai, tang kuei, tang kwei, Chinese angelica.
Note: The phonetic "dong quai" Romanization is not the correct Pinyin transliteration, which is "dang gui." "Tang kuei" is the earlier Wade Giles transliteration, less used today.

HERB CHARACTERISTICS

Family

Apiaceae.

Related Species

In East Asian commerce, several species may be traded as substitutes. *Levisticum officinale* Koch., or lovage, sometimes known as "European dang gui," is a recorded adulterant, not a substitute.

Parts Used

Root; in East Asian traditional medicine, the head, body, and tail of the root are regarded as having different medicinal properties.

Common Forms

Dried: Prepared root, smoke-dried; baked in wine.
Fluid Extract: 1:1 70% ethanol, according to the *Pharmacopoeia of the People's Republic of China (PPRC)*.
Standardized Extract: Liquid or dry extracts may be standardized to ligustilide content (0.8%-1.0%) and to ferulic acid (0.05%-0.01%).

INTERACTIONS REVIEW

Strategic Considerations

One of the better known herbs from the materia medica of classical Chinese medicine, dang gui (in traditional terms) *supplements* (nourishes) *xue* (blood), moves and dispels blood stasis, and regulates menses. It is also used for moistening dry conditions, dispersing swelling, and promoting the discharge of pus.[1] The herb has been incorporated into Western herbal medicine, primarily as a women's tonic herb for menstrual disorders and infertility. Dang gui use for menopausal issues is not currently supported by clinical trial data.[2] The herb is also used for its cardioprotective, hepatoprotective, and mild immunomodulatory effects. In the contemporary practice of Chinese medicine, it is widely used in many herbal formulae, as well as in combination with conventional treatments, such as myelosuppressive chemotherapy.[3]

Much of the literature on dang gui is in Chinese-language journals, and many reports relate to formulae involving several ingredients, including dang gui. Few controlled trials are available, but there is a large body of traditional-use data, as well as a considerable number of uncontrolled trials in the East Asian medical literature. Many of the available studies, animal and human, involve parenteral administration, which cannot be readily extrapolated to oral administration used in the West. The herb is not referenced in official Western pharmacopoeias (although it was briefly in the *USD* in 1937) but has been official in the *PPRC* since 1977. The *American Herbal Pharmacopoeia* has produced a Western-oriented monograph, including a supplement on traditional Chinese usage,[4] and McKenna et al.[5] have reviewed much of the literature. Chen and Chen[6] have reviewed both the pharmacology and the traditional uses of the herb.

Interactions concerns about dang gui are largely the result of extrapolations from experimental pharmacological data of isolated ingredients, such as ferulic acid, ligustilide, or polysaccharide fractions of the herb, and usually stress the risks of concomitant use with anticoagulants. The traditional precautions and contraindications for dang gui, which include bleeding disorders, hemorrhagic disease, excessive menses, and first-trimester pregnancy, may be seen as equally appropriate in Western contexts.

Effects on Drug Metabolism and Bioavailability

Minimal data are available on the effects of dang gui on the different aspects of drug detoxification. Two Japanese studies are available. One screened a number of umbelliferous crude drugs in vitro for general cytochrome P450 (CYP450) inhibitory effects and found weak but measurable inhibition by dang gui, as well as other *Angelica* spp. After high-performance liquid chromatography analysis, the authors attributed this to the activity of a coumarin-derivative constituent, imperatorin.[7] A more specific in vitro study using rodent hepatic microsomes with various drug substrates found partial inhibition by dang gui extracts of CYP450 3A4, 2C9, and 2D6.[8] A Chinese study examined the effects of dang gui polysaccharide administration in normal and liver-damaged (by prednisolone) rodents and found that the herb fraction increased hepatic microsomal CYP450, glutathione-*S*-transferase, and reduced-glutathione content.[9] Pharmacokinetic interactions have not been reported, and in the case of warfarin have been ruled out as a mechanism of interaction[10] (see following discussion). Nonetheless, such effects seem theoretically possible, and further research is required to clarify the extent and significance of any potential pharmacokinetic interactions.

HERB-DRUG INTERACTIONS

Warfarin and Related Oral Vitamin K Antagonist Anticoagulants

Evidence: Warfarin (Coumadin, Marevan, Warfilone).
Extrapolated, based on similar properties: Anisindione (Miradon), dicumarol, ethyl biscoumacetate (Tromexan), nicoumalone (acenocoumarol; Acitrom, Sintrom), phenindione (Dindevan), phenprocoumon (Jarsin, Marcumar); other drugs affecting hemostasis.

Interaction Type and Significance

✗✗ **Minimal to Mild Adverse Interaction—Vigilance Necessary**

Probability:
4. Plausible

Evidence Base:
▽ **Mixed**

Effect and Mechanism of Action

Addition of dang gui to previously stabilized warfarin anticoagulation regimens may require the dose of oral anticoagulant to be adjusted to prevent excessive anticoagulation. Only one report is available, suggesting the interaction is unlikely to be clinically significant. Dang gui has multiple effects on hemorheological parameters, the mechanisms of which are not fully elucidated, and whether this is a strict interaction or merely an additive common pharmacodynamic effect has not been established.

Research

The literature on hemorheological activities of dang gui is dominated by an emphasis on isolated constituents (e.g., ferulate, butylidenephthalide) with parenteral administration at high dose levels in animal and human studies. The trend of the data supports a possible antiplatelet effect, probably operating through arachidonic acid metabolism.[11-17] Other hemorheological effects were observed in a study using parenteral dang gui (200 mL aqueous solution, intravenous administration daily for 20 days), in a group of 50 patients after acute ischemic stroke, where administration resulted in significant reductions (p <0.001) in platelet adhesion, red blood cell (RBC) and platelet electrophoresis times, erythrocyte sedimentation rate (ESR) and serum fibrinogen, and blood and plasma adhesion ratios.[18] Oral administration of an aqueous decoction of dang gui and the related *Angelica acutiloba* were given to six healthy patients, and whole-blood viscosity was reduced (p <0.05) after 180 minutes compared with controls.[19]

A study of warfarin and dang gui coadministration in rabbits investigated the effect of adding single-dose warfarin to animals pretreated with dang gui, as well as addition of dang gui to warfarin-stabilized animals, as measured by coagulation parameters. In the first case, adding warfarin to a dang gui pretreated group led to a (p <0.05) lowering of prothrombin time (PT) compared with warfarin alone. Pharmacokinetic parameters of warfarin were not changed in the presence of dang gui pretreatment. Addition of dang gui to stable, warfarinized animals led to no significant change in PT or warfarin levels. In this study, warfarin was given at high dose levels subcutaneously, and a 2:1 extract of dang gui was given at 2 g/kg orally. The implication of this study appears to be that adding dang gui to stabilized warfarin is less problematic than adding drug to stabilized dang gui (in rabbits), although pharmacokinetic interactions were not observed.[10]

Reports

In a single but much-cited report, a 46-year-old female warfarinized patient experienced an unexplained rise in international normalized ratio (INR) to 4.05. Investigations revealed no identifiable cause, and she was advised to discontinue her 5-mg warfarin dose for 24 hours. The INR remained elevated on retesting 1 week later. The patient admitted taking a herbal preparation (Nature's Way brand of dang gui), 565 mg twice daily. She was advised to stop the herb, and the INR declined to 3.41, then to 2.48 after 1 week. Concomitant medications included digoxin and furosemide.[20] Fugh-Berman and Ernst[21] evaluated the interaction as "likely," scoring 8 of 10 on their report reliability scale.

Clinical Implications and Adaptations

The lack of reports of spontaneous bleeding associated with dang gui consumption alone, with only one report of the warfarin–dang gui interaction to date, suggests that concerns about the incidence and severity of the interaction are exaggerated. As always, self-prescription is a separate issue, and many warfarinized patients are poorly compliant with their monitoring test schedules. As a guideline, prescribing dang gui to warfarinized patients should generally be avoided unless there are compelling reasons for coadministration. In such cases, close monitoring of INR is required.

However, as is often the case from an integrative perspective, the potential interaction may be beneficial under specific circumstances. Dang gui has cardioprotective and thrombolytic effects that may be beneficial depending on the situation.[6,22] For example, patients receiving a typical 1 mg/day oral dose of Coumadin after temporary installation of vascular access ports/catheters for prevention of thrombosis at the catheter tip may benefit from the addition of dang gui, combined with natural antiplatelet and fibrinolytic agents, particularly if there are other indications for prescribing the herb. However, checking PT/INR weekly would be appropriate if coadministration is considered, because 1 mg Coumadin could affect PTs if circumstances altered (e.g., vitamin K deficiency).

Erythropoiesis-Stimulating Agents

Epoetin alpha (EPO, epoetin alfa, recombinant erythropoietin; Epogen, Eprex, Procrit), epoetin beta (NeoRecormon), darbepoetin alpha (darbepoetin alfa; Aranesp).

Interaction Type and Significance

⊕ **Potential or Theoretical Beneficial or Supportive Interaction, with Professional Management**

Probability:
4. Plausible

Evidence Base:
☐ **Inadequate**

Effect and Mechanism of Action

Recombinant analogs of endogenous erythropoietin are used parenterally to correct anemia in seriously ill patients (cancer and chronic renal failure). The interaction is a pharmacodynamic additive effect on hematopoiesis. Dang gui may also help facilitate responsiveness to the drug.

Research

Several Chinese experimental studies have examined the effects of dang gui, particularly the polysaccharide fraction, in stimulating hematopoiesis and erythropoiesis. Hemoglobin, RBC count, and progenitor cells were all increased by the administration of the herb in normal and anemic mice as well as in cell culture systems.[23-25] Murine studies have demonstrated myeloprotective effects of dang gui and its polysaccharide fractions against cyclophosphamide-induced and radiation-induced leukopenia.[26,27]

Reports

Bradley et al.[28] reported a single case of an anemic hemodialysis patient who was apparently resistant to the recombinant drug. The patient started self-prescription of a decoction of dang gui and *Paeonia lactiflora,* and after 1 month the hematocrit increased from 29.7% to 34.4%, and the amount of the drug was reduced by more than 90%. The effect of the other component of the formula cannot be ascertained.

Integrative Therapeutics, Clinical Concerns, and Adaptations

Published data substantiating this interaction are currently inadequate. However, the Chinese materia medica for *Supplementing the Xue/Blood* is an established part of protocols for supporting patients undergoing myelosuppressive chemotherapies in Chinese medicine. Dang gui is incorporated into many of these formulae, which are based on different patterns of bone marrow suppression according to traditional diagnostic criteria. Specialist review of these formulae is available from clinical texts, including Peiwen.[3] The risk/benefit ratios of this approach are favorable, and the combination requires further investigation by preclinical and controlled clinical studies.

THEORETICAL, SPECULATIVE, AND PRELIMINARY INTERACTIONS RESEARCH, INCLUDING OVERSTATED INTERACTIONS CLAIMS

Acetaminophen

APAP, paracetamol (Tylenol); combination drugs: acetaminophen and codeine (Capital with Codeine, Phenaphen with Codeine, Tylenol with Codeine); acetaminophen and hydrocodone (Anexsia, Anodynos-DHC, Co-Gesic, Dolacet, DuoCet, Hydrocet, Hydrogesic, Hy-Phen, Lorcet 10/650, Lorcet-HD, Lorcet Plus, Lortab, Margesic H, Medipain 5, Norco, Stagesic, T-Gesic, Vicodin, Vicodin ES, Vicodin HP, Zydone); acetaminophen and oxycodone (Endocet, Percocet 2.5/325, Percocet 5/325, Percocet 7.5/500, Percocet 10/650, Roxicet 5/500, Roxilox, Tylox); acetaminophen and pentazocine (Talacen); acetaminophen and propoxyphene (Darvocet-N, Darvocet-N 100, Pronap-100, Propacet 100, Propoxacet-N, Wygesic).

Dang gui extracts and polysaccharide fractions have been shown to have some moderate hepatoprotective activity. One study examined CCl4 and acetaminophen-induced hepatotoxicity and found that hepatoprotective effects for dang gui extracts were more pronounced in the case of acetaminophen, suggesting a glutathione-dependent mechanism for the protective effects.[29,30] The "interaction" of acetaminophen with dang gui described by Chen and Chen[6] is thus more likely an effect of general antioxidant hepatoprotective activity mediated by glutathione.

Cycloheximide, Scopolamine

Cycloheximide (Acti-aid, ActiDione, Actispray, actidone, hizaricin, kaken, naramycin, naramycin A, neocycloheximide), scopolamine (Scopace Tablet, Transderm Scop Patch).

A study with a rodent behavioral model examined the effects both hexane and methanol extracts of dang gui on amnesia induced by scopolamine and cycloheximide and *p*-chloroamphetamine. High doses of the hexane extract (1 g/kg) appeared to attenuate the amnesia induced by scopolamine and cycloheximide but not by chloramphetamine in this model. The authors suggest this implies an effect on memory function, but the significance of this for therapeutic doses of conventional extracts of dang gui in humans remains unclear.[31]

Nifedipine

Nifedipine (Adalat, Adalat CC, Nifedical XL, Procardia, Procardia XL); combination drug: nifedipine and atenolol (Beta-Adalat, Tenif).

Coadministration of nifedipine and dang gui in 40 patients with chronic obstructive pulmonary disease (COPD) led to a greater degree of reduction of pulmonary arterial pressure than in untreated controls or those treated with nifedipine alone.[32] Dose of dang gui was high (250 mL 25% solution/day) and was administered parenterally, which makes extrapolation from this study problematic, although some clinical evidence suggests that dang gui alone may have a vasodilator effect on the pulmonary circulation. More investigation is needed before this is confirmed as a clinically consequential interaction, particularly in light of the in vitro evidence suggesting a pharmacokinetic reduction of nifedipine level by inhibition of CYP450 3A4 and 2D6 by dang gui.[8]

Oral Contraceptives and Related Estrogen-Containing and Synthetic Estrogen and Progesterone Analog Medications

Oral contraceptives: monophasic, biphasic, and triphasic estrogen preparations:
Ethinyl estradiol and desogestrel (Desogen, Ortho-TriCyclen).
Ethinyl estradiol and ethynodiol (Demulen 1/35, Demulen 1/50, Nelulen 1/25, Nelulen 1/50, Zovia).
Ethinyl estradiol and levonorgestrel (Alesse, Levlen, Levlite, Levora 0.15/30, Nordette, Tri-Levlen, Triphasil, Trivora).
Ethinyl estradiol and norethindrone/norethisterone (Brevicon, Estrostep, Genora 1/35, GenCep. 1/35, Jenest-28, Loestrin 1.5/30, Loestrin1/20, Modicon, Necon 1/25, Necon 10/11, Necon 0.5/30, Necon 1/50, Nelova 1/35, Nelova 10/11, Norinyl 1/35, Norlestin 1/50, Ortho Novum 1/35, Ortho Novum 10/11, Ortho Novum 7/7/7, Ovcon-35, Ovcon-50, Tri-Norinyl, Trinovum).
Ethinyl estradiol and norgestrel (Lo/Ovral, Ovral).
Mestranol and norethindrone (Genora 1/50, Nelova 1/50, Norethin 1/50, Ortho-Novum 1/50).
Related, internal application: Etonogestrel/ethinyl estradiol vaginal ring (Nuvaring).
Hormone replacement therapy, estrogens: Chlorotrianisene (Tace); conjugated equine estrogens (Premarin); conjugated synthetic estrogens (Cenestin); dienestrol (Ortho Dienestrol); esterified estrogens (Estratab, Menest, Neo-Estrone); estradiol, topical/transdermal/ring (Alora Transdermal, Climara Transdermal, Estrace, Estradot, Estring FemPatch, Vivelle-Dot, Vivelle Transdermal); estradiol cypionate (Dep-Gynogen, Depo-Estradiol, Depogen, Dura-Estrin, Estra-D, Estro-Cyp, Estroject-LA, Estronol-LA); estradiol hemihydrate (Estreva, Vagifem); estradiol valerate (Delestrogen, Estra-L 40, Gynogen L.A. 20, Progynova, Valergen 20); estrone (Aquest, Estragyn 5, Estro-A, Estrone '5', Kestrone-5); estropipate (Ogen, Ortho-Est); ethinyl estradiol (Estinyl, Gynodiol, Lynoral).
Hormone replacement therapy, estrogen/progestin combinations: Conjugated equine estrogens and medroxyprogesterone (Premelle cycle 5, Prempro); conjugated equine estrogens and norgestrel (Prempak-C); estradiol and dydrogesterone (Femoston); estradiol and norethindrone, patch (CombiPatch); estradiol and norethindrone/norethisterone, oral (Activella, Climagest, Climesse, FemHRT, Trisequens); estradiol valerate and cyproterone acetate (Climens); estradiol valerate and norgestrel (Progyluton); estradiol and norgestimate (Ortho-Prefest).
Hormone replacement therapy, estrogen/testosterone combinations: Esterified estrogens and methyltestosterone (Estratest, Estratest HS).
Selective estrogen response modulators (SERMs): Raloxifene (Evista), tamoxifen (Nolvadex), toremifene (Fureston).

Partly because of its reputation as a "female tonic" herb, some sources suggest interaction of dang gui with female sex hormones (ERT, HRT) or hormone-modulating drugs (e.g., SERMs, aromatase inhibitors). Known phytoestrogenic compounds have not been recorded in the root, and a controlled clinical trial of postmenopausal women found no changes in endometrial thickness or vaginal cell proliferation after 24 weeks' administration of a standardized extract of dang gui.[33] However, a cell line model found some evidence for both estrogen-dependent and estrogen-independent proliferative activity by a water extract of dang gui.[34] Recent reviews of botanicals for menopause have found no positive evidence of effects of dang gui alone on menopausal symptoms.[2,34,35] In the absence of estrogenic clinical effects or pharmacological estrogen receptor binding, suggestions of female hormone interactions with dang gui by some authors are unsupported at this time.[36]

Ouabain and Related Cardiac Glycosides and Antiarrhythmic Drugs

Evidence: Ouabain (g-strophanthin).
Extrapolated, based on similar properties: Amiodarone (Cordarone, Pacerone), deslanoside (cedilanin-D), digitoxin (Cystodigin), digoxin (Digitek, Lanoxin, Lanoxicaps, purgoxin), disopyramide (Norpace), dofetilide (Tikosyn), flecainide (Tambocor), ibutilide (Corvert), procainamide (Pronestyl, Procan-SR), quinidine (Quinaglute, Quinidex, Quinora), sotalol (Betapace, Betapace AF, Sorine).

Some experimental evidence exists for an antiarrhythmic effect of parenteral dang gui extracts, in animal models, including ouabain-induced ventricular fibrillation, as well as in digitalis- and epinephrine-induced arrhythmias.[37] Some secondary sources suggest that the herb must interact adversely with antiarrhythmic drugs, but logically a beneficial interaction would be suggested, and clinical reports of the adverse interaction are lacking.

The 37 citations for this monograph are located under Dang Gui on the CD at the back of the book.

Devil's Claw

Botanical Name: *Harpagophytum procumbens*, DC ex Meissner.
Pharmacopoeial Name: Harpagophyti radix.
Common Names: Devil's claw, grapple plant, Cape grapple plant.

HERB DESCRIPTION

Family
Pedaliaceae.

Parts Used
Secondary roots (tuber).

Common Forms
Dried: Cut/powdered secondary root, containing not less than 1.2% harpagoside.
Tincture, Fluid Extract, Hydroethanolic extracts 1:2, 1:3, 1:5 in 25% ethanol.
Standardized Extract: Tablets or capsules, standardized 6:1 to 9:1 on 8.5% harpagoside. (WS 1531, Schwabe GmbH) or 1.5:1 to 2.5:1 standardized at 2.5% harpagoside (Doloteffin, Ardeypharm GmbH).

INTERACTIONS REVIEW

Strategic Considerations

Devil's claw, a South African native, has been used in Western Europe for chronic arthritic conditions for several decades. The root tubers are bitter, containing iridoid glycosides, principally harpagoside.[1] The bitter nature of the remedy, suggested by Weiss[2] as comparable to gentian, led the German Commission E to approve its use for dyspepsia and loss of appetite.[3] In practice, however, it is only used for atonic digestion secondary to or associated with a primary arthritic condition. The European Scientific Cooperative on Phytotherapy (ESCOP) indications are for low back pain and osteoarthritis.[4,5] There is positive clinical trial evidence as well as pharmacological support for the use of the herb in painful, chronic arthritic conditions. Most of the trials to date have been German or French and recently reviewed.[6-8] Neither of the European therapeutic monographs notes any interactions between devil's claw and pharmaceutical drugs.

Pharmacologically, devil's claw has three principal areas of action: anti-inflammatory and analgesic, antiarrhythmic and hypotensive, and bitter tonic. Data regarding mechanism of the anti-inflammatory action has been conflicting, with initial studies suggesting a nonecosanoid mechanism because animal models of inflammation did not respond to the extract, although some direct effect on lipoxygenase and cyclooxygenase (COX) pathways was noted.[9-11] More recent studies suggest that there may be a downregulation of inducible COX-2 and inducible nitric oxide synthase (iNOS), as well as a similar effect on tumor necrosis factor alpha (TNF-α) transcription, probably resulting from upstream effects on activating protein-1 (AP-1).[12-15] This is consistent with the efficacy of the herb as a chronic, rather than acute, anti-inflammatory and analgesic agent operating through different pathways than the nonsteroidal anti-inflammatory drug (NSAID)–type direct effects on arachidonic acid metabolism.[16] Parallels with other botanical derivatives exist, and evidence is emerging for modulation of nuclear factor kappa B (NF-κB),[17] as well as the metalloproteinase TIMP-2.[18]

Mechanism aside, clinical trials on the anti-inflammatory effects of devil's claw have revealed useful data relating to coadministration with several different NSAIDs and in clinical populations with chronic arthritic complaints using long-term NSAID therapy for management. This is a primary area for integrative use of the herb.

The cardiovascular effects of devil's claw have not been studied in humans, although studies of ex vivo Langendorff preparations (rabbit heart) and live rats strongly suggest the potential for protection against arrhythmias, including those induced by digoxin, together with a biphasic dose-response on heart rate.[19-21] Interestingly, harpagoside did not reproduce the electrophysiological effects of whole-plant extract. The same researchers noted a hypotensive reaction to the extract in normotensive rats, but only with intraperitoneal administration of high doses. Further studies on this aspect of the herb's pharmacology have not been published, and devil's claw clearly is a complex remedy that is not fully understood. Traditional South African indications include seizures, and some scientific corroboration of this has been found in a murine model.[22] Meanwhile, monitoring heart rate and blood pressure in patients with either preexisting hypotension or disturbances of rate or rhythm during early stages of administration of the herb may be prudent.

Effects on Drug Metabolism and Bioavailability

The bitter tonic aspects of the herb suggest that a potential for stimulation of hepatobiliary activity, but studies of the generic effect of bitters on drug metabolism and detoxification systems are unavailable, and pharmacokinetic interactions with devil's claw have not been reported to date. A single in vitro screening study of the effect of the herb on a mixture of human recombinant drug–metabolizing enzymes derived from baculovirus-infected insect cells suggested a potential inhibition of cytochrome P450 (CYP450) by devil's claw extracts.[23]

HERB-DRUG INTERACTIONS

Nonsteroidal Anti-Inflammatory Drugs and Related Antiarthritic Medications

Nonsteroidal anti-inflammatory drugs (NSAIDs):
COX-1 inhibitors: Diclofenac (Cataflam, Voltaren), combination drug: diclofenac and misoprostol (Arthrotec), diflunisal (Dolobid), etodolac (Lodine), fenoprofen (Dalfon), furbiprofen (Ansaid), ibuprofen (Advil, Excedrin IB, Motrin, Motrin IB, Nuprin, Pedia Care Fever Drops, Provel, Rufen); combination drug: hydrocodone and ibuprofen (Reprexain, Vicoprofen), indomethacin (indometacin; Indocin, Indocin-SR), ketoprofen (Orudis, Oruvail), ketorolac (Acular ophthalmic, Toradol), meclofenamate (Meclomen), mefenamic acid (Ponstel), meloxicam (Mobic), nabumetone (Relafen), naproxen (Aleve, Anaprox, Naprosyn), oxaprozin (Daypro), piroxicam (Feldene), salsalate (salicylic acid; Amigesic, Disalcid, Marthritic, Mono Gesic, Salflex, Salsitab), sulindac (Clinoril), tolmetin (Tolectin).

COX-2 inhibitors: Celecoxib (Celebrex).

Acetylsalicylic acid: acetosal, acetyl salicylic acid, ASA, salicyl-salicylic acid; Arthritis Foundation Pain Reliever, Ascriptin, Aspergum, Asprimox, Bayer Aspirin, Bayer Buffered Aspirin, Bayer Low Adult Strength, Bufferin, Buffex, Cama Arthritis Pain Reliever, Easprin, Ecotrin, Ecotrin Low Adult Strength, Empirin, Extra Strength Adprin-B, Extra Strength Bayer Enteric 500 Aspirin, Extra Strength Bayer Plus, Halfprin 81, Heartline, Regular Strength Bayer Enteric 500 Aspirin, St. Joseph Adult Chewable Aspirin, ZORprin; combination drugs: ASA and caffeine (Anacin); ASA, caffeine, and propoxyphene (Darvon Compound); ASA and carisoprodol (Soma Compound); ASA, codeine, and carisoprodol (Soma Compound with Codeine); ASA and codeine (Empirin with Codeine); ASA, codeine, butalbital, and caffeine (Fiorinal); ASA and extended-release dipyridamole (Aggrenox, Asasantin).

Interaction Type and Significance

⊕⊕⊕ **Beneficial or Supportive Interaction, Not Requiring Professional Management**

☼ **Prevention or Reduction of Drug Adverse Effect**

Probability:	Evidence Base:
1. Certain	◉ Emerging

Effect and Mechanism of Action

Additive pharmacodynamic anti-inflammatory effect enables reduced drug dose and reduction in drug adverse effects for a range of NSAIDs.

Research

Chrubasik et al.[24-29] have conducted several trials with a proprietary extract of devil's claw (Doloteffin) in various arthritic conditions, comparing both drug versus herb and drug in combination with various NSAIDs, including the COX-2 inhibitor rofecoxib (Vioxx). The general conclusions of this (ongoing) series of controlled trials and qualitative investigations are (1) for acute exacerbations of chronic arthritic conditions, including low back pain, knee pain, and hip pain, devil's claw extract is associated with fewer adverse effects than NSAIDs; (2) coadministation allows a lower dose of NSAIDs (or of opioid rescue medications in trials where these were allowed); and (3) for longer periods of administration, devil's claw was associated with almost twice the incidence of pain-free outcomes than rofecoxib. This latter result was from a subsequent pilot study, which, although it lacked the statistical power to establish the result as significant due to sample size, was interesting because the trial dropouts were almost all in the NSAID group, resulting from adverse effects of the drug.[26] In a qualitative study after coadministration of devil's claw with NSAIDs, the respondents were using a range of drugs that included aspirin, celecoxib, diclofenac, ibuprofen, indomethacin, ketoprofen, metazoal, naproxen, piroxicam, propyphenazon, and rofecoxib. This suggests that the effects observed in the controlled trials may be reasonably extrapolated to a number of anti-inflammatory drugs. In this connection, a 4-month trial compared diacerhein (an unrelated drug of the slow-acting drug for osteoarthritis–[SADOA] class) to devil's claw in 122 osteoarthritis patients. Diacerhein (a prodrug of the anthraquinone rhein, which is an interleukin-1 [IL-1] inhibitor), found fewer adverse effects and less rescue medication needed by the devil's claw group, although the degree of pain reduction was not significantly different.[30] Lipopolysaccharide (LPS)–stimulated COX-2 (and iNOS) messenger ribonucleic acid (mRNA) increases were inhibited by harpagoside through blocking of NF-κB activation of LPS in a human hepatoma cell line model, although the detailed mechanism of inhibition has not been established.[17]

Integrative Therapeutics, Clinical Concerns, and Adaptations

The NSAIDs, including selective COX-2 inhibitors, remain widely used for management of arthritic pain. The adverse effect profile of nonselective NSAIDs is a well-known problem, with gastropathies resulting in considerable expense for hospital care and responsible for about 17,000 deaths per year in the United States from major gastrointestinal bleeding. Emerging data also suggest that the COX-2 inhibitors are not as free from adverse effects as initially believed.[31,32] Recently, it has become clear that if aspirin (including low dose, i.e., 80 mg/day) or any classic NSAIDs are combined with COX-2 inhibitors, the risk of bleeding is higher than for classic NSAIDs alone. On the economic cost side of the equation, standardized devil's claw and COX-2 inhibitors are probably equal in cost. At this stage, however, the use of devil's claw as adjunctive, or even where possible as an alternative, medication in acute exacerbations of long-standing arthritis should be actively considered. Given that the adverse effect profile of the herb is benign, coadministration may not require professional management because symptom relief is the determining factor for the patient.

THEORETICAL, SPECULATIVE, AND PRELIMINARY INTERACTIONS RESEARCH, INCLUDING OVERSTATED INTERACTIONS CLAIMS

Warfarin and Related Oral Vitamin K Antagonist Anticoagulants

Anisindione (Miradon), dicumarol, ethyl biscoumacetate (Tromexan), nicoumalone (acenocoumarol; Acitrom, Sintrom), phenindione (Dindevan), phenprocoumon (Jarsin, Marcumar), warfarin (Coumadin, Marevan, Warfilone).

A secondary survey of plant toxicology in the United Kingdom over a 5-year period included reference to a single case in which there was an alleged adverse interaction between devil's claw and warfarin.[33] However, the details of this case were completely unavailable, rendering it impossible to evaluate, a conclusion confirmed by Fugh-Berman and Ernst.[34] Nonetheless, a persistent repetition of this unsubstantiated interaction occurs in the secondary literature despite the lack of verifiability of the original source and an absence of preclinical or clinical evidence for its existence.

The 34 citations in this monograph are located under Devil's Claw on the CD at the back of the book.

Echinacea

Botanical Names: The three principal species used commercially are *Echinacea angustifolia* DC, *Echinacea purpurea* (L.) Moench, and *Echinacea pallida* (Nutt.) Nutt.
Pharmacopoeial Names: Echinaceae radix, Echinaceae herba.
Common Names: Echinacea; *E. angustifolia:* narrow-leaved coneflower, Western echinacea; *E. purpurea:* purple coneflower, purple echinacea; *E. pallida:* pale coneflower echinacea, pale echinacea.

SUMMARY

Drug/Class Interaction Type	Mechanism and Significance	Management
Cyclosporine Allograft immunosuppressive agents ✗	Theoretically, long-term concomitant use might require increased levels of immunosuppression in allograft patients. Inadvertent use without professional care may cause drug failure.	Avoid, except for short-term acute coadministration, with professional monitoring.
Cyclophosphamide ?/⊕/✗	Immunotherapeutic outcomes of low-dose drug protocols (*not* cytotoxic schedules) may be enhanced by concomitant administration. High-dose drug effects on myelosuppression may be reduced.	Adopt; coadminister only with integrative oncologist supervision.
Myelosuppressive Antineoplastic Chemotherapies ⊕/☼	Echinacea may help protect white blood cell (WBC) counts in chemotherapy-induced myelosuppression. Natural killer (NK) cell number and activity increased by long-term administration.	Adopt; coadminister with related myeloprotective agents. Continue herb after chemotherapy.
Interferon, interleukin-2 (IL-2) Immunotherapeutic BRMs ?/⊕	Possible additive effects of herb and drug allow sparing of drug, reduction of drug side effects, and enhanced therapeutic responses.	Consider adopting; professional management required.
Tumor necrosis factor-alpha antagonists Immunosuppressive BRMs ?/⊕/✗	Echinacea may theoretically be used to enhance cellular immunity during temporary drug withdrawal mandated by opportunistic infection.	Stop drug; administer herb short-term only, before recommencing drug therapy.

*BRM*s, Biological response modifiers.

HERB DESCRIPTION

Family

Asteraceae.

Related Species

The *Echinacea* genus contains about 12 species, depending on the taxonomic authority consulted, although three major species (*E. angustifolia, E. purpurea, E. pallida*) are used in commerce. The minor taxa are sometimes classed as variants of the principal species. The minor species are confined to relatively small wild populations and include *Echinacea paradoxa, E. simulata,* and *E. atrorubens;* the Eastern species *E. tenneseensis* and *E. laevigata* are endangered.

Habitat and Cultivation

Echinacea angustifolia is native to the Great Plains and Atlantic drainage areas of the United States (U.S.) and Canada. *Echinacea purpurea* was introduced from the U.S. to Germany by Dr. Madaus before World War II and became cultivated on a large scale in Western Europe, where it is the dominant species of commerce.

Parts Used

Root and aerial flowering herb; commercially, the roots of Western echinacea *(E. angustifolia)* are preferred in the U.S.; aerial parts of purple echinacea *(E. purpurea)* are the principal part used in Europe.

Common Forms

Dried: Root powder and aerial parts.
Fluid Extract or Tinctures: Any of the above, 45% ethanol.
Fresh Stabilized Juice: Echinacin is a German preparation (Madaus AG) that consists of *E. purpurea* flowering tops' succus stabilized in 22% ethanol.
Solid Extracts, Tableted, or Encapsulated: Combinations of the above in different concentrations are available.
Standardized Extracts: In the U.S., echinacosides have been used as a marker; however, agreement on standardization is lacking, and manufacturers' preparations may vary.

HERB IN CLINICAL PRACTICE

Overview

The medicinal use of echinacea derived from indigenous Native American medicine. Widely used in the U.S. in the preantibiotic era for infectious diseases of all types, the modern view of the herb is narrower in focus, corresponding to the influence of European phytotherapy. An influential German clinical literature primarily employed aerial parts of *E. purpurea*, usually the stabilized fresh-juice preparation, administered both orally and parenterally. Historically, this resulted from the widespread cultivation of *E. purpurea* in Germany, which lacks native populations of echinacea. The roots of *E. angustifolia* are the preferred medicinal species in North American use. Modern clinical trials of echinacea focus largely on its use in prophylaxis and treatment of common colds and flu, whereas other therapeutic aspects of the herb remain underinvestigated by clinical researchers.

In popular use, echinacea is usually associated with prophylaxis and self-treatment of mild respiratory infections such as the common cold. However, the trial evidence for echinacea's efficacy for this indication remains conflicting and is perennially controversial in part because of the different *Echinacea* spp., different plant parts used in preparations, and different dosing regimens, as well as varying study design, methodology, and power.[1,2] The debate regarding the efficacy of echinacea in relation to the common cold has unfortunately become emblematic of divisions between advocates of natural medicine and those of conventional medicine. Arguably, this detracts from issues of more practical concern to clinicians, who likely are more focused on the general immunomodulating properties of the herb rather than on whether a trial shows "it works" for the common cold.

The detailed pharmacological mechanisms of action of echinacea remain to be fully characterized. It is well established, however, that the herb enhances cell-mediated immunity, particularly phagocytosis, and has moderate anti-inflammatory as well as beneficial wound-healing and connective tissue effects. Different constituent groups are thought to act in concert to affect immune parameters. Although there have been many studies of the herb, variations in the form of preparation, including differing plant parts and plant species used, as well as dose ranges and routes of administration, have contributed to a surprising lack of cohesive understanding of the pharmacology of echinacea. Novel discoveries about the immunological properties of echinacea emerge as research into this complex herb continues; recent examples include the discovery of a "melanin"-like constituent that activates nuclear factor kappa B (NF-κB) via a toll-like receptor (TLR2) mechanism, as well as a cannabinoid receptor–dependent pathway of immunoactivation unique to the alkylamide fraction.[3,4]

Historical/Ethnomedicine Precedent

Echinacea was used by Native American peoples as a medicinal agent for a wide variety of ailments, both topically and internally, including for snakebites, enlarged glands, and septic conditions. It was introduced into mainstream herbal medicine as a component of "Meyer's Blood Purifier" in the 1870s, where it came of the attention of the Eclectics, particularly John Uri Lloyd and John King. In the 1880s, Eclectic physicians started using echinacea, and the herb rapidly became a mainstay of their practice. Eclectic indications included carbuncles, furunculosis, abscesses, nasopharyngeal and respiratory catarrh, dysentery, syphilis, snakebites, sepsis, and cancer; their empirical reports constitute detailed, comprehensive, and authoritative contributions to the literature on echinacea.[5,6] Echinacea was official in the *National Formulary* from 1916 to 1946. Brinker[7] has systematically detailed the divergent historical, cultural, and pharmacological aspects of the two major medicinal *Echinacea* species, *E. angustifolia* and *E. purpurea,* in the U.S. and Europe.

Known or Potential Therapeutic Uses

Internal: Immunomodulation and promotion of cell-mediated immunity, particularly increasing phagocytosis by macrophages and monocytes, in a wide range of bacterial and viral conditions; chemotherapy-induced immunosuppression; recurrent candidiasis, sinusitis, etc.; upper respiratory tract infections (URIs); prophylaxis of URIs and infection in general.

Topical: Wound healing and connective tissue repair, venomous bites, including snakebites and spider bites.

Key Constituents

Caffeic acid derivatives, alkylamides, flavonoids, polyacetylenes, essential oil, polysaccharides, alkaloids. *Echinacea angustifolia* root contains isobutylamides; *E. pallida* lacks these compounds but contains polyacetylenes, which appear to have similar pharmacological effects on immune parameters. Constituent profiles also vary according to part used (root vs. herb) and the method of extraction; for example, immunoactive polysaccharides are not present in most hydroethanolic preparations because of their insolubility in ethanol. "Melanin" has recently been identified in phenolic extractions.[4]

Therapeutic Dosing Range

Suggested therapeutic dose ranges of the herb vary widely. Western echinacea root preparations are often administered at lower doses than *E. purpurea* aerial parts. Acute and chronic dose ranges also widely vary, as do posological approaches, which include the homeopathic through supraphysiological. The following are composite figures based on several sources.[8-13]

Chronic Dose Range
Dried Root: 1 to 5 g/day
Dried Aerial Parts: 2.5 to 6 g/day
Fluid Extract (1:1) 3 to 5.5 mL/day
Fresh Juice: 8 to 9 mL/day

Acute Dose
The chronic doses may be significantly increased for short-term administration in acute conditions; 10 to 15 g/day or equivalent in liquid preparations is common.

INTERACTIONS REVIEW
Strategic Considerations

Authoritative monographs for *Echinacea* spp. generally list no known interactions.[10,11,13,14] The German Commission E listed certain contraindications "in principle" that have been challenged as speculative (see Theoretical, Speculative, and Preliminary Interactions Research). Because the mechanisms of action of different constituents of echinacea are not fully characterized, extrapolations from the available data to in vivo interactions involve a degree of speculation, although consideration of specific clinical contexts of herb/drug administration can clarify potential interaction issues.

Self-prescribing consumers may administer echinacea for more serious conditions than colds and flu, as shown by a recent survey of nonconventional therapy use by cancer patients.[15] Echinacea is anecdotally used by herbalists as an immune stimulant for various indications, including immunosuppressive or immunosupportive pharmacotherapies, and for patients with immunodeficiency or autoimmune conditions and cancer. Possible interactions in these contexts are addressed later, despite lack of published data and inherent problems of extrapolating from limited experimental data to in vivo clinical practice. Echinacea in these settings is established in herbal practice, however, and this implies a wider concept of the therapeutic value of echinacea than the cold and flu treatment that dominates mainstream perceptions and publications among conventional health care professionals and the lay public.[16,17]

As a nonspecific cell-mediated immunomodulator, echinacea has been combined with anti-infective pharmacotherapies, either to increase net antimicrobial effect or to provide a similar degree of antimicrobial action at a lower drug dose. Few studies support this type of strategic interaction, although a study showing that a combination of *E. purpurea* intravenously with econazole was more efficacious than econazole alone in preventing recurrent candidal infection over a 6-month period is an often-cited example.[18] Some secondary sources evaluate this single study as evidence for a specific econazole-echinacea interaction. However, it is probably more appropriate to consider it as a specific instance of a general additive combination with converging antimicrobial effects leading to an enhancement of T helper cell type 1 (Th1) immunity; this interaction could arguably be extrapolated to several classes of anti-infective drugs for which evidence is not currently available.

The emerging use of pharmaceutical *biological response modifiers* (BRMs) that target different molecular aspects of the inflammatory process constitutes a challenging and complex scenario for clinicians considering the use of immunomodulating herbs. Several such agents are approved in a variety of chronic inflammatory conditions, including psoriasis, inflammatory bowel disease, and rheumatoid arthritis, as well as spondylosing arthropathies. Currently, the most frequently used class of these drugs targets tumor necrosis factor alpha (TNF-α) through a variety of mechanisms. Although necessarily speculative at this stage, the interactions between echinacea and these important emerging agents are considered later. A related consideration that should not be overlooked is that herbs influence human physiology differently than drugs, even when the apparent effects are convergent, as with echinacea and recombinant interleukin-2 (rIL-2).[19]

Incorporation of echinacea as an ingredient in Western botanical formulae for bone marrow recovery after myelosuppressive chemotherapies is consistent with known pharmacology of the herb. At this time, coadministration with pharmaceutical colony-stimulating factors such as Neupogen lacks published support, although adverse event reports from concomitant administration are lacking. Related botanical strategies for protection of white blood cell (WBC) counts during chemotherapy are found in both Chinese and Western botanical integrative oncological settings.[19,20]

Effects on Drug Metabolism and Bioavailability

Until recently, data on the effects of echinacea on drug-metabolizing systems were unavailable. An in vitro fluorometric screening study by Budzinski et al.[21] suggested moderate in vitro inhibition of cytochrome P450 (CYP450) 3A4 by echinacea extracts, implying a potential for pharmacokinetic interactions with substrates of this drug-metabolizing enzyme, but such interactions have not been reported to date in the clinical literature. No other potentially significant pharmacokinetic interactions with drug absorption, distribution, metabolism, and excretion (ADME) parameters have been reported. An in vitro study using a Ca-co cell membrane model examined differential transport of the caffeic acid derivatives and alkylamides, the principal components of hydroethanolic extracts of echinacea, and found that the apparent intestinal permeability for the alkyl amides was significantly greater than that for the caffeic acid compounds.[22] Another in vitro study found no inhibition of CYP2D6 and mild to moderate inhibition of CYP3A4 that was, unusually, dependent on the

substrate, but marked inhibition of CYP2C9.[23] Currently, minimal data exist on echinacea and drug-transporter proteins. An experimental model of the human organic anion-transporting polypeptide-B (OATP-B) revealed a moderate inhibitory effect on estrone-3-sulfate uptake after echinacea addition. However, the number of known OATP-B substrates in humans is limited at present, although it does include DHEA-S and estrone.[24] The in vivo relevance of these data remains to be established.

A clinical study by Gorski et al.[25] used in vivo CYP450 substrate specific probe techniques to examine the effect of echinacea on several drug-metabolizing enzymes in healthy volunteers. After a washout period following baseline probe administration, using as probe drugs caffeine (1A2), tolbutamide (2C9), dextromethorphan (2D6), and midazolam (hepatic and intestinal 3A4), echinacea was administered at 400 mg of dried root four times daily for 8 days; the probes then were readministered and blood samples taken. The echinacea appeared to have no effect on 2D6 but exerted moderate inhibition on 2C9 and 1A2 and a complex effect on 3A4 involving a near–self-canceling inhibition of intestinal 3A4 with induction of hepatic 3A4 (see Theoretical, Speculative, and Preliminary Interactions Research). Notably, the Gorski study used powdered *E. purpurea* root for 8 days, although aerial herb is the more typical form of purple coneflower preparation, and the healthy volunteers were not phenotyped for polymorphisms of the P450 enzymes studies, which is particularly relevant for 2C9. A wide range of intersubject variability in pharmacokinetic responses was noted, in line with predictable levels of individual variation known to be partly associated with genetic, genomic, and metabolomic differences.

More research with larger populations is required to examine the in vivo effects of echinacea on drug-metabolizing systems. Inhibition of drugs metabolized by CYP2C9 may be a potential risk. Principal among these would be the *S*-warfarin isomer, phenytoin, and the sulfonylureas. These interactions have not been observed or reported to date.

HERB-DRUG INTERACTIONS

Cyclosporine and Related Immunosuppressants

Evidence: Cyclosporine (Ciclosporin, cyclosporin A, CsA; Neoral, Sandimmune, SangCya).
Extrapolated, based on similar properties: Azothioprine (asathioprine; Azamun, Imuran, Thioprine), cyclophosphamide (Cytoxan, Endoxana, Neosar, Procytox), prednisolone oral (Delta-Cortef, Orapred, Pediapred, Prelone), prednisone oral (Deltasone, Liquid Pred, Meticorten, Orasone), tacrolimus (FK-506, fujimycin; Prograf).

Interaction Type and Significance
✗ Potential or Theoretical Adverse Interaction of Uncertain Severity

Probability:
4. Plausible

Evidence Base:
☐ **Inadequate**

Effect and Mechanism of Action
Enhancement of cell-mediated immunity by echinacea administration holds the potential to cause a shift in the level of immunosuppression required to maintain host-graft adaptation in transplant recipients. Arguably, this proposed phenomenon represents a "contraindication" rather than interaction.

Research

Studies have shown phagocytic activity of human peripheral blood monocytes can be stimulated by echinacea polysaccharide fractions.[26-31] Resistance to systemic infection in immunosuppressed animals was enhanced by echinacea.[32] Natural killer (NK) cell activity from human peripheral blood monocytes drawn from immunodeficient patients (AIDS, CFIDS) compared with normal subjects showed that cell-mediated immune activity was significantly enhanced after echinacea administration to the immunodeficient groups.[33] More controversially, a "melanin"-like compound from echinacea has been shown to activate NF-κB through a toll-like receptor (TLR) mechanism (involving TLR2), resulting in increased Th1 cytokine levels.[4] At this time the clinical role, if any, of plant melanins as immunomodulating agents remains to be established.

Integrative Therapeutics, Clinical Concerns, and Adaptations

Immunosuppressed allograft recipients are more vulnerable to minor infection than normal individuals. Acute use of echinacea at the onset of symptoms (e.g., common cold, acute URIs) is preferred by some allograft patients and practitioners to antibiotic therapies, because preexisting susceptibility to opportunistic infection (e.g., *Candida*) is likely to be exacerbated by antibiotics. Assuming prior stable immunosuppression within accepted safety margins, as reflected in serum immunosuppressive drug levels, there seems no reason to oppose the use of echinacea acutely for prophylaxis or treatment of mild infection. However, compelling reasons would be needed to extend echinacea treatment to chronic use in this patient population. Clinical features of graft rejection must be treated by aggressive intensification of immunosuppressive therapy.

Cyclophosphamide

Cyclophosphamide (Cytoxan, Endoxana, Neosar, Procytox).

Interaction Type and Significance

? **Interaction Likely but Uncertain Occurrence and Unclear Implication**

⊕/✗ Bimodal or Variable Interaction, with Professional Management

Probability:
4. Plausible

Evidence Base:
○ **Preliminary**

Effect and Mechanism of Action

This complex interaction may depend on the dose of drug and the clinical context. In cancer, low doses of cytotoxic agents such as cyclophosphamide have been found to have "paradoxical" immunostimulatory effects despite their myeloablative effects at high dose levels. Echinacea appears to increase the immunity-dependent anticancer effects of low-dose cyclophosphamide when given concurrently. In autoimmune disease, cyclophosphamide may be used at noncytotoxic doses to achieve immunosuppression, in which context echinacea would be theoretically contraindicated.

Research

Emerging interest in the anticancer effects of nontoxic doses of cyclophosphamide and other agents (e.g., vinca alkaloids) has established an immunity-dependent mechanism of action. Although not fully understood, it is considered that T-regulatory cells are effectively disabled by low doses of the drug. Interleukin-10 (IL-10) and TNF-α have also been implicated as possibly mediating the effect in animal studies.[34-37] Echinacea administration is associated with increases in interleukin-1

(IL-1), IL-10, and TNF-α by macrophages, although other mechanisms may be, and likely are, involved in echinacea effects.[28,38] Cytokine and chemokine cascades are interrelated, complex, and difficult to study, in that they occur rapidly and are often confined to a small cellular compartment and not reflected in serum levels of these compounds. At the current level of scientific knowledge, such interactions are best gauged clinically, although continued research is essential to improving our ability to understand, predict, and utilize the potential value of this botanical-pharmaceutical interaction.

Lersch et al.[39,40] investigated the effects of combining echinacea in the form of intramuscularly administered Echinacin and concurrent thymostimulin (a thymic peptide preparation) with low-dose cyclophosphamide (300 mg/m² intravenously, every 28 days) in two small groups of patients, one with advanced hepatocellular carcinoma and the other with advanced colorectal carcinoma. Numbers of CD4+ and NK cells as well as lymphokine-activated killer (LAK) cell activity increased significantly in the hepatoma patients. In the colorectal patients, all of whom had previous surgery and progressive disease, partial regression was noted in one patient and stabilization in six others, with a decrease in tumor markers and tumor volume (by ultrasonography).

Steinmuller et al.[32] used a rodent model of cyclophosphamide-induced immunosuppression and found that resistance to opportunistic infection by *Candida albicans* or *Listeria monocytogenes* was restored in echinacea polysaccharide–treated animals compared with controls. They also found an increase in TNF-α and enhanced cytotoxic activity in macrophages from the echinacea polysaccharide–treated animals.

Integrative Therapeutics, Clinical Concerns, and Adaptations

Although published data are tentative, the possibility of strategic enhancement of responsiveness to immunotherapeutic agents (e.g., low-dose Cytoxan) and recombinant agents (e.g., IL-2, interferons) by concurrent echinacea administration will be of interest to integrative practitioners attempting to address modulation of immunoreactivity.[19] Although parenteral preparations were used in the studies, as typical in Germany, most intravenous echinacea effects apply also to oral administration. (See also Astragalus monograph, as well as following section on myelosuppressive chemotherapy.) Because the therapeutic objectives of cyclophosphamide treatment vary in different situations and the effects may vary with different doses (biphasic responses), experienced professional management is required for coadministration of cyclophosphamide with echinacea.

Interferon Alpha (IFN-α), Interleukin-2, and Other Immunotherapeutic Biological Response Modifiers

Aldesleukin (IL-2, recombinant interleukin-2 (rIL-2); Proleukin), GCSF/filgrastim (Neupogen), GMCSF/sargramostim (Granulocyte-Macrophage Colony-Stimulating Factor), interferon alpha (IFN-α; Alferon N, Intron A, Roferon-A), interferon gamma-1b levamisole (Ergamisol), oprelevkin (Neumega), pegfilgrastim (PEG-filgrastim; Neulasta), pegylated interferon alfa-2b (PEG-Intron).

Interaction Type and Significance

? **Interaction Likely but Uncertain Occurrence and Unclear**

⊕ Potential or Theoretical Beneficial or Supportive Interaction, with Professional Management

Probability:
4. Plausible

Evidence Base:
☐ **Inadequate**

Effect and Mechanism of Action

Echinacea may increase endogenous interferon production by leukocytes and potentiate the effects of therapeutic recombinant interferon administration. It also increases NK cell number and activity, a target of IL-2 treatment.

Research

Research on the coadministration of echinacea and interferon is lacking, although preliminary positive data exist for astragalus, another interferon-enhancing herb (see also Astragalus monograph, aldesleukin/IL-2 discussion). However, in vitro, ex vivo, and in vivo evidence indicates that echinacea extracts increase IFN-α, which is consistent with its antiviral effect.[41,42] Miller[19] has used murine models to compare echinacea effects on NK cells to IL-2.

Integrative Therapeutics, Clinical Concerns, and Adaptations

Combining immunomodulating BRMs with echinacea has not been studied. At this time, extrapolations from echinacea pharmacology merely suggest the possibility of an additive enhancement (or sparing); data are insufficient to make clear recommendations.

Myelosuppressive Antineoplastic Chemotherapy

Alkylating agents: Busulfan (Myleran), carboplatin (Paraplatin), chlorambucil (Leukeran), cisplatin (cis-diaminedichloroplatinum, CDDP; Platinol, Platinol-AQ), cyclophosphamide (Cytoxan, Endoxana, Neosar, Procytox), dacarbazine (DIC, DTIC, DTIC-Dome, imidazole carboxamide), ifosfamide (Ifex, Mitoxana), mechlorethamine (Mustargen, nitrogen mustard), melphalan (Alkeran), oxaliplatin (Eloxatin), phenylalanine mustard (Melphalan), pipobroman (Vercyte), streptozocin (Zanosar), temozolomide (Temodar), thiotepa (Thioplex), uracil mustard (uramustine).
Cytotoxic antibiotics: Bleomycin (Blenoxane), dactinomycin (Actinomycin D, Cosmegen, Cosmegen Lyovac), mitomycin (Mutamycin), plicamycin (Mithracin).
Antimetabolites: Agalsidase beta (Fabrazyme), capecitabine (Xeloda), cladribine (Leustatin), cytarabine (ara-C; Cytosar-U, DepoCyt, Tarabine PFS), floxuridine (FUDR), fludarabine (Fludara), fluorouracil (5-FU, Adrucil, Efudex, Efudix, Fluoroplex), gemcitabine (Gemzar), lometrexol (T64), mercaptopurine (6-mercaptopurine, 6-MP, NSC 755; Purinethol), methotrexate (Folex, Maxtrex, Rheumatrex), pentostatin (Nipent), pemetrexed (Alimta), raltitrexed (ZD-1694; Tomudex), thioguanine (6-thioguanine, 6-TG, 2-amino-6-mercaptopurine; Lanvis, Tabloid), ZD9331.
Mitotic inhibitors: Docetaxel (Taxotere), paclitaxel (Paxene, Taxol), paclitaxel, protein-bound (Abraxane), vinblastine (Alkaban-AQ, Velban, Velsar), vincristine (Leurocristine, Oncovin, Vincasar PFS), vinorelbine (Navelbine).
Similar natural compounds.

Interaction Type and Significance

⊕ **Potential or Theoretical Beneficial or Supportive Interaction, with Professional Management**
☼ **Prevention or Reduction of Drug Adverse Effect**

Probability:	Evidence Base:
3. Possible	○ Preliminary

Effect and Mechanism of Action

Echinacea may help support and protect bone marrow myelopoiesis during chemotherapy, thereby ameliorating toxic effects of these agents on white blood cell counts.

Research

In animal studies, echinacea has proliferative effects at both spleen and bone marrow levels in rodents, although this study was confined to examining elevations in NK cells.[43] The same group examined the effects of echinacea on myeloid progenitor cells in spleen and marrow and found that echinacea did not significantly increase granulocyte precursors.[44] Weight loss was reduced and recovery from cisplatin administration was increased in rodents pretreated with *E. pallida* extracts intraperitoneally.[45] A German study on 70 breast cancer patients post-chemoradiotherapy found that a formula containing extracts of *E. angustifolia* and *E. purpurea* root with *Thuja occidentalis* and *Baptisia tinctoria* exhibited a limited ability to protect peripheral blood counts, although the doses of preparation were low at 1.25 mL of the formula per day.[46] A subsequent study involving 15 patients with advanced gastric cancer undergoing palliative chemotherapy with 5-FU, leucovorin, and etoposide received 2 mg daily of intravenous *E. purpurea* polysaccharide extract for 10 days total (3 days before chemotherapy) showed significant increases in leukocyte numbers compared with controls.[47]

Integrative Therapeutics, Clinical Concerns, and Adaptations

Many classes of antineoplastic agents exhibit dose-limiting toxicities on myelopoiesis, involving some or all cell lines, to the extent that leukopenia, thrombocytopenia, and anemia may prevent continued administration of chemotherapy. Nutritional status and general health of patients undergoing myelosuppressive chemotherapy are recognized as important factors in successful treatment toleration. A number of herbal and nutritional agents have been used as myeloprotective influences during chemotherapy, including echinacea extracts. These agents are often combined with other herbs directed at minimizing related chemotherapy-induced toxicities. Chinese medicine has explored these strategies more fully than Western herbal medicine to date, although echinacea can be incorporated into Western formulae for this purpose. Additionally, anecdotal clinical experience suggests that use of recombinant agents such as granulocyte colony-stimulating factor (G-CSF) would not be compromised by such approaches, and concomitant administration may potentially be beneficial. The additional effects of Th1 cytokine promotion (cell-mediated immunity) further support the rationale of using echinacea, particularly in combination formulae, in this context.[48]

Tumor Necrosis Factor-Alpha (TNF-α) Antagonists

Adalimumab (Humira), infliximab (Remicade), etanercept (Enbrel).

Interaction Type and Significance

? **Interaction Likely but Uncertain Occurrence and Unclear**
⊕/✗ **Bimodal or Variable Interaction, with Professional Management**

Probability:	Evidence Base:
6. Unknown	○ Preliminary

Effect and Mechanism of Action

At this time, the interaction is a theoretical concern but with important implications. Approved BRMs targeting the cytokine TNF-α reduce chronic inflammatory processes but increase susceptibility to infection. Echinacea extracts, administered short-term in acute doses, upregulate cell-mediated immunity to enhance drug-induced depression in mounting endogenous immune responses to pathogenic agents.

Research

Some experimental pharmacological in vitro and in vivo evidence suggests that fresh-pressed juice extracts of echinacea may increase TNF-α.[28-30,38,41] These results have not been replicated with hydroethanolic echinacea root extracts (which lack in polysaccharides) or with oral administration to healthy human subjects.[42,49,50] Immunosuppressed animals (with cyclophosphamide or cyclosporine) given echinacea respond to opportunistic infection more effectively than untreated animals.[32]

Integrative Therapeutics, Clinical Concerns, and Adaptations

Despite their common ability to inhibit cytokine bioactivity, the molecular structures and mechanisms of action of the various anti–TNF-α drugs currently approved for different conditions are in turn significantly different. For example, the TNF-binding moiety of etanercept is derived from soluble TNF receptor subunits; infliximab is a chimeric (mouse-human) monoclonal antibody to TNF, and adalimumab is a fully human anti-TNF monoclonal antibody.[51] A significant side effect of these agents is an increase in susceptibility to opportunistic infections, including by potentially ominous pathogenic agents such as tuberculosis.[52]

Current manufacturer recommendations suggest the cessation of TNF-α antagonists at the onset of self-limiting infections such as influenza, to allow for resolution of the infection, before recommencing drug therapy. The shortest half-life among this class of drug is etanercept (5 days). This window would be a time to use echinacea as a short-term immunostimulant, in acute doses, to enhance cell-mediated immune responses to accelerate resolution of infection before resumption of the anti-inflammatory therapy. The kinetics of echinacea effects on immune cells is known to be rapid. At this time, use of echinacea and other herbal immunomodulators in patients using BRMs as chronic anti-inflammatories remains problematic due to lack of data, partly because of the novelty of the TNF-α antagonist drugs, but is likely to become an increasingly important therapeutic concern for integrative practitioners with the increasing adoption of such agents.

THEORETICAL, SPECULATIVE, AND PRELIMINARY INTERACTIONS RESEARCH, INCLUDING OVERSTATED INTERACTIONS CLAIMS

Antimicrobials Such as Antibiotic, Antifungal, Antimycobacterial, and Antiretroviral Agents

Evidence: Econazole (Ecostatin, Spectazole).

Because of its ability to stimulate nonspecific immunity, echinacea, when taken alone, can be beneficial in a wide range of infectious conditions. Echinacea may also be helpful when coadministered with many antimicrobial drugs. Studies specifically examining the possible benefits of coadministration are rare. Coeugniet and Kuhnast[18] compared topical econazole nitrate in 60 patients with recurrent candidiasis with econazole and *E. purpurea* given orally, subcutaneously, or intravenously. Rate of recurrence dropped from 60.5% with econazole alone to 15% to 16% for the echinacea plus econazole groups (oral and parenteral), and *Candida* recall antigen sensitivity was increased two to three times for all echinacea groups. Although some authors describe this as an echinacea-econazole

interaction, there would appear to be reasonable grounds, derived from the known immunostimulating pharmacology of echinacea, for regarding it as one example of how echinacea may be beneficially combined with antimicrobial agents. Trials combining nonspecific immunomodulating herbs such as echinacea with different antimicrobials are required for evidential support of such a generic interaction claim. Well-designed and adequately powered clinical trials using combination botanicals and drugs methodology are, unfortunately, likely to remain the exception rather than the rule in the short term because of the limited interest in such integrative strategies. However, this may change with the increasing concerns over issues such as the rise of drug-resistant strains, hospital-acquired infections, and high drug development costs.

A recent trial on echinacea in the treatment of the common cold in children failed to account for a substantial proportion of the children in both the placebo and the echinacea group taking a variety of over-the-counter (OTC) medications, as well as various dietary supplements, presumably assuming that these would not have any effect when combined with the echinacea.[53] The trial has also been criticized on other methodological grounds.[54,55] Meanwhile, although integrative practitioners might find that coadministration has multiple benefits, this sweeping generic interaction is classified here as "speculative."

Cytochrome P450 1A2 Substrates, Including Clozapine and Related Atypical Antipsychotics, Cyclobenzaprine, Tacrine, and Tertiary Tricyclic Antidepressants

Atypical antipsychotics: Aripiprazole (Abilify, Abilitat), clozapine (Clozaril), olanzapine (Symbyax, Zyprexa), quetiapine (Seroquel), risperidone (Risperdal), ziprasidone (Geodon). Cyclobenzaprine (Flexeril), tacrine (tetrahydroaminoacridine, THA; Cognex).

Tertiary tricyclic antidepressants: Amitriptyline (Elavil), combination drug: amitriptyline and perphenazine (Etrafon, Triavil, Triptazine), clomipramine (Anafranil), doxepin (Adapin, Sinequan), imipramine (Janimine, Tofranil), trimipramine (Surmontil).

Recent in vivo human pharmacokinetic data suggest that echinacea may inhibit CYP1A2.[25] (See Strategic Considerations earlier.) Interactions between echinacea and 1A2 substrates have not been reported to date. A low-affinity, high-throughput CYP450 isoform, 1A2 is subject to induction by a range of environmental and dietary factors, including caffeine, brassicaceous vegetables, charbroiled foods, and tobacco smoking. Theoretically, the predominant patterns of echinacea prescription (i.e., short-term acute dosing for URIs) may mitigate any tendency to generate significant interactions caused by CYP450 effects. Until further data are available, however, a few critical substrates of 1A2 should be noted for potential interactions with prolonged echinacea use. These include the cholinesterase inhibitor tacrine (also a 1A2 inhibitor), the methylxanthines theophylline and caffeine, cyclobenzaprine, clozapine, and related antipsychotics. Tertiary tricyclics are cosubstrates of 1A2 and 3A4, which may be relevant if 3A4 is also inhibited by echinacea.

Cytochrome P450 3A4 Substrates

At present, interactions between narrow-therapeutic-index CYP3A4 drugs and echinacea have not been reported. Budzinski et al.[21] originally reported in vitro evidence for inhibition of 3A4. Gorski et al.[25] found that echinacea inhibited intestinal 3A4 and induced hepatic 3A4 in a manner that tended to offset the net effects on availability of 3A4 substrates. Yale and Glurich[23] found that in vitro, *E. purpurea* extracts moderately inhibited one 3A4 model substrate but did not affect another. This suggests that predicting the effect of echinacea on 3A4 substrates is likely to be complex, and that the actual effects will be variable. Further research is required to clarify whether echinacea administration will in lead to any significant 3A4 substrate drug interactions.

Warfarin

Coumadin, Marevan, Warfilone.

Warfarin is metabolized by both CYP1A2 (the *R*-enantiomer) and 2C9 (the *S*-enantiomer). The Gorski study on echinacea inhibition of P450 enzymes found a significant inhibition of 1A2 and a moderate inhibition of 2C9.[25] Yale and Glurich[23] confirmed 2C9 inhibition in vitro. This suggests that warfarin levels may theoretically be increased in susceptible individuals (2C9-poor metabolizers) because of lowered clearance after coadministration with echinacea; however, this interaction has not been reported clinically. Theoretically, normal monitoring and adjustment of warfarin levels would preclude the potential for increased risk of bleeding resulting from elevated drug levels.

Related Issues

Duration of Use, Hepatotoxicity, Autoimmunity, and Interactions with Hepatotoxic Drugs, Including Anabolic Steroids, Amiodarone, Methotrexate, and Ketoconazole

It has been asserted that echinacea administration exceeding 8 weeks induces hepatotoxicity, which leads to adverse interactions with a variety of hepatotoxic drugs, including anabolic steroids, amiodarone, methotrexate, and ketoconazole.[56] This assertion may be based on the presence of trace amounts of pyrrolizidine alkaloids (PAs) ($\sim 0.0006\%$ of tussilagine and isotussilagine) in the roots of *E. pallida* and *E. angustifolia*.[57] These PAs in fact lack the necessary necine macrocyclic ring structure of the hepatotoxic PAs that are metabolized into intermediate compounds, which form covalent adducts in hepatocytes, leading to the characteristic veno-occlusive disease toxicity.

The issue of limits to duration of use originated from Commission E, who stated that oral preparations of *E. purpurea* herb and *E. pallida* root should be consumed for no longer than 8 weeks.[13] No evidence exists for imposing restrictions on duration of use, either from adverse effects, suppression of immune function, or tachyphylaxis, and this assertion has been refuted in recent literature.[16,58] Miller[19] used a murine model to demonstrate that long-term administration actually *increases* health and longevity, with sustained improvements in immunological parameters.

Echinacea was also stated by Commission E "in principle" to be contraindicated in "progressive systemic diseases" such as tuberculosis, "leucosis" (sic), collagenosis, multiple sclerosis, acquired immunodeficiency syndrome (AIDS), human immunodeficiency virus (HIV) infection, and other autoimmune diseases. In fact, phytotherapists regularly use echinacea in several autoimmune conditions, with studies on its use in HIV infection and AIDS, as well as a report of extended administration in chronic lymphocytic leukemia.[59,60]

Historically, Eclectic physicians used echinacea to treat thousands of patients with tuberculosis. Among professional herbalists and naturopathic physicians, possible aggravations of autoimmune disease have been extensively discussed, and although the consensus is that a blanket contraindication is generally unsupported, isolated incidents of symptom flare-up in patients with systemic lupus erythematosus (SLE) associated with echinacea use have been informally reported.

Given the heterogenous and multifactorial mechanisms of autoimmunity and the currently available data, a prudent conclusion at this time would be to approach echinacea use with caution in patients with serious or progressed autoimmune disease, especially those who are susceptible to symptom flare, as in lupus (SLE) and some forms of multiple sclerosis.

Allergenicity

A review by Parnham[61] of echinacea adverse event data in Germany from 1989 to 1995 found 13 adverse drug reactions (ADRs) possibly related to oral Echanacin use, of which four were attributed to echinacea exposure. All were allergic reactions with skin manifestations. In the study period, an unknown number of doses of echinacea were consumed in Germany, but Dr. Bauer, an acknowledged echinacea expert, estimates that 10 million doses are sold annually in Germany; allowing for a degree of underreporting of herbal ADRs, frequency of allergic response would appear to be low.

An Australian report of an atopic female patient who experienced allergic symptoms requiring emergency room attention was followed by a review of Australian safety data by the investigator.[62] The author concluded that 26 patients, of whom more than half were known to be atopic, had experienced echinacea-related allergic symptoms, and that IgE-mediated ADRs are possible from echinacea exposure among susceptible individuals.[63] The national usage data for echinacea in Australia were not given, but if the figures are of the same order of magnitude as in Europe and the U.S., the risk/benefit ratio would appear to be lower rather than higher. This is corroborated by a skin test study of sensitivity to various herbal preparations involving more than 1000 subjects, in which echinacea caused dermatological reactions in only two subjects.[64]

Probiotics

In a 10-day randomized trial involving 15 healthy adults, Hill et al.[65] observed potentially problematic changes in intestinal microbiota after *Echinacea* administration. Standardized *E. purpurea* (1000 mg daily) stimulated the growth of certain *Bacteroides* spp. of intestinal bacteria, which may act as pathogens, particularly when the gut ecology has been disrupted. In stool samples, *Echinacea* use was associated with increased counts for three groups of organisms: the total group of aerobic bacteria, the anaerobic *Bacteroides* in general, and *Bacteroides fragilis* in particular. The authors concluded that the "health consequences associated with this change are unknown."[65] Notably, reports of potentially related adverse events associated with *Echinacea* use are lacking, such as irritable bowel syndrome or other pathological responses that might be predicted to result from such unfavorable alterations.

Although similar findings for echinacea or other herbs (e.g., goldenseal, isatis) often used as antimicrobial or immunostimulant agents are generally absent in the scientific literature, such effects from chronic use at high doses would not necessarily be unexpected. Further research and judicious pharmacovigilance are appropriate and necessary as the use of botanical medicine grows within the consumer self-care market and professional therapeutic application.

The 65 citations for this monograph are located under Echinacea on the CD at the back of the book.

Eleuthero

Botanical Name: *Eleutherococcus senticosus* (Rupr. and Maxim.) Maxim.
Pharmacopoeial Name: Radix Eleutherococci.
Synonym: *Acanthopanax senticosus* (Rupr. and Maxim.) Maxim.
Common Names: Eleuthero, Siberian ginseng.

SUMMARY

Drug/Class Interaction	Mechanism and Significance	Management
Antineoplastic treatments Myelosuppressive chemotherapies Radiation ⊕/☼	Eleuthero promotes myelopoiesis, helps protect white blood cell (WBC) counts during cyclophosphamide or other myelosuppressive chemotherapies. May synergize with radioprotective agents. Laboratory support and limited clinical evidence; controlled studies lacking, but interaction likely.	Pretreat, coadminister, and continue after chemo/radiotherapy until WBC count normalized (use with related adaptogenic herbs).

HERB DESCRIPTION

Family

Araliaceae.

Habitat and Cultivation

Native to northern and eastern Russia, northern China, Korea, and Japan; commercially grown in Siberia, as well as parts of China.

Parts Used

Root; the leaf is also used in Russia.

Common Forms

Dried: Powdered root.
Tincture: 1:5.
Fluid Extract: 1:1, 33% to 40% ethanol.
Standardized Preparations: Usually based on eleutheroside E > 1.0% and/or eleutheroside B.

HERB IN CLINICAL PRACTICE

Overview

Eleuthero is considered one of the defining adaptogen medicinal plants. *Adaptogens* have no equivalent among conventional pharmaceutical agents. The term was coined by Soviet researcher Lazarev in 1947 and subsequently defined by Brekhman in terms of three salient qualities: *nonspecific* (in relation to a wide range of stressor stimuli), *nontoxic* (cause minimal disturbance to normal physiological function), and *normalizing* (direction of action varies depending on the prior state of response to stressor and always normalizes).[1,2] The properties of adaptogens have been reviewed recently by Panossian[3] and Wagner.[4] Panossian and Wagner[5] also recently published an important paper distinguishing between the adaptogenic effects of the herb resulting from chronic dosing protocols compared with the stimulating effect of single acute doses.

With more than 1000 studies, eleuthero was initially the most widely studied adaptogenic herb, although *Panax ginseng* has a more voluminous literature. Eleuthero has established immunomodulating, anabolic, radioprotective, chemoprotective, antiviral, gonadotrophic, antiviral, and insulinotropic/antidiabetic effects; enhances learning, memory, visual and auditory acuity, and exercise endurance and recovery; and has antitoxic and antialcohol effects, as well as a range of antineoplastic actions.

Western reviews of some of the literature are available by Wagner and Norr,[4] Farnsworth et al.,[6] McKenna et al.,[7] Davidov and Krikorian,[8] and Baranov.[9] Therapeutic monographs are available from the European Scientific Cooperative on Phytotherapy,[10] World Health Organization (WHO),[11] German Commission E,[12] and British Herbal Medical Association.[13]

Confusion over nomenclature for the herb exists both with the binomial name (it is known as *Acanthopanax senticosus* in Chinese medicine) and the common name; the previous name "Siberian ginseng" implies similarity with "true" *Panax ginseng*. The current common name "eleuthero" was recently adopted in commerce to emphasize that although both plants are adaptogenic, eleuthero is pharmacologically distinct from *Panax ginseng* in terms of both constituents and activity profile. Medical reports often fail to use the correct binomial designation to identify herbal ingredients, and eleuthero has notoriously been confused with the entirely different species *Panax ginseng* (see Ginseng monograph).

Historical/Ethnomedicine Precedent

Eleuthero root (*Ci Wu Jia*) has been used in traditional Chinese medicine as a spleen (*Pi*) and kidney (*Shen*) qi tonic and is claimed to calm the Spirit/Mind (*Shen*). The root bark is considered a separate remedy. Eleuthero was incorporated into Western medicine in Russia in the early 1960s after two decades of Soviet research to locate more economic adaptogenic species than the slow-growing *Panax ginseng*, and it was introduced to the U.S. market in the 1970s.[9] As with many herbs used in Chinese medicine, *Ci Wu Jia* is used in complex formulae corresponding to specific classical diagnostic patterns and is prescribed in higher typical dose levels than in Western usage.[14]

Known or Potential Therapeutic Uses

Stress reduction and neuroendocrine balancing (e.g., dysglycemia, adrenal deficiency); fatigue, convalescence; enhancement of stamina, exercise, athletic, and work capacity and performance; increasing mental alertness and cognitive performance (e.g., memory, visual acuity); adjunctive to radiation and chemotherapy treatment; various psychological complaints (e.g., insomnia, depression); immunoprotection and immunomodulation; prophylaxis of infection, especially viral infection; antineoplastic.

Key Constituents

Lignans and other phenylpropanoids.
A series of "eleutheroside" compounds have been identified (eleutherosides A-M), but none of these is unique to eleuthero, and not all are the eleutheroside homologous compounds.
Oleanic acid derivatives (eleutherosides I-M), senticosides A-F, and polysaccharides, including glycans (eleutherans A-G); miscellaneous sterols, saponins, vitamins, and carbohydrates.

Therapeutic Dosing Range

Dried Root: 2 to 3 g daily (Western); 9 to 30 g daily (Chinese).
Tincture: 3.0 to 12.0 mL daily (equivalent 1:1).
Standardized Dry Extract: 150 to 300 mg three times daily; 10:1 extracts standardized to eleutherosides B and E.

INTERACTIONS REVIEW

Strategic Considerations

Authoritative monographs on eleuthero do not list any known interactions between eleuthero and pharmaceuticals.[10-13] The WHO monograph does refer to a case report that suggested eleuthero extracts interacted with digoxin. This case is considered likely an issue of adulteration or of interference between certain constituents of the herb and the digoxin assay and is discussed later (see Theoretical, Speculative, and Preliminary Interactions Research).

The general adaptogenic properties of eleuthero (according to the criteria of Lazarev and Breckhman) have been substantiated by a number of indexed Western studies, particularly regarding performance enhancement, although the bulk of the supporting literature, both experimental and clinical, is in Russian-language journals, much of it dating from the 1950s through the 1970s. Authoritative evaluations of the original literature in terms of study design, statistics, methods, and materials are not generally available. In the 1980s, Farnsworth et al.[6] and Baranov[9] attempted to summarize a number of eleuthero studies from the earlier Russian literature.

From an integrative perspective, the use of eleuthero in oncological settings is of particular interest because of the putative protective effects against chemotherapy- and radiation-induced toxicity suggested by the Russian research. Unfortunately, little corroborative work has been undertaken in the West to support the Soviet-era data. This is discussed later as a generic interaction.

As with other adaptogenic herbs, the nonspecific immunomodulating properties may bring about beneficial interactions with antimicrobial agents, although for eleuthero there are minimal data on this application.[15] (See also Ginseng [*Panax ginseng*] monograph.)

Effects on Drug Metabolism and Bioavailability

An in vitro fluorometric probe study failed to detect any effect of eleutherosides E and B on a battery of recombinant human cytochrome P450 (CYP450) isoforms (1A2, 2C9, 2C19, 2D6, and 3A4).[16] A "before and after" study on 12 healthy human volunteers failed to establish any effect of standardized *Eleutherococcus* extract (485 mg twice daily) with dextromethorphan and alprazolam probes. The authors concluded

that the extract is likely to alter disposition of drugs metabolized by 3A4 and 2D6.[17] From the limited data currently available, pharmacokinetic interactions caused by eleuthero effects on phase-one drug-metabolizing enzymes seems unlikely, and clinical reports of such interactions have not to date been made.

HERB-DRUG INTERACTIONS

Antineoplastic Chemotherapy, Including 6-Mercaptopurine, Cyclophosphamide

Cyclophosphamide (Cytoxan, Endoxana, Neosar, Procytox), mercaptopurine (6-mercaptopurine, 6-MP, NSC 755; Purinethol).

Interaction Type and Significance

⊕ **Potential or Theoretical Beneficial or Supportive Interaction, with Professional Management**
☼ **Prevention or Reduction of Drug Adverse Effect**

Probability:	Evidence Base:
2. Probable	○ Preliminary

Effect and Mechanism of Action

Eleuthero extracts are used to reduce adverse effects of antineoplastic therapies through a variety of mechanisms, including protection against and reversal of leukopenia, reduction of chemical toxicities, and enhancement of general stress resistance.

Research

In vitro and animal studies confirm that eleuthero extracts can modulate the immune system through a variety of mechanisms. These include increases in phagocytosis, natural killer (NK), and cytotoxic T-cell activity; modulation of T helper cell types 1 and 2 (Th1 and Th2) cytokines; and increased endogenous granulocyte colony-stimulating factor (G-CSF) production.[18-28] Two human studies are available. A flow-cytometry study was performed by Bohn et al.[21] on healthy human volunteers, who consumed 10 mL of eleuthero extract three times daily for 4 weeks. Significant increases in Th1 and NK cell numbers were observed, with increased activity of T cells. Russian researchers Kupin et al.[29,30] reported stimulation of immunological reactivity in breast cancer patients treated with eleuthero extracts. Although limited, these studies suggest that eleuthero has immunostimulating and immunomodulating activities in humans.

Coadministration of eleuthero with various antineoplastic agents (as well as radiation) has been reported in a number of Russian studies. Farnsworth et al.[6] report several animal studies in the Russian literature by Monakhov[31,32] and other researchers that involved a variety of antitumor agents, including 6-mercaptopurine, cyclophosphamide, and ethydimine. An in vitro study by Hacker and Mendon[33] found that eleuthero extracts at 75 µg/mL potentiated the effects of antileukemic agents cytarabine and N6-adenosine against murine L1210 leukemia cells. In a controlled study, Brekhman[34] reported a reduction of adverse effects in a controlled study of 80 breast cancer patients undergoing chemotherapy and/or radiation treatment when treated concurrently with eleuthero extracts, compared with controls not treated with eleuthero. Radioprotective effects of the herb have also been documented.[35,36] A rodent study by Minkova and Pantev[37] found that a radioprotective drug known as "adenturone" was potentiated by prophylactic pretreatment with eleuthero, although the dose of herb used was very high (5 g/kg orally).

Integrative Therapeutics, Clinical Concerns, and Adaptations

The documented evidence supporting benefits of coadministration of eleuthero with chemotherapy and/or radiation in oncology patients is limited, but sufficient data exist to justify the inclusion of eleuthero with other adaptogenic herbs in protective protocols designed to minimize myelosuppressive side effects of cancer treatment. (See also Ginseng monograph.)

THEORETICAL, SPECULATIVE, AND PRELIMINARY INTERACTIONS RESEARCH, INCLUDING OVERSTATED INTERACTIONS CLAIMS

The lack of equivalent pharmaceutical agents corresponding to herbal adaptogens may confound "theoretical" extrapolated interactions based on in vitro pharmacology, if adaptogens are "normalizing" as claimed.[38,39] Such extrapolations have been attempted, however, as in an adverse interaction with alcohol (from prolonged sleeping time with hexobarbital in a rodent model) and with oral hypoglycemics (from a rodent study suggesting alloxan-induced diabetic rats' blood glucose is lowered by eleuthero). In fact, eleuthero has been used anecdotally both for treatment of alcoholic toxicity and withdrawal and for "balancing" blood sugar, depending on whether the prior state was hypoglycemic or hyperglycemic.[40] The herb has more recently been shown to be more stimulating than sedative, at least in single doses.[5]

Digoxin and Related Cardiac Glycosides

Digoxin (Digitek, Lanoxin, Lanoxicaps; purgoxin).
Extrapolated, based on similar properties: Deslanoside (cedilanin-D), digitoxin (Cystodigin), ouabain (g-strophanthin).

An isolated case report describes a 74-year-old man with atrial fibrillation, stable on taking digoxin, who was tested for excessively high serum digoxin levels during routine monitoring, although he was asymptomatic. The digoxin was stopped, but the elevated level persisted. The patient disclosed self-administration of eleuthero. The product was not specified, and no analysis was performed to confirm the identity of the commercial preparation reported as consumed. After cessation of the supplement, digoxin levels normalized, and the patient resumed digoxin therapy.[41] Because eleuthero contains no cardiac glycosides, two hypotheses have been advanced to explain the apparent interaction. First, variation in eleuthero commercial products is well known.[42] Second, commercial samples of eleuthero, especially those sourced from China, have been documented on occasion as being contaminated with the species *Periploca sepium* Bge., a different Chinese herbal substance whose bark resembles that of eleuthero. *Periploca* is cardiotoxic in the doses that equate to nontherapeutic levels of eleuthero because of the presence of cardiac glycosides.[43] Given the failure to test the composition of the suspected eleuthero product involved in the case, Awang[44] postulated that adulteration with *Periploca* could explain the apparent test elevations.

An alternative explanation is that the botanical preparation may have interfered with the digoxin assay, causing falsely elevated readings. A recent investigation by Dasgupta et al.[45] supports this possibility, showing in vitro, as well as in vivo with human subjects, that eleuthero extracts can interfere with fluorescence polarization, creating false elevations in digoxin assay readings. The modest "false" elevated digoxin test readings caused by eleuthero may not explain the total apparent increase found in the case reported by McRae,[41] and combination factors still may have been involved. Finally, it has not been established that eleuthero is without effect on the P-glycoprotein transporter, of which digoxin is a substrate.

In summary, currently available data do not support the existence of any interaction between eleuthero and cardiac glycosides.

Antimicrobial Agents, Including Aminoglycoside Antibiotics

Evidence: Kanamycin (Kantrex), paromomycin (monomycin; Humatin).

An uncontrolled study by Vereshchagin et al.[15] suggests that coadministration of eleuthero with antibiotics (monomycin/paromomycin or kanamycin) in the treatment of children with *Shigella*- or *Proteus*-related gastrointestinal infections was more effective than treatment with antibiotic alone. As discussed by Brinker,[46] this possible interaction is circumstantially supported by some experimental data on the effects of eleuthero on increasing lymphocyte and NK cell activity.[21] Full evaluation of the original Russian-language study in unavailable in English, and the absence of corroborative data on antimicrobial-eleuthero combinations indicates that the potential interaction required may best be categorized as "overstated" at this time. It is theoretically arguable that such an interaction may be of widespread clinical applicability with a variety of antimicrobial drug classes, but this hypothesis remains to be tested. (See also interactions between *Panax ginseng* and beta-lactam antibiotics as discussed in the Ginseng monograph.)

Monoamine Oxidase-B (MAO-B) Inhibitors

Isocarboxazid (Marplan), moclobemide (Aurorix, Manerix), phenelzine (Nardil), procarbazine (Matulane), tranylcypromine (Parnate).

Reports of a ginseng-phenelzine interaction persist in the literature on *Panax ginseng*. These reports have been shown to be incorrect, arising from a confusion of *Panax ginseng* with eleuthero.[47] In any event, the reports contained insufficient or inadequate data for evaluation.

The 47 citations for this monograph are located under Eleuthero on the CD at the back of the book.

Ephedra

Botanical Names: *Ephedra sinica* Stapf., *Ephedra equisetina* Bunge., *Ephedra intermedia* Shenk and CA Meyer.
Pharmacopoeial Name: Ephedrae herba.
Common Names: Ephedra, *Ma-huang*, *Ma huang*, jointfir.

SUMMARY

Drug/Class Interaction Type	Mechanism and Significance	Management
Acetazolamide Urinary pH modifiers ◇/?	Probable pharmacokinetic interaction. Significance not established. Drug may increase herb levels by renal retention.	Avoid.
Caffeine, Theophylline Methylxanthines ✗✗	Well-established additive increase in sympathetic adverse events by multiple mechanisms.	Coadministration requires professional assessment and monitoring.
Dexamethasone Corticosteroids, oral glucocorticosteroids ?	Possible pharmacokinetic increase in drug clearance during coadministration. Significance and applicability to other steroidal drugs unknown.	Avoid.
Guanethidine Peripheral adrenergic blockers ✗✗✗	Herb reduces drug action and may greatly increase hypertension when coadministered.	Avoid.
Phenelzine MAO inhibitors ✗✗✗	Potential for increased sympathetic adverse effects by multiple mechanisms.	Avoid.
Reserpine, clonidine Sympatholytics ✗✗✗	Herb and drug have directly conflicting pharmacodynamic mechanisms. Coadministration (unlikely) will impair therapeutic efficacy of drug or herb.	Avoid.

MAO, Monoamine oxidase.

HERB DESCRIPTION

Related Species

The three main *Ephedra* spp. (*E. sinica, E. equisetina, E. intermedia*) are official in the Chinese and Japanese pharmacopoeias. Commercial sources also include *E. distachya* L. and *E. geradiana* Wall. ex Stapf. The latter is common in medicinal use in India. The North American species known as Mormon or Brigham Tea (*E. nevadensis* S. Wats.) contains little or no alkaloid and is not used medicinally.

Habitat and Cultivation

Widespread perennial shrub native to China, Mongolia, Tibet, Siberia, Japan, India, Pakistan, and Afghanistan; it is also extensively cultivated.

Parts Used

Dried aerial parts (stems); the roots and rhizomes, known as *Ma Huang gen*, are a separate medicinal agent in Chinese medicine with distinct actions and uses.

Common Forms

Dried: Powdered stems.
Tincture: 1:4, 45% alcohol (BHP).
Standardized Extracts: Unavailable.

Alkaloid content of ephedra-containing dietary supplement combinations in the United States and elsewhere are often not accurately labeled, and significant product variability has been demonstrated.[1-3] Crude herb extracts are subject to seasonal and species variations in alkaloid content.[4] Ephedra is a component of several commercially available Chinese standard formulae.

HERB IN CLINICAL PRACTICE

Overview

Ephedra has a long history of use in Chinese medicine, dating from 3100 BCE. Some authorities consider ephedra to be the mythical *soma* plant of the Vedas.[5,6] Traditionally, ephedra, or *Ma Huang*, has been used as a bitter warming herb for feverish and catarrhal conditions of the respiratory tract. Currently, regulatory restrictions permitting, it continues to be used clinically for its traditional indications, including bronchial asthma, allergic rhinitis, and as a diaphoretic in colds and influenza in both Western and Chinese medical formulations.

The activity of the crude herb is dominated by sympathomimetic phenethylamine alkaloid constituents, principally ephedrine and pseudoephedrine. Synthetic (racemic) ephedrine itself was produced by Merck in 1926 and introduced into clinical medicine as a treatment for pediatric asthma in 1927; thereafter it rapidly replaced epinephrine because it could be orally administered. Then, as now, the undesirable central stimulating effects of ephedrine were considered limiting factors on its clinical use.

Ephedra monographs by both the World Health Organization (WHO)[7] and the German Commission E support its traditional use for catarrhal conditions of the respiratory tract.[8] The clinical literature on ephedra appears extensive but actually is dominated by a persistent confusion of the crude herb with isolated ephedrine alkaloid. To a limited degree, pharmacokinetic and pharmacodynamic data suggest a similarity between crude ephedra and ephedrine, and the general sympathomimetic activity of ephedra is broadly correlated with ephedrine content. However, aspects of ephedra pharmacology, such as cytotoxicity or phosphodiesterase inhibition, cannot be attributed to ephedrine alone.[9-11] In answer to the question of whether there is full equivalence between synthetic ephedrine and ephedra, eminent German phytotherapist Weiss replied, "On the whole yes, but not quite."[5]

The problems of literature interpretation and data comparison are compounded by the variable ingredients and combinations of agents contained in dietary supplements marketed as "weight loss" products that have been used in clinical trials.[2,9] Caffeine or caffeine-containing herbs such as guaraná (*Paullinea cupana*) may be present, with aspirin or salicylate-containing herbs such as willow bark (*Salix alba*) sometimes combined with micronutrients such as trivalent chromium. Most recent trials have invariably examined these combination products and often incorrectly describe the results as referring to "ephedra." This in turn casts some methodological doubts on metastudies such as the Cantox and RAND reports, and although both reviews acknowledged the problem, their conclusions should be critically qualified in this regard.[12,13]

In the U.S., ephedra-containing supplements previously permitted under the Dietary Supplement Health and Education Act (DSHEA) have been banned since 2003, largely because of inappropriate consumption of ephedrine-containing weight loss and "natural stimulant" products resulting in a significant number of adverse events (see Note: Regulation, Safety, and Ephedra Weight Loss Products).

Historical/Ethnomedicine Precedent

Chinese traditional uses include acute wind-cold syndromes (characterized by chills, mild headaches, fevers without sweating, runny or stuffy nose, and body or joint aches) as well as bronchial asthma and allergic rhinitis. Several millennia-old classical Chinese formulae contain Ma Huang, including *Ma Huang Tang* (ephedra decoction), *She Gan Ma Huang Tang* (belamcanda and ephedra decoction), *Ge Gan Tang* (pueraria decoction), and *Xiao Qing Long Tang* (minor blue dragon decoction). In these combinations, ephedra comprises 15% to 25% of the total prescription, delivering 60 to 90 mg total alkaloid daily at normal adult dose levels.

In Chinese medicine, a further distinction is made between the stems of the plant, *Ma Huang,* and the root, *Ma Huang gen.* The roots contain dimeric flavonols and macrocyclic alkaloids not found in the aerial parts. In Chinese medicine the root is considered antisudorific, used for night sweats and excessive perspiration, whereas the stem is diaphoretic.

Known or Potential Therapeutic Uses

Asthma, coryza of common colds, fevers, allergic and vasomotor rhinitis, hives, and topical use for insect bites, stings, and allergic irritations of the skin and enuresis.

A recent comprehensive meta-analysis of these trials supports a moderate short-term weight loss effect from ephedra alkaloids when combined with stimulants such as caffeine.[14,15] Ephedrine and pseudoephedrine are approved for use in over-the-counter (OTC) bronchodilator and nasal decongestant products. Ephedrine has limited use in the hospital setting for the management of hypotension during epidural block and inhalational anesthesia in the operating room (intravenous

and intramuscular). Ephedrine has been historically used as a mydriatic and also as a pharmacotherapeutic agent for Stokes-Adams heart block, for enuresis, and for myasthenia gravis, in which latter its mechanism of action is unclear.[16] Some herbal texts also mention the latter two indications, but these are not general practice today, although some urologists continue to investigate the use of ephedrine for enuresis.[17]

Key Constituents

Phenylethylamine alkaloids, from approximately 0.5% to more than 2.4% total. (See Note.)
Catechin tannins, including epicatechin and epigallocatechin as well as catechin and gallocatechin.
Volatile oil, including terpinol, cineole, and tetramethylpyrazine; biflavonols.
The roots contain dimeric flavonols and spermine alkaloids not found in the stems.

Note: Proportions of the different alkaloids vary. The majority is 1R,2S-ephedrine (up to 80%), which occurs alongside the optical isomer 1S,2S-pseudoephedrine and their corresponding nor- and methyl- derivatives. The ratio of ephedrine to pseudoephedrine is variable and even reversed in some minor species of *Ephedra.*[4] Alkaloid composition can be used to "fingerprint" product samples containing ephedra herb because of the four possible optical isomers of ephedrine, only 1R,2S-ephedrine and 1S,2S-pseudoephedrine occur naturally.[18]

Therapeutic Dosing Range

Adults

Dried prepared herb for traditional decoction: 3 to 9 g daily. Typical recommended doses in Chinese and Western herbal practice deliver between 60 to 90 mg total alkaloid daily.
Commission E: 15 to 30 mg single dose and maximum of 300 mg daily total ephedra alkaloid.
OTC ephedrine: Up to 150 mg alkaloid daily.
OTC pseudoephedrine: Up to 240 mg alkaloid daily.

Children

Not to be administered to children under 6 years of age. Pediatric dose up to 0.5 mg total alkaloid per kg body weight daily; according to Commission E and WHO figures.[7,8]

INTERACTIONS REVIEW
Strategic Considerations

Ephedra alkaloids act as combination direct and indirect sympathomimetic agents at all alpha and beta adrenoceptor subtypes and have multiple effects on catecholamine pathways.[19] As a result, ephedra may interact with a variety of drugs that directly target the sympathetic nervous system. They may also indirectly interact with other classes of drug, such as antihypertensives or antiarrhythmics that do not directly affect the adrenergic pathways.

Within an integrative medical setting, however, the use of ephedra-containing formulae for traditional indications is limited and largely unproblematic when used by professionals trained in botanical medicine. Using traditional formulation models, ephedra is combined with other herbs that mitigate its "warming" energetics and the central nervous system (CNS) stimulatory aspects of its actions. The proportion of ephedra in a given formula is rarely more than approximately 15% to 20% of the total. Administered at therapeutic doses for traditional indications, ephedra is generally considered safe. This is supported by the complete absence of adverse event reports associated with administration of the crude herb or crude herb extracts either alone or in traditional formulations, as opposed to isolated alkaloid in multi-ingredient commercial preparations. Ephedra alkaloids are not degraded by monoamine oxidase, lacking the necessary hydroxyl configuration, and are excreted almost entirely unchanged renally, with a half-life of 3 to 5 hours.[20]

Adverse effects of the herb result from the CNS stimulatory actions and sympathomimetic actions and include insomnia, anxiety, tachycardia, tremors, and at higher doses, arrhythmias and increased blood pressure. Prolonged and repetitive use may induce tachyphylaxis, but suggestions of "dependency" are not corroborated by clinical reports. Nonclinical toxicological data is based on studies of the isolated alkaloids, principally ephedrine. Clinical data on safety are derived from adverse drug reactions (ADRs) noted in clinical trials on weight loss, and anecdotal reports following initial use or with abuse of ephedrine-containing combination weight loss products.

Assuming normal clinical practice and basic professional physiology and pharmacology knowledge, ephedra herb and its crude extracts do not present any hazardous interactions issues, despite the recent increases in adverse reports related to weight loss dietary supplements and isolated alkaloids (see Note: Regulation, Safety; and Ephedra Weight Loss Products). Professional management of ephedrine interactions for therapeutic purposes also occurs within the hospital setting, typically in relation to management of anesthesia-induced hypotension.

HERB-DRUG INTERACTIONS

Acetazolamide and Other Urinary PH Modifiers

Acetazolamide (Diamox, Diamox Sequels), aluminum hydroxide, ammonium chloride, kaolin clay, sodium bicarbonate.

Interaction Type and Significance

◈ **Adverse Drug Effect on Herbal Therapeutics—Strategic Concern**
? **Interaction Likely but Uncertain Occurrence and Unclear Implications**

Probability:	Evidence Base:
4. Plausible	◉ **Emerging**

Effect and Mechanism of Action

This pharmacokinetic interaction causes retention of ephedrine and pseudoephedrine (and amphetamine) by means of reduced urinary elimination under alkaline conditions. As pH rises, the pKa of ephedrine favors the nonionic association form, which is more lipophilic and reabsorbable at the nephron. This effectively reduces clearance and increases half-life.

Research

The mechanism of this interaction has been experimentally established in animals and humans using ephedrine and ammonium chloride,[21] as well as with pseudoephedrine and ammonium hydrochloride.[22]

Reports

Reports of this ADR in patients are rare. After encountering the interaction in a patient with persistently alkaline urine,

Brater et al.[23] studied ephedrine and pseudoephedrine excretion in normal patients and those with renal acidosis. They concluded that the rate of flow of urine as well as pH affected the elimination of ephedrines.

Clinical Implications and Adaptations

Although acetazolamide is usually listed as the interacting agent, this is an extrapolation from the studies with inorganic alkalizing compounds. The further extension from ephedra alkaloids to ephedra herb adds an additional layer of imponderability to the clinical significance and implications of this interaction, which is therefore of unknown or problematic status.

Caffeine, Theophylline, and Other Methylxanthines

Caffeine (Cafcit, Caffedrine, Enerjets, NoDoz, Quick Pep, Snap Back, Stay Alert, Vivarin); combination drugs: acetylsalicylic acid and caffeine (Anacin); ASA, caffeine, and propoxyphene (Darvon Compound); ASA, codeine, butalbital, and caffeine (Fiorinal); acetaminophen, butalbital, and caffeine (Fioricet).
Theophylline/aminophylline (Phyllocontin, Slo-Bid, Slo-Phyllin, Theo-24, Theo-Bid, Theocron, Theo-Dur, Theolair, Truphylline, Uni-Dur, Uniphyl); combination drug: ephedrine, guaifenesin, and theophylline (Primatene Dual Action).

Interaction Type and Significance

✗✗ **Minimal to Mild Adverse Interaction—Vigilance Necessary**

Probability:	Evidence Base:
1. Certain	● **Consensus**

Effect and Mechanism of Action

The effects of ephedrine on weight loss through thermogenesis, lipolysis, and appetite suppression are potentiated by caffeine. Frequency and severity of sympathomimetic adverse events, principally palpitations, tachycardia, agitation, and insomnia, are also increased when theophylline or caffeine are coadministered with ephedrine.

Research

Numerous studies have shown the combination of caffeine and ephedrine moderately increases weight loss, whereas the agents administered separately show little or no effect.[15,24-31] The mechanism of the interaction is multifactorial. Methylxanthines antagonize adenosine receptors and are phosphodiesterase (PDE) inhibitors. Their action on the cardiovascular system is complex, mediated by brainstem vasomotor and vagal centers as well as by direct effects on the vascular and cardiac tissues, mediated by both catecholamines and the renin system. At higher doses, caffeine and theophylline definitely induce tachycardia and are proarrhythmic, with sensitive individuals likely to experience premature ventricular contractions (PVCs). As with the ephedra alkaloids, caffeine is also centrally stimulating, and in methylxanthine-naive individuals, administration of caffeine or theophylline can cause elevation of circulating epinephrine and initial hypertension; however, tolerance rapidly develops.[32-35] Caffeine alone is not associated with increased frequency of arrhythmia in normal subjects or those with history of ventricular ectopy.[36]

In a recent study on a proprietary formulation (Metabolife 356) containing 12 mg ephedra extract and 48 mg caffeine, among several other ingredients, single dosing caused significant prolongation of QTc interval, at levels associated with possible torsades de pointes arrhythmia in conventional drugs (~30 msec prolongation).[37] However, a long-term rodent study showed no effects on metabolic cardiac parameters after 1 year of ephedrine-caffeine administration at 10 times the normal human dose.[38] Interestingly, crude ephedra has been shown to have PDE inhibitory activity that is not exhibited by pure ephedrine.[11,39] Theophylline is generally more potent than caffeine in its effects; it was often combined with ephedrine in nasal decongestant products before more selective adrenergic blockers became available. An early study found the theophylline-ephedrine combination no more effective than theophylline alone in 23 asthmatic children, whereas the ADR rate was higher for the combination than for theophylline.[40] Another study of asthmatic children, however, showed no additional adverse effects from the combination.[41]

Reports
Shekelle et al.[13] reviewed hundreds of ADR reports from the ephedrine-caffeine combination in the RAND study and concluded the quality of data was too poor to draw conclusions about a causal association of the ADRs with the combination. At the same time, they noted that clinical data suggest that the combination is associated with a significant risk of nausea, vomiting, anxiety, mood changes, autonomic hyperactivity, and palpitations. Other researchers, however, have concluded that adverse effects during trials involving the combination are not significant.[31,42]

Clinical Implications and Adaptations
Any synergy of effect on weight loss from the ephedrine-caffeine combination is largely offset by associated increase in adverse effects. Professional management, screening of at-risk patient groups, and therapeutic monitoring might largely preclude the development of serious adverse effects from the combination. However, pharmacotherapy for obesity does not generally favor use of herbal combination products, and integrative approaches to obesity do not emphasize pharmacotherapy.[43] In traditional use, ephedra is not combined with other stimulants, and obesity is not considered an indication for ephedra herb. Therefore the notoriety attached to the interaction of these agents is incommensurate with the significance of the issue in informed clinical practice.

Dexamethasone and Other Oral Corticosteroids

Evidence: Dexamethasone (Decadron).
Related but evidence lacking for extrapolation: Betamethasone (Celestone), cortisone (Cortone), fludrocortisone (Florinef), hydrocortisone (Cortef), methylprednisolone (Medrol), prednisolone (Delta-Cortef, Orapred, Pediapred, Prelone), prednisone (Deltasone, Liquid Pred, Meticorten, Orasone), triamcinolone (Aristocort).

Interaction Type and Significance
? Interaction Likely but Uncertain Occurrence and Unclear Implications

Probability: Evidence Base:
3. Possible   ◉ Emerging

Effect and Mechanism of Action
A pharmacokinetic interaction is possible whereby the clearance of dexamethasone is increased during concurrent ephedrine administration.

Research
The mechanism of this interaction was experimentally established in nine asthmatic patients, comparing the effects of ephedrine, theophylline, and placebo on airway symptoms. The interaction apparently does not occur between theophylline and dexamethasone. This finding helped tilt bronchodilator products for asthmatic patients away from ephedrine and toward theophylline.[44]

Reports
Despite some cautions in the drug interactions literature,[45] the importance and significance of this interaction remain problematic, and extension to other glucocorticoids has not been established.

Clinical Implications and Adaptations
The implications of this interaction are unclear, other than monitoring concurrent corticosteroid and ephedra use.

Guanethidine and Related Peripheral Adrenergic Blocking Agents

Evidence: Guanethidine (Apo-Guanethidine, Ismelin).
Similar properties but evidence lacking for extrapolation: Betanidine (Esbatal, Regulin), bretylium, debrisoquine, guanadrel (Hylorel).

Interaction Type and Significance
✗ ✗ ✗ Potentially Harmful or Serious Adverse Interaction—Avoid

Probability: Evidence Base:
1. Certain   ● Consensus

Effect and Mechanism of Action
Guanethidine and related drugs are prevented from entering, and are displaced from adrenergic neurons by, sympathomimetics. This abolishes the hypertensive effect of the blockading drug and also results in superadditional hypertensive effects because of the release of norepinephrine from the presynaptic terminal by ephedrine-induced indirect stimulation.

Research
The mechanism of this established interaction has been confirmed experimentally in humans and cats with amphetamine.[46] In a clinical study involving 16 hypertensive patients maintained on 25 to 35 mg guanethidine, Gulati et al.[47] observed abolition of the effects of guanethidine, as well as hypertension in excess of the treatment level, when subjects were treated concurrently with a range of oral sympathomimetics, including ephedrine.[47]

Reports
Despite clinical confirmation of the underlying mechanism of the interaction, recent reports of its occurrence are lacking.[48] Also, it is unclear to what extent this is an issue with the combination of sympathomimetic alkaloids in ephedra herb or crude extracts. The German Commission E suggests that the interaction may "enhance the sympathomimetic effect," which presumably refers to the experimentally confirmed fact that peripheral adrenergic blockade causes a hypersensitization of the postsynaptic receptors to *direct* sympathomimetic stimulation.[8] The significance of this in practice with mixed sympathomimetics is unknown, although guanethidine and epinephrine are known to result in exaggerated pressor and mydriatic responses.[49]

Clinical Implications and Adaptations

Although this must be viewed as a serious and an established interaction, the poorly tolerated guanethidine is no longer in widespread use for hypertension as it was in the 1970s. The newer derivatives are restricted to use in cases where other blocking agents (e.g., reserpine, methyldopa) have unacceptable CNS adverse effects. The clinical significance of the interaction is therefore limited in practice, although it is usually often cited without qualification as a principal ephedra-drug interaction in the herbal literature.

Phenelzine and Other Monoamine Oxidase Inhibitors (MAOIs)

MAO-A inhibitors: Isocarboxazid (Marplan), moclobemide (Aurorix, Manerix), phenelzine (Nardil), procarbazine (Matulane), tranylcypromine (Parnate).

MAO-B inhibitors: Selegiline (deprenyl, L-deprenil, L-deprenyl; Atapryl, Carbex, Eldepryl, Jumex, Movergan, Selpak); pargyline (Eutonyl), rasagiline (Azilect).

Interaction Type and Significance

✗✗✗ **Potentially Harmful or Serious Adverse Interaction—Avoid**

Probability:
1. Certain

Evidence Base:
● Consensus

Effect and Mechanism of Action

As indirect and direct sympathomimetics, ephedra alkaloids have "double" potential to cause rapid elevations of epinephrine at adrenergic and noradrenergic terminals if cytosolic monoamine oxidase (MAO) is inhibited. Monoamine oxidase inhibitors (MAOIs) cause presynaptic epinephrine accumulation. Ephedra will both promote release of the accumulated presynaptic epinephrine and simultaneously have a direct stimulating effect on the postsynaptic receptors itself. Exaggerated pressor responses will result, with possible hypertensive crisis or hemorrhagic stroke.

Research

The sympathomimetic action of ephedra alkaloids is well established.[50,51] However, the literature seldom mentions that ephedrine, pseudoephedrine, and norephedrine are themselves all unlabeled MAOIs, although weak and reversible in character.[52,53] Thus, they may also affect levels of 5-hydroxytryptamine (5-HT, serotonin) and dopamine both centrally and peripherally, as well as interact with tyramine-containing foods such as aged cheese and red wine. The manufacturers of serotonin agonists such as sibutramine caution against combining with ephedra alkaloids. Although a theoretical basis for this may exist because of the MAOI-like action of ephedra, the risk of serotonin syndrome is apparently low, and reports are lacking. Theoretically the newer, selective MAO-A or MAO-B drugs should be less interactive, but reports show that moclobemide increases the pressor action of ephedrine twofold to fourfold in healthy volunteers.[54] On the other hand, a recent case report describes ephedrine and phenylephrine being used uneventfully to control hypotension during epidural anesthesia in a patient taking moclobemide.[55]

Reports

The standard drug interactions literature through the 1960s and 1970s contains isolated reports of fatal intracranial and subarachnoid hemorrhage, but these refer to amphetamines combined with older MAOI drugs.[49] More recently, concerns have been raised about a renewed increase in occurrence of this interaction caused by the increased use of ephedrine-containing weight loss products.[56]

Clinical Implications and Adaptations

The older, nonselective, irreversible MAOIs, whether prescribed for hypertension or depression, should never be combined with indirect sympathomimetics. Even the newer, selective, reversible MAOIs should not be combined with sympathomimetics. This established and serious drug interaction can be plausibly extended to ephedra. After use of irreversible MAOIs, renewed MAO synthesis takes time, and 2 weeks has been suggested as a safe period after which ephedrine can be administered.[56]

Sympatholytic Agents, Including Clonidine, Methyldopa, Opioids, Reserpine

Clonidine (Apo-Clonidine, Catapres Oral, Catapres-TTS Transdermal Dixarit, Duraclon, Novo-Clonidine, Nu-Clonidine); combination drug: clonidine and chlorthalidone (Combipres); methyldopa (Aldomet); combination drugs: methyldopa and chlorothiazide (Aldoclor), methyldopa and hydrochlorothiazide (Aldoril); reserpine (Harmonyl).

Interaction Type and Significance

✗✗✗ **Potentially Harmful or Serious Adverse Interaction—Avoid**

Probability:
3. Possible

Evidence Base:
◉ Emerging

Effect and Mechanism of Action

Although each of these agents has somewhat different mechanisms of action, they can be considered as a group because their interaction is theoretically likely to induce the adverse effect of hypertension. The rauwolfia alkaloids exert their sympatholytic effects through depletion of epinephrine and norepinephrine at the presynaptic vesicles. This has the dual effect of sensitizing the postsynaptic receptors to direct sympathomimetics and rendering indirect (presynaptic) sympathomimetics ineffective. Mixed direct and indirect sympathomimetics are likely to have mixed effects in combination with reserpine. Clonidine is a central alpha agonist that reduces peripheral sympathetic outflow; methyldopa may act in a similar manner.[50]

Research

Early experiments in dogs, in vivo and in vitro, suggest that the pressor effects of indirect sympathomimetics are reduced or abolished by reserpine.[57] Human data are sparse, but patients undergoing ocular surgery who were already taking reserpine were found to have blood pressure elevations of +30/+13 mm Hg after administration of phenylephrine eyedrops.[58] There are no data on the methyldopa-ephedrine combination; however, an 80-patient trial, in which subjects were pretreated with clonidine, showed a blood pressure augmentation when given intravenous ephedrine at 0.1 mg/kg in both anesthetic and waking control groups.[59]

Reports

Clinical reports of ADRs from interactions involving these combinations are unavailable.

Clinical Implications and Adaptations

There are obvious pharmacological implications of combining sympatholytics with sympathomimetics. Concurrent prescription would be unusual, which may account for the lack of adverse effect reports. Reserpine is rarely used in hypertension treatment, although rauwolfia herbal extracts are frequently used in natural medicine as short-term hypotensives, usually with a holding strategy while implementing long-term lifestyle and dietary changes. The methyldopa interaction remains speculative, and the clonidine interaction is of questionable practical importance.

THEORETICAL, SPECULATIVE, AND PRELIMINARY INTERACTIONS RESEARCH, INCLUDING OVERSTATED INTERACTIONS CLAIMS

The principal scientific and clinical literature base describing ephedra interactions is almost entirely synonymous with the literature on the interactions of ephedrine, pseudoephedrine, and related indirect sympathomimetics, including phenylpropanolamine. Extrapolations to the herb are plausible and may provide useful guidance to practice. Although the data could be regarded as theoretical, the advantage is that the pure-alkaloid safety data will provide a conservative assessment when applied to the crude herb.

A low frequency of reported ephedrine interactions in the mainstream drug interactions literature may reflect the historic decrease in the clinical use of ephedrine in favor of more receptor-selective adrenergic agents. This is in stark contrast to the increase in anecdotal reports of self-prescribed ephedrine-containing weight loss combinations, most of which are technically caffeine-ephedrine interactions, or multiple interactions involving the caffeine-ephedra combination with other agents.

Likewise, the herbal and phytotherapeutic literature on ephedra interactions is also controversial. The German Commission E posits certain interactions, without substantiation of mechanism or context, which have been widely repeated by derivative sources.[8]

Cardiac Glycosides

Deslanoside (cedilanin-D), digitoxin (Cystodigin), digoxin (Digitek, Lanoxin, Lanoxicaps; purgoxin), ouabain (g-strophanthin).

Commission E suggests the interaction between ephedra and cardiac glycosides, citing increased risk of arrhythmias.[8] Despite the large repertoire of known interactions associated with digoxin, there are no reported interactions between digoxin (or other cardiac glycosides) and ephedrine (or other sympathomimetics) in the drug interaction literature. In clinical practice the interaction is unlikely.

Halothane and Other Halogenated Inhalational Anesthetic Agents

Desflurane (Suprane), enflurane (Ethrane), halothane (Fluothane), isoflurane (Forane), sevoflurane (Sevorane, Ultane).

Commission E warns that ephedra interacts with halothane.[8] Halothane was a primary inhalational anesthetic for more than 25 years. It has largely been replaced by related halogenated derivatives (enflurane, isoflurane, desflurane, sevoflurane) because of concerns of postoperative hepatic necrosis associated with halothane. The ability of these agents to sensitize the myocardium to arrhythmia is well known in anesthesiology and probably underlies Commission E's position, although this is not stated.

The halothane "interaction" is arguably a misleading one, especially in the context of consumer-oriented literature. Administration of intramuscular or intravenous ephedrine remains the best choice in management of anesthetic-induced hypotension, both for epidural block and with propofol and sevoflurane.[60-62] In other words, the interaction is beneficial with appropriate management. Advice to disclose ephedra use, along with any other relevant herbs and supplements, before surgery is more appropriate to anesthesia management issues than repeating solemn warnings to the general public about the danger of interactions with an inhalational anesthetic that is no longer generally used.[63]

Oxytocin

Oxytocin (Pitocin, Syntocinon).

Commission E lists the interaction between ephedra and oxytocin.[8] Oxytocin causes vascular relaxation and hypotension with reflex tachycardia. There are no reports of oxytocin and ephedrine interactions, and the probability of concurrent administration clinically is remote because induction of labor is an unlikely context for ephedrine use. This interaction may be regarded as speculative.

Oral Hypoglycemic Agents and Insulin

Buformin (Andromaco Gliporal, Buformina), chlorpropamide (Diabinese), glimepiride (Amaryl), glipizide (Glucotrol; Glucotrol XL), glyburide (glibenclamide; Diabeta, Glynase, Glynase Prestab, Micronase, Pres Tab), insulin (animal-source insulin: Iletin; human analog insulin: Humanlog; human insulin: Humulin, Novolin, NovoRapid, Oralin), metformin (Dianben, Glucophage, Glucophage XR); combination drugs: glipizide and metformin (Metaglip), glyburide and metformin (Glucovance); phenformin (Debeone, Fenformin), tolazamide (Tolinase), tolbutamide (Orinase, Tol-Tab).

An antagonistic interaction between ephedra and hypoglycemics such as insulin has been implied by some secondary sources. There is no evidence for this interaction, and, in fact, ephedra extracts have hypoglycemic activity and pancreatic islet regenerative effects.[64,65]

Secale Alkaloids

Commission E suggests an interaction between ephedra and "secale alkaloids" (i.e., ergotamine derivatives from the rye grass fungus *Claviceps* spp.), presumably based on theoretical additive pressor effects.[8] Because ergotamine derivatives are primarily used in postpartum hemorrhage or as migraine prophylaxis, the interaction is clinically improbable. The drug interactions literature lacks any reports of this interaction, and its repetition by secondary sources is presumably derived from the original, unsubstantiated claim in Commission E.

Note: Regulation, Safety, and Ephedra Weight Loss Products

Ephedrine-containing dietary supplements sold as weight loss aids have been associated with numerous adverse event reports in the U.S., including hypertension, tremors, myocardial infarction and hemorrhagic stroke. After a long controversy, this led the Food and Drug Administration (FDA) to invoke a sweeping restriction on the public sale of ephedra-containing products in 2003, directed specifically at commercial weight loss supplements. Subsequent clarification has effectively granted limited access to licensed practitioners of Chinese medicine. As of 2007, this regulation remains in force. In the context of practitioner-level information, political and regulatory concerns over weight loss products containing ephedra alkaloids are of secondary importance; the primary interactions issue is the underlying ephedra alkaloids–methylxanthine interaction.

Two major comprehensive reviews of safety and toxicity data on ephedrine-containing weight loss products are available.[12,13] The RAND report of Shekelle et al.[13] also reviewed efficacy trials for weight loss and athletic performance enhancement. None of these clinical trials or case reports involved ephedra crude herb alone, but only combinations of herbal extracts or isolated ephedrine with stimulants such as caffeine. The RAND report analyzed adverse event data from both clinical trial reports and postmarketing pharmacosurveillance sources, including reports to the FDA's MEDWATCH, and data from the customer files of a major weight loss product manufacturer (HerbaLife). The reviewers concluded that ephedrine-containing formulations are associated with a significant risk of nausea, vomiting, anxiety, mood changes, autonomic hyperactivity, and palpitations. Their meta-analysis of the clinical trials on weight loss confirmed that products combining ephedrine with caffeine were capable of producing short-term weight loss of about 1 kg (2.2 lb) per month compared with placebo.[13]

The possible role of adrenoceptor (AR) polymorphisms as an explanatory factor in the variability of weight loss data has not been considered by these reviewers, despite its known relevance to obesity. The precise contribution of direct receptor interaction, indirect release of endogenous catecholamines, or reuptake inhibition to the overall action of ephedrine remains unclear. Recently, ephedrine has been shown to act directly on the human beta-3 AR, which is involved in lipolysis in human brown adipose tissue as well as thermogenesis, which may explain the moderate effects on short-term weight loss, especially combined with the central anorectic properties of the phenylethylamines.[66,67] The emerging pharmacogenomic data on AR polymorphisms may partially explain the variable results with obesity and could theoretically support more effective drug targeting of ephedrine in obese patient populations.[68] However, the "therapeutic gap" between current AR polymorphism data and their implications for clinical practice remains sizable.[66,69]

Several sympathomimetic agents are licensed as prescription medications for short-term use (< 12 weeks) in weight loss, including benzphetamine and phendimetrazine, both of which are FDA Schedule III because of their abuse potential. Phenylpropanolamine (PPA), which is identical to norpseudoephedrine found in ephedra, was recently withdrawn from the market because of concerns about hemorrhagic stroke in women.[70] However, the norpseudoephedrine content in ephedra is generally very low, and although a small proportion of ephedrine may also be metabolized to norephedrine, the threshold dose of PPA considered to constitute a risk for hemorrhagic

stroke is 75 mg/day.[70] A recent case-control study found no association between ephedrine use and hemorrhagic stroke.[71]

Meanwhile, research and trials continue on new pharmacological interventions for obesity, with recent emphasis on selective beta-3 AR agonist drugs. Despite the prevalence of overweight and obesity and the alarming rate of increase in obesity-related conditions, the overall understanding of this multifactorial condition and the efficacy of current pharmacological treatments remain limited.[43]

The adverse events reviewed by RAND and others can be extrapolated to ephedra herb with some minor qualifications. The crude herb contains tannin constituents that have angiotensin-converting enzyme (ACE)–inhibiting activity, as well as multiple constituents that include organic acids, flavonoids, and volatile oils that will modulate the alkaloid-fraction effects.[72] It is plausible that extrapolations from ephedrine effects will be overly conservative with respect to the crude herb.[72] Again, these studies used combinations with caffeine or caffeine-containing herbs.

Classic pressor responses have been established for the crude herb, but the dose-response kinetics are significantly slower than for pure ephedrine, and the pressor response is small, with considerable individual variation.[73] Nephrolithiasis has been reported recently after crude herb consumption; the urologists' search of the Louis C. Herring and Company kidney stone database show that this is an endemic complication of ephedrine, with hundreds of previous episodes.[74] At the same time, one experimental study has showed a significant reduction of uremic toxins after administration of aqueous crude herb extract in an animal model of renal failure.[75]

The recent banning of ephedra-containing weight loss products by the FDA has changed the degree to which undisclosed use of ephedra may be a potential danger in most cases. The market for weight loss products remains active, and "ephedra-free" formulations are available to the public that attempt to circumvent regulatory restrictions, based on extracts of *Citrus aurantium* (bitter orange), which contains the mildly sympathomimetic alkaloid synephrine. Lipolytic effects in human adipocytes have been demonstrated, but convincing evidence for efficacy of the extract as a weight loss aid is not currently available.[76-78]

The 78 citations for this monograph are located under Ephedra on the CD at the back of the book.

Feverfew

Botanical Name: *Tanacetum parthenium* (L.) Schultz Bip.
Pharmacopoeial Name: Tanaceti partheni herba.
Synonyms: *Matricaria parthenium* L.; *Chrysanthemum parthenium* (L.) Bernh.;
Leucanthemum parthenium (L.) Gren. and Godron; *Pyrethrum parthenium* L. Sm.
Common Name: Feverfew.

HERB DESCRIPTION

Family
Asteraceae.

Parts Used
Aerial herb.

Common Forms
Fresh leaf.
Dried leaf, freeze-dried leaf.
Tincture: 1:5 25% ethanol.[1]
Standardized Extract: Not less than 0.2% parthenolide content.

INTERACTIONS REVIEW

Strategic Considerations

The modern use of feverfew as a specific for migraines followed its adoption by physicians at the London Migraine Clinic in the early 1980s, who investigated anecdotal reports of the effectiveness of the fresh leaf as a migraine prophylactic and treatment.[2,3] Following initial studies, its use spread rapidly to North America, and today the herb hovers in the lower ranks of the top-20 best-selling botanicals in the United States, partly because of the large number (29 million) of migraine sufferers seeking effective treatment for the often-refractory condition. This indication was never prevalent in Germany, and the herb is not mentioned by Weiss,[4] Wichtl,[5] or the German Commission E.[6] The first modern-use therapeutic monograph was in the *British Herbal Compendium*[1]; this has been superseded by a comprehensive monograph from the European Scientific Cooperative on Phytotherapy (ESCOP)[7] and recent reviews from Mills and Bone[8] and McKenna et al.[9]

Despite its current public popularity, recent systematic reviews of the available controlled trial data suggest that the effectiveness of feverfew for migraine prophylaxis is not conclusively established beyond reasonable doubt, although most trials favor the herb against placebo and suggest it has a good safety profile.[10,11]

Interpretations of the pharmacodynamics of feverfew extracts that stress only the sesquiterpene lactone *parthenolide* as the active constituent responsible for the anti-inflammatory and antimigraine actions of the herb have been described as controversial, particularly the so-called serotonin-parthenolide hypothesis of migraine prophylaxis.[12] The recent ESCOP monograph asserts that connections between the constituents of the herb and its migraine prophylactic action should be considered as complex and not definitively established.[7] However, a clearer picture may be emerging from recent studies.

Currently, the pharmacology of feverfew is being intensively reexamined after the discovery of the anti–nuclear factor kappa B (NF-κB) properties of parthenolide.[13-15] From an interactions perspective, given the pluripotent activities governed by this transcription factor, inhibition of NF-κB suggests several potentially valuable strategic interactions; these include modulation of adhesion molecule expression,[16] inhibition of inducible nitric oxide synthase (iNOS),[17,18] and possible targeting of antireperfusion injury,[19] as well as induction of apoptosis and modulation of drug resistance.[20,21] Parthenolide also appears to be a thiol depleter, which may be part of the mechanism underlying its antiaggregatory effect.[22,23] The induction of apoptosis by parthenolide also involves thiol antioxidant modulation.[21,24] The presence of NF-κB in platelets also suggest that this factor may have a role in aggregation, independently of gene regulation.[25]

Parthenolide has recently been shown to be a selective inducer of apoptosis in cells from chronic lymphocytic leukemia (CLL) patients at the relatively low median inhibitory concentration (IC_{50}) of 6.2 μmol.[26] Increasing research interest in the anticancer properties of feverfew and parthenolide are expanding the "herb for migraine" conception of the botanical that characterized feverfew in the late twentieth century.

The official ESCOP monograph lists no known interactions between feverfew and pharmaceuticals, and interactions reports are absent from the literature, although some secondary sources persistently assert an interaction between feverfew and warfarin[7,27] (see Theoretical, Speculative, and Preliminary Interactions Research). An interaction with drugs targeting hemostasis is theoretically more likely with antiplatelet thrombolytics, but depending on context and intent, such interactions are as likely to be beneficial as adverse. Protection against gastropathies induced by nonsteroidal anti-inflammatory drugs (NSAIDs) is a more than theoretically possible interaction, and although evidence for adjunctive interactions in oncological therapies (involving NF-κB–mediated activities) is preliminary, this may be an area of future interest as research evidence continues to emerge.

Pharmacokinetic data on the herb are meager; a recent report suggests that parthenolide and other sesquiterpene lactones exhibit a high degree of protein binding in human plasma.[28] The metabolic fate of parthenolide and its possible modulation of the cytochrome P450 (CYP450) system is unknown, but to date the herb does not appear to be associated with any obvious pharmacokinetic interactions.

HERB-DRUG INTERACTIONS

Indomethacin and Related Nonsteroidal Anti-Inflammatory Drugs (NSAIDs)

Evidence: Indomethacin (indometacin; Indocin, Indocin-SR). Extrapolated, based on similar properties: Nonsteroidal anti-inflammatory drugs (NSAIDs):

COX-1 inhibitors: Diclofenac (Cataflam, Voltaren), combination drug: diclofenac and misoprostol (Arthrotec), diflunisal (Dolobid), etodolac (Lodine), fenoprofen (Dalfon), furbiprofen (Ansaid), ibuprofen (Advil, Excedrin IB, Motrin, Motrin IB, Nuprin, Pedia Care Fever Drops, Provel, Rufen), combination drug: hydrocodone and ibuprofen (Reprexain, Vicoprofen), indomethacin (indometacin; Indocin, Indocin-SR), ketoprofen

(Orudis, Oruvail), ketorolac (Acular ophthalmic, Toradol), meclofenamate (Meclomen), mefenamic acid (Ponstel), meloxicam (Mobic), nabumetone (Relafen), naproxen (Aleve, Anaprox, Naprosyn), oxaprozin (Daypro), piroxicam (Feldene), salsalate (salicylic acid; Amigesic, Disalcid, Marthritic, Mono Gesic, Salflex, Salsitab), sulindac (Clinoril), tolmetin (Tolectin).

COX-2 inhibitor: Celecoxib (Celebrex).

Interaction Type and Significance

☼ **Prevention or Reduction of Drug Adverse Effect**

Probability:	Evidence Base:
3. Possible	○ **Preliminary**

Effect and Mechanism of Action
The anti-inflammatory effects of feverfew may protect against gastropathic adverse effects of indomethacin and possibly other NSAIDs occurring with chronic use of these agents.

Research
In a rodent model of experimentally induced gastric ulceration by ethanol, oral pretreatment with either feverfew extract or parthenolide 24 hours before ethanol administration created protective effects ranging between 34% and 100% for the extract and 27% and 100% for parthenolide. At doses of 40 mg/kg body weight, the mean ulcer index declined from 4.8 (control) to 1.4 for the extract and 0.5 for parthenolide.[29] The researchers used *Tanacetum larvatum* (Grisb. ex Pant), a related feverfew species with a higher parthenolide content (1.1%) than *T. parthenium*, to examine the ulceroprotective effects of the herb against indomethacin-induced ulcers in rodents. They concluded that there was significant reduction of the ulcerogenic effect at 50 mg/kg orally, given after indomethacin (not pretreatment). The same extract significantly reduced NF-κB activation in two assay methods, at levels of 20 μg/mL. They also examined the anti-inflammatory effect of combining indomethacin and the herbal extract on the rat-paw carrageenan model and concluded that although there was slight synergy of effect for the combination, it was not significant.[29]

Previous studies on the ulceroprotective effects of dihydroleucodine, a sesquiterpene lactone from *Artemisia douglasiana,* support the hypothesis that the protective effects are caused by increased mucus secretion, which is significantly reduced by indomethacin.[30] More recently, unrelated investigations have shown that indomethacin markedly activates mucosal NF-κB 48 hours after administration, lending indirect support to the hypothesis that the therapeutic effects of feverfew are mediated through inhibition of this transcription factor.[31]

Integrative Therapeutics, Clinical Concerns, and Adaptations
The protective effectiveness of feverfew extracts in ameliorating NSAID-induced gastropathy is experimentally established, and positive data are available relating to indomethacin. In practice, unless feverfew is an agent of choice for therapeutic reasons, primarily migraine or arthritis, other botanical agents, such as licorice or aloe, may have a superior cost/risk profile to feverfew for this purpose. Toxicological data on possible mutagenicity of feverfew is controversial, although otherwise the extract has a good safety profile. In addition, additive or synergistic anti-inflammatory effects are therapeutically preferable, and in the case of feverfew and NSAIDs, this synergism has not been clearly demonstrated; a controlled trial of 50 migraine patients found no significant difference between placebo and control

groups.[32] However, use of anti-inflammatory medications by patients in the feverfew group showed a decline over the 9-month trial period.

Taxanes: Paclitaxel, Docetaxel

Evidence: Docetaxel (Taxotere), paclitaxel (Paxene, Taxol), paclitaxel, protein-bound (Abraxane).
Extrapolated, based on similar properties: Chemotherapeutic agents that activate NF-κB:

Cisplatin (*cis*-diaminedichloroplatinum, CDDP; Platinol, Platinol-AQ), daunorubicin (Cerubidine, DaunoXome), doxorubicin (Adriamycin, Rubex), doxorubicin, pegylated liposomal (Caelyx, Doxil, Myocet), epirubicin (Ellence, Pharmorubicin), etoposide (Eposin, Etopophos, Vepesid, VP-16), idarubicin (Idamycin, Zavedos), irinotecan (camptothecin-11, CPT-11; Campto, Camptosar), tamoxifen (Nolvadex), topotecan (Hycamtin), vinblastine (Alkaban-AQ, Velban, Velsar), vincristine (Leurocristine, Oncovin, Vincasar PFS), vinorelbine (Navelbine).

Interaction Type and Significance

⊕ **Potential or Theoretical Beneficial or Supportive Interaction, with Professional Management**

Probability:	Evidence Base:
4. Plausible	○ **Preliminary**

Effect and Mechanism of Action
Parthenolide experimentally increases the sensitivity of breast cancer cells with constitutively active NF-κB expression to apoptosis-inducing effects of taxanes. This is likely a specific case of general chemosensitization by naturally occurring NF-κB inhibitors to chemotherapeutic agents known to have antiapoptotic effects of NF-κB. Clinical support for the interaction is not available.

Research
Parthenolide and feverfew extracts both exhibit NF-κB inhibitory actions.[13-15] This transcription factor is involved in multiple effects in cancer biology, including cell survival, adhesion, inflammation, proliferation, and metastasis, as well as chemoresistance, and its expression can be modulated by a range of chemopreventive natural compounds.[33,34] Paradoxically, a number of cytotoxic chemotherapeutic agents activate NF-κB, leading to chemoresistance.[35,36] Cory and Cory[37] found that parthenolide acted as an augmenter of apoptosis through NF-κB inhibition in a leukemia cell line, and later they studied an NF-κB–expressing subset of breast cancer cells that were chemoresistant to paclitaxel. The sensitivity to the chemotherapeutic agent could be increased in the malignant cells both by I-κB-α superrepressor and parthenolide. The effect was not replicated in nonmalignant cells. The authors suggest that the active ingredients of herbs may be useful in increasing the chemosensitivity of cancers with constitutively active NF-κB.[20,37]

An in vivo and in vitro study using three breast cancer lines found that parthenolide combined with docetaxel increased the antiapoptotic and antimetastatic effects of the taxane, and that the effect was accompanied by lower tumor levels of NF-κB.[38] Another NF-κB–related effect has been demonstrated with tamoxifen resistance reduction and parthenolide in MCF7 cells.[39] Thiol and redox status may also relate to the important differential effects of parthenolide on apoptosis between malignant and normal cells.[21,24] Parthenolide acted as an in vitro sensitizer to the NSAID sulindac in a pancreatic carcinoma cell line. The effect of the combination was synergistic (greater than either agent alone), suggesting possible preclinical support for combining parthenolide with other NF-κB inhibitors in chemotherapy.[40] For example, parthenolide combined with dehydroepiandrosterone (DHEA) attenuated tumor growth in vivo in a murine model compared to either agent alone.[41] Weak synergistic effects of parthenolide with other constituents of the whole herb on growth inhibition for two breast and one endometrial cancer cell lines were found in the case of the flavonoids apigenin and luteolin by Wu et al.[42]

Integrative Therapeutics, Clinical Concerns, and Adaptations

This potential interaction may be of considerable significance, although it currently lacks clinical support and must be regarded as preliminary. Incorporation into chemotherapy protocols at this time should be considered only by practitioners with solid clinical grounding in integrative oncology and may be specifically limited to issues related to chemotherapy-induced NF-κB activation.

Acetylsalicylic Acid, Clopidogrel, Ticlopidine, and Other Antiplatelet Thromboprophylactics

Evidence: Acetylsalicylic acid (acetosal, acetyl salicylic acid, ASA, salicylsalicylic acid; Arthritis Foundation Pain Reliever, Ascriptin, Aspergum, Asprimox, Bayer Aspirin, Bayer Buffered Aspirin, Bayer Low Adult Strength, Bufferin, Buffex, Cama Arthritis Pain Reliever, Easprin, Ecotrin, Ecotrin Low Adult Strength, Empirin, Extra Strength Adprin-B, Extra Strength Bayer Enteric 500 Aspirin, Extra Strength Bayer Plus, Halfprin 81, Heartline, Regular Strength Bayer Enteric 500 Aspirin, St. Joseph Adult Chewable Aspirin, ZORprin); combination drugs: ASA and caffeine (Anacin); ASA, caffeine, and propoxyphene (Darvon Compound); ASA and carisoprodol (Soma Compound); ASA, codeine, and carisoprodol (Soma Compound with Codeine); ASA and codeine (Empirin with Codeine); ASA, codeine, butalbital, and caffeine (Fiorinal).

Extrapolated, based on similar properties: Cilostazol (Pletal), clopidogrel (Plavix), dipyridamole (Permole, Persantine), ticlopidine (Ticlid), combination drug: ASA and extended-release dipyridamole (Aggrenox, Asasantin).

Interaction Type and Significance

✗ **Potential or Theoretical Adverse Interaction of Uncertain Severity**

Probability:
5. Improbable

Evidence Base:
☐ **Inadequate**

Effect and Mechanism of Action

Aspirin (acetylsalicylic acid, ASA) is a well-documented antiplatelet agent acting through inhibition of cyclooxygenase production of thromboxane A_2 (TXA_2). Ticlopidine interacts with glycoprotein IIb/IIIa to inhibit fibrinogen binding to activated platelets and has been used for prevention of thrombosis when aspirin is poorly tolerated. Because of reports of hematological adverse effects associated with ticlopidine, clopidogrel (Plavix) is currently the preferred antiplatelet agent in such cases. As with ticlopidine, clopidogrel is another irreversible antiplatelet drug operating through adenosine diphosphate (ADP) receptor antagonism. The potential interaction is thus a theoretical additive pharmacodynamic increase in antiplatelet activity. Such an additive effect may theoretically increase the likelihood of bleeding disorders related to disturbances of primary hemostasis.

Research

In vitro investigations have demonstrated antiaggregatory actions of feverfew extracts and isolated parthenolide. Several aggregatory stimuli are inhibited by parthenolide, including ADP, collagen, and arachidonate.[43-46] Platelet secretory activity is also inhibited by parthenolide, reducing 5-hydroxytryptamine (5-HT, serotonin) release.[44,47,48] Thiol depletion plays a significant role in the mechanism.[22,49,50] Interestingly, the antiaggregatory effects of feverfew extracts and isolated parthenolide appear to be equivalent in magnitude.[51]

In a comprehensive review of antiplatelet activity of plant compounds, Venton et al.[52] stressed that because the relevant assay technologies are currently quite straightforward, many plant extracts and isolated compounds have been screened in vitro for platelet-inhibiting properties. Although many potentially active compounds that inhibit activation by one or more agonists have been identified, none has yet been transformed into a clinically effective antithrombotic drug.[52] Other than the pharmacokinetic modeling studies by Boik,[33] there has been little attempt to create meaningful algorithms to extrapolate in vitro IC_{50} values from the different study methods into meaningful estimates of likely therapeutic levels of the compounds after therapeutic oral doses of herb.

Reports

There are no preclinical studies or clinical reports confirming this interaction. On the contrary, the original clinical investigators of feverfew at the London Migraine Clinic reported to the *Lancet* in 1982 that they had tested 10 patients who had taken feverfew for 3½ to 8 years and assayed dose–aggregatory response curves to several platelet agonists, including ADP, thrombin, serotonin, and a prostaglandin analog (U46619). Aggregation responses to ADP and thrombin were identical to controls who had not taken feverfew for 6 months.[53] This was in direct conflict with in vitro findings of Makheja and Bailey[43] published earlier in 1982, confirming that extrapolation from in vitro activity to in vivo effects is problematic.

Clinical Implications and Adaptations

At present, this potential interaction can be considered clinically insignificant, if in fact it exists. Monitoring migraine or arthritis patients who may be combining substantial doses of feverfew chronically with antiplatelet drugs for signs relating to disturbances of primary hemostasis may be prudent (e.g., petechiae, ecchymoses, superficial bleeds at mucous membranes).

THEORETICAL, SPECULATIVE, AND PRELIMINARY INTERACTIONS RESEARCH, INCLUDING OVERSTATED INTERACTIONS CLAIMS

5-Hydroxytryptamine Receptor Agonists (Triptans)

Almotriptan (Axert), eletriptan (Relpax), frovatriptan (Frova), naratriptan (Amerge), rizatriptan (Maxalt), sumatriptan (Imitrex), zolmitriptan (Zomig).

There is no evidence of interaction between feverfew and the triptan drugs used for prophylaxis and treatment of migraine. Triptans are potent 5-HT agonists, and most triptans undergo metabolism by either monoamine oxidase A or CYP450 1A2 or 3A4. The serotonin hypothesis of feverfew pharmacology is no longer considered credible, and although direct evidence is lacking, obvious effects of the herb on CYP450 enzymes appear unlikely, therefore currently ruling out plausible pharmacokinetic and pharmacodynamic mechanisms for a feverfew-triptan interaction.

Warfarin and Related Oral Vitamin K Antagonist Anticoagulants

Anisindione (Miradon), dicumarol, ethyl biscoumacetate (Tromexan), nicoumalone (acenocoumarol; Acitrom, Sintrom), phenindione (Dindevan), phenprocoumon (Jarsin, Marcumar), warfarin (Coumadin, Marevan, Warfilone).

Although denied by authoritative secondary sources, a warfarin-feverfew interaction has been suggested by some derivative sources, based on in vitro antiplatelet activity previously discussed. Clinical evidence for this interaction is currently lacking.

The 53 citations for this monograph are located under Feverfew on the CD at the back of the book.

Garlic

Botanical Name: *Allium sativum* L.
Pharmacopoeial Name: Alii sativi bulbus.
Synonym: Porvium sativum Rehb.
Common Names: Garlic, stinking rose.

SUMMARY

Drug/Class Interaction Type	Mechanism and Significance	Management
Acetaminophen ⊕⊕⊕/☼	Potential pharmacokinetic interaction caused by garlic inhibition of cytochrome P450 2E1 may reduce hepatoxic metabolite NAPQI formation. Not clinically demonstrated.	Not applicable for management of acute acetaminophen toxicity.
Dipyridamole Antiplatelet thromboprophylactics ⊕✗/✗/⊕	Possible additive increased antiplatelet activity with dipyridamole. Not established with other antiplatelet agents. Clinical significance not established; increased risk of bleeds likely overstated.	Avoid *or* adopt and monitor bleed times. Combine garlic in antithrombotic protocols.
Doxorubicin Anthracycline chemotherapy ⊕/☼	Garlic protects against and reduces drug-induced cardiotoxicity through multiple mechanisms, including increasing myocardial antioxidant status. Not clinically demonstrated.	Pretreat, coadminister, and continue herb postchemotherapy in cardioprotective protocols.
HMG-CoA reductase inhibitors (statins) ⊕/☼	Additive inhibition of HMG-CoA theoretically allows lowered statin dose and reduction of drug adverse effects. Plausible but not clinically established.	Consider adopting if statin-induced ADRs (myalgias, fatigue, etc.); trial if symptomatic.
Methotrexate Fluorouracil (5-FU) Chemotherapy associated with mucositis ⊕/☼	Garlic may prevent and reduce chemotherapy-induced mucositis through anti-inflammatory and antioxidant mechanisms. Not clinically established.	Consider incorporating garlic with other agents in protective protocols for chemotherapy-induced mucositis.
Saquinavir Protease inhibitor antiretrovirals ✗/◇◇	Possible pharmacokinetic interaction with saquinavir; reduces drug bioavailability; does not occur with ritonavir. Unknown significance and applicability to related protease inhibitors.	Monitoring serum drug levels advisable if coadministered.
Warfarin Oral vitamin K antagonist anticoagulants ✗/⊕	Theoretical additive effects on hemostasis caused by possible platelet inhibition. Clinical studies suggest interaction insignificant.	If coadministered, monitor INR and check for peripheral bleed symptoms.

HMG-CoA, Hydroxymethylglutaryl coenzyme A; *ADRs*, adverse drug reactions; *INR*, international normalized ratio.

HERB DESCRIPTION

Family

Liliaceae.

Related Species

Allium cepa L. (onion), *Allium schoenoprasum* L. (chives).

Habitat and Cultivation

Originally native to central Asia; commercially cultivated for 5000 years as a food and medicinal herb worldwide.

Parts Used

Fresh or dried bulb.

Common Forms

Fresh bulb.
Dried bulb.
Dried powder (allicin-stabilized).
Aged garlic extract (AGE).
Garlic oil (steam-distilled).
Garlic oil (macerated).

HERB IN CLINICAL PRACTICE

Overview

Garlic dietary supplements consistently occupy second or third place of the top-selling botanical products in the United States, quite apart from the widespread availability and use of garlic cloves as a dietary/culinary herbal ingredient. Scientific studies and numerous clinical trials support the following three primary areas of use in modern practice:

1. For cardiovascular disease prevention and treatment as a hypolipidemic, antiatherosclerotic, hypotensive, antiplatelet, and fibrinolytic agent.
2. For infectious conditions as a broad-spectrum antibiotic, antifungal, antiviral, and anthelmintic agent.
3. As a chemopreventive and anticancer agent; antioxidant and immunostimulant properties impact each of these areas.

The pharmacology of the herb derives from its organosulfur constituents (OSCs), although the chemistry of these is extremely complex and has not been fully characterized. Importantly, different garlic preparations may have significantly different constituent profiles; the principal compounds in the intact bulb are gamma-glutamyl cysteine peptides and the cysteine sulfoxide alliin. The enzyme allinase (released by damage to intact cells) converts alliin to the thiosulfinate allicin. Allicin is unstable and degrades to various volatile sulfide congeners, depending on the conditions applied.

Steam distillation converts water-soluble thiosulfinates to oil-soluble diallyl sulfides, whereas oil maceration produces ajoenes and vinyldithins.

Similarly, pharmacokinetic differences exist among the various preparations and their components. Metabolic transformation of various sulfides leads to the formation of compounds that have modulating effects on the cytochrome P450 (CYP450) system. Enteric-coated preparations have been shown to release only a fraction of their active allicin content.

These differences complicate attempts to compare data from various experimental and clinical trials using different garlic preparations. More than 45 randomized clinical trials have been conducted with garlic preparations. Metastudies have concluded that these trials show positive, although limited, short-term benefits of garlic on serum cholesterol and some coagulation parameters, but no significant effect on hypertension or blood glucose levels.[1-4] Some authors have criticized the meta-analyses, noting the lack of equivalence between preparations and inadequate definition or characterization of active principles in the trials, which seriously limits the clinical conclusions that can be drawn from the majority of trials to date.[5,6] Epidemiological studies of the cancer-protective effects of garlic consumption have also been subject to meta-analysis, and positive effects were found for stomach and colon cancers from raw and cooked garlic consumption.[7,8]

Garlic has not been official in the *U.S. Pharmacopoeia* since 1900, but it is listed in the 2002 edition of the *National Formulary* as "fresh or dried compound bulbs containing not less than 0.5% alliin." The German Commission E approved the use of "fresh or carefully dried bulbs" as "supportive to dietary measures at elevated levels of lipids in the blood" and as a "preventative for age-dependent vascular changes."[9] The European Scientific Cooperative on Phytotherapy (ESCOP) monograph indicates garlic for "treatment of elevated blood lipid levels insufficiently influenced by diet" and mentions the traditional indication for upper respiratory tract infections and catarrhal conditions while also noting that these lack trial support.[10] The World Health Organization (WHO) also includes mild hypertension as an indication.[11] Both ESCOP and McKenna et al.[12] provide comprehensive reviews of the recent scientific literature.

Historical/Ethnomedicine Precedent

In Europe, garlic has been used for millenia. It was a staple of the Roman army, Pliny recorded more than 60 uses for garlic, and Galen first recorded its use as a disinfectant before and after surgery. More recent folk use centers on respiratory conditions, including coughs, colds, flus, sinus and bronchial infections, pneumonia and tuberculosis, and the elimination of worms and other parasites. As an external treatment, garlic has been used as a "counterirritant" for rheumatic and arthritic conditions, as well as for earache, skin infections, and snakebites. Topical applications are also used in respiratory conditions. Garlic has been employed in all major world systems of medicine for many years. In China, garlic use was recorded in texts from the fifth century CE, principally as an antidote for poisons as well as a treatment for infectious and parasitical intestinal conditions such as diarrhea, dysentery, and diphtheria.

Known or Potential Therapeutic Uses

Antimicrobial, antifungal, atherosclerosis, bronchial and upper respiratory conditions, catarrh, colds, coughs, flu, gastric and colon carcinomas (prevention), hyperlipidemia, hypertension, hyperviscosity, immunostimulation, peripheral arterial occlusive disease, rhinitis, sinusitis, thrombosis.

Key Constituents

Organosulfur compounds (OSCs), principally alliin [(+)-S-allyl-L-cysteine sulfoxide] and gamma-L-glutamyl peptides. Alliin is transformed into allicin by allinase, and depending on physicochemical conditions, various derivatives may be formed. Flavonoids and saponins are also present.

Therapeutic Dosing Range

Fresh Garlic: 2.7 to 4.0 g daily.
Dried Powder: 0.4 to 1.2 g daily.
Tincture (1:5): 20 mL daily.
Oil: 2 to 5 mg daily.
Standardized Extracts:
    Garlic powder (Kwai): 200 to 300 mg three times daily.
    Aged garlic extract (AGE, Kyolic): 300 to 800 mg three times daily.
    Other preparations: Corresponding to 4 to 12 mg alliin, or 2 to 5 mg allicin-equivalent daily.

INTERACTIONS REVIEW

Strategic Considerations

The German Commission E did not list any known interactions for garlic in its 1998 monograph.[9] However, the later monographs by WHO and ESCOP both list a possible interaction between garlic and warfarin.[10,11] Although garlic consumption is usually assumed to be a risk to anticoagulated patients, reliable reports of such interactions are not available.[13]

As with ginkgo, garlic and several of its constituents have established antiplatelet activity in vitro. Using aggregometry in response to platelet-stimulating factors such as collagen and adenosine diphosphate (ADP), three clinical trials have demonstrated modest effects on platelet aggregation in vivo by AGE extracts[14,15] and garlic powder.[16,17] Bleed times and international normalized ratio (INR) were not measured, and the clinical significance of the antiaggregatory effects of garlic remains to be established. Three reports associate garlic alone with spontaneous bleeding, but none of these allows causality to be attributed to the herb[18-20] (see later discussion on garlic and antiplatelet thromboprophylactics). Cessation of high levels of garlic consumption before elective surgery may be prudent, but on the basis of currently available evidence, the risk of garlic-induced bleeding and interactions with drugs affecting hemostasis appears to be very low.[21]

On the other hand, inclusion of garlic in protocols for patients at risk of thrombosis, particularly those with history of atherosclerotic disease, offers multiple "collateral" benefits due to the pleiotropic actions of the herb on several cardiac risk factors.[22-27] The lipid-lowering effect of garlic extracts operates by several mechanisms, including the inactivation of hydroxymethylglutaryl coenzyme A (HMG-CoA) reductase. This has led at least one author to suggest the potential value of combining garlic with pharmaceutical HMG-CoA reductase inhibitors for hyperlipidemia to reduce the risk of adverse effects such as rhabdomyolysis in sensitive populations, such as renal transplant patients.[28] This potentially beneficial interaction is proposed later, although previously undefined in the literature.

Effects on Drug Metabolism and Bioavailability

Experimental, animal, in vitro, and ex vivo human data suggest that garlic OSCs may be substrates, inducers, and/or inhibitors of various CYP450 enzymes. As with the pharmacodynamic effects of garlic, there are differences in effect among the different OSCs, different dose/duration regimens, and different species (mouse, rat, rabbit, human). The full spectrum of effects of OSCs on drug metabolism in humans is not well understood, but in vivo evidence is compelling for an inhibition of CYP450 2E1 by OSCs.

Diallyl sulfide (DAS) is converted by CYP2E1 to diallyl sulfoxide (DASO) and sequentially to diallyl sulfone (DASO$_2$).[29] These derivatives are competitive inhibitors of 2E1, and DASO$_2$ is also an irreversible (suicide) inhibitor of 2E1.[30,31] This is a typical example of 2E1 activity, which shares with CYP450 1A1 and 1A2 the role of metabolizing potentially carcinogenic aromatic hydrocarbons, and which may also bioactivate certain substrates to toxic or reactive intermediates (e.g., acetaminophen; see later discussion).[32,33] Loizou and Cocker[34] found that both DAS and garlic oil extract showed significant inhibition of 2E1 in eight healthy human volunteers with the 2E1 probe chlorzoxazone. Gurley et al.[35] also found significant inhibition of 2E1 after 28 days of garlic oil administration in healthy human volunteers using the same chlorzoxazone probe methodology. Davenport and Wargovich[36] found that single-dose in vivo OSCs in a rodent model decreased 2E1 protein but not its messenger ribonucleic acid (mRNA) levels. They also noted a slight increase in 1A1 and 1A2 levels.

Inhibition of CYP450 2E1 is considered one of the major mechanisms by which garlic consumption reduces mutagenesis and carcinogenesis and exerts hepatoprotective effects.[37,38] Other mechanisms may be involved, including OSC induction of glutathione transferases as well as scavenging of carcinogenic free-radical species.[39,40] Recent studies suggest that a number of complex effects on signal-transduction pathways may be involved in the chemopreventive effects of garlic OSCs.[41] Garlic-drug interactions with 2E1 substrates caused by inhibition by garlic OSCs have not yet appeared to be a clinically significant issue, and case reports are lacking. Drug substrates that theoretically may be affected by inhibition of 2E1 are verapamil, the halogenated anesthetics, and (a minor pathway) theophylline. In a clinical study restricted to older volunteers (mean age, 67 years), Gurley et al.[42] found a 22% inhibition of 2E1 by garlic oil administered for 28 days. The authors suggested that age-related changes in CYP450 activity are significant and should be factored into drug dose and potential interactions calculations.

Garlic is not the only dietary substance to modulate 2E1 expression. Inducers include ethanol, lettuce, and above all, increased body weight or obesity, whereas inhibitors include watercress and elements of *Camellia sinensis* (both green tea and black tea), especially epigallocatechin-3-gallate. If polymorphisms are taken into account, the total contribution of these variables to individual response variation in 2E1-mediated clearance of the probe substrate chlorzoxazone is 73%, with body weight alone accounting for 43% of the phenotypical variability in 2E1 activity.[43,44]

The effect of garlic on CYP450 enzymes other than 2E1 is less clear. A "before and after" probe study with healthy volunteers examined the effect of Kwai (aged) garlic consumption (600 mg three times daily for 14 days) on probe drugs for CYP3A4 (alprazolam) and CYP2D6 (dextromethorphan) pharmacokinetics and found no significant effects after garlic administration.[45] The authors concluded that aged (Kwai) garlic is unlikely to cause 3A4-modulated or 2D6-modulated drug interactions. Gurley et al.[35] found no effect of garlic oil on 3A4, 2D6, or 1A2 in healthy volunteers using a midazolam, debrisoquin, and caffeine cocktail in the study previously mentioned that demonstrated 2E1 inhibition.

Foster et al.[46] conducted an in vitro study using recombinant human CYP450 enzymes that investigated the effects of 10 different garlic products (including aged, odorless, oil, freeze-dried, and three fresh forms: common, Chinese, and elephant) on enzyme activity. The authors found that 2D6 was unaffected, but that 2C9*1, 2C19, 3A4, 3A5, and 3A7 were all inhibited by fresh garlic, whereas 2C9*2 was actively stimulated by fresh garlic. These authors concluded that pharmacokinetic interactions with narrow-therapeutic-range drugs may result from garlic consumption, affecting metabolism of drug substrates mediated by 2C9, 2D6, and 3A4. The same extracts were tested against an in vitro model of P-glycoprotein (P-gp) based on an adenosinetriphosphatase (ATPase) colorimetric assay, using verapamil as a positive control. (Stimulation of the ATPase assay is correlated with increased inhibitory activity of P-gps.) Aqueous extracts of aged garlic preparations exerted a very low to moderate inhibition of P-gp in the assay used.[46] In another in vitro model based on human KB-C2 cells, Nabekura et al.[47] found no effect of OSCs on the P-gp–mediated transport of daunorubicin and rhodamine 123. Greenblatt et al.[48] used an in vitro human hepatocyte model to test possible activity of different water-soluble compounds in garlic for CYP inhibitory activity and found negligible effect, except for high concentrations (100 µmol/L) of S-methyl-L-cysteine and S-allyl-L-cysteine, both of which produced modest inhibition of CYP3A. The authors concluded that CYP3A interactions with garlic and prescription drugs were unlikely.

Pharmacokinetic data for garlic (other than those related to drug-metabolizing systems) are minimal. However, one rodent study examined the effect of the saponin constituents of garlic and concluded that these compounds may contribute to the lipid-lowering activity of garlic by reducing lipid absorption levels at the intestinal wall.[49] Studies are required to delineate human pharmacokinetics of garlic and OSC preparations in order to determine the extent to which many of the important effects of OSCs described in vitro in animal models can be replicated in vivo at micromolar concentrations that correspond to those employed in the experimental models. Further research is also required to establish the full spectrum of effects of different forms of garlic and OSCs on drug metabolism and potential pharmacokinetic interactions. Inconclusive data are available relating to garlic and the human immunodeficiency virus type 1 (HIV-1) protease inhibitors, saquinavir and ritonavir (discussed later). Patients with HIV infection are likely to take garlic products or preparations, and physicians specializing in this patient population are usually aware of the complexities of managing polypharmaceutical regimens and empirically monitoring possible interactions. Other than this clinically circumscribed area, currently no compelling data exist on adverse pharmacokinetic interactions between pharmaceuticals and garlic preparations. The established inhibition of CYP450 2E1 underlies a major part of the hepatoprotective and chemoprotective benefits of garlic consumption.

HERB-DRUG INTERACTIONS

Acetaminophen

Acetaminophen (APAP, paracetamol; Tylenol); combination drugs: acetaminophen and codeine (Capital with Codeine;

Phenaphen with Codeine; Tylenol with Codeine); acetaminophen and hydrocodone (Anexsia, Anodynos-DHC, Co-Gesic, Dolacet, DuoCet, Hydrocet, Hydrogesic, Hy-Phen, Lorcet 10/650, Lorcet-HD, Lorcet Plus, Lortab, Margesic H, Medipain 5, Norco, Stagesic, T-Gesic, Vicodin, Vicodin ES, Vicodin HP, Zydone); acetaminophen and oxycodone (Endocet, Percocet 2.5/325, Percocet 5/325, Percocet 7.5/500, Percocet 10/650, Roxicet 5/500, Roxilox, Tylox); acetaminophen and pentazocine (Talacen); acetaminophen and propoxyphene (Darvocet-N, Darvocet-N 100, Pronap-100, Propacet 100, Propoxacet-N, Wygesic).

Interaction Type and Significance

⊕⊕⊕ **Beneficial or Supportive Interaction, Not Requiring Professional Management**
☼ **Prevention or Reduction of Drug Adverse Effect**

Probability:
3. Possible

Evidence Base:
◉ **Emerging**

Effect and Mechanism of Action
This is primarily a pharmacokinetic interaction, whereby garlic extracts inhibit the CYP450 2E1 isoform that mediates the production of the hepatotoxic metabolite of acetaminophen (NAPQI). Although experimentally validated, the clinical significance of the interaction is not established.

Research
Acetaminophen is extensively metabolized through glucuronidation and sulfation as well as oxidation by CYP450 1A2, 3A4, and 1E2.[50-52] Oxidative metabolism by 2E1 forms the reactive intermediate NAPQI (N-acetyl-p-benzoquinone imine), which is subsequently conjugated by glutathione. Under normal circumstances, little NAPQI is formed, but if 2E1 undergoes induction, typically by alcohol consumption, NAPQI may be formed in greater-than-usual quantities. In turn, if glutathione capacity is exceeded at the same time, clinical hepatotoxicity may result, with significant risk of fulminant hepatic failure. Deliberate overdose with acetaminophen is the major cause of drug-related liver failure and emergency liver transplants in the United States and until recently in the United Kingdom (when measures to restrict OTC availability of the drug were implemented).[53,54] Emergency treatment of acetaminophen poisoning with N-acetylcysteine (NAC) can help regenerate glutathione stores and prevent further NAPQI formation, but NAC is usually effective only in the earliest stages of intoxication.

Extensive in vitro and in vivo evidence exists for the ability of garlic preparations in the form of fresh garlic, garlic oil, and AGE to inhibit human CYP450 2E1[30,35,46] (see also pharmacokinetics earlier). A number of rodent studies have established that pretreatment with different garlic preparations exerts a protective effect against single-dose–induced acetaminophen toxicity according to a number of endpoints, including hepatic histology, aminotransferase and lactate dehydrogenase levels, 2E1 levels, reduced glutathione levels, and cataracts.[55] Studies have been performed with ajoene,[56] S-allylmercaptocysteine (SAMC),[57,58] DAS and fresh garlic,[37,39] DASO₂,[59] and diallyl disulfide (DADS)[60] and garlic oil.[61] Although the animal evidence appears substantial, doses in these experimental studies are often high, from 5 g/kg body weight for fresh garlic extracts to between 25 and 200 mg/kg for isolated OSCs. These do not translate into typical dietary doses of garlic or normal supplemental or therapeutic intake using garlic extracts.

The only available human study, conducted by Gwilt et al.,[62] examined the effects of 3 months' pretreatment with AGE at a dose equivalent to six to seven cloves of garlic daily in healthy volunteers. A 1-g dose of acetaminophen was given before garlic treatment, and at the end of each month for 3 months, urinary and plasma measurements levels of acetaminophen and its conjugates were taken. A slight increase in sulfate conjugates was found, but no significant reduction in acetaminophen or its metabolites was noted. This study did not directly examine toxic doses of acetaminophen, but rather was seeking to determine effects of garlic on subtoxic levels of the drug, which may be different from effects at higher exposure levels.

Further human studies are required to establish whether the data from rodent experiments can be extrapolated to clinical practice.

Integrative Therapeutics, Clinical Concerns, and Adaptations
Despite the experimental demonstration of garlic-acetaminophen interaction in animal models and the known inhibition of CYP450 2E1 in humans by garlic OSCs, garlic's clinical and therapeutic significance is not established. Disulfiram, a pharmaceutical inhibitor of 2E1, has been shown to reduce the formation of NAPQI in healthy volunteers pretreated with a single dose, 10 hours before receiving 500 mg acetaminophen toxicity from overdose or from chronic alcohol consumption.[50] In the study previously described, Gwilt et al.[62] failed to find similar effects exerted by garlic in healthy volunteers. Given that acetaminophen poisoning is a serious condition requiring intensivist management, garlic use as an acute management strategy would be inappropriate in this context. For alcoholic patients with any degree of compliance, however, the addition of garlic by diet or supplementation would appear to be a logical counter to the chronic effects of alcohol on 2E1 induction.

Dipyridamole and Related Antiplatelet Thromboprophylactics

Evidence: Dipyridamole (Permole, Persantine).
Extrapolated, based on similar properties: Antiplatelet thromboprophylactics: Acetylsalicylic acid (acetosal, acetyl salicylic acid, ASA, salicylsalicylic acid; Arthritis Foundation Pain Reliever, Ascriptin, Aspergum, Asprimox, Bayer Aspirin, Bayer Buffered Aspirin, Bayer Low Adult Strength, Bufferin, Buffex, Cama Arthritis Pain Reliever, Easprin, Ecotrin, Ecotrin Low Adult Strength, Empirin, Extra Strength Adprin-B, Extra Strength Bayer Enteric 500 Aspirin, Extra Strength Bayer Plus, Halfprin 81, Heartline, Regular Strength Bayer Enteric 500 Aspirin, St. Joseph Adult Chewable Aspirin, ZORprin); combination drugs: ASA and caffeine (Anacin); ASA, caffeine, and propoxyphene (Darvon Compound); ASA and carisoprodol (Soma Compound); ASA, codeine, and carisoprodol (Soma Compound with Codeine); ASA and codeine (Empirin with Codeine); ASA, codeine, butalbital, and caffeine (Fiorinal); cilostazol (Pletal), clopidogrel (Plavix), ticlopidine (Ticlid); combination drug: ASA and extended-release dipyridamole (Aggrenox, Asasantin).

Interaction Type and Significance

⊕✗ **Bimodal or Variable Interaction, with Professional Management**
✗ **Potential or Theoretical Adverse Interaction of Uncertain Severity** *or*
⊕ **Potential or Theoretical Beneficial or Supportive Interaction, with Professional Management**

Probability:
2. Probable

Evidence Base:
◉ **Emerging**

Effect and Mechanism of Action

Garlic extracts and OSC compounds have established antiaggregatory effects. Coadministration of garlic with dipyridamole results in synergistically increased antiplatelet effects. Although related antiplatelet agents may operate through different mechanisms, net disabling of platelets is likely to be increased. Professional monitoring and management of this theoretical additive interaction are required.

Research

A number of in vitro and animal experiments suggest that garlic and certain garlic OSCs, particularly ajoene, exert significant antiplatelet activity through a variety of routes, including inhibition of ADP-induced aggregation.[63-70] Multiple mechanisms are involved and include membrane fluidity changes, inhibition of phospholipase C, inhibition of calcium mobilization, increase in nitric oxide and cyclic adenosine monophosphate (cAMP) production, and inhibition of thromboxane A_2 (TXA_2), all of which are antiaggregatory in effect.[71,72] Human studies have demonstrated antiaggregatory and antithrombotic activity in vivo with various forms of garlic, in healthy individuals as well as patients with atherosclerotic disease.[15-17,63,67,73-75]

Apitz-Castro et al.[76] employed ajoene, a garlic OSC found in oil preparations but not in AGE or powdered garlic, in an aggregometric investigation of the effects of the garlic compound on collagen-evoked platelet aggregation on the blood of healthy volunteers. The investigators also examined the effects of indomethacin, dipyridamole, and forskolin alone, as well as in combination with the ajoene. The effects of coadministration were found to be a synergistic (i.e., greater than additive) increase in aggregation for the combinations. In the case of dipyridamole, the median inhibiting dose ID_{50} was decreased fourfold with garlic. Harenberg et al.[77] found that although fibrinolysis increased after 4 weeks of garlic consumption in healthy volunteers, collagen-evoked and ADP-evoked aggregation remained unchanged.

Integrative Therapeutics, Clinical Concerns, and Adaptations

Dipyridamole is primarily used in conjunction with coumarin anticoagulants in cardiac valve replacement patients and seldom used as a primary antiplatelet drug, compared with the commonplace "baby aspirin" or clopidogrel, as well as the emerging oral glycoprotein IIb/IIIa receptor–binding drugs. Although direct clinical data on the interaction are lacking for most antiplatelet agents, extrapolation appears warranted by the existing pharmacological data. Determination of context will define whether coadministration should be adopted or avoided within specific patient populations. For example, within an integrative therapeutic context, hyperlipidemic patients with or without a history of thrombosis or coronary artery disease (CAD) would benefit from addition of garlic consumption, with monitoring of the levels of coadministered antiplatelet pharmaceuticals and close attention to symptoms, including peripheral bleeds and INR increases. Patients at risk of thromboembolism invariably receive several drugs in combination to achieve anticoagulation and thromboprophylaxis. With professional management, the addition of garlic to these regimens may improve overall outcomes, as well as enable lower doses of the drugs, which may decrease the likelihood of adverse drug effects.[78,79]

Doxorubicin and Related Anthracycline Chemotherapy Agents

Evidence: Doxorubicin (Adriamycin, Rubex).

Extrapolated, based on similar properties: Daunorubicin (Cerubidine, DaunoXome), epirubicin (Ellence, Pharmorubicin), idarubicin (Idamycin, Zavedos), mitoxantrone (Novantrone, Onkotrone).

Similar properties but evidence indicating no or reduced interaction effects: Doxorubicin, pegylated liposomal (Caelyx, Doxil, Myocet).

Interaction Type and Significance

⊕ **Potential or Theoretical Beneficial or Supportive Interaction, with Professional Management**
☼ **Prevention or Reduction of Drug Adverse Effect**

Probability:
3. Possible

Evidence Base:
○ Preliminary

Effect and Mechanism of Action

Anthracyclines generate free radicals that cause oxidative damage, particularly microsomal lipid peroxidation, through an iron-dependent process, which results in cardiotoxicity and adverse effects on other tissues, distinct from their antitumor actions. Garlic extracts exert a protective effect against cardiotoxicity from doxorubicin by specific enhancement of endogenous myocardial antioxidants and possibly by additional, unknown mechanisms. The interaction has been demonstrated in animal experiments; clinical studies and reports are unavailable to date.

Note: Cardiotoxicity is similar between equipotent doses of doxorubicin and daunorubicin, slightly lower for epirubicin, and only one-sixth that of doxorubicin for equipotent doses of mitoxantrone. Doxil (liposome-encapsulated doxorubicin) has negligible cardiotoxicity, presumably because of negligible cardiac exposure to the active drug with the pharmacokinetics of the liposome-encapsulated preparation.

Research

Doxorubicin is a highly effective antineoplastic agent, but acute and chronic cardiotoxicity is an adverse effect occurring in up to one third of the patients treated after a cumulative dose of 300 mg/m^2, and increasing sharply beyond a cumulative dose of 360 mg/m^2. The resultant irreversible and dose-dependent cardiomyopathy limits its clinical usefulness. The chronic form of anthracycline-induced cardiotoxicity may only manifest years after initial exposure, after an apparently asymptomatic interval, and has been documented two decades after treatment.[80] Cardiotoxicity of anthracycline chemotherapy agents is multifactorial and partly involves oxidative stress mediated by an iron-catalyzed Fenton reaction; iron-chelating agents such as dexrazoxane have been shown to decrease doxorubicin cardiac toxicity. The mechanisms of cardiotoxicity are considered to be distinct from the tumoricidal activity of the compounds.[81]

Several animal studies have examined the effects of garlic and OSCs on doxorubicin-induced cardiotoxicity. Intraperitoneal administrations of AGE[82] and DADS[83] were found to exert cardioprotective effects. Oral doses of garlic extracts (20 and 100 mg/kg) induced significant changes in the redox status of mouse red blood cells (measured by MDA generation and glutathione peroxidase activity) after doxorubicin exposure.[84] Mukherjee et al.[85] used fresh garlic homogenate administered to rats at oral does of 250 and 500 mg/kg daily for 30 days, followed by a single dose of Adriamycin, 30 mg/kg. Cardiotoxicity was reduced according to histopathological criteria. In addition, myocardial redox enzyme activity (catalase, superoxide dismutase, glutathione peroxidase) was increased, and tumor necrosis factor alpha (TNF-α) expression was reduced.

These experimental studies provide preliminary support for the potential interaction, but it remains to be established whether oral doses of garlic extracts or purified OSCs in humans can generate sufficient concentrations in vivo to correspond to the micromolar levels employed in the in vitro and animal models. Research into garlic and OSC pharmacokinetics in vivo is required to establish dose parameters for the interaction in clinical practice. Nonetheless, the multifactorial antioxidant effects of garlic are being increasingly understood, with extensive implications for inflammatory and cardiovascular diseases as well as cancer.[41,86]

Integrative Therapeutics, Clinical Concerns, and Adaptations

Acute cardiotoxicity can be evaluated by creatine kinase, particularly the cardiac specific MB isoenzyme. Chronic cardiotoxicity can be monitored using electrocardiography and left ventricular performance monitored by computerized M-mode echocardiography measuring the ejection fraction and/or MUGA scan (nuclear medicine technique for measuring cardiac ejection fraction), both of which are reliable and highly sensitive noninvasive parameters for evaluating myocardial contractility.

Anecdotal clinical experience has indicated that therapeutic benefit can be obtained in patients with existing doxorubicin-induced cardiomyopathy and clinical congestive heart failure using L-carnitine, coenzyme Q10, taurine, fish oil, magnesium, and hawthorn *(Crataegus)* leaf/flower and berry extracts, at least in some cases. Given the additional pluripotent effects of garlic OSCs on signal transduction in cancer cells, including cell cycle arrest, induction of apoptosis, and inhibition of inflammatory cytokines, as well as inhibition of multidrug (P-gp) resistance, there would appear to be good grounds for incorporating garlic extracts into prechemotherapy protocols for prophylaxis of anthracycline-induced cardiotoxicity.[41,87,88] Integrative management with these nutrients, botanicals, and appropriate pharmaceuticals may be of greatest clinical benefit, when applied by health care professionals trained and experienced in both nutritional therapeutics and conventional medicine. Randomized controlled clinical trials in this area would be of great interest.

Hydroxymethylglutaryl Coenzyme A (HMG-CoA) Reductase Inhibitors (Statins)

Atorvastatin (Lipitor), fluvastatin (Lescol, Lescol XL), lovastatin (Altocor, Altoprev, Mevacor), combination drug: lovastatin and niacin (Advicor), pravastatin (Pravachol), rosuvastatin (Crestor), simvastatin (Zocor), combination drug: simvastatin and extended-release nicotinic acid (Niaspan).

Interaction Type and Significance

⊕ **Potential or Theoretical Beneficial or Supportive Interaction, with Professional Management**

☼ **Prevention or Reduction of Drug Adverse Effect**

Probability:
4. Plausible

Evidence Base:
○ Preliminary

Effect and Mechanism of Action

The mechanism of garlic-induced hypocholesterolemic activity is multifactorial but includes inhibition of cholesterol synthesis at the level of 3-hydroxy-3-methylglutaryl coenzyme A (HMG-CoA) reductase. Coadministration of garlic with

pharmaceutical HMG-CoA reductase inhibitors may enable lower statin drug doses, resulting in reduced risk of drug-related adverse effects.

Research

The pharmacology of garlic's cholesterol-lowering action is multifactorial, and remains to be fully characterized.[89] In vitro studies with rodent and human hepatocyte models of cholesterol synthesis have demonstrated that HMG-CoA reductase inhibition is a significant but not the sole mechanism.[90-93] More recent data implicate inhibition of sterol-4α-methyl oxidase as being the major enzyme involved.[94]

Integrative Therapeutics, Clinical Concerns, and Adaptations

Although efficacy has been established by numerous clinical trials, the magnitude and clinical significance of the hypocholesterolemic effects of garlic extracts are controversial, according to meta-analyses of the available trial data.[1,3,95] In clinical practice, however, incorporation of garlic and garlic extracts into integrative hypolipidemic protocols with a variety of nutritional and botanical agents is commonplace. The increasingly widespread prescription of HMG-CoA reductase inhibitors by primary health care providers for relatively moderate cholesterol elevations (or previously normal-range values) has raised concerns about the potential long-term effects of depletion of coenzyme Q10 by these agents, particularly in populations with history of serious CAD and myocardial infarction.[96] Degree of coenzyme Q10 depletion by statins depends on several factors, including patient age, but a positive correlation exists between level of dosage and level of depletion (see Coenzyme Q10 monograph).

For patients experiencing adverse effects of statin drug therapy, such as myalgias and fatigue, it is possible that drug dose levels may be lowered without loss of efficacy by combination with garlic. For patients with a previous history of cardiac disease also prescribed statin therapy, prudence would suggest that prophylaxis of cardiomyopathy should not only include coadministration of coenzyme Q10 to appropriate levels, but also incorporate integrative hypocholesterolemic protocols that may allow exposure levels to statins to be lowered or, in some cases, the drug to be replaced by nonpharmaceutical interventions. Other groups at specific risk, such as renal allografts, may also be considered for this approach.[28]

Mucositis-Inducing Chemotherapeutic Agents, Including Fluorouracil, Bleomycin, Doxorubicin, and Ethanol

Evidence: Fluorouracil (5-FU; Adrucil, Efudex, Efudix, Fluoroplex), methotrexate (Folex, Maxtrex, Rheumatrex).
Extrapolated, based on similar properties: Bleomycin (Blenoxane), doxorubicin (Adriamycin, Rubex), and others.

Interaction Type and Significance

⊕ **Potential or Theoretical Beneficial or Supportive Interaction, with Professional Management**

☼ **Prevention or Reduction of Drug Adverse Effect**

Probability:
4. Plausible

Evidence Base:
☐ Inadequate

Effect and Mechanism of Action

Mucositis (oral and intestinal) can be a dose-limiting adverse effect of certain chemotherapies. Preliminary evidence suggests that garlic extracts may exert a protective activity at the mucosa, which may reduce mucositis and increase ability to sustain required doses of chemotherapy. The clinical significance of the interaction remains to be established. A possible ulceroprotective effect against ethanol-induced gastropathy has been noted, which may be considered a related interaction.

Research

Garlic and OSCs are known to have antioxidant and anti-inflammatory effects. Recent evidence has indicated garlic modulates of inflammatory cytokines in various tissues, including intestinal epithelia. Spontaneous secretion of TNF-α in Caco-2 cells was inhibited by allicin, which also suppressed interleukin-8 (IL-8) and interleukin-1 (IL-1), while inhibiting degradation of INF-κ (thus increasing NF-κ inhibition).[97] Together with multiple effects of OSCs on redox status and eicosanoid metabolism, several plausible mechanisms underlie the potential protective effects against chemotherapy-induced mucositis, as demonstrated in animal models for both methotrexate and 5-FU using dietary AGE.[98,99] Related oxidative mechanisms are involved in ethanol-induced gastric ulceration. Another rodent study observed that an oral garlic oil preparation (0.25 and 0.5 mg/kg) administered 30 minutes before ingestion of ethanol (1 mL) reduced the ulcer index, increased antioxidant enzyme levels, and reduced lipid peroxidation compared with controls.[100] Extrapolation from these studies to in vivo human oral consumption ultimately depends on a fuller understanding of OSC pharmacokinetics than is currently available.

Integrative Therapeutics, Clinical Concerns, and Adaptations

Treatment of chemotherapy- or radiation-induced mucositis (oral and intestinal) is particularly amenable to integrative strategies employing combinations of botanicals agents (see also Aloe and Licorice Root monographs) and nutrients such as glutamine, vitamin E, and beta-carotene. Combination protocols are often used in integrative oncology environments, despite the lack of published trial support at present. The possible inclusion of garlic/OSC extracts in such protocols is an interesting possibility because similar to capsicum, the herb is popularly considered to have a gastroirritant potential, and as with capsaicin, garlic in fact can exert gastroprotective effects. Additionally, garlic OSCs interact with a number of molecular targets with a resultant anticancer action. At present the optimal form and dose of garlic extracts in any such protocol need to be established empirically; ultimately, clinical trials are required to establish the benefits of adding garlic for treatment of chemotherapy-related mucositis.

Saquinavir and Related Antiretroviral Protease Inhibitors

Evidence: Saquinavir (Fortovase, Invirase).
Extrapolated, based on similar properties: Amprenavir (Agenerase), atazanavir (Reyataz), brecanavir, darunavir (Prezista), fosamprenavir (Lexiva), indinavir (Crixivan), nelfinavir (Viracept), tipranavir (Aptivus); combination drug: lopinavir and ritonavir (Kaletra).
Similar properties but evidence indicating no or reduced interaction effects: Ritonavir (Norvir).

Interaction Type and Significance

✗ **Potential or Theoretical Adverse Interaction of Uncertain Severity**

◇◇ Impaired Drug Absorption and Bioavailability, Precautions Appropriate

Probability:
3. Possible

Evidence Base:
☐ **Inadequate**

Effect and Mechanism of Action

Saquinavir, like all protease inhibitors, is a cosubstrate of CYP3A4 and P-gp. A pharmacokinetic interaction has been demonstrated in healthy volunteers, in whom garlic significantly reduced drug bioavailability. Further data are needed to establish the precise mechanism and clinical significance before extrapolations to other antiretrovirals and to HIV-1 patient populations are fully warranted.

Research

Piscitelli et al.[101] administered garlic extracts, with an allicin content equivalent to four to six garlic cloves per day, to 10 healthy volunteers for 3 weeks. Before and after the garlic treatment period, saquinavir was administered for 3 days (1200 mg three times daily), and blood samples were taken to measure pharmacokinetic parameters. After a 10-day washout period, the saquinavir dose was repeated and a further sample measured. Peak concentration and AUC (area under curve) of saquinavir were reduced by 54% and 51%, respectively, and after the washout period, levels did not return to baseline but were approximately 60% to 70% of the pretreatment values. The authors suggested that either induction of intestinal 3A4 reduced the bioavailability or P-gp may be involved, rather than changes in systemic clearance. Failure to return to baseline levels after the washout period is unexplained. A further finding that complicates interpretation of this study was the separation of the small number of subjects into two distinct groups. The first group had no significant change in saquinavir AUC with garlic, but exhibited a drop in AUC after the washout period. The other group had a significant drop in saquinavir AUC with garlic, but postwashout AUC was less than baseline. This bimodal pharmacokinetic result awaits a satisfactory explanation.

Garlic administration does not significantly affect the single-dose pharmacokinetics of the related protease inhibitor ritonavir in healthy volunteers after 4 days of acute dosing with garlic, according to a study by Gallicano et al.[102] However, the dose of garlic in this study was relatively low (10-mg odorless capsules daily), and a trend was noted to decreased bioavailability. Ritonavir powerfully inhibits and induces CYP3A4, and a single dose cannot be extrapolated to steady-state kinetics of therapeutic administration. Available experimental studies implicate both P-gp and intestinal 3A4 in ritonavir and saquinavir clearance modulation. An in vitro investigation using a MDR1-transfected MDCK cell model for assaying P-gp efflux activity found that allicin inhibited P-gp–mediated efflux of ritonavir in a dose-dependent fashion.[103] Mouly et al.[104] used another in vitro model, the Caco-2 cell, to examine the kinetics of saquinavir in relation to 3A4, P-gp, and serum protein binding and implicated both 3A4 and P-gp, but not serum albumin, in saquinavir availability.

Case reports are lacking.

Clinical Implications and Adaptations

Patients with HIV/AIDS are likely to use garlic preparations. Such use, if self-prescribed, should be disclosed to the prescribing physician or specialist team managing the patient's drug regimen. However, blanket cautions regarding dangers of herbal modulation of antiviral drug therapy for HIV patients are arguably inappropriate, although frequently made in the literature. It is well known that long-term retroviral agents in HIV-infected patients exhibit kinetic differences that are not necessarily revealed by short-term studies in healthy volunteers. Both saquinavir and ritonavir are known to exhibit decreases in AUC over several months of administration in infected patients.[105] The interactivity of the antiretroviral drugs with each other and with unrelated drugs is well known among HIV/AIDS specialist providers and most patients. Polypharmacy is common, and viral load is invariably monitored as an indicator of antiviral therapeutic efficacy. Serum drug levels should be monitored directly; serum dosage, timing of administration, and drug combinations may need to be adjusted accordingly and frequently. (See also St. John's Wort monograph, Indinavir section.)

Warfarin and Related Oral Vitamin K Antagonist Anticoagulants

Anisindione (Miradon), dicumarol, ethyl biscoumacetate (Tromexan), fluindione, nicoumalone (acenocoumarol; Acitrom, Sintrom), phenindione (Dindevan), phenprocoumon (Jarsin, Marcumar), warfarin (Coumadin, Marevan, Warfilone).

Interaction Type and Significance

✗ Potential or Theoretical Adverse Interaction of Uncertain Severity

⊕ Potential or Theoretical Beneficial or Supportive Interaction, with Professional Management

Probability:
4. Plausible

Evidence Base:
▽ Mixed

Effect and Mechanism of Action

A theoretical additive effect between coumarin anticoagulants and garlic upon hemostasis is hypothesized to increase INR and/or increase risk of bleeding. Reliable reports of the interaction are unavailable, and direct pharmacodynamic interaction is contradicted by the clinical data.

Research

Substantial data suggest that garlic and OSC components of garlic exert in vitro and in vivo antiaggregatory effects (see Antiplatelet Thromboprophylactics earlier). However, data demonstrating effects of garlic on coagulation proper (i.e., secondary hemostasis), through interference with the production or action of soluble coagulation factors, are unavailable.

Reports of bleeding induced by garlic alone are rare, and of the three reports available, none appears to demonstrate a causal link between garlic consumption and hemorrhagic episodes. Spontaneous spinal epidural hematoma in an 87-year-old man who consumed an average of four garlic cloves daily for an unstated duration was attributed to garlic.[19] In their review of the evidence for interactions between warfarin and garlic, however, Vaes and Chyka[13] noted that such epidural hematomas are rare, and the cause is unknown in 40% of cases.[13] Another anecdotal report involved postoperative bleeding following mammoplasty; atypical "bloody oozing" was noted during surgery, and a 200-mL hematoma developed postoperatively and was later evacuated. The patient had apparently had a "heavy garlic intake" preoperatively, although preparation, dose, and duration of intake were not specified. At a second, later mammoplasty, after discontinuation of garlic, the bleeding did not recur.[20] A third case involved a 72-year-old man who experienced

postoperative hemorrhage after a standard transurethral prostate resection procedure. He required transfusion with 4 units of blood. The patient later admitted habitual garlic consumption, the preparation and dose of which were not stated.[18]

A warfarin-garlic interaction is suggested by authoritative secondary sources, such as the ESCOP[10] and WHO[11] therapeutic monographs, both of which base this claim on a single anecdotal report by Sunter in 1991. The report underlying this apparent interaction was a short letter from Sunter containing inadequate information that failed to mention the form, preparation, dose, duration of administration, comedications, or case history details, or even the magnitude of the apparent INR change.[106] This report has been challenged as "unreliable," scoring zero in the scale of report reliability devised by Fugh-Berman and Ernst.[107] Meanwhile, unsupported claims that garlic prolongs INR are repeated by derivative sources without substantiation.[108] A controlled trial using AGE at 1200 mg/day for 4 weeks versus placebo in eight patients, all stable taking warfarin, found no significant changes between garlic and placebo when INR was compared to baseline levels after garlic administration.[109] Another trial with 48 patients monitored potential bleeding and thromboembolic episodes during anticoagulant therapy with warfarin while consuming AGE at 5 mL twice daily for 12 weeks. No adverse events or changes in hemostatic or platelet parameters were noted.[21]

Reports

Pathak et al.[110] reported a case in which garlic tablets consumed at 600 mg/day for 12 days apparently reduced the INR of an 82-year-old patient previously stable taking fluindione. The case reporting seems reliable, and the report is somewhat unexpected because fluindione is an indanedione derivative similar to phenindione, which is used as vitamin K antagonist anticoagulant, mainly in France. Cessation of garlic tablets restored the INR within 4 days. The authors suggested a possible pharmacokinetic induction by garlic compounds of the CYP450 enzymes responsible for metabolizing the drug, or a possible effect on serum protein binding.[110] Assessment of the case is problematic; fluindione is known to exhibit extreme individual variation in pharmacokinetics, and the pathways of its metabolism are not definitely established.[111]

Clinical Implications and Adaptations

The 4-hydroxycoumarin compound warfarin is the most widely used anticoagulant drug in the Western world. It is known for a high variability in interindividual and intraindividual response. The primary individual factors affecting response variability are age and polymorphisms of CYP450 2C9.[112] The incidence of warfarin-related bleeding complications is difficult to estimate because of methodological issues surrounding data collection and interpretation. Recent calculations suggest that improved anticoagulation control has reduced the serious adverse drug reaction (ADR) category of "major bleeds, non-fatal" incidence to approximately 2.5% to 8.0%, with a "minor bleed" incidence of about 15% per year. Fatal bleed estimates vary from 1% to 4.8% per year.[113] Warfarin interacts with a wide range of drugs, including antibiotics, central nervous system agents, and cardiac drugs, as well as many dietary ingredients, most of which increase anticoagulation.[114]

All this confounds the already-complex situation of determining the medical appropriateness, form, and level of anticoagulation, especially in older individuals with multiple risk factors for bleeding, such as unstable INR, comorbidities (especially bleeding related), polypharmacy (especially with NSAIDs), advanced age, and difficulty in compliance with requirements of coagulation control.

Synergistic or additive interaction between warfarin and garlic is effectively unproven. It has been well argued that anticoagulation and antithrombotic therapy exemplifies the methodological and theoretical limits that pervade the discussion of interactions in general; in particular, the development of more precise tools to test for potential interactions is needed.[115,116] Meanwhile, candidates for garlic coadministration with warfarin might best be reviewed on a case-by-case basis before using garlic extracts, and if appropriate, they should be monitored for signs of increased peripheral bleeding after initiating coadministration.

THEORETICAL, SPECULATIVE, AND PRELIMINARY INTERACTIONS RESEARCH, INCLUDING OVERSTATED INTERACTIONS CLAIMS

Chlorzoxazone

Chlorzoxazone (Paraflex, Parafon Forte, Relaxazone, Remular-S).

Several pharmacokinetic studies examining the effect of garlic and its OSCs on CYP450 2E1 have used chlorzoxazone probe methodology (see Effects on Drug Metabolism and Bioavailability). Because a degree of 2E1 inhibition has been established by these studies, this finding is "reversed" by some authors into a presumed or purported interaction. However, the therapeutic index of chlorzoxazone is not such to warrant a particular caution, and in practice, drug dose levels and frequency of this antispasmodic are often adjusted to the required level of symptom relief. Given the lack of reports of the interaction and its likely minimal significance, it is currently classified here as "overstated."

Isoproterenol

Isoproterenol (Isoprenaline; Isuprel, Medihaler-Iso).

The nonselective beta-adrenergic receptor agonist isoprenaline was originally used in inhalant form for asthma and parenterally for cardiac resuscitation. In most applications, it has now been replaced by more selectively acting agents. Coadministration of garlic with isoprenaline in animal models has shown that garlic may reduce the proarrhythmic adverse effects associated with the drug, as well as minimize or prevent ischemic and necrotic damage to the heart (and other organs) that can result from exposure to excessively high doses of the drug.[117-119] Some secondary sources list this as an established interaction, based on the animal evidence.[120] In everyday practice, the drug is little used, and in any event it is improbable that isoproterenol would be administered at doses that might induce necrotic organic toxicities. Of interest, however, are related animal studies that have demonstrated an

antiarrhythmic activity in garlic extracts in experimentally induced models of ventricular and supraventricular arrhythmias.[121-123]

Oral Hypoglycemic Agents and Insulin

Buformin (Andromaco Glliporal, Buformina), chlorpropamide (Diabinese), glimepiride (Amaryl), glipizide (Glucotrol; Glucotrol XL), glyburide (glibenclamide; Diabeta, Glynase, Glynase Prestab, Micronase, Pres Tab), insulin (animal-source insulin: Iletin; human analog insulin: Humanlog; human insulin: Humulin, Novolin, NovoRapid, Oralin), metformin (Dianben, Glucophage, Glucophage XR); combination drugs: glipizide and metformin (Metaglip), glyburide and metformin (Glucovance); tolazamide (Tolinase), phenformin (Debeone, Fenformin), tolbutamide (Orinase, Tol-Tab).

A handful of early studies conducted in the 1960s and 1970s suggested hypoglycemic activity in experimental or animal models, and these data have been used to suggest a speculative interaction with insulin.[124,125] Of the few human investigations that examined blood sugar parameters in response to garlic or OSCs, most have failed to detect significant hypoglycemic activities resulting from garlic consumption, although some trials have noted trends toward lowered blood glucose levels.[2,16,74] One study noted bimodal gender differences in glycemic responses to garlic, with females experiencing elevation and males reduction of blood sugar.[126] Recent evidence suggests that garlic extracts may be protective against diabetes-induced sequelae by inhibiting glycation.[127,128] Antioxidant cardioprotective and vasodilatory effects are also relevant in diabetic patients. However, significant reduction of blood glucose levels does not appear to be a viable therapeutic strategy in management of diabetes, and interactions with oral hypoglycemics would seem to be speculative based on current data.

Surgery

The literature contains two reports of postoperative bleeding purported to be associated with garlic use, as discussed earlier under Warfarin and related Oral Vitamin K Antagonist Anticoagulants. However, the data in both cases are inadequate to ascribe causality to the herb. Given the lack of reports of either spontaneous or postoperative bleeding associated with garlic use, it would appear that moderate garlic use is generally safe for those undergoing elective surgery. Preoperative measurement of bleed times or temporary cessation of garlic consumption may be prudent management strategies, depending on individual circumstances. It is axiomatic that herb and nutrient intake are disclosed before surgery; however, the general risk associated with garlic appears to be overstated in the secondary and derivative literature.

The 128 citations for this monograph are located under Garlic on the CD at the back of the book.

Ginger

Botanical Name: *Zingiber officinale* Roscoe.
Pharmacopoeial Name: Zingeribis rhizoma.
Synonym: *Amomum zingiber* L.
Common Names: Ginger, zingiber.

SUMMARY

Drug/Class Interaction Type	Mechanism and Significance	Management
Anesthesia, general ⊕⊕/☼	Herb reduces postoperative nausea and vomiting (PONV) caused by anesthetic. Possible alternative to pharmaceuticals in moderate PONV. Insufficient activity for emetic rescue in acute cases.	Consider pretreatment in elective surgery patients. Postoperative treatment may help moderate cases.
Antiplatelet agents ✗	Theoretical interaction based on "NSAID-like" properties of ginger. Clinical occurrence and significance not established. Increased risk of bleed negligible.	Preferably avoid; if coadministration compelling, professional monitoring advised.
Cisplatin Emetogenic chemotherapy ⊕⊕/☼	Ginger reduces acute nausea associated with cisplatin and other emetogenic antineoplastic chemotherapies.	Consider pretreatment, and posttreatment (up to 24 hours) for nausea.
Nonsteroidal anti-inflammatory drugs (NSAIDs) Antiarthritic analgesics ⊕⊕⊕/☼	Herb used as adjuvant with antiarthritic NSAIDs increases symptom relief and reduces side effects of drug by allowing lower doses.	Consider coadministration in appropriate populations.
Phenprocoumon Oral vitamin K antagonist anticoagulants ✗	Theoretical additive effects on hemostasis (similar to aspirin/warfarin combinations). One case report, conflicts with clinical data; suggests risk generally overstated.	Preferably avoid; if coadministered, maintain stable regimen and monitor INR.

PONV, Postoperative nausea and vomiting; *INR*, international normalized ratio.

HERB DESCRIPTION

Family

Zingiberaceae.

Habitat and Cultivation

Perennial, with tuberous rhizomes, native to Southeast Asia, and cultivated in tropical regions, including India, West Indies, Jamaica, Africa, and China.

Parts Used

Rhizome.

Common Forms

Fresh or Dried Rhizome: considered different agents in Chinese practice.
Dried Powdered Rhizome.
Tincture (1:5), Fluid Extract (1:1), 90% ethanol, fresh or dried rhizome.
Standardized Extracts: Various, including EV.EXT 33 (Ferrosan) standardized to hydroxy-methoxy phenols; Zintona standardized to 1.4% volatiles and minimum of 2.0 mg gingerols and shogoals per 250-mg capsule.

HERB IN CLINICAL PRACTICE

Overview

Best known as a pungent spice and dietary ingredient, ginger is among the top-20 dietary supplements in retail sales in the United States. Primarily viewed by conventional medicine as an antiemetic for motion sickness, the nausea of pregnancy, and postoperative nausea, the herb has many more, diverse therapeutic applications in both Western and Asian botanical medicine. It has potent anti-inflammatory effects on eicosanoid metabolism, circulatory and digestive tonic actions, and metabolic, endocrine, antimicrobial, antipyretic, antioxidant, and antineoplastic activities. Toxicity is minimal, and ginger is free of adverse effects at therapeutic doses.

Therapeutic monographs for ginger generally limit the indications to recent clinical trial–driven applications. Ginger was approved by the German Commission E in 1988 for dyspepsia and motion sickness, although not for morning sickness.[1] The European Scientific Cooperative on Phytotherapy (ESCOP)[2] recently reviewed much of the research but also suggested only motion sickness and postoperative nausea prevention as clinical uses. Broader authoritative surveys of the herb can be found in literature reviews by Mills and Bone[3] and McKenna et al.[4] Recent interest in the cancer chemopreventive properties has provided a new emphasis in pharmacological research into ginger and its constituent compounds.[5,6]

Historical/Ethnomedicine Precedent

Ginger has been used for centuries in Ayurvedic and Chinese medicine, where it is a major ingredient in innumerable formulae for many treatment indications. In India, ginger is not only widely used as a spice and meat preservative and antimicrobial digestive tonic, but also considered to have aphrodisiac and cognitive-enhancing effects, especially on memory, and has also been used as a narcotic antagonist. In classical Chinese medicine, the fresh rhizome *(Sheng Jiang)* is distinguished from the dried and processed rhizome *(Gan Jiang)*. In light of modern precautions suggesting elevated risk of bleeding with ginger consumption, an interesting Chinese medical use of dried ginger is to arrest bleeding, especially bleeding associated with "Deficiency" and "Cold."[7] Doses of the herb in Chinese practice are considerably higher than in modern phytotherapy, maximum dosage for Sheng Jiang is 30 g.[7] Traditional Western botanical medicine considers ginger to be a "diffusive stimulant," to be added to formulae to enhance the bioavailability of other herbs, as well to support diffusive physiological processes (e.g., expectoration, diaphoresis).[3]

Known or Potential Therapeutic Uses

Appetite stimulation, dyspepsia, flatulence, digestive/choleretic secretory stimulation, increasing bioavailability of foods and medicines, ulceroprotection, circulatory stimulation, thermogenesis, menstrual flow irregularities, colds, influenza, fevers, atherosclerosis, hypercholesterolemia, hyperviscosity, hepatic protection, pain relief in osteoarthritis and rheumatoid arthritis, Kawasaki's disease, antiemesis in nausea of motion, pregnancy, drug withdrawal, and chemotherapy; antineoplastic adjuvant.

Key Constituents

Pungent oleoresin containing phenolic gingerols and their dehydration derivatives, shogoals (formed by drying); volatile oil (variable composition of monoterpenes and sesquiterpenes depending on botanical chemotypes and physical methods of preparation).

Therapeutic Dosing Range

Fresh or Dried Rhizome: 2 to 4 g daily.
Tincture 1:5 (90% ethanol): 1.25 to 3.0 mL three times daily.
Fluid Extract 1:1 (90% ethanol): 0.25 to 0.75 mL three times daily.
Standardized Extract: Dose equivalent to 2 to 4 g dried rhizome daily.

INTERACTIONS REVIEW

Strategic Considerations

The available therapeutic monographs on ginger minimize suggestions of herb-drug interactivity. The German Commission E listed ginger interactions under "none known,"[1] ESCOP[2] mentions only the possible increase in bioavailability of sulfaguanide, and the World Health Organization (WHO)[8] monograph suggests an "enhancement" of pharmaceutical anticoagulant therapy, adding that the clinical significance of the possible interaction has not been evaluated. By contrast, secondary literature and commentators in both professional and popular press emphasize potential anticoagulant effects of ginger and freely extrapolate to hypothetical interactions with drugs affecting hemostasis.

The presumed mechanism of interference with normal hemostasis by ginger is based on in vitro studies that suggest the herb may affect platelet aggregation, primarily through inhibition of eicosanoid metabolism and specifically reduction of thromboxane levels.[9] However, the experimental support is inconclusive, and to date the balance of in vivo studies suggest a lack of effect of ginger on thromboxane-induced platelet aggregation in humans.[10-15] Until recently, clinical reports were based only on a questionable single case report of platelet aggregation inhibition apparently attributed to the consumption of ginger marmalade.[16] A recent single report of elevated international normalized ratio (INR) and epistaxis in a patient

previously stable on phenprocoumon anticoagulant therapy is discussed later.[17] However, no pharmacological data show that ginger affects the coagulation pathways reflected by the INR, so this case remains an isolated and unexplained interaction, its significance unclear. The existence of only two somewhat controversial reports in a quarter century suggests that portentous warnings about risks of combining ginger with anticoagulants may be overstated.

The activity of the herb as an anti-inflammatory, analgesic, and circulatory stimulant has led to its incorporation in protocols for arthritis. Coadministration of ginger in combination regimens with nonsteroidal anti-inflammatory drugs (NSAIDs) or analgesics for arthritis has been examined indirectly in trials that permitted NSAID/analgesic rescue or in one trial where patients added ginger to an existing NSAID regimen.[18-20] Although further investigations are warranted, there may be neither significant additive effect between NSAIDs and ginger alone in arthritis nor any significant difference between NSAIDs and ginger alone for arthritic symptom relief. However, ginger's adverse effect profile is superior to conventional NSAID drugs, and ginger could be incorporated into combination protocols for botanical cyclooxygenase-2 (COX-2) inhibition in arthritis and related inflammatory conditions to maintain integrity of the protective, constitutive gastric cyclooxygenase and prostaglandin E_2 (PGE_2). Common compound formulations with ginger include herbs such as rosemary, *Boswellia,* and the plant-derived compound resveratrol, which act as COX-2 inhibitors at the receptor level and also downregulate inducible COX-2 transcription. Ginger extracts have been shown to exert an ulceroprotective effect against aspirin and indomethacin, implying the pharmacology of ginger-containing combination protocols targeting COX-2 could be applied to a variety of inflammatory conditions, including malignancy.[21]

The established antiemetic effects of ginger, well proven for motion sickness and morning sickness of pregnancy, have also been found to be helpful in drug-induced nausea and vomiting. The strong association of certain antineoplastic chemotherapies (e.g., cisplatin) with acute nausea, as well as postoperative nausea and vomiting (PONV) associated with emetogenic anesthetics, constitute beneficial interactions with ginger (see anesthetics and chemotherapies later). Ginger may well find application in the treatment of other cases of drug-induced nausea when symptom occurrence is not inevitable; one report suggests that it can be used for nausea relating to symptoms of disequilibrium after discontinuation of serotonin-inhibiting drugs.[22]

Effects on Drug Metabolism and Bioavailability

An experimental study found that ginger enhanced the absorption of sulfaguanidine across the small intestine in rodents.[23] Secretory increases by the pancreas and bile are also associated with ginger administration.[24] An early study suggests glucuronide conjugation and renal and biliary excretion are involved in elimination of the volatile component zingerone.[25] In rats, [6]-gingerol was eliminated partly by hepatic metabolism, and the gingerol was more than 90% bound to serum protein.[26]

Traditionally, ginger has been used to promote the absorption of herbs in multiherb botanical prescriptions. The Ayurvedic *Trikatu* formula is a mixture of ginger with long-pepper and black pepper that has been shown to increase the bioavailability of several pharmaceuticals.[27] A more recent study of the effect of Trikatu on the kinetics of sodium diclofenac found the opposite effect: a significant reduction of bioavailability.[28] These studies are not applicable directly to ginger alone, and the piperine ingredient of the other herbs in the formula are known to have modulating effects on several cytochrome P450 isoforms.[29]

Data on potential effects of ginger and its constituents on drug-metabolizing enzymes are largely unavailable at this time. Although traditional botanical prescribing conventions may use ginger for increasing bioavailability of other herbs, the effects on pharmaceutical drug absorption are not predictable on the basis of the current data. One study has documented an inhibitory effect on P-glycoprotein (P-gp). Accumulation of daunorubicin was increased in a multidrug-resistant cell line in the presence of [6]-gingerol, which also appeared to increase the cytotoxicity of vinblastine, suggesting an inhibition of P-gp–mediated efflux of the cytotoxic drug from the cells.[30] Until further data are available, the prediction of P-gp–mediated drug-ginger interactions remains speculative, if theoretically possible.

HERB-DRUG INTERACTIONS

Anesthesia, General

Evidence: Atracurium (Tracrium), fentanyl (Actiq Oral Transmucosal, Duragesic Transdermal, Fentanyl Oralet, Sublimaze Injection), hyoscine hydrobromide, combination drug: morphine hydrochloride, codeine hydrochloride, and papaverine hydrochloride (Papaveretum); suxamethonium (scoline, succinylcholine; Anectine), thiopentone (Thiopental), vecuronium (Norcuron).
Extrapolated, based on similar properties: Emetogenic anesthetics.

Interaction Type and Significance

⊕⊕ **Beneficial or Supportive Interaction, with Professional Management**
☼ **Prevention or Reduction of Drug Adverse Effect**

Probability:	Evidence Base:
3. Possible	▽ **Mixed**

Effect and Mechanism of Action

Anesthesia-induced PONV may be reduced by pretreatment with ginger extracts, which probably act at both central serotonergic and peripheral gastric levels to inhibit emesis.

Research

Six trials performed over 15 years specifically examined the effects of ginger pretreatment on the severity and incidence of PONV.[31-36] All trials involved gynecological settings, and the majority (five of six) involved laparoscopic outpatient procedures, with a total of 668 subjects across all the studies. Powdered ginger in capsules was used in all cases, with oral doses ranging from 0.5 to 2.0 g of herb, administered 1 to 3 hours before the procedure, although one trial also administered ginger both before and after the procedure.

In a meta-analysis of only three of the trials, Ernst and Pittler[37] concluded that the evidence for ginger efficacy in PONV was positive. However, a more recent meta-analysis by Morin et al.[38] that included all six trials available to date concluded that the antiemetic effects of ginger were insufficient to consider the incorporation of the herb into the PONV clinical setting.

Visalyputra et al.[35] examined 111 women undergoing laparoscopic gynecological diagnostic procedures, divided into placebo, ginger-only, droperidol, and droperidol/ginger groups. The dose of ginger was divided into 1.0 g before the procedure and another 1.0 g 30 minutes before discharge. No significant differences were found between placebo and the other groups.[35] The only notably positive study was by Phillips et al.,[36] who used 1 g ginger 1 hour before anesthesia. The ginger appeared to be equally effective to metoclopramide (10 mg) in reducing nausea, both being significantly better than placebo.[36]

A recent meta-analysis of these trials concluded that there was definite evidence for a positive effect of ginger at 1.0 g per day for PONV.[39]

Integrative Therapeutics, Clinical Concerns, and Adaptations

Although the trial evidence is not conclusive, there would appear to be reasonable grounds for patients undergoing elective procedures who may prefer nonpharmaceutical options, when available, to utilize ginger pretreatment before procedures involving anesthesia. Data are not available for emetic rescue, and conventional use of metoclopramide or dexamethasone may be required after exposure to emetogenic anesthetics. The risks of bleeding to anticoagulant effects of the herb are discussed in the following sections on antiplatelet agents and phenprocoumon. Theoretical cautions against combining ginger with anesthetics have also been made on the basis of a single rodent study in which administration of isolated [6]-gingerol and [6]-shogoal at doses of 3.5 mg/kg induced increases in hexobarbital sleep time in rats.[40] Equivalent human doses of ginger powder or fresh ginger would be orders of magnitude higher than normal therapeutic dose levels of the herb.

Antiplatelet Agents

Antiplatelet thromboprophylactics: Acetylsalicylic acid (acetosal, acetyl salicylic acid, ASA, salicylsalicylic acid; Arthritis Foundation Pain Reliever, Ascriptin, Aspergum, Asprimox, Bayer Aspirin, Bayer Buffered Aspirin, Bayer Low Adult Strength, Bufferin, Buffex, Cama Arthritis Pain Reliever, Easprin, Ecotrin, Ecotrin Low Adult Strength, Empirin, Extra Strength Adprin-B, Extra Strength Bayer Enteric 500 Aspirin, Extra Strength Bayer Plus, Halfprin 81, Heartline, Regular Strength Bayer Enteric 500 Aspirin, St. Joseph Adult Chewable Aspirin, ZORprin); combination drugs: ASA and caffeine (Anacin), ASA, caffeine, and propoxyphene (Darvon Compound); ASA and carisoprodol (Soma Compound); ASA, codeine, and carisoprodol (Soma Compound with Codeine); ASA and codeine (Empirin with Codeine); ASA, codeine, butalbital, and caffeine (Fiorinal); cilostazol (Pletal), clopidogrel (Plavix), dipyridamole (Permole, Persantine), ticlopidine (Ticlid); combination drug: ASA and extended-release dipyridamole (Aggrenox, Asasantin).
Monoclonal antibody antiplatelet agents: Abciximab (ReoPro), eptifibatide (Integrelin), tirofiban (Aggrastat).

Interaction Type and Significance

✗ **Potential or Theoretical Adverse Interaction of Uncertain Severity**

Probability:	Evidence Base:
6. Unknown	▽ **Mixed**

Effect and Mechanism of Action

A theoretical interaction extrapolated from the ''NSAID-like'' activity of ginger and its active compounds through inhibition of thromboxane-evoked platelet aggregation, creating an assumed additive disabling of platelets. The interaction has not been clinically demonstrated to date.

Research

Equivocal results have been obtained in experimental and in vitro studies attempting to characterize effects of ginger extracts and isolated ginger compounds on platelet aggregation, although there is evidence for a dual inhibitory effect on eicosanoid synthesis, with lipoxygenase as well as cyclooxygenase subject to inhibition.[14,15,41-43] COX-2 effects may be mediated by the effect of [6]-gingerol on nuclear factor kappa B (NF-κB) activation. Kim et al.[44] used a mouse skin model and found evidence of the ginger compound blocking phosphorylation of I-κBα as well as p65. This was reversed by a p38 mitogen-activating protein (MAP) kinase inhibitor, implicating the p38 MAP kinase signaling pathway of NF-κB as the upstream mediator of COX-2 downregulation.[44]

Four human studies have investigated the effects of ginger on platelet aggregation. Verma et al.[45] examined the effects of a fatty diet (100 g butter for 7 days) on platelet aggregation in 20 healthy volunteers. Ten individuals also consumed 5 g dried ginger with the fatty meal. Adenosine diphosphate (ADP) and epinephrine-induced platelet aggregation was significantly lower in the butter-plus-ginger group than in the butter-only group. Lumb[12] conducted a small, double-blind randomized trial with eight healthy volunteers who consumed 2 g ginger or placebo. No effect was found on any parameters of platelet activity (samples taken 3 and 24 hours after ginger administration), including bleed time, aggregometry, and platelet count. Srivastava[10] measured platelet thromboxane in human volunteers before and after 7 days consumption of 5 g/day fresh garlic or 70 g/day raw onion. Thromboxane B$_2$ (TXB$_2$) levels (measured after sample clotted by incubation for 1 hour) were reduced by approximately one third in the ginger group ($n = 7$). The small sample size was statistically underpowered ($p < 0.1$). The onion-consuming group exhibited a trend to increased TXB$_2$ after clotting.

Another study investigated the effects of ginger on TXB$_2$ with higher doses of ginger administered by vanilla custard, with 15 g raw ginger daily or 40 g cooked stem ginger for 2 weeks, in 18 healthy volunteers of both genders. There was no washout period in the crossover design, and when venous blood samples were taken on both day 12 and day 14, no significant change in TXB$_2$ levels was detected between either form of ginger and placebo. In contrast, an earlier pilot study by the same researchers had detected significant (39%) TXB$_2$ reduction after only 3 mg/day administration of acetylsalicylic acid (ASA).[13] Bordia et al.[11] used a placebo-controlled trial to examine the effects of powdered ginger administered at 4 g daily for 3 months in 60 patients with a history of coronary artery disease. Blood lipids and glucose, plasma fibrinogen, and fibrinolytic activity, as well as ADP and epinephrine-induced platelet aggregation, were measured at 1½ and 3 months. No significant differences were found between the placebo and ginger groups in any of the parameters measured. However, a single 10-g dose of ginger did produce significant reduction in platelet aggregation evoked by the two test agonists measured 4 hours after ginger administration.

Jiang et al.[46] conducted a small, open-label trial (12 healthy male volunteers) and examined a range of pharmacokinetic and hemostasis parameters after administration of ginger or ginkgo, alone or with warfarin. Aggregation, INR, warfarin enantiomer concentrations in plasma and urine, and warfarin enantiomer binding were all measured at day 1 and day 7. The dose of ginger was three tablets of 0.4 g powdered rhizome three times for 1 week. Neither ginger nor ginkgo produced significant effect on clotting status or the pharmacokinetics and pharmacodynamics of warfarin.

Clinical Implications and Adaptations

The quality of the evidence is variable, partly because of small sample sizes, different forms of ginger tested (or different purified compounds), and differing doses used. However, the balance of available data suggests that the effects of ginger compounds on cyclooxygenase and lipoxygenase inhibition do not appear to have detectable clinical effects on primary hemostasis. By extension, it appears that ginger can be safely utilized at therapeutic doses along with antiplatelet and anticoagulant medications. Theoretically, for certain individuals with unique pharmacogenomic susceptibility or subclinical platelet disorders, ginger preparations might interact adversely with either antiplatelet or anticoagulant agents.

Cisplatin and Emetogenic Antineoplastic Chemotherapies

Evidence: Cisplatin (*cis*-diaminedichloroplatinum, CDDP; Platinol, Platinol-AQ), cyclophosphamide (Cytoxan, Endoxana, Neosar, Procytox).

Extrapolated, based on similar properties: Carboplatin (Paraplatin), mechlorethamine (nitrogen mustard; Mustargen), oxaliplatin (Eloxatin), phenylalanine mustard (Melphalan), uracil mustard (uramustine).

Interaction Type and Significance

⊕⊕ **Beneficial or Supportive Interaction, with Professional Management**

☼ **Prevention or Reduction of Drug Adverse Effect**

Probability:	Evidence Base:
2. Probable	○ **Preliminary**

Effect and Mechanism of Action

Nausea and vomiting are predictable adverse effects of certain chemotherapies, typically cisplatin and nitrogen mustards, and often occur with various other agents. The established antiemetic activity of ginger may be effective against acute (<24 hours) chemotherapy-induced nausea and vomiting, possibly through serotonergic mechanisms.

Research

Morrow[47] surveyed 442 oncology outpatients receiving consecutive chemotherapy and found that 16% who reported susceptibility to motion sickness were more likely to experience nausea and vomiting after chemotherapy than matched controls. Ginger has been investigated in numerous trials for the treatment of various kinds of nausea, including motion sickness, postoperative nausea, and morning sickness. The majority of studies have been positive, and a meta-analysis of six randomized double-blind placebo-controlled trials concluded that ginger was a "promising antiemetic remedy" in 2000, although more data are required to draw firm conclusions.[37] Sharma et al.[48,49] investigated preadministration of acetone and alcoholic extracts of ginger in rodent and canine models of cisplatin-induced emesis. Cisplatin inhibits gastric emptying, and the endpoint used is the delay in gastric emptying associated with the antiemetic agent. Acetone ginger extracts (200 and 500 mg/kg orally) were more significantly effective than the 5-hydroxytryptamine (5-HT$_3$) receptor antagonist ondansetron in delaying gastric emptying in rodents. In canines, researchers using a similar procedure, but with the ginger extracts (25-200 mg/kg) given 30 minutes after cisplatin, also caused a dose-dependent reduction in emesis and increase in emetic latency compared with controls. Aqueous extracts were ineffective. The acetone extract of ginger was more effective than the alcoholic extract, preventing emesis in 20% of dogs, compared to none for the alcoholic extract. Yamahara et al.[50] found that oral administration of [6]-gingerol (25 or 50 mg/kg orally) or an acetone extract of ginger (150 mg/kg orally) pretreatment could completely prevent cyclophosphamide-induced emesis in a rodent model.

The antiemetic mechanisms of ginger compounds were investigated by Abdel-Aziz et al.[51] using three different molecular models. They concluded that although an effect on 5-HT$_3$ receptor ion-channel complex was definitely implicated, there were also indirect effects, possibly through substance P and muscarinic receptors.[51] Finally, in a wider context but still within the oncology setting, a rodent model was used to demonstrate that ginger may also be effective in radiation-induced taste aversion.[52]

Integrative Therapeutics, Clinical Concerns, and Adaptations

Three temporal phases of chemotherapy-induced nausea are distinguished: *anticipatory* (occurring before exposure), *acute* (onset within or lasting up to 24 hours of exposure), and *delayed* (onset more than 24 hours after exposure, typically 48 to 72 hours, with variable duration). The anticipatory type is independent of the specific agent of both the type of cancer and the chemotherapy regimen, essentially a conditioned response. The acute form is most susceptible to treatment with antiemetic agents, whereas delayed symptoms are less susceptible to antiserotonergic agents, suggesting that different mechanisms may be involved.[53,54] Although human studies are lacking, ginger extracts have been used clinically by practitioners versed in botanical medicine to prevent and treat the acute phases of chemotherapy-induced nausea typified by the emetic effects of cisplatin.

Nonsteroidal Anti-Inflammatory Drugs (NSAIDs) and Analgesic Antiarthritics

COX-1 inhibitors: Diclofenac (Cataflam, Voltaren), combination drug: diclofenac and misoprostol (Arthrotec), diflunisal (Dolobid), etodolac (Lodine), fenoprofen (Dalfon), furbiprofen (Ansaid), ibuprofen (Advil, Excedrin IB, Motrin, Motrin IB, Nuprin, Pedia Care Fever Drops, Provel, Rufen); combination drug: hydrocodone and ibuprofen (Reprexain, Vicoprofen), indomethacin (indometacin; Indocin, Indocin-SR), ketoprofen (Orudis, Oruvail), ketorolac (Acular ophthalmic, Toradol), meclofenamate (Meclomen), mefenamic acid (Ponstel), meloxicam (Mobic), nabumetone (Relafen), naproxen (Aleve, Anaprox, Naprosyn), oxaprozin (Daypro), piroxicam (Feldene), salsalate (salicylic acid; Amigesic, Disalcid, Marthritic, Mono Gesic, Salflex, Salsitab), sulindac (Clinoril), tolmetin (Tolectin).
COX-2 inhibitors: Celecoxib (Celebrex).

Interaction Type and Significance

⊕⊕⊕ **Beneficial or Supportive Interaction, Not Requiring Professional Management**
☼ **Prevention or Reduction of Drug Adverse Effect**

Probability:
2. Probable

Evidence Base:
○ **Preliminary**

Effect and Mechanism of Action

Ginger and ginger extracts exert anti-inflammatory effects through multiple mechanisms, including cyclooxygenase and lipoxygenase inhibition. Adjuvant combination of ginger with NSAIDs for arthritis leads to increased symptom relief and allows the NSAID dose to be lowered and in some cases discontinued. Ginger has a superior adverse effect profile to known NSAIDs, and coadministration reduces adverse effects through lower NSAID dose or eventual substitution.

Research

In vitro evidence has established that ginger and some of its constituent compounds are effective inhibitors of cyclooxygenase and lipoxygenase and may downregulate transcription of cyclooxygenase and inducible nitric oxide synthase (iNOS) by inhibition of NF-κB.[21,42-44] Two randomized placebo-controlled clinical trials have demonstrated small but significant effects for ginger treatment of osteoarthritis, although in the study by Bliddal et al.[19] the effect was small compared with ibuprofen and was confined to a first period of treatment in a crossover design. The trial by Altman and Marcussen[20] showed a significant effect in 261 patients with osteoarthritis of the knee, although the ginger extract was administered in combination with the herb galangal (*Alpinia galangia*). Acetaminophen was permitted as a rescue medication in both studies. The ginger group had less use of rescue medication than the placebo group. Additionally, several rodent experimental model studies have shown that ginger extracts are directly protective against NSAID-induced gastric ulcers in a rodent model.[55-58]

Reports

Srivastafa and Mustafa[59] reported a case series of seven patients who used ginger extracts combined with NSAIDs, but who were not taking other antiarthritic medications (e.g., gold) or steroids. Six patients were taking NSAIDs for 3 months but failed to experience symptom relief. After 3 months of oral ginger administration (up to 5.0 g fresh rhizome or 1.0 g powdered rhizome daily), while continuing NSAID therapy, the patients all experienced reduction in pain symptoms and improved range of motion, and two patients also experienced relief of myalgia. After 3 months of coadministration the NSAIDs were stopped; the patients continued with ginger alone and were able to maintain the same degree of symptom relief.

Integrative Therapeutics, Clinical Concerns, and Adaptations

The adverse effect profile of NSAIDs, including the COX-2 specific inhibitors, continues to present significant problems to the pharmaceutical anti-inflammatory strategies for arthritis. Ginger extracts may additively combine with NSAIDs and after a period of coadministration can substitute for them in some cases. Health care professionals versed in botanical medicine are more likely to incorporate ginger into polyherbal anti-inflammatory formulae rather than use it as a single agent. Typical associated ingredients might include curcumin, *Boswellia serrata*, resveratrol, and the salicylate-containing *Salix* spp.

Phenprocoumon and Related Oral Vitamin K Antagonist Anticoagulants

Evidence: Phenprocoumon (Jarsin, Marcumar).
Extrapolated, based on similar properties: Anisindione (Miradon), dicumarol, ethyl biscoumacetate (Tromexan), nicoumalone (acenocoumarol; Acitrom, Sintrom), phenindione (Dindevan), warfarin (Coumadin, Marevan, Warfilone).

Interaction Type and Significance

✗ Potential or Theoretical Adverse Interaction of Uncertain Severity

Probability:	Evidence Base:
4. Plausible	▽ **Mixed**

Effect and Mechanism of Action

A theoretical additive effect between coumarin anticoagulants and ginger on hemostasis is hypothesized to increase INR and risk of bleeding. Unsupported by the currently known pharmacology of the herb, a single report of the possible interaction is available. The clinical significance of the proposed interaction is minimal.

Research

There are no human studies investigating pharmacodynamic effects of ginger on the vitamin K–dependent clotting factors II, VII, IX, and X. Weidener and Sigwart[60] conducted a series of experimental investigations with EV.EXT 33 ginger extracts on Wistar rats, including a study of the effects of oral warfarin (0.25 mg/kg daily) alone and in combination with the ginger extract. Warfarin significantly increased prothrombin time (PT) and activated partial thromboplastin time (APTT) compared with normal controls. Coadministration of ginger extract at 100 mg/kg for 4 days had no effect on warfarin-induced changes in PT and APTT and did not alter these coagulation parameters in a control group receiving no warfarin.[60]

In a recent study described earlier under Antiplatelet Agents, Jiang et al.[46] found that ginger and ginkgo had no significant effect on clotting status or the pharmacological profile of warfarin.

Pharmacokinetic data demonstrating any effect of the herb on drug-metabolizing enzymes mediating coumarin drug metabolism (cytochromes P450 1A2 and 2C9) are also unavailable. Further studies are required to establish definitively an absence of effect of ginger on coagulation, but the balance of currently available evidence suggests such effects are unlikely.

Reports

A single German case involving ginger and phenprocoumon was reported by Krüth et al.[17] in 2004. A 76-year-old woman with a history of mitral insufficiency, atrial fibrillation, congestive heart failure, and osteoporosis who was taking concurrent cholecalciferol, captopril, piretanide, digoxin, and a nitrate vasodilator was maintaining a stable INR (range, 2.0 to 3.0) while receiving long-term phenprocoumon therapy. Because of a peripheral bleed incident (epistaxis), she was admitted to hospital, and INR was greater than 10. Phenprocoumon was stopped, and she received three doses of vitamin K_1 (initially 10 mg intravenously, then 5.0 mg and 3.0 mg orally after 3 and 6 days, respectively). By day 6, the INR and PTT normalized and phenprocoumon was resumed, with INR maintained at normal levels by the same dose used before the bleeding episode. A detailed history revealed "a regular ginger intake (pieces of dried ginger and tea from ginger powder)" for several weeks before the bleeding incident occurred. The patient was advised to refrain from ginger use, and no further episodes of bleeding were noted. The authors note that the current pharmacological data on ginger do not provide any obvious mechanism for the observed effects.

The report, although complete in some respects, lacks vital information. The exact form, amount, dose, frequency, and duration of ginger administration are not given, making the incident impossible to evaluate. Further, "Dried ginger pieces"

is an unusual form of ingesting the herb given its pungent and acrid taste, and "ginger tea" does not exclude the presence of nonginger ingredients. The ginger was apparently consumed for several weeks before the INR elevation. Case data show a rapid elevation of INR between two measurements 7 days apart. Relating this to an unstated dose of ginger consumed several weeks earlier does not constitute a reasonable association by timing for the INR effect to be causally associated with the herb consumption. The INR plots show values maintained within therapeutic range for more than a week before the bleed episode, presumably during the "several weeks" consumption of ginger. The observed INR increase might be explained by excessive phenprocoumon levels caused by inadvertent drug misadministration, a dietary pharmacokinetic interaction, or sudden decrease in dietary intake of vitamin K–containing foods, none of which was considered by the authors.[17]

Clinical Implications and Adaptations

The single available case report is insufficient to confirm the existence of a ginger–oral anticoagulant interaction, especially with the lack of a plausible pharmacological mechanism and inadequacies in the report data. In addition, some controlled trial evidence suggests that ginger has no measurable effect on warfarin pharmacokinetics or pharmacodynamics. Until further data are available, it cannot be assumed that moderate ginger consumption exerts clinically significant effects on the coagulation cascade and INR values. As normally occurs with coumarin-effected anticoagulation, monitoring of INR and alerting patients to report early signs of bleeding (e.g., epistaxis, ecchymoses) remain essential elements of vitamin K antagonist therapy. Possible antiplatelet activity cannot be ruled out completely at this time (see Antiplatelet Agents), but epistaxis or other serious bleeding episode would be expected with an INR higher than 10.

The use of cured ginger in Chinese medicine to arrest bleeding in certain conditions has already been mentioned. Anecdotal clinical experience also suggests that at normal therapeutic dose ranges for appropriate indications, ginger and ginger extracts present no significant risk of bleeding in patients on oral vitamin K antagonist anticoagulation.

THEORETICAL, SPECULATIVE, AND PRELIMINARY INTERACTIONS RESEARCH, INCLUDING OVERSTATED INTERACTIONS CLAIMS

Aminoglycoside Antibiotics

Amikacin (Amikin), gentamicin (G-mycin, Garamycin, Jenamicin), kanamycin (Kantrex), neomycin (Mycifradin, Myciguent, Neo-Fradin, NeoTab, Nivemycin), netilmicin (Netromycin), paromomycin (monomycin; Humatin), streptomycin, tobramycin (AKTob, Nebcin, TOBI, TOBI Solution, TobraDex, Tobrex).

A preliminary in vitro study by Nagoshi et al.[61] found a potential synergy between aminoglycoside antibiotics and [10]-gingerol against vancomycin-resistant enterococci. The authors suggested that this may be caused by detergent-like effect of the gingerol increasing membrane permeability. Whether this preliminary finding can be replicated in vivo remains to be established.

Sulfaguanidine

Sulfaguanidine

Using an experimental rat intestine model, Sakai et al.[23] demonstrated that ginger extracts enhanced the absorption of sulfaguanidine by 150% compared with controls. This has been identified as the sole possible ginger-drug interaction by two authoritative secondary reviews.[2,62] Whether or not this is an example of general effects of ginger on intestinal absorption in rodents (see pharmacokinetics discussion earlier), the likelihood of this being a clinically significant interaction, given the limited contemporary use of this agent for enteric infections and the lack of human data, suggests that the interaction is overstated, particularly when identified as the only interaction of ginger with any pharmaceutical agent.

The 62 citations for this monograph are located under Ginger on the CD at the back of the book.

Ginkgo

Botanical Name: *Ginkgo biloba* L.
Pharmacopoeial Name: Ginkgo folium
Common Names: Ginkgo, maidenhair tree.

SUMMARY

Drug/Class Interaction Type	Mechanism and Significance	Management
Anesthesia, general ?	Possible increased sleeping time: mechanism unknown; significance unclear; inadequate data.	Management: same as surgery; eliminate potential interaction.
Acetylsalicylic acid/aspirin Ticlopidine, clopidogrel Antiplatelet agents ✗	Theoretical additive antiplatelet activity; significance not established, likely overstated. Ginkgo may allow lower dose of drug, reducing drug adverse effects.	Avoid or adopt and monitor bleed times.
Cisplatin ⊕⊕/☼	Ginkgo may help reduce platinum drug toxicities (renal, neural).	Consider coadministration.
Cyclosporine ⊕⊕/☼	Ginkgo may help reduce PAF-mediated drug nephrotoxicity. Potentially important for allograft patients.	Consider coadministration.
Doxorubicin Anthracycline chemotherapy ⊕/☼	Ginkgo protects against and reduces drug-induced cardiotoxicity through multiple mechanisms.	Pretreat, coadminister, and continue herb postchemotherapy.
Fluorouracil (5-FU) ?	Suggested additive therapeutic effect caused by increase in drug disposition by circulatory effects of ginkgo.	Coadministration could be beneficial, unlikely to be harmful. Professional advice mandatory.
Fluoxetine SSRI antidepressants ⊕⊕/☼	Ginkgo reduces sexual dysfunction adverse effects (including erectile dysfunction in men) of drug through multiple mechanisms; may have additive antidepressant effects.	Consider trial if symptomatic.
Gentamicin Aminoglycoside antibiotics ⊕/☼	Herb may reduce drug induced ototoxicity through neuroprotective and neuroreparative mechanisms.	Consider trial adoption. Continue herb if symptomatic after antibiotic therapy.
Halperidol Neuroleptics ⊕/☼	Herb may reduce drug-induced tardive dyskinesia adverse effects through neuroprotective and neuroreparative actions.	Consider adopting. Continue herb if tardive dyskinesia symptoms persist.
Surgery ✗✗✗/⊕✗/⊕	Ginkgo may decrease hemostasis via antiplatelet effects presurgically. Anti-ischemic and neuroreparative postsurgically.	Stop ginkgo 1 week before surgery. Adopt postsurgically if indicated.
Trazodone ?	Mechanism unknown; significance unclear; inadequate data.	Avoid until further data available.
Warfarin Oral vitamin K antagonist anticoagulants ✗	Theoretical additive effects on hemostasis caused by potential platelet inhibition; similar to aspirin/warfarin combinations. Inadequate data; incidence and significance unknown. General risk overstated.	Audit elderly populations for undisclosed herb use. If coadministered, maintain regimen, monitor INR. Hold if INR supratherapeutic or signs of abnormal bleeding occur.

PAF, Platelet aggregation (platelet-activating) factor; *SSRI*, selective serotonin reuptake inhibitor; *INR*, international normalized ratio.

HERB DESCRIPTION

Family

Ginkgoaceae.

Habitat and Cultivation

Sole survivor of an ancient botanical taxon (Ginkgoales), the ginkgo tree is now widely cultivated as an urban ornamental because of its pollution resistance. Considered a "native" to China, large commercial plantations in the temperate areas of the United States and Western Europe provide most crude herb for medicinal extracts.

Parts Used

Leaf.

Common Forms

Dried Leaf: Powdered.
Tincture, Fluid Extract: 50% ethanol.
Standardized Dry Extract: 22% to 27.0% flavonoids and 5.0% to 7.0% terpene ginkgolides. Dry extract preparations usually stipulate maximum permitted levels of ginkgolic acid (<5 ppm).

HERB IN CLINICAL PRACTICE

Overview

Ginkgo leaf extract is unusual in that its current use originates entirely from European pharmacological studies in the 1960s rather than a long history of traditional use. Notably, many secondary sources incorrectly claim ginkgo has been used for centuries; the fruit or nut, not the leaf, is the traditional medicine in Chinese herbal practice. Positive clinical trials demonstrating efficacy of ginkgo leaf extract for Alzheimer's disease and other age-related dementias have helped position it as a consistent top-10 best seller throughout Europe and North America in recent years. In the United States, retail sales of ginkgo surpassed $36 million in 2002, and in the same year an estimated 1.375 billion *daily* single treatments of ginkgo were prescribed in Germany alone. This constitutes a substantial volume of post-marketing surveillance data, which generally confirms the minimal toxicity and adverse effect profile of the extract. Adverse effect incidence corresponds to the low levels noted in clinical trials (< 1.5%).

The chemistry of ginkgo leaf extract is complex and includes several unique terpenoid compounds. Research has centered on these compounds' pharmacology, including inhibition of platelet aggregation by ginkgolide B, which is an unusually high-affinity ligand for the platelet aggregation (platelet-activating) factor (PAF) receptor. However, the known pharmacodynamics of the herb are generally considered a synergistic result of multiple constituents, including flavonol glycosides and oligomeric proanthocyanidins, as well as the terpenoids. Almost all the clinical research has been conducted with the concentrated (50:1) standardized *Ginkgo biloba* extracts, EGb 761 and LI 1370. Partly because of interest in potential antiplatelet therapeutic agents, several studies have employed isolates of the diterpene trilactones, either ginkgolide B (BN 52021) alone or a combination of ginkgolides A, B, C, and J (BN 52063); however, these data may have limited application to whole-leaf dry extract. In turn, botanical practitioners often use hydroethanolic liquid extracts of whole leaf when preparing blended individual prescriptions. Such extracts have been poorly investigated compared to the standardized dry-extract material, to which they should not be regarded as therapeutically equivalent. Ginkgo folium has therapeutic monographs by the German Commission E (1998)[1] and World Health Organization (WHO, 1999)[2] and subsequent monographs (2003) by the European Scientific Cooperative on Phytotherapy (ESCOP)[3] and *American Herbal Pharmacopoeia*.[4] Longer works by DeFeudis[5] and van Beek[6] provide more comprehensive and in-depth reviews of the extensive literature.

Historical/Ethnomedicine Precedent

Traditional Western therapeutic indications for ginkgo leaf are absent because of its historically recent incorporation into the materia medica, although seeds have been used in Chinese medicine for centuries.

Known or Potential Therapeutic Uses

Altitude sickness, asthma, Alzheimer's disease and multi-infarct dementia; cerebral insufficiency and associated impairments of memory, learning, attention, and cognitive function (enhancement of these functions in healthy and in aging adult populations, as well as after head trauma); depression, dysmenorrhea, hypoxia; neuroprotection, ischemic protection (cardiac, cerebral, renal), and neurorestoration of disease and iatrogenic nerve damage; macular degeneration, neurosensory deficits including tinnitus, cochlear hearing impairment, oxidative stress, peripheral vascular disorders including intermittent claudication and Raynaud's disease; reduced retinal blood flow, vertigo.

Key Constituents

Terpenes: Ginkgolides A, B, C, and J (diterpene trilactones); bilobalide (sesquiterpene).

Flavonoids: Glycosides of quercitin, kaempferol, and isorhamnetin; (+)-catechin, (−)-epicatechin, (−)-epigallocatechin, and (+)-gallocatechin; oligomeric and polymeric procyanidins. Phenolic acids, including ginkgolic acid; essential oil.

Therapeutic Dosing Range

Fluid Extract: 1:1, 3.0 to 8.0 mL/day.
Standardized Extract: 120 to 240 mg/day in divided doses.

Note: Unless otherwise stated in this monograph, ginkgo leaf and ginkgo leaf extract refer to the standardized solid extract preparations that have formed the basis of almost all studies of ginkgo leaf.

INTERACTIONS REVIEW
Strategic Considerations

The consensus of the authoritative botanical monographs is that there are no established interactions between ginkgo leaf (or its standardized extracts) and prescription drugs. Some secondary sources suggest that interaction with anticoagulants is theoretically possible.[3,4] From the conventional side, *Stockley's Drug Interactions* cites several herbs that interact with anticoagulants, but does not include ginkgo.[7] Given the widespread use of ginkgo and its multisystem actions, classified by DeFeudis[5] into four broad categories (vasoregulation, cognition-enhancement, stress alleviation, gene regulation), the range of possible interactions may be larger and more complex than suggested by the current literature and reports.

The literature is uneven in quality, leading to interpretive problems. Botanical monographs have distinguished between effects of traditional forms of ginkgo leaf preparations (and the properties of the 50:1 standardized extracts) and effects of isolated constituents (e.g., terpenoid ginkgolides). Conventional sources frequently fail to distinguish form, dose, and duration of administration of ginkgo extracts in their reporting; often also misspelling the name of the herb as "gingko."[8-16] Despite the low quality of reports, some trends emerge when reviewing secondary literature.

A tendency of ginkgo extract alone to induce spontaneous bleeding (i.e., in healthy individuals) is often assumed in mainstream reports of ginkgo interactions; this is controversial. Relative to its high level of use, very few reports of spontaneous bleeding are actually attributable to ginkgo use.[16-19] The poor standard of adverse event reporting of ginkgo-associated bleeds has been criticized both in journal correspondence and in several review articles.[20,21] The apparent consensus of the reports on bleeding is that although ginkgo leaf extracts may have been associated with some hemorrhagic episodes, particularly ophthalmic neurovascular bleeds, causality is not established, and the general risk is probably overstated. At least three trials in healthy volunteers have failed to demonstrate any significant effect of ginkgo on platelet and coagulation parameters in healthy humans.[22-24] Larger-scale trials are needed to investigate potential hematological effects of the extract, particularly in older populations. Several reports of postoperative bleeding are described later in the discussion of surgery.

Coadministration of ginkgo extracts with drugs affecting hemostasis presents questions with no simple evidence-based answers at present. Careful individual assessment and monitoring, with case-by-case therapeutic choices, remain the best practice. Given that the herb has been confirmed by meta-analysis of clinical trials to be effective for peripheral arterial disease, the precise populations that may choose gingko self-prescription may also be those more at risk of potential interactions because of their use of prescription drugs affecting hemostasis. (See further discussion later in the sections on interactions involving antiplatelet agents and warfarin.)

A number of the beneficial interactions of ginkgo listed later relate to its anti-ischemic, antioxidant, neuroprotective/neuroreparative, and chemoprotective effects. Typically, these interactions involve reduction of drug-induced toxicities, such as nephrotoxicity or neurotoxicity, through multiple mechanisms. these protective effects against drug toxicities most likely apply to numerous medications other than those for which preliminary evidence already exists; see doxorubicin, cyclosporine, gentamicin, and haloperidol later. Integrative oncological applications for ginkgo may include radiation sensitization as well as chemoprotection.[25] The role of ginkgo extracts in integrative oncological protocols is a new area of study.[5,26]

Pharmacokinetics

There are some pharmacokinetic data on ginkgo extracts in both animal models and humans. Bioavailability of both the triterpene lactones and flavonol glycosides is high, with figures up to eighty per cent for some ginkgolide fractions. The flavonol glycosides are rapidly absorbed, but are extensively metabolized in humans, whilst the terpenoids are excreted unchanged, with overall half-life of about six hours.[27-30] There is animal and human evidence that the extract constituents can cross the blood-brain barrier.[31-33] The ginkgo flavonoids quercitin, kaempferol, and isorhamnetin are themselves substrates of P-glycoprotein (P-gp).[34]

Effects on Drug Metabolism and Bioavailability

Until recently, the question of whether *Ginkgo biloba* extracts significantly affect drug-metabolizing systems had not been systematically investigated. Initial data from in vitro studies was typically inconclusive or conflicting, but results of more recent in vivo human trials now suggest minimal effects of the herb on cytochrome P450 (CYP450) activity.

Gurley et al.[35,36] studied the effects of ginkgo in both young adults and, interestingly, older populations (60-76 years) using the probe—drug cocktail methodology they helped establish as a standard technique for evaluating CYP450 induction and inhibition effects. They found no significant effects of ginkgo extracts on CYP450 1A2, 3A4, 2E1, or 2D6. This corroborates the previous results of Duche et al.,[37] as well as Markowitz et al.,[38] who found no in vivo effect of ginkgo on CYP2D6 or CYP3A4. A negative study with donepezil (Aricept) and ginkgo coadministration in human volunteers failed to find any effects of ginkgo on the pharmacokinetics of the cholinesterase inhibitor.[39] Donepezil is metabolized by 2D6 and 3A4 and is conjugated by uridine glucuronosyltransferase (UGT) enzymes. Two different trials with separate probe substrates have demonstrated a lack of effect on CYP2C9, the warfarin S-enantiomer—metabolizing enzyme.[40,41] This corroborates Jiang et al.,[24] who found a lack of pharmacokinetic interaction between warfarin and ginkgo[24] (see warfarin discussion later). A subsequent in vivo trial did detect effects of ginkgo administration on phenotyped variants of CYP2C19 using omeprazole as a substrate; however, this drug is also a potent inhibitor of 2C19, so the general applicability of these results is problematic.[42] At this stage, the possibility of 2C19 interactions remains to be corroborated.

Reliable case reports suggestive of pharmacokinetic interactions between ginkgo and prescription drugs mediated by CYP450 effects are unavailable. Meanwhile, in vitro studies on ginkgo and CYP450 using various models, including rodent and human hepatocytes as well as recombinant enzymes, continue to provide prospective data for in vivo investigations. however, the in vitro models do not correlate well with in vivo data.[43-47]

The issue of possible ginkgo effects on drug transporters has not been well studied to date. Absence of any observed effect of the herb on digoxin levels suggests a probable lack of effect on P-gp.[48] Certain ginkgo flavonoids such as quercitin and kaempferol, which are ubiquitous ingredients, have been shown to inhibit P-gp in vitro, as well as being substrates for P-gp themselves.[49,50]

HERB-DRUG INTERACTIONS

Anesthesia, General

Anesthesia, General

Interaction Type and Significance

? **Interaction Likely but Uncertain Occurrence and Unclear Implications**

Probability:
6. Unknown

Evidence Base:
☐ **Inadequate**

Effect and Mechanism of Action

Anesthetic-induced sleeping time may be altered by pretreatment with ginkgo. The mechanism of action is unknown.

Research

Ginkgo leaf extracts are known to cross the physiological intact blood-brain barrier (BBB) in a rodent model. A shortening effect on narcosis-induced sleeping times was demonstrated when a single intraperitoneal dose of EGb 761 at 25 and 50 mg/kg body weight or ginkgolide B at 1 and 5 mg/kg was administered before sodium barbital—induced narcosis.[31] Ginkgolide A was ineffective. A similar study also found shortening of sleeping time after intraperitoneal administration of hexobarbital, α-chloralose, and urethane in mice.[32] However, these researchers found that ginkgolide A isolate and bilobalide isolate could reproduce the shortening effects of the whole-leaf extract. A human study using quantitative electroencephalographic (EEG) data established that a single 240-mg dose of EGb 761 induced a significant increase in EEG activity 3 hours later, corresponding to that associated with "cognitive activator drugs." This suggests effective penetration of the human BBB.[33]

Clinical Implications and Adaptations

In the absence of reports, and given the small number of rodent studies, this interaction cannot be characterized clearly at this time. The pharmacological evidence for a mechanism is circumstantial, but the prospect that EGb 761 extracts may cross the intact BBB and interact with medications affecting neurotransmission is finite. More research is required to understand the effects of ginkgo extracts on increasing brain activity in opposition to anesthesia.

Given the additional possibility of antiplatelet effects on primary hemostasis during surgical procedure (see surgery), elective surgery patients should be carefully questioned regarding disclosure of self-administered herb use and advised to refrain from ginkgo consumption before surgery, to prevent possible interactions with anesthetics.

Antiplatelet Thromboprophylactics

Acetylsalicylic acid (acetosal, acetyl salicylic acid, ASA, salicyl-salicylic acid; Arthritis Foundation Pain Reliever, Ascriptin, Aspergum, Asprimox, Bayer Aspirin, Bayer Buffered Aspirin, Bayer Low Adult Strength, Bufferin, Buffex, Cama Arthritis Pain Reliever, Easprin, Ecotrin, Ecotrin Low Adult Strength, Empirin, Extra Strength Adprin-B, Extra Strength Bayer Enteric 500 Aspirin, Extra Strength Bayer Plus, Halfprin 81, Heartline, Regular Strength Bayer Enteric 500 Aspirin, St. Joseph Adult Chewable Aspirin, ZORprin); combination drugs: ASA and caffeine (Anacin); ASA, caffeine, and propoxyphene (Darvon Compound); ASA and carisoprodol (Soma Compound); ASA, codeine, and carisoprodol (Soma Compound with Codeine); ASA and codeine (Empirin with Codeine); ASA, codeine, butalbital, and caffeine (Fiorinal).

Clopidogrel (Plavix), Ticlopidine (Ticlid)

Extrapolated, based on similar properties: Cilostazol (Pletal), dipyridamole (Permole, Persantine); combination drug: ASA and extended-release dipyridamole (Aggrenox, Asasantin).

Interaction Type and Significance

✗ **Potential or Theoretical Adverse Interaction of Uncertain Severity**

Probability: Evidence Base:
3. Possible   ▽ **Mixed**

Effect and Mechanism of Action

A theoretical pharmacodynamic convergence exists between the inhibitory effects of ginkgo leaf dry extracts on platelet aggregation and the antiplatelet effects of drugs affecting primary hemostasis at the platelet level. The significance of the interaction is unknown but appears to be both overstated and controversial. It may also be regarded as a "contraindication" rather than an interaction, depending on circumstances.

The presumed mechanism is a suggested convergence on platelet disabling by various pathways. Acetylsalicylic acid (aspirin/ASA) is a well-documented antiplatelet agent acting through inhibition of cyclooxygenase production of thromboxane A_2 (TXA_2). Ticlopidine (Ticlid) interacts with glycoprotein IIb/IIIa to inhibit fibrinogen binding to activated platelets and has been used to prevent thrombosis when aspirin is poorly tolerated. After reports of hematological adverse effects associated with ticlopidine, clopidogrel (Plavix) is currently the preferred antiplatelet agent in such cases. As with ticlopidine, clopidogrel is an irreversible antiplatelet drug operating through adenosine diphosphate (ADP) receptor antagonism.

Research

Experimental evidence indicates that the components of ginkgo leaf extract can cause in vitro and ex vivo inhibition of platelet aggregation, probably through several mechanisms. These include increase in endogenous aggregation inhibitors such as nitric oxide (NO) and prostaglandin I_2 (PGI_2), as well as direct inhibition of PAF.[51] However, the evidence for clinically significant effects of ginkgo extracts on platelet aggregation in humans is not available. In fact, Koch[52] showed that the concentrations of ginkgolides required to inhibit human (vs. rabbit) aggregation induced by PAF were more than 100 times greater than the levels demonstrated by pharmacokinetic measurements in humans after normal dosing at 120 to 240 mg EGb 761 daily. In other words, inhibition of PAF (itself a weak aggregatory factor) requires such high concentrations of ginkgolides that clinical effects of ginkgo consumption on platelet aggregation mediated by PAF seem improbable.

Preclinical investigations by European manufacturers of their ginkgo leaf extracts, as part of the toxicological and related regulatory requirements for medicinal product licensing, have been accessed and reported indirectly by DeFeudis[5] and in the 2003 *American Herbal Pharmacopoeia* monograph of the dry extract.[4] Unpublished preclinical studies by Schwabe apparently failed to find any effect of EGb 761 on bleed times at 240 mg/day for 7 days in healthy volunteers, either alone or in combination with acetyl salicylate. The Beaufort-IPSEN-Pharma group sponsored a double-blind trial with 32 healthy volunteers and found no effect on bleed time or other hemostatic parameters after administration of 120 to 480 mg/day for 2 weeks.

A small preclinical study in France administered EGb at three dose levels (120, 240, and 480 mg/day) to 23 normal males for 2 weeks and found no effect on platelet function or coagulation.[23] Another study with healthy volunteers examined the effect of ginkgo extract administration on peripheral microcirculation in normal volunteers with a variety of red blood cell (RBC) and platelet parameters. No effect on platelet aggregation was noted, but a significant increase in RBC aggregation was found.[53] A study with 50 healthy volunteers found no significant effects on coagulation or clotting parameters after 240 mg/day EGb 761 versus placebo for 7 days in a crossover design trial.[22] The same study group continued the investigation into a second phase using the same subjects and assays and found no discernible effect of ginkgo when combined with aspirin, this time versus ASA alone in the same crossover design.

A brief report compared the arterial antithrombotic effect of EGb 761 and aspirin in an animal model using laser-induced emboli. Both aspirin and EGb 761 pretreatment reduced the number and duration of emboli compared with controls. They were not significantly different from each other in antiembolic effect.[54] A rodent study found a potentiation of the effect of ticlopidine by coadministering ginkgo in thrombosis-induced rats, such that 50 mg/kg ticlopidine with 40 mg/kg oral ginkgo was equivalent to 200 mg/kg ticlopidine in inhibition of ADP-dependent platelet aggregation.[55]

Jiang et al.[24] conducted an open-label trial (12 healthy male volunteers) and examined a range of pharmacokinetic and hemostasis parameters after administration of ginger or ginkgo, alone or with warfarin (see later section). Aggregation, international normalized ratio (INR), warfarin enantiomer concentrations in plasma and urine, and warfarin enantiomer binding were all measured at day 1 and day 7. The dose of ginkgo was two tablets of EGb 761 standardized 24/6 three times daily for 1 week. Ginkgo had no significant effect on clotting status or the pharmacokinetics and pharmacodynamics of warfarin.

Reports

Only one report of bleeding associated with aspirin and ginkgo concurrent administration is available. A case of hyphema (retinal bleed) reported in a 70-year-old man with a history of coronary bypass and 3 years of aspirin use at 325 mg/day. One week after commencing standardized ginkgo at 40 mg twice daily, he had a spontaneous bleed in the anterior chamber of the right eye. This resolved on cessation of ginkgo, and there was no recurrence after cessation.[17] This case was classified as a "possible" interaction by Fugh-Berman and Ernst.[20]

Although not involving aspirin, in a related report a 71-year-old man in Germany had taken 40 mg ginkgo extract twice daily for 30 months and started to take 600 mg ibuprofen daily for osteoarthritic pain. After 4 weeks of concurrent use, the patient was found comatose and died the next day from a massive intracerebral bleed. The authors suggest that TXA_2-dependent platelet aggregation was inhibited by the ibuprofen, and that this combined with the antiplatelet effect of ginkgo. Concurrent medications were not recorded.[56]

Integrative Therapeutics, Clinical Concerns, and Adaptations

The frequent suggestions in both professional and consumer literature that the ginkgo-aspirin combination is responsible for significant incidence of major hemorrhagic adverse events are unsubstantiated at this time. A single report and the failure to demonstrate any effects of the combination on bleed times in preclinical studies suggest that potential clinical problems associated with interaction are considerably overstated. Recent trial evidence demonstrating no effects of EGb 761 alone on hemostasis in healthy volunteers suggests that the potential interaction should probably be reclassified as "speculative."[22] However, pending large-scale trials, prudence may warrant a degree of caution.

The mechanism of prophylaxis of cerebrovascular accident (CVA, stroke) by antiplatelet agents is poorly understood. Certain individuals may exhibit "aspirin resistance",[57,58] one study suggested the incidence may be as high as 40%.[59] Also, any prophylactic benefit of aspirin may be caused by secondary rather than primary mechanisms, because hyperactivity of the anucleated platelet is predetermined to a degree at the megakaryocyte level during hematopoiesis.[60,61]

Given the favorable profile of ginkgo extract effects on ischemic reperfusion injury, as well as the demonstrated neuroprotective and neuroreparative properties, there is a supportable argument for the benefits of ginkgo leaf extract as a prophylactic for stroke in *healthy* elderly populations. For those subpopulations with definite indications for prophylactic ASA administration, the combination with ginkgo is unlikely to disrupt hemostasis and may permit the lower dose range of aspirin to be administered, thereby reducing the incidence and severity of gastric mucosal damage. Definitive consensus on the dose of ASA required for effective thromboprophylaxis is not available, but the lower dose of 75 mg/day may suffice in combination with concurrent ginkgo extract use, with less potential gastric mucosal irritation and damage than the higher doses of ASA monotherapy.[62,63] Recent epidemiological evidence suggests that the 75-mg dose of ASA is responsible for the largest number of drug/adverse drug reaction (ADR)–related hospital admissions in the United Kingdom.[64] In this light, the recent (animal) evidence that ginkgo exerts ulceroprotective and cytoprotective effects against inflammation and duodenal ulcers is particularly relevant.[65,66]

Cisplatin and Related Platinum Chemotherapy Compounds

Evidence: Cisplatin (*cis*-diaminedichloroplatinum, CDDP; Platinol, Platinol-AQ).
Extrapolated, based on similar properties: Carboplatin (Paraplatin), oxaliplatin (Eloxatin).

Interaction Type and Significance

⊕⊕ **Beneficial or Supportive Interaction, with Professional Management**
☼ **Prevention or Reduction of Drug Adverse Effect**

Probability:
4. Plausible

Evidence Base:
○ **Preliminary**

Effect and Mechanism of Action

Platinum compounds have well-documented neurological and renal toxicities. Pretreatment, coadministration, and posttreatment use of ginkgo extracts with platinum chemotherapy may exert protection against drug toxicities. The interaction is unsupported by human evidence.

Research

Two preliminary experimental studies have investigated whether the established neuroprotective and renal-protective properties of ginkgo might be active against platinum toxicity. One rodent study demonstrated that pretreatment with ginkgo reduced cisplatin ototoxicity, as measured by compound action potential–determined auditory threshold and reduced hair cell damage on scanning electron microscopy, compared with cisplatin alone. Blood urea nitrogen (BUN) and creatinine levels were also lower in the pretreatment group, and histological renal damage was lower than in the nonginkgo group. Finally, rates of tumor growth were unaffected by ginkgo-pretreatment versus cisplatin-alone animals inoculated with squamous cell carcinoma SCC-158 line.[67] Another study examined the effects of coadministration (rather than pretreatment) with ginkgo and cisplatin in mice. Sensory nerve conduction velocity and the growth of dorsal root ganglia neurons in culture were superior in the ginkgo coadministration group.[68]

Integrative Therapeutics, Clinical Concerns, and Adaptations

In both animal studies, oral ginkgo dose was moderately high, approximately 100 mg/kg. Assuming known interspecies pharmacokinetic scaling algorithms, this is approximately equivalent to a daily human dose of 1000 mg, which is higher than the normal therapeutic range for ginkgo extracts. However, acute toxicity of ginkgo is low, and the interaction is plausible. Thrombocytopenia should be monitored because the antiplatelet effects of high doses of ginkgo have not been studied. However, human studies are needed to determine the effectiveness of ginkgo against platinum-induced toxicity.

Cyclosporine

Cyclosporine (Ciclosporin, cyclosporin A, CsA; Neoral, Sandimmune, SangCya).

Interaction Type and Significance

⊕⊕ **Beneficial or Supportive Interaction, with Professional Management**
☼ **Prevention or Reduction of Drug Adverse Effect**

Probability:
4. Plausible

Evidence Base:
○ **Preliminary**

Effect and Mechanism of Action

Nephrotoxicity is the principal adverse effect of cyclosporine. Ginkgo may significantly ameliorate cyclosporine-induced nephrotoxicity. In addition, acute rejection responses in cyclosporine-immunosuppressed patients may lead to ischemic damage to the graft organ. Ginkgo offers an additional degree of protection from such damage, which is also mediated in part through PAF.

Research

Cyclosporine is known to increase PAF. Rodent studies with ginkgolide B in cyclosporine-immunosuppressed animals have shown that the hemodynamic renal damage induced by the drug can be reversed by BN 52021 administration.[69] A rodent study of skin allograft in mice found that whole-leaf ginkgo extract could reproduce the effect of BN 52021 in prolonging allograft survival, although the effect was less than with the ginkgolide B isolate.[70] Animal studies have also suggested a protective effective for cardiac allografts and against cardiac ischemic-reperfusion injury.[71,72] A Japanese in vitro study of the interaction between cyclosporine and BN 52021 in human monocytes from asthma patients suggested that the two agents may be synergistic in reducing inflammatory cytokine production.[73] Another in vitro study, using human liver microsomes, found that EGb 761 abolished cyclosporine-induced lipid peroxidation.[74]

A double-blind pilot study ($n = 20$) examined the effects of pretreatment with BN 52021 both in renal graft donors before harvesting and in recipients before grafting, versus placebo. Immunosuppression was with cyclosporine and prednisone. Posttransplant renal failure was 33% in the placebo group and 0% in the BN 52021 group, who also had better serum creatinine values after transplantation than the controls.[75]

Integrative Therapeutics, Clinical Concerns, and Adaptations

The pharmacological data, although mostly experimental, suggest several potential benefits from the concurrent administration of ginkgo with cyclosporine in immunosuppressed graft patients. The mechanisms underlying improved graft survival and protection against ischemic-reperfusion injury are likely multifactorial. Renal graft patients must confront the paradox that cyclosporine, as well as tacrolimus, is nephrotoxic. Naturopathic physicians and other practitioners of botanical medicine have incorporated ginkgo, along with related renal-protective herbs, into protocols for protective support of renal graft patients.[76] Cyclosporine being a substrate of CYP3A4 should not cause concern in that the pharmacokinetic effects of ginkgo on this enzyme are not considered significant.[36,37] This infrequently discussed interaction could be of great potential value to renal allograft patients, whether using cyclosporine or unrelated immunosuppressants.[77] On a cautionary note, one transplant team reported undisclosed use of ginkgo as being responsible for postoperative bleeding after a hepatic transplant.[13]

Doxorubicin and Related Anthracycline Chemotherapy

Evidence: Doxorubicin (Adriamycin, Rubex).
Extrapolated, based on similar properties: Daunorubicin (Cerubidine), epirubicin (Ellence, Pharmorubicin), idarubicin (Idamycin, Zavedos), mitoxantrone (Novantrone, Onkotrone). Similar properties but evidence lacking for extrapolation: Daunorubicin, liposomal (DaunoXome); doxorubicin, pegylated liposomal (Caelyx, Doxil, Myocet).

Interaction Type and Significance

⊕ **Potential or Theoretical Beneficial or Supportive Interaction, with Professional Management**
☼ **Prevention or Reduction of Drug Adverse Effect**

Probability:
4. Plausible

Evidence Base:
○ **Preliminary**

Effect and Mechanism of Action

Doxorubicin is known to induce dose-related cumulative cardiotoxicity (short term and long term). This may be reduced by concurrent ginkgo administration.

Research

Few studies have directly examined the possibility that ginkgo and its constituents may ameliorate anthracycline-associated cardiopathy. One rodent study examined the effects of concurrent EGb 761 and doxorubicin administration in mice, one group of which was also pretreated with ginkgo before induction of gastric tumors with benzo(a)pyrene. The ginkgo-pretreated animals had a lower tumor incidence and had higher hepatic glutathione and glutathione-S-transferase levels. Concurrent doxorubicin and oral EGb 761 did not additively increase the antitumor effect, compared with doxorubicin alone, but reduced cardiotoxic markers, both histological damage and lipid peroxidation levels.[78] Another study examined the effects of EGb 761 on various parameters of doxorubicin cardiotoxicity in otherwise-normal animals. The EGb-treated animals had significantly lower mortality, ascites, myocardial lipid peroxidation, normalization of antioxidant enzymes, reversal of electrocardiographic (ECG) changes, and minimal ultrastructural damage of the heart, compared with doxorubicin alone.[15] In unrelated studies, ginkgo has been shown to ameliorate the adverse effects of bleomycin.[79,80] Antioxidant protectant effects have also been shown for other drugs, including acetaminophen and vancomycin.[81,82]

Integrative Therapeutics, Clinical Concerns, and Adaptations

Doxorubicin is one of the most widely used antineoplastic agents, but its effectiveness is limited by well-documented cardiotoxic adverse effects, which can manifest decades after cessation of treatment.[83] The pathogenetic mechanisms of anthracycline cardiotoxicity are not fully understood, although the ultimate clinical presentation is indistinguishable from typical congestive heart failure. Although an early toxicity may be observed, shortly after commencement of administration (especially in elderly patients), the symptoms of progressive heart failure can appear months or even years after conclusion of the treatment, and the cardiomyopathy initially may be quite asymptomatic. Several possible cardiac protection agents have been examined, but none has been found effective, including vitamin E and N-acetyl cysteine. The iron-chelating agent dexrazoxane (Zinecard) reduces cardiotoxicity but has been associated with possible reduction in antitumor effects; part of the doxorubicin toxicity may be caused by FeII-dox-complex free-radical formation.[84]

Based on the preliminary animal evidence, and considering the known pharmacology of ginkgo, patients receiving doxorubicin may benefit from a cardioprotection protocol incorporating ginkgo extracts, together with related herbal agents such as hawthorn and nutritional supplements such as coenzyme Q10 and acetyl-carnitine. Further studies are required to examine the potential benefits of this interaction.

Fluorouracil

Fluorouracil (5-FU; Adrucil, Efudex, Efudix, Fluoroplex).

Interaction Type and Significance

?   Interaction Possible but Uncertain Occurrence and Unclear Implications

Probability:
6. Unknown

Evidence Base:
□ **Inadequate**

Effect and Mechanism of Action

A possible effect of EGb 761 on fluorouracil administration in combination with immediate ginkgo pretreatment has been proposed. This may enhance distribution of the chemotherapeutic agent to tumor sites and reduce side effects.

Research

Ginkgo and 5-FU have been concomitantly administered on colorectal patients[85] and pancreatic cancer patients.[86] These studies used a parenteral preparation (EGb 761 ONC) as a 30-minute intravenous-push pretreatment before administration of 5-FU (500 mg/m^2/day) for 6 days. These were effectively phase II trials. No adverse effects of the combination were noted, and some improvement was recorded in two patients, with a cessation of cancer progression in several who had previously failed the 5-FU. Quality-of-life parameters and median survival times were not altered. The authors suggest further combination investigation may be warranted. The present studies suggest that the combination is safe and does not lead to increased toxicity.

Integrative Therapeutics, Clinical Concerns, and Adaptations

Although the data are preliminary, corresponding to a phase II trial, the effects of ginkgo extracts as a combination agent in chemotherapy not only have the potential to ameliorate drug-induced toxicities (see Doxorubicin), but also may have anticancer effects. This is a promising topic for integrative oncology that requires research and clinical investigation.[87]

Fluoxetine and Related Selective Serotonin Reuptake Inhibitor (SSRI) Antidepressants

Evidence: Fluoxetine (Prozac).
Extrapolated, based on similar properties: Citalopram (Celexa), escitalopram (S-citalopram; Lexapro), fluoxetine (Prozac, Sarafem), fluvoxamine (Faurin, Luvox), paroxetine (Aropax, Deroxat, Paxil, Seroxat), sertraline (Zoloft).
Similar properties but evidence lacking for extrapolation: Serotonin-norepinephrine reuptake inhibitor (SSRI/SNRI) antidepressants: Duloxetine (Cymbalta), venlafaxine (Effexor).

Interaction Type and Significance

⊕⊕ **Beneficial or Supportive Interaction, with Professional Management**
☼ **Prevention or Reduction of Drug Adverse Effect**

Probability:　　　　　　Evidence Base:
3. Possible　　　　　　∇ **Mixed**

Effect and Mechanism of Action

Sexual dysfunction is a well-documented adverse effect of SSRI antidepressant therapy. Ginkgo leaf extract may be useful in ameliorating such adverse effects by various mechanisms, including NO-dependent vasorelaxation.

Research

A small number of studies have investigated this possible beneficial interaction, but the evidence is mixed. In a negative study, Kang et al.[88] found an unusually large placebo effect in a 2-month double-blind randomized controlled trial of SSRI-induced sexual dysfunction after ginkgo administration in increasing doses up to 240 mg/day for 8 weeks total. There was no difference between the EGb 761 and control groups, both reporting significant decrease in symptoms of dysfunction. An open trial of men and women using a variety of antidepressant medications with an unspecified ginkgo extract for 4 weeks at an average dose of 209 mg/day reported effectiveness in reducing SSRI-related symptoms, more so in women ($n = 33$) than men ($n = 30$).[89] The study was subsequently criticized for

methodological weaknesses and inadequate statistical analysis by more than one correspondent.[90,91] A small ($n = 22$), positive study by Ashton et al.[92] found a slight but incomplete reversal of SSRI-induced sexual dysfunction in men and women after higher-dose ginkgo administration, although the extract product details were not disclosed.

Report

A single case report exists of a woman taking fluoxetine who experienced relief from fluoxetine-induced genital anesthesia after concurrent administration of EGb 761, 180 to 240 mg/day for 2 weeks.[93]

Integrative Therapeutics, Clinical Concerns, and Adaptations

This interaction is plausible but cannot be regarded as firmly substantiated. However, the prevalence of SSRI-related sexual dysfunction and excellent safety and toxicological profile of ginkgo leaf extract, whether alone or in combination, may prompt integrative practitioners to conduct an empirical trial with affected patients. Circumstantial support for this approach derives from the known antidepressant effects of ginkgo and its general effectiveness in combination with a variety of antidepressant medications.[94]

Gentamicin and Related Aminoglycoside Antibiotics

Evidence: Gentamicin (G-mycin, Garamycin, Jenamicin), amikacin (Amikin).
Extrapolated, based on similar properties: Kanamycin (Kantrex), neomycin (Mycifradin, Myciguent, Neo-Fradin, NeoTab, Nivemycin), netilmicin (Netromycin), paromomycin (monomycin; Humatin), streptomycin, tobramycin (AKTob, Nebcin, TOBI, TOBI Solution, TobraDex, Tobrex).

Interaction Type and Significance

⊕ **Potential or Theoretical Beneficial or Supportive Interaction, with Professional Management**
☼ **Prevention or Reduction of Drug Adverse Effect**

Probability:　　　　　　Evidence Base:
3. Possible　　　　　　∇ **Mixed**

Effect and Mechanism of Action

Gentamicin and the aminoglycoside antimicrobials have well-documented adverse effects of ototoxicity and nephrotoxicity. Concurrent administration of ginkgo leaf extract may modulate these toxicities, through multiple mechanisms.

Research

The same researchers who examined protective effects of ginkgo leaf extract against Adriamycin-induced cardiotoxicity (see Doxorubicin) also performed a rodent study to investigate the effects of ginkgo on gentamicin-induced nephrotoxicity. After 2 days of pretreatment with EGb 761 (300 mg/kg op) and 8 days of concurrent administration with 80 mg/kg gentamicin, serum markers of kidney function and histopathology in Wistar rats demonstrated significant protective effects for the ginkgo-combination versus gentamicin-alone group.[95] Another animal study examined neurosensory cochlear damage induced by gentamicin using both electrosensory and histopathological criteria in guinea pigs. Pretreatment with ginkgo extract reduced the level of acute toxic changes.[96] However, in conflict with these studies, another rodent study of ototoxicity induced by the related aminoglycoside alizarin (amikacin, Amikin) suggested that ototoxicity may be increased by concurrent administration of EGb 761 and alizarin versus alizarin alone.[97]

Integrative Therapeutics, Clinical Concerns, and Adaptations

This potential interaction is an extrapolation from the known neuroprotective and neuroreparative effects of ginkgo extracts. Protection against the neurosensory toxicity and nephrotoxicity of gentamicin is a plausible beneficial interaction with some evidence from animal experiments, but clinical reports and studies are not available. The rodent studies are also open to methodological criticism, particularly the high dosage levels of EGb 761 used, which do not readily translate to normal human dose schedules for the extract.

Based on current data, concurrent administration of gentamicin or aminoglycoside and ginkgo cannot be recommended without qualification. However, if clinical symptoms of cochlear toxicity or vestibular toxicity persist after cessation of aminoglycoside therapy, subsequent ginkgo leaf extract administration likely would be beneficial in helping reverse the symptoms, although in some cases, certain forms of damage (i.e., to hair cells) may be irreversible. Nephrotoxicity caused by aminoglycosides is considered more reversible than ototoxicity, although the evidence from other forms of drug-induced nephrotoxicity would support the use by extrapolation of ginkgo leaf extract in this context. Until further data are available, firm clinical directions about this interaction are not possible.

Haloperidol and Related Antipsychotics

Evidence: Haloperidol (Haldol).
Similar properties but evidence lacking for extrapolation: Chlorpromazine (Largactil, Thorazine), clozapine (Clozaril), fluphenazine (Permitil, Prolixin, Prolixin Decanoate, Prolixin Enanthate), olanzapine (Zyprexa), prochlorperazine (Compazine, Stemetil), quetiapine (Seroquel), risperidone (Risperdal).

Interaction Type and Significance

⊕ **Potential or Theoretical Beneficial or Supportive Interaction, with Professional Management**
☼ **Prevention or Reduction of Drug Adverse Effect**

Probability:
4. Plausible

Evidence Base:
☐ **Inadequate**

Effect and Mechanism of Action

Haloperidol is a heterocyclic antipsychotic drug associated with adverse effects of akathisia and tardive dyskinesia common to the thorazine group of neuroleptics. A beneficial reduction in adverse effects and an increase in drug efficacy, possibly associated with antioxidant activity of the ginkgo extract, may take place with concomitant administration.

Research

A double-blind trial with refractory schizophrenia patients ($n = 109$) compared haloperidol, 25 mg/day, alone to the same dose of haloperidol with EGb 761, 360 mg/day, for 12 weeks. Both groups showed some improvement in psychobehavioral scores, although the ginkgo group improved more than the haloperidol-only group. Extrapyramidal symptoms were significantly reduced in the combination group.[98] In two related studies, the same authors repeated these findings and also measured the levels of superoxide dismutase (SOD) before and after treatment with the combination; SOD levels were maintained in the ginkgo group more than the controls. The improvements in psychobehavioral assessment scores were positively correlated with SOD levels.[99,100]

Integrative Therapeutics, Clinical Concerns, and Adaptations

The initial studies by one group of researchers provide an intriguing insight into the possible benefits of combining ginkgo with antipsychotic drugs. The prominent extrapyramidal adverse effects of these agents have long been a cause for concern, particularly during long-term neuroleptic administration, during which tardive dyskinesia symptoms may become irreversible. This has caused some controversy in psychiatric circles, with critics such as Breggin[101] and others suggesting that the *modus operandi* of the neuroleptics in psychotic patients is "brain disabling" by causing cellular damage at the neuronal level.

Although the newer neuroleptic drugs have less severe adverse effects than haloperidol and the thorazine-related heterocyclics, the problem remains significant. The possibility that the established neuroprotective and neuroreparative effects of ginkgo leaf extracts may minimize drug toxicity deserves further investigation. Until more data are available, this must be classed as a "theoretical but plausible" beneficial interaction.

Surgery

Surgery

Interaction Type and Significance

✗✗✗ **Potentially Harmful or Serious Adverse Interaction—Avoid**
⊕✗ **Biomodal or Variable Interaction, with Professional Management**
⊕ **Potential or Theoretical Beneficial or Supportive Interaction, with Professional Management**

Probability:
3. Possible

Evidence Base:
☐ **Inadequate**

Effect and Mechanism of Action

Perioperative administration of ginkgo leaf is suggested to increase the likelihood of surgery-related and postoperative bleeding. Ginkgo leaf concentrated extracts have inhibitory effects on platelet aggregation in vitro and ex vivo. Antiplatelet activity may operate not only through inhibition of PAF, but also through other aggregation inducers such as thrombin, ADP, collagen, and arachidonic acid. However, clinically significant in vivo antiplatelet effects have not been established in vivo.

Research

Epidemiological and survey data suggest that consumption of herbal and dietary supplements among preoperative patients is common.[11] Failure to disclose herbal medicine usage may be as high as 70% of patients.[10] Norred et al.[102] surveyed 500 elective surgery patients, of whom 51% used herbal and nutritional products in the 2 weeks before surgery. Of surveyed patients, 24% consumed 50 different herbs; classification by potential adverse effects revealed that 27% of surgical patients consumed natural pharmacological agents that may inhibit coagulation, affect blood pressure (12%), cause sedation (9%), have cardiac effects (5%), or alter electrolytes (4%). Direct studies of ginkgo use in the preoperative scenario are unavailable.

Reports

Several case reports of excessive postoperative bleeding are available, varying in quality from low to unassessable. Fessenden et al.[12] reported a case after laparoscopic cholecystectomy in a patient using an unidentified "gingko" (sic) peparation.[12] The patient was apparently also taking a "multivitamin," the ingredients of which were not disclosed.

The report is impossible to evaluate due to lack of information about the form and dose of the herb.

A report by Norred and Finlayson[103] of postsurgical bleeding following mastectomy after use of high doses of ginkgo extract (375 mg four times daily) involved polypharmacy and thus confounds simple interpretation. The patient was also taking vitamin E (800 IU/day for 10 years) and ginseng (300 mg four times daily for 6 weeks), along with bilberry, astragalus, and several prescription medications, although none that directly affects coagulation.[103] Although a typical "real life" scenario, the case report is difficult to evaluate, particularly the role of ginkgo extract in the adverse event.

Bebbington et al.[104] also reported a case of apparently persistent postoperative bleeding after a hip arthroplasty. The 77-year-old woman was concurrently taking aspirin and "simple anti-inflammatories." Allegation of ginkgo use (120 mg/day) was made by a relative, and the authors attribute the excessive bleeding to the herb. Given the concurrent use of ASA and unspecified anti-inflammatory medications, any single causal attribution seems unwarranted.

Destro et al.[105] report two similar histories of 50-year-old women undergoing plastic surgery who both experienced diffuse perioperative bleeding and subsequent bilateral hematoma after their rhytidoplasty and blepharoplasty procedures. Medical history, concurrent medications, and validation of ginkgo involvement were not given, although apparently both cases were "linked by chronic auto medication with a commercial extract of ginkgo."

Yagmur et al.[106] made a better-documented report of postoperative bleeding with thorough assessments of various coagulation parameters. A 75-year-old woman was taking an 80-mg/day dose of a commercial preparation for more than 1 year before an ambulatory procedure that was followed by extensive bleeding. Postoperative aggregation tests showed a decreased level of aggregation in response to collagen, although ADP, adrenaline, and ristocetin stimuli all resulted in normal aggregation. The patient discontinued the ginkgo postoperatively. Bleed times in response to collagen were reduced from 228 seconds to 168 seconds at 10 days after cessation of the ginkgo.

Clinical Implications and Adaptations

Dire warnings about the dangers of postoperative bleeding with concomitant use of ginkgo extracts are controversial. Norred and Brinker[107] noted that given the established reluctance of patients to disclose herbal medication usage, overzealous admonitions to "discontinue all herbs prior to surgery" may have the effect of further encouraging clandestine herb use by surgical patients, thus hindering patient communication and rapport and compromising patient safety.

Patient safety mandates a preoperative screening for herb-nutrient-drug interactions as a required element of admission. Ginkgo should be included in advisories to elective surgery patients about potential adverse effects of herbs and nutritional supplements on hemostasis, particularly older women undergoing plastic surgery involving ocular areas, based on the limited case reports. The potential interaction should be presented as a possibility that can be sensibly averted by avoiding ginkgo leaf extract consumption preoperatively. However, the stress-alleviating aspects of ginkgo could also be of therapeutic benefit in the postoperative period, and the acute stress of surgery may be ameliorated by ginkgo administration.[87,108]

Trazodone (Desyrel).

Interaction Type and Significance

? Interaction Likely but Uncertain Occurrence and Unclear Implications

Probability:	Evidence Base:
6. Unknown	☐ Inadequate

Effect and Mechanism of Action

Trazodone, an antidepressant 5-hydroxytryptamine (5-HT$_2$) receptor blocker, can cause heavy sedation at antidepressant doses of approximately 400 mg/day. Concurrent ginkgo use could potentiate sedation. The interaction cannot be considered established.

Report

An 80-year-old patient with Alzheimer's disease taking nonsedative doses (20 mg at night) of trazodone commenced ginkgo (form unspecified) at 80 mg twice daily. After 3 days the patient became comatose and was revived by 1 mg of intravenous flumazenil. Both the ginkgo and the trazodone were being used at low levels; concurrent medications were not disclosed. The authors suggest that because of the flumazenil response, benzodiazepine mechanisms were involved (since flumazenil is often used to reverse benzodiazepine-induced intoxication).[9] This single report is insufficient basis to consider the interaction between trazodone and ginkgo extract as established. From the known pharmacodynamics of trazodone, concurrent ginkgo must have been potentiating trazodone effects by at least twentyfold because the patient was taking a nonsedating dose. Some sources include this report under a heading of "possible interactions with benzodiazepines," which is also difficult to justify.[4]

Research

Current research data do not help elucidate the mechanism or likelihood of this interaction. In vitro effects on neuronal transmission and activity remain poorly understood and are undoubtedly complex, as well as unknown in vivo.[109,110] Also, the antidoting mechanism of flumazenil and its principal active metabolite 1-methyl-chlorophenyl-piperazine (mCPP) on benzodiazepines is not fully understood, although it may be independent of the benzodiazepine site.[111] Extrapolations from the available data to support the interaction report are speculative.

Clinical Implications and Adaptations

These are unclear at this time. For older patients (> 75 years) using central nervous system drugs, cautious commencement of ginkgo administration would be prudent. Titration of ginkgo dose toward the desired end-dose range can be made gradually over weeks while monitoring for adverse effects.

Evidence: Warfarin (Coumadin, Marevan, Warfilone).
Extrapolated, based on similar properties: Anisindione (Miradon), dicumarol, ethyl biscoumacetate (Tromexan), nicoumalone (acenocoumarol; Acitrom, Sintrom), phenindione (Dindevan), phenprocoumon (Jarsin, Marcumar).

Interaction Type and Significance

✗ Potential or Theoretical Adverse Interaction of Uncertain Severity—Avoid

Probability: Evidence Base:
3. Possible   ▽ **Mixed**

Effect and Mechanism of Action

Theoretical pharmacodynamic convergence occurs between the inhibitory effects of ginkgo leaf dry extracts on platelet aggregation and the hypoprothrombinemic effects of warfarin. The interaction is theorized to increase overall risk of bleeding, although no compelling evidence exists for the clinical occurrence of the interaction, and a single isolated report is contradicted by limited available trial evidence, which suggests the risk may be overstated.

Research

Experimental evidence indicates that the components of ginkgo leaf extract can cause in vitro and ex vivo inhibition of platelet aggregation, probably through several mechanisms, including increase in endogenous aggregation inhibitors such as NO and PGI_2, as well as direct inhibition of PAF.[51] However, the evidence for clinically significant effects of ginkgo extracts on platelet aggregation in humans is mixed.

As discussed under Clopidogrel, preclinical investigations by European manufacturers of their ginkgo leaf extracts for medicinal product licensing have been reviewed by DeFeudis[5] and in the *American Herbal Pharmacopoeia* monograph.[4] Schwabe (the German producers of EGb 761) failed to find any effect on bleed times at 240 mg EGb 761 daily for 7 days in healthy volunteers, either alone or in combination with acetyl salicylate. The Beaufort-IPSEN-Pharma group's double-blind trial with 32 healthy volunteers found no effect on bleed time or other hemostatic parameters after 2 weeks of 120 to 480 mg/day.

In the French study cited earlier (see Clopidogrel), EGb at 120, 240, or 480 mg/day in 23 normal males for 2 weeks had no effect on platelet function or coagulation.[23] A trial of 50 healthy volunteers found no significant effect of ginkgo on clotting and bleed time parameters when administered alone for 7 days, versus placebo in a crossover design.[22] Another study with healthy volunteers examined the effect of ginkgo extract on peripheral microcirculation and found no effect on platelet aggregation but a significant increase in RBC aggregation.[53]

A small clinical study examined the effects of ginkgo on INR in warfarin-anticoagulated patients. The small crossover trial examined the effects of ginkgo leaf dry extract (100 mg/day orally) and coenzyme Q10 on INR values in 14 outpatients (average age, 64.5 years) maintained on warfarin anticoagulation. INR was not affected, and the mean warfarin dose remained unchanged.[112]

Also as previously discussed, Jiang et al.[24] conducted a open-label trial with 12 healthy male volunteers and examined pharmacokinetic and hemostasis parameters after administration of ginger or ginkgo, alone or with warfarin. Aggregation, INR, warfarin enantiomer concentrations in plasma and urine, and warfarin enantiomer binding were measured at days 1 and 7. The ginkgo dose was two tablets of EGb761 standardized 24/6 three times daily for 1 week. Neither ginger nor ginkgo produced any significant effect on clotting status or on the pharmacokinetics and pharmacodynamics of warfarin.

Report

A single report is available that associates concurrent warfarin and ginkgo use with intracerebral hemorrhage. A 78-year-old woman with a history of dementia, myocardial infarction,

hypertension, and atrial fibrillation had used warfarin for 5 years since a coronary bypass procedure. She also had a pacemaker. Sudden-onset apraxia was followed by a computed tomography (CT)–based diagnosis of left parietal hemorrhage; her prothrombin time (PT) was 16.9 and partial thromboplastin time (PTT) 35.5. Ginkgo use was discovered (dose, form, and regimen unstated) for the preceding 2 months. Anticoagulation reversed after cessation of warfarin and ginkgo, without vitamin K administration; however, the patient remained apraxic.[113] Fugh-Berman and Ernst[20] characterized this case as "possible," but a single-point score above "unevaluable."

Clinical Implications and Adaptations

The 4-hydroxycoumarin compound warfarin is the most widely used anticoagulant drug in the Western world. It is known for a high variability in interindividual and intraindividual response. The primary individual factors affecting response variability are age and polymorphisms of CYP450 2C9.[114] The incidence of warfarin-related bleeding complications is difficult to estimate because of methodological issues surrounding data collection and interpretation. Recent calculations suggest that improved anticoagulation control has reduced the serious ADR category of "major bleeds, non-fatal" incidence to approximately 2.5% to 8.0%, with a "minor bleed" incidence of about 15% per year. Fatal bleed estimates vary from 1% to 4.8% annually.[63] Warfarin interacts with a wide range of drugs, including antibiotics, central nervous system agents, and cardiac drugs, as well as dietary substances, many of which increase anticoagulation.[115]

All this confounds the already-complex situation of determining the medical appropriateness, form, and level of anticoagulation, especially in older individuals with multiple risk factors for bleeding, such as unstable INR, comorbidities (especially bleeding related), polypharmacy (especially with NSAIDs), advanced age, and difficulty in compliance with requirements of coagulation control.

From an integrative perspective, the patient populations who might benefit most from the neuroprotective and anti-ischemic effects of ginkgo, such as older (>75 years) individuals with a history of dementia or cerebral ischemia, are also much more likely to be anticoagulated with warfarin.[116] Because no way currently exists to identify those who might be at risk of a ginkgo-induced adverse event, let alone a warfarin-ginkgo interaction, integrative practitioners are arguably confronted by a more complex choice than their conventional care counterparts. This includes whether to switch to different forms of antithrombotic therapy, including strategies based on natural agents such as garlic and nattokinase, to gain benefits from ginkgo administration against possible ischemic damage. (Use of warfarin alternatives is normally restricted to those who have a demonstrated intolerance for the drug.) A case-by-case evaluation, coupled with vigilant monitoring, is essential. Recently available laboratory tests that examine genetic parameters of hypercoagulability, as well as soluble fibrin monomer and dimer, can provide useful information in this regard.

THEORETICAL, SPECULATIVE, AND PRELIMINARY INTERACTIONS RESEARCH, INCLUDING OVERSTATED INTERACTIONS CLAIMS

Anticonvulsant Medications

Carbamazepine (Carbatrol, Tegretol), clonazepam (Klonopin), clorazepate (Tranxene), divalproex semisodium, divalproex sodium (Depakote), ethosuximide (Zarontin), ethotoin (Peganone), felbamate (Felbatol), fosphenytoin (Cerebyx, Mesantoin), levetiracetam (Keppra), mephenytoin, mephobarbital (Mebaral), methsuximide (Celontin), oxcarbazepine (GP 47680, oxycarbamazepine; Trileptal), phenobarbital (phenobarbitone; Luminal, Solfoton), phenytoin (diphenylhydantoin; Dilantin, Phenytek), piracetam (Nootropyl), primidone (Mysoline), sodium valproate (Depacon), topiramate (Topamax), trimethadione (Tridione), valproate semisodium, valproic acid (Depakene, Depakene Syrup), vigabatrin (Sabril), zonisamide (Zonegran).

Some secondary reviewers recommend avoidance of ginkgo with anticonvulsants because of the presence of a "neurotoxin" in the seed and the extracts.[117,118] This refers to a specific anti–vitamin B_6 compound, 4'-O-methylpyridoxine (MPN), present only in the seeds and thought to be responsible for causing convulsions after intoxication following seed (nut) consumption in China and Japan.[119] Levels of MPN in ginkgo leaf (1-5 µg per leaf) are much lower than in seed (80 µg per seed), and neurotoxic effects, including convulsions, occur at oral levels of 11 mg/kg (LD_{50} of 50 mg/kg) in guinea pigs. The amount of MPN in a typical human therapeutic daily dose of EGb 761 would be about 10 to 50 µg/day, suggesting that intoxication and interaction are unlikely.[4] Van Beek has reviewed MPN toxicity in depth.[6] Clinical reports of MPN intoxication from ginkgo leaf consumption are absent. A recent speculative case report alleging fatal ginkgo-induced seizures, possibly from MPN intoxication or pharmacokinetic interaction with valproate and phenytoin, was unreliable. The authors failed even to confirm the use of the herb, much less mention dose, frequency of administration, and so on, while including comments about ginkgo nut toxicity and suggesting unproven pharmacokinetic interactions with anticonvulsants through CYP450 2C9 induction.[120]

Monoamine Oxidase (MAO) Inhibitors

MAO-A inhibitors: Isocarboxazid (Marplan), moclobemide (Aurorix, Manerix), phenelzine (Nardil), procarbazine (Matulane), tranylcypromine (Parnate).
MAO-B inhibitors: Selegiline (deprenyl, L-deprenil, L-deprenyl; Atapryl, Carbex, Eldepryl, Jumex, Movergan, Selpak); pargyline (Eutonyl), rasagiline (Azilect).

Evidence from in vitro and ex vivo rodent studies on MAO-A and MAO-B inhibitory activity does not suggest central MAO inhibition by ginkgo. A human study using radiolabeled l-deprenyl and clorgyline (which inactivate MAO-A and -B isoforms, respectively) after 1 month of pretreatment with 60 mg EGb 761 twice daily in 10 normal subjects showed no effect on MAO activity in any brain region imaged by positron emission tomography (PET).[121] Peripheral MAO inhibition is not precluded by these studies.

Oral Hypoglycemic Agents and Insulin

Buformin (Andromaco Gliporal, Buformina), chlorpropamide (Diabinese), glimepiride (Amaryl), glipizide (Glucotrol, Glucotrol XL), glyburide (glibenclamide; Diabeta, Glynase, Glynase Prestab, Micronase, Pres Tab), insulin (animal-source insulin: Iletin; human analog insulin: Humanlog; human insulin: Humulin, Novolin, NovoRapid, Oralin), metformin (Dianben, Glucophage, Glucophage XR); combination

drugs: glipizide and metformin (Metaglip), glyburide and metformin (Glucovance); phenformin (Debeone, Fenformin), tolazamide (Tolinase), tolbutamide (Orinase, Tol-Tab).

Data are conflicting on the possible effects of ginkgo on pancreatic beta-cell activity, as well as on oral hypoglycemic agents. In a study on the effects of EGb 761 in patients with non-insulin-dependent diabetes mellitus (NIDDM, diet and medication controlled), Kudolo[122] suggests that hyperinsulinemic (insulin-resistant) patients should avoid EGb 761 because of an increase in insulin level on an oral glucose tolerance test (OGTT). Kudolo et al.[123] performed a later study that found no effect of EGb 761 on pancreatic beta-cell activity. A Japanese group performed several rodent studies that suggest possible biphasic effects of ginkgo extracts on 2C9, the p450 enzyme that metabolizes sulfonylurea and "glitazone" oral hypoglycemic agents.[46,124] The relevance of these data to humans is unknown. Suggestions of clinically significant interactions between oral hypoglycemics and ginkgo extracts are not warranted by the available data at this time.

Thiazide Diuretics

Bendroflumethiazide (bendrofluazide; Naturetin), combination drug: bendrofluazide and propranolol (Inderex); benzthiazide (Exna), chlorothiazide (Diuril), chlorthalidone (Hygroton), cyclopenthiazide (Navidrex), combination drug: cyclopenthiazide and oxprenolol hydrochloride (Trasidrex); hydrochlorothiazide (Aquazide, Esidrix, Ezide, Hydrocot, HydroDiuril, Microzide, Oretic); combination drugs: hydrochlorothiazide and amiloride (Moduretic); hydrochlorothiazide and captopril (Acezide, Capto-Co, Captozide, Co-Zidocapt); hydrochlorothiazide and enalapril (Vaseretic); hydrochlorothiazide and lisinopril (Prinzide, Zestoretic); hydrochlorothiazide and losartan (Hyzaar); hydrochlorothiazide and metoprolol (Lopressor HCT); hydrochlorothiazide and spironolactone (Aldactazide); hydrochlorothiazide and triamterene (Dyazide, Maxzide); hydroflumethiazide (Diucardin), methyclothiazide (Enduron), metolazone (Zaroxolyn, Mykrox), polythiazide (Renese), quinethazone (Hydromox), trichlormethiazide (Naqua).

A paradoxical report in a secondary source suggests that a hypertensive patient receiving a thiazide diuretic took ginkgo (unspecified) and experienced a rise in blood pressure, which was reversed only by cessation of both agents.[125] Given the vasorelaxant effects of ginkgo extracts, this interaction appears improbable, and the report is not reinforced by any other data at this time.

The 125 citations for this monograph are located under Ginkgo on the CD at the back of the book.

Ginseng

Botanical Name: *Panax ginseng* C.A. Meyer.
Pharmacopoeial Name: Radix ginseng.
Synonym: *Panax ginseng* T. Nees.
Common Names: Ginseng, Korean ginseng, Chinese ginseng, Asian or Oriental ginseng.

SUMMARY

Drug/Class Interaction Type	Mechanism and Significance	Management
Amoxicillin Beta-lactam antibiotics ⊕⊕⊕	Ginseng increases T helper cell typ. 1 (Th1) immunity and may enhance effectiveness of many antimicrobial agents, although evidence of interaction is specific to amoxicillin. Clinical significance: possibly widely applicable, although currently unknown.	Consider coadministration, especially in antibiotic-resistant conditions or immunocompromised patients.
Chemotherapy Radiotherapy ⊕/☼	Ginseng may decrease drug toxicities and increase drug efficacy through multiple mechanisms, including immunomodulation, chemosensitization, and specific toxicity reduction. Western clinical trial support negligible, despite anecdotal clinical support.	Pretreatment and coadministration with chemotherapy and radiation recommended, with appropriately experienced professional management.
Ethanol Antiarthritic analgesics ◇/☼/⊕⊕⊕	Clearance of alcohol may be increased by herb pretreatment. Interaction of questionable clinical value.	None.
Narcotics, opioids, central stimulants ?	Ginseng may reduce drug-induced tolerance development and decrease adverse effects of drug use. Clinical significance not established.	Consider possible use as additional support for adverse effect reduction in analgesia or withdrawal from narcotic/opioid abuse.
Phenelzine Monoamine oxidase inhibitors (MAOIs) ✗	Ginseng effect on neurotransmitters not considered physiologically significant. Current low use of nonselective MAOIs renders clinical significance marginal. Interaction overstated.	Normal precautions regarding nonselective MAOI advice for patients adequate.
Vaccine immunotherapies ⊕	Ginseng extracts may increase antibody response and effectiveness of some vaccine therapies by enhancing antigen-presenting cell (APC) activity. In particular, ginsenosides may be a useful pretreatment and adjuvant for improving potency and immunogenicity of vaccines.	Pretreatment and coadministration worthy of consideration.
Warfarin Oral vitamin K antagonist anticoagulants ✗	International normalized ratio (INR) reduction in a single report, probably idiosyncratic. Significance unknown, likely minimal.	Observe normal INR monitoring, especially if adding or removing any drug/herb to stable anticoagulation.

HERB DESCRIPTION

Family

Araliaceae.

Related Species

Panax quinquefolius L. (American ginseng) or *Xi Yang Shen.*

Habitat and Cultivation

Slow-growing woodland perennial native to northern China and Korea, now widely cultivated in those countries and in Japan.

Parts Used

Main and lateral roots.

Common Forms

Dried peeled root (white ginseng); steamed dried root (red ginseng) by decoction, or infusion if powdered.
Tincture or Fluid extract.
Standardized Extract: Dried concentrates, typically standardized to 4% to 5% ginsenosides (with ginsenosides Rg1/Rb1 ratio ≥ 0.5).

HERB IN CLINICAL PRACTICE

Overview

Ginseng is economically the most important herb in world commerce and has generated more scientific studies and a larger general literature than any other herb. Although used in Asia for more than 2000 years, ginseng has now become widely incorporated into consumer products as well as the herbal materia medica in the West. Ginseng is the archetypal adaptogenic herb. *Adaptogens* have no equivalent among conventional pharmaceutical agents. The term was coined by Soviet researcher Lazarev in 1947 and subsequently defined by Brekhman in terms of three salient qualities. Adaptogens are *nonspecific* (in relation to a wide range of stressor stimuli), *nontoxic* (cause minimal disturbance to normal physiological function), and *normalizing* (direction of action varies depending on the prior state of response to stressor and always normalizes).[1] The general properties of adaptogens have been reviewed by Panossian et al.[2] and Wagner and Norr.[3] As with its companion adaptogen eleuthero (see Eleuthero monograph), ginseng and its constituent ginsenosides have a broad range of immunomodulating, chemopreventive, neuroendocrine, and antineoplastic activities, as well as behavioral effects on athletic, sexual, and cognitive performance.

The literature on ginseng is voluminous; recent accessible Western resources include therapeutic monographs by the World Health Organization (WHO),[4] British Herbal Medical

Association (BHMA),[5] and European Scientific Cooperative on Phytotherapy (ESCOP),[6] as well as literature reviews by McKenna et al.[7] and Court.[8] Recent monographs from the Chinese medicine perspective include Bensky et al.[9] and Chen and Chen.[10] *Ren shen* is a transliteration of the Chinese name for "peeled, dried root," also known as "white ginseng." *Hong shen*, or "red ginseng," is the root steamed before drying. Red ginseng is considered more *Yang* (i.e., warmer and stronger) than white ginseng. The ginsenoside profile of the two forms is different. The separate species *Panax quinquefolius* L. (American ginseng or wild American ginseng) is known as *Xi Yang Shen* and is regarded as closer to Japanese-cultivated *Panax ginseng*, or *Dong Yang Shen*, and has less warming properties than *Ren shen*.[10] The Western literature does not usually observe these energetic distinctions, although *P. quinquefolius* and *P. ginseng*, despite similarities, are not considered interchangeable by most authoritative Western sources, and the scientific literature on *P. quinquefolius* is considerably less than that for *P. ginseng*.

In consumer product marketing, the term "ginseng" has been confusingly used to refer to related species such as American ginseng *(P. quinquefolius)* as well as unrelated species such as Siberian ginseng (now known as eleuthero). Correct recording of the Latin binomial is always essential to identify an herb accurately, and failure to properly identify the species is a persistent defect of mainstream medical discussions of ginseng-related adverse events and drug interactions. A further problem, endemic to the dietary supplement market, is the variable quality and composition of commercial products containing, or claiming to contain, ginseng.[11] Because of the high price of the root, adulteration can occur, and several contaminating species have been identified in China.[9]

Historical/Ethnomedicine Precedent

In classical Chinese medicine, ginseng is a major *qi* tonifying herb, addressing general deficiencies of *yuan qi* ("source qi") to replenish *jing* ("vital essence"), as well as deficiencies of blood *(xue)*, spleen *(Pi)*, lung *(Fei)*, and kidney *(Shen)* qi. As a *shen* herb, it also calms the "Spirit/Mind" and improves mental function. Ginseng has been progressively integrated into Western use in the last 30 years, primarily as an adaptogenic tonic herb to treat fatigue and neurasthenia, enhance general wellness, and improve physical, sexual, and cognitive performance. As in China, ginseng is now increasingly seen as a potentially valuable agent in Western integrative cancer protocols.[12,13]

Known or Potential Therapeutic Uses

Stress reduction and neuroendocrine balancing (dysglycemia, adrenal insufficiency); fatigue, chronic fatigue immune dysfunction syndrome (CFIDS); convalescence; enhancement of exercise, athletic and work capacity, and performance; increasing mental alertness and cognitive performance; adjunct to radiation and chemotherapy treatment; immunoprotection and immunomodulation, chemoprevention, cardiotonic, hepatoprotective, hyperlipidemic, hypoglycemic.

Key Constituents

Steroidal saponins, known as *ginsenosides* (up to 3.0%). The ginsenosides are based on three sapogenin aglycones: 20(S)-protopanaxodiol, 20(S)-protopanaxotriol, and oleanic acid. Ginsenosides are designated by the letter "R" followed by various subscripts. The total number of ginsenosides has not been definitively determined; more than 30 have been described. Ginsenosides are present as a complex mixture, and the composition may vary with conditions of cultivation and processing.

Polyacetylene compounds, peptidoglycans, volatile oil, polysaccharides, and lipids.

Therapeutic Dosing Range

Dried root: Western—up to 2 g daily; Chinese—up to 9 to 10 g daily.

Tincture/Fluid extract: Up to 3 mL/day, 1:1 equivalent.

Standardized Extract: 100 mg 5:1 4% ginsenosides (e.g., G115, Pharmaton S.A.) solid extract twice daily, i.e., 8 mg ginsenosides total daily.

INTERACTIONS REVIEW
Strategic Considerations

The "normalizing" effect of ginseng on homeostatic parameters, coupled with a broad spectrum of activities and minimal toxicity, underlies a lack of pronounced pharmacodynamic drug interactions with the herb at therapeutic doses. In a recent review of the safety and toxicity of ginseng, including adverse drug interactions, Coon and Ernst[14] concluded that the herb was rarely associated with adverse events or drug interactions. Authoritative monographs either report no interactions (German Commission E)[15] or cite the often-repeated but unlikely adverse interaction with phenelzine (see later discussion) and a possible interaction with warfarin (WHO, ESCOP).[4,6]

Secondary sources often suggest theoretical or speculative interactions based on extrapolations from the pharmacology of the herb. However, pharmacological data for ginseng often reveal apparently opposing effects, such as hypertensive/hypotensive, central nervous system (CNS) stimulant/CNS depressant, and antihistamine/histamine-like actions.[16] These opposing effects extend to genomic activity.[17] Such apparently conflicting data and the correlation of the direction of many ginseng effects with baseline physiological state before consumption are explained partly by the opposing action of the separate ginsenoside components of the herb.[18] This also applies to more complex processes, such as angiogenesis; ginseng can promote angiogenesis in wound healing but inhibit it in tumorigenesis.[19,20] As with steroidal hormones, the ginsenosides are capable of exerting complex actions at genomic and proteomic levels, exhibiting membrane intercalation and nuclear localization, as well as more rapid actions at a signal transduction and second-messenger level.[18] Many of the observed downstream effects of ginsenosides may result from these levels of activity. There is evidence that ginsenosides may reverse the classic downregulation of glucocorticoid receptor (GR) by dexamethasone, although evidence for direct binding to the GR is equivocal.[21] This should not be read so much as evidence for a "dexamethasone-ginseng" interaction, but rather as an indication of the complexity of actions of the herb. For example, diverse effects of the ginsenosides may be downstream consequences of GR modulation, including several antineoplastic effects.[22] Similarly, putative estrogenic activity by some ginsenosides[23] may be caused by crosstalk between GR and ER,[24] rather than direct "phytoestrogen" effects, which have not historically been attributed to the herb, in contrast to recent data on isolated ginsenoside components.[25,26]

In conclusion, the documented literature on ginseng interactions largely fails to account for the complex, pleiotropic and nonspecific effects of the herb, particularly on stress-related homeostasis and neuroendocrine and immune parameters. Practitioners versed in botanical medicine are likely to emphasize precisely these adaptogenic aspects in therapeutic practice, whereas the mainstream view continues to regard ginseng narrowly as some type of mild stimulant, although an exotic one.

Effects on Drug Metabolism and Bioavailability

The effects of ginseng (and isolated ginsenosides) on cytochrome P450 (CYP450) has not been fully characterized, but the balance of available data from rodent, in vitro, and preclinical in vivo studies suggests that the herb has minimal effects on the mixed-function oxidase system, lacking pronounced induction or inhibition effects that may contribute to metabolic drug interactions.[27] Two in vivo human CYP450 studies are available to date. Anderson et al.[28] found no effect of 14 days' administration of standardized (G115) ginseng in 20 healthy volunteers on urinary 6-β-OH cortisol/cortisol ratios, suggesting lack of induction of the herb on CYP3A4. Gurley et al.[29] used a probe cocktail methodology in 12 healthy volunteers to examine the effects of 28 days' administration of *Panax ginseng* at a high dose of 500 mg three times daily. They found no significant changes in CYP450 1A2, 2D6, 2E1, or 3A4.[29] Two recombinant human CYP450 enzyme studies suggest a possible weak inhibition of isoforms 1A1, 1A2, and 1B1 by G115 extract.[30] Another study using isolated component ginsenosides found that R_d, R_c, and R_f exerted a very weak effect on 1A2, 2C9, 2C19, 2D6, and 3A4. Ginsenosides R_c and R_f also exerted activation effects on 2C9 and 3A4, respectively, but only at concentrations of 200 μM. The authors concluded that these small effects would be unlikely to have in vivo effects on coadministered medications.[31] Rodent models have also failed to reveal significant effects on CYP450 enzymes 1A2, 2B1, and 3A23.[32-34]

In contrast to the Phase II drug metabolism, there is preliminary experimental evidence for a modulating effect of ginseng on P-glycoprotein (Phase III drug metabolism), and substrates of this transporter protein may be subject to pharmacokinetic interactions.[35] The mechanisms of drug resistance modulation have not been fully characterized; cell line evidence examining the effects of ginsenoside components on drug efflux with vinblastine and doxorubicin suggests a competitive inhibition mechanism rather than transcriptional induction/inhibition.[36-39] Confirmed clinical correlations of drug resistance modulation or other efflux pump-mediated interactions with ginseng or ginsenosides are not available to date, although doxorubicin (Adriamycin) cardiotoxicity was reduced in a rodent model when ginseng was coadministered with the drug.[40]

Finally, evidence suggests that in both rodents and humans, certain intestinal bacteria may hydrolyze ginseng saponins into novel ginsenoside metabolites with antineoplastic activity, suggesting a prodrug bioactivation aspect to the action of the herb under certain circumstances.[41,42] The clinical significance of this bioactivation mechanism has not been established.

HERB-DRUG INTERACTIONS

Amoxicillin and Related Beta-Lactam Antibiotics

Evidence: Amoxicillin (Amoxicot, Amoxil, Moxilin, Trimox, Wymox); combination drug: amoxicillin and clavulanic acid (Augmentin, Augmentin XR, Clavulin, Nuclav).

Extrapolated, based on similar properties: Beta-lactam antibiotics: Methicillin (Staphcillin); aztreonam (Azactam injection); carbapenem antibiotics: meropenem (Merrem I.V.); combination drug: imipenem and cilastatin (Primaxin I.M., Primaxin I.V.); cephalosporin antibiotics; penicillin antibiotics: ampicillin (Amficot, Omnipen, Principen, Totacillin); combination drug: ampicillin and sulbactam (Unisyn); bacampicillin (Spectrobid), carbenicillin (Geocillin), cloxacillin (Cloxapen), dicloxacillin (Dynapen, Dycill), mezlocillin (Mezlin), nafcillin (Unipen), oxacillin (Bactocill), penicillin G (Bicillin C-R, Bicillin L-A, Pfizerpen, Truxcillin), penicillin V (Beepen-VK, Betapen-VK, Ledercillin VK, Pen-Vee K, Robicillin VK, Suspen, Truxcillin VK, V-Cillin K, Veetids), piperacillin (Pipracil); combination drug: piperacillin and tazobactam (Zosyn); ticarcillin (Ticar); combination drug: ticarcillin and clavulanate (Timentin).

Interaction Type and Significance

⊕⊕⊕ **Beneficial or Supportive Interaction, Not Requiring Professional Management**

Probability:
2. Probable

Evidence Base:
○ Preliminary

Effect and Mechanism of Action

A synergistic effect between amoxicillin (plus clavulanic acid) and coadministered ginseng results in increased antibacterial effect. The mechanism is likely caused by increased cellular immunity (Th1) induction by ginseng.

Research

A group of 75 patients with acute bronchitis received 875 mg amoxicillin and 12 mg clavulanic acid twice daily for 9 days. They were then randomized into two groups; one received additional ginseng (G115, 200 mg/day) and the other antibiotic only for the 9 days. On days 4 to 7 the ginseng group had significantly lower bacteria counts than the antibiotic-only group, although this became a nonsignificant trend after day 8. The authors of this pilot study suggested that ginseng may be a particularly useful adjunct in cases of acute bronchitis.[43] (Arguably, however, most infectious disease experts would agree that antibiotic treatment of this condition is not necessary or indicated in patients who are not debilitated or immunosuppressed.)

Integrative Therapeutics, Clinical Concerns, and Adaptations

The effect of ginseng extracts in enhancing cell-mediated immunity, particularly natural killer (NK) cell activity, has been documented. The combination of natural compounds with beta-lactam antibiotics to deal with refractory conditions or bacterial resistance is also documented (e.g., see Green Tea monograph). The interaction identified by the previous study is more likely a specific instance of the general enhancement of immune responses by ginseng. Such an effect is probable in combination with a wide variety of antimicrobial agents, rather than as a specific interaction couplet between amoxicillin or beta-lactam agents, implying a broader clinical significance than suggested by the specific report.

Antineoplastic Chemotherapy and Radiotherapy

Bleomycin (Blenoxane), carboplatin (Paraplatin), cisplatin (*cis*-diaminedichloroplatinum, CDDP; Platinol, Platinol-AQ), cytarabine (ara-C; Cytosar-U, DepoCyt, Tarabine PFS), dactinomycin (Actinomycin D, Cosmegen, Cosmegen Lyovac), daunorubicin (Cerubidine, DaunoXome), docetaxel

(Taxotere), doxorubicin (Adriamycin, Rubex), etoposide (Eposin, Etopophos, Vepesid, VP-16), mitomycin (Mutamycin), oxaliplatin (Eloxatin), paclitaxel (Paxene, Taxol), paclitaxel, protein-bound (Abraxane), vinblastine (Alkaban-AQ,Velban, Velsar), vincristine (Leurocristine, Oncovin, Vincasar PFS), vinorelbine (Navelbine).

Interaction Type and Significance
⊕ **Potential or Theoretical Beneficial or Supportive Interaction, with Professional Management**
☼ **Prevention or Reduction of Drug Adverse Effect**

Probability: Evidence Base:
4. Plausible   ○ **Preliminary**

Effect and Mechanism of Action
Coadministered ginseng may potentially act as both a chemosensitizer and a protector against antineoplastic drug toxicities, particularly antitumor antibiotics and platinum compounds. Mechanisms may include multidrug resistance disabling, potentiation of cytotoxic activity with some drugs, protection of healthy cells, and enhancement of immune system activity during myelosuppression. These potential interactions have not been subject to Western clinical trials at this time, although they are supported by anecdotal clinical practice and preliminary pharmacological data.

Research
Experimental and animal data supporting the general use of ginseng extracts, particularly red ginseng, in association with antineoplastic agents are available. Most reports are in original Asian literature, which is only briefly summarized here.

Isolated triterpene (ginsenoside) fractions have been shown to reverse drug resistance to daunomycin, doxorubicin (Adriamycin), and vinblastine in resistant leukemia cell line P388/ADM, with Adriamycin sensitivity increasing the most.[36] Inhibition of leukemic progenitor cells cultured from bone marrow of patients with acute myelogenous leukemia (AML) increased significantly when cytotoxic drugs (homoharringtonine, cytarabine, Adriamycin, etoposide) were coadministered with a complete saponin extract of *Panax ginseng* (20 µg/mL); a total of 17 of 72 drugs tested exhibited resistance reversal.[44] A Chinese formula with ginseng as the main ingredient reduced the cardiotoxic effects of Adriamycin in rabbits compared with controls.[45] Combination treatment with a sapogenin metabolite of ginseng (50 mg/kg) in mice orally administered with doxorubicin (3 mg/kg) significantly reduced germ cell injury and other parameters (e.g., serum LDH, CPK) to the level of control animals.[46]

The effects of extracts of both red and white ginseng were compared in the activity of mitomycin C in vitro against Ehrlich ascites sarcoma cells. The ginsenosides Rh2 and Rg3 promoted mitomycin uptake by the tumor cells, and when an in vivo comparison was performed in mouse Ehrlich ascites sarcoma and rat ascites hepatoma, the red ginseng extracts showed a stronger effect in combination with mitomycin than the white ginseng extract.[47-49] Conducting in vitro studies with ginsenoside Rg(3), Kim et al.[39] showed that inhibition of multidrug resistance was caused by competitive inhibition of binding with P-glycoprotein (P-gp), rather than by transcription effects on MDR1 gene or P-gp levels. Ginsenoside Rh2 from red ginseng demonstrated a synergistic effect with cisplatin in vitro and in vivo (when inoculated into mice) against growth of a cell line derived from a human ovarian adenocarcinoma.[50] A cisplatin-resistant subline of human

lung cancer cells was also shown to undergo resistance reversal in vitro when cisplatin was coadministered with IH-90 (intestinal metabolite of Rb1 and Rd).[37,51]

Shin et al.[52] used a rodent model to demonstrate that red ginseng polysaccharide had a synergistic effect with paclitaxel against the proliferation of implanted sarcoma and melanoma cancer cell lines. The extract also restored NK cell activity suppressed by the drug. Radioprotective effects of ginseng pretreatment have also been demonstrated in rodent models.[53-59] Immunomodulation effects of ginseng have been shown to preserve bone marrow function and CD4 cell activity during exposure to chemotherapeutic agents.[60] A small trial (*n* = 42) with stage III gastric cancer patients found that CD3/CD4 cell activity was preserved, with positive effects on survival, when red ginseng was combined with postoperative adjuvant chemotherapy.[61]

Integrative Therapeutics, Clinical Concerns, and Adaptations
Clinical research is needed to corroborate these interactions in vivo. Given the pleiotropic anticancer effects of ginseng extracts, multiple rationales exist for incorporation of the herb into integrative protocols in the oncology setting. The antifatigue and immunomodulating effects of ginseng are likely to add to its usefulness, particularly for later-stage cancers. Modern Chinese medicine has incorporated herbal and conventional treatments to a higher degree than current Western practice, with ginseng a primary ingredient in compound formulations designed to address specific clinical circumstances.[62] At present, further clinical data are required to substantiate the use of ginseng in this context; however, its value as an adjuvant in oncology is beginning to be recognized in the West.[12]

Ethanol

Ethanol

Interaction Type and Significance
◈ **Impaired Drug Absorption and Bioavailability, Negligible Effect**
☼ **Prevention or Reduction of Drug Adverse Effect**
⊕⊕⊕ **Beneficial or Supportive Interaction, Not Requiring Professional Management**

Probability: Evidence Base:
2. Probable   ○ **Preliminary**

Effect and Mechanism of Action
Ginseng appears to increase the metabolic clearance of ethanol and lower blood alcohol level, possibly by delaying gastric emptying. The clinical significance of the interaction is low.

Research
A much-quoted but methodologically limited preclinical study used 14 healthy males in an open-label and uncontrolled design that compared blood alcohol levels 40 minutes after ingestion for alcohol given alone and for the same dose of alcohol combined with 3 g *Panax ginseng*. Blood alcohol levels were 32% to 51% lower when ginseng was coadministered. Full pharmacokinetic measurements were not made, with no data on maximum concentration (C_{max}) or area under curve (AUC).[63]

Animal experiments have confirmed the general finding that alcohol clearance is increased by ginseng coadministration. Pretreatment with ginseng in a rat model (200 mg/kg) reduced ethanol AUC by 21% compared with controls.[64] Pretreatment with ginseng and ginsenosides reduced the onset of loss of the righting reflex in mice treated with ethanol, but did not affect ethanol-induced sleeping time in the animals.[65] Presence of a pharmacodynamic element in the effect of the ginseng/alcohol combination is uncertain. In a rodent model, however, red ginseng extracts reduced ethanol's impairment of a behavioral task, and administration of neurotropic agents suggested that this effect may be mediated by an adrenergic pathway.[66] Another rodent study found that an ethanol-induced decrease in brain weight in neonatal rats was reduced by administration of ginsenosides, suggesting a neuroprotective effect against alcohol damage.[67]

Integrative Therapeutics, Clinical Concerns, and Adaptations

The ramifications of pharmacokinetic lowering of ethanol blood levels by ginseng are arguably of less clinical significance than interest for recreational alcohol consumers. This interaction should be clinically distinguished from potential neuroprotective activities of the ginseng saponins that may partly underlie the beneficial effects of the herb on cognitive function.[68,69]

Narcotic Analgesics (Opiates) and Psychostimulants

Evidence: Cocaine, methamphetamine, morphine sulfate (Astramorph PF, Avinza, Duramorph, Infumorph, Kadian, MS Contin, MSIR, Oramorph SR, RMS; Roxanol, Roxanol Rescudose, Roxanol T).

Extrapolated, based on similar properties: Narcotic analgesics: Butorphanol (Stadol, Stadol NS), codeine, fentanyl (Actiq Oral Transmucosal, Duragesic Transdermal, Fentanyl Oralet, Sublimaze Injection), hydrocodone, hydromorphone (Dilaudid), levorphanol (Levo-Dromoran), meperidine (Demerol), methadone (Dolophine, Methadose), opium tincture, oxycodone (Endocodone, OxyContin, OxyIR, Percolone, Roxicodone), oxymorphone (Numorphan), paregoric, pentazocine (Talwin, Talwin NX), propoxyphene (Darvon, Darvon-N).

Combination drugs: buprenorphine and naloxone (Suboxone); codeine and acetaminophen (Capital with Codeine; Phenaphen with Codeine; Tylenol with Codeine); codeine and acetylsalicylic acid (Empirin with Codeine); codeine, acetylsalicylic acid, caffeine, and butalbital (Fiorinal); hydrocodone and acetaminophen (Anexsia, Anodynos-DHC, Co-Gesic, Dolacet, DuoCet, Hydrocet, Hydrogesic, Hy-Phen, Lorcet 10/650, Lorcet-HD, Lorcet Plus, Lortab, Margesic H, Medipain 5, Norco, Stagesic, T-Gesic, Vicodin, Vicodin ES, Vicodin HP, Zydone); hydrocodone and acetylsalicylic acid (Lortab ASA); hydrocodone and ibuprofen (Reprexain, Vicoprofen); opium and belladonna (B&O Supprettes); oxycodone and acetaminophen (Endocet, Percocet 2.5/325, Percocet 5/325, Percocet 7.5/500, Percocet 10/650, Roxicet 5/500, Roxilox, Tylox); oxycodone and acetylsalicylic acid (Endodan, Percodan, Percodan-Demi); pentazocine and acetaminophen (Talacen); pentazocine and acetylsalicylic acid (Talwin Compound); propoxyphene and acetaminophen (Darvocet-N, Darvocet-N 100, Pronap-100, Propacet 100, Propoxacet-N, Wygesic); propoxyphene and acetylsalicylic acid (Bexophene, Darvon Compound-65 Pulvules, PC-Cap); propoxyphene, acetylsalicylic acid, and caffeine (Darvon Compound).

Interaction Type and Significance

?   Interaction Likely but Uncertain Occurrence and Unclear Implications

Probability:	Evidence Base:
3. Possible	**○ Preliminary**

Effect and Mechanism of Action

Ginseng extracts may interfere with analgesic effects of morphine and related opioids while preventing or reversing drug-induced tolerance, according to animal data. The mechanism and clinical significance of the interaction are not established, although theoretically the herb may be of value in preventing or modulating drug adverse effects, including drug tolerance.

Research

Investigators have conducted experimental studies into the effects of ginseng pretreatment and coadministration with psychostimulant and opioid drugs, principally morphine but also methamphetamine and cocaine, in rodent behavioral models (conditioned–place preference tests). The general conclusions were that drug-induced hyperactivity was reduced by ginseng, with ginsenosides fractions Rg1 and Rb1 being primarily responsible for the antiopioid activity. The effect may be related to dopaminergic pathway modulation but has not been established.[70-76]

Clinical Implications and Adaptations

At least one author has suggested that ginseng extracts hold the potential to prevent and treat the effects of abuse of cocaine, methamphetamine, and morphine.[77] These extrapolations from rodent models to drug abuse behavior and tolerance mechanisms in humans require supporting clinical data, which are unavailable at present.

Phenelzine and Other Monoamine Oxidase (MAO-A) Inhibitors

Evidence: Phenelzine (Nardil).

Extrapolated, based on similar properties, as MAO-A inhibitors: Isocarboxazid (Marplan), moclobemide (Aurorix, Manerix), procarbazine (Matulane), tranylcypromine (Parnate).

Interaction Type and Significance

✗   Potential or Theoretical Adverse Interaction of Uncertain Severity

Probability:	Evidence Base:
5. Improbable	**☐ Inadequate**

Effect and Mechanism of Action

Possible hypomania or hypermania and exacerbation of CNS adverse effects normally associated with phenelzine alone have been reported during ginseng coadministration. Report reliability is low, the mechanism unknown, and the existence of the interaction improbable.

Research

Some data from in vitro and animal studies suggest effects of ginseng modulation on CNS neurotransmitters, but the clinical implications of such data are unknown, and extrapolations to in vivo interactions with effects on the monoamine oxidase system are unwarranted at this time. Tsang et al.[78] showed that ginseng extracts dose-dependently inhibited uptake of gamma-aminobutyric acid (GABA), glutamate, dopamine, norepinephrine, and serotonin in rat brain synaptosomes. Ginsenosides compete with agonists for binding to GABA-A and GABA-B receptors.[79] *Panax quinquefolius* extracts are also known to exert GABA-A modulating effects.[80]

Reports

The claimed interaction between phenelzine and ginseng is listed in both conventional sources, such as Stockley,[81] and in authoritative monographs on *Panax ginseng*, including WHO.[4] This interaction is also reiterated by innumerable secondary and derivative sources, apparently based on two case reports, discussed here in depth.

The first documented report was a brief mention in a 1985 editorial by the then-editors of the *Journal of Clinical Psychopharmacology*, Shader and Greenblatt.[82] The case involved a 64-year-old woman who took an undisclosed dose for an undisclosed period of the combination dietary supplement product "Natrol High" while taking phenelzine, 60 mg/day. She then experienced symptoms of "insomnia, headache, and tremulousness." Unfortunately, the authors failed to include any medical details or to identify the ingredients of the Natrol product, which contains no *Panax ginseng*, but rather some *Eleutherococcus senticosus* (previously known as Siberian ginseng), in combination with several micronutrients (e.g., niacin, vitamin B_6, thiamine) and other herbs, including ginger, mallow, licorice root, and winter berry.[83]

In 1988, Shader and Greenblatt[84] speculated further on the topic, relating to a further episode with the same patient.[84] Now 67 years old and taking 45 mg phenelzine per day, the patient had been prescribed a herbal tea formula and some "ginseng" capsules "for energy." The ingredients of the prescription tea formula and capsules were not identified and the dose not disclosed. She experienced similar symptoms as in the previous episode, but this time associated with increased depression. After cessation of the tea formula and "ginseng" capsules, she "felt better."

The only other report on phenelzine is a letter from Jones and Runikis[85] in 1987 commenting on the case in the original Shader-Greenblatt editorial. They briefly describe a 42-year-old female patient taking 45 mg phenelzine per day, along with 0.5 mg triazolam at night and 1 mg lorazepam four times daily. The patient concurrently consumed an unspecified amount of "ginseng and bee pollen." The species and form of ginseng, the dose, and other constituents of the product were not disclosed. During coadministration of the herbal products and phenelzine, the patient became "extremely active and optimistic," her sleep was decreased, and she did not "feel tired." She also was irritable and had tension headaches and "occasional vague hallucinations," which she attributed to the phenelzine, and she therefore ceased both the drug and the herbs. Her depressive symptoms then began to return, so she restarted the phenelzine at 45 mg/day. This time she experienced no therapeutic benefit from the drug (without the "ginseng and bee pollen"), although she did experience headache with the phenelzine alone.

The persistent citation of these two cases as evidence of a phenelzine-ginseng interaction is remarkable, given that ginseng was not even involved in the first case and not identified as the herb involved in the second. No dose was given, and concurrent multi-ingredient supplements were used, as well as psychiatric comedications in the second case. In addition, the adverse effects described are consistent with well-known adverse effects of phenelzine alone, which in both cases was used at doses higher (60 mg/day, 45 mg/day) than usual for maintenance therapy of 15 mg/day. Also, the Jones and Runikis case report[85] seems to imply that the supplements were responsible for improved therapeutic outcome of the MAO inhibitor therapy, as opposed to the authors' interpretation of an adverse effect, because rechallenge by phenelzine alone without the herbal agents failed to have a beneficial effect on depression.

An unrelated but possibly relevant case report from Italian psychiatrists Gonzales-Seljo and others claimed that ginseng alone is associated with mania. In fact, the patient had been taking lithium carbonate, 1200 mg/day, and amitriptyline, 75 mg/day, for 6 years. She abruptly ceased this regimen, then started taking one "ginseng tablet" (brand, form, dose, and other ingredients unidentified). Ten days after the cessation of lithium and amitriptyline, she became "manic," including being sleepless, irritable, aggressive, and hyperactive. The authors suggested this must have been caused by the "ginseng." Abrupt withdrawal symptoms from both lithium and tricyclics are well known, and relapse into mania after lithium withdrawal has been documented in at least 14 studies.[86]

Clinical Implications and Adaptations

The suggested ginseng-phenelzine interaction is in the "speculative-overstated" category. At least one of the three case reports relates to eleuthero (previously Siberian ginseng); this basic error was documented by Treasure and also by Chen, who notes this is the case in several of the infamous "ginseng abuse syndrome" reports.[87-89] In the other reports the herb is simply unidentified. Neither the reports nor the known pharmacology of the herb lend significant support to the existence of an adverse interaction.

The declining use of phenelzine as a therapeutic intervention for depression (largely because of the lethal nature of interactions of this class of drugs with such common agents as dextromethorphan in OTC cough syrup) suggests that future routine pharmacosurveillance reports are unlikely to be forthcoming or to generate further clarification. The persistent tendency for secondary sources to repeat uncritically the interaction merits the full discussion here, but the clinical significance can be regarded as negligible. However, prudence still suggests great care be exercised when combining classic MAO inhibitors with botanicals or drugs known to interact in any significant way with neurotransmitter function.

Vaccine Immunotherapies

Interaction Type and Significance

⊕ **Potential or Theoretical Beneficial or Supportive Interaction, with Professional Management**

Probability:
2. Probable

Evidence Base:
○ **Preliminary**

Effect and Mechanism of Action

Ginseng extracts may increase the effectiveness of some vaccine therapies. This synergy has been observed both directly, when vaccines are prepared with the addition of parenteral ginseng saponin ingredients, and indirectly with oral pretreatment with ginseng before vaccination. The mechanism of the increased antibody response may be improved immunogenicity from enhanced antigen-presenting cell (APC) activity. The clinical significance remains to be established.

Research

Scaglione et al.[90] followed 227 patients attending a primary care practice who were scheduled to receive a polyvalent influenza vaccine. They were divided into two groups; one received G115, 100 mg ginseng per day, and the other placebo for 12 weeks. The vaccine was administered on week 4. There was a statistically greater incidence of subsequent influenza in the placebo group. At week 8, antibody titers and NK cell activity were much ($p < 0.0001$) higher in the verum group.

In the veterinary setting, Rivera et al.[91] examined the effects of adding a ginsenoside preparation into a conventional porcine parvovirus (PPV) vaccine in a guinea pig model.

They also injected ginseng and vaccine at separate sites, as well as providing ginseng pretreatment, followed by immunization. An aluminum hydroxide vaccine co-ingredient was also tested with and without ginsenosides. The Al(OH)$_3$ with ginseng mixture vaccine produced a 20-fold increase in immunoglobulin G (IgG) response to the PPV antigen, a synergistic effect greater than adding either Al(OH)$_3$ or ginsenosides alone. Rivera et al.[92] also conducted in vivo investigations with pigs and the commercial PPV vaccine, adjuvated with Al(OH)$_3$, supplemented with ginseng versus vaccine alone. Vaccines with ginseng resulted in higher immunogenicity (higher IgG values by ELISA) than without ginseng. The authors suggest that ginseng may be a useful adjuvant for improving the potency and immunogenicity of commercial vaccine preparations.

Integrative Therapeutics, Clinical Concerns, and Adaptations

Ginseng saponins have well-established immunomodulatory effects. It appears likely that vaccine immunogenicity can be significantly enhanced by ginseng pretreatment and, more interestingly, perhaps by adding ginsenosides as a co-adjuvant to the vaccine mixture itself. The clinical benefits of using immunomodulating herbs for populations at risk of infection, whether alone or combined with conventional therapies, is an established practice among practitioners of botanical and natural medicine. Wider adoption of such integrative strategies may be predicated on currently emerging research data.

The increasing interest in vaccines in oncological settings may provide such a stimulus, and a recent study of relevance to the ginseng-vaccine interaction issue has come from this field. The priming of cell cultures with specific ginseng saponin metabolites (M1 and M4 being bacterial hydrolysis products of ginsenosides) has been shown to increase the ability of dendritic cells to induce differentiation of T cells (i.e., to enhance Th1 responses), and ginseng may be a useful adjuvant in the emerging dendritic cell cancer vaccine field.[93] However, future research is needed to clarify the full potential of ginseng in vaccine immunotherapies.

Warfarin and Related Oral Vitamin K Antagonist Anticoagulants

Evidence: Phenprocoumon (Jarsin, Marcumar), warfarin (Coumadin, Marevan, Warfilone).
Extrapolated, based on similar properties: Anisindione (Miradon), dicumarol, ethyl biscoumacetate (Tromexan), nicoumalone (acenocoumarol; Acitrom, Sintrom), phenindione (Dindevan).

Interaction Type and Significance

✗ **Potential or Theoretical Adverse Interaction of Uncertain Severity**

Probability: Evidence Base:
5. Improbable   ▽ **Mixed**

Effect and Mechanism of Action

The mechanism of this suggested interaction, based on a single case report of INR reduction in a patient previously stable on warfarin, is unknown. The proposed interaction seems improbable or idiosyncratic.

Research

Zhu et al.[94] investigated the potential warfarin-ginseng interaction in a rodent model. They examined pharmacokinetic and pharmacodynamic parameters in both single-dose and steady-state warfarin dosing regimens using plasma warfarin AUC and prothrombin time (PT) measurements. No significant effects were found on either single or multiple warfarin doses, either in terms of warfarin AUC or PTs. An open-label human study, using a randomized crossover design in 12 healthy subjects who had 7 days of pretreatment with high-dose ginseng (3.0 g/day, equivalent ~ 45.0 mg ginsenosides/day), found no effect of ginseng coadministration on S-warfarin or R-warfarin enantiomer clearance and no significant effect on platelet aggregation or INR.[95] By contrast, an in vitro study using human platelet aggregation assay resulted in significant reduction of thrombin- and collagen-induced aggregation in response to a red ginseng extract.[96] The human data contrast with the available animal studies. In rodent models, ginseng administration led to a significant increase in PT and partial thromboplastin time (PTT) of rats treated with various anticoagulants.[96,97]

A recent clinical study used the related species *P. quinquefolius* (American ginseng) to examine potential interactions with warfarin. The study gave 12 healthy volunteers warfarin for 3 days at 5 mg/day, followed by 4 weeks of American ginseng (1.0 g twice daily), with a repeat 3 days of warfarin during the fourth week. Parameters measured were peak warfarin and peak INR, as well as INR AUC and warfarin AUC. Compared to controls, there were modest reductions in INR (except in one patient who showed an INR increase, as well as small but significant reductions in warfarin AUC and peak plasma levels).[98] However, the variability of the results was very high, and there was no pharmacokinetic phenotyping of the healthy volunteers. Cytochrome P450 2C9 polymorphisms are known to be a critical factor associated with warfarin response variability. The ethnic composition of the study group suggested possible CYP450 2C9 phenotype variations as an explanation for the wide variability of the data, which were not controlled for by the investigators.[99-102] The investigators' comment that their study was conducted to clarify the matter of the Janetzky case report[103] (see next) seems curious given the investigators choice of *P. quinquefolius* rather than *P. ginseng*, which was the subject of the warfarin-ginseng case report.

Reports

The case report on which this potential interaction was based concerned a 47-year-old male with a history of hypertension, thrombosis, angina, and osteoarthritis. He was stabilized on warfarin at 5.0 mg/day and an INR of 3.0 to 4.0 for 9 months before commencing a ginseng preparation (Pharmaton 100-mg capsules, unspecified number, three times daily) for 4 weeks. He was comedicated with diltiazem at 30 mg three times daily, nitroglycerin as needed, and salsalate at 500 mg three times daily. After 4 weeks of ginseng coadministration, his INR was found to be 1.5. Two weeks after cessation of the herbal product, the INR returned to 3.3. The patient denied other changes to his dietary regimen, herb intake, or drug protocols. He did not experience a thrombotic episode during the period of reduced INR, but because of his history, a rechallenge was not performed. The authors noted that ginseng appeared to be associated with the INR change, but that the mechanism was not obvious.[103]

A similar report from Rosado[104] involved a prosthetic aortic valve patient who failed to maintain his INR while taking warfarin and was admitted to a hospital with an acute myocardial infarction and diabetic ketoacidosis. The author suggested that self-treatment with an unconfirmed "ginseng" commercial product for an unspecified period was likely the cause of his INR decrease.

Both these reports remain as isolated examples, and given the poor level of documentation, they cannot be taken as reliable support for the interaction.

Clinical Implications and Adaptations

The weight of the currently available research data suggests that the reported ginseng-warfarin interaction is not a clinically significant problem. Further studies of more effective design should be conducted to examine possible differences between American and Asian ginseng species on hemostatic parameters and possible interactions with clinical anticoagulation. Because Coumadin interacts with a wide variety of substances, sometimes unpredictably, it is prudent to measure the INR at least twice weekly in the weeks after starting or stopping any another therapy, including other drugs, nutraceuticals, and botanicals. Only in recent years have the significant interactions of Coumadin with acetaminophen and cranberry juice been recognized, despite both these having been coadministered with Coumadin for many years before recognition of the interaction.

THEORETICAL, SPECULATIVE, AND PRELIMINARY INTERACTIONS RESEARCH, INCLUDING OVERSTATED INTERACTIONS CLAIMS

Furosemide and Related Loop Diuretics

Bumetanide (Bumex), ethacrynic acid (Edecrin), furosemide (Lasix), torsemide (Demadex).

A frequently cited letter in *JAMA* suggested that the development of refractory response to diuretic therapy in a 63-year-old man with membranous glomerulonephritis on a regimen that included cyclosporine and furosemide was caused by "germanium" content of a "ginseng" preparation.[105] The ginseng species, dose, and duration of administration were not identified (nor were the other "daily nutritional supplements"). The basis for the authors' supposition that the ginseng product contained germanium is therefore unclear; regardless, the "interaction" was attributed to germanium toxicity, not "ginseng," and therefore describing it a "ginseng interaction" is incorrect by the author's own account. Without any corroboratory data, this interaction report is unevaluable and unsupported.

Oral Hypoglycemic Agents and Insulin

Buformin (Andromaco Gliporal, Buformina), chlorpropamide (Diabinese), glimepiride (Amaryl), glipizide (Glucotrol; Glucotrol XL), glyburide (glibenclamide; Diabeta, Glynase, Glynase Prestab, Micronase, Pres Tab), insulin (animal-source insulin: Iletin; human analog insulin: Humanlog; human insulin: Humulin, Novolin, NovoRapid, Oralin); metformin (Dianben, Glucophage, Glucophage XR); combination drugs: glipizide and metformin (Metaglip), glyburide and metformin (Glucovance); phenformin (Debeone, Fenformin), tolazamide (Tolinase), tolbutamide (Orinase, Tol-Tab).

Several secondary sources claim that there is a potential adverse interaction between ginseng and antidiabetic drugs. This appears to be a typical speculative "reverse extrapolation" based on the established property of American ginseng *(P. quinquefolius)* to induce postprandial glucose level lowering in animal and human studies.[106,107] The use of other ginseng species, including *P. ginseng*, as adjuvants for glycemic control is not currently indicated by the available data, which are confined to parenteral administration in rodent models of polysaccharide compounds, "panaxans," rather than ginsenosides.[108,109]

Clinical application of ginseng-related herbs in diabetes has been well reviewed by Sievenpiper et al.[110-113] Relevant issues concerning commercial product variability, dose, and ginsenoside composition are raised in the context of safety and efficacy of these agents as potential antihyperglycemics. However, speculative assertions of adverse interactions are unwarranted by the data and represent a poorly informed clinical appreciation of the general clinical context of using herbal adjuvants in glycemic control.

The 113 citations in this monograph are located under Ginseng on the CD at the back of the book.

Gotu Kola

Botanical Name: *Centella asiatica* (L.) Urban.
Pharmacopoeial Name: Herba centellae.
Synonym: *Hydrocotyl asiatica* L.
Common Names: Centella, gotu kola, Indian pennywort, Indian water navel wort.

HERB DESCRIPTION

Family

Apiaceae.

Parts Used

Aerial parts (or entire plant).

Common Forms

Dried leaves, by infusion.
Tincture, Fluid extract: 45% alcohol.
Standardized Extracts: Triterpene fraction gotu kola (TFGC); titrated extract *Centella asiatica* (TECA); total triterpene fraction of *Centella asiatica* (TTFCA) based on total triterpenes (typically 40% asiaticosides, 30% madecassic acid, 30% asiatic acid). Manufacturers' preparations may vary.

INTERACTIONS REVIEW

Strategic Considerations

In Ayurvedic medicine, centella (gotu kola) is regarded as a *Rasayana* herb (*rasa*, "essence," and *ayana*, "enters").[1] Rasayana tonic herbs are believed to rejuvenate and revitalize mind-body-spirit.[1] Centella has been used in traditional South Asian medicine as a topical remedy for leprosy, eczema, psoriasis, and ulcerous skin conditions, as well as a depurative and tonic. Western uses of gotu kola reflect the traditional indications, with primary emphasis on topical effects, including prevention of keloids and hypertrophic scars, treatments of burns, general acceleration of cicatrization and wound healing after surgery or trauma, and treatment for venous insufficiency, leg ulcers, and varicose and postthrombotic issues. The Rasayana aspects of the herb, in Western terms *adaptogenic,* such as its effects on stress and cognitive performance, resulted in increased popularity and widespread adoption of the remedy by Western herbal practitioners, despite only moderate support in the clinical literature for adaptogenic effects.

Despite its recent popularity, gotu kola is underrepresented in modern therapeutic literature. In the 1983 *British Herbal Pharmacopoeia,* gotu kola was mentioned only for its topical dermatological and vulnerary actions.[2] A more recent monograph by the World Health Organization (WHO)[3] restricts supported therapeutic indications to topical use for wounds, burns, and ulcerous skin ailments, as well as internal use for venous disorders and treatment of stress-induced ulcers.

Much of the literature on gotu kola draws on data from earlier studies (1950s through 1970s), primarily from the Indian and other Asian (Thai, Vietnamese, Indonesian) sources, supported by secondary reviews from African ethnobotany and ethnopharmacological sources. The pharmacological and clinical findings extrapolated from this earlier and limited research have not generally been replicated and can be considered problematic. As a result, depending on the variable emphasis placed on these sources by different reviewers, differing portrayals of the herb have appeared in the secondary literature.

The monograph by WHO[3] tends to underemphasize the earlier data and paints a narrow, but evidentially accurate, picture of gotu kola primarily as a dermatological agent. Other, secondary sources accept the earlier data without qualification.[4] Predictably, however, more derivative sources have the extrapolated further from this secondary literature to suggest interactions that are entirely speculative and unrelated to present clinical uses of the herb.[5] In the authoritative botanical literature, however, gotu kola has no known listed interactions with pharmaceuticals.[3] Clinical reports of any interactions with either galenical extracts or triterpene-enriched preparations are unavailable. From an integrative perspective and drawing on more recent research, interactions between gotu kola and pharmaceuticals (and other natural agents) must be considered in the clinical areas of (1) wound healing in relation to trauma and surgery; (2) venous insufficiency and related issues, such as varicosities, ulcers, and diabetic microangiopathy; and (3) cognitive dysfunction, integrative oncology, and toxic metal chelation.

Several experimental and clinical studies support topical use of gotu kola as a wound-healing and cicatrizing agent.[6-8] A tertiary review (Cochrane) examined trials of topical preparations for striae gravidarum and found at least one combination preparation had significant results for this condition.[9] Although the underlying mechanisms for this activity have not been fully elucidated, recent experimental data suggest effects on fibroblast gene expression modulating connective tissue matrix formation and angiogenesis, including by fibroblast growth factor.[10,11] This is consistent with previous animal studies that showed increases in collagen strength and extracellular matrix collagen content in animal wound-healing models, although the involvement of an antioxidant mechanism is also possible.[6,7,12,13] The mechanisms of wound healing suggest that combinations with nutritional and herbal agents directed toward promotion of wound healing are likely to be a fruitful area of interaction research. For example, Cesarone, Belcaro, Incandela, De Sanctis, and others have conducted numerous small clinical trials with oral gotu kola extracts (particularly Centellase, a preparation standardized to 40% asiaticosides, 30% madecassic acid, 30% asiatic acid) for venous insufficiency, varicose veins, and diabetic microangiopathy, with positive results.[14-23] The Cochrane review of trials of topical preparations for treatment of striae gravidarum found that the most effective preparation was a combination product in which the centella extract was combined with α-tocopherol and collagen hydrolysates, suggesting that the combination with vitamin E was more effective than preparations based on the herb alone.[9]

Adaptogenic herbs such as the ginsengs (e.g., *Panax ginseng* C.A. Meyer) have been incorporated in several ways into integrative cancer protocols. Evidence for possible roles for gotu kola interacting with conventional treatments in the integrative oncological environment is limited, however, and its use needs to be approached with caution. Discounting antiproliferative effects on keratinocytes in psoriasis, few studies show direct cytotoxic effects on cell lines (Ehrlich ascites and Dalton's lymphoma ascites, MCF-7 and MDA-MB231 breast cancer) and in vivo (mouse lung fibroblast) models.[24,25]

One caveat for use of gotu kola in the oncology setting is that the wound-healing activity of the herb is associated with promotion of angiogenesis.[11] Arguably, in metastatic disease treated with antiangiogenic agents, theoretical antagonism with these agents, such as bevacizumab (Avastin), is possible. Many antiangiogenic drugs are investigational at present but are likely to expand significantly as a drug class in the near future.

Oral extracts of gotu kola appear to have potential for protection against radiation-induced dermatitis in animal models, as well as for reduction of radiation-induced changes in taste-related behavior and protection of healthy cells against damage by radiation.[26-29]

Combinations with cytotoxic chemotherapeutic drugs have recently been investigated in a few experimental studies. In a colon cancer line, asiatic acid dose-dependently synergized with irinotecan (CPT-11).[30] Oral pretreatment with *Centella asiatica* ameliorated doxorubicin-induced cardiomyopathy in a rodent model.[31]

In another study, asiaticoside enhanced the cytotoxicity of vincristine in four cell lines.[32] Such data are preliminary, but taken together with the general antioxidant, neuroprotective, and immunomodulating properties of the herb, suggest promise for its possible incorporation into integrative oncological protocols.

There are few leads to suggest mechanisms of neurocognitive pharmacology of gotu kola, despite its traditional reputation for cognitive enhancement and as a longevity tonic.[33,34] In vitro the herb appears to promote neurite growth and nerve regeneration.[35] Experimental studies suggest some modulation of streptozocin-induced "models" of Alzheimer's disease,[36] and semisynthetic asiaticoside derivatives have been tested positively against beta-amyloid neurotoxicity.[37] Centella extracts may protect against glutamate-induced excitotoxicity in cortical neuron culture systems, an effect considered to be mediated by antioxidant mechanisms.[38] Modulation of the acoustic startle responses in rodents (resembling similar effects induced by anxiolytic drugs) has been demonstrated after oral administration of the extracts and is thought to be mediated by a cholecystokinin (CCK) mechanism.[39,40] Another rodent study examined the effect of oral gotu kola on the course of kindling development, kindling-induced learning deficit, and oxidative stress markers in pentylenetetrazole (PTZ)–induced kindling in rats. The authors suggested a possible interaction role for combining gotu kola with antiepileptic medications to help prevent kindling-promoted learning deficits.[41]

At present the available data, mostly derived from in vitro and animal tests, are not sufficiently coherent for a meaningful analysis of potential interactions with psychiatric or neurological drugs. Nonetheless, research in the role of gotu kola extracts in neurocognitive conditions may lead to their use in psychopharmacological integrative strategies as more data become available.

HERB-DRUG INTERACTIONS

Acetylsalicylic Acid and Nonsteroidal Anti-Inflammatory Drugs (NSAIDs) and Other Ulcerogenic Agents

Acetylsalicylic acid (acetosal, acetyl salicylic acid, ASA, salicylsalicylic acid; Arthritis Foundation Pain Reliever, Ascriptin, Aspergum, Asprimox, Bayer Aspirin, Bayer Buffered Aspirin, Bayer Low Adult Strength, Bufferin, Buffex, Cama Arthritis Pain Reliever, Easprin, Ecotrin, Ecotrin Low Adult Strength, Empirin, Extra Strength Adprin-B, Extra Strength Bayer Enteric 500 Aspirin, Extra Strength Bayer Plus, Halfprin 81, Heartline, Regular Strength Bayer Enteric 500 Aspirin, St. Joseph Adult Chewable Aspirin, ZORprin); combination drugs: ASA and caffeine (Anacin); ASA, caffeine, and propoxyphene (Darvon Compound); ASA and carisoprodol (Soma Compound); ASA, codeine, and carisoprodol (Soma Compound with Codeine); ASA and codeine (Empirin with Codeine), ASA, codeine, butalbital, and caffeine (Fiorinal); ASA and extended-release dipyridamole (Aggrenox, Asasantin).

COX-1 inhibitors: Diclofenac (Cataflam, Voltaren), combination drug: diclofenac and misoprostol (Arthrotec); diflunisal (Dolobid), etodolac (Lodine), fenoprofen (Dalfon), furbiprofen (Ansaid), ibuprofen (Advil, Excedrin IB, Motrin, Motrin IB, Nuprin, Pedia Care Fever Drops, Provel, Rufen); combination drug: hydrocodone and ibuprofen (Reprexain, Vicoprofen); indomethacin (indometacin; Indocin, Indocin-SR), ketoprofen (Orudis, Oruvail), ketorolac (Acular ophthalmic, Toradol), meclofenamate (Meclomen), mefenamic acid (Ponstel), meloxicam (Mobic), nabumetone (Relafen), naproxen (Aleve, Anaprox, Naprosyn), oxaprozin (Daypro), piroxicam (Feldene), salsalate (salicylic acid; Amigesic, Disalcid, Marthritic, Mono Gesic, Salflex, Salsitab), sulindac (Clinoril), tolmetin (Tolectin).

COX-2 inhibitor: Celecoxib (Celebrex).

Interaction Type and Significance

⊕ **Potential or Theoretical Beneficial or Supportive Interaction, with Professional Management**

Probability:	Evidence Base:
4. Plausible	○ **Preliminary**

Effect and Mechanism of Action

Ulcerogenic agents such as NSAIDs induce or exacerbate gastric mucosal damage. Concomitant administration of gotu kola reduces gastropathic adverse effects by several protective mechanisms, including increased mucosal secretion and angiogenesis.

Research

Experimental rodent models of gastric ulcers induced by both physical methods and pharmacological agents, including aspirin and ethanol, have demonstrated ulceroprotective effects, with increased mucous secretion and proliferation of epithelial cells of the mucosa as well as increased angiogenesis by oral gotu kola extracts, fresh juice, and purified asiaticide preparations.[11,42,43] Treatment of gastric and duodenal ulcers in humans has been supported by three Korean studies (unavailable for review) cited in the WHO monograph.[3] In one of these, an open-label trial, 15 patients with either peptic or duodenal disease received 60 mg gotu kola extract orally per day. Endoscopic and radiological parameters suggested that 73% of ulcers were healed by the treatment, and 93% of patients reported subjective symptom improvement.

Clinical Implications and Adaptations

Given that a variety of well-documented natural agents are protective against aspirin- and NSAID-induced gastropathy, such as deglycyrrhizinated licorice (DGL) and aloe-based preparations (see Licorice and Aloe monographs), in the West this interaction is unlikely to be considered a significant addition to existing integrative strategies of ulceroprotection by botanicals.

THEORETICAL, SPECULATIVE, AND PRELIMINARY INTERACTIONS RESEARCH, INCLUDING OVERSTATED INTERACTIONS CLAIMS

Central Nervous System (CNS) Depressants: Alcohol, Barbiturates, Benzodiazepines, Opioids, and Sedative-Hypnotics

One 1970s rodent study from the Indian literature attributed sedative effects to gotu kola, and a more recent study of stress-induced ulcers in a rodent model concluded that the ulceroprotective effects of gotu kola could be abolished by pretreatment with bicuculline methiodide, a known gamma-aminobutyric acid (GABA) antagonist.[42] Extrapolations from these limited data to suggest additive interactions with CNS sedatives have been made but do not appear justified.

Oral Hypoglycemic, Hypolipidemic, and Hypocholesterolemic Drugs

Two small preclinical studies on gotu kola from the 1960s Indian literature by Appa Rao and co-workers have been cited by various secondary authors.[4,44] These studies found a tendency for oral administration of the extracts to be associated with elevations in blood sugar, serum cholesterol, and red blood cells in normal subjects. The elevations in the first two parameters were not statistically significant. Nonetheless, these findings have been used speculatively to suggest possible interactions between cholesterol-lowering and antidiabetic pharmaceuticals.[45] No recent work on metabolic effects of gotu kola has substantiated these proposed actions.

The 45 citations for this monograph are located under Gotu Kola on the CD at the back of the book.

Green Tea

Botanical Name: *Camellia sinensis* L. Kuntze.
Pharmacopoeial Name: Folium Camellia sinensis (Theae folium).
Synonym: *Thea sinensis* L.
Common Names: Tea, cha. Various prefixes, such as the country name (e.g., Ceylon), district (e.g., Assam), grade or part (e.g., pekoe [buds]), or degree of fermentation (e.g., green, oolong, black), are used to differentiate various commercial tea products by common name.

Summary

Drug/Class Interaction Type	Mechanism and Significance	Management
Corticosteroids, topical ⊕⊕⊕/☼	Tea additively increases anti-inflammatory effects of drug in refractory atopic dermatitis. Coadministration enables lower dose. May apply to tacrolimus/steroid combinations.	Include green tea extract (GTE) in integrative protocols for refractory atopic dermatitis.
Doxorubicin Anthracycline chemotherapy ⊕/☼	Chemosensitization by L-theanine and polyphenols; cardioprotection by polyphenols. Experimentally demonstrated, not clinically established.	Coadminister GTE and L-theanine during anthracycline chemotherapy.
Iron salts, nonheme ◇	Concurrent consumption of tea with iron salts may reduce bioavailability of iron. Only significant in patient groups with, or at high risk of, iron deficiency anemia.	Use heme iron where supplementation necessary, or temporally separate tea and iron salt dosing and use Fe-absorption enhancers.
Methicillin Beta-lactam and other antibiotics ⊕	Coadministration with beta-lactam antibiotics reverses MRSA resistance. May be of more general clinical significance, synergism demonstrated for various antibiotics.	Coadminister GTE with beta-lactam antibiotics to increase efficacy, especially for suspected drug-resistant strains.
SERMs Aromatase inhibitors ⊕	GTE enhances tamoxifen-induced apoptosis in vitro and inhibits aromatase. Interactions not clinically established.	Consider GTE coadministration with adjuvant endocrine therapies in estrogen-dependent malignancy.
Trastuzumab ⊕	Possible additive effects on HER-2/neu inhibition; not clinically established. Tyrosine kinase inhibition may have more general significance.	Consider coadministration in integrative protocols for HER-2/neu—overexpressing cancers.
Warfarin Anticoagulant or antiplatelet agents ?	Possible antiplatelet effects; one unreliable report of warfarin interaction. Clinical significance unknown, probably minor.	Monitor INR; monitor for signs of bleeding. Low levels of GTE unlikely to be problematic.

MSRA, Methicillin-resistant *Staphylococcus aureus*; *SERMs*, selective estrogen response modulators; *INR*, international normalized ratio.

HERB DESCRIPTION

Family

Theaceae (Ternstroemiaceae).

Related Species

At least one subspecies and several cultivars are described.

Habitat and Cultivation

Tea plants are actually evergreen trees maintained as tea bushes by pruning in cultivation to shrub height to enable hand harvesting of the young leaves. Tea *(Cha)* originally was native to the Yunnan province in southwestern China and initially spread to several different areas in China and India, but it has been in cultivation for so long in rain forest zones throughout many Southeast Asian countries that wild-type plants are now rare. China and India are the largest cultivators, and India is the largest exporter. Pu'erh tea *(Pu Erh Cha)* is derived from the leaves of old tea trees on six specific mountains in Yunnan, fermented and aged through specific processes, and is considered a separate beverage with significantly different characteristics and medicinal actions.

Parts Used

Young leaves, tips, and leaf buds.

Common Forms

Dried Leaf.
Powdered Green Tea Leaf.
Dry Extracts: Derived from ethanolic extracts, preparations may vary; some may be decaffeinated, standardized to total catechins of greater than 25%. Concentrates of specific tea polyphenols, up to 97% catechins, and other compounds, such as L-theanine (analog of L-glutamine), are marketed as nutrient preparations and therapeutic agents. L-Theanine is also produced in high yield by microbial fermentation for use in nutriceutical products.

HERB IN CLINICAL PRACTICE

Overview

Tea is the most common beverage in the world (other than water). Tea belongs to the universally popular category of xanthine-containing beverages, such as coffee, cola, maté, and cocoa, the popularity of which is partly related to their caffeine content. Commercially, the principal types are green tea and black tea. Green tea is stabilized and dried immediately after harvesting, then rolled. This processing method means the crude herb approximates as closely as possible to its natural state at harvesting; thus green tea is designated as the "medicinal" form of the herb, as derived from tea bushes. Black teas are dried after the rolling process, allowing oxidative enzymatic changes to take place, principally polymerization of the flavan-3-ols into the characteristic oligomeric red-brown theaflavins and thearubigins, as well as the polymeric tannins, which are absent from green tea.

Research interest in green tea compounds has accelerated dramatically in the last decade, with epidemiological, experimental, and clinical evidence for chemopreventive, antiproliferative, and cardioprotective benefits of tea polyphenols. These activities are the result of a variety of pharmacological mechanisms, including antioxidant effects, cell cycle effects, and signal transduction effects.[1-4]

Green tea has not traditionally been considered part of the Western herbal materia medica until the rather recent interest in its chemopreventive properties. The usual authoritative sources of botanical medicine have not, to date, produced therapeutic monographs on the plant. In herbal medicine, tea has primarily been regarded as a dietary source of caffeine and astringent tannins and is regarded as a milder stimulant than the caffeine-containing cola and guaraná, which have been preferred when caffeine-containing herbs were indicated. McKenna et al.[5] reviewed the general literature on tea in 2002. Interest in the chemopreventive and cardioprotective properties of tea polyphenols have led to the manufacture of concentrated preparations of these compounds. Tea leaf is regulated as a food beverage ("generally recognized as safe," GRAS) in the United States, whereas isolated and concentrated green tea polyphenols are classified as dietary supplements.

Historical/Ethnomedicine Precedent

Traditional Chinese use of green tea leaf (*Lu Cha*) is primarily for gastrointestinal complaints, for which it is combined with other herbs to treat nausea and vomiting and as an antidiarrheal (astringent). It is also used for headaches and dispelling "damp." In Ayurvedic medicine, green tea is similarly considered a diuretic, astringent, and mild stimulant. As noted, Pu'erh tea (*Pu Erh Cha*) is considered a separate medicinal agent, significantly rarer and highly valued, with distinct qualities and uses. *Pu Erh Cha* is considered "Earth" in nature and *Lu Cha* "Wood" in nature.

Known or Potential Therapeutic Uses

Atherosclerosis; adjunct to some antimicrobial and antineoplastic pharmacotherapies for microbial infections; cardioprotection and reduction of cardiovascular risk factors; chemoprotection; chemoprevention of colon, pancreatic, esophageal, and other cancers; central nervous system (CNS) stimulation; gingival and periodontal infection; headache; hypercholesterolemia; mild diarrhea; thermogenesis (and weight loss); renal insufficiency.

Key Constituents

Methylxanthines, principally caffeine (2%-4%); polyphenols (30%-40%), four principal compounds: (−)-epicatechin (EC), (−)-epigallocatechin (EGC), (−)-epicatechin gallate (ECG), and (−)-epigallocatechin gallate (EGCG).

Other constituents include various flavonols, including proanthocyanidins, amino acids (principally L-theanine), protein, vitamins (ascorbate, B group), minerals, and organic acids.

Note: The abbreviations EC, EGC, ECG, and EGCG are used throughout this monograph to designate the four principal catechin compounds.

Therapeutic Dosing Range

Infusion of Dried Leaf: 1.0 to 3.0 g as required; 1 cup delivers 300 to 400 mg of polyphenols; up to 5 cups per day as a beverage.
Powder: 4 to 12 g by decoction, typical modern Chinese dosing.
Standardized Extract: Polyphenols range from 25% (Exolise, Arktopharma) to 97% (Tegreen, Pharmanex LLC) polyphenols to deliver up to approximately 750 mg of polyphenols per dose.

INTERACTIONS REVIEW
Strategic Considerations

Beverage consumption of tea needs to be delineated from therapeutic administration of polyphenol-rich green tea extracts (GTEs). The popularity of beverage tea consumption, particularly in the form of black tea, is often considered to be based primarily on its caffeine content. Caffeine, an ingredient of hundreds of over-the-counter (OTC) medications, is well known for its CNS-stimulating and adenosine receptor–mediated effects. In beverage use, green tea delivers only 50 to 100 mg caffeine per cup, about half (or less) the quantity of caffeine in a cup of coffee. Some authors, when reviewing green tea interactions, have resorted to listing well-known caffeine-drug interactions without contextualization of beverage versus therapeutic use of tea, or distinction between green tea and black tea forms, and despite the lack of evidence that normal dietary tea consumption induces caffeine-drug interactions.

Caffeine interactions are properly classified in the domain of the drug-drug interaction literature; for example, *Stockley's Drug Interactions*[6] lists more than 70 interactions between caffeine and other drugs. Caffeine, along with related methylxanthines such as theophylline, is cleared oxidatively by cytochrome P450 (CYP450) 1A2, so drugs that strongly inhibit 1A2 (e.g., fluvoxamine, quinolone antibiotics) can accentuate the adverse effects of caffeine consumption in chronic high-level tea consumption. The clinical importance of these effects is not established, however, and case reports are lacking. Caffeine has been shown to contribute to chemopreventive effects of GTEs in the few studies that have made direct comparisons among tea, decaffeinated tea, and caffeine.[7-9]

The principal health benefits of chemoprevention and cardioprotection associated with dietary tea consumption are related to its polyphenol content. The amount of polyphenols in green tea infusions is about 300 to 400 mg per cup, whereas standardized GTEs can contain up to 97% polyphenols, and some may be decaffeinated. Relatively high doses of green tea infusion are required for therapeutic use because of the poor intrinsic oral bioavailability of the polyphenols; 10 cups of green tea per day (not uncommon in Japan) could arguably be considered the transition between beverage and therapeutic dose exposure. Black tea contains considerably less flavan-3-ol catechins, which are transformed by fermentation into oligomeric derivatives, the thearubigins and theaflavins, which are not found in unfermented green tea products.[10]

Typical concerns about potential adverse effects of cardio-protective herbs on hemostasis and possible interactions with anticoagulants are discussed later in relation to tea compounds. The mechanisms underlying the chemopreventive and anticancer effects of green tea are currently subject of much investigation, and emerging data on tea polyphenols' synergistic effects with chemotherapy, modification of drug resistance, and multiple effects on signal transduction are emerging from in vitro and cell-line studies, with potentially valuable implications for integrative cancer therapeutics. These potential interactions are reviewed here, although clinical data are currently anecdotal. However, at least two significant caveats must be considered when in vivo extrapolations are made from the experimental findings. Current epidemiological data on the chemopreventive effects of green tea are positive, at least for breast cancer, although the data are limited and clinical trial evidence is lacking.[11]

First, cell-line studies using concentrations of tea polyphenols in the 100 to 1000 micromolar (μM) range cannot be extrapolated to beverage consumption because of the low oral bioavailability of these compounds. The different polyphenols and their metabolites do have differing bioavailabilities; EGCG is less bioavailable than the other compounds, possibly because it is the only tea polyphenol that is a substrate as well as inhibitor of intestinal P-glycoprotein; P-gp is inhibited by all the tea polyphenols, with EGCG being the most potent inhibitor.[12] A human study of single–oral dose kinetics of EGCG found that higher doses (800 mg) achieved significantly greater area under curve (AUC) and maximum concentration (C_{max}) levels than lower doses (200 and 400 mg), suggesting a saturable first-pass mechanism.[13] Biotransformation of green tea polyphenols is complex and involves glucuronidation, sulfation, and methylation by catechol-O-methyltransferase (COMT) as well as intestinal flora–mediated ring fission products that are further metabolized to phenylacetic and phenylpropionic acids. The activities of the different intermediate metabolites remain unclear, although their bioavailability is higher than that of EGCG.[14] Preliminary evidence also suggests that significant differences may exist between rodent and human microsomal metabolism of tea polyphenols.[15]

Second, although derivative literature often ascribes the effects of green tea polyphenols to their antioxidant properties, some of their in vitro activity may result from pro-oxidant actions. EGCG is unstable in cell culture conditions and tends to undergo auto-oxidation, producing superoxide radicals and hydrogen peroxide (H_2O_2).[16] Hou et al.[17] suggested that EGCG-related peroxide formation may underlie cell-line effects such as apoptosis induction and that free radicals may be responsible for the observed EGCG-induced inhibition of growth factor receptors EGFR and PDGR. It is unclear whether such pro-oxidative reactions occur in vivo as a result of the low oxygen partial pressures and high antioxidant capacity found in vivo.

The phenomenon of in vitro pro-oxidant effects is likely an artifact of the in vitro absence of antioxidant networks. Logically, only in vitro systems that include physiological levels of albumin, glucose, uric acid, and glutathione and typical serum levels of diet-derived antioxidants would be reasonable in terms of extrapolating to the in vivo situation. Most in vitro systems do not attempt to replicate in vivo antioxidant networks.

Effects on Drug Metabolism and Bioavailability

Green tea compounds may affect all three phases of drug transport and metabolism and thus potentially participate in pharmacokinetic interactions with drugs. Animal and in vitro evidence suggests that polyphenols inhibit Phase I drug metabolism by CYP450 enzymes 1A1 and 1A2.[18-23] One study using recombinant human CYP450 in a genetically engineered bacterial model found EGCG appears to have nonspecific inhibitory effects on 1A1, 1A2, 2A6, 2C19, 2E1, and 3A4.[24] Different forms of tea exhibit different effects on rat liver enzyme activity in a study of rats fed different teas for 4 weeks; for example, oolong and Earl Grey tea induced increases in 3A4 activity but green tea did not, and 1A2 was unaffected by any tea, but 1A1 was affected by both green and fermented teas.[25] These studies suggest that different tea compounds may exert different effects on various drug-metabolizing enzymes, especially those involved in carcinogen metabolism. At this time, however, the clinical effects in humans remain to be established.

Phase II conjugation reactions are mediated by conjugases and transferases. Tea polyphenols not only are substrates for glucuronidation and sulfation, but also have demonstrated significant induction effects on uridine diphosphate (UDP) glucuronosyltransferase (UGT) and sulfotransferase isoforms (SULTs) as well as glutathione transferase in rodent models and in vitro.[15,26-32] Again, these effects have not been studied in vivo in humans, although it is plausible that they may underlie the chemopreventive effects of green tea against certain carcinogenic and tumorigenic agents.

Phase III, mediated by drug transporters, principally P-gp, is also modulated by all the tea polyphenols, but EGCG appears to be the most potent inhibitor.[12,16,33-38] There is some evidence that additional drug transporter proteins, including the organic anion-transporting polypeptide (OATP), may be inhibited by tea polyphenols.[39-41] No single polyphenol component appears to be responsible for the inhibitory effect of GTE on multidrug resistance–associated protein 2 (MRP-2), found in intestinal cells.[42] The amino acid theanine has specific effects on the glutamate transporter, which is considered to be the mechanism underlying an interaction between theanine (and whole green tea) and anthracycline agents such as doxorubicin.[43-46] At this time, the firmest evidence that tea polyphenols may exhibit significant pharmacokinetic interactions with prescription drugs relates to effects on Phase III drug transporters. Further studies are required to elucidate the details of their effects on Phase I and Phase II enzymes, for which in vivo human data are currently lacking.

Theanine

The amino acid constituent L-theanine (δ-glutamylethylamide) is the primary amino acid constituent of green tea and constitutes 1% to 3% of the dry weight of the dry leaf. L-Theanine has recently become available as a separate nutrient product after research suggested that it underlies the synergistic interactions of GTEs with anthracycline chemotherapeutic drugs, as well as having neuroregenerative and mood-elevating effects that may have applications in Alzheimer's disease and affective disorders. The currently known L-theanine interactions are included in the next section (see Doxorubicin).

HERB-DRUG INTERACTIONS

Corticosteroids, Topical

Alclometasone (Aclovate, Modrasone), amcinonide (Cyclocort), beclomethasone, betamethasone dipropionate/valerate (betamethasone topical; Alphatrex, Beta-Val, Betaderm, Betanate, Betatrex, Diprolene AF, Diprolene,

Diprosone, Luxiq, Maxivate, Teladar, Uticort, Valisone), clobetasol (clobetasol topical; Cormax, Dermoval, Dermotyl, Dermovate, Dermoxin, Eumosone, Lobate, Olux, Temovate, Temovate E, Topifort), clobetasone (Eumovate), clocortolone (clocortolone pivalate topical; Cloderm), desonide (DesOwen, Tridesilon), desoximetasone (Topicort, Topicort LP), desoxymethasone, dexamethasone (Aeroseb-Dex, Decaderm, Decadron, Decaspray), diflorasone (Apexicon, Florone, Maxiflor, Psorcon), diflucortolone (Nerisona, Nerisone), fluocinolone (Derma-Smoothe/FS, Fluonid, Synelar, Synemol), fluocinonide (Fluonex, Lidex, Lidex-E, Lonide, Vanos), fludroxycortide (flurandrenolone), fluocortolone (Ultralan), flurandrenolide (Cordran, Drenison), fluticasone (Cutivate), halobetasol (Ultravate), halcinonide (Halog), hydrocortisone 17-butyrate/acetate/probutate/valerate (hydrocortisone topical; Acticort100, Aeroseb-HC, Ala-Cort, Ala-Scalp HP, Allercort, Alphaderm, Bactine, Beta-HC, Caldecort Anti-Itch, Cetacort, Cort-Dome, Cortaid, Cortef, Cortifair, Cortizone, Cortone, Cortril, Delacort, Dermacort, Dermarest, DriCort, DermiCort, Dermtex HC, Epifoam, Gly-Cort, Hi-Cor, Hydro-Tex, Hytone, LactiCare-HC, Lanacort, Lemoderm, Locoid, MyCort, Nutracort, Pandel, Penecort, Pentacort, Proctocort, Rederm, S-T Cort, Synacort, Texacort, Westcort), mometasone (Elocon, mometasone topical), triamcinolone (Aristocort, Triderm, Kenalog, Flutex, Kenonel, triamcinolone topical); combination drug: triamcinolone and nystatin (Mycolog II).

Interaction Type and Significance

⊕⊕⊕ **Beneficial or Supportive Interaction, Not Requiring Professional Management**
☼ **Prevention or Reduction of Drug Adverse Effect**

Probability:	Evidence Base:
3. Possible	○ **Preliminary**

Effect and Mechanism of Action

Coadministration of tea with topical steroids improves dermatological response to these drugs in refractory atopic dermatitis. This may allow reduction of corticosteroid dose and lowered adverse drug effects.

Research

Uehara et al.[47] conducted an open trial of 118 patients with refractory atopic dermatitis, who were instructed to continue with their pharmacological treatments, primarily topical steroids. Some patients (not specified) were taking oral histamines. An infusion of oolong tea was consumed three times a day, the beverage being made from 10 g dried tea infused in 1000 mL water for 5 minutes. After 1 month a significant improvement in skin lesions was recorded in 63% of patients. Benefits appeared after 1 to 2 weeks of treatment, and at 6 months, 54% of patients reported persistent improvement. The authors suggest that oolong tea extracts have antiallergenic properties and improve response to topical steroid pharmacotherapy.[47] The mechanisms of the effect of tea polyphenols on atopic inflammatory responses are not known but may involve antioxidant effects.

Clinical Implications and Adaptations

The small study reporting beneficial effects of coadministration of tea with topical steroids is interesting for the low dose of tea used. Reduction of steroid anti-inflammatory dose is always a desirable goal when these agents are administered chronically. Increasingly, however, the treatment of choice in atopic dermatitis are the topical immunosuppressive agents (e.g., tacrolimus), which are often combined with topical corticosteroids in refractory cases of atopic dermatitis.[48] Effects of tea polyphenols on this combination are unknown.

Doxorubicin and Related Anthracycline Chemotherapy

Evidence: Doxorubicin (Adriamycin, Rubex).
Extrapolated, based on similar properties: Cisplatin (*cis*-diaminedichloroplatinum, CDDP; Platinol, Platinol-AQ), daunorubicin (Cerubidine, DaunoXome), epirubicin (Ellence, Pharmorubicin), irinotecan (camptothecin-11, CPT-11; Campto, Camptosar), mitoxantrone (Novantrone, Onkotrone).
Related but evidence lacking for extrapolation: Doxorubicin, pegylated liposomal (Caelyx, Doxil, Myocet).

Interaction Type and Significance

⊕ **Potential or Theoretical Beneficial or Supportive Interaction, with Professional Management**
☼ **Prevention or Reduction of Drug Adverse Effect**

Probability:	Evidence Base:
4. Plausible	○ **Preliminary**

Effect and Mechanism of Action

Tea polyphenols appear to reduce doxorubicin-induced cardiotoxicity by modifying lipid peroxidation and cardiomyocyte–fatty acid metabolism patterns. EGCG also increases tumor sensitivity to doxorubicin by inhibiting P-gp, which promotes efflux of the drug from malignant cells. Theanine further enhances the efficacy of doxorubicin through inhibition of glutamate transporters and modulation of the glutathione-*S* conjugate exporter pump (GS-X). Preliminary data suggest that related anthracyclines and possibly unrelated classes of chemotherapy agents such as cisplatin and irinotecan may behave similarly when coadministered with tea polyphenols and theanine.

Research

Sugiyama, Sadzuka, and colleagues have conducted a series of investigations on the effects of theanine and EGCG on the modulation of sensitivity to doxorubicin in different cell lines, including Ehrlich ascites carcinoma cells,[35,49] and in an animal model using M5076 ovarian sarcoma tumor–bearing mice,[44-46,50,51] as well as in P388 leukemia cell–bearing animals.[35] The effect of theanine at 10 mg/kg/day intraperitoneally in the animal model was a significant increase (2.9 times) in intratumor doxorubicin concentration and a significant decrease in hepatic metastasis development. Oral administration of green tea/theanine at 100 mg/kg/day for 4 days also led to a 55% reduction in tumor size compared with doxorubicin-only control animals. Theanine reduced concentrations of doxorubicin in normal tissues (lung, liver, kidney) but was found to increase doxorubicin concentration in hepatic metastases. Theanine also reduced myocardial lipid peroxidation. Theanine, itself a glutamate derivative, inhibits glutamate transporters, and this is now considered to be one mechanism for doxorubicin concentrations to be increased in tumor cells. The experimental findings are reviewed by Sugiyama and Sadzuka.[46]

Tea polyphenols also modulate P-gp by inhibiting the membrane adenosinetriphosphatase (ATPase).[34,38] The well-documented cardioprotective effects of green tea polyphenols have been shown to reduce the toxicity of doxorubicin in cultured cardiomyocytes, as measured by fatty acid composition, conjugated diene concentration, and lactate dehydrogenase

(LDH) release. The primary mechanism is antioxidant prevention of lipid peroxidation by the doxorubicin-induced superoxide and peroxide radicals. However, there is also a direct effect on unsaturated fatty acid metabolism involving the desaturating/elongating enzymes.[52]

Because iron-chelating compounds are also protective against anthracycline-induced cardiac damage, chelation by tea polyphenols may be an additional mechanism, but evidence for this is not available.

Clinical Implications and Adaptations

Experimental data suggest that anthracycline cardiotoxicity can be reduced by green tea polyphenols, and that the green tea component theanine can increase sensitivity to doxorubicin in drug-resistant cell lines. Clinical studies are required to confirm these effects in human patients; however, given the lack of adverse effects of theanine and the green tea polyphenols, employment of these natural compounds as adjuncts to anthracycline chemotherapy should be considered for inclusion in integrative support protocols during anthracycline chemotherapy.

Iron Salts (Nonheme Iron)

Interaction Type and Significance

◈ Impaired Drug Absorption and Bioavailability, Negligible Effect

Probability:
3. Possible

Evidence Base:
● Consensus

Effect and Mechanism of Action

Tea polyphenols have been shown to form chelates with nonheme iron. A pharmacokinetic interaction may occur if green tea is coadministered with food containing nonheme iron, which may reduce the level of iron absorption. The clinical significance of this interaction on iron status is considered minimal.

Research

Samman et al.[53] performed a small open trial using radiolabeled iron added to meals over 4 days in healthy young women. The meals were identical except that green tea polyphenol extract or rosemary extract was added to the baseline test meal. A standard reference dose of an iron salt was also administered to examine variation in iron absorption characteristics. Addition of either natural agent to the meal caused a small decrease in iron absorption, slightly more with green tea than rosemary, a relative absorption decrease of 28% ($p < 0.01$).

A systematic review of available data on the inverse association between tea consumption and iron status examined 16 studies, including subgroups with high and low anemia risk status. Following adjustment for dietary factors there was no association between tea consumption and ferritin and hemoglobin status.[54] Another systematic review of observational studies examining the effects of tea drinking on iron consumption concluded that restrictions on tea drinking were unnecessary in healthy people with no risk of iron deficiency.[55] One often-quoted study suggests that infants age 6 to 12 months consuming 250 mL tea per day (median value) had a higher incidence of microcytic anemia than those who did not drink tea.[56]

Integrative Therapeutics, Clinical Concerns, and Adaptations

Standard medical advice for groups at risk of iron deficiency anemia is to drink tea between meals, waiting at least 1 hour after eating.[57] Iron absorption enhancers such as ascorbic acid can be used in at-risk individuals, and administration of supplementary iron in the form of heme iron will tend to avoid any chelation problems based on the simple salts (e.g., ferrous sulfate, gluconate).

Methicillin and Related Beta-Lactam Antibiotics

Evidence: Methicillin (Staphcillin); beta-lactamase–resistant penicillins: cloxacillin (Cloxapen), dicloxacillin (Dynapen, Dycill), oxacillin (Bactocill); carbapenem antibiotics: meropenem (Merrem I.V.); combination drug: imipenem and cilastatin (Primaxin I.M., Primaxin I.V.).
Extrapolated, based on similar properties: Cephalosporin antibiotics, ciprofloxacin and other fluoroquinolone antibiotics, ketaconazoles, macrolide antibiotics, other penicillin antibiotics; combination drugs: amoxicillin and clavulanic acid (Augmentin, Augmentin XR, Clavulin, Nuclav); clavulanic acid and ticarcillin (Timentin).

Interaction Type and Significance

⊕ Potential or Theoretical Beneficial or Supportive Interaction, with Professional Management

Probability:
1. Certain

Evidence Base:
○ Preliminary

Effect and Mechanism of Action

A synergistic interaction between tea polyphenols when combined with a broad range of beta-lactam antibiotics that appears to reverse beta-lactam resistance by modulating the bacterial phenotype in methicillin-resistant strains of *Staphylococcus aureus* (MRSA). The interaction may be an example of a general interaction between tea polyphenols and antimicrobial drugs.

Research

A number of experimental studies have demonstrated significant reductions in minimum inhibitory concentration (MIC) of methicillin, penicillin, oxacillin, and other beta-lactam antibiotics by two orders of magnitude. This effectively reverses resistance in several isolated MRSA strains by lowering MIC to below the resistance breakpoint.[58-61] Initial studies used either EGCG or ECG, and there were discrepancies regarding the relative potencies of the two catechins, as well as a lack of data on the mechanisms involved and as to whether related polyphenolic compounds might exert similar effects. The mechanism of modulation of resistance may be multifactorial, including efflux pump disabling[62] and penicillinase inhibition,[63] as well as direct binding to peptidoglycan in the bacterial membrane and intercalation in the membrane lipid layer.[64,65]

Stapleton et al.[66] systematically tested ECG, EGCG, and several other gallates and catechins, measuring oxacillin activity against different MRSA isolates, and established that ECG has a greater capacity to modulate beta-lactam resistance than EGCG. They also found that the gallate moiety was essential for activity, and that ECG was also effective with the carbapenem antibiotics imipenem and meropenem. Recent investigations suggest that the synergistic effects with antimicrobials may extend to other drug-microbial combinations, such as macrolides with *Helicobacter pylori*, ketaconazoles with *Candida albicans*, and fluoroquinolones and *Escherichia coli*.[67-71] A rodent model of prostatitis was used to demonstrate a synergistic effect between ciprofloxacin and green tea catechin.[72]

One small, controlled trial examined the effects of inhalation of tea catechins (2 mL containing 7.4 mg polyphenols with 3.7 mg EGCG via nebulizer three times daily for 4 weeks) in 12 elderly patients with confirmed MRSA titer in sputum samples versus 12 similar controls. Classification of MRSA was defined as cultured *S. aureus* showing an oxacillin MIC of more than 4 mg/L. The trial included patients who had been treated with antibiotics, but during the trial period the catechins were administered alone. After 1 week the number of patients in the catechin group with detectable MRSA was significantly less than that of the controls. Hospital stay was also significantly reduced for the catechin group compared with controls.[73] This trial suggests benefits to catechins taken alone in MRSA-positive patients, but did not investigate the effects of coadministration.

To date, clinical trials on combinations are unavailable.

Integrative Therapeutics, Clinical Concerns, and Adaptations

Methicillin-resistant *S. aureus* is a widespread cause of nosocomial infection. Experimental evidence strongly supports the use of tea catechins, particularly EGC, in combination with beta-lactam antibiotics. Although most relevant to the hospital setting, studies have yet to be undertaken. However, integrative practitioners dealing with community-acquired infections in vulnerable populations suspected of demonstrating antibiotic resistance might choose to coadminister tea polyphenol extracts to modulate the antibiotic resistance.

Selective Estrogen Response Modulators (SERMs), Aromatase Inhibitors

Evidence: Tamoxifen (Nolvadex).
Extrapolated, based on similar properties: Anastrozole (Arimidex), exemestane (Aromasin), letrozole (Femara), raloxifene (Evista), toremifene (Fareston).

Interaction Type and Significance

⊕ Potential or Theoretical Beneficial or Supportive Interaction, with Professional Management

Probability: Evidence Base:
6. Unknown   ○ Preliminary

Effect and Mechanism of Action

A possible interaction is based on in vitro evidence that tamoxifen-induced apoptosis is increased by EGCG, possibly mediated by inhibitory effects on tumor necrosis factor alpha (TNF-α). Additional evidence suggests that tea polyphenols may also have aromatase inhibitor–like activity. The interaction is not clinically established.

Research

In a series of studies using human lung cancer PC-9 and breast cancer MCF-7 cell lines, Suganuma et al.[74,75] investigated the induction of apoptosis by different tea polyphenols alone and in combination. They found that EC (which lacks the galloyl moiety and has no effect on apoptosis alone) synergistically increased the apoptotic effects of ECGC in a dose-dependent manner. Parallel effects were found on BALB/C-3T3 cells in which EC synergistically increased the effect of EGCG on inhibition of TNF-α (IC$_{50}$ reduced from 60 to 7 μM), leading the investigators to posit a TNF-α–mediated mechanism. Using the same technique, they examined the effects of adding either sulindac (a classic NSAID) or tamoxifen to EGCG in the PC9 cell model and found that cotreatment by EGCG with either agent induced apoptosis

more than when EGCG was given alone. The effect was smaller with tamoxifen than with sulindac. They replicated the effects of the combination on TNF-α inhibition in the BALB/C-3T3 cells, as well as in MCF7 cells, although these data were not presented.

Way et al.[76] conducted a series of investigations into the mechanisms of EGCG and three black tea theaflavin compounds effects on HER-2/neu transfected MCF7 breast cells. They demonstrated that both EGCG and theaflavins inhibited tyrosine kinase phosphorylation, and further that EGCG/theaflavins could modulate the resistance of the HER-2/neu transfected cells to tamoxifen. The same study series also found the tea compounds showed significant aromatase inhibitory activity in rat ovarian and human placental microsomes. Aromatase inhibition by tea polyphenols has also been confirmed in a human placenta microsome assay, using a combination polyphenol extract (P-60) (IC$_{50}$ = 28 μM).[77] Because aromatase enzymes, predominantly in fat tissue, synthesize estrogen from adrenal androgens, pharmaceutical aromatase inhibitors are widely used in treatment of estrogen-dependent breast cancer in women without active ovarian function, to reduce estrogen levels further.

As a footnote, a rodent model found that GTE reduced tamoxifen-induced hepatic injury, following 7 days of tamoxifen at 45 mg/kg intraperitoneally, as indexed by transaminase levels as well as increases in glutathione and other antioxidant enzymes.[78]

Integrative Therapeutics, Clinical Concerns, and Adaptations

The current experimental data for possible synergy between tamoxifen and tea polyphenols are preliminary, and extrapolations cannot be reliably made until confirmation of the effects by human and clinical studies. The suggestions that TNF-α pathways may be modulated by estrogen, and that the activity of tamoxifen involves interaction with this and related factors, are supported in the literature, although the mechanisms are not fully understood.[79,80] Given the activities of tea compounds on multiple molecular targets of the cancer process, coadministration of GTEs in hormone-dependent and hormone-independent mammary carcinoma with adjuvant chemotherapeutic agents warrants further study.

Trastuzumab

Trastuzumab (Herceptin).

Interaction Type and Significance

⊕ Potential or Theoretical Beneficial or Supportive Interaction, with Professional Management

Probability: Evidence Base:
4. Plausible   ⊕ Preliminary

Effect and Mechanism of Action

Potential additive or synergistic interaction occurs between tea polyphenols, especially EGCG, and trastuzumab because of convergent pharmacodynamic HER-2/neu inhibition effects, probably associated with receptor tyrosine kinase activity. The interaction has been experimentally demonstrated, but clinical support is currently not available.

Research

The chemopreventive effects of tea polyphenols have been demonstrated in various animal models as well as by human epidemiological studies. The mechanisms are multifactorial and have been studied in a variety of cell culture models.[1-4,14,17,81-83]

The tea polyphenol EGCG inhibits receptor tyrosine kinase activity (IC_{50} = 1-2 µM).[84] Masuda et al.[85] demonstrated EGCG inhibition of EGFR autophosphorylation in head and neck squamous cell carcinoma and breast cancer cell lines. The same investigators later demonstrated significant inhibition of HER-2/neu activation in the same cell lines, although at high concentrations (10 and 30 µg); also, the sensitivity of both cell lines to paclitaxel (Taxol) was significantly increased by much lower doses of (0.1-1.0 µg/mL) of EGCG.[86]

Way et al.[76] conducted a series of investigations into the effects of EGCG and three black tea theaflavin compounds on HER-2/neu transfected MCF7 breast cells. They demonstrated that both EGCG and theaflavins inhibited tyrosine kinase phosphorylation, and further that EGCG/theaflavins could modulate the resistance of the HER-2/neu transfected cells to tamoxifen. The same study series also found the tea compounds showed significant aromatase inhibitory activity in rat ovarian and human placental microsomes.[76] The authors concluded that tea polyphenols could be useful in HER-2/neu–overexpressing cancers. Shimizu et al.[87] used a colon cancer line overexpressing HER-3 and cyclooxygenase-2 (COX-2) and found that very low doses of ECGC inactivated EGFR, HER-2, and HER-3; decreased COX-2 and Bcl-xL proteins; and induced apoptosis.

Integrative Therapeutics, Clinical Concerns, and Adaptations

Concentrated tea polyphenol extracts are typically combined with other chemopreventive compounds in botanical and nutritional components of integrative cancer therapeutic protocols. Despite the preliminary nature of the experimental data, the available studies suggest tyrosine kinase inhibition is one of the pluripotent therapeutic activities of tea polyphenols, and that these may be effective in combination with trastuzumab (Herceptin) in diseases that overexpress the HER-2/neu receptor. Because this receptor is also present on myocardial cells, trastuzumab is associated with cardiotoxicity, which is exacerbated when combined with anthracycline agents, themselves cardiotoxic.[68,88,89] Coadministration of anthracycline chemotherapy agents and trastuzumab is contraindicated because of the high incidence of clinical congestive heart failure that occurred in clinical trials of the combination. Even patients who have received anthracycline chemotherapy many years previously have an increased sensitivity to cardiotoxic effects of trastuzumab. In patients undergoing chemotherapy with trastuzumab, especially in patients who have previously received doxorubicin, coadministration of green tea polyphenol extracts in sufficient doses may ameliorate cardiotoxicity and increase drug effectiveness. Previous reservations about the applicability of cell-line studies with tea compounds are particularly pertinent to these extrapolations (see Strategic Considerations).

Warfarin and Related Oral Vitamin K Antagonist Anticoagulants

Evidence: Warfarin (Coumadin, Marevan, Warfilone).
Similar properties but evidence indicating no or reduced interaction effects: Anisindione (Miradon), dicumarol, ethyl biscoumacetate (Tromexan), nicoumalone (acenocoumarol; Acitrom, Sintrom), phenindione (Dindevan), phenprocoumon (Jarsin, Marcumar).

Interaction Type and Significance
? **Interaction Possible but Uncertain Occurrence and Unclear Implications**

Probability:
5. Improbable

Evidence Base:
▽ Mixed

Effect and Mechanism of Action
An interaction was originally suggested by an isolated case report of significant INR reduction after consumption of green tea (beverage) in a patient stable on warfarin. The hypothesized mechanism of vitamin K content of green tea counteracting the effects of warfarin on vitamin K–dependent coagulation factor synthesis is unlikely. Antiplatelet rather than anticoagulant effects are more plausible.

Research
Kang et al.[90] investigated the in vitro effects of tea catechins and EGCG on human platelet aggregation induced by adenosine, epinephrine, collagen, and calcium ionophore A23187 and found a dose-dependent inhibition of platelet aggregation but no change in any coagulation parameters. This confirmed an earlier report by Sagesaka-Mitane et al.[91] that the hot-water extracts of tea and EGCG inhibited collagen-induced aggregation in rabbit platelets. Son et al.[92] performed a series of tests on rabbit and rodent platelets with GTE and concluded that the antiplatelet activity observed in vitro was caused by inhibition of thromboxane A_2 (TXA_2) and prostaglandin D_2 resulting from inhibition of arachidonic acid liberation and of inhibition of TXA_2 synthase in response to collagen-induced aggregation.

Few human studies to date have examined the effects of tea on platelet aggregation. In a randomized crossover study, Duffy et al.[93] examined the effects of acute and chronic black tea beverage consumption versus water placebo on 49 patients with coronary artery disease (CAD). They failed to detect any effects on platelet aggregation induced by adenosine diphosphate (ADP) or thrombin receptor activating peptide by the tea infusions at either acute or chronic doses. However, most patients in this study apparently continued with aspirin antithrombotic therapy, which confounds interpretation of the results. Wolfram et al.[94] found that with 1 month of black tea consumption, healthy volunteers displayed gender differences in effect, with only females showing a slight decrease in ADP-induced platelet aggregation. Hodgson et al.[95] examined a wide range of hemostasis parameters before and after the consumption of black tea (five cups per day for 4 weeks) by 22 volunteers. Platelet aggregation did not differ for collagen or ADP stimulation, and no differences in coagulation or fibrinolytic factor were observed after tea consumption. The same researchers performed a similar study on acute, single-dose tea consumption and similarly found no effects on postprandial platelet aggregation.[96] The available evidence therefore suggests that although in vitro studies show a potential for antiaggregatory activity, these have not been reliably reproduced in vivo. Currently, no evidence exists for any effect on coagulation (as opposed to platelet) parameters of hemostasis.

Reports
Taylor and Wilt[97] reported a case of a 44-year-old man with Marfan's syndrome who was receiving Coumadin (7.5 mg daily) to establish an international normalized ratio (INR) of 2.5 to 3.5 after a mechanical aortic valve replacement procedure. He had been on this regimen for 14 months, although with a history of fluctuation in INR that was countered by anticoagulant dose adjustment. The patient presented for routine primary care and was found to have an INR of 3.79. He was advised to stabilize his intake of vitamin K–containing foods and was retested 22 days later without warfarin dose adjustment. The INR was 1.37. The patient could not be contacted but returned 1 month later for regular INR testing,

when his INR was 1.14. He denied changes in diet, disease, medication, or warfarin dose, but he later admitted that he had commenced drinking green tea, between half and one gallon daily, before the previous INR of 1.37. He was instructed to discontinue the tea, and 1 week later the INR was 2.55. The authors suggested that the only explanation for the INR decrease was antagonism of warfarin by vitamin K in the green tea.[97] This explanation seems improbable, however, because with the lipophilicity of phylloquinone, the vitamin K content of brewed tea is negligible, at 0.05 µg/100 g, versus the 1.43 mg/100 g of green tea leaf (USDA Nutrient Data Research figures).[98] The possibility of tea inhibiting CYP450 1A2, which metabolizes the weaker R-enantiomer of warfarin, was not discussed. If the patient were a poor metabolizer at 2C9 (which metabolizes the more active S-warfarin enantiomer), this could have been a contributory factor. The report remains difficult to interpret and an isolated case without corroborative data.

Clinical Implications and Adaptations

Given the widespread consumption of tea as a beverage, any impact on hemostasis would be consequential from a public health point of view. The balance of data currently available suggests that the cardioprotective effects of tea polyphenols are unrelated either to vitamin K–dependent coagulation factor modulation or to in vivo antiplatelet effects. Nonetheless, standard practice is for patients using oral anticoagulation and antithrombotic therapies to avoid excessive tea beverage consumption.

Whether concentrated tea polyphenol extracts contain significant amounts of vitamin K is not currently known. In cases of intended coadministration of high doses of such extracts with anticoagulant drugs, standard monitoring of INR should be vigilantly followed, particularly before and immediately after commencement of the extract administration.

The 98 citations in this monograph are located under Green Tea on the CD at the back of the book.

Hawthorn

Botanical Name: *Crataegus laevigata* (Poir) DC, *Crataegus monogyna* Jacq.
(Lindm.).
Pharmacopoeial Name: Folium cum Flore Crataegi.
Synonym: *Crataegus oxyacantha* L. (for C. laevigata). Also as *Crategus* spp.
Common Names: Hawthorn, English hawthorn, whitethorn, may flower.

SUMMARY

Drug/Class Interaction Type	Mechanism and Significance	Management
Digoxin, digitoxin Cardiac glycosides ⊕/☼	Plausible additive inotropic and antiarrhythmic effects. Interaction not established, possibly overstated. *Crataegus* may enable lower drug levels, reducing digoxin toxicity.	Coadminister with professional management and monitoring.
Doxorubicin Anthracycline chemotherapy ⊕/☼	Theoretical reduction of drug-induced cardiotoxicity.	Adopt, and continue *Crataegus* long-term postchemotherapy.
Hydrochlorothiazide Thiazide diuretics ⊕⊕/☼	Additive beneficial effects on heart failure parameters.	Adopt. Coadminister.

HERB DESCRIPTION

Family

Rosaceae.

Related Species

Crataegus apiifolia Medik. non Michx., *Crataegus piperi* Britton, *Crataegus rivularis* Nutt.
In Chinese herbal medicine, *Crataegus pinnatifida* Bunge.; the fruit has traditionally been used.

Habitat and Cultivation

Thorny shrub or small tree, widespread throughout northern and eastern Europe and northeastern America in temperate zones. Hawthorn species hybridize freely, and in commerce, several related species may be used.

Parts Used

Leaf, flower.

Note: Hawthorn fruits, berries, or haws (Fructus Crataegi) are also traditionally used but lack comprehensive pharmacological and clinical data and are not considered separately here. The fruit is monographed separately in the official *European Pharmacopoeia* and the unofficial *American Herbal Pharmacopoeia*[1] and is "unapproved" by the German Commission E.[2]

Common Forms

Dried leaf and flower.
Tincture: 40% to 60% alcohol
Standardized Extracts: 30 mg 5:1 5% oligomeric proanthocyanidins (OPCs) (Crataegutt, W Schwabe Pharmaceuticals); 80 mg 5:1 18.75% OPCs, ethanol extracted (Crategutt forte WS1442, W Schwabe); 300 mg 4:1 to 7:1 standardized to 2.25% flavonoids (Faros LI 132, Lichtwer Pharma AG).

Note: Oligomeric procyanidins, oligomeric proanthocyanidins, procyanidins, procyanidolic oligomers, and pycnogenols are synonymous terms, with the last also being a trademarked brand name for pine bark extract.

HERB IN CLINICAL PRACTICE

Overview

Hawthorn is currently one of the most popular herbal remedies in Europe and is among the top-20 best-selling botanical products in the United States. In the past 20 years, hawthorn has been studied primarily as an adjuvant therapy for early congestive heart failure (New York Heart Association [NYHA] stage I-II), which is currently one of the principal clinical trial–driven indications for the herb. However, because of the broad spectrum of its pharmacology, resulting in part from the characteristic properties of the flavonoid and oligomeric procyanidin constituents, and its negligible toxicity and favorable adverse effect profile, practitioners of botanical medicine have long regarded hawthorn as a pivotal "all-round cardiovascular wellness remedy," as well as the most significant herb for ischemic heart disease. It has antioxidant, anti-inflammatory, hypocholesterolemic, cardioprotective, angioprotective, hypotensive, antiarrhythmic, and positively inotropic properties, with additional beneficial actions on the digestive system and peripheral circulation, including collagen stabilization.

Hawthorn is suitable for extended duration of consumption, and official sources specify a minimum 4 to 6 weeks of administration to obtain maximum benefits in cardiac insufficiency. The German Commission E,[2] European Scientific Cooperative on Phytotherapy (ESCOP),[3] *American Herbal Pharmacopoeia*,[4] and World Health Organization (WHO)[5] provide monographs on hawthorn leaf and flower.

Historical/Ethnomedicine Precedent

Historically, hawthorn fruits were used for hundreds of years before the incorporation of the leaf and flower into medicinal usage. The modern use of hawthorn as a cardiac remedy began with the later Eclectics. Both Ellingwood[6] and Felter[7] experimented in the early 1900s with hawthorn fruit, flowers, and bark for functional heart conditions, along with their primary repertoire of cardiac glycoside–containing plants and their favored heart cardiac remedy *Selenicereus grandiflorus*. By the mid-twentieth century, a clinical understanding had developed of the differential indications of various cardiac glycoside–containing plants for congestive heart failure (CHF). German phytotherapist Rudolf Weiss's 1960 review of the cardiac glycoside herbs, including *Digitalis, Strophanthus, Convallaria, Urginea,* and *Adonis,* remains a classic bridging text to the present. For Weiss, as with the Eclectics, hawthorn was a mild remedy essentially indicated for functional heart problems, especially the "senile heart," with the glycoside-containing plants reserved for treatment of organic heart disease.[8]

As purified pharmaceutical digitaloids replaced the routine use of crude herbal drug cardiac glycoside–containing botanicals in heart failure, the German phytopharmaceutical manufacturers repositioned *Crataegus* as a CHF "adjunctive" remedy; backed by a shift in research emphasis based on Schwabe's proprietary (Crataegutt and WS 1442) hawthorn preparations for CHF. In this context, the contemporary emphasis on hawthorn as a CHF treatment is a rather recent and restrictive view of hawthorn, dominated by phytopharmaceutical industry priorities rather than the inherent properties of the remedy.

Known or Potential Therapeutic Uses

Cardiotonic and cardiopreventive for the "senile heart," i.e., mild symptoms, including early angina, nervous heart complaints, myocardial weakness after serious illness, circulatory support, arteriosclerosis, hypertension, low heart rate variability, and peripheral arterial disorders.
Early CHF corresponding to NYHA stages I-II, possibly III. Feelings of congestion and oppression in the precordium; protection against drug-induced cardiotoxicity.

Key Constituents

Flavonoids, glycosides (e.g., vitexin, vitexin-2-rhamnoside, rutin, quercitin), and related anthocyanidins (cyanidin and others) and oligomeric proanthocyanidins (catechin and epicatechin derivatives).
Triterpenes (crataegolic acid and others), phenylpropanoids, several amino acids, and various monoamines.

Therapeutic Dosing Range

Dried Leaf and Flower: Up to 1.5 g, three to four times daily, by infusion.
Tincture: 3 to 7 mL 1:2 daily.
Standardized Extract: 600 to 900 mg daily.

INTERACTIONS REVIEW
Strategic Considerations

Pharmacopoeial sources, including the 1994 German Commission E monograph, deny any interactions between hawthorn and prescription pharmaceuticals.[2] However, the secondary literature persistently suggests that hawthorn may potentiate digoxin and other cardiac glycoside–containing herbs[4,9] (see later discussion).

Cumulative cardiac drug polypharmacy is a familiar clinical presentation, especially among elder patients, often combined with one or more psychiatric drugs, such as anxiolytics and sedatives. Such patients constitute a "red flag" population for potential interactions of all permutations (i.e., drug-drug, herb-drug, drug-nutrient). It is relevant to consider the possible benefits of hawthorn in such populations. Is hawthorn beneficial and safe in the cardiac polypharmacy environment?

The indirect evidence, especially from clinical trial data, is reassuring. Pittler et al.[10] conducted a meta-analysis of clinical trials of hawthorn extract for treatment of chronic heart failure. Eight of 13 of the qualifying studies specifically allowed concomitant medications for CHF, including diuretics, angiotensin-converting enzyme (ACE) inhibitors, and calcium channel blockers, in their inclusion criteria. The remaining trials did not specify concomitant medications in their eligibility criteria. The majority of studies were therefore actually "interaction" trials between hawthorn and various cardiac medications in a substantial cohort of NYHA stage I-III CHF patients. The meta-analysis concluded there was a better-than-placebo effect on the surrogate endpoints (maximum workload, pressure–heart rate product, left ventricular ejection fraction) for the reviewed studies. Quality of life was tested by subjective questionnaire in only one of the smaller trials (30 patients) and was significantly improved in the verum over the placebo group.[11]

Overall, adverse events were zero in five trials and minimal in the others. Vertigo and dizziness was the most common adverse event, followed by gastrointestinal symptoms. Only two patients (632 total) reported electrocardiologically related symptoms (i.e., palpitations and tachycardia). The implication is that hawthorn is beneficial in the cardiac polypharmacy patient. This is confirmed by the methodological approach of an international multicenter trial examining actual mortality outcomes in NYHA stage II-III CHF patients (*n* = 2300). The study is investigating Crataegus WS1442 extract versus placebo and various conventional therapies, with cardiac glycosides, beta blockers, diuretics, and ACE inhibitors accepted in the inclusion criteria.[12]

The conclusions from concurrent drug-herb trial data are that addition of hawthorn extracts may be beneficial and may interact positively or at worst may be neutral with a range of cardiac medications in CHF without adverse effects. As Zick et al.[13] indicated in a survey, however, patients in these trials may also be consuming unrelated dietary supplements, some of which may interact with their medications.

Cardiac conduction disturbances are a similar critical area of potential drug interaction. Electrophysiologically, hawthorn corresponds most closely to the Vaughan-Williams class III drugs such as amiodarone (i.e., increase of action potential duration, usually by K^+ channel block).[14-16] Hawthorn extracts have positive inotropic effects, decrease atrioventricular (A-V) conduction time, increase coronary blood flow, and decrease myocardial energy utilization.[17-19] However, intracellular recordings of rodent myocytes demonstrate that the effective refractory period (ERP) is prolonged by hawthorn extracts, not shortened as in class III agents.[20] Confirmation of increased ERP has been shown in the ex vivo Langendorff model (perfused guinea pig heart) by Joseph et al.[15]

Conventional treatment of arrhythmias with pharmacotherapeutic antiarrhythmic agents remains largely empirical and is confounded by several problems, including the proarrhythmic properties of many of the drugs; also, left untreated, arrhythmias may resolve over time.[14] The post–Cardiac Arrhythmia Suppression Trial (CAST) era has seen a reevaluation of the advisability of treating nonlethal disturbances in cardiac rhythm versus preventing lethal ventricular tachycardia or ventricular fibrillation and sudden cardiac death.[21,22] The antiarrhythmic properties of hawthorn make it a suitable agent for mild arrhythmias before empirical treatment with pharmaceutical antiarrhythmic agents.[23] This is further supported by hawthorn's positive effects on coronary flow and reduction of ischemic reperfusion injury, because transient ischemic events often trigger rhythm disturbances.[24,25] The high morbidity associated with arrhythmias and CHF make hawthorn an outstanding remedy for this patient group.

Further indirect evidence for the pluripotent cardiovascular effects of hawthorn comes from the pharmacology of isolated constituents, particularly the oligomeric cyanidins and flavonoids. In vitro work has demonstrated nitric oxide (NO)–mediated endothelial relaxation by vitexin-rhamnoside. Phosphodiesterase-inhibiting activity, thromboxane A_2 (TXA_2) inhibition of adenosine $5'$-diphosphate–induced platelet aggregation, ACE inhibition, and phospholipase A_2 inhibition, as well as antioxidant, hypolipidemic, and antiatherosclerotic properties, have all been shown by in vitro studies.[25-33]

Weiss's summary remains a succinct statement of the strategic framework for hawthorn administration. He contrasts it to digitalis, noting that "the two drugs are at opposite poles of heart therapy; hawthorn's gentle and long lasting action, lacking risks and unpleasant side effects, [means] that patients can on the whole be left to use it without constant supervision." It is "particularly suitable for long-term prophylactic use in middle aged patients, . . . and in follow up therapy for myocardial infarction."[8]

HERB-DRUG INTERACTIONS

Digoxin, Digitoxin and Related Cardiac Glycosides

Evidence: Digoxin (Digitek, Lanoxin, Lanoxicaps, purgoxin). Extrapolated, based on similar properties: Deslanoside (cedilanin-D), digitoxin (Cystodigin), ouabain (g-strophanthin).

Interaction Type and Significance
⊕ **Potential or Theoretical Beneficial or Supportive Interaction, with Professional Management**
☼ **Prevention or Reduction of Drug Adverse Effect**

Probability: Evidence Base:
3. Possible   ○ **Preliminary**

Effect and Mechanism of Action
Hawthorn extracts have positive inotropic properties and could be used to potentiate digoxin and theoretically may lower the risk of digoxin toxicity by enabling a lower therapeutic dose because of additive inotropic effects.

Research
This interaction has been persistently suggested since animal work in the 1950s by Semm, Bersin, and others that suggested pretreatment of cardiac tissue with hawthorn or cardiac glycoside could act mutually as a sensitizer to the other agent. Extrapolating from this finding, a synergistic effect in vivo was hypothesized that might enable reduced dose of digoxin and a lesser risk of toxicity. This early work has never been repeated and has been criticized as methodologically flawed in design and an inappropriate basis for extrapolating to human use.[34]

The positive inotropic effect of hawthorn extracts has been demonstrated in isolated rodent ventricular myocytes and by guinea pig heart (Langendorff) preparations.[15,20] Trunzler and

Schuler[35] used a modified Langendorff model to record contractile amplitude and coronary flow variation with digoxin, digitoxin, g-strophanthinin, and hawthorn extracts (Crataegutt) separately and in combination. The combination of digoxin and Crataegutt showed an increase in both parameters compared with digoxin alone.[35] The mechanism of contractility increase caused by hawthorn extracts is not fully understood, but there is evidence of a similar pharmacodynamic mechanism to the cardiac glycosides with action at the sarcolemmal sodium-potassium adenosinetriphosphatase (Na^+, K^+-ATPase) pump in human cardiac muscle ex vivo.[36] In addition, *Crataegus* does not cause adrenergic blockade at levels that are negatively chronotropic.[37] In summary, the principal cardiac effects of the two agents can be tabulated as follows:

	Digoxin	Hawthorn
Contractility	↑	↑
Spontaneous rate	↑	←→
A-V conduction time	↑	↑
Refractory period	↓	↑
Coronary flow	↑	↑

Modified from references 15 and 19.

Despite widespread suggestions in the secondary literature about the interaction between *Crataegus* extracts and digoxin, case reports are entirely lacking, with negligible pharmacokinetic or pharmacodynamic data. Tankanow et al.[38] examined the possibility of both pharmacokinetic and pharmacodynamic interactions between digoxin and *Crataegus* WS1442 extracts in a preclinical, open-label crossover study of eight healthy subjects, male and female. WS 1442 did not interfere with the digoxin assay, and there was no significant difference in pharmacokinetic parameters (AUC, C_{max}, C_{min}, $t_{1/2}$) between the digoxin and the digoxin plus hawthorn group. However, the trend was for a reduction in digoxin levels in the presence of hawthorn, but the small number of participants rendered the difference statistically insignificant. The authors postulated that this effect resulted from mild induction of P-glycoprotein (P-gp) by quercitin and other flavonoids in the WS 1442 preparation. Electrocardiographic (ECG), heart rate, and blood pressure parameters did not suggest a pharmacodynamic interaction. The principal limitation was the application of a single dose of hawthorn, which is likely inadequate to modify pharmacodynamic parameters.[38]

Integrative Therapeutics, Clinical Concerns, and Adaptations
Digoxin is infamous for its narrow therapeutic index and potential for toxicity. Natural agents, including flavonoid extracts, have been found to modulate P-gp, of which digoxin is a substrate.[39] This is the basis of the pharmacokinetic interaction between St John's wort and digoxin, which can cause a clinically significant decrease in serum digoxin levels.[40] The concurrent administration data from clinical trials of hawthorn extracts and the previous preclinical study[38] suggest that pharmacokinetic interactions between hawthorn extract and digoxin are not clinically significant. Strategic evaluation of the pharmacodynamic interaction between hawthorn and digoxin needs to consider the context of digoxin prescription.

In patients with CHF, digoxin use remains controversial, except in those with atrial flutter or other arrhythmias associated with heart failure.[41-43] In this setting, digoxin is likely to be prescribed additively after first-line measures such as salt restriction, limitation of physical activity, and vasodilation

(ACE inhibitor) have failed to halt progression of symptoms. Diuretics are usually also prescribed in combination. The NYHA functional class for this patient population is typically advanced stage II, or stage III, more progressed than that suggested by clinical trial data for hawthorn use in CHF. However, given the high morbidity associated with dysrhythmias in CHF patients, the lack of adverse effects associated with the digoxin-hawthorn combination, and the potential benefits of the interaction, coadministration would likely be beneficial in this setting.

When digoxin is prescribed for heart rate control in supraventricular arrhythmias outside CHF, the potential benefits of concurrent administration of hawthorn could be greater than for digoxin alone, given the pluripotent cardiac effects of the herb. These multivalent actions suggest that hawthorn may effectively stabilize "cardiac excitability," an arrhythmogenic mechanism added to the basic concept of altered automaticity or impulse propagation by Arnsdorf.[44-46] Another view would be that the multiple effects of hawthorn might maintain or enhance the degree of nonlinearity of cardiac rate and rhythm, which is known to decrease with aging and CHF.[47-50]

The most effective interaction between hawthorn and digoxin may be "prophylactic," in the sense that hawthorn pretreatment or maintenance is the botanical medicine foundation of integrative strategies aimed at prophylaxis of, or intervention and reversal of, early heart failure. In combination with other strategies, such as dietary improvements, smoking cessation, weight loss, stress reduction, exercise, and selective nutritional support, hawthorn may prevent or at least delay the need for digoxin.

Doxorubicin and Related Anthracycline Chemotherapy

Evidence: Doxorubicin (Adriamycin, Rubex).
Extrapolated, based on similar properties: Daunorubicin (Cerubidine), epirubicin (Ellence, Pharmorubicin), idarubicin (Idamycin, Zavedos), mitoxantrone (Novantrone, Onkotrone). Similar properties but evidence lacking for extrapolation: Daunorubicin, liposomal (DaunoXome), doxorubicin, pegylated liposomal (Caelyx, Doxil, Myocet).

Interaction Type and Significance

⊕ **Potential or Theoretical Beneficial or Supportive Interaction, with Professional Management**
☼ **Prevention or Reduction of Drug Adverse Effect**

Probability:	Evidence Base:
6. Unknown	☐ Inadequate

Effect and Mechanism of Action

Doxorubicin is known to induce dose-related cumulative cardiotoxicity (short and long term). This may be reduced by concurrent hawthorn administration.

Research

Doxorubicin is one of the most widely used antineoplastic agents, but its effectiveness is in part limited by well-documented cardiotoxic adverse effects, which can manifest long after cessation of treatment. The pathogenetic mechanisms of anthracycline cardiotoxicity are not fully understood, although the ultimate clinical presentation is indistinguishable from typical CHF. Although an early toxicity may be observed, shortly after initiation of administration (especially in older patients), the symptoms of progressive heart failure can appear months or even years after treatment, and the cardiomyopathy initially may be quite asymptomatic.[51] Several possible cardiac protective agents have been examined, but none found to be

effective, including vitamin E and *N*-acetylcysteine. The iron-chelating agent dexrazoxane (Zinecard) reduces cardiotoxicity but has been associated with possible reduction in antitumor effects (doxorubicin toxicity partly may be caused by FeII-dox-complex free-radical formation).[52]

Integrative Therapeutics, Clinical Concerns, and Adaptations

Based on the known pluripotent cardioprotective effects of hawthorn, its efficacy for CHF, benign safety profile, and suitability for long-term administration, cardioprotection protocols for oncology patients using doxorubicin might beneficially incorporate hawthorn extracts, together with related herbal agents (e.g., ginkgo) and nutrients (e.g., coenzyme Q10, acetylcarnitine). Direct studies are required to establish the potential benefits of this strategic interaction with doxorubicin (see also Ginkgo monograph).

Hydrochlorothiazide and Related Thiazide Diuretics, Combined with Triamterene

Evidence: Hydrochlorothiazide (Aquazide, Esidrix, Ezide, Hydrocot, HydroDiuril, Microzide, Oretic); combination drug: hydrochlorothiazide and triamterene (Dyazide, Maxzide). Extrapolated, based on similar properties: Bendroflumethiazide (bendrofluazide; Naturetin), combination drug: bendrofluazide and propranolol (Inderex); benzthiazide (Exna), chlorothiazide (Diuril), chlorthalidone (Hygroton), cyclopenthiazide (Navidrex), combination drug: cyclopenthiazide and oxprenolol hydrochloride (Trasidrex); hydrochlorothiazide combination drugs: hydrochlorothiazide and amiloride (Moduretic); hydrochlorothiazide and captopril (Acezide, Capto-Co, Captozide, Co-Zidocapt); hydrochlorothiazide and enalapril (Vaseretic); hydrochlorothiazide and lisinopril (Prinzide, Zestoretic); hydrochlorothiazide and losartan (Hyzaar); hydrochlorothiazide and metoprolol (Lopressor HCT); hydrochlorothiazide and spironolactone (Aldactazide); hydroflumethiazide (Diucardin), methyclothiazide (Enduron), metolazone (Zaroxolyn, Mykrox), polythiazide (Renese), quinethazone (Hydromox), trichlormethiazide (Naqua).

Interaction Type and Significance

⊕⊕ **Beneficial Supportive Interaction, with Professional Management**
☼ **Prevention or Reduction of Drug Adverse Effect**

Probability:	Evidence Base:
2. Possible	◉ Emerging

Effect and Mechanism of Action

Addition of hawthorn extract to existing diuretic therapy in CHF patients leads to improved symptom reduction and reduction in adverse effects through a general additive effect compared with diuretic therapy alone.

Research

In a randomized trial by Tauchert[53] of 209 patients with NYHA stage III heart failure, inclusion criteria included only preexisting diuretic or ACE inhibitor therapy. A pretreatment combination of thiazide diuretic and the antikaliuretic triamterene was given for 4 weeks, and patients were then randomized to into two dose groups of hawthorn extract WS 1442 (450 or 900 mg twice daily) versus placebo for 16 weeks while the preexisting combination was also continued. A dose-dependent improvement in exercise capacity and reduction in symptom severity was noted over the placebo (diuretic-only) group. However, the HERB-CHF trial, which involved adding hawthorn to ACE inhibitor and beta blocker–treated NYHA II-III patients for 6 weeks, found negligible difference between the control drug group and the drug-herb combination group, although in the latter group left ventricular function (LVF) was stable and in the drug-only group the trend was for LVF to decline.[54]

Integrative Therapeutics, Clinical Concerns, and Adaptations

As previously suggested (see Strategic Considerations), inclusion criteria in hawthorn clinical trials suggest that the weight of indirect evidence for the safety of hawthorn in cardiac polypharmacy favors the view of hawthorn as a beneficial interactor. The Tauchert trial[53] comparison with thiazide diuretic therapy supports this view more directly.

THEORETICAL, SPECULATIVE, AND PRELIMINARY INTERACTIONS RESEARCH, INCLUDING OVERSTATED INTERACTIONS CLAIMS

Derivative sources have suggested several possible interactions based on overenthusiastic extrapolations from pharmacological data without clinical contextualization. These include

suggestions that the vasodilatory effects of hawthorn extracts could interact positively with coronary vasodilators or negatively with topical inhalant vasoconstrictors.[9] Such assertions lack clinical foundation, given the framework of hawthorn administration as a gentle, long-term remedy, as well as any plausible supporting data. The proposal that hawthorn, taken as a beverage tea, may adversely affect the absorption of iron salts lacks evidence and merit.[55]

The 55 citations for this monograph are located under Hawthorn on the CD at the back of the book.

Horse Chestnut

Botanical Name: *Aesculus hippocastanum* L.
Pharmacopoeial Name: Hippocastani semen.
Common Names: Horse chestnut, chestnut.

HERB DESCRIPTION

Family

Sapindaceae (classified in Hippocastanaceae until 1998).

Parts Used

Seeds.
The bark and leaf of the tree are separate remedies, little used today.[1,2]

Common Forms

Tincture: Fresh or dried seed, 65% alcohol.
Standardized Extract: Horse chestnut standardized extract (HCSE)—5:1 to 8:1 standardized to 16% to 20% triterpene glycosides, tablets or capsules (Aesculoforce, Bioforce AG; Venostat, Pharmaton Natural Health Products).
Topical: Ointments, gels containing extracts at 2% aescin.

INTERACTIONS REVIEW

Strategic Considerations

Horse chestnut preparations have been popular in Europe for several decades, used for a variety of conditions of the venous system, both chronic (venous insufficiency, varicosities, hemorrhoids, leg ulcers, and edema) and acute (postoperative and posttraumatic edema, including elevated intracranial pressure, traumatic hematoma, contusions, and soft tissue swelling; sports injuries, especially involving edema). *Aesculus* seed is well described by Weiss[3] under diseases of the venous system and has monographs by the German Commission E[4] (1994, revised from an earlier unapproved monograph of leaf and flower in 1984), World Health Organization (WHO) in 2002, and European Scientific Cooperative on Phytotherapy (ESCOP) in 2003, as well as a recent literature review by McKenna et al.[7] Clinical trials for horse chestnut in chronic venous insufficiency (CVI) have been subjected to meta-analysis for the Cochrane database by Pittler and Ernst,[8] who found positive evidence for short-term efficacy in treating CVI.

Pharmacological attention has focused on the activity of the triterpene saponin fraction, a complex mixture of triterpenoids usually described as escin *(aescin)*, which has venoactive anti-inflammatory and antiedematous properties, with some in vitro antioxidant, antiproliferative, and immunomodulatory activities.[9,10] Available controlled clinical trials (13 total, 8 placebo controlled) of HCSE for venous insufficiency were systematically reviewed by Pittler and Ernst,[11] who concluded HCSE was safe, effective, and superior to placebo for short-term treatment of CVI. European use has also involved parenteral preparations of aescin (sodium escinate) and extensive use of a proprietary topical product Essaven which is a combination of aescin with pharmaceutical ingredients, heparin and phospholipids.

The monographs by German Commission E[4] and ESCOP[6] list no known interactions between horse chestnut seed and pharmaceutical drugs. (See, however, the later precaution regarding gentamicin from WHO.) Interactions reports in the literature are lacking. Positive clinical reports and trials of the topical combination product Essaven since the 1970s suggest a potential benefit of the combination in a wide range of conditions, and this is therefore accorded the status of a beneficial interaction (heparin + phospholipid; see later). Earlier European studies provide some basis for considering a potentially beneficial interaction with corticosteroid therapy; this is also assigned a potential interaction status here despite a lack of recent data. Speculative interactions include warfarin and hypoglycemics. Pharmacokinetic data are not currently available, and effects on drug-metabolizing enzymes, if any, have not been established.

HERB-DRUG INTERACTIONS

Corticosteroids, Oral

Betamethasone (Celestone), cortisone (Cortone), dexamethasone (Decadron), fludrocortisone (Florinef), hydrocortisone (Cortef), methylprednisolone (Medrol) prednisolone (Delta-Cortef, Orapred, Pediapred, Prelone), prednisone (Deltasone, Liquid Pred, Meticorten, Orasone), triamcinolone (Aristocort).

Interaction Type and Significance

⊕ **Potential or Theoretical Beneficial or Supportive Interaction, with Professional Management**

Probability:	Evidence Base:
2. Probable	☐ **Inadequate**

Effect and Mechanism of Action

Adrenocortical steroids and analogs combined with HCSE or aescin may provide additive beneficial antiedematous effects, particularly in cerebral edema. This interaction, which has been used in neurosurgical environments, is of unknown significance beyond that specialized clinical context.

Research

Rodent studies in the 1960s on adrenalectomized or hypophysectomized rodents showed that normal corticosteroid levels are required for the antiedematous effects of aescin.[12,13] The combination of sodium aescinate and corticosteroids was more effective than steroids alone in reducing cerebral edema in a study of 142 patients with acute motor vehicle crash–related cerebral trauma.[14] Aescin has been used alone and in combination with steroids in a wide range of neurological situations.[15] A rodent model using cortically injured animals found that aescin dramatically lowered nuclear factor kappa B (NF-κB) activation and tumor necrosis factor alpha (TNF-α) levels and alleviated brain edema after injury.[16]

Integrative Therapeutics, Clinical Concerns, and Adaptations

This interaction is related to use of parenteral horse chestnut saponin preparations in acute surgical situations, and extrapolations are problematic. Single-dose and two-dose pharmacokinetic studies on oral aescin preparations suggest a very low bioavailability, with reduction of absorption by food.[10,17-19] Bowel flora hydrolysis of the glycosides hypothetically may result in longer-term release of the aglycone or its metabolites, but studies are lacking.[13] Although specific blood-brain barrier data are not available, the established general systemic effects on edema suggest that circulating levels of the saponin aglycones should theoretically be available to cerebral circulatory system. Comparative data on serum levels (AUC) of intravenous (IV) versus oral administration are not available. The possible benefits of the combination using oral HCSE remain to be established.

Heparin Sodium + Phosphatidylcholine + Aescin

Heparin sodium, phosphatidylcholine, and aescin (Essaven, topical).

Interaction Type and Significance

⊕⊕ **Beneficial or Supportive Interaction, with Professional Management**

Probability:	Evidence Base:
1. Certain	● Consensus

Effect and Mechanism of Action

Proprietary combination that synergistically enhances anti-inflammatory, antiedematous, antiexudative effects of the herb.

Research

The antiedematous effects of topical aescin-based HCSE preparations combined with heparin and phospholipids have been well documented since the 1970s. Reports include use for preventing and treating acute injuries from sports injuries, blunt trauma, mastectomy-related lymphedema, thrombophlebitis, hematoma, oral surgery, varicosities, hemorrhoids, and diabetic microangiopathy.[20-45]

Integrative Therapeutics, Clinical Concerns, and Adaptations

Clinically, this interaction inevitably results from an established proprietary phytonutripharmaceutical combination and is as relevant as an example of effective integrative combination as for the inherent importance of interaction.

THEORETICAL, SPECULATIVE, AND PRELIMINARY INTERACTIONS RESEARCH, INCLUDING OVERSTATED INTERACTIONS CLAIMS

Gentamicin and Related Aminoglycoside Antibiotics, and Other Potentially Nephrotoxic Agents

Amikacin (Amikin), gentamicin (G-mycin, Garamycin, Jenamicin), kanamycin (Kantrex), neomycin (Mycifradin, Myciguent, Neo-Fradin, NeoTab, Nivemycin), netilmicin (Netromycin), paromomycin (monomycin; Humatin), streptomycin, tobramycin (AKTob, Nebcin, TOBI, TOBI Solution, TobraDex, Tobrex).

WHO[5] suggests a potential interaction based on a report of nephrotoxicity after excessive doses of aescin with gentamicin. The report, dating from 1978, involved a combination of aescin, an IV preparation of purified saponin compounds,

with the known nephrotoxic antibiotic gentamicin.[46] McKenna et al.[7] cite an earlier Italian report by Grasso and Corvaglia[47] (text and abstract unavailable for inspection) of two cases of toxic nephropathy associated with high dose of aescin (i.e., intoxication), not interaction. These two cases both involved IV saponin fraction in the clinical context of acute postsurgical edema. Sirtori[10] reports that at the time of these warnings of potential nephrotoxicity, three trials examined the renal function in 83 patients who had preexisting kidney disease and in healthy volunteers who received 10 mg IV aescin per day. No worsening of renal impairment in the renal patients or effect on the healthy individuals was noted.

Oral Hypoglycemic Agents and Insulin

Buformin (Andromaco Gliporal, Buformina), chlorpropamide (Diabinese), glimepiride (Amaryl), glipizide (Glucotrol; Glucotrol XL), glyburide (glibenclamide; Diabeta, Glynase, Glynase Prestab, Micronase, Pres Tab), insulin (animal-source insulin: Iletin; human analog insulin: Humanlog; human insulin: Humulin, Novolin, NovoRapid, Oralin); metformin (Dianben, Glucophage, Glucophage XR); combination drugs: glipizide and metformin (Metaglip); glyburide and metformin (Glucovance); tolazamide (Tolinase), phenformin (Debeone, Fenformin), tolbutamide (Orinase, Tol-Tab).

Based on two rodent studies, claims of interactions with hypoglycemic agents have been speculatively suggested. One study did not use an experimentally induced model of diabetes but compared glucose levels in glucose-loaded normal rats to normal controls.[48] A hypoglycemic effect was observed only in the glucose-loaded rats after administration of purified aescin compounds. A second study found no effect in alloxan-induced diabetic rats.[49] There are no human reports of HCSE disturbing glucose levels in euglycemic or dysglycemic individuals or of interactions with oral hypoglycemics.

Warfarin and Related Oral Vitamin K Antagonist Anticoagulants

Evidence: Warfarin (Coumadin, Marevan, Warfilone).
Related: Anisindione (Miradon), dicumarol, ethyl biscoumacetate (Tromexan), nicoumalone (acenocoumarol; Acitrom, Sintrom), phenindione (Dindevan), phenprocoumon (Jarsin, Marcumar).

It has been suggested that horse chestnut or HCSE potentiates the anticoagulant effect of warfarin.[50] This is based on two erroneous assumptions: the seeds contain coumarins, and coumarins inevitably interact with warfarin. In fact, esculin and its 6-glycoside esculetin have only been reported in bark of the tree, and this coumarin derivative lacks the 4-OH minimal structural activity for anti–vitamin K activity, although some in vitro evidence suggests it may inhibit platelet lipoxygenases.[51] The suggested interaction has not been clinically reported and lacks foundation in the known pharmacology of HCSE.

The 51 citations for this monograph are located under Horse Chestnut on the CD at the back of the book.

Kava

Botanical Name: *Piper methysticum* G. Forster.
Pharmacopoeial Name: Piperis methystici rhizoma.
Common Names: Kava, kava-kava, kawa, 'awa.

Summary

Drug/Class Interaction Type	Mechanism and Significance	Management
Alprazolam Triazolobenzodiazepines **✗/?**	Possible pharmacokinetic and pharmacodynamic interaction resulting in increased central nervous system effects. General significance not established. (May be significant for intravenous midazolam preoperatively.)	Avoid coadministration, except during withdrawal from drug under professional supervision.
Dopamine agonists Dopamine antagonists **?**	Herb may have mixed/paradoxical actions on central dopaminergic pathways. Poorly understood and significance unknown, but may be useful in reducing antipsychotic drug-induced tardive dyskinesia.	Avoid coadministration, except under close professional supervision.
Ethanol **?/✗**	Potential interaction resulting in increased toxicity of either herb or drug, or both. Mechanism and significance not established.	Avoid.

HERB DESCRIPTION

Family

Piperaceae.

Habitat and Cultivation

Piper methysticum is a vegetatively propagated cultivar, and botanical authorities believe it was derived from wild species (e.g., *Piper wichmanni* C. DC). Historically, kava was widely domesticated throughout the Pacific regions of Polynesia, Micronesia, and Melanesia. Currently, commercial cultivation of the major chemotypic variants occurs principally in Fiji, Vanuatu, and Hawaii.

Parts Used

Rootstock, lateral roots. Notably, the outer root bark/peelings and base stem are not used traditionally, although these have been exported for commercial use.

Common Forms

Fresh or dried peeled rootstock and lateral roots, some lower stem.
Tincture, Fluid Extract: Greater than 60% alcohol.
Standardized Solid Extract: Often acetone extracted, in tablets or encapsulated powder form, usually standardized to 70% total kavalactones. Because chemotypic variants exist, this form of standardization is not necessarily a reliable guide to consistency.
Synthetic Kavain: Racemic D,L-kavain has been incorporated into certain proprietary medications in Germany but is not in common use.

HERB IN CLINICAL PRACTICE

Overview

Medically, kava is currently regarded mainly as a herbal anxiolytic agent. Several positive clinical trials suggest kava root extracts may be a safe and effective alternative to benzodiazepine pharmacotherapy for mild anxiety. Recent systematic reviews, including a Cochrane database review, support the efficacy of kava extracts for anxiety and have emphasized their favorable safety profile.[1-3] The "anxiolytic" indication has overshadowed its wider uses in traditional cultural practice and contemporary herbal medicine. Practitioners of botanical medicine consider the herb useful for urogenital indications, including interstitial and infective cystitis, prostatitis, painful micturition from any cause, nocturnal enuresis, as well as for menopausal symptoms, and value it for its musculorelaxant and sedative effects as much as its anxiolytic indications.[4]

The German Commission E[5] approved the use of kava for anxiety in 1990, listing no known adverse effects, but suggested a limitation to duration of use of 3 months and contraindication in "endogenous depression." The 2002 World Health Organization (WHO) monograph[6] echoes the Commission E. The 2003 therapeutic monograph by the European Scientific Cooperative on Phytotherapy (ESCOP)[7] indicates the use of the herb for anxiety, tension, and restlessness, considering it safe when used as a short-term monotherapy, but contraindicating in cases of preexisting liver disease and alcohol abuse. A 2004 comprehensive overview of the literature from ethnology to pharmacology, edited by kava authority Singh,[8] updates and complements the classic monograph by Lebot.

Commencing in 1998, isolated case reports of possible kava-related hepatoxicity began to emerge.[9-15] On the basis of 28 case reports, the German Bundesinstitut für Arzneimitttel und Medizinprodukte (BfArM; Federal Institute for Drugs and Medical Devices) withdrew product licenses in 2002 from all kava products. Several other countries, including Canada and France took similar action, in 2002 the British Medicines Control Agency (MCA) announced a complete kava product ban, and in 2003 Swissmedic (formerly the Swiss IKS) followed suit. The U.S. Food and Drug Administration (FDA) issued a public advisory in 2001 about concerns of potential kava hepatoxicity, but kava products remain on sale in the United States at this time. A comprehensive review of the controversy is beyond the scope of this monograph; Schmidt[16] reviews each BfArM case (continuously updated on the internet), and in Mills and Bone's comprehensive 2005 survey, Schmidt et al.[17] discuss the 82 cases cited by regulatory authorities, with risk-benefit analysis of kava. The ongoing debate over kava hepatoxicity is discussed later under interactions.

Historical/Ethnomedicine Precedent

Indigenous use of kava, practiced for centuries throughout Polynesia and Micronesia, continues in the South Pacific islands. Kava is consumed regularly, primarily as a diluted fresh (on some islands, dried) root juice extract (succus), both as a relaxing social beverage and as a component of traditional ceremony. Folk healers in these communities use various parts of the plant for treating a wide range of ailments, including urogenital and menstrual problems, headaches, respiratory conditions, sleeping difficulties, and many skin problems.[8] Western therapeutic use began at the end of the nineteenth century, although the crude drug was available on both sides of the Atlantic several decades earlier. In 1892, Cerna[18] described kava's anti-inflammatory and analgesic effects on the male and female urinary tract, also noting its central nervous system (CNS) intoxicant properties. The Eclectics tended to underemphasize the CNS effects but described indications for trigeminal and other neuralgias.[19]

The dual affinities of the herb for the CNS and urogenital tract were retained until the late twentieth century, with Weiss[20] classifying kava both as a tranquilizer and as a treatment for "neurogenic" disorders of the bladder in women and prostatitis in men. The increasing promotion of standardized extracts, especially WS1490 (70% kavalactones; Willmar Schwabe), and the adoption of this extract in clinical studies for anxiety in the 1980s and 1990s coincided with the emergence of the now-dominant psychiatric indications of kava as an anxiolytic and a corresponding deemphasis of its other indications.

Known or Potential Therapeutic Uses

Internal Use: Anxiety; benzodiazepine drug withdrawal; headache; insomnia; irritable bladder; menopausal symptoms; nervous and muscular tension; neuralgia; prostatitis; restlessness of nonpsychotic origin; rheumatism; urinary tract inflammation, infection, and pain.

External Use: Analgesic for joint pain, mouth sores, wounds, and skin conditions.

Key Constituents

Alpha-pyrones known as *kavalactones*: total content varies according to cultivar type, growing conditions, age, and part used, from a typical range of 5.5% to 8%,[21] up to a recorded maximum of 21%.[22] Approximately 18 kavalactones have been described, of which six are considered important: kawain (kavain), dihydrokawian, methysticin, dihydromethysticin, yangonin, and desmethoxyyangonin. Other constituents include the alkaloid pipermethysticine in the leaf and bark, chalcones (flavokavins A-C), and cinammalketone.[23]

Therapeutic Dosing Range

Dried Plant: 6 to 12 g/day by cold maceration, or decoction.
Tincture, Fluid Extract: Based on 1:1, 6 to 12 mL/day.
Standardized Extract: Typically 100 mg, 70% kavalactones, three times daily (i.e., 210 mg total kavalactones daily).

Traditional South Sea beverage use dosage of kavalactones is controversial, given use of local chemotypes and varying preparation methods, but has been estimated as high as 2500 mg of lactones in one "session," or 10 cups at approximately 250 mg of lactones per cup. Most ethnobotanical authorities agree, however, that the traditional dose can be significantly greater than that used in botanical medicine.

INTERACTIONS REVIEW

Strategic Considerations

Before the recent concerns over the potential hepatoxicity of kava extracts, specific interactions of kava with pharmaceutical drugs had not been identified as a significant problem, and the safety of the herb in the preceding decade was considered excellent. The Commission E had pointed out that pharmacodynamic interactions with psychoactive medications, particularly CNS depressants such as barbiturates and alcohol, were theoretically possible.[5] WHO mentioned the alprazolam-kava interaction report (see later) but suggested that it was unconfirmed.[6] Systematic experimental or clinical investigations of pharmacodynamic kava-drug interactions are not available. Extrapolations have been made from limited pharmacological data and the few available case reports, indicating potential interactions issues with CNS depressants and other centrally acting agents, such as alcohol, alprazolam, and levodopa. These data are reviewed later.

Practitioners versed in botanical prescribing view the coadministration of synthetic drugs with herbs that have identical indications as unnecessary and undesirable, if not frankly contraindicated. (This is independent of underlying pharmacological mechanism because there is rarely a simple homology between the effects of herbal extracts and pharmaceuticals.) A good example is St. John's wort (SJW; see monograph) and the serotonin reuptake inhibitors (SRIs) for depression, or kava and benzodiazepine anxiolytics. Exception may be made in particular clinical circumstances, such as elective withdrawal from the drug. Anecdotal clinical experience is available for use of SJW in SRI drug withdrawal, and kava can be used to support benzodiazepine withdrawal.[24]

Hepatotoxicity Controversy and Kava-Drug Interactions

The status of the case reports gathered by Swissmedic, the German BfArM, British MCA, U.S. FDA, and other national bodies to support claims of kava hepatoxicity have been critically reviewed by several authors.[16,17,25-28] Full case details were not initially released for public or expert review, and it subsequently was found that much of the original data were incomplete or defective. Documents from different regulatory authorities contained duplicate cases, errors, and inconsistencies, and in most cases the information provided was significantly below the minimum standards required for rigorous evaluation of potential causality. The emerging expert consensus is that the case for inherent kava hepatoxicity remains unproven, and by implication, the complete banning kava products was precipitous given the clinical trial–demonstrated efficacy and adverse effects profile of the herb for anxiety and its favorable risk-benefit comparison to benzodiazepines.[17,28] Interestingly, the former German Commission E members, generally known for their cautious perspective, unanimously expressed unease at their government's (BfArM) decision to ban kava.[29] A similar statement was made by the Society for Medicinal Plant Research.[30]

Various theories of mechanisms have been proposed to account for the case reports of hepatotoxicity, including idiosyncratic drug reactions, immunoallergic responses, pharmacogenetic variation in drug-metabolizing enzymes and metabolic bioactivation to toxic intermediates, glutathione depletion, differences between commercial kava preparations in terms of plant parts used, possible contamination with the alkaloid pipermethysticine present in stem peelings, possible adulteration with known hepatotoxic species such as germander, contamination by extracting solvents such as acetone, consumption of pure synthetic kavain preparations versus natural kavalactone mixtures, excessive total kavalactone dose, and variance in kavalactone composition of products.[17,26,28,31-33] The overall incidence of verifiable kava-associated hepatotoxic events, estimated on the basis of 3 years' usage data to be 0.1 case per million daily doses, is very low and compares favorably with the relative incidence of suspected hepatotoxic reactions for common benzodiazepines (diazepam: 2.12 cases per million doses).[17] Epidemiologically, this is typical of idiosyncratic hepatotoxic drug responses; the apparently low frequency rate partly results from the multifactorial determinants involved in their causation, with the net probability of a critical adverse event occurrence being the sum of all the discrete probabilities of each determinant factor.[34]

Logically, in the context of potential kava-drug interactions, several of the hepatoxicity cases determined by reviewers as being unable to support claims of inherent kava hepatotoxicity because of concurrent comedication are de facto cases of potential kava-drug interactions. Unfortunately, the well-described problems of report quality and reliability also confound reanalysis of these cases as interactions data. Nonetheless, the hypothesis that kavalactones might pharmacokinetically increase the plasma concentrations of drugs associated with idiosyncratic or inherent hepatotoxicity requires evaluation, because several of the cases involved comedication with such agents. These drugs included fluoxetine, paroxetine, acetylsalicylic acid, thiazide diuretics, oral contraceptives, nonsteroidal anti-inflammatory drugs (NSAIDs) including celecoxib and diclofenac, antidiabetic agents, and benzodiazepines.[16] Most of these are also known substrates, inducers, or inhibitors of drug-metabolizing enzymes, and most have been associated to varying degrees with hepatic adverse reactions.

As with pharmacodynamic interactions, direct studies on kava-drug pharmacokinetic interactions are not currently available. However, experimental data on the effect of kavalactones on cytochrome P450 (CYP450) mixed oxidases suggest a potential for pharmacokinetic herb-drug interactions.

Effects on Drug Metabolism and Bioavailability

Several in vitro studies have determined that both kava preparations and individual kavalactones can exert inhibitory effects on CYP450 isoforms.[35-39] Zou et al.[37,38] compared activity of both recombinant human CYP450 enzymes and human hepatocytes with standard control compounds and addition of kava. They found that an ethanolic extract of kava containing 28% total kavalactones significantly inhibited (in descending order of effect size) CYP450 2C9, 2C19, 3A4, 2D6, 2E1, and 1E2 at both 100 micromolar (μM) and also at lower concentrations of approximately 10 μM. There was good agreement between the two methods used, and the experiments were repeated with individual kavalactones. Of these, desmethoxyyangonin and methysticin were found to be the most potent inhibitors of 1A2, 2C9, 2C19, 2E1, and 3A4 (median inhibition concentration [IC_{50}] <10 μM). At higher doses the authors also established toxic effects on hepatocyte viability, although the concentrations were 100 μM and therefore 10 to 20 times that likely attainable in vivo.[38]

Mathews et al.[35] also used a human hepatocyte test system to analyze the in vitro effects of kava extracts (40% lactones) at 100 μM on human P450 enzyme activity compared with positive control substrates. At these high concentrations they found a significant inhibition of 2C9, 2C19, 3A4, 2D6, and 4A9/11. At lower concentrations of 10 μM, individual lactones were tested; 2C9 was significantly inhibited by

desmethoxyyangonin, methysticin, and dihydromethysticin; 2C19 by desmethoxyyangonin; 3A4 by desmethoxyyangonin, methysticin, and dihydromethysticin; and 2D6 by meythysticin.

Unger et al.[36] examined the effect of different fractions of a crude ethyl acetate extract of kava root powder for inhibitory activity using a testosterone hydroxylation system to assay 3A4 activity with kava compared to ketoconazole as a positive control.[36] They found a significant inhibition of 3A4 with different solvents used for the kava extract. Using high-performance liquid chromatography (HPLC) fractionation, they established that kavain, dihydrokavain, methysticin, dihydromethysticin, and dihydroyangonin were the most active lactones. However, IC_{50} values were not recorded.

Cote et al.[39] used a standard fluorescence screening assay method to compare traditional water extracts of kava with various commercial solvent extracts against the activity of 1A2, 2C9, 2C19, and 3A4. Kavalactones were present at highest levels in the acetone extracts, which also had the highest CYP450 inhibitory activity. The authors found that 3A4 and 2C19 were inhibited most actively, with IC_{50} values of approximately 1 μg/mL, or about 1 μM. A poster report of a study in six healthy volunteers tested with a probe cocktail for 1A2, 2D6, 2C19, 2E1, and 3A4 found that traditional aqueous extracts only significantly inhibited 1A2.[40]

Raucy[41] used an unrelated approach and screened the mechanisms of 3A4 *induction* by various drugs and natural compounds by examining 3A4 messenger ribonucleic acid (mRNA) values in human hepatocytes incubated with various inducers. Raucy also used a luciferase assay for pregnane X receptor (PXR) activation after transfecting HepG2 cells with plasmids containing hPXR and distal CYP3A4 promoters to assess the possible involvement of PXR in the enzyme induction mechanisms. She found that only kava (of various natural compounds tested) dramatically affected luciferase values consistent with activation of PXR.[41] However, the concentrations of the kava extract were 100 μM, and lower values were not tested.

Gurley et al.[42] performed an in vivo human study with 12 healthy volunteers to investigate the effects of 28 days' administration of several herbal extracts on probe drug cocktail administered before and after supplementation, designed to test the effects of the herb on single-point CYP450 kinetics.[42] In contrast to the in vitro studies, they found no measurable effects with kava on 3A4, 1A2, or 2D6, but pronounced inhibitory effects on 2E1. No elevations of serum hepatic transaminases were noted during the study. 2E1 shares with 1A1 and 1A2 the role of metabolizing aliphatic and aromatic hydrocarbons, but in particular, 2E1 is known to generate carcinogenic intermediates from simple organic compounds (e.g., nitrosamines in cigarette smoke).

Mathews et al.[35] also found evidence for an unidentified metabolic intermediate when methysticin and dihydromethysticin were incubated with human liver microsomes.[35] Zou et al.[43] found the first metabolic intermediate to be identified, dubbed 6-PHO (or 6-phenyl-3-hexen-2-one), demonstrating the reactivity of 6-PHO with reduced glutathione in vitro and also establishing its presence in human urine as a mercapturic (i.e., sulfhydryl) conjugate. The authors speculated that theoretically a nucleophilic compound could conjugate with such metabolic intermediates to form complexes that induce immune-mediated hepatotoxic reactions or direct hepatotoxicity through deoxyribonucleic acid (DNA) alkylation. Tarbah et al.[44] examined the metabolism of D,L-kavain (the synthetic racemate) after oral doses in humans and found that hydroxylation (probably by CYP2D6) was the initial metabolic transformation step, and that sulfated and glucuronated conjugates were found in serum and urine. Full details of the metabolic degradation of the kavalactones remain to be elucidated.

Russmann et al.[45] reported an interesting analysis on six healthy subjects who were chronic kava consumers. The subjects gave up kava (traditional aqueous extract) for 30 days, undergoing metabolic phenotyping for CYP450 using five probe substrates at days 1 and 31. Kava abstinence led to a "deinhibition" of CYP1A2, suggesting that the extract normally inhibits this enzyme. The authors suggest this may explain the observed inverse association between kava consumption and cancer through prevention of environmental carcinogen activation.[46] However, kava was recently shown to have nuclear factor kappa B (NF-κB) inhibitory properties, and hypothetically this may also confer cancer prevention benefits on the regular traditional kava consumer.[47]

Collectively, the currently available data on kavalactone effects on CYP450 suggest possibly significant inhibitory effects in vivo. This implies the possibility of pharmacokinetic interactions between kava and drug substrates of CYP450.[48] Estimates from existing pharmacokinetic data suggest that the in vitro inhibitory effects at $10\text{-}\mu M$ concentrations are commensurate with in vivo concentrations after typical kava administration of oral doses at 200 to 250 mg kavalactones.[49] Whether biphasic effects are caused by PXR-mediated induction of 3A4 subsequent to mechanism based inhibition effects is not known, but is a possibility. This would be parallel to the effects of SJW extracts, which initially inhibit then induce 3A4 via PXR-mediated transcription (see St. John's Wort monograph). Since CYP450 2C9, 2C19, 2D6, and 2E1 are inhibited by kavalactones and are also subject to common polymorphisms, a level of pharmacogenetic variability in response to kavalactones is supported by the data. A deficiency in 2D6 was identified in one case of hepatotoxicity associated with kava and alcohol use.[9] Interestingly, the 2D6 polymorphisms that are prevalent at about ten per cent in Caucasians are absent from Polynesian populations.[50]

Formation of potentially reactive intermediates from kavalactones during metabolism under certain circumstances cannot be excluded, although currently the potential reactivity or toxicity is not known. Systematic studies of the effects of kava consumption on plasma levels of various medications are urgently needed to clarify all the in vivo implications of the in vitro data. At present, compelling reasons would be required to coadminister kava extracts with narrow-therapeutic-range drugs that are substrates of CYP450 3A4, 2C9, 2C19, 2D6, and 2E1, particularly in polypharmaceutical combination with other drugs that are noted substrates, inhibitors, or inducers of the same enzymes. (Note that the benzodiazepines are primarily metabolized by 3A4 and 2C19 and the halogenated anesthetics by 2E1.) If such coadministration is required, pharmacokinetic interaction management precautions should be taken, such as plasma drug monitoring with clinical correlation, especially during the periods of addition or withdrawal of any of the agents to a regimen. Ideally, phenotyping of "poor metabolizers" should also be conducted.

The potential for additive pharmacodynamic effects with CNS-active drugs, as well as the possibility of pharmacokinetic interactions mediated by CYP450 modulation and the small but finite risks of idiosyncratic hepatotoxicity, all suggest that adoption of comprehensive history taking, identification of proper clinical indications, monopharmacy prescription, and vigilant monitoring for hepatic signs and symptoms are prudent and appropriate with kava use.

HERB-DRUG INTERACTIONS

Alprazolam and Related Triazolobenzodiazepines

Evidence: Alprazolam (Xanax).
Extrapolated, based on similar properties: Adinazolam (Deracyn), brotizolam (Lendormin), estazolam (ProSom), midazolam (Hypnovel, Versed), triazolam (Halcion).

Interaction Type and Significance

✗   **Potential or Theoretical Adverse Interaction of Uncertain Severity**

?   **Interaction Likely but Uncertain Occurrence and Unclear Implications**

Probability:	Evidence Base:
3. Possible	▽ Mixed

Effect and Mechanism of Action

A single case report suggests an additive pharmacodynamic interaction between sedative and hypnotic effects of kava with alprazolam, although it may be partly a pharmacokinetic interaction. Clinical significance is not established.

Research

Two lines of evidence have been invoked to support possible pharmacodynamic interactions between kavalactones and CNS depressants. The first is derived from early animal studies showing synergistic enhancement of sleeping times after administration of combination of kavalactones with the barbiturates pentobarbital and hexobarbital. Klohs et al.[51] found extension of pentobarbital-induced sleeping times increased 410% in mice after 60 mg/kg coadministration of oral dihydromethysticin. Other kavalactones had lesser effects at higher doses of 160 mg/kg. Meyer[52] repeated these findings and found that intraperitoneal dihydromethysticin at 20 mg/kg increased sleeping time induced by hexobarbital significantly. Neither study measured blood levels, and thus pharmacokinetic interactions are not ruled out. These results are in conflict with a small, randomized crossover trial with 18 healthy volunteers that investigated the effects of combining 240 mg kavalactones per day with bromazepam (9 mg daily) versus bromazepam alone. This failed to reveal any additive or synergistic effects or any significant effects on performance measures, such as motor coordination, stress tolerance, or vigilance.[53]

The second line of evidence comes from "reverse" extrapolations based on receptor binding and neurotransmitter-mediated studies with kava extracts. However, the available evidence is inconsistent, and kavalactones appear to exhibit inconsistent and weak (if any) binding to gamma-aminobutyric acid (GABA) and benzodiazepine receptors.[54-58] In a multicenter placebo-controlled clinical trial of alprazolam for panic attacks, the safety profile of the drug was revealing: 10 patients of the 263 in the verum group reported serious adverse effects. Of these, three were acute intoxication and two were hepatitis; one hepatitis patient developed jaundice and hepatomegaly, which were reversed on discontinuation of the drug, and the other had elevated transaminase levels, which were reversed by cutting the alprazolam dose by 50%.[59]

Reports

A single case report in a letter from Almeida and Grimsley[60] entitled "Coma from the health food store" in 1996 involved an apparent kava-alprazolam interaction. the report was correctly dismissed as "unevaluable," according to the

Fugh-Berman and Ernst criteria.[61] The form and dose of kava administration were not identified, nor was the dose of alprazolam. The symptoms of the 54-year-old man were not clearly described; a "lethargic and disorientated" state on admission to hospital does not correspond to "coma," according to diagnostic criteria such as the Glasgow scale. Comedications apparently included cimetidine and terazosin, and the authors failed to consider alternative explanations; cimetidine, a potent CYP3A4 inhibitor, may have affected alprazolam levels because the triazolobenzodiazepines are all exclusively substrates of 3A4 (differing from other benzodiazepines, which are metabolized through multiple pathways). The report has no evidential value regarding a possible interaction.[61]

A single case in the hepatoxicity report series (German BfArM reference #93015209, also British MCA case #13) involved a woman who developed cholestatic jaundice symptoms after 3 months' use of kavalactones at 210 mg/day, while also taking diazepam (for 6 months, dose unknown), a combination oral contraceptive, and L-thyroxine.[16] Viral hepatitis was apparently a possible etiological factor. Diazepam is metabolized by 2C19, which is also inhibited in vitro by kavalactones. Schmidt et al.[17] categorized this case as "possible" kava hepatoxicity but conceded that concomitant medications or other etiologies might also be involved.

Clinical Implications and Adaptations

Benzodiazepines are prescribed as hypnotic/anxiolytic agents, which is identical to the principal clinical trial–supported indication for kava. As previously discussed, general prescribing guidelines followed by practitioners versed in use of botanical medicines discourage coadministration of an herbal and pharmaceutical agent taken concurrently for the same indication. It is also well established that kava extracts are comparable in efficacy for mild anxiety states to benzodiazepines, but with a better safety profile; thus "standard of care" botanical practice would be to prescribe kava as a preliminary trial alternative, not an addition, to benzodiazepines.[1,2] Patients should be advised not to self-prescribe kava while using prescription anxiolytics or other CNS-depressant agents.

With appropriately qualified professional management, exceptions to generic cautions are possible under certain circumstances. For example, kava extracts have been used anecdotally by natural health care providers to assist in tapered-withdrawal protocols in patients attempting to break long-term dependencies on benzodiazepines.[24] Combinations with other, mild herbal sedatives such as passionflower (*Passiflora incarnata*) are likely to be synergistic and lack potentially problematic interactions that may occur with pharmaceuticals.[62]

Dopamine Agonists and/or Antagonists

Evidence: Levodopa (L-dopa, Dopar, Larodopa), haloperidol (Haldol).
Extrapolated, based on similar properties: Carbidopa (Lodosyn), levodopa combination drugs: levodopa and benserazide (co-beneldopa; Madopar); levodopa and carbidopa (Atamet, Parcopa, Sinemet, Sinemet CR); levodopa, carbidopa, and entacapone (Stalevo); neuroleptics (i.e., agents inducing extrapyramidal symptoms); dopamine agonists other than levodopa.

Interaction Type and Significance

? **Interaction Likely but Uncertain Occurrence and Unclear Implications**

Probability:
4. Plausible

Evidence Base:
▽ Mixed

Effect and Mechanism of Action

Kavalactones may have mixed effects on central dopaminergic pathways, but the mechanism and effect of the interaction(s) are not established. This is reflected clinically in apparent kava-induced "parkinsonian" symptoms reversed by anticholinergics, as well as in experimental evidence that tardive dyskinesia induced by the neuroleptic agent haloperidol is reversed by kava.

Research

The multiple effects of kava cannot be attributed to a simple or single neurotransmitter mechanism, and the effect of kavalactones on dopaminergic pathways is not fully understood. Baum et al.[63] used intraperitoneal administration of kava extracts at two doses (20 and 120 mg/kg) as well as separate kavalactones in a rodent model to examine resultant behavioral and changes and their correlation with dopamine concentrations in the nucleus accumbens. Their results indicated both dopamine-agonist and dopamine-antagonistic effects, with yangonin decreasing dopamine concentrations, whereas D,L-kavain and desmethoxyyangonin increased the neurotransmitter levels; dihydrokavain, methysticin, and dihydromethysticin had no effect on dopamine. About half the animals also showed increased 5-hydroxytryptamine (5-HT, serotonin) levels, whereas the others showed no change or decreased 5-HT levels. The authors speculated that yangonin may limit the euphoric or dopaminergic actions of the other lactones.[63]

Noldner and Chatterjee[64] investigated the effect of kava on haloperidol-induced catalepsy in a rodent model, established as a validated test system for detecting compounds with extrapyramidal symptom liability in humans. They found no cataleptogenic effect of kava extract administered alone, and in a second series of experiments they found pretreatment or coadministration of kava (WS1490 at 100 mg/kg orally) completely abolished the cataleptic effects of 0.2 mg/kg haloperidol subcutaneously. They also found that dihydrokavain was the only isolated kavalactone that exerted similar actions, but the effect of the whole extract was greater than that of kavain alone.[64]

Reports

Schelosky et al.[65] described four patients with suspected central dopamine antagonism after kava ingestion. One patient, a 76-year-old woman taking levodopa for Parkinson's disease for more than 8 years, presented at the hospital with an acute attack of involuntary neck extension and forced upward gaze of the eyes, which commenced 90 minutes after ingesting a single dose of 100 mg of standardized kava. The symptoms resolved after 40 minutes without treatment. However, the same patient had a history of acute dystonic symptoms induced by promethazine and fluspirilene for anxiety, which were reversed by treatment with biperiden (anticholinergic). The other cases were not parkinsonian patients, and levodopa was not involved; however, all three had developed various acute-onset dyskinetic symptoms while using kava standardized extracts, and all were successfully treated with 5 mg biperiden intravenously.[65] The authors' suggestion that kava may induce Parkinson-like symptoms led to the Noldner and Chatterjee[64] investigation with kava previously discussed.

Meseguer et al.[66] reported another case of spontaneous tremor, in a 45-year-old woman using kava for anxiety; again the patient improved with anticholinergic treatment. The authors suggested that a genetic susceptibility may explain the apparent induction of parkinsonian symptoms in some individuals using kava.

Clinical Implications and Adaptations

There appears to be a small but finite likelihood that kava extracts spontaneously induce either Parkinson-like or related dystonic symptoms in some patients, reversible by anticholinergics. In one case report a direct interaction seemed to occur with levodopa. Interestingly, the extrapyramidal effects of antipsychotic drugs are known to be related to dopamine antagonism, but there are no reports of worsening of tardive dyskinesia from kava-neuroleptic combinations, and experimental evidence suggests the opposite, that kava may ameliorate such effects. This might also be theoretically predicted from the clinical observations of the muscular relaxant properties of the herb. Parenthetically, in a secondary review of kava, Pepping[67] suggested that the in vitro inhibition of platelet monoamine oxidase (MAO-B) by kavalactones might theoretically display additive effects with selegiline or related MAO-B inhibitors used in the treatment of Parkinson's disease.

At present, evidence is insufficient to determine the predisposing factors for the direction of kava effects in combination with drugs that directly or indirectly affect dopaminergic pathways. Professionally monitored exposure to a trial challenge with the herb might be considered when compelling reasons exist for coadministration with such agents, because the reported apparent dystonic reactions were acute in onset after single doses. Tardive dyskinesia symptoms arising from neuroleptic drug exposure are persistent after cessation of the drug, so kava use for extrapyramidal sequelae to antipsychotic therapy may be appropriate, with professional management. Clinical studies are needed to validate the theoretical benefits of the herb in this context.

Ethanol

Ethanol

Interaction Type and Significance

? Interaction Likely but Uncertain Occurrence and
   Unclear Implications

✗ Potential or Theoretical Adverse Interaction of
   Uncertain Severity

Probability: Evidence Base:
4. Plausible   ∇ Mixed

Effect and Mechanism of Action

A suggested interaction, either pharmacodynamic or pharmacokinetic or both, between alcohol and kava theoretically could increase the toxicity of either agent under certain circumstances.

Research

Experiments by Jamieson and Duffield[68] are often cited as support for a possible alcohol-kava interaction. Using a rodent model, these researchers found that alcohol coadministered intraperitoneally with oral lipophilic kava extracts resulted in dose-dependent increase in sleeping times. However, the doses of both alcohol (up to 4 g/kg) and kava extracts (350 or 450 mg/kg) were much higher than those used therapeutically or in indigenous social/ceremonial consumption. The combined doses also proved to have high levels of lethal toxicity in the study animals. Also, the data appear to have little relevance to human clinical or social contexts, although arguably the toxicity of the combination was demonstrated to be greater than the inherent toxicity of either agent alone.

In contrast to the animal findings, Herberg[69] conducted a human study using a typical therapeutic kava dose of 300 mg/day (70% standardized extract). The placebo-controlled, randomized trial with 20 healthy volunteers examined the effects of WS1490 at 100 mg three times daily over 8 days, combined with oral ethanol administered to a blood level of 0.05% concentration, on seven performance parameters (e.g., concentration, vigilance, motor coordination tasks) on days 1, 4, and 8. No multiplicative negative effects of the combination were found. In the concentration test the combination group showed an actual improvement over alcohol alone ($p < 0.01$). On the other hand, Foo and Lemon[70] conducted a series of four trials with 40 healthy subjects, comparing the effects of aqueous kava extract (1 g/kg) alone with alcohol at a "social" dose of 0.75 g/kg alone, alcohol and kava combined, and placebo. In most performance tests, kava alone had little effect, but when combined with ethanol, performance deteriorated, to a greater degree than with ethanol alone.

The available data do not appear to resolve whether there is a pharmacokinetic or pharmacodynamic effect of the kava-alcohol combination, or whether the combination actually has any significant effect on cognitive function at "normal" dose levels. Gurley et al.[42] demonstrated in vivo inhibition of CYP2E1 by kava, but this is not the only pathway for alcohol metabolism. Anke et al.[71] showed that in vitro the four major kavalactones failed to exert detectable inhibition on alcohol dehydrogenase, even at 1 μM; as the authors noted, this suggests lack of pharmacokinetic interaction but does not preclude a pharmacodynamic effect. Further studies are required to clarify the occurrence, effects, and mechanism of the suggested interaction.

Reports

Alcohol was a factor in a detailed adverse event report from Russmann and Lauterburg[9] involving necrotizing hepatitis in a 34-year-old woman who had been consuming 210 mg kavalactones daily for 3 weeks. After consumption of 60 g alcohol, she became icteric, and laboratory values for transaminases and bilirubin were elevated. Biopsy confirmed the histopathological damage. She screened negatively for viral hepatitis but had low titers of Epstein-Barr virus. She recovered 8 weeks after cessation of the kava. She was phenotyped as a 2D6-poor metabolizer by debrisoquine challenge, and a lymphocyte transformation test revealed a strong T-cell reactivity to the kava extract. The authors suggested this was a case of immune-mediated hepatotoxicity, and that 2D6 phenotype may be important in the etiology of such reactions.

Clinical Implications and Adaptations

Evidence for an adverse interaction between alcohol and kava is inconclusive. Hepatoxicity from pharmacokinetic issues may be increased by the combination, particularly when one or both agents are taken at excessive levels. The clinical significance of the potential interaction is arguably less than its possible social implications, given that both kava and alcohol are subject to abuse, and a history of combined abuse of both agents has been recorded in some cases.[72] The interaction appears to be of low significance at therapeutic and socially acceptable doses.

THEORETICAL, SPECULATIVE, AND PRELIMINARY INTERACTIONS RESEARCH, INCLUDING OVERSTATED INTERACTIONS CLAIMS

Anticonvulsant Medications

Carbamazepine (Carbatrol, Tegretol), clonazepam (Klonopin), clorazepate (Tranxene), divalproex semisodium, divalproex sodium (Depakote), ethosuximide (Zarontin), ethotoin (Peganone), felbamate (Felbatol), fosphenytoin (Cerebyx, Mesantoin), levetiracetam (Keppra), mephenytoin, mephobarbital (Mebaral), methsuximide (Celontin), oxcarbaze-pine (GP 47680, oxycarbamazepine; Trileptal), phenobarbital (phenobarbitone; Luminal, Solfoton), phenytoin (diphenylhy-dantoin; Dilantin, Phenytek), piracetam (Nootropyl), primi-done (Mysoline), sodium valproate (Depacon), topiramate (Topamax), trimethadione (Tridione), valproate semisodium, valproic acid (Depakene, Depakene Syrup), vigabatrin (Sabril), zonisamide (Zonegran).

Limited experimental studies in rodent models suggest that kava extracts have a potential for antiseizure effects.[73,74] D,L-kavain had only a weak effect against strychnine-induced seizure in mice.[75] Electrophysiological studies show kava induces an increase in slow-wave activity in rodents and humans.[57,76] Human data for antiseizure effects are not available, although Spinella[77] suggested that kava extracts may potentiate anticonvulsants and increase adverse effects, such as lethargy and cognitive impairment. This hypothetical inter-action should be avoided and is subsumed under the general contraindication of not coadministering a herb (kava) and drug (anticonvulsant) for the same indication (epilepsy).

Caffeine

Caffeine

Donadio et al.[78] reported a case of acute rhabdomyolysis in a 29-year-old man after ingestion of a single dose of a com-pound herbal supplement containing 500 mg guaraná, 200 mg ginkgo, and 100 mg kava. The precise dose of the product was not revealed, and neither were comedications and medical his-tory, other than that the patient was a regular weight trainer who had just resumed weight training after 2 years. The patient was hospitalized with myoglobinuria and elevated creatine kinase (CK) and myoglobin levels. He developed no renal com-plications and recovered fully after 6 weeks. Treatment, if any, was not detailed. The authors speculate that the antidopami-nergic and neuromuscular-blocking properties of kava were pathogenetically relevant, along with the methylxanthine effects of caffeine from guaraná. Given the single dose of the supplement and the relatively small amounts of caffeine, equivalent to one or two cups of coffee, the authors' explana-tion is not readily plausible. The complete lack of additional reports of myoglobinuria in association with caffeine-kava con-sumption, which is likely a common combination, further detracts from the credibility of this suggested interaction.

Monoamine Oxidase (MAO-B) Inhibitors

Selegiline (deprenyl, L-deprenil, L-deprenyl; Ataptyl, Carbex, Eldepryl, Jumex, Movergan, Selpak); pargyline (Eutonyl), rasa-giline (Azilect).

Uebelhack et al.[79] conducted in vitro tests for MAO-B inhi-bitory activity by kava extracts and kavalactones in a human platelet system, both with intact and homogenized platelets. They found an IC_{50} of 24 µM for intact platelets, with substantially lower values for platelet homogenate.[79] MAO inhibitor activity has not been reported for kavalactones in

neurotransmitter studies, and the in vivo effects of the herb are not commensurate with selective MAO-B inhibition. Suggestions have been made of theoretical interactions with MAO inhibitors[67]; these are speculative.

Proton Pump Inhibitors

Evidence: Omeprazole (Losec, Prilosec).
Extrapolated, based on similar properties: Esomeprazole (Nexium), lansoprazole (Prevacid, Zoton), pantoprazole (Protium, Protonix, Somac), rabeprazole (AcipHex, Pariet).

Of the cases of hepatoxicity reported by BfArM, 21 included comedications with several prescription or over-the-counter (OTC) pharmaceuticals. Notably, the proton pump inhibitor (PPI) omeprazole (or rabeprazole) was involved in chronic use in four cases, two of which involved liver failure and transplant; one of these patients died after transplantation.[16] None of the cases was well documented, and all involved additional poly-pharmacy (see hepatotoxicity and interactions section earlier). Omeprazole (and all other PPIs) are metabolized by CYP450 3A4 and 2C19, both of which are inhibited by kava, with 2C19 subject to a poor-metabolizer polymorphism. Omeprazole alone is known to be associated with reports of acute hepatitis, transaminitis, and hepatic failure.[80-83]

Reliable data on the kava-omeprazole interaction are not available. However, given that omeprazole is often used for periods considerably longer than the manufacturer's recom-mended 4-week limit, pharmacokinetic interactions with kava are possible, resulting in elevated plasma levels of the drug. Therefore, increased risk of hepatic side effects may be of more than theoretical concern.

Warfarin and Related Oral Vitamin K Antagonist Anticoagulants

Warfarin (Coumadin, Marevan, Warfilone).
Related: Anisindione (Miradon), dicumarol, ethyl biscoumace-tate (Tromexan), nicoumalone (acenocoumarol; Acitrom, Sintrom), phenindione (Dindevan), phenprocoumon (Jarsin, Marcumar).

A human platelet aggregometry study by Gleitz et al.[84] established that isolated kavain could suppress arachidonic acid–induced aggregation at IC_{50} of 78 µM/L. This figure is an order of magnitude in excess of in vivo–attained concentra-tions after oral administration of kavalactones. Reports of inter-actions with drugs affecting hemostasis are unavailable. The S-enantiomer of warfarin is metabolized by CYP2C9 and the less active R-enantiomer by CYP1A2; both are inhibited by kavalactones at therapeutic dose levels (see pharmacokinetics discussion earlier).[35-40] Pharmacokinetic interactions with warfarin are therefore theoretically possible, although no inter-actions with anticoagulants have been reported, and no bleed-ing adverse effects have been attributed to kava.[85]

The 85 citations for this monograph are located under Kava on the CD at the back of the book.

Licorice

Botanical Name: *Glycyrrhiza glabra* L.
Pharmacopoeial Names: Liquiritae radix, Radix glycyrrhizae
Synonym: *Glycyrrhiza glandulifera* Walst. and Kit.
Common Names: Licorice, licorice root; U.K. spelling = liquorice; literally, "sweet root."

Summary

Drug/Class Interaction Type	Mechanism and Significance	Management
Acetaminophen UGT1A substrates ⊕⊕/☼	Licorice induces UGT1A and increases clearance of acetaminophen. Minor significance for acetaminophen due to multiple pathways of the drug's metabolism.	None relevant; vigilance with drugs exclusively conjugated by UGT.
Acetylsalicylic acid gastroirritant and ulcerogenic agents ⊕⊕	Licorice helps reduce gastroirritant adverse effects of aspirin. Clinically significant; anecdotally applicable to other drugs, such as NSAIDs, mucositis-inducing chemotherapy agents, and ethanol.	Coadministration preferred. Deglycyrrhizinated licorice (DGL) is effective.
Antibiotics ◇	Activation by hydrolysis of licorice glycoside (GL) to aglycone (GA) depends on bowel flora. Antibiotics reduce bowel flora number and function and may reduce herb bioavailability.	If coadministration necessary, use probiotics or DGL, if appropriate.
Beta-lactam antibiotics ⊕	Licorice constituents reduce or reverse drug resistance in MRSA when combined with beta-lactam antibiotics.	Coadminister licorice with drug in diagnosed MRSA.
Cimetidine Histamine (H₂) receptor antagonists ⊕	Synergistic increase in ulceroprotective and ulcer-healing properties suggested by combination of drug with DGL.	Coadminister.
Cortisol Prednisolone Corticosteroids, oral ⊕⊕/☼	Licorice spares steroid by inhibiting metabolic degradation, potentiates anti-inflammatory effects; reduced adverse effects because lower drug doses permitted by combination.	Combination used to minimize steroid doses; assist in tapered steroid drug withdrawal.
Digoxin Cardiac glycosides ✗✗	Supratherapeutic doses of licorice may induce hypokalemia, which has been associated with potential digitalis toxicity. Clinical significance low if drug and herb correctly prescribed and monitored, with electrolyte monitoring.	Avoid excessive doses and herb administration. Monitor electrolytes, and supplement with K⁺/Mg⁺⁺ if coadministration indicated.
Furosemide Potassium-depleting diuretics ✗✗/◇	Additive hypokalemic toxicity possible. In practice, reported cases all caused by unwitting or inappropriate self-administration of licorice-containing products.	Avoid. Caution patients to monitor labels of candy, laxatives, and other possible licorice-containing products.
Spironolactone Aldosterone antagonists ?	Complex interaction involving opposition of hypokalemia by drug at mineralocorticoid receptor, and possible reduction in licorice adverse effect of hypertension. Significance not established.	Avoid until further data available.
Nitrofurantoin Nitrofuran urinary antiseptics ☼	Reduction of gastroirritant side effects of drug. Clinically less relevant due to replacement of nitrofurans with ciprofloxacin, etc. Arguably same interaction as with aspirin, i.e., generic gastroprotective effect of herb.	Coadminister DGL with gastroirritant drugs known to cause adverse effects.

UGT1A, Uridine diphosphate (UDP) glucuronosyltransferase; *NSAIDs*, nonsteroidal anti-inflammatory drugs; *MRSA*, methicillin-resistant *Staphylococcus aureus*.

HERB DESCRIPTION

Family

Fabaceae.

Related Species

Glycyrrhiza uralensis Fisch ex DC (*Gan cao*). The favored Chinese species, *Gan cao* is pharmacologically similar to *Glycyrrhiza glabra*.[1]

Habitat and Cultivation

A perennial shrub in the pea family, *G. glabra* is a Mediterranean native, but more than 20 related species are distributed throughout Europe, Asia, the Americas, and Australia. *Glycyrrhiza uralensis* and *G. glabra* are both widely cultivated in warmer zones throughout Eurasia.

Parts Used

Root, stolons.

Common Forms

Dried Root: Whole dried root, and powdered dried root without bark.
Tincture, Fluid Extract: 15% to 20% alcohol.
Standardized Extracts: Up to 20% glycyrrhizin.
Deglycyrrhizinated Licorice (DGL): 0.5% to 2.0% flavonoids as liquiritigenin.

HERB IN CLINICAL PRACTICE

Overview

Licorice is one of the most ubiquitous herbs in Asian medicine and has been an important remedy in Western herbalism since

Greco-Roman times. Licorice is a complex and clinically valuable herb that, without substantial justification, has acquired an uneven reputation in conventional medicine. In part, confusion arises from the many different forms of the herb, its constituents, concentrates, and derivatives, such as the antiulcer drug carbenoxolone sodium, deglycyrrhizinated licorice (DGL), or parenteral products such as SNMC (no longer available) from Japan. These preparations were developed after the emergence of scientific interest in the pharmacology of the herb because of its unusually broad range of effects, including multiple actions on steroid metabolism and inflammatory pathways; hepatoprotective, chemopreventive, and antitumorigenic properties; and pronounced antiviral activities (e.g., glycyrrhizin is the most potent SARS antiviral agent currently known).[2,3]

A significant proportion of "bad press" associated with licorice root is attributable to the use of concentrated glycyrrhizin in the processed food and tobacco industries as a flavoring agent because of its characteristic intense sweetness. "Licorice" is also used to describe a range of widely available popular confectionery products; notably, in the United States, these are more often flavored with anise rather than real licorice or glycyrrhizin. Reports in the medical literature of licorice-related adverse events are invariably associated with the use/abuse of such products, rather than therapeutic doses of the crude herb or its extracts in a clinical setting.

Therapeutic monographs on licorice root are available by the European Scientific Cooperative on Phytotherapy (ESCOP),[4] British Herbal Medical Association (BHMA),[5] World Health Organization (WHO),[6] and German Commission E.[7] The herb is official in the 2003 *United States Pharmacopoeia–National Formulary*, the *European Pharmacopoeia*, and the 1997 *Pharmacopoeia of the People's Republic of China*.

Historical/Ethnomedicine Precedent

Licorice has been used for food and medicine around the world since ancient Egyptian and Assyrian records were first written on papyri and clay tablets. It was one of the riches stored in King Tutankhamen's tomb. Scythians near the Sea of Azov knew the sweet root to be a successful treatment for people with asthma and dry cough. Documented in the third century BCE by the Greek Theophrastus, this use is still common with many herbalists today. Medicinal uses of licorice are recorded from every dynasty of Chinese history. The herb is one of the most frequently used in Chinese formulae, often included as an adjuvant in prescriptions to harmonize other herbs, and thus esteemed as the "Great Harmonizer"; it is primarily considered to tonify spleen (*Pi*) and stomach (*Wei*) *qi* deficiencies, moisten the lungs (*Fei*), relieve pain, clear "Heat" and "Toxins."[8] The herb is also used widely in other Asian traditions, including Kampo and Ayurvedic medicine.

In Western use, licorice attracted medical interest when the Dutch physician Revers discovered at the end of World War II that some of his patients were using licorice as a home remedy to treat their ulcers successfully. This led to the development of semisynthetic antiulcer medication called *carbenoxolone*, long since replaced by newer classes of drug, such as histamine (H$_2$) blockers and proton pump inhibitors. Deglycyrrhizinated licorice was a byproduct of carbenoxolone manufacture, and DGL is currently used to deliver high levels of anti-inflammatory licorice flavonoid compounds with significantly lower levels of glycyrrhetinic acid (GA), reducing the risk of GA-induced pseudoaldosteronism. The effects of the herb on glucosteroid metabolism simultaneously led to medical interest in its use for Addison's disease.[9,10] This is reflected in the incorporation of licorice into prescriptions for (functional) "adrenal insufficiency" and chronic fatigue conditions by modern herbalists and naturopathic physicians. In botanical medicine the herb continues to be valued for its general tonic properties as well as for its more specific indications (e.g., peptic ulcers).

Known or Potential Therapeutic Uses

Addison's disease, adrenal insufficiency, asthma, bronchitis, cancer chemoprevention, chronic fatigue, constipation, cough, hepatoprotection against toxicity, herpes simplex infection (topically), human immunodeficiency virus (HIV) infection, inflammations of the gastric and urinary tracts, joint inflammation, mouth ulcers, peptic ulcers, polycystic ovarian syndrome, sudden acute respiratory syndrome (SARS), sore throat, stress, viral hepatitis.

Key Constituents

Triterpene saponins, principally glycyrrhizin 2% to 6% (aglycone = glycyrrhetin or glycyrrhetinic acid).
Polysaccharides, flavonoids (approximately 1.0%) including liquiritin, chalcones including isoliquiritin, isoflavonoids, sterols.

Note: Nomenclature for the glycyrrhizin and its aglycone varies. This monograph adopts the abbreviation "GL" for the *glycoside* (glycyrrhizin, glycyrrhizic acid, glycyrrhizinic acid) and "GA" for the *aglycone* (glycyrrhetinic acid).

Therapeutic Dosing Range

Dried Root: By decoction, 3 to 10 g/day; typical maximum Chinese dose: 15 to 30 g/day.
Tincture/Fluid Extract: Based on 1:1, 2 to 5 mL three times daily.
Standardized Extract: Up to 20% glycyrrhizin, equivalent to 5 to 15 g/day DGL—0.5% to 2.0% flavonoids, chewable tablets approximately 380 mg three times daily.

INTERACTIONS REVIEW
Strategic Considerations

The major therapeutic monographs for licorice root vary slightly in their accounts of potential interactions between licorice root preparations and prescription drugs, but the general theme is consistent. The German Commission E maintains that "potassium loss due to other drugs may be increased," and suggests that "with potassium loss, sensitivity to digitalis glycosides may be increased."[7] The same warning is repeated by ESCOP,[4] who include other "antiarrhythmic drugs or drugs which induce reversion to sinus rhythm such as quinidine" in their precautions about hypokalemia, as well as repeating the warnings of Commission E about combining licorice with potassium depleters, including stimulant laxatives and loop or thiazide diuretics. ESCOP also notes a possible alteration of prednisolone pharmacokinetics (i.e., glucocorticoid-sparing effect) with licorice. The WHO monograph[6] includes a further precaution about combining aldosterone antagonists such as spironolactone or amiloride with licorice.

These warnings are representative of most discussions on licorice's interactions with prescription drugs. Strictly speaking, these are better classified as drug "contraindications" based on the known pharmacological property of GL to induce a syndrome known as *pseudoaldosteronism* or "apparent mineralocorticoid excess." The first report of licorice-induced hypokalemia was unwittingly made by London physician de Cayley in 1950, who recorded the three cases of hypokalemic arrhythmia associated with p-aminosalicylic acid (PAS) therapy for tuberculosis.[11] De Cayley did not detect the connection to licorice, but the following year, Strong[12] realized that PAS was in fact flavored with licorice root extract. In 1979, Ulick et al.[13] used "apparent mineralocorticoid excess" (AME) to describe the congenital pediatric syndrome of hypertension, hypokalemia, suppressed renin-angiotensin-aldosterone axis, and increased urinary ratio of 11β-hydroxy to 11-oxo metabolites of cortisol (suggesting a failure of conversion of cortisol to cortisone).[14,15]

Subsequently, the ability of licorice extracts to inhibit the enzyme 11β-hydroxysteroid dehydydrogenase (11β-HSD) became established through in vitro, animal, and human experiments, and the resultant effects are usually termed licorice-induced "pseudoaldosteronism" to distinguish it from congenital AME.[16-19] Renal 11β-HSD-2 normally serves to "protect" local mineralocorticoid receptors from activation by cortisol by metabolizing the endogenous glucocorticoid locally to its inactive form. That is, the enzyme confers aldosterone specificity on intrinsically nonspecific renal mineralocorticoid receptors. When this enzyme is inhibited, the resulting excess cortisol stimulates both the glucocorticoid and the "unprotected" renal mineralocorticoid receptors, promoting potassium loss. If unchecked, this can lead to sodium retention and hypokalemia, with possible sequelae of hypertension, myopathy, rhabdomyolysis with potential renal failure from myoglobinemia, and cardiac rhythm disturbances.[17-27] The corollary impression that licorice is thus associated with potentially life-threatening toxicities pervades secondary accounts of the herb and reports of its interactions.

In practice, the situation is less clear-cut. First, the theoretical potential of licorice and its derivatives (except DGL) to induce pseudoaldosteronism is well known to practitioners of natural medicine who regularly use the herb and has been documented in conventional medical literature for over half a century. Coadministration of licorice with potassium-depleting drugs such as thiazide or loop diuretics, especially in patients vulnerable to electrolyte disturbance or using narrow-therapeutic-index antiarrhythmics, is a contraindication and clear departure from the standard of care. If two separate agents possessing similar toxicities are coadministered, there is risk of additive toxicity. This is not strictly speaking an interaction, unless there is evidence for unexpected "synergistic" or nonlinear increases in toxicity resulting from the combination. In botanical medicine settings, high doses of licorice are never prescribed for prolonged periods, and when used at normal therapeutic doses for 6 to 8 weeks, the adverse sequelae of pseudoaldosteronism are rarely observed. Blood pressure is usually monitored during higher-dose licorice prescription. There are no published reports of licorice-induced pseudoaldosteronism arising from practitioner-administered use of licorice; all published reports relate to either unwitting or deliberate consumption of products such as licorice candy, chewing tobacco, or flavored and sweetened beverages and laxatives. The risks of adverse events from self-administration are small but finite, given the public availability of these products, but it is appropriate to distinguish these concerns from clinical practice.[28]

Second, inhibition of renal 11β-HSD-2 by licorice and resulting mineralocorticoid receptor–mediated effects do not appear to account fully for the known features of the pseudoaldosteronism syndrome, particularly the varying individual expressions of both hypertension and edema. There is evidence of central nervous system (CNS) involvement unrelated to the renin-angiotensin axis, as well as local renovascular nitric oxide (NO)–mediated endothelial effects in addition to direct mineralocorticoid effects.[29,30]

The impact of licorice on steroid metabolism is complex and not fully understood. Inactivation of cortisol by 11β-HSD-2 is reversible because the enzyme is a bidirectional oxidoreductase. There are at least two isoforms of the enzyme; 11β-HSD-1 is widely distributed in peripheral tissues and the brain and acts predominantly as a reductase (i.e., reactivating glucocorticoids); 11β-HSD-2 is also bidirectional, but a higher-affinity enzyme that predominantly inactivates glucocorticoids, and it is co-localized with mineralocorticoid receptors (e.g., in the kidney).[31] Evidence for a third isoform, found in choriocarcinoma cells, has also been presented.[32] Glucocorticoid receptors are also subject to polymorphisms that contribute to individual variability in responses. There appears to be pronounced sexual dimorphism in humans between the relative contributions to cortisol inactivation by the A-ring reductases and 11β-HSD-1.[33,34] Licorice and GA also inhibits the A-ring reductases (5α- and 5β-reductase); both these enzymes irreversibly inactivate glucocorticoids.[35,36] The relationship between relative activities of the irreversible A-ring reductases and bidirectional oxidoreductases appears to vary widely and independently, depending on metabolic conditions.[37,38]

Data from animal studies used to explore the steroid biology must be extrapolated with caution to humans because definite species differences exist in the enzymatic determinants of steroid metabolism, which have diverged throughout mammalian evolution.[36,39-42] Pharmacokinetic variation in the bioavailability of GA has been demonstrated, and given the dependence of GL hydrolysis and release of GA on intestinal flora, this factor may be highly significant.[43-46] (See later discussion on the interaction between licorice and antibiotics.) Other compounds in food or herbal medicines may also inhibit 11β-HSD-1, notably grapefruit juice.[47,48]

In the final analysis, the inhibition of 11β-HSD isoenzymes by licorice arguably underlies only one clinically significant drug interaction, which is the consequent ability of licorice to "spare" prescription glucocorticoids (see licorice-prednisone/corticosteroid interaction). This interaction is not emphasized by secondary sources or the general literature. Licorice dosage required to effect a sustained inhibition of 11β-HSD have been estimated in a human pharmacokinetic study by Krahenbul et al.[49] to be 1000 to 1500 mg GA per day, whereas dose levels of less than 500 mg GA/day did not appear to be able to sustain levels of inhibition. Similar results were established by Bernardi et al.,[50] who found mild adverse effects only at the highest dose (814 mg GL/day) in a trial of healthy volunteers taking different daily doses for 2 weeks, although measurable renin depression occurred at lower-dose groups of 217 and 380 mg GL daily.[50]

The modulation by licorice of multiple steroid-metabolizing enzymes has some impact on sex hormones as well as glucocorticoids. Reports have suggested mild antitestosterone effects and weak estrogen receptor (ER) binding by licorice, and pronounced biphasic phytoestrogenic activity for the flavonoid compounds isoliquiritigen and glabidrin.[51-63] Speculations about interactions between licorice and prescription steroid sex hormones have inevitably been made but are currently unsupported by clinical data. The only available trial was a small, open-label study with 15 women and 21 men that examined the effects of 4 weeks' daily consumption of 9 g licorice (150 mg GA) on steroidal hormone levels. Negligible effects were found in the androgens, but in men a slight decrease in dehydroepiandrosterone sulfate (DHEAS) was observed[64] (see Theoretical, Speculative, and Preliminary Interactions Research).

Effects on Drug Metabolism and Bioavailability

Effects of licorice on the major drug-metabolizing and xenobiotic-metabolizing enzymes and effects of its compounds have not been fully characterized. Kent et al.[65] tested recombinant human cytochrome P450 (CYP450) enzymes in vitro for inhibition by whole-licorice-root extract and the licorice flavonoid glabidrin and found significant inhibition of 3A4 and 2B6 by both licorice extract and glabidrin. The effects were mechanism based and dose dependent but were demonstrated at plausible concentrations of licorice extract, with 6.9 micromolar (μM) achieving more than 50% inhibition of 3A4. CYP 2C9 was competitively inhibited by the licorice flavonoid glabidrin, whereas 2D6 and 2E1 did not appear to be affected by either licorice extract or isolated glabidrin.[65] Using a live rodent model, however, Jeong et al.[66] demonstrated that CYP450 2E1 inhibition was a component part of the mechanism underlying carbon tetrachloride hepatotoxicity prevention by oral pretreatment with GA.[66]

Paolini et al.[67,68] found that single doses of licorice extract or GL had no effect on mixed oxidases in a murine model. However, prolonged administration of 240 or 480 mg/kg GA resulted in significant increases of CYP450 3A4 activity, also shown to result from changes in messenger ribonucleic acid (mRNA), denoting increased induction of the enzyme. Smaller increases in 2A1, 2B1, 1A2, and 2B9 were also noted. A much-quoted in vitro fluorometric screening assay by Budzinski et al.[69] of several commercial herbal extracts and compounds on human 3A4 suggests that licorice extract was a moderate inhibitor of 3A4. However, the concentrations used were effectively in the 5-millimolar range, far in excess of attainable in vivo levels. Also, the relationship between in vitro fluorometric data and in vivo activity has not been demonstrated to have any consistent correlation.

The current picture of licorice effects on phase I drug metabolism remains incomplete. Clinical studies are required to establish how the preliminary and inconclusive experimental data may translate into significant drug-herb interactions. One rodent study suggests a possible enhancement effect of licorice on the phase II conjugase enzyme uridine diphosphate (UDP) glucuronosyltransferase (UGT1A), which did not appear to be an induction (mRNA) effect.[70] Additional evidence suggests possible effects of licorice on drug transporters of the organic anion peptide subfamily.[71] Finally, some animal data suggest that steroid drug distribution may be affected by licorice modulating steroid-binding globulins; however, the clinical significance of these data is not known.[72,73]

In conclusion, preliminary evidence exists that licorice may exert pharmacokinetic interaction effects on phases I, II, and III of drug metabolism, as well as some aspects of drug distribution. A preliminary report based on Chinese licorice (*Gan cao*) suggests the possibility that *Glycyrrhiza uralensis* compounds may bind to the pregnane X receptor (PXR).[74] If corroborated for licorice root, such effects might indicate a more significant potential for pharmacokinetic interactions than has been established to date. At present, however, clinical reports suggestive of pronounced pharmacokinetic interactions between licorice and pharmaceutical drugs are absent, and the complex effects on steroid-metabolizing enzymes dominate the considerations of the herb from an interactions perspective.

HERB-DRUG INTERACTIONS

Acetaminophen

Evidence: Acetaminophen (APAP, paracetamol; Tylenol); combination drugs: acetaminophen and codeine (Capital with Codeine; Phenaphen with Codeine; Tylenol with Codeine); acetaminophen and hydrocodone (Anexsia, Anodynos-DHC, Co-Gesic, Dolacet, DuoCet, Hydrocet, Hydrogesic, Hy-Phen, Lorcet 10/650, Lorcet-HD, Lorcet Plus, Lortab, Margesic H, Medipain 5, Norco, Stagesic, T-Gesic, Vicodin, Vicodin ES, Vicodin HP, Zydone); acetaminophen and oxycodone (Endocet, Percocet 2.5/325, Percocet 5/325, Percocet 7.5/500, Percocet 10/650, Roxicet 5/500, Roxilox, Tylox); acetaminophen and pentazocine (Talacen); acetaminophen and propoxyphene (Darvocet-N, Darvocet-N 100, Pronap-100, Propacet 100, Propoxacet-N, Wygesic). Extrapolated, based on similar properties: Substrates of glucuronosyltransferase (UGT1A).

Interaction Type and Significance

$\oplus\oplus$ **Beneficial or Supportive Interaction, with Professional Management**

☼ **Prevention or Reduction of Drug Adverse Effect**

Probability:	Evidence Base:
4. Plausible	○ **Preliminary**

Effect and Mechanism of Action

In this pharmacokinetic interaction, acetaminophen clearance is increased by the induction of glucuronosyltransferase activity by licorice.

Research

Moon and Kim[70] used a rodent model to investigate the effects of licorice root on acetaminophen pharmacokinetics. Pretreatment with glycyrrhizin (1 g/kg) for 6 days increased biliary and urinary excretion of glucuronic conjugates, but not of sulfate or thioether conjugates. Acetaminophen is also conjugated by sulfurotransferases and oxidized by CYP450 3A4.

Clinical Implications and Adaptations

Because acetaminophen is metabolized by multiple pathways, the significance of this interaction is low. Notably, the critical factors in acetaminophen toxicity are the extent of the hepatotoxic metabolite NAPQI formation by CYP 2E1 and the availability of glutathione for its conjugation.

Acetylsalicylic Acid and Other Gastroirritant and Ulcerogenic Agents

Evidence: Acetylsalicylic acid (acetosal, acetyl salicylic acid, ASA, salicylsalicylic acid; Arthritis Foundation Pain Reliever, Ascriptin, Aspergum, Asprimox, Bayer Aspirin, Bayer Buffered Aspirin, Bayer Low Adult Strength, Bufferin, Buffex, Cama Arthritis Pain Reliever, Easprin, Ecotrin, Ecotrin Low Adult Strength, Empirin, Extra Strength Adprin-B, Extra Strength Bayer Enteric 500 Aspirin, Extra Strength Bayer Plus, Halfprin 81, Heartline, Regular Strength Bayer Enteric 500 Aspirin, St. Joseph Adult Chewable Aspirin, ZORprin); combination drugs: ASA and caffeine (Anacin); ASA, caffeine, and propoxyphene (Darvon Compound); ASA and carisoprodol (Soma Compound); ASA, codeine, and carisoprodol (Soma Compound with Codeine); ASA and codeine (Empirin with Codeine); ASA, codeine, butalbital, and caffeine (Fiorinal); ASA and extended-release dipyridamole (Aggrenox, Asasantin).

Extrapolated, based on similar properties: Ulcerogenic/gastropathic drugs of several unrelated classes, including NSAIDs, ethanol, and antineoplastic chemotherapy agents.

Interaction Type and Significance

⊕⊕ **Beneficial or Supportive Interaction, with Professional Management**

Probability:	Evidence Base:
1. Certain	◉ Emerging

Effect and Mechanism of Action

The antiulcer and gastroprotective effects of licorice and DGL reduce the incidence of aspirin-induced gastric irritation and bleeding. The mechanism is multifactorial, including increase of mucin secretion to restore the gastric mucosal barrier, together with probable inhibition of gastric acid secretion; anti-inflammatory and cell proliferation effects may also be involved.

Research

A rodent study demonstrated that ulcer lesion scores and bleeding severity after gastric tube administration of ASA at 64 mg/kg were reduced significantly by coadministration of DGL at 2000 mg/kg. However, pretreatment with DGL did not have the same protective effect.[75] Other rodent studies found a protective reduction in bile acid and aspirin-induced ulceration in rats with DGL coadministration and a reduction in ulcer index using oral aspirin with a licorice coating.[76,77] The mechanism appears to be primarily related to increased mucin production.[78] Only one human study has examined the effects of coadministering aspirin with DGL. Rees et al.[79] performed a placebo-controlled, double-blind crossover study with patients who received either aspirin alone (325 mg three times daily) or aspirin (325 mg) plus DGL (175 mg three times daily). Fecal blood loss was significantly lower in the combination group, and the authors believed the result would have been more marked with higher doses of DGL.

Clinical Implications and Integrative Therapeutics

Aspirin-induced (and NSAID-induced) gastropathy is a well-documented and widespread problem and the cause of a significant number of serious drug-related adverse events, even at cardioprotective doses of 80 mg ASA/day.[80,81] Coadministration with proton pump inhibitors (PPIs) is considered a pharmaceutical management approach. An alternative is cotreatment with DGL, which appears to provide substantial protection while avoiding the adverse effects of long-term PPI use. Anecdotal clinical uses of the gastroprotective effects of licorice and DGL include prophylaxis and treatment of antineoplastic chemotherapy–induced mucositis.

Antibiotics and Antimicrobial Agents (Systemic)

Aminoglycoside Antibiotics: Amikacin (Amikin), gentamicin (G-mycin, Garamycin, Jenamicin), kanamycin (Kantrex), neomycin (Mycifradin, Myciguent, Neo-Fradin, NeoTab, Nivemycin), netilmicin (Netromycin), paromomycin (monomycin; Humatin), streptomycin, tobramycin (AKTob, Nebcin, TOBI, TOBI Solution, TobraDex, Tobrex).

Beta-Lactam Antibiotics: Methicillin (Staphcillin); aztreonam (Azactam injection); carbapenem antibiotics: meropenem (Merrem I.V.); combination drug: imipenem and cilastatin (Primaxin I.M., Primaxin I.V.); penicillin antibiotics:

amoxicillin (Amoxicot, Amoxil, Moxilin, Trimox, Wymox); combination drug: amoxicillin and clavulanic acid (Augmentin, Augmentin XR, Clavulin); ampicillin (Amficot, Omnipen, Principen, Totacillin); combination drug: ampicillin and sulbactam (Unisyn); bacampicillin (Spectrobid), carbenicillin (Geocillin), cloxacillin (Cloxapen), dicloxacillin (Dynapen, Dycill), mezlocillin (Mezlin), nafcillin (Unipen), oxacillin (Bactocill), penicillin G (Bicillin C-R, Bicillin L-A, Pfizerpen, Truxcillin), penicillin V (Beepen-VK, Betapen-VK, Ledercillin VK, Pen-Vee K, Robicillin VK, Suspen, Truxcillin VK, V-Cillin K, Veetids), piperacillin (Pipracil); combination drug: piperacillin and tazobactam (Zosyn); ticarcillin (Ticar); combination drug: ticarcillin and clavulanate (Timentin).

Cephalosporin Antibiotics: Cefaclor (Ceclor), cefadroxil (Duricef), cefamandole (Mandol), cefazolin (Ancef, Kefzol), cefdinir (Omnicef), cefepime (Maxipime), cefixime (Suprax), cefoperazone (Cefobid), cefotaxime (Claforan), cefotetan (Cefotan), cefoxitin (Mefoxin), cefpodoxime (Vantin), cefprozil (Cefzil), ceftazidime (Ceptaz, Fortaz, Tazicef, Tazidime), ceftibuten (Cedax), ceftizoxime (Cefizox), ceftriaxone (Rocephin), cefuroxime (Ceftin, Kefurox, Zinacef), cephalexin (Keflex, Keftab), cephapirin (Cefadyl), cephradine (Anspor, Velocef), imipenem combination drug: imipenem and cilastatin (Primaxin I.M., Primaxin I.V.); loracarbef (Lorabid), meropenem (Merrem I.V.).

Fluoroquinolone (4-Quinolone) Antibiotics: Cinoxacin (Cinobac, Pulvules), ciprofloxacin (Ciloxan, Cipro), enoxacin (Penetrex), gatifloxacin (Tequin), levofloxacin (Levaquin), lomefloxacin (Maxaquin), moxifloxacin (Avelox), nalidixic acid (Neggram), norfloxacin (Noroxin), ofloxacin (Floxin, Ocuflox), sparfloxacin (Zagam), trovafloxacin (alatrofloxacin; Trovan).

Macrolide Antibiotics: Azithromycin (Zithromax), clarithromycin (Biaxin), dirithromycin (Dynabac), erythromycin oral (EES, EryPed, Ery-Tab, PCE Dispertab, Pediazole), troleandomycin (Tao).

Sulfonamide Antibiotics: Sodium sulfacetamide (AK-Sulf, Bleph-10, Sodium Sulamyd), sulfamethoxazole (Gantanol), sulfanilamide (AVC), sulfasalazine (salazosulfapyridine, salicylazosulfapyridine, suphasalazine; Apo-Sulfasalazine, Azulfidine, Azulfidine EN-Tabs, PMS-Sulfasalazine, Salazopyrin, Salazopyrin EN-Tabs, SAS), sulfisoxazole (Gantrisin); combination drug: sulfamethoxazole and trimethoprim (cotrimoxazole, cotrimoxazole, SXT, TMP-SMX, TMP-sulfa; Bactrim, Bactrim DS, Cotrim, Septra, Septra DS, Sulfatrim, Uroplus); triple sulfa (Sultrin Triple Sulfa).

Chemotherapy, Cytotoxic Antibiotics: Bleomycin (Blenoxane), dactinomycin (Actinomycin D, Cosmegen, Cosmegen Lyovac), mitomycin (Mutamycin), plicamycin (Mithracin).

Miscellaneous Antibiotics: Bacitracin (Caci-IM), chloramphenicol (Chloromycetin), chlorhexidine (Peridex), colistimethate (Coly-Mycin M), dapsone (DDS, diaminodiphenylsulphone; Aczone Gel, Avlosulfon), furazolidone (Furoxone), lincomycin (Lincocin), linezolid (Zyvox), nitrofurantoin (Macrobid, Macrodantin), oral clindamycin (Cleocin), trimethoprim (Proloprim, Trimpex), vancomycin (Vancocin).

See also Beta-Lactam Antibiotics.

Interaction Type and Significance

◈ **Adverse Drug Effect on Herbal Therapeutics, Strategic Concern**

Probability:	Evidence Base:
2. Probable	☐ Inadequate

Effect and Mechanism of Action

Bioavailability of licorice root metabolites is partially dependent on bacterial flora which hydrolyze glycyrrhizic acid (GL) to its aglycone form. Oral antibiotic therapy suppresses normal bowel commensal flora and may reduce bioavailability of glycyrrhetinic acid (GA).

Research

The involvement of bowel flora in hydrolysis of GL to GA was first demonstrated in humans by Hattori et al.[44,45] Animal studies suggest significant species differences in stomach and bowel formation of licorice metabolites.[46] A rodent study showed that coadministration of a licorice-containing Chinese formula to rats with triple anti–*Helicobacter pylori* drug combination (omeprazole, amoxicillin, and metronidazole) significantly reduced the AUC of GA compared with administration of the formula alone. The authors attribute the effect to loss of GL-hydrolysis activity through reduction of bowel flora caused by the antimicrobials.[82]

Human data are equivocal. Cantelli-Forti et al.[43] showed little difference between the bioavailability of GL and GA up to 36 hours after single dosing.[43] A human pharmacokinetic study by Krahenbuhl et al.[83] demonstrated that GL and GA both undergo biliary elimination; GL is recycled enterohepatically, whereas GA is conjugated as a glucuronide before removal in the bile. Almost all orally administered GL reaches systemic circulation as GA after bowel flora hydrolysis.

Integrative Therapeutics, Clinical Concerns, and Adaptations

No studies are available demonstrating decreased bioavailability of GA in patients with reduced bowel flora after antibiotic therapy. Based on current information, however, antibiotics may reduce GA plasma levels if coadministered. This would not affect DGL preparations.

Beta-Lactam Antibiotics

Evidence: Oxacillin (Bactocill).
Extrapolated, based on similar properties: Methicillin (Staphcillin); beta-lactamase–resistant penicillins: cloxacillin (Cloxapen), dicloxacillin (Dynapen, Dycill); carbapenem antibiotics: meropenem (Merrem I.V.); combination drug: imipenem and cilastatin (Primaxin I.M., Primaxin I.V.); cephalosporin antibiotics, ciprofloxacin and other fluoroquinolone antibiotics, ketaconazoles, macrolide antibiotics, other penicillin antibiotics; combination drugs: amoxicillin and clavulanic acid (Augmentin, Augmentin XR, Clavulin, Nuclav); clavulanic acid and ticarcillin (Timentin).

Interaction Type and Significance

⊕ **Potential or Theoretical Beneficial or Supportive Interaction, with Professional Management**

Probability:
4. Plausible

Evidence Base:
○ **Preliminary**

Effect and Mechanism of Action

Licorice constituents may reduce or reverse drug resistance of methicillin-resistant *Staphylococcus aureus* (MRSA) to beta-lactam antibiotics.

Research

Experimental data are accumulating that a variety of natural compounds can effectively reverse drug resistance in various phenotypes of resistant *S. aureus*.

Licorice compounds have shown this potential with oxacillin against MRSA in vitro.[84] Mechanisms are not fully understood, but direct binding to bacterial wall peptidoglycans by the flavonoids is considered likely, and the effect is synergistic, not additive.[85]

Clinical Implications and Integrative Therapeutics

Clinical implementation of this potential interaction by combining licorice extracts with antibiotic therapy in MRSA has not been institutionally implemented. Substantial in vitro evidence also exists for green tea polyphenols and other natural compounds that exhibit similar resistance-reversing potential (see Green Tea monograph). Despite current lack of clinical support in the literature, integrative practitioners encountering MRSA infection, whether hospital or community acquired, should consider empirical trials of potentially synergistic herb-drug combinations given the serious nature of these infections.

Cimetidine and Related Histamine (H₂) Receptor Antagonists

Evidence: Cimetidine (Tagamet; Tagamet HB).
Extrapolated, based on similar properties: Famotidine (Pepcid RPD, Pepcid, Pepcid AC), nizatidine (Axid, Axid AR), ranitidine (Zantac); ranitidine, bismuth, and citrate (Tritec).
Interaction Type and Significance
⊕ **Potential or Theoretical Beneficial or Supportive Interaction, with Professional Management**

Probability:
4. Plausible

Evidence Base:
○ **Preliminary**

Effect and Mechanism of Action

Cimetidine and DGL combined are reported experimentally to exert synergistic antiulcer effects greater than either agent used alone.

Research

The efficacy of licorice derivatives in the form of DGL (Caved-S) has been compared to cimetidine in several clinical trials.[86-88] On balance, the evidence suggests that the botanical and the pharmaceutical are comparable in their ulcer-healing effects, possibly with slightly more rapid results achieved by cimetidine. Relapse rates are also no different between the two agents. A single study by Bennet et al.[89] suggested that in a rat model of aspirin-induced mucosal damage, coadministration of DGL and cimetidine resulted in greater gastroprotection than either agent given alone.

Clinical Implications and Integrative Therapeutics

The clinical significance of this possible synergy is not established, although it presents an "integrative" treatment choice that may be superior to the use of either herb or drug alternative alone.

Cortisol, Prednisolone, and Related Corticosteroids (Oral and Topical)

Evidence: Hydrocortisone oral (Cortef), methylprednisolone oral (Medrol), prednisolone oral (Delta-Cortef, Orapred, Pediapred, Prelone); topical hydrocortisone 17-butyrate/acetate/probutate/valerate (Acticort100, Aeroseb-HC, Ala-Cort, Ala-Scalp HP, Allercort, Alphaderm, Bactine, Beta-HC, Caldecort Anti-Itch, Cetacort, Cort-Dome, Cortaid, Cortef, Cortifair, Cortizone, Cortone, Cortril, Delacort, Dermacort, Dermarest, DriCort, DermiCort, Dermtex HC, Epifoam, Gly-Cort, Hi-Cor, Hydro-Tex, Hytone, LactiCare-HC, Lanacort, Lemoderm, Locoid, MyCort, Nutracort, Pandel,

Penecort, Pentacort, Proctocort, Rederm, S-T Cort, Synacort, Texacort, Westcort).

Similar properties but evidence indicating no or reduced interaction effects: Cortisone and prednisone (semisynthetic steroids with an 11-keto substitution), including prednisone oral (Deltasone, Liquid Pred, Meticorten, Orasone); triamcinolone oral (Aristocort).

Extrapolated, based on similar properties: Topical corticosteroids: Alclometasone (Aclovate, Modrasone), amcinonide (Cyclocort), beclomethasone, betamethasone dipropionate/valerate (betamethasone topical; Alphatrex, Beta-Val, Betaderm, Betanate, Betatrex, Diprolene AF, Diprolene, Diprosone, Luxiq, Maxivate, Teladar, Uticort, Valisone), clobetasol (clobetasol topical; Cormax, Dermoval, Dermotyl, Dermovate, Dermoxin, Eumosone, Lobate, Olux, Temovate, Temovate E, Topifort), clobetasone (Eumovate), clocortolone (clocortolone pivalate topical; Cloderm), desonide (DesOwen, Tridesilon), desoximetasone (Topicort, Topicort LP), desoxymethasone, dexamethasone (Aeroseb-Dex, Decaderm, Decadron, Decaspray), diflorasone (Apexicon, Florone, Maxiflor, Psorcon), diflucortolone (Nerisona, Nerisone), fluocinolone (Derma-Smoothe/FS, Fluonid, Synalar, Synemol), fluocinonide (Fluonex, Lidex, Lidex-E, Lonide, Vanos), fludroxycortide (flurandrenolone), fluocortolone (Ultralan), flurandrenolide (Cordran, Drenison), fluticasone (Cutivate), halcinonide (Halog), halobetasol (Ultravate), mometasone (Elocon, mometasone topical), triamcinolone (Aristocort, Triderm, Kenalog, Flutex, Kenonel, triamcinolone topical); combination drug: triamcinolone and nystatin (Mycolog II).

Interaction Type and Significance

⊕⊕ **Beneficial or Supportive Interaction, with Professional Management**

☼ **Prevention or Reduction of Drug Adverse Effect**

Probability:
1. Certain

Evidence Base:
◉ **Emerging**

Effect and Mechanism of Action

Licorice pharmacokinetically potentiates prednisone and cortisol and spares endogenous cortisol through inhibition of the enzymatic degradation by A-ring reductase and oxidoreductase enzymes. Steroid side effects may be reduced indirectly through sparing of the drug, allowing lower doses, and directly through pharmacodynamic mechanisms, including increased anti-inflammatory effects.

Research

The inhibitory effects of GL and GA on 11β-SDH isoforms, A-ring reductases, and other steroid-metabolizing enzymes are well documented (see Strategic Considerations). An interesting rodent study by Whorwood et al.[90] found that the inhibition of 11β-HSD by licorice derivatives combined with exogenous cortisol resulted in large changes in mRNA of the enzyme, indicating pretranslational inhibition significantly greater than that observed with either cortisol or GA alone. Inhibition of endogenous cortisol breakdown by GA in humans has been confirmed by Mackenzie et al.[23] in a small ($n = 10$) open-label study. Another small ($n = 6$) crossover human study examined the effect of oral pretreatment with GL (50 mg four times daily) on the pharmacokinetics of a single-dose infusion of prednisolone. The AUC of free plasma prednisolone was significantly increased and clearance significantly decreased by the GL pretretament.[91] In a skin vasoconstrictor assay, topical GA potentiated the action of hydrocortisone on

human skin.[92] An unrelated study examined the effects of GA on the antiproliferative activity of glucocorticoids against breast cancer cell lines MCF-7 and ZR-75-1; GA significantly increased the degree of antiproliferative activity by the steroids.[93]

Clinical Implications and Integrative Therapeutics

The sparing effect of GL and GA on glucocorticoids is well established and follows from the same enzyme inhibition mechanisms that underlie licorice-induced pseudoaldosteronism. Unlike the latter, this potentially beneficial interaction is not generally recognized in the conventional literature. A primary area of application of the sparing effect of licorice on corticosteroids has been in the context of tapered steroid drug withdrawal.[94] Anecdotally, this is an important clinical use of the herb in botanical medicine, along with the related ability to minimize steroid daily-dose levels required for maintenance of chronic inflammatory conditions such as temporal arteritis. The inhibitory effects of GA and GL persist after cessation of administration, at least 2 to 4 weeks.[95] This partly results from a transcriptional component in the lowering of the enzyme activity, evidenced in rodent studies by reduced mRNA levels for the enzyme after GA administration.[90] A possibly relevant point in consideration of this interaction is that the semisynthetic steroids with an 11-keto substitution (e.g., cortisone, prednisone) require initial activation by reduction, which is effected through hepatic 11β-HSD (i.e., the enzyme inhibited by GL). Therefore, if coadministration is proposed, it would be preferable to use steroids that do not require enzymatic activation, such as cortisol and prednisolone.

Digoxin and Related Cardiac Glycosides

Evidence: Digoxin (Digitek, Lanoxin, Lanoxicaps, purgoxin). Extrapolated, based on similar properties: Cardiac glycosides and antiarrhythmics including deslanoside (cedilanin-D), digitoxin (Cystodigin), ouabain (g-strophanthin)

Interaction Type and Significance

✗✗ **Minimal to Mild Adverse Interaction—Vigilance Necessary**

Probability:
4. Plausible

Evidence Base:
○ **Preliminary**

Effect and Mechanism of Action

Licorice extracts in supratherapeutic doses may induce hypokalemia, which theoretically may increase toxicity of antiarrhythmic drugs such as digitalis. Arguably, this is more an avoidable toxicity than an interaction. A single case report is available, but this fails to establish the interaction because of confounding factors.

Research

Potential hypokalemic effects consequent to licorice inhibition of renal 11β-HSD-2 are described in Strategic Considerations. A recent experimental study may have bearing on the kinetics of the licorice and digoxin combination. Ismair et al.[71] demonstrated that GL is both a substrate and inhibitor of several organic anion-transporting polypeptides (OATPs) localized in human hepatocytes, including OATP-8. Digoxin is known to be transported by OATP-8.[96] Whether and how this may affect the bioavailability of digoxin coadministered with licorice remains to be clarified.

Report

A single, well-documented report is available.[97] An 84-year-old man with a history of mitral regurgitation and atrial fibrillation was prescribed furosemide (80 mg/day) and digoxin (0.125 mg/day; plasma digoxin level of 1.0 ng/mL). The patient took a Chinese herbal laxative formula containing licorice root (400 mg) and rhubarb root (1600 mg) three times daily for 7 days. By day 7 he complained of fatigue, appetite loss, and dependent edema. On examination he had a heart rate of 30 beats per minute, blood pressure of 120/60, enlarged heart and lung congestion on radiograph, digoxin level of 2.9 ng/mL, and potassium of 2.9 mEq/L. Renin activity and aldosterone were low normal. Both the digoxin and the laxative were discontinued; 18 days later his pulse was 60 beats per minute, potassium 4.3 mEq/L, and renin and aldosterone levels midrange. Digoxin was restarted, and the plasma level was 0.6 ng/mL.

This report cannot be used to infer any direct causal support for a licorice-digoxin interaction. Furosemide, a potassium depleter, was already coadministered with digoxin in this patient. However, the case illustrates the possible risks of drug toxicity in at-risk patient populations when narrow-therapeutic-index drugs are combined with inappropriate herbal formulae added to polypharmacy. Rhubarb root (*Rheum palmatum*) is an anthraquinone-containing stimulant laxative, typically regarded as having the potential to induce electrolyte imbalance and volume depletion (both demonstrated in this case report). In this case, *three* potassium-depleting agents are involved: the furosemide, the rhubarb root, and the licorice. Finally, regarding the digoxin-licorice interaction, this patient, although bradycardic, was only mildly hypokalemic and did not display signs of more extreme digitalis intoxication, such as bigeminy, or require treatment with digoxin Fab.

Clinical Implications and Adaptations

The effects of potassium depletion on digitalis toxicity are not established. Stockley[98] reviewed data from several retrospective studies for evidence of a connection between potassium-depleting diuretics and digitalis toxicity and concluded that a link is not established beyond reasonable doubt, with several studies failing to demonstrate any connection. Nonetheless, the apparent consensus is that concurrent use of potassium-depleting diuretics with cardiac glycosides may result in digitalis intoxication. One management solution is the use of potassium-sparing diuretics, such as spironolactone or triamterene.[99] However, spironolactone interacts with licorice, as discussed later.

Complications of drug therapy in elderly patients with heart failure are common, particularly with the cardiac glycosides.[100,101] Digoxin itself causes increased renal magnesium excretion, and magnesium depletion also increases digitalis toxicity.[102] Elderly cardiac patients, especially those on polypharmacy regimens, should have their drugs regularly reviewed. Use of cardiac glycosides with potassium-depleting agents should ideally be accompanied by monitoring of drug and electrolyte levels, and where appropriate, patients should be supplemented with both potassium and magnesium.

Cases of licorice root–induced hypokalemia have been described only after self-administration of licorice-containing products by consumers. No reports support an interaction between licorice and digitalis. Hypokalemia resulting from therapeutic-dose levels of licorice is unlikely in clinical practice. The licorice–cardiac glycoside combination is better regarded as a contraindication because of additive adverse effects, and unless compelling reasons exist for coadministration, it should be avoided. Notably, this warning would not apply to the use of DGL.

Evidence: Furosemide (Lasix).
Extrapolated, based on similar properties:

Loop diuretics: Bumetanide (Bumex), ethacrynic acid (Edecrin), torsemide (Demadex).

Thiazide diuretics: Bendroflumethiazide (bendrofluazide; Naturetin), benzthiazide (Exna), chlorothiazide (Diuril), chlorthalidone (Hygroton), cyclopenthiazide (Navidrex), hydrochlorothiazide (Aquazide, Esidrix, Ezide, Hydrocot, HydroDiuril, Microzide, Oretic); hydroflumethiazide (Diucardin), methyclothiazide (Enduron), metolazone (Zaroxolyn, Mykrox), polythiazide (Renese), quinethazone (Hydromox), trichlormethiazide (Naqua).

Related but evidence lacking for extrapolation: Combination drugs: bendrofluazide and propranolol (Inderex); cyclopenthiazide and oxprenolol (Trasidrex); hydrochlorothiazide and amiloride (Moduretic); hydrochlorothiazide and captopril (Acezide, Capto-Co, Captozide, Co-Zidocapt); hydrochlorothiazide and enalapril (Vaseretic); hydrochlorothiazide and lisinopril (Prinzide, Zestoretic); hydrochlorothiazide and losartan (Hyzaar); hydrochlorothiazide and metoprolol (Lopressor HCT); hydrochlorothiazide and amiloride (Moduretic); hydrochlorothiazide and enalapril (Vaseretic); hydrochlorothiazide and lisinopril (Prinzide, Zestoretic); hydrochlorothiazide and spironolactone (Aldactazide); hydrochlorothiazide and triamterene (Dyazide, Maxzide).

Interaction Type and Significance

✗✗   **Minimal to Mild Adverse Interaction—Vigilance Necessary**

◇   **Adverse Drug Effect on Herbal Therapeutics, Strategic Concern**

Probability:	Evidence Base:
2. Probable	● **Consensus**

Effect and Mechanism of Action

Inhibition of renal 11β-HSD-2 by licorice may induce hypokalemia, especially at excessive doses administered for chronic periods. In combination with potassium-depleting diuretics such as furosemide, additive hypokalemic toxicity results. Myopathy and acute renal failure resulting from rhabdomyolysis and myoglobinuria have been recorded in settings of consumer self-administration of licorice.

Research

The pseudoaldosterone effects of licorice have been documented for more than 50 years in the medical literature (see Strategic Considerations). Potential adverse renal and muscular sequelae have been reviewed.[95] Importantly, furosemide, as with GL and GA, inhibits renal 11β-HSD-2 directly, thus sharing (at least in part) the same mechanism of potassium depletion.[47]

Reports

Shintani et al.[103] reviewed 57 published case reports of glycyrrhizin-induced hypokalemic myopathy in the literature from the 1960s to 1980s. Two salient features emerged from their review.

First, the reports appeared linked to different historical "fashions" of licorice consumption by the public. Initially, cases in the 1950s were from England and Australia related to PAS in the treatment of tuberculosis. In the 1960s, case reports predominantly originated from France and were associated with excessive consumption of a licorice-flavored alcoholic beverage, "Boisson de Coco." From the 1970s on, the emphasis shifted to Chinese herbal medicines and various commercial products for gastrointestinal complaints, including antiulcer medications and laxatives; more recently, a variety of licorice-flavored products (e.g., chewing tobacco) as well as licorice confectionary (e.g., "pontefract cakes") have been implicated. Notably, the cases reviewed were associated with self-administration of licorice compounds, often at supratherapeutic doses, and often for extended periods.

Second, the overwhelming associated factor in the reports of licorice-induced hypokalemia was the concurrent use of potassium-depleting diuretics. Also, the majority of patients belonged to the older-age demographic of 60 to 89 years.[103]

Another effect of prolonged hypokalemia is rhabdomyolysis. Chandler[95] analyzed three available case reports linking glomerulopathy, tubulopathy, and acute renal failure to myoglobinemia resulting from rhabdomyolysis induced by licorice consumption. In all three cases, furosemide was in concurrent use and regarded as a contributing factor in the renal reactions. Recent reports of hypokalemic myopathy or renal complications are extremely rare. Chubachi et al.[104] reported a case of renal failure associated with both furosemide and licorice ingestion. Elinav and Chajek-Shaul[105] reported an unusual case of licorice-induced myopathy related to use of licorice as a sweetener and not associated with furosemide.

Clinical Implications and Adaptations

No therapeutic rationale exists for coadministration of licorice root extracts with potassium-depleting diuretics. The potential additive hypokalemic effects amount to a contraindication for the combination, particularly in vulnerable demographics such as older cardiac patients. The availability of the potassium-sparing diuretics, together with the licorice derivative DGL, which lacks the mineralocorticoid effects of the parent herb for use in peptic ulcer treatment, provides alternative management strategies. Patients prescribed potassium-depleting agents should be warned of the possible risks of unwitting consumption of licorice as an ingredient of commercial products.

Spironolactone

Evidence: Spironolactone (Aldactone).
Extrapolated, based on similar properties: combination drug: spironolactone and hydrochlorothiazide (Aldactazide).

Interaction Type and Significance
? Interaction Likely but Uncertain Occurrence and Unclear Implications

Probability:
2. Probable

Evidence Base:
○ Preliminary

Effect and Mechanism of Action
Spironolactone is classified as a potassium-sparing diuretic but is a competitive inhibitor of aldosterone at the mineralocorticoid receptor, used clinically to oppose hypokalemia. Experimental evidence suggests spironolactone appears to normalize licorice-induced hypertension by restoring

endothelial-dependent vascular relaxation function. The clinical significance of this is not established.

Research
Quaschning et al.[106,107] investigated renovascular hemodynamics in a rodent model of hypertension. Rats were fed GA for 21 days to induce hypertension through 11β-HSD-2 inhibition by the licorice derivative. The resulting hypertension was causally related to the renovascular nitric oxide (NO) system as well as mineralocorticoid receptor–mediated effects. The GA administration reduced endothelial NO synthase (eNOS) and endothelin-1 levels, which were restored by spironolactone. There is emerging evidence that 11β-HSD activity may be depressed in essential hypertension.[108]

Clinical Implications and Adaptations
The reversal of GA-induced hypertension by spironolactone suggests a therapeutic potential for treatment of 11β-HSD deficiency–related cardiac disease. However, the implications of the interaction are unclear, given that coadministration of licorice and spironolactone would generally be avoided because of their opposing effects on kaliuresis.

Nitrofurantoin and Related Nitrofuran Antibiotics

Evidence: Nitrofurantoin (Furadantin, Macrobid, Macrodantin).
Extrapolated, based on similar properties: Nitrofuran antibiotics: Furazolidone (Furasian, Furoxone), furaltadone, nitrofurazone (Actin-N, Furacin).

Interaction Type and Significance
☼ **Prevention or Reduction of Drug Adverse Effect**

Probability:
4. Plausible

Evidence Base:
○ Preliminary

Effect and Mechanism of Action
The urinary antibiotic nitrofurantoin is associated with pronounced adverse effects. It has been suggested that coadministration with DGL reduces nausea and vomiting. The mechanism is not established but is probably related to the established gastroprotective effects of DGL.

Research
The nitrofurans were important urinary antiseptics, particularly for treatment of infection by *Escherichia coli* and other enterococci in the 1970s and 1980s. Despite concentration by the renal tubules and localization in the bladder, nitrofurantoin is associated with pronounced systemic adverse effects, including nausea and vomiting, and possible serious pulmonary fibrosis. Two studies performed more than 25 years ago suggested that coadministration with DGL led to increased clearance and a reduction in nausea and vomiting, together with improved effects on pyelonephritis.[109,110]

Clinical Implications and Adaptations
Nitrofuran treatment of urinary tract infection is less common now, partly because of the resistance of many strains of bacteria to the drug and its poor adverse effects profile. Fluoroquinolones (e.g., ciprofloxacin) have a superior oral bioavailability and fewer adverse effects and are now the preferred agents. The apparently beneficial DGL-nitrofurantoin interaction was established at the time of widespread prescription of the drug and is likely to receive minimal further investigation. However, a number of drugs

with pronounced gastroirritant properties may be better tolerated with coadministration by DGL.

THEORETICAL, SPECULATIVE, AND PRELIMINARY INTERACTIONS RESEARCH, INCLUDING OVERSTATED INTERACTIONS CLAIMS

Cyclophosphamide

Cyclophosphamide (Cytoxan, Endoxana, Neosar, Procytox).

A single animal study examined the effects of several herbal preparations, including licorice, coadministered with cyclophosphamide on mice inoculated with Lewis lung carcinoma and found reduction in tumorigenesis and metastasis compared with cyclophosphamide alone, although quantitative and statistical details were not available.[111] Suggestions of a synergistic interaction with cyclophosphamide or related antineoplastic chemotherapy have not been made to date and would be premature.

Insulin

Animal-source insulin (Iletin); human analog insulin (Humanlog); human insulin (Humulin, Novolin, Novo-Rapid, Oralin).

A human study suggested that carbenoxolone may improve insulin sensitivity in healthy individuals.[112] Another study, however, indicated coadministration of parenteral (SNMC) licorice with insulin in diabetic patients led to hypokalemia, sodium retention, and suppression of the renin-angiotensin axis, which the authors claimed was not caused by the pseudoaldosterone effects of SNMC because of normal urinary potassium levels.[113] The implications of these two studies are unclear but insufficient to support the claim of an insulin-licorice interaction.

Interferon and Related Antiviral Immunotherapy

Interferon alpha (Alferon N, Intron A, Roferon-A); combination drug: interferon alpha-2b and ribavirin (Rebetron).

Licorice is an established component of botanical medical treatment of viral hepatitis B and C, and GA has demonstrated potent antiviral activity against SARS.[2,3] In vitro evidence suggests that GL and GA can increase endogenous interferon production by lymphocytes and macrophages in response to concanavalin A.[114] A human study with hepatitis patients using SNMC (parenteral GA) in combination with interferon demonstrated a significant effect on normalization of alanine transaminase (ALT) compared with interferon alone.[115] Related experimental data support a possible role for licorice in stimulation of interferon production and efficacy against viral hepatitis.[116-118] Although the data suggest a possible interaction between licorice and recombinant interferon immunotherapies, this remains speculative pending further studies, particularly with oral rather than parenteral preparations.

Laxatives

Two reports indicated hypokalemia after use of licorice-containing laxatives.[97,119] Both preparations included anthraquinone-containing laxative herbs, which are also associated with potential electrolyte disturbances, especially when abused. Harada et al.[97] reported concurrent administration with a potassium-depleting diuretic (see licorice-furosemide interaction under Digoxin). Generic cautions about laxative use interactions with licorice are overstated.

Monoamine Oxidase (MAO) Inhibitors

MAO-A inhibitors: Isocarboxazid (Marplan), moclobemide (Aurorix, Manerix), phenelzine (Nardil), procarbazine (Matulane), tranylcypromine (Parnate).

MAO-B inhibitors: Selegiline (deprenyl, L-deprenil, L-deprenyl; Ataptryl, Carbex, Eldepryl, Jumex, Movergan, Selpak); pargyline (Eutonyl), rasagiline (Azilect).

An in vitro study demonstrated that the licorice isoflavone isoliquiritigenin from *G. uralensis* exhibited MAO-inhibition activity (IC_{50} = 17.3 millimolar).[120] Hatano recorded moderate in vitro MAO-inhibiting activity by a number of licorice compounds, including coumarins such as licocoumarone. The in vivo significance of these studies is unclear, and suggestions of potential interactions between licorice root and MAO inhibitors or biogenic amines is unsupported by clinical reports or pharmacological data. Recently, however, licorice isoflavonoids were shown to inhibit serotonin reuptake in vitro.[121]

Oral Contraceptives: Monophasic, Biphasic, and Triphasic Estrogen Preparations (Synthetic Estrogen and Progesterone Analogs)

Ethinyl estradiol and desogestrel (Desogen, Ortho-TriCyclen).
Ethinyl estradiol and ethynodiol (Demulen 1/35, Demulen 1/50, Nelulen 1/25, Nelulen 1/50, Zovia).
Ethinyl estradiol and levonorgestrel (Alesse, Levlen, Levlite, Levora 0.15/30, Nordette, Tri-Levlen, Triphasil, Trivora).
Ethinyl estradiol and norethindrone/norethisterone (Brevicon, Estrostep, Genora 1/35, GenCep 1/35, Jenest-28, Loestrin 1.5/30, Loestrin1/20, Modicon, Necon 1/25, Necon 10/11, Necon 0.5/30, Necon 1/50, Nelova 1/35, Nelova 10/11, Norinyl 1/35, Norlestin 1/50, Ortho Novum 1/35, Ortho Novum 10/11, Ortho Novum 7/7/7, Ovcon-35, Ovcon-50, Tri-Norinyl, Trinovum).
Ethinyl estradiol and norgestrel (Lo/Ovral, Ovral).
Mestranol and norethindrone (Genora 1/50, Nelova 1/50, Norethin 1/50, Ortho-Novum 1/50).
Related, internal application: Etonogestrel/ethinyl estradiol vaginal ring (Nuvaring).

Suggestions of potential interactions between licorice and oral contraceptives (OCs) have been made speculatively. Pharmaceutical drug induction of UGT1A and CYP3A4 (e.g., by griseofulvin, rifampin) has been documented to lead to increased clearance of ethinyl estriol and progestins, with potential breakthrough bleeding and loss of clinical efficacy. Evidence for UGT and CYP3A4 induction by licorice is confined to murine and in vitro models at this time. Healthy volunteers consuming 9 g licorice/day for 4 weeks exhibited no changes in androgens or DHEAS.[64] Additionally, biphasic dose-related phytoestrogenic effects have been observed with licorice isoflavones, and GL inhibition of 17β-hydroxylase and modulation of sex steroid–binding globulin contribute to the difficulty of extrapolating from the complex pharmacological data to an in vivo interaction. Until clinical reports are available, the potential interaction with OCs should be classified as speculative.

Oral Vitamin K Antagonist Anticoagulants

Anisindione (Miradon), dicumarol, ethyl biscoumacetate (Tromexan), nicoumalone (acenocoumarol; Acitrom, Sintrom), phenindione (Dindevan), phenprocoumon (Jarsin, Marcumar), warfarin (Coumadin, Marevan, Warfilone).

A licorice coumarin derivative was demonstrated in vitro to have antiplatelet activity, mediated through cyclic adenosine monophosphate, and GL has been shown to have in vitro antithrombin properties.[122,123] Currently, no support exists for interactions between licorice and anticoagulant drugs, and clinical reports are unavailable.

The 123 citations for this monograph are located under Licorice on the CD at the back of the book.

Milk Thistle

Botanical Name: *Silybum marianum* (L.) Gaertner.
Pharmacopoeial Name: Fructus silybi mariae.
Synonyms: *Carduus marianus* L., *Cnicus marianus* L., *Cnicus benedictus* L.
Common Names: Milk thistle, St. Mary's thistle, holy thistle, wild artichoke.

Summary

Drug/Class Interaction Type	Mechanism and Significance	Management
Cisplatin Platinum chemotherapy Alkylating agents ⊕⊕/☼	Silymarin reduces drug-induced nephrotoxicity by countering lipid peroxidation and cell membrane destabilization. Silymarin may additively increase anticancer effects of platinum compounds.	Coadminister during and after platinum chemotherapy. May be restorative retroactively.
Doxorubicin Anthracycline chemotherapy ⊕⊕/☼	Drug cardiotoxicity reduced by silymarin. Possible chemosensitization of resistant cells to anthracyclines. Drug transporter inhibition may be involved.	Coadminister silymarin as adjunctive to support protocols during and after anthracycline chemotherapy.
Hepatotoxic substances; various agents and classes ⊕⊕⊕/☼	General drug-induced hepatotoxicity countered by silymarin coadministration through multiple mechanisms, including free-radical scavenging, reduced lipid peroxidation, membrane stabilization, and cirrhosis/fibrosis inhibition. Demonstrated for numerous drugs and xenobiotic toxins. Wide clinical significance probable.	Coadminister especially in hepatically compromised patients requiring drugs that stress liver function.
Insulin ⊕	Silymarin normalizes glycemic control, maintains islet integrity, reduces insulin requirement. May protect against diabetic sequelae, especially in cirrhotic patients.	Coadminister, long term.
Metronidazole Nitroimidazole antiprotozoals ◇◇/⊕✗/☼	Coadministration of herb with drug may reduce drug availability by induction of drug-metabolizing enzymes.	Avoid coadministration. Preexisting herb use may require higher drug dose for therapeutic efficacy.

HERB DESCRIPTION

Family

Asteraceae.

Related species

Silybum eburneum Coss and Dur.

Habitat and Cultivation

Originally a Mediterranean native, milk thistle is now naturalized in many parts of Europe and North America, in drier sunny soils. Considered an invasive weed in some areas, it is widely cultivated for commercial use.

Parts Used

Fruit, typically described as milk thistle seed.

Common Forms

Powdered or whole dried hulled seed.
Tincture, Fluid Extract: 50% ethanol.
Standardized Extract: Solid concentrate 70:1, standardized to 70% to 80% silymarin (as silibinin).

HERB IN CLINICAL PRACTICE

Overview

Long known as a liver remedy in European and American botanical medicine, milk thistle is now well documented as a hepatoprotective herb and is used as an antidote to liver intoxication with chemical and biological toxins, including alcohol and a range of hepatotoxic drugs. After German researchers identified the flavolignan complex "silymarin" as the active component of the ripe seeds in the late 1960s, silymarin became available as a purified concentrate, and pharmacological research focused on the effects of silymarin on the liver. Silymarin was found to have antioxidant properties and was able to reverse glutathione depletion; it stabilized cell membranes and modulated efflux pumps such as P-glycoprotein (P-gp); it promoted hepatic ribosomal ribonucleic acid (rRNA) synthesis and liver regeneration; and it exerted anticirrhotic effects through inhibition of the transformation of stellate hepatocytes into fibroblasts. Several controlled clinical trials have found silymarin increases survival in alcohol-induced cirrhosis. It is widely prescribed for these indications, particularly in Germany.

The herb is well tolerated, with negligible toxicity and an excellent safety record. In the United States the herb typically ranks just under the "top 10" in retail sales. The German Commission E approved the whole herb for dyspeptic complaints and separately approved silymarin isolates for toxic liver damage and supportively for chronic inflammatory liver disease and hepatic cirrhosis.[1] The World Health Organization (WHO) monograph approves the herb for supportive treatment of acute and chronic hepatitis and cirrhosis induced by alcohol, drugs, or toxins.[2] A survey in 1998 showed that milk thistle was the most common hepatoprotectant used by outpatients in gastroenterological clinics.[3] A recent Cochrane systematic review of 13 trials of milk thistle extracts for alcoholic or hepatitis B/C virus–related liver disease found that liver-related mortality across all trials was significantly reduced. However, the methodological quality of the trials was poor, and the highest-quality data did not support the efficacy of the herb by criteria of overall mortality, liver histology, or liver-related complications.[4] Recent research has focused more on the anticancer effects of silymarin, but at present, despite promising basic science results with silymarin, clinical trial evidence in the oncological setting is lacking.[5]

It is important to distinguish among milk thistle seed extracts (whole herb), the flavolignan complex or "silymarin" present in small quantities in the whole herb but available as a concentrated solid extract, and *silybin* (also called silibinin), the predominant component among the flavolignan constituents, used as a reference for standardization. Most preclinical and clinical trials have used silymarin concentrate (see Key Constituents).

Historical/Ethnomedicine Precedent

Dioscorides mentions milk thistle use for snakebite, and the herb and seeds were used in Europe in the Middle Ages for liver conditions. The leaves have been used as a food, according to Culpeper, especially as a cleansing spring vegetable when well cooked, and were also considered to enhance milk production in nursing mothers. The ethanolic seed extract, which included the husks, was first promoted in the United States by Rademacher in 1841. The homeopathic physicians in the U.S. were enthusiastic about the remedy, which was included in the U.S. *Homeopathic Pharmacopeia* in 1878, where it is indicated for melancholy as well as varicose ulcers, among other uses. The Eclectic physician Ellingwood used the extract for hepatic indications closer to contemporary use, although other Eclectics viewed the seeds extracts as an "alterative." Brinker[6] provides a comprehensive historical review of the migration of the herb into American botanical medicine.

Known or Potential Therapeutic Uses

Amanita mushroom poisoning, amenorrhea, chemotherapy adjunctive, cholestasis, cirrhosis, constipation, diabetic complications, dyspepsia, fatty liver, gallstones, hepatitis (drug, alcohol, or chemical induced), hepatoprotection, protective against skin cancer (phototherapy, ultraviolet B, or radiation induced), right-upper-quadrant pain (associated with jaundice, hepatomegaly, or gallstones), uterine hemorrhage, varicose veins, venous congestion/stasis.

Key Constituents

1.5% to 3.0% silymarin, a flavolignan complex of silybin and isosilybin (its stereoisomer), silychristin, and silydianin. Silybin is also called silibinin. Other flavolignans are present, but silibinin is the primary compound.
Flavonoids: Quercetin, taxifolin, and dehydrokaempferol.
Lipids: 20% to 30% of the fruit is a lipid fraction, including linoleic acid and beta-sitosterol. Silymarin concentrates do not incorporate the broad spectrum of ingredient compounds, including the lipid fraction.

Therapeutic Dosing Range

Dried seed by infusion or decoction: Up to 15 g per day.
Tincture/Fluid Extract: Up to 8.5 mL 1:1 per day.
Standardized Extract: Concentrated 200 to 800 mg 70% to 80% silymarin per day. Clinical trial doses have typically been 420 mg/day in divided dose. The most common proprietary form is a 140 mg per dose 36:1 to 44:1 extract (from an ethyl acetate extraction), known as Thisilyn in the United States or Legalon in Europe, standardized to approximately 80% silymarin as silibinin. Bioavailability of oral silymarin is very low, and preparations complexed with lipids such as phosphatidylcholine have been developed.

INTERACTIONS REVIEW
Strategic Considerations

Therapeutic monographs for milk thistle are notable for an absence of established interactions with drugs. Herbalists regard the seeds as among the more benign, neutral, nontoxic foodlike botanicals in the materia medica; this is supported by the clinical trial data, which report negligible adverse effects, other than minimal incidence of mild gastric discomfort.[4] Toxicity studies corroborate this, with median lethal dose (LD_{50}) tests failing to produce mortality at oral doses of 20 g/kg in rodents.

In practice, the herb is used to ameliorate the adverse effects of xenobiotics, including pharmaceuticals, particularly on the liver. These beneficial effects of milk thistle were first discovered through its ability to antidote to *Amanita* mushroom intoxication.[7] Subsequently, similar hepatoprotective effects were established for a wide range of industrial chemicals and poisons, including carbon tetrachloride (CCl_4), tyramine beta-hydroxylase (TBH), and heavy metals.[8-15] The mechanisms underlying these effects are multifactorial; they include antioxidant activity through free-radical scavenging, prevention of glutathione depletion and enhancement of superoxide dismutase (SOD) activity, prevention of lipid peroxidation, stabilization of hepatocyte cell membranes, stimulation of liver regeneration, promotion of hepatocyte protein and glycoprotein synthesis, and antifibrotic effects from prevention of collagen formation by stellate hepatocytes. Silymarin also chelates metals such as lead and thallium, exhibits anti-inflammatory effects (by lipoxygenase inhibition and other mechanisms), and has chemopreventive influences through its inhibition of intestinal beta-glucuronidase, modulation of carcinogen-metabolizing enzymes, and signal transduction effects (notably epidermal growth factor receptor [EGFR] inhibition) and kinase inhibition. Recent research on the pharmacology of silymarin has been reviewed.[16-22]

The multiple mechanisms underlying the hepatoprotective properties of milk thistle seed connect a number of documented beneficial interactions between silymarin and hepatotoxic drugs. These are considered here as thematically related and are described later.

Effects on Drug Metabolism and Bioavailability

In vitro, silymarin has been shown to have some modulating effects on phase I and phase II drug-metabolizing enzymes, but the relevance of the limited available data is unclear. The few in vivo studies that have been performed suggest that clinically significant modulation of drug availability by silymarin on cytochrome P450 (CYP450) is *unlikely*. For example, the disposition of indinavir (a well-known substrate of both CYP3A4 and P-gp) is unaffected by milk thistle coadministration in healthy volunteers despite in vitro evidence of CYP3A4 and P-gp inhibition by silymarin.[23,24] Effects on phase II drug conjugation through induction of glutathione-S-transferase and inhibition of beta-glucuronidase (affecting conjugated drug–glucuronides subject to enterohepatic recycling) are also possible.[25,26] Effects on phase III (transporter proteins) may be significant, although at present this is extrapolated from in vitro data.

A universal problem, discussed throughout this text, is the issue of validity of such extrapolations, especially from nonphysiological concentrations used in vitro to in vivo clinical practice. This is particularly acute with silymarin, which has very low bioavailability and may only attain nanogram levels in the plasma after oral administration.[27] Weyhenmeyer et al.[28] found that at high oral doses (1270 mg silymarin per day, or approximately two to three times the normal therapeutic dose), peak plasma concentration of silibinin isomers in healthy volunteers was only 2.0 μg/mL. Preparations that complex silymarin with phosphatidylcholine (or lecithin) have superior bioavailability.[29-31]

In vitro CYP450 modulation data can be summarized as follows: Beckmann-Knopp et al.[32] found no significant effect on 2E1, 2C19, 1A2, or 2A6 but significant inhibition of 3A4 and 2C9 (at IC_{50} of 29-45 micromolar [μM]) with human liver microsomes and silibinin. Budzinski et al.[33] used dilutions of milk thistle whole-seed extract and found no significant effect on 3A4 using fluorometric assays with recombinant human enzymes. Venkataramanan et al.[34] used human hepatocytes and determined that 0.25 millimolar (a very high concentration) silymarin effected 100% inhibition of 3A4 and uridine glucuronosyltransferase (UGT1A). Zuber et al.[35] found that all three flavolignan components of silymarin exhibited dose-dependent competitive inhibition of 2D6, 2E1, and 3A4; however, doses were in excess of physiological levels in vivo, and interactions caused by enzyme inhibition were unlikely. Raucy[36] found that silymarin caused no significant changes in CYP3A4 messenger ribonucleic acid (mRNA) levels of human hepatocytes, suggesting that silymarin did not induce 3A4. Patel et al.[37] found a similar lack of effect on CYP3A4 mRNA and MDR1 mRNA in a CaCo-2 cell-line model. Sridar et al.[38] used recombinant enzymes and established that purified silibinin could effect a dose-dependent inhibition in vitro of 3A4 and 2C9. The potassium iodide (KI) values for 3A4 (166 μM) were not comparable to in vivo levels, although the lower value of 5.0 μM for 2C9 may be more clinically significant. Another rodent model was used to examine the effects of silymarin on drug-induced increases in 2E1 following chronic exposure to three 2E1 inducers. When the drugs were coadministered (for 12 weeks) with 50 mg/kg silymarin orally, 2E1 levels were not elevated.[39]

Extrapolation from data that employ different milk thistle preparations or compounds (silibinin, silymarin, whole-seed extract) in a range of experimental models at widely varying concentrations is problematic. The significance of the lack of effect on in vivo indinavir pharmacokinetics has already been noted.[23,24] This suggests that CYP3A4 is not inhibited in vivo despite the in vitro inhibition data. In fact, a small clinical trial by Rajnarayana et al.[40] suggested that silymarin pretreatment for 9 days at 140 mg/day significantly *increased* the clearance of 3A4/2C9 cosubstrate metronidazole, suggesting an in vivo *induction* effect. In a clinical study, Gurley et al.[41] examined the effects of herbal compounds on CYP450 in healthy volunteers by means of probe cocktails administered after 28 days of pretreatment with each botanical. Milk thistle was administered at 175 mg, standardized to 80% silymarin, twice daily. No significant changes were found in 1A2, 2D6, 2E1, or 3A4. The authors concluded that pharmacokinetic interactions with prescription pharmaceuticals were unlikely. Van Erp et al.[42] examined the effects milk thistle on the pharmacokinetics of irinotecan in six cancer patients. Irinotecan is a known substrate of CYP3A4 and UGT1A1. The administration of milk thistle (for 4 or 12 days) did not produce any significant change in irinotecan disposition.

The principal drug-metabolizing enzymes of phase II drug transformation are the uridine-5′-diphosphate glucuronosyltransferases (UGTs). This family of enzymes is primarily hepatic but is also distributed intestinally; it plays a key part in first-pass metabolism of drugs. Glucuronide conjugates are eliminated in the bile and, when hydrolyzed by beta-glucuronidase, undergo enterohepatic recirculation while the glucuronic acid recycles for use in further conjugation. There is in vitro evidence for silymarin-induced inhibition of UGT enzyme inhibition in a recombinant human enzyme model.[34,38] However, a study with rodent hepatocyte model and in vivo liver models showed that UGT inhibition induced by galactosamine might be reversed by silymarin.[43] Some inhibitory effects have also been found on the glutathione-S-transferases (GSTs), also involved with phase II metabolism, in the rodent hepatocyte model.[44] These GST inhibition effects have not been identified in vivo, where the main action of silymarin is on the prevention of thiol depletion and promotion of thiol replenishment, particularly in conjunction with cysteine donors.[45] On balance, induction of GST seems probable, and enzyme increase has been demonstrated in rodent liver, lung, stomach, skin, and small bowel after systemic administration of silibinin at 50 mg/kg orally.[26] These authors suggest that phase II enzyme induction may underlie the chemopreventive properties of silymarin, as demonstrated especially with skin cancers.[18,46,47]

Several herbal agents are now known to modulate drug transporters (phase III) at transcriptional and posttranscriptional levels.[48] Experimental data suggest that milk thistle flavolignans inhibit P-gp. This has been shown using the standard Caco-2 model in vitro, with drugs that are substrates of P-gp, such as digoxin, doxorubicin, vinblastine, and ritonavir.[37,49,50] Nguyen et al.[51] used a pancreatic cell-line (Panc-1) that overexpresses the MRP-1 transporter protein to examine the effects of flavonoids on the accumulation of transporter substrates daunorubicin and vinblastine. Silymarin significantly inhibited transport of these drugs. Because of the interest in potential modulators of drug resistance in cancer therapy, structure/function studies have examined the effects of different compounds on transporter proteins. Semisynthetic derivatives of silibinin have been tested to be even more effective P-gp inhibitors than the natural parent compound.[52-54] Combinations of flavonoid molecules in a "cocktail" from different botanicals, including silymarin sources, appear to have additive effects on inhibition of resistance to mitoxantrone in an MCF-7 in vitro model.[55] Once again, in vitro and in vivo data appear to be in conflict. For example, Gurley et al.[56] found that milk thistle supplementation for 2 weeks in healthy volunteers had no significant effect on any pharmacokinetic parameters of digoxin compared with rifampin and clarithromycin, used as positive controls for P-gp induction and inhibition, respectively.

In summary, in vivo pharmacokinetic interactions caused by milk thistle seem improbable, despite suggestions from in vitro studies. The case of metronidazole is a possible exception, as discussed later.

HERB-DRUG INTERACTIONS

Cisplatin and Related Platinum-Based Chemotherapy

Evidence: Carboplatin (Paraplatin), cisplatin (*cis*-diaminedichloroplatinum, CDDP; Platinol, Platinol-AQ).
Extrapolated, based on similar properties: Oxaliplatin (Eloxatin).

Interaction Type and Significance

⊕⊕ **Beneficial or Supportive Interaction, with Professional Management**

☼ **Prevention or Reduction of Drug Adverse Effect**

Probability:
2. Probable

Evidence Base:
◉ Emerging

Effect and Mechanism of Action

Silymarin (pretreatment or coadministration) reduces the nephrotoxicity of cisplatin and carboplatin without reducing and possibly increasing the antitumor effects of these agents in certain malignancies.

Research

Rodent studies using parenteral silibinin pretreatment have demonstrated protective effects against a nephrotoxic dose of cisplatin. Bokemeyer et al.[57] established that pretreatment with pure silibinin by infusion before cisplatin treatment significantly reduced nephrotoxicity, as measured by excretion of brush border enzymes and magnesium. Silibinin alone had no effect on renal function. The authors then used a human testicular cancer cell line to establish that silibinin did not lower the cytotoxicity of either cisplatin or ifosfamide. A similar model was used by Gaedeke et al.,[58] who employed a single-dose pretreatment of silibinin (200 mg/kg intravenously) 1 hour before a single dose of cisplatin. The silibinin pretreatment completely prevented any decrease in creatine clearance or proteinuria, and enzymuria and magnesium wasting were significantly reduced. The nephroprotective effect was correlated with histological findings of decreased tubular morphology changes.

Karimi et al.[59] found that both silymarin and a methanoic extract of milk thistle seeds could provide protection against tubular damage induced by cisplatin. Pretreatment was more effective than administering the milk thistle or silymarin 2 hours after cisplatin. Doses of silymarin were lower in this study (50 mg/kg).

In addition to protection against platinum-induced renal damage, a synergistic effect between silibinin and platinum compounds has been reported in which drug cytotoxicity was increased or potentiated by the flavolignan compound. Apoptosis in MCF-7 cells was increased by a combination of carboplatin and silibinin (but not by cisplatin and silibinin).[60] Silibinin and cisplatin exerted dose-dependent synergistic effects on platinum-resistant ovarian cancer cell lines at low concentrations of 0.1 to 20 μM.[61] Giacomelli et al.[62] performed in vitro experiments that showed silibinin alone had no activity against a human ovarian cancer line, A2780, but that it produced a dose-dependent increase in the cytotoxicity of cisplatin against these cells at 1-μM and 10-μM levels. In vivo, tumors induced in rodents by xenografts of the same cell line were treated by cisplatin alone and in combination with silibinin (450 mg/kg orally) in the form of a phosphatidylcholine-complexed preparation, IdB 1016; the combination therapy produced a statistically significant increase in treatment efficacy, as measured by tumor size. Interestingly, the combination-treatment groups recovered more rapidly from cisplatin treatment, as measured by body weight, than the cisplatin-only group. Finally, the researchers found a statistically significant in vivo antiangiogenic effect of the combination on the xenografted animals. Silibinin doses used in this experiment were considerably higher than therapeutic equivalents in humans.[62]

Dhanalakshmi et al.[63] used a prostate cancer cell-line model to examine the effects of silibinin combined with carboplatin or cisplatin on cell growth and apoptosis. At 50- to 100-μg additions of silibinin in combination with the platinum drugs, significant increases in cell growth inhibition were found. The mechanisms included increased apoptosis for both platinum agents, increased G2–cell cycle arrest for cisplatin, and complete S-phase arrest for carboplatin.[63]

Integrative Therapeutics, Clinical Concerns, and Adaptations

The purely experimental data are supportive of nephroprotective effects of silymarin or silibinin when coadministered with platinum compounds. Because tubular damage can be a dose-limiting toxicity of platinum chemotherapy, this is a potentially valuable beneficial interaction, although it remains to be clinically demonstrated. The data also suggest that silibinin may sensitize certain malignancies to platinum treatment; this may have importance in ovarian cancer, for which platinum is a common treatment. The observed sensitization effects of silibinin and platinum on prostate cell lines may simply be additive, not synergistic, because independent activity of silymarin against prostate lines has been demonstrated by several studies.[17,64-69]

Pharmacokinetic and pharmacodynamic studies are needed to determine the clinical significance of all these effects, particularly because the dose levels of silymarin/silibinin used experimentally are relatively high, and the preparation typically employed was pure silibinin. There may also be important differences among malignancies in terms of chemosensitization effects induced by silibinin.

Doxorubicin and Related Anthracycline Chemotherapy

Evidence: Doxorubicin (Adriamycin, Rubex).
Extrapolated, based on similar properties: Daunorubicin (Cerubidine), epirubicin (Ellence, Pharmorubicin), idarubicin (Idamycin, Zavedos), mitoxantrone (Novantrone, Onkotrone). Similar properties but evidence lacking for extrapolation: Daunorubicin, liposomal (DaunoXome); Doxorubicin, pegylated liposomal (Caelyx, Doxil, Myocet).

Interaction Type and Significance

⊕⊕ **Beneficial or Supportive Interaction, with Professional Management**

☼ **Prevention or Reduction of Drug Adverse Effect**

Probability:
2. Probable

Evidence Base:
○ Preliminary

Effect and Mechanism of Action

Milk thistle or silymarin may reduce adverse effects of anthracyclines through reduction of lipid peroxidation and membrane stabilization. The herb may also sensitize drug-resistant cells by inhibition of P-gp to increase drug cytotoxicity.

Research

In a rat cardiomyocyte model, co-incubation of silymarin (and component flavolignans) with doxorubicin resulted in dose-dependent reductions in cardiotoxicity, with silydianin exerting the most significant effects.[70] Psotova et al.[71] demonstrated that the protective effects of silymarin flavolignans against doxorubicin-induced rat cardiomyocyte mitochondrial and microsomal damage were related to free-radical scavenging rather than iron chelation. Tyagi et al.[60,72] have demonstrated additive cytotoxic effects against a prostate cancer cell line when doxorubicin and silibinin are coadministered. P-glycoprotein inhibition may play a part in the sensitization of anthracycline-resistant cells because silymarin has been demonstrated to be an inhibitor of the efflux pump. This is supported by the work of Zhang and Morris,[49] who used MCF-7 cells to demonstrate the effects of silymarin co-incubation on increasing intracellular daunorubicin and dox-orubicin accumulation. In a pancreatic cancer model, intracellular daunorubicin accumulation was also significantly increased by silymarin.[51]

Integrative Therapeutics, Clinical Concerns, and Adaptations

Direct support for the cardioprotective effects of silymarin is limited. However, given the general protective effects of the herb against parenchymal damage to hepatic, renal, and pan-creatic tissue, there would seem to be circumstantial support for including silymarin in protective protocols during and after anthracycline chemotherapy administration. Currently, evi-dence for possible modulation of resistance to anthracycline chemotherapeutic drugs is preliminary, but the underlying mechanics have been established as inhibition of P-gp. Clinical studies are required to establish the significance of this potentially useful interaction.

> **Hepatotoxic Substances, Including Acetaminophen, Acetylsalicylic Acid, Antitubercular Agents, Butyrophenone and Phenothiazine Neuroleptics, Ethyl Alcohol, Halothane, Methandienone, Methotrexate, Nortriptyline, and Phenytoin**

Evidence: Acetaminophen (APAP, paracetamol; Tylenol); acet-ylsalicylic acid (acetosal, acetyl salicylic acid, ASA, salicylsalicylic acid; Arthritis Foundation Pain Reliever, Ascriptin, Aspergum, Asprimox, Bayer Aspirin, Bayer Buffered Aspirin, Bayer Low Adult Strength, Bufferin, Buffex, Cama Arthritis Pain Reliever, Easprin, Ecotrin, Ecotrin Low Adult Strength, Empirin, Extra Strength Adprin-B, Extra Strength Bayer Enteric 500 Aspirin, Extra Strength Bayer Plus, Halfprin 81, Heartline, Regular Strength Bayer Enteric 500 Aspirin, St. Joseph Adult Chewable Aspirin, ZORprin); amitriptyline (Elavil).

Antitubercular agents: Isoniazid (isonicotinic acid hydrazide; INH, Laniazid, Nydrazid), pyrazinamide (PZA; Tebrazid), rifampicin (Rifadin, Rifadin IV); combination drugs: isoniazid and rifampicin (Rifamate, Rimactane); isonia-zid, pyrazinamide, and rifampicin (Rifater); chlorpromazine (Largactil, Thorazine); ethyl alcohol; halothane (Fluothane); methandienone, methandrostenolone (Dianabol); metho-trexate (Folex, Maxtrex, Rheumatrex); nortriptyline (Aventyl, Pamelor); phenytoin (diphenylhydantoin; Dilantin, Phenytek).

Extrapolated, based on similar properties: See table for classes.

Acetaminophen combination drugs: Acetaminophen and codeine (Capital with Codeine; Phenaphen with Codeine; Tylenol with Codeine); acetaminophen and hydrocodone (Anexsia, Anodynos-DHC, Co-Gesic, Dolacet, DuoCet, Hydrocet, Hydrogesic, Hy-Phen, Lorcet 10/650, Lorcet-HD, Lorcet Plus, Lortab, Margesic H, Medipain 5, Norco, Stagesic, T-Gesic, Vicodin, Vicodin ES, Vicodin HP, Zydone); acetaminophen and oxycodone (Endocet, Percocet 2.5/325, Percocet 5/325, Percocet 7.5/500, Percocet 10/650, Roxicet 5/500, Roxilox, Tylox); acetaminophen and pentazocine (Talacen); acetaminophen and propoxyphene (Darvocet-N, Darvocet-N 100, Pronap-100, Propacet 100, Propoxacet-N, Wygesic).

Acetylsalicylic acid/aspirin combination drugs: ASA and caffeine (Anacin); ASA, caffeine, and propoxyphene (Darvon Compound); ASA and carisoprodol (Soma Compound); ASA, codeine, and carisoprodol (Soma Compound with Codeine); ASA and codeine (Empirin with Codeine); ASA, codeine, butalbital, and caffeine (Fiorinal); ASA and extended-release dipyridamole (Aggrenox, Asasantin).

Anticonvulsant medications: Carbamazepine (Carbatrol, Tegretol), clonazepam (Klonopin), clorazepate (Tranxene), divalproex semisodium, divalproex sodium (Depakote), etho-suximide (Zarontin), ethotoin (Peganone), felbamate (Felbatol), fosphenytoin (Cerebyx, Mesantoin), levetiracetam (Keppra), mephenytoin, methsuximide (Celontin), oxcarbaze-pine (Trileptal), phenobarbital (Luminal, Phenobarbitone, Solfoton), piracetam (Nootropyl), primidone (Mysoline), sodium valproate (Depacon), topiramate (Topamax), trimetha-dione (Tridione), valproate semisodium, valproic acid (Depakene, Depakene Syrup), vigabatrin (Sabril), zonisamide (Zonegran).

Butyrophenone neuroleptics: Benperidol (Anquil, Benperidol-neuraxpharm, Frenactil, Glianimon), droperidol (Dridol, Inapsine), haloperidol (Haldol), melperon (Buronil), triperidol (Trifluperidol).

Halogenated inhalational anesthetic agents: Desflurane (Suprane), enflurane (Ethrane), isoflurane (Forane), sevoflur-ane (Sevorane, Ultane).

Phenothiazines: Acetophenazine (combination drug: Tindal, with hydrocodone), fluphenazine (Permitil, Prolixin, Prolixin Decanoate, Prolixin Enanthate), mesoridazine (Serentil), methotrimeprazine (levomepromazine; Nozinan), perphenazine (Trilafon); combination drugs: Etrafon, Triavil, Triptazin), prochlorperazine (Stemetil), promazine (Sparine), promethazine (Phenergan), propiomazine (Largon), thiethyl-perazine (Torecan), thioridazine (Mellaril), trifluoperazine (Stelazine), triflupromazine (Vesprin).

Tricyclic antidepressants: Amoxapine (Asendin), clomipramine (Anafranil), desipramine (Norpramin, Pertofrane), doxepin (Adapin, Sinequan), imipramine (Janimine, Tofranil), protriptyline (Vivactil), trimipramine (Surmontil).

Interaction Type and Significance

☼ **Prevention or Reduction of Drug Adverse Effect**
⊕ **Beneficial or Supportive Interaction, Not Requiring Professional Management**

Probability:
1. Certain

Evidence Base:
● **Consensus**

Effect and Mechanism of Action

Coadministration of milk thistle extracts or silymarin with hepatotoxic drugs reduces biochemical and histopatho-logical markers of drug-induced hepatocellular toxicity. The mechanism is multifactorial, including antioxidant free-radical scavenging, prevention of lipid peroxidation, stabiliz-ation of cell membranes, prevention of fibrosis, increase in hepatocellular regeneration, prevention of thiol depletion, induction of GST, and possibly inhibition of CYP2E1 activation of procarcinogens.

Research

Most data, except for ethanol-induced damage, are derived form preclinical evidence using a wide range of experimental models. (See table.)

Drug	Model (Citation)	Mechanism (or Finding)
Acetaminophen	Rodents, acute intoxication[73,74] Rat hepatocytes[9] Human hepatocytes[75] Human cell lines A431 and Hep G2[76]	Prevention of glutathione (GSH) depletion and lipid peroxidation. Prevention of GSH depletion. Downregulation TNF-α. Increase in GSH, mitochondrial membrane stabilization.
Acetylsalicylic acid, aspirin	Rodent CCl$_4$-induced cirrhosis, + ASA[77] Rodent portal vein ligation (PVL)—induced portal hypertension[78]	ASA pharmacokinetics normalized by silymarin coadministration. ASA pharmacokinetics normalized in PVL by silymarin coadministration.
Anabolic steroids	Rodents, coadministration of methandienone and silymarin[79]	Improved hepatocyte histochemical parameters.
Anticonvulsants (phenytoin)	Human case report[80] Observational study, psychiatric patients[81]	Decrease serum cholinesterase. Reduction of elevated transaminases, normalized bromsulphalein levels.
Antitubercular agents (isoniazid, rifampicin, and pyrazinamide)	Rodents, chronic intoxication[39,82]	Reversal of lipid peroxidation and GSH depletion, CYP2E1 activation, and transaminase normalization.
Ethanol	Rodents, acute intoxication[83-85] Rat behavioral model to assess effects of ethanol fetotoxicity[86] Rodents, acute intoxication[74] Placebo-controlled double-blind clinical trials of alcohol-induced liver disease treated with silymarin (420 mg/day)[87-90]	Antioxidant activity on alcohol metabolism and inhibition of lipid peroxidation. Reduction of ethanolic natal induced learning deficits by coadministration silymarin. Prevention of GSH depletion and lipid peroxidation. Various improvements, including reduction of transaminase elevation, decreased bilirubin, increased GSH levels, general symptom improvement, increase in survival rates.
Halothane	Rodents, acute intoxication[91] Hypoxic rodents, acute intoxication[92]	Prevention microsomal activity suppression by silibinin. Transaminase reduction.
Methotrexate, 6-MP	Case report, AML patient during chemotherapy[93]	Silymarin coadministration reduced transaminase elevation.
Narcotics (unspecified)	Clinical trial, cholecystectomy patients[94]	Serum cholinesterase reductions with silymarin before and after surgery.
Neuroleptics (butyrophenones and phenothiazines)	Double-blind clinical trial in long-term patients[95] Comparative study, long-term chlorpromazine patients[96]	Decreased serum malondialdehyde levels, decreased transaminases. Silymarin decreased or normalized drug-induced transaminase elevations.
Tricyclics (amitriptyline, nortriptyline)	Neonatal rodent hepatocytes[12]	Reduction of histopathological changes, lower transaminase alterations.

Integrative Therapeutics, Clinical Concerns, and Adaptations

Most evidence for hepatoprotective effects of milk thistle with specific pharmaceuticals has been derived from experimental models. However, the clinical use of milk thistle in alcohol and *Amanita* intoxication has clinical support, and in well-established experimental models of hepatocellular damage such as CCl$_4$ intoxication, silymarin has shown pronounced hepatoprotective effects. Several of the contributing mechanisms may apply to the parenchyma of other organs besides the liver, including pancreas and kidney, in relation to various drug-induced toxicities.[97-100]

Hepatoprotection may be conferred by "concurrent" or "retroactive" administration, depending on whether silymarin is coadministered with drugs known to be hepatotoxic or administered in response to an unanticipated hepatotoxic reaction or an "idiosyncratic" hepatotoxic reaction. Anecdotally, in clinical practice, milk thistle is widely used in various situations of compromised liver function, and the primary markers or endpoints of efficacy are usually transaminase levels, because the establishment of precise differentials in apparent hepatotoxicity cases often remains unknown.

Insulin

Animal-source insulin (Iletin), human analog insulin (Humanlog), human insulin (Humulin, Novolin, Novo-Rapid, Oralin).

Interaction Type and Significance

⊕ **Potential or Theoretical Beneficial or Supportive Interaction, with Professional Management**

Probability:
3. Possible

Evidence Base:
◉ **Emerging**

Effect and Mechanism of Action

Exogenous insulin requirements in insulin-dependent diabetes may be reduced by silymarin coadministration. Clinical trial evidence is available for type 2 diabetic patients with liver cirrhosis. Therefore, extension to other diabetic groups (e.g., type 1 without liver disease, otherwise-normal type 2) is not possible, although experimental evidence supports a hypoglycemic and islet-protective activity by silymarin.

Research

Soto et al.[99,101,102] conducted a series of experiments in the rodent model of alloxan-induced diabetes and found that islet damage can be reversed by silymarin. Three antioxidative enzymes—SOD, glutathione peroxidase, and catalase—were all increased as a result of silymarin administration, and when alloxan was followed by prolonged silymarin treatment (200 mg/kg/day orally for 9 weeks), the animals became normoglycemic, with insulin and glucagon levels comparable to untreated controls, and showed normal islet histology.

A controlled but open clinical trial was conducted over 12 months with insulin-dependent (type 1) diabetic patients who also had biopsy-confirmed liver cirrhosis. After 4 months' administration of silymarin (600 mg/day), glycemic control significantly improved, and exogenous insulin requirements and fasting insulin levels were reduced. All other parameters (HbA$_{1c}$, C-peptide, malondialdehyde, transaminases, bilirubin, total and HDL cholesterol, triglycerides, creatinine, microalbuminuria) continued to improve throughout the 12 months.[103] Unfortunately, lack of placebo control, together with progressive improvement of hepatic function in the cirrhotic patient population, confounds a generalization of the results to noncirrhotic patients. Further studies with different patient groups would help establish the significance and mechanisms of the observed results.

Integrative Therapeutics, Clinical Concerns, and Adaptations

Lipid peroxidation and cell membrane damage are associated with ineffective antioxidant defense in type 1 and type 2 diabetic patients and also with sequelae such as microangiopathy. Therefore the potential of silymarin in preserving pancreatic function and glycemic control in these populations is important. Adjunctive use of silymarin at relatively high doses (600 mg/day) in combination protocols may be a useful option in integrative strategies targeting normalization of glycemic and oxidative stress parameters.

Metronidazole and Related Nitroimidazole Antiprotozoals

Evidence: Metronidazole (Flagyl).
Extrapolated, based on similar properties: Ornidazole (Tiberal), secnidazole (Pronil), tinidazole (Fasigyn, Tindamax).

Interaction Type and Significance

◇◇ **Impaired Drug Absorption and Bioavailability, Precautions Appropriate**

⊕/✗ **Bimodal or Variable Interaction, with Professional Management**

☼ **Prevention or Reduction of Drug Adverse Effect**

Probability:	Evidence Base:
3. Possible	○ **Preliminary**

Effect and Mechanism of Action

In this combination interaction, milk thistle may reduce the bioavailability of the drug, as well as reduce drug-induced adverse effects.

Research

Metronidazole is a cosubstrate of CYP450 3A4 and 2C9. In a study discussed earlier under Effects on Drug Metabolism and Bioavailability, Rajnarayana et al.[40] administered 140 mg silymarin to 12 healthy volunteers for 9 days. The silymarin pretreatment increased the clearance of the drug by 30%. The time scale suggests an induction of the metabolizing enzymes. Unfortunately, the subjects of this small trial were not phenotyped by 2C9 polymorphism. A canine study found that coadministration of silymarin with metronidazole increased the efficacy of drug treatment (measured by fecal cyst count) and improved a number of metabolic parameters compared with metronidazole alone.[104]

Integrative Therapeutics, Clinical Concerns, and Adaptations

Efficacy of metronidazole therapy is determined by clearance of parasite. The drug is generally considered to be poorly tolerated, but addition of milk thistle to ameliorate hepatic side effects during therapy should be avoided because decreased plasma levels are possible, based on the limited available data. The use of silymarin posttherapeutically to normalize liver function can be considered. Addition of metronidazole to patients who are chronic milk thistle users may require increased drug dose levels, although as

in all such cases, the pharmacokinetics of the drug will be subject to individual variability, which is often not considered in prescribing.

THEORETICAL, SPECULATIVE, AND PRELIMINARY INTERACTIONS RESEARCH, INCLUDING OVERSTATED INTERACTIONS CLAIMS

Oral Contraceptives and Related Estrogen-Containing and Synthetic Estrogen and Progesterone Analog Medications

Ethinyl estradiol and desogestrel (Desogen, Ortho-TriCyclen).
Ethinyl estradiol and ethynodiol (Demulen 1/35, Demulen 1/50, Nelulen 1/25, Nelulen 1/50, Zovia).
Ethinyl estradiol and levonorgestrel (Alesse, Levlen, Levlite, Levora 0.15/30, Nordette, Tri-Levlen, Triphasil, Trivora).
Ethinyl estradiol and norethindrone/norethisterone (Brevicon, Estrostep, Genora 1/35, GenCep 1/35, Jenest-28, Loestrin 1.5/30, Loestrin1/20, Modicon, Necon 1/25, Necon 10/11, Necon 0.5/30, Necon 1/50, Nelova 1/35, Nelova 10/11, Norinyl 1/35, Norlestin 1/50, Ortho Novum 1/35, Ortho Novum 10/11, Ortho Novum 7/7/7, Ovcon-35, Ovcon-50, Tri-Norinyl, Trinovum).
Ethinyl estradiol and norgestrel (Lo/Ovral, Ovral).
Mestranol and norethindrone (Genora 1/50, Nelova 1/50, Norethin 1/50, Ortho-Novum 1/50).
Related, internal application: Etonogestrel/ethinyl estradiol vaginal ring (Nuvaring).
Hormone replacement therapy (HRT), estrogens: Chlorotrianisene (Tace); conjugated equine estrogens (Premarin); conjugated synthetic estrogens (Cenestin); dienestrol (Ortho Dienestrol); esterified estrogens (Estratab, Menest, Neo-Estrone); estradiol: topical, transdermal, ring (Alora Transdermal, Climara Transdermal, Estrace, Estradot, Estring FemPatch, Vivelle-Dot, Vivelle Transdermal); estradiol cypionate (Dep-Gynogen, Depo-Estradiol, Depogen, Dura-Estrin, Estra-D, Estro-Cyp, Estroject-LA, Estronol-LA); estradiol hemihydrate (Estreva, Vagifem); estradiol valerate (Delestrogen, Estra-L 40, Gynogen L.A. 20, Progynova, Valergen 20); estrone (Aquest, Estragyn 5, Estro-A, Estrone '5', Kestrone-5); estropipate (Ogen, Ortho-Est); ethinyl estradiol (Estinyl, Gynodiol, Lynoral).
HRT, estrogen/progestin combinations: Conjugated equine estrogens and medroxyprogesterone (Premelle cycle 5, Prempro); conjugated equine estrogens and norgestrel (Prempak-C); estradiol and dydrogesterone (Femoston); estradiol and norethindrone, patch (CombiPatch); estradiol and norethindrone/norethisterone, oral (Activella, Climagest, Climesse, FemHRT, Trisequens); estradiol valerate and cyproterone acetate (Climens); estradiol valerate and norgestrel (Progyluton); estradiol and norgestimate (Ortho-Prefest).
HRT, estrogen/testosterone combinations: Esterified estrogens and methyltestosterone (Estratest, Estratest HS).
It has been speculated that silymarin may interfere with oral contraceptive therapy, with the theoretical consequence of possible contraceptive failure. This proposed interaction is presumably based on an extrapolation from an assumption of increased clearance of estrogenic compounds caused by altered hepatic metabolism, or beta-glucuronidase—mediated effect on enterohepatic recirculation of estrogen conjugates. One study reported silymarin inhibition of human beta-glucuronidase, but evidence for pharmacokinetic effects on reproductive steroid metabolism is not available.[25]

A recent study with recombinant estrogen receptors (ERs) has demonstrated that silymarin appears to exert a selective estrogen response modulator (SERM)–like effect by acting as a selective ligand for ER-beta receptors while lacking an effect on ER-alpha receptors; however, the in vivo consequences of these activities remain to be demonstrated.[105] A single adverse event report in Australia involved a reaction in a 57-year-old woman taking ethinylestradiol as HRT, co-prescribed with amitriptyline. On taking a supplement that included silymarin, among other ingredients, she had acute gastrointestinal (GI) symptoms, including nausea and vomiting, colicky cramping, and diarrhea. The GI symptoms were repeated on rechallenge with the supplement. Although recording this as an adverse reaction to milk thistle, the report concedes that causality was not established.[106]

Tacrine

Tacrine (Tetrahydroaminoacridine, THA; Cognex).

A small clinical trial was conducted with Alzheimer's patients using tacrine to determine if silymarin might reduce the hepatic transaminase elevation typically associated with long-term administration of the drug. The study failed to reveal a significant effect of milk thistle on hepatic parameters, but the authors maintained that nonhepatic drug adverse effects (e.g., GI symptoms) were lower in the verum group than the control group.[107] The significance of this is unclear because milk thistle itself has been associated with mild GI adverse effects.

The 107 citations for this monograph are located under Milk Thistle on the CD at the back of the book.

Red Clover

Botanical Name: *Trifolium pratense* L.
Pharmacopoeial Name: Trifolii flos.
Common Names: Red clover, purple clover, trefoil.

HERB DESCRIPTION

Family

Fabaceae.

Parts Used

Flowers (traditional); "leaf" (standardized isoflavone preparations).

Common Forms

Dried flowering tops.
Tincture, Fluid Extract: Flowers, ethanol 25% to 35%, typically 1:2 to 1:5.
Standardized Extract: Standardized to 40 mg total isoflavones (Promensil, Trinovin); note: these are not red clover flowers (see following discussion).

INTERACTIONS REVIEW

Strategic Considerations

Current mainstream perceptions of red clover are dominated by the view of the herb as a source of phytoestrogenic isoflavones. This contrasts with traditional medicine's view of red clover flowers as having "alterative" (i.e., normalizing and "blood cleansing") properties. Historically, red clover flowers have been used internally as an alterative, antiscrofulous, antispasmodic, expectorant, and topically as a poultice for acne, ulcers, and cancerous growths.

Red clover flowers were a key ingredient of a famous Eclectic medical formulation "Trifolium Compound." Other ingredients included compound fresh extracts of *Stillingia sylvatica*, *Lappa minor*, *Phytolacca decandra*, *Cascara amarga*, *Berberis aquifolium*, *Podophyllum peltatum*, *Xanthoxylum carolinianum*, and potassium iodide. It was intended for administration "in syphilis, scrofula, chronic rheumatism, glandular and various skin affections."[1] The popularization of red clover as a cancer treatment in the first half of the twentieth century derived from various sources, including Jethro Kloss and the controversial Harry Hoxsey, whose anticancer "Hoxsey Formula" incorporated most of the herbs of the original Trifolium Compound, including red clover flowers.[2] Hoxsey formula–type products persist in the retail marketplace today. Red clover flowers remain in widespread use by modern herbalists, particularly in women's health care, despite the rise of interest in standardized leaf extracts, based on isoflavones.[3]

Interactions reports for red clover flower are not available. Extrapolations from the available pharmacological literature encounter difficulties. First, there is the difference between traditional red clover flower preparations and isoflavone standardized extracts. Bone[4] suggests that the traditional 25% alcohol extracts of red clover flowers have a very different constituent profile than the leaf-based standardized extracts. Analytical data suggest that the isoflavone content of clover flowers is 25% that of the leaves. Thus the flower heads have

relatively small quantities of isoflavones, and only formononetin has been positively demonstrated.[5] In addition, the traditional pharmacopoeial remedy Trifollii flos is based on *Trifolium pratense* inflorescence (flowers). The literature on red clover flowers itself is not extensive. The herb is monographed in the *British Herbal Compendium*[5] and *British Herbal Pharmacopoeia*[6] but has received scant attention from other pharmacopoeial sources.

Second, much of the related research and literature focuses on the two soy-derived isoflavones, genistein and daidzein. These occur naturally as free compounds and as glycosides, genistin and daidzin. Red clover primarily contains biochanin A and formononetin, which are not present in soy. For example, a recent patent registered by Novogen Research Pty., the manufacturers of Promensil, for "therapy of estrogen associated disorders," cites the use of "clovers" (*Trifolium* spp.) and "chick peas" (*Cicer arietinum* L., Fabaceae) as sources of isoflavones. The clover species in the patent include *Trifolium repens* and *T. subterranean*, as well as "any clover related species or chick pea variety." The use of multiple leguminous sources for the isoflavone content of standardized extracts is controversial from a traditional pharmacopeial perspective, and such extracts are likely to include high concentrations of materials not present in red clover flowers. However, significant differences in effect are likely with the different proportions of different isoflavone ingredients.

Booth et al.[7] analyzed the estrogenicity and estrogen receptor (ER)–binding properties of different isoflavone compounds in a "preformulated red clover clinical extract." All the isoflavones, except formononetin, showed binding activity to one or other recombinant ER type. Analytical methods have been developed that allow accurate characterization of the isoflavone content of clover products.[8,9] Given the use of semipurified extracts containing isoflavones from multiple sources in commercial preparations used in controlled trials on "red clover" and available commercially for menopausal symptom relief, the interactions relating to these products are closer to those relating to soy isoflavones, isolates that are not a food, nutrient, or herb in any commonly accepted sense, than to red clover.

Pharmacokinetics and Effects on Drug Metabolism

Setchell et al.[10] reviewed the complex metabolism of these compounds and analyzed 33 commercial isoflavone-containing supplements. They concluded that the ingredients showed considerable variation and demonstrated that pharmacokinetics of different preparations were not at all equivalent. The naturally occurring form of the isoflavones is glycosidic, as genistin and daidzin. In vivo, the glycosides undergo bacterial hydrolysis in the large bowel to release the aglycones genistein and daidzein. Availability of appropriate bacterial enzymes for hydrolysis of glycosidic isoflavones may also vary widely based on varying endogenous bacterial ecologies, which may lead to large variations in bioavailability of the aglycone forms.

The red clover isoflavones include biochanin A and formononetin, which are not present in soy; these are partially metabolized in vivo to the estrogenic metabolite equol. Polymorphisms between "fast" and "slow" equol producers have been described, and equol also undergoes enterohepatic recirculation.[11] Biochanin A and formononetin may also be metabolized in hepatocytes to genistein and daidzein.[12] The modulation of cytochrome P450 (CYP450) enzymes by isoflavones has been a topic of research interest; the inhibition of CYP450 1A2 partly explains the chemopreventive properties of the compounds.[13] Biochanin A and formononetin may also modulate P-glycoprotein.[14] Budzinski et al.[15] showed that an unidentified commercial ethanolic red clover extract was a potential inhibitor of CYP3A4 in a high-throughput in vitro screening assay of various compounds and commercial extracts. However, no reports of interactions with CYP3A4-metabolized pharmaceuticals have been made to date. Meanwhile, Kroyer[16] established that the total polyphenolic content and antioxidant activity of ethanolic extracts of red clover leaf were significantly higher than those of comparable soybean-based extracts.

A double caveat must therefore be applied in evaluating the literature pertaining to red clover. Not only are red clover flower extracts significantly different from standardized red clover preparations, but data derived from isolated soy isoflavones such as genistein and daidzein are not directly applicable to red clover isoflavone extracts.

THEORETICAL, SPECULATIVE, AND PRELIMINARY INTERACTIONS RESEARCH, INCLUDING OVERSTATED INTERACTIONS CLAIMS

Warfarin and Related Oral Vitamin K Antagonist Anticoagulants

Anisindione (Miradon), dicumarol, ethyl biscoumacetate (Tromexan), nicoumalone (acenocoumarol; Acitrom, Sintrom), phenindione (Dindevan), phenprocoumon (Jarsin, Marcumar), warfarin (Coumadin, Marevan, Warfilone).

Diverse secondary sources repeat the persistent claim that the presence of coumarin compounds in *Trifolium* spp. may cause interaction with anticoagulant drugs such as warfarin. Not only are reports of this interaction entirely lacking, but this assertion is based on incorrect pharmacological assumptions. The coumarin content of red clover is in the form of coumestrol, a molecule lacking the 4-hydroxylation structure required for anticoagulant effects of dicoumarol and never associated with clinically significant modification of coagulation parameters. Fermentation (decomposition) is the only natural method whereby coumarin can become transformed into a congener of dicoumarol, and red clover extracts are not made from composted crude herb.

Simple coumarins are widespread constituents of numerous vegetable roots, such as carrots, parsnips, and celery.[17]

The 17 citations for this monograph are located under Red Clover on the CD at the back of the book.

Reishi

Botanical Name: *Ganoderma lucidum* (W. Curtis.: Fr.) P. Karst.
Pharmacopoeial Name: Fructus ganodermi.
Synonym: *Boletus lucidus* Fr.
Common Names: Reishi, reishi mushroom, red reishi; Ling Zhi. (*Ganoderma japonicum* = black reishi; *Ganoderma applanatum* = artist's conk).

Summary

Drug/Class Interaction Type	Mechanism and Significance	Management
Acyclovir, cefazolin Antimicrobials Antivirals ⊕	Synergistic effects (greater than additive) have been observed with antimicrobial and antiviral combinations. Significance not established generally.	Consider coadministration, especially for immunocompromised patients with chronic viral and microbial infection.
Immunosuppressive, myelosuppressive chemotherapy ⊕/☼	Multifactorial interaction between reishi and chemotherapy; combination may improve therapeutic outcomes. Clinical significance anecdotally established. Related mushroom polysaccharides also effective.	Consider pretreatment, coadministration, and posttreatment with chemotherapy.

HERB DESCRIPTION

Family

Ganodermataceae (Polyporaceae).

Related Species

Ganoderma japonicum (Fr.) Lloyd. (synonym, *G. sinense* Zhao, Xu et Zhang.), *Ganoderma applanatum* (Pers.) Pat, *Ganoderma tsugae* Murrill.

Habitat and Cultivation

A woody shelf-fungus that grows on rotting tree stumps and fallen logs in temperate forests throughout much of North America, most of Europe, South America and Asia, typically affecting oak trees. Reishi is now rare in the wild in China and rarer in Japan but has been under widespread industrial-scale cultivation in China for several years, which constitutes the bulk of commercial reishi supply internationally.

Parts Used

Fruiting body. Spore and mycelium preparations exist but have limited commercial availability; they are not identical to the fruiting body in composition or activity.

Common Forms

Dried whole fruiting body, by decoction (or very finely powdered).
Tincture: Traditionally, rice wine extract.
Standardized Solid Extract: Concentrates available greater than 20:1.

INTERACTIONS REVIEW

Strategic Considerations

Traditional Chinese use of reishi includes stand-alone herb for various conditions (Chinese syndrome-patterns), including heart *(Xin) qi* and lung *(Fei) qi* deficiencies.[1] In modern Western usage, reishi is primarily considered as a safe and virtually nontoxic immunomodulatory agent. It is primarily used in the clinical context of immunocompromise, such as chronic fatigue immune dysfunction syndrome (CFIDS), or as an adjunct in integrative cancer protocols to support patients undergoing myelosuppressive conventional therapies. Pharmacological data suggest four primary areas of activity for reishi extracts: immune enhancing and antitumorigenic, cardiovascular regulatory, hypoglycemic, and hepatoprotective.[2] Of these, interactions with pharmaceuticals are suggested primarily by the immunomodulatory data.

Support for use of reishi in oncological settings is largely derived from experimental studies on the biological activities of its polysaccharide and triterpene compounds. These have direct antitumor activity mediated by several pathways, notably the inhibition of the key transcription factors nuclear factor-kappa B (NF-κB) and activating protein 1 (AP-1). The indirect anticancer effects are mediated by promotion of mixed-lymphocyte responses, including enhancement of cytotoxic activity of monocyte-macrophages, natural killer (NK) cells, and lymphokine-activated killer (LAK) cells and increased secretion of cytokines such as interleukin-1 (IL-1), IL-6, and interferon gamma (IFN-γ).[3-5] Protection against myelosuppression from chemotherapeutic agents and radiation therapy has moderate experimental and anecdotal clinical support; however, clinical trials are required to establish the efficacy of reishi for this purpose. Although some sources have cited Chinese-language clinical studies in support of these uses, full translations are unavailable, and evaluation of these trials by these secondary sources is typically schematic.[6]

More substantial clinical data are available for related mushrooms, such as *Coriolus, Polyporus,* and *Lentinus,* and medicinal mushroom polysaccharides, particularly the branched (1→3)-beta-D glucans, are thought to be broadly similar in their general immunomodulatory and anticancer effects.[7,8] Additive interactions with antimicrobial pharmaceutical agents have been reported (see later), but these probably are also indirect results from a general enhancement of cell-mediated immunity and antiviral activity by reishi compounds, rather than specific herb-drug interactions. The long-term use of immunomodulating herbs in patient populations dependent on immunosuppressive therapies (e.g., to prevent graft rejection) is de facto contraindicated, and reishi extracts have been shown to reverse immunosuppressive effects of morphine.[9]

Cardiovascular drug interactions seem unlikely given the mild cardiotonic effects of reishi despite suggestions in secondary literature of possible potentiating interactions with cholesterol-lowering and anticoagulant drugs. These interactions have not been demonstrated or reported, and claims of their likelihood are classified as "speculative" here, along with equally hypothetical suggestion of interactions with hypoglycemic drugs, as discussed later.

Effects on Drug Metabolism and Bioavailability

Pharmacokinetic interactions between reishi and pharmaceutical drugs have not been reported, and studies on the effects of the herb on drug-metabolizing systems have not been conducted to date. Induction of human hepatic glutathione-S-transferase in vitro by reishi polysaccharide has been recorded in one in vitro study.[10] Inhibition of beta-glucuronidase in vitro by the triterpene constituent ganoderenic acid A was demonstrated in vitro, and the same constituent had a potent inhibitory effect against carbon tetrachloride (CCl_4)–induced hepatotoxicity in a rodent model.[11]

The hepatoprotective effects of the herb may counter solvent and other chemical or solvent-induced hepatotoxicity.[12,13] These effects on drug-metabolizing enzymes may contribute, along with the antioxidant effects of the herb, to the established hepatoprotective properties of reishi observed in some studies. From these limited data, the potential theoretically exists for some modulation of clearance of glucuronide prodrugs, as well as accelerated clearance of glutathione and glucuronated drug conjugates. The effects of variation in activity of beta-glucuronidase on drug metabolism have not been systematically studied to date, but it may be a clinically significant determinant of variability of individual response to pharmaceuticals.[14]

HERB-DRUG INTERACTIONS

Antimicrobial and Antiviral Therapies

Evidence: Acyclovir (Zovirax), cefazolin (Ancef, Kefzol).
Extrapolated, based on similar properties: Cephalosporin antibiotics: Aztreonam (Azactam injection), cefaclor (Ceclor), cefadroxil (Duricef), cefamandole (Mandol), cefdinir (Omnicef), cefepime (Maxipime), cefixime (Suprax), cefoperazone (Cefobid), cefotaxime (Claforan), cefotetan (Cefotan), cefoxitin (Mefoxin), cefpodoxime (Vantin), cefprozil (Cefzil), ceftazidime (Ceptaz, Fortaz, Tazicef, Tazidime), ceftibuten (Cedax), ceftizoxime (Cefizox), ceftriaxone (Rocephin), cefuroxime (Ceftin, Kefurox, Zinacef), cephalexin (Keflex, Keftab), cephapirin (Cefadyl), cephradine (Anspor, Velocef), imipenem combination drug: imipenem and cilastatin (Primaxin I.M., Primaxin I.V.); loracarbef (Lorabid), meropenem (Merrem I.V.); possibly many other antimicrobial and antiviral agents.
Similar properties but evidence lacking for extrapolation: Nucleoside (analog) reverse-transcriptase inhibitors (NRTIs or NNRTIs): Abacavir (Ziagen), didanosine (ddI, dideoxyinosine; Videx); dideoxycytidine (ddC, zalcitabine; Hivid), lamivudine (3TC, Epivir), stavudine (D4T; Zerit), tenofovir (Viread), zidovudine (azidothymidine, AZT, ZDV,

zidothymidine; Retrovir); combination drugs: zidovudine and lamivudine (Combivir); abacavir, lamivudine and zidovudine (Trizivir).
Similar properties but evidence indicating no or reduced interaction effects: Vidarabine (Ara-A, arabinoside; Vira-A).

Interaction Type and Significance

⊕ **Potential or Theoretical Beneficial or Supportive Interaction, with Professional Management**

Probability:
4. Plausible

Evidence Base:
○ **Preliminary**

Effect and Mechanism of Action

Synergy between reishi extracts or polysaccharides with acyclovir and cefazolin have been demonstrated in vitro. These effects are greater than linear additive effects but may be augmented in vivo by general enhancement of T helper cell type 1 (Th1) immune responses by reishi. The clinical significance of the interaction or general applicability to other antimicrobial or antiviral agents has not been established.

Research

An in vitro study measured the minimum inhibitory concentration (MIC) of an aqueous extract of Ganoderma alone and in combination with several antibiotics (ampicillin, cefazolin, oxytetracycline, chloramphenicol) against a variety of gram-negative and gram-positive bacteria. In combination with cefazolin against *Klebsiella oxytoca* and *Bacillus subtilis*, synergistic versus linear additive reductions in MIC were observed.[15] Oh et al.[16] used an in vitro model of human herpes simplex virus type 1 (HSV-1) and type 2 (HSV-2) in culture and examined the effects of acyclovir and vidarabine nucleoside agents, alone and in combination, on viral plaque size with an acidic protein-bound polysaccharide extract of reishi. They found a synergistic antiviral effect with acyclovir and reishi extract against both types. With vidarabine, however, there was an antagonistic effect against HSV-2 but a synergistic effect against HSV-1, suggesting that results may not generally be applicable to other nucleoside antivirals or specific viruses. Several reishi triterpene compounds have also been found to exhibit anti–human immunodeficiency virus (HIV) activity in one in vitro study.[17]

Clinical Implications and Integrative Therapeutics

Reishi extracts alone have in vitro antiviral effects against both HSV-1 and HSV-2.[18,19] The antiviral effects mechanism is not thought to directly involve cytokine such as IFN, but rather an interaction between reishi polysaccharides and the HSV glycoproteins involved in binding to host cell membranes.[19] In addition, reishi polysaccharides enhance Th1 immunity, including the promotion of Th1 cytokines such as IFN-γ and IL-12, as well as NK cell activity.[20-22] Clinically, the experimental data suggest that herpetic viral conditions may benefit from reishi coadministered with acyclovir, but extrapolations to other antivirals or other viral infections cannot reliably be made. However, reishi polysaccharides enhance cell-mediated immunity, tending to induce increased antimicrobial and antiviral aspects of immune responses, and can be administered to maintain immunocompetence before or after drug administration. Also, reishi extracts are effective in controlling postherpetic pain.[23]

Antineoplastic Therapies, Including Anthracyclines, Radiotherapy, and Surgery

Evidence: Cyclophosphamide (Cytoxan, Endoxana, Neosar, Procytox), doxorubicin (Adriamycin, Rubex).
Extrapolated, based on similar properties: Daunorubicin (Cerubidine, DaunoXome), epirubicin (Ellence, Pharmorubicin), idarubicin (Idamycin, Zavedos), mitoxantrone (Novantrone, Onkotrone).

Interaction Type and Significance

⊕ **Potential or Theoretical Beneficial or Supportive Interaction, with Professional Management**
☼ **Prevention or Reduction of Drug Adverse Effect**

Probability:	Evidence Base:
4. Plausible	○ Preliminary

Effect and Mechanism of Action

Reishi extracts may protect against immunosuppressive aspects of antineoplastic therapies and improve therapeutic outcomes. Mechanisms are multifactorial and include protection against specific toxicities, reversal of leukopenia, and preservation of cell-mediated immune responses; antioxidant scavenging of free radicals; inherent anticancer activity resulting from inhibition of transcription factors NF-κB, AP-1, and free-radical reactive oxygen species (ROS); and other mechanisms.

Research

Reishi (Ganoderma japonicum) increased white blood cell (WBC) count in 72.5% of 175 leukopenic patients, according to a Chinese study cited by Chen and Chen.[6] A Chinese rodent study of doxorubicin (Adriamycin) toxicity by Hongwei and colleagues, cited in detail by Upton,[2] found that oral pretreatment with reishi extract at 500 mg/kg body weight for 14 days significantly reduced histological parameters of doxorubicin-induced toxicity in cardiac, hepatic, and renal cells, compared with controls receiving doxorubicin alone. An unrelated study demonstrated dose-dependent cardioprotective activity of hot-water reishi extracts against ethanol-induced heart toxicity in rodents through antioxidative protection against lipid peroxidation.[24] This is the established mechanism of anthracycline-induced cardiotoxicity. Lu and Lin[9] demonstrated reversal of B-cell and T-cell response suppression by morphine after administration of a polysaccharide reishi extract to morphine-dependent mice. Animal studies have demonstrated radioprotective effects of reishi in recovering immunocompetence after radiation exposure.[25,26] However, this includes protection against deoxyribonucleic acid (DNA) strand breakage.[27] A murine model showed that oral pretreatment with reishi enabled a significant reduction in cyclophosphamide toxicity in terms of preventing leukopenia. An in vitro study found that reishi may inhibit the angiogenic vascular endothelial growth factor (VEGF), and theoretically, angiogenesis inhibition may interfere with postsurgical wound repair.[28]

McKenna et al.[29] reviewed two small human studies from conference reports relating to Ganoderma use in a clinical oncology setting. The first, an open-label trial by Kupin[30] of 48 patients with advanced cancer (renal, gastric, breast), examined the effects of coadministering reishi extracts during chemotherapy and radiation. The WBC levels were normalized in those taking reishi compared with controls, and treatment-induced leukopenia was rapidly ameliorated in the reishi group, who also had greater appetite and higher levels of

general vigor than the controls. Of those patients requiring surgery, the reishi subjects experienced faster recovery and improved wound healing compared with the control group surgical candidates. A smaller study of patients with acute myelogenous leukemia (AML) or nasopharyngeal carcinoma who were pretreated with reishi extracts for 1 week before chemo/radiotherapy, contining the extracts for 3 months after the treatments, reported similar findings in terms of increased efficacy of treatment and reduction of treatment-induced adverse effects.[31]

Clinical Implications and Integrative Therapeutics

The pluripotent anticancer effects of reishi polysaccharides and triterpenes have been subject of extensive experimental study, but to date, clinical trials have not confirmed these in vivo. Evidence for other mushroom beta-glycans is perhaps more compelling, but reasonable rationale appears to exist for combining reishi extracts into protocols designed for therapeutic protection against myelosuppression as a dose-limiting toxicity of chemotherapy. If the antiangiogenic effects of reishi are confirmed, combination with monoclonal antibody drugs targeting VEGF is theoretically a reasonable strategy.

THEORETICAL, SPECULATIVE, AND PRELIMINARY INTERACTIONS RESEARCH, INCLUDING OVERSTATED INTERACTIONS CLAIMS

Anticoagulants, Oral Vitamin K Antagonists

Anisindione (Miradon), dicumarol, ethyl biscoumacetate (Tromexan), nicoumalone (acenocoumarol; Acitrom, Sintrom), phenindione (Dindevan), phenprocoumon (Jarsin, Marcumar), warfarin (Coumadin, Marevan, Warfilone).

Limited experimental data from aggregometry studies suggest that water extracts of reishi have some potential to induce aggregation in vitro, possibly because of an adenosine component in the extracts.[32] The effects may be related to anti-inflammatory properties of reishi acting through a thromboxane A₂ (TXA₂) pathway.[33,34] One small human study showed inhibition of adenosine diphosphate (ADP)–induced aggregation in healthy volunteers, as well as antithrombotic potential (measured by size of extracorporeal thrombi) resulting from oral administration of reishi extracts in atherosclerotic patients. The authors did not speculate on the possible mechanisms of these observed results.[35] This has led to cautions about possible interactions with anticoagulants.[2] However, recent data suggest a lack of effect on hemostatic parameters in healthy volunteers, and adverse interaction with antiplatelet or anticoagulant drugs seems unlikely.[36]

Central Stimulants; Chlorpromazine, Phenobarbital, Reserpine

Amphetamine aspartate monohydrate, amphetamine sulfate, dextroamphetamine saccharate, dextroamphetamine sulfate; D-amphetamine, Dexedrine.
Methylphenidate (Metadate, Methylin, Ritalin, Ritalin-SR; Concerta); combination drug, mixed amphetamines: amphetamine and dextroamphetamine (Adderall; dexamphetamine); chlorpromazine (Largactil, Thorazine); phenobarbital (phenobarbitone; Luminol, Solfoton); reserpine (Harmonyl).

There are limited reports that reishi extracts may exert a partial antagonism to the central stimulant effects of amphetamines as well as potentiation of the sedating effects of reserpine and chlorpromazine and increase phenobarbital-induced sleeping times.[2] Reishi is not known clinically for its sedative effects in Western use, although it is incorporated into formulae for certain patterns of insomnia in Chinese herbal medicine. The limited available data do not suggest a straightforward pharmacological mechanism that enables extrapolation to an interaction at this time.

HMG-CoA Reductase Inhibitors (Statins) and Other Cholesterol-Lowering Drugs

Atorvastatin (Lipitor), fluvastatin (Lescol, Lescol XL), lovastatin (Altocor, Altoprev, Mevacor), combination drug: lovastatin and niacin (Advicor); pravastatin (Pravachol), rosuvastatin (Crestor), simvastatin (Zocor), combination drug: simvastatin and extended-release nicotinic acid (Niaspan).

Recent experimental evidence has confirmed the modern Chinese medical use of reishi extracts for reducing cholesterol levels, although this is not an established use in Western botanical medicine.[37,38] The mode of action is partially through the mevalonate pathway, possibly at the level of 3-hydroxy-3-methylglutaryl (HMG)–coenzyme A (CoA), but is likely multifactorial, with a beta-sitosterol–like effect on cholesterol absorption. These data have been used by secondary sources to suggest an interaction with HMG-CoA reductase inhibitor drugs (statins).[2] Reverse extrapolation from a therapeutic effect to suggest that drugs with the same action may be clinically problematic is not evidence of an interaction. The combination of statins and reishi has not been studied, although Shiao[38] suggests this combination may have an anticancer effect (presumably via farnesyl protein transferase). If used for hypocholesterolemia, the statin-reishi combination would probably have an additive effect on cholesterol levels, but to date an interactive synergy has not been demonstrated.

Insulin and Oral Hypoglycemic Agents

Evidence: Animal-source insulin (Iletin); human analog insulin (Humanlog); human insulin (Humulin, Novolin, NovoRapid, Oralin).

Extrapolated, based on similar properties: Buformin (Andromaco Gliporal, Buformina), chlorpropamide (Diabinese), glimepiride (Amaryl), glipizide (Glucotrol; Glucotrol XL), glyburide (glibenclamide; Diabeta, Glynase, Glynase Prestab, Micronase, Pres Tab), metformin (Dianben, Glucophage, Glucophage XR); combination drugs: glipizide and metformin (Metaglip), glyburide and metformin (Glucovance); phenformin (Debeone, Fenformin), tolazamide (Tolinase), tolbutamide (Orinase, Tol-Tab).

Hypoglycemic effects of reishi triterpenes have been established in animal studies.[39] The effect partly results from reishi-induced increases in insulin secretion and partly from effects on hepatic glucose metabolism.[40,41] An open-label study in eight diabetic patients reported by Teow[31] and reviewed by McKenna[29] apparently found that 1 g reishi extract daily was comparable in effect to the hypoglycemic effect of insulin (100 IU/mL) or oral hypoglycemic agents. Details were not supplied, and additional human trials are unavailable. Corroboration of hypoglycemic effects in vivo by controlled studies is required, together with analysis of the mechanism, before theoretical extrapolations to interactions can be considered more than speculative.

The 41 citations for this monograph are located under Reishi on the CD at the back of the book.

Saw Palmetto

Botanical Name: *Serenoa repens* (W. Bartram) Small.
Pharmacopoeial Name: Fructus serenoae repentis.
Synonyms: *Sabal serrulata* (Michaux) Nuttall ex Schultes.
Common Names: Saw palmetto, sabal.

HERB DESCRIPTION

Family

Arecaceae (Palmae).

Habitat and Cultivation

Native to coastal regions of southeastern United States, especially Florida; also found in the West Indies and parts of Central America, southern Spain, and North Africa.

Parts Used

Berries. Botanically, the fruit is a drupe with single seed; the oily flesh, not the seed, is used; the fruits are often called "berries."

Common Forms

Fresh or dried, whole or ground fruit, including powders or tablets.

Hydroethanolic Tincture and Fluid Extracts: 70% to 95% alcohol.

Lipid/Sterol Extract (LESP): Hexane or supercritical carbon dioxide (CO_2) extraction. LESP may be standardized to "total fatty acid content" between 70% and 95%; however, manufacturers' preparations may vary.[1]

INTERACTIONS REVIEW

Strategic Considerations

Serenoa berries have monographs by the German Commission E[2] and World Health Organization (WHO)[3] and are described in virtually all authoritative literature of Western herbal medicine. In 2002, the *United States Pharmacopeia* (*USP*)[4] reinstated an official monograph on saw palmetto, which had been deleted from editions after 1916. The primary modern use of saw palmetto extracts is for lower urinary tract symptoms (LUTS) related to benign prostatic hyperplasia (BPH). More than 20 clinical trials have now been conducted to examine the efficacy of saw palmetto for BPH and LUTS. Meta-analyses of 19 of these trials have concluded that the extract is effective for these indications.[5] Saw palmetto berries are typically used in combination with root of *Urtica dioica* L. and *Urtica urens* L. (stinging nettles) for mild BPH.[6] *Urtica radix* is indicated in monographs by the European Scientific Cooperative on Phytotherapy (ESCOP)[7] and WHO[8] for conditions of mild prostatic hyperplasia. A clinical trial using a proprietary blended product (Nutrilite) has established a slight increase in effectiveness for LUTS for the blend versus placebo, although studies comparing the combination product directly with single components are not available.[6]

The trial-supported uses of the herb are restricted, in contrast with the original uses of the plant by the indigenous cultures of the southeastern United States, who exploited all parts of the saw palmetto dwarf palm extensively, including as a food for animals and humans, as a fiber source, as well for medical purposes (although the latter are not well documented).[9] Early Western medical uses included as a digestive and respiratory remedy; nutritive to build tissues; reproductive remedy for various male and female conditions, including atrophy of the breasts, dysmenorrhea, irritation, and relaxation of the prostate; aphrodisiac; and sexual vigor and sperm production enhancer.[10,11] Modern herbalists have emphasized its anabolic nutritive properties, and general effects that extend beyond the limited view of the herb as a "BPH remedy" for men.[12]

There are no direct clinical data on interactions between saw palmetto berries and pharmaceutical drugs, nor are any interactions suggested by the major therapeutic monographs on saw palmetto. Because of the widespread use of the herb in benign prostatic hypertrophy (BPH), as well as an ingredient of herbal formulations for prostate cancer, the potential for interaction with coadministered drugs such as anti-androgens is considerable. These two clinical settings are briefly discussed here.

For mild BPH, a trial course of saw palmetto (in combination with related botanicals) may be used prior to considering drug therapy to examine whether symptoms can be controlled by herbal medication alone. If the lower urinary tract symptoms (LUTS) are refractory to botanical protocols, 5-alpha-reductase (5-AR; 5-α-reductase) inhibition drug therapy (Avodart, Proscar) might be initiated, but combination herb-drug treatments have not been demonstrated to be additive and are unlikely to be beneficial.

In prostate cancer, androgen-deprivation therapy (ADT) is a conventional approach involving one or more endocrine approaches, including luteinizing hormone–releasing hormone (LHRH) agonism (Lupron, Trelstar, Viadur, Zoladex). After causing an initial (several-week) surge in testosterone levels, LHRH agonism subsequently results in castrate levels of testosterone as long as the agent is continued. Alternately, ADT includes LHRH antagonism (Abarelix, Centrilex), antiandrogenics (Androcur, Casodex, Eulexin, Nilandron), and 5-AR inhibition (Avodart, Proscar). *Serenoa* has been anecdotally incorporated into adjunctive botanical protocols combined with ADT because the herb exhibits antiproliferative effects, such as cyclooxygenase-2 (COX-2) inhibition, as well as inhibition of insulin-like growth factor-1 (IGF-1)–mediated kinase activation that are not dependent on its antiandrogenic effects[13,14] (see PC-SPES).

Effects on Drug Metabolism and Bioavailability

Pharmacokinetic interactions between saw palmetto and prescription drugs resulting from herbal modulation of drug-metabolizing systems have not been reported. Two separate controlled trials using healthy volunteers have examined the effects of saw palmetto administration at 320 mg standardized extract daily on cytochrome P450 3A4 (CYP3A4) and CYP2D6 (14 days' administration)[15] and on CYP1A2, 2D6, 2E1, and 3A4 (28 days' supplementation).[16] Both studies used probe drug methodology to compare preadministration and postadministration pharmacokinetics of the test substrates, and both failed to find significant differences before and after saw palmetto administration compared with controls, suggesting that the herb poses negligible risk for pharmacokinetic interactions. By contrast, an in vitro study using purified recombinant (i.e., nonhuman) CYP3A4, 2D6, and 2C9 examined the effect of a commercial saw palmetto extract on the kinetics of test substrates of these enzymes. The herb was a potent in vitro inhibitor of all three CYPs tested.[17] These researchers did not analyze the content of the saw palmetto product used in the study, and accurate molecular concentration and composition of the material were not established. Conflict between in vitro and in vivo data in this area is not uncommon, but until/unless further data to the contrary become available, saw palmetto is unlikely to exhibit marked pharmacokinetic interactions with pharmaceutical substrates of the principal CYP enzymes.

THEORETICAL, SPECULATIVE, AND PRELIMINARY INTERACTIONS RESEARCH, INCLUDING OVERSTATED INTERACTIONS CLAIMS

Steroidal Sex Hormones

5-Alpha (5-α)-reductase (5-AR) inhibitors: Dutasteride (Avidart, Avodart, Avolve, Duagen, Dutas, Dutagen, Duprost), finasteride (Propecia; Proscar).
Alpha-1(α_1)-adrenoceptor (A1A) antagonists: Doxazosin (Cardura), prazosin (Minipress), tamsulosin (Flomax, Flomaxtra), terazosin (Hytrin).

Various secondary sources have proposed interactions between saw palmetto and prescription medications affecting steroidal sex hormones, presumably based on extrapolations from the clinical effects of the herb. However, the precise pharmacological mechanisms by which saw palmetto berries influence the clinical course of lower urinary tract symptoms remain elusive, and plausible mechanisms underlying antiandrogenic effects (e.g., steroid 5-AR inhibition, A1A antagonism), experimentally demonstrated in vitro, have not been corroborated in human studies.[18] As a result, suggestions of interactions between saw palmetto and antiandrogenic pharmaceutical agents, such as the 5-AR inhibitor finasteride (Proscar) or A1A agents such as tamsulosin (Flomax), must be classified as "speculative." In the case of the tamsulosin, the only study that directly compared the effects of tamsulosin alone and in combination with saw palmetto extract (LESP) demonstrated an absence of additive effects for the combination.[19]

Anticoagulants, Oral Vitamin K Antagonists

Anisindione (Miradon), dicumarol, ethyl biscoumacetate (Tromexan), nicoumalone (acenocoumarol; Acitrom, Sintrom), phenindione (Dindevan), phenprocoumon (Jarsin, Marcumar), warfarin (Coumadin, Marevan, Warfilone).

A suggested interaction between anticoagulant drugs and saw palmetto[20] is hypothesized in a case report claiming a possible connection between a patient's undisclosed saw palmetto use and increased intraoperative bleeding time during brain surgery.[21] This report not only fails to identify the saw palmetto product used, but does not record the dose and duration of administration or its temporal association with the adverse event. The suspected cause of the adverse event was not confirmed by rechallenge, and alternative explanations (e.g., undisclosed or forgotten aspirin or NSAID use) were not discounted; thus the report does not meet minimal criteria to substantiate an association between the adverse bleeding and saw palmetto consumption. To extrapolate this further to an interaction between saw palmetto and anticoagulant therapy is unwarranted, as confirmed by the widespread use

of saw palmetto extracts, which has not yet revealed any pattern of adverse effects related to platelet dysfunction or bleeding. Another vascular adverse event was a single cerebral hemorrhage in the verum group during one clinical trial of Permixon (a hexane liposterolic extract standardized to 90% free fatty acids) for BPH, which the investigators considered not to be attributable to saw palmetto.[22]

At this time, given the absence of validated reports in the literature, the suggestion of possible interactions between anticoagulant agents and saw palmetto can be considered at best to be speculative.

Related Issue

PC-SPES

PC-SPES

A combination preparation of eight herbs including saw palmetto (PC-SPES) used in several clinical trials for prostate cancer was associated with reduction in prostate-specific antigen (PSA) in several trials for both androgen-independent and androgen-dependent prostate cancer.[23-26] The herbs in the formula were *Ganoderma lucidum* (Leyes.ex Fr) P.Karst, *Scutellaria baicalensis* Georgi., *Rabdosia rubescens*, *Isatis tinctoria* L., *Panax notoginseng* Burk., *Dendranthema morifolium* Tzvel., and *Glycyrrhiza uralensis* Fisch. The saw palmetto content (< 10%) was less than any other ingredient of the mixture. The product was manufactured in China and distributed by BotanicLab of California.

Sold as a dietary supplement, PC-SPES became popular but controversial because its mechanism, although partly estrogenic, was unclear. Adverse effects after long-term administration of PC-SPES included reports of gynecomastia, mastalgia, and decreased libido, as well as transient gastrointestinal symptoms (diarrhea, dyspepsia). Deep vein thrombosis, stroke, and pulmonary embolism were reported in patients with advanced prostate cancer while taking the preparation. Such patients are at increased risk for abnormal thrombus formation and its sequelae, and no studies were done to determine whether frequency of these effects was increased by use of PC-SPES. Several of the herbal ingredients of PC-SPES, as well as unlisted ingredients and contaminants, may have contributed to its toxicity. Small amounts of warfarin, indomethacin, diethylstilbestrol (DES), and ethinyl estradiol were found in some samples after testing by the California Department of Health Services using mass spectrometry with chromatographic techniques.[27] In February 2002, BotanicLab voluntarily withdrew PC-SPES from the market, and the product is no longer available. After several other BotanicLab products tested positively for contamination with pharmaceuticals, the company ceased trading in June 2002.

Despite this, PC-SPES still poses a complex challenge, and several issues remain. Most of the ingredients were imported from China, where combining pharmaceutical and herbal ingredients into a product is "integrative" practice. The pharmacodynamic mechanism of the formula cannot be reduced to any single component ingredient or entirely attributed to contamination with estrogenic compounds. An in vitro study on lymph node carcinoma of prostate (LNCaP) cells comparing PC-SPES with DES showed that DES could not account for the different antiproliferative actions of PC-SPES.[28] A randomized clinical trial initiated by urologic oncologist Eric Small and associates at the University of California–San Francisco (UCSF) compared treatment of patients with metastatic androgen-independent prostate cancer with PC-SPES to DES. The trial was halted on discovery of the pharmaceuticals in PC-SPES; up to that point, however, the results suggested superior activity of PC-SPES over DES. Small et al.[23] had already published preliminary positive trial results with the extract in 2000.

The herbal combination of ingredients in PC-SPES, without pharmaceutical adulterants, still could be a synergistic mixture with in vivo activity against prostate cancer. Arguably, the combination of the herbs with estrogenic compounds, nonsteroidal anti-inflammatory drugs (NSAIDs; e.g., indomethacin), and warfarin may have increased effectiveness of the formula. In turn, this suggests a theoretically beneficial interaction between the herbal formula and these pharmaceuticals in prostate cancer, although it appears unlikely that this proposition will be investigated in the near future.

The 28 citations for this monograph are located under Saw Palmetto on the CD at the back of the book.

St. John's Wort

Botanical Name: *Hypericum perforatum* L.
Pharmacopoeial Name: Hyperici herba.
Common Names: St. John's wort, Klamath weed (historic: Fuga daemonum, herba solus).

Summary

Drug/Class Interaction Type	Mechanism and Significance	Management
Alprazolam Triazolobenzodiazepines ◇ ◇	Drug is 3A4 substrate. St. John's wort (SJW) lowers bioavailability by inducing 3A4 enzyme production. Interaction proved experimentally; no clinical reports. May be significant for intravenous midazolam preoperatively.	Coadministration usually contraindicated. Avoid.
Amitriptyline Tertiary tricyclic antidepressants ◇ ◇ ◇	Drug 3A4/P-glycoprotein (P-gp) cosubstrate. Herb lowers bioavailability. Interaction proved experimentally; no clinical reports.	Coadministration usually contraindicated. Avoid.
Anesthesia, general ✗/?	Potential pharmacokinetic and pharmacodynamic interactions with premedications and anesthetics. Reports scarce.	Cessation SJW 1 to 2 weeks before procedure suggested. Disclosure essential.
Antiretrovirals Indinavir, nevirapine Protease inhibitors NNRTIs ✗ ✗/✗ ✗ ✗/◇ ◇	Most antiretroviral agents are 3A4/P-gp cosubstrates. Decreased bioavailability demonstrated. No clinical reports.	Generally avoid. Coadministration requires specialist supervision and monitoring of drug levels.
Cyclosporine Immunosuppressive agents ✗ ✗ ✗/◇ ◇ ◇	Cyclosporine A is cosubstrate of 3A4/P-gp. Decreased bioavailability demonstrated. Numerous serious reports of graft rejection.	Avoid.
Digoxin Cardiac glycosides ✗ ✗/◇ ◇	Drug is P-gp substrate. Possible biphasic response, short-term increase, long-term decrease in bioavailability. Isolated report of bigeminy, short term.	If coadministered, ramp/taper the addition/cessation of herb, and monitor drug levels with vigilance during transition.
Etoposide Topoisomerase II inhibitors ✗ ✗/◇ ◇/?	Possible combination pharmacokinetic and pharmacodynamic interaction, decreased availability (drug is 3A4 substrate), and interference with therapeutic action by hypericin, blocking topo II inhibition.	Avoid.
Fexofenadine Histamine H1-receptor antagonist antihistamine ✗/◇	Drug is P-gp substrate. Decreased bioavailability demonstrated. No clinical reports; minimal significance.	Unlikely to cause problems.
Imatinib Tyrosine kinase inhibitors ◇ ◇ ◇	Gleevec is 3A4 substrate; decreased drug bioavailability demonstrated. Possible compromise to targeted anticancer therapy. No case reports.	Avoid.
Irinotecan Camptothecin analogs ✗/◇ ◇ ◇	Variable pharmacokinetic interaction probable. Significance unknown. Camptothecin-11 responses subject to high inherent variability.	Avoid.
Omeprazole Benzimidazole Proton pump inhibitors ✗/◇ ◇	Prilosec is 3A4/2C19 substrate; SJW reduces bioavailability, as experimentally demonstrated. No clinical reports, although large size of effect may be clinically significant.	Avoid, or monitor and increase dose drug.
Oral contraceptives (OCs) ✗/◇ ◇	Steroids hormones are 3A4 substrates. SJW increases breakthrough bleeding, may reduce OC compliance. OC failure not established despite theoretical risk.	Avoid, or adopt barrier methods during coadministration.
Paclitaxel, docetaxel Taxanes ?/◇ ◇ ◇	Theoretically, induction of CYP3A4 and P-gp could influence drug disposition. Significance not established. Drug mostly eliminated via CYP2C8.	Avoid.
Paroxetine, trazodone SSRI and SSRI/SNRI antidepressants ?	Herb may lead to varying combined pharmacokinetic and pharmacodynamic interactions, at least with some SSRI/NSRI drugs. Mild symptoms of serotonergic excess possible. Several reports of varying reliability. Significance not established.	Avoid, except with professional monitoring during drug taper.
Simvastatin HMG-CoA reductase inhibitors (statins) ◇	Some older statins are cosubstrates of 3A4/P-gp. Minimal significance; no reports available.	Consider newer statins if coadministration indicated.
Tacrolimus ✗ ✗ ✗/◇ ◇ ◇	Cyclosporine A is a cosubstrate of 3A4/P-gp. Experimental evidence that tacrolimus is also 3A4 substrate, but no interactions reports for tacrolimus.	Avoid.
Verapamil Calcium channel blockers ✗/◇ ◇	Verapamil (and all calcium channel blockers) are 3A4 substrates. SJW induces intestinal 3A4 and increases drug clearance. No reports. Interaction significance not established.	Monitored coadministration unlikely to be problematic.

Summary

Drug/Class Interaction Type	Mechanism and Significance	Management
Voriconazole Triazole antifungals X/◇ ◇	Drug is 3A4/2C19/2C9 substrate. SJW reduces bioavailability, as experimentally demonstrated. No clinical reports, although large size of effect may be clinically significant.	Avoid.
Warfarin, Phenprocoumon Oral vitamin K antagonist anticoagulants X X	Mechanism not established. Possible pharmacokinetic effect; may lead to reduced INR. Significance minimal to moderate. Reliable clinical reports or trials unavailable.	Unlikely to cause problems. If coadministered, monitor INR once or twice weekly, and titrate anticoagulant dosage when starting or stopping SJW therapy, until INR stable.

NNRTIs, Nonnucleoside reverse-transcriptase inhibitors; *SSRI*, selective serotonin reuptake inhibitor; *SNRI*, serotonin-norepinephrine reuptake inhibitor; *HMG-CoA*, 3-hydroxy-3-methylglutaryl–coenzyme A; *INR*, international normalized ratio.

HERB DESCRIPTION

Family

Clusiaceae (Guttiferae, Hypericaceae).

Habitat and Cultivation

Perennial; native in Europe Asia and North Africa; naturalized in the United States and considered a noxious weed in many areas; widespread in temperate zones, favoring disturbed ground.

Parts Used

Flowering tops.

Common Forms

Dried Plant: Flowering tops.
Tincture: 60% ethanol, 1:2 to 1:5 weight/volume.
Standardized Extract: 0.3% hypericin, 2.0% to 4.5% hyperforin.
Infused Oil: Fresh flowers, for external use.

HERB IN CLINICAL PRACTICE

Overview

A well-documented botanical medicine since Greco-Roman times, St. John's wort (SJW) has a long history of folk and traditional use as a *vulnerary* ("wound healer") and for banishing mental afflictions, particularly melancholy. For example, Gerard[1] (1633) described its use as a balm for wounds, burns, ulcers, and bites as being without equal. The oil made from the macerated flowers was listed in the first *Pharmacopoeia Londinensis* (1618). *Hypericum perforatum* was proved and introduced into the homeopathic materia medica by Muller in the mid-1800s and has been included in the *Homeopathic Pharmacopoeia of the United States* since that era, with primary indications focusing on nerve pain and traumatic injuries (e.g., concussion, coccygeal impact, sequelae).

More recently, clinical trial evidence accumulated through the 1980s and 1990s established the efficacy and safety of standardized SJW extracts for treating mild to moderate depression, and the "natural antidepressant" label propelled the herb to second-best-selling supplement in the United States by the late 1990s. In 2000, reports of serious interactions with prescription drugs began to appear, and the resulting adverse publicity caused sales of the herb to fall significantly, although SJW remains one of the top-selling U.S. botanicals. It was approved by the German Commission E for "depressive moods" (internally) and "contused injuries" (externally) in 1984.[2] The pharmacology and clinical effects of the herb are currently the focus of considerable research interest and, because of rapid accumulation of data, relatively recent literature reviews (e.g., 1997 *American Herbal Pharmacopoeia* monograph) are in some respects dated.[3] More recent reviews of the extensive literature include the 2003 European Scientific Cooperative on Phytotherapy (ESCOP) monograph[4] and a comprehensive monograph by McKenna et al.[5]

Historical/Ethnomedicine Precedent

Traditionally, SJW was used as a calming herb for symptoms of nervous tension, including anxiety and insomnia, as well as a restorative for melancholic conditions that might currently be diagnosed as depression. Folk use attributed the herb with properties of protection against enchantments, including demonic possession, and it was used for warding off evil spirits. *Hypericum* was characterized as "hot and dry" in the Galenic humoral system of medicine and has classically been associated with the liver and spleen, as well as the Sun. Historically considered a "woundwort," SJW is still used both internally and externally for pain relief, particularly neuralgic pain, shingles, mild contusions, and burns to the skin. For external use, the fresh flowers, traditionally harvested on St. John's Day (immediately following Summer Solstice), are the basis of a macerated oil, which is usually red (by the dianthrone hypericin). This red color was considered an indication of its vulnerary nature (likened to blood) by the Doctrine of Signatures. Before the modern clinical trial–driven indications of the herb for "mild to moderate depression," the nervous system indications were less clearly defined and included "psychovegetative" disorders, as well as such conditions as nocturnal enuresis and night terrors. Its psychological effects were considered much less pronounced than those of prescription medications; Weiss[6] classified the herb as a "mild (i.e., gentle) psychotropic" agent.

Known or Potential Therapeutic Uses

Analgesic, antiviral, anti-inflammatory, anxiety, coccygeal impact, concussion depression (mild to moderate), hepatoprotection, herpes simplex infection (orofacial and genital), herpes zoster (shingles and postherpetic neuralgia), menopause-related psychological symptoms, psychosomatic and somatiform disorders (mild), nervousness, neuralgia, nocturnal enuresis, photodynamic antitumor activity, premenstrual syndrome, restlessness, sacral irritation and spinal injuries, sciatica, seasonal affective disorder, tissue healing and wound repair.

Key Constituents

Characteristic napthodianthrones, including hypericin; phloroglucinols, including hyperforin and adhyperforin.
Flavonoids, including proanthocyanidin polymers of catechin and epicatechin; flavonols; phenylpropanoids; essential oil; amino acids; xanthones.

Therapeutic Dosing Range

Dried Plant: 2 to 5 g/day.
Tincture and Fluid Extract: As 1:1 equivalents, 1 to 3 mL/day.
Standardized Extracts: 900 mg/day in divided doses.
Topical: *Oleum hyperici*, oily macerate from fresh flowering tops (applied as needed).
Also used in ultradilute succussed preparations based on homeopathic indications.

INTERACTIONS REVIEW
Strategic Considerations/Background

Although an old medicine, SJW has a pivotal place in the relatively recent field of herb-drug interactions. The publication of convincing reports of interactions between SJW and digoxin[7] in 1999 and cyclosporine[8] and indinavir[9] in 2000 was seminal, initiating a widespread reevaluation of the safety of this popular herb, previously considered to be benign, in the context of conventional medications.[10] It also propelled the issue of potential interactions between botanicals and pharmaceuticals into media prominence and research focus. The subsequent years have seen increased understanding of the pharmacology of SJW, and the herb is now known to be associated with a number of clinically significant pharmacokinetic interactions, as suggested by the original reports. These interactions are mediated by its effects on several key components of drug metabolism, including the cytochrome P450 (CYP450) mixed-oxidase system, various conjugases and transferases, as well as the transporter proteins that modulate drug efflux across intestinal, renal, and biliary epithelia. These systems compose what are now often referred to as phases (or stages) I, II, and III of drug metabolism/detoxification.

The initial reports of SJW interactions with narrow-therapeutic-range drugs prompted sweeping warnings in professional and consumer media about the dangers of SJW herb-drug interactions (and often of herb-drug interactions in general). At the time, however, the actual number of reports of documented SJW-related drug interactions was, and in fact remains, relatively small, with data of widely varying reliability. Surveying the available cases in 2001, Fugh-Berman and Ernst[11] found 54 published reports claiming SJW interactions. Of these, 29 were rejected as unclassifiable, and the remaining 25 were evaluated for reliability according to the authors' "reliability rating score" system. Of these, 12 were classified as "unreliable," 11 as "possible," and only two as "likely." More recently, Meyer et al.[12] analyzed six documented potential herb-drug interactions, including SJW-cyclosporine and SJW-digoxin, across a wide range of "tertiary sources" and found high variability in the reporting of the data, with only three sources even mentioning all six known interactions. Interestingly, as recently reviewed by Izzo,[13] clinical reports of SJW-drug interactions seem to be decreasing rather than increasing in frequency.

Mills et al.[14] recently conducted a systematic review of trials investigating SJW pharmacokinetic interactions with conventional drugs. The authors found the methodological quality of the studies was limited; in particular lacking accepted controls such as correct randomization, observance of established blinding procedures, and allowance for time-dependent effects. They also found that only 15 of the 22 available studies assayed the SJW content of the preparations used, and that varied dosing regimens and duration of exposure to the herb were common, without presenting a rationale for the tested dosing patterns. These limitations mean that most trials on SJW interactions do not appear to conform to the U.S. Food and Drug Administration (FDA)–recommended standards for safeguards against bias in pharmacokinetic trials.[15] This in turn results in questions about the interpretation and applicability of the available data that can only be resolved by more and better-designed studies, as well as consistent application of necessary standards in pharmacovigilance.

Official and regulatory reaction was also triggered by the initial SJW interaction reports. In 2000 the U.K. Committee on Safety of Medicines (CSM)[16] issued a general advisory letter on SJW interactions to all physicians and pharmacists. This included a fact sheet listing medications for which SJW might interact and advised patients to "stop taking St John's Wort," while warning against immediate discontinuation in the event that drug levels might rise, causing serious adverse effects. Lists of drugs that might interact with SJW, causing "serious adverse interactions," were provided, including selective serotonin reuptake inhibitors (SSRIs), anticonvulsants, and triptans. In 2001 the Irish Medical Board (IMB)[17] restricted SJW to physician prescription only, effectively removing the herb (along with ginkgo and several others) from general public access, citing the monoamine oxidase inhibitor (MAOI) activity of SJW as potentially interacting with tyramine foods and potentiating MAOI drugs, as well as claiming SJW caused phototoxicity and other (unspecified) adverse effects. The FDA issued an advisory to health care professionals warning about the SJW-indinavir interaction in 2000, also suggesting physicians alert patients about potential drug interactions involving "any drug metabolized via the cytochrome P450 pathway."[18]

Effects on Drug Metabolism and Bioavailability
Cytochrome P450

The complete spectrum of induction and inhibition effects of SJW on the CYP450 system in vivo in humans is not yet fully characterized. Possibly because of a number of differing investigative methodologies, as well as differences between the various types of extracts used, the available studies are inconclusive. In vitro evidence exists for *inhibition* effects by crude SJW extracts, its flavonoid components, and hypericin and hyperforin on CYP450 1A2, 2C9, 2C19, 2D6, and 3A4.[19,20] In vivo studies using single probe drugs that are specific CYP substrates have found *induction* effects by SJW on 3A4,[21] and with multiprobe drug "cocktails," for 3A4, 2E1, 1A2, and 2D6[22] and 2C19.[23] By contrast, no significant effects on 2D6 and 3A4 were found by two other groups,[24,25] and a further probe cocktail study found no effect on 1A2, 2C9, or 2D6.[26] More recent studies have confirmed in vivo coordinate induction effects by SJW on hepatic and intestinal 3A4 and P-glycoprotein (P-gp).[27,28]

Summarizing the data available at this time, SJW definitely induces human 3A4; probably induces 1A2, 2C19, and 2E1; and probably does *not* significantly affect 2C9 or 2D6. It also induces P-gp and possibly other, related transporters. There is a degree of tissue specificity, with induction of both hepatic and intestinal 3A4, as well as a possible biphasic effect, at least on 3A4 and P-gp, with short-term *inhibition* followed by an *increasing induction* of enzymes over 7 to 10 days. However, evidence from isolated constituent studies suggests that hyperforin plays the main role in induction activity.[23,29-34] The initial inhibition may be caused by hypericin, but also by flavonoid constituents; a number of flavonoids are known to inhibit 3A4, with those from grapefruit and other citrus-derived flavonoids being the best-known examples.[35,36] This "biphasic" effect of a short-term enzyme inhibition succeeded by longer-term induction has recently been demonstrated in a clinical study of voriconazole pharmacokinetics. This open-label study with 16 healthy male volunteers determined that that SJW coadministration with voriconazole (a substrate of CYP2C19) led to a short-term but clinically insignificant increase in the area under curve (AUC) of 22%, and after 15 days, AUC was reduced by 59% compared with controls.[37,38]

Pregnane X Receptor

The recent finding that hyperforin, an active phloroglucinol constituent compound of SJW, acts as a high-affinity ligand for the orphan nuclear receptor pregnane X receptor (PXR) is highly significant.[39,40] The PXR and related nuclear receptors, such as the constitutive androstane receptor (CAR) and the retinoid X receptor (RXR), have been described as "promiscuous" because of the unprecedented structural diversity of compounds that interact with their ligand-binding domain (LBD).[41-43] Activation of the PXR leads to upregulation of genes controlling multiple aspects of xenobiotic metabolism, including phase I (CYP450 1A1, 1A2, 2B6, 2C9, and 3A4) mixed oxidases, phase II conjugases (uridine diphosphate [UDP] glucuronosyltransferases, glutathione-S-transferases, sulfonyltransferases), and phase III drug transporters (MDR1/P-gp, MDR2, organic anion-transporting polypeptides [OATPs]).*

The implication is that the PXR and related nuclear receptors may effectively act to coordinate xenobiotic detoxification.[41-43,52-56] The PXR itself is subject to a degree of genetically determined polymorphism, the importance of which remains to be clarified, but pronounced interspecies differences are known to exist in activator compounds, with marked differences among rodent, rabbit, and human ligands.[41,57,58] Pascussi et al.[59] have aptly described expression of the genes controlling xenobiotic metabolism as a "tangle of networks of nuclear and steroid receptors, where receptors share partners, ligands, DNA response elements and target genes and where the different pathways exhibit cross-talk at several levels."

A broader view of SJW emerges from these recent developments. The herb can be conceptualized as a master inducer of detoxification, or more accurately as a *xenosensory activator,* capable of triggering the complex adaptive system evolved to metabolically eliminate toxic compounds, both endogenous and xenobiotic.[60,61] The downstream consequences of PXR activation on drug metabolism suggest that, to some extent, SJW interactions may be predicted (and thus managed) on the basis of whether a given coadministered drug is a substrate of the enzymes or transporters induced by PXR activation, particularly 3A4 and P-gp.[55,62]

P-Glycoprotein

Induction of P-gp by SJW further complicates the picture and may confound attempts to predict interactions. P-glycoprotein is a membrane-associated, adenosine triphosphate (ATP)–dependent "pumping" protein that ejects foreign or toxic compounds from cells and mediates "multidrug resistance" when induced in cancer cells. Durr et al.[28] estimated the induction of intestinal P-gp by SJW at a 1.5-fold increase in healthy human volunteers. Ernst[63] noted drugs that are dual substrates of both P-gp and CYP3A4 likely present an increased risk of pharmacokinetic interaction as a result of

*References 19, 26, 29, 30, 32, 33, 44-51.

co-induction by SJW. However, the relative contributions of P-gp and 3A4 to drug efflux appear to be complex and differ for different agents that are dual substrates.[64]

The existence of several polymorphisms in P-gp phenotypes affects normal levels of expression of both hepatic and intestinal P-gp. These polymorphisms are known to exhibit variation with racial and gender characteristics.[65,66] As with P450 enzymes, dietary food ingredients may also affect P-gp expression; known examples include piperine from black pepper and some citrus flavonoids.[67,68] Alpha-tocopherol can also influence P-gp, probably through PXR activation.[52] Finally, the role of non–P-gp drug transporters, such as the OATP family, has recently emerged as another potential mechanism in controlling drug bioavailability, although modulating influences on OATP expression are not currently well characterized.

Overall, the interplay between CYP3A4 and P-gp (and other transporters) is not well understood, but this "drug-efflux metabolism alliance," as aptly named by Benet and Cummins,[69] remains of a crucial research area for future elucidation of drug interactions.[70,71]

Managing Pharmacokinetic Interactions

Numerous pharmaceuticals are metabolized by CYP3A4, which is a low-affinity, high-throughput P450 enzyme expressed primarily in the small intestinal mucosa and liver. This has led to suggestions that SJW may interact with more than 50% of all known drugs. Indeed, evidence is now rapidly accumulating from preclinical screening studies that confirms SJW induction effects on a range of drugs, particularly 3A4 substrates, often in the absence of any clinical interactions data. However, the magnitude of SJW induction effects is considerably less than that of other known PXR ligands, the best-known example being rifampin, a mainstay of conventional tuberculosis therapy. Rifampin is a coordinate inducer of P-gp and 3A4 with an induction effect on midazolam (a 3A4-specific substrate) that is 25 times that of SJW.[72] Red wine has similar order-of-magnitude effects as SJW on oral clearance of cyclosporine (a dual substrate).[73]

Theoretical predictions should be confirmed by clinical data before an interaction can be assumed inevitable. For example, carbamazepine is a well-known substrate and inducer of 3A4. When SJW was given for 14 days to patients previously stabilized on carbamazepine, no effect of SJW on carbamazepine kinetics or drug levels was observed.[74] This suggests that close attention must be paid to the precise metabolic pathways involved for each specific drug and to the associated effects on induction or inhibition of P450, enzymes, transferases, and transporters. Unfortunately, older drugs were not always well characterized by their manufacturers in terms of their interaction with the P450 metabolizing enzymes, leading to obvious problems for prediction and management of metabolic interactions.

Proposed coadministration should also consider different temporal patterns of combining herb and pharmaceutical agents. Three alternative scenarios are possible. First, adding an inducer (SJW) to a substrate (drug) will induce a lowering of previously stable drug levels over 1 to 2 weeks through increased drug metabolism, risking consequent loss of therapeutic efficacy. Moreover, in the case of SJW, initial inhibition may complicate this pattern, creating an apparent biphasic effect. Second, if the substrate (drug) is added to inducer (SJW), standard drug-dosing levels may be inadequate and may result in failure of therapy. Notably, this would not apply to drugs whose level is established by monitoring and titration to a therapeutic endpoint (e.g., coumarin/INR value). Third, *withdrawal* of an inducer (SJW) from a regimen of previously stable coadministration with a substrate drug will reverse induction and possibly cause rebound toxicity from elevated drug levels. Theoretically, this series of patterns would be "reversed" if the drug concerned was a prodrug, depending on activation for the metabolic transformation by the CYP450 induced. Armstrong et al.[75] well describe this schema of possible pharmacokinetic interaction patterns among inducers, inhibitors, and substrates of CYP450 drug-metabolizing enzymes.

In summary, if appropriate data about metabolic pathways of a drug are available, the pharmacokinetics of any drug proposed for coadministration with SJW should be reviewed before prescription and, wherever possible, drugs metabolized by multiple routes selected. If this is not possible, and if compelling reasons exist for coadministration of the herb with the drug, precautionary measures should be adopted; this is mandatory for any drug with narrow therapeutic indices. Introduction or cessation of SJW should be ramped or tapered, respectively, and serum levels of the pharmaceutical need to be monitored to titrate drug levels and thus counter increased clearance rates. When factors such as financial cost or intermediate metabolite toxicity militate against compensatory increases in drug doses, avoidance of coadministration is the optimum management solution.

The literature on SJW interactions continues to expand, with persistent calls in secondary sources for large-scale in vitro screening of herbs to establish the "risk" of potential (pharmacokinetic) interactions with drugs. These calls ignore that drug disposition is unpredictably mediated by a wide variety of dietary[62] compounds, foods, herbs, beverages, and lifestyle products and also affected by a wide range of individual variables, from genomics through biological, lifestyle, and socioeconomic factors, all of which render meaningful screening virtually impossible.

One study analyzing responses of six different ethnic groups to SJW did not uncover significant differences in induction effects on CYP3A4 and P-gp.[76] However, Gurley et al.[77] examined CYP450 phenotypes in elderly versus younger subjects and found age-related differences in responsiveness to botanical agents regarding CYP3A4 induction, concluding that population vulnerabilities may exist in elders. The results of in vitro tests are often contradictory and may be at odds with clinical reality because of the inherent differences between experimental systems and the in vivo complexities of herbal administration; therefore these tests have limited predictive value. Butterweck et al. pointed out that logically, systematic screening for pharmacokinetic interactions should first be applied to narrow-therapeutic-index drugs.[78,79]

Some argue that understanding and managing variability in drug responses would be better than scaremongering about overstated adverse effects of herbs.[80,81] More recent mainstream papers suggest that the emphasis is beginning to shift in a more constructive direction.[62,82] Equally, the development of "low-hyperforin" extracts of SJW may provide efficacy in antidepressant indications without invoking PXR-mediated downstream effects on drug disposition.[34,83] However, hyperforin confers numerous other properties on SJW whole-plant extracts, including anti-inflammatory, antitumor, and antiangiogenic effects.[84]

Pharmacodynamic Interactions

In addition to pharmacokinetic interactions, pharmacodynamic interactions based on the antidepressant activity of SJW have been widely suggested, principally when combined with the SSRI antidepressants. The evidence for pharmacodynamic interactions is more problematic than that supporting the metabolic interactions, partly related to the general unreliability of SJW case reports, as previously noted.[11,14] Qualitative data sources such as postal surveys of psychiatrists have been used to suggest adverse reports and interactions that in effect are unassessable.[85] Safety and efficacy data from clinical trials of SJW suggest that adverse effects of the herb are an order of magnitude less (1%-3%) than those of pharmaceutical antidepressants.[86] Despite the known interactions issues, SJW remains a first-line treatment for mild to moderate depression in Europe.[87] Significantly, the adverse effect data from clinical trials of the herb suggest a completely different profile of adverse effects than with common antidepressant drugs. This correlates with current understanding of the underlying mechanisms of SJW's observed antidepressant effects. The herb is now believed to work through novel and apparently complex mechanisms, dissimilar to those of known pharmaceutical antidepressants.

Initial research presumed a typical druglike biogenic amine mechanism for SJW, but early in vitro data suggesting MAOI activity have not been substantiated by in vivo studies. Reports of hypertensive MAOI-SJW interactions are lacking, as are reliable reports of interactions between SJW and tyramine-containing food substances[88,89] (see also Theoretical, Speculative, and Preliminary Interactions Research later). Extensive research in vitro and on animals has examined the effects of both full-spectrum SJW extracts and isolated constituents on neurotransmitter uptake for serotonin, dopamine, noradrenaline, gamma-aminobutyric acid (GABA), and L-glutamate.[90-100] The emerging conclusion is that the phloroglucinol-derivative hyperforin acts as a synaptosomal uptake inhibitor for all five of these neurotransmitters. Müller[97] has described this effect as "broad-band" reuptake inhibition. The molecular mechanism of the "pseudo-nonselective reuptake" effect is thought to be related to activation by hyperforin of a sodium ion channel that causes an increase in intracellular sodium content, modifying the sodium gradient that is the common basis of all neuronal neurotransmitter transport proteins.[90,92,99,100]

Although hyperforin appears to be unique in having an approximately equal inhibitory effect on all five neurotransmitters, its effects also are at least an order of magnitude less than that of pharmaceutical antidepressants when quantified in vitro.[97] The improbability of achieving in vivo concentrations of hyperforin from oral SJW consumption that could correspond to effects of synthetic neurotransmitter uptake inhibitors is rarely considered when suggestions of "serotonin syndrome" are made relating to SJW interactions.[89] Serotonin syndrome, first characterized by Sternbach[101] in 1991, was initially described as the result of the adverse interaction of SSRIs with MAOI drugs. The clinical concept of serotonin syndrome has been overused and frequently misapplied in the drug interactions literature.[102] The concept has been reviewed and revised by Radomski et al.,[103] who found a high level of misdiagnosis and distinguished several subsets of the serotonin syndrome based on symptom severity, from transient mild symptoms to fatal toxic states. The latter must also be differentiated from neuroleptic malignant syndrome.[104]

Although hyperforin appears to be the only constituent that can affect uptake of all five neurotransmitters, it cannot be considered responsible for all the observed antidepressant effects of SJW. In some animal behavioral models of depression (e.g., the Porsolt test), hyperforin-free extracts exhibited significant activity, suggesting that other constituents have an effect. Clinical trials with a low-hyperforin extract also demonstrated antidepressant activity against placebo, fluoxetine, and imipramine.[105,106] Furthermore, methodological controversy continues to surround clinical trials comparing SJW with placebo and pharmaceutical antidepressants, particularly because of the well-documented, powerful placebo responses associated with these trials.[107-109]

Despite the absence of definitive understanding of the mechanism of SJW antidepressant activity, caution regarding potential interactions with pharmaceutical antidepressants is more than warranted. Also, several classes of psychiatric drugs are substrates or inhibitors of CYP3A4 and P-gp, suggesting combined pharmacokinetic and pharmacodynamic interactions with SJW. Common agents likely to be encountered in general and psychiatric practice include triazolobenzodiazepines (alprazolam, estazolam, midazolam, triazolam), which are substrates of 3A4, as are the nonbenzodiazepine hypnotics zolpidem and zaleplon and the "atypical" anxiolytic buspirone.

HERB-DRUG INTERACTIONS

Alprazolam, Midazolam, and Related Triazolobenzodiazepines

Evidence: Alprazolam (Xanax), midazolam (Hypnovel, Versed). Extrapolated based on similar properties: Adinazolam (Deracyn), brotizolam (Lendormin), estazolam (ProSom), triazolam (Halcion).

Interaction Type and Significance
◈◈ **Impaired Drug Absorption and Bioavailability, Precautions Appropriate**

Probability:
2. Probable

Evidence Base:
◉ **Emerging**

Effect and Mechanism of Action
Alprazolam, midazolam, and related triazolobenzodiazepines are specific substrates of CYP450 3A4, which is induced by SJW. If the drug is added to SJW, standard dosing levels may be ineffectively low. Conversely, if SJW is added to the drug, plasma levels will be reduced after 7 to 10 days.

Research
Markowitz et al.[110] conducted an open-label preclinical study with 12 healthy volunteers using dextromethorphan and alprazolam probes as markers of CYP2D6 and CYP3A4 activity. Alprazolam was chosen because it is metabolized specifically by 3A4 and is not known to be a cosubstrate of P-gp. The oral preparation of SJW, LI60, was standardized to 0.3% hypericins and administered at 300 mg three times daily for 14 days; the probe was a single oral dose of 2 mg generic alprazolam. The measurements showed a twofold decrease in AUC for alprazolam versus time and shortening of mean half-life to 50% of the baseline. No significant differences were found between baseline and post-SJW maximum plasma levels or time taken to attain them. The kinetics of 2D6, as measured by urinary dextromethorphan, were unaffected by SJW. The study did not distinguish between intestinal mucosa and hepatic 3A4 effects. This result contrasted with an earlier study by the same group in 2000 that failed to demonstrate significant effects of SJW coadministration on alprazolam kinetics; however, the SJW administration period in that trial was only 3 days.[24]

Wang et al.[26] also studied midazolam, using both oral and intravenous doses of the drug before and after 14 days of SJW administration. They found a comparable 50% reduction in oral AUC, corresponding to a twofold clearance increase.

Intravenous bioavailability was reduced 21%, suggesting significant intestinal as well as hepatic 3A4 effects.[26] Considerable interindividual variability in the level of 3A4 induction was noted in this study, and another study found a significant difference between healthy female and male subjects in the level of induction of 3A4 by SJW. This second study used a single time point, "phenotypic ratio" methodology and a drug cocktail probe that included midazolam, after 28 days of SJW administration.[22]

Although they did not find the same gender differences, Dresser et al.[64] established oral and parenteral values for midazolam kinetics after 12 days of pretreatment with SJW in 21 healthy subjects; however, interindividual differences were higher for oral than intravenous route. Their data confirmed the large decreases (55%) in oral bioavailability after SJW pretreatment reported by other investigators.

Clinical Implications and Adaptations
There are no clinical reports of this interaction, which was experimentally established by pharmacokinetic "probe" studies of P450 effects with the drug. Theoretically, the consequences of adding triazolobenzodiazepines to a stable SJW regimen are that normal drug-dosing levels will result in insufficient sedation. Conversely, inhibition rather than induction of 3A4 can cause enhanced effects, such as delirium and excessive sedation; for example, grapefruit juice with midazolam or triazolam.[111] In practice, the interaction is probably of minimal clinical significance. Intravenous midazolam is extensively used in preoperative sedation, and SJW use by elective surgical patients should be checked routinely.

Amitriptyline and Related Tertiary Tricyclic Antidepressants

Evidence: Amitriptyline (Elavil).
Extrapolated, based on similar properties: Amitriptyline combination drug: amitriptyline and perphenazine (Etrafon, Triavil, Triptazine), clomipramine (Anafranil), doxepin (Adapin, Sinequan), imipramine (Janimine, Tofranil), trimipramine (Surmontil).

Interaction Type and Significance
◈◈◈ **Impaired Drug Absorption and Bioavailability, Avoidance Appropriate**

Probability:
3. Possible

Evidence Base:
○ **Preliminary**

Effect and Mechanism of Action
A complex pharmacokinetic interaction occurs between the tertiary tricyclic amitriptyline and its metabolites, including the active secondary tricyclic metabolite nortriptyline, with involvement of P450 and P-gp, resulting in decreased oral bioavailability of the drug.

Research
One preclinical study examined the effect of adding SJW at 900 mg once daily for 14 days to 12 healthy subjects pretreated with 12 days of oral amitriptyline at 75 mg twice daily. The AUC values for amitriptyline were reduced by 22% and for nortriptyline by 41%. The reduction in nortriptyline was evident after only 3 days of SJW administration. Urinary and plasma amounts of amitriptyline and metabolites varied directly with administration of its SJW. The authors suggested a P450 and P-gp mechanism would explain the observed decreases in AUC.[112]

Clinical Implications and Adaptations

There are no clinical reports of this interaction. The metabolism of tricyclic antidepressants (TCAs) is rather complex; amitriptyline is initially hydroxylated by CYP2D6 to nortriptyline, a secondary TCA which is further demethylated by other P450 enzymes before conjugation. However, nortriptyline is also an inhibitor of 2D6, which is a high-affinity, low-capacity enzyme and the rate-limiting step in transformation of TCAs. SJW is not known to affect 2D6. CYP3A4 may play a secondary "backup" role in hydroxylation. Both amitriptyline and nortriptyline are also P-gp substrates, whereas amitriptyline is a P-gp inhibitor. Polymorphisms in 2D6 are well known, and the complexity of the metabolic picture suggests that clinical consequences of coadministration are unpredictable. The conventional drug-drug interactions literature has established the potential seriousness of 2D6 *inhibition* (e.g., by fluoxetine) as a potentially serious interaction with TCAs; however, there is no obvious drug-drug precedent for P-gp/3A4 *induction*-driven interactions with TCAs. Given the unpredictable outcome of coadministration, avoiding this interaction would be a prudent strategy.

Anesthesia, General

Anesthesia, General
Related but evidence lacking for extrapolation: Halogenated inhalational anesthetic agents: Desflurane (Suprane), enflurane (Ethrane), halothane (Fluothane), isoflurane (Forane), sevoflurane (Sevorane, Ultane).

Interaction Type and Significance

✗ Potential or Theoretical Adverse Interaction of Uncertain Severity

? Interaction Likely but Uncertain Occurrence and Unclear Implications

Probability:	Evidence Base:
6. Unknown	☐ Inadequate

Effect and Mechanism of Action

Theoretically, variable pharmacokinetic and interactions with common preoperative and anesthetic agents are possible, depending on the particular agent and individual factors. Central pharmacodynamic effects have also been suggested, based on animal data for sedation times. The incidence, effects, and significance of the potential interactions are unknown.

Research

Evidence for pharmacokinetic interactions with anesthetic agents is mixed, but circumstantially compelling. The CYP3A4 probe midazolam (Versed) is used preoperatively, and its metabolism is significantly affected by SJW. The halogenated anesthetics are metabolized by CYP2E1, which has more recently been demonstrated subject to SJW induction.[22] Pharmacodynamic effects are not established, although an animal study suggested that ethanolic extracts of SJW prolong sleeping time induced by phenobarbital in rats.[113]

Reports

A patient experienced a severe episode of hypotension during a routine surgical procedure and was initially unresponsive to intravenous epinephrine, which the author attributed to SJW after the patient admitted to regular SJW use in the 6 months before the procedure (dose and preparation unspecified). The author suggested that adrenergic modulation by the herb had affected the sympathetic responsiveness to the drug, and that the herb was the only logical "offending agent," having failed to find alternative explanations for the mechanism of circulatory collapse.[114] This speculation does not appear to have any foundation in the known pharmacology of the herb, and attributing causation involves implausible logic. Further investigations in animal models would be appropriate.

Clinical Implications and Adaptations

Disclosure of all herbal and nutrient consumption is accepted as mandatory before elective surgery, the primary objective being to audit for possible disturbances in normal hemostasis induced by herbal medicines and similar agents before the procedure.

Induction effects of SJW on P450 and P-gp may be considered sufficiently complex by some anesthesiologists to mandate patient cessation of SJW before surgery, which would require at least 10 days for complete reversal of enzyme induction. This is arguably a judgment call that could be made on the basis of individual case history and indications for antidepressant therapy, as well as expert knowledge of the pharmacokinetics of the drugs to be used. Exaggeration of possible dangers from herbal consumption may be counterproductive by reinforcing patient reluctance to disclose usage. Pharmacodynamic interactions with central sedation from SJW seem improbable from the known pharmacology of the herb, and any minor effects would be unlikely to present untoward management issues in the context of high-profile inpatient clinical settings such as surgical procedures.

Antiretrovirals: Protease Inhibitors and Nonnucleoside Reverse-Transcriptase Inhibitors

Evidence: Indinavir (Crixivan); nevirapine (Viramune).
Similar properties but evidence lacking for extrapolation:
Protease inhibitors: Amprenavir (Agenerase), atazanavir (Reyataz), brecanavir, darunavir (Prezista), fosamprenavir (Lexiva), nelfinavir (Viracept), ritonavir (Norvir), saquinavir (Fortovase, Invirase), tipranavir (Aptivus); combination drugs: lopinavir and ritonavir (Aluvia, Kaletra), saquinavir and ritonavir (SQV/RTV).
Nonnucleoside reverse-transcriptase inhibitors (NNRTIs): Delavirdine (Rescriptor), efavirenz (Sustiva).

Interaction Type and Significance

✗✗ Minimal to Mild Adverse Interaction—Vigilance Necessary

✗✗✗ Potentially Harmful or Serious Adverse Interaction—Avoid

◇◇ Impaired Drug Absorption and Bioavailability, Precautions Appropriate

Probability:	Evidence Base:
2. Probable	○ Preliminary (although apparently ● Consensus)

Effect and Mechanism of Action

All known protease inhibitors and nonnucleoside reverse-transcriptase inhibitors (NNRTIs) are metabolized by CYP3A4 and are also probable cosubstrates of P-gp. It is established that SJW increases oral clearance of the typical representative of both classes of antiretrovirals (indinavir and nevirapine), although evidence for other drugs in either class is lacking. Theoretically, this may lead to decreased therapeutic efficacy; however, case reports are lacking.

Research

The first study to investigate this interaction remains the most quoted. Piscitelli et al.[9] reported a small, open-label "before and after" trial in 2000, in which eight healthy male volunteers were administered 800 mg oral indinavir for 2 days to establish baseline kinetics of the protease inhibitor. From day 3, participants were given SJW (0.3% hypericin) 300 mg three times daily for 14 days, then another 800 mg oral dose of indinavir was given, for which AUC of the drug decreased by 57% compared to baseline.[9] The authors did not comment on indinavir being both a highly potent inhibitor of 3A4, which it also moderately induces, and an inhibitor of intestinal P-gp.[115,116] These factors suggest that extrapolation from this study to in vivo steady-state coadministration is not possible.

A case-series analysis by de Maat et al.[117] used retrospective nonlinear analysis of variance on a cohort of human immunodeficiency virus (HIV) patients whose serum nevirapine had been checked routinely every 3 months. The authors reviewed five patients who admitted concomitant use of SJW (dose and preparation not specified), with at least one serum reading reflecting a period of SJW coadministration and one of nevirapine alone. These patients showed a significant increase in oral clearance (35%; $p = 0.02$) of nevirapine during SJW use. Nevirapine is also a moderate autoinducer of the two P450 enzymes of which it is a substrate, 3A4 and 2B6.

Clinical Implications and Adaptations

The interaction with indinavir was highly publicized, and advisories from regulatory bodies in the United Kingdom and United States recommended that coadministration of all antiretrovirals with SJW be avoided.[16,18] Management by avoidance may be an appropriate strategy to eliminate interaction, but this official consensus was based on a single preclinical study of one protease inhibitor. The authorities did not mention that the clinical pharmacology of HIV and acquired immunodeficiency syndrome (AIDS) is a field in which complex interactions are the norm. The antiretrovirals in particular display a wide range of highly volatile and variable interactions, both pharmacokinetic and pharmacodynamic, with other drugs as well as with each other. Pharmacogenomic factors also play a major but currently little-acknowledged role in treatment of individuals with HIV/ AIDS.[118]

This interactivity of the antiretroviral drugs is well known among HIV/AIDS specialist providers and many HIV/AIDS patients. The pharmacokinetic effects of the drugs on P450 enzymes are extensive and vary considerably between different drugs; for example, indinavir potently inhibits and induces 3A4, whereas ritonavir is a powerful pan-inhibitor of most P450 enzymes and a specific inducer of 3A4, 1A2, 2C9, and 2C19. Pronounced interactions of antiretrovirals with each other and many drugs are well established, and prescribing regimens for HIV and AIDS patients often involve empirical antiretroviral drug cocktails. Additional polypharmacy with other drugs is also likely, depending on individual status. Viral load is invariably monitored as an indicator of antiviral therapeutic efficacy. Serum drug levels are often monitored directly, and serum dosage, timing of administration, and drug combinations may be adjusted accordingly and frequently. Extrapolation from the one available (and limited) study on one agent to all known antiretrovirals is at best an oversimplification, at worst a suspect (and potentially counterproductive) judgment call.

St. John's wort aroused interest in the late 1980s and early 1990s because of its potential as an antiretroviral agent, but preliminary studies with both the herb and synthetic hypericin (the purportedly active anti-HIV constituent) were disappointing. Nonetheless, patients may incorporate SJW by self-prescription into their treatment protocols for indications such as depression. Such cases would require vigilant attention to viral load monitoring or (preferably) serum drug levels before and after initiation of SJW. Theoretically, once a stable level of SJW administration was established, long-term management issues of coadministration would be routine for clinicians experienced in the field, although financial costs may also be a significant factor if substantial increases in drug dose were required to maintain therapeutic levels.

Cyclosporine

Cyclosporine (Ciclosporin, cyclosporin A, CsA; Neoral, Sandimmune, SangCya).

Interaction Type and Significance

✗✗✗ Potentially Harmful or Serious Adverse Interaction—Avoid

◇◇◇ Impaired Drug Absorption and Bioavailability, Avoidance Necessary

Probability:
1. Certain

Evidence Base:
● Consensus

Effect and Mechanism of Action

Cyclosporin A (CsA) is a dual substrate of both P-glycoprotein and of CYP450 3A4, both of which are induced by SJW. Addition of SJW to previously stable cyclosporine patients will result in significant reductions in drug levels and the possibility of therapeutic failure of immunosuppression. The interaction is well documented and considered established.

Research

The induction effects of SJW on 3A4 and P-gp are established. Cyclosporine is a cosubstrate whose disposition is controlled by both proteins, with P-gp (MDR1) affecting intestinal absorption and biliary excretion, and intestinal and hepatic 3A4 both contributing to first-pass metabolism.[119-121] Bauer et al.[122] recently described a case series of 11 renal graft patients maintained with immunosuppressive regimens incorporating CsA who were administered relatively low doses of SJW (600 mg once daily) for 14 days. Dose-corrected CsA levels decreased more than 40%, and CsA had to be increased from 2.7 to 4.1 mg/kg/day to maintain therapeutic levels. Interestingly, these figures correspond closely to the increase in clearance for cyclosporine found by Dresser et al.[27] in a preclinical study designed to quantify the relative levels of P-gp and 3A4 induction in the effects of SJW. They estimated induction effects of SJW on cyclosporine to be 1.6-fold after oral administration.[27] The authors note that unexplained discrepancies remain in data on the effects of coordinate induction on dual-substrate compounds. According to their results, increased cyclosporine clearance caused by SJW is not only less than that of a unique 3A4 substrate, such as midazolam, but also an order of magnitude less than that induced by pretreatment with rifampin, also a SXR/PXR ligand, as is hyperforin.[72] Dresser et al.[27] conclude that other, as yet undefined, mechanisms (e.g., OATPs) may be involved.

Reports

The multiple case reports of the cyclosporine-SJW interaction make it the best documented of the SJW pharmacokinetic interactions. The initial *Lancet* report in early 2000 by Ruschitzka et al.[8] described two cardiac transplant patients who developed acute rejection responses after starting SJW. Serum levels of cyclosporine were depressed, and after intensification of immunosuppressive therapy and cessation of the herb, the acute rejection responses were reversed, and plasma cyclosporine levels returned to normal. Fugh-Berman and Ernst[11] rated this report as "likely" with a maximum score of 9/9 points on their reliability rating scale; however, other reports have been poorly documented, providing minimal data for evaluation. In a more recent review of 11 available reports, Ernst[63] concluded that the clinical evidence for actual decreases in cyclosporine levels in transplant patients was conclusive, and that the risk of acute rejection was significant. Several reports noted decreased serum levels of cyclosporine after SJW administration in renal and cardiac graft patients, fortunately before rejection episodes.[122-125] Since the original Ruschitzka report,[8] two other cases of acute rejection have been documented, one involving a renal-pancreatic graft and the other a hepatic graft patient.[126,127]

Clinical Implications and Adaptations

The addition of SJW to previously stable regimens of immunosuppression based on CsA will clearly cause serum levels of the drug to fall, approximately 1.5-fold according to the available data. This is considerably less than the effect of known pharmaceutical inducers and about equivalent to the effect of consuming red wine.[73] Cyclosporine levels are regularly monitored in transplant patients, so theoretically, coadministration with professional management does not present insurmountable problems. Upward adjustment in oral dosing of the drug sufficient to maintain effective plasma levels to compensate for the metabolic induction by the herb should, all other factors being equal, maintain immunosuppression if coadministration were to be adopted. However, because the metabolites of cyclosporine also exhibit nephrotoxicity, increased drug ingestion to maintain therapeutic levels may risk increased toxic effects; furthermore, because the drug is expensive, cost factors would not favor this approach.

In reality, risks from the cyclosporine interaction are most likely with undisclosed self-prescription of the herb by allograft patients unaware of the potential dangers; this has been the case with all the reported cases of graft rejection to date. The real risk of acute rejection in such patients has led to publicity emphasizing the need for disclosure and the counseling of transplant patients on potential dangers of adding SJW to immunosuppressive protocols. (See also Tacrolimus later.)

Digoxin, Digitoxin, and Related Cardiac Glycosides

Evidence: Digoxin (Digitek, Lanoxin, Lanoxicaps, purgoxin), digitoxin (Cystodigin).
Related but evidence lacking for extrapolation: Deslanoside (cedilanin-D), ouabain (g-strophanthin).

Interaction Type and Significance

✗✗ **Potentially Harmful or Serious Adverse Interaction—Vigilance Necessary**
◇◇ **Impaired Drug Absorption and Bioavailability, Precautions Appropriate**

Probability:
1. Certain

Evidence Base:
▽ Mixed

Effect and Mechanism of Action

A pharmacokinetic interaction arises because digoxin is a specific substrate for P-gp, which is induced by SJW. The effects of coadministration may be biphasic, depending on the sequence and manner of combining herb and drug. The clinical significance of the interaction is not established.

Research:

The induction effects of SJW on intestinal P-gp are known (see Strategic Considerations earlier). Digoxin and related cardiac glycosides are substrates of P-gp, and the inhibition of P-gp by cardiac drugs such as verapamil and quinidine is the known mechanism of several well-established drug interactions involving digoxin that lead to increased cardiac glycoside toxicity. The original study by Johne et al.,[7] implicating SJW in a pharmacokinetic interaction with digoxin, found a 25% decrease in digoxin AUC after 10 days of treatment with oral SJW, 900 mg once daily, in healthy subjects with previously stabilized digoxin levels by serum monitoring. Importantly, a 10% increase in digoxin levels was found with single-dose addition of SJW, but this value was not statistically significant and is never reported in the secondary literature. A subsequent "before and after" study by Durr et al.[28] examined the induction effects of SJW on intestinal P-gp/MDR1 and intestinal and hepatic 3A4. After 14 days of SJW administration in healthy volunteers, SJW increased intestinal P-gp by 1.4-fold and decreased the AUC of a standard 0.5-mg digoxin dose by 18% compared with baseline.[28]

Although these two studies are in broad agreement about the long-term effects of SJW on digoxin kinetics, it is possible that the effect of SJW on digoxin may be biphasic, mirroring the behavior of fexofenadine (Allegra), another P-gp specific substrate that has been used as a probe in experimental investigations of P-gp. Wang et al.[26] investigated this hypothesis in a study that confirmed the biphasic effects of SJW on drug transporter kinetics. They found the effect of a single oral dose of SJW (900 mg) administered within 1 hour of 60 mg fexofenadine decreased the clearance of the drug by 20%, resulting in a 45% *increase* in serum drug level ($p < 0.05$). Long term, however, there was a 35% *decrease* in maximum plasma concentrations after 14 days of SJW administration at 900 mg once daily.[26]

A recent study by Mueller et al.[128] examined the effects of 10 forms of SJW preparation and different doses of several forms on digoxin kinetics. The preparations included SJW dried herb tea, powdered crude herb, fresh plant juice, standardized extracts with high and low hyperforin content (LI60, Ze 117), and infused oil, as well as a placebo control. Healthy volunteers ($n = 93$) were stabilized on digoxin at 0.2 to 0.3 mg three times daily for 1 week, followed by adding SJW concurrently for 14 days. Only two of the SJW preparations tested, the LI60 and high dose of *Hypericum* powder (4 g once daily, with comparable hyperforin content to LI60), produced comparable and significant reductions in digoxin maximum concentration (C_{max}) and AUC_{0-24}. The reductions in AUC were approximately 25% and in C_{max} approximately 37%, with 95% confidence interval (CI). The dose of the SJW preparations that failed to generate significant changes in digoxin pharmacokinetics correspond to dosage levels given for traditional use in therapeutic monographs, such as Commission E and ESCOP (2-4 g crude herb daily),[2,4] suggesting a probable difference in the capability to induce interaction effects between traditional herbal prescription and hyperforin/hypericin standardized concentrated extracts.

At present, data are insufficient to characterize fully the mechanisms of the interaction. However, the OATP family, in addition to P-gp, may be implicated. There is a specific transporter for digoxin (OATP-8),[129] and digoxin transport was shown to be more affected by naturally occurring bioflavonoids operating on P-gp than on OATP in an in vitro model.[130] In a recent poster study, SJW completely abolished P-pg–mediated digoxin transport in vitro.[50] A recent immunohistochemical study identified another transporter, OATP-4C1, that mediates digoxin, ouabain, triiodothyronine, and methotrexate transport in a sodium-dependent manner and is located in the proximal tubule of the human nephron.[131] Further research is required to fully elucidate the various mechanisms of digoxin disposition.

Reports

Case reports of subtherapeutic digoxin levels after addition of SJW to previously stable digitalized patients are unavailable. A single report is available that describes the predicted pattern of cessation of an inducer (SJW) causing rebound drug toxicity. An 80-year-old man stable on digoxin consumed 2000 mL of SJW tea daily. On cessation of the tea, he developed nodal bradycardia and bigeminy, which was treated successfully with digoxin (FAB). The original report is in Serbian and unavailable for full evaluation.[132]

Clinical Implications and Adaptations

Addition of SJW to a stable digoxin level may result in a short-term increase in drug levels potentially capable of inducing classic digitalis toxicity. However, longer-term coadministration risks inducing a decline in drug levels after induction of transporter proteins. This could theoretically lead to therapeutic failure if not corrected.

Introduction of SJW to patients already stabilized on digoxin should therefore initially follow a ramped dose increase of the herb over several days, rather than starting at 100% of the target dose, to avoid possible short-term inhibitory effects on drug transport. Once stable therapeutic doses are attained, serum digoxin level monitoring should drive any adjustment in cardiac glycoside dosage to compensate for transporter induction. Discontinuation of the herb must also be tapered, to avoid rebound digitalis intoxication resulting from the reversal of induction.

Patients stable on cardiac glycoside therapy must be counseled on the potential risks of unsupervised addition or withdrawal of SJW. However, the order of magnitude of these effects is similar to that resulting from dietary ingredients, particularly citrus bioflavonoids and red wine,[35,51,130,133] and is not itself a compelling reason to avoid coadministration if clinically indicated.

Etoposide and Related Topoisomerase II Inhibitors

Evidence: Etoposide (Eposin, Etopophos, Vepesid, VP-16). Extrapolation based on similar properties: DNA topoisomerase II inhibitors: Daunorubicin (Cerubidine, DaunoXome), doxorubicin (Adriamycin, Rubex), doxorubicin, pegylated liposomal (Caelyx, Doxil, Myocet), epirubicin (Ellence, Pharmorubicin), idarubicin (Idamycin, Zavedos), mitoxantrone (Novantrone, Onkotrone), teniposide (Vumon).

Interaction Type and Significance

✗ **Potential or Theoretical Adverse Interaction of Uncertain Severity**

◇◇ **Impaired Drug Absorption and Bioavailability, Precautions Appropriate**

? **Interaction Likely but Uncertain Occurrence and Unclear Implications**

Probability:
4. Plausible

Evidence Base:
☐ **Inadequate**

Effect and Mechanism of Action

Combined pharmacokinetic and pharmacodynamic interaction is possible. Etoposide is partially metabolized through CYP3A4 and is therefore subject to SJW induction, while the naphthadianthrone constituent hypericin pharmacodynamically interferes with the etoposide-mediated cytotoxicity in vitro. The clinical significance of this plausible interaction is not established.

Research

Peebles et al.[134] investigated the mechanism of action by which hypericin interfered with the topoisomerase (topo) II poisons, using an HL-60 cell-line model. The study was partially motivated by the initial hypothesis that hypericin may exhibit leukemogenic toxicities, because these are known to be associated with topo II agents. The mechanism of action of hypericin was unlike that of etoposide (and amsacrine), resembling the effect of topo II catalytic inhibitors that operate upstream of etoposide to inhibit etoposide effects, protecting the HL-60 cells from etoposide-mediated damage.[134] Methodologically, extrapolations are not directly possible to in vivo situations with oncology patients, and the dose-response curves of the hypericin effects were not established. However, as Block and Gyllenhaal[135] noted in a review of herb-drug interactions in cancer chemotherapy, etoposide is also metabolized by 3A4 before renal elimination.

Clinical Implications and Adaptations

Cancer patients are likely candidates for self-prescription of SJW, and concurrent use of botanical and dietary agents during chemotherapy should be audited closely. Information about putative antitumor activity of hypericin is available on the Internet, and purified hypericin can currently be obtained as a "dietary supplement," suggesting the possibility of undisclosed self-prescription. At present, insufficient data are available to establish the in vivo effects of hypericin and SJW interactions with any chemotherapy agents (see also Irinotecan [CPT-11] discussion), although the potential clearly exists for a reduction of cytotoxic efficacy through several pharmacokinetic mechanisms, and in the case of etoposide, additional pharmacodynamic factors may be involved. Combining nutritional and botanical agents with chemotherapy is a specialist field, and professionals experienced in integrative oncology should be involved in any decisions on coadministration.

Fexofenadine

Fexofenadine (Allegra)

Interaction Type and Significance

✗ **Potential or Theoretical Adverse Interaction of Uncertain Severity**

◇ **Impaired Drug Absorption and Bioavailability, Negligible Effect**

Probability:
3. Possible

Evidence Base:
● **Consensus**

Effect and Mechanism of Action

The histamine H_1-receptor antagonist fexofenadine hydrochloride is a documented substrate of P-gp that is induced by SJW, and the herb is known to be capable of modifying fexofenadine levels. The clinical effect and significance are likely minimal because of the wide therapeutic index of the drug.

Research

Fexofenadine is a specific substrate of P-gp and is eliminated without undergoing significant metabolism. It has been used as a probe drug in preclinical investigations of P-gp pharmacokinetics because of its high specificity for the transporter and because it is relatively well tolerated, with few adverse effects over a widely varying dose range. Notably, the manufacturer's information suggests an absence of effects on QT interval for doses ranging from 60 to 400 mg twice daily in healthy individuals. The innocuous characteristics of the drug have been used to analyze the behavior of P-gp substrates with a much narrower therapeutic index, such as digoxin (see previous SJW-digoxin section).[27,51,133,136]

Clinical Implications and Adaptations

Despite substantial evidence of the ability of SJW to affect fexofenadine levels, the interaction itself lacks case reports and is probably of minimal clinical significance. Given the wide therapeutic index of the drug in clinical practice, as well as the likelihood of patient self-adjustment of drug dosage levels to treat allergic symptoms as required, coadministration with SJW appears unproblematic. The inclusion of this interaction in lists of SJW interactions without qualification in the secondary literature is arguably a case of "overstatement." (See Theoretical, Speculative, and Preliminary Interactions Research later.)

Imatinib

Imatinib (Gleevec, Glivec)

Interaction Type and Significance

◇◇◇ **Impaired Drug Absorption and Bioavailability, Avoidance Appropriate**

Probability:	Evidence Base:
3. Possible	☐ Inadequate

Effect and Mechanism of Action

A pharmacokinetic interaction in which SJW may reduce serum levels of the active metabolite of the tyrosine kinase inhibitor, causing possible decrease in drug exposure. Preliminary evidence supports the interaction, and imatinib is known to be metabolized by 3A4.

Research

A study recently reported by Frye et al.[137] investigated the possible interaction of SJW and the 3A4 substrate imatinib with 12 healthy volunteers, comparing single-dose oral clearance of the drug (400 mg) before and after 14 days of SJW (300 mg three times daily) pretreatment. Clearance was increased by 44%, AUC decreased by 30%, and the half-life and C_{max} were also decreased. Cytochrome P450 3A4 is the primary metabolic pathway that has been described for the drug, although individual variability in response to the drug (resistance) may result from pharmacogenomic mechanisms not yet adequately described. The 3A4-inducer phenytoin has also been shown to reduce AUC of imatinib to about 20% of the typical AUC_{24}, and this was reversed by ketaconazole.[138]

Clinical Implications and Adaptations

Given the serious indications for Gleevec, including chronic myelogenous leukemia (CML) and gastrointestinal stromal tumors (GIST), accurate dosage levels should be confidently maintained for the clinical populations involved. Cancer patients are arguably likely to self-prescribe with SJW for depression and should be cautioned to avoid the herb during Gleevec treatment. Alternatively, if preexisting treatment with SJW has had significant positive impact on quality of life, and if alternative approaches have been poorly tolerated, higher doses of imatinib, with serum drug level monitoring, would be indicated.

Irinotecan

Irinotecan (Camptothecin-11, CPT-11; Campto, Camptosar).

Interaction Type and Significance

✗ **Potential or Theoretical Adverse Interaction of Uncertain Severity**

◇◇◇ **Impaired Drug Absorption and Bioavailability, Avoidance Appropriate**

Probability:	Evidence Base:
4. Plausible	☐ Inadequate

Effect and Mechanism of Action

SJW may reduce serum levels of the active metabolite of the camptothecin analog CPT-110. The mechanism of interaction is complex, and pharmacogenetic factors can cause high individual variability in drug levels. A resultant decrease in tumor cytotoxic exposure is possible. Because of the known complexity of irinotecan metabolism and the wide variability in individual responses to the drug, the clinical significance of the interaction is not known.

Research

One small, unblended, crossover study involved five cancer patients treated with intravenous CPT-11 before and after SJW administration for 18 days at 900 mg once daily. Serum concentrations of the active cytotoxic metabolite SN38 (7-ethyl-10-hydroxy CPT) were reduced by a mean of 42% after SJW administration. Myelosuppression was less in the SJW phase, indicating a reduced chemotoxicity. This is significant because toxicity (NCI Common Toxicity Grading Criteria) often governs dose adjustment in irinotecan chemotherapy regimens. In fact, the statistical mean of this small sample of patients was derived from a range of 14% to 79%, typical of the wide interindividual variation in responses to the drug.

Clinical Implications and Adaptations

Irinotecan pharmacokinetics have been well documented and are known to be highly complex.[139-141] The prodrug is converted to the active compound SN38 by serum carboxylases; subsequent metabolism is through hepatic UGT1A1 glucuronidation and biliary excretion, which depends on a canalicular multispecific transporter (cMOATP). The conjugated form undergoes enterohepatic recirculation. The prodrug is secondarily transformed by 3A4 into two inactive metabolites, APC and ANC, which form 2% to 8% of the eliminated compounds. Finally, SN38 is 94% albumin bound in plasma. Considerable potential metabolic variability exists; hepatic microsomes display a thirteenfold variation in rate of SN38 formation, and genetically determined polymorphisms of UGT1A1 play a role in response variation. Significant pharmacokinetic interactions with conventional drugs have been observed with competitors and inducers of the glucuronidation process more than with 3A4-specific inducers, and P-gp induction (biliary) may also play a part in irinotecan interactions.[142]

More data are required before the effects of SJW on irinotecan metabolism can be accurately identified. Several authors have raised important questions about the possibility of SJW interactions with chemotherapeutic agents through induction of metabolism and transport.[135,143,144] The area is important, especially because of the possible effects of SJW on multidrug resistance through P-gp; oncologists, as well as integrative primary care providers supporting cancer patients undergoing conventional chemotherapies, should be cognizant of the issues, despite the lack of definitive data. Dosing of these agents by body surface area seems a seriously outmoded practice, given the narrow therapeutic index of cytotoxic chemotherapy agents, the well-established wide variations in serum drug levels caused by genetic polymorphisms of drug-metabolizing enzymes, and the potential interactions with other drugs and dietary components as well as with herbal and nutritional agents (many as yet unknown), often unreported by patients to their oncologists.

The development of widely available clinical laboratory tests for cytotoxic chemotherapy drug levels and their routine utilization should be encouraged to enhance efficacy and reduce toxicity in the clinical practice of medical oncology. Such tests have been routinely used for decades with agents of much larger therapeutic indices, such as phenytoin (Dilantin) and digoxin. Development and utilization of serum chemotherapy drug levels tests would greatly simplify management of the underlying genetic polymorphisms affecting these levels and would help uncover covert use of self-prescribed herbal and nutritional agents, as well as allowing prescribers to compensate for such coadministration when indicated or reasonable.

Omeprazole and Related Proton Pump Inhibitors

Evidence: Omeprazole (Losec, Prilosec).
Extrapolated, based on similar properties: Esomeprazole (Nexium), lansoprazole (Prevacid, Zoton), pantoprazole (Protium, Protonix, Somac), rabeprazole (AcipHex, Pariet).

Interaction Type and Significance

✗ **Potential or Theoretical Adverse Interaction of Uncertain Severity**

◇◇ **Impaired Drug Absorption and Bioavailability, Precautions Appropriate**

Probability: Evidence Base:
2. Probable   ○ **Preliminary**

Effect and Mechanism of Action

A pharmacokinetic interaction occurs between SJW and omeprazole, and possibly with related benzimidazole drugs, which are metabolized by 3A4 and 2C19, resulting in a lowering of drug levels caused by enzyme induction by SJW. The interaction is experimentally confirmed, but clinical reports are lacking to date.

Research

A recent, randomized, crossover trial examined the effects of SJW pretreatment (300 mg three times daily) for 14 days on the single-dose kinetics of 20 mg oral omeprazole and its metabolites.[23] The 12 healthy volunteers were phenotyped for 2C19 polymorphisms because these are known to affect the metabolism of the substrate omeprazole. The drug is metabolized by two routes, involving sulfoxidation by 3A4 and hydroxylation by 2C19, so the separate metabolites (5-hydroxymeprazole and omeprazole sulfone) were measured in plasma by high-performance liquid chromatography (HPLC) along with the parent drug. Substantial decreases in omeprazole C_{max} (37.5%) and AUC (49.6%) [$p < 0.001$] were found with SJW pretreatment. The wild-type variants of 2C19 or "extensive metabolizers" (EMs) also displayed significant increases in 5-hydroxy metabolite levels, but "poor metabolizer" (PM) phenotypes showed lower effects. Xie[145] elaborated on the authors' interpretation of this study, noting that the 3A4 pathway is a minor metabolic route, and

because omeprazole is also a competitive inhibitor of 2C19, as well as a substrate and inhibitor of the efflux transporter P-gp, that the disposition of the drug involves integrated effects of multiple pathways.

Clinical Implications and Adaptations

The authors of the previous study suggest that SJW induces 3A4 and also 2C19, the latter in a genotype-dependent manner, to the extent that significant increases in drug doses would be necessary during herb-drug coadministration to compensate for the induction effects by the herb.[23] The benzimidazoles do not have a narrow therapeutic index, and there are currently no clinical reports of this interaction; however, the size of the observed experimental effects suggests that the interaction could be clinically significant. Physicians prescribing proton pump inhibitors must consider the need for increased dose levels if there is prior stable usage of SJW, and adding SJW to omeprazole may significantly reduce previously stable drug levels.

Oral Contraceptives and Related Estrogen-Containing and Synthetic Estrogen and Progesterone Analog Medications

Evidence: Oral contraceptives: monophasic, biphasic, and triphasic estrogen preparations:
Ethinyl estradiol and desogestrel (Desogen, Ortho-TriCyclen).
Ethinyl estradiol and ethynodiol (Demulen 1/35, Demulen 1/50, Nelulen 1/25, Nelulen 1/50, Zovia).
Ethinyl estradiol and levonorgestrel (Alesse, Levlen, Levlite, Levora 0.15/30, Nordette, Tri-Levlen, Triphasil, Trivora).
Ethinyl estradiol and norethindrone/norethisterone (Brevicon, Estrostep, Genora 1/35, GenCept 1/35, Jenest-28, Loestrin 1.5/30, Loestrin1/20, Modicon, Necon 1/25, Necon 10/11, Necon 0.5/30, Necon 1/50, Nelova 1/35, Nelova 10/11, Norinyl 1/35, Norlestin 1/50, Ortho Novum 1/35, Ortho Novum 10/11, Ortho Novum 7/7/7, Ovcon-35, Ovcon-50, Tri-Norinyl, Trinovum).
Ethinyl estradiol and norgestrel (Lo/Ovral, Ovral).
Mestranol and norethindrone (Genora 1/50, Nelova 1/50, Norethin 1/50, Ortho-Novum 1/50).
Related, internal application: Etonogestrel/ethinyl estradiol vaginal ring (Nuvaring).
Related but evidence lacking for extrapolation:
Progestin-only oral contraceptives, implants, and post-coital contraceptives: Etonogestrel, implant (Implanon); levonorgestrel, implant (Jadelle, Norplant; Norplant-2); levonorgestrel, oral postcoital contraceptive (Duofem, Escapelle, Levonelle, Levonelle-2, Microlut, Microval, Norgeston, NorLevo, Plan B, Postinor-2, Vika, Vikela); medroxyprogesterone, injection (Depo-Provera, Depo-subQ Provera 104); medroxyprogesterone, oral (Cycrin, Provera); NES progestin, implant (ST-1435, Nestorone); norethindrone, oral (norethisterone; Aygestin, Camila, Errin, Jolivette, Micronor, Nor-QD, Ortho-Micronor); norethindrone, injectable (NET EN; Noristerat); norgestrel, oral (Ovrette).
Hormone replacement therapy (HRT), estrogens: Chlorotrianisene (Tace); conjugated equine estrogens (Premarin); conjugated synthetic estrogens (Cenestin); dienestrol (Ortho Dienestrol); esterified estrogens (Estratab, Menest, Neo-Estrone); estradiol, topical/transdermal/ring (Alora Transdermal, Climara Transdermal, Estrace, Estradot, Estring FemPatch, Vivelle-Dot, Vivelle Transdermal); estradiol cypionate (Dep-Gynogen, Depo-Estradiol, Depogen, Dura-Estrin, Estra-D, Estro-Cyp, Estroject-LA, Estronol-LA); estradiol hemihydrate (Estreva, Vagifem); estradiol valerate

(Delestrogen, Estra-L 40, Gynogen L.A. 20, Progynova, Valergen 20); estrone (Aquest, Estragyn 5, Estro-A, Estrone '5', Kestrone-5); estropipate (Ogen, Ortho-Est); ethinyl estradiol (Estinyl, Gynodiol, Lynoral).

HRT, estrogen/progestin combinations: Conjugated equine estrogens and medroxyprogesterone (Premelle cycle 5, Prempro); conjugated equine estrogens and norgestrel (Prempak-C); estradiol and dydrogesterone (Femoston); estradiol and norethindrone, patch (CombiPatch); estradiol and norethindrone/norethisterone, oral (Activella, Climagest, Climesse, FemHRT, Trisequens); estradiol valerate and cyproterone acetate (Climens); estradiol valerate and norgestrel (Progyluton); estradiol and norgestimate (Ortho-Prefest).

HRT, estrogen/testosterone combinations: Esterified estrogens and methyltestosterone (Estratest, Estratest HS).

Interaction Type and Significance

✗   **Potential or Theoretical Adverse Interaction of Uncertain Severity**

◇◇ **Impaired Drug Absorption and Bioavailability, Precautions Appropriate**

Probability:	Evidence Base:
3. Possible	○ Preliminary

Effect and Mechanism of Action

A pharmacokinetic interaction may theoretically result from SJW induction of estrogen and progestin metabolism, causing increased clearance and lowered serum drug levels, resulting in "breakthrough bleeding" and theoretically a risk of contraceptive failure, although failure is not established. Variability in oral contraceptive (OC) product formulations and known interindividual variability of responses to exogenous hormones confounds simple interpretation of the currently available data. Clinical significance of the interaction is not established.

Research

The metabolism of OCs is highly complex and incompletely characterized; the pharmacokinetics of steroidal hormones is subject to considerable interindividual variability because of the sheer complexity and number of metabolic pathways involved and the polymorphisms they exhibit. Also, significant differences in formulation exist between different OC products. By consensus, 3A4 is considered to the major P450 enzyme for metabolic transformation of both estrogens and progestins. However, the original OC estrogenic compound mestranol is in fact activated by 2C9 to ethinyl estradiol (EE). Similarly, the common progestin ingredient desogestrel is also a prodrug, metabolized by 2C9 to the active metabolite 3-ketodesogestrel. Glucuronidation and sulfation by the relevant transferase enzymes adds further variability because of polymorphisms in the transferase enzyme systems, which are also subject to induction and inhibition. Finally, conjugated EE is also hydrolyzed by bowel flora and undergoes enterohepatic recirculation, unlike the progestins. In turn, OCs themselves are mild inhibitors of 3A4 and more pronounced inhibitors of 1A2 and 2C19, although their effects on the clearance of other drug substrates of these enzymes are not well researched.

One pilot study has examined the effects of SJW on concentrations of circulating androgens by immunoassay after administration of the herb to healthy volunteers (six female, six male) for a 14-day period sufficient for CYP3A4 induction. No significant changes in androgen levels resulted from SJW administration, although there was a small reduction in the level of 5α-reduced androgens, more so in women than in men.[146]

Two recent controlled studies addressed the effects of SJW on combination OC therapy with regard to ovarian activity, the possibility of contraceptive failure, and the kinetics of the steroidal components of the OC products used.[147,148] The clinical findings of both trials were similar and confirmed that SJW coadministered with combination OCs increased breakthrough bleeding but did not result in ovulation (as recorded by endosonographic measurement). The studies differed significantly in other findings.

Pfrunder et al.[148] found no changes in ethinyl estradiol AUC with SJW coadministration, at either 600 mg or 900 mg SJW daily doses with a combination OC (EE/desogestrel), but the progestin metabolite 3-ketodesogestrel decreased significantly at both these dosage levels. This metabolite is generated by 2C9 (and possibly 2C19), then further metabolized by 3A4. The authors suggested that 2C9 may be inhibited by hyperforin or apigenin constituents of SJW because of in vitro evidence for 2C9 inhibition,[19] or that 3A4 induction was responsible for the decrease, despite the apparent lack of effect on EE. This study did not examine hyperforin or hypericin levels, although the extract used (LI60) had high hypericin and hyperforin content.

Hall et al.[147] coadministered 900 mg SJW once daily for two cycles with Ortho-Novum (a combination OC containing EE/norethindrone) and examined a more comprehensive set of parameters. These included hyperforin levels, follicle-stimulating hormone (FSH), luteinizing hormone (LH), progesterone, pharmacokinetic parameters for norethindrone and EE, and oral and intravenous values for the 3A4 probe midazolam.[147] The clearance of EE was increased by 47% by SJW coadministration, but this was not deemed significant ($n = 12$). Norethindrone clearance increased by 16%. The midazolam probe data suggested that the changes were caused by intestinal rather than hepatic 3A4 induction, since systemic clearance was not changed but oral clearance increased by 50%. Hyperforin levels averaged a steady-state level of 20 ng/mL; however, a large (threefold) variation was noted between the subjects in hyperforin levels, which may reflect the variability in response rates. Breakthrough bleeding was positively correlated with significantly higher midazolam oral clearance. Larger studies are needed to confirm definitively whether SJW will permit ovulation during OC therapy, but both trials suggest that this is unlikely.

Reports

Despite media publicity, anecdotal reports of "miracle babies" born to women using SJW concurrently with OC therapy remain unsubstantiated.[149] Reports in the professional literature are sparse and contribute no useful data to establishing the incidence and significance of the possible SJW-OC interaction. The earliest report was in correspondence to the *Lancet* in 1999 that gave no details for three purported cases of breakthrough bleeding associated with combination OCs and SJW coadministration.[10] Another *Lancet* letter contained a report from Sweden by Yue et al.[150] (see also warfarin-SJW later) that mentioned "eight cases of intermenstrual bleeding and one report of changed menstrual bleeding from manufacturers of SJW products."[121] Patient history, details of the OC preparation, and SJW form and dose were not given. No contraceptive failure was mentioned. Fugh-Berman and Ernst[11] later classified the Yue reports as "unreliable."

A single case of contraceptive failure involved a 36-year-old patient with a history of depression and use of pharmaceutical antidepressants who stopped all pharmaceutical treatment in favor of SJW (1700 mg once daily, a high dose). After 3 months, while still taking a combination OC (EE/dienogestrel), she conceived unexpectedly.[64] A midwifery magazine article also reports unwanted pregnancies as occurring while SJW was used, citing cases drawn from several government agency reports: from the U.K. Medicines Control Agency (MCA; seven cases) and from Sweden and Germany (four cases). None of these has been documented in professional literature, except the Swedish reports already mentioned, although the British MCA warned that the SJW-OC interaction would result in risk of unintended pregnancy in its advisory letter to practitioners and pharmacists.[16]

Clinical Implications and Adaptations

In the conventional drug interactions literature, induction of CYP450 3A4 and uridine glucuronosyltransferase (UGT) has been shown to increase EE and progestin clearance and is typically associated with increased symptoms of breakthrough bleeding. Ovulation parameters have not been well studied in this area, but ovulation with pharmaceutical 3A4/UGT inducers has not been reported.[151,152] The few reports of pregnancies resulting from combining conventional drugs with OCs are rare and almost impossible to evaluate. The situation appears similar with SJW-OC interactions. The risk of actual unwanted pregnancy seems small, but unquantifiable, at present.

Breakthrough bleeding, although associated with initial phases of OC therapy alone, appears to be increased by SJW coadministration. Bleeding is also associated with decreased compliance with OC therapy and thus indirectly with increased risk of contraceptive failure as other, less reliable alternative forms of contraception are adopted to avoid undesirable symptoms. Despite the lack of solid evidence for failure of contraception due to SJW, women using OCs concurrently with the herb should be advised about the risks and should consider the simultaneous use of barrier methods.

Given the contemporary trend toward "ultra-low" dosage of EE in commercial OC preparations because of concerns over adverse effects, the risks of contraception failure may be marginally higher than with the earlier, higher-dose products. Most available data relate only to combination products. Extrapolations to progestin-only minipills, to implants, and to postcoital "morning-after" pills cannot be drawn from current data.

The effect of SJW on hormone replacement therapy (HRT) has not been studied, although SJW is likely to have some impact on estrogen clearance in HRT. Because this population has no vulnerability to unwanted pregnancy, it would appear to be a lower priority for further research. The complex field of sex steroid molecular biology and metabolism will presumably yield more conclusive data in the future.

Paclitaxel, Docetaxel: Taxane Microtubule-Stabilizing Agents

Evidence: Docetaxel (Taxotere), paclitaxel (Paxene, Taxol). Similar properties but evidence lacking for extrapolation: Paclitaxel, protein-bound (Abraxane).

Interaction Type and Significance

✗   **Potential or Theoretical Adverse Interaction of Uncertain Severity**

◇◇◇ **Impaired Drug Absorption and Bioavailability, Avoidance Necessary**

Probability:
3. Possible

Evidence Base:
○ **Preliminary**

Effect and Mechanism of Action

This possible pharmacokinetic interaction could influence drug availability, although biotransformation of taxanes is primarily through CYP2C8. Multiple mechanisms are thought to underlie response variability and drug resistance to taxanes.

Research

Komoroski et al.[153] used a human hepatocyte model to test the effects of rifampin and hyperforin on the induction of docetaxel metabolism compared with controls. Hyperforin addition increased metabolism of the drug in a dose-dependent manner, with 1.5-micromolar hyperforin causing a sevenfold increase over control. The rifampin increased drug metabolism by a factor of 32. The authors concluded that chronic coadministration of SJW with docetaxel may reduce drug bioavailability to subtherapeutic levels. Wada et al.[154] used an MDR1-overexpressing line of HeLa cancer cell model and found that both hypericin and SJW lowered the antiproliferative activity of paclitaxel while inhibiting MDR1-mediated drug transport.

Clinical Implications and Adaptations

The taxanes are widely used in the treatment of breast, prostate, lung, and ovarian cancers. Body surface area (BSA) dosing is standard practice, but variability in responsiveness and resistance to the drugs is well documented. Paclitaxel is metabolized by CYP2C8, with minor CYP3A4 and CYP3A5 involvement, whereas docetaxel is primarily metabolized by 3A4 and 3A5. Administration of docetaxel with ketoconazole leads to a significant decrease in drug clearance (49%), suggesting that docetaxel disposition will be affected by 3A4 inducers and inhibitors in vivo.[155] Paclitaxel, although primarily metabolized by 2C8, has been shown to be influenced by 3A4 induction.[138] Further complexity arises when considering taxane resistance, which is thought to be at least partly caused by drug efflux pump mechanisms.

At present, avoidance of SJW with taxane administration is indicated. Modulation of taxane metabolism by induction of CYP450 by SJW has been emphasized as a problem (e.g., see Sparreboom et al.[144]). In context, however, there is considerable potential for improving the taxane-based pharmacotherapy by application of pharmacogenomics data to dosing.[156] Information about the difference, if any, between the traditional taxane drugs and the novel liposomal forms in terms of their metabolic degradation pathways is unavailable at this time.

Paroxetine and Related Selective Serotonin Reuptake Inhibitor and Serotonin-Norepinephrine Reuptake Inhibitor (SSRI and SSRI/SNRI) Antidepressants and Nonselective Serotonin Reuptake Inhibitors (NSRIs)

Evidence: Paroxetine (Aropax, Deroxat, Paxil, Seroxat); nefazodone (Serzone), trazodone (Desyrel).
Extrapolated, based on similar properties: Bupropion (Wellbutrin), citalopram (Celexa), duloxetine (Cymbalta), escitalopram (S-citalopram; Lexapro), fluoxetine (Prozac, Sarafem), fluvoxamine (Faurin, Luvox), mirtazapine (Remeron), sertraline (Zoloft), venlafaxine (Effexor).

Interaction Type and Significance

?   **Interaction Likely but Uncertain Occurrence and Unclear Implications**

Probability:
3. Possible

Evidence Base:
○ **Preliminary** (arguably ☐ Inadequate)

Effect and Mechanism of Action

These complex, potential interactions involve variable pharmacokinetic and pharmacodynamic factors, depending on the specific serotonin uptake drug, the timing and manner of herb-drug coadministration, concurrent comedications, and individual factors. "Serotonin syndrome" has been suggested as a possible clinical outcome of the interaction, but this is controversial and poorly documented, and precise mechanisms for such effects are not consistent with known SJW pharmacology. Few clinical reports are available and are of variable quality. Overall, the clinical significance of the interaction may be overstated.

Research

This proposed interaction was originally based on early assumptions about SJW pharmacology that have not been confirmed by recent research. The first was the erroneous belief that SJW functions as a MAOI-like agent, and the interaction with SSRIs was simply an assumed extrapolation from the known drug-drug MAO-A inhibitors and serotonin reuptake agents. The in vitro findings of MAO inhibition have not been replicated and have been suggested by Cott[89] to be artifactual (see Theoretical, Speculative, and Preliminary Interactions Research later). The second assumption was that SJW exerts its antidepressant effects through a druglike serotonin uptake inhibition, thus leading to excessive serotonin levels, and the possibility of serotonin syndrome if combined with a pharmaceutical SSRI. As previously noted, the neurotransmitter effects of SJW do not appear to be homologous to any pharmaceutical drug action on specific neurotransmitter pathways; rather, this appears to be a "broad-band" effect on the reuptake of all five main central neurotransmitters.[94] Finally, "serotonin syndrome" may have been overenthusiastically reported; a significant proportion of cases probably resulted from misdiagnosis, according to Radomski et al.[103] (see Reports).

Given the likelihood that SJW extracts may act biphasically, inhibiting 3A4 in acute short-term doses, with progressive induction of P-gp and 3A4 at 7 to 10 days, adverse reactions caused by the addition of SJW to preexisting SSRI regimens may be the result of a short-term pharmacokinetic interaction, parallel to the digoxin-SJW interaction. This hypothesis might help explain the effects reported by Lantz (see Reports), which are more like enhanced adverse effects of the drug than "serotonin syndrome." Because each of the six principal SSRI drugs has different routes of metabolism, as well as different inhibitory profiles on P450 enzymes, the situation becomes more complex if the interaction is indeed pharmacokinetic. The respective CYP450 metabolic properties and pathways of the selective and nonselective serotonin uptake drugs are listed in the table.[157]

As data in the table show, none of the serotonin reuptake inhibitor (SRI) drugs is an exclusive substrate of 3A4; that nefazodone and norfluoxetine (the active metabolite of fluoxetine) are potent inhibitors of 3A4; and that nefazodone, trazodone, and venlafaxine also induce P-gp. It therefore seems unlikely that short-term inhibition would inevitably produce excessive serotonin levels, whereas the predominant effect of long-term coadministration should be for SSRI drug levels to be lowered by SJW induction, with a consequent decrease in serotonin levels. Further research is needed to clarify the precise extent and role of pharmacokinetic factors in different SJW-SRI drug combinations.

Reports

Reports of serotonin syndrome (SS) arising from the coadministration of SJW and SSRI/NSRI drugs are rare, particularly in Europe.[86] However, ominous warnings of the potentially fatal consequences of SS often accompany secondary accounts of SJW interactions in the United States. This appears unnecessarily alarmist because all six of the known fatalities in the toxicology literature for SS were caused by toxic encephalopathy (on postmortem examination), and five were deliberate drug overdoses involving the MAO-A inhibitor moclobemide with citalopram or clomipramine.[158] Other severe symptoms of toxic SS include disseminated intravascular coagulation (DIC), resulting in renal failure. These should be distinguished from the common symptoms of mild SS, which include myoclonus, tremor, diaphoresis, and restlessness, all of which are transient and self-limiting and do not usually require medication changes or supportive treatment.[103]

A frequently cited U.S. case series is from a geriatric care facility reported by Lantz in 1999; four elderly patients

Metabolism of Serotonin Reuptake Inhibitor Drugs

Drug	Major P450 Metabolism Site(s)	Inhibits	Induces
Selective Serotonin Reuptake Inhibitors (SSRIs)			
Citalopram	2C19, 2D6, 3A4	2D6	
Escitalopram	2C19, 2D6, 3A4	2D6	
Fluoxetine	2C9, 2C19, 2D6, 3A4	1A2, 2B6, 2C9, **2C19**, **2D6**, 3A4 (+ norfluoxetine)	
Fluvoxamine	1A2, 2D6	**1A2**, 2B6, 2C9, **2C19**, 2D6, 3A4	
Paroxetine	2D6	1A2, **2B6**, 2C9, 2C19, **2D6**, 3A4	
Sertraline	2B6, 2C9, 2C19, 2D6, 3A4	1A2, 2B6, 2D6, glucuronidation	
Nonselective Serotonin Reuptake Inhibitors (NSRIs)			
Bupropion	2B6	**2D6**	
Mirtazapine	1A2, 2D6, 3A4		
Nefazodone	3A4, 2D6	**3A4**, P-gp (acute)	P-gp
Trazodone	3A4, 2D6		P-gp
Venlafaxine	2D6	2D6	P-gp

Modified from Cozza.[157]
Bold-face text denotes pronounced effects; *P-gp*, P-glycoprotein.

who were stable on sertraline commenced SJW and experienced symptoms diagnosed by the author as "central serotonergic syndrome." However, the data for at least one of the four cases were inadequate, according to the Ernst and Fugh-Berman criteria (failure to list comedications), and in none of the cases was the herbal preparation fully identified.[11] The primary symptoms for all four were nausea and in three, vomiting. These symptoms alone are atypical of SS; according to a detailed review of all 62 published cases from 1982 to 1995 by Radmoski et al.,[103] nausea occurred in only 6%, and vomiting was never recorded. The fifth elderly woman in the same series was stable on nefazodone and experienced the same symptoms after adding SJW. The case presents problems of interpretation, even assuming a short-term pharmacokinetic inhibition of CYP 3A4. Nefazodone is a powerful 3A4 inhibitor and only likely to exhibit interactions with a more potent inhibitor than itself,[157] which rules out a SJW effect. Sertraline is cometabolized by multiple P450 CYPs (2B6, 2C9, 2C19, 2D6, *and* 3A4; see table), which suggests it would only be vulnerable to pharmacokinetic interactions with pan-inhibitors or pan-inducers, which excludes SJW. This suggests that the interaction may have been pharmacodynamic, but the antidepressant effects of SJW in vivo are mild, take several weeks to manifest, and are not equivalent to the pharmaceutical SSRI/NSRI drug mechanisms. Despite its frequent invocation as confirming the SJW-SSRI interaction, the Lantz report is inconclusive, and the authors' explanations are not consistent with the currently understood pharmacology of SJW.

Another case report involved a woman who became lethargic, having discontinued paroxetine (40 mg once daily) after 8 months, and who began 600 mg of SJW powdered herb daily (preparation unspecified) 10 days later. On the second day of this regimen she also took a single dose of paroxetine (20 mg) to help with insomnia. The next day she was almost unable to rise from bed and was groggy and incoherent but arousable. Two hours later she still complained of fatigue, weakness, and nausea, although her vital signs and mini–mental status examination were normal. Twenty-four hours later she had no remaining ill effects.[159] The reporting physician described this as resembling a "sedative/hypnotic syndrome" intoxication. Interpretation of this case must account for paroxetine being a potent inhibitor of 2D6, the enzyme of which it is a substrate; the 10-day washout after the prolonged paroxetine therapy may have caused 2D6 to rebound, rendering the patient hypersensitive to a subsequent repeat dose of the SSRI. CYP2D6 is well known to exhibit "slow" and "fast" polymorphisms. This report is probably a case of excessive sedation resulting from enhanced effects of the drug, rather than a pharmacodynamic SJW interaction. Several in vivo studies have examined short-term and long-term effects of SJW on 2D6, the current consensus being a lack of observable effect for short-term inhibition or longer-term 2D6 induction.[24,26,31,29]

Nirenberg et al.[160] recorded mania in two depressive patients in temporal association with SJW consumption. Both patients had initially been diagnosed with major depression, and before initiating prescription psychiatric drugs, they had experimented with SJW. In an interesting conjecture, the authors suggested the resulting manic episodes were caused by an "unmasking" of rapid-cycling bipolar disorder, supported by both patients subsequently responding to lithium therapy. The authors advise that patients should be screened for episodes of hypomania and mania by their physician before the recommendation of SJW for depression.

A brief French report, drawn from the official Marseilles pharmacovigilance database, described a 32-year-old man with a history of depression who added SJW "mother tincture" to his regimen of venlaxafine.[161] In herbal pharmacy practice, "mother tincture" refers to 1:10 hydroethanolic extract of crude fresh herb. After 3 days of SJW at 200 drops three times daily, the patient developed symptoms of anxiety, hyperhydrosis, and tremor. These reversed on cessation of the SJW tincture. The authors note that the normal dose of this type of SJW preparation is 160 drops total per day, and the dose taken was 600 drops, more than triple the recommended level. The symptoms, however, do correspond to those described for mild SS. Venlafaxine is also a potent inhibitor not only of serotonin reuptake, but also of dopamine, which might make it more prone to interact with the pan-neurotransmitter reuptake inhibitor effects of SJW.

Integrative Therapeutics, Clinical Concerns, and Adaptations

The nature of the SJW-SRI interaction remains controversial, although enhanced serotonin effects appear probable under some circumstances. Further data are required before the mechanisms, incidence, and clinical significance can be adequately characterized. Physicians and psychiatrists experienced in psychopharmacology are usually aware of potential drug-drug interactions. The notoriety of SJW as a potential interactor with antidepressants is well known among mental health professionals, many of whom prescribe SJW alone as first-line therapy for mild depression, particularly in Europe.[85]

At a professional level, SJW coadministered for specific therapeutic goals does not present significant problems, given appropriate monitoring. Specifically, SJW may be used empirically before starting pharmaceutical antidepressant therapy, or it may be used to assist tapered withdrawal from antidepressant therapy, particularly with SSRIs, which are subject to withdrawal symptoms of varying severity. An alternative viewpoint adopted by some providers is to "err on the side of caution," refrain from using SJW to support withdrawal, and only commence herbal therapy following a suitable washout period after cessation of the SRI, usually 3 weeks. Polypharmacy presents challenges that are unpredictable, as illustrated in the report by Spinella and Eaton[162] involving ginkgo, SJW, fluoxetine, and buspirone (see Buspirone later).

Simvastatin and Related HMG-COA Reductase Inhibitors (Statins)

Evidence: Simvastatin (Zocor).

Extrapolated, based on similar properties: Atorvastatin (Lipitor), lovastatin (Altocor, Altoprev, Mevacor); combination drug: lovastatin and niacin (Advicor); simvastatin combination drug: simvastatin and extended-release nicotinic acid (Niaspan).

Similar properties but evidence indicating no or reduced interaction effects: Fluvastatin (Lescol, Lescol XL), pravastatin (Pravachol), rosuvastatin (Crestor).

Interaction Type and Significance

◈ **Impaired Drug Absorption and Bioavailability, Negligible Effect**

Probability:
3. Possible

Evidence Base:
○ **Preliminary**

Effect and Mechanism of Action

Simvastatin is a prodrug and cosubstrate for 3A4 and P-gp. Serum levels of active metabolite may be lowered by concomitant administration with SJW because of the induction of drug efflux and metabolism. Clinical effects of the interaction have not been established. Different statins are metabolized quite differently, and the interaction cannot be extrapolated to all 3-hydroxy-3-methylglutaryl–coenzyme A (HMG-CoA) reductase inhibitors as a class.

Research

A single, small, double-blind crossover trial used two groups of eight healthy volunteers to investigate the effects of SJW versus placebo pretreatment on single-dose simvastatin (10 mg) and pravastatin (20 mg) kinetics. SJW was administered at 300 mg three times daily for 14 days and 24-hour blood samples taken. No changes were found for pravastatin, but the active metabolite simvastatin hydroxy acid (SVA) showed a significant decrease in AUC after SJW compared with placebo.[163] Simvastatin, lovastatin, and atorvastatin are all similar lactone prodrugs and cosubstrates of P-gp and 3A4, showing similar responses to 3A4/P-gp inhibitors such as itraconazole. CYP3A4 is probably only involved with a minor degree of transformation of pravastatin and fluvastatin, neither of which are prodrugs, and which do not appear to affect P-gp.[164]

Clinical Implications and Adaptations

Lowering of SVA levels by concomitant administration with SJW suggests theoretically that lipid-lowering targets may not be achieved because of underexposure to the drug. Clinical data are not available and would not necessarily be expected to emerge from case reports, given other known issues for statin therapy failure, such as poor long-term compliance. Duration of SJW administration, if taken for mild depression indications, can be many months, and statin therapy is often similarly continued for extended periods. If long-term coadministration is proposed, statins such as pravastatin or fluvastatin should be selected because these do not share the 3A4/P-gp characteristics of simvastatin and lovastatin. Newer statin drugs such as rosuvastatin have different P450/P-gp characteristics and may also be selected over simvastatin or lovastatin.

Tacrolimus

Tacrolimus (FK-506, fujimycin; Prograf).

Interaction Type and Significance

✗✗✗ Potentially Harmful or Serious Adverse Interaction—Avoid

◇◇◇ Impaired Drug Absorption and Bioavailability, Avoidance Necessary

Probability:
1. Certain

Evidence Base:
◉ Emerging

Effect and Mechanism of Action

Tacrolimus is a macrolide immunosuppressant that is a dual substrate of P-gp and 3A4, both of which are induced by SJW. Addition of SJW to previously stable tacrolimus regimens will result in significant reductions in serum drug levels and the risk of therapeutic failure and nephrotoxicity because of its narrow therapeutic and toxicological indices.

Reports

A single case report suggested that a renal graft patient previously stable on tacrolimus took SJW, 600 mg once daily for a month, and serum drug levels were depressed, reversing after cessation of the herb.[165]

Research

Two studies have confirmed this important interaction. A small preclinical "before and after" investigation on 10 healthy volunteers examined tacrolimus single oral doses before and after 18 days of SJW administration at 300 mg three times daily. Oral tacrolimus clearance was significantly increased by 59% and AUC significantly reduced by 50% after SJW administration.[166] Mai et al.[167] studied a case series of renal graft patients stable on a combination of tacrolimus and mycophenolic acid to examine the effects of adding SJW (300 mg twice daily, a lower-than-usual dose); after 14 days of SJW administration, tacrolimus levels decreased significantly from 180 to 75.9 ng/mL/hour. The median dose adjustment of tacrolimus to correct the herb induction effects was almost double, from 4.8 to 8.0 mg once daily.[167] Mycophenolic acid levels were unaffected.

Clinical Implications and Adaptations

The tacrolimus interaction is analogous to that of SJW-cyclosporine, as discussed earlier. Both agents are used in allograft patients for suppression of cell-mediated immunity, and the risks of therapeutic failure (acute graft rejection) are potentially fatal. Clinical case reports of rejection reactions caused by SJW interactions with tacrolimus are lacking. Whether this is caused by widespread avoidance of coadministration following publicity of the SJW-cyclosporine interaction is unknown.[63] The nephrotoxicity of tacrolimus is high, and upward adjustment of dose to compensate for pharmacokinetically induced increases on oral clearance will increase risks of toxicity.[165] This toxicity potential as well as the increased financial cost of higher dose regimens suggests that despite the theoretical possibility of steady-state coadministration with SJW being managed using routine serum monitoring of drug levels, in practice this is not a feasible option, and the combination should be avoided.

Verapamil and Related Calcium Channel Blockers

Evidence: Verapamil (Calan, Calan SR, Covera-HS, Isoptin, Isoptin SR, Verelan, Verelan PM).

Extrapolated, based on similar properties: Amlodipine (Norvasc); combination drug: amlodipine and benazepril (Lotrel); bepridil (Bapadin, Vascor), diltiazem (Cardizem, Cardizem CD, Cardizem SR, Cartia XT, Dilacor XR, Diltia XT, Tiamate, Tiazac), felodipine (Plendil), combination drugs: felodipine and enalapril (Lexxel), felodipine and ramipril (Triapin); gallopamil (D600), isradipine (DynaCirc, DynaCirc CR), lercanidipine (Zanidip), nicardipine (Cardene, Cardene I.V., Cardene SR), nifedipine (Adalat, Adalat CC, Nifedical XL, Procardia, Procardia XL); combination drug: nifedipine and atenolol (Beta-Adalat, Tenif); nimodipine (Nimotop), nisoldipine (Sular), nitrendipine (Cardif, Nitrepin); verapamil combination drug: verapamil and trandolapril (Tarka).

Interaction Type and Significance

✗ Potential or Theoretical Adverse Interaction of Uncertain Severity

◇◇ Impaired Drug Absorption and Bioavailability, Precautions Appropriate

Probability:
2. Probable

Evidence Base:
○ Preliminary

Effect and Mechanism of Action

A pharmacokinetic interaction between SJW and verapamil may be by induction of presystemic drug metabolism at the intestinal mucosa by SJW. The interaction is experimentally confirmed with verapamil, but clinical reports are lacking to date. The interaction is likely to occur with related calcium channel blockers, most of which are substrates of CYP450 3A4.

Research

A pharmacokinetic study used a jejunal perfusion technique to examine the pharmacokinetics of racemic verapamil before and after SJW treatment (14 days, 300 mg three times daily) in eight healthy volunteers.[168] By comparing the levels of verapamil and its 3A4 metabolite norverapamil in perfusate and plasma, the investigators were able to localize the site and mechanism of the interaction. They concluded that the notable reduction in AUC (approximately 80%) of both *R*- and *S*-enantiomers of verapamil after pretreatment with the herb was caused by presystemic metabolism by 3A4, primarily at the intestinal wall.

Clinical Implications and Adaptations

Verapamil is a well-known substrate of 3A4, as are the majority of calcium channel blockers. *R*-/*S*-verapamil is also metabolized to some extent by 2C9 and by 2E1, unlike most other calcium channel blockers. Verapamil is also an inhibitor of 3A4, although not as potent as diltiazem. The related calcium channel blocker mibefradil was withdrawn because of the severity of its 3A4 and 2D6 inhibition-related adverse interaction effects. Verapamil is also an inhibitor of P-gp. The single available study does not illuminate the kinetics of sustained in vivo coadministration of SJW and the drug, and predicting the net results of combined autoinhibition of 3A4 and P-gp by the drug, with SJW induction of the same metabolic factors, is problematic.

Verapamil is well known in the conventional literature to exhibit metabolic interactions with digoxin, beta blockers, antineoplastic agents, and alcohol. Theoretically, coadministration with SJW may increase drug levels required for management of the condition, typically angina (including variant or Prinzmetal's angina), hypertension, atrial flutter or fibrillation, and supraventricular tachycardia. At present, given the lack of reports of the interaction, normal standards of vigilance and monitoring relating to calcium channel blocker polypharmacy are probably adequate until evidence to the contrary becomes available.

Voriconazole and Related Triazole Antifungal Agents

Evidence: Voriconazole (Vfend).
Extrapolated, based on similar properties: Fluconazole (Diflucan), itraconazole (Sporanox), posaconazole (Noxafil).

Interaction Type and Significance

✗ **Potential or Theoretical Adverse Interaction of Uncertain Severity**

◇◇ **Impaired Drug Absorption and Bioavailability, Precautions Appropriate**

Probability:
2. Probable

Evidence Base:
○ Preliminary

Effect and Mechanism of Action

A pharmacokinetic interaction between SJW and voriconazole, which are metabolized by CYP450 3A4, 2C9, and 2C19, resulting in a lowering of drug levels due to enzyme induction by SJW. The interaction is experimentally confirmed, but clinical reports are lacking to date.

Research

Rengelshausen et al.[37] examined the disposition of single doses of voriconazole in 16 healthy male volunteers stratified by CYP2C19 genotype on day 1 and day 15 of concomitant SJW administration (300 mg three times daily, extract LI160). They found an overall decrease in AUC at day 15 of up to 59%, broadly equivalent to the effect of SJW on tacrolimus and cyclosporine. In addition, they found that 2C19 wild type (extensive metabolizer) exhibited the lowest exposure to the antifungal drug. The clearance data revealed an initial but insignificant increase in plasma levels of the drug after onset of SJW administration. This is a predictable result of the "biphasic" effect of SJW flavonoids mechanistically inhibiting CYP450, followed by a more potent effect of induction (see Effects on Drug Metabolism and Bioavailability).[38]

Clinical Implications and Adaptations

The novel antifungal voriconazole is used in patients with invasive aspergillosis and other serious fungal invasions. Therapeutic dosing is critical and, in SJW coadministration, should be avoided. The manufacturer's data on voriconazole do not recommend 2C19 phenotyping, although the wild-type polymorphism would appear to be at risk for lowered drug exposure.

Warfarin and Oral Vitamin K Antagonist Anticoagulants

Evidence: Phenprocoumon (Jarsin, Marcumar), warfarin (Coumadin, Marevan, Warfilone).
Extrapolated, based on similar properties: Anisindione (Miradon), dicumarol, ethyl biscoumacetate (Tromexan), nicoumalone (acenocoumarol; Acitrom, Sintrom), phenindione (Dindevan).

Interaction Type and Significance

✗✗ **Minimal to Mild Adverse Interaction—Vigilance Necessary**

Probability:
5. Improbable

Evidence Base:
▽ **Mixed**

Effect and Mechanism of Action

This suggested pharmacokinetic interaction could result in a pharmacodynamic decrease in the international normalized ratio (INR) because of lowered drug levels. Theoretically, the risk is decreased anticoagulation, but clinical reports of thrombosis caused by coadministration are lacking. The incidence and significance of the interaction are not established.

Research

A poster study examined the kinetics of single-dose oral phenprocoumon after SJW administration in 10 healthy males age 18 to 50 years.[169] SJW was given at 300 mg three times daily for 10 days, and the dose of phenprocoumon was 12 mg on day 11. AUC of phenprocoumon was significantly decreased ($p = 0.0007$) in the SJW group. Phenprocoumon is a warfarin analog unavailable in the United States but widely used in Europe. It is pharmacodynamically identical in action to warfarin but is well known to have different pharmacokinetics, its half-life being considerably longer than that of warfarin.[170] As with *S*-warfarin, it is metabolized by 2C9, but evidence indicates that the active sites on the 2C9 enzyme are different for warfarin and phenprocoumon, which may account for the difference in kinetics.[171] Currently available direct evidence suggests SJW in vivo lacks effect on either 1A2 or 2C9.[26] Cott[89] suggested that P-gp effects may cause a reduction in absorption at the enterocyte level, resulting in reduced drug levels. Circumstantial support for this hypothesis comes from a rodent model in which oral warfarin levels were reduced after

SJW treatment, but hepatic microsomal levels of CYP450 were unaltered.[172]

A human study examining warfarin pharmacogenomics showed that a specific haplotype for ABC1 (the *mdr*1 gene encoding for P-gp) was consistently overexpressed in a "low-dose" warfarin group; at present, however, it is not clear whether warfarin isomers are substrates of P-gp transporters or other, as-yet uncharacterized transporters.[173] It is known that the principal pharmacogenetic determinants of variability in warfarin kinetics are older age and the common 2C9 polymorphisms, 2C9*2 and 2C9*3.[174-177] A subsequent open-label trial examined the effects of ginseng and SJW pretreatment on warfarin kinetics in 12 healthy volunteers, using laboratory parameters (INR, derived from prothrombin time) and pharmacokinetic data (plasma levels of *S*- and *R*-enantiomers of warfarin and urinary *S*-7-hydroxywarfarin levels). Pretreatment with SJW resulted in significant effects on clearance of warfarin and reduction in INR.[178] However, the INR changes were a mean of 21%, well below the value suggested by Wells et al.[179] for "level 1 evidence" of a substantive interaction between warfarin and another agent. The ginseng pretreatment had no effect.

Reports

The only available and often-cited report of warfarin-SJW interaction is a case series summarized in a 2000 letter to the *Lancet* from Yue and colleagues[150] of the Swedish Medical Products Agency in a correspondence generated by the commentary on SJW safety by Ernst.[10] The series involved seven patients (six elderly, three male and four female) who apparently experienced reductions in previously stable INR after starting SJW (preparation, dose, and duration unspecified). None of the patients experienced thromboembolic episodes, and dose adjustment or cessation of herb apparently restabilized INR in all cases, although details were not given. Fugh-Berman and Ernst[11] later reviewed this report in their survey of interaction report reliability and found the Swedish reports scored "unreliable" and were effectively unevaluable. In an original and rigorous literature survey of warfarin drug-food interactions, Wells et al.[179] suggested that because of the variability of warfarin responses, only twofold INR changes (i.e., 50% or 200% stable value) should be admitted as "level 1 evidence" of an interaction on warfarin induced by another agent. In fact, three of seven INR values in the Swedish series met this criterion. However, comedications, comorbidities, and patient histories, as well as dose, preparation form, and duration of SJW administration, were not recorded, and the report must remain classified as unreliable.[11]

Clinical Implications and Adaptations

The absence of reliable reports of the interaction, especially given that warfarin is the most widely prescribed anticoagulant in the Western world and SJW remains a popular herbal medication, suggests that the interaction has minimal clinical significance, if it indeed exists. The phenprocoumon trial indicates some effect in younger healthy patients, but the use of this drug in Germany (Jarsin) has not been associated with adverse reports in combination with SJW, at an incidence level of two cases per million prescriptions of Jarsin, according to figures given at a recent ESCOP symposium.[180] If SJW has an induction effect on warfarin pharmacokinetics, there may be some reduction in drug levels if SJW is added to stably warfarinized patients. The degree of INR change is probably relatively small, about 20%, according to available preclinical data (males). Because INR monitoring is essential as a concomitant of warfarin therapy, however, management of coadministration should theoretically present no problems if monitoring procedures are maintained or increased, with dose-adjustment

corrections made accordingly. Discontinuation of SJW from a stable regimen of coadministration would be more critical, potentially resulting in excessive anticoagulation and the risk of bleeds. However, this appears to be a theoretical concern at present, particularly compared to the many known determinants of anticoagulation variability in response to warfarin, from 2C9 polymorphisms through dietary factors and numerous drug-drug interactions.

THEORETICAL, SPECULATIVE, AND PRELIMINARY INTERACTIONS RESEARCH, INCLUDING OVERSTATED INTERACTIONS CLAIMS

Buspirone

Buspirone (Buspar).

In a survey of SJW interactions by Izzo,[13] buspirone-SJW was listed as an interaction. This was based on an isolated case report by Spinella and Eaton,[162] reporting "hypomania" after the addition of both SJW and ginkgo to buspirone. The patient was in fact comedicated with fluoxetine, and paradoxical interactions between fluoxetine and buspirone have been recorded in the conventional drug literature, including adverse reactions, the mechanism of which is not understood.[111] Although buspirone is metabolized by CYP3A4, the interaction cannot be reliably deduced from this report. Fluoxetine is also well known to precipitate manic episodes in patients with bipolar disorders misdiagnosed as unipolar depressive disorders.

Chlorzoxazone

Chlorzoxazone (Paraflex, Parafon Forte, Relaxazone, Remular-S).

The antispasmodic skeletal muscle relaxant chlorzoxazone is metabolized exclusively by CYP2E1 and used experimentally as a probe for phenotyping poor and fast metabolizing expressions of this enzyme. The recent investigation of the effect of several herbs on P450 phenotyping probes by Gurley et al.[22] was the first demonstration of a possible in vivo induction of 2E1 by SJW using chlorzoxazone as a probe drug. Interactions of the drug are rare, and human case reports are lacking. The induction of 2E1 by SJW appears unlikely to constitute a clinically significant interaction. The effect of SJW is probably no greater than induction of 2E1 by chronic ethanol consumption or tobacco use. The most significant established interaction involving induction of 2E1 is in the production of *N*-acetyl-*p*-benzoquinone imine (NAPQI), the hepatotoxic metabolite of acetaminophen. NAPQI is produced when acetaminophen intoxication exceeds available glutathione stores and is metabolized by 2E1 instead of glutathione-*S*-transferase, resulting in fulminant hepatic failure. At present, however, the SJW-chlorzoxazone interaction is overstated, and potential for SJW involvement in acetaminophen hepatotoxicity remains conjectural.

Loperamide

Loperamide (Imodium A-D, Imodium A-D Caplets, Kaopectate 1-D, Maalox Anti-Diarrheal, Pepto Diarrhea Control).

Loperamide is an opioid derivative lacking central nervous system (CNS) effects that is used for treatment of diarrhea. It is metabolized by CYP3A4 and is a substrate of P-gp (thus does not cross the blood-brain barrier). A letter described a single case of delirium in a 39-year-old woman with a history of migraines and depression, apparently stable on a regimen of "two tablets of St. John's wort and a valerian tablet daily" (preparation and dose not specified) for 6 months. She was admitted to the emergency room in a confused, disoriented state. She was afebrile and tachycardic with elevated blood pressure, and a toxicology screen was positive for opioids. Subsequent history revealed she had taken loperamide for diarrhea. The patient had a previous history of admission because of Demerol (meperidine) intoxication. The authors suggested that the interaction was a MAOI type between SJW and loperamide.[181] This is speculation unsupported by the known pharmacology of SJW; further aspects of the report are "unreliable" in that doses of SJW and loperamide were not given, and the access of the patient to Demerol and her history of drug use increase the possibility of covert meperidine use. Pharmacokinetic interaction with SJW can be ruled out; it would have decreased rather than increased drug toxicity. Nonetheless, this speculative interaction is usually included without comment in secondary reviews.[78]

Monoamine Oxidase (MAO) Inhibitors

MAO-A inhibitors: Isocarboxazid (Marplan), moclobemide (Aurorix, Manerix), phenelzine (Nardil), procarbazine (Matulane), tranylcypromine (Parnate).
MAO-B inhibitors: Selegiline (deprenyl, L-deprenil, L-deprenyl; Ataptryl, Carbex, Eldepryl, Jumex, Movergan, Selpak); pargyline (Eutonyl), rasagiline (Azilect).

Early recommendations that SJW should not be coadministered with MAO inhibitors were based on extrapolation of putative MAOI and catechol-O-methyltransferase (COMT) activity from in vitro studies, which have not been substantiated experimentally or demonstrated in vivo (see Strategic Considerations earlier). In a survey, 862 psychiatrists in Australia and New Zealand were questioned about SJW use and adverse effects. No cases of hypertension were noted, although two (<1%) claimed reports of palpitations as an adverse effect of SJW alone. Five reports of interaction with moclobemide were noted, but these could not be evaluated due to lack of details.[85]

There is a brief report of otherwise-unexplainable hypertension associated with prescribed SJW alone (Ze 1117, 250 mg twice daily for 1 week) that reversed on cessation of the herb. The herb was self-prescribed for stress, and the patient lacked previous cardiovascular history and took no other drugs.[182] The correspondent speculatively attributed this episode to norepinephrine uptake inhibition by SJW. Another case described a 41-year-old man admitted to the emergency room with confusion, disorientation, tachycardia, and hypertension (blood pressure, 210/140) who was negative for toxicology screen and numerous other laboratory and diagnostic tests, which ruled out pathological causes. He apparently took no concurrent medications or nutritional supplements. History revealed use of SJW (dose and preparation not specified) and consumption of cheese and red wine immediately before the episode.[183] This report is the only one suggesting a tyramine food interaction with SJW, but unfortunately the dose and preparation of the herb (and possible other ingredients) were not identified, and thus the report is not evaluable. At this time, advice to avoid tyramine-containing foods with SJW seems unnecessary.

Photosensitizing Agents

Delta-aminolevulinic acid (d-ALA)
Phototoxicity is frequently suggested as a possible adverse effect of SJW, although published human case reports are lacking. According to official German adverse drug interaction (ADR) data reviewed by Schulz,[86] reversible skin photosensitization responses have been reported at a rate of less than one per 300,000 doses of SJW between October 1991 and December 1999, during which an estimated 8 million patients were treated

with SJW. Hypericin, the naphthodianthrone constituent of SJW, in fact exhibits photodynamic properties, and it has been used in oncological research as an investigational cytotoxic agent in photodynamic therapy (PDT) and as an imaging agent in photodiagnosis (PD).[184]

Delta-aminolevulinic acid (d-ALA) is a precursor compound used to enhance endogenous synthesis of the photosensitizer protoporphyrin IX through the heme pathway. There is one report of a possible interaction between d-ALA and SJW in a dermatological case in which excessive skin erythema occurred after topical irradiation.[185] Currently, these uses of ALA are confined to specialized clinical environments.[186] If the photosensitizer d-ALA becomes more generally used in photodynamic imaging studies, potential interactions with SJW should be considered, and avoidance may be prudent pending further data.

Theophylline/Aminophylline

Theophylline/aminophylline (Phyllocontin, Slo-Bid, Slo-Phyllin, Theo-24, Theo-Bid, Theocron, Theo-Dur, Theolair, Truphylline, Uni-Dur, Uniphyl); combination drug: ephedrine, guaifenesin, and theophylline (Primatene Dual Action).

Several secondary sources have repeated a suggested interaction between theophylline and SJW. However, the suggestion is derived from a single case reported in a letter from Nebel et al.[187] in 1999. Theophylline is metabolized by CYP1A2 and has a relatively narrow therapeutic index in that toxicity can arise from marginally supranormal plasma levels. The patient in the case report smoked half a pack of cigarettes daily (tobacco smoke induces 1A2 via the arylcarbon receptor) and was taking 11 concurrent prescription medications, including the leukotriene antagonist zafirlukast, which is a 1A2 inhibitor and interacts with theophylline.[111] Other medications included morphine, amitriptyline, valproate, and zolpidem. With a polypharmaceutical regimen that includes multiple substrates, inducers, and inhibitors of multiple metabolic enzymes and transporters, several of which are known to interact with each other, the report is unevaluable as evidence of a putative SJW-theophylline interaction, despite the authors' suggestion that theophylline levels increased after cessation of SJW (dose and preparation unrecorded).

A recent study by Morimoto et al.[188] has confirmed the lack of clinically significant interaction with theophylline. After 15 days of pretreatment with 300 mg SJW three times daily, healthy Japanese male volunteers showed no significant change in urinary concentrations of theophylline or its metabolites after a single 400-mg oral dose.

The 188 citations for this monograph are located under St. John's Wort on the CD at the back of the book.

Turmeric/Curcumin

Botanical Name: *Curcuma longa* L.
Pharmacopoeial Name: Curcumae longae rhizome.
Synonym: *Curcuma domestica* Valeton.
Common Names: Turmeric, Indian saffron.

Summary

Drug/Class Interaction Type	Mechanism and Significance	Management
Bleomycin Cytotoxic antibiotics ⊕/☼	Herb may reduce drug-induced pulmonary toxicity. Clinical significance not established.	Consider coadministration only under specialist professional management.
Cisplatin Platinum chemotherapy compounds ⊕	Herb may reduce drug-induced renal and neurotoxicities. Clinical significance not established.	Consider coadministration only under specialist professional management.
Cyclophosphamide Alkylating agents ?	Herb may reduce drug-induced toxicity but may also reduce effectiveness of drug. Conflicting data; clinical significance not established.	Avoid until further data available.
Cyclosporine Immunosuppressive agents ⊕✗/◇◇/⊕	Herb may enhance immunosuppressive efficacy of drug, but also risks possible reduction in drug bioavailability. Clinical significance not established.	Consider coadministration only under specialist professional management with serum monitoring of drug levels.
Doxorubicin Anthracycline chemotherapy ?/⊕✗	Herb protects against and reduces drug-induced cardiotoxicity and may reduce drug-induced resistance. Effect on drug efficacy controversial. Clinical significance not established.	Avoid coadministration, until further data available. Consider before and after chemotherapy.
Ethanol ☼/⊕⊕	Herb reduces alcohol-related pathologies in liver, pancreas, and central nervous system. Clinical significance not established.	Incorporate into natural treatment protocols for alcohol-related conditions.
Indomethacin Nonsteroidal anti-inflammatory drugs (NSAIDs) ⊕/☼	Herb may reduce incidence and promote healing of drug-induced gastric ulceration. Clinical trial suggests turmeric no different than antacids for healing ulcers.	Consider coadministration with ulcerogenic NSAIDs to prevent gastropathies.
Paclitaxel Taxanes ⊕	Herb may chemosensitize malignant cells to drug. Clinical significance not established.	Consider coadministration only under specialist professional management.
Vinblastine Vinca alkaloids ⊕	Herb may reduce drug resistance by inhibition of efflux mechanisms.	Consider coadministration only under specialist professional management.

HERB DESCRIPTION

Family

Zingiberaceae.

Related Species

Curcuma aromatica Salisbury, *Curcuma xanthorrhiza* Roxb.

Habitat and Cultivation

Native to tropical zones in India and Southeast Asia; cultivated for culinary and medicinal purposes for many centuries; now imported principally from India, China, and Indonesia.

Parts Used

Rhizome.

Common Forms

Dried: Rhizome, powdered.
Oleoresin or essential oil.
Tincture, Fluid Extract: Dried or fresh rhizome, 45% ethanol.

Standardized Extract: Solid extracts, concentrated and standardized to 95% curcuminoids, as curcumin.

Note: Experimental studies often use purified laboratory-grade diferuloylmethane or curcumin-I only; semisynthetic derivatives are also available.

HERB IN CLINICAL PRACTICE

Overview

Although in medicinal use in Asia for more than a millennium, turmeric is probably better known in the West as a common yellow spice from the ginger family, used as a pungent flavoring ingredient in curries, which is also widely used in the U.S. food industry as a coloring agent. Until recently, Western medicine viewed turmeric primarily as a spice with minor aromatic digestive stimulant and hepatic stimulant properties, indicated but little used for functional hepatobiliary disorders. In 1985 the German Commission E approved "Turmeric Root" for dyspeptic conditions,[1] although the herb was absent from both the 1983 and the 1996 edition of the *British Herbal Pharmacopoeia*. The World Health Organization (WHO) monograph repeats the Commission E indications.[2]

Pharmacological investigations into the anticancer and anti-inflammatory properties of the herb and its constituents began to attract research interest in the 1980s. Currently, curcumin is regarded as a natural compound of great interest and of considerable therapeutic potential because of its multiple properties, which include antioxidant, anti-inflammatory, chemopreventive, antimutagenic, anticarcinogenic, antimetastatic, antiangiogenic, and cardioprotective activities. Although this research currently constitutes a rapidly expanding body of literature, a 2003 therapeutic monograph on turmeric by the European Scientific Cooperative on Phytotherapy (ESCOP)[3] echoes the original 1985 Commission E indications for "symptomatic treatment of mild digestive disturbances and minor biliary dysfunction." Aggarwal et al.[4] recently reviewed the chemopreventive and anticancer molecular biology of curcumin. The majority of recent scientific studies on turmeric employed purified laboratory-grade diferuloylmethane or curcumin-I, which should be noted before extrapolating to mixtures of curcuminoids or to crude whole-herb extracts.

Historical/Ethnomedicine Precedent

In Ayurveda, turmeric is used internally for digestive problems and is considered a blood purifier and antimicrobial. Externally it is used for skin problems, as well as for sprains and strains. The powdered herb is often administered in a base of dietary ingredients, such as milk or honey, or in slaked lime for topical applications.[5] In classical Chinese medicine, turmeric invigorates the *xue* (blood) and relieves pain, especially related to liver *(Gan);* it clears heat and cools the blood, clears the heart *(Xin)* (which helps with psychological problems), and benefits the gallbladder *(Dan)* and treats jaundice.[6]

Known or Potential Therapeutic Uses

Abdominal pain, adjunctive cancer treatment, antimicrobial, arthritis, cardiovascular disease prophylaxis, chemoprevention, chemosensitization, cholestasis, dyspepsia, ethanol-related hepatic conditions, hyperlipidemia, inflammation, jaundice, radiosensitization.
Topically for skin conditions, sprains, and strains.

Key Constituents

Curcuminoids (diferuloylmethanes), including curcumin and its methoxylated derivatives (2%-5%), are the yellow pigments and principal actives. Sometimes designated as curcumins I to IV: I, curcumin; II, desmethoxycurcumin; III, bisdesmethoxycurcumin; and IV, cyclocurcumin.
Essential oil (3% and 5%), including sesquiterpene ketones and monoterpenes.

Therapeutic Dosing Range

Powdered Rhizome: Up to 12 g daily by decoction.
Tincture, Fluid Extract: 5 to 15 mL daily (as 1:1 equivalent).
Standardized Extract: Equivalent of 400 to 600 mg curcumin three times daily.

INTERACTIONS REVIEW
Strategic Considerations

No interactions with prescription drugs are noted in the available therapeutic monographs on turmeric. Both Western and

Chinese herbal authorities have advised using caution when coadministering turmeric with antiplatelet or anticoagulant drugs and avoiding higher doses of the herb in such settings.[7,8] No interaction with anticoagulant or antiplatelet medications has been reported clinically or described experimentally, and the suggested interaction is classified here as "overstated/speculative" (see Theoretical, Speculative, and Preliminary Interactions Research).

The primary clinical context for current use of curcumin extracts is inflammatory conditions and the integrative oncology setting. Curcumin has innumerable effects on a wide range of signal transduction pathways and molecular targets affecting cell growth, multiplication, differentiation, and apoptosis, including inhibition of nuclear factor kappa B (NF-κB) and activating protein-1 (AP-1).[4,9-13] Experimental evidence is emerging for potential interactions with a variety of cytotoxic drugs, as well as radiotherapy. A novel interactions issue, unaddressed by research to date, is how curcumin, known to inhibit a number of molecular targets involved in angiogenesis, including vascular endothelial growth factor (VEGF), might interact with the newer generation of antiangiogenic agents such as the monoclonal antibody bevacizumab (Avastin).[14,15] Despite the rapidly expanding basic science research on the molecular targets affected by curcumin, extrapolation to clinical settings is problematic given the lack of large-scale trial evidence. Curcumin is incorporated with other natural compounds into adjunctive anticancer protocols on an anecdotal clinical basis, and preliminary data support synergistic combination of curcumin with genistein.[16-18]

Although several potentially beneficial interactions with chemotherapeutic agents are listed later, these interactions have not been well studied, particularly in vivo. One research group has questioned the advisability of combining curcumin with alkylating agents such as cyclophosphamide, which induces apoptosis through activation of Janus kinase (JNK), which may be inhibited by relatively low doses of curcumin.[19] The same authors raised concerns about the advisability of coadministering curcumin with chemotherapy agents, which increase activation of NF-κB. Even though this may reduce drug-induced NF-κB—mediated drug resistance, the activation of NF-κB may be an important (but not exclusive) part of the cytotoxic mechanism of these drugs (e.g., doxorubicin), although this study has been criticized.[20] However, until further data are available with respect to specific chemotherapy agents and specific malignancies, decisions regarding coadministration of curcumin with chemotherapy need to be made in conjunction with practitioners experienced in the integrative oncological setting. There is also evidence, not detailed here, that curcumin may have beneficial interactions with radiotherapies.[21-23]

Effects on Drug Metabolism and Bioavailability

Turmeric potentially exerts concerted effects on all three phases of drug metabolism. As with many herbs, the clinical implications of in vitro data remain to be established, and the interpretation of some studies is particularly controversial because of the extremely low bioavailability of curcumin. Biphasic effects have also been reported. In a Phase I study of 25 patients with various premalignant diagnoses, Cheng et al.[24] established that single oral doses of 8000 mg curcumin resulted in peak plasma concentrations of only 1.77. In colorectal adenocarcinoma patients who were administered curcumin for 7 days at 3600 mg/day, levels of curcumin were 2.5 times higher in malignant colorectal cells than in normal colon tissue, at 12.7 nmol/g in the form of sulfate and glucuronide conjugates. The effect of curcumin was to decrease levels of an oxidative deoxyribonucleic acid (DNA) adduct marker of cyclooxygenase-2 (COX-2) expression, which was not affected.[25,26] In a rodent model, Shoba et al.[27] showed that coadministration of piperine (20 mg/kg) with curcumin increased the bioavailability of the herb by a factor of 154% in a single-dose pharmacokinetic study; in humans, 20 mg piperinen increased the bioavailability of curcumin by 2000%.[27] The low bioavailability results from rapid glucuronidation both hepatically and directly at the intestinal wall.

Effects on cytochrome P450 (CYP450) enzymes have been documented. Two different research groups used a rodent hepatocyte model to demonstrate curcumin inhibited both the induction and the activity of CYP450 1A1and 1A2, 2B1 and 2B2, and 2E1.[28-30] The inhibitory effects were weak to moderate, except for 1A1/1A2, for which inhibition was more potent. These CYP450 enzymes are particularly related to metabolism of carcinogens, including the polycyclic aromatic hydrocarbons (PAHs). Using human oral mucosa cells and oral squamous cell carcinoma (SCC) cells, Rinaldi et al.[31] demonstrated induction of the nuclear translocation of the aryl hydrocarbon receptor (AhR), a process that leads to downstream activation of phase I and phase II AhR-responsive carcinogen-metabolizing enzymes. They also demonstrated increased CYP1A1 activity in oral SCC cells, combined with a decrease in carcinogen bioactivation, as well as an increase in intracellular reduced-glutathione (GSH) levels. The authors concluded that curcumin has a significant ability to modulate carcinogen activation in the human oral cavity. In a study by Raucy[32] using human hepatocytes, curcumin did not demonstrate any induction effects on CYP3A4, suggesting negligible interactions with the many drugs metabolized by this enzyme. Animal studies corroborate a significant effect of curcumin on phase II enzymes, particularly glutathione-S-transferase, and the ability of the curcuminoids to increase intracellular glutathione has been documented in several experimental models.[30,33,34]

Several studies have demonstrated pronounced inhibitory effects of curcumin on P-glycoprotein (P-gp) in several cell lines, with dose-dependent effects at concentrations between 1 and 15 micromolar (μM).[35,36] Anuchapreeda et al.[37] found that in human cervical carcinoma cells (KB-VI), pretreatment with curcumin at 1 to 10 μM for up to 72 hours significantly lowered MDR1 gene expression. Curcumin also inhibited rhodamine-123 efflux from these cells but had no effect on wild-type KB-3 cells that do not overexpress P-gp. The same research group later established that curcumin-I was the most effective inhibitory compound among the curcuminoids I to III, and that vinblastine sensitivity was increased in the homologous but drug-resistant KB-V1 line.[38] Nabekura et al.[36] established similar results for daunorubicin accumulation in the same drug-resistant cell line.

HERB-DRUG INTERACTIONS

Bleomycin

Bleomycin (Blenoxane).

Interaction Type and Significance
⊕ Potential or Theoretical Beneficial or Supportive
   Interaction, with Professional Management
☼ Prevention or Reduction of Drug Adverse Effect

Probability: Evidence Base:
4. Plausible   ○ Preliminary

Effect and Mechanism of Action
Curcumin reduces the characteristic bleomycin-induced pulmonary fibrosis toxicity, according to animal data. The mechanism is not understood but may result from antioxidant and anti-inflammatory effects of curcumin.

Research
Two studies using rodent models have demonstrated that oral curcumin pretreatment for 10 days before bleomycin, and continued during the drug treatment for up to 1 month, reduces pulmonary fibrosis, inflammation, and other markers of lung toxicity, including alveolar macrophage tumor necrosis factor alpha (TNF-α) release and superoxide and nitric oxide induction. Total lung hydroxyproline was also significantly reduced with curcumin coadministration. In both studies the oral doses of curcumin were high, 300 mg/kg/day and 550 nmol/kg/day.[39,40]

Clinical Implications and Integrative Therapeutics
Pulmonary fibrosis is a well-documented adverse effect of bleomycin. Data are lacking on whether curcumin will affect the cytotoxic action of bleomycin. However, because the agent is often administered in combination with doxorubicin and vinblastine, and in vitro data suggest these agents may be more effective with curcumin administration, it may be beneficial to incorporate curcumin as an adjuvant/protective in protocols such as ABVD (Adriamycin, Blenoxane, vinblastine, dacarbazine), but clinical trial support is unavailable.

Cisplatin and Related Platinum Chemotherapy Compounds

Evidence: Cisplatin (cis-diaminedichloroplatinum, CDDP; Platinol, Platinol-AQ).
Extrapolated, based on similar properties: Carboplatin (Paraplatin), oxaliplatin (Eloxatin).

Interaction Type and Significance
⊕ Potential or Theoretical Beneficial or Supportive
   Interaction

Probability: Evidence Base:
4. Plausible   ○ Preliminary

Effect and Mechanism of Action
Curcumin combined with cisplatin results in synergistic antitumor activity in experimental models.

Research
Navis et al.[41] analyzed tumor markers in liver and kidney homogenates of rats with experimentally induced fibrosarcoma that was treated with cisplatin or a cisplatin-curcumin combination versus controls. Cisplatin alone reduced the markers, but the effect of the combination was to restore markers to control levels. Notarbartolo et al.[42] examined the antitumor effects of curcumin alone and in combination with cisplatin on a hepatocellular carcinoma line that constitutively overexpressed NF-κB. They found a sequence-dependent synergy effect of the herb-drug combination on apoptosis, which depended on pretreatment with curcumin and was not observed during simultaneous coadministration. The effect was partially reversed by adding the antioxidant N-acetylcysteine (NAC) and involved caspase-dependent and caspase-independent mechanisms, as well as reduction in the gene expression of several inhibitor of apoptosis proteins (IAPs). Interestingly, the effects of curcumin alone on NF-κB were

temporally biphasic, with an initial increase followed by a decrease. The concentrations of curcumin that were effective ranged from 10 to 25 µM.

Clinical Implications and Integrative Therapeutics

Preliminary evidence suggests that curcumin pretreatment may act as a chemosensitizer to cisplatin therapy. The clinical significance of this potentially beneficial interaction, demonstrated in vitro for hepatocellular carcinoma, remains to be established.

Cyclophosphamide

Evidence: Cyclophosphamide (Cytoxan, Endoxana, Neosar, Procytox).

Extrapolated, based on similar properties: Irinotecan (camptothecin-11, CPT-11; Campto, Camptosar); bleomycin (Blenoxane; see earlier section).

Interaction Type and Significance

? Interaction Likely but Uncertain Occurrence and Unclear Implications

Probability:
4. Plausible

Evidence Base:
▽ Mixed

Effect and Mechanism of Action

An experimental reduction in cyclophosphamide-induced lung toxicity is likely mediated by the anti-inflammatory and antioxidant effects of curcumin. The interaction parallels that between bleomycin and curcumin. However, curcumin may reduce the effects of alkylating agent–induced apoptosis mediated through the JNK pathway.

Research

Venkatesan and Chandrakasan[43] used a rodent model to show that 7 days of pretreatment with curcumin in healthy rats prevented lung damage from one intraperitoneal dose of cyclophosphamide, measured by bronchopulmonary lavage fluid levels of angiotensin-converting enzyme (ACE), lactate dehydrogenase (LDH), alkaline phosphatase, lipid peroxide, glutathione, and ascorbate. Somasundaram et al.[19] questioned the advisability of combining curcumin with alkylating agents such as cyclophosphamide, which induces apoptosis through activation of the JNK pathway, based on preliminary in vivo rodent data. Using human MCF-7 and BT-474 breast cancer cells xenografted into nude mice, oral feeding of low doses of curcumin prevented cyclophosphamide (single dose intraperitoneally) from decreasing tumor size after 24 and 48 hours. This study has been criticized for the short duration of administration of both curcumin and cyclophosphamide and the low doses of curcumin used.[20] (See also Theoretical, Speculative, and Preliminary Interactions Research.)

Clinical Implications and Adaptations

Further research is needed to establish whether the potential reduction of cyclophosphamide toxicity by curcumin is demonstrable in vivo without any countervailing reduction of therapeutic effect of the compound.

Cyclosporine and Related Immunosuppressive Agents

Evidence: Cyclosporine (Ciclosporin, cyclosporin A, CsA; Neoral, Sandimmune, SangCya).

Extrapolated, based on similar properties: Mycophenolate (CellCept).

Interaction Type and Significance

⊕✗ **Bimodal or Variable Interaction, with Professional Management**

◇◇ **Impaired Drug Absorption and Bioavailability, Precautions Appropriate**

⊕ **Potential or Theoretical Beneficial or Supportive Interaction, with Professional Management**

Probability:
4. Plausible

Evidence Base:
○ Preliminary

Effect and Mechanism of Action

In a mixed pharmacodynamic and pharmacokinetic interaction, curcumin may enhance immunosuppressive activity of cyclosporine while reducing its bioavailability. The interaction has not been demonstrated clinically to date.

Research

Chueh et al.[44] used a rodent cardiac allograft model to demonstrate that curcumin could effectively synergize with cyclosporine. Curcumin alone prolonged survival time of allograft rats compared with controls, but when combined with subtherapeutic doses of cyclosporine, the recipient animals survived longer than those with curcumin alone. Cytokine analysis suggested reduced levels of interleukin-2 (IL-2), interferon gamma (IFN-γ), and granzyme B in both the combination and the curcumin-only animals versus controls. Ranjan et al.[45] showed in vitro with human lymphocytes that curcumin inhibits T-cell activation through the CD28/B7 co-stimulation pathway. This pathway is resistant to cyclosporine suppression and synergistic suppression of T-cell responses. In a later study the same group showed curcumin suppressed NF-κB–mediated IL-2 release in response to mitogen activation by various stimuli.[46]

Additional, if circumstantial, evidence for immunosuppressive effects comes from the ability of curcumin extracts to inhibit experimental allergic encephalomyelitis (a standard animal model of multiple sclerosis); this was mediated by interleukin-12–signaling blockade, resulting in decreased T-cell proliferation and T helper cell type 1 (Th1) differentiation.[47] A complication of any in vivo coadministration of cyclosporine with curcumin is that the drug is a substrate of P-gp, which is inhibited by curcumin, thus potentially decreasing bioavailability of cyclosporine. This was demonstrated, as an incidental finding, in an animal study examining the (lack of) effect of curcumin on cyclosporine-induced cholestasis and hypercholesterolemia.[48]

Clinical Implications, Adaptations, and Integrative Therapeutics

Insufficient data are available to establish the clinical significance of this interaction. However, given the practice of measuring serum values for cyclosporine concentration during immunosuppressive therapy, the problems of adjusting to pharmacokinetic variation caused by P-gp inhibition are theoretically manageable. At present, the beneficial effect of the combination shown experimentally remains to be confirmed by clinical studies. Other evidence suggests a renal-protective effect of curcumin, renal toxicity being a known effect of cyclosporine.

Jones and Shoskes[49] showed that several plant-derived compounds reversed renal ischemia and reperfusion injury induced by mycophenolate (CellCept). Coadministration should be considered only with profession management, including monitoring of serum cyclosporine levels by the transplant providers.

Doxorubicin and Related Anthracycline Chemotherapy

Evidence: Doxorubicin (Adriamycin, Rubex).
Extrapolated, based on similar properties: Daunorubicin (Cerubidine, DaunoXome), epirubicin (Ellence, Pharmorubicin), idarubicin (Idamycin, Zavedos), mitoxantrone (Novantrone, Onkotrone).
Similar properties but evidence lacking for extrapolation: Doxorubicin, pegylated liposomal (Caelyx, Doxil, Myocet).

Interaction Type and Significance

?   **Interaction Likely but Uncertain Occurrence and Unclear Implications**
⊕✗   **Bimodal or Variable Interaction, with Professional Management**

Probability: Evidence Base:
4. Plausible   ▽ **Mixed**

Effect and Mechanism of Action

In this complex multifactorial interaction, curcumin may reduce the known cardiotoxicity of doxorubicin and may also counter the development of drug resistance by inhibiting doxorubicin-induced NF-κB activation. However, curcumin may lower drug efficacy under some circumstances.

Research

Rodent studies demonstrated that both acute cardiotoxicity (measured by serum creatine kinase, LDH, and malondialdehyde levels) and nephrotoxicity (measured by proteinuria, albuminuria, hypolipemia, and urinary N-acetyl-β-glucosaminidase excretion) caused by single-dose intraperitoneal Adriamycin (30 mg/kg) were significantly reduced by oral curcumin pretreatment (200 mg/kg) 7 days before and 2 days after drug administration.[50,51] The mechanism likely involves antioxidant effects of the curcuminoids, particularly the lowering of lipid peroxidation in cardiomyocytes. Chuang et al.[52] used multiple human cancer cell lines to examine the various chemotherapeutic drugs clinically associated with the ability to induce drug resistance (doxorubicin, 5-fluorouracil, cisplatin, paclitaxel). Drug resistance was accompanied by transient increases in NF-κB. When doxorubicin (1 μM) was combined with curcumin (10 μM), NF-κB production was inhibited significantly more than by curcumin alone. The effect was not mediated by TNF-α, and the authors suggested that the effect of curcumin on NF-κB may be important in overcoming drug resistance. Other mechanisms, including glutathione-S-transferase modulation, may be important to the inhibition of doxorubicin resistance by curcumin.[53]

Another study provides conflicting data. Somasundaram et al.[19] found that doxorubicin-induced apoptosis of MCF-7 cells may be significantly reduced by curcumin at low levels in a time- and dose-dependent manner (1.0-10.0 μM). Because the curcumin concentrations used approach those found in human pharmacokinetic studies, the authors advise that patients with breast cancer (and other malignancies) should not concurrently use curcumin with chemotherapy until further investigations clarify the situation. These conclusions have been criticized as generalizations that disregard the methodology of the in vitro model, particularly the temporal kinetics based on very-short-term effects, low doses of curcumin, and a failure to account for the multifactorial mechanisms involved.[20] The issues remain unresolved.

Notarbartalo et al.[42] examined the complexity of this interaction in relation to the relative role of NF-κB and other factors using a hepatic cancer cell line. Messenger ribonucleic acid (mRNA) analysis suggested that expression of multiple genes in various pathways is modulated by the combination of agents, with effects that are in part additive and in part antagonistic.

Clinical Implications and Adaptations

Although the protective action of curcumin against doxorubicin toxicity is plausible, the effects on drug efficacy have been questioned. Extrapolations from limited in vitro data to clinical settings (especially on dose levels) are problematic, and further data are needed to characterize the interaction. Curcumin may in addition have a role in anthracycline protocols that have exhibited the emergence of drug resistance. Decisions whether to adopt concurrent use of curcumin will also likely depend on the role assigned to dietary antioxidants (vitamins A, C, and E; carotenoids) during anthracycline chemotherapy, itself a controversial topic.

Ethanol

Ethanol

Interaction Type and Significance

☼   **Prevention or Reduction of Drug Adverse Effect**
⊕⊕   **Beneficial or Supportive Interaction, with Professional Management**

Probability: Evidence Base:
1. Certain   ○ **Preliminary**

Effect and Mechanism of Action

In an experimentally demonstrated interaction, curcumin treatment prevents or reduces ethanol-induced toxicities in various organs and tissues (e.g., hepatic, neural, pancreatic) through multiple mechanisms.

Research

Rodent models of experimentally induced alcoholic liver disease demonstrate the efficacy of curcumin in prevention of ethanol-induced pathology.[54-56] Similar studies show related effects in ethanol-induced and non-ethanol-induced pancreatitis, as well as in ethanol-induced neural damage.[57,58] Along with several in vitro investigations, these studies reveal a variety of mechanisms involved in mediating the protective effects. These include suppression of NF-κB activated proinflammatory genes, including inducible nitric oxide synthase (iNOS) and COX-2, as well as antioxidant activity and matrix metalloproteinase (MMP) inhibition.[54,59-61]

Clinical Implications and Integrative Therapeutics

Turmeric extracts and curcumin may be useful adjuncts in the treatment of acute and chronic alcohol-related liver and pancreatic disease.

Indomethacin, Related Nonsteroidal Anti-Inflammatory Drugs (NSAIDs), and Other Ulcerogenic Substances

Evidence: Indomethacin (indometacin; Indocin, Indocin-SR).
Extrapolated, based on similar properties: NSAIDs:
  COX-1 inhibitors: Diclofenac (Cataflam, Voltaren), combination drug: diclofenac and misoprostol (Arthrotec), diflunisal (Dolobid), etodolac (Lodine), fenoprofen (Dalfon), furbiprofen (Ansaid), ibuprofen (Advil, Excedrin IB, Motrin, Motrin IB, Nuprin, Pedia Care Fever Drops, Provel, Rufen);

combination drug: hydrocodone and ibuprofen (Reprexain, Vicoprofen); ketoprofen (Orudis, Oruvail), ketorolac (Acular ophthalmic, Toradol), meclofenamate (Meclomen), mefenamic acid (Ponstel), meloxicam (Mobic), nabumetone (Relafen), naproxen (Aleve, Anaprox, Naprosyn), oxaprozin (Daypro), piroxicam (Feldene), salsalate (salicylic acid; Amigesic, Disalcid, Marthritic, Mono Gesic, Salflex, Salsitab), sulindac (Clinoril), tolmetin (Tolectin).

COX-2 inhibitor: Celecoxib (Celebrex).
Ethanol (see earlier section).

Interaction Type and Significance

⊕⊕ **Beneficial or Supportive Interaction, with Professional Management**
☼ **Prevention or Reduction of Drug Adverse Effect**

Probability:	Evidence Base:
1. Certain	○ **Preliminary**

Effect and Mechanism of Action

This interaction was serendipitously discovered while using indomethacin as an ulcerogenic agent in a rodent model of acute gastric ulceration. Curcumin prevents indomethacin ulceration and accelerates ulcer healing. The mechanism is multifactorial and includes suppression of MMP-9 and iNOS (regulated by NF-κB activation).

Research

In a rodent model, turmeric extracts at an oral dose of 500 mg/kg produced significant antiulcerogenic activity in animals subjected to a variety of ulcer-inducing agents, including indomethacin and reserpine.[62] The mechanism has recently been shown to involve the inhibition of MMP-9 and MMP-2.[63] A clinical open-label trial attempting to establish the efficacy of turmeric (1000 mg/day) compared with antacids in 50 patients over 6 weeks found that the antacid was superior to turmeric in inducing ulcer healing. However, this trial was not related to indomethacin-induced ulcers, and the mechanism may be relatively specific to ulcers caused by chemical agents (involving MMP-9 inhibition).

Clinical Implications and Integrative Therapeutics

This interaction has been cited as a demonstration of the anti-ulcerogenic effects of curcumin, but the available clinical trial evidence shows turmeric ineffective in healing gastric ulcers.[64] The interaction appears is specific to ulcers caused by iatrogenic agents such as NSAIDs. Involvement of the MMPs (especially MMP-9) would predict that curcumin likely has antimetastatic activity, which has indeed been demonstrated.[65] Similar mechanisms are involved in the protective effects of curcumin against ethanol-induced toxic damage. (See also previous ethanol-curcumin discussion.) If ulcerogenic drugs likely to induce gastropathic ulceration are administered chronically, turmeric coadministration would appear to be warranted, despite the lack of evidence for turmeric effect on stress ulcers.

Further evidence for the general applicability of these findings to iatrogenic mucosal damage is provided by a study of intestinal mucositis induced by methotrexate. The villous atrophy that resulted from methotrexate damage was partially inhibited by curcumin coadminstration.[23] This suggests a possible role for curcumin in the amelioration of cytotoxic chemotherapy-induced mucositis.

Paclitaxel and Related Taxanes

Evidence: Paclitaxel (Paxene, Taxol).
Extrapolated, based on similar properties: Docetaxel (Taxotere); paclitaxel, protein-bound (Abraxane).

Interaction Type and Significance

⊕ **Potential or Theoretical Beneficial or Supportive Interaction, with Professional Management**

Probability:	Evidence Base:
4. Plausible	○ **Preliminary**

Effect and Mechanism of Action

An experimentally demonstrated chemosensitization by curcumin to paclitaxel (Taxol)–induced cytotoxicity; the mechanism is independent of microtubule polymerization.

Research

Bava et al.[66] tested HeLa cells with paclitaxel (Taxol) alone and Taxol in combination with curcumin and found that the combination exerted synergistic effects on cell kill, and that this was accompanied by caspase activation and cytochrome c release. Taxol-induced NF-κB activity was reduced by curcumin coadministration. There appeared to be no effect on tubulin polymerization or cyclin-dependent CdC2 activation induced by Taxol.

Clinical Implications and Integrative Therapeutics

Coadministration of curcumin with taxanes may result in increased efficacy of the drug. Clinical trial support is not available. The known pharmacology of curcumin does not suggest interference with microtubule mechanisms affected by the taxane class of chemotherapy agents.

Vinblastine, Related Vinca Alkaloids, and Platinum Chemotherapy Compounds

Evidence: Vinblastine (Alkaban-AQ, Velban, Velsar).
Extrapolated, based on similar properties: Vincristine (Leurocristine, Oncovin, Vincasar PFS), vinorelbine (Navelbine); Platinum chemotherapy compounds: Carboplatin (Paraplatin), cisplatin (cis-diaminedichloroplatinum, CDDP; Platinol, Platinol-AQ), oxaliplatin (Eloxatin).

Interaction Type and Significance

⊕ **Potential or Theoretical Beneficial or Supportive Interaction, with Professional Management**

Probability:	Evidence Base:
4. Plausible	○ **Preliminary**

Effect and Mechanism of Action

In this experimentally demonstrated pharmacokinetic interaction, curcumin may increase the bioavailability of vinblastine by inhibition of P-glycoprotein.

Research

The inhibition of P-gp by curcuminoids is well documented (see Effects on Drug Metabolism and Bioavailability). Anuchapreeda et al.[37] tested the ability of curcumin to decrease P-gp–mediated drug resistance in a human cervical carcinoma line and established that curcumin increased their sensitivity to vinblastine, which was consistent with an observed intracellular increase in rhodamine-123 (a P-gp sub-strate).[37] The same group later established that curcumin-I was more effective than curcumin-II and -III in causing retention of vinblastine by the same cell line. There was no effect on a wild-type variation of the same cell line that lacked drug resistance.[38]

Clinical Implications and Integrative Therapeutics

There is growing interest in the potential of natural com-pounds as potential modulators of drug resistance mediated by the ABC (ATP-binding cassette) family of drug transpor-ters. Coadministration of curcumin with vinca alkaloids may reduce drug resistance to these agents, and the curcuminoids are not known to interfere with the activity of microtubule inhibitors. In vivo studies are necessary to confirm the clinical efficacy of the combination, but curcumin administration may be considered if drug resistance appears responsible for lack of efficacy in malignancies previously responsive to vinblastine.

THEORETICAL, SPECULATIVE, AND PRELIMINARY INTERACTIONS RESEARCH, INCLUDING OVERSTATED INTERACTIONS CLAIMS

Anticoagulants and Antiplatelet Drugs

Several experiments using animal models (rodents and simians), as well as one study with washed human platelets, have demonstrated that curcumin can inhibit platelet aggrega-tion induced by arachidonate, adrenaline, collagen, and platelet-activating factor (PAF) through modulation of eicosa-noid biosynthesis, particularly prostaglandin I_2 (PGI_2; prosta-cyclin) and thromboxane A_2 (TXA_2) inhibition.[67-69] Doses of curcumin used in rats and monkeys were between 100 and 300 mg/kg orally, and no measurements were made of bleed times or other coagulation parameters. Shah et al.[70] found that 20- to 25-μM concentrations were effective at inhibiting PAF and arachidonic acid (AA)–induced aggregation, but that much higher doses were needed for collagen and adrenaline.[70] These doses are higher than those likely to be attained in vivo. Studies testing combinations of turmeric or curcumin coadministration with antiplatelet or anticoagulant drugs are unavailable to date. In the absence of corroboration, extrapo-lated warnings that turmeric should be avoided with antiplate-let drugs can be considered speculative and overstated.[7]

Irinotecan/Camptothecin, Mechlorethamine

Irinotecan (camptothecin-11, CPT-11; Campto, Camptosar). Mechlorethamine (nitrogen mustard; Mustargen).

These two agents were included the in vitro but not in vivo rodent phase of a group of tests conducted by Somasundaram et al.[19] No other data are available on these particular drugs, although countervailing data exist for other agents included in this study. Apoptosis induced by the drugs was reduced by addition of curcumin. As noted earlier, because the curcumin concentrations used approach those found in human pharma-cokinetic studies, the authors suggest that patients with breast cancer (and other malignancies) should not concurrently use curcumin with these chemotherapies until further studies clar-ify the situation.[19] Derivative sources have repeated these con-clusions as definitive interactions without qualification. The Somasundaram study conclusions have been criticized as being generalizations that disregard the methodology employed in the in vitro model, particularly the temporal kinetics based on very-short-term effects, low doses of curcu-min, and a failure to account for the multifactorial mechan-isms.[20] The situation is complex, as illustrated by the analysis of Notarbartolo et al.[42] (see Cyclophosphamide and Doxorubicin).

Oral Hypoglycemic Agents and Insulin

Buformin (Andromaco Gliporal, Buformina), chlorpropamide (Diabinese), glimepiride (Amaryl), glipizide (Glucotrol; Glucotrol XL), glyburide (glibenclamide; Diabeta, Glynase, Glynase Prestab, Micronase, Pres Tab), insulin (animal-source insulin: Iletin; human analog insulin: Humanlog; human insulin: Humulin, Novolin, NovoRapid, Oralin), met-formin (Dianben, Glucophage, Glucophage XR); combination drugs: glipizide and metformin (Metaglip), glyburide and met-formin (Glucovance); phenformin (Debeone, Fenformin), tolazamide (Tolinase), tolbutamide (Orinase, Tol-Tab).

Experimental data on diabetic mice suggest that chronic curcuminoid consumption may have beneficial effects on blood glucose levels.[71,72] These data have been "reverse extrapolated" to imply an adverse interaction with oral hypo-glycemics. The possibility of interaction may be different in acute administration versus chronic dietary curcumin con-sumption, and diabetic patients monitoring blood glucose are generally familiar with compensating for dietary-induced variations in blood sugar. In fact, a more appropriate charac-terization would be that turmeric and curcumin as dietary ingredients are protective against pathological diabetic sequelae and help maintain glucose homeostasis, as well as being hypocholesterolemic.[73-75]

The 75 citations for this monograph are located under Turmeric/Curcumin on the CD at the back of the book.

Valerian

Botanical Name: *Valeriana officinalis* L.
Pharmacopoeial Name: Valerianae radix.
Common Name: Valerian.

Summary

Drug/Class Interaction Type	Mechanism and Significance	Management
Diazepam Benzodiazepines ☼/⊕	Herb may reduce side effects of benzodiazepine withdrawal acting as partial agonist at GABA$_A$-benzodiazepine receptor complex, as well as antidepressant, muscle relaxant, and other effects.	Consider incorporating valerian into nutritional/botanical support protocols for drug tapers.
Barbiturates Central nervous system (CNS) depressants ✗	Herb will combine additively with centrally acting depressants at multiple receptor subtypes (5-HT, GABA$_A$, H$_1$, D$_2$, and adenosine). Effects shown to be additive not supra-additive.	Avoid herb-drug coadministration except in short-term/acute circumstances or specialized settings with professional management. (See benzodiazepines.)

GABA, Gamma-aminobutyric acid; *5-HT*, hydroxytryptamine (serotonin); *H*, histamine; *D*, dopamine.

HERB DESCRIPTION

Family

Valerianaceae.

Related Species

There are several hundred members of the *Valeriana* genus, and several species are traded as medicinal valerian root. In North America these include Mexican valerian (*V. edulis* Nutt.); Indian valerian (*V. wallichi* DC) and Pacific valerian (*V. sitchensis* Bong). Ornamental Valerianaceae genera such as *Centranthus* may sometimes be called "valerians," but these are nonmedicinal.

Habitat and Cultivation

Valerian is cultivated widely in Europe and North America and Russia, with Europe providing the bulk of the commercial material.

Parts Used

Fresh or dried rhizomes, roots, and stolons.

Common Forms

Dried Root: Cut or powdered.
Tincture, Fluid Extract: 70% ethanol.
Solid Concentrates: Between 4:1 and 7:1. Standardization to total valerenic acid (0.8%) has been suggested, but a consistent standard has not been established to date. Manufacturers' preparations may vary.

HERB IN CLINICAL PRACTICE

Overview

Valerian root is widely known as a mild sedative-hypnotic herb with a strong, characteristic odor when dried. It is used medicinally to reduce sleep latency, to treat mild to moderate insomnia, and to relieve spasmodic conditions of the smooth muscle. The herb is chemically and pharmacologically complex, and its sedative mechanisms are not fully understood. Herbalists consider that valerian is capable of producing paradoxical effects, but it is not established whether this is caused by the variability in constituent composition resulting from differences in growing conditions, harvesting times, and preparation methods or by constitutional variability among patients or consumers, or both. There is known chemotypic variation in the quantity and distribution of sesquiterpenes and valepotriates among different species, and polyploidal variants exist within species, including *V. officinalis*. Chemical differences between fresh and dried root preparations caused by the instability of the monoterpene valepotriates add to the overall variability. In clinical practice, valerian is usually combined with other sedative herbs, such as hops, passionflower, or lemon balm, rather than used alone.

Valerian has therapeutic monographs from the German Commission E,[1] World Health Organization (WHO),[2] European Scientific Cooperative on Phytotherapy (ESCOP),[3] and the *American Herbal Pharmacopoeia* (*AHP*).[4] Literature reviews are available by Houghton,[5] Morazzoni and Bombardelli,[7] and McKenna et al.[8] The established indications for valerian root are sleep promotion, relief of temporary mild anxiety, and reduction of sleep latency. More than a dozen clinical trials support the use of valerian for insomnia, although a systematic review found the overall evidence for efficacy of the herb was inconclusive based on nine trials included in the metastudy.[9]

Historical/Ethnomedicine Precedent

Valerian has been in documented use in Western herbal medicine since Greco-Roman times. It was initially used as an aromatic and digestive remedy and subsequently became known as a treatment for epilepsy and for various nervous disorders. It was listed in the *United States Pharmacopeia* (*USP*) from 1820 to 1930 and continues to be listed in the *British Pharmacopoeia* and the major homeopathic materia medicas.[10] The Eclectic physicians used valerian for patients with impaired cerebral circulation associated with depression.[11] It has a traditional history of popular use in the United Kingdom, reputedly for treatment of "shell shock" in both world wars and as a home remedy for promotion of sleep, without addictive effects or cognitive impairment.[12] Valerian root is unusual in that the traditional alcoholic tincture remains a favored preparation, partly because of the complex chemistry of the root, which defies straightforward standardization to a unique "active" ingredient.

Known or Potential Therapeutic Uses

Anxiety; epileptic seizure; fibromyalgia; gastric spasm and colic hyperactivity; infantile convulsions; insomnia; menstrual cramps; mild tremor; nervous asthma; nervous tension; post-traumatic stress disorder (PTSD), including "combat fatigue;" sleep disturbances; spasmodic conditions of the gastrointestinal and urogenital tracts.

Key Constituents

Essential oil (0.1%-2.0%), containing three classes of sesquiterpenes (kessane, valerenic aid, valeronone skeletons) and monoterpenes, principally bornyl acetate.
Valepotriates (0.5%-14.5%): epoxy iridoid esters and their degradation products (baldrinals).
Amino acids, including arginine, γ-aminobutyric acid (GABA), glutamine.
Alkaloids (0.01% to 0.05%), lignans, and flavonoids.

Therapeutic Dosing Range

Dried Root: 3 to 9 g daily
Tincture: Based on 1:1 equivalent, 1 to 3 mL three times daily
External (Bath): 100 g per bath

INTERACTIONS REVIEW
Strategic Considerations

The majority of authoritative monographs on valerian maintain that the herb does not exhibit any notable interactions with pharmaceutical drugs. This is corroborated by an absence of any clear-cut case reports in the literature. However, the central nervous system (CNS) depressant properties of the herb have been substantiated, and as a result, several secondary sources including the *USP*, suggest that the herb may potentiate the effects of a variety of CNS depressant drugs.[12,13] Also, valerian may interfere with antiepileptic medications[14]; this speculation has been eloquently refuted by Eadie[15] in a historical review that concluded valerian is in fact antiepileptic. Although inconclusive, experimental data from the 1980s and 1990s tended to favor a GABAergic mechanism of the sedative effects of the herb.[16] Reverse extrapolations from this putative pharmacological mechanism have also been used to support suggestions of interactions with CNS depressants that act at the GABA-benzodiazepine-chloride channel complex.[13] This includes speculations that the herb will interact with anesthetics.[17] Such reverse extrapolations are better described as "potential contraindications" rather than interactions. Although the possibility of additive effects with CNS depressant drugs is examined as a potential interaction here, the available evidence suggests that synergistic interactions (vs. simple additive effects) between valerian and pharmaceutical sedatives do not exist.

The more recent ligand-binding studies suggest multiple possible actions at different neural receptors, including melatonin and serotonin subtypes, as well as partial GABA$_A$ receptor agonism and H$_1$ histamine and D$_2$ dopamine receptor binding.[18-24] In clinical practice, valerian has been used, as with kava, to facilitate withdrawal from benzodiazepenes.[25] In this context the clinical coadministration of herb and drug is a valid exception to the general rule of avoiding concomitant use of herbs and drugs that have similar neurotransmitter effects. (See also benzodiazepines section of the Kava monograph.)

The "psychiatric" indications for valerian are anecdotally well known by the herb-consuming public. Populations who have previously used psychiatric drugs such as sedatives and anxiolytics are arguably more likely to self-prescribe valerian. This may lead to inadvertent additive effects from what would be regarded as contraindicated herb-drug combinations in a professional setting. Unfortunately, literature reviews such as the recent survey by Ernst[26] suggest valerian is ineffective as an anxiolytic, confusing the issue, even if strictly correct in terms of meta-analysis methodology. The poor quality of trials on valerian as a single agent is likely to produce such a conclusion; in practice, valerian is used in combination with other sedative or anxiolytic herbs. Generally, combinations of "nervine herbs," such as hops, lemon balm, and passionflower, with valerian demonstrate greater efficacy than single agents.[27-29]

Effects on Drug Metabolism and Bioavailability

Several in vitro studies have examined the effects of valerian extracts on cytochrome P450 (CYP450) enzymes. Strandell et al.[30] used fluorometric screening methodology and found a moderate inhibition of recombinant human microsomal CYP450 3A4 with a dimethyl sulfoxide (DMSO) extract derived from one of two valerian preparations tested, whereas no effect was found on CYP450 2C19 or 2D6. The effect was not observed when an ethanol extract rather than DMSO was used, and the second valerian product exhibited no inhibitory effects on CYPs. Lefebvre et al.[31] also used fluorometric assay methodology to examine the effects of 14 different commercial preparations of valerian on CYP3A4. They noted wide variation in the composition of the valerian products, with valerenic acid content varying from 21 to 2661 ppm. They found an inhibitory effect on CYP3A4 and also on P-glycoprotein (P-gp), using an ATPase-dependent assay system with a verapamil control. The effect varied with solvents used, with water being the least inhibitory and acetonitrile the most inhibitory. By contrast, earlier fluorometric study of 3A4 inhibition by Budzinski et al.[32] found that both valerian extract and pure valerenic acid were unable to inhibit 3A4 at clinically relevant concentrations and were the weakest inhibitors of the various herbs and pure compounds tested.

Gurley et al.[33,34] performed a study on valerian (and three other herbs) with 12 healthy volunteers consuming the extract for a month. Preadministration and postadministration data for a variety of probe substrates relating to CYP450 3A4, 1A2, 2E1, and 2D6 were determined. No significant changes were found for valerian (125 mg three times daily for 28 days), and the authors concluded that valerian is unlikely to cause pharmacokinetic interactions mediated by the major CYP450 enzymes. Donovan et al.[35] used higher doses of herb (1000 mg containing 11 mg valerenic acid) taken every night for 14 days by 12 healthy volunteers. They used probe drugs (dextromethorphan and alprazolam) to test for effects on CYP2D6 and CYP3A4. No significant changes in baseline preadministration levels were found.

From the available data, clinically significant pharmacokinetic interactions between valerian and prescription drugs appear to be unlikely despite conflicting results from in vitro studies.

HERB-DRUG INTERACTIONS

Benzodiazepines

Evidence: Diazepam (Valium).
Extrapolated, based on similar properties: Alprazolam (Xanax), bromazepam (Lexotan), chlordiazepoxide (Librium),

clonazepam (Klonopin, Rivotril), clorazepate (Gen-Xene, Tranxene), estazolam (ProSom), flurazepam (Dalmane), lorazepam (Ativan), medazepam (Nobrium), midazolam (Versed, Hypnovel), oxazepam (Serax), prazepam (Centrax), quazepam (Doral), temazepam (Restoril), triazolam (Halcion).

Interaction Type and Significance

☼ **Prevention or Reduction of Drug Adverse Effect**

⊕ **Potential or Theoretical Beneficial or Supportive Interaction, with Professional Management**

Probability:
3. Possible

Evidence Base:
○ **Preliminary**

Effect and Mechanism of Action

In a beneficial interaction specific to settings of withdrawal from benzodiazepine drugs, the effects of valerian reduce benzodiazepine withdrawal symptoms. A GABAergic mechanism has been proposed. The herb also has other potentially beneficial effects on typical withdrawal symptoms, such as antidepressant and antispasmodic activity.

Research

Andreatini et al.[36] used a behavioral test with a rodent model designed to differentiate between anxiolytic and anxiogenic responses to study the effects of a valepotriate preparation (80% dihydrovaltrate, 15% valtrate, 5% acetovaltrate) on the effects of benzodiazepine withdrawal. After treating a group of animals for 28 days with diazepam intraperitoneally (IP), withdrawal symptoms were induced by complete cessation of the drug. Low-dose diazepam (2.5 mg/kg IP) was compared to both 6 mg and 12 mg/kg valepotriates IP. The withdrawal groups given low-dose diazepam and high-dose valepotriates were comparable and exhibited significantly lower anxiety response rates than the control or low-dose valepotriate groups. The authors concluded that valepotriates may be useful in benzodiazepine withdrawal.[36]

A review article by Rasmussen[25] reported clinical work in a drug detoxification setting using botanicals as adjunctive treatment for withdrawal. Valerian and kava were both used extensively in benzodiazepine tapers. The author suggested that duration of use should be limited to 2 to 3 months of continuous administration, although valerian extracts are free from the dependency issues associated with benzodiazepines.

Reports

One case report suggests the "reverse" interaction, in which a patient taking valerian extracts (unspecified) up to five times daily for many years presented with delirium and cardiac failure. The valerian was stopped, and the patient was treated successfully with midazolam and lorazepam, followed by clonazepam (0.5 mg twice daily), and was stable at 8 and 20 weeks after discharge on this regimen.[37] The case is impossible to evaluate, however, because the patient was concurrently taking numerous drugs, including digoxin, benazepril, furosemide, ibuprofen, nitrates, and multiple vitamin and mineral supplements.

Clinical Implications and Integrative Therapeutics

A case can be made for using valerian extracts in clinical settings of benzodiazepine withdrawal to reduce the severity of withdrawal symptoms and increase the likelihood of successful treatment. Long-term dependency on benzodiazepines constitutes a significant problem and is also likely to be seen in the drug detoxification setting. Anecdotal evidence suggests

that valerian (as well as kava and other sedative herbs) may be of use in this context where substitution of another, potentially dependency-inducing drug, would be undesirable. Outside the drug taper-withdrawal setting, coadministration of valerian and benzodiazepines is arguably contraindicated because of additive sedative effects, although there is no evidence for synergistic interaction. (See next section.)

Barbiturates and Other Central Nervous System Depressants

Evidence: Phenobarbital (phenobarbitone; Luminal, Solfoton), thiopental (Pentothal).
Extrapolated: CNS depressants, sedative-hypnotics, anticonvulsants, preanesthetics, adrenergic antagonists and related agents.

Interaction Type and Significance

✗ **Potential or Theoretical Adverse Interaction of Uncertain Severity**

Probability:
6. Unknown

Evidence Base:
▽ **Mixed**

Effect and Mechanism of Action

Extrapolating from experimental extension of barbiturate sleeping times by valerian extracts administered IP in rodent experiments and the clinically established sedative effects of the herb, potentiation of various classes of CNS depressants has been hypothesized. Available evidence suggests predictable additive effects, but synergistic interactions have not been demonstrated.

Research

Animal studies have shown moderate increases in sleeping time when barbiturates were administered with valerian ingredients. However, doses were relatively high and administered IP (50 and 100 mg/kg valerenic acid).[38,39] Hiller and Zetler[40] found that valerian extract at 100 mg/kg IP was equivalent to diazepam at 0.2 mg/kg IP in prolonging anesthesia in mice induced by thiopental. A controlled clinical trial by Kohnen and Oswald[41] examined the effects of valerian extracts (100 mg orally) compared with valerian extracts combined with propranolol (20 mg) in 48 healthy volunteers subjected to stress-inducing tests. No drug interaction was found with the combination, and the researchers concluded that the agents had independent but similar actions, based on the objective and subjective measures used. Low doses of valerian were used in this trial because the researchers decided that higher doses would be excessively sedative, as opposed to lower doses being anxiolytic.

Ugalde et al.[42] used a rigorous experimental design to examine the possible interactions between hydroethanolic extracts of *Valeriana edulis* and six common CNS depressant drugs (diazepam, ethanol, pentobarbital, buspirone, haloperidol, diphenhydramine). The median effective dose (ED_{50}) for dose-dependent sedative effects was established in the rodent model for each drug and for the valerian extracts. Equally effective doses of each drug were then combined with valerian extract in fixed 1:1 ratio, and the combined drug-herb effects were analyzed by isobolographic methodology. This simple mathematical method analyzes fixed-ratio combinations of agents in terms of whether their combined effects are linearly additive (noninteractive) or superadditive (interactive, synergistic) across a range of dose-response data.[43] The researchers found that the combinations of valerian coadministered with each of the six classes of CNS drugs exhibited only linear additive effects. From this point of view, valerian can be said not to display interactions (in a strict supra-additivity sense) with the CNS drugs used. In addition, valerian may be hypothesized to have multiple mechanisms across a range of receptors, as represented by the diverse neurotransmitter and receptor mechanisms of the six drugs employed. Isobolographic analysis has been theoretically established as a tool for inferring pharmacological mechanisms from dose-response relations of drug combinations.[44]

Clinical Implications and Adaptations

From a clinical perspective, valerian extracts may have additive effects with a range of CNS depressant drugs, although these are not strictly classifiable as interactions, but rather simple linear effects. Warnings to avoid valerian before anesthesia are appropriate, although risks in this setting are unlikely to be significant. Chronic coadministration with sedative-hypnotic, anxiolytic, or anticonvulsant medications is contraindicated.

THEORETICAL, SPECULATIVE, AND PRELIMINARY INTERACTIONS RESEARCH, INCLUDING OVERSTATED INTERACTIONS CLAIMS

Anticonvulsants

Some suggest that valerian may exacerbate seizures, thus compromising efficacy of anticonvulsant medications.[14] Not only is there no experimental or clinical evidence for this speculation, but traditional use and neuropharmacology suggest that the herb has anticonvulsive properties.[15] (See Barbiturates.)

Anesthesia

Related but evidence lacking for extrapolation: Halogenated inhalational anesthetic agents: Desflurane (Suprane), enflurane (Ethrane), halothane (Fluothane), isoflurane (Forane), sevoflurane (Sevorane, Ultane).

Concerns regarding use of herbal sedatives before surgical procedure are based on presumptions of the risk of excessive sedation. Given the mild effects of valerian and the high level of available technical monitoring in the operative setting, these risks may be overstated.[45] Reports of perioperative problems with valerian are not available. The use of low doses of herbal anxiolytics before elective surgery could even be argued as potentially beneficial for stress reduction, with minimal effects on sedation.

The 45 citations for this monograph are located under Valerian on the CD at the back of the book.

Vitex

Botanical Name: *Vitex agnus-castus* L.
Pharmacopoeial Name: Agni casti fructus.
Common Names: Chaste tree, chaste berry, agnus-castus, vitex, monk's pepper.

HERB DESCRIPTION

Family

Verbenaceae.

Related Species

Vitex negundo L., *V. trifoliate* L., *V. rotundifolia* L., *V. pediuncularis* Wall., *V. jeguado* L. var *cannabifolia*.[1]

Parts Used

Fruit.

Common Forms

Dried or fresh ripe fruit for decoction.
Tincture, Fluid Extract: Of dried or fresh fruit, 50% to 70% alcohol.
Standardized Extract: 6:1 to 12:1 standardized to casticin 0.6% (e.g., PreMens by Zeller AG).

INTERACTIONS REVIEW

Strategic Considerations

Vitex has an ancient reputation as a "galactogue" and long been considered to suppress sexual excitability. It was more recently popularized in Germany and approved by the Commission E in 1985 for menstrual irregularities.[2,3] Vitex is currently used primarily as a gynecological herb for cyclical problems, including dysmenorrhea, amenorrhea, oligomenorrhea, corpus luteum insufficiency (and infertility related to luteal insufficiency), hyperprolactinemia, premenstrual syndrome (PMS), acne, mastalgia and mastodynia, and lactation issues. The constituents of the fruit are complex, including diterpenes, irdoid glycosides, lipophilic flavonoids, triglycerides, and essential oil. The active constituents are poorly characterized, although the lipophilic components, especially diterpenoids such as rotundifuran, are thought to be important for its effects. Several significant research reports are in German; comprehensive reviews of the data have been published by the *American Herbal Pharmacopoeia (AHP)*,[4] McKenna et al.,[1] and European Scientific Cooperative on Phytotherapy (ESCOP).[5]

No interactions for vitex are documented; this was confirmed by a recent survey on the safety of the herb.[6] The authors confirmed, however, the cautionary note originating from the 1992 revised Commission E monograph, that because of recorded dopaminergic effects in animal experiments, vitex may interact with pharmaceutical dopamine receptor agonists. The Commission E also noted there were no reports of such interactions.[3] The dopamine-binding caution is now widely repeated in the derivative interactions literature, and some sources also suggest that interactions may occur with oral contraceptives (OCs) and hormone replacement therapy (HRT) or with monoamine oxidase inhibitors (MAOIs), selective serotonin reuptake inhibitors (SSRIs), and tricyclic antidepressants (TCAs). However, no interactions reports are associated with vitex. Reviewing the known pharmacology from an integrative perspective will contextualize these speculations.

The emerging consensus is that dopaminergic effects of vitex may be partly responsible for its prolactin-inhibiting actions. Several experimental studies using rodent striatum, calf striatum, and human recombinant dopamine D_2 receptors with two different ligand probes, sulpiride and spiroperidol, suggest that a variable degree of binding occurs between crude extracts and diterpene fractions of vitex.[7,8] However, reviews of all the data, including German unpublished material, suggest an order of magnitude variation (IC_{50} 40-500 µg/mL) in dose required for receptor binding for whole-plant extracts.[1,4,5] Additionally, isolated constituent studies for the diterpene rotundifuran (considered by some to be the most important dopaminergic compound in the crude herb) show an order of magnitude or more difference, with 100 micromolar (µM) rotundifuran about equivalent to 1 µM dopamine (data from Christoffel et al., 1999; reviewed by Upton[4]). It is also unclear whether the receptor binding is in fact agonistic or antagonistic in vivo, and evidence suggests that dose-response kinetics are biphasic. Weak binding also takes place with other receptor subtypes, including mu (µ) and kappa (κ) opioid receptors, as well as to estrogen receptors.[7,9,10] In clinical practice, vitex seems to effect moderate prolactin inhibition and may be clinically appropriate in mild hyperprolactinemia, and the herb will have fewer adverse effects than bromocriptine for such indications.[11]

The D_2 family of receptors are also targets for neurological drugs (antiparkinsonian) and psychiatric (antipsychotic) drugs, such as L-dopa and haloperidol. This has given rise to more speculation on possible interactions between vitex and such psychopharmaceuticals. Clinically, the most typical prescribing patterns for vitex extracts by English-speaking herbal practitioners involve the use of small doses, 0.5 to 5.0 mL crude herb in a single dose, taken in the morning on rising. With this approach, the latency of herb effects on cyclical irregularities and related menstrual problems is extended, typically requiring at least three menstrual cycles to achieve a stable situation.[12,13] This is also seen in the results of clinical trials, where herb effects on both symptom reduction and prolactin secretion became significant over three cycles.

The relation between this pattern of moderate vitex prescription and a slow modulation of cyclical irregularity (or prolactin level normalization) interacting with pharmaceutical agents is difficult to assess. A German report of a trial by Wuttke and colleagues in 1997 is discussed at length in the AHP monograph[4]; measurable reductions of prolactin levels were achieved after 3 months with vitex preparations compared to placebo. However, metoclopramide-induced prolactin secretion did not differ between the treatment and placebo groups. A 2-week trial in 20 healthy males (presumed to lack the cyclical hormone fluctuations in women) found a biphasic response to thyrotropin-releasing hormone (TRH)–stimulated prolactin levels among three groups administered vitex extract at different doses. A low dose (120 mg/day) increased the area under curve (AUC) for prolactin, a high dose (240 mg/day) reduced AUC, but a median dose (240 mg/day) did not differ from controls.[14] Therefore, the simple view of vitex having a "bromocriptine"-like dopamine agonism apparently is inappropriate, and extrapolating interactions on the assumption that it is a pharmaceutical-level agent is not justifiable. Also, the pharmacology of the herb remains incompletely characterized. Emerging experimental data suggest that vitex extracts may act as agonists to the μ-opiate receptor, although the levels required to achieve median inhibition concentration (IC_{50}) were higher than those likely to be attained in vivo; at this time a role for opiate receptor agonism for vitex in vivo cannot be considered established.[15]

Given that the median age of onset for Parkinson's disease is 57 years, it is unlikely a significant population of female parkinsonian patients would present with typical gynecological indications for vitex. In the psychiatric category, the effects of various antipsychotics and neuroleptics on in vivo dopamine remains poorly understood. The "dopamine hypothesis" of schizophrenia is increasingly considered a controversial over-simplification. Because of the high frequency of pharmacokinetic and pharmacodymamic interactions exhibited by many classes of psychiatric medications, prudence would suggest monitoring usage of all coadministered herbs, and vitex interactions with neuroleptic agents having dopamine D_2, D_3, and D_4 subtypes must remain speculative at this time.

The currently known pharmacology of the herb suggests that the common interactions extrapolated from putative pharmacology between pharmaceuticals and vitex should be considered unproven, or overstated until substantial evidence becomes available.

THEORETICAL, SPECULATIVE, AND PRELIMINARY INTERACTIONS RESEARCH, INCLUDING OVERSTATED INTERACTIONS CLAIMS

Analgesic and Anticonvulsant Medications

A research group from India published two related reports in which an extract of *Vitex negundo* was found to

potentiate the effects of the anticonvulsant drugs valproate and dihydrophenytoin against electrically induced seizures in a murine model. The same group also established a potentiating effect of the same extract with analgesics drugs (meperidine and aspirin) in an animal test. Until further corroboration of these preliminary reports is available, this cannot be considered an established interaction; it is nonetheless interesting in relation to the different central effects of vitex.[16,17]

Dopamine Agonists and/or Antagonists

Although vitex is sometimes cited as interacting with, for example, anti-Parkinson's medications, reports are absent. (See Strategic Considerations for a discussion of neurotransmitter data.)

Oral Contraceptives and Related Estrogen-Containing and Synthetic Estrogen and Progesterone Analog Medications

Early suggestions that vitex had significant effects on follicle-stimulating hormone (FSH) and luteinizing hormone (LH) have not been substantiated. The herb has been described as "progesteronic," but this is clearly a result of multifactorial effects, including on hypophyseal dopamine levels. Extremely weak binding to recombinant human estrogen receptor (ER) alpha and ER beta has been noted, with IC_{50} levels of 46 and 64 μg/mL, respectively. Weak activity was also found with Ishekawa endometrial carcinoma cell line (ER/PR+).[10] The controlled trial on vitex for PMS symptoms by Berger et al.[18] included 13 subjects concurrently using OCs. No effects were noted on any parameters in the study that were confined to the OC subjects.[18] Suggestions of interactions are hypothetical, and the available evidence would suggest that this is unlikely. In any event, for the majority of situations, coadministration of vitex with exogenous sex hormones could be described as "clinically inappropriate" and does not constitute normal practice.

The 18 citations for this monograph are located under Vitex on the CD at the back of the book.

Beta-Carotene

Nutrient Name: Beta-Carotene

Synonyms: β-carotene, b-carotene, *trans* beta-carotene, provitamin A, betacarotenum.

Related Substances: Other provitamin A carotenoids: alpha-carotene, cryptoxanthin, lutein, lycopene, zeaxanthin; retinol (preformed vitamin A).

Summary

Drug/Class Interaction Type	Mechanism and Significance	Management
Anthelmintic drugs ⊕⊕⊕	Vitamin A deficiencies are associated with increased risk of parasitic infections. Combining anthelmintic agents with increased beta-carotene (and vitamin A) intake can reduce symptoms of intestinal parasites while supporting epithelial integrity and immune response, especially when combined with increased fat intake.	Coadminister beta-carotene and/or vitamin A and/or foods with accompanying lipid intake. Follow with improved nutrient intake (quality and quantity) to reduce susceptibility.
Chemotherapy Cytotoxic agents ☼/⊕⊕/✗/⊕✗	Administration of beta-carotene before, during, and/or after cytotoxic chemotherapy can mitigate adverse effects (particularly oral mucositis) and may enhance outcomes. Risk of interference of cytotoxic action through antioxidant effects increasingly appears less likely but remains contentious; evidence inconclusive and not likely to be uniform for all agents, conditions, or patients.	Coadministration may be appropriate in some cases. Carotenoid use requires supervision by experienced clinicians collaborating in applying an integrative strategy, particularly given significant risk of toxicity. Multiple nutrients providing a network effect are preferred when antioxidants deemed appropriate.
Cholestyramine Colestipol bile acid sequestrants ≈≈≈/◇	By reducing fat absorption, bile acid sequestrants can significantly reduce absorption, assimilation and transport of beta-carotene and, to varying degrees, other fat-soluble nutrients. Beta-carotene absorption appears more likely than vitamin A (and less likely than other nutrients) to be adversely effected to a clinically significant degree, though that may vary depending upon the agent used, diet and supplemental intake, and patient characteristics. Available research inconclusive and limited by subject population characteristics, duration and scope; further research warranted.	During extended therapy, concurrent administration of multivitamin formulation providing modest levels of carotenoids, along with vitamins A, D, E, and K, folate, and mixed tocopherols, can counter potential adverse effects with little risk and minimal expense. Separate intake.
Colchicine ≈≈≈/◇	Oral colchicine may induce intestinal malabsorption of beta-carotene (and other nutrients) and block hepatic release of retinol-binding protein. Clinical trials warranted to assess frequency and circumstances of occurrence and determine clinical significance.	During extended therapy, coadministration of multivitamin formulation including carotenoids can counter potential adverse effects with little risk and minimal expense.
Medroxyprogesterone ≈≈/☼	Medroxyprogesterone as injectable contraceptive or oral HRT, may elevate serum retinol levels, possibly also retinol-binding protein. Clinical significance of elevated levels and possible alteration in vitamin A function is unclear; however, serum carotenoids may decrease as a result of competition and/or altering vitamin A transport. Response likely to depend on multiple factors including diet and patient characteristics. Further research warranted.	Conservative practice suggests carotenoid support may be indicated. Generally avoid high-dose retinol unless otherwise indicated; if used, monitor carefully when patient has compromised liver function.
Methyltestosterone ◇≈≈/≈≈	Single case report suggests methyltestosterone may impair visual function by altering serum levels and metabolism of beta-carotene and vitamin A. This minimal evidence may represent atypical pharmacogenomic response but indicates need for further investigation, including potential benefit of nutrient supplementation.	Discontinuation of drug therapy indicated on appearance of adverse effects.
Mineral oil ✗/≈≈≈	Mineral oil may interfere with or otherwise alter absorption of many nutrients, especially with simultaneous intake and extended use. Mixed evidence suggests impact on various nutrients may vary, possibly decreasing beta-carotene levels and elevating serum retinol levels. Further research warranted; timing, dosage, duration, diet, and other factors likely to influence degree of clinical significance.	Separate intake of mineral oil from meals and beta-carotene administration. Avoid extended use of mineral oil internally.
Neomycin ≈≈≈/◇	Oral neomycin, particularly high doses over extended periods, may impair absorption and increase elimination of beta-carotene through adverse effects on digestive tract; this could potentially contribute to depletion pattern. Preliminary evidence suggests further research warranted to assess degree of and factors influencing clinical significance.	Coadminister beta-carotene and/or vitamin A with oral neomycin use of 2 days or longer.
Omeprazole Proton pump inhibitors (PPIs) ≈≈≈	Inhibition of gastric acid production may reduce absorption of beta-carotene. Dose response to beta-carotene administration observed after gastric acid inhibition by omeprazole. Further research warranted to assess degree of and factors influencing clinical significance, especially with extended suppression of gastric parietal cell function by antacid therapy.	Encourage increased dietary consumption of carotenoid-rich fruits and vegetables, possibly with beta-carotene or mixed carotenoid supplementation, during extended PPI therapy. Monitoring of blood carotenoid levels may be appropriate.

Continued

Summary

Drug/Class Interaction Type	Mechanism and Significance	Management
Orlistat ≈≈≈	Orlistat may interfere with absorption of beta-carotene and other fat-soluble nutrients. Mixed evidence suggests degree of impact on various nutrients may vary, with findings ranging from no observed effect to depletion despite concurrent supplementation. Further research warranted; timing, dosage, duration, diet, and other factors likely to influence degree of clinical significance.	Coadministration of a multivitamin formulation providing modest levels of carotenoids, along with vitamins A, D, E, and K and mixed tocopherols, may counter possible depletion pattern with little risk and minimal expense.
Probucol ◇≈≈/≈≈/✗/◇	Preliminary research indicates that probucol may interfere with absorption and activity of beta-carotene and other carotenoids, by competing for incorporation into VLDL. Conversely, beta-carotene might potentially interfere with probucol absorption, but evidence is lacking. Further research warranted.	Supplementation with beta-carotene and increased consumption of carotenoid-rich foods may be appropriate. Monitoring may be advisable to ensure drug efficacy.

HRT, Hormone replacement therapy; *VLDL*, very-low-density lipoprotein.
Note: See also monograph for Vitamin A (Retinol).

NUTRIENT DESCRIPTION

This monograph reviews interactions issues relating to and deriving from intake of beta-carotene and other forms of provitamin A, as dietary components and supplements, and the metabolic processes of these substances within physiological/healthy, dysfunctional, and pathological processes and states. The related monograph for Vitamin A (Retinol) focuses on interactions issues involving intake, assimilation, and metabolic processes of the class of compounds that exhibit the biological activity of retinol. Inherently, interactions with some pharmaceutical agents involve both substances and their respective class of related substances.

Chemistry and Forms

Beta-carotene is the most well-known carotenoid, a class of related compounds found exclusively in plants (fruit and vegetable), where they are recognizable as brightly colored red, orange, and yellow pigments. Approximately 600 carotenoids have been identified, and about 50 are known to exert provitamin A activity; that is, they can serve as a naturally occurring precursor to vitamin A. Thus, "provitamin A" is the name of beta-carotene (and related compounds) that most directly describes its primary function in human physiology as viewed by conventional medicine. Alpha-carotene, lutein, lycopene, cryptoxanthin, and zeaxanthin are the most frequently occurring members of the group classified as "provitamin A carotenoids," as is all-*trans* (i.e., synthetic) beta-carotene, which is actually the most active in terms of potential for conversion to vitamin A on a weight basis.

Beta-carotene consists of two retinol molecules. Bonds within beta-carotene are cleaved to form all-*trans* retinol (and possibly *retinal*, the aldehyde form of vitamin A); divergent theories exist regarding the site of this cleavage, the product(s) and their proportion, though molecular structures suggest that one molecule of beta-carotene would result in two molecules of retinol. It is not reasonable, however, to equate the predicted retinol yield of the various provitamin A carotenoids, then add these to provide units of "vitamin A equivalents," because in non–vitamin A–deficient humans, only a small proportion of provitamin A carotenoids are actually converted to retinol or retinal. The supplement labeling convention of stating provitamin A carotenoid content in units of "retinol equivalents" has led to a widespread misperception among the lay public and many medical professionals alike, that such products contain potentially toxic levels of vitamin A. Potential toxicity of carotenoids, such as synthetic beta-carotene supplements in smokers, derives from the bimodal antioxidant/pro-oxidant phenomenon demonstrated by beta-carotene and is unrelated to issues of vitamin A toxicity.

Physiology and Function

In 1913, vitamin A was the first fat-soluble vitamin to be isolated. In 1929, Moore demonstrated that beta-carotene was converted into vitamin A, and 2 years later the chemical structures of both vitamin A and beta-carotene were determined. In 1932, beta-carotene (provitamin A) was discovered to be the precursor to vitamin A. Initially beta-carotene was considered to have the exclusive function in human physiology of serving as a source compound for conversion into vitamin A. The primary physiological functions of carotenoids include exerting antioxidant activity and deoxyribonucleic acid (DNA) protection, enabling both cell-mediated and humoral immunity, and feeding into the metabolic pathways of retinol, which is required for maintenance of all epithelial tissues.

The issue of bioavailability and conversion of beta-carotene and other provitamin A carotenoids to retinol remains contentious, evolving and often confusing because of uncertainty about the functional meaning of "bioavailability" and the inadequacy of the indicators used in its determination. Animal studies of the mechanism of carotenoid conversion to vitamin A indicate that before absorption, the two linked retinol molecules constituting beta-carotene can be converted to vitamin A in the wall of the small intestine. They are hydrolyzed in the gastrointestinal (GI) tract and absorbed into the mucosal cells of the small intestine, where they can be oxidized to retinoic acid and retinol in the presence of fat and bile acids. Carotenoids alpha, gamma, and beta are converted to vitamin A primarily in the intestinal mucosa. Theoretically, beta-carotene should be twice as active as the alpha and gamma carotenoids because it is composed of two potential molecules of retinol, and the others contain only one potential molecule of retinol. Both thyroxine and vitamin E enhance the conversion of carotene to retinol. Diabetes and hypothyroidism are two conditions that may impair conversion of carotenes to vitamin A. In non–vitamin A–deficient humans, it appears that the bulk of provitamin A carotenoids are absorbed intact and are not converted to vitamin A in significant quantities.

Absorption of beta-carotene and other carotenoids is influenced significantly by dietary intake, nutritional status, and storage levels, with efficiency of assimilation and utilization increasing in deficiency states and dropping with saturation of retinol and its metabolites. Beta-carotene and the other primary carotenoids with provitamin A activity demonstrate less bioavailability than retinol, also known as *preformed vitamin A*.

Retinol itself is absorbed two to four times as efficiently as beta-carotene. Carotene relies much more on bile salts for absorption than retinol. Although retinol can also be absorbed from a micelle in the presence of any nonionic detergent, carotenoids can only be absorbed from a micelle in the presence of bile salts. Furthermore, carotenoids are absorbed by passive absorption regardless of their concentration, whereas retinol is absorbed by diffusion when present in high doses but is carrier mediated at low doses.

For all these reasons, only one third of ingested beta-carotene is absorbed, as much as 75% of which can be converted into retinyl esters and retinol, with 25% remaining intact as beta-carotene. Small amounts are then stored in the liver as active retinol. Beta-carotene is approximately one-sixth as biologically active as pure retinol. The resulting convention of 6 micrograms (μg) of beta-carotene being equivalent to 1 μg of retinol is generally accepted, but absorption, conversion, and utilization of carotenoids are highly variable. As the daily intake of carotene rises above 5000 international units (IU; on the basis of theoretical conversion to retinol), the percentage absorption rate decreases significantly. Ultimately, absorption is typically 20% to 50% but can be as low as 10% when intake is elevated.

Storage of beta-carotene and most carotenoids occurs primarily in adipose tissue, the adrenals, epidermal and dermal layers, and the corpus luteum, in contrast to vitamin A, which is predominantly stored in the liver. Minor amounts of beta-carotene are conjugated with glucuronic acid and converted to retinol in the liver; small amounts are also stored in the lungs. Colostrum also contains relatively high levels of carotenoids. Very-low-density lipoprotein (VLDL) or low-density lipoprotein (LDL) cholesterol transports intact beta-carotene in the blood, with blood levels varying according to intake levels. Serum levels of beta-carotene directly reflect daily consumption, not storage. Elimination of beta-carotene is primarily through the feces, but conjugated water-soluble forms are also excreted through the urine.

In plants the antioxidant effects of carotenoids enable these compounds to play a crucial role in protecting plant organisms against damage during photosynthesis. Beta-carotene functions as a chain-breaking antioxidant; rather than preventing initiation of lipid peroxidation, it stops the chain reaction by trapping free radicals, which halts the progression of free-radical activity. Many consider beta-carotene to be the most effective natural agent for quenching single-oxygen free radicals in humans. However, beta-carotene and other carotenoids exhibit a bimodal functionality characteristic of many "antioxidant" agents in that it can act either as an antioxidant or a pro-oxidant, depending on availability of other antioxidant compounds, and the level of oxidative stress present in the compartment in which it is acting.

The *cis* isomers of beta-carotene, which occur only in natural source, as opposed to synthetic all-*trans* beta-carotene, are the most potent scavengers of singlet-oxygen radicals. Under high-oxidative-stress conditions, such as in the lungs of smokers who have a poor dietary intake of other antioxidants, large quantities of beta-carotene, particularly of the all-*trans* isomer, can generate long-lived all-*trans* beta-carotene free radicals, which set in motion their own cell-damaging chain reactions, thus functioning as pro-oxidants rather than antioxidants. The presence of multiple antioxidant substances appearing together in their natural context emphasizes the interdependent network effect of diet-derived antioxidants and suggests that they provide optimal benefit when consumed together rather than as individual, isolated nutrients.

Both beta-carotene and retinyl esters from the diet are converted to retinal (11 *cis* isomer). Retinal is combined with the protein *opsin* to form rhodopsin in the rods of the retina and iodopsin in the cones. Light hitting the retina causes visual excitation and changes the *cis* configuration into the all-*trans* form of retinaldehyde. The rods are particularly sensitive to vitamin A deficiency. When retinol is in low supply, the all-*trans* form generated during the light reaction cannot be converted back to the active rhodopsin, which is why natural sources of carotenes and preformed vitamin A, which provide *cis* isomers, are needed in some cases to prevent or correct night blindness.

The roles and effects of retinol and the various metabolites of vitamin A are reviewed in the Vitamin A (Retinol) monograph and derive, at least in part, from the presence of beta-carotene and the other provitamin A carotenoids.

NUTRIENT IN CLINICAL PRACTICE
Known or Potential Therapeutic Uses

Until recently, conventional medicine has largely treated beta-carotene as simply a precursor of vitamin A (and assigned similar subsidiary roles to the other carotenoids). Over the past decade, beta-carotene and related carotenoids have been increasingly recognized as independent nutrients of physiological significance with parallel development of recommended intake levels. A small amount of beta-carotene is converted into vitamin A in the body, but beta-carotene and other carotenoids act independently from vitamin A as antioxidants as well as in other roles. Preliminary and experimental studies, as well as significant epidemiological data, suggest that a higher dietary intake of carotenes offers protection against developing certain malignancies (e.g., GI tract, lung, skin, cervix, uterus), macular degeneration, cataracts, and other health conditions linked to oxidative or free-radical damage.

Historical/Ethnomedicine Precedent

Some Western medical traditions, particularly naturopathic medicine, and many indigenous folk and professional traditions of plant medicine (i.e., food and herbs) have emphasized the importance of foods containing carotenoids, readily identifiable through their signature pigments, as important to supporting health and beneficial in treating disease. Mothers and grandmothers have long advocated the consumption of carrots, collards, spinach, and sweet potatoes as "good for you"; they may not have known the mechanisms involved, but they paid attention to outcomes. Modern research into the manifold benefits of the Mediterranean diet increasingly points to the significant contributions of colorful vegetables and fruits and healthy oils from olives and fish toward its salubrious effects.

Possible Uses

Alcohol withdrawal support, asthma, atherosclerosis, cancer (risk reduction), cataracts, cervical dysplasia, cognitive decline (protective; APOE 4 allele), coronary heart disease (risk reduction; in combination), gastritis, heart attack, human immunodeficiency virus (HIV) support, immune support, leukoplakia, lung cancer, macular degeneration, night blindness, osteoarthritis, photoprotection (erythropoietic protoporphyria), photosensitivity, pancreatic insufficiency, scleroderma, sickle cell anemia.

Deficiency Symptoms

Deficiencies of beta-carotene are associated with increased free-radical activity and a weakened immune system. However, comprehensive analysis of deficiency patterns is limited by a narrow conception of its physiological function and subsequent inadequacies in available research data. Scientific research into the deficiency patterns associated with compromised beta-carotene intake has largely been lacking, and specific symptoms attributable to deficiency have not been characterized. Much of the conventional medical literature has focused almost exclusively on beta-carotene's role as a dietary precursor of vitamin A, and as a result, framed deficiencies of this nutrient as largely synonymous with the symptoms of vitamin A deficiency. Inadequate dietary intake of fruits and vegetables rich in carotenoids, signaled by their bright orange, red, and yellow pigments, constitutes the primary cause of beta-carotene deficiency.

Dietary Sources

Beta-carotene occurs exclusively in plant foods (vegetables and fruits). Foods containing high amounts of beta-carotene are yellow and dark leafy green vegetables, especially carrots, collards, sweet potatoes, squash, spinach, and green, yellow, and red peppers, and yellow fruit such as apricot, cantaloupe, and peach.

Mild cooking of food sources (e.g., carrot) for short periods can significantly increase bioavailability compared with raw forms. However, beta-carotene is quite unstable, and exposure to oxygen reduces its potency. Frying, freezing, microwaving, and canning can reduce stable beta-carotene content of foods, whereas overcooking can significantly reduce bioavailability.

Continued uncertainty about the meaning of bioavailability of carotenoids, shortcomings in methods for determining bioavailability and absorption, and emerging knowledge of numerous factors in individual variability reveal fundamental inadequacies and inaccuracy in current systems for evaluating and comparing various forms of vitamin A, particularly those from dietary intake of carotenoid-containing foods. Given the wide range of reported conversion ratios of beta-carotene to vitamin A in humans, including the ratio of 6:1 for beta-carotene and 12:1 for alpha-carotene and cryptoxanthin devised by the World Health Organization (WHO), it appears prudent to consider all such approaches as, at best, providing only an estimate that is not applicable to all diets or individuals.

Dosage Forms Available

Capsule, liquid, tablet.

Source Materials for Nutrient Preparations

Naturally occurring beta-carotene contains 40% of the nutrient as the all-*trans* isomer and 38% in a form designated 9-*cis*. In contrast, synthetic beta-carotene is 97% "all-*trans*" with virtually none of the "9-*cis*" isomer. Absorption of 9-*cis* molecule from food sources may be less than the *trans* isomers, and it can be converted to all-*trans* beta-carotene quickly after assimilation, although actual in vivo fates of the various isomers are complex and uncertain.

Natural beta-carotene supplements can be derived from a variety of sources, such as the sea algae *Dunaliella salina*, and usually contains small amounts of other carotenoids, such as alpha-carotene, lycopene, and cryptoxanthins. However, most commercial products contain synthetic beta-carotene.

Many supplements provide a combination of retinol and beta-carotene to increase carotenoid benefits and mitigate risks associated with vitamin A excess. Combinations of mixed carotenoids, along with other naturally occurring antioxidants, are favored by some health care professionals experienced in nutritional therapeutics.

Dosage Range

Dietary: 2 to 6 mg/day.
Supplemental/Maintenance: No recommended dietary allowance (RDA) has been established for beta-carotene. The most common supplemental dose range of beta-carotene is 5000 to 25,000 IU (3-15 mg).
Pharmacological/Therapeutic: 25,000 to 75,000 IU (15-45 mg).
Toxic: No toxic dose has been established.

One IU of beta-carotene is equivalent to one IU of vitamin A; 1 mg of beta-carotene is equivalent to 500 µg of vitamin A, although, as noted previously, these equivalencies are on a theoretical basis only.

> 1000 retinol equivalents (RE)
> = 1 mg retinol
> 6 mg beta-carotene
> 12 mg other provitamin A carotenoids
> 3330 international units (IU) vitamin A

Note: Further discussion of dosage issues and retinol equivalents is provided in the Vitamin A (Retinol) monograph.

Laboratory Values

Plasma beta-carotene: Normal: 0.3 to 0.6 mmol/L

SAFETY PROFILE

Overview

In general, carotenoids are nontoxic, even when consumed in large amounts. Beta-carotene has a high safety profile, and documented reports of serious adverse effects are generally lacking. Absorption and assimilation are self-regulating, and beta-carotene is not stored to a significant degree. Conversion to retinol is tightly regulated.

Nutrient Adverse Effects

Supplemental intake of beta-carotene is not normally associated with adverse effects. However, excessive intake of beta-carotene or other carotenoids in very high amounts (> 100,000 IU, or 60 mg, per day) may result in hypercarotenemia and reversible yellow-orange discoloration of the skin. This can be distinguished from jaundice by the absence of scleral pigmentation.

Beta-carotene may have antagonistic effects on vitamin E status. Thus, it may be advisable to supplement vitamin E if large doses of beta-carotene are given for prolonged periods. In fact, it may be judicious to coadminister the entire range of fat-soluble nutrients to an individual who is taking large doses of beta-carotene for prolonged periods.[1] There have been some reports of women who consume large amounts of carotenoids from foods becoming amenorrheic.

Hypercarotenemia can be associated with hypothyroidism, diabetes mellitus, liver/hepatic disease, and renal disease. It can also result from a rare genetic variation that reduces the ability to convert beta-carotene to vitamin A.

The most well-known, controversial, and misunderstood concern with potential adverse effects associated with beta-carotene intake derives from its bimodal relationship to oxidative stress. This paradoxical effect was highlighted in the Finnish Alpha Tocopherol Beta Carotene (ATBC) trial, conducted between 1985 and 1993. In this study, more than 29,000 middle-aged men in Finland, who smoked over a pack of cigarettes daily for an average of 36 years each, were divided into four groups and followed for 5 to 8 years. One group received 20 mg (or 33,000 units) of synthetic beta-carotene daily. A second group received 50 mg of synthetic vitamin E, in the form of D,L-alpha tocopherol acetate. A third group received both these vitamins, and a fourth group received a placebo. The results of the study indicated a statistically significant 18% increase in incidence of lung cancer in the group receiving only beta-carotene,[2] which may have been due to the beta-carotene functioning as a pro-oxidant under these conditions. Average consumption of fruits and vegetables in Finland is low, and average consumption of alcohol (another source of oxidative stress) is high. The soil (and thus food produced from it) is very low in selenium, an important antioxidant trace mineral that cofunctions with vitamin E.

In another large study, the U.S. Carotene and Retinol Efficacy Trial (CARET), investigators administered 30 mg of synthetic beta-carotene and 25,000 IU of vitamin A daily to half of a group of 18,000 participants, a fourth of whom were asbestos-exposed men, while the rest were either former or present smokers. The other half of the group received placebo. In this trial, the beta-carotene and vitamin A group had 28% more lung cancers and 17% more deaths than the placebo group.[3] That study was discontinued early because of this trend. Notably, there was no evidence of increased incidence of other forms of cancer related to beta-carotene administration. Beta-carotene may decrease levels of other carotenes, such as lycopene, lutein, and canthaxanthin, in the body. In smokers and people exposed to asbestos, these carotene levels may already be low. Some clinicians have suggested clinical trials with multiple carotenes as well as vitamin E and with vitamin E alone to differentiate the effects of these nutrients, which should prove beneficial; comparisons between supplements from natural sources versus those from synthetic sources and between food sources and supplements are also warranted.[4]

In addition to the pro-oxidant effect associated with using high doses of synthetic beta-carotene in a population likely depleted of antioxidant reserves and under high oxidative stress, *synthetic* versus natural beta-carotene is also an issue. A 1989 Israeli study showed a 10-fold higher accumulation of natural beta-carotene versus synthetic beta-carotene in the livers of laboratory animals. The researchers stated, "Attention should be paid to the different sources of beta-carotene when testing their efficacy ... such as in their possible role in the prevention of some types of cancer."[5] Even more significantly, natural beta-carotene has shown the ability to reverse premalignant gastric lesions, whereas synthetic beta-carotene had no activity of this sort.[6]

General Adverse Effects

Hypercarotenemia caused by excessive intake is nonthreatening and reflects high concentrations of carotenoids in the plasma and characteristic tissues. The yellowish discoloration of the skin, often most noticeable on the palms and soles, and without yellowing of the whites of the eyes (in contrast to jaundice), is harmless and will gradually recede after excess intake has been halted.

Hypervitaminosis A is not associated with intake of beta-carotene or other carotenoids alone because efficiency of absorption decreases rapidly as intake dose rises, and because the relatively slow rate of conversion to vitamin A is usually inadequate to induce vitamin A accumulation and toxicity.

Diarrhea, dizziness, and arthralgia have been associated with high intake of carotenoid supplements on rare occasions. Reports of allergic reactions, amenorrhea, and leukopenia also appear in the literature, but their incidence appears to be rare.

Adverse Effects Among Specific Populations

Individuals with *erythropoietic protoporphyria* and related disorders may develop canthaxanthin retinopathy with extended intake of 50 to 100 mg of canthaxanthin, a relative of beta-carotene used therapeutically in such patients because it reduces the severe skin photosensitivity.

Hypercarotenemia can also result from a rare genetic variation that reduces the ability to convert beta-carotene to vitamin A.

Synthetic beta-carotene has been associated with increased risk of lung cancer in smokers. This pattern of risk also extends to those with high alcohol intake and increases further when both lifestyle stressors are combined.[3,7,8]

Pregnancy and Nursing

Beta-carotene is not known to increase the risk of birth defects. Animal studies indicate beta-carotene is not toxic to a fetus or a newborn; evidence of adverse effects from human trials or case reports is lacking.

Excretion in breast milk is unconfirmed but probable, given the fat-soluble nature of carotenoids. Caution and professional supervision may be appropriate with high-dose administration during lactation.

Infants and Children

No particular adverse effects or toxicity related to beta-carotene has been indicated for infants or children.

Contraindications

Smokers and other individuals with high oxidative stress, especially involving respiratory exposure, are strongly advised to avoid consumption of synthetic beta-carotene. Similar cautions may be appropriate for individuals with high alcohol intake. Ethanol can interact with beta-carotene and interfere with its conversion to retinol. Furthermore, ethanol can promote a deficiency of vitamin A while also increasing toxicity of both vitamin A and beta-carotene. Some evidence indicates that combining beta-carotene and ethanol may increase the risk of hepatotoxicity.[8] Moreover, in smokers who also consume alcohol, beta-carotene supplementation may further exacerbate oxidative stress to promote pulmonary cancer and, possibly, cardiovascular complications. This narrowed therapeutic window for beta-carotene (and retinol) needs to be considered when formulating treatments for vitamin A deficiency in populations with high ethanol consumption.

Caution may be appropriate in individuals with renal or hepatic impairment.

Although preformed vitamin A intake in excess of 1500 µg/day (5000 IU/day) has been associated with increased risk of osteoporotic fracture and decreased bone mineral density

(BMD) in older men and women, no evidence or underlying pattern indicates that beta-carotene might induce such adverse effects on bone health.

INTERACTIONS REVIEW

Strategic Considerations

Interactions issues involving beta-carotene focus on three primary themes: antioxidant activity, decreased absorption and potential depletion, and purposeful coadministration. Patterns of clinical evidence are emerging in each of these areas, but scientific knowledge and clinical understanding are still limited, and further research is warranted through well-designed trials based on a clear understanding of the physiologic function of beta-carotene and related carotenoids and their roles in clinical practice.

Evidence suggests that mixed carotenes found in food can protect against cancer, cataracts, osteoarthritis, and heart disease.[9-15] Food rich in carotenoids (i.e., colorful vegetables and fruits) are generally considered more beneficial than isolated beta-carotene supplements. Furthermore, products containing only purified beta-carotene, especially of synthetic origin, may actually increase risk for or counter therapeutic measures against these conditions.[2,7,16-19] Thus, for physiological support, disease prevention, and therapeutic application, administration of a group of antioxidant nutrients, including carotenoids, is safer and more efficacious than administration of a single one, thus paralleling the natural pattern of diverse nutrient intake from nutritious food sources. Furthermore, although the body can convert beta-carotene into retinoids, the extent of that conversion is limited. Consequently, consumption of high doses of beta-carotene does not provide the same effect as intake of vitamin A itself.

NUTRIENT-DRUG INTERACTIONS

Note: Some interactions described in the Vitamin A (Retinol) monograph are relevant to the subject of beta-carotene but are presented there without replication here. Although interactions issues for retinoids and beta-carotene usually diverge when examining administration and its effects, directly or concomitantly with pharmaceutical agents, the interactions issues characterized by nutrient depletion are inherently synonymous in most cases. Issues of absorption and assimilation may coincide for these two primary forms of vitamin A, within food or administered as nutritional supplements or therapeutic agents.

Anthelmintic Drugs

Albendazole (Zentel), levamisole (Ergamisol), praziquantel (Biltricide).

Interaction Type and Significance

⊕⊕⊕ **Beneficial or Supportive Interaction, Not Requiring Professional Management**

Probability:	Evidence Base:
2. Probable	●●● Consensus

Effect and Mechanism of Action

Helminth infections, particularly roundworms, can interfere with vitamin A absorption, partly through their effect on intestinal epithelial cells, and thereby deplete bodily stores of vitamin A. Vitamin A deficiencies are also associated with increased risk of parasitic infections. Increased intake of vitamin A sources, whether through diet or supplementation, can counter this adverse effect of intestinal parasites and can be further enhanced by coadministration of antihelminthic (anthelmintic) agents. Enhanced vitamin A status may then help prevent or reduce symptoms associated with intestinal worms, especially roundworm. Furthermore, beta-carotene and vitamin A supplementation has often been suggested for its physiological role in maintaining epithelial integrity, its ability to stimulate specific and nonspecific immune functions, and its beneficial effects on diarrhea. Absorption of beta-carotene and vitamin A can also be supported by increasing levels of dietary fat intake because both beta-carotene and retinoids are fat soluble.

Research

Depressed iron status and serum retinol have been associated with infections involving intestinal helminths, particularly *Ascaris lumbricoides* and hookworm, in South Asian and African children.[20] Deworming can contribute significantly to the prevention of morbidity and mortality associated with vitamin A deficiency among children in rural communities where intestinal helminth infection is prevalent.[21]

Jalal et al.[22] conducted a study of the effect of food sources of beta-carotene, increased dietary fat, and *A. lumbricoides* infection on serum retinol concentrations in children, 3 to 6 years of age, in Sumatra, Indonesia. Some children were administered levamisole for deworming before the feeding period, and others were untreated and remained infected. These researchers found that the incorporation of beta-carotene sources (primarily as red sweet potatoes) into the diet significantly increased serum retinol concentrations, with the greatest rise occurring when meals contained both additional beta-carotene sources and extra fat and the children had been dewormed. Adding more fat to the meal and deworming caused a rise in serum retinol similar to that observed when the diet included additional beta-carotene. Furthermore, the combined effects of dietary fat and deworming were additive to the effects of dietary additional beta-carotene sources. When the meal contained additional beta-carotene sources, added fat caused a further improvement in serum retinol concentrations, but only if *A. lumbricoides* infection was low.

In a study involving 977 Kenyan children, Mwaniki et al.[23] found that the combination of multi-micronutrient supplementation, including 1000 μg (3300 IU) vitamin A, and multihelminth chemotherapy, using albendazole and praziquantel, reduced egg output of *Schistosoma mansoni*, a species of trematode blood flukes, and increased serum retinol, regardless of initial serum retinol.

Nutritional Therapeutics, Clinical Concerns, and Adaptations

Increasing vitamin A or beta-carotene intake through beta-carotene–rich dietary sources and administration of supplements, especially with additional dietary fat intake, can reduce susceptibility to and adverse outcomes from intestinal helminth infections and work synergistically with anthelmintics to eradicate such infections. Health care professionals treating such infections or supporting preventive measures in at-risk populations can improve clinical outcomes by increasing dietary sources of vitamin A, through plant foods rich in beta-carotene and other nutrients, or through administration of broad-based nutritional supplements. Dosing levels for supplements should be based on intake needs and safety restrictions, as determined by age, weight, and other relevant factors.

Chemotherapy (Cytotoxic Agents)

Evidence: Cisplatin (*cis*-diaminedichloroplatinum, CDDP; Platinol, Platinol-AQ), cyclophosphamide (Cytoxan, Endoxana, Neosar, Procytox), docetaxel (Taxotere), fluorouracil (5-FU; Adrucil, Efudex, Efudix, Fluoroplex), methotrexate (Folex, Maxtrex, Rheumatrex), paclitaxel (Paxene, Taxol).

Interaction Type and Significance

☼ **Prevention or Reduction of Drug Adverse Effect**
⊕⊕ **Beneficial or Supportive Interaction, with Professional Management**
✗ **Potential or Theoretical Adverse Interaction of Uncertain Severity**
⊕✗ **Bimodal or Variable Interaction, with Professional Management**

Antioxidant Activity
Probability:
3. Possible and
2. Probable

Evidence Base:
◎◎ Emerging and
▽ Mixed

Oral Mucositis
Probability:
2. Probable to 1. Certain

Evidence Base:
●●● Consensus

Effect and Mechanism of Action

Beta-carotene can reduce adverse effects of chemotherapy, particularly oral mucositis (i.e., mouth sores), by reducing drug-induced oxidative stress and free-radical damage. Similarly, beta-carotene may reduce oral mucositis caused by radiotherapy. Such antioxidant activity carries the potential risk of interfering with the free-radical–based mechanism of action of radiotherapy, as well as of drugs such as docetaxel and methotrexate, which require oxidation for activation, particularly when administered within 24 hours of such therapies.

Research

Kennedy et al.[24] conducted a 6-month observational study of 103 children with acute lymphoblastic leukemia treated with chemotherapy. They reported that a large percentage of children undergoing treatment for acute lymphoblastic leukemia (ALL) have inadequate intakes of antioxidants and vitamin A, and lower intakes of antioxidants are associated with increases in the adverse side effects of chemotherapy. In particular, greater beta-carotene intakes at 6 months after beginning therapy were associated with a decreased risk of toxicity.

Mills[25] gave chemotherapy patients approximately 400,000 IU of beta-carotene per day for 3 weeks and then 125,000 IU/day for an additional 4 weeks. Those taking beta-carotene still had mouth sores, but these developed later and tended to be less severe than the sores in patients receiving the same chemotherapy without beta-carotene.

In animal tumor models, beta-carotene has been associated with reduction of 5-fluorouracil (5-FU) activity, but an increase in cytotoxic activity of alkylating chemotherapy agents, etoposide and doxorubicin.

Teicher et al.[26] compared the effect of treatment with beta-carotene alone and in combination with minocycline (a tetracycline antibiotic), as chemotherapy modulators, along with several different chemotherapeutic agents in two murine solid tumors, the FSaII fibrosarcoma and the SCC VII carcinoma. Administration of the modulators alone or in combination did not alter the growth of either tumor. Whereas increases in tumor growth delay (indicative of increased chemotherapy

effect) occurred with the antitumor alkylating agents and beta-carotene as well as with minocycline and beta-carotene, a diminution in tumor growth delay (indicative of decreased chemotherapy effect) produced by 5-FU in the presence of these modulators. The modulator combination also resulted in increased tumor growth delay with doxorubicin and etoposide. Tumor-cell survival assay showed increased killing of FSaII tumor cells with the modulator combination and melphalan or cyclophosphamide, compared with the drugs alone. In vitro experiments can be used only as hypothesis generators to test in clinical trials; the results cannot be reliably extrapolated to in vivo effects in human patients.

Beta-Carotene, Antioxidants in General, and Chemotherapy/Radiotherapy

Oxygen radicals have increasingly come under investigation as highly toxic stressors contributing to the causes of many diseases, including many forms of cancer. Beta-carotene is among the nutrients well known as antioxidant agents. Antioxidants protect the body against cellular oxidative damage and thus some of the adverse effects induced by cisplatin and other cytotoxic drugs. Many nutritionally oriented health care professionals regard the oxidative damage caused by chemotherapy as a particularly troublesome adverse effect because evidence increasingly indicates that oxidative damage is a contributing factor in many cancers. Some oncologists consider antioxidants as potentially contraindicated with some agents or during some phases of chemotherapy based on the premise that many chemotherapeutic agents attack cancer cells by inducing oxidative damage, mediated by free radicals. No substantial clinical research in humans has emerged to support this speculation or to warrant considering antioxidants as inherently contraindicated during chemotherapy, and the trend in reviews and meta-analyses increasingly suggests a lack of adverse effect and possible evidence of benefit in some circumstances.[27]

The interactions between chemotherapeutic agents and antioxidant nutrients display some patterns of similarity, but also other aspects of diversity in usage, action, and attention by researchers. The issue of antioxidants in oncology remains controversial, with a small but slowly growing body of clinically based evidence. In general, clinicians and researchers most familiar with antioxidants consistently emphasize the importance of using antioxidant agents in clusters capable of creating an antioxidant network to avert the potential for individual nutrients to act as pro-oxidants under conditions of high oxidative stress, particularly in individuals with multiple biochemical stressors and compromised physiology. Furthermore, high-quality randomized trials that control for the antioxidant contribution of diet, which may well confound the contribution of antioxidant supplements, have not been performed, and this key issue of study design has not been adequately addressed by those presenting their findings as conclusive.

See also Vitamin E or Melatonin monograph for further discussion of antioxidants in relation to radiotherapy.

Nutritional Therapeutics, Clinical Concerns, and Adaptations

The coordinated use of beta-carotene and some chemotherapeutic agents may play a valuable role in an integrative approach to oncology care. Consistent evidence supports benefit from beta-carotene in preventing or remediating treatment-induced oral mucositis. Broader use of beta-carotene, alone or with other antioxidants, requires close supervision and regular monitoring and is most appropriate in the context of collaborative care involving health care

Nutrient-Drug Interactions and Drug-Induced Nutrient Depletions

professionals trained and experienced in both conventional oncology and nutritional therapeutics. In many cases the timing of such nutritional interventions in the therapeutic sequence is critical to its safety, effectiveness, and synergy. In particular, practitioners who judiciously use antioxidants during chemotherapy or other conventional cancer treatments are advised to question patients about self-prescribing of antioxidants. Such concomitant use could be problematic and contraindicated, beneficial and appropriate, or both, for certain patients with individualized dosage at coordinated intervals. In almost all cases the administration of multiple antioxidant agents, such as mixed tocopherols, vitamin C, N-acetylcysteine, parenteral glutathione, coenzyme Q10, and proanthocyanadins, is more likely to be appropriate, safe, and effective than the use of single agents in high doses. Further research through well-designed human trials is necessary to inform this evolving debate.

Cholestyramine, Colestipol, and Related Bile Acid Sequestrants

Evidence: Cholestyramine (Locholest, Prevalite, Questran), colestipol (Colestid).
Extrapolated, based on similar properties: Colesevelam (WelChol).

Interaction Type and Significance

≈≈≈ **Drug-Induced Nutrient Depletion, Supplementation Therapeutic, Not Requiring Professional Management**
◇ **Adverse Drug Effect on Nutritional Therapeutics, Strategic Concern**

Probability:
3. Possible

Evidence Base:
◉◉ Emerging and/or ▽ Mixed

Effect and Mechanism of Action

Absorption of dietary sources of beta-carotene requires bile. Bile acid sequestrants, such as cholestyramine and colestipol, can decrease lipid digestion and absorption, as well as absorption of beta-carotene and other fat-soluble nutrients.[28-33] Furthermore, VLDL or LDL cholesterol transport intact beta-carotene in the blood, with blood levels varying according to intake levels; consequently, decreased lipid levels may impair beta-carotene transport. Conversely, both beta-carotene and vitamin A may increase triglycerides.

Carotenes rely on bile salts for absorption much more than retinol. Retinol can also be absorbed from a micelle in the presence of a nonionic detergent, but carotenoids can only be absorbed from a micelle in the presence of bile salts. Furthermore, carotenoids are absorbed by passive absorption regardless of the concentration, whereas retinol is absorbed by diffusion when present in high doses, but is carrier mediated at low doses.

Research

A general consensus has emerged over the past 40 years: Drugs that alter fat absorption and bile function will disrupt absorption and assimilation of fat-soluble nutrients. However, the evidence on the degree of such impairment, the nutrients affected, and the clinical significance of the phenomena is mixed, inconclusive, and still emerging. Using early research by Longnecker and Basu[28] and later by West and Lloyd,[29] reviews posited a general impairment of absorption of vitamin A and the range of fat-soluble nutrient caused by bile acid sequestrants and other antilipidemic agents. Subsequent human trials have investigated the significance of these effects

on various nutrients for different medications used in various patient populations.

West and Lloyd[29] studied the effects cholestyramine (mean dosage, 0-6 g/kg/day) on 18 children with familial hypercholesterolemia over 1 to 2½ years. In addition to a major reduction in serum folate concentration and red blood cell folate, these researchers also noted "a significant decrease in the mean serum concentrations of vitamins A and E and of inorganic phosphorus over the first two years of treatment, although values remain within the normal range." They concluded that "routine administration of fat-soluble vitamins appears unnecessary, but it is prudent to measure prothrombin time [to assess vitamin K status] and serum vitamins A and E at intervals."

Knodel and Talbert[33] reported that large doses of cholestyramine (>32 g/day) may be associated with malabsorption of fat-soluble vitamins but concluded that impaired absorption of vitamins D and K presented the most significant clinical risk with long-term therapy, with bone loss and bleeding disorders being the potential adverse outcomes. However, in a 3-year, double-blind randomized trial involving 303 hypercholesterolemic subjects, Elinder et al.[34] demonstrated that cholestyramine lowered serum concentrations of beta-carotene by 40% "due to impairment of gastrointestinal absorption and to serum cholesterol lowering"; likewise, vitamin E and lycopene were reduced by 7% and 30%, respectively.

In a study involving type IIa hyperlipoproteinemic patients, Probstfield et al.[35] observed that serum total carotenoid levels fell by 30% after administration of colestipol (30 g/day) for 6 months, most likely as a result of decreased absorption of carotenoids induced by bile acid sequestrant administration, but that serum vitamin A levels were not significantly altered. Tonstad et al.[36] investigated the effects of colestipol granules (10 g/day), along with a low-fat diet, in an 8-week, double blind placebo-controlled trial, followed by open treatment for 44 to 52 weeks, on LDL cholesterol levels in 37 boys and 29 girls, age 10 to 16 years, with familial hypercholesterolemia. Serum concentrations of vitamins A and D, as well as other relevant nutrient parameters, were not affected significantly in the colestipol group even though levels of serum folate, vitamin E, and carotenoids were significantly reduced. Thus, although these researchers did not suggest a need for compensatory enhancement of fat-soluble nutrients in general or vitamin A in particular, they did recommend supplementation with folate and "possibly vitamin D." They also noted the high degree of noncompliance among the adolescents in the study.[36]

This trend toward a significant interaction raises serious questions given the ongoing debate regarding the correlation between nutrient status, particularly dietary antioxidants, and long-term risk of coronary heart disease. Most importantly, the limited scope of the research available and lack of follow-through investigation of long-term effects (i.e., decades) of such drug-induced nutrient depletion patterns on nutrient status, healthy cardiovascular function, and ultimate outcomes render the data suggestive but inconclusive in answering the fundamental questions of benefit and risk.

Nutritional Therapeutics, Clinical Concerns, and Adaptations

Although not always necessary, supplementation with beta-carotene, as well as other affected nutrients, in the form of a multivitamin-mineral formulation can provide a safe and inexpensive means of avoiding adverse effects from these medications without interfering with (and perhaps enhancing) the therapeutic goal of supporting healthy cardiovascular function and reducing risk. Beta-carotene and other fat-soluble nutrients (as well as folic acid and many medications) should be taken

1 hour before or 4 to 6 hours after bile acid sequestrants for optimal absorption. Characteristics of the individual being treated will influence the need for compensatory nutrient administration, particularly age, typical diet, digestive function, comorbid conditions, and pharmacogenomic response to the medication being used. Increased consumption of red, orange, and yellow fruits and vegetables, which may also contribute to cholesterol lowering, as well as providing increased dietary intake of carotenoids, should be encouraged.

Colchicine

Colchicine

Interaction Type and Significance

≈≈≈ **Drug-Induced Nutrient Depletion, Supplementation Therapeutic, Not Requiring Professional Management**

◇ **Adverse Drug Effect on Nutritional Therapeutics, Strategic Concern**

Probability:	Evidence Base:
4. Plausible or 2. Probable	○ Preliminary

Effect and Mechanism of Action

Oral colchicine may impair absorption of beta-carotene and other nutrients.[37,38] Colchicine also blocks hepatic release of retinol and retinol-binding protein (RBP) and thereby impairs upregulation of serum retinol and interferes with its homeostasis.

Research

Race et al.[37] reported that oral colchicine can induce intestinal malabsorption, affecting beta-carotene and other nutrients.

Nutritional Therapeutics, Clinical Concerns, and Adaptations

Physicians prescribing colchicine for extended regular use should suggest the likely benefit of using a high-potency multivitamin/mineral supplement to compensate for potential drug-induced depletion of beta-carotene and other nutrients. Further research through well-designed human trials is warranted to determine the severity, frequency, and clinical implications of this probable interaction and to identify characteristics of individuals most susceptible to clinically significant adverse effects and the circumstances involved.

Medroxyprogesterone

Conjugated equine estrogens and medroxyprogesterone (Premelle cycle 5, Prempro); medroxyprogesterone, oral (Cycrin, Provera); medroxyprogesterone, injection (Depot medroxyprogesterone acetate, DMPA; Depo-Provera, Depo-subQ Provera 104); progestin and estrogen injectable: estradiol cypionate and medroxyprogesterone acetate (Cyclofem, Lunelle).

Interaction Type and Significance

≈≈ **Drug-Induced Nutrient Depletion, Supplementation Therapeutic, with Professional Management**

☼ **Prevention or Reduction of Drug Adverse Effect**

Probability:	Evidence Base:
3. Possible or 2. Probable	◉◉ Emerging

Effect and Mechanism of Action

Medroxyprogesterone acetate (MPA) use is associated with elevations in serum retinol levels. Exogenous estrogen and progestin increase hepatic synthesis of RBP, thus increasing the export of RBP-retinol complex in the blood.

Research

Numerous clinical trials have investigated the effect of medroxyprogesterone administration, whether for contraception or as a component of menopausal hormone replacement therapy (HRT), on blood levels of vitamin A and its metabolites as well as other nutrients. Elevations in serum retinol levels have been observed in most studies, with 40% mean increases in some trials; RBP elevations were also noted in one study.[39-43] In a trial involving 12 healthy, nonlactating Thai women, Amatayakul et al.[39] found no significant changes in serum levels of several nutrients, including vitamin A, before and with daily coadministration of a vitamin-mineral supplement, including beta-carotene and vitamin A, in association with 1 year's continual use of MPA as an injectable contraceptive (150 mg intramuscularly every 90 days). In a subsequent study focusing on the effect of 1 year of oral contraceptive (OC) use on liver vitamin A storage, as assessed by the relative dose response (RDR) test, daily (one capsule) or periodic (two capsules 7 days per month) multivitamin supplementation, including 1700 μg vitamin A per capsule, did not significantly influence vitamin A serum values. After 13 cycles, however, the RDR test was elevated in one individual who had taken OCs and the periodic multivitamin supplement, returning to normal after supplementation with vitamin A.[41]

Given the inadequate nutritional intake or compromised nutrient status of the women in some of these studies, the researchers have interpreted the phenomena of elevated serum retinol as beneficial. However, in the study of Nigerian women, whose diet is typically high in carotenoids, Wien and Ojo[44] reported that serum carotene was lower in OC users (combination estrogen-progestogen) than in groups using intrauterine devices (IUDs) or injectable progestogen. These researchers concluded that "more detailed study of plasma transport forms of vitamin A is needed to determine if the very high serum vitamin A levels seen in some OC users in this population are potentially harmful." The role of dietary and supplemental beta-carotene in this interaction pattern deserves further research through well-designed human trials to determine the severity, frequency, and clinical implications of this probable interaction and to identify characteristics of individuals most susceptible to clinically significant adverse effects and the circumstances involved. Studies of tissue levels of retinol and carotenoids in these populations would also be useful.

Nutritional Therapeutics, Clinical Concerns, and Adaptations

Physicians prescribing medroxyprogesterone, for contraception or as a component of menopausal HRT, are advised to consider monitoring blood levels of vitamin A in patients, particularly those with compromised liver function. Enhanced carotenoid intake may be beneficial, through diet and supplementation, and is unlikely to contribute significantly to further elevation of vitamin A levels, given the body's limited ability to convert carotenoids to vitamin A. In some individuals, vitamin A supplementation may need to be avoided; in others it might be indicated, depending on individual patient characteristics and response to the medication. Dietary intake of provitamin A carotenoids and preformed vitamin A, nutritional status, age and menstrual status, dose, form, and therapeutic intent are all important factors that appear to influence the degree to which medroxyprogesterone administration alters beta-carotene and vitamin A levels and functions and whether that effect is beneficial, adverse, or insignificant.

Methyltestosterone

Methyltestosterone (Android, Methitest, Testred, Virilon). Related but evidence lacking for extrapolation: Methyltestosterone combination drug: methyltestosterone and esterified estrogens (Estratest, Estratest HS); testolactone (testolacton, HSDB 3255, SQ 9538; Fludestrin, Teolit, Teslac, Teslak).

Interaction Type and Significance

◇≈≈ Drug-Induced Adverse Effect on Nutrient Function, Coadministration Therapeutic, with Professional Management

≈≈ Drug-Induced Nutrient Depletion, Supplementation Therapeutic, with Professional Management

Probability:	Evidence Base:
6. Unknown	☐ Inadequate

Effect and Mechanism of Action

The mechanisms involved in the report examined are not established, and research has not specifically focused on this potential interaction, its mechanisms, susceptibility factors, or clinical implications.

Report

Nisbett et al.[45] reported the case of a 59-year-old man who presented with a 3-month history of night blindness and a 9-month history of steatorrhea after initiating therapy with methyltestosterone. Low serum levels of carotene (0.1 mmol/L) and vitamin A were accompanied by numerous changes in visual function. The symptoms and the biochemical and electrophysiological abnormalities resolved within 9 months of the discontinuation of methyltestosterone.

Nutritional Therapeutics, Clinical Concerns, and Adaptations

Although this report may represent an anomalous phenomenon, resulting from pharmacogenomic variability and/or other factors, it still suggests a need for further research. Physicians prescribing methyltestosterone (an anabolic steroid, not testosterone replacement) may find it prudent to assess patients for beta-carotene and vitamin A status and recommend concomitant supplementation with beta-carotene and/or vitamin A as indicated.

Mineral Oil

Mineral Oil (Agoral, Kondremul Plain, Liquid Parafin, Milkinol, Neo-Cultol, Petrogalar Plain).

Interaction Type and Significance

✗ Potential or Theoretical Adverse Interaction of Uncertain Severity

≈≈≈ Drug-Induced Nutrient Depletion, Supplementation Therapeutic, Not Requiring Professional Management

Probability:	Evidence Base:
4. Plausible or 2. Probable	○ Preliminary

Effect and Mechanism of Action

Mineral oil, as a lipid solvent, may absorb many substances and interfere with normal absorption of beta-carotene, retinol, and other nutrients.

Research

Some disagreement exists, but most research has found that mineral oil can interfere with the absorption of, and thus contribute to a depletion of, many nutrients, including beta-carotene, calcium, phosphorus, potassium, and vitamins A, D, K, and E. One study involving 25 children with chronic constipation found that a short course of mineral oil can reduce serum levels of beta-carotene while elevating serum retinol levels modestly.[46]

Nutritional Therapeutics, Clinical Concerns, and Adaptations

As a preventive and protective measure, health care professionals are advised to recommend regular use of a multivitamin supplement to individuals using mineral oil for an extended period. Malabsorption of fat-soluble vitamins from ingestion of mineral oil can be minimized by administering mineral oil on an empty stomach or administering vitamin or mineral supplements at least 2 hours before or after the mineral oil. In general it is advisable to limit the internal use of mineral oil to less than 1 week.

Neomycin

Neomycin (Mycifradin, Myciguent, Neo-Fradin, NeoTab, Nivemycin).
Combination drugs: Adcortyl with Graneodin, Betnovate-N, Dermovate-NN, Gregoderm, Synalar N, Tri-Adcortyl, Trimovate.

Interaction Type and Significance

≈≈≈ Drug-Induced Nutrient Depletion, Supplementation Therapeutic, Not Requiring Professional Management

◇ Adverse Drug Effect on Nutritional Therapeutics, Strategic Concern

Probability:	Evidence Base:
2. Probable	●●● Consensus or ○ Preliminary

See also Vitamin A (Retinol) monograph.

Effect and Mechanism of Action

Neomycin may damage the structure and adversely affect the function of the lining of the digestive tract. In many individuals this reduces the absorption and increases the elimination of beta-carotene from the body.[30,38] Neomycin may also reduce the bioavailability of vitamin A.

Research

Orally administered neomycin can impair absorption of beta-carotene (and vitamin A).[47-50]

Nutritional Therapeutics, Clinical Concerns, and Adaptations

Physicians prescribing neomycin internally for more than 2 or 3 days can advise patients of the probable benefit of supplementing with beta-carotene (25,000 IU or 15 mg daily) or vitamin A (25,000 IU or 7.5 mg daily). Individuals using neomycin topically will not experience problems related to malabsorption; likewise, adverse effects are unlikely to result from a single dose of oral neomycin as part of surgery preparation.

Omeprazole and Related Proton Pump Inhibitors

Evidence: Omeprazole (Losec, Prilosec).
Extrapolated, based on similar properties: Esomeprazole (Nexium), lansoprazole (Prevacid, Zoton), pantoprazole (Protium, Protonix, Somac), rabeprazole (AcipHex, Pariet).

Interaction Type and Significance

≈≈≈ **Drug-Induced Nutrient Depletion, Supplementation Therapeutic, Not Requiring Professional Management**

Probability:	Evidence Base:
4. Plausible	○ Preliminary

Effect and Mechanism of Action

Proton pump inhibitors (PPIs) impair production of stomach acid by inhibiting the hydrogen-potassium–adenosine triphosphate (ATP) enzyme system in gastric parietal cells. This change in the gastric environment and its effect on subsequent digestive chemistry may adversely affect absorption of beta-carotene, as well as other nutrients.

Research

In a crossover trial involving 12 normal adults, Tang et al.[51] administered omeprazole for 7 days to block gastric acid secretion and raise gastric pH from the normal postprandial level of between 1 and 2 to greater than 4.5. They then measured blood levels of beta-carotene after a single dose of 120 mg beta-carotene before starting omeprazole (low gastric pH phase), then again after administering omeprazole for 9 or 26 days (high gastric pH phase). Increases in serum concentrations of both *trans* and *cis* beta-carotene at 6 and 24 hours after the beta-carotene dose were significantly greater at a low gastric pH phase (i.e., without omeprazole) than at a high gastric pH phase (i.e., with omeprazole). Likewise, 24 hours after beta-carotene administration, the area under the blood beta-carotene response curve (*trans* plus *cis* beta-carotene) was significantly greater at a low gastric pH than at a high gastric pH. Results after 9 days of omeprazole were the same as those after 26 days. Although expressing uncertainty as to the mechanisms underlying the observed phenomenon, the researchers concluded that "suppressed blood response of beta-carotene at a high intraluminal pH may have been due to the slower movement of negatively charged micelles through the unstirred water layer and cell membrane."[51]

This test demonstrated that almost complete loss of stomach acid in healthy subjects can interfere with the digestive absorption of single-dose beta-carotene. However, its limited design did not address the response to repeated administration of supplemental beta-carotene or carotenoids from food sources in determining whether continued use of PPIs might induce beta-carotene depletion. The results do suggest that testing blood carotenoid levels in patients receiving extended PPI therapy might be useful and, if low, dietary or supplemental therapy instituted.

Nutritional Therapeutics, Clinical Concerns, and Adaptations

Physicians prescribing PPIs for extended periods are advised to recommend that these patients increase their dietary intake of fruits and vegetables rich in carotenoids and consider supplementation with naturally occurring forms of beta-carotene. Monitoring of blood levels of carotenoids could be used to detect and forestall nutrient depletion, if suspected. Further research through well-designed human trials is warranted to determine the severity, frequency, and clinical implications of this plausible nutrient depletion pattern and to develop guidelines for protecting nutrient status.

Orlistat

Orlistat (alli, Xenical).

Interaction Type and Significance

≈≈≈ **Drug-Induced Nutrient Depletion, Supplementation Therapeutic, Not Requiring Professional Management**

Probability:	Evidence Base:
3. Possible (short term) or	○ Preliminary or
2. Probable (long term)	◉◉ Emerging

Effect and Mechanism of Action

As a GI lipase inhibitor, and thus an inhibitor of dietary fat absorption, orlistat may also decrease absorption of beta-carotene and other fat-soluble nutrients. Carotenes rely on bile salts for absorption to a much greater extent than retinol does. Furthermore, in contrast to retinol, carotenoids are absorbed by passive absorption and are not stored to the extent of retinol.

Research

Clinical trials investigating the short-term pharmacokinetic effects of orlistat on beta-carotene, vitamin A, and other nutrients have shown reductions in nutrient absorption but no significant depletion in the time frame studied. In an open-label, parallel, placebo-controlled, randomized, two-way crossover study involving 48 healthy subjects in 1996, Zhi et al.[52] demonstrated that simultaneous intake of orlistat and beta-carotene can reduce beta-carotene by approximately one-third. They concluded that two thirds of a dose of beta-carotene will still be absorbed during orlistat treatment, and that such intake levels would generally be sufficient to achieve physiological levels of beta-carotene with an appropriate dose, when coadministered to prevent or respond to orlistat-induced beta-carotene deficiency. Also in 1996, in a small, open-label, placebo-controlled, randomized, two-way crossover trial, Melia et al.[53] investigated the effect of orlistat on the absorption of sequential single oral doses of vitamins A (25,000 IU) and E (400 IU) in 12 healthy volunteers. Based on subsequent analysis of serum concentrations of retinol, they found no significant effect on absorption of vitamin A during oral administration of 120 mg orlistat or placebo three times daily for 9 days, although absorption of vitamin E was reduced significantly (about 43% according to maximum concentration and 60% according to area under the concentration-time curve). Beta-carotene was not directly studied in this experiment, but general pharmacological principles suggest that its absorption would be more susceptible to impairment than that of vitamin A.

Longer trials indicate that regular use of orlistat can exert a continued effect on nutrient absorption, but the cumulative effects of this pharmacokinetic phenomenon have not been studied for more than 1 year. In a multicenter, randomized, double-blind, parallel-group clinical trial involving 676 obese male and female subjects, van Gaal et al.[54] demonstrated reduced blood levels of vitamin A (and vitamin D) after administration of orlistat for 6 months in conjunction with a mildly hypocaloric diet. However, mean levels of beta-carotene, as well as of vitamins A, D, and E, remained within the clinical reference ranges in all treatment groups. A small percentage of patients developed levels deemed low enough to require supplementation. However, at the end of a 1-year, randomized, double-blind, placebo-controlled, multicenter trial involving 228 obese adult patients, Finer et al.[55] also reported that orlistat decreased plasma levels of beta-carotene (and vitamin E) compared with placebo.

They concluded, "Fat-soluble vitamin supplements may be required during chronic therapy."

Nutritional Therapeutics, Clinical Concerns, and Adaptations

Research into the efficacy and tolerability of orlistat indicates that it can be an effective tool in treating obesity. However, further research is warranted to investigate the probable risk of long-term nutrient depletion as a result of known adverse effects on absorption of beta-carotene and other fat-soluble nutrients. Pending conclusive evidence of a lack of cumulative effect, physicians prescribing orlistat for longer than 3 months can recommend to their patients that they take a multivitamin supplement containing naturally occurring forms of beta-carotene, alpha-tocopherol, and other potentially affected nutrients, at least 2 hours after orlistat or at bedtime.

Further research through long-term, well-designed human trials can determine the severity, frequency, and clinical implications of this probable nutrient depletion pattern and identify characteristics of individuals most susceptible to clinically significant adverse effects and the circumstances involved.

Probucol

Probucol (Bifenabid, Lesterol, Lorelco, Lurselle, Panesclerina, Superlipid).

Interaction Type and Significance

◇≈≈ **Drug-Induced Adverse Effect on Nutrient Function, Coadministration Therapeutic, with Professional Management**

≈≈ **Drug-Induced Nutrient Depletion, Supplementation Therapeutic, with Professional Management**

✗ **Potential or Theoretical Adverse Interaction of Uncertain Severity**

◇ **Adverse Drug Effect on Nutritional Therapeutics, Strategic Concern**

Probability: Evidence Base:
2. Probable   ○ Preliminary; possibly
                            ◉◉ Emerging

Effect and Mechanism of Action

Probucol is lipid soluble and can interfere with absorption and activity of beta-carotene and other carotenoids, at least in part, through competition for incorporation into VLDL during hepatic synthesis.

Research

In a 3-year, double-blind randomized trial involving 303 hypercholesterolemic subjects, Elinder et al.[34] demonstrated that probucol reduced serum carotenoids by 30% to 40%, "most probably due to reductions in lipoprotein particle size and to competition with these substances for incorporation into VLDL during its assembly in the liver." Similarly, serum vitamin E decreased 14% secondary to cholesterol and triglyceride lowering.

Nutritional Therapeutics, Clinical Concerns, and Adaptations

The available research, although limited, provides strong preliminary evidence that use of probucol, a lipid-soluble antioxidant and cholesterol-lowering drug, may have adverse effects on blood levels of beta-carotene and other diet-derived antioxidants. Supplementation with affected nutrients may be judicious to prevent or reverse depletion, and regular monitoring is appropriate to confirm that such increased nutrient intake does not interfere with drug efficacy by the same apparent mechanism of competition that contributes to the decrease in nutrient levels. Further research through well-designed human trials is warranted to determine the severity, frequency, and clinical implications of this probable nutrient depletion pattern and to develop guidelines for protecting nutrient status while maintaining drug efficacy.

THEORETICAL, SPECULATIVE, AND PRELIMINARY INTERACTIONS RESEARCH, INCLUDING OVERSTATED INTERACTIONS CLAIMS

HMG-CoA Reductase Inhibitors (Statins)

Atorvastatin (Lipitor), fluvastatin (Lescol, Lescol XL), lovastatin (Altocor, Altoprev, Mevacor), combination drug: lovastatin and niacin (Advicor), pravastatin (Pravachol), rosuvastatin (Crestor), simvastatin (Zocor); combination drug: simvastatin and extended-release nicotinic acid (Niaspan).

It is known that 3-hydroxy-3-methylglutaryl–coenzyme A (HMG-CoA) reductase inhibitors may increase serum retinol levels.[56] However, the question of how HMG-CoA reductase inhibition might influence beta-carotene metabolism or alter liver regulation of vitamin A has not been investigated.

Very-low-density lipoprotein cholesterol or LDL cholesterol transports intact beta-carotene in the blood, with blood levels varying according to intake levels; consequently, decreased lipid levels may impair beta-carotene transport. Conversely, both beta-carotene and vitamin A may increase triglycerides.

Further research through well-designed human trials is warranted to determine the severity, frequency, and clinical implications of this potential interaction and to identify characteristics of individuals most susceptible to clinically significant adverse effects and the circumstances involved.

Retinoids: Isotretinoin, Tretinoin

Acitretin (Soriatane), bexarotene (Targretin), etretinate (Tegison), isotretinoin (Accutane), tretinoin (all-*trans* retinoic acid, ATRA; Atragen, Avita, Renova, Retin-A, Vesanoid, Vitinoin).

The concomitant use of retinoids and supplemental vitamin A is generally considered contraindicated based on additive toxicity of the two structurally similar substances. However, no such risk pertains to coadministration of pharmaceutical retinoids and beta-carotene. Some retinol is metabolized into retinoic acid, but in the absence of retinol deficiency, very little beta-carotene (or other provitamin A carotenoid) is metabolized into retinol.

Quinidine

Quinidine (Quinaglute, Quinidex, Quinora).

Quinidine therapy is associated with the development of sensitivity to ultraviolet radiation from the sun (photosensitivity) in certain individuals. Preliminary research by Fisher[57] involving three subjects indicates that patients with skin inflammation caused by quinidine may experience greater tolerance of intense sun exposure without recurrence of the rash when supplemented with 90 to 180 mg beta-carotene daily.

Although data are promising, further research is necessary to confirm that individuals taking quinidine can prevent adverse effects by supplementing with beta-carotene.

NUTRIENT-NUTRIENT INTERACTIONS

Carotenoids

Antheraxanthin, astaxanthin, canthaxanthin, alpha-carotene, beta-carotene, epsilon-carotene, gamma-carotene, zeta-carotene, alpha-cryptoxanthin, diatoxanthin, 7,8-didehydroastaxanthin, fucoxanthin, fucoxanthinol, lactucaxanthin, lutein, lycopene, neoxanthin, neurosporene, peridinin, phytoene, rhodopin, rhodopin glucoside, siphonaxanthin, spheroidene, spheroidenone, spirilloxanthin, uriolide, uriolide acetate, violaxanthin, zeaxanthin.

Large doses of beta-carotene could theoretically reduce bioavailability, assimilation, and utilization of other carotenoids. In one small study with two healthy subjects, White et al.[16] observed that ingestion of beta-carotene concurrently with the carotenoid canthaxanthin reduced the peak serum canthaxanthin concentration by 38.8% and the 72-hour area under the serum canthaxanthin concentration-time curve by 34.4%. These results suggest that administration of beta-carotene inhibits the bioavailability of canthaxanthin. Although canthaxanthin had no effect on the bioavailability of beta-carotene, these findings suggest that administration of beta-carotene alone might promote deficiencies of other carotenoids. Further research is necessary to draw any reliable conclusions regarding bioavailability interactions between provitamin A carotenoids.

Vitamin E (Alpha-Tocopherol)

A competitive relationship between beta-carotene and alpha-tocopherol has been suggested, but evidence is lacking. Generally, health care professionals experienced with antioxidant nutrients recommend that multiple antioxidant agents be coadministered to achieve a network effect that would enhance beneficial effects and prevent the agents from exerting pro-oxidant activity.

The 57 citations for this monograph, as well as additional reference literature, are located under Beta-Carotene on the CD at the back of the book.

Folic Acid

Nutrient Name: Folic acid; folate, folinic acid.
Synonyms: Folacin; folate triglutamate, folicin, pteroyltriglutamate, pteroylglutamic acid, vitamin B₉, vitamin Bc, vitamin M; 5-formyltetrahydrofolate (5-FTHF), 5-methyltetrahydrofolate (5-MTHF), 6(S) 5-MTHF, L-methylfolate; calcium folinate, calcium levofolinate, citrovorum factor, sodium folinate.

Summary

Drug/Class Interaction Type	Mechanism and Significance	Management
Acetylsalicylic acid (ASA, aspirin) Salsalate ≈≈/≈≈≈/☼/⊕⊕⊕	Aspirin and salicylic acid can inhibit folate-dependent enzymes, interfere with folate metabolism, and increase urinary excretion of folate. Drug-induced impairment well-documented, but degree of adverse effects variable depending on dose, duration, and patient characteristics. Evidence lacking that coadministration of folic acid might interfere with drug activity. Synergy probable with low-dose ASA in stroke prevention.	Supplement folic acid with chronic and high-dose ASA or salsalate.
Antacids Histamine (H₂) antagonists Gastric acid—suppressive medications ≈≈≈/≈≈/☼/◇	Agents that interfere with normal acidic-alkaline balance in gastrointestinal environment, particularly alkalinization of jejunum, can impair folic acid absorption and availability. Mineral-containing antacids can reduce absorption by binding folate. Adverse effects on vitamin B₁₂ assimilation may also impair folate function. Possible clinically significant folate deficiency (and B₁₂ depletion), which may not parallel degree of change in pH, especially in compromised patients, MTHFR and CYP2C19 polymorphisms, compromised gut ecology, Zollinger-Ellison syndrome, and atrophic gastritis.	Coadminister folic acid, as well as a cobalamin intramuscularly or orally (>500 µg/day), during extended antacid therapy.
Anticonvulsant medications Antiepileptic drugs (AEDs) ☼/◇≈≈/≈≈/◇◇/ ≈◇◇/⊕ ✗/✗✗/✗✗✗	Adverse effects of anticonvulsants on folate are documented and well known, especially with multiple agents. AEDs decrease absorption of folate (and cobalamin); all except valproic acid induce CYP450. Anemia common from drug-induced folic acid and B₁₂ deficiency, also elevated homocysteine. Teratogenic effects may be particularly severe, even months before pregnancy. Evidence conclusive, but variable probability of clinically significant effect. Folic acid may decrease phenytoin levels and increase risk of seizure activity; unlikely with <1 mg/day folic acid. Folate mouthwash protects against gingival hyperplasia.	Supplement folic acid and B₁₂ during extended or multidrug anticonvulsant therapy. Monitor folate, homocysteine, and cobalamin status and medication levels. Avoid pregnancy; otherwise, supplement or change medication. Genomic testing may be warranted.
Antifolates, antimetabolites Lometrexol, methotrexate, pemetrexed ✗✗✗/⊕⊕/◇≈/≈≈/☼/ ⊕✗/◇◇	Antifolates competitively inhibit folate and interfere with folate-related enzyme systems; thus they inherently carry significant risk of folate deficiency and attendant toxicity. Folic acid or 5-MTHF may impair antineoplastic activity but is often appropriate for reducing adverse effects and sometimes critical against toxicity. Significant effect axiomatic, and coherent pattern of evidence emerging as to coadministration.	Pharmacogenomic assessment helpful in predicting drug efficacy and tolerance. Folic acid or 5-MTHF generally warranted in treating inflammatory conditions; only with close supervision and active management in integrative oncology setting. Monitor folate status and medication levels.
Bile acid sequestrants ≈≈≈/◇/⊕⊕	Bile acid sequestrants likely to impair absorption and reduce bioavailability of folic acid and B₁₂, as well as fat-soluble nutrients. Coadministration suggested for comprehensive cardiovascular support strategy. Further research warranted. Cholestyramine and folinic acid may be used together to reduce methotrexate toxicity.	Folic acid recommended as prudent and proactive, especially in children and with MTHFR C677T mutation. Fat-soluble nutrients warranted. Separate intake of drug and nutrients.
Chloramphenicol ◇≈≈/☼/⊕⊕⊕/◇	Chloramphenicol interferes with hematopoietic processes and may cause aplastic anemia. Folic acid may prevent or reduce such adverse effects. Drug activity may impair therapeutic action of folic acid. Significant effect probable but specific evidence lacking; broad agreement on mechanisms.	Coadministration of folic acid prudent with extended chloramphenicol. Monitor hematological parameters.
Colchicine ◇≈≈/☼/⊕⊕⊕/◇	Colchicine may decrease folate levels. Minimal evidence. Significant effect plausible. Evidence lacking to confirm benefit of concomitant folic acid. Research may be warranted.	Coadminister folic acid during extended colchicine therapy. Monitor folate and homocysteine levels.
Fibrates Fenofibrate, bezafibrate ≈≈/☼/⊕⊕⊕	Fenofibrate, bezafibrate, and to lesser degree other fibrates are known to elevate total plasma homocysteine (Hcy), but primarily nonatherogenic protein-bound Hcy. Observed effect most likely from mechanisms other than folate depletion. Concomitant folic acid may lower Hcy and enhance therapeutic strategy, but evidence mixed as to whether drug-induced effects on Hcy are clinically significant.	Administration of folic acid, B₆, and B₁₂ may be appropriate, if only for strategic considerations. Monitor folate, Hcy, and lipid levels.
Fluoxetine Selective serotonin reuptake inhibitor and serotonin-norepinephrine reuptake inhibitor (SSRI and SSRI/SNRI) antidepressants ⊕⊕	Folate plays important roles in synthesis of S-adenosylmethionine (SAMe) and tetrahydrobiopterin; deficiency may be associated with depressive disorders and lack of response to SSRIs. Concomitant folic acid may enhance response to fluoxetine therapy by improving tryptophan, phenylalanine, and serotonin status; improvements in Hcy levels may also support strategic outcomes.	Coadminister folic acid with SSRI therapy. Monitor tissue folate and plasma Hcy levels. Genetic assessment often relevant.
Isoniazid (INH), rifampin Antitubercular agents ☼/◇≈≈	Generally accepted that isoniazid and related antitubercular medications adversely affect action of folate and potentially induce depletion. Multiple mechanisms likely, including interference with B₆ and B₁₂, but knowledge incomplete.	Broad nutrient support, including folic acid, B₃, B₆, and B₁₂, judicious during antitubercular therapy. Supervise closely and monitor regularly.

Summary

Drug/Class Interaction Type	Mechanism and Significance	Management
	Numerous reports of adverse effects, but evidence inconclusive and further research needed.	
Levodopa Antiparkinsonian medications ☼/⊕⊕/◇≈≈	Levodopa can elevate Hcy in Parkinson's patients, particularly in the context of compromised B-vitamin status, caused by competition at site of methylation. Folic acid, with B_6 and B_{12}, may help prevent Parkinson's, maintain healthy Hcy levels, and reduce adverse effects of levodopa therapy. Evidence of folate's effects on Hcy is well-established. However, evidence of benefit from folate during levodopa therapy limited. Genomic factors may significantly influence pathology, folate levels, nutrient activity, and drug response.	Supplement folic acid (and B_{12}) during levodopa therapy. Monitor folate, Hcy, and L-dopa levels. Caution appropriate regarding high-dose B_6 use with carbidopa or benserazide.
Lithium ⊕⊕	Higher folate levels may be associated with better clinical response to lithium. Coadministration of folic acid may enhance therapeutic efficacy of lithium therapy. Evidence lacking to suggest that lithium depletes folate or folic acid reduces lithium adverse effects.	Concomitant folic acid may be beneficial, but drug dose may need to be modified. Monitor folate status and lithium levels.
Mercaptopurine, azathioprine, and thioguanine Thiopurines ✗/⊕✗/⊕	Thiopurines are cytotoxic antimetabolites used predominantly in cancer and autoimmune disease therapies where they act as purine antagonists and tend to induce myelosuppression and macrocytic nonmegaloblastic anemia. Genetic variation in folate handling may influence drug efficacy and toxicity. Limited evidence indicates that concomitant folate may protect bone marrow, moderate drug adverse effects, and enhance tolerance.	Consider folic acid or 5-MTHF coadministration. Monitor folate and hematological status. Pharmacogenomic evaluation may be warranted.
Metformin Biguanides ≈≈/☼/⊕⊕/◇	Metformin is known to elevate Hcy, but evidence not conclusive as to degree to which biguanides deplete folate. Metformin impairs vitamin B_{12} absorption through calcium-dependent mechanism, which may be corrected with concomitant calcium. Maintaining low Hcy levels important to therapeutic strategy of reducing cardiovascular risk.	Coadminister folic acid B_{12}, B_6, and calcium, especially in women with PCOS. Encourage exercise and folate-rich diet. Monitor folate, Hcy, serum holotranscobalamin II, and glucose levels.
Neomycin ≈≈≈/☼	Neomycin can decrease absorption and increase elimination of folate and numerous other nutrients. Interaction accepted as consensus but evidence limited. Extended use or high dosage can further disrupt gut ecology and impair synthesis of folate and B_{12} by eliminating probiotic flora.	Daily multivitamin and mineral formulation, and probiotic flora, recommended during extended neomycin therapy. Separate nutrient intake from neomycin.
Nitroglycerin Nitrates ⊕⊕	Folate-dependent activities involving NADPH, tetrahydrobiopterin, and nitric oxide synthase appear to play key roles in tolerance to nitroglycerin, although mechanisms not yet fully elucidated. Coadministration of folic acid can attenuate tolerance by enhancing regeneration and bioavailability of tetrahydrobiopterin; it also supports therapeutic strategy of reducing cardiovascular risk.	Coadminister folic acid during nitrate therapy. Monitor folate and cobalamin status and medication levels.
Nitrous oxide (N_2O) ☼/⊕⊕	Nitrous oxide can interfere with activity of folate and vitamin B_{12}, potentially depleting both; in particular, resultant methyl trap can decrease mitochondrial folates. Significant effect plausible but remains controversial. Duration and extent of exposure, as well as individual patient characteristics, may determine degree of effect and attendant risk.	Prudence suggests supplementation with acid or 5-MTHF (and B_{12}) starting 1 week before major N_2O anesthesia. Medical and dental personnel may also benefit from prophylactic nutrient support; consider periodic B_{12} assessment.
Nonsteroidal anti-inflammatory drugs (NSAIDs) ≈≈≈/≈≈/◇/☼	Many NSAIDs exert antifolate activity by impairing or competitively interfering with folate absorption, metabolism, and transport. Chronic use, especially at high doses, could potentially decrease serum folate concentrations and cause deficiency. Limited evidence suggests need for further human research. Evidence lacking to confirm benefits of folate coadministration or to suggest interference with drug activity.	Concomitant folic acid may be prudent during extended high-dose NSAID therapy.
Oral contraceptives (OCs) ≈≈≈/≈≈/☼	Birth control pills, especially with higher estrogen doses, can impair folate metabolism and may cause depletion, especially in women with compromised folate status; these effects may play a role in known OC risks. Evidence is mixed and controversy continues regarding probability of occurrence and clinical significance of adverse effects. Folic acid particularly important with cervical dysplasia and possibility of pregnancy after OC termination.	Concomitant folic acid and vitamin B_6 recommended as prudent, especially in smokers. Consider assessing folate, platelets, and Hcy, initially and periodically.
Pancreatic enzyme Proteolytic enzymes ≈≈≈	Simultaneous intake of pancreatin and other proteolytic enzymes may impair folic acid absorption. Research involving patients with pancreatic insufficiency indicates higher serum folate levels before treatment. Significant effect plausible; evidence inconclusive.	Consider supplementing folic acid with extended use of pancreatic extracts, especially with history of insufficiency.
Pyrimethamine ◇≈≈/≈≈/⊕✗/✗	Pyrimethamine is competitive inhibitor of dihydrofolate reductase that acts as folic acid antagonist and inhibits biosynthesis of tetrahydrofolic acid; it depletes serum folic acid levels and interferes with hematopoiesis, especially in combination with other antifolates (sulfadiazine, sulfadoxine, methotrexate). Bone marrow suppression, neutropenia, thrombocytopenia, and megaloblastic anemia are among clinically significant adverse effects resulting from drug-induced folate deficiency.	Coadminister folic acid acid or 5-MTHF, as well as oral or intramuscular cobalamin. Monitor cobalamin and folate levels, as well as hematological parameters. Extra caution with G6PD deficiency or hepatic or renal impairment.
Sulfasalazine ≈≈≈/≈≈/◇/☼	Sulfasalazine and other sulfonamides interfere with absorption, bioavailability, and activity of folic acid, most likely acting as competitive inhibitor and impairing activity of folate-dependent enzymes. Adverse effects of sulfasalazine on	Encourage diet rich in high-folate foods. Coadminister folic acid acid or 5-MTHF. Monitor red blood cell (RBC)/tissue folate and Hcy levels.

Continued

Nutrient-Drug Interactions and Drug-Induced Nutrient Depletions

Summary

Drug/Class Interaction Type	Mechanism and Significance	Management
	folate are generally recognized. However, no evidence-based consensus as to influence of various factors, including drug dosage, polymorphisms, nutritional deficiencies, and comorbid conditions. Tissue depletion and elevated Hcy more likely than frank deficiency with maintenance sulfasalazine. Increased risk of colon cancer in patients with irritable bowel and colitis.	
Tetracycline antibiotics ⊕⊕/⊕✗/◇◇/◇≈≈	Folic acid and tetracyclines may bind and inhibit absorption and availability of both agents when ingested simultaneously. These antibiotics can also interfere with activity of and potentially induce depletion of folic acid and other nutrients. Extended use or high dosage can further disrupt gut ecology and impair synthesis of folate and B_{12} by eliminating probiotic flora. Coadministration of tetracycline and folate, often with B_{12}, is recommended treatment for tropical sprue.	Daily multivitamin formulation, and probiotic flora, recommended during repeated or extended tetracycline therapy. Separate intake. Monitor cobalamin and folate status.
Triamterene Potassium-sparing diuretics ◇≈≈/≈≈≈/◇/⊕⊕	Triamterene impairs folate absorption and bioavailability, possibly by acting as competitive inhibitor of folate intestinal absorption. It may contribute to folate depletion and thereby contribute to teratogenesis and hyperhomocysteinemia. Triamterene may decrease biologically active folates by acting as relatively weak folate antagonist through dose-related inhibitory effect on dihydrofolic reductase. Evidence indicates variable risk of clinically significant adverse effect, but concomitant folic acid may mitigate such effects. Also contributes to strategic goal of reducing cardiovascular and stroke risk by lowering Hcy level.	Encourage diet rich in high-folate foods. Coadminister folic acid or 5-MTHF. Monitor RBC/tissue folate and Hcy levels.
Trimethoprim-sulfamethoxazole Sulfonamide antibiotics ≈≈/◇≈≈/☼/⊕✗/✗	Trimethoprim and sulfamethoxazole inhibit dihydrofolic reductase to block conversion of unreduced dietary folates into tetrahydrofolate. Co-trimoxazole—induced folate deficiency possible, especially with underlying folate deficiency, and teratogenicity and macrocytic anemia are known adverse effects, particularly with high dose and prolonged use. However, clinically significant anemia is considered rare. Folic acid coadministration could theoretically interfere with drug activity, but evidence indicates that interference is unlikely with low-dose intake.	Concomitant folic acid or 5-MTHF, with probiotic flora, may be prudent during extended therapy.
Zidovudine/AZT Reverse-transcriptase inhibitor (nucleoside) antiretroviral agents ◇≈≈/≈≈/☼	Macrocytosis, anemia, and granulocytopenia are common adverse effects associated with AZT therapy. However, coadministration of vitamin B_{12} and folinic acid may not prevent or reduce drug-induced myelotoxicity. Modification of drug regimen often necessary to reverse toxic effects.	Coadminister folic acid acid or 5-MTHF as well as oral or intramuscular cobalamin. Closely monitor cobalamin and folate status.

5-MTHF, 5-Methyltetrahydrofolate; *MTHFR*, methylenetetrahydrofolate reductase; *CYP*, cytochrome P450; *NADPH*, reduced nicotinamide-adenine dinucleotide phosphate; *IM*, intramuscular; *PCOS*, polycystic ovary syndrome; *G6PD*, glucose-6-phosplate dehydrogenase; *RBC*, red blood cell.

NUTRIENT DESCRIPTION

Chemistry and Forms

The Latin word for leaf, *folium*, was chosen to designate the nutrient present in green leafy vegetables and originally isolated from four tons of spinach leaves in 1946. The terms "folic acid" and "folate" are often used interchangeably for this water-soluble B-complex vitamin. However, *folate* is the preferred term for the mixture of related compounds occurring naturally in foods, whereas *folic acid* is the more stable form and is used in supplements and added to fortified foods, but rarely occurs in foods or the human body. Thus, forms are preferentially referred to on this basis in most usages within this monograph, with deference to nomenclature of original sources.

Folic acid may be more specifically identified as pteroylmonoglutamate or pteroylglutamic acid (PGA). Described chemically as *N*-[4-[[(2-amino-1,4-dihydro-4-oxo-6-pteridinyl)methyl]amino]benzoyl]-L-glutamic acid, it is comprised of *para*-aminobenzoic acid (PABA) linked at one end to a pteridine ring and at the other end to glutamic acid. Its molecular formula is $C_{19}H_{19}N_7O_6$, and its molecular weight is 441.40 daltons. Folic acid forms yellowish orange crystals. The color is imparted by the pteridine ring of folic acid. Pteridine also imparts color to the wings of certain butterflies.

Pteroylmonoglutamate (PGA) is the parent compound for many structurally related, derivative compounds that exhibit the biological activity of folic acid and are collectively referred to by the generic term *folate*. Most naturally occurring folates are pteroylpolyglutamate derivatives, containing two to seven glutamates joined in amide (peptide) linkages to the gamma-carboxyl of glutamate, with folylpoly-γ-glutamates being the predominant, naturally occurring form of dietary folates. Naturally occurring folates include 5-methyltetrahydrofolate (5-MTHF), 5-formyltetrahydrofolate (5-formyl-THF), 10-formyltetrahydrofolate (10-formyl-THF), 5,10-methylenetetrahydrofolate (5,10-methylene-THF), 5,10-methenyltetrahydrofolate (5,10-methenyl-THF), 5-formiminotetrahydrofolate (5-formimino-THF), 5,6,7,8-tetrahydrofolate (THF), and dihydrofolate (DHF). The term *folate* is also used specifically to designate the anionic form of folic acid.

Physiology and Function

Folate, usually present as pteroylpolyglutamate derivatives in food, is hydrolyzed to pteroylmonoglutamate forms by folyl conjugase (also known as folate conjugase or γ-glutamylhydrolase) from the pancreas and mucosal conjugase from the intestinal wall before absorption from the small intestine. The monoglutamate forms of folate, including folic acid, are transported across the proximal small intestine, primarily the jejunum, by both active transport and diffusion. This is a saturable pH-dependent process, so absorption is decreased in an alkali medium and in the presence of added zinc. When ingested on an empty stomach, folic acid is generally twice as available as dietary sources of folate; folic acid consumed with food is 1.7 times as available as folate in food.

Following absorption of physiological amounts of folic acid into the enterocytes, a certain percentage undergoes reduction. Folic acid (PGA) is the inactive precursor of tetrahydrofolic acid (THFA) and methyltetrahydrofolate; it is converted to THFA, its biologically active form, with the participation of niacin and vitamin C, as well as several coenzymes and other nutrients. However, a functional methionine synthase deficiency can develop within the context of vitamin B_{12} deficiency so that essentially all the folate becomes trapped as the N5-methyl THF derivative, thus preventing the synthesis of other THF derivatives required for the purine and thymidine nucleotide biosynthesis pathways. Reduced folate is transported to the liver via the portal circulation, where it is metabolized to polyglutamate derivatives by the action of folyl-polyglutamate synthase. These pteroylpolyglutamate forms are the active cellular cofactor forms of folate.

The total body store of folate is about 12 to 28 mg. All tissue forms of folate are polyglutamates, with pteroylpentaglutamates being the principal type of intracellular folates. Approximately two thirds of folate in plasma is protein bound. Circulating forms of folate are monoglutamates, with pteroylmonoglutamates as the principal extracellular folates and 5-MTHF in its monoglutamate form being the principal folate in the plasma. The liver contains approximately 50% of the body stores of folate, or about 6 to 14 mg. Folate is excreted in the bile, and much of it is reabsorbed through the enterohepatic circulation. This enterohepatic recycling is important for modulating serum levels. Folate is also synthesized by the gut microflora, and as a result, some folates may be eliminated in the feces. However, the kidneys provide the predominant route for folate excretion. Folate enters the glomerulus intact and is reabsorbed into the proximal renal tubule. It is excreted in the urine primarily as folate cleavage products, with only a small amount of intact folate. The excretion of folates found through the breast milk represents a critical pathway for folate activity by providing availability for infant development.

The functions of folate in human physiology are relatively simple, but the implications of their activity (and dysfunction) can be profound and far-reaching. Through its coenzymes, folate plays an essential role in synthesis of nucleic acids, interconversion of amino acids, and single-carbon metabolism. Mediation of single-carbon transfer reactions is considered the primary and possibly exclusive function of folate coenzymes involved in a variety of reactions critical to the metabolism of nucleic acids and amino acids, especially the synthesis of purines and pyrimidines, glycine, and methionine. Thus, through its role in the synthesis of nucleotides from guanine, adenine/pyrimidine, and thymine, folate is required for the synthesis, methylation, and repair of deoxyribonucleic acid (DNA) and is involved in the synthesis of transfer ribonucleic acid (tRNA). This role in cell division is critical in cellular development and maturation, including tissue regeneration, but especially fetal growth and development in general and healthy formation of the nervous system in particular.

Folate plays a fundamental role in synthesis and interconversion of amino acids and the formation and utilization of formate. Folate is involved in the synthesis of glutamic acid, norepinephrine, and serotonin and the detoxification of homocysteine (Hcy) to methionine. Notably, several genetic mutations, including the 677CT polymorphism, influence Hcy metabolism by their effect on the activity of 5,10-methylenetetrahydrofolate reductase, the gene that provides instructions for making *methylenetetrahydrofolate reductase* (MTHFR), a critical enzyme (requiring flavin adenine dinucleotide [FAD] as a cofactor) that converts 5,10-methylenetetrahydrofolate to 5-methyltetrahydrofolate, which is required for the conversion of Hcy to methionine. Consequently, individuals who are homozygous (TT) for the abnormal gene have lower levels of the MTHFR enzyme and a marked tendency to hyperhomocysteinemia. Improved folate nutriture appears to stabilize the MTHFR enzyme, as does adequate riboflavin nutriture (the source of FAD), resulting in improved enzyme levels and lower Hcy levels. Methionine synthase (another enzyme requiring folate and B_{12} as cofactors) combines Hcy with the 5-MTHF produced in the reaction catalyzed by MTHFR so that the Hcy becomes methionine and the 5-MTHF becomes MTHF. Thus, this folate coenzyme plays a critical role in the synthesis of methionine, which is required for the synthesis of *S*-adenosylmethionine (SAMe), the universal methyl donor essential to many biological methylation reactions.

Folate is also essential for the formation and maturation of red blood cells (RBCs) and white blood cells (WBCs). Folic acid is required for nucleoprotein synthesis and maintenance in erythropoiesis and is the single carbon carrier in the formation of heme; it also stimulates WBC and platelet production. Folate deficiency anemia is one of the megaloblastic anemias and is clinically and pathologically indistinguishable from vitamin B_{12} deficiency anemia (pernicious anemia).

Impairment of any of these activities of folate, whether caused by genetic mutations, dietary deficiency, or drug-induced depletion, can produce a cascade of adverse effects directly influencing fetal development, DNA replication, healthy cellular and system function, and development of atherosclerosis, heart disease, and cancer.

NUTRIENT IN CLINICAL PRACTICE
Known or Potential Therapeutic Uses

Within conventional practice, supplemental folic acid and dietary folate are used exclusively for the prevention of neural tube defects (NTDs; e.g., spina bifida, anencephaly) during in utero development and the treatment of demonstrated folate deficiency, primarily manifesting as megaloblastic and macrocytic anemias. However, epidemiological and clinical evidence continues to emerge regarding the preventive and therapeutic efficacy of enhanced folate intake in reducing atherogenic Hcy levels and improving endothelial function to modify cardiovascular risks, supporting neurotransmitter levels in relation to mood disorders and neurodegenerative processes, and preventing cancers, particularly breast, pancreatic, and colon cancers.

Broad efforts at preventing NTDs through dietary fortification have produced mixed benefits. Thus, although largely successful, these programs have exhibited varied penetration of key susceptible populations, and controversy as to their adequacy continues regarding both NTDs and other epidemiological patterns.[1-9] For example, a 2006 survey showed that, even after mandatory fortification of U.S. cereals and grains with folic acid in 1998, women in racial and ethnic minority groups had lower serum folate levels than non-Hispanic white women.[10] Thus, pregnant women who do not regularly take folic acid–containing supplements are eight times more likely to have low serum folate values, despite eating folate-fortified foods.[11] Additionally, expanding knowledge of the multiple polymorphisms affecting folate metabolism is providing a working understanding of susceptibilities to folate-related pathologies and is highlighting the influence of individual genomic variability in the effectiveness of preventive measures and therapeutic applications.

Historical/Ethnomedicine Precedent

The long-standing adages declaring the value of leafy green vegetables in health maintenance and disease prevention may be a result, at least in part, of their being rich in folates.

Possible Uses

Acquired immunodeficiency syndrome and human immunodeficiency virus (AIDS/HIV) support, age-related hearing loss (reduction), Alzheimer's disease, anemia (thalassemia, if deficient), anger (hyperhomocysteinemia associated with MTHFR mutations), atherosclerosis, bipolar disorder, breast cancer prevention (risk reduction in women who consume alcohol), canker sores (with deficiency), cardiac events and death (risk reduction after first stroke), celiac disease (deficiency only), cervical cancer prevention, cervical dysplasia (abnormal Pap test), Crohn's disease, colon cancer prevention, depression, dermatitis herpetiformis (deficiency), diarrhea, Down syndrome, epilepsy, folate metabolism polymorphisms, gingivitis (as rinse), gout, hemorrhagic stroke (risk reduction), hypercholesterolemia, hyperhomocysteinemia, hypertension (risk reduction), laryngeal leukoplakia (risk reduction), lung cancer (risk reduction), malabsorption and gastrointestinal inflammation, megaloblastic anemia, migraine headaches, myocardial infarction, neural tube defect (prevention), osteoarthritis (with vitamin B_{12}), osteoporosis, periodontal disease, peripheral vascular disease, postpartum support, preeclampsia, pregnancy (potential or known), psoriasis, restless legs syndrome, rheumatoid arthritis, schizophrenia (deficiency or hyperhomocysteinemia associated with MTHFR mutations), seborrheic dermatitis, second stroke (risk reduction), seizure disorders, sickle cell anemia (hyperhomocysteinemia), skin ulcers, ulcerative colitis, vitiligo.

Deficiency Symptoms

Folate deficiency results in reduction of DNA synthesis and thus in reduction of cell division. Because the main metabolic consequences of folic acid deficiency are changes in cellular nuclear morphology, rapidly multiplying cells are most affected, such as fetal tissue, erythrocytes, and the epithelial cells of the stomach, intestines, vagina, and cervix. Thus, folate deficiencies result in neural tube and other birth defects, impaired infant development, poor growth, megaloblastic (macrocytic) anemia and other blood disorders, fatigue, weakness, frequent infections, insomnia, irritability, paranoid behavior, mental confusion, hostility, forgetfulness, depression, syncope, headache, palpitations, elevated Hcy level, atherosclerosis, dyspnea, anorexia, glossitis, nausea, dyspepsia, constipation, diarrhea, cervical dysplasia, and hair loss. Gastrointestinal (GI) disturbances are common, resulting from atrophy of digestive tract epithelium. Reduced production of platelets can increase risk of abnormal bleeding. Likewise, impairments in WBC development reduce immune response and increase susceptibility to infections.

Folate deficiency is common, and folate activity is subject to many stressors. Intake of dietary folate and supplemental folic acid is inadequate for a significant proportion of the population, and mild folic acid deficiencies are often undetected. Populations particularly at risk for compromised folate nutriture include alcoholics, the elderly, impoverished people, women using birth control pills, and individuals with malabsorption disorders. Some conditions, such as chronic alcohol consumption and celiac disease, are associated with both low dietary intake and diminished absorption. Tobacco decreases the absorption of folic acid. Certain conditions, such as pregnancy, lactation, hemolytic anemia, leukemia, and other cancers, result in increased rates of cell division and metabolism, leading to an increase in the body's demand for folate. In 1975, folate deficiency during pregnancy was estimated as high as 60%; programs of folate fortification of grains have not been consistently effective in eliminating this significant risk factor. Finally, numerous medications can interfere with folate metabolism, deplete folate (especially with long-term use), or exacerbate folate deficiency in those with other factors adversely influencing folate status.

Several genetic mutations may directly impair folate activity, with profound implications only beginning to be understood. Most prominently, the C677T MTHFR polymorphism, a common variation involving the gene for methylenetetrahydrofolate reductase (MTHFR), can adversely affect folate metabolism and function, particularly the conversion of 5,10-methylene-THF to 5-methyl-THF. Elevated Hcy levels and increased risk for vascular disease are strongly associated with these MTHFR mutations because methyl-THF is the predominant circulatory form of folate and the main carbon donor for the remethylation of homocysteine to methionine. A mutation in the MTHFR gene leading to mild to moderate hyperhomocysteinemia has been found in 15% of patients with premature cerebrovascular disease. Individuals with severe MTHFR deficiency (0%-20% residual activity) present in infancy or adolescence with developmental delay, motor and gait dysfunction, seizures, schizophrenic disturbances, and other neurological abnormalities; they are also at risk of vascular complications.

Homocysteic acid, the oxidation product of Hcy, exerts potent excitatory effects and may be associated with anger, hostility, schizophrenia-like psychosis, depression, and bipolar disorder, particularly in individuals with the homozygous TT genotype of the thermolabile C677T MTHFR polymorphism. The risk of elevated serum levels of total homocysteine (tHcy) is increased in individuals with the combination of the MTHFR 677TT and RFC1 80GG genotypes. Devlin et al.[12] conducted a study of interactions among polymorphisms in folate-metabolizing genes and serum tHcy concentrations in a healthy elderly population. They found that folate and tHcy concentrations were not affected individually by the MTHFR 1298AC, RFC1 80GA, or GCPII 1561CT polymorphisms or by combinations of the MTHFR 677CT and MTHFR 1298AC genotypes. However, individuals with the combination of MTHFR 677TT and RFC1 80GG genotypes exhibited higher serum tHcy.

Inherited defects in methionine synthase, dihydrofolate reductase, and glutamate formiminotransferase, as well as congenital conditions affecting folate absorption and membrane transport, can also influence vascular and mental health through their impact on folate metabolism.

Administration of folic acid will produce marked alleviation of pernicious anemia (the megaloblastic anemia related to vitamin B_{12} deficiency), but the GI signs and symptoms and the neurological lesions continue to progress. For this reason, supplements of 1000 μg (1 mg) or greater of folic acid require a prescription in the United States and some other Western countries. Combining 1 mg or more of oral vitamin B_{12} with

1 mg or more of folic acid would obviate this problem; 1 mg or more of vitamin B_{12} will reliably correct B_{12} deficiency, even in the presence of pernicious anemia, atrophic gastritis, chronic proton pump inhibitor therapy, or other B_{12} malabsorption syndromes.

Dietary Sources

Foods rich in folates include dark-green leafy vegetables (spinach, kale, mustard greens, turnip greens, escarole, chard, arugula, beet greens, bok choy, dandelion green, mache, radicchio, rapini or broccoli de rabe, Swiss chard), liver (beef or chicken) and other organ meats, egg yolk, and brewer's yeast. Folylpoly-γ-glutamates are the predominant form of folates occurring naturally in foods. Other good sources are beets, broccoli, brussel sprouts, cabbage, cauliflower, asparagus, orange juice, cantaloupe, kidney and lima beans, pinto beans, garbanzo beans, black-eyed peas, lentils, soybeans, soy flour, potato, wheat germ, and whole-grain cereals and breads. Fortified cereals made from processed grains can also serve as sources of folic acid. The symbiotic flora comprising the intestinal microbiota, if intact, also synthesize a significant amount of folate.

Folic acid is water soluble, with some forms stable to heat and others heat sensitive. Some forms are stable to acid and others destroyed. Vegetables stored at room temperature undergo considerable loss of folic acid. Virtually all the folate in dried milk has been destroyed.

The absorption efficiency of natural folates is approximately 50% that of folic acid in supplements or fortified foods. The model of *dietary folate equivalents* (DFEs) has been introduced to account for the difference in absorption efficiency between natural food folate and folic acid. Thus, DFEs can be calculated as follows:

$$1 \text{ microgram } (\mu g) \text{ of DFEs} = 1\mu g \text{ food folate}$$
$$= 0.5 \ \mu g \text{ folic acid taken on empty stomach}$$
$$= 0.6 \ \mu g \text{ folic acid taken with meals}$$

Nutrient Preparations Available

The principal form of supplemental folate is folic acid, as a single ingredient or in combination products such as B-complex formulations. Folate triglutamate (pteroyltriglutamate) is also used. 5-Methyl folate and 5-formyl folate are commercially available reduced folates.

5-formyltetrahydrofolate (5-FTHF) and 5-methyltetrahydrofolate (5-MTHF) are the reduced and metabolically active forms of folic acid. Folinic acid, the free acid of calcium folinate, is the more frequently used form and is also known as calcium folinate (Leucovorin Calcium, Leukovorin, Wellcovorin), calcium levofolinate (Isovorin), citrovorum factor (Citrovorum), and sodium folinate (Sodiofolin). Folinic acid is a racemic mixture of levorotatory and dextrorotatory isomers. The levo-isomer is the metabolically active moiety. These calcium or sodium salts are used for parenteral or oral administration.

Metafolin, Merck's patented synthetic form of 6(S) 5-MTHF, or L-methylfolate, is the only form available (for the duration of Merck's patent) of the levorotatory (L) chiral isomer of 5-MTHF, which is the chiral isomer made by human metabolism from folic acid, and also the chiral form found in foods which contain 5-MTHF. It is derived from commercially available B-complex vitamin folic acid, which is reduced to tetrahydrofolate in a process that leads to the formation of a new chiral center and two diastereoisomers in an equimolar

ratio. The L isomer (6S-isomer) of methylfolate is then isolated by selective crystallization. Metafolin is promoted as a form of folate that requires no reduction steps once absorbed and that is immediately bioavailable and thus unaffected by the MTHFR C→T polymorphism.[14] L-Methylfolate also bypasses most folate-interfering compounds, such as those that inhibit dihydrofolate reductase (e.g., methotrexate, pemetrexed, EGCG).

Dosage Forms Available

Oral: Capsule, liposomal spray, liquid, tablet, tablet (effervescent).
Injection: Deep intramuscular, subcutaneous, or intravenous; sodium folate solution (0.1 mg folic acid per 1 mL), usually 5 mg/mL (10 mL), contains benzyl alcohol.

Source of Materials for Nutrient Preparations

Folic acid used in supplements, prescriptions, and food fortification (e.g., wheat flour) is synthesized from guanidine and glutamic acid as starting materials. The chemical synthesis of L-5-MTHF (Metafolin) starts from the commercially available vitamin folic acid, which is chemically reduced to tetrahydrofolate (THF). This reduction step leads to the formation of a new chiral center and two diastereoisomers in an equimolar ratio. In nature, reduced folates consist only of the pure levo (L) isomer (corresponding to the 6S isomer for methylfolate); thus, processes were developed allowing the isolation of the natural L form by selective crystallization.[13]

Dosage Range
Adult

Dietary: 300 μg folic acid daily for adults. In United Kingdom, average adult daily diet for women provides 224 μg, and for men, 322 μg.
Supplemental/Maintenance: 400 μg daily for adults.

The U.S. Food and Drug Administration (FDA) recommends 600 μg folic acid for pregnant women and 500 μg for nursing women. Based on survey data published in 1996, Lawrence et al.[10] recommend, "Until the optimal folate level is identified that confers maximum protection against neural tube defects, health care providers and women's health advocates should continue to encourage women who can become pregnant to take a vitamin containing 400 micrograms of folic acid every day." Women who could become pregnant are advised to take 400 to 800 μg of folic acid per day in anticipation of the possibility of conceiving because folic acid deficiency is most critical during the initial stages of pregnancy, when many women are not yet aware of their being pregnant.

The folic acid dose in over-the-counter (OTC) nutritional supplements is limited to 900 μg. Doses of 1 mg or greater require a prescription. Folic acid is best taken between or with meals, preferably with the dose divided throughout the day.
Pharmacological/Therapeutic:
   500 to 800 μg/day is common.
   Pregnant and lactating women: 0.8 mg/day
   Pharmacological dosages in scientific literature: 400 to 4000 μg

Administration of 5 to 10 mg daily may occur in research or other specialized settings, including treatment of severe deficiency. Men show a smaller increase in folate and decrease in Hcy to a given dose of folic acid than women.[15]

Toxic: Folic acid is essentially nontoxic, even at very high doses. The tolerable upper intake level (UL) established by the U.S. Institute of Medicine's Food and Nutrition Board is 1000 µg/day (based on synthetic folic acid). This UL is based on folic acid doses of 1 mg or more masking an undiagnosed vitamin B_{12} deficiency (by correcting the anemia that occurs with B_{12} deficiency, which is often the sole sign that alerts health care providers to the presence of an underlying B_{12} deficiency).

Pediatric (<18 Years)
Dietary:
Infants, birth to 6 months: 25 µg/day
Infants, 7 to 12 months: 35 µg/day
Children, 1 to 3 years: 150 µg/day
Children, 4 to 8 years: 200 µg/day
Children, 9 to 13 years: 300 µg/day
Adolescents, 14 to 18 years: 300 µg/day
Supplemental/Maintenance:
Infants, birth to 12 months: 0.1 mg/day
Children, 1 to 3 years: up to 0.3 mg/day
Children, 4 years and older: 0.4 mg/day
Pharmacological/Therapeutic: None specifically established at this time.
Toxic: None specifically established at this time.

Laboratory Values
Serum Folate
Serum folate reflects recent dietary intake and is most useful when combined with assays of vitamin B_{12} and red blood cell (RBC) folic acid. However, serum folate and serum vitamin B_{12} can be normal in mild folate and vitamin B_{12} deficiencies. Homocysteine (folate and B_{12}) and methylmalonic acid (B_{12} only) are more sensitive indicators of mild folate and vitamin B_{12} deficiencies.
Normal levels: 4.5 to 30 nmol/L or 5.4 to 24 µg/mL.

Red Blood Cell Folate (Erythrocyte Folate)
The RBC folate levels reflect body folate stores. RBCs are generally macrocytic when folate and/or B_{12} deficiency states are present except in combined deficiencies of both folate and iron, common in malnourished individuals.
Normal levels: 280 to 790 ng/mL RBCs.
Levels < 312 nmol/L can indicate deficiency.

Note: Different laboratories use different reference ranges for serum folate and RBC folate because their analytical assays vary. Many antibiotics may interfere with the microbiological assay for serum and erythrocyte folic acid and can produce falsely low results.

Neutrophilic Hypersegmentation Index (NHI)
The *neutrophilic hypersegmentation index* (NHI) can identify the earliest stages of folate insufficiency. Deficiency indicated when the ratio of neutrophils with five or more lobes to those with four or fewer lobes is greater than 30%. Hypersegmentation can also result from vitamin B_{12} deficiency and is not reliable during pregnancy.

Serum Methylmalonic Acid
Methylmalonic acid (MMA) is useful in differentiating folate and cobalamin deficiency. L-Methylmalonyl coenzyme A (CoA mutase is a vitamin B_{12}–dependent enzyme; therefore a B_{12} deficiency, but not a folate deficiency, will lead to an increase in MMA.

Total Homocysteine
Total homocysteine (tHcy) concentration indicates folate and/or cobalamin deficiency and serves as predictor of risk for arterial stiffness, ischemic stroke, and myocardial infarction. Homocysteine levels can also be elevated by genetic polymorphisms that result in greater requirements of pyridoxine (vitamin B_6), as well as deficiencies of pyridoxine and methyl donor nutrients in general.

A plasma tHcy concentration exceeding 15 µmol/L indicates hyperhomocysteinemia, although many investigators propose that achieving much lower levels (7-10 µmol/L) is necessary for decreasing vascular disease risk.

If anticoagulated blood tubes are allowed to sit longer than 10 minutes before spinning, the tHcy level can be falsely elevated. Pharmacological doses of niacin also falsely elevate tHcy levels and should be held for 24 hours before drawing blood to determine tHcy levels.

Serum Homocysteine
Serum Hcy indicates folate or cobalamin deficiency and serves as predictor of risk for ischemic stroke and myocardial infarction. It is used to assess homocystinuria.
Normal levels: Male: 4.3-11.4 micromol/L
Female: 3.3-10.4 micromol/L

Emerging and Related Tests
- Tetrahydrofolate (THF) concentrations.
- Whole-blood folate may also be valuable in some settings, but standards have only recently been established.
- Fluorescence polarization immunoassay (FPIA) can be performed for the quantitation of total human L-homocysteine in serum or plasma.
- Methylene-THFR identifies normal, heterozygous, and homozygous genotypes.
- 5,10-Methylene-THFR C677T polymorphism identifies the mutation and provides preliminary evaluation of associated increased thrombotic risk and obstetrical risk.

Emerging research indicates the need to test for MTHFR 1298AC, RFC1 80GA, and GCPII 1561CT polymorphisms in establishing cardiovascular risk.[12]

Analysis of both the C677T mutation and the A1298C mutation is recommended for evaluation of obstetrical risk in patients with recurrent fetal loss. Patients who are heterozygous for the C677T mutation are reflex-tested for the A1298C mutation. Only C677T homozygotes and C677T/A1298C compound heterozygotes are at increased risk for thrombotic events.

Note: S-adenosylmethionine (SAMe) has a similar molecular form to S-adenosylhomocysteine, and exogenous intake, at therapeutic levels, may interfere with this assay.

SAFETY PROFILE
Overview
Supplemental folic acid is essentially nontoxic, even at high doses, and extremely safe at nutritional doses. Folic acid doses up to 1 mg daily are well tolerated. Substantive and consistent evidence of adverse effects attributable to folic acid supplementation is lacking. Adverse effects attributed to folic acid primarily derive from issues of diagnosis and clinical management.

Health care professionals are advised to counsel patients to avoid supplementing with 800 µg or more of folic acid daily unless they have been evaluated for vitamin B_{12} deficiency or they coadminister 1 mg or more of B_{12}. Inappropriate use of folic acid in large doses could precipitate neuropathy in individuals with undiagnosed B_{12} deficiency (usually from pernicious anemia). More than 100 cases have been reported in which vitamin B_{12}–deficient subjects receiving oral folic acid at 5 mg or more daily experienced progression of neurological symptoms and signs. Reports are rare of such complications in individuals receiving doses of folic acid less than 5 mg daily. Consequently, the U.S. Food and Nutrition Board advises that all adults limit their intake of folic acid to 1000 µg daily. The concerns regarding safety underlying dose restrictions are limited to synthetic folic acid intake through supplements and fortification. Folate from food sources is generally considered highly unlikely to mask vitamin B_{12} deficiency.

Aggravations of seizure disorders have been reported in patients who initiated folic acid supplementation while undergoing anticonvulsant therapy. Such reactions may result from folic acid interfering with the activity of antiepileptic drugs.

Nutrient Adverse Effects

General Adverse Effects

Sleep disturbances, mental changes, and GI effects have been associated with high-dose folic acid intake, greater than 10 mg daily. Doses greater than 5 mg (5000 µg) daily may cause digestive upset in some individuals. Wheezing, dyspnea, fever, erythema, skin rash, itching, and other symptoms of allergic reactions have been reported on rare occasions.

Some secondary sources suggest that extended intake of high doses may cause uricosuria or produce folacin crystals in the kidney. Dialysis patients have increased requirements for folic acid and vitamin B_6, needing at least 800 µg to 1 mg or more of folic acid and 10 mg or more of B_6 each day.

Adverse Effects Among Specific Populations

Folic acid supplementation, without vitamin B_{12}, is contraindicated in patients with B_{12} deficiency, especially pernicious anemia.

The effects of folate on cognitive function have generally been considered salubrious, particularly in elderly persons. However, a single study in 2005 produced the unexpected finding that high folate intake was associated with more rapid cognitive decline in older adults, particularly men and women taking supplemental folic acid at levels greater than 400 µg/day. Subjects in the top quintile of folate intake (> 700 µg/day) exhibited twice the rate of mental decline over 6 years as those who with the lowest folate intake. Although suggesting caution in routine use of folic acid supplements (without vitamin B_{12}), the authors emphasized that evidence was lacking to confirm that folate itself caused the cognitive deterioration seen in some study participants and noted that high folate intake might be masking a vitamin B_{12} deficiency in some individuals.[16] No other research has pointed to similar patterns. An intervention trial administering folate supplements, B_{12} supplements (in equivalent doses to the folate), and both folate and B_{12} together, with single and double placebo control groups, to elderly subjects over 5 years would be required to address the issues conclusively. Notably, in the subsequent Veterans Affairs Normative Aging Study, Tucker et al.[17] found that high Hcy and low B-vitamin plasma levels predicted cognitive decline in aging men. Moreover, folate (plasma and dietary) "remained independently protective against a decline in spatial copying score after adjustment for other vitamins and for plasma homocysteine."

Preschool children administered folic acid (and iron) may be at higher risk of severe illness and death in a high-malaria-transmission setting. Routine prophylactic supplementation should be avoided pending further research. However, within the context of an active program "to detect and treat malaria and other infections, iron-deficient and [anemic] children can benefit from supplementation."[18]

Haggarty et al.[19] reported that high levels of serum folate appear to increase the risk of a dizygotic twin birth after women are impregnated through in vitro fertilization (IVF) or intracytoplasmic sperm injection (ICSI). In particular, the rate of twins was associated with elevated levels of plasma and RBC folate (odds ratio [OR] 1.27 for each 100-g change in folate intake). However, the authors noted that "there was no significant association between folate and vitamin B_{12} intake, or blood levels, and pregnancy or rate of live births or pregnancy loss after IVF."

Pregnancy and Nursing

Enhancement of dietary folates and supplemental folic acid is recommended for any woman of childbearing age who might become pregnant, and this is specifically required during pregnancy. Folate enters breast milk and is beneficial. Folic acid and folate are specifically recommended to prevent developmental birth defects, particularly neural tube defects. Specific maximum safe dosages have not been established for pregnant or nursing women. (See, however, previous discussion on possible effects of high folate levels in relation to assisted reproduction.)

Infants and Children

No adverse effects have been reported in children or would be predicted.

Contraindications

Folic acid at doses greater than 800 µg/day is contraindicated when vitamin B_{12} status is uncertain. Doses greater than 1 mg/day may obscure pernicious anemia, with irreversible progression of neuropathy, unless the B_{12} deficiency is corrected with high-dose (1-2 mg/day) oral or parenteral B_{12}.

Prophylactic folic acid (and iron) may be contraindicated for children in malarial environments.[18]

Some clinicians have suggested that individuals with elevated blood levels of histamine (i.e., histadelia) should avoid supplemental folic acid because it can produce further histamine excess and aggravate a tendency to depression, schizophrenia, or other adverse effects purported to be associated with elevated histamine levels.

Precautions and Warnings

Self-administration of folic acid at levels greater than 400 µg/day is inadvisable in individuals being treated with anticonvulsants, antifolates, and other medications with a mechanism of action based on interfering with folate activity.

INTERACTIONS REVIEW

Strategic Considerations

Folate is a vital nutrient for everyone, as evidenced by universal recommendation to eat bountiful amounts of dark-green leafy vegetables and other folate-rich foods. Overwhelming evidence indicates that folate deficiency is widespread, even among those presumed to have adequate diets, but particularly among the elderly population, malnourished individuals, tobacco smokers, and those who excessively consume alcohol or processed foods. Furthermore, the folate that is consumed in the diet, produced endogenously, and ingested as a supplement is fragile, or at least vulnerable to a wide range of stressors, most notably pharmacological agents.

Healthy levels of folate in the blood and target tissues enable many key physiological functions, such as normal DNA synthesis and healthy cell division, homocysteine regulation, and endothelial function, and thus play a key role in preventing many pathological processes, including carcinogenesis and atherogenesis. However, polymorphisms in the genes coding for key folate metabolism enzymes, such as MTHFR, thiopurine methyltransferase (TPMT), and inosine triphosphate pyrophosphatase (ITPase), play a key role in folate status, susceptibility to folate-related pathologies, response to folate administration, and tolerance of and therapeutic response to medications affecting folate.

Conventional medicine does not generally employ laboratory tests adequately sensitive for detecting compromised folate status, particularly depletion patterns and deficiency states at the tissue and mitochondrial level, before they reach pathological proportions at a system-wide level. Unless specifically contraindicated, folic acid supplementation could reasonably be recommended for everyone as basic nutritional support for health maintenance and prevention of many pathological and degenerative processes, especially if the person is taking one of the medications discussed later. The supervising caregiver then focuses on carefully monitoring the patient in specific situations requiring closer clinical management. The implications of folate deficiency can be profound and severe, from teratogenesis during pregnancy to stroke later in life, and constitute the primary clinically significant influence of drug interactions involving folate and folic acid for both short-term medical management and long-term strategies of wellness and prevention.

The main caution against folic acid administration is that vitamin B_{12} deficiency, especially severe deficiencies such as those associated with pernicious anemia, might be masked. This warning, however, seems misplaced or at least uninformed because almost every folic acid product on the market is formulated with vitamin B_{12}, at a minimum, or a comprehensive range of synergistic nutrients, as in a multivitamin or B-complex formulation. All health care providers experienced in nutritional therapeutics routinely coadminister folic acid and vitamin B_{12} as a matter of safety, synergy, and efficacy. The more significant (and sometimes controversial) question centers on appropriate dosage levels, and emerging evidence is clarifying this clinical picture. Generous quantities of B_{12} may be critical to effectiveness much more often than previously thought, especially in older people. Generally, conventional nutritional education has framed folate dosing in hundreds of micrograms and B_{12} in single-digit micrograms because of the difference in quantity that prevents serious deficiency states. However, a pivotal clinical trial by Eussen et al.[20] showed that once deficient (by MMA levels), at least 500 to 600 μg of oral vitamin B_{12} is required to correct an established pattern of "mild" depletion. Thus it is advisable always to give equivalent amounts of B_{12} with folate.

Folic acid interacts with and is depleted by a wide range of medications. Some agents incidentally impair folate absorption and transport, but others rely on competitive inhibition and other means of directly interfering with folate activation and folate-dependent enzymes as central to their mechanism of action. In most cases, coadministration of folic acid offers a safe, easy, and inexpensive means of preventing, reducing, or reversing drug-induced adverse reactions, particularly folate deficiency at blood, tissue, and cellular levels, and interference with physiological activities of folate and related enzymes.

Folate coadministration is contraindicated only in patients being treated with antifolate medications for tumors, and then primarily in doses greater than 1000 μg/day. Moreover, when the toxic effects of these medications exceed tolerance or safety limits, folic acid, or more often folinic acid, the activated form, is applied "to pull the situation back from the brink" (so-called rescue). Such contraindications are generally not applicable when the same medications, particularly methotrexate, are used for reasons other than antineoplastic activity.

Research and clinical experience increasingly indicate significant clinical benefits from use of 5-FTHF (folinic acid) and 5-MTHF as sources of activated folate in light of impaired enzyme activity, especially MTHFR, as a result of drug interference and genetic polymorphisms. For many years the use of folinic acid (5-FTHF) has largely been restricted to rescue use with methotrexate and other antifolate medications. The therapeutic significance of this and other forms of folate administration that bypass enzymatic inhibition (e.g., 5-MTHF) becomes more apparent, with growing awareness of the potential adverse implications of unintended decreases in functional folate levels.

Along with the major risk of neural tube defects from folate deficiency during early gestation, homocysteine (Hcy) regulation appears as the most recurrent theme in reviewing the strategic significance of drug interactions with dietary folate and supplemental folic acid. The pervasive and destructive effects of elevated Hcy levels are well documented and widely known. Methionine synthase, the enzyme that metabolizes Hcy to methionine, uses 5-MTHF and vitamin B_{12} as cofactors. Folic acid may have antiatherogenic mechanisms independent of lowering Hcy levels. Besides effects on the vascular system, plasma tHcy level and low serum folate concentrations are independent risk factors for dementia as well as low bone mineral density, particularly among women.[17,21-26] In a randomized, placebo-controlled trial involving 46 Taiwanese subjects (42 men, average age 73), Lin et al.[27] demonstrated that low-dose folic acid (400 μg daily) supplementation reduces Hcy concentration in hyperhomocysteinemic coronary artery disease (CAD) patients and could also reduce CAD risk. Compliance was assessed over 8 weeks by 24-hour diet recalls at week 0 and week 8. Notably, although the low-dose folic acid supplements had no significant effect on Hcy concentrations in the general study population, levels did significantly decrease in hyperhomocysteinemic subjects, by 1.8 μmol/L, especially for carriers of the T-allele.

The evolving debate as to whether Hcy represents a causal or coincident factor in heart disease, cerebrovascular accident (stroke), and related conditions shifted to a new level with publication of the Vitamin Intervention for Stroke Prevention (VISP) trial. When the VISP intention-to-treat analysis failed to show efficacy of combined vitamin therapy for recurrent vascular events in patients with nondisabling stroke, Spence et al.[27a] conducted an "efficacy analysis limited to patients most likely to benefit from the treatment, based on hypotheses arising from evidence developed since VISP was initiated." After excluding "patients with low and very high B_{12} levels at baseline," they found "a 21% reduction in the risk of events in the high-dose group compared with the low-dose group." Also, "patients with a baseline B_{12} level at the median or higher randomized to high-dose vitamin had the best overall outcome, and those with B_{12} less than the median assigned to low-dose vitamin had the worst." They concluded: "In the era of folate fortification, B_{12} plays a key role in vitamin therapy for total homocysteine. Higher doses of B_{12}, and other treatments to lower total homocysteine, may be needed for some patients."

Subsequently, the Women's Antioxidant and Folic Acid Cardiovascular Study (WAFACS), NORVIT, and HOPE-2 trials supported research demonstrating that these nutrients help lower Hcy levels. However, these trials failed to support the hypothesis that lowering Hcy levels alone will provide protection against a future cardiovascular event in high-risk patients with established cardiovascular disease. For example, in the Norwegian study of post–myocardial infarction (MI) patients randomized to a folate-B_{12}-B_6 formulation or placebo, Bønaa et al.[28,29] observed a pattern of increased risk of a second MI in the intervention group, despite a lowering of Hcy. Although relevant to certain patient populations, the findings from these trials suggest that such a study of secondary prevention (patients with previous MI) have limited applicability to primary prevention (individuals without previous vascular events) in healthy individuals and in those with elevated risk. Notably, the HOPE-2 study demonstrated a statistically significant 25% reduction in nonfatal strokes.[30]

Nevertheless, the current data are incomplete because all patients were taking standard post-MI medications (e.g., beta blockers, ACE inhibitors, aspirin). Also, investigators did not monitor drug levels to see if the B vitamins were depleted by the medications or, conversely, if the medications were impaired or levels lowered by the nutrients, as may occur if the nutrients (e.g., vitamin E) induce the pregnane X receptor (PXR). Such potentially significant variables, which were not assessed or factored in, might explain the unexpected "increased risk" associated with the B vitamins, which would actually be analogous to poor compliance with medication. Research into PXR is in preliminary stages, and a focus on its relevance to B vitamins may be warranted and could clarify these and other findings. More broadly, such findings do not detract from other potential benefits derived from lowering Hcy levels, or at least reversing processes associated with elevated Hcy.

An ongoing dialectic between reviews and meta-analyses continues and is unlikely to produce definitive conclusions and more precise recommendations until large-scale, long-term, and well-designed prospective interventional clinical trials are conducted. In reviewing the data from numerous cohort studies, Wald et al.[31] (2006) determined that despite controversy and apparently conflicting evidence in reports of the benefits of folate consumption on cardiovascular disease risk, the weight of evidence supports recommending folic acid for cardiovascular health. Their meta-analysis showed that a 3-μmol/L decrease in serum Hcy levels, considered achievable with a daily folic acid intake with 0.8 mg, lowers the risk of heart attack and stroke by 15% and 24%, respectively. Furthermore, in studies focusing on MTHFR genotypes, the investigators reported that high Hcy levels were associated as "causal" for the risk of stroke and that the "dose-response relation in the genetic studies is particularly relevant in suggesting a causal effect." Overall, the estimate from the trials was consistent with a short-term protective effect of 12% on ischemic heart disease episodes and 22% on stroke, or a greater long-term effect. The degree that folic acid reduces Hcy concentration depends on background folate levels, so increasing folic acid consumption should reduce the risk of heart attack and stroke to a degree related to the Hcy reduction. The authors concluded "that the evidence is now sufficient to justify action on lowering homocysteine concentrations, although the position should be reviewed as evidence from ongoing trials emerges."[31]

Conversely, in a meta-analysis, Bazzano et al.[32] evaluated the effects of folic acid supplementation on risk of cardiovascular diseases and mortality in randomized controlled trials among persons with preexisting cardiovascular or renal disease.

They concluded that folic acid supplementation "has not been shown to reduce risk of cardiovascular diseases or all-cause mortality among participants with prior history of vascular disease," but noted that "ongoing trials with large sample sizes might provide a definitive answer to this important clinical and public health question."

The issue of whether the potential benefits of folic acid and related nutrients that affect Hcy derive from other functions and effects, beyond lowering Hcy, appears increasingly important given the controversial findings and disappointed expectations of Hcy-centered interventional trials and meta-analyses. The role of folic acid in reversing endothelial dysfunction may be central to these protective effects. In a small but potentially pivotal study involving 128 patients with CAD, Moat et al.[33] found that high-dose folic acid (5 mg/day) for 6 weeks significantly improved endothelial function, independent of its effect on lowering plasma Hcy levels. Notably, these investigators observed that subjects administered folate at either 400 μg/day or 5 mg/day had significant increases in plasma folate and significant decreases in plasma Hcy, whereas only subjects who received 5 mg/day exhibited significant improvements in flow-mediated dilation. Another subgroup of subjects, administered betaine (3 g twice daily), showed significant impairment in flow-mediated dilation, despite a reduction in plasma Hcy. The authors' conclusion that their findings suggest that folic acid "dose-dependently improves endothelial function in CAD via a mechanism independently of Hcy lowering" may portend a significant evolution in this body of research.

In a related experiment focused on the mechanism(s) underlying such observed phenomena, Moat et al.[34] demonstrated that folic acid can reverse "both the endothelial dysfunction and increased production of superoxide following depletion of rabbit aortic ring tetrahydrobiopterin (BH4) levels with 2,4-diamino-6-hydroxy-pyrimidine (DAHP) and N-acetyl-5-hydroxy-tryptamine (NAS)." Thus, they concluded that "folic acid reverses the endothelial dysfunction induced by BH4 depletion independently of either the regeneration or stabilization of BH4 or an antioxidant effect."

Emerging evidence indicates that the influence of elevated Hcy levels extends beyond risk of stroke and heart disease, and that folate and other B vitamins have an important role in preventing or reducing other degenerative processes, especially those associated with aging. The literature associating hyperhomocysteinemia with dementia is well known and suggests a broader focus for future research and preventive nutritional support. For example, in a 3-year, randomized, placebo-controlled trial involving 728 subjects age 50 to 72, Durga et al.[35] found that folate (800 μg/day) may reduce age-associated hearing loss, particularly in individuals with elevated Hcy levels. The interconnections between Hcy, folate nutriture, and degenerative processes will undoubtedly be the subject of continued investigation.

The causes of hyperhomocysteinemia are broadly categorized as "inherited" and "acquired." Many causes involve folate nutriture, metabolism, and function. The inherited causes include MTHFR deficiency or defect, methionine synthase defect, vitamin B_{12} transport defect, vitamin B_{12} coenzyme synthesis defect, and cystathionine-β-synthase deficiency. The acquired causes can be grouped as vitamin deficiencies, chronic diseases, and medication effects. Nutritional deficits of folic acid, vitamin B_{12}, and vitamin B_6 can usually be remedied by ensuring adequate dietary sources and administering supplements that provide these synergistic nutrients. Enhanced folate intake may be of direct and indirect benefit for patients with chronic renal failure, hypothyroidism, psoriasis, and malignancies (including acute lymphoblastic leukemia). Notably, conventional treatment of these conditions often involves drug therapies that deplete or interfere with folate. Also, medications that adversely affect folate status and function constitute one of the primary risk factors for hyperhomocysteinemia. Fortunately, this last factor may be the most amenable to clinician intervention, with this monograph being a tool in providing safe and effective medical management by employing an evidence-based, integrative approach to health care delivery.

NUTRIENT-DRUG INTERACTIONS

Acetylsalicylic Acid (Aspirin) and Salsalate

Acetylsalicylic acid (acetosal, acetyl salicylic acid, ASA, salicylsalicylic acid; Arthritis Foundation Pain Reliever, Ascriptin, Aspergum, Asprimox, Bayer Aspirin, Bayer Buffered Aspirin, Bayer Low Adult Strength, Bufferin, Buffex, Cama Arthritis Pain Reliever, Easprin, Ecotrin, Ecotrin Low Adult Strength, Empirin, Extra Strength Adprin-B, Extra Strength Bayer Enteric 500 Aspirin, Extra Strength Bayer Plus, Halfprin 81, Heartline, Regular Strength Bayer Enteric 500 Aspirin, St. Joseph Adult Chewable Aspirin, ZORprin); combination drugs: ASA and caffeine (Anacin); ASA, caffeine, and propoxyphene (Darvon Compound); ASA and carisoprodol (Soma Compound); ASA, codeine, and carisoprodol (Soma Compound with Codeine); ASA and codeine (Empirin with Codeine), ASA, codeine, butalbital, and caffeine (Fiorinal); ASA and extended-release dipyridamole (Aggrenox, Asasantin). Salsalate (salicylic acid; Amigesic, Disalcid, Marthritic, Mono Gesic, Salflex, Salsitab).
See also Nonsteroidal Anti-inflammatory Drugs (NSAIDs).

Interaction Type and Significance

≈≈ **Drug-Induced Adverse Effect on Nutrient Function, Coadministration Therapeutic, Not Requiring Professional Management**
≈≈≈ **Drug-Induced Nutrient Depletion, Supplementation Therapeutic, Not Requiring Professional Management**
☼ **Prevention or Reduction of Drug Adverse Effect**
⊕⊕⊕ **Beneficial or Supportive Interaction, Not Requiring Professional Management**

Probability: Evidence Base:
3. Possible   ○ Preliminary

Effect and Mechanism of Action
Aspirin and salicylic acid, its metabolite, can inhibit folate-dependent enzymes and interfere with folate metabolism. Increased urinary excretion of folate has been associated with chronic ASA use in patients with rheumatoid arthritis (RA).[36] Administration of exogenous folic acid may compensate for and reverse these adverse effects on endogenous folate metabolism.

Research
In 1971, Alter et al.[37] initiated the discussion of reduced blood levels of folate among individuals with rheumatoid arthritis taking aspirin chronically.[37] Lawrence et al.[38] conducted in vivo and in vitro studies of serum binding and urinary excretion of endogenous folate caused by aspirin ingestion. They analyzed serum and blood samples during two series of experiments involving one healthy woman following a fixed diet for 11 days and taking 650 mg aspirin orally every 4 hours during the middle 3 days. They found that "aspirin induced a brisk,

significant but reversible fall in total and bound serum folate and a small but insignificant rise in urinary folate excretion." Furthermore, aspirin in vitro also displaced significant amounts of bound serum folate. The authors concluded that "aspirin in therapeutic doses can contribute to subnormal serum folate values, and if it increases urinary folate excretion even slightly, may impair folate balance."[38]

Baggott et al.[39] found that salicylic acid was a competitive inhibitor (with respect to folate) of avian liver phosphoribosylaminoimidazolecarboxamide formyltransferase (AICAR transformylase, EC 2.1.2.3) and bovine liver dihydrofolate reductase (EC 1.5.1.3), whereas aspirin (as well as the antipyretic-analgesic drugs acetaminophen and antipyrine) were weak inhibitors of these enzymes. Their research suggests that, based on a structure-activity correlation, an aromatic ring with a side chain containing a carboxylic acid is a requirement for competitive inhibition of the transformylase. Thus, "aspirin exerts its anti-inflammatory effects after its conversion into salicylic acid, which possesses greater antifolate activity than its parent compound."[39] They also noted that sulindac, sulphasalazine, naproxen, and ibuprofen are the NSAIDs possessing more potent antifolate activity.

The evidence demonstrating interference with folate metabolism by aspirin is direct and incontrovertible, but the clinical significance of such interference and subsequent folate depletion appears to depend on dosage, duration of intake, and individual variability and susceptibility. High aspirin dosage levels over extended periods can produce adverse effects that are potentially significant and can increase the metabolic needs for folic acid. Further research is warranted given the broad use of ASA, especially over long periods.

Nutritional Therapeutics, Clinical Concerns, and Adaptations
Physicians and other health care providers are advised to ask patients regarding their patterns of aspirin use, prescribed and self-administered, and to counsel folate supplementation as a prudent protective measure against potential adverse effects from long-term intake. The body of evidence indicates that although interference with folate metabolism is probable and cumulative depletion of folate possible, the effects of such processes will vary among individuals depending on other factors, such as age, gender, nutritional intake, supplement use, genomic variability, and drug depletion. Supplementation with a minimum of 400 µg folate daily represents a judicious intervention, given the multiple stressors affecting folate status and the low cost and strong safety profile of folic acid. The necessary amount of daily folic acid support can usually be obtained in a multivitamin formula. However, 800 µg/day is probably appropriate in some individuals, such as pregnant women and those with other risk factors. Low-dosage, chronic ASA intake, as in stroke prevention, is unlikely to contribute to significant compromise of folate status and function, barring other major influences. However, given its potential beneficial impact on homocysteine, supplementation with folic acid and allied nutrients is generally warranted in such patients to reduce risk of atherosclerosis and stroke.

Antacids, Histamine (H₂) Antagonists, and Related Gastric Acid—Suppressive Medications

Antacids

Evidence: Aluminum hydroxide (Alternagel, Amphojel).
Extrapolated, based on similar properties: Aluminum carbonate gel (Basajel), aluminum hydroxide combination

drugs: aluminum hydroxide, magnesium carbonate, alginic acid, and sodium bicarbonate (Gaviscon Extra Strength Tablets, Gaviscon Regular Strength Liquid, Gaviscon Extra Strength Liquid); aluminum hydroxide and magnesium hydroxide (Advanced Formula Di-Gel Tablets, Co-Magaldrox, Di-Gel, Gelusil, Maalox, Maalox Plus, Mylanta, Wingel); aluminum hydroxide, magnesium trisilicate, alginic acid, and sodium bicarbonate (Alenic Alka, Gaviscon Regular Strength Tablets), calcium carbonate (Titralac, Tums); magnesium hydroxide (Phillips' Milk of Magnesia MOM); combination drugs: magnesium hydroxide and calcium carbonate (Calcium Rich Rolaids); magnesium hydroxide, aluminum hydroxide, calcium carbonate, and simethicone (Tempo Tablets); magnesium trisilicate and aluminum hydroxide (Adcomag trisil, Foamicon); magnesium trisilicate, alginic acid, and sodium bicarbonate (Alenic Alka, Gaviscon Regular Strength Tablets); combination drug: sodium bicarbonate, aspirin, and citric acid (Alka-Seltzer).

Cimetidine and Related Histamine (H₂) Receptor Antagonists

Evidence: Cimetidine (Tagamet; Tagamet HB).
Extrapolated: Famotidine (Pepcid RPD, Pepcid, Pepcid AC), nizatidine (Axid, Axid AR), ranitidine (Zantac), combination drug: ranitidine, bismuth, and citrate (Tritec).

Proton Pump Inhibitors

Similar properties but evidence lacking for extrapolation: Esomeprazole (Nexium), lansoprazole (Prevacid, Zoton), omeprazole (Losec, Prilosec), pantoprazole (Protium, Protonix, Somac), rabeprazole (AcipHex, Pariet).

Interaction Type and Significance

≈≈≈ Drug-Induced Nutrient Depletion, Supplementation Therapeutic, Not Requiring Professional Management

≈≈ Drug-Induced Adverse Effect on Nutrient Function, Coadministration Therapeutic, Not Requiring Professional Management

☼ Prevention or Reduction of Drug Adverse Effect

◇ Adverse Drug Effect on Nutritional Therapeutics, Strategic Concern

Probability: Evidence Base:
4. Plausible or 3. Possible   ⊙ Emerging

Effect and Mechanism of Action

The influence of gastric acid sets the stage for folate absorption, which is maximal in the jejunum. Thus, medications that interfere with the normal pH of the gastrointestinal (GI) environment, particularly alkalinization of the proximal small intestine, can impair folic acid absorption and may cause low or deficient plasma and erythrocyte folate.[40] However, some evidence indicates the degree to which a medication alters pH does not always parallel the degree to which it adversely affects folic acid absorption.[40,41] Additionally, antacids containing aluminum hydroxide, magnesium hydroxide, or other minerals may bind to folate and reduce its absorption.[41,42] These pharmacokinetic interactions may produce secondary metabolic effects because folic acid is required for proper metabolic function of vitamin B_{12}.

Research

A review of the available literature indicates medications that suppress gastric acidity can reduce folate bioavailability and absorption to a degree that might not affect most individuals but are of increased clinical significance in populations who use such medications frequently for extended periods and who also have compromised folate nutriture or increased metabolic demands, both of which are relatively common situations.

Cimetidine and ranitidine are H_2 antagonists known to reduce folate absorption because of their effect on pH in the GI tract, although this is generally minor and unlikely to be of clinical significance in most individuals. Russell et al.[41] conducted two experiments investigating these issues. First, in vitro studies showed that neither cimetidine nor ranitidine physically bound folate or interfered with its metabolism (as indicated by a lack of inhibition of dihydrofolate reductase at concentrations of 5 and 50 μmol/L). Subsequently, 30 participants followed a standard regimen of either cimetidine or ranitidine and then were fed a specially formulated liquid meal containing 200 μg of folate. Monitoring of pH values at the ligament of Treitz showed that the slight acidity existing before consumption of the liquid meal was generally maintained during the 2-hour period after food intake. Folate absorption was 50% with the formula meal alone versus 45.8% with the formula meal plus cimetidine. The decrease in folate absorption with ranitidine did not attain statistical significance. Although drug-induced effect on intestinal pH was the focus, the observation that cimetidine reduced folate absorption more than ranitidine suggests a more complex interaction because ranitidine increased intestinal pH to a greater degree.

Russell et al.[41] also observed that aluminum with magnesium hydroxide reduces folate absorption to a small extent, apparently by adsorbing the nutrient, rather than through its effect on gastric acid. These researchers tested dietary folate absorption in 30 subjects by administering the antacid 1 hour and 3 hours after a specially formulated liquid meal containing 200 μg of folate. Folate absorption was 50.6% with the formula meal alone versus 43.1% when the antacid was administered after the formula meal. Acidity actually increased slightly during the 2-hour period after the liquid meal, as indicated by monitoring of pH values at the ligament of Treitz, despite the activity of the antacid.

Further research indicates that the aluminum hydroxide component of the antacid adsorbs folate onto its surface, as gel particles agglomerate and hydroxide begins to precipitate from the gel state (characteristic at pH range of ~3.7-10), and removes it from contact with the aqueous phase.[42]

Evidence regarding the effects of proton pump inhibitors (PPIs) on folate and folic acid is lacking, but these agents might be expected to have a similar effect. This possible interaction poses significant risk because such medications are often prescribed for patients in populations most susceptible to folate deficiency, such as the elderly. The PPIs have clearly been shown to interfere with vitamin B_{12} absorption.

Reports

Ruscin et al.[42a] reported on a 78-year-old, nonvegetarian Caucasian woman with symptomatic gastroesophageal reflux who had vitamin B_{12} deficiency associated with long-term use (~4½ years) of cimetidine and a PPI; serum folate was within the normal range at 4.9 ng/mL. The patient responded to oral B_{12} replacement, thus demonstrating that she could adequately absorb non–protein-bound vitamin B_{12} from the GI tract and suggesting her deficiency was a result of food-cobalamin malabsorption. This case report suggests that long-term H_2/PPI antagonist therapy (≥4 years) may adversely impact vitamin B_{12} status but is unlikely to influence folate.

Nutritional Therapeutics, Clinical Concerns, and Adaptations

Most medications that suppress gastric acid appear to impact folate (and vitamin B_{12}) absorption to some degree by at least one mechanism. The severity of such effect may vary based on individual physiological characteristics, diet, pathophysiology, and specific factors relating to particular drug agents or classes. Although the effects on folate absorption and nutriture are often dismissed as "marginal," they may produce significant adverse effects, especially in undernourished populations and individuals with increased metabolic needs (e.g., pregnancy). Prudence suggests that physicians prescribing such medications advise patients to supplement with a folic acid/B_{12} combination. Increasing folate intake without accompanying B_{12} can stimulate systems that also use B_{12} and can result in lower B_{12} levels. Such preventive measures should also be communicated to patients who may be self-administering antacids on a chronic basis, especially if they are at risk of folate deficiency from dietary factors or depletion from medications.

Anticonvulsant Medications, Including Phenobarbital, Phenytoin, and Valproic Acid

Evidence: Carbamazepine (Carbatrol, Tegretol), divalproex semisodium, divalproex sodium (Depakote), fosphenytoin (Cerebyx, Mesantoin), phenobarbital (phenobarbitone; Luminol, Solfoton), phenytoin (diphenylhydantoin; Dilantin, Phenytek), primidone (Mysoline), sodium valproate (Depacon), valproate semisodium, valproic acid (Depakene, Depakene Syrup).

Extrapolated, based on similar properties: Ethosuximide (Zarontin), ethotoin (Peganone), felbamate (Felbatol), levetiracetam (Keppra), mephenytoin, mephobarbital (Mebaral), methsuximide (Celontin), phensuximide (Milontin), tiagabine (Gabitril), topiramate (Topamax), trimethadione (Tridione), zonisamide (Zonegran).

Similar properties but evidence lacking for extrapolation: Acetazolamide (Diamox, Diamox Sequels), gabapentin (Neurontin), pheneturide (ethylphenacemide), piracetam (Nootropyl), vigabatrin (Sabril).

Similar properties but evidence indicating no or reduced interaction effects: Clonazepam (Klonopin), clorazepate (Tranxene), diazepam (Valium), lamotrigine (Lamictal), lorazepam (Ativan), oxcarbazepine (GP 47680, oxycarbamazepine; Trileptal).

Interaction Type and Significance

☼   **Prevention or Reduction of Drug Adverse Effect**

◇≈≈   **Drug-Induced Adverse Effect on Nutrient Function, Coadministration Therapeutic, with Professional Management**

≈≈   **Drug-Induced Nutrient Depletion, Supplementation Therapeutic, with Professional Management**

◇◇   **Drug-Induced Effect on Nutrient Function, Supplementation Contraindicated, Professional Management Appropriate**

≈◇◇ **Drug-Induced Nutrient Depletion, Supplementation Contraindicated, Professional Management Appropriate**

⊕✗   **Bimodal or Variable Interaction, with Professional Management**

✗✗   **Minimal to Mild Adverse Interaction—Vigilance Necessary**

✗✗✗ **Potentially Harmful or Serious Adverse Interaction—Avoid**

Probability:
2. Probable

Evidence Base:
● Consensus

Effect and Mechanism of Action

Antiepileptic drugs (AEDs) and related medications interact with supplemental folic acid and dietary folate through several mechanisms to produce varied, complex, reinforcing, and sometimes countervailing effects. Most drugs in this broad class interfere with folate function and cause folate depletion by inhibiting nutrient absorption, inducing microsomal oxidase enzymes (cytochrome P450) to increase hepatic folate metabolism, and adversely impacting the microbiota of symbiotic flora in the gut.[43-45] Furthermore, the recycling of folate cofactors depends on vitamin B_6 and riboflavin, and riboflavin is necessary for activating vitamin B_6 to pyridoxal 5'-phosphate (PLP).[46] Thus, induction of enzymes by anticonvulsants may strain available folate resources and limit synthesis of the cytochromic enzymes responsible for AED metabolism.

Numerous factors can adversely influence folate metabolism in individuals being treated with anticonvulsant medications. Decreased MTHFR activity in some individuals reduces conversion of folate to active forms. Primidone and phenobarbital, its metabolite, may both decrease folate absorption and increase its hepatic metabolism while also inhibiting the growth of folate-dependent symbiotic microflora.[47] Valproic acid may interfere with folate absorption but may not induce enzymes; decreased folate levels are found after long-term valproate therapy. Carbamazepine can reduce folate absorption, but evidence is conflicting as to whether this enzyme inducer (CYP450) actually produces any significant effect on hepatic metabolism of folate.[48,49] Many AEDs are metabolized through arene oxides, which are highly reactive intermediates and generally considered to be teratogenic.[50] By impairing the action of epoxide hydrolase (the enzyme system responsible for detoxifying arene oxides), inadequate folate levels could result in incomplete metabolism of anticonvulsants and the accumulation of highly reactive epoxides and thus could contribute to fetal abnormalities.[43,51] For example, the teratogenicity of carbamazepine appears to derive, at least in part, from the formation of the 10,11-epoxide metabolite, which may act as a free radical, binding to proteins and nucleic acids and disrupting DNA, RNA, and protein synthesis.[52] In contrast to carbamazepine, oxcarbazepine undergoes reduction of the carbonyl group to form MHD, which subsequently undergoes glucuronidation, and thus does not form the epoxide.[53] However, such effects constitute only one of several factors in the significant rate of major malformations in offspring exposed to these medications during pregnancy.[54-58] Anticonvulsant-induced low serum folate levels can also elevate homocysteine (Hcy) levels and thereby increase risk of cardiovascular disease, particularly atherosclerosis.[59-61] Elevated Hcy levels are associated with pregnancy complications, neural tube defects (NTDs), and other birth defects. Notably, Hcy has been used as an experimental convulsant.

Conversely, folate may decrease serum levels of some medications (e.g., phenytoin), possibly by acting as a cofactor for the enzyme epoxide hydrolase, or otherwise increasing metabolism of the anticonvulsants and reducing serum drug levels, possibly to subtherapeutic levels. Thus, increased intake of supplemental folic acid, and/or theoretically of dietary folate, could impair the therapeutic activity of AEDs and could increase the incidence of seizure activity. In particular, folate in doses greater than 1 mg daily can compromise phenytoin seizure control by creating a "pseudo–steady state" in which phenytoin appears to be at steady state but actually is not; this effect may be due to competition for brain-cell surface receptors.[43]

Research

Although the issues of folate deficiency and depletion may have significant effects on the health and disease susceptibility of broad sections of the general population, their impact is perhaps most dramatic among individuals being treated with AEDs for seizure disorders and related conditions. Decades of research have demonstrated low folate levels (and increased Hcy levels) in patients treated with AEDs, particularly as polypharmacy.[45,59-67] Nevertheless, although the interaction between AEDs and folates is well documented and potentially clinically important, its clinically significant incidence is uncertain and subject to many variables.

In their landmark 1966 study, Reynolds et al.[68] examined folate status in 62 patients with epilepsy, 54 of whom were taking phenobarbital, primidone, or phenytoin singly or in various combinations, with eight serving as untreated controls. Serum folate concentrations in 76% of treated patients were below the range found in control subjects, and average folate concentration for the treated patients was 3.7 ng/mL, versus 6.4 ng/mL for the controls. Of 45 with bone marrow examination, 17 exhibited megaloblastic hematopoiesis, even though none of the treated patients was anemic, and only 7 of the 54 treated patients showed macrocytosis.

In a survey of the red blood cell (RBC) folate status of 200 patients with epilepsy and 72 controls, Goggin et al.[69] found that median RBC folate levels were reduced significantly in patients treated with phenytoin or carbamazepine alone. Also, patients administered AED polypharmacy had reduced levels, with 22% in the group taking more than one drug showing reduced levels of RBC folate compared with 17% of those receiving carbamazepine monotherapy, 13% taking phenytoin only, and 9% taking sodium valproate only. Notably, patients treated with sodium valproate alone exhibited no significant decrease in RBC folate levels (compared to controls). Dietary folate intake was significantly reduced in all the patient groups compared with controls, but there was no significant correlation between RBC folate levels and dietary folate. The investigators concluded that "all anticonvulsant drugs interfere with folate metabolism."[69]

Kishi et al.[45] measured serum folate concentrations in epileptic outpatients treated with a single anticonvulsant drug, including carbamazepine, phenobarbital, and valproate, and in age-matched controls without anemia. They used a protein-binding radioassay to demonstrate that reduced serum folate was associated with hepatic CYP450 enzyme induction by carbamazepine and phenobarbital, but not valproate, compared with controls.

The influences of AEDs and the MTHFR genotype further complicate the research exploring the powerful relationship between folate status and homocysteine and its profound implications for health and disease. The methylenetetrahydrofolate reductase (MTHFR) genotype appears to modulate depletion of active folate and contribute directly to an increased incidence of hyperhomocysteinemia. Elevated Hcy levels have been documented after anticonvulsant treatment with phenytoin, carbamazepine, phenobarbital, and primidone, agents that induce CYP450.[59-61,66,67,70-72] Likewise, in addition to impairing folate status, long-term treatment with valproate also increases Hcy levels.[67,72] Yoo and Hong[73] demonstrated that the TT allele of the MTHFR C677T polymorphism, a common mutation in the MTHFR gene, is a significant determinant of hyperhomocysteinemia in epileptic patients receiving anticonvulsants.

The concerns raised by high Hcy levels extend beyond cardiovascular risk. In their study of 130 epileptic patients taking anticonvulsant monotherapy or multidrug polytherapy (including carbamazepine and/or phenytoin), Ono et al.[59] noted that individuals diagnosed with megaloblastic anemia as a result of folate deficiency exhibit a high incidence of neuropsychiatric illness and elevated plasma total homocysteine (tHcy) levels. The four folate-deficient patients had received long-term treatment (>7 years) with multiple anticonvulsants. Their tHcy levels were higher than the 90th percentile of those in control subjects. Folate therapy normalized their Hcy and folate levels. Notably, disturbances of the remethylation pathway of Hcy can significantly impact numerous physiological activities, thereby influencing fetal development and contributing to malformations such as NTDs, spontaneous abortions, and other pregnancy complications. Dean et al.[74] found that the MTHFR C677T polymorphism is associated with fetal anticonvulsant syndrome in the offspring of mothers administered AEDs during pregnancy.

The impact of anticonvulsant medications on folate status has been a concern since the introduction of AEDs, and thus research has focused most on the consequences of drug-induced folate deficiency, especially during pregnancy, and the clinical implications of compensatory folic acid coadministration. The strong association between increased risk of birth defects and treatment with AEDs is well established by a consistent body of epidemiological evidence.[75-79] Hydantoins such as phenytoin are most frequently associated with teratogenesis.[55,80] Valproic acid (VPA), divalproex, and valproate sodium have all been reported to cause birth defects when administered during the first 3 months of pregnancy. Specifically, VPA use during early pregnancy can result in a 1% to 2% incidence of spina bifida aperta in humans, a closure defect of the posterior neural tube.

Hendel et al.[48] conducted research on the effect of carbamazepine and valproate treatment on folate metabolism in 11 epileptic patients and interpreted their findings as an inhibition of intestinal folic acid absorption caused by the antiepileptic therapy. However, Kishi et al.[45] examined the role of induction of liver enzymes by AEDs in folate depletion and determined that patients treated with valproate, a non–enzyme inducer, exhibited serum folate levels that did not differ significantly from values in controls. Furthermore, NTDs in humans and rodents associated with VPA do not seem to be related to folate deficiency, and NTD incidence has not changed with administration of folic acid or its activated form, folinic acid.[80] Several other studies have indicated that VPA has the least antifolate action of the major AEDs, and that folate is probably not involved in the mechanism of VPA-induced embryotoxicity. One study found that the consumption of ethanol potentiated VPA-induced NTDs in mice resulting from toxicokinetic interactions.[81] Subsequently, however, findings from a Finnish population-based study by Artama et al.[82] confirmed the teratogenicity of valproate. "The offspring of women with epilepsy on valproate [at doses >1500 mg/day] during the first trimester of pregnancy have a substantially increased risk for congenital malformations." They also reported that the risk for teratogenic malformations is not elevated in offspring of mothers using carbamazepine, oxcarbazepine, or phenytoin (as monotherapy or polytherapy without valproate). This study is notable in being one of the few large studies on the teratogenic effects of AEDs to include a reference group of untreated women with epilepsy.

The incidence of NTDs, such as spina bifida and anencephaly, may dominate broad awareness of adverse effects, but cardiovascular defects, oral clefts, and urinary tract defects are also reported. Likewise, a Danish study by Fonager et al.[77] found that the risks of low birth weight and preterm delivery were increased by 50% and 60%, respectively, in women exposed to anticonvulsant drugs. In another Danish study, Hvas et al.[78] observed that the infants of women with drug-treated epilepsy exhibited a lower birth weight, shorter length, and a smaller head circumference than infants of untreated subjects.

For years clinicians and investigators were unsure as to whether the incidence of fetal abnormalities in mothers with seizure disorders was a result of the condition itself or of their medications. Kaneko et al.[83] prospectively analyzed 983 offspring born in Japan, Italy, and Canada to identify the major risk factors for the increased incidence of congenital malformations in offspring of mothers being treated for epilepsy with AEDs during pregnancy and to determine the relative teratogenic risk of AEDs. The incidence of congenital malformations in offspring with drug exposure was 9.0%, versus an incidence without drug exposure of 3.1%. The highest incidence among offspring exposed to a single AED occurred with primidone (14.3%), followed by valproate (11.1%), phenytoin (9.1%), carbamazepine (5.7%), and phenobarbital (5.1%). The incidence of malformations was positively associated with the total daily dose and number of drugs, with specific combinations of AEDs (e.g., valproate and carbamazepine; phenytoin, primidone, and phenobarbital) producing a higher incidence of congenital malformations. Moreover, the presence of malformations in siblings was the only background factor associated with the incidence of malformations. These authors concluded that "the increased incidence of congenital malformations was caused primarily by AEDs, suggesting that malformations can be prevented by improvements in drug regimen, and by avoiding polypharmacy and high levels of VPA (more than 70 µg/mL) in the treatment of epileptic women of childbearing age."[83]

In a multicenter study, Holmes et al.[56] screened 128,049 pregnant women at delivery to investigate the frequency of anticonvulsant embryopathy (i.e., major malformations, growth retardation, hypoplasia of midface and fingers) and determine whether the abnormalities are caused by the maternal epilepsy itself or by exposure to anticonvulsant drugs in utero. They reported that the combined frequency of anticonvulsant embryopathy was higher in 223 infants exposed to one anticonvulsant drug than in 508 control infants (20.6% vs. 8.5%) and that the frequency was higher in 93 infants exposed to two or more anticonvulsant drugs than in the controls (28.0% vs. 8.5%). Moreover, the 98 infants born to the mothers with a history of epilepsy but no use of anticonvulsants during pregnancy did not exhibit a higher frequency of abnormalities than control infants.[56]

In 2003, Kaaja et al.[84] prospectively followed up 970 pregnancies in women with epilepsy at a single maternity clinic from 1980 through 1998. Of the 979 total offspring, 740 were exposed to maternal AEDs during the first trimester, and 239 were not exposed. Serum folate concentrations were measured at the end of the first trimester, as were maternal AED levels (to minimize exposure). Major malformations were detected in 28 fetuses (3.8%) exposed to maternal AED and in two (0.8%) not exposed. Eight of the 28 cases had NTDs, which is fourteenfold the national rate. Seven had oral clefts, six had cardiovascular malformations, four had visceral malformations, and three exhibited miscellaneous malformations. Logistical regression analysis revealed that the occurrence of major malformations was independently associated with use

of carbamazepine (odds ratio [OR] 2.5), valproate (OR 4.1), and oxcarbazepine (OR 10.8); low serum folate concentration; and low maternal level of education. Also, the authors found no association between major malformations and seizures during the first trimester. None of these women reported preconception use of folate, but all were advised to take multivitamins containing 0.1 to 0.8 mg of folate at the first antenatal visit, usually between the eighth and twelfth week of gestation.[84]

The risks of AED-induced folate deficiency on fetal development also involve the effect of AEDs on the efficacy of birth control. The most common AEDs induce the CYP450 enzymes that metabolize estrogens (e.g., ethinyl estradiol, mestranol), causing up to a 40% reduction in serum levels.[85-88] Oral contraceptives (OCs) can also interfere with folate cofactor interactions, causing impaired DNA synthesis. Thus the use of OCs or Norplant does not reduce the need for folic acid coadministration in women of childbearing age and may actually increase such need because increased clearance of the contraceptive agents may impair their efficacy.

Compared with older anticonvulsants, particularly hydantoin derivatives, newer AEDs may exert less adverse effect on fetal development because of lesser adverse influence on vitamin status, among other reasons.[89] Such probabilities, their implications, and clinical responses have yet to be adequately researched and supported by conclusive evidence.

The coadministration of folic acid to counterbalance the adverse effects of AEDs on folate nutriture has been investigated and refined to a point where broad parameters of efficacy and guidelines for clinical implementation now have general consensus. In a long-term study, Reynolds[90] investigated the effects of 1 to 3 years of folate coadministration on the "mental state and fit-frequency" in 26 chronic epileptic patients with AED-induced folic-acid deficiency treated with one or more anticonvulsants. Mental state improved in 22 patients, but seizure frequency or severity was aggravated in 13 patients (50%). Reynolds concluded that "folic acid partially reverses both the therapeutic (antiepileptic) and retarding effects of phenobarbitone, phenytoin, and primidone."[90] Baylis et al.[91] assessed the effects of folic acid administration in 50 folate-deficient epileptic patients taking phenytoin, primidone, and phenobarbital in various combinations. Serum phenytoin levels fell from 20 to 10 µg/mL in a group of 10 patients after 1 month's treatment with folic acid, 5 mg/day. Likewise, serum phenytoin levels fell from 14 to 11 µg/mL in a second group of 40 patients administered 15 mg/day of folic acid. "In one patient the fall was to below the therapeutic range and was associated with deterioration in fit control."[91] Phenobarbital levels were unchanged in the presence of folate supplementation.

In a randomized, double-blind trial, Gibberd et al.[92] tested the effects of folic acid coadministration on seizure frequency in a group of outpatients with epilepsy treated with phenytoin for at least 1 year. Although the group receiving folic acid in the treatment period showed a significant improvement in seizure frequency, the authors suggested that "subjective well-being of patients was not influenced by folic acid therapy" and concluded that "the improvement while on folic acid was not due to the folic acid treatment alone."[92] Biale and Lewenthal[93] conducted a study to determine the frequency of malformations among newborn infants of mothers receiving anticonvulsive therapy with and without folate supplementation. In the retrospective portion of the study involving 24 women not receiving folate, 10 children among the 66 newborns (15% frequency) exhibited congenital malformations, including congenital heart disease, cleft lip and palate, NTDs, and skeletal abnormalities; 3 of the 10 were stillborn or died immediately after delivery. In the prospective portion of the study, involving 22 women receiving folate, all 33 infants were born alive, and no congenital malformations occurred. The authors concluded that the "teratogenic activity of anticonvulsant drugs seems to be mediated by interference with folic acid metabolism, and such activity might be influenced by hereditary and environmental factors."[93] They recommended folic acid coadministration to epileptic women intending to become pregnant.

Berg et al.[43] (1995) demonstrated the interdependence of the phenytoin-folate interaction by showing that the addition of folic acid to phenytoin therapy improved phenytoin pharmacokinetics and produced changes in blood levels of phenytoin. In a randomized crossover study involving six women of childbearing age, they compared outcomes of two groups of women, both receiving 300 mg phenytoin daily. Both groups had essentially equivalent dietary folate intake, but the subjects in the second treatment group also received 1 mg folic acid daily. The no–folic acid group exhibited a 38% reduction in serum folate level, with a serum phenytoin concentration in the low therapeutic range. The folic acid/phenytoin group showed a 26% increase in serum folate level, with a phenytoin level similar to that in phenytoin-only subjects. Notably, only one woman achieved phenytoin steady state during phenytoin-only treatment, but four women achieved steady state during treatment with both folic acid and phenytoin (PHT). The authors concluded that their findings suggest "an interdependence between PHT and folic acid and supports the observation that fertile women treated with PHT require folic acid supplementation to maintain a normal serum folate level."[43]

Later in 1995, in their review of the literature on phenytoin-folate interactions, Lewis et al.[44] proposed that folic acid should always be prescribed with phenytoin because of a synergistic effect. Folic acid supplementation in folate-deficient patients with epilepsy can change the pharmacokinetics of phenytoin and, without appropriate clinical management, may increase risk of possible seizure breakthrough by leading to lower serum phenytoin concentrations. Folate is hypothesized to be a cofactor in phenytoin metabolism and may be able to assist in obtaining a concentration where phenytoin appears to be at steady state but actually is not. Phenytoin and folic acid therapy initiated concomitantly with monitoring and titration can prevent decreased folate and obtain steady-state phenytoin concentrations sooner. The authors concluded that folic acid supplementation should be initiated concomitantly with phenytoin therapy because of the hypothesized cofactor mechanism, decreased adverse effects associated with folate deficiency, and better seizure control with no perturbation of phenytoin pharmacokinetics.

Subsequently, in a controlled trial, Eros et al.[94] reported that both healthy and epileptic women taking less than 1 mg of folic acid daily had no increased risk of seizures. Of 60 epileptic women with periconception multivitamin supplementation with 800 μg of folic acid, none developed epilepsy-related side effects during the periconception period. One epileptic woman delivered a newborn with cleft lip and palate. However, a 22-year-old epileptic woman receiving carbamazepine, as well as taking a daily multivitamin supplement with 1.0 mg of folic acid from the twentieth week of gestation, exhibited a cluster of seizures after the periconception period. Furthermore, she developed status epilepticus and symptoms of systemic lupus erythematosus; this pregnancy ended with stillbirth. The authors concluded that an autoimmune disease (probably drug-induced lupus) had emerged in this epileptic patient and damaged the blood-brain barrier, so the 1-mg (or greater)

therapeutic dose of folic acid may have triggered a cluster of seizures. Overall, they noted that administration of a physiological dose (<1 mg) of folic acid to women without autoimmune disease did not increase the risk of epileptic seizures.

Evidence is mixed as to what dosage level and form of folic acid coadministration is necessary to reverse adverse AED effects on folate metabolism yet avoid interfering with the therapeutic activity of the medications. A review of the evidence generally indicates that the levels of folic acid in typical multivitamin formulations (e.g., 400 μg/day) may be adequate for folate nurture during pregnancy in healthy, nonmedicated women. Some sources, such as Hiilesmaa et al.,[95] suggest that "low-dose" folic acid (100-1000 μg/day) is sufficient to prevent deficiency during pregnancy in women treated with AEDs. In contrast, most authorities now report that 800 to 1000 μg/day is required for effective protection within the context of folate-depleting medications. Nulman et al.[88] advise that "seizure control should be achieved at least six months prior to conception and, if clinically possible, by the lowest effective dose of a single anticonvulsant according to the type of epilepsy." Moreover, they recommend that women undergoing AED polytherapy supplement with 5 mg of folic acid daily, for 3 months before conception and during the first trimester, to prevent malformations caused by drug-induced folic acid deficiency.[88] Thus, based on individual variability and the medication involved, folate coadministration is simply not adequate for some women, and a change in AED regimen, such as eliminating valproate, may be necessary for a safe pregnancy. Furthermore, administration of 5-methyltetrahydrofolate (5-MTHF), such as folinic acid, may be required to counterbalance the adverse effects of folate-depleting medications as well as concurrent factors such as inadequate nutritional status, smoking, alcohol intake, and genetic variability.

Gingival hyperplasia is a common adverse effect associated with some AEDs, particularly phenytoin and valproic acid. The topical application of folate is generally helpful in the treatment of gingival overgrowth, especially in pregnant women, outside the context of anticonvulsants.[96-98] Folate mouthwash appears to have an influence on gum health through local rather than systemic influence. Most research on phenytoin-induced changes in the gums indicates that daily rinses with a folate-based mouthwash may also inhibit gum disease caused by phenytoin. Notably, the level of dietary folate did not correlate with changes in hyperplasia in experimental subjects.[99-101]

The broad context of diet, lifestyle, economic status, and education frames the more narrow clinical issues of folic acid coadministration, Hcy status, and genomics. Lower economic status and educational levels are both associated with increased risk of birth defects in general and AED-induced malformations in particular. Likewise, children of women with epilepsy who smoked had lower gestational age and were at 3.4-fold increased risk of preterm delivery compared with infants of nonepileptic women who smoked.[78] However, the findings of a 2002 British questionnaire-based survey of 795 women of childbearing age with epilepsy revealed significant shortcomings in education and awareness regarding pregnancy and childbearing. Of those women surveyed who considered the questions personally relevant, 38% to 48% recalled receiving information about contraception, pre-pregnancy planning, folic acid, and teratogenicity; overall, proportions were lower among adolescent women.[102]

Researchers and public health experts predict that the policies of dietary folate fortification and associated nutrition education programs adopted during the 1990s will have a significant, but not optimal, effect in preventing folate-related birth defects among healthy women, even those eating foods fortified with folic acid.[1,5,10,11,103] However, these folate intake recommendations, typically a 400 µg daily dose before and during pregnancy, as adopted by the U.S. FDA in 1998, and folate fortification of grains and other foods, estimated to increase actual daily intake of folic acid by approximately 78 µg, do not provide adequately for woman with compromised folate metabolism, particularly those taking folate-depleting medications.[104]

Botto et al.[105] conducted an international retrospective cohort study of NTDs in relation to folic acid recommendations and found limited effect in Europe. After examining 13 birth defects registries, they reported that "the issuing of recommendations on folic acid was followed by no detectable improvement in the trends of incidence of neural tube defects" from 1988 to 1998. They concluded that dietary recommendations alone did not seem to influence trends in NTDs up to 6 years after clinical trials confirmed the effectiveness of folic acid, and that "cases of neural tube defects preventable by folic acid continue to accumulate."[105] Perhaps even more disturbing, evidence suggests that enrichment of foods with folic acid may not be circumventing widespread deficits in nutritional awareness and a related lack of proactive behavioral changes, to serve as an effective preventive measure.[11] However, in reviewing results from the National Health and Nutrition Examination Survey (1999–2000), Pfeiffer et al.[1] concluded: "Every segment of the US population appears to benefit from folic acid fortification." Some commentators have also raised troubling yet essential questions about strong genetic selection pressure and potential adverse effects on the human genome from such public policy.[106]

More immediately, the policy of food fortification with folic acid expands the long-standing issue of folic acid supplementation with vitamin B_{12} supplementation from clinical management to unsupervised mass intervention into nutrient interrelationships. Thus, researchers might find it worthwhile to study the real potential of introducing a relative excess of folate into well-nourished populations who do not necessarily need it, while failing to enhance the nutrient intake of less well-fed populations and failing to consider B_{12} deficiencies, both relative and absolute.

Reports

A long-standing body of literature in case reports and scientific reviews documents the relatively high incidence of megaloblastic anemia and other hematological disorders among individuals undergoing long-term, and sometimes even short-term, therapy with AEDs.[107-117]

Guidolin et al.[118] reported on a 26-year-old woman being treated with carbamazepine for symptomatic partial epilepsy with simple and complex seizures. She experienced an increase in seizure frequency and severity after initiation of folic acid prophylaxis at 800 µg/day in anticipation of pregnancy.

Torres et al.[119] reported three cases of neonates with seizures who were unresponsive to one or more anticonvulsant medications but demonstrated immediate relief after administration of folinic acid.

When viewed within the context of relevant research literature, these reports reflect the broad trends and illustrate the need for further research into the individual variations in folate coadministration requirements, permutations of clinical response, and close supervision and regular monitoring during such coadministration, particularly on initiation or modification.

However, coadministration of preconception folic acid may not be protective for women with epilepsy. Craig et al.[120] described a young woman whose seizures were controlled for 4 years by of valproic acid (2000 mg/day). Even though she supplemented with 4.0 mg of folic acid daily for 18 months before her pregnancy, she delivered a child with a lumbosacral NTD, a ventricular and atrial septal defect, cleft palate, and bilateral talipes. Likewise, two Canadian women delivered children with NTDs despite folate supplementation. One taking folic acid (3.5 mg/day) for 3 months before conception and valproic acid (1250 mg) aborted a child with lumbosacral spina bifida, Arnold Chiari malformation, and hydrocephalus. Another woman who supplemented with folic acid (5.0 mg/day) experienced one spontaneous abortion of a fetus with an encephalocele and two therapeutic abortions of fetuses with lumbosacral spina bifida.[121] It would be of interest to know if these women carried MTHFR genetic polymorphisms and might have been unable to properly metabolize and activate folic acid in its usual form.

Nutritional Therapeutics, Clinical Concerns, and Adaptations

Physicians prescribing anticonvulsants and related medications are advised to educate their patients regarding implications of drug-induced depletion of folate and other nutrients and to assess their serum B_{12} and Hcy levels. The available evidence indicates that valproic acid, as monotherapy or a component of polytherapy, carries significantly greater risk of teratogenicity than other AEDs administered during pregnancy. Coadministration of folic acid and enhancement of dietary intake of folate-rich foods are almost always appropriate to prevent a drug-induced deficiency. Nevertheless, the data remain unclear and the benefits uncertain as to whether folate coadministration in women with epilepsy taking AEDs will reduce their risk. Further research using L-5-methyl folate is needed. Coadministration of folic acid (800 µg/day) and vitamin B_{12} (6 µg/day) may be sufficient in some cases, but levels typical of multivitamins have proved inadequate for many individuals. Dose titration enables reduction of adverse effects while minimizing the risk of interfering with the therapeutic activity of the AED(s). Special attention should be given to the possibility of decreased seizure control as folic acid supplementation is initiated, as well as to possible increased AED toxicity when administration of additional folic acid is halted.

The critical importance of ongoing supervision, nutritional assessment, and lifestyle education within the context of a frank and supportive therapeutic relationship cannot be overstated in the care of patients undergoing long-term therapy with AEDs. Close supervision and regular monitoring of serum levels of the medication(s) and clinical effects, as well as monitoring of folate and Hcy levels, are essential, especially with patients receiving long-term multidrug therapy. Although folate is generally considered nontoxic, large doses of folic acid may precipitate clinical B_{12} deficiency, especially if vitamin B_{12} status was already impaired. Spontaneously or iatrogenically hypochlorhydric patients may require much more than 6 µg of B_{12} for adequate function. Urinary and serum MMA levels may be the most reliable way of assessing functional B_{12} status. Beyond the concerns of folate deficiency and Hcy-associated risk in the general population, thrombosis from hyperhomocysteinemia in epileptic patients taking anticonvulsants represents a significant risk responsive to proactive clinical management. Genetic testing for folate polymorphisms may provide an especially valuable tool in risk assessment and clinical management of Hcy status in relation to folate nutriture during treatment with AEDs. Patients with a TT allele of the

MTHFR C677T polymorphism, particularly in combination with the RFC1 80GG genotype, may have an even higher folate requirement than other patients treated with AEDs because of their significantly increased risk of elevated Hcy from compromised folate metabolism.

The dosage and number of folate-lowering drugs should be minimized and folic acid coadministration initiated in women with epilepsy who are contemplating pregnancy.

Seizure control should be achieved at least 6 months before conception and, if clinically possible, by the lowest effective dose of a single anticonvulsant individualized according to the type of epilepsy. Substitution of another agent is strongly indicated in women being treated with valproic acid, as monotherapy or a component of polytherapy. Folic acid at 5 mg/day (along with vitamins B_6 and B_{12}) should be administered starting 3 months before conception and during the first trimester to prevent folic acid deficiency–induced malformations. Strong consideration should be given to using the activated form (L-5-methyl or 5-formyl) of folate in this setting, unless genetic testing has ruled out MTHFR genetic polymorphisms. The addition of folic acid to a prenatal regimen becomes even more imperative for women using OCs while undergoing anticonvulsant therapy when they choose to become pregnant, because OCs also tend to adversely affect folate status. Some clinicians consider benzodiazepines or phenytoin to be effective for seizure cessation during labor and delivery. Administration of vitamin K immediately after birth is prudent. Furthermore, the neonate should be thoroughly assessed for epilepsy and anticonvulsant-associated dysmorphology.

Antifolates and Related Antimetabolites, Including Lometrexol, Methotrexate, Pemetrexed

Evidence: Lometrexol (T64), methotrexate (Folex, Maxtrex, Rheumatrex), pemetrexed (Alimta), raltitrexed (ZD-1694; Tomudex).

Similar properties but evidence lacking for extrapolation: Agalsidase beta (Fabrazyme), capecitabine (Xeloda), cladribine (Leustatin), cytarabine (ara-C; Cytosar-U, DepoCyt, Tarabine PFS), floxuridine (FUDR), fludarabine (Fludara), fluorouracil (5-FU, Adrucil, Efudex, Efudix, Fluoroplex), gemcitabine (Gemzar), mercaptopurine (6-mercaptopurine, 6-MP, NSC 755; Purinethol), methotrexate (Folex, Maxtrex, Rheumatrex), pentostatin (Nipent), thioguanine (6-thioguanine, 6-TG, 2-amino-6-mercaptopurine; Lanvis, Tabloid), ZD9331, Trimetrexate (Neutrexin).

See also Mercaptopurine (and Thioguanine) later, as well as Raltitrexed under Theoretical, Speculative, and Preliminary Interactions Research.

See also Pyrimethamine.

Interaction Type and Significance

✗✗✗   **Potentially Harmful or Serious Adverse Interaction—Avoid**

⊕⊕   **Beneficial or Supportive Interaction, with Professional Management**

◇≈≈   **Drug-Induced Adverse Effect on Nutrient Function, Coadministration Therapeutic, with Professional Management**

☼   **Prevention or Reduction of Drug Adverse Effect**

⊕✗   **Bimodal or Variable Interaction, with Professional Management**

◇◇   **Drug-Induced Effect on Nutrient Function, Supplementation Contraindicated, Professional Management Appropriate**

Nutrient Depletion

Probability:
2. **Probable** to 1. **Certain**

Evidence Base:
● **Consensus**

Coadministration Benefit
Probability:
2. **Probable** or 3. **Possible**

Evidence Base:
◉ **Emerging** to
● **Consensus**

Effect and Mechanism of Action

By definition, the agents in this drug class share the central mechanism of being "antifolate" as well as several key characteristics that influence folate metabolism and affect clinical implications of depletion. However, they differ in their pharmacological characteristics and mechanisms, therapeutic applications and effects, and characteristic patient populations, all of which influence their safety profile, adverse effects, and approaches to coadministration of folic acid.

Methotrexate is the prototype antifolate, used in oncology for decades before it was introduced to rheumatology, and still used in both specialties. The cancer chemotherapeutic agent lometrexol [(6R)-5,10-dideaza-5,6,7,8-tetrahydrofolate] is a representative later generation folate antimetabolite. Used mainly in treating solid tumors, lometrexol targets the de novo purine nucleotide biosynthesis pathway and limits DNA synthesis by inhibiting glycinamide ribonucleotide formyltransferase (GARFT), the first folate-dependent enzyme in de novo purine synthesis; it is avidly polyglutamated and retained in tissues expressing folylpolyglutamate synthetase.[122-125] Lometrexol pharmacokinetics are often described by a three-compartment model and are considered independent of either lometrexol or folic acid dose. The cumulative hematological toxicity of lometrexol is related to cellular pharmacokinetics and tissue concentration and not plasma pharmacokinetics.[126]

Methotrexate is a folic acid antagonist used in the treatment of several types of cancer, rheumatoid arthritis (RA), psoriasis, and other conditions. Many of the adverse effects associated with methotrexate are similar to those of severe folate deficiency. Methotrexate produces its immunosuppressant and antineoplastic effects by binding to and reversibly inhibiting the activity of dihydrofolate reductase, which reduces folate to active tetrahydrofolate.[127] By thus restricting levels of tetrahydrofolate, methotrexate decreases the availability of single-carbon fragments required for biosynthesis of purines, DNA, and cellular proteins. Perhaps the most widely used folate antagonist, methotrexate has varying patterns of use for different conditions, and the relationship of folic acid to the drug mechanism changes accordingly. This difference is especially important in individuals using methotrexate as a chemotherapeutic agent and those taking it for RA.

As with other antifolates, pemetrexed exerts its antineoplastic activity by inhibiting multiple tetrahydrofolate cofactor-requiring enzymes involved in the de novo biosynthesis of purine, thymidine, and pyrimidine nucleotides, thus interfering with folate-dependent metabolic processes critical to cell replication. Pemetrexed also inhibits dihydrofolate reductase. Its greater potency, compared with other antifolates, is related to its transport into cells by both the reduced–folate carrier system and the membrane folate-binding protein transport system. The enzyme folylpolyglutamate synthetase then intracellularly converts pemetrexed to polyglutamate forms, which are retained in cells and act as inhibitors of thymidylate synthase (TS) and GARFT. Thus, functionally, pemetrexed acts as a prodrug for its polyglutamate forms. Polyglutamation occurs more rapidly and extensively in tumor cells than in healthy tissues, and polyglutamated metabolites exhibit a prolonged intracellular retention in malignant cells and a 60-fold increase in inhibition of TS compared with the monoglutamated form. Pemetrexed has demonstrated significant antineoplastic activity against a variety of tumor types, including lung, breast, colon, mesothelioma, pancreatic, gastric, bladder, head and neck, and cervix. Tumors with codeletion of the methylthioadenosine phosphorylase gene, as a consequence of p16 deletions, may be particularly sensitive to pemetrexed. Attention has also focused on its ability to enhance the cytotoxicity and tolerability of doxorubicin, paclitaxel, cisplatin, gemcitabine, and other important chemotherapeutic agents.[128-132]

Raltitrexed is a quinazoline folate analog that selectively inhibits TS and thereby causes DNA fragmentation and cell death. Raltitrexed is transported into cells through a reduced folate carrier, where it is extensively polyglutamated. As with pemetrexed, polyglutamation enhances potency and extends half-life to increase the duration of TS inhibition and raltitrexed's antitumor activity.

In summary, the finding that folate intake does not seem to interfere with efficacy of these drugs, both in autoimmune disease and cancer applications, is both intriguing and clinically significant, suggesting these agents may have other mechanisms besides folate antagonism or being "antifolate."

Research

Researchers and clinicians generally agree that impaired folate status plays a major role in the activity and toxicity of methotrexate and other antifolates.[127] The degree of folate depletion during methotrexate therapy for autoimmune disease depends primarily on the weekly administered dose. The risk of adverse effects from interference with folic acid utilization is particularly significant with high dose and prolonged use. Folic acid (or 5-MTHF) coadministration can usually mitigate adverse effects of antifolates, but their ability to do so without impairing drug efficacy may vary significantly in low-dose treatment (e.g., methotrexate for RA or psoriasis) versus high-dose administration (e.g., cancer therapy). Furthermore, emerging trends suggest research may be warranted to explore the clinical potential of antifolates whose pharmacodynamic effects are less affected by variations in folate status among different patients.

The coadministration of folinic acid (Leucovorin) is well established in conventional practice as an adjunctive therapy to mitigate toxic effects of methotrexate, lometrexol, and related agents, particularly in the context of high-dose antineoplastic chemotherapy. Folinic acid (5-FTHF) is the most well-known reduced form of folic acid, available as a calcium salt for parenteral or oral administration, which competes with methotrexate for entry into cells and repletes intracellular pools of tetrahydrofolate. Overall, findings from studies conducted in the late 1980s and early 1990s were mixed as to both the effects of folinic acid coadministration in reducing methotrexate toxicity and drug-induced adverse effects and the possible impairment of methotrexate efficacy and therapy outcomes.[133-140] Nevertheless, folinic acid has been used as a rescue agent throughout the history of clinical trials and has become part of conventional practice in the clinical application of antifolates, such as after high-dose methotrexate in the treatment of osteosarcoma.[141] For many years, folinic acid has been coadministered as part of a standard therapy using 5-fluorouracil for metastatic colorectal cancer (5-FU/leukovorin), at least in part because of its ability to increase the affinity of fluorouracil for TS. More recently, with raltitrexed, intravenous folinic acid,

25 mg/m^2 every 6 hours, can reduce intestinal damage and improve recovery of neutrophil and platelet levels.[142] As a form of 5-formyltetrahydrofolate (5-FTHF), folinic acid's ability to bypass dihydrofolate reductase contributes both to its rapid action and therapeutic efficacy and its potential to reduce drug activity.

In certain circumstances, folic acid may be capable of reducing the symptoms of antifolate toxicity without interfering with clinical effectiveness. Evidence consistently demonstrates the safety and efficacy of folate coadministration with methotrexate in the treatment of RA, psoriasis, and similar autoimmune conditions. In contrast to folinic acid or 5-MTHF, folic acid still requires reduction by dihydrofolate reductase, a factor that may reduce its potency and the probability of it interfering with antifolate drug efficacy.

As the use of methotrexate for the treatment of RA has evolved, so has the understanding of the use of folic acid by individuals undergoing therapy. Although use of methotrexate for RA treatment has grown in recent years, more than 30% of patients abandon treatment because of drug-related adverse effects. Initially, researchers assumed that methotrexate's effects on folic acid were the source of its presumed benefits in cases of rheumatoid arthritis, as in chemotherapeutic uses. However, with time and further research, practice has shifted to support the coadministration of folic acid to counter the adverse effects of methotrexate in these cases for several reasons: (1) its well-proven ability to reduce toxic effects of methotrexate; (2) methotrexate causes folate deficiency, and the folate status of patients taking even low-dose methotrexate declines precipitously without adjunctive folic acid; and (3) plasma Hcy levels can increase significantly in those taking methotrexate but not folate, thereby significantly increasing risk of cardiovascular disease. These and other benefits are gained with no apparent loss of antirheumatic effect. Most researchers have found that folic acid levels were not related to parameters of disease activity and concluded that methotrexate does not exert its action in RA primarily by inhibiting dihydrofolate reductase.[143-148]

In 1993, Duhra[149] studied 78 patients with psoriasis to determine the frequency, severity, and dose relationship of GI symptoms induced by low-dose, once-weekly oral methotrexate (MTX) therapy and the response to concomitant folic acid administration. After initiation of MTX, 32% of subjects reported GI symptoms, with nausea accounting for 80%. The author reported that the "onset and severity of symptoms were related to the weekly dose of methotrexate but not to the cumulative dose or to the duration of methotrexate therapy." Folic acid, 5 mg daily, eliminated these adverse effects without impairing the therapeutic effect of the medication. Likewise, Morgan et al.[138] found that "5 mg or 50 mg/week dose of folic acid supplementation does not alter the efficacy of methotrexate treated rheumatoid arthritis patients." In a double-blind, placebo-controlled trial of 79 patients over 1 year, Morgan et al.[148] demonstrated that folic acid coadministration (5 or 27.5 mg/week) prevents deficient blood folate levels and hyperhomocysteinemia, thus providing cardiovascular disease prevention, during long-term, low-dose MTX therapy for RA. Folate nutriture declined in patients administered low-dose MTX without adjunctive folic acid. The authors observed that "low blood folate levels and increased mean corpuscular volumes were associated with substantial methotrexate toxicity, whereas daily dietary intakes of more than 900 nmol (400 micrograms) of folic acid were associated with little methotrexate toxicity." Plasma Hcy levels increased significantly and hyperhomocysteinemia occurred more often in the placebo group than in the folic acid–supplemented groups. The authors concluded that for long-term, low-dose MTX therapy, "there are now at least three reasons to consider supplementation with folic acid (a low cost prescription): (1) to prevent MTX toxicity, (2) to prevent or treat folate deficiency, and (3) to prevent hyperhomocysteinemia."[148]

Suzuki et al.[150] retrospectively analyzed 66 RA patients to assess the incidence and risk factors for elevation of serum hepatic alanine (ALT) and aspartate (AST) aminotransferases during MTX therapy. The frequency of elevation of serum AST or ALT was four to five times greater than in patients taking other disease-modifying antirheumatic drugs (DMARDs). Subsequently, the authors prospectively evaluated the effect of adjunctive folic acid on serum ALT and RA activity in 14 patients who exhibited sustained, high serum ALT levels. The ALT levels decreased with folic acid coadministration in all patients within 3 months. Eleven patients treated with folic acid showed no change in RA symptomatology, but three exited the study because of exacerbation of their RA symptoms. These researchers advised that "careful monitoring of serum hepatic aminotransferases is necessary in patients with predisposing factors, especially those receiving more than 0.15 mg/kg of MTX weekly."[150] They cautioned that although folic acid coadministration can reverse the sustained elevation of ALT, it might also exacerbate RA in some patients.

In a prospective, randomized, double-blind, placebo-controlled study, Griffith et al.[151] (2000) tested the benefits of folate support in RA patients receiving ongoing MTX treatment (<20 mg weekly) by withdrawing folic acid (5 mg/day) from one group and substituting a placebo. The authors monitored all toxicity (including absolute changes in hematological and liver enzyme indices), recorded patient reports of changes in drug efficacy, and tracked discontinuation of MTX over 1 year. Among the 25 subjects who concluded the study early, a significantly larger proportion (17; 46%) of those receiving MTX alone discontinued the drug, versus eight (21%) in the group remaining on folic acid. The placebo/MTX group reported an increased incidence of nausea (45% vs. 7%) at 9 months, and two patients in that group discontinued because of neutropenia. Although subjects in the placebo group exhibited significantly lower disease activity on several of the variables measured, the researchers adjudged that "these were probably not of clinical significance." Overall, these findings indicate that folic acid coadministration reduced adverse effects and enabled patient tolerance and compliance without significantly interfering with MTX's therapeutic activity.[151]

Also in 2000, van den Berg et al.[152] showed that 83.5% of patients (61 of 85) treated with concomitant folic acid during low-dose MTX therapy for RA continued treatment for more than 1 year, compared with 53.1% of patients (23 of 49) not receiving folic acid support. The authors attributed this pattern of decreased patient discontinuation of MTX to folic acid's effects in reducing adverse effects from the medication.

In a 48-week, randomized, double-blind, placebo-controlled clinical trial involving 434 RA patients, van Ede et al.[153] compared the effects of MTX plus placebo, folic acid (1 mg/day), or folinic acid (2.5 mg/week) with regard to discontinuation of MTX because of adverse effects and MTX dosage, efficacy, and toxicity. The initial MTX dosage was 7.5 mg/week; dosage increases were allowed up to a maximum of 25 mg/week for insufficient responses. Folate dosages were doubled once the dosage of MTX reached 15 mg/week. These researchers reported that parameters of disease activity improved equally in all groups, although subjects in both folate groups required slightly higher dosages of MTX to

obtain similar symptomatic improvement. However, only 17% of the folic acid group and 12% of the folinic acid group discontinued MTX therapy because of toxicity-related adverse effects, in contrast to 38% of the placebo group. The authors attributed these between-group differences to a decreased incidence of elevated liver enzyme levels in the folate groups. No other between-group differences were found in the incidence, severity, or duration of other adverse events, including GI and mucosal effects.

Hoekstra et al.[154] analyzed data from a 48-week, multicenter, randomized clinical trial involving 411 patients with RA treated with MTX, comparing folates and placebo to assess factors associated with toxicity, final dose, and drug efficacy. Coadministration of folates and MTX was strongly related to the lack of hepatotoxicity, as well as reduced levels of drug discontinuation and efficacy of MTX therapy. Reaching a final dose of MTX of 15 mg/week or more was related to folate supplementation and the absence of prior GI events. Other baseline characteristics predictive of MTX treatment outcome included body mass index, gender, use of nonsteroidal anti-inflammatory drugs (NSAIDs), and creatinine clearance.

Khanna et al.[155] examined the effect of folic acid on the efficacy of MTX treatment in RA patients at 12 months in two Phase III, randomized controlled trials of leflunomide in which MTX was used as a comparator. A U.S. study involved 482 patients with active RA; of these, 179 received at least one dose of MTX, and all were mandated to receive 1 mg of oral folic acid once or twice daily. A multinational European study involved 999 patients with active RA; of these, 489 received at least one dose of MTX, and oral folic acid was not required, although 50 received folate after developing an adverse event. After using propensity scores to adjust for differences in the baseline characteristics of folic acid users and non–folic acid users, the authors concluded that 9% to 21% fewer MTX-treated RA patients taking folic acid had 20%, 50%, or 70% improvement, according to American College of Rheumatology (ACR) standards, at 52 weeks compared with those who did not receive folic acid. Thus, 17% more patients in the group who did not receive folic acid met ACR improvement criteria, whereas ACR 50% responses were 14% higher in the non–folic acid group and ACR 70% responses 12% higher; such findings suggest that adjunctive folic acid may impair the efficacy of MTX in such patients. Furthermore, they reported relatively similar rates of adverse events among U.S. and European subjects, 93% and 94%, respectively, but a significantly higher occurrence of elevated liver transaminase levels among European subjects (62%), most of whom were not taking folic acid, in contrast to 29% of U.S. study patients, most of whom were taking folic acid. The authors also emphasized that physicians should consider a possible exacerbation when their RA patients taking MTX are started on folic acid, suggesting these patients may require a higher MTX dose.[155]

Kirby et al.[156] investigated folic acid–prescribing patterns among dermatologists in the United Kingdom treating psoriasis patients with MTX. Of the 153 physicians who responded to the survey, 75% reported that they coadministered folic acid, 46% considered folic acid effective in reducing drug-induced nausea, and 60% reported that such nutrient support did not impair MTX efficacy in the treatment of psoriasis.

The efficacy of and tolerance for MTX therapy varies from patient to patient. Pharmacogenomic variability represents one important factor influencing clinical response and patient compliance. For example, the ability of leukemia cells to accumulate methotrexate polyglutamate (MTXPG) is an important determinant of the antileukemic effects of MTX. Kager et al.[157]

measured in vivo MTXPG accumulation in leukemia cells from 101 children with acute lymphoblastic leukemia (ALL) to determine distinct mechanisms of subtype-specific differences in MTXPG. They determined that "B-lineage ALL with either TEL-AML1 or E2A-PBX1 gene fusion, or T-lineage ALL, accumulate significantly lower MTXPG compared with B-lineage ALL without these genetic abnormalities or compared with hyperdiploid (fewer than 50 chromosomes) ALL." They analyzed expression of 32 folate pathway genes in diagnostic leukemia cells from 197 children using oligonucleotide microarrays and found that ALL subtype-specific patterns of folate pathway gene expression were significantly related to MTXPG accumulation. Numerous studies have documented the incidence of increased intolerance to MTX and related antifolate therapies among individuals with genetic polymorphisms affecting folate metabolism.[158-164] The utility of folic acid coadministration in such individuals, once identified, may appear self-evident, but well-designed clinical trials are warranted and surely will be forthcoming.

For example, ongoing research by Sanderson and colleagues at St. Thomas' Hospital in London is focusing on new tools for predictive pharmacogenomics of antifolates, with a focus on treatment of inflammatory bowel disease. They have observed an association between genetic variation in levels of the enzyme thiopurine methyltransferase (TPMT) and inosine triphosphate pyrophosphatase (ITPase) and a significant risk of adverse responses (or lack of response) to these antifolate agents. (See later Mercaptopurine, Azathioprine, and Thioguanine [Thiopurines] section for further discussion.) Pretreatment assessment of these enzyme levels can provide a valuable tool in either avoidance of the drug or use at a lower dose to avoid adverse effects.

In a multicenter, cross-sectional study involving 226 adult patients treated with weekly MTX for more than 3 months, Dervieux et al.[165] investigated the contribution of red blood cell (RBC) MTXPGs, RBC folate polyglutamates, and a pharmacogenetic index to the clinical status of RA patients. They calculated a composite pharmacogenetic index comprising low-penetrance genetic polymorphisms in reduced folate carrier (RFC-1 G80A), AICAR transformylase (ATIC C347G), and thymidylate synthase (TSER*2/*3). Using a multivariate analysis, they found that lower RBC MTXPG levels (median, 40 nmol/L) and a lower pharmacogenetic index were associated with a higher number of joint counts, higher disease activity, and Health Assessment Questionnaire (HAQ). An RBC MTX PG level below 60 nmol/L and a low pharmacogenetic index were associated with an increased likelihood of poor therapeutic response to MTX. These authors concluded that "therapeutic drug monitoring of methotrexate treatment combining pharmacogenetic and intracellular metabolite measurements may be useful to optimize methotrexate treatment" by enabling "more sophisticated" methods for optimizing dosing, personalizing care, and minimizing adverse effects. They also suggested that "prospective studies are warranted to investigate the predictive value of these markers for MTX efficacy."[165]

Myelosuppression, neutropenia, and mucositis are among the most common and serious toxicities of pemetrexed, a newer antifolate drug developed for cancer treatment. Emerging evidence from research and clinical practice indicates that coadministration of oral folic acid or intramuscular vitamin B_{12} mitigates the toxicity profile of pemetrexed and clinical outcomes in difficult-to-treat cancers without impairing drug pharmacokinetics or compromising its antitumor effect, even over multiple treatment cycles.[131,166-169] For example, in a Phase III study involving 456 chemotherapy-naive patients

with malignant pleural mesothelioma, Vogelzang et al.[170] found that the combination of pemetrexed and cisplatin improved survival time, time to progression, and response rates compared with controls treated with cisplatin alone. Notably, after 117 patients had enrolled, "folic acid and vitamin B_{12} were added to reduce toxicity, resulting in a significant reduction in toxicities in the pemetrexed/cisplatin arm ... without adversely affecting survival time." Furthermore, in a review of pemetrexed's pharmacology, Calvert[132] noted that multivariate analyses have "demonstrated that pretreatment total plasma homocysteine levels significantly predicted severe thrombocytopenia and neutropenia, with or without associated grade 3/4 diarrhea, mucositis, or infection." She concludes: "Routine vitamin B_{12} and folic acid supplementation have resulted in decreased frequency/severity of toxicities associated with pemetrexed without affecting efficacy, making this novel antifolate a safe and efficacious anticancer agent."

Nutritional Therapeutics, Clinical Concerns, and Adaptations

Tolerance, safety, and compliance issues are significant in clinical management of patients treated with methotrexate and other antifolates. Physicians prescribing or administering these medications are strongly advised to inform patients regarding the high probability of drug-induced adverse effects on folate status and the clinical implications. Pharmacogenomic assessment (e.g., MTHFR, TPMT) can play a critical role in predicting drug efficacy and tolerance, especially with regard to folate metabolism and probable requirements, and in crafting an individualized treatment strategy. In most individuals, measured folic acid coadministration may enhance treatment efficacy and outcomes by reducing toxicity and adverse effects and increasing tolerance and compliance.

In treating patients with methotrexate for rheumatoid arthritis, psoriasis, and inflammatory bowel disease, large doses of folic acid can reduce adverse effects without compromising therapeutic activity. However, close supervision and regular monitoring of plasma drug levels and folate status, as well as plasma Hcy levels, are essential to safe and effective clinical management.

Concomitant use of folic acid during maintenance-phase antifolate treatment for leukemia and other forms of cancer is more controversial and requires a more careful, individualized, and closely managed approach to clinical care. Excessive repletion of folate may interfere with the intended therapeutic action of the medication in suppressing DNA synthesis and cellular proliferation of the malignant clone.

The administration of 5-FTHF (folinic acid) or 5-MTHF may be more efficacious in patients with high Hcy levels despite folic acid, B_{12}, pyridoxine, and methyl donor supplementation; in patients with low levels of dihydrofolate reductase enzyme activity; in those taking medications or supplements that suppress dihydrofolate reductase activity; and in patients with compromised liver or bone marrow function who might not reduce folate adequately.

Bile Acid Sequestrants

Evidence: Cholestyramine (Locholest, Prevalite, Questran), colestipol (Colestid).
Extrapolated, based on similar properties: Colesevelam (Welchol).

Interaction Type and Significance

≈≈≈ **Drug-Induced Nutrient Depletion, Supplementation Therapeutic, Not Requiring Professional Management**

◇ **Adverse Drug Effect on Nutritional Therapeutics, Strategic Concern**
⊕⊕ **Beneficial or Supportive Interaction, with Professional Management**

Nutrient Depletion
Probability:
2. Probable

Evidence Base:
● **Consensus**

Coadministration Benefit
Probability:
2. Probable

Evidence Base:
○ **Preliminary**

Effect and Mechanism of Action
Through their intended effect of limiting absorption and assimilation of dietary lipids, bile acid sequestrants may prevent absorption and reduce bioavailability of folic acid as well as other nutrients, such as the fat-soluble vitamins, A, D, E, and K.[57,171-174]

Through complementary mechanisms, folinic acid and cholestyramine can be used together to counter methotrexate toxicity.

Research
In 1979, Leonard et al.[175] demonstrated that cholestyramine and colestipol bound, to a great extent, vitamin B_{12}–intrinsic factor complex, folic acid, and iron citrate in vitro. Likewise, in studying the mechanisms of intestinal folate transport, Strum[176] found that cholestyramine (20 mg) adsorbs 95% of pteroylglutamate (folate) in vitro.

Using a rodent model, Hoppner and Lampi[177] observed that cholestyramine significantly reduced the intestinal deconjugation, absorption, and bioavailability of folic acid compared with brewer's yeast folate.

Several human studies have specifically documented the effects of bile acid sequestrants on folate absorption and bioavailability. In a trial involving 20 children and young adults with familial hypercholesterolemia, Farah et al.[178] investigated the effects of cholestyramine in the context of a diet low in cholesterol and high in polyunsaturated fats. Cholestyramine administration was associated with a significant decrease in mean serum folate levels in female patients. Tonstad et al.[179] conducted a study involving 37 boys and 29 girls age 10 to 16 years with familial hypercholesterolemia, first in an 8-week, double blind, placebo-controlled protocol, then in open treatment for 44 to 52 weeks. Levels of serum folate, vitamin E, and carotenoids were reduced in the colestipol group. Only a minority of adolescents adhered to the new formulation of orange-flavored "colestipol granules" for the full year. Nevertheless, the authors concluded that "folate and possibly vitamin D supplementation is recommended." Subsequently, in a randomized controlled trial involving children with familial hypercholesterolemia, Tonstad et al.[180] and another Norwegian team of investigators found that heterozygosity and homozygosity for the C677T mutation in the MTHFR gene was associated with low serum folate and increased susceptibility to elevation of plasma tHcy during cholestyramine treatment. These authors recommended folic acid coadministration as "prudent in these children" because of the independent relationship between elevated plasma tHcy and cardiovascular disease.

The ability of hypocholesterolemic resins to adsorb and reduce bioavailability of both folic acid and methotrexate (MTX) may be relevant in countering the toxicity of this potent antimetabolite, well-known for a range of adverse effects influencing tolerance and compliance. Interestingly,

cholestyramine may be used to enhance the biliary excretion of MTX, which acts as an antifolate through competitive inhibition.[181] Based on multiple experiments examining the relative adsorption of MTX and calcium leucovorin (folinic acid) onto cholestyramine in vitro, Merino-Sanjuan et al.[182] suggested that "cholestyramine may be a potentially useful adjunctive therapy in the treatment of an overdose of MTX." Fernandez et al.[183] described severe MTX-induced toxicity secondary to renal failure in a patient with non-Hodgkin's lymphoma. "Corrective measures included folinic acid rescue therapy, cholestyramine resin administration, hydration and urine alkalinization, urine pH monitoring, and extracorporeal clearance techniques."

Nutritional Therapeutics, Clinical Concerns, and Adaptations
Physicians prescribing bile acid sequestrants are advised to coadminister folic acid, vitamins B_{12} and B_6, mixed tocopherols and tocotrienols, vitamin D, coenzyme Q10, and other synergistic nutrients within a comprehensive and individualized strategy of integrative therapeutics for the prevention and treatment of cardiovascular disease. The relationship between folate status and homocysteine would be adequate by itself to justify increased intake of dietary folate and supplemental folic acid, of at least 800 μg/day, in such a patient population. The probable interference with absorption and bioavailability of folate and other relevant nutrients by these hypocholesteremic resins further heightens the imperative for enhanced nutriture. Daily administration of a high-potency multivitamin/mineral combination will replace the nutrients impeded by the drug. Folic acid (as well as other nutrients and medications) should be taken 1 hour before or 4 to 6 hours after bile acid sequestrants to reduce impairment of absorption and obtain optimal bioavailability.

Chloramphenicol

Chloramphenicol (Chloromycetin).

Interaction Type and Significance
◇≈≈ **Drug-Induced Adverse Effect on Nutrient Function, Coadministration Therapeutic, with Professional Management**
☼ **Prevention or Reduction of Drug Adverse Effect**
⊕⊕ **Beneficial or Supportive Interaction, Not Requiring Professional Management**
◇ **Adverse Drug Effect on Nutritional Therapeutics, Strategic Concern**

Probability:
2. Probable to
1. Certain

Evidence Base:
● **Consensus** but
○ **Preliminary**

Effect and Mechanism of Action
Drug-induced anemia is well established as an adverse effect of chloramphenicol.[110] Aplastic anemia has resulted from chloramphenicol in a small percentage of patients. Folic acid administration may reduce adverse effects of chloramphenicol to some degree. In patients prescribed folic acid for preventive benefits or therapeutic effects, concurrent administration of chloramphenicol for an extended period (or sometimes only a short period) can interfere with the hematopoietic response to folic acid and reduce effectiveness of folic acid in the treatment of anemias.

Research
Specific research on the interaction between chloramphenicol and dietary folate or supplemental folic acid is lacking.

However, consensus as to probable effects and outcomes is based on widely recognized functions and activities of the two substances.

Nutritional Therapeutics, Clinical Concerns, and Adaptations
Physicians are advised to monitor closely all major hematological parameters in patients prescribed chloramphenicol. Known toxicity has generally led to its disuse, except when no suitable alternative is available or the mortality of the treated disease is high.

Colchicine

Interaction Type and Significance
◇≈≈ Drug-Induced Adverse Effect on Nutrient Function, Coadministration Therapeutic, with Professional Management
☼ Prevention or Reduction of Drug Adverse Effect
⊕⊕⊕ Beneficial or Supportive Interaction, Not Requiring Professional Management
◇ Adverse Drug Effect on Nutritional Therapeutics, Strategic Concern

Probability:	Evidence Base:
4. Plausible to 2. Probable	○ Preliminary

Effect and Mechanism of Action
Colchicine is reported to depress blood folate levels.

Research
Depression of whole-blood folate activity by colchicine was demonstrated in 1965 and has not since been the subject of direct research.[184] No clinical trials have been published on the mitigation of adverse effects through folic acid coadministration. Further research through well-designed clinical trials may be warranted.

Nutritional Therapeutics, Clinical Concerns, and Adaptations
Physicians prescribing colchicine should closely monitor both folate and Hcy levels in patients. Pending substantive research through well-designed clinical trials, coadministration of folic acid, 800 µg/day, can provide a safe and potentially effective means of compensating for drug-depletion effects and may support the clinical strategies toward reducing cardiovascular risk.

Fenofibrate, Bezafibrate, and Related Fibrates

Evidence: Bezafibrate (Bezalip), fenofibrate (Lofibra, Tricor, Triglide).
Extrapolated, based on similar properties: Ciprofibrate (Modalim), clofibrate (Atromid-S).
Related but evidence against extrapolation: Gemfibrozil (Apo-Gemfibrozil, Lopid, Novo-Gemfibrozil).

Interaction Type and Significance
≈≈ Drug-Induced Adverse Effect on Nutrient Function, Supplementation Therapeutic, Not Requiring Professional Management
☼ Prevention or Reduction of Drug Adverse Effect
⊕⊕⊕ Beneficial or Supportive Interaction, Not Requiring Professional Management

Reduction of Drug-Induced Adverse Effect
Probability:	Evidence Base:
4. Plausible or 2. Probable	◉ Emerging, ▽ Mixed

Coadministration Benefit
Probability:	Evidence Base:
2. Probable to 1. Certain	● Emerging to ◉ Consensus

Effect and Mechanism of Action
A consistent body of evidence demonstrates that fibrates, particularly fenofibrate and bezafibrate, cause marked elevations in total plasma homocysteine (tHcy) levels. The molecular mechanisms involved have not been elucidated, but multiple mechanisms may contribute to this effect. Numerous studies show that coadministration of folic acid, especially with synergistic nutrients, can mitigate this particular adverse drug effect, but such intervention does not appear to alter clinical outcomes and thus may not constitute an "adverse clinical event."

Nutrient depletion resulting from hypolipidemic drugs, as indicated by plasma levels, appears to be lacking, a secondary factor of lesser clinical significance, or simply one that has not been adequately demonstrated within the design and time frame of the available clinical trials.[185] Impairment of renal function, alteration of creatine-creatinine metabolism, and changes in methyl transfer are regarded as more probable mechanisms.[186,187] Many of the effects of fibrates are known to be mediated by the peroxisome proliferator-activated receptor alpha (PPAR-α), a transcription factor belonging to the nuclear receptor family, and fibrates appear to increase homocystinemia through a PPAR-α–mediated mechanism.[188,189] For example, bezafibrate is a known activator of PPARs that can activate both PPAR-α and PPAR-β.

These and other findings suggest that the Hcy form elevated by fibrates may be protein-bound Hcy rather than atherogenic, reduced Hcy. Furthermore, although folic acid effectively reduces the fibrate-induced elevation of tHcy and creatinine, it does not affect the drug-induced elevation of total plasma cysteine (tCys).[190]

Research
An extensive body of scientific research has explored the effects of fibrates on Hcy levels, the role of folate in these effects, and the impact of such adverse effects and compensatory folate support within the overall strategy of cardiovascular risk reduction and outcomes. Fibrates are among the drugs of choice in conventional treatment of hypertriglyceridemia and low levels of high-density lipoprotein (HDL) cholesterol, both recognized as significant risk factors for cardiovascular disease. Increased blood levels of homocysteine, an amino acid derived from the methionine cycle, are generally associated with increased risk of endothelial damage, atherosclerosis, and coronary, cerebral, or peripheral vascular disease, although it is uncertain whether such elevations in Hcy represent a cause or a consequence of the pathological process. Some fibrates, particularly fenofibrate and bezafibrate, raise tHcy levels by 20% to 40%, but evidence from human research is still lacking to demonstrate that agents in this drug class induce depletion of folic acid or other nutrients known to modulate Hcy. Notably, multiple studies have found that gemfibrozil does not increase Hcy. Thus the overall trend in the literature shows that fibrate administration, particularly fenofibrate and bezafibrate, causes often-dramatic elevations in Hcy levels and that folic acid coadministration can neutralize this adverse effect, but suggests cardiovascular outcomes are unaffected by fibrate-induced hyperhomocysteinemia.

Significant evidence demonstrates that fenofibrate, bezafibrate, and potentially other frequently prescribed fibrates greatly increase plasma Hcy levels, and that coadministration of folate and synergistic nutrients can reduce this effect, even though fibric acid derivatives apparently do not reduce blood concentrations of these key nutrients. De Lorgeril et al.[191] reported a 46% increase in plasma Hcy in patients treated with fenofibrate for 12 weeks. Later in 1999, Dierkes et al.[192] reported that fenofibrate (200 mg) and bezafibrate (400 mg) significantly reduced triglycerides but also increased plasma Hcy by 44% and 17.5%, respectively, in 20 male patients (age 39-56) with hypertriglyceridemia but normal renal and thyroid function after 6 weeks of therapy. In discussing the underlying mechanisms, the authors noted that "the vitamin status does not appear to be involved in the first line, because folate, cobalamin, and vitamin B_6 (in the bezafibrate group) remained unaltered." In contrast, they emphasized that "creatinine and cystatin C increased, suggesting an alteration of renal function." The tHcy concentrations increase as renal function deteriorates, and fibrates increase serum creatinine moderately and reversibly.

In 2001, Dierkes et al.[193] conducted a randomized, double-blind crossover study involving hyperlipidemic men for 6 weeks to investigate the ability of nutrient coadministration to mitigate the Hcy elevation induced by fenofibrate. Subjects administered fenofibrate plus folic acid (650 μg), vitamin B_6 (5 mg), and vitamin B_{12} (50 μg) demonstrated an increase in Hcy concentration of 13% ± 25%, whereas those given fenofibrate plus placebo exhibited an increase of 44% ± 47%. The authors advised that "fenofibrate may counteract the cardioprotective effect of lipid lowering" and that nutrient coadministration "may therefore be warranted for routine use." Folic acid supplementation in patients treated with fenofibrate significantly reduced the increase in plasma Hcy levels.

In 2003, in a randomized, open-label study of 22 patients with mixed hyperlipidemia, Melenovsky et al.[190] compared the effect of micronized fenofibrate (200 mg daily) alone versus fenofibrate plus folic acid (10 mg every other day) on plasma Hcy levels over a 9-week treatment period. Overall, plasma Hcy levels increased by 6.85 μmol/L in subjects treated with fenofibrate only, but increased by 2.01 μmol/L in the group treated with both fenofibrate and folic acid, a statistically significant difference.

Although they arrived at similar conclusions, none of these studies were designed to determine whether amelioration of this adverse effect increases the clinical benefit of fibrates.[190-193]

Bissonnette et al.[185] investigated tHcy levels as a post hoc analysis after testing the effect of micronized fenofibrate on postprandial lipemia in the fasted and fed states. The randomized, placebo-controlled, double-blind study involved 20 men with established coronary artery disease (CAD), or at least two cardiovascular risk factors, who had elevated plasma triglyceride levels and reduced HDL cholesterol levels, and in whom a fibrate was clinically indicated. As expected, fenofibrate caused a marked reduction in all triglyceride-rich lipoprotein parameters, but administration was also associated with an increase in fasting tHcy and fed tHcy levels, 6 hours after the fat load. The fenofibrate-induced changes in tHcy level were not associated with changes in plasma levels of folate, vitamins B_6 or B_{12}, or creatinine, but methionine and cysteine were significantly increased.

Thus, several research teams have concluded that the effects of fibrates, particularly fenofibrate, in elevating plasma tHcy levels could compromise their putative cardioprotective properties, and that concomitant support with folate and related nutrients may contribute to the overall clinical strategy.

Among conventional hypolipidemic agents, statin drugs have exhibited a significant lack of adverse effects on folate relative to fibrates. In response to concern that elevated tHcy could compromise the cardiovascular benefit from lipid lowering by fibrates, Mayer et al.[193a] conducted an open, randomized, prospective crossover study to investigate the effects of fenofibrate. The 24 volunteers had total cholesterol of 6 mmol/L or higher and triglycerides less than 5 mmol/L, with normal blood pressure, normal blood glucose, and without any pharmacotherapy or clinical vascular or metabolic disease. In successive 6-month phases, the researchers measured lipids, tHcy, folate, vitamin B_{12}, and renal function markers after diet, after 200 mg of fenofibrate (3 months in monotherapy followed by 3 months in combination with 10 mg folate), and then after fluvastatin (3 months of 40 mg followed by 3 months of 80 mg). They found that fenofibrate monotherapy increased tHcy from 10.0 to 14.2 μmol/L while coadministration of folate decreased tHcy to 10.6 μmol/L. Fuvastatin, however, did not significantly influence the tHcy concentrations. In a trial involving 128 patients with primary hyperlipidemia, Milionis et al.[194] compared the effects of atorvastatin, simvastatin, and fenofibrate on serum Hcy levels. Although neither statins nor fenofibrate had any effect on serum vitamin B_{12} and folic acid levels, Hcy levels were significantly increased only by fenofibrate and did not change from baseline after statin treatment.

Emerging research into the molecular mechanisms underlying the differential effects of fibrates on Hcy subfractions may help to understand their tendency to increase tHcy, establish the relative benefits of their hypolipidemic effects, and elucidate the strategic implications of such factors in preventing cardiovascular disease. Plasma tHcy comprises both reduced, free oxidized Hcy and protein-bound Hcy; the reduced Hcy is thought to be the atherogenic, but minor, subfraction. In a set of animal experiments, Luc et al.[189] demonstrated that activation of PPAR-α mediates the effect of fenofibrate on gene expression and modulates the effect of fenofibrate on Hcy levels. In particular, the usual fenofibrate-induced increase in Hcy levels was completely abolished in PPAR-α–deficient mice. Likewise, Legendre et al.[188] applied a rodent model in investigating the effects of fibrates known to be mediated by the nuclear receptor PPAR-α. Using PPAR-α–deficient mice, they found that fenofibrate increases serum tHcy by inducing a selective increase of the protein-bound fraction. Furthermore, in comparing the effects of fenofibrate versus fenofibrate plus folate in rats, they observed that fenofibrate increased serum tHcy by 69%, whereas the coadministration of folate with fenofibrate increased tHcy by only 7%. Nevertheless, as with the mice, only the protein-bound fraction of Hcy was increased in the rats administered fenofibrate; the atherogenic, reduced Hcy was unaffected.

Thus, both studies concluded that fenofibrate and other fibrates increase homocystinemia in a PPAR-α–dependent manner, and that such findings constitute a valid animal model for analyzing the molecular mechanisms of fibrate-induced elevations in dyslipidemic patients.[188,189] Findings from animal studies can be taken only as provisional, but they suggest a more complete and clinically effective knowledge of cardiovascular risk factors requires that research fully account for the specific variables within each physiological parameter (e.g., forms of Hcy or cholesterol), the interplay among multiple risk factors, and the influences of individual genomic variability on susceptibility and therapeutic response.

Nutrient-Drug Interactions and Drug-Induced Nutrient Depletions

Nutritional Therapeutics, Clinical Concerns, and Adaptations

Physicians prescribing fibrates, particularly fenofibrate and bezafibrate, are advised to coadminister folic acid, vitamin B_{12}, vitamin B_6, and riboflavin based on their synergistic role in the comprehensive strategy of preventing and treating cardiovascular disease. Even though evidence indicates that these hypolipidemic agents do not deplete these nutrients, coadministration is prudent based on their beneficial effect in lowering Hcy levels and otherwise countering the disease process. Such modulation of hyperhomocysteinemia is generally a clinically appropriate tactic, even if, as suggested by the animal research just discussed, fibrate-induced Hcy elevation is of the non-atherogenic form. Thus, regular monitoring of tHcy levels is essential in patients taking fibrates, with special attention to subfractions. Evidence indicates that such nutrient administration carries a high safety profile and does not interfere with the therapeutic activity of the medication.

Multiple interventions, coordinated and evolving within an integrative strategy, can often provide the most effective means of preventing and treating the pathophysiological processes of endothelial damage, atherosclerosis, and coronary, cerebral, or peripheral vascular disease. Within the standards of conventional practice, gemfibrozil or statins represent the other primary options for addressing hypertriglyceridemia or dyslipidemia, respectively. Concomitant use of L-carnitine, coenzyme Q10, magnesium, fish oils (omega-3 fatty acids), mixed tocopherols and tocotrienols, and vitamin D may also be appropriate, according to the characteristics and needs of the individual patient, any comorbid conditions, and medications. The research regarding fibrates and their effects on folate and Hcy illustrates the need for further studies and evolution of clinical practice in assessing cardiovascular risk. Refined laboratory evaluation of complex and interdependent biomarkers should not only include C-reactive protein and Hcy, but also further develop the implications of variations, such as free versus bound Hcy.

Fluoxetine and Related Selective Serotonin Reuptake Inhibitor and Serotonin-Norepinephrine Reuptake Inhibitor (SSRI and SSRI/SNRI) Antidepressants

Evidence: Fluoxetine (Prozac, Sarafem).
Extrapolated, based on similar properties: Citalopram (Celexa), duloxetine (Cymbalta), escitalopram (S-citalopram; Lexapro), fluvoxamine (Faurin, Luvox), paroxetine (Aropax, Deroxat, Paxil, Seroxat), sertraline (Zoloft), venlafaxine (Effexor).

Interaction Type and Significance

⊕⊕ **Beneficial or Supportive Interaction, with Professional Management**

Probability:
2. Probable

Evidence Base:
○ **Preliminary** to
◉ **Emerging**

Effect and Mechanism of Action

Affective disorders such as depression are caused, at least in part and in certain individuals, by a deficiency of serotonin (5-hydroxytryptamine, 5-HT), noradrenaline (norepinephrine), dopamine, or a combination of these key monoamines. Folate and vitamin B_{12} are major determinants of one-carbon metabolism, in which S-adenosylmethionine (SAMe), a key methyl donor in numerous methylation reactions, is synthesized from methionine. Folate plays a pivotal role in the synthesis of tetrahydrobiopterin, which is the cofactor for the hydroxylation of phenylalanine and tryptophan and is the rate-limiting step in the synthesis of these and related neurotransmitters. Thus, coadministration of folic acid (or enhancement of dietary intake of folates) in conjunction with fluoxetine or other conventional antidepressants may produce an additive or synergistic effect, particularly on serotonin.

Research

Folate deficiency, impaired methylation, and hyperhomocysteinemia have been associated with depression and related mood disorders in many studies. In individuals with certain genomic characteristics, folate deficiency may play an even greater role in impaired metabolism of serotonin, SAMe, dopamine, and noradrenaline. Poor therapeutic response to antidepressants may be related to depressed folate status. Both gender and certain polymorphisms (e.g., MTHFR C677T polymorphism) influence folate and homocysteine (Hcy) metabolism and their relationship to depression and response to antidepressants.[195] In a systematic review and meta-analysis of randomized controlled trials involving treatment of depression with folic acid, Taylor et al.[196] concluded that "limited available evidence suggests folate may have a potential role as a supplement to other treatment for depression," but that it is "currently unclear if this is the case both for people with normal folate levels, and for those with folate deficiency." Folic acid administration can be beneficial in many individuals, and coadministration has enhanced efficacy of antidepressants in certain cases. Enhanced folate nurture may also help reduce the cardiovascular risk factors associated with the hyperhomocysteinemia prevalent in one third or more of individuals diagnosed with depression.

Decreased serum/RBC folate and serum vitamin B_{12} and an increase in plasma Hcy have been associated with greater susceptibility to depression and poorer response to antidepressant treatment. According to a review by Coppen and Bolander-Gouaille,[197] Hong Kong and Taiwan populations with traditional Chinese diets (rich in folate), including patients with major depression, have high serum folate concentrations. However, these countries have very low lifetime rates of major depression. In a large population-based study, Norwegian researchers observed an association between depression and hyperhomocysteinemia and the 677CT polymorphism in the MTHFR gene. For the TT MTHFR genotype, the odds ratio for depression was 1.69 compared with the CC genotype. Folate and vitamin B_{12} were not associated with anxiety disorder or depression in general, but the risk of depression was tripled in middle-aged women with serum folate less than 5 nmol/L.[198] Likewise, in geriatric populations, both depression and dementia have been associated with lower folate levels.[199,200]

In a study on the effects of folic acid fortification of flour in the United States since 1998, Ramos et al.[201] report that plasma folate concentrations are associated with depressive symptoms in elderly Latina women despite dietary folic acid fortification. Notably, using radioassay to determine plasma folate concentrations, these researchers reported that the prevalence of folate deficiency (plasma folate ≤6.8 nmol/L) in the cohort of elderly Latinos (age 60 or older) in the Sacramento, California, area as less than 1%, significantly lower than almost every other estimate of folate deficiency in the general population, let alone the elderly. The possible inconsistencies in these findings indicate the need for continued research into both the adequacy of standard methods of testing for folate deficiency and the effectiveness of folic acid fortification of foods. Overall the assembled data and clinical prudence suggest the need for folic acid supplementation at a significantly higher dosage level than typically attainable through such policies and methods.

A series of clinical trials have consistently found that patients with low folate status are more susceptible to depression, slower to respond to antidepressant medications, and more refractory to fluoxetine treatment. In an experiment involving 213 depressed adults treated with fluoxetine, 20 mg/day, Mischoulon et al.[202] found that "neither macrocytosis nor anemia predicted low serum folate/B_{12}, or antidepressant refractoriness." Fava et al.[203] investigated folate, vitamin B_{12}, and homocysteine status in 213 outpatients with major depressive disorder taking 20 mg/day of fluoxetine for 8 weeks. Subjects with low serum folate levels were more likely to be diagnosed with melancholic depression and were significantly more likely not to respond to fluoxetine. Also, Hcy and B_{12} levels were not associated with depressive subtype or treatment response. Similarly, in a double-blind trial involving 55 patients with major depressive disorder, Papakostas et al.[195] found that low serum folate levels, but not elevated Hcy or low vitamin B_{12} levels, were associated with poorer response to fluoxetine treatment. In a related study, these researchers measured serum folate, vitamin B_{12}, and Hcy at baseline and followed 71 outpatients with remitted major depressive disorder for 28 weeks of continued treatment with fluoxetine (40 mg/day) to monitor for depressive relapse. The presence of low serum folate levels, but not low B_{12} or elevated Hcy level, was associated with relapse during continued treatment with fluoxetine.[204] In a third study involving 110 outpatients with major depressive disorder (MDD) who responded to an 8-week trial of fluoxetine, Papakostas et al.[205] observed that subjects with low folate levels (≤ 2.5 ng/mL) were more likely to experience a later onset of clinical improvement by an average 1½ weeks than eufolatemic patients. They noted a lack of association between B_{12} and Hcy levels and time to clinical improvement.

Coadministration of folic acid appears to enhance the antidepressant action of fluoxetine. In a randomized, placebo-controlled trial involving 127 patients diagnosed with major depression, Coppen and Bailey[206] demonstrated enhancement of the antidepressant action of fluoxetine (20 mg/day) by concomitant folic acid (500 µg/day). Subjects administered folic acid showed a significant increase in plasma folate. However, among the fluoxetine plus folate group, increases in plasma folate levels, decreases in Hcy levels, and improvements in depression scores were all significantly stronger in women than in men. Reports of adverse effects were significantly higher in the fluoxetine plus placebo group than in those given folic acid. These authors concluded: "Folic acid is a simple method of greatly improving the antidepressant action of fluoxetine and probably other antidepressants." They recommend a folic acid dosage sufficient to decrease plasma Hcy and note the higher dose requirements for folic acid in men to obtain a therapeutic response; as to the exact dose, they suggest that further research is required "to ascertain the optimum dose of folic acid."[206]

Nutritional Therapeutics, Clinical Concerns, and Adaptations

Physicians treating individuals susceptible to or diagnosed with depressive disorders are advised to discuss the potential benefits of folic acid supplementation and enhancing dietary folate intake. In patients for whom prescribing an antidepressant such as fluoxetine is appropriate, concomitant folic aid (800 µg/day), preferably with vitamin B_{12} (1 mg daily), can often enhance the action of the medication with no attendant risk. Assessment of folate, B_{12}, and Hcy status is warranted and may be clinically useful, as might testing for MTHFR polymorphisms, because those with low activity of MTHFR may be more responsive to L-5-methyl folate than to folic acid.

Evidence: Isoniazid (isonicotinic acid hydrazide; INH, Laniazid, Nydrazid), pyrazinamide (PZA; Tebrazid), rifampicin (Rifadin, Rifadin IV); combination drugs: isoniazid and rifampicin (Rifamate, Rimactane); isoniazid, pyrazinamide, and rifampicin (Rifater).

Similar properties but evidence lacking for extrapolation: Cycloserine (Seromycin), ethambutol (Myambutol), ethionamide (2-ethylthioisonicotinamide; Ethide, Ethiocid, Ethomid, Etomide, Mycotuf, Myobid, Trecator SC).

Interaction Type and Significance

☼   **Prevention or Reduction of Drug Adverse Effect**

◇≈≈ **Drug-Induced Adverse Effect on Nutrient Function, Coadministration Therapeutic, with Professional Management**

Probability: Evidence Base:
3. Possible to   ◉ **Emerging**, but generally
2. Probable   presented as ● **Consensus**

Effect and Mechanism of Action

Isoniazid is generally considered the most potent antitubercular medication and is always used in conjunction with other drugs to prevent development of resistance. These drugs appear to adversely affect the action of folate and potentially induce depletion. However, the incomplete evidence thus far available suggests that such effects may be indirect, through the metabolic interrelationships among various vitamins, rather than direct effects on folate itself.

Isoniazid, the hydrazide derivative of isonicotinic acid, interferes with the synthesis of lipids, nucleic acids, and the mycolic acid of the cell walls of pathogenic mycobacteria such as *Mycobacterium tuberculosis*. Although its precise mode of action is not known, many of the adverse effects associated with isoniazid, such as peripheral neuropathy, result from its activity as a synthetic analog of pyridoxine and the subsequently induced relative pyridoxine deficiency. This interference of isoniazid with vitamin B_6 appears to be the primary mechanism for its well-known interference with the synthesis of vitamin B_{12}; both effects will interfere with the synthesis and activity of folate.[171] In individuals being treated with phenytoin, isoniazid may also adversely affect folate by decreasing the excretion of the anticonvulsant or enhancing its activity. Notably, isoniazid can induce seizures in susceptible individuals.

Rifampin blocks RNA synthesis by binding to the beta subunit of the bacterial DNA-dependent RNA polymerase.

Research and Reports

Drug-drug interactions involving isoniazid and rifampin are widely known, but systematic research into interactions between these agents and nutrients, specifically folate, is lacking. Numerous studies and case reports, primarily from the 1960s and 1970s, suggest that isoniazid and rifampin can interfere with the synthesis or activity of folate and have the potential to induce depletion.[207-216] Many secondary sources present such drug-induced adverse effects as though they were well documented. Such assertions are plausible, and the general consensus appears to approach the likelihood of a clinically significant interaction as "probable." Low serum folate levels have been reported in patients undergoing isoniazid therapy. Nevertheless, evidence from large, well-designed clinical trials is lacking to support these attributions, and the reports available primarily describe the adverse effects of these agents in the context of multiple interdependent nutrients, particularly vitamins B_3, B_6, and B_{12}, rather than folate or folic acid per se. Furthermore, a renewal of research would be necessary to determine the frequency, severity, and circumstances of clinically significant adverse reactions due to drug-induced effects upon folate, and thus refine the general occurrence or peculiar conditions needed to substantiate a conclusive interactions assessment.

In a randomized, placebo-controlled trial involving children age 1 to 35 months living in Zanzibar, Sazawal et al.[18] found that "supplementation with iron and folic acid in preschool children in a population with high rates of malaria can result in an increased risk of severe illness and death." Routine prophylactic folate supplementation in such situations should be avoided pending further research. However, within the context of an active program "to detect and treat malaria and other infections, iron-deficient and anaemic children can benefit from supplementation."

The effect of isoniazid or rifampin, alone or in combination with other antituberculosis drugs, on the human fetus is not known. Safety for use during pregnancy has not been established. No isoniazid-related congenital anomalies have been found in reproduction studies in mammalian species (mice, rats, and rabbits). However, offspring of rodents given oral doses of 150 to 250 mg/kg/day of rifampin during pregnancy have exhibited an increase in congenital malformations, primarily spina bifida and cleft palate.

Note: Therapeutic levels of rifampin interfere with standard laboratory assays for serum folate and vitamin B_{12}.[217] Alternative testing methods, such as the neutrophilic hypersegmentation index (NHI), need to be considered when assessing folate and vitamin B_{12} concentrations in individuals being treated with rifampin, although if abnormal, the NHI cannot distinguish between a B_{12} deficiency and a folate deficiency. It can be used, however, as an indication to administer both nutrients, which regardless is sound practice.

Nutritional Therapeutics, Clinical Concerns, and Adaptations

Physicians prescribing antitubercular drugs as monotherapy or in combination should be aware of potential adverse effects on folate status caused by these medications, directly or more likely indirectly. In particular, long-term administration of isoniazid may lead to pyridoxine deficiency and may prevent isoniazid-induced niacin deficiency. Some physicians may choose to monitor folate, B_3, B_6, and B_{12} status and coadminister a multivitamin only if deficiency is observed. Given the high safety profile, low cost, and minimal potential for significant adverse effects, prudence suggests that prophylactic supplementation may be judicious. Many experienced practitioners of nutritional therapeutics prescribe nutrients in higher dosage levels to patients undergoing isoniazid or rifampin therapy, for example, folic acid (800 µg/day) and vitamin B_6 (50-100 mg/day). Nevertheless, prophylactic folic acid (and iron) may be contraindicated for children in malarial environments.

These potent antitubercular agents should be prescribed during pregnancy only when therapeutically absolutely necessary. Likewise, given the high degree of uncertainty and the severity of teratogenic potential, their use in women capable of bearing children should be carefully weighed against the benefits of therapy. Coadministration of folic acid (800 µg/day) is appropriate in the event that administration of antitubercular drugs is required.

Levodopa and Related Antiparkinsonian Agents

Carbidopa (Lodosyn), levodopa (L-dopa; Dopar, Larodopa); combination drugs: levodopa and benserazide (co-beneldopa; Madopar); levodopa and carbidopa (Atamet, Parcopa, Sinemet, Sinemet CR); levodopa, carbidopa, and entacapone (Stalevo).

Interaction Type and Significance

☼   **Prevention or Reduction of Drug Adverse Effect**
⊕⊕   **Beneficial or Supportive Interaction, with Professional Management**
◇≈≈ **Drug-Induced Adverse Effect on Nutrient Function, Coadministration Therapeutic, with Professional Management**

Probability: Evidence Base:
2. Probable   ◉ Emerging to ● Consensus

Effect and Mechanism of Action

Homocysteine (Hcy) is often elevated in individuals with Parkinson's disease, and levodopa can aggravate this pathological tendency. Metabolism of levodopa requires vitamin B_6 and can induce B_6 depletion if available supplies are inadequate. Coadministration of dopa decarboxylase inhibitors such as carbidopa limits peripheral degradation of levodopa and prevents vitamin B_6 depletion, but also increases conversion of levodopa to 3-O-methyldopa (3-OMD) by catechol-O-methyltransferase (COMT), the key enzyme in the metabolism of Hcy. COMT requires magnesium (Mg^{++}) and S-adenosylmethionine (SAMe), which is synthesized from adenosine triphosphate (ATP) and methionine, as a methyl donor and yields S-adenosylhomocysteine (SAH), which is converted to total homocysteine (tHcy). Plasma tHcy depends on folic acid and vitamins B_2, B_6, and B_{12}, which work together to support remethylation from tHcy to methionine.[218] However, methylation of levodopa (and dopamine) by COMT interferes with this process by consuming methyl groups in the transmethylation reaction, thereby causing significant increases of SAH concentrations in tissues, which is rapidly converted to Hcy, as well as significant decreases of SAMe.

Folate intake, in conjunction with vitamin B_6, may contribute to the prevention or treatment of Parkinson's disease and other forms of dementia, or folate and B_6 may work with antiparkinsonian medications by enhancing their therapeutic effects or reducing their adverse effects.

Research

The high occurrence of elevated Hcy levels in parkinsonian patients has attracted the attention of clinicians and researchers since the 1990s.[219,220] In addition to being a major risk factor for atherothrombotic disease, hyperhomocysteinemia is also strongly associated with an increased risk of dementia and cognitive impairment, both of which are common in the course of Parkinson's disease. Growing evidence indicates that Hcy may damage DNA in the substantia nigra, the area of the brain affected in Parkinson's disease. Kuhn et al.[219] observed significantly elevated plasma Hcy levels in subjects with Parkinson's disease and speculated that Hcy may be an independent risk factor for vascular disease in Parkinson's disease. However, they cautioned that this pattern of "elevated levels of homocysteine may be either caused by an unknown endogenous metabolic disturbance or by antiparkinsonian treatment, because no association to severity or duration of disease was found."

Emerging but mixed evidence indicates that the effect of L-dopa on plasma Hcy is accentuated under conditions of impaired Hcy metabolism and may be influenced by B-vitamin status, including folate deficiency. Animal studies have indicated that levodopa-induced hyperhomocysteinemia is a consequence of significant O-methylation and that the COMT inhibitors can prevent such elevation of Hcy concentrations by reducing the O-methylation of levodopa.[221,222] Using a rat model, Daly et al.[223] demonstrated that plasma Hcy concentration was significantly higher in male rats 1 hour after intraperitoneal injection with 100 mg L-dopa/kg, and this increase was greater in the folate-deficient rats than in the replete controls. In a second experiment involving nondeficient female rats, such drug-induced elevations of Hcy persisted with daily L-dopa injections over 17 days, although less so than in animals treated with L-dopa for only 1 day. In a 1999 letter, Muller et al.[224] reported increased Hcy levels in parkinsonian patients undergoing long-term L-dopa therapy compared with previously untreated parkinsonian patients and controls. The authors expressed concern that L-dopa was promoting atherosclerosis and vascular disease. Other letters from clinicians, such as Yasui et al.,[225] have also reported levodopa-induced hyperhomocysteinemia in patients with Parkinson's disease. Muller et al.[226] reported a decrease in methionine and SAMe levels and increased Hcy in a study involving 20 Parkinson's patients treated with levodopa and dopa decarboxylase inhibitors and corresponding controls. These same researchers investigated O-methylation in treated parkinsonian subjects and found that Hcy was significantly elevated in the group with higher 3-OMD concentrations and positively correlated to 3-OMD.[227]

Rogers et al.[228] investigated the influence of L-dopa on elevated plasma Hcy levels and CAD in a study involving 235 patients with Parkinson's disease, 201 of whom had been treated with levodopa, with the remaining 34 levodopa naive. Mean plasma Hcy levels were significantly higher in patients treated with levodopa, and patients with Hcy levels in the higher quartile had increased prevalence of CAD compared with levodopa-naive patients. However, the authors observed no difference in the plasma concentration of folate, cobalamin, or MMA between the two groups and concluded that folate or vitamin B_{12} deficiency does not explain the elevated Hcy levels. In contrast, a study involving 40 subjects diagnosed with idiopathic Parkinson's disease, 20 of whom were taking levodopa and the other 20 levodopa naive, Miller et al.[229] observed that mean plasma Hcy concentration was higher in the treatment group than in the controls and correlated with plasma folate, vitamin B_{12}, and pyridoxal-5'-phosphate (B_6) concentrations in the treatment group, but not in the controls. They concluded that the extent to which L-dopa caused hyperhomocysteinemia in Parkinson's patients is influenced by B-vitamin status, and that increased B-vitamin intake is necessary to maintain normal plasma Hcy concentrations in patients treated with L-dopa. In a review, Lokk[229a] (2003) concluded that levodopa therapy can affect latent folic acid and vitamin B_{12} deficiency and further contribute to risk of elevated Hcy levels in patients with Parkinson's disease.

These findings indicate that levodopa-induced hyperhomocysteinemia, of varying degree, can be caused by competition at the site of methylation, rather than by a deficiency of folate or other B vitamins, but that coexisting risk factors for elevated Hcy (e.g., smoking) or compromised nutrient status can contribute to an additive effect.

Clinical outcomes with Parkinson's disease, hyperhomocysteinemia, and nutrient status vary among individuals, and the mixed research findings suggest the need for research into the influences of such underlying genetic variation. Yasui et al.[230] measured plasma Hcy and cysteine levels in 90 Parkinson's patients with the MTHFR C677T (TT) genotype. The authors not only found that Hcy levels were elevated by 60% in levodopa-treated Parkinson's patients, but also observed that TT-genotype patients exhibited the most marked Hcy elevation, and their Hcy and folate levels were inversely correlated. Subsequently, Woitalla et al.[218] compared plasma folic acid, B_6, B_{12}, and tHcys levels in 83 levodopa-treated Parkinson's patients and 44 controls. Patients with the CT (heterozygous) or TT (homozygous) genotype had significantly higher tHcy levels than controls or Parkinson's patients with the CC (wild-type) allele. Furthermore, although concentrations of B_6 or B_{12} did not differ, folic acid was significantly higher in parkinsonian patients with the CT mutation.

Levodopa-induced hyperhomocysteinemia can aggravate the neurodegenerative processes contributing to dementia, depression, vascular disease, and Parkinson's disease. O'Suilleabhain et al.[231] conducted neuropsychometric tasks and tested plasma Hcy levels in 97 patients with a mean Parkinson's duration of 3.6 years to determine if hyperhomocysteinemia in Parkinson's patients is associated with depression or with cognitive or physical impairments. Subjects with elevated Hcy level were slightly older (68 vs. 62 years), were more depressed, had worse cognition, and performed worse on neuropsychometric tasks than normohomocysteinemic patients. Notably, those with hyperhomocysteinemia had similar plasma concentrations of vitamin B_{12} and folate. In a study involving 31 levodopa-treated patients with Parkinson's disease and 27 control subjects, Muller et al.[232] investigated peripheral neuronal dysfunction, specifically sural nerve axonal neurodegeneration, in patients treated with antiparkinsonian drugs using electrophysiological sural nerve conduction assessment. Sensory nerve action potentials significantly differed between Parkinson's patients and controls, but sensory nerve conduction velocity results showed no significant differences. Daily levodopa/dopa decarboxylase inhibitor intake was significantly related to tHcy levels, with significant associations between tHcy levels and sensory nerve action potentials. The authors suggested that sensory nerve action potentials might serve as a surrogate marker for the levodopa metabolism–induced elevation of Hcy levels.

Use of other pharmacological therapies for Parkinson's disease, such as COMT inhibitors (COMT-I) or dopamine agonists, may provide an effective alternative to levodopa-induced Hcy elevation and attendant risks, including decreased folate levels. O'Suilleabhain et al.[233] prospectively measured the effects of levodopa initiation on plasma tHcy and B-vitamin status, as well as the effects of levodopa dose changes and treatment with dopamine agonists and entacapone. They compared vitamin B_{12}, folate, and tHcy concentrations, at baseline and after several months of treatment, in 30 patients initiating levodopa, 15 whose L-dopa dose was doubled, 14 whose L-dopa dose was halved or stopped, 15 starting or stopping entacapone, and 16 patients initiating or doubling dopamine agonist monotherapy. The tHcy concentration increased from 8.7 to 10.1 µmol/L, and average vitamin B_{12} concentration decreased from 380 to 291 pmol/L an average of 94 days after initiation of 604 (240-1050) mg/day of L-dopa. Furthermore, although subjects who doubled their daily L-dopa dose exhibited tHcy elevations from 9.5 to 11.1 µmol/L, no significant effects were observed with L-dopa reduction, agonist treatment, and entacapone treatment. Thus, these authors concluded that initiation of L-dopa "elevates tHcy and lowers

Nutrient-Drug Interactions and Drug-Induced Nutrient Depletions

vitamin B_{12} concentration to modest degrees,"[233] but that clinical implications, if any, were uncertain.

An Italian research team has been conducting ongoing research into the effects of various antiparkinsonian drugs on Hcy. In 2005, Lamberti et al.[234] compared plasma levels of Hcy, B_{12}, and folate in 26 Parkinson's patients treated with levodopa, 20 treated with levodopa plus a COMT-I, and 32 controls. Plasma Hcy was increased significantly in the two Parkinson's groups and significantly lower in the group treated with levodopa plus COMT-I. Folate concentrations were significantly lower in the levodopa-treated group, but statistical analysis indicated that the difference in mean Hcy levels observed among Parkinson's patients was associated with COMT-I coadministration rather than folate concentrations. No significant differences were observed in vitamin B_{12} levels. In a parallel study, Zoccolella et al.[220] compared Hcy, B_{12}, and folate levels in 45 Parkinson's patients (15 in each of three groups receiving dopamine agonists, L-dopa, or L-dopa plus a COMT-I) and in 15 controls. They determined that "L-dopa administration significantly increases Hcy concentrations and that the addition of COMT-I effectively reduces the homocysteinemia." Also in 2005, Valkovic et al.[235] found that mean plasma Hcy concentration was higher in 19 Parkinson's patients receiving levodopa monotherapy than in subjects receiving a combination of levodopa and the COMT-I entacapone or in a control group of 17 subjects receiving dopamine agonists.

Even though the relationship between folate (and vitamin B_{12}) and Hcy and the effects of levodopa on Hcy are well established, evidence from human trials specifically investigating the potential benefits of nutrient coadministration are limited. Chen et al.[236] prospectively investigated intake of folate, vitamin B_6, or vitamin B_{12} in 248 men and 167 women with documented Parkinson's disease diagnoses to determine whether higher nutrient intake was related to a lower risk of disease. Folate intake was not associated with the risk of Parkinson's disease, nor was intake of vitamins B_6 or B_{12}. The authors concluded that their data "does not support the hypothesis that higher intake of folate or related B vitamins lowers the risk of Parkinson's disease." However, in an Italian study related to those previously cited, Lamberti et al.[237] compared plasma Hcy, folate, and cobalamin levels in 20 Parkinson's patients treated with L-dopa at baseline and after 5 weeks of treatment with cobalamin and folate with levels in 35 controls. Hcy levels were higher in Parkinson's patients treated with L-dopa compared with age and gender–matched controls, and coadministration of cobalamin and folate was effective in reducing Hcy concentrations.

Further research involving well-designed clinical trials, especially long-term prospective cohort studies, is warranted to establish further the efficacy of folate (and B_{12}) administration in patients undergoing levodopa therapy, alone in or in combination with other antiparkinsonian drugs, as a countermeasure against drug-induced hyperhomocysteinemia, and to formulate therapeutic strategies for safe and effective coadministration.

Nutritional Therapeutics, Clinical Concerns, and Adaptations

Physicians treating individuals with Parkinson's disease or related conditions are advised to prescribe concomitant folic acid, cobalamin (B_{12}), and pyridoxal-5'-phosphate (B_6), especially in light of the high incidence of strokes among such patients. MTHFR genotyping and regular tHcy monitoring are also recommended in Parkinson's patients. Although conclusive evidence is lacking to support claims that increased folate intake might prevent the onset of Parkinson's disease, folic acid supplementation is safe and inexpensive and may support healthy neurological function, counter Hcy elevation, and reverse adverse effects of levodopa, especially in those with the MTHFR C677T (TT) genotype or other factors increasing susceptibility to folate deficiency and hyperhomocysteinemia.

No evidence yet indicates that coadministration of folic acid or vitamin B_{12} would impair the therapeutic activity of levodopa or related medications. However, supplemental B_6 at levels greater than 10 to 15 mg/day could override the ability of carbidopa or benserazide (in Sinemet and Madopar, respectively) to limit the effects of vitamin B_6 on levodopa. The levels of B_6 found in most multivitamins are unlikely to interfere with the medication's therapeutic activity. In general, nutrients administered concomitantly with antiparkinsonian medications are best ingested with meals at least 2 hours before or after levodopa or at bedtime with a small amount of food.

Lithium Carbonate

Lithium Carbonate (Camcolit, Carbolith, Duralith, Eskalith, Li-Liquid, Liskonum, Litarex, Lithane, Lithobid, Lithonate, Lithotabs, PMS-Lithium, Priadel).

Interaction Type and Significance

$\oplus\oplus$ **Beneficial or Supportive Interaction, with Professional Management**

Coadministration Benefit Probability:	Evidence Base:
3. Possible or 2. Probable	◉ **Emerging** to ● **Consensus**

Nutrient Depletion Probability:	Evidence Base:
5. Improbable	◉ **Emerging** to ● **Consensus**

Effect and Mechanism of Action

Folate and vitamin B_{12} play major roles in one-carbon metabolism, in which SAMe is formed and methyl groups are made available for neurological function.

Research

Limited research suggests that low folate levels do not appear to characterize patients treated with lithium, but folate status may influence therapeutic response to lithium therapy. Stern et al.[238] measured serum and RBC folate levels in 17 outpatients receiving prophylactic lithium carbonate for recurrent major affective disorder. They observed "no evidence for low folate concentrations or for any significant correlation between folate levels and affective morbidity." Subsequently, a team of Chinese researchers investigated whether folate concentrations were lower in patients undergoing long-term lithium therapy, and if the medication might play a role in decreasing such levels. Lee et al.[239] found that serum folate correlated negatively with lithium dose and serum level among 46 Chinese and mostly manic-depressive (85%) outpatients attending a lithium clinic in Hong Kong. However, mean folate levels in the lithium-treated patients did not differ from lithium-free outpatients, and "virtually no patients had low serum (0%) or erythrocyte (2%) folate." Nevertheless, they noted that patients "with a good response to lithium in the previous one year had a higher mean serum folate level than those with unsatisfactory response." They concluded that "folate at high concentrations enhances lithium prophylaxis," even though "data suggest that folate deficiency is uncommon among Chinese psychiatric outpatients."[239] Notably, neither of these studies specifically focused on whether increased folate intake (food or supplements) might enhance the efficacy of lithium therapy, decrease adverse effects, or allow reductions of therapeutic lithium dose.

The general finding in human trials indicates that concomitant folic acid administration can enhance the therapeutic efficacy of lithium. In a 1982 study involving 107 patients receiving long-term lithium, Coppen and Abou-Saleh[240] found that "those with lower plasma folate concentration had a higher affective morbidity than those with higher folate, both at the time and during the previous two years." In 1986, Coppen et al.[241] determined that folic acid enhances lithium prophylaxis in reducing affective morbidity. In a double-blind trial, they administered folic acid (200 μg/day) or placebo to 75 patients receiving lithium therapy. Patients with the highest plasma folate concentrations exhibited a significant reduction in their affective morbidity, with a 40% reduction in affective morbidity among subjects in whom plasma folate increased to 13 ng/mL or higher. Based on these findings, the authors suggested that a daily dose of 300 to 400 μg folic acid would be useful in long-term lithium prophylaxis.

Nutritional Therapeutics, Clinical Concerns, and Adaptations

Physicians prescribing lithium therapy, especially on a long-term basis, are advised to discuss with patients the potential therapeutic benefit of concomitant folic acid administration, typically 200 to 400 μg/day or more. Higher folic acid dosage may be appropriate in some patients, based on diet, comorbid conditions, other medications, and genomic variability (e.g., MTHFR genotype). Evidence is lacking to suggest that lithium use depletes folate, or that folic acid reduces adverse effects associated with lithium. Given the probability of an additive or synergistic effect from coadministration, close supervision, regular monitoring, and dose titration are warranted, particularly with introduction of folate or change in dose of either agent.

Mercaptopurine, Azathioprine, and Thioguanine (Thiopurines)

Mercaptopurine (6-mercaptopurine, 6-MP, NSC 755; Purinethol), azathioprine (asathioprine; Azamun, Imuran, Thioprine), thioguanine (6-thioguanine, 6-TG, 2-amino-6-mercaptopurine; Lanvis).

Interaction Type and Significance

✗ Potential or Theoretical Adverse Interaction of Uncertain Severity
⊕✗ Bimodal or Variable Interaction, with Professional Management
⊕ Potential or Theoretical Beneficial or Supportive Interaction, with Professional Management

Probability:
4. Plausible to 2. Probable

Evidence Base:
▽ Mixed and ○ Preliminary

Effect and Mechanism of Action

Mercaptopurine, azathioprine, and thioguanine are cytotoxic antimetabolites used in the treatment of irritable bowel syndrome, leukemia, and some cancers. The mechanisms involved in their therapeutic activity have not been fully elucidated. Thiopurine S-methyltransferase (TPMT) catalyses the S-methylation of all three drugs. Mercaptopurine requires intracellular anabolism by hypoxanthine guanine phosphoribosyltransferase (HGPTPT, or HGPRT) to become cytotoxic. Likewise, azathioprine is an immunosuppressive prodrug, the

S-imidazole precursor of 6-mercaptopurine, converted to 6-MP in the liver by TPMT. Intracellular activation of thioguanine, a 6-thiopurine analog of the naturally occurring purine bases hypoxanthine and guanine, results in incorporation into DNA as a false purine base.

Mercaptopurines act through purine antagonists and consequently tend to induce macrocytic nonmegaloblastic anemia. Serum folate levels are typically low in patients treated with these medications. Folate coadministration may moderate the adverse effects of these agents, thereby enhancing tolerance and facilitating efficacy. However, determining whether folate also interferes with the anticancer efficacy of this class of drugs requires further clinical research.

Research

Many patients are intolerant or resistant to thiopurine drugs, and their clinical management remains a challenge. Myelosuppression is the major dose-limiting effect with these agents. Hematopoietic toxicity, rapid bone marrow suppression, and leukopenia present a particularly significant risk in individuals with an inherited deficiency of TPMT or HGPTPT, even at normal dose levels.[242-249] Notably, relative leukopenia is typically not associated with clinical response.[250] Adverse drug reactions and intolerance to azathioprine, occurring in 15% to 28% of patients, may be attributable more often to polymorphism in the ITPA gene and inosine triphosphate pyrophosphatase (ITPase) deficiency, which results in the benign accumulation of the inosine nucleotide ITP; preliminary evidence, however, is mixed.[251-253] All these enzymes are involved in folate handling.

Genetic variation in the way individuals handle folate can be predicted to influence activity of the TPMT enzyme, which may assist in predicting adverse drug reactions in some patients. For example, polymorphisms in the gene encoding MTHFR may have an indirect impact on thiopurine drug methylation by influencing levels of the methyl donor SAMe.[253] As a result of genetic variation, 1 in 300 of the Caucasian population have a total lack of TPMT and are at high risk of severe toxicity if given azathioprine; 1 in 10 individuals have half the level and are also at increased risk of side effects. With prior knowledge of such genetic polymorphisms and related enzyme levels, the drug can be avoided or used at a lower dose, or other strategies can be used to minimize adverse effects.

The available findings of drug-induced depletion of folate are limited but consistent with scientific knowledge of renal transplant patients in general and patients treated with azathioprine in particular. In assessing the impact of renal transplant and azathioprine on folate status, Zazgornik et al.[254] monitored serum folic acid levels in 26 chronic hemodialysis patients, 52 renal transplant recipients, and 20 healthy controls using radioimmunoassay. Diminished serum folic acid levels were found not only in patients shortly after surgery, but also in patients with excellent graft function up to 6 years after transplantation. The mean serum folic acid level was significantly lower in both the dialyzed patients and the renal transplant recipients than in the controls. The highest serum folic acid level was observed in a transplant patient who had not taken azathioprine for 2 years. Macrocytosis was found in 52% of the renal transplant patients and was observed only in patients with good graft function treated with azathioprine. Serum vitamin B_{12} levels were within the normal range in both dialyzed and renal transplant patients. No intervention trials of folic acid administration in renal transplant patients taking azathioprine have been done, so the question remains whether folate replacement might improve clinical outcomes or increase risk of graft rejection by interfering with azathioprine-induced immune suppression.

Concomitant folic acid may protect proliferative capacity of the bone marrow and moderate hematological parameters of drug toxicity in patients treated with these purine antagonists. In a retrospective longitudinal study, Lennard et al.[255] investigated myelosuppression and the effect of folate coadministration on 6-mercaptopurine (6-MP) remission maintenance therapy in 10 children with acute lymphoblastic leukemia (ALL). During the control period they observed significant correlations between 6-MP dose and 6-thioguanine (6-TG) nucleotide concentration, the active cytotoxic metabolite of 6-MP, and also between 6-TG nucleotide concentrations and the peripheral neutrophil count at 14 days. With the introduction of folic acid these relationships were no longer evident, and the children tolerated significantly higher doses of 6-MP longer before neutropenia developed. Although folate does not affect the conversion of 6-MP to 6-TG, white blood cell (WBC) counts were elevated for a longer period despite the same exposure to 6-TG, indicating possible interference with the cytotoxicity of 6-TG on neutrophils. Thus, although they reported "no significant difference in red cell 6-thioguanine nucleotide concentration in the absence and presence of folate supplements," the authors expressed concern that "folate supplements may interfere with remission maintenance therapy in ALL."[255] Similarly, in a trial involving 53 children with ALL in maintenance treatment with methotrexate (MTX) and 6-MP, Schroder et al.[255a] administered daily folic acid (75-200 μg) in vitamin tablets to 25 subjects for at least the preceding 3 months. Compared with children who received no folic acid, subjects receiving folic acid exhibited improved proliferative capacity of the bone marrow, as demonstrated by significantly higher erythrocyte folate (ery-folate) concentration, higher platelet counts, higher leukocyte counts, higher neutrophil counts, and lower erythrocyte mean cell volumes. Nevertheless, these authors recommended that "since none of the children was folate deficient as judged by the ery-folate [level],... vitamins given to children in maintenance treatment with MTX and 6-MP for ALL should not contain folic acid."

The present data indicate that folic acid appears to protect normal neutrophils from 6-TG and antagonize the effects of MTX and 6-MP on normal hematopoiesis. However, folate may or may not antagonize these antimalignancy effects; that is, folate may or may not protect leukemia (ALL) cells, even though it appears to protect normal neutrophils from the cytotoxic effect of these drugs. Schroder et al.[255a] assumed that folic acid protects normal WBCs from the cytotoxic effect of 6-TG and therefore might protect leukemia cells as well. Such speculation may or may not be well founded. Folate coadministration also might actually improve clinical outcomes. There have been documented instances of natural products that kill cancer cells without affecting normal cells or, conversely, protect normal cells from cytotoxic agents without protecting malignant cells. Such determinations could only be made in this case by investigating relapse of ALL as the endpoint of the trial. This would require a fairly large study, giving half the children folic acid and the other half placebo (and control for dietary folate, not easy in adults, let alone children), and using relapse of leukemia as the endpoint. Institutional review boards (IRBs) might consider this an unethical experiment, even though risk of missing a clinical benefit must be balanced against risk of losing therapeutic efficacy. The question arises whether folic acid might have an opposite effect on 6-TG and ALL cells versus its effect on 6-TG and normal neutrophils. At least this issue should be further studied in vitro and in animal models. The possibility of increased tolerance of maintenance chemotherapy by folate supplementation leading to improved clinical outcomes in childhood ALL warrants further investigation.

Regular monitoring, with periodic blood counts every 2 weeks initially and then every 3 months thereafter, is required given the action of these drugs in interrupting production of RBCs, WBCs, and platelets. In a study of 57 patients with inflammatory bowel disease treated with low-dose 6-MP, Bernstein et al.[256] determined that "leukopenia was not uncommon in patients treated with low-dose 6-MP, but was not clinically significant." Furthermore, macrocytosis may occur in the absence of vitamin B_{12} and folate deficiencies. The authors thus concluded that, despite the risk of myelosuppression, weekly blood count monitoring was not necessary when administering low-dose 6-MP therapy.

Evidence is lacking from large prospective or population-based studies on the use of these immunosuppressants during pregnancy. Effects on folate metabolism could play a potentially significant role in pregnant women.

Nutritional Therapeutics, Clinical Concerns, and Adaptations

Physicians prescribing purine antagonists such as mercaptopurine, azathioprine, or thioguanine are advised to investigate the patient's folate status and coadminister folic acid as indicated. The evidence for benefit from such nutrient support is preliminary and inconclusive and suggests that concomitant folate administration might impair the therapeutic activity of these medications. Screening for polymorphisms and gene promoter activity, particularly the TPMT gene, before initiation of azathioprine therapy may be valuable in predicting pharmacogenomic responses and assisting drug tolerance. Close supervision, regular monitoring, and a coordinated strategy involving health care professionals experienced in both conventional pharmacology and nutritional therapeutics are essential to providing safe and effective individualized treatment within such an integrative approach.

Metformin and Related Biguanides

Evidence: Metformin (Dianben, Glucophage, Glucophage XR). Extrapolated, based on similar properties: Buformin (Andromaco Gliporal, Buformina); combination drugs: glipizide and metformin (Metaglip), glyburide and metformin (Glucovance); phenformin (Debeone, Fenformin).

Interaction Type and Significance

≈≈   **Drug-Induced Nutrient Depletion, Supplementation Therapeutic, with Professional Management**

☼   **Prevention or Reduction of Drug Adverse Effect**

⊕⊕   **Beneficial or Supportive Interaction, with Professional Management**

◇   **Adverse Drug Effect on Nutritional Therapeutics, Strategic Concern**

Probability:	Evidence Base:
2. Probable	◉ Emerging or ● Consensus

Effect and Mechanism of Action

Metformin can reduce the absorption and lead to lower serum levels of folate, total vitamin B_{12}, and transcobalamin II (TCII)–B_{12} complex levels. Metformin interferes with calcium-dependent membrane action and impairs B_{12}–intrinsic factor complex uptake by ileal cell surface receptors.[257,258] Although this involves at least one mechanism, food-cobalamin malabsorption or drug-induced changes in intestinal bacterial flora have also been suggested.[259,260] The available evidence is insufficient to determine whether the reported increase in total homocysteine (tHcy) levels is secondary to reduced folate levels, vitamin B_{12} levels, or a combination of both.

Decreased nutrient bioavailability plays a central role in the moderate elevations in plasma Hcy levels observed with long-term metformin therapy. Hyperhomocysteinemia is more prevalent in diabetic populations, women with polycystic ovary syndrome, and other patients likely to be prescribed biguanide therapy than among the general population.[174,261,262] Drug-induced elevations would further increase the risk of diabetes-associated conditions, such as coronary artery disease (CAD), vascular disease, and hypertension resulting from adverse effects on platelets, clotting factors, and endothelium, although not necessarily retinopathy or albuminuria.[263-266]

Note: The biguanide class was introduced when metformin and phenformin were developed in 1957. Metformin first became available in France in 1979 and has been widely used in Europe since that time. Phenformin and buformin, other biguanides, are well-established causes of lactic acidosis and have been removed from the U.S. market because of the high incidence of this adverse effect. Metformin was eventually found to be 20 times less likely to cause lactic acidosis and was cleared for use in the treatment of type 2 diabetes in the United States in 1994. Nevertheless, phenformin and buformin are still available internationally as oral agents for the treatment of diabetes and have reportedly been used in the United States.

This discussion focuses on metformin, and the evidence presented is based primarily on research involving metformin. Some studies mentioned also include phenformin and buformin or provide findings that may reasonably be extrapolated to these related biguanides.

Research

Long-term use of metformin has largely been associated with elevated Hcy levels in a wide range of human trials, although findings regarding the severity and clinical significance of this effect have varied.

The initial research into metformin-induced adverse effects on nutritional status focused on vitamin B_{12}. Carpentier et al.[267] compared the hematological effects in 30 diabetic patients treated with metformin versus those in 27 patients treated with insulin and 13 treated with sulfonylureas. Compared with the other groups, serum levels of vitamin B_{12} were significantly lower in patients receiving metformin, with five subjects exhibiting serum levels of vitamin B_{12} below 270 pg/mL and five others with borderline values. However, no differences were observed between the three groups in the mean serum folic acid levels, RBC counts, RBC volumes, or hemoglobin concentrations. These authors noted that the study period was not long enough to determine accurately whether vitamin B_{12} deficiency would develop. In a 1980 case report, Callaghan et al.[268] reported that megaloblastic anemia caused by vitamin B_{12} malabsorption was associated with long-term metformin treatment.

DeFronzo and Goodman[268a] observed effects on serum vitamin B_{12} and folic acid in two large, randomized, parallel-group, double-blind controlled studies comparing metformin, glibenclamide, and diet over 29 weeks in moderately obese patients with non–insulin-dependent diabetes mellitus (NIDDM) whose diabetes was inadequately controlled by diet alone. They reported that "serum folate concentrations

did not change in either the metformin or placebo groups" but that "serum vitamin B_{12} concentration at week 29 was lower in the metformin group (by 22 percent) but did not change in the placebo group." No changes were observed in hematocrit or hemoglobin in either group.

Drug-induced depletion of folate and vitamin B_{12} appears to play a key role in biguanide-induced hyperhomocysteinemia, but testing methodology and patient variables may influence the occurrence and severity of this adverse effect. In 1997, Hoogeveen et al.[269] investigated fasting serum tHcy level in a cross-sectional study involving 40 NIDDM patients who had received treatment with metformin (500-2550 mg/day) for at least 6 months and 71 matched NIDDM metformin-naive patients. Mean serum tHcy level was 11.5 μmol/L in the metformin-exposed patients, "slightly higher" than the 10.6 μmol/L in the nonexposed patients. Also in 1997, in an open, prospective, randomized study involving 60 nondiabetic male patients with coronary heart disease, Carlsen et al.[270] compared the effects of metformin on serum tHcy and related parameters with or without metformin (up to 2000 mg/day) in the context of diet and lifestyle advice and lovastatin (40 mg/day). After 12 and 40 weeks of metformin treatment, tHcy levels increased moderately but significantly in the metformin group relative to the control group while serum vitamin B_{12} levels decreased, with both trends greater over time. Serum folate levels did not change after 12 weeks, but decreased by 8.0% after 40 weeks compared to controls. However, serum levels of tHcy and methylmalonic acid (MMA) did not change. Based on this last variable, the authors concluded that "it remains an open question whether the increase in tHcy levels is secondary to reduced vitamin B_{12} levels, folate levels or a combination of both."[270]

Similarly, Hermann et al.[271] reported that serum B_{12} remained unchanged in a 12-month, placebo-controlled, double blind trial investigating glycemic improvement from coadministration of metformin in 16 insulin-treated, obese type 2 diabetes patients. However, comparing the effects of metformin and sulfonylurea therapy, Bauman et al.[258] reported that metformin induced a 29% decline in serum levels of vitamin B_{12} but a 36.6% drop in serum holotranscobalamin II (holo-TCII). Similarly, in a subsequent cross-sectional cohort study, Hermann et al.[272] found that by "considering the four variables reflecting vitamin B_{12} status, apart from MMA there were more patients in the metformin group with abnormalities indicating vitamin B_{12} deficiency." Moreover, such effects were exhibited "most clearly for holotranscobalamin," for which none of the control subjects had values less than the lower reference value, whereas eight (16%) of the metformin-treated subjects had reduced levels.

In an epidemiological study, Smulders et al.[264] applied multiple-regression analysis to 85 NIDDM subjects. In a subset of 31 subjects treated with metformin, levels of Hcy and vitamin B_{12} were similar to those without metformin. Also, low-normal values of folate (<20 nmol/L), vitamin B_{12} (<350 pmol/L), and creatinine clearance, as well as postmenopausal status in women, were significant predictors of fasting Hcy level, whereas B_6 levels (<80 nmol/L), creatinine clearance, and female gender were determinants of postmethionine load Hcy levels.

In a randomized, placebo-controlled trial, Wulffele et al.[273] investigated the effects of metformin therapy (vs. placebo) for 16 weeks on serum concentrations of Hcy, folate, and vitamin B_{12} in 353 patients treated with insulin for type 2 diabetes mellitus. Compared with placebo, metformin was associated with a "modest" increase in serum Hcy levels (4%; 0.2-8 μmol/L), and decreases in folate (−7%) and vitamin B_{12} (−14%). Furthermore, applying structural equation modeling, they demonstrated that the increase in Hcy was an indirect effect mediated by direct effects on folate and vitamin B_{12}, rather than a direct effect on Hcy by metformin. The authors concluded that a persistent increase in serum Hcy of 3 μmol/L was associated with an increased risk of coronary heart disease and stroke in nondiabetic individuals, and that available evidence indicates that this risk may be even greater in diabetic patients.

Wolever et al.[259] found that miglitol (Glyset), an alpha-glucosidase or alpha-amylase inhibitor, prevents the metformin-induced fall in serum folate and vitamin B_{12} in subjects with type 2 diabetes. Keeping dietary folate intake consistent, they observed that "serum folate and vitamin B_{12}, respectively, did not change on placebo, but fell by 14% and 15% on metformin and rose by 12% and 23% on miglitol." Notably, with the combination of metformin and miglitol, "both folate and vitamin B_{12} tended to rise, but the difference from metformin was only significant for folate." These authors concluded that "that increased carbohydrate delivery to the colon increases intestinal biosynthesis of folate."

In a study involving nine women with polycystic ovary syndrome (PCOS) conducted at the Center for Perinatal Studies at Swedish Medical Center in Seattle, Vrbikova et al.[262] found that a second-trimester Hcy elevation was associated with a 3.2-fold increased risk of preeclampsia. The authors noted that women with PCOS were already at increased risk for atherosclerosis, and that elevated Hcy could also contribute to pregnancy complications.

The adverse effects of metformin on folate and vitamin B_{12} status, Hcy levels, and related cardiovascular risk can often be mitigated by coadministration of folate, B_{12}, and calcium. In a 12-week, prospective, randomized, double-blind placebo-controlled study, Aarsand and Carlsen[274] studied whether administration of folate reduces serum tHcy levels in patients receiving long-term metformin treatment. All subjects who had been receiving metformin (minimum of 1000 mg/day) for at least 1 year were included, and all baseline serum tHcy levels were within the reference range. In addition to metformin, one group received concomitant folate (0.25 mg/day) in addition to iron (Fe^{++}; 60 mg/day), whereas the placebo group received only 60 mg/day of Fe^{++}. Of the 28 subjects who finished the trial, 26 had been diagnosed with NIDDM, two with hyperlipidemia. Subjects in the folate group demonstrated reduced serum levels of tHcy (vs. placebo group) by 13.9% and 21.7% at weeks 4 and 12, respectively, as well as increased serum levels of vitamin B_{12} (9.9% and 9.6%) and folate (96.9 and 89.9%). In the trial cited earlier, Bauman et al.[258] investigated the effects of metformin antagonism on B_{12}–intrinsic factor complex uptake by ileal cell surface receptors, a calcium-dependent membrane action. After observing "diminished B_{12} absorption and low serum total vitamin B_{12} and TCII-B_{12} levels" in patients receiving metformin therapy, they found that calcium coadministration reverses metformin-induced B_{12} malabsorption.

In a related study with uncertain clinical implications, Child et al.[275] investigated the effect of oral folic acid on Hcy, glutathione, glycemia, and lipids in type 2 diabetic patients. After administering folic acid (10 mg daily) for 3 months to 27 diabetic patients (26 male, one female; age 48-68) with microalbuminuria, they observed an increase in RBC folate that correlated with a reduction in microalbuminuria. Notably, "plasma glutathione increased despite reduction in its precursor Hcy," but correlated with levels of vitamin B_6;

however, this change in glutathione correlated inversely with change in hemoglobin A_{1c} (HbA_{1c}), total cholesterol, and triglycerides and positively with HDL cholesterol. Thus, oral folic acid supplementation reduced plasma Hcy level and increased glutathione level in subjects with type 2 diabetes, but levels of HbA_{1c}, triglycerides, and HDL cholesterol deteriorated. In addition, the authors noted that "some aspects of the response to folate may be different in patients on metformin."[275]

Lifestyle interventions can be more effective than metformin for curbing the incidence of diabetes in individuals at high risk. Continued research emerging from the work of the Diabetes Prevention Program (DPP) Research Group emphasizes that although metformin can be effective, a broader strategic approach emphasizing diet and exercise can produce more fundamental benefits. Analyzing DPP trial data in the *New England Journal of Medicine*, Knowler et al.[276] showed that, overall, metformin reduced the risk of diabetes by about 31%, compared with a 58% reduction for those assigned to intensive nutrition and exercise counseling. The study's 3234 participants were significantly overweight and had "impaired glucose tolerance." Approximately 1000 subjects were put on a low-fat diet (25% of overall calories), told to engage in moderate physical exercise, such as walking for 30 minutes, received training in goal setting and problem solving, and were invited to participate in group events. In addition to reducing diabetes risk, the lifestyle intervention group exhibited reduced body weight by 5% to 7%. In a subsequent analysis, Molitch et al.[277] concluded that, on the basis of these rates, the estimated number of persons who would need to be treated for 3 years to prevent one case of diabetes during this period is 6.9 for the lifestyle intervention versus 13.9 for metformin. Likewise, Orchard et al.[278] calculated that "diet and exercise delayed the onset of type 2 diabetes by about 11 years, while metformin delayed the onset by about three years." Increased dietary intake of folate-rich foods, especially dark-green leafy vegetables, would fit well within such an approach.

Nutritional Therapeutics, Clinical Concerns, and Adaptations

Physicians treating patients with dysglycemia, diabetes, PCOS, or related conditions using metformin are advised to integrate such biguanide therapy within a comprehensive therapeutic strategy. Regular exercise and a diet emphasizing low-glycemic-load carbohydrates and healthy sources of fats (such as olive oil or fish oils) can provide the most effective foundation for such an approach. Coadministration of folic acid (400 μg once or twice daily), vitamins B_{12} and B_6, and calcium can help reduce associated risks and adverse effects attributable to the medication, particularly cardiovascular risks linked to elevated Hcy levels.

Close supervision, active support for lifestyle changes, and regular monitoring are all essential to successful intervention. Folate and Hcy levels, as well as liver function, should be checked regularly. Total serum cobalamin is not sufficiently specific and does not reflect intracellular B_{12} deficiency. Screening for genetic polymorphisms, especially MTHFR genotype, affecting folate status and Hcy susceptibility may be appropriate because interindividual variability may be significant for both therapeutic response to biguanides and folate metabolism. Serum holo-TCII is a sensitive marker of cobalamin balance, more accurately assessing B_{12} availability for the cells, but this analysis may not be feasible in routine clinical practice. MMA and tHcy can reflect intracellular B_{12} deficiency, but these metabolites may also increase in various clinical conditions, most notably with impaired renal function.

Neomycin

Neomycin (Mycifradin, Myciguent, Neo-Fradin, NeoTab, Nivemycin).

Interaction Type and Significance

≈≈≈ **Drug-Induced Nutrient Depletion,**
Supplementation Therapeutic, Not Requiring
Professional Management
☼ **Prevention or Reduction of Drug Adverse Effect**

Probability:	Evidence Base:
5. Improbable or	○ Preliminary, but
2. Probable (depending on duration)	generally regarded as ● Consensus

Effect and Mechanism of Action

Oral neomycin can decrease absorption and/or increase elimination of folic acid and other nutrients, including beta-carotene, calcium, carbohydrates, fats, iron, magnesium, potassium, sodium, and vitamins A, B_{12}, D, and K.[279,280] These effects increase with time in long-term neomycin therapy and can be most significant in elderly persons.[281]

Research

In 1966, Faloon et al.[282] documented the adverse effects of neomycin on intestinal absorption of nutrients.[282] In 1969, Hardison and Rosenberg[283] further elucidated the effect of neomycin on bile salt metabolism and fat digestion in humans. Subsequently, the adverse effects of neomycin on nutrient status were explored extensively in the pioneering work of D.A. Roe (1923–1993) of Cornell University, Division of Nutritional Sciences, through publications such as "Drug-Induced Nutritional Deficiencies" (1976). As such, this characterization has largely become the "consensus" of the literature documenting adverse drug effects and drug-induced nutrient depletions, without passing through the stages of published case reports, human trials, reviews, and so on, which constitute the emerging standard within the scientific literature of drug-nutrient interactions. Further research may be warranted.

Nutritional Therapeutics, Clinical Concerns, and Adaptations

Physicians prescribing a course of oral neomycin longer than a few days are advised to coadminister a multivitamin-mineral supplement containing folic acid. Depletion is improbable with short-term use of oral neomycin associated with surgery or perioperative care. A course of probiotic flora is also appropriate following broad-spectrum antibiotics to restore normal gut ecology and prevent sequelae adversely affecting vitamin B_{12} synthesis and folate metabolism.

Nitroglycerin and Related Nitrates

Nitroglycerin (glyceryl trinitrate, GTN; Deponit, Minitran, Nitrek, Nitro-Bid, Nitro-Dur, Nitro-Time, Nitrodisc, Nitrogard, Nitroglyn, Nitrolingual, Nitrol, Nitrostat, Transderm-Nitro, Tridil).
Extrapolated, based on similar properties: Isosorbide dinitrate (ISDN, Isordil, Sorbitrate); combination drug: hydralazine and isosorbide dinitrate (BiDil); isosorbide mononitrate (Imdur, ISMN, ISMO, Isotrate, Monoket).

Interaction Type and Significance

⊕⊕ **Beneficial or Supportive Interaction, with**
Professional Management

Probability:	Evidence Base:
2. Probable	◉ Emerging

Effect and Mechanism of Action

Nitroglycerin and other organic nitrates have been used clinically as nitric oxide (NO)–donating agents for more than 100 years in cardiovascular therapeutics and continue to be widely used in ischemic heart disease, even though knowledge of their intimate mechanism of action is incomplete. Progressive attenuation of their efficacy (tolerance) is a frequent problem in patients with acute coronary syndromes undergoing continuous, long-term therapy, as is cross-tolerance to endothelial NO; tolerance can also occur within 24 to 48 hours after administration of a nitrate medication.

Nitrate medications appear to cause tolerance by inducing nitric oxide synthase (NOS) dysfunction, probably as a result of reduced bioavailability of tetrahydrobiopterin. This metabolic syndrome is characterized by mitochondrial dysfunction and mediated significantly by inhibition of vascular aldehyde dehydrogenase (ALDH-2).[284] Also, Loscalzo[285] suggests that nitrate "depletes NADPH and an NADPH-dependent cofactor essential for the enzymatic activity of endothelial nitric oxide synthase." Several mechanisms may explain this phenomenon, including nitrate-mediated depletion of intracellular thiols, enhanced mitochondrial reactive oxygen species (ROS) formation, and increased superoxide production. Endothelial nitric oxide synthase (eNOS) is an enzyme that predominantly produces NO under normal physiological conditions, controlled by the regulatory coenzyme calmodulin, the substrate L-arginine, and the cofactor tetrahydrobiopterin. However, in the context of dyslipidemia and other pathophysiological conditions, eNOS production shifts from NO to superoxide. Thus, increased intracellular oxidative stress appears to be a mechanism for nitrate tolerance.

Folic acid can prevent nitroglycerin-induced nitrate tolerance and cross-tolerance to endothelial NO by enhancing the regeneration and bioavailability of tetrahydrobiopterin in the context of the oxidative stress associated with long-term nitroglycerin administration. The mechanisms of this activity have not been fully elucidated. Dihydrofolate reductase reduces dietary folate to tetrahydrofolate using reduced nicotinamide-adenine dinucleotide phosphate (NADPH) as a cofactor. NADPH is also a required cofactor for NOS activity and for the synthesis of tetrahydrobiopterin from the direct and salvage pathways. However, NOS is unable to function either as an L-arginine oxidase or as an oxygen reductase when supplies of NADPH are compromised. "Thus, one plausible argument for the benefits of folate in nitrate tolerance is that it [nitrate] depletes NADPH and an NADPH-dependent cofactor essential for the enzymatic activity of endothelial nitric oxide synthase."[285] However, evidence is lacking to confirm or refute this proposed mechanism.

Folic acid and its active form, 5-methyltetrahydrofolate (5-MTHF), have been shown in some studies to prevent uncoupling of the eNOS, reduce eNOS-mediated superoxide production, enhance NO synthesis by NOS, and restore impaired NO bioavailability, particularly in dyslipidemic conditions.[286-292] Such inhibition of eNOS uncoupling could contribute to improved endothelial function. The tetrahydrobiopterin radical appears to be directly involved in the facilitated catalysis of eNOS by 5-MTHF and thus the formation of NO.[293] Related research showing the benefits of ascorbic acid in potentiating eNOS activity, by increasing intracellular tetrahydrobiopterin, complements the hypothesis that the tetrahydrobiopterin radical plays a role in NO synthesis by mediating reductive activation of the ferrous heme-O_2 moiety of the eNOS enzyme.[294] Other research indicates that the pteridine-binding domain in NOS is similar to the folate-binding site of dihydrofolate reductase.[295]

Continued research will determine the validity and significance of each of these hypotheses and clarify the relative role of each mechanism in folate's apparent ability to improve endothelial function and ameliorate nitrate tolerance.

Research

Clinical research investigating therapeutic synergies using folic acid in concert with nitrate preparations is only in the initial phases. Although a body of research exists on the mechanisms in the relationship between nitrates and nitric acid, including the potential roles of folates, a comprehensive model of folate and its activities has yet to be elucidated.

In an animal study, Gruhn et al.[296] found that administration of tetrahydrobiopterin improves endothelium-dependent vasodilation in nitroglycerin-tolerant rats and concluded that "altered bioavailability of tetrahydrobiopterin is involved in the pathophysiology of endothelial dysfunction seen in nitroglycerin tolerance." Subsequently, Sydow et al.[284] observed decreases in vascular mitochondrial aldehyde dehydrogenase (ALDH-2) activity, nitroglycerin (GTN) biotransformation, and cyclic guanosine monophosphate (cGMP)–dependent kinase activity in rats treated for 3 days with GTN infusions. Multiple inhibitors and substrates of ALDH-2 had little effect on tolerant vessels, whereas these agents reduced both GTN stimulation of cGKI and GTN-induced vasodilation in control vessels. Furthermore, "GTN increased the production of reactive oxygen species (ROS) by mitochondria," and "antioxidants/reductants decreased mitochondrial ROS production and restored ALDH-2 activity." These findings indicate that mitochondrial ROS and inhibition of vascular ALDH-2 play a significant role in mediating nitrate tolerance.

In a small, randomized, double-blind trial, Gori et al.[297] tested the effects of concomitant folic acid (10 mg daily for 1 week, a relatively high dose) on development of tolerance to continuous transdermal GTN (0.6 mg/hour) in 18 healthy male volunteers (age 19-32). In measurements taken on the return visit, folic acid "prevented GTN-induced endothelial dysfunction, as assessed by responses to intraarterial acetylcholine and N-monomethyl-L-arginine." The authors also noted that "responses to intraarterial GTN were significantly greater than those observed after transdermal GTN plus placebo" in the subjects treated with folic acid plus transdermal GTN. Thus, they concluded that "oxidative stress contributes to nitrate tolerance," and that "supplemental folic acid prevents both nitric oxide synthase dysfunction induced by continuous GTN and nitrate tolerance in the arterial circulation of healthy volunteers."

These data are consistent with the mechanisms previously discussed and provide a foundation for continued research into an expanded role for folic acid coadministration in preventing nitrate tolerance and enhancing the therapeutic effects of nitrate therapy. Confirmatory findings in high-powered, well-designed clinical trials would have major implications for the treatment of atherothrombotic vascular disease.

Nutritional Therapeutics, Clinical Concerns, and Adaptations

Physicians prescribing nitroglycerin or related nitrate preparations are advised to coadminister folic acid to prevent tolerance to the medication over time and as part of the broader strategy for reduction of cardiovascular risk. Evidence from complementary research suggests that such patients might also benefit from concomitant L-arginine, vitamin C, coenzyme Q10,

vitamin B_{12}, and magnesium. Implementation of such an integrative strategy requires close supervision and regular monitoring, most effectively by a multidisciplinary team incorporating health care professionals trained and experienced in both conventional pharmacology and nutritional therapeutics.

Nitrous Oxide

Nitrous Oxide

Interaction Type and Significance

☼ **Prevention or Reduction of Drug Adverse Effect**
⊕⊕ **Beneficial or Supportive Interaction, with Professional Management**

Probability:	Evidence Base:
5. Improbable or **3. Possible**	◉ **Emerging** to ● **Consensus**

Effect and Mechanism of Action

Exposure to nitrous oxide (N_2O) can produce megaloblastic anemia, neuropathy, and birth defects, all caused primarily by induced deficiency of vitamin B_{12} and secondarily by the effects of vitamin B_{12} deficiency on folate metabolism. Such adverse effects of N_2O were well established long before the mechanisms of its effects on folate and vitamin B_{12} were elucidated. Nitrous oxide can significantly interfere with activity of vitamin B_{12}, alter intracellular folate coenzyme levels, perturb the normal pathways of folic acid metabolism by oxidizing the enzyme-B_{12} (Co+) complex formed during catalysis, and thereby inactivate methionine synthase.[298-300] Anesthesia with N_2O may also impair DNA synthesis in bone marrow cells.[301] Notably, researchers have often employed N_2O as a probe for investigating the folate–vitamin B_{12} interrelationships because of these well-known effects.[302]

Thus, N_2O exposure can cause an accumulation of cytosolic 5-methyltetrahydrofolate (5-MTHF; e.g., in liver and pancreas), at the expense of other reduced folates, specifically tetrahydrofolate (THF) and 5-formyltetrahydrofolate (5-FTHF), which in turn can lead to significantly lower total mitochondrial folates.[303,304] This phenomenon is known as the *methyl trap hypothesis,* first presented in 1962, which states that, in the context of methionine synthase inactivation resulting from vitamin B_{12} deficiency, folates are trapped as 5-MTHF, the synthesis of which is not reversible in vivo.[305,306]

Research

Researchers have studied the adverse effects of N_2O on folate activity and the benefits of folic acid administration for more than 20 years. Using the deoxyuridine (dU) suppression test in 1985, Amos et al.[301] investigated secondary development of folate deficiency and delayed recovery after N_2O anesthesia in 48 patients admitted to an intensive care unit (ICU). The pattern of correction of the abnormal dU suppression tests on admission to the ICU, after N_2O anesthesia, was "typical of that seen in vitamin B_{12} deficiency"; 3 days later "the pattern had changed to that usually seen in folate deficiency." Likewise, "serum folate levels fell to subnormal values," and although elevated after N_2O administration, urinary folate excretion was "insufficient by itself to explain the development of folate deficiency." Moreover, administration of physiological amounts of folic acid accelerated the recovery of the bone marrow abnormalities present after N_2O anesthesia.

In a 1986 rat study, Keeling et al.[307] found that coadministration of folinic acid provided protection against N_2O teratogenicity. "The incidence of major skeletal abnormalities in the untreated nitrous oxide group was significantly increased to five times that of the control groups, whereas the incidence in the nitrous oxide group receiving folinic acid was not significantly different from control."

Two teams of researchers conducted parallel experiments investigating the short-term effects of N_2O on folate and vitamin B_{12} metabolism in rats and human patients. Koblin et al.[308] found that exposure to nitrous oxide (60% N_2O, 40% O_2) in rats of various ages greatly enhanced urinary excretion of formic acid and formiminoglutamic acid (FIGLU), compounds that are elevated in the urine of mammals with a deficiency in folate. Urinary formic acid excretion increased threefold to 25-fold the first day after 6 hours of N_2O exposure and returned to background levels by the second day after exposure in all age groups. Urinary FIGLU excretion increased 100-fold to 300-fold the first day after N_2O exposure, with the highest FIGLU excretion rates in the elderly rats and the lowest in the young rats. FIGLU excretion rates returned to baseline levels by the second day after N_2O exposure in all age groups. Increasing age was progressively associated with decreased plasma folate, but no age-dependent changes were observed in RBC folate, liver folate, or plasma vitamin B_{12} levels.

Subsequently, Koblin et al.[309] investigated folic acid metabolism in 49 surgical patients exposed to isoflurane alone or combined with N_2O. They found no increase in urinary formic acid and FIGLU in 23 patients exposed to N_2O for total hip replacement. However, patients undergoing resection of acoustic neuromas (with mean duration of anesthesia of 9.3 hours) exhibited a small, transient increase in the FIGLU/creatinine ratio, which peaked at the end of anesthetic exposure and returned toward control levels by the first day after anesthesia and surgery. The researchers noted a lack of predictive association between low preoperative levels of RBC folate and low-normal levels of serum vitamin B_{12} and an increase in formic acid or FIGLU in response to N_2O. They concluded: "Although an occasional patient may prove highly susceptible to and develop signs of severe vitamin B_{12} and folic acid deficiency after exposure to N_2O, our findings suggest that this is a rare event."[309]

In a study involving 40 patients under N_2O anesthesia for 70 to 720 minutes, Ermens et al.[310] demonstrated that postoperative plasma levels of folate and homocysteine (Hcy) increased up to 220% and 310%, respectively, in a manner correlating significantly with exposure time. This response appeared rapidly, after 75 minutes of N_2O exposure, and required several days to return to normal levels. Plasma Hcy levels had not returned to preoperative levels within 1 week in eight patients receiving N_2O anesthesia. Based on these findings, the authors suggested that elevated plasma Hcy levels may be used for monitoring N_2O-induced cobalamin inactivation and the resultant disturbance of Hcy and folate metabolism.

In related 1991 in vitro research using blast cells from leukemia patients, Ermens et al.[303] found that 8 hours' exposure to N_2O caused an equal decrease of 10-FTHF and 5-FTHF in both acute myeloid leukemia (30%) and acute lymphoid leukemia (45%), whereas 5-MTHF increased (130%). They concluded that N_2O treatment of leukemic cells causes an accumulation of 5-MTHF at the expense of other folate forms. In a similar 1997 experiment, Horne et al.[304] investigated the effects of N_2O inactivation of methionine synthase on the compartmentation of folate metabolism in rat pancreas. Rats exposed to N_2O exhibited cytosolic 5-MTHF concentrations that were significantly greater (59% of total folates) and

THF concentrations significantly lower (32%) than those in controls. Exposure to N_2O was associated with significantly lower activity of methionine synthase and concentration of THF and 5-FTHF, but not 5-MTHF or 10-FTHF, thus leading to significantly lower total mitochondrial folates. These findings are consistent with emerging knowledge of the mechanisms involved.

Issues of adverse effects of N_2O may represent a significant risk to medical and dental personnel exposed daily to low levels of anesthetic. Salo et al.[311] gathered peripheral blood samples from eight anesthetists and seven internists in a survey of potential occupational health hazard to operating theater personnel chronically exposed to trace N_2O concentrations. They observed no definite signs of B_{12}-N_2O interaction in peripheral blood counts or films, serum vitamin B_{12} or plasma, or erythrocyte folate concentrations.

The issue of how this interaction might affect individuals abusing nitrous oxide has not been addressed in a systematic or direct manner and deserves consideration as a potential area of concern.

Reports

Nunn et al.[312] reported the case of a "seriously ill patient" who exhibited "megaloblastic changes in his bone marrow" following N_2O anesthesia for 105 minutes. After a 7-hour delay and administration of folinic acid (30 mg), a second round of N_2O was administered; 4 hours later his marrow was normal.

Flippo and Holder[299] reviewed five cases in which "patients unsuspected of having vitamin B_{12} deficiency developed subacute combined degeneration of the spinal cord following nitrous oxide anesthesia." They attributed these adverse effects to N_2O-induced "irreversible oxidation to the Co++ and Co forms that renders vitamin B_{12} inactive" and that impairs DNA synthesis and the methylation of myelin basic protein involved in the maintenance of the myelin sheath. They cautioned that "patients with vitamin B_{12} deficiency are exceedingly sensitive to neurologic deterioration" after N_2O anesthesia, which, if unrecognized, could cause "irreversible" deterioration and "may result in death."

Nutritional Therapeutics, Clinical Concerns, and Adaptations

Physicians are advised to consider assessment of vitamin B_{12} and folate status as part of preoperative care in patients who will be receiving major anesthesia that includes N_2O. Administration of folic acid (1000 µg/day) and vitamin B_{12} (100 µg/day), beginning 1 week before and extending through 1 week after prolonged exposure to N_2O, is prudent if the patient is susceptible to or has a history of nutrient deficiency and if N_2O exposure will be of extended duration. Such concerns are amplified and further monitoring and compensatory nutrient support warranted in pregnant women because of the significantly greater risk inherent in transient depletion of folate levels, particularly in early gestation. Patients with normal vitamin B_{12} and folate levels who undergo N_2O anesthesia for less than 2 hours generally do not require supplementation; however, such prophylaxis would be safe, compatible, and inexpensive.

Evidence is lacking to support a recommendation for routine supplementation by medical or dental staff regularly exposed to N_2O. However, consideration should be given to the need for B_{12} and folate administration to individuals who have a recent history of, or are known to be currently engaged in, the habitual use of N_2O as a recreational drug. Urinary MMA level and plasma tHcy determination might be sensitive markers for monitoring in both situations.

Nonsteroidal Anti-Inflammatory Drugs (NSAIDs)

COX-1 inhibitors: Diclofenac (Cataflam, Voltaren); combination drug: diclofenac and misoprostol (Arthrotec); diflunisal (Dolobid), etodolac (Lodine), fenoprofen (Dalfon), furbiprofen (Ansaid), ibuprofen (Advil, Excedrin IB, Motrin, Motrin IB, Nuprin, Pedia Care Fever Drops, Provel, Rufen); combination drug: hydrocodone and ibuprofen (Reprexain, Vicoprofen); indomethacin (indometacin; Indocin, Indocin-SR), ketoprofen (Orudis, Oruvail), ketorolac (Acular ophthalmic, Toradol), meclofenamate (Meclomen), mefenamic acid (Ponstel), meloxicam (Mobic), nabumetone (Relafen), naproxen (Aleve, Anaprox, Naprosyn), oxaprozin (Daypro), piroxicam (Feldene), salsalate (salicylic acid; Amigesic, Disalcid, Marthritic, Mono Gesic, Salflex, Salsitab), sulindac (Clinoril), tolmetin (Tolectin).
COX-2 inhibitor: Celecoxib (Celebrex).
See also Acetysalicylic Acid and Sulfasalazine.

Interaction Type and Significance

≈≈≈ **Drug-Induced Nutrient Depletion, Supplementation Therapeutic, Not Requiring Professional Management**

≈≈ **Drug-Induced Nutrient Depletion, Supplementation Therapeutic, with Professional Management**

◇ **Impaired Drug Absorption and Bioavailability, Negligible Effect**

☼ **Prevention or Reduction of Drug Adverse Effect**

Probability: Evidence Base:
5. **Improbable** or   ○ **Preliminary**
3. **Possible**

Effect and Mechanism of Action

In vitro and animal research indicates that the "antifolate activity of NSAIDs, and hence cytostatic consequences, are important factors in producing anti-inflammatory activity."[39] Some NSAIDs, such as sulindac and sulfasalazine (SASP), are known antifolates. With chronic use and when taken in high doses, many NSAIDs may exert antifolate activity by impairing folate absorption and transport, which could decrease serum folate concentrations and cause deficiency.[38,39,313-315] Furthermore, many NSAIDs (including ibuprofen, indomethacin, mefenamic acid, naproxen, piroxicam, salicylic acid, sulindac, and sulphasalazine) and NSAID-like drugs act as competitive inhibitors of enzymes involved in folate metabolism and transport, including phosphoribosyl aminoimidazolecarboxamide formyltransferase transformylase (AICAR transformylase), dihydrofolate reductase, methylenetetrahydrofolate reductase, and serine transhydroxymethylase. Other in vitro experiments indicate that these NSAIDs can act as folate antagonists and inhibit the THF-dependent biosynthesis of serine from glycine and formate (i.e., C1 index) by human blood mononuclear cells (BMCs). In contrast, aspirin, acetaminophen, and antipyrine were weak inhibitors of these enzymes; acetaminophen exerted a weak inhibitory effect on the C1 index. Notably, both aspirin and salsalate exert anti-inflammatory effects after conversion to salicylic acid, which possesses greater antifolate activity than either parent compound.[39,314]

Other NSAIDs, such as p-aminosalicylic acid (an older antituberculosis agent), may decrease folic acid absorption in the GI tract and decrease serum folate concentrations.[316] Furthermore, p-aminosalicylic acid is also a structural analog of p-aminobenzoic acid (PABA) and thus inhibits de novo folate synthesis.

Research

Most evidence regarding the effects of NSAIDs on folate comes from in vitro and animal research, as previously reviewed. Some of these studies derive from human studies, but not clinical trials. Thus, although a coherent body of data indicates that NSAIDs exert multiple actions that may be deleterious to folate levels and functions, only preliminary evidence is available from human trials to confirm these phenomena and delineate the associated factors or determine their clinical significance.

Baggott et al.[39] observed in vitro that the C1 index of BMCs from rheumatoid arthritis (RA) patients receiving drugs with minimal antifolate activity (e.g., acetaminophen) is higher than the C1 index from RA patients receiving NSAIDs with more potent antifolate activity (e.g., sulindac, sulfasalazine, naproxen, ibuprofen). "The mean activity of the transformylase in BMCs taken from healthy humans was 1.98 nmol of product/h per 10^6 cells and the activity was positively correlated with BMC folate levels."

Analyzing serum and blood samples from a healthy female subject following a fixed diet for 11 days and taking 650 mg aspirin orally every 4 hours during the middle 3 days, Lawrence et al.[38] observed a "brisk, significant but reversible fall in total and bound serum folate and a small but insignificant increase in urinary folate excretion." Noting also that aspirin in vitro "displaced significant amounts of bound serum folate," they concluded that "aspirin in therapeutic doses can contribute to subnormal serum folate values, and if it increases urinary folate excretion even slightly, may impair folate balance." (See also Acetylsalicylic Acid.)

No direct evidence has confirmed that folate coadministration is beneficial for individuals taking most NSAIDs. Conversely, no evidence to date has suggested that concomitant folate administration might interfere with the therapeutic activity of such NSAIDs, although this may be possible given the role of antifolate activity in the mechanisms of action observed in many of these drugs. Nevertheless, the positive clinical outcomes regarding coadministration of folate with methotrexate in autoimmune arthritides indicates that folate does not necessarily interfere with the therapeutic action of antifolate drugs.

Nutritional Therapeutics, Clinical Concerns, and Adaptations

Physicians prescribing NSAIDs should consider discussing with patients the potential benefits of concomitant folic acid (400 μg once or twice daily) and increased dietary folate intake with frequent, long-term, or high-dose NSAID therapy. Monitoring for folate deficiency using serum/RBC folate levels and plasma Hcy may be advisable.

Substantive evidence is lacking to confirm, or even suggest, that routine low-dose NSAID use is likely to affect folate status adversely in most individuals. The available evidence indicates that the adverse effect may be marginal in some cases and could be severe in a few patients, particularly with chronic use at higher dosage levels. Such concerns may be particularly relevant in pregnant women and in patients with compromised dietary folate status or susceptibility caused by individual genomic variability.

Oral Contraceptives: Monophasic, Biphasic, and Triphasic Estrogen Preparations (Synthetic Estrogen and Progesterone Analogs)

Ethinyl estradiol and desogestrel (Desogen, Ortho-TriCyclen). Ethinyl estradiol and ethynodiol (Demulen 1/35, Demulen 1/50, Nelulen 1/25, Nelulen 1/50, Zovia).

Ethinyl estradiol and levonorgestrel (Alesse, Levlen, Levlite, Levora 0.15/30, Nordette, Tri-Levlen, Triphasil, Trivora).
Ethinyl estradiol and norethindrone/norethisterone (Brevicon, Estrostep, Genora 1/35, GenCept 1/35, Jenest-28, Loestrin 1.5/30, Loestrin 1/20, Modicon, Necon 1/25, Necon 10/11, Necon 0.5/30, Necon 1/50, Nelova 1/35, Nelova 10/11, Norinyl 1/35, Norlestin 1/50, Ortho Novum 1/35, Ortho Novum 10/11, Ortho Novum 7/7/7, Ovcon-35, Ovcon-50, Tri-Norinyl, Trinovum).
Ethinyl estradiol and norgestrel (Lo/Ovral, Ovral).
Mestranol and norethindrone (Genora 1/50, Nelova 1/50, Norethin 1/50, Ortho-Novum 1/50).
Related, internal application: Etonogestrel/ethinyl estradiol vaginal ring (Nuvaring).
See also Medroxyprogesterone.

Interaction Type and Significance

≈≈≈ **Drug-Induced Nutrient Depletion,**
Supplementation Therapeutic, Not Requiring
Professional Management
≈≈ **Drug-Induced Nutrient Depletion,**
Supplementation Therapeutic, with
Professional Management
✧ **Prevention or Reduction of Drug Adverse Effect**

Probability: Evidence Base:
5. Improbable or   ○ **Preliminary** to
3. Possible   ● **Emerging**

Effect and Mechanism of Action

Oral contraceptives (OCs) may lower serum and RBC folate, but such changes do not appear to induce folate deficiency or cause anemia or megaloblastic changes under most circumstances. OCs are also associated with lowered levels of cyanocobalamin, which in turn can adversely affect folate status and related hematological parameters.[317,318] The mechanisms of such possible effects have not been elucidated. In 1968, Shojania et al.[319] noted the high incidence of folate deficiency in pregnancy and proposed that "one would expect a similar effect in women on longterm oral contraceptives, which are known to produce a pseudopregnancy state."

Folic acid may protect against precancerous cervical dysplasia in women, especially those taking OCs.

Research

It has been well established that birth control pills, especially those containing higher estrogen doses, impair folate metabolism and tend to deplete folic acid, with several possible adverse repercussions, especially increased risk of cervical dysplasia and vascular thrombosis. However, evidence is mixed regarding the probability of occurrence and clinical significance of such an adverse effect; the issue remains contentious. Differing estrogen doses in various OC formulations, as well as such confounding variables as dietary folate intake and genetic polymorphisms affecting folate, may account for some of the inconsistency in research findings.[320]

Folic acid deficiency enhances OC-induced platelet hyperactivity and oxidative stress. In various studies in female rats and also in women, OCs were found to induce a platelet hyperactivity related to increased oxidative stress. Many researchers suspect that OCs deplete folate stores and point to cases of megaloblastic anemia reported to occur in women taking OCs.

Using a rat model, Durand et al.[321] determined that dietary folic acid deficiency contributed to the thrombogenicity of OCs and "magnified OC-induced oxidative stress, which resulted in platelet hyperactivity by elevating the pro-oxidant

homocysteine plasma concentration." Animals were fed for 6 weeks with either a folic acid–deficient diet (250 μg/kg folic acid) or a control diet (750 μg/kg folic acid). Half the animals in each group received an OC (ethinyl estradiol plus lynestrenol). The authors observed that folic acid deficiency and OCs "individually potentiated platelet aggregation in response to thrombin and ADP [adenosine diphosphate] and the release and metabolism of arachidonic acid, in particular, the biosynthesis of thromboxane. These platelet activities were further enhanced in animals given both the folic acid–deficient diet and the OC treatment." Furthermore, folic acid deficiency "enhanced the pro-oxidant state in OC-treated rats characterized by (1) a fall in platelet and plasma n-3 fatty acids, (2) an increase in plasma lipid peroxidation products such as conjugated dienes, lipid peroxides, and thiobarbituric reactive substances, [and] (3) a rise in *ex vivo* erythrocyte susceptibility to free radicals." Also, OC administration "led to a reduction of plasma and erythrocyte folate concentrations associated with a moderate hyperhomocysteinemia." Despite the limitations of this animal model, the authors concluded that their findings "suggest that in addition to cigarette smoking, inadequate folic acid intake might predispose those taking OC to vascular thrombosis."[321]

Most human studies have found that OC use adversely affects folate status, but conclusions vary depending on estrogen dose levels, methods of assessing folate levels, and duration of trial period. In a preliminary 1968 study of 86 women (24 normal nonpregnant women of childbearing age and 62 women taking OCs), Shojania et al.[319] determined that the OC group showed, on average, a significantly lower serum folate level than the control group, with 30% (19) of the OC women exhibiting a serum folate level lower than the lowest value in the control group. The authors recommended that the "serum folate level of women on long-term oral contraceptives be determined, especially when they stop the medication and plan for conception."

Subsequently, in a 1975 review, Lindenbaum et al.[322] reported that "in some series, but not in others, serum and/or red cell folate concentrations have been reduced in oral contraceptive users" but that "a disturbance in folate balance serious enough to cause symptoms (i.e., megaloblastic anemia) occurs very rarely." In a 1991 study, Mooji et al.[323] compared folate concentration in serum and RBCs, as well as other nutrient levels, over four cycles in 29 women taking OCs (containing 30 μg of ethinyl estradiol) and 31 women serving as non-OC controls, with both groups administered a multivitamin and folic acid supplement. OCs did not lower serum and RBC folate levels or induce folate deficiency, at least within the limited time frame of the trial. The authors concluded that "supplementation during OC use or just after discontinuing treatment cannot be justified for healthy young women," but added that, "in the case of women with a critical vitamin balance or higher folate needs, multivitamin supplementation may be considered."

In 1993, Steegers-Theunissen et al.[324] compared serum folate levels after oral folate loading in a study of the kinetics of folic acid monoglutamate involving 29 users of OCs containing less than 50 μg of estrogen and in 13 women serving as controls. Median serum folate concentrations after oral folate loading were decreased in OC users, reaching statistically significant lower levels after 210 minutes (260 nmol/L) compared with controls (400 nmol/L). Apparently, OCs with less than 50 μg estrogen significantly affected folate kinetics and vitamin B_{12} levels. Even so, the authors concluded that "folate and vitamin B_{12} status does not seem to be at risk."

In 1998, Green et al.[325] investigated the impact of "currently available" OCs, as well as smoking and alcohol, on serum and RBC folate and serum B_{12} and homocysteine in 229 adolescent females (age 14-20) in Canada. Use of OCs was associated with an estimated 33% lower serum B_{12} level than nonuse, but OC use (as well as alcohol use and smoking) was not significantly associated with lower serum or RBC folate levels, after controlling for folate intake.

The investigators in many of these studies concluded that the effect of OCs on folate is not clinically significant, but their findings are generally limited by the parameters employed to assess folate status and the short duration of the trials.

A "rigorous meta-analysis" of 14 studies by Baillargeon et al.[326] found that "current use" (i.e., use at the time of the event or within 3 months) of low-dose OCs "significantly increases the risk of both cardiac and vascular arterial events," including vascular arterial complications with third-generation OCs. Overall, the use of low-dose OCs was associated with a doubling of the risk of cardiovascular outcomes (myocardial infarction or ischemic stroke), with both second-generation and third-generation OCs being associated with a significantly increased risk of ischemic stroke (relative risk, 2.12). The association between third-generation OC use and myocardial infarction proved nonsignificant.

Researchers often allude to but generally do not directly address the implications for women who might subsequently become pregnant. To address this critical issue, Martinez and Roe[327] investigated residual effects of OCs on the folate status of pregnant women who had discontinued intake of these drugs within 6 months of conception. They found that OC users demonstrated "lower plasma and red blood cell folate values than did the respective control subjects." Factoring in seasonal variability in RBC folate values, which were lower in the winter months, RBC folate values were more affected by previous drug use in the winter group than in the summer group. Also, dietary folate exhibited a significant effect on plasma and RBC folate, and blood folate values were significantly lower in OC users for any given level of folate intake. Correlation of post–OC use folate levels versus non-OC users and risk of subsequent neural tube defect (NTD) pregnancies would be useful.

Researchers and clinicians have long debated the role of folate in the relationship between OC use and the occurrence of cervical dysplasia and cancer. In 1973, Whitehead et al.[328] reported megaloblastic changes in the cervical epithelium in association with OC therapy and reversal with folic acid. In 1982, Butterworth et al.[329] published promising initial research from a 3-month, double-blind placebo-controlled trial where megadoses of folic acid (10 mg daily) were associated with regression of cervical intraepithelial neoplasia (CIN) among OC users. In a 1975 review, Lindenbaum et al.[322] concluded that "about 20 percent of women taking contraceptive hormones manifest mild megaloblastic changes on Papanicolaou smears of the cervicovaginal epithelium which disappear after folic acid therapy," but that (then) "current evidence, however, would not indicate that any significant benefit would ensue from routine folate supplementation in women on oral contraceptives."

In 1996, Zarcone et al.[330] found that folic acid supplements did not alter the course of established cervical dysplasia. Further, at this time, no substantial evidence has been published to support the view that folic acid supplementation alone can play a significant role in the treatment of cervical cancer. In related research concerning human papillomavirus (HPV), often associated with cervical dysplasia, Kwasniewska

et al.[331] determined that statistically lower levels of folic acid were found in the women with CIN-HPV (+) and cited other studies showing that lower levels of antioxidants coexisting with low levels of folic acid increase the risk of CIN development. In contrast, Sedjo et al.[332] found "no significant associations ... between HPV persistence and dietary intake of folate, vitamin B_{12}, vitamin B_6, or methionine from food alone or from food and supplements combined or from circulating folate" in 201 women with a persistent or intermittent HPV infection. Moreover, among women not using OCs, folic acid has not been found to improve abnormal Pap smears. However, folate replacement in the range of 5 to 20 mg has been associated with reversal of dysplasia, particularly HPV-related dysplasia (which is the vast majority). The older literature was unaware of the relationship between HPV and cervical dysplasia, and some of the negative studies may have used too low a folic dose. There may also have been disproportionate numbers of MTHFR mutations in the negative studies. Studies should be repeated that control for these factors, with either genetic testing or use of activated folate.

Nutritional Therapeutics, Clinical Concerns, and Adaptations

Physicians prescribing OCs are advised to discuss with their patients the potential adverse effects of these exogenous hormones on the status of folate and other nutrients, especially vitamin B_6. Folate testing may be warranted, but coadministration of folic acid (400-800 µg/day) with vitamin B_6 (50-100 mg/day) can provide safe and inexpensive support against cardiovascular and other potential adverse effects without interfering with the intended contraceptive effect. Enhanced dietary folate intake and folic acid supplementation are especially important for women who stop using OCs with the intention (or simply the possibility) of becoming pregnant. Those who are diagnosed with cervical dysplasia or who are concerned with increased risks of stroke might particularly benefit from incorporating folic acid into a therapeutic program under the care of a nutritionally trained health care professional. Vitamin B_{12} status should also be checked by serum B_{12} levels or serum/urine MMA levels and corrected as necessary whenever high-dose folic acid therapy is implemented.

Pancreatic Enzymes, Pancreatin, and Related Proteolytic Enzymes

Pancreatic enzymes, pancreatin, proteolytic enzymes.

Interaction Type and Significance

≈≈≈ **Drug-Induced Nutrient Depletion, Supplementation Therapeutic, Not Requiring Professional Management**

Probability:	Evidence Base:
4. Plausible	○ **Preliminary**

Effect and Mechanism of Action

Proteolytic enzymes, including pancreatin, have been reported to form insoluble complexes with folate and interfere with absorption. Diminished absorption of dietary folate could lead to folate deficiency.[333]

Research

In vitro and human studies have reported impairment of folic acid absorption in the presence of oral pancreatic extracts. Russell et al.[334] described higher serum folate levels "among newly diagnosed, untreated patients with pancreatic insufficiency than among treated patients despite greater fat malabsorption in the former group." Further, in vivo experiments involving "folate absorption tests using tritium-labeled pteroylmonoglutamatic acid showed folate absorption to be enhanced in pancreatic insufficiency patients as compared to control subjects." Also, "pancreatic extract significantly inhibited folate absorption" in both normal subjects and patients with pancreatic insufficiency. The authors recommended that "folate status should be monitored in patients being treated for pancreatic insufficiency," especially when pancreatic extract and bicarbonate are coadministered. Further research is warranted.

Nutritional Therapeutics, Clinical Concerns, and Adaptations
Health care professionals prescribing pancreatin and other proteolytic enzymes are advised to suggest concomitant supplementation with folic acid (400 µg/day) to counteract any resultant decrease in folate absorption and prevent diminished folate status. Monitoring of folate levels may be appropriate in patients with susceptibility to or history of folate deficiency or comorbid conditions, in whom folate deficiency could cause enhanced risk. Administering folate supplements several hours before or after intake of pancreatic enzyme preparations would also appear prudent.

Pyrimethamine

Pyrimethamine (Daraprim); combination drug: sulfadoxine and pyrimethamine (Fansidar).

Interaction Type and Significance
◇≈≈   Drug-Induced Adverse Effect on Nutrient Function, Coadministration Therapeutic, with Professional Management
≈≈   Drug-Induced Nutrient Depletion, Supplementation Therapeutic, with Professional Management
⊕✗   Bimodal or Variable Interaction, with Professional Management
✗   Potential or Theoretical Adverse Interaction of Uncertain Severity

Probability:
3. Possible or
2. Probable

Evidence Base:
◉ Emerging to
● Consensus

Effect and Mechanism of Action
Pyrimethamine is a competitive inhibitor of dihydrofolate reductase that acts as a folic acid antagonist and can reduce serum folic acid levels. Pyrimethamine is widely recognized as a cause of megaloblastic anemia resulting from a folate deficiency. In combination with sulfadiazine, it is often used in the treatment of toxoplasmosis. However, bone marrow suppression, resulting predominantly from depression of folate metabolism and causing neutropenia and thrombocytopenia, is a frequent toxic adverse effect. Coadministration of folic acid (or more often, 5-MTHF as folinic acid) can mitigate adverse effects on folate levels and function but could decrease pyrimethamine efficacy because of pharmacodynamic antagonism.

Fansidar, an antimalarial agent, is a combination of sulfadoxine and pyrimethamine that inhibits sequential steps involved in the biosynthesis of tetrahydrofolic acid. Thus, interference with protozoal nucleic acid and protein production is achieved by depleting folic acid, an essential cofactor in the biosynthesis of nucleic acids. Sulfadoxine competitively inhibits the enzyme dihydropteroate synthetase; it is a structural analog of PABA. The dual sequential action of these two agents creates a synergistic effect that enables reduction of the minimum effective dose of each medication but amplifies the antifolate effects.

Research
Although the mechanism of action of pyrimethamine and its adverse effects on folate status are widely acknowledged, the frequency and conditions of clinically significant interactions are not well known. At lower doses the need for folic acid coadministration has not been researched adequately to enable well-founded conclusions. The risk of bone marrow suppression can increase significantly with concurrent use of pyrimethamine and other antifolates, such as methotrexate or sulfa antibiotics. At higher doses, such as used in treatment of toxoplasmosis and *Pneumocystis carinii* pneumonia, folate support may be necessary. However, such concurrent administration may impair the therapeutic activity of pyrimethamine, although this has not been established with careful clinical research.

Of several dihydrofolate reductase inhibitors tested against *P. carinii* in a rat model, Walzer et al.[335] noted that "all drugs were well tolerated except pyrimethamine, which caused bone marrow depression; folinic acid ameliorated this adverse reaction but did not interfere with *P. carinii* treatment." This suggests that the previous caution regarding potential interference with therapeutic activity of pyrimethamine by at least some forms of folic acid may not be a concern.

Nutritional Therapeutics, Clinical Concerns, and Adaptations
Physicians prescribing pyrimethamine, alone or in combination with other agents, are advised to consider coadministration of folic acid or 5-MTHF as a preventive measure. Folinic acid is the form of 5-MTHF most often used in conventional practice, 5 to 15 mg/day (orally, intravenously, or intramuscularly) until normal hematopoiesis restored, although L-5-MTHF (Metafolin) may be preferable, because it is the chiral form used by the body. Folate and pyrimethamine levels should be monitored regularly. Pyrimethamine dose may also need to be reduced or the medication discontinued if folate deficiency develops, depending on patient response. Caution is also warranted in patients with hepatic or renal impairment. Pyrimethamine may precipitate hemolytic anemia in patients with glucose-6-phosphate dehydrogenase (G6PD) deficiency.

Although the safety of pyrimethamine in pregnancy has not been well researched, prudence suggests that increased folic acid supplementation may be warranted with female patients who are or might become pregnant.

Sulfasalazine and Related Sulfonamide Antibiotics (Systemic)

Sulfasalazine (salazosulfapyridine, salicylazosulfapyridine, suphasalazine; Apo-Sulfasalazine, Azulfidine, Azulfidine EN-Tabs, PMS-Sulfasalazine, Salazopyrin, Salazopyrin EN-Tabs, SAS).
Extrapolated, based on similar properties: Sodium sulfacetamide (AK-Sulf, Bleph-10, Sodium Sulamyd), sulfamethoxazole (Gantanol), sulfanilamide (AVC), sulfisoxazole (Gantrisin), triple sulfa (Sultrin Triple Sulfa).
See also Trimethoprim-Sulfamethoxazole and Nonsteroidal Anti-Inflammatory Drugs (NSAIDs).

Interaction Type and Significance
≈≈≈   Drug-Induced Nutrient Depletion, Supplementation Therapeutic, Not Requiring Professional Management
≈≈   Drug-Induced Adverse Effect on Nutrient Function, Coadministration

◇   Therapeutic, Not Requiring Professional
       Management

◈   Adverse Drug Effect on Nutritional
       Therapeutics, Strategic Concern

☼   Prevention or Reduction of Drug Adverse Effect

Probability: Evidence Base:

5. Improbable or   ◉ Emerging to
   3. Possible   ● Consensus

Effect and Mechanism of Action

Sulfonamides, including sulfasalazine, interfere with the absorption, bioavailability, and activity of folic acid, as well as adversely affecting vitamin B_6 and vitamin K. Sulfasalazine can impair absorption and transport of folic acid and dietary folate, most likely acting as a competitive inhibitor.[314,336-338] The target of sulfonamides, and the basis for their selectivity, is the enzyme dihydropteroate synthase (DHPS) in the folic acid pathway.[339] Sulfasalazine also inhibits other folate-dependent enzymes, particularly dihydrofolate reductase, methylenetetrahydrofolate reductase, and serine transhydroxymethylase, as discussed earlier with interactions involving NSAIDs as a class. Animal research indicates that "sulfasalazine interferes with a folate recognition site which is common to these enzymes and to the intestinal transport system."[313] Sulfasalazine-induced blood dyscrasias might involve folic acid depletion. "The mechanisms by which sulfasalazine antagonizes folate metabolism are dose-dependent and, consequently, higher doses might precipitate folate deficiency."[340]

Research

Sulfasalazine is well known for adversely affecting folate, but some controversy exists as to whether the drug by itself can cause clinically significant deficiencies of folic acid. Megaloblastic anemia caused by sulfasalazine has responded to drug withdrawal alone.[341] However, a high proportion of the literature indicates a multifactorial causality for folate depletion in the affected populations, with the adverse effects of sulfasalazine being an important but not necessarily adequate stress. The conditions for which sulfasalazine is typically prescribed are often associated with malabsorption, poor diet, old age, and chronic inflammation. For example, a high proportion of individuals with inflammatory bowel disease and ulcerative colitis exhibit compromised folate status.[342]

In addition to the increased risks associated with hyperhomocysteinemia resulting from drug-induced folate deficiency, the association between folate status and colorectal cancer risk may be especially relevant to individuals in such populations. Ulcerative colitis, folate-related polymorphisms, and folate deficiency have all been linked to an increased risk for colon cancer.[343-348] A wide range of authors further suggest that increased folate intake may play a preventive (and/or therapeutic) role against some colorectal cancers.[348-354] Significant research demonstrates the contributory role of sulfasalazine in the etiology of folate deficiency among patients treated for ulcerative colitis. However, other evidence suggests that although sulfasalazine impairs folate absorption among such patients, "this only becomes significant if other reasons for folate deficiency are also present."[336,355] Thus, optimal folate status represents an important factor in the therapeutic strategy for care of patients with ulcerative colitis and irritable bowel disease and increased risk for colorectal cancer.

The available evidence indicates that the risk of clinically significant folate deficiency may not be high among patients treated with sulfasalazine generally, but that high doses increase adverse effects, including deficiency, and that folate deficiency could play a significant role in both GI and overall disease risk. However, a review of the range of human studies in this area also suggests that the researchers' choices for laboratory measures to assess absorption and metabolism folate and their implications may be influential in shaping the findings and conclusions.

In 1981, Halsted et al.[336] found that sulfasalazine inhibits the absorption of folates in patients with ulcerative colitis. In 1982, Longstreth and Green[342] analyzed hematological data, including serum and RBC folate assays, from 45 outpatients with chronic colitis, 27 of whom were receiving maintenance doses of sulfasalazine. Mean hemoglobin, hematocrit, serum folate, and RBC folate levels were similar overall in sulfasalazine users and nonusers. However, among the sulfasalazine users, "RBC folate was inversely correlated with drug dose; serum folate was not," and those "taking 2 g or more of sulfasalazine daily had lower mean RBC folate levels (221.2 ± 27.3 ng/mL) than patients either taking less (371.7 ± 35.0 ng/mL) or nonusers (330.3 ± 30.3 ng/mL)." Also, mean RBC corpuscular volume (MCV) was related to drug dose but not to RBC folate. The authors concluded: "Although maintenance sulfasalazine use rarely causes clinically significant folate deficiency, subclinical tissue depletion occurs as a dose-related effect."[342]

In a case-control study of patients with chronic ulcerative colitis, Lashner et al.[356] found a 62% lower risk of colon cancer with folate supplementation, compared to ulcerative colitis patients who did not supplement with folic acid. In a later study involving 98 patients with ulcerative colitis, Lashner and a different team[357] found that individuals who have ulcerative colitis and who supplement folic acid had a 55% lower risk of developing colon cancer. The dose of folate varied with the risk of neoplasia, and folate use also varied with the degree of dysplasia. Although these findings were not statistically significant, the authors concluded that daily folate supplementation may protect against the development of dysplasia or neoplasia in ulcerative colitis patients. Although diverse factors contribute to colon cancer, many researchers suggest that folic acid deficiency may increase susceptibility, and that folic acid supplementation and enhanced dietary folate intake may have a preventive effect.

The implications of sulfasalazine therapy on folate status in patients treated for rheumatoid arthritis (RA) parallel those of patients with bowel disorders. In a prospective study of 30 subjects, Grindulis and McConkey[340] investigated the effects of sulfasalazine on folate deficiency in RA patients, who often have low serum and RBC folate concentrations. Pretreatment serum and RBC folate concentrations were low-normal. They administered 2 g sulphasalazine over 24 weeks, using 500 mg penicillamine daily for controls, although knowledge of possible interactions between folate status and penicillamine is incomplete. No change was observed in serum and RBC folate concentrations in either group. However, MCV increased only in patients taking sulfasalazine, possibly reflecting reticulocytosis secondary to drug-induced hemolysis. Measurement of reticulocyte counts might clarify any future investigation in this area.

In 1996, Krogh Jensen et al.[315] analyzed plasma total homocysteine (tHcy, as a sensitive marker of folate deficiency), serum folate, erythrocyte (RBC) folate, serum cobalamin, and routine indices of hemolysis in 25 arthritis outpatients treated with sulfasalazine, to assess the frequency of folate deficiency and hemolysis among such patients. Notably, none of the subjects had taken folate-containing vitamins for at least 8 weeks preceding the trial; it is unclear whether this was by exclusion design or simply reflective of the patient population. The control group consisted of 72 healthy hospital staff. The patient group exhibited median plasma tHcy that was significantly higher than controls, with five patients (20%) having plasma tHcy levels that exceeded the upper-normal limit. Median serum folate was significantly lower in the patient group, with 11 patients (40%) exhibiting depressed serum folate. Notably, there was no difference in the levels of RBC folate between the two groups, and only three patients (12%) had RBC folate values below the reference interval. Furthermore, no patient had cobalamin deficiency, as assessed by serum cobalamin and methylmalonate, but the treated group exhibited significantly lower S-cobalamin levels. These findings also indicate it is "unlikely that any patient had increased plasma tHcy due to cobalamin deficiency." The authors also reported that 12 of the 24 treated subjects in whom HbA_{1c} was measured had decreased levels indicating chronic hemolysis. They proposed that the chronic hemolysis caused by sulfasalazine "might explain the similar RBC folate values in the two groups because of a relatively higher folate content of young erythrocytes." The authors concluded that observed patterns in plasma tHcy among those treated with sulfasalazine "suggest that a substantial number of patients may have folate deficiency at the tissue level."[315] Their findings also demonstrate the need for determination of and testing with sensitive indicators of folate status, which RBC folate does not appear to be.

Initial research indicates that drug-induced effects on folate are not likely to have teratogenic effects, but evidence is limited and inconclusive. In a population-based case-control study of the safety of sulfasalazine use during pregnancy, Norgard et al.[357a] found no significant increased prevalence of selected congenital abnormalities in the children of women treated with sulfasalazine during pregnancy. Further research is warranted.

Reports
In 1986, Logan et al.[358] reported that sulfasalazine-associated pancytopenia may be caused by acute folate deficiency. They described three patients who, after taking sulfasalazine for more than 2 years, "suddenly developed severe pancytopenia with gross megaloblastic changes in the marrow." Administration of "high dose oral folic acid" achieved a "good response" in two patients, "but the third required folinic acid." The authors proposed acute folate deficiency as the apparent mechanism involved, noting that "the requirement for folinic acid in one case suggests that the known inhibition of folate metabolism by sulphasalazine also contributes." Furthermore, they observed that "the syndrome appears to be associated with high dosage and slow acetylator status." Subsequently, therapy was well tolerated in two patients after the drug was "restarted at reduced dosage with folate supplements"; both patients were "slow acetylators." The progression of disease in the third patient, however, led to colectomy, and her acetylator status was not determined.

In a 1999 review, Hoshino et al.[359] reported a case of ulcerative colitis with folate-deficient megaloblastic anemia induced by sulfasalazine.

Nutritional Therapeutics, Clinical Concerns, and Adaptations
Physicians prescribing sulfasalazine for longer than 2 weeks should be alert to risk factors for compromised folate status,

monitor blood and tissue folate levels using sensitive indicators, and coadminister folic acid, typically 500 to 600 µg twice daily, when appropriate. Folate has no known risks at the suggested levels and can potentially provide a number of benefits to those taking sulfasalazine. In particular, folate supplementation during sulfasalazine administration is recommended, especially to reduce the risk of dysplasia or cancer in patients with ulcerative colitis. Recommendations within conventional practice have favored high-folate foods rather than folic acid supplements, but increased intake through both forms seems reasonable and more likely to be effective. Clinically significant adverse effects are improbable with sulfasalazine therapy of 2 weeks or less. Even though evidence of heightened risks during pregnancy is lacking, prudence suggests that all women undergoing sulfasalazine therapy supplement with 1000 µg or more of folic acid for 6 months before becoming pregnant and continuing throughout pregnancy.

The available research consistently demonstrates that sulfasalazine exerts multiple adverse effects on folate and suggests that such antagonistic effects on folate metabolism are dose dependent. Consequently, higher doses (and longer duration of treatment) will tend to increase risk and degree of adverse effects and might precipitate folate deficiency. Such risks increase in patients with genetic predispositions to folate metabolism dysfunctions or other factors contributing to compromised folate status. Given the low cost and nontoxic nature of folic acid, enhanced intake (via supplements or foods) represents a simple, low-risk adjunctive therapy for every patient taking sulfasalazine, unless otherwise indicated.

Tetracycline Antibiotics (Systemic)

Demeclocycline (Declomycin), doxycycline (Atridox, Doryx, Doxy, Monodox, Periostat, Vibramycin, Vibra-Tabs), minocycline (Dynacin, Minocin, Vectrin), oxytetracycline (Terramycin), tetracycline (Achromycin, Actisite, Apo-Tetra, Economycin, Novo-Tetra, Nu-Tetra, Sumycin, Tetrachel, Tetracyn); combination drugs: chlortetracycline, demeclocycline, and tetracycline (Deteclo); bismuth, metronidazole, and tetracycline (Helidac).

Interaction Type and Significance

⊕⊕   **Beneficial or Supportive Interaction, with Professional Management**

⊕✗   **Bimodal or Variable Interaction, with Professional Management**

◇◇   **Impaired Drug Absorption and Bioavailability, Precautions Appropriate**

◇≈≈   **Drug-Induced Adverse Effect on Nutrient Function, Coadministration Therapeutic, with Professional Management**

Probability:
5. Improbable or
3. Possible

Evidence Base:
◉ **Emerging** to
● **Consensus**

Effect and Mechanism of Action
The several mechanisms of interaction between the tetracycline class of antibiotics and folic acid are complex and conflicting, depending on dose, duration, timing, and patient characteristics. Folic acid may interfere with the absorption and effectiveness of tetracycline antibiotics if ingested simultaneously, and vice versa.[360] Tetracyclines inhibit bacterial protein synthesis by binding to the 30S ribosome, blocking access of the aminoacyl tRNAs at the "A" acceptor site on the mRNA-ribosome complex. These drugs may interfere with the activity

and induce the depletion of folic acid and other nutrients, particularly other B vitamins.[361] Additionally, extended or recurrent use of antibiotics can cause folate depletion by eliminating the healthy intestinal flora, a major source of endogenous biosynthesis of folate (and B_{12}).[362,363] Many patients with conditions for which tetracyclines are prescribed have depleted folate nutriture.

Research

Omray and Varma[360] demonstrated that oral administration of a vitamin C– and vitamin B–complex formulation could impair absorption and reduce bioavailability of tetracycline hydrochloride through pharmacokinetic interference. However, numerous clinicians and authors fail to mention such risks or advise appropriate corrective measures in discussions of coadministration of these agents.

Some patient populations receiving antibiotic therapy have pathophysiological conditions, medical history, and lifestyle/dietary factors characterized by malnutrition, malabsorption, or nutrient depletion. For example, evidence spanning four decades indicates that tetracyclines and folic acid may provide enhanced therapeutic efficacy in many situations (e.g., treatment of tropical sprue), but that separation of oral intake may be essential to efficacy.[364] Westergaard[365] summarizes the evolution and rationale of the primary treatment strategy as follows:

> Patients with tropical sprue typically present with macrocytic anemia due to malabsorption of folate and/or vitamin B_{12}. Treatment of tropical sprue with folic acid replacement was introduced more than 50 years ago and has become standard medical treatment. Vitamin B_{12} replacement is usually added if there is evidence of B_{12} deficiency or malabsorption. Treatment of tropical sprue with folate and B_{12} cures the macrocytic anemia and the accompanying glossitis, and often results in increased appetite and weight gain. However, even prolonged treatment with these vitamins fails to restore villus atrophy, and malabsorption usually persists. The benefit of antibiotic treatment of tropical sprue was first documented during World War II, when sulfonamides were used to treat epidemics of tropical sprue in British and Italian troops in India. Antibiotic treatment has since become the standard treatment, and tetracycline has replaced sulfonamides. The recommended length of treatment with tetracycline is 6 months and it is given in combination with folate.

Reports

Similarly, in a discussion of several cases of tropical sprue among indigenous patients in Australia, with a history of excessive alcohol intake and characterized by alteration in the intestinal microflora, overgrowth of coliform bacteria, mucosal damage and malabsorption, and protein loss, Hanson[366] recommended that concomitant tetracycline use, specifically doxycycline, and folic acid therapy "can be rapidly and dramatically effective, although the tetracycline course should continue for 3-6 months."

Note: Falsely low serum folate concentrations may occur with the *Lactobacillus casei* assay method in patients receiving tetracycline therapy.

Nutritional Therapeutics, Clinical Concerns, and Adaptations

Physicians prescribing tetracycline antimicrobials, repeatedly or for more than 2 weeks, are advised to coadminister folic acid; a moderate supplemental dose of 400 to 800 μg/day typically is adequate. These levels may also be obtained through a diet rich in leafy green vegetables, beans, beets, citrus, meat, and wheat germ. The importance of such nutrient support is

amplified in pregnant women and individuals with compromised nutritional status or a history of high alcohol intake.

No evidence demonstrates an increased risk for major birth defects in children exposed to tetracycline in the first trimester of pregnancy. Nevertheless, tetracyclines are generally contraindicated after the first trimester of pregnancy (and in children <8 years old) because they tend to cause staining of teeth, hypoplasia of dental enamel, and abnormal bone growth in children and in the fetuses of pregnant women.

Coadministration of probiotic flora along with vitamins B_{12} and K is usually appropriate. The aim of an integrative approach combining tetracycline, folate, and vitamin B_{12} is to restore intestinal mucosal structure, normalize absorptive function, correct folate and B_{12} deficiencies, and correct any macrocytic anemia.

In most patients, only the probiotic flora are appropriate when a shorter course of a tetracycline (7-10 days) is administered as a countermeasure to the antibiotic-induced disruption of healthy intestinal ecology. Regular supplementation with vigorous cultures of *Lactobacillus acidophilus, Bifidobacterium bifidus,* and other probiotic bacteria for 2 to 4 weeks can safely and effectively preclude or reverse subsequent antibiotic-induced folate depletion; up to 6 months of probiotic intake may be necessary to fully reestablish the symbiotic intestinal flora in patients receiving more than one course of antibiotics.

Tetracycline should be administered at least 2 hours before or 4 hours after oral intake of folic acid, alone or as part of a B-complex or multivitamin formulation, to avoid interference with gastric absorption. Evidence for such an adverse interaction is minimal, but prudence suggests that such simple precautions may be beneficial.

Triamterene and Related Potassium-Sparing Diuretics

Evidence: Triamterene (Dyrenium).
Extrapolated, based on similar properties: Amiloride (Midamor), spironolactone (Aldactone); combination drugs: amiloride and hydrochlorothiazide (Moduretic); spironolactone and hydrochlorothiazide (Aldactazide); triamterene and hydrochlorothiazide (Dyazide, Maxzide).

Interaction Type and Significance

◇≈≈ **Drug-Induced Adverse Effect on Nutrient Function, Coadministration Therapeutic, with Professional Management**

≈≈≈ **Drug-Induced Nutrient Depletion, Supplementation Therapeutic, Not Requiring Professional Management**

◇ **Adverse Drug Effect on Nutritional Therapeutics, Strategic Concern**

⊕⊕ **Beneficial or Supportive Interaction, with Professional Management**

Probability:	Evidence Base:
3. Possible	◉ **Emerging** to
	● **Consensus**

Effect and Mechanism of Action

Triamterene impairs folate absorption and bioavailability and may contribute to folate depletion, at least in part because of its structural similarity to folic acid. Animal research also found that triamterene acted as a competitive inhibitor of folate absorption in the rat intestine.[367] Triamterene also acts as a relatively weak folate antagonist by inhibiting dihydrofolate reductase, which is necessary to converting unreduced dietary folates into tetrahydrofolates, the biologically active folates. Triamterene has been known to contribute to the appearance of megaloblastosis in patients with decreased folic acid stores.[114,368-370]

Research

For more than four decades, researchers have investigated the mechanisms as well as the frequency and circumstances of clinically significant triamterene-induced adverse effects on folate, particularly teratogenesis and hyperhomocysteinemia. In 1967, Maass et al.[371] first investigated the effect of triamterene on folic reductase activity and reproduction in the rat. In 1986, Zimmerman et al.[367] investigated the effect of triamterene on folic acid absorption in the rat jejunum. Applying an in vivo intestinal loop method, triamterene inhibited the intestinal absorption of folic acid in a dose-dependent fashion, with 50% inhibition of systemic absorption occurring at a luminal concentration of 0.01 mmol/L of triamterene. However, animal studies are not always predictive of human response.

Schalhorn et al.[368] documented the dose-related inhibitory effect of triamterene and its metabolites on human leukocyte dihydrofolate reductase. The authors concluded by emphasizing the potential significance of these findings in relation to "the possible toxic side effects of long-term triamterene treatment in patients suffering from alcoholic cirrhosis, who may have impaired metabolism of triamterene and a concomitant severe folate deficiency."

Mason et al.[372] studied 272 elderly individuals in two free-living populations receiving chronic diuretic therapy and found normal folic acid levels and no signs of folic acid deficiency among 32 patients who used triamterene at unknown dose levels on a long-term basis, but lacked additional risks for folic acid deficiency. The possibility of confounding variables limits the strength of findings from this observational study.

The administration of multivitamin supplements containing folic acid appears to diminish the occurrence of birth defects associated with periconception exposure to triamterene and other folic acid antagonists.[373] Hernández-Díaz et al.[76] investigated possible adverse effects of a broad range of folic acid antagonists (including trimethoprim, triamterene, carbamazepine, phenobarbital, and primidone) during pregnancy in an ongoing case-control study of birth defects (1979–1998) in the United States and Canada. First, they studied the exposure to folic acid antagonists that act as dihydrofolate reductase inhibitors (including triamterene) and to certain antiepileptic drugs in 3870 infants with cardiovascular defects, 1962 infants with oral clefts, and 1100 infants with urinary tract defects; the control group consisted of 6249 infants with structural defects and 2138 infants with chromosomal or mendelian defects. The authors determined that the "relative risks of cardiovascular defects and oral clefts in infants whose mothers were exposed to dihydrofolate reductase inhibitors during the second or third month after the last menstrual period, as compared with infants whose mothers had no such exposure, were 3.4 and 2.6 respectively." Furthermore, they observed that the "use of multivitamin supplements containing folic acid diminished the adverse effects of dihydrofolate reductase inhibitors, but not that of antiepileptic drugs."[76] Subsequently, these researchers examined related data to determine whether periconception exposure to folic acid antagonists (FAAs) might increase the risk of neural tube defects (NTDs), specifically spina bifida, anencephaly, and encephalocele. Their findings suggest that "a number of FAAs may increase NTD risk, and they provide estimates of risk for selected drugs."[79] However,

these data concerned a number of folate antagonists and, as such, are limited in their applicability to triamterene.

A probable link between hypertension and folate deficiency, via homocysteine (Hcy), suggests that any adverse effects by diuretics on folate status could contribute to increased risk for cardiovascular disease. Comparing blood samples from 17 hypertensive patients receiving long-term diuretic therapy and 17 hypertensive patients not taking diuretics, Morrow and Grimsley[374] observed that, in general, long-term diuretic therapy (>6 months) is associated with a significant increase in serum Hcy concentration and a significant decrease in RBC folate concentration. In 2005, Forman et al.[266] found that higher total folate intake was associated with a decreased risk of incident hypertension, particularly in younger women.

Reports

Case reports in the literature describe patients, particularly with cirrhosis or otherwise-compromised liver function, who developed megaloblastic anemia while being treated with triamterene, most often at higher doses (150-600 mg/day).[114,375]

Nutritional Therapeutics, Clinical Concerns, and Adaptations

Patients receiving antihypertensive therapy using triamterene or related diuretics may benefit from the Hcy-lowering effects of folic acid, particularly if they have a history of, or significant risk factors for, inadequate folate intake, nutrient depletion, or hyperhomocysteinemia. Such concomitant nutrient support may be prudent, even though evidence indicates that triamterene at typical doses is not likely to affect folate status to a clinically significant degree in most patients. Folate supplementation during (or before) pregnancy is essential, and an increased dose may be warranted in women treated with triamterene; other treatment options might also need to be considered.

Even though the research thus far indicates adverse effects from triamterene in patients with folate deficiency, it is important to note that the diet of a significant portion of the population in the United States, Canada, the United Kingdom, and similar settings does not provide the recommended levels of folate. Assessment of tissue folate and plasma tHcy levels, within the context of the individual patient's risk factors including (e.g., diet, family history, genomic polymorphisms), is essential to shaping a customized and evolving integrative strategy for prevention and treatment of cardiovascular disease.

A therapeutic strategy incorporating coadministration of folic acid might require using 5-MTHF, the vitamin's activated form, such as folinic acid, in some patients, because triamterene interferes with the vitamin's activation, thus rendering common folic acid supplements potentially ineffective. Research is lacking to confirm or disprove this possibility.

Trimethoprim-Sulfamethoxazole

Cotrimoxazole and related trimethoprim-containing antibiotics: Trimethoprim (Proloprim, Trimpex); combination drug: trimethoprim and sulfamethoxazole (cotrimoxazole, co-trimoxazole, SXT, TMP-SMX, TMP-sulfa; Bactrim, Bactrim DS, Cotrim, Septra, Septra DS, Sulfatrim, Uroplus). Related drugs: Dapsone (DDS, diaminodiphenylsulphone; Aczone; Avlosulfon), sulfonamides, sulfones.

Interaction Type and Significance

≈≈ **Drug-Induced Nutrient Depletion,**
       Supplementation Therapeutic, with
       Professional Management

◇ ≈ ≈   Drug-Induced Adverse Effect on Nutrient
         Function, Coadministration Therapeutic, with
         Professional Management
☼   Prevention or Reduction of Drug Adverse Effect
⊕✗   Bimodal or Variable Interaction, with
         Professional Management
✗   Potential or Theoretical Adverse Interaction of
         Uncertain Severity

Probability: Evidence Base:
3. Possible to 2. Probable   ◉ Emerging to ●
                                  Consensus

Effect and Mechanism of Action

Trimethoprim and sulfamethoxazole (cotrimoxazole) interfere with the bacterial biosynthesis of folic acid by inhibiting tetrahydrofolate synthesis.[376] Trimethoprim acts as folate antagonist by inhibiting dihydrofolate reductase, which is necessary to converting unreduced dietary folates into tetrahydrofolates, the biologically active form.[377,378] It is generally considered that trimethoprim inhibits the bacterial enzyme more efficiently than the human enzyme (sensitivity of bacterial enzyme 10000-fold > mammalian), and therefore the drug theoretically has only a minimal risk of adverse effects on biosynthesis of folic acid in humans. However, the risk of folate depletion and inhibition of granulopoiesis can be significant with high-dose or prolonged use, presumably more so in the presence of folate deficiency; neutropenia may result. Sulfamethoxazole and other sulfonamides interfere with folate by competitively displacing PABA from its binding site on dihydropteroate synthase, the enzyme that catalyzes a key step in the biosynthesis of folic acid.[379] Teratogenicity and macrocytic anemia are known adverse effects associated with cotrimoxazole-induced folate deficiency.

Concomitant intake of folic acid at high doses could theoretically decrease efficacy of trimethoprim and sulfamethoxazole because of antagonistic effects. Coadministration of 5-methyltetrahydrofolate (5-MTHF), such as folinic acid (leucovorin calcium), instead of folic acid, is usually appropriate given the inhibition of dihydrofolate reductase by the antibiotics.

Research

Sulfamethoxazole and trimethoprim are known inhibitors of tetrahydrofolate synthesis and may partially deplete reduced folate levels.[376,377] Furthermore, folic acid deficiency increases risks of toxicity from these agents. This interaction is widely acknowledged. Trimethoprim-sulfamethoxazole (TMP-SMX) is associated with folic acid deficiency anemia, but the incidence of this adverse effect is generally believed to be rare. Overall, consensus has yet to emerge as to the frequency, severity, and circumstances of clinically significant events or management of potential interference between trimethoprim and folic acid.

Kahn et al.[377] found that administration of trimethoprim (1 g/day) for more than 14 days appears to impair folate utilization to some extent, which may lead to hematological changes reversible with folic acid (400 µg/day). Bjornson et al.[380] conducted two linked studies investigating the antifolate action contributing to the neutropenia occasionally observed in patients treated with TMP-SMX. First, they administered TMP-SMX to 12 healthy adults and observed that the "number of circulating granulocytes and granulocyte progenitors was not significantly altered by a 5-day course of therapy." However, they conducted experiments that simulated the in vivo condition of folate deficiency to investigate the antifolate action of these drugs on circulating granulocyte precursors

(CFU-C) from normal donors and the mechanism of inhibition on granulopoiesis. Trimethoprim (8 µg/mL) resulted in a 47% decrease in the total number of colonies, whereas the combination of 8 µg/mL trimethoprim and 40 µg/mL sulfamethoxazole resulted in a 52% decrease in the number of colonies. In both situations, adding folinic acid to the culture prevented this inhibitory effect. In contrast, sulfamethoxazole (40 µg/mL) alone exerted "no discernible effect on granulopoiesis."[380]

In a study of 12 AIDS/HIV patients with or suspected of *Pneumocystis carinii* pneumonia, Bygbjerg et al.[381] found that neither folic acid nor folinic acid reversed cotrimoxazole-induced cytopenia. They concluded, however, that although "routine prescription of folinic acid is not recommended," supplementation with folic acid is inexpensive and "may be beneficial and should be prescribed." Subsequently, Safrin et al.[382] reported that coadministration of folinic acid with TMP-SMX for *P. carinii* pneumonia in AIDS patients is associated with an increased risk of therapeutic failure and decreased survival rate.

No evidence has appeared to support the proposition that administration of folic acid or an activated 5-MTHF might significantly impair the therapeutic activity of trimethoprim or sulfamethoxazole. It is now generally accepted that concomitant folic acid, in typical doses, does not interfere with the antibacterial activity of trimethoprim or TMP-SMX.[383,384]

Reports

Numerous case reports have described "neutropenia developing during even brief periods of oral therapy, particularly in individuals with either folate deficiency or increased folate requirements."[380]

Nutritional Therapeutics, Clinical Concerns, and Adaptations

Physicians prescribing trimethoprim and sulfamethoxazole, alone or in combination, should be aware that these agents may impair folate metabolism to a clinically significant extent. Concomitant folate may prevent or reverse adverse effects on folate activity and hematopoietic processes but generally is not necessary unless the patient has a preexisting folate deficiency, increased folate requirements, or otherwise-compromised folate status. Trimethoprim and TMP-SMX should be prescribed with caution in patients with known or potential folic acid deficiency; close supervision and regular monitoring of folate status are warranted.

Although some researchers and clinicians suggest that administration of folinic acid (leucovorin calcium) may be necessary to achieve such effects, because of drug-induced inhibition of dihydrofolate reductase, others have found that folic acid can usually achieve a therapeutic response. Pharmacogenomic variants related to folate metabolic pathways may also influence which form is required. Other forms of 5-methyltetrahydrofolate, such as 6(S) 5-MTHF (L-methyl folate or Metafolin), would be expected to be equally efficacious.

Many authorities caution against use of trimethoprim and sulfamethoxazole during pregnancy. Concomitant folic acid becomes imperative if such medications are necessary during pregnancy, with a dose of at least 800 µg/day being appropriate.

Zidovudine/AZT

Zidovudine (azidothymidine, AZT, ZDV, zidothymidine; Retrovir); combination drugs: zidovudine, and lamivudine (Combivir); abacavir, lamivudine, and zidovudine (Trizivir).

Interaction Type and Significance

⬦≈≈ Drug-Induced Adverse Effect on Nutrient
      Function, Coadministration Therapeutic, with
      Professional Management

≈≈   Drug-Induced Nutrient Depletion,
      Supplementation Therapeutic, with
      Professional Management

☼   Prevention or Reduction of Drug Adverse Effect

Probability: Evidence Base:
2. Probable to 1. Certain   ● Consensus

Effect and Mechanism of Action

Hematological toxicity is the most common adverse effect related to long-term administration of zidovudine (AZT), with macrocytosis developing in a large majority of AZT-treated subjects, despite folate and vitamin B_{12} supplementation. The macrocytosis is caused by AZT interfering with DNA replication in bone marrow RBC precursors. As a nucleoside analog, AZT interferes with HIV DNA production by reverse transcriptase, but also with non-HIV DNA as well. Folate and B_{12} deficiency leads to RBC macrocytosis, also by interfering with DNA synthesis, but based on deficiency versus toxicity. Consequently, administration of folate/B_{12} may fail to ameliorate AZT's hematological toxicity.

Research

In a rodent model using CBA/Ca mice, Cronkite et al.[385] found that "higher doses of folate given daily" resulted in partial amelioration of AZT-induced macrocytic anemia. A B_{12}/folate regimen was ineffectual.

In several placebo-controlled studies, macrocytosis, anemia, and granulocytopenia were the most significant adverse effects associated with zidovudine use, especially among patients with advanced, symptomatic HIV disease. Significant anemia most often occurred after 4 to 6 weeks of therapy and in many cases required dose adjustment, discontinuation of zidovudine, or blood transfusions.[386] In 2002, Romanelli et al.[387] conducted a retrospective chart review in an outpatient HIV clinic and concluded that "macrocytosis may be useful in assessing adherence to zidovudine-containing antiretroviral regimens."

Manfredi et al.[388] investigated the kinetics of modifications of some hematological parameters of erythroid series in 65 patients with HIV infection treated with AZT for a mean duration of 7.6 months and correlated the observed evolution of these laboratory changes with the onset of severe anemia. They reported "no correlation between an elevated mean corpuscular volume and the development of severe anaemia (Hb less than or equal to 9 g/dL) in an individual patient; a fall in the reticulocyte count appears to be the earliest peripheral blood sign of the development of bone marrow toxicity."

In 1993, Snower and Weil[389] studied 100 consecutive inpatients in a large metropolitan urban hospital with mean corpuscular volumes greater than 110 fL. Of these, 44% were AIDS patients receiving zidovudine, 19% were alcoholic patients, and 12% had malignant neoplasms. Only 3% were folate deficient and 4% vitamin B_{12} deficient by conventional measures. The authors concluded that "zidovudine has become the most common cause of macrocytosis in the hospitalized urban patient population," and "vitamin B_{12} and folate deficiencies have decreased in proportion."

However, in a prospective, randomized study involving 60 HIV-infected patients receiving zidovudine, Falguera et al.[390] compared hematological toxicity of either ZDV (AZT, 500 mg daily) alone or in combination with folinic acid (15 mg daily)

and intramascular vitamin B_{12} (1000 µg monthly). During the study, vitamin B_{12} and folate levels were significantly higher in vitamin-treated patients, but no differences in hemoglobin, hematocrit, mean corpuscular volume, or white cell, neutrophil, or platelet count were observed between groups at 3, 6, 9, and 12 months. Moreover, they observed "severe hematologic toxicity" in four zidovudine-only patients and seven assigned to the vitamin-treated group. They reported "no correlation between vitamin B_{12} or folate levels and development of myelosuppression." The authors concluded that coadministration of vitamin B_{12} and folinic acid with AZT therapy "does not seem useful in preventing or reducing ZDV-induced myelotoxicity in the overall treated population, although a beneficial effect in certain subgroups of patients cannot be excluded."[390]

Nutritional Therapeutics, Clinical Concerns, and Adaptations

Physicians prescribing zidovudine/AZT are advised to monitor closely the folate and vitamin B_{12} status of patients, using sensitive indicators capable of accurately assessing hematological and tissue levels of these vitamins and their functional surrogates, such as homocysteine and methylmalonate. Concomitant administration of folic acid (or 5-MTHF) and B_{12} may be appropriate to prevent or reverse adverse effects, with prophylactic measures generally being prudent in patients with a history of folate deficiency, compromised nutritional status, or other risk factors for susceptibility. However, clinical experience and research indicate that such nutrient support is often inadequate in reducing macrocytosis and marrow suppression in many patients, and that modification of the drug regimen is often necessary.

THEORETICAL, SPECULATIVE, AND PRELIMINARY INTERACTIONS RESEARCH, INCLUDING OVERSTATED INTERACTIONS CLAIMS

Acyclovir

Acyclovir (Zovirax)

Acyclovir is a synthetic purine nucleoside analog that achieves its antiviral activity by acting as a purine antagonist, and it is known to induce macrocytic nonmegaloblastic anemia. The mechanism of interaction with folic acid, when it occurs, appears to be direct bone marrow toxicity, rather than being mediated through a folate interaction. However, concomitant folate deficiency would very likely compound any drug toxicity and should therefore be avoided.

Close monitoring of folate status through sensitive indicators is prudent, especially in patients on long-term acyclovir therapy who have a history of folate deficiency, compromised nutritional status, or other risk factors for susceptibility.

Antibiotics

Antibiotics

See also individual agents or classes.

Along with the serious issue of multidrug antibiotic resistance, the loss or impairment of endogenous production of B vitamins, including folate, is one of the most important adverse effects resulting from a substantial course of antibiotics, by significantly damaging or destroying the symbiotic bacterial flora of the intestinal microbiota. *Acidophilus*, bifidobacteria, and other enteral bacteria manufacture folic acid and other B vitamins, such as niacin, biotin, and vitamin B_6.[391-401]

The effects of antibiotics as a broad grouping of agents and drug classes on folate status is more accurately described as "unresearched" rather than unproven. Although knowledge and appreciation of the manifold functions of healthy bacteria have grown exponentially in recent years, the full clinical significance is not yet understood. Continued research into the systemic long-term effects of broad-spectrum antimicrobials is warranted, with implications on the functions and activity of folic acid deserving special attention.

Concomitant or subsequent administration of folic acid, vitamin B$_{12}$, and large doses of vigorous variegated probiotic flora provides a safe and inexpensive means of supporting healthy gut ecology and nutrient metabolism to prevent or correct direct and indirect adverse effects from antibiotic therapy, particularly in high doses or with repeated or long-term courses.

Beta-Adrenergic Blocking Agents and Calcium Channel Blockers (Systemic)

Beta-1-adrenergic blocking agents (beta-1 antagonists): Acebutolol (Sectral), atenolol (Tenormin); combination drugs: atenolol and chlorthalidone (Co-Tendione, Tenoretic), atenolol and nifedipine (Beta-Adalat, Tenif); betaxolol (Kerlone), bisoprolol (Zebeta), carteolol (Cartrol), esmolol (Brevibloc), labetalol (Normodyne, Trandate), metoprolol (Lopressor, Toprol XL); combination drug: metoprolol and hydrochlorothiazide (Lopressor HCT); nadolol (Corgard), nebivolol (Nebilet), oxprenolol (Trasicor), penbutolol (Levatol), pindolol (Visken), propranolol (Betachron, Inderal LA, Innopran XL, Inderal); combination drug: propranolol and bendrofluazide (Inderex); sotalol (Betapace, Betapace AF, Sorine), timolol (Blocadren).
Similar properties but evidence indicating no or reduced interaction effects:

Beta-adrenergic blocking eyedrops (ophthalmic forms): Betaxolol (Betoptic), carteolol (Cartrol, Ocupress), levobunolol (Betagan), metipranolol (OptiPranolol), timolol (Timoptic).

Calcium channel blockers: Amlodipine (Norvasc); combination drug: amlodipine and benazepril (Lotrel); bepridil (Bapadin, Vascor), diltiazem (Cardizem, Cardizem CD, Cardizem SR, Cartia XT, Dilacor XR, Diltia XT, Tiamate, Tiazac), felodipine (Plendil); combination drugs: felodipine and enalapril (Lexxel), felodipine and ramipril (Triapin); gallopamil (D600), isradipine (DynaCirc, DynaCirc CR), lercanidipine (Zanidip), nicardipine (Cardene, Cardene I.V., Cardene SR), nifedipine (Adalat, Adalat CC, Nifedical XL, Procardia, Procardia XL); combination drug: nifedipine and atenolol (Beta-Adalat, Tenif); nimodipine (Nimotop), nisoldipine (Sular), nitrendipine (Cardif, Nitrepin), verapamil (Calan, Calan SR, Covera-HS, Isoptin, Isoptin SR, Verelan, Verelan PM); combination drug: verapamil and trandolapril (Tarka).

Folate is essential for the metabolism of the atherogenic amino acid homocysteine (Hcy). The reduction of plasma and erythrocyte folate concentrations is also associated with a moderate hyperhomocysteinemia. Moderate hyperhomocysteinemia is an independent risk factor for cardiovascular disease that may be causal. Numerous studies have confirmed a strong association between lower folate levels and elevated Hcy and the efficacy of enhanced folate intake in the reduction of Hcy levels.[402-417]

The coadministration of folic acid with a beta blocker or calcium channel blocker may provide a synergistic effect in an integrative approach to prevention and treatment of cardiovascular disease involving atherosclerosis, especially coronary artery disease. For example, Landgren et al.[418] studied the effect on plasma Hcy of 6 weeks' treatment with daily oral folic acid doses of 2.5 or 10 mg, compared with no treatment, in patients with a recent history of myocardial infarction (MI). Folic acid lowered plasma Hcy in all but 2 of 33 treated

patients, with no difference between the effect of 2.5 and 10 mg of folic acid. In the untreated group, plasma Hcy increased in the post-MI period. Thus far, no clinical trials are available that specifically investigate the efficacy of an integrative approach combining beta blockers with nutrients such as folic acid. Such research is warranted.

Several calcium channel blockers are known to produce "clinically and histologically similar gingival enlargements in certain susceptible patients."[419] Disturbances in folate uptake are among the factors contributing to such drug-induced adverse effects. As with other drugs, the coadministration of folic acid, prophylactically or in response to symptoms, may play a role in preventing and correcting these events.

Supplementation with folic acid could lower Hcy levels and thereby reduce the risk of the cardiovascular conditions for which these medications are usually prescribed on a systemic basis. Although folic acid is essentially nontoxic, physician supervision is appropriate when introducing any new elements into the therapeutic regimen. A moderate supplemental dose of folic acid is usually about 400 µg/day, in the form of a folic acid supplement or as part of a multivitamin formula. These levels can also be obtained through a diet rich in beets, leafy green vegetables, beans, citrus, meat, and wheat germ. A higher intake level, in the range of 650 to 800 µg or greater, may be more efficacious in individuals with preexisting cardiovascular disease, a significant family history, less responsive hyperhomocysteinemia, or other risk factors. Furthermore, enhanced intake of vitamins B$_6$ and B$_{12}$, as well as betaine, is also essential because these nutrients work with folate to metabolize homocysteine.

Corticosteroids, Oral, Including Prednisone

Betamethasone (Celestone), cortisone (Cortone), dexamethasone (Decadron), fludrocortisone (Florinef), hydrocortisone (Cortef), methylprednisolone (Medrol) prednisolone (Delta-Cortef, Orapred, Pediapred, Prelone), prednisone (Deltasone, Liquid Pred, Meticorten, Orasone), triamcinolone (Aristocort). Similar properties but evidence lacking for extrapolation: Inhaled or topical corticosteroids.

Oral corticosteroids, particularly when administered for extended periods or at high dosage levels, can both decrease the activity and effects of folic acid and cause depletion of folate. Such drug-induced adverse effects on folate status may contribute to the hyperhomocysteinemia observed in some patients with autoimmune diseases, such as Crohn's disease and systemic lupus erythematosus (SLE, lupus), undergoing long-term steroid therapy.[420,421] Further research through well-designed clinical trials is warranted.

Physicians prescribing extended courses of oral corticosteroids are advised to monitor all major folate and Hcy levels in these patients. Pending substantive research through clinical trials, coadministration of folic acid, 800 µg/day, can provide a safe and potentially effective means of compensating for drug-related interference and depletion effects and can support clinical strategies toward reducing cardiovascular risk. The probability that inhaled or topical corticosteroids might cause such adverse effects is low or nonexistent, and reports or warnings are lacking in the scientific literature.

Cycloserine

Cycloserine (Seromycin).

For decades researchers have reported that cycloserine may interfere with the absorption and activity of folic acid (as well as of vitamins B$_6$ and B$_{12}$).[171,422] Case reports of folate deficiency induced by antitubercular drugs, including cycloserine, were published in the 1960s.[211] Well-designed clinical trials are lacking to confirm these preliminary and anecdotal findings, assess their clinical implications, and determine whether folic acid coadministration would effectively counter such adverse effects without impairing the therapeutic activity of the medication. Such research may be warranted. Pending further studies, coadministration of folic acid and vitamin B_{12} may be prudent with close supervision and regular monitoring.

Fluorouracil

Fluorouracil (5-FU; Adrucil, Efudex, Efudix, Fluoroplex).
See also Antifolates and Related Antimetabolites.

Folinic acid (leucovorin or Leukovorin) is a form of 5-MTHF often administered in conventional oncology care, particularly to treat metastatic colorectal cancer, enhancing the binding affinity of 5-FU to its target enzyme, thymidylate synthase (TS). In breast and other cancers, for which 5-FU is used as part of combination chemotherapy (e.g., CMF, platinum/5-FU), leucovorin is generally not used because of its increased toxicity in this context. However, leucovorin has continued to be used with 5-FU in the emerging combination chemotherapies for gastrointestinal (GI) cancers (e.g., with oxaliplatin, irinotecan). Evidence is mixed as to whether polymorphisms in the TS and dihydropyrimidine dehydrogenase (DPD) genes contribute to interpatient variability in 5-FU pharmacokinetics, response, and toxicity, although significant DPD deficiency is a well-established cause of life-threatening 5-FU toxicity.[423,424]

In 1995, Mainwaring and Grygiel[425] published case reports describing severe fluorouracil toxicity in two patients coincident with taking multivitamins containing folic acid. One patient, a woman with carcinoma of the rectum, was treated with intravenous fluorouracil (500 mg/m²) daily for 5 days, commencing a month after surgery. She was admitted at the end of the chemotherapy exhibiting numerous signs interpreted as fluorouracil toxicity, including anorexia, severe mouth ulcerations, bloody diarrhea, and vaginal bleeding. An inventory of her oral intake revealed that she was taking 5 mg folic acid within a B-complex multivitamin, as well as loperamide, sulfasalazine, hormone replacement therapy (HRT), and vitamins K and B_{12}. A month later, when chemotherapy was resumed after discontinuation of folic acid, she tolerated the treatment well, and signs of toxicity were absent. Similarly, the second patient, a man, experienced severe mouth ulceration and bloody diarrhea 2 days after starting treatment with fluorouracil for colon cancer. Discontinuation of his daily multivitamin preparation, containing 500 μg folic acid, allowed resumption of 5-FU with no such adverse effects during subsequent courses at the same dosage level. Apparently, the elevated folate levels caused by supplementation had increased the inhibition of thymidine synthesis by fluorouracil and increased the toxicity of the chemotherapeutic agent. Thus the adverse reaction in these cases resulted more from shortcomings in physician-patient communication and lack of supervision than from an irresolvable incompatibility, especially because a 5-MTHF agent such as folinic acid is much more potent than folic acid.

Although these reports do not meet the full standards of qualification, the observed events are consistent with the effects of folinic acid. Patients undergoing chemotherapy with 5-FU should be advised to avoid folic acid intake, and supplements should be inspected for its presence; a trusting therapeutic relationship and frank communication are necessary to obtain full disclosure from many patients using nutritional supplements. Although use of folic acid in the form of leucovorin

or other L-methyl folates may be plausible, research on coadministration in such cases is lacking and may be warranted. Close supervision and regular monitoring would be essential in any such application, as indicated by the risks of self-administration detailed in these case reports.

Furosemide and Related Loop Diuretics

Bumetanide (Bumex), ethacrynic acid (Edecrin), furosemide (Lasix), torsemide (Demadex).
See also Triamterene and Related Potassium-Sparing Diuretics.

Decreased folic acid levels and increased Hcy levels are associated with long-term furosemide therapy for hypertension.[374] Higher total folate intake is associated with a decreased Hcy levels and decreased risk of incident hypertension, particularly in younger women.[266,320,426] Conversely, elevated plasma Hcy levels are associated with increased risk of atherosclerosis and cardiovascular disease.[402,427-430]

In general, patients receiving antihypertensive therapy using furosemide or related loop diuretics are likely to benefit from the Hcy-lowering effects of folic acid and vitamin B_{12}, as well as concomitant magnesium, coenzyme Q10, and mixed tocopherols. Assessment of the individual patient's risk factors, including diet, family history, and genomic polymorphisms, is essential to crafting a customized and evolving integrative strategy for prevention and treatment of cardiovascular disease.

Coadministration of folic acid may be prudent, safe, and inexpensive but has not been specifically investigated. Well-designed and adequately powered clinical trials are warranted.

Medroxyprogesterone

Conjugated equine estrogens and medroxyprogesterone (Premelle cycle 5, Prempro); medroxyprogesterone, oral (Cycrin, Provera); medroxyprogesterone, injection (depot medroxyprogesterone acetate, DMPA; Depo-Provera, Depo-subQ Provera 104); progestin and estrogen injectable: estradiol cypionate and medroxyprogesterone acetate (Cyclofem, Lunelle).
See also Oral Contraceptives.

In a 1-year study of predominantly malnourished women from two urban centres in India (Bombay/Mumbai and Hyderabad) and one rural center in Thailand (Chiang Mai), Joshi et al.[431] found that 3-month injectable depot medroxyprogesterone acetate (DMPA) used for contraception was associated with increased blood folate and serum vitamin A. The clinical implications of these findings are unclear, and further research is warranted.

Raltitrexed

Raltitrexed (ZD-1694; Tomudex).
See also Antifolates and Related Antimetabolites.

Raltitrexed is a quinazoline folate analog indicated in the treatment of advanced colorectal cancer. It causes DNA fragmentation and cell death, selectively inhibiting TS and thereby interfering with the de novo synthesis of thymidine triphosphate (TTP) and DNA synthesis. The manufacturer and some researchers have cautioned that concomitant folic acid may interfere with the action and reduce the efficacy of raltitrexed and recommended that folic acid intake be avoided immediately before or during raltitrexed administration.[432-434] Coadministration of leucovorin is similarly contraindicated. These interactions have been proposed on theoretical grounds and have not been confirmed by clinical trials or systematic review of qualified case reports. Raltitrexed is contraindicated during pregnancy and for at least 6 months after discontinuation of treatment if either partner is receiving raltitrexed.[434]

Pemetrexed (Alimta), a similar drug, has shown no decrease in efficacy but a significant decrease in toxicity when coadministered with folate and vitamin B_{12}. Thus the earlier antifolates discussion may be relevant in extrapolating speculative approaches to the interactions involving folate and raltitrexed.

Thiazide Diuretics

Bendroflumethiazide (bendrofluazide; Naturetin); combination drug: bendrofluazide and propranolol (Inderex); benzthiazide (Exna), chlorothiazide (Diuril), chlorthalidone (Hygroton), cyclopenthiazide (Navidrex); combination drug: cyclopenthiazide and oxprenolol hydrochloride (Trasidrex); hydrochlorothiazide (Aquazide, Esidrix, Ezide, Hydrocot, HydroDiuril, Microzide, Oretic); combination drugs: hydrochlorothiazide and amiloride (Moduretic); hydrochlorothiazide and captopril (Acezide, Capto-Co, Captozide, Co-Zidocapt); hydrochlorothiazide and enalapril (Vaseretic); hydrochlorothiazide and lisinopril (Prinzide, Zestoretic); hydrochlorothiazide and losartan (Hyzaar); hydrochlorothiazide and metoprolol (Lopressor HCT); hydrochlorothiazide and spironolactone (Aldactazide); hydrochlorothiazide and triamterene (Dyazide, Maxzide); hydroflumethiazide (Diucardin), methyclothiazide (Enduron), metolazone (Zaroxolyn, Mykrox), polythiazide (Renese), quinethazone (Hydromox), trichlormethiazide (Naqua).
See also Furosemide and Related Loop Diuretics and Triamterene and Related Potassium-Sparing Diuretics.

Some derivative sources have suggested that coadministration of folic acid with thiazide diuretics could reduce adverse drug effects and enhance the efficacy of the broader therapeutic aims. Specific evidence is lacking to substantiate such interactions. However, patients receiving thiazide therapy are likely to benefit from the homocysteine-lowering effects of folic acid and vitamin B_{12}, as well as concomitant magnesium, coenzyme Q10, and mixed tocopherols. Assessment of the individual patient's risk factors, including diet, family history, and genomic polymorphisms, is essential to shaping a customized and evolving integrative strategy for prevention and treatment of cardiovascular disease.

NUTRIENT-NUTRIENT INTERACTIONS

B Vitamins

Vitamin B_2 (riboflavin); vitamin B_6 (pyridoxine); vitamin B_{12} (cobalamin).

The B vitamins work synergistically, so adequate and proportionate amounts of all B vitamins need to be available for optimal functioning. Deficiency (or excess) of any single nutrient can lead to abnormalities in the metabolism, interrelationships, and activity of one or more of the other B vitamins. In particular, vitamins B_2, B_6, and B_{12} work with folate in maintaining healthy homocysteine (Hcy) levels.[417,435,436] Riboflavin (B_2) is the precursor for FAD, the cofactor for methylenetetrahydrofolate reductase (MTHFR).[437,438] For example, Schnyder et al.[439] found that a combination of folate (1 mg), vitamin B_{12} (400 µg), and B_6 (10 mg) significantly reduces Hcy levels and decreases the rate of restenosis after coronary angioplasty. A synergy between vitamin D and mecobalamin (B_{12}) appears to play a preventive role in risk of hip fracture among stroke patients, with Hcy as a predictive factor.[440,441] Combinations of these nutrients are used in health optimization, disease prevention, and therapeutic interventions related to a wide range of body systems and medical conditions, including bronchial dysplasia in smokers, chronic fatigue, and vitiligo.

The emergent trend in the scientific research and clinical practice among providers experienced in nutritional therapeutics suggests that it is important to match generous quantities of B_{12} with folate administration, especially in older people. Supplementing folic acid without B_{12} can stimulate systems that also use B_{12} and result in lower B_{12} levels. Assessment of B_{12} status and concomitant administration of B_{12} with folate are generally advisable to enhance physiological synergies and to prevent masking of B_{12} deficiency. Furthermore, recent research indicates that a fundamental reconfiguration of assessment standards and therapeutic strategy is necessary to achieve correction of serious or even mild deficiency states. Conventional guidelines have recommended folate doses in hundreds of micrograms and B_{12} in single-digit micrograms. However, a landmark study (2005) showed that once individuals become B_{12}-deficient (by MMA levels), they typically require 500 to 600 µg at least (i.e., >200 times the RDA) to correct mild vitamin B_{12} deficiency, particularly elderly patients.[20] Thus, equivalent amounts of B_{12} are generally advisable with folate administration.

Pancreatin and Proteolytic Enzymes

See Pancreatic Enzymes under Nutrient-Drug Interactions.

Vitamin C

Vitamin C
Vitamin C plays a key role in the conversion of folic acid to its active form and helps to reduce folic acid excretion.

Zinc

Zinc

An interaction between zinc and folic acid has often been suggested, at least partly because bioavailability of dietary folate is increased by the action of folate conjugase, a zinc-dependent enzyme. Therefore, low zinc intake or zinc deficiency could impair absorption of food pteroylpolyglutamates and decrease folate bioavailability. Conversely, some studies and many derivative sources have suggested that folic acid may reduce zinc absorption and impair zinc utilization in individuals, particularly with high folate doses in those with marginal zinc status.[442-444] However, Butterworth and Tamura[445] reviewed the mixed findings in the research literature, as of 1989, and concluded that the "weight of current evidence favors the view that daily supplements of 5 to 15 mg folic acid do not have significant adverse effects on Zn nutriture in healthy nonpregnant subjects." Subsequently, in a trial involving 12 men (age 20-34) fed low-zinc diets (3.5 mg/day), Kauwell et al.[446] found that administration of folic acid at 800 µg/day, a relatively high dose, for 25 days did not alter zinc status, nor did zinc intake impair folate utilization.

HERB-NUTRIENT INTERACTION

Coffee

Coffee (*Caffea arabica, Caffea canephora, Caffea robusta*).
In a randomized, placebo-controlled study, Strandhagen et al.[447] found that administration of folic acid decreases the homocysteine-increasing effect normally associated with coffee prepared by the filter method.

The 453 citations for this monograph, as well as additional reference literature, are located under Folic Acid on the CD at the back of the book.

Vitamin A (Retinol)

Nutrient Names: Vitamin A, retinol.
Synonym: Preformed vitamin A.
Related Substances: Retinal (retinaldehyde); retinoic acid; retinyl esters, such as retinyl acetate, retinyl palmitate, and retinyl propionate; all-trans dehydroretinol, vitamin A2; beta-carotene (provitamin A) and other provitamin A carotenoids: alpha-carotene, cryptoxanthin, lutein, lycopene, zeaxanthin.

Summary

Drug/Class Interaction Type	Mechanism and Significance	Management
Antacids ⊕⊕	Vitamin A coadministration exerts cytoprotective effect and enhances healing of gastric ulcers.	Coadminister.
Anthelmintic drugs ⊕⊕⊕	Vitamin A deficiencies are also associated with increased risk of parasitic infections. Combining anthelmintic agents with increased vitamin A intake can reduce symptoms of intestinal parasites while supporting epithelial integrity and immune response, especially when combined with increased fat intake.	Coadminister vitamin A and/or beta-carotene supplements/foods with accompanying lipid intake. Follow with improved nutrient intake (quality and quantity) to reduce susceptibility.
Chemotherapy Cytotoxic Agents ✗/⊕✗/⊕⊕	Chemotherapeutic agents interact with vitamin A in various ways, from adjunctive vitamin A for nutritive support and amelioration of adverse drug effects to cotherapy using retinoids as chemotherapeutic agents. Pattern of interaction varies depending on patient characteristics, form of cancer, and agents involved. Risk of interference with cytotoxic action through antioxidant effects contentious, but evidence inconclusive and likely not uniform for all agents, conditions, or patients.	Coadministration appropriate in some cases. Retinoid use requires close monitoring by experienced clinicians collaborating on integrative strategy, particularly given significant risk of toxicity. Multiple nutrients providing a network effect are preferred when antioxidants deemed appropriate.
Cholestyramine, colestipol Bile acid sequestrants ≈≈≈/◇	By reducing fat absorption, bile acid sequestrants tend to reduce absorption and assimilation of vitamin A and other fat-soluble nutrients. Significant adverse effects on vitamin A absorption appear less likely than for other nutrients, although may depend on agent used, diet and supplemental intake, and patient characteristics. Available research inconclusive and limited by subject population characteristics, duration, and scope; further research warranted.	Concurrent supplementation with multivitamin providing modest levels of A, D, E, and K with folate, carotenoids, and mixed tocopherols can counter potential adverse effects with little risk and minimal expense.
Colchicine ≈≈≈	Colchicine may impair vitamin A absorption and can interfere with retinol homeostasis by blocking release of retinol–retinol binding protein (RBP).	Coadminister vitamin A, beta-carotene, and other potentially affected nutrients.
Corticosteroids, oral ☼/⊕/✗	Exogenous steroid administration may cause transient increases in levels vitamin A and retinol-binding protein (RBP), whereas extended use may reduce levels of vitamin A and metabolites in plasma and tissues. Concomitant use may enhance drug efficacy by mobilizing hepatic stores and elevating plasma concentrations, particularly in very-low-birth-weight (VLBW) neonates with bronchopulmonary dysplasia. Further research into protective and synergistic effects of coadministration warranted.	Supplement during and after extended steroid administration. Monitor vitamin A and RBP levels.
HMG-CoA reductase inhibitors (statins) ◇◇	Statin therapy may elevate serum retinol levels, possibly by altering liver function; clinical implications unclear and research preliminary. Clinical trials warranted.	Caution advised with retinol intake during statin therapy. Monitoring (or alternatives to statins) appropriate with compromised liver function.
Medroxyprogesterone ◇◇/◇≈≈/⊕✗	Medroxyprogesterone, as injectable contraceptive or oral hormone replacement therapy (HRT), may elevate serum retinol levels, possibly RBP. Clinical significance, with possible underlying alteration in vitamin A function, is unclear, but serum carotenoids may decrease because of competition and altering vitamin A transport. Response likely to depend on multiple factors, including diet and patient characteristics. Further research warranted.	Conservative practice suggests avoiding retinol administration at high doses unless otherwise indicated. Carotenoid support may be indicated. Monitor with compromised liver function.
Methyltestosterone ◇≈≈/≈≈	Single case report indicates that methyltestosterone may impair visual function by altering serum levels and metabolism of vitamin A and beta-carotene. This minimal evidence may represent an atypical pharmacogenomic response but suggests the need for further investigation, including potential benefit of nutrient supplementation.	Discontinuation of drug therapy indicated on appearance of adverse effects.
Mineral oil ✗/≈≈≈	Mineral oil may interfere with or otherwise alter absorption of many nutrients, especially with simultaneous intake and extended use. Mixed evidence suggests that impact on various nutrients may vary, possibly elevating serum retinol levels and decreasing beta-carotene levels. Further research warranted; timing, dosage, duration, diet, and other factors likely influence clinical significance.	Separate intake of mineral oil from meals, and supplement administration. Avoid extended use of mineral oil internally.
Neomycin ≈≈≈	Oral neomycin, particularly high doses over extended periods, may impair vitamin A absorption and could contribute to depletion pattern. Preliminary evidence suggests further research warranted to assess clinical significance.	Coadminister vitamin A and/or beta-carotene with high-dose internal neomycin use of 2 days or longer.
Oral contraceptives (OCs) ◇◇/⊕/✗	OCs (exogenous estrogen and progestin formulations) associated with increased serum levels of vitamin A, at least in part due to increased hepatic synthesis of RBP and elevated export of RBP-retinol complex; lower carotenoid	Conservative practice suggests avoiding retinol administration at high doses unless otherwise indicated. Carotenoid support may be indicated. Monitor with compromised liver function.

Continued

Summary

Drug/Class Interaction Type	Mechanism and Significance	Management
	levels may result from competition and alterations of vitamin A transport. Clinical implications of this apparent drug effect on nutrient function uncertain, but further research warranted to investigate this emerging pattern of evidence.	
Orlistat ≈≈≈	Orlistat may interfere with absorption of vitamin A and other fat-soluble nutrients. Mixed evidence suggests that impact on various nutrients may vary, with findings ranging from no observed effect to depletion despite concurrent supplementation. Further research warranted; timing, dosage, duration, diet, and other factors likely influence clinical significance.	Concurrent supplementation with multivitamin providing modest levels of vitamins A, D, E, and K with carotenoids and mixed tocopherols may counter possible depletion pattern with little risk and minimal expense.
Retinoids ✗✗✗	Concomitant use of supplemental vitamin A and pharmaceutical retinoids not formally investigated, and evidence of clinical significance lacking. Nevertheless, "consensus" considers additive effect inevitable and inherently risky. This conclusion may be reasonable, but clinical trials providing conclusive findings are unlikely.	Avoid supplementation of more than 5000 IU vitamin A during retinoid therapy.
Tetracycline antibiotics ✗✗/✗✗✗	Concurrent use of vitamin A/retinoids and tetracycline antibiotics associated with severe adverse effects, particularly headaches and pseudotumor cerebri (benign intracranial hypertension). Consensus exists on clinical significance of risk of interaction and contraindication against concurrent use. Effects may be sudden and severe.	Avoid concomitant retinoids, including vitamin A at doses above 10,000 IU/day, during antibiotic therapy employing tetracyclines. Discontinue use immediately if symptoms appear.

Note: See also Beta-Carotene monograph.

NUTRIENT DESCRIPTION

This monograph reviews interactions issues relating to and deriving from intake of retinol and other forms of preformed vitamin A and the metabolic processes of these substances within physiological/healthy, dysfunctional, and pathological processes and states. The monograph for beta-carotene focuses on interactions issues involving intake, assimilation, and metabolic processes that constitute provitamin A activity and affect retinol and its metabolic activity. Interactions with some pharmaceutical agents inherently involve both substances and their respective class of related substances.

Chemistry and Forms

Vitamin A is a generic term used to describe the class of compounds that exhibit the biological activity of retinol. The two main sources of vitamin A in foods are retinol and the provitamin A carotenoids. *Retinol* (an alcohol), *retinal* (an aldehyde), and *retinoic acid* are collectively known as "retinoids"; they naturally occur only in animal products and can be classified as "preformed vitamin A." Some structurally related synthetic analogs (e.g., tretinoin) are also considered retinoids and may exhibit significant, partial, or no retinol-like activity.

Carotenoids are a class of related compounds found exclusively in plants (fruits, vegetables, algae, phytoplankton) and animals that feed directly on high-carotenoid plant sources, such as krill, small saltwater and freshwater crustaceans that accumulate astaxanthin from phytoplankton. Approximately 600 carotenoids have been identified thus far. Beta-carotene, alpha-carotene, lutein, lycopene, cryptoxanthin, and zeaxanthin are principal among those specifically classified as "provitamin A carotenoids"; they are so named because humans can metabolically convert them into retinol. Bonds within beta-carotene are cleaved to form all-*trans* retinol (and possibly retinal); divergent theories exist regarding the site of this cleavage, the products, and their proportion, although molecular structures suggest that one molecule of beta-carotene would result in two molecules of retinol. It is unreasonable, however, to equate the predicted retinol yields of the various provitamin A carotenoids, then add these to provide units of "vitamin A equivalents," because in non–vitamin A–deficient humans, only a small proportion of provitamin A carotenoids are actually converted to retinol or retinal.

The dietary supplement labeling convention of stating provitamin A carotenoid content in units of "retinol equivalents" (REs) or international units (IUs) of vitamin A activity has led to a widespread misperception among the lay public and many medical professionals alike, that such supplements contain potentially toxic levels of vitamin A. Potential toxicity of carotenoids such as synthetic beta-carotene in smokers is another issue, unique to beta-carotene, and unrelated to issues of vitamin A toxicity (see section on beta-carotene and other provitamin A carotenoids).

Physiology and Function

In 1913, vitamin A was the first vitamin to be isolated, thus the nomenclature "A". Researchers initially focused on its key role in vision, particularly in preventing night blindness and xerophthalmia. In 1929, Moore demonstrated that beta-carotene was converted to vitamin A, and 2 years later the chemical structures of both vitamin A and beta-carotene were determined.

Vitamin A is readily absorbed in the duodenum and jejunum in the presence of gastric secretions, bile salts, pancreatic and intestinal lipase, protein, and dietary fat. More than 90% of all dietary retinol is in the form of esters, usually retinyl palmitate. These esters must be hydrolyzed in the intestinal lumen by pancreatic enzymes and within the brush border of the intestinal epithelial cells before absorption. Retinol can be absorbed from a micelle in the presence of bile salts or a nonionic detergent. Retinol is absorbed by diffusion when present in high doses, but at low doses its transport across intestinal epithelial cells is mediated by cellular *retinol-binding protein* (RBP). In average doses, retinol is almost entirely absorbed, with peak concentrations in 4 hours. Retinol is absorbed two to five times more efficiently than beta-carotene, the bioavailability and absorption of which are also influenced by multiple factors, including the amount of carotenoid in the diet, interactions with other carotenoids, dietary fat and fiber, nutritional deficiencies of zinc and protein, and other disease states.

Excess retinol is converted to retinyl esters again and stored in the liver. Retinol binds to RBP, which serves as the carrier associated with vitamin A transport in the blood. When the amount of vitamin A exceeds the capacity of RBP to bind to it, the excess retinol binds to lipoproteins, and in this form it has toxic effects. The liver holds 90% (or more) of the body's vitamin A stores, which typically approximate 2 years' requirement for an adult; consequently, it generally does not need to be consumed daily. The lungs and kidneys also store retinol in small amounts. Retinol in storage has a half-life of 50 to 100 days. Vitamin A is present in breast milk. Vitamin A metabolites are eliminated in the bile and urine. When large amounts of retinol are ingested, a portion can be excreted in the feces, independent of biliary absorption and excretion.

Vitamin A is a key micronutrient needed to combat infection and maintain immunity and epithelial cell differentiation and turnover. Retinol and retinoic acid are necessary for maintenance of the structural and functional integrity of epithelial tissue and the immune system, cellular differentiation and proliferation, bone growth, gonadal (testicular and ovarian) function, and embryonic development. Vitamin A also acts as a cofactor in numerous biochemical reactions. A single effect or mechanism cannot account for the diverse vitamin A actions on the immune system.

Retinal is essential for the normal function of the retina, particularly visual adaptation to darkness. Both retinyl esters and beta-carotene from the diet are converted to retinal (11-*cis* isomer). Retinal is combined with the protein opsin to form rhodopsin in the rods of the retina and iodopsin in the cones. Light hitting the retina causes visual excitation and changes the *cis* configuration into the all-*trans* form of retinaldehyde. The rods are particularly sensitive to vitamin A deficiency. When in low supply, the all-*trans* form generated during the light reaction cannot be converted back to the active rhodopsin. Retinal can be also converted to retinoic acid, the form of vitamin A most directly involved in gene transcription. Approximately 20% to 35% of the retinol in food sources (e.g., cod and other fish liver oils) is in the *cis* configuration, whereas virtually all the vitamin A in supplements and vitamin A–fortified foods (e.g., dairy products) is in the all-*trans* configuration. Some evidence suggests that the *cis* configuration may be essential to certain visual and brain functions, at least in certain individuals.

A small amount of beta-carotene is converted into vitamin A in the body, but beta-carotene and the other carotenoids act independently from vitamin A as antioxidants. Only 30% to 50% of the more than 600 known carotenoids are thought to be converted into vitamin A by the body, with alpha-carotene, beta-carotene, and cryptoxanthin the most widely distributed of the provitamin A carotenoids.

NUTRIENT IN CLINICAL PRACTICE
Known or Potential Therapeutic Uses

In conventional practice, supplemental vitamin A is generally thought to have no established therapeutic uses other than correcting frank deficiencies. The evidence for efficacy from administration of exogenous vitamin A (as retinol) is often considered "mixed" and "preliminary." However, both natural and synthetic retinoids have been used as pharmacological agents to treat dermatological disorders, with their action most likely deriving from their effect on the transcription of skin growth factors and their receptors. Acitretin (and previously etretinate) has been employed in the treatment of psoriasis,

and tretinoin (Retin-A) and isotretinoin (Accutane) are typically used to treat severe cases of acne vulgaris; tretinoin is also used cosmetically to reduce signs of skin aging. Most oncology uses of retinoids involve retinoic acid, including 13-*cis*, 9-*cis*, and all-*trans* forms.

Historical/Ethnomedicine Precedent

Vitamin A (retinol) is not used historically as an isolated nutrient.

Possible Uses

Acne vulgaris, acute promyelocytic leukemia, alcohol withdrawal support, Alzheimer's disease, anemia (associated with deficiency), autism (*cis*-containing fish liver–derived form only), blepharitis, breast cancer, bronchitis, burns, cataracts, celiac disease, cervical dysplasia, childhood diseases, colorectal cancer, conjunctivitis, Crohn's disease (associated with deficiency), cystic fibrosis, diabetes mellitus, diabetic retinopathy (in combination with selenium, vitamins C and E), diarrhea, diverticulitis, eczema, fibrocystic breast disease, food poisoning, gastritis, glaucoma, goiter, hemorrhoids, human immunodeficiency virus and acquired immunodeficiency syndrome (HIV/AIDS) support, hypothyroidism, ichthyosis (noninflammatory skin peeling), immune function, intestinal parasites, iron deficiency anemia (with iron), keratosis follicularis (Darier's disease), leukoplakia, lichen planus pigmentosus, lung cancer, menorrhagia, mucopolysaccharidosis (Hurler syndrome), myocardial infarction, myeloproliferative disorders, night blindness (nyctalopia), osteoarthritis, osteoporosis, peptic ulcer, peritonitis, pityriasis rubra pilaris, premenstrual syndrome, psoriasis, respiratory syncytial virus (RSV), retinitis pigmentosa, retinopathy (in combination with selenium, vitamins C and E), rosacea, roundworms, rubeola (measles, severe cases, with deficiency, especially to reduce measles mortality in developing countries), seborrhea, sickle cell anemia, skin cancer, sprains and strains (associated with deficiency), surgery (preparation and recovery), tuberculosis, ulcerative colitis, urinary tract infection, varicella (chickenpox), vaginitis, warts, wound healing, xerophthalmia (classic manifestation of vitamin A deficiency).

Vitamin A deficiency is widespread, in association with general malnutrition, in developing countries, particularly among young children. Frank deficiencies are generally considered uncommon in developed countries, especially in adults, but marginal intake and deficiency status are known to occur with inadequate and poor-quality diet, especially in children and elderly persons. Furthermore, individuals who restrict their dietary intake of liver, dairy products, and vegetables rich in beta-carotene increase their risk of developing vitamin A deficiency. Chronic consumption of alcohol can deplete liver stores of vitamin A, which can be further complicated by alcohol-induced liver damage. Chronic consumption of alcohol and acetaminophen can greatly increase the hepatotoxicity of vitamin A supplements (but not of provitamin A carotenoid supplements).

Special Populations

Extremely low-birth-weight infants (≤1 kg [2.2 lb]) are at high risk of a deficiency at birth. Individuals with vitamin A deficiency caused by abnormal storage and transport conditions, including abetalipoproteinemia, diabetes mellitus, fever, hyperthyroidism, cystic fibrosis (with liver involvement), liver disease, and protein deficiency.

Nutrient-Drug Interactions and Drug-Induced Nutrient Depletions

Deficiency Symptoms

Blindness, defective tooth and bone formation, diarrhea, diminished immune function, dry skin, increased susceptibility to respiratory and urinary tract infections, loss of appetite, metaplasia and keratinization of respiratory tract cells and other systems/organs, night blindness (nyctalopia), papular eruptions, reduced synthesis of steroid hormones, visual impairment, xerophthalmia.

Dietary Sources

Free retinol is not generally found in foods.

The richest readily available dietary source of vitamin A is fish liver oil, especially cod liver oil. In particular, all-*trans* dehydroretinol, previously known as vitamin A$_2$, is a vitamin A–related compound found in freshwater fish flesh and liver and, to a lesser extent, in some marine fish; it is estimated to have 40% to 50% of the vitamin A activity of all-*trans* retinol. Likewise, *cis* isomers of retinol, exhibiting up to 75% relative activity of all-*trans* retinol, can account for up to 35% of preformed vitamin A measured in fish liver oils. Oily fish such as herring, pilchards, tuna, and sardines are considered rich sources. *Retinyl palmitate*, a precursor and storage form of retinol, is found in foods from animal sources and is, along with the acetate ester, the most common form in dietary supplements. Good food sources of vitamin A include liver, kidney, butter, egg yolk, whole milk and cream, whole-milk yogurt, and fortified skim milk. Cod liver oil and halibut fish oil contain high levels of vitamin A and have been used therapeutically.

Carotenoid sources are reviewed in the Beta-carotene monograph.

Nutrient Preparations Available

Many supplements provide a combination of retinol and beta-carotene. Some individuals appear to be able to absorb water-soluble forms of vitamin A supplements better than fat-soluble vitamin A, particularly those with compromised biliary function.

Dosage Forms Available

Capsule, liquid, tablet.

Source Materials for Nutrient Preparations

The primary forms of preformed vitamin A (retinol) in supplements are the vitamin A esters retinyl palmitate and retinyl acetate. Vitamin A can be produced by extraction from fish liver oil, although the more common process is synthesis from beta-ionone.

Dosage Range

One international unit (1 IU) of beta-carotene is equivalent to 1 IU of vitamin A; 1 mg (1000 micrograms [μg]) of beta-carotene is equivalent to 500 μg of vitamin A.

Nutrient values of preformed vitamin A and provitamin A carotenoids are often combined into a single numerical value designating functional vitamin A activity. Originally, the internationally accepted values were international units, with 1 IU being defined as 0.30 μg of all-*trans* retinol, or 0.60 μg of all-*trans* beta-carotene. Although the system of retinol equivalents has become the accepted standard, these earlier

are still found in many food composition tables and scientific publications.

Strong evidence for lower bioavailability of beta-carotene than previous estimates led to revision of the values for the biological activity of various forms of vitamin A and carotenoids. On the basis of rodent studies, the other provitamin A carotenoids have an estimated 50% of the growth-promoting activity of beta-carotene. Although further research has revealed greater diversity in bioavailability, absorption, and differential biological activity, the initial proportional estimates resulted in units of expression for vitamin A activity called *retinol equivalents* (REs). Retinol equivalents are now used as the internationally accepted units for vitamin A activity and can be summarized as follows:

$$
\begin{aligned}
1000 \text{ REs} &= 1 \text{ mg all-trans retinol} \\
&= 6 \text{ mg all-trans beta-carotene} \\
&= 12 \text{ mg other provitamin A carotenoids} \\
&= 3330 \text{ IU vitamin A (retinol)} \\
&= 10{,}000 \text{ IU carotene}
\end{aligned}
$$

However, differences in equivalency when converting beta-carotene to retinol has produced persistent confusion between IU and RE. Calculating total vitamin A activity using the RE system reduces the contribution of provitamin A compared with the IU system. The resultant formula for interconversion follows:

$$
\begin{aligned}
\text{RE} &= \text{IU retinol}/3.33 + \text{IU beta-carotene}/10.0 \\
&= \mu g \text{ retinol} \\
&= \mu g \text{ beta-carotene}/6 + \mu g \text{ other provitamin A carotenoids}/12
\end{aligned}
$$

Continued uncertainty about the meaning of bioavailability of carotenoids, shortcomings in methods for determining bioavailability and absorption, and emerging knowledge of numerous factors in individual variability reveal fundamental inadequacies and inaccuracy in current systems for evaluating and comparing various forms of vitamin A, particularly those from dietary intake of carotenoid-containing foods. Given the wide range of reported conversion ratios of beta-carotene to vitamin A in humans, including the ratio of 6:1 for beta-carotene and 12:1 for alpha-carotene and cryptoxanthin devised by the World Health Organization (WHO), it appears prudent to consider all such approaches as, at best, providing only an average estimate that is not applicable to all diets or individuals. Furthermore, isomerization remains a largely unaddressed issue in quantifying provitamin A activity in processed forms of plant products.

Adult

Dietary: 2333 IU/day for women and 3000 IU/day for men, from dietary sources of both vitamin A and beta-carotene, will generally be adequate to support normal gene expression, immune function, and vision. Breast-feeding women: 4000 to 4333 IU (1200-1300 μg) daily.

Supplemental/Maintenance: 2500 IU of vitamin A as retinol, or 5000 IU of vitamin A, total, with at least 50% in the form of beta-carotene.

Pharmacological/Therapeutic: 25,000 IU (7500 μg) of vitamin A daily is typically used. Doses of 100,000 to 400,000 IU/day have been used for limited periods in the treatment of certain conditions with professional supervision. A maximum of 15,000 IU/day may be more appropriate for individuals over age 65 and those with liver disease outside the context of professional supervision.

Toxic: Doses greater than 50,000 IU/day have resulted in toxicity. Adverse effects may occur in adults at intake levels above 25,000 IU (7500 μg) daily, with higher levels, at or above 100,000 IU/day, more likely to result in cumulative toxicity. Pregnant women (or those who could become pregnant during or shortly after extended supplementation) should not exceed 10,000 IU (3000 μg) daily because of the risk of birth defects, less if foods fortified with vitamin A are consumed to a significant degree with any regularity.

Pediatric (<18 years)
Dietary and Supplemental (combined):
Infants, birth to 6 months: 1333 IU (400 μg), or retinol equivalent (RE) (AI, adequate intake).
Infants 7 to 12 months: 1667 IU (500 μg), or retinol equivalent (RE) (AI)
Children, 1 to 3 years: 1000 IU (300 μg)/day (AI)
Children, 4 to 8 years: 1333 IU (400 μg)/day (RDA)
Children, 9 to 13 years: 2000 IU (600 μg)/day (RDA)
Adolescents, females, 14 to 18 years: 2333 IU (700 μg)/day
Adolescents, male, 14 to 18 years: 3000 IU (900 μg)/day (RDA)

Note: Supplementation often advised for children 6 months to 5 years of age (unless diet known to provide adequate intake)

Pharmacological/Therapeutic: 10,000 IU or greater daily for a child is considered high-dose therapy
Toxic: 10,000 IU (3000 μg) daily

Laboratory Values

Plasma retinol: levels less than 1.05 mmol/L indicate deficiency.

Note: Plasma retinol levels are maintained at the expense of liver stores of vitamin A. Thus, a decline in plasma retinol levels appears only when vitamin A deficiency is progressed to a severe degree.

Liver vitamin A content (biopsy): Levels less than 0.07 mmol/g indicate deficiency.

Note: Liver biopsy provides an accurate assessment of body stores of vitamin A.

SAFETY PROFILE
Overview

Vitamin A toxicity is relatively rare. Hypervitaminosis A is caused by excessive intake of preformed vitamin A and has never been attributed to consumption of carotenoids. Preformed vitamin A is rapidly absorbed and slowly cleared from the body. The risk of developing hypervitaminosis A is derived from total cumulative vitamin A intake rather than a specific daily dosage level, and dosage levels necessary to induce hypervitaminosis A vary significantly among individuals. Thus, vitamin A toxicity can occur in two forms: acute and chronic; that is, toxicity may result acutely from high-dose exposure over a short time, or chronically from lower intake.

Acute hypervitaminosis A results from ingestion of a very high dose of vitamin A over a brief period. Typical symptoms include bulging fontanels in infants and headache in adults, nausea, vomiting, fever, vertigo, and visual disorientation. Peeling of the skin may also occur. Chronic hypervitaminosis A is more common than the acute form and results from

continued ingestion of high doses for months or even years. Symptoms include anorexia, dry itchy skin, alopecia, increased intracranial pressure, fatigue, irritability, somnolence, pronounced craniotabes (congenital cranial osteoporosis) and occipital edema, skin desquamation, fissuring of the lips, pain in the legs and forearms, neurological disturbances, and lethargy. Elevated blood lipids are also common. Furthermore, because vitamin A is fat soluble, excesses tend to accumulate in fatty tissues.

Doses up to 25,000 units (U) per day of vitamin A are generally regarded as safe, although toxicity has been associated with doses as low as 20,000 IU/day. Alleged toxicity at this lower dose has occurred in persons with liver dysfunction caused by drugs, chronic alcohol intake, viral hepatitis, aging, or protein-calorie malnutrition. Most cases of toxicity in nonpregnant females result from more than 200,000 IU/day supplementation for at least 6 to 8 months. Although widely discussed, the teratogenic risks of vitamin A intake appear to occur rarely; however, the teratogenic risk associated with ingestion of the synthetic retinoids (e.g., all-*trans* and 13-*cis* retinoic acid) during pregnancy appears to be much higher.

Reports of adverse effects are associated with doses and durations as low as 20,000 IU/day supplementation for 4 to 6 months. However, doses as high as 500,000 to 1 million IU/day over several years have not caused adverse effects in many people.

Nutrient Adverse Effects
General Adverse Effects

Typical symptoms, especially in children, include drowsiness, fatigue, irritability, vomiting, and bulging of the fontanel. In adults, headaches, dry itchy or scaly skin, brittle nails, alopecia, fatigue, anorexia, diarrhea, gingivitis, cheilosis, bone pain, hepatosplenomegaly, abnormal liver function, and visual disturbances have been reported. Severe cases of hypervitaminosis A may result in hemorrhage, liver damage, and coma.[1]

Generally, discontinuation of vitamin A intake causes symptoms to disappear within a few days with no permanent repercussions, although permanent liver injury has been reported.

Findings from several recent prospective studies suggest that long-term intake of preformed vitamin A in excess of 1500 μg (5000 IU) per day are associated with decreased bone mineral density (BMD) and increased risk of osteoporotic fracture in older men and women, particularly a greater risk of hip fractures in women.[2-6] However, because vitamin D deficiency (defined as a serum 25-hydroxyvitamin D level <20 mg/mL) appears to be relatively common in the general population (particularly older age groups), because vitamin A may antagonize the effects of vitamin D,[7] and because vitamin D status was not investigated in any of these reports, the role (if any) of vitamin D status in the higher fracture risk associated with higher intakes of vitamin A is unclear.

Adverse Effects Among Specific Populations

Lower dosage levels are generally recommended in elderly individuals because of increased risk of compromised liver function and attendant increased risk of toxicity, as well as potentially elevated risk of osteoporosis. Individuals with liver disease or diabetes may also have diminished ability to release vitamin A stored in the liver and therefore an elevated risk of toxic accumulation. Individuals with a genetic predisposition to hypercholesterolemia may also be more susceptible to toxicity at lower doses.

Nutrient-Drug Interactions and Drug-Induced Nutrient Depletions

Pregnancy and Nursing

The greatest concerns about toxicity are the embryotoxic effects that may occur during early pregnancy. Large doses of vitamin A and most of the retinoids can interfere with normal fetal cell development and cause birth defects, although this is usually observed with other retinoids (compounds related to vitamin A, such as retinoic acid), rather than for vitamin A itself. Thus, excessive dietary intake of vitamin A has been associated with birth defects in humans in fewer than 20 reported cases over the past 30 years.[8,9] Other studies combining human and animal data suggest that up to 30,000 U/day is safe in pregnancy.[10] Nevertheless, until more conclusive, large-scale data are available, most experts suggest limiting vitamin A intake from food and supplements combined to 10,000 U during pregnancy. This standard recommendation of a 10,000 IU safe limit became institutionalized after the 1995 *New England Journal of Medicine* report on vitamin A–related teratogenicity.[11]

However, a subsequent report by Mastroiacovo et al.[12] observed only three major malformations among several hundred women exposed to 10,000 to 300,000 IU (median exposure of 50,000 IU) per day, a typical rate of occurrence regardless of vitamin A intake. Furthermore, congenital malformations were lacking in any of the 120 infants exposed to maternal intakes of vitamin A greater than 50,000 IU/day, and this high-exposure group actually demonstrated a 50% decreased risk for malformations, compared with infants not exposed to vitamin A, and a risk level lower than those exposed to midlevel doses (10,000-40,000 IU/day).[12] Other research has found a beneficial effect of vitamin A supplements in reducing free-radical–induced lipid peroxidation associated with third-trimester pregnancy–induced hypertension,[13] thus demonstrating this vitamin's antioxidant activity in an important clinical situation.

In a randomized clinical trial, Fawzi et al.[14] found that a multivitamin supplement reduced death and prolonged HIV-free survival significantly among children born to women with low maternal immunological or nutritional status. Vitamin A alone, however, was associated with increased risk of HIV transmission from mother to child while nursing. Further research is inappropriate, but prudence advises limited use of vitamin A by HIV-infected women who are nursing or susceptible to pregnancy.

Contraindications

Retinol is contraindicated in patients with compromised liver, hepatitis, or any liver disease. High alcohol intake can induce vitamin A deficiency, but ethanol and retinol may interact to increase oxidative stress and the risk of hepatotoxicity.[15]

Precautions and Warnings

High doses (>10,000 IU/day) of supplemental retinol are contraindicated in women who are or might become pregnant. This upper level may be reduced to 1500 μg (5000 IU) of vitamin A per day if foods fortified with preformed vitamin A constitute a significant component of their diet.

High doses should not be administered to older men and women, especially those with decreased BMD and corresponding increased risk of osteoporotic fractures.

At high dosage levels, especially outside the context of broad-based antioxidant nutrient networks, both vitamin A and synthetic beta-carotene have the potential to elevate triglycerides and increase oxidative stress and thereby increase risk of death from heart disease, particularly in smokers. Supplementation with synthetic all-*trans* beta-carotene has also been associated with an increased risk of lung cancer in smokers. Notably, however, retinoid therapy in former smokers, using 9-*cis*-retinoic acid, reverses loss of retinoic acid receptor-beta expression in the bronchial epithelium and may help prevent lung cancer.[16]

INTERACTIONS REVIEW

Strategic Considerations

Vitamin A is generally used in supporting healthy function and treating disorders of the tissues for which it has the greatest affinity: eyes and vision, skin and mucous membranes, cell regeneration and immune function. Both animal and plant foods can serve as dietary sources of vitamin A, but only the preformed vitamin A (primarily retinyl esters and retinol) can contribute to toxicity from excessive dietary intake.

As a nutritional supplement or as a pharmaceutical agent, retinol is primarily administered for its pharmacological activity and not as an antioxidant, as might be a primary intended function of beta-carotene and other carotenoids. In general, retinoids, whether synthetic or natural in origin, should be considered as prescription drugs because their typical use in high doses will usually override normal physiological regulatory mechanisms, thus introducing the risk of accumulation, toxicity, and adverse effects. Apart from application in supporting development and immune function in infants and children, vitamin A has largely been displaced by synthetic retinoids in conventional practice.

Vitamin A continues to play a limited role in oncology therapeutics. In some cases, particularly involving squamous tumors, up to 1 million units/day emulsified vitamin A (the preferred form because of lower hepatic accumulation) is administered daily until significant cheilosis develops, then lowered to 100,000 IU/day and gradually increased again. With such use, experienced physicians follow the blood retinol level, pushing it to the upper limit of normal, and take care to monitor hepatic enzymes, symptoms, and skeletal metabolism and adjust as needed to prevent bone loss. It is important to remain aware that liver damage may result from long-term use of 25,000 IU nonemulsified A, especially in conjunction with chemotherapeutic agents such as tamoxifen. Within conventional oncology practice, all-*trans* retinoic acid (ATRA), combined with chemotherapy, has become standard treatment for promyelocytic leukemia over the past 10 years. In contrast to such uses within conventional pharmacology, retinol and its esters are really the only "nutrient" forms of vitamin A.

NUTRIENT-DRUG INTERACTIONS

Antacids

Aluminum carbonate gel (Basajel), aluminum hydroxide (Alternagel, Amphojel); combination drugs: aluminum hydroxide, magnesium carbonate, alginic acid, and sodium bicarbonate (Gaviscon Extra Strength Tablets, Gaviscon Regular Strength Liquid, Gaviscon Extra Strength Liquid); aluminum hydroxide and magnesium hydroxide (Advanced Formula Di-Gel Tablets, co-magaldrox, Di-Gel, Gelusil, Maalox, Maalox Plus, Mylanta, Wingel); aluminum hydroxide, magnesium trisilicate, alginic acid, and sodium bicarbonate (Alenic Alka, Gaviscon Regular Strength Tablets); calcium carbonate (Titralac, Tums); magnesium hydroxide (Phillips' Milk of Magnesia MOM); combination drugs: magnesium hydroxide and calcium carbonate (Calcium Rich Rolaids); magnesium hydroxide, aluminum hydroxide, calcium carbonate, and simethicone (Tempo Tablets); magnesium trisilicate and aluminum hydroxide (Adcomag trisil, Foamicon); magnesium trisilicate, alginic acid, and sodium bicarbonate (Alenic Alka, Gaviscon Regular Strength Tablets); combination drug: sodium bicarbonate, aspirin, and citric acid (Alka-Seltzer).

Interaction Type and Significance

⊕⊕   **Beneficial or Supportive Interaction, with Professional Management**

Probability:
2. Probable

Evidence Base:
○ Preliminary

Effect and Mechanism of Action

Vitamin A provides nutritive support for tissue regeneration within the context of suppression of irritative gastric secretions by antacids.

Research

Patty et al.[17] investigated the combined effects of vitamin A and antacids on ulcer healing in a multiclinical, multicenter, randomized, prospective trial involving 60 patients with chronic gastric ulcer divided into three groups; they also studied the basal and maximal gastric secretory responses of 12 patients. For 4 weeks, subjects in the first group were treated with antacids only, in the second group with antacids plus vitamin A (50,000 IU orally three times daily), and in the third group the combination of antacids, vitamin A, and cyproheptadine (4 mg orally three times daily). Endoscopic analysis and planimetric measurement of ulcer sizes revealed a significant pattern of enhanced healing associated with concomitant use of vitamin A. Gastric ulcers were completely healed in 15 of 40 individuals who received vitamin A. The reduction in ulcer size was greater in the group receiving vitamin A plus antacids after both 2 and 4 weeks of use. Furthermore, vitamin A (given in doses of 100,000 IU intramuscularly) decreased neither basal nor maximal gastric secretory responses. These findings demonstrate a cytoprotective effect of vitamin A and suggest that coadministration with vitamin A and antacids may be more effective than antacids alone in healing ulcers.

Nutritional Therapeutics, Clinical Concerns, and Adaptations

Patients with gastric ulcers being treated with antacid medications may derive enhanced clinical outcomes through coadministration of vitamin A. Further research is warranted to determine safe and effective dosage levels, define parameters for establishing appropriate treatment period, and shape clinical guidelines for phased withdrawal of antacids on resolution of ulcerations. Concomitant administration of nutrients adversely affected by suppression of gastric acidity, such as vitamin B_{12}, folic acid, beta-carotene, and vitamin D, may also be warranted depending on the actions of the particular agent used, duration of use, and patient characteristics. It is not known whether similar synergy might exist between vitamin A and H_2 blockers and/or proton pump inhibitors. The relationship between vitamin A supplementation and *Helicobacter pylori* infection has also not yet been systematically investigated.

Anthelmintic Drugs

Albendazole (Zentel), levamisole (Ergamisol), praziquantel (Biltricide).

Interaction Type and Significance

⊕⊕⊕   **Beneficial or Supportive Interaction, Not Requiring Professional Management**

Probability:
2. Probable

Evidence Base:
● Consensus

Effect and Mechanism of Action

Helminth infections, particularly roundworms, can interfere with vitamin A absorption, partly through their effect on intestinal epithelial cells, thus depleting body stores of vitamin A. Vitamin A deficiencies are also associated with increased risk of parasitic infections. Increased intake of vitamin A sources, whether through diet or supplementation, can counter this adverse effect of intestinal parasites and can be further enhanced by coadministration of anthelmintic agents. Enhanced vitamin A status may then help prevent or reduce symptoms associated with intestinal worms, especially roundworm. Furthermore, vitamin A supplementation has often been suggested for its physiological role in maintaining epithelial integrity, its ability to stimulate specific and nonspecific immune functions, and its beneficial effects on diarrhea. Absorption of vitamin A can also be supported by increasing levels of dietary fat intake, because both retinoids and beta-carotene are fat soluble.

Research

Depressed iron status and serum retinol have been associated with infections involving intestinal helminths, particularly *Ascaris lumbricoides* and hookworm, in South Asian and African children.[18] Deworming can contribute significantly to the prevention of morbidity and mortality associated with vitamin A deficiency among children in rural communities where intestinal helminth infection is prevalent.[19]

Jalal et al.[20] studied the effect of food sources of beta-carotene, increased dietary fat, and *A. lumbricoides* infection on serum retinol concentrations in children, 3 to 6 years of age, in Sumatra, Indonesia. Some children were administered levamisole for deworming before the feeding period; others were untreated and remained infected. Incorporation of beta-carotene sources (primarily as red sweet potatoes) into the diet significantly increased serum retinol concentrations, to the greatest degree when meals contained both additional beta-carotene sources and extra fat and the children had been dewormed. Adding more fat to the meal and deworming the children caused a rise in serum retinol similar to that observed when the diet included additional beta-carotene. Furthermore, the combined effects of fat and deworming were additive to the effects of additional beta-carotene sources. When the meal contained additional beta-carotene sources, added fat further improved serum retinol concentrations, but only with low-grade *A. lumbricoides* infection.

In a study involving 977 Kenyan children, Mwaniki et al.[21] found that the combination of multi-micronutrient supplementation, including 1000 μg (3300 IU) vitamin A, and multihelminth chemotherapy, using albendazole and praziquantel, reduced egg output of *Schistosoma mansoni*, a species of trematode blood flukes, and increased serum retinol, regardless of initial serum retinol.

Nutritional Therapeutics, Clinical Concerns, and Adaptations

Increasing vitamin A or beta-carotene intake through beta-carotene–rich dietary sources and administration of supplements, especially with additional dietary fat intake, can reduce susceptibility to and adverse outcomes from intestinal helminth infections and work synergistically with anthelmintics to eradicate such infections. Health care professionals treating such infections or supporting preventive measures in at-risk populations can improve clinical outcomes by increasing dietary sources of vitamin A, through plant foods rich in beta-carotene and other nutrients, or through administration of broad-based nutritional supplements. Dosing levels for supplements would be based on intake needs and safety restrictions, as determined by age, weight, and other relevant factors.

Chemotherapy (Cytotoxic Agents)

Evidence: Cisplatin (*cis*-diaminedichloroplatinum, CDDP; Platinol, Platinol-AQ), cyclophosphamide (Cytoxan, Endoxana, Neosar, Procytox), docetaxel (Taxotere), fluorouracil (5-FU; Adrucil, Efudex, Efudix, Fluoroplex), methotrexate (Folex, Maxtrex, Rheumatrex), paclitaxel (Paxene, Taxol), tamoxifen (Nolvadex).
See also Tamoxifen later.

Interaction Type and Significance

✗　　**Potential or Theoretical Adverse Interaction of Uncertain Severity**

⊕✗　　**Bimodal or Variable Interaction, with Professional Management**

⊕⊕　　**Beneficial or Supportive Interaction, with Professional Management**

Probability:	Evidence Base:
3. Possible or	◉ Emerging
2. Probable	▽ Mixed

Effect and Mechanism of Action

Vitamin A has been used concurrently with chemotherapy or other forms of oncological care in many ways, and the patterns of interaction involved are not characterized by a singular or consistent mechanism of action or therapeutic strategy. All forms of cytotoxic chemotherapy are fundamentally aimed at killing dividing cells, but each class of agents clearly has different modes of action. For example, cyclophosphamide (Cytoxan) is an alkylating agent, 5-FU is an antimetabolite, and taxanes are mitosis disruptors that bind the mitotic spindle structures. Vitamin A (as retinol or retinyl esters) has its own antioxidant activity, although it is generally considered not as potent as that of the provitamin A carotenoids, which have a larger electron cloud of conjugated double bonds to utilize. In oncology, however, retinol/retinoid activities more likely are related to cell signaling (through retinoid-responsive elements of nuclear DNA), which involves cellular/tissue differentiation and induction of apoptosis.

Vitamin A with Chemotherapy in Treatment of Late-Stage Breast Cancer. An additive or synergistic effect has been reported and is presumed to be the underlying effect of concomitant use.

Antioxidants and Chemotherapy. Oxygen radicals have increasingly come under investigation as highly toxic stressors contributing to the causes of many diseases, including many forms of cancer. Vitamin A is among the nutrients well known as antioxidant agents. Antioxidants protect the body against cellular oxidative damage and thus some of the adverse effects induced by cisplatin and other cytotoxic drugs. Many nutritionally oriented health care professionals consider the oxidative damage caused by chemotherapy to be a particularly troublesome adverse effect given that evidence increasingly points to oxidative damage as a contributing factor in the causation of many cancers. However, many oncologists reason that antioxidants might be contraindicated with some agents or during some phases of chemotherapy because many chemotherapeutic agents attack cancer cells by inducing oxidative damage. For example, activation of cyclophosphamide requires hepatic oxidation, a process with which antioxidant nutrients could theoretically interfere. However, no substantial clinical research in humans has yet emerged to support this speculation or to warrant considering antioxidants as inherently contraindicated during chemotherapy.

Research

Sacks et al.[22] have conducted a number of experiments into the effects of retinoids on cancer cells, directly and in conjunction with chemotherapeutic agents. In 1990 they demonstrated that beta-ATRA inhibits macrocellular growth of a multicellular tumor spheroid model for squamous carcinoma, but allows for continuing DNA synthesis and cell cycle progression, with these two effects reconciled by a cell death effect. In 1995 these investigators used eight squamous carcinoma cell lines and reported that retinoic acid worked synergistically with chemotherapy to modulate cell growth and proliferation.[23] Although suggesting the clinical value of vitamin A as a component of integrative oncological therapeutics, such research typically evolves from nutrient administration to cotherapies using retinoids as pharmacological agents.

In a randomized controlled trial involving 100 women with late-stage metastatic breast cancer, Israel et al.[24] found that postmenopausal women experienced enhanced remission rates, duration of response, and projected survival, compared with controls, when administered 350,000 to 500,000 IU of vitamin A daily (according to body weight, given indefinitely) with their chemotherapy. Serum retinol levels were significantly increased only in the subgroup of postmenopausal women given high-dose vitamin A. Premenopausal women did not demonstrate significant elevations of serum retinol levels or significantly improved outcomes from the combined therapy.

The interactions between chemotherapeutic agents and antioxidant nutrients display similar patterns but also diversity in usage, action, and attention by researchers. The issue of antioxidants in oncology remains controversial, with conjecture on both sides and a slowly emerging body of clinically based evidence. In general, clinicians and researchers most familiar with antioxidants consistently emphasize the importance of using antioxidants in clusters capable of creating an antioxidant network, as a means of averting the potential for individual nutrients to act as pro-oxidants under conditions of high oxidative stress, particularly in individuals with multiple biochemical stressors and compromised physiology; higher doses are often recommended as more efficacious than lower doses. Furthermore, high-quality randomized trials that control for the antioxidant contribution of diet, which may well confound the contribution of supplements, have not been performed and this key issue of study design not adequately addressed by those with "conclusive" findings.

Animal research indicates that vitamin A may enhance antitumor effect of 5-fluorouracil.[25]

Besides no research linking antioxidant vitamins to reduced cyclophosphamide effectiveness in cancer treatment, Ghosh and Das[26] found that vitamin A supplementation *enhanced* the therapeutic action of cyclophosphamide in mice with vitamin A deficiency. Preliminary studies on humans undergoing chemotherapy with cyclophosphamide have indicated promise of increased survival rates when supplemented with antioxidant nutrients, including vitamin A. Nevertheless, although antioxidants might have many benefits as cotherapies, evidence as to their effectiveness in patients taking cyclophosphamide is inconclusive.[27-30] On the other hand, no conclusive evidence has confirmed concerns of a potential adverse interaction resulting from antioxidant coadministration interfering with activation of cyclophosphamide (since it requires oxidation in the liver) and its effectiveness.[31] Thus, such concern remains speculative at this time.

A variety of studies, primarily in vitro and animal, have found vitamins A, C, and E; N-acetylcysteine; and other antioxidants to increase the effectiveness of and reduce adverse effects of chemotherapy in several types of cancer.[27,32-43] In a review of 71 scientific papers, Prasad et al.[44] found no evidence to support the proposition that antioxidants interfere with the therapeutic effect of chemotherapy. To the contrary, the data suggest that such combinations would do more to increase efficacy. The authors express caution, but their review indicates a low risk that these antioxidants prevent the therapeutic activity of chemotherapy, and more likely that antioxidants enhance the action of chemotherapeutic agents. Simone et al.[45a-b] arrived at parallel conclusions in a similar review of 280 peer-reviewed papers. Prasad et al.[45c] conclude the following:

> Antioxidants such as retinoids, vitamin E, vitamin C and caro-tenoids inhibit the growth of cancer cells. These antioxidants individually, and in combination, enhance the effects of x-irradiation, chemotherapeutic agents, and certain biological response modifiers such as hyperthermia, sodium butyrate and interferon, on cancer cells. Antioxidants individually protect normal cells against some of the toxicities produced by these therapeutic agents. Therefore, the fear of oncologists and radi-ation therapists that these antioxidants may protect cancer cells against free radicals that are generated by these agents is unfounded. It should be pointed out that other antioxidants such as sulfhydryl compounds will protect cancer cells at least against radiation damage. This is not true for any of the proposed antioxidant vitamins and carotenoids.

Several researchers have offered the seemingly paradoxical conclusion that the appropriate administration of antioxidant inhibitors and free-radical–generating compounds may be a useful strategy in the treatment of solid tumors. However, reports at the 1999 American Society of Cell Biology annual meeting suggested that vitamin A and E–deficient mice were less susceptible to brain tumor progression than non–vitamin-deficient control animals. Salignik et al.[46] suggested that suppression of free radicals by the antioxidant vitamins may suppress apoptosis (programmed cell death). After reviewing the relationship between chemotherapy and antioxidants, Weijl et al.[38] rebuffed warnings to avoid antioxidants during che-motherapy, but also determined that no substantive evidence supported the use of antioxidants to provide relief from the adverse side effects of chemotherapy. Although most preclinical evidence and the limited clinical evidence suggest a greater like-lihood of benefit than harm from coadministration of antioxi-dants with radiotherapy and chemotherapy to treat human cancer, existing evidence is just beginning to answer the ques-tion,[46a] and large, well-designed clinical trials are needed for definitive answers. This question is important to public health because most mainstream medical and radiation oncology practi-tioners routinely proscribe concurrent use of antioxidant supple-ments, but many cancer patients use them covertly, based on the available information, accessible through the internet and other sources. Diet and antioxidant content vary among cancer patients, which confounds clinical trial design and has not been adequately addressed.

Interactions from coadministration of antioxidants and nutrients other than vitamin A are reviewed in the monographs of those nutrients.

Nutritional Therapeutics, Clinical Concerns, and Adaptations

The use of high doses of vitamin A to complement conven-tional chemotherapy offers significant potential for clinical benefit. The levels of vitamin A administered as part of the French research reviewed are much higher than levels generally considered toxic.

Physicians prescribing chemotherapy for breast cancer may want to discuss with patients the potential therapeutic value of adding vitamin A to their treatment regimen. Close supervision and regular monitoring of serum retinol levels, hepatic enzymes, and symptoms (e.g., cheilosis, headache) are required for proper dosing of vitamin A at high levels and for evaluation of efficacy, potential adverse effects, and the disease process itself.

The use of vitamin A as a chemotherapeutic agent, alone or in combination with conventional chemotherapy, involves potential risks and requires supervision by health care profes-sionals experienced in both conventional pharmacology and nutritional therapeutics, preferably collaborating in a mul-tidisciplinary approach to integrative oncology care. Likewise, practitioners who judiciously use antioxidants during chemo-therapy or other conventional cancer care are advised to ques-tion patients about self-prescribing of antioxidants. Such concomitant use could be problematic and contraindicated, beneficial and appropriate, or both, for certain patients taking individualized and evolving dosage levels at coordinated inter-vals and durations. In almost all cases the administration of multiple antioxidants, such as mixed tocopherols, vitamin C, N-acetylcysteine, parenteral glutathione, coenzyme Q10, and proanthocyanadins, is more likely to be appropriate, safe, and effective than single agents in high doses.

High doses of vitamin A carry significant potential risks of toxicity, particularly with extended use. As noted previously, some physicians experienced in nutritional therapeutics and integrative oncology have employed dosage levels of up to 1 million units per day, using emulsified vitamin A for short periods, typically followed by reductions to 100,000 IU/day. Development of significant cheilosis can be used as a physio-logical monitor for toxicity and the need to reduce dosage levels until it resolves, then consider dose escalation again, based on clinical status and response.

Because the emulsified form of vitamin A is water soluble, it is absorbed directly into the lymphatics of the small intestine, thus obviating the need for micelle formation by bile salts and avoiding immediate processing by the liver ("first pass" metab-olism of food components that form micelles and are trans-ported through the portal vein to the liver). This allows larger amounts of vitamin A to reach the peripheral tissues and decreases hepatic accumulation.

Women who could become pregnant should avoid vitamin A doses greater than 10,000 IU (3000 µg) per day because it can be teratogenic, even though typical chemotherapeutic agents present significant risks for causing birth defects, partic-ularly in the first trimester of gestation. Generally, for pharma-cological action rather than supplementation support, vitamin A doses up to 25,000 IU (7500 µg) per day are considered safe for postmenopausal women and males. Nevertheless, the risk of liver damage should always be considered when administering retinoids, especially in patients with compromised liver function or chronic infection with hepatitis B or C or who are regularly ingesting hepatic toxins such as alcohol or large doses of acetaminophen. Likewise, it is also important to mon-itor skeletal metabolism, optimize vitamin D status by moni-toring the 25-hydroxyvitamin D blood level, and adjust vitamin A dosage and serum retinol levels as appropriate to prevent bone loss.

Cholestyramine, Colestipol, and Related Bile Acid Sequestrants

Evidence: Cholestyramine (LoCholest, Prevalite, Questran), colestipol (Colestid).
Extrapolated, based on similar properties: Colesevelam (WelChol).

Interaction Type and Significance

≈≈≈≈Drug-Induced Nutrient Depletion, Supplementation Therapeutic, Not Requiring Professional Management

◇   Adverse Drug Effect on Nutritional Therapeutics, Strategic Concern

Probability:	Evidence Base:
3. Possible	◉ Emerging and/or ▽ Mixed

Effect and Mechanism of Action

Absorption of dietary (and supplemental) sources of vitamin A requires bile salts and the presence of lipids. Bile acid sequestrants, such as cholestyramine and colestipol, decrease lipid digestion and absorption. In the process, they also reduce absorption of the fat-soluble vitamins (e.g., vitamin A) and other nutrients.[47-51] Vitamin A (and beta-carotene) may also increase triglyceride levels.

Research

The general consensus over the past 40 years is that drugs that alter fat absorption and bile function will disrupt absorption and assimilation of fat-soluble nutrients. However, the evidence on the degree of such impairment, the nutrients affected, and the clinical significance is mixed, inconclusive, and still emerging. Early research by Longneck and Basu and later by West and Lloyd[52] informed several review articles that posited a general impairment of absorption of vitamin A and fat-soluble nutrients by bile acid sequestrants and other anti-lipidemic agents. Subsequent human trials have investigated the significance of these effects on nutrients for various medications in different patient populations.

West and Lloyd[52] (1975) studied the effects of cholestyramine (mean dosage, 0-6 g/kg/day) on 18 children with familial hypercholesterolemia over 1 to 2½ years. In addition to a major reduction in serum folate concentration and red blood cell (RBC) folate, these researchers also noted "a significant decrease in the mean serum concentrations of vitamins A and E and of inorganic phosphorus over the first two years of treatment, although values remain within the normal range." They concluded that "routine administration of fat-soluble vitamins appears unnecessary but it is prudent to measure prothrombin time [to assess vitamin K status] and serum vitamins A and E at intervals."[52]

In a study of type IIa hyperlipoproteinemic patients, Probstfield et al.[53] observed that serum total carotenoid levels fell by 30% after administration of colestipol (30 g/day) for 6 months, most likely from decreased absorption of carotenoids by bile acid sequestrant administration, but that serum vitamin A levels were not significantly altered.

In 1987, Knodel and Talbert[50] reported that "large doses of cholestyramine (>32 g/day) may be associated with malabsorption of fat-soluble vitamins," but concluded that impaired absorption of vitamins D and K presented the most significant clinical risk with long-term therapy, with bone loss and bleeding disorders being the potential adverse outcomes.

Tonstad et al.[54] investigated the effects of colestipol granules (10 g/day) and low-fat diet in an 8-week, double blind, placebo-controlled trial, followed by open treatment for 44 to 52 weeks, on low-density lipoprotein (LDL) cholesterol levels in 37 boys and 29 girls, age 10 to 16 years, with familial hypercholesterolemia. Serum concentrations of vitamins A and D, as well as other relevant nutrient parameters, were not affected significantly in the colestipol group, even though levels of serum folate, vitamin E, and carotenoids were significantly reduced. Thus, although these researchers did not suggest a need for compensatory enhancement of fat-soluble nutrients in general or vitamin A in particular, they did recommended supplementation with folate and "possibly vitamin D." They also noted the high degree of noncompliance among the adolescents in the study.

This trend toward a significant interaction raises serious questions given the ongoing debate on the correlation between nutrient status, particularly antioxidants, and long-term risk of coronary heart disease. Most importantly, with limited research and no follow-up investigation of long-term effects (i.e., decades) of such drug-induced nutrient depletion patterns on nutrient status, healthy cardiovascular function, and ultimate outcomes, the data are suggestive but inconclusive in regard to benefit versus risk.

Nutritional Therapeutics, Clinical Concerns, and Adaptations

Although not always necessary, multivitamin/mineral supplementation with vitamin A and other affected nutrients can provide a safe and inexpensive means of avoiding adverse effects from these medications without interfering with (and perhaps enhancing) the therapeutic goal of supporting healthy cardiovascular function and reducing risk. Vitamin A and other fat-soluble nutrients (as well as folic acid and many medications) should be taken 1 hour before or 4 to 6 hours after bile acid sequestrants for optimal absorption. It may be more effective to coadminister water-miscible vitamin A to patients undergoing long-term bile acid sequestrant therapy. Patient characteristics will influence the need for compensatory nutrient administration, particularly age, typical diet, digestive function, comorbid conditions, and pharmacogenomic response to the medication.

Colchicine

Colchicine

Interaction Type and Significance

≈≈≈≈ Drug-Induced Nutrient Depletion, Supplementation Therapeutic, Not Requiring Professional Management

Probability:	Evidence Base:
4. Plausible or 2. Probable	○ Preliminary

Effect and Mechanism of Action

Oral colchicine may impair absorption of vitamin A and other nutrients.[55,56] Colchicine also blocks hepatic release of retinol-RBP and thereby impairs upregulation of serum retinol and interferes with serum retinol homeostasis.

Research

Race et al.[55] reported that oral colchicine can induce intestinal malabsorption, affecting beta-carotene and other nutrients.

Nutritional Therapeutics, Clinical Concerns, and Adaptations

Physicians prescribing colchicine for an extended period can suggest to patients the likely benefit of supplementing with a high-potency multivitamin/mineral supplement to compensate for potential drug-induced depletion of vitamin A, beta-carotene, and other nutrients. Further research through well-designed human trials is warranted to determine the severity, frequency, and clinical implications of this probable interaction and to identify characteristics of individuals most susceptible to clinically significant adverse effects.

Corticosteroids, Oral

Betamethasone (Celestone), cortisone (Cortone), dexamethasone (Decadron), fludrocortisone (Florinef), hydrocortisone (Cortef), methylprednisolone (Medrol) prednisolone (Delta-Cortef, Orapred, Pediapred, Prelone), prednisone (Deltasone, Liquid Pred, Meticorten, Orasone), triamcinolone (Aristocort).

Interaction Type and Significance

☼ **Prevention or Reduction of Drug Adverse Effect**

⊕ **Potential or Theoretical Beneficial or Supportive Interaction, with Professional Management**

✗ **Potential or Theoretical Adverse Interaction of Uncertain Severity**

Probability:
4. Plausible

Evidence Base:
○ **Preliminary**

Effect and Mechanism of Action

Extended use of oral corticosteroids can impair immune function and wound healing. The nutritive effect of vitamin A on immune function and tissue regeneration could prevent and support recovery from such adverse drug effects. Evidence indicates that oral corticosteroids may deplete tissue levels of vitamin A. However, some oral steroids may stimulate transient increases in plasma concentrations of vitamin A and RBP in some circumstances.

Research

Hunt et al.[57] observed that administration of topical or internal vitamin A reversed the inhibitory effect of cortisone on healing of open wounds and improved wound healing in 8 of 10 patients receiving corticosteroid therapy. Theoretically, concomitant vitamin A supplementation might interfere with the therapeutic action of corticosteroids in some patients, but evidence is lacking.[58]

Steroidal anti-inflammatory drugs may contribute to depletion of vitamin A. Using adult male rats, Atukorala et al.[59] found that the administration of large doses of corticosterone resulted in a rapid loss of vitamin A from the plasma, liver, adrenals, and thymus. Of the organs studied, the thymus appeared to be the most sensitive to treatment. Subsequent coadministration of vitamin A with corticosterone reversed the steroid-mediated depression of vitamin A levels in plasma and tissue. Also using a rat model, Georgieff et al.[60] found significant reductions in liver and lung tissue concentrations of vitamin A, retinol, and individual retinyl esters in animals treated with dexamethasone, including those assessed as "vitamin A sufficient" at the onset and demonstrating transient elevations in serum retinol levels in response to the drug.

In a prospective cohort study involving very-low-birth-weight (VLBW) neonates with bronchopulmonary dysplasia (BPD), Shenai et al.[61] investigated the effects of a 7-day course of dexamethasone to test the hypothesis that vitamin A status is critical for the therapy's beneficial pulmonary response. They measured plasma concentrations of vitamin A and RBP at baseline, then during and after dexamethasone treatment, and

graded pulmonary response to dexamethasone daily. A "significant, yet short-term, increase in plasma concentrations of both vitamin A and RBP was observed in most infants treated with dexamethasone." Also, "plasma vitamin A and RBP responses to dexamethasone tended to be higher in infants with a positive pulmonary response than in those with a negative response. Accounting for gender, a vitamin A response with each 10.0 microg/dL increment in plasma vitamin A concentration was associated with a 60% increase in the odds favoring a positive pulmonary response to dexamethasone." They attributed the observed increase in plasma concentrations of both vitamin A and RBP to endogenous mobilization of hepatic vitamin A stores and concluded their findings "suggest that the beneficial pulmonary response to dexamethasone in infants with BPD is influenced, at least in part, by the vitamin A status."[61] Potential synergy derived from coadministration of vitamin A was not investigated in relation to this research but may warrant investigation, given the evidence that vitamin A and its active metabolites are important to premature infants in general and support healthy respiratory epithelial differentiation and growth in particular.

Nutritional Therapeutics, Clinical Concerns, and Adaptations

Physicians prescribing oral corticosteroids, especially for extended periods, are advised to consider coadministration of or subsequent supplementation with vitamin A. Daily doses of up to 25,000 IU (7500 µg) of vitamin A are considered safe for men and postmenopausal women for limited periods. However, women who may become pregnant should restrict their daily intake of vitamin A to less than 5000 IU (1500 µg) in supplemental form. Alternatively, when beta-carotene is used as the supplemental source, daily doses of 25,000 IU (15 mg), or even as high as 100,000 IU (60 mg), are considered safe, except in smokers (see Beta-carotene monograph). The temporary elevations of serum levels reported in the literature may not be problematic and may be beneficial in some patients but could be inappropriate for others, especially those with compromised liver function. Whenever administering vitamin A, especially in doses over 50,000 IU/day, it is important to monitor serum levels for inappropriate excess and to advise patients to report headaches or other signs of toxicity promptly. Likewise, with drugs such as steroids, it is equally important to be alert for depleted vitamin A status.

HMG-CoA Reductase Inhibitors (Statins)

Atorvastatin (Lipitor), fluvastatin (Lescol, Lescol XL), lovastatin (Altocor, Altoprev, Mevacor), combination drug: lovastatin and niacin (Advicor), pravastatin (Pravachol), rosuvastatin (Crestor), simvastatin (Zocor); combination drug: simvastatin and extended-release nicotinic acid (Niaspan).

Interaction Type and Significance

◇◇ **Drug-Induced Effect on Nutrient Function, Supplementation Contraindicated, Professional Management Appropriate**

Probability:
4. Plausible

Evidence Base:
○ **Preliminary**

Effect and Mechanism of Action

The 3-hydroxy-3-methylglutaryl–coenzyme A (HMG-CoA) reductase inhibitors may increase serum retinol levels. The question of how HMG-CoA reductase inhibition might alter liver regulation of vitamin A has not been investigated.

Research

Muggeo et al.[62] observed a pattern of elevation in serum retinol levels over 2 years of therapy in 37 hypercholesterolemic patients treated with diet modification and HMG-CoA reductase inhibitors.

Nutritional Therapeutics, Clinical Concerns, and Adaptations

Pending further research with well-designed clinical trials of sufficient size, physicians prescribing HMG-CoA reductase inhibitors should monitor blood levels of vitamin A in patients also taking this nutrient, particularly those with compromised liver function, and consider alternatives to statins in compromised patients. Furthermore, regular monitoring of liver function, especially enzyme levels, is important for prudent management of all patients taking statin drugs. Coadministration of coenzyme Q10 is also appropriate to prevent adverse effects upon endogenous coenzyme Q10 synthesis by HMG-CoA reductase inhibition.

Medroxyprogesterone

Conjugated equine estrogens and medroxyprogesterone (Premelle cycle 5, Prempro); medroxyprogesterone, oral (Cycrin, Provera); Medroxyprogesterone, injection (Depot medroxyprogesterone acetate, DMPA; Depo-Provera, Depo-subQ Provera 104); progestin and estrogen injectable: estradiol cypionate and medroxyprogesterone acetate (Cyclofem, Lunelle).
See also Oral Contraceptives below.

Interaction Type and Significance

◇◇ **Drug-Induced Effect on Nutrient Function, Supplementation Contraindicated, Professional Management Appropriate**
◇≈≈ **Drug-Induced Adverse Effect on Nutrient Function, Coadministration Therapeutic, with Professional Management**
⊕✗ **Bimodal or Variable Interaction, with Professional Management**

Probability: Evidence Base:
3. Possible or **2. Probable**   ◉◉ **Emerging**

Effect and Mechanism of Action

Medroxyprogesterone acetate (MPA) use is associated with elevations in serum retinol levels. Exogenous estrogen and progestin increase hepatic synthesis of RBP, thus increasing the export of RBP-retinol complex in the blood.

Research

Numerous clinical trials have investigated the effect of medroxyprogesterone administration, whether for contraception or in menopausal hormone replacement therapy (HRT), on blood levels of vitamin A and its metabolites as well as other nutrients. Most studies report increased serum retinol levels, with 40% mean increases in some trials; one study also noted RBP elevations.[63-67] In 12 nonlactating healthy Thai women, Amatayakul et al.[63] found no significant changes in levels of several nutrients, including vitamin A serum levels, before and with daily coadministration of a vitamin-mineral formulation that included vitamin A and beta-carotene, in association with 1 year of MDA use as an injectable contraceptive (150 mg intramuscularly every 90 days). In a subsequent study on the effect of 1 year of oral contraceptive (OC) use on liver vitamin A storage, as assessed by the relative dose response (RDR) test, these researchers reported that daily (one capsule) or periodic (two capsules 7 days per month) multivitamin

supplementation, including 1700 µg vitamin A per capsule, did not significantly influence vitamin A serum values. However, the RDR test after 13 cycles was elevated in one woman who had taken OCs and the periodic multivitamin supplement; it reverted to normal after supplementation with vitamin A.[65]

Given the inadequate nutritional intake or compromised nutrient status of the women in some of these studies, the researchers have interpreted the phenomena of elevated serum retinol as beneficial. However, in the study of Nigerian women, whose diet is typically high in carotenoids, Wien and Ojo[68] reported that serum carotene was lower in OC users (combination estrogen-progestogen) than in groups using intrauterine device (IUD) or injectable progestogen. These researchers concluded that "more detailed study of plasma transport forms of vitamin A is needed to determine if the very high serum vitamin A levels seen in some OC users in this population are potentially harmful."

Nutritional Therapeutics, Clinical Concerns, and Adaptations

Physicians prescribing medroxyprogesterone for contraception or menopausal HRT should consider monitoring blood levels of vitamin A, particularly in patients with compromised liver function. vitamin A supplementation may need to be avoided in some patients; in others it might be indicated, depending on patient characteristics and response to the medication. Enhanced carotenoid intake (diet, supplementation) may be beneficial. Dietary intake of preformed vitamin A and provitamin A carotenoids, nutritional status, age and menstrual status, dose, form, and therapeutic intent all influence how much medroxyprogesterone alters vitamin A levels and function and whether this is beneficial, adverse, or insignificant.

Methyltestosterone

Methyltestosterone (Android, Methitest, Testred, Virilon); combination drug: methyltestosterone and esterified estrogens (Estratest, Estratest HS).
Related but evidence lacking for extrapolation: Fluoxymesterone (Halotestin); testolactone (testolacton; HSDB 3255, SQ 9538; Fludestrin, Teolit, Teslac, Teslak); testosterone cypionate.

Interaction Type and Significance

◇≈≈ **Drug-Induced Adverse Effect on Nutrient Function, Coadministration Therapeutic, with Professional Management**
≈≈ **Drug-Induced Nutrient Depletion, Supplementation Therapeutic, with Professional Management**

Probability: Evidence Base:
6. Unkown   ☐ **Inadequate**

Effect and Mechanism of Action

The mechanism involved in the following report is not known.[69] Also, no research has focused on this potential interaction, its mechanisms, susceptibility factors, or clinical implications.

Report

Nisbett et al.[69] reported the case of a 59-year-old man with a 3-month history of night blindness and a 9-month history of steatorrhea subsequent to his initiation of therapy with methyltestosterone. Low serum levels of carotene (0.1 mmol/L) and vitamin A were accompanied by numerous changes in visual function. The symptoms and the biochemical and electrophysiological abnormalities resolved within 9 months of the discontinuation of methyltestosterone.

Nutritional Therapeutics, Clinical Concerns, and Adaptations

Although this report may represent an anomalous phenomenon, it still suggests a need for further research. Physicians prescribing methyltestosterone (an anabolic steroid, not testosterone replacement) may find it prudent to assess patients for vitamin A status and recommend concomitant supplementation with vitamin A and/or beta-carotene as indicated.

Mineral Oil

Agoral, Kondremul Plain, Liquid Parafin, Milkinol, Neo-Cultol, Petrogalar Plain.

Interaction Type and Significance

✗   **Potential or Theoretical Adverse Interaction of Uncertain Severity**

≈≈≈   **Drug-Induced Nutrient Depletion, Supplementation Therapeutic, Not Requiring Professional Management**

Probability:
4. Plausible

Evidence Base:
○ **Preliminary**

Effect and Mechanism of Action

Mineral oil, as a lipid solvent, may absorb many substances and interfere with normal absorption of retinol, beta-carotene, and other nutrients.

Research

Some disagreement exists, but most research has found that mineral oil can interfere with the absorption of, and thus contribute to a depletion of, many nutrients, including beta-carotene, calcium, phosphorus, potassium, and vitamins A, D, K, and E. One study involving 25 children with chronic constipation found that a short course of mineral oil can reduce serum levels of beta-carotene while elevating serum retinol levels modestly.[70]

Nutritional Therapeutics, Clinical Concerns, and Adaptations

As a preventive and protective measure, health care professionals are advised to recommend regular use of a multivitamin supplement to patients using mineral oil for any extended period. Malabsorption of fat-soluble vitamins caused by ingestion of mineral oil can be minimized by administering mineral oil on an empty stomach or taking vitamin or mineral supplements at least 2 hours before or after the mineral oil. In general, internal use of mineral oil should be limited to less than 1 week.

Neomycin

Neomycin (Mycifradin, Myciguent, Neo-Fradin, NeoTab, Nivemycin); combination drugs: Adcortyl with Graneodin, Betnovate-N, Dermovate-NN, Gregoderm, Synalar N, Tri-Adcortyl, Trimovate.

Interaction Type and Significance

≈≈≈   **Drug-Induced Nutrient Depletion, Supplementation Therapeutic, Not Requiring Professional Management**

Probability:
2. Probable

Evidence Base:
●●● **Consensus** or
○ **Preliminary**

Effect and Mechanism of Action

Oral neomycin impairs absorption of vitamin A, especially in large doses.[48,56]

Research

In a rat model, Favaro et al.[71] observed that neomycin reduced the bioavailability of vitamin A by approximately 13% in both vitamin A–deficient and normal animals. In a double-blind trial involving five healthy male subjects, Jacobson et al.[72] observed a significantly reduced increase in plasma vitamin A levels in all study subjects subsequent to consuming a standard meal containing vitamin A (300,000 IU) when followed by neomycin sulfate (2 g) versus placebo.

The significance of this interaction on daily supplementation of vitamin A has not undergone further research and remains unknown. Nevertheless, this interaction hypothesis has largely settled into the status of consensus, even though evidence from clinical trials is minimal.

Nutritional Therapeutics, Clinical Concerns, and Adaptations

Physicians prescribing neomycin internally for more than 2 to 3 days can advise patients of the probable benefit of supplementing with vitamin A (25,000 IU or 7.5 mg daily) or beta-carotene (25,000 IU or 15 mg daily). Individuals using neomycin topically will not experience problems related to malabsorption; likewise, adverse effects are unlikely to result from a single dose of oral neomycin as part of surgery preparation.

Oral Contraceptives: Monophasic, Biphasic, and Triphasic Estrogen Preparations (Synthetic Estrogen and Progesterone Analogs)

Ethinyl estradiol and desogestrel (Desogen, Ortho-TriCyclen).
Ethinyl estradiol and ethynodiol (Demulen 1/35, Demulen 1/50, Nelulen 1/25, Nelulen 1/50, Zovia).
Ethinyl estradiol and levonorgestrel (Alesse, Levlen, Levlite, Levora 0.15/30, Nordette, Tri-Levlen, Triphasil, Trivora).
Ethinyl estradiol and norethindrone/norethisterone (Brevicon, Estrostep, Genora 1/35, GenCept 1/35, Jenest-28, Loestrin 1.5/30, Loestrin1/20, Modicon, Necon 1/25, Necon 10/11, Necon 0.5/30, Necon 1/50, Nelova 1/35, Nelova 10/11, Norinyl 1/35, Norlestin 1/50, Ortho Novum 1/35, Ortho Novum 10/11, Ortho Novum 7/7/7, Ovcon-35, Ovcon-50, Tri-Norinyl, Trinovum).
Ethinyl estradiol and norgestrel (Lo/Ovral, Ovral).
Mestranol and norethindrone (Genora 1/50, Nelova 1/50, Norethin 1/50, Ortho-Novum 1/50).
Related, internal application: Etonogestrel/ethinyl estradiol vaginal ring (Nuvaring).
See also Medroxyprogesterone earlier.

Interaction Type and Significance

◇◇   **Drug-Induced Effect on Nutrient Function, Supplementation Contraindicated, Professional Management Appropriate**

⊕   **Potential or Theoretical Beneficial or Supportive Interaction, with Professional Management**

✗   **Potential or Theoretical Adverse Interaction of Uncertain Severity**

Probability:
3. Possible or **2. Probable**

Evidence Base:
◉◉ **Emerging**

Effect and Mechanism of Action

Oral contraceptive use has been associated with increased blood levels of vitamin A (and copper).[73-75] Exogenous estrogen and progestin increase hepatic synthesis of retinol-binding protein (RBP), thus increasing the export of RBP-retinol complex in the blood.

Research

Several studies have reported an association between the use of OCs and increased serum levels of vitamin A.[73,76,77] Horwitt et al.[78] found that women using OCs had the lowest average levels of carotenoids corresponding to the highest average levels of vitamin A in the serum, and that estrogens seemed to increase the rate of conversion of carotene to vitamin A. The clinical implications of this potential interaction are uncertain at this time.

Nutritional Therapeutics, Clinical Concerns, and Adaptations

Physicians prescribing exogenous estrogen and progestins for contraception may consider monitoring blood levels of vitamin A in patients, particularly in individuals with compromised liver function. Vitamin A supplementation may need to be avoided in some women; in others it might be indicated, depending on patient characteristics and response to the medication. Enhanced carotenoid intake (diet, supplementation) may be beneficial. Dietary intake of preformed vitamin A and provitamin A carotenoids, nutritional status, age and menstrual status, dose, form, and therapeutic intent all affect the degree to which OC administration alters vitamin A levels and function and whether this is beneficial, adverse, or insignificant.

Orlistat (Xenical)

Orlistat (alli, Xenical)

Interaction Type and Significance

≈≈≈ **Drug-Induced Nutrient Depletion, Supplementation Therapeutic, Not Requiring Professional Management**

Probability:
3. **Possible** (short term) or
   4. **Plausible** (long term)

Evidence Base:
◎◎ **Emerging**

Effect and Mechanism of Action

As a gastrointestinal (GI) lipase inhibitor that reduces dietary fat absorption, orlistat can reduce the absorption of vitamin A and other fat-soluble nutrients.

Research

Melia et al.[79] reported that orlistat had no significant short-term effect on blood levels of vitamin A in a small, open-label, placebo-controlled, randomized, two-way crossover study involving 12 healthy volunteers. Each participant received a single oral dose of 25,000 IU vitamin A, followed 24 hours later by a single oral dose of 400 IU vitamin E, on two separate occasions during oral administration of 120 mg orlistat or placebo three times daily for 9 days. A washout period of at least 2 weeks separated the two treatments. Based on subsequent analysis of serum concentrations of retinol, no significant effect was found on absorption of vitamin A during oral administration of 120 mg orlistat or placebo, although absorption of vitamin E was reduced significantly (by ~43% on C_{max} and ~60% on AUC). In a multicenter, randomized, double-blind, parallel-group clinical trial involving 676 obese male and female subjects, Van Gaal et al.[79a] examined dose parameters, tolerability, and effects of orlistat over 6 months. Mean levels of vitamins A, D, and E and beta-carotene remained within the

clinical reference ranges in all treatment groups and rarely required supplementation.

In a year-long multicenter study assessing the efficacy and tolerability of orlistat (120 mg three times daily) on weight loss in 228 obese adult patients Finer et al.[80] coadministered vitamins A, D, and E to a small proportion of subjects "to maintain normal plasma levels of fat-soluble vitamins" and concluded that "fat-soluble vitamin supplements may be required during chronic therapy." In a clinical trial involving seventeen obese African-American and Caucasian adolescents receiving orlistat, 120 mg three times daily, McDuffie et al.[81] observed several significant nutrient depletion patterns despite coadministration of a daily multivitamin supplement containing vitamin A (5000 IU), vitamin D (400 IU), vitamin E (300 IU), and vitamin K (25 µg). However, during 3 to 6 months of orlistat treatment, acute absorption of retinol was not significantly altered, and serum levels of vitamin A did not change significantly. In contrast, mean vitamin D levels were significantly reduced compared with baseline after 1 month of orlistat, despite multivitamin supplementation, and alpha-tocopherol absorption was significantly reduced, although serum levels were not significantly altered.

Nutritional Therapeutics, Clinical Concerns, and Adaptations

Although alpha-tocopherol, vitamin D, and beta-carotene status may be adversely affected by orlistat, the emerging evidence indicates it does not impact absorption enough to deplete serum retinol levels to a clinically significant degree, at least not in most patients over periods up to 12 months. The average hepatic storage of vitamin A can prevent deficiency for 2 years with no vitamin A intake and may significantly confound attempts to assess such interactions. Nevertheless, physicians prescribing orlistat may find it prudent to monitor relevant nutrient status, as well as suggest regular use of a multivitamin containing low to moderate dosages levels of vitamin A and other fat-soluble nutrients, when treating patients likely deficient in such nutrients and for whom extended use (>1 year) increases the risk of cumulative adverse effects.

Retinoids

Acitretin (Soriatane), bexarotene (Targretin); etretinate (Tegison), isotretinoin (13-*cis* retinoic acid; Accutane), tretinoin (all-*trans* retinoic acid, ATRA; Atragen, Avita, Renova, Retin-A, Vesanoid, Vitinoin).

Interaction Type and Significance

✗✗✗ **Potentially Harmful or Serious Adverse Interaction—Avoid**

Probability:
2. **Probable** or
   1. **Certain**

Evidence Base:
●●● **Consensus** (extrapolated);
□ **Inadequate** (direct)

Effect and Mechanism of Action

Tretinoin and other pharmaceutical retinoids are modified versions of the vitamin A molecule. For example, isotretinoin is an isomer of all-*trans* retinoic acid (ATRA), a metabolite of retinol. A high dose intake of any retinoid (e.g., >50,000 IU daily) can result in accumulation and toxicity. An additive effect is predicted from concurrent intake of pharmaceutical retinoids and vitamin A supplements, based on structural similarities and known toxicities.

Research

Clinical research into interactions between and combined toxicity of retinol and retinoids has generally been avoided, regarded as unethical because of the apparently self-evident risk of clinically significant adverse effects. However, clinical trials do provide evidence of the impact of exogenous retinol sources on internal levels.

Rollman and Vahlquist[82] administered oral isotretinoin (0.5 mg/kg/day) for 3 months to 17 patients with severe acne vulgaris, then continued isotretinoin at a higher dose (0.75 mg/kg/day) to a subset of eight patients for an additional 3 months. After 3 months of therapy, epidermal retinol content increased by 53%, whereas dehydroretinol decreased by 79%. The researchers concluded that isotretinoin therapy interferes with the endogenous vitamin A metabolism in the skin. In a subsequent trial by this team involving 22 subjects with severe acne, administration of isotretinoin (1 mg/kg/day) for 4 months produced a marked increase in retinol and a decrease in dehydroretinol content in the skin.[83]

Clinical Implications and Adaptations

Even though no studies have confirmed adverse interactions, the structural similarities between and significant toxicities of both pharmaceutical retinoids and naturally occurring forms of vitamin A warrant caution. Consequently, supplementation of vitamin A by anyone using Accutane or related substances should be undertaken only under the supervision of an appropriately trained health care professional. These concerns are amplified for women of childbearing age because the risk of birth defects inherent to either substance is increased by their simultaneous use.

Physicians prescribing retinoids are advised to ask patients about use of vitamin supplements. Conservative practice suggests avoidance of supplemental vitamin A (particularly >10,000 IU/day) while taking Accutane or other retinoids. Most multivitamin formulations will be within the range generally considered as safe. Nevertheless, patients should watch for signs of toxicity. Headache is a common adverse effect associated with vitamin A toxicity; bone pain, dry scaly skin, and hair loss are other potential symptoms.

Some retinol is metabolized into retinoic acid, but in the absence of retinol deficiency, minimal beta-carotene (or alpha-carotene) is metabolized into retinol. Thus, current knowledge indicates that beta-carotene supplementation introduces no known risk of contributing to cumulative retinol toxicity through an additive interaction.

Tetracycline Antibiotics

Evidence: Minocycline (Dynacin, Minocin, Vectrin).
Extrapolated: Demeclocycline (Declomycin), doxycycline (Atridox, Doryx, Doxy, Monodox, Periostat, Vibramycin, Vibra-Tabs), oxytetracycline (Terramycin), tetracycline (Achromycin, Actisite, Apo-Tetra, Economycin, Novo-Tetra, Nu-Tetra, Sumycin, Tetrachel, Tetracyn); combination drugs: chlortetracycline, demeclocycline, and tetracycline (Deteclo); bismuth, metronidazole, and tetracycline (Helidac).

Interaction Type and Significance

✗✗ **Minimal to Mild Adverse Interaction—Vigilance Necessary**

✗✗✗ **Potentially Harmful or Serious Adverse Interaction—Avoid**

Probability:
2. Probable or **1. Certain**

Evidence Base:
◉◉◉ **Consensus** (extrapolated);
● **Preliminary** (direct)

Effect and Mechanism of Action

Benign intracranial hypertension and pseudotumor cerebri (PTC) have been associated with both hypervitaminosis A and tetracycline use independently. Vitamin A may potentiate the development of intracranial hypertension when taken in combination with tetracycline antibiotics. The development of severe headaches and PTC (or benign intracranial hypertension) have been associated with such concurrent use.[84,85]

Reports

Use of retinoids, particularly Accutane, has been associated with a number of cases of pseudotumor cerebri, some of which involved concomitant use of tetracyclines. First described by Gerber et al.[86] in 1954, PTC or benign intracranial hypertension has long been associated with vitamin A administration.[87,88] PTC occurs in 30% to 50% of patients with hypervitaminosis A and has been associated with isotretinoin therapy and etretinate in particular.[85,89-91] Combination therapy with tetracyclines may increase the risk of occurrence. Typical symptoms include papilledema, vision problems, nausea, and severe headaches. However, three specific criteria constitute its clinical characterization: (1) neurological and ocular symptoms and signs of increased intracranial pressure, which may include headache, nausea, transient visual obscurations, sixth-nerve palsies, and papilledema; (2) radiologically demonstrable normal or small cerebral ventricles; and (3) elevated cerebrospinal fluid (CSF) pressure.[92,93]

Moskowitz et al.[94] published a case report describing a 16-year-old girl who developed headaches and double vision after starting treatment for acne with vitamin A and minocycline; these adverse effects resolved once the compounds were discontinued. Further research is warranted to determine whether the symptoms could have been caused by an interaction between vitamin A and the drug.

Nutritional Therapeutics, Clinical Concerns, and Adaptations

Despite minimal direct evidence, conservative practice warrants avoidance of concomitant treatment with tetracycline antibiotics and vitamin A, based on functional equivalence of vitamin A and pharmaceutical retinoids and standard contraindications against coadministration of tetracyclines and such agents. Physicians prescribing antibiotics, particularly tetracyclines, need to ask patients about supplement use, particularly self-administration of vitamin A; tetracycline antibiotics and vitamin A are both used for acne vulgaris. Patients should be advised to limit supplemental retinol to 10,000 IU or less and to watch for signs of toxicity. Headache is a common adverse effect associated with vitamin A toxicity, as are bone pain, dry scaly skin, and hair loss.

Erythromycin can serve as an effective alternative to the tetracycline family and is less likely to produce serious adverse interactions, when antibiotic therapy is considered imperative.

Current knowledge indicates that in the absence of retinol deficiency, minimal beta-carotene (or alpha-carotene) is metabolized into retinol. Thus, beta-carotene supplementation does not contribute to cumulative retinol toxicity, although evidence of its efficacy in treating acne vulgaris is relatively weak compared with that supporting the use of retinol and related substances.

THEORETICAL, SPECULATIVE, AND PRELIMINARY INTERACTIONS RESEARCH, INCLUDING OVERSTATED INTERACTIONS CLAIMS

Antibiotics

Concomitant use of vitamin A with antibiotics has been proposed as efficacious in the treatment of shigellosis. Compromised nutritional status can play a significant role in susceptibility to many infections, and vitamin A is well known for its ability to reduce risk and assist treatment of many viral and bacterial infections. The use of vitamin A with antibiotic therapy represents an area of potential synergy in integrative therapeutics. However, systematic research is only beginning, and a wide range of clinical trials will be necessary before substantive conclusions can be made on nutritional synergies in antibiotic-treated bacterial infections.

In a randomized, double-blind, controlled clinical trial involving 83 children in Bangladesh, age 1 to 7 years, with acute shigellosis but no clinical signs of vitamin A deficiency, Hossain et al.[95] investigated the efficacy of a single, large oral dose of vitamin A. Nalidixic acid (55 mg/kg/day, every 6 hours), or an alternative determined by sensitivity test, was administered to all subjects. Of these, 42 received a single oral dose of 200,000 IU of water-miscible vitamin A as retinyl palmitate plus 25 IU of vitamin E; the 41 subjects in the control group received 25 IU of vitamin E. Subjects were evaluated after 5 days for evidence of "bacteriological cure." The researchers concluded that a single oral dose of 200,000 IU vitamin A can hasten clinical cure in acute shigellosis, can reduce its severity by promoting repair of the colonic mucosa and stimulating the immune system, and was especially relevant for children in areas with widespread vitamin A deficiency.

Salam et al.[96] criticized the previous study's design and the interpretation of the findings, emphasizing that the antibiotic used did not provide adequate antimicrobial treatment for most of the patients. They stated that the original authors' conclusions were not supported by the data, and that the potential clinical benefit of adjuvant vitamin A administration could not be proved without significant changes in study design and further research.

See also Tetracycline Antibiotics and Neomycin sections.

Anticonvulsant Medications, Including Phenobarbital, Phenytoin, and Valproic Acid

Evidence: Carbamazepine (Carbatrol, Tegretol), divalproex semisodium, divalproex sodium (Depakote), ethosuximide (Zarontin), phenobarbital (phenobarbitone; Luminal, Solfoton), phenytoin (diphenylhydantoin; Dilantin, Phenytek), sodium valproate (Depacon), valproic acid (Depakene, Depakene Syrup), valproate semisodium.
Extrapolated, based on similar properties: Clonazepam (Klonopin), clorazepate (Tranxene), ethotoin (Peganone), felbamate (Felbatol), fosphenytoin (Cerebyx, Mesantoin), gabapentin (Neurontin), lamotrigine (Lamictal), levetiracetam (Keppra), mephobarbital (Mebaral), methsuximide (Celontin), oxcarbazepine (Trileptal), pentobarbital (Nembutal), piracetam (Nootropyl), primidone (Mysoline), topiramate (Topamax), trimethadione (Tridione), vigabatrin (Sabril), zonisamide (Zonegran).

Conventional practice regards both vitamin A and anticonvulsant drugs as carrying significant risks of teratogenic adverse effects, especially when taken in high doses during pregnancy, although the mechanism involved has thus far eluded researchers. Preliminary evidence suggests that anticonvulsant medications can significantly alter endogenous retinoid metabolism in several ways. In particular, numerous studies have found that antiepileptic drugs (AEDs) alter endogenous retinoid concentrations, and that this effect could provide a possible mechanism for the pattern of teratogenesis observed with anticonvulsant therapy.

Although birth defects have been presented as a significant risk of high levels of vitamin A intake, other research indicates that supplemental vitamin A might prevent birth defects in children born to women receiving multiple-anticonvulsant therapy. All-*trans* retinoic acid (ATRA) and other vitamin A metabolites significantly influence embryonic development (e.g., growth, differentiation, morphogenesis), and imbalances in vitamin A status, both excess and deficiency, have been associated with teratogenic effects. Thus, medications such as AEDs that disrupt healthy levels of plasma retinoids could result in adverse effects, which could vary depending on the pathophysiology of the patient's underlying disorder(s), the medications and dosage levels being used, as well as the clinical response, nutritional status, general state of health, and other characteristics of the mother.

Evidence indicates that the toxicity of anticonvulsant drugs, and most likely some of their teratogenic effect, may be related to low blood levels of vitamin A. Nau et al.[97] measured plasma levels of retinol and its oxidative metabolites all-*trans*, 13-*cis*, and 13-*cis*-4-oxo retinoic acid in 75 infants and children treated with various AEDs for seizures and in 29 untreated controls of comparable age. Retinol levels increased with age, whereas the concentrations of retinoic acid compounds did not exhibit age dependency. Valproic acid monotherapy increased retinol levels in the young age group, and a trend toward increased retinol concentrations was seen in all other patient groups. The authors also noted significant declines in plasma levels of 13-*cis* and 13-*cis*-4-oxo retinoic acid in all patient groups treated with phenytoin, phenobarbital, carbamazepine, and ethosuximide, in combination with valproic acid, to levels below one third and one tenth of corresponding control values, respectively. Only minor changes were observed with ATRA, except in one patient group treated with valproic acid plus ethosuximide who demonstrated increased levels of this retinoid.

The available research does not conclusively answer whether coadministration of anticonvulsants and vitamin A inherently results in adverse effects or increases the risk of birth defects when taken during pregnancy. Because both retinoids and AEDs are highly associated with teratogenicity, clinical trials adding retinoid to AEDs in pregnant epileptic women are unlikely and inadvisable. Ultimately, characterization of these interactions remains important for understanding pharmacology and physiology, but it does little to change the recommendations of clinicians for their female patients of childbearing age; that is, neither anticonvulsants nor moderate to high doses of vitamin A should be considered as safe during pregnancy; and alternative therapeutic strategies of lesser toxicity are required.

Furthermore, these cautions need to be extended because of "off-label" prescribing of medications broadly classified as "anticonvulsants." These medications may be more often prescribed for pain, insomnia, anxiety, migraines, postherpetic neuralgia, and conditions other than seizure disorders. For example, up to 90% of gabapentin (Neurontin) is prescribed for off-label purposes, which are aggressively promoted by drug manufacturers and marketers. Such off-label use, however, is generally for conditions with less serious consequences than uncontrolled seizure disorders, and thus continued medication use during pregnancy is less likely to occur for such conditions.

Arachidonic Acid Cascade Inhibitors

5,8,11,14-Eicosatetraenoic acid, curcumin, indomethacin, l-phenyl-3-pyrazolidone (phenidone), nordihydroguaiaretic acid (NDGA).

Based on the findings of previous in vivo research Spingarn et al.[98] conducted in vitro studies on the potential synergistic effects of combining 13-cis retinoic acid (a retinoid, Accutane) and arachidonic acid cascade inhibitors (AACIs) on growth of head and neck squamous cell carcinoma (HNSCC). First, they investigated the effects of several AACIs (indomethacin, curcumin, phenidone, nordihydroguaiaretic acid, and 5,8,11,14-eicosatetraenoic acid) and 13-cis retinoic acid on the growth of two HNSCC cell lines and found that AACIs caused dose-dependent growth inhibition of both cell lines. When they combined these substances with 13-cis retinoic acid, they found that, except for indomethacin, they were able to inhibit HNSCC cell growth at lower concentrations of these drugs.

Although provocative and encouraging, this initial research has not yet matured to the level necessary for practical implementation in a clinical setting. Furthermore, because this research involved 13-cis retinoic acid, rather than a standard supplemental form of vitamin A, any extrapolation to such forms of vitamin A are not directly supported by the available evidence. Oncologists might consider discussing the potential benefit of such experimental adjunctive treatment options with patients. Such coadministration would necessitate close monitoring in conjunction with health care professionals trained and experienced in nutritional therapeutics, preferably within the context of a coordinated integrative care facility. Further research is warranted.

Methotrexate

Methotrexate (Folex, Maxtrex, Rheumatrex).

Vitamin A plays an important role in the function of healthy skin and proper function of the immune system. Both vitamin A and methotrexate are used in the treatment of psoriasis; methotrexate is also used against many other conditions, including malignant tumors. Nakagawa et al.[25] found that coadministration of methotrexate and retinyl palmitate enhanced antitumor activity in mice bearing ascites sarcoma 180 or P388 leukemia.

These preliminary findings suggest potential value in further study using well-designed research. Physicians prescribing methotrexate might consider coadministration of vitamin A within the context of close supervision and regular monitoring by health care professionals experienced in both conventional pharmacology and nutritional therapeutics.

Tamoxifen

Tamoxifen (Nolvadex).

Tamoxifen is an estrogen antagonist, specific for estrogen-driven cancers, and not a form of cytotoxic chemotherapy per se. Thus it needs to be treated separately from the agents discussed earlier under chemotherapy.

Some clinical oncologists experienced in the treatment of breast cancer patients with integrative therapeutics have used high-dose emulsified vitamin A in conjunction with tamoxifen.

This form of vitamin A is significantly less likely to produce as much hepatic retinyl ester accumulation, with dosage levels as high as 1 million U/day administered until significant cheilosis developed, then cut to 100,000 IU/day and gradually increased again. Close monitoring of the blood retinol level is essential, especially since it is typically pushed to or slightly beyond the upper limit of normal. Likewise, it is necessary to monitor skeletal metabolism and adjust vitamin A intake as needed to prevent bone loss. In an anecdotal report, one patient developed liver damage from long-term use of 25,000 IU nonemulsified vitamin A along with tamoxifen.[99] Further research into efficacy, safety, and factors influencing individual appropriateness is warranted through well-designed clinical trials, preferably within the context of integrative oncology care involving health care professionals trained and experienced in conventional pharmacology and nutritional therapeutics.

Thioridazine

Thioridazine (Mellaril).

Curtis and Swicord[100] stated that patients taking thioridazine exhibited elevated plasma vitamin A concentrations compared with individuals not using the medication. The clinical implications of this reported phenomenon, as well as its frequency and patterns of individual susceptibility, remain to be investigated. Well-designed clinical trials and thorough documentation of case reports are needed to determine whether this potential interaction might result in clinically significant effects. Pending such evidence, physicians prescribing thioridazine, and possibly other phenothiazines, are advised to ask patients about supplement intake, educate regarding signs and symptoms of vitamin A toxicity, and monitor those individuals for whom concurrent use appears appropriate but risky.

Warfarin and Related Oral Vitamin K Antagonist Anticoagulants

Anisindione (Miradon), dicumarol, ethyl biscoumacetate (Tromexan), nicoumalone (acenocoumarol; Acitrom, Sintrom), phenindione (Dindevan), phenprocoumon (Jarsin, Marcumar), warfarin (Coumadin, Marevan, Warfilone).

Vitamin A may increase the anticoagulant effects of warfarin or related anticoagulant medications. Physicians are advised to ask all patients about supplement intake, and vitamin A dosage should be noted. Despite minimal corroborating evidence, doses of vitamin A greater than 750 μg (2500 IU) have been reported to induce a hypoprothrombinemic response.[101] Long-term use of vitamin A or use of high doses may lead to an increased risk of bleeding for those taking anticoagulant medications, particularly warfarin.

The clinical significance and frequency of occurrence of this possible interaction are uncertain, even with several case reports. Physicians prescribing warfarin need to be aware of the risk of altered treatment effect when vitamin A is coadministered and closely monitor such patients for increased effects. International normalized ratio (INR) levels and prothrombin time (PT) need to be checked with greater frequency during the first 2 weeks after either starting or stopping vitamin A, particularly at high doses, to verify that the risk of bleeding or clotting (as reflected by the INR value) is not being affected by the nutrient. In general, it is important always to monitor PT twice weekly when medications, supplements, and diet are changed; this is the safest and most reliable method of compensating for unexpected or idiosyncratic interactions in patients undergoing treatment with coumarin derivatives.

NUTRIENT-NUTRIENT INTERACTIONS

Calcium

Because growing evidence indicates that excessive vitamin A intake may promote bone loss, the concomitant increase of calcium intake in conjunction with vitamin D support (through diet, supplements, and sunlight, titrating to blood level of 25-hydroxyvitamin D) is to be encouraged with high-dose administration of retinoids more than briefly.

Iron

Vitamin A deficiency may exacerbate iron deficiency anemia. Research involving anemic children indicates that concomitant intake of iron and vitamin A supplements enhances treatment of iron deficiency more effectively than iron supplementation alone.[102] Suharno et al.[103] reported similar findings in research involving treatment of pregnant women with "nutritional anemia" in West Java, Indonesia. Vitamin A supplementation can also improve iron status in populations, especially children, when poor nutritional status, including iron deficiency, is related to helminthiasis, as discussed earlier.[18] Conversely, Muñoz et al.[104] found that supplementation with iron and zinc improved indicators of vitamin A status in Mexican preschoolers.

Vitamin D

Vitamin A may antagonize the action of vitamin D.[7]

Vitamin E

Large doses of vitamin E can interfere with the absorption of vitamin A.

Zinc

Zinc deficiency appears to interfere with vitamin A metabolism through several mechanisms, including its absorption, transport, and utilization. Zinc binds with the transporter protein RBP, which is then able to transport vitamin A from liver stores to cells and tissues of numerous organs. Consequently, zinc deficiency results in decreased synthesis of RBP, thus affecting transport of retinol to target tissues. Zinc deficiency results in decreased activity of retinyl-palmitate esterase, the hepatic enzyme that releases retinol from retinyl palmitate, its storage form. Zinc is also required for retinol dehydrogenase, the enzyme involved in the oxidative conversion of retinol into retinal.[1,105]

As noted, Muñoz et al.[104] found that administration of zinc and iron improved indicators of vitamin A status in Mexican preschoolers. However, most human studies have shown only a weak link between vitamin A and zinc status. Thus far, animal and human studies have not conclusively differentiated responses related to zinc deficiency from generalized protein-energy deficiency. In disease states in which liver function is severely compromised and both zinc and vitamin A metabolism and transport are impaired, serum zinc and vitamin A concentrations tend to be positively correlated. More research is warranted to understand further the apparent synergy between these two nutrients, its mechanisms, and contextual influences, particularly individual variations and coexisting, moderate to severe, zinc and vitamin A deficiencies.

The 108 citations for this monograph, as well as additional reference literature, are located under Vitamin A (Retinol) on the CD at the back of the book.

Vitamin B₁ (Thiamine)

Nutrient Name: Vitamin B₁, thiamine.
Synonyms: Thiamin, thiamine.
Related Substances: Aneurine hydrochloride, thiamine hydrochloride, thiaminium chloride hydrochloride; benfotiamine; tetrahydrofurfuryl disulfide (TTFD).

Summary

Drug/Class Interaction Type	Mechanism and Significance	Management
Antacids ≈≈≈	Antacids interfere with the absorption of thiamine and other nutrients.	Separate intake of thiamine sources and antacids by at least 2 hours.
Antibiotics ≈≈≈	Repeated or protracted administration of broad-spectrum antibiotics can destroy beneficial intestinal flora and disrupt healthy gut ecology, including production of B vitamins. Mechanism is widely recognized, but clinical significance and long-term implications are just beginning to be acknowledged and understood.	Administration of diverse probiotic is judicious after significant antibiotic therapy. Multivitamin supplementation may be indicated if deficient.
Fluorouracil (5-FU) Antimetabolite chemotherapeutic agents ◇◇/⊕✗/◇≈≈	Fluorouracil interferes with conversion of thiamine to thiamine pyrophosphate as a means of inhibiting DNA and RNA synthesis and tumor cell proliferation. Mechanism and probability of this interaction are axiomatic, and its clinical significance is fundamental to use as chemotherapeutic strategy.	Thiamine restriction and depletion essential, but intermittent dietary enhancement or supplementation may be appropriate. Supervision and monitoring critical.
Furosemide Loop diuretics ≈≈≈/☼/◇	Furosemide and other loop diuretics can increase urinary thiamine excretion and induce thiamine depletion, which can contribute to cardiac insufficiency and aggravate congestive heart failure. With mechanism and prevalence of this adverse effect reaching consensus, so has appreciation of its profound clinical significance and long-term implications. Changes in medical practice are emerging.	Coadminister with diuresis longer than 1 month. Monitor for deficiency symptoms.
Nortriptyline Tricyclic antidepressants (TCAs) ≈≈≈/⊕⊕⊕	Response improved with coadministration of antidepressants, including nortriptyline and TCAs, and B vitamins, particularly thiamine. Mechanism undetermined: prevention of nutrient depletion or promotion of active synergistic effect, or both. Evidence preliminary but with strong positive trend. Clinical significance and individual patient factors still undefined.	B-complex coadministration judicious and considered safe, especially with probable deficiency.
Oral contraceptives (OCs) ≈≈≈/☼	Variable decreases in levels of thiamine and other nutrients associated with OC use. Clinical significance controversial; evidence mixed.	B-complex coadministration judicious and considered safe, especially with probable deficiency.
Phenytoin Anticonvulsant medications ≈≈≈/☼	Phenytoin interferes with thiamine function, particularly in brain, CNS, and CSF. Antiepileptic drugs may deplete thiamine (and folate), and supplementation may enhance therapeutic effect.	Coadminister with anticonvulsant therapy longer than 1 month. Monitor for deficiency symptoms.
Scopolamine ⊕⊕/☼	Scopolamine may interfere with CNS functions of thiamine, particularly involving acetylcholine. Preliminary evidence of reduced adverse effects with thiamine coadministration. Clinical significance probable.	Coadminister; may require high doses under supervision.
Stavudine Reverse-transcriptase inhibitor (nucleoside) antiretroviral agents ≈≈≈/☼	Thiamine used to counter severe lactic acidosis associated with stavudine, alone or with HAART protocols, particularly in patients with genetic susceptibility or preexisting vitamin deficiency. Evidence from anecdotal reports, but pattern consistent.	Preventive B-complex coadministration prudent. Intravenous thiamine administration indicated in critical cases. Close supervision, monitoring.
Tetracycline Tetracycline antibiotics ◇◇	Thiamine and other B-complex vitamins may interfere with tetracycline pharmacokinetics. Concomitant intake may significantly impair bioavailability. Evidence minimal but not controversial.	Avoid thiamine and B vitamins. If necessary, separate intake by 4 hours.

CNS, Central nervous system; *CSF*, cerebrospinal fluid; *HAART*, highly active antiretroviral therapy.

NUTRIENT DESCRIPTION

Chemistry and Forms

In 1926, thiamine was the first B vitamin isolated, as a crystalline, water-soluble, yellowish white powder with a salty, slightly nutty taste. By 1936 it had been synthesized and its chemical structure determined. This substance is heat and oxygen stable in its dry form, heat and alkali reactive in solution, and stabilized by acid.

Physiology and Function

Thiamine uptake by active transport is highest in the jejunum and ileum, with both passive diffusion and active, carrier-mediated transport. Throughout the small intestine, and generally by cells in various organs, absorption is mediated by a saturable, high-affinity transport system, and once absorbed, thiamine is primarily transported in the serum bound to albumin. In humans, thiamine can be synthesized in the large intestine as *thiamine pyrophosphate* (TPP). Too large a molecule to be absorbed across the intestinal mucosa, TPP requires the use of an enzyme to cleave the smaller thiamine molecule out of the compound. Skeletal muscle, heart, liver, kidneys, and the brain are sites of particularly high concentrations, although only small amounts of thiamine (30-70 mg) are typically stored in the body.

Thiamine is required for all tissues as a coenzyme in the metabolism of carbohydrates and branched-chain amino acids, particularly in the tricarboxylic acid (TCA) cycle and pentose phosphate shunt. Thiamine needs to be phosphorylated to become metabolically active, and thiamine diphosphate is its active form. Thiamine diphosphate is a cofactor for several important enzymes involved in the biosynthesis of neurotransmitters and various cell constituents, for the production of reducing equivalents used in oxidative stress responses, and for the biosyntheses of pentoses (e.g., ribose, deoxyribose) used as nucleic acid precursors. When it combines with two molecules of phosphoric acid, thiamine will form TPP. Functioning as a co-carboxylase, TPP is required for the oxidative decarboxylation of pyruvate to form active acetate and acetyl coenzyme A. It is also required for the oxidative decarboxylation of other alpha keto acids such as α-ketoglutaric acid and the 2-keto-carboxylates derived from the amino acids methionine, threonine, leucine, isoleucine, and valine. TPP is also involved as a coenzyme for the transketolase reaction, which functions for the pentose monophosphate shunt pathway. With a specific role in neurophysiology separate from its coenzyme function, TPP works at the nerve cell membrane to allow displacement so that sodium ions can freely cross the membrane. Although thiamine is needed for the metabolism of carbohydrates, fat, and protein, it is especially central to carbohydrate metabolism in the brain. In addition to providing TPP, thiamine becomes part of thiamine triphosphate, which appears to have an important function in brain cell viability. Thiamine is also required in acetylcholine and fatty acid synthesis.

Research is ongoing into the genetic and biochemical factors contributing to interindividual differences in susceptibility to development of disorders related to thiamine deficiency, as well as the differential vulnerabilities of various tissues and cell types.

NUTRIENT IN CLINICAL PRACTICE
Known or Potential Therapeutic Uses

Thiamine deficiency manifests primarily as disorders of the nervous, cardiovascular, muscular, and gastrointestinal systems. Deficiency symptoms include: fatigue, weight loss, depression, irritability, memory loss, mental confusion, heart palpitations, tachycardia, anorexia, indigestion, edema, neuritis, neuropathies, paresthesia, hyporeflexia (especially of legs), defective muscular coordination, muscular weakness, and sore muscles (especially calves).

Historical/Ethnomedicine Precedent

Beriberi, the classic thiamine deficiency disease.

Possible Uses

Alcoholism, Alzheimer's disease, anxiety, atherosclerosis, canker sores, chronic dieting, congestive heart failure (CHF), Crohn's disease, depression, diabetes mellitus, dysmenorrhea, fibromyalgia, glaucoma, hepatitis, human immunodeficiency virus and acquired immunodeficiency syndrome (HIV/AIDS) support, insomnia, Kearns-Sayre syndrome, Leigh's disease, minor injuries, mosquito repellant, multiple sclerosis, neuropathy (especially benfotiamine), roundworms, sciatica, sensory neuropathy (diabetic), trigeminal neuralgia, Wernicke-Korsakoff syndrome; diets consisting primarily of highly processed, refined foods; treatment of thiamine deficiency–related disorders, including cardiovascular (wet) beriberi, nervous (dry) beriberi, Wernicke's encephalopathy syndrome, and peripheral neuritis associated with pellagra (vitamin B₃ deficiency); alcoholic patients with altered sensorium; various genetic metabolic disorders, such as thiamine-responsive megaloblastic anemia.

Dietary Sources

Pork, liver, chicken, fish, beef, wheat germ, dried yeast, cereal products, lentils, potatoes, brewer's yeast, rice polishings, most whole-grain cereals (especially wheat, oats, and rice), all seeds and nuts, beans (especially soybeans), milk and milk products, vegetables such as beets, green leafy vegetables.

Most plant and animal foods contain some thiamine, but the richest dietary sources are brewer's yeast and organ meats.

Thiamine deficiency is one of the most common nutritional deficiency patterns in modernized societies. Almost half the U.S. population consumes less than half the recommended daily allowance (RDA) of thiamine, according to the U.S. Department of Agriculture. Although whole grains may be rich in thiamine, processing of grains significantly reduces their thiamine content. Likewise, because thiamine is water soluble and heat sensitive, cooking largely results in the loss or destruction of this vitamin, especially when chlorinated water is used.

Clinical signs of thiamine deficiency primarily involve the nervous, cardiovascular, muscular, and gastrointestinal systems. Adults have the following symptoms:

- Mental confusion, anorexia, muscle weakness, calf muscle tenderness, ataxia, indigestion, constipation, tachycardia with palpitations.
- *Wet beriberi:* edema starting in the feet and progressing upward into the legs, trunk, and face, eventually resulting in death from cardiac enlargement and CHF.
- *Dry beriberi:* worsened polyneuritis in early stages (particularly peripheral neuritis), difficulty walking, and muscle wasting, especially atrophy of the legs.

The distinction between wet (cardiovascular) and dry (neuritic) manifestations of beriberi usually relates to the duration and severity of the deficiency, the degree of physical exertion, and the caloric intake. The wet or edematous condition results from severe physical exertion and high carbohydrate intake. The dry or polyneuritic form stems from relative inactivity with caloric restrictions during the chronic deficiency.

Wernicke-Korsakoff syndrome is the classical manifestation of central nervous system (CNS) deficiency of thiamine caused by alcoholism. Patients present with impaired memory and cognitive function, irritability, and nystagmus caused by weakness in the sixth cranial nerve; coma is a common end state. Vitamin B₁ is necessary for the metabolism of alcohol, but alcohol interferes with its absorption, making malnourished alcoholics often severely thiamine deficient. Alcoholics given intravenous (IV) glucose without thiamine are at high risk of developing Wernicke-Korsakoff syndrome and sustain permanent neurological damage, because the glucose, which also requires thiamine for its metabolism, rapidly depletes remaining tissue levels of brain thiamine. For this reason, an IV "cocktail" of glucose, thiamine, and a narcotic antagonist is typically administered in emergency rooms to unconscious patients who present with unconsciousness of unknown etiology.

Infant symptoms appear suddenly and severely, involving cardiac failure and cyanosis.

The etiology of thiamine deficiency can be traced to an exclusive diet of milled, nonenriched rice or wheat, raw fish consumption (microbial thiaminases), large amounts of tea, alcoholism (impaired absorption and storage, poor nutrition, increased thiamine utilization), use of loop diuretics, and several inborn errors of metabolism.

Special Populations

Individuals with alcoholism, anorexia, CHF, Crohn's disease, folate deficiency, malabsorption syndrome, and multiple sclerosis are at increased risk of developing thiamine deficiency, as are those undergoing long-term diuretic therapy, hemodialysis, or peritoneal dialysis.

Alcoholic individuals frequently develop a deficiency of thiamine because the vitamin is a necessary cofactor in the metabolism of alcohol. Because many alcoholics tend to eat less and drink more, and usually their alcohol-based drinks are low in thiamine, they frequently develop a thiamine deficiency. In hospitals it is routine for alcoholics to receive intramuscular (IM) injections of thiamine on admission.

Elderly persons demonstrate a general decline in thiamine levels that is apparently related more to age than to coexisting illness or health status. This increased susceptibility enhances the risk for adverse effects of drug-induced depletion, especially in regard to cardiovascular health and cognitive stability.[1]

Nutrient Preparations Available

Thiamine, water soluble. *Thiamine hydrochloride* is generally considered the preferred supplemental form of thiamine. Thiamine mononitrate is also available. Thiamine supplementation is usually provided in vitamin B–complex formulations, in most multivitamin preparations, and in vitamin-enriched foods, such as breakfast cereals.

Benfotiamine is a lipid-soluble form of thiamine developed and patented in Japan, now widely used in neuropathy therapies.

Dosage Forms Available

Capsule, liquid, tablet, effervescent tablet; liposomal spray. Parenteral form may be administered by IM or slow IV injection.

Source Materials for Nutrient Preparations

Synthesized.

Dosage Range

The RDA for thiamine varies slightly with gender and life stage.

Men (> 19 years): 1.2 mg/day
Women (> 19 years): 1.1 mg/day
Pregnancy and breastfeeding (any age): 1.4 mg/day

Adults

Supplemental/Maintenance: Dependent on dietary intake, usually 1 to 2 mg/day. A paper on the "ideal" daily thiamine intake reported that the healthiest people consumed more than 9 mg/day.[2]

Pharmacological/Therapeutic: 1.5 to 200 mg/day. In research studies, therapeutic dosage for most conditions ranges from 10 to 100 mg/day, in divided doses. In clinical practice, 200 to 600 mg/day may be given, and some clinicians have used oral dosages as high as 8 g/day, in divided doses, for a variety of metabolic disorders.

Thiamine deficiency (beriberi): 5 to 30 mg per dose, intramuscularly (IM) or intravenously (IV), three times daily (if critically ill); then orally 5 to 30 mg/day in single or divided doses, three times daily for 1 month.

Wernicke's encephalopathy: 100 mg IV initially, then 50 to 100 mg/day IM or IV until consuming a consistently balanced and nutritious diet.

Toxic: There is no defined upper limit (UL) for thiamine because of its relative safety.

Pediatric (<18 years)
Supplemental/Maintenance:
   Infants: 0.3 to 0.5 mg/day
   Children: 0.5 to 1 mg/day
Pharmacologic/Therapeutic, for thiamine deficiency (beriberi): 10 to 25 mg per dose, IM or IV, daily (if critically ill), or 10 to 50 mg per dose orally every day for 2 weeks, then 5 to 10 mg per dose orally daily for 1 month.
Toxic: No toxic intake level known to date.

SAFETY PROFILE

Overview

Thiamine is generally considered virtually nontoxic, even in very high doses orally. Being water soluble, thiamine excretion is rapid; the vitamin is not stored in the body, and accumulation to toxic levels is highly improbable using oral intake. No adverse effects associated with thiamine intake from food sources or nutritional supplements have been reported. Rare occurrences of adverse effects of thiamine have been documented, although they appear to be largely associated with allergic reactions to thiamine injections.

Nutrient Adverse Effects
General Adverse Effects

Adverse effects are theoretically possible but rare with oral supplemental thiamine intake. Oral doses greater than 200 mg have been reported to cause drowsiness in some individuals. In a study of 989 patients, 100 mg/day IV thiamine hydrochloride resulted in a burning effect at the injection site in 11 subjects and pruritus in one.[3]

Large doses of vitamin B₁ over an extended period may cause imbalance among various B vitamins.

Administration of IV or IM thiamine warrants caution because anaphylactic or allergic reaction infrequently occurs. Allergic reactions to thiamine injections are rare (< 1%) but can be severe and include cardiovascular collapse and death, angioedema, paresthesia, warmth, and rash.

Adverse Effects Among Specific Populations

High oral intakes might have some unknown potential for adverse reactions in select, metabolically compromised populations because of pharmacogenomic susceptibility, but such data are only recently under consideration.

Pregnancy and Nursing

A review of the medical literature reveals no substantial reports of adverse effects related to fetal development during pregnancy or to breast-fed infants.

Infants and Children

A review of the medical literature reveals no substantial reports of adverse effects specifically related to the use of thiamine in infants and children.

Contraindications

No contraindications are known to date, except hypersensitivity to thiamine or to any component of any compound formulation. Some clinicians and researchers are proposing that cancer patients undergoing chemotherapy may benefit from restricted thiamine intake during treatment.

Precautions and Warnings

Use with caution with parenteral administration, especially with IV administration.

Laboratory Values

Whole-blood thiamine: Level less than 70 nmol/L indicates deficiency.

Erythrocyte transketolase (EKTA): Low activity of EKTA (< 5 U/mmol hemoglobin) indicates deficiency, as does increase in EKTA (> 16 U/mmol) after stimulation by the addition of TPP.

Therapeutic reference range: 1.6-4.0 mg/dL.

INTERACTIONS REVIEW

Strategic Considerations

Thiamine plays a critical role in a range of metabolic processes, especially the Krebs cycle and adenosine triphosphate (ATP) synthesis. Vitamin B$_1$ depletion by diet, lifestyle, or medications increases several risk factors, especially for the cardiovascular and nervous systems. Although thiamine is central to metabolic vitality and cardiovascular health, the use of loop diuretics increases the risk of clinically significant thiamine depletion. However, adverse effects caused by drug depletion can be safely and effectively treated with thiamine supplementation, while further supporting healthy cardiac function. Thiamine intake during chemotherapy is challenging, and personalized integrative care may clarify paradoxical data. In other, simpler situations, the potential for adverse effects from unintentional depletion of thiamine by pharmacological agents can be corrected through supplementation at typical therapeutic levels.

NUTRIENT-DRUG INTERACTIONS

Antacids, Including Aluminum Hydroxide and Magnesium Trisilicate

Aluminum carbonate gel (Basajel), aluminum hydroxide (Alternagel, Amphojel); combination drugs: aluminum hydroxide, magnesium carbonate, alginic acid, and sodium bicarbonate (Gaviscon Extra Strength Tablets, Gaviscon Regular Strength Liquid, Gaviscon Extra Strength Liquid); aluminum hydroxide and magnesium hydroxide (Advanced Formula Di-Gel Tablets, co-magaldrox, Di-Gel, Gelusil, Maalox, Maalox Plus, Mylanta, Wingel); aluminum hydroxide, magnesium trisilicate, alginic acid, and sodium bicarbonate (Alenic Alka, Gaviscon Regular Strength Tablets); calcium carbonate (Titralac, Tums), magnesium hydroxide (Phillips' Milk of Magnesia MOM); combination drugs: magnesium hydroxide and calcium carbonate (Calcium Rich Rolaids); magnesium hydroxide, aluminum hydroxide, calcium carbonate, and simethicone (Tempo Tablets); magnesium trisilicate and aluminum hydroxide (Adcomag trisil, Foamicon); magnesium trisilicate, alginic acid, and sodium bicarbonate (Alenic Alka, Gaviscon Regular Strength Tablets); combination drug: sodium bicarbonate, aspirin, and citric acid (Alka-Seltzer).

Interaction Type and Significance

≈≈≈ **Drug-Induced Nutrient Depletion, Supplementation Therapeutic, Not Requiring Professional Management**

Probability:	Evidence Base:
3. Possible	○ **Preliminary**

Effect and Mechanism of Action

Antacids interfere with the absorption of many nutrients, including thiamine. Thiamine is alkali reactive in solution and stabilized by acid. Thiamine absorption in the human small intestinal brush-border membrane vesicle is pH dependent.[4] In particular, aluminum-based antacids may lower thiamine absorption.

Report

Majoor and de Vries[5] described a patient who developed cardiac beriberi with polyneuritis after chronic use of large amounts of magnesium trisilicate.

Nutritional Therapeutics, Clinical Concerns, and Adaptations

The adverse effect on absorption of thiamine can be reduced by separating antacid use by at least 2 hours from intake of thiamine supplements or foods relied on as primary thiamine dietary sources.

Antibiotics and Antimicrobial Agents (Systemic)

Aminoglycoside antibiotics: Amikacin (Amikin), gentamicin (G-mycin, Garamycin, Jenamicin), kanamycin (Kantrex), neomycin (Mycifradin, Myciguent, Neo-Fradin, NeoTab, Nivemycin), netilmicin (Netromycin), paromomycin (monomycin; Humatin), streptomycin, tobramycin (AKTob, Nebcin, TOBI, TOBI Solution, TobraDex, Tobrex).

Beta-lactam antibiotics: Methicillin (Staphcillin); aztreonam (Azactam injection); carbapenem antibiotics: meropenem (Merrem I.V.); combination drug: imipenem and cilastatin (Primaxin I.M., Primaxin I.V.); penicillin antibiotics: amoxicillin (Amoxicot, Amoxil, Moxilin, Trimox, Wymox); combination drug: amoxicillin and clavulanic acid (Augmentin, Augmentin XR, Clavulin); ampicillin (Amficot, Omnipen, Principen, Totacillin); combination drug: ampicillin and sulbactam (Unisyn); bacampicillin (Spectrobid), carbenicillin (Geocillin), cloxacillin (Cloxapen), dicloxacillin (Dynapen, Dycill), mezlocillin (Mezlin), nafcillin (Unipen), oxacillin (Bactocill), penicillin G (Bicillin C-R, Bicillin L-A, Pfizerpen, Truxcillin), penicillin V (Beepen-VK, Betapen-VK, Ledercillin VK, Pen-Vee K, Robicillin VK, Suspen, Truxcillin VK, V-Cillin K, Veetids), piperacillin (Pipracil); combination drug: piperacillin and tazobactam (Zosyn); ticarcillin (Ticar); combination drug: ticarcillin and clavulanate (Timentin).

Cephalosporin antibiotics: Cefaclor (Ceclor), cefadroxil (Duricef), cefamandole (Mandol), cefazolin (Ancef, Kefzol), cefdinir (Omnicef), cefepime (Maxipime), cefixime (Suprax), cefoperazone (Cefobid), cefotaxime (Claforan), cefotetan (Cefotan), cefoxitin (Mefoxin), cefpodoxime (Vantin), cefprozil (Cefzil), ceftazidime (Ceptaz, Fortaz, Tazicef, Tazidime), ceftibuten (Cedax), ceftizoxime (Cefizox), ceftriaxone (Rocephin), cefuroxime (Ceftin, Kefurox, Zinacef), cephalexin (Keflex, Keftab), cephapirin (Cefadyl), cephradine (Anspor, Velocef), imipenem combination drug: imipenem and cilastatin (Primaxin I.M., Primaxin I.V.); loracarbef (Lorabid), meropenem (Merrem I.V.).

Fluoroquinolone (4-Quinolone) antibiotics: Cinoxacin (Cinobac, Pulvules), ciprofloxacin (Ciloxan, Cipro), enoxacin (Penetrex), gatifloxacin (Tequin), levofloxacin (Levaquin), lomefloxacin (Maxaquin), moxifloxacin (Avelox), nalidixic acid (Neggram), norfloxacin (Noroxin), ofloxacin (Floxin, Ocuflox), sparfloxacin (Zagam), trovafloxacin (alatrofloxacin; Trovan).

Macrolide antibiotics: Azithromycin (Zithromax), clarithromycin (Biaxin), dirithromycin (Dynabac), erythromycin oral (EES, EryPed, Ery-Tab, PCE Dispertab, Pediazole), troleandomycin (Tao).

Sulfonamide antibiotics: Sodium sulfacetamide (AK-Sulf, Bleph-10, Sodium Sulamyd), sulfamethoxazole (Gantanol), sulfanilamide (AVC), sulfasalazine (salazosulfapyridine, salicylazosulfapyridine, suphasalazine; Apo-Sulfasalazine, Azulfidine, Azulfidine EN-Tabs, PMS-Sulfasalazine, Salazopyrin, Salazopyrin EN-Tabs, SAS), sulfisoxazole (Gantrisin); combination drug: sulfamethoxazole and trimethoprim (cotrimoxazole, cotrimoxazole, SXT, TMP-SMX, TMP-sulfa; Bactrim, Bactrim DS, Cotrim, Septra, Septra DS, Sulfatrim, Uroplus); triple sulfa (Sultrin Triple Sulfa).

Chemotherapy, cytotoxic antibiotics: Bleomycin (Blenoxane), dactinomycin (Actinomycin D, Cosmegen, Cosmegen Lyovac), mitomycin (Mutamycin), plicamycin (Mithracin).

Miscellaneous antibiotics: Bacitracin (Caci-IM), chloramphenicol (Chloromycetin), chlorhexidine (Peridex), colistimethate (Coly-Mycin M), dapsone (DDS, diaminodiphenylsulphone; Aczone Gel, Avlosulfon), furazolidone (Furoxone), lincomycin (Lincocin), linezolid (Zyvox), nitrofurantoin (Macrobid, Macrodantin), oral clindamycin (Cleocin), trimethoprim (Proloprim, Trimpex), vancomycin (Vancocin). See also Tetracycline later.

Interaction Type and Significance

≈≈≈ **Drug-Induced Nutrient Depletion, Supplementation Therapeutic, Not Requiring Professional Management**

Probability:	Evidence Base:
3. Possible	○ **Preliminary**

Effect and Mechanism of Action
The B vitamins, including thiamine, are produced in appreciable amounts by probiotic microorganisms as part of their synergistic role within the healthy intestinal microecology.

Research
Repeated or chronic use of antimicrobial agents can deplete or functionally eliminate these beneficial flora and contribute to depleted status of thiamine and other important nutrients.[6,7]

Nutritional Therapeutics, Clinical Concerns, and Adaptations
The severity of disruption to the intestinal microecology will vary depending on many factors, including an individual's diet, medical history, health status, and co-morbid conditions. Potential adverse effects of antibiotics on thiamine status can be safely and effectively prevented or reversed through supplementation with thiamine and related nutrients at standard supplemental levels, along with replenishment of flora through consumption of high doses of vigorous and variegated probiotic microorganisms. Duration of such restorative nutritional therapy depends on the individual's health status as well as the dosage, duration, and type of antibiotic medications(s) being administered. Individuals not undergoing diuretic therapy, suffering from alcoholism, or characterized by other high-risk factors will generally not require, although they may benefit from, increased thiamine supplementation during or after a single course of antibiotics; a short course of probiotic therapy is still recommended as supportive in such circumstances.

Fluorouracil and Related Antimetabolite Chemotherapeutic Agents

Evidence: Fluorouracil (5-FU; Adrucil, Efudex, Efudix, Fluoroplex).

Extrapolated, based on similar properties: Agalsidase beta (Fabrazyme), capecitabine (Xeloda), cladribine (Leustatin), cytarabine (ara-C; Cytosar-U, DepoCyt, Tarabine PFS), floxuridine (FUDR), fludarabine (Fludara), gemcitabine (Gemzar), lometrexol (T64), mercaptopurine (6-mercaptopurine, 6-MP, NSC 755; Purinethol), methotrexate (Folex, Maxtrex, Rheumatrex), pentostatin (Nipent), pemetrexed (Alimta), raltitrexed (ZD-1694; Tomudex), thioguanine (6-thioguanine, 6-TG, 2-amino-6-mercaptopurine; Lanvis, Tabloid), ZD9331.

Interaction Type and Significance

◇◇ **Drug-Induced Effect on Nutrient Function, Supplementation Contraindicated, Professional Management Appropriate**

⊕✗ **Bimodal or Variable Interaction, with Professional Management**

◇≈≈ **Drug-Induced Adverse Effect on Nutrient Function, Coadministration Therapeutic, with Professional Management**

Probability:	Evidence Base:
3. Probable	◉ **Emerging**

Effect and Mechanism of Action
Fluorouracil is an antimetabolite of the pyrimidine analog type. In the form of its active metabolite, 5-FU inhibits the conversion of thiamine to TPP and inhibits DNA and RNA synthesis. The cofactor of transketolase, TPP promotes nucleic acid ribose synthesis and tumor cell proliferation through the nonoxidative transketolase (TK) pathway.[8-10]

Research
The research on the role of thiamine during chemotherapy is complex and seemingly contradictory, but an emerging consensus may clarify clinical options for integrative therapies within a strategic framework. Thiamine deficiency frequently occurs in patients with advanced cancer, particularly within the context of drug-induced nutrient depletion, and therefore thiamine supplementation has often been used for nutritional support.[9] In vitro research and clinical observations suggest that fluoropyrimidines may increase cellular thiamine metabolism and depletion.[10-12] This has raised concern of possible thiamine deficiency and indicated a potential beneficial role for increased dietary intake and supplementation of thiamine.[13] Lactic acidosis caused by thiamine deficiency is known to complicate chemotherapy and radiotherapy of malignant tumors. However, clinical and experimental data demonstrate both increased thiamine utilization by tumor cells and thiamine's interference with certain types of anti-neoplastic chemotherapy.[13] In particular, metabolic control analyses predict that, by supporting a high rate of nucleic acid ribose synthesis, thiamine and other stimulators of transketolase enzyme synthesis contribute to tumor cell survival, chemotherapy resistance, and cancer cell proliferation.[13-15] Both human and animal studies support these hypotheses.

Nutritional Therapeutics, Clinical Concerns, and Adaptations
Scientific research and clinical experience suggest that no static and generic protocol is possible for thiamine support or restriction in patients undergoing antineoplastic chemotherapy, especially involving 5-FU. Integrating the findings of the research literature into a clinical context requires an individualized and evolving approach to the therapeutic process, tactical emphases, and the patient's general health status. Ultimately,

it is critical to determine whether the benefits of thiamine administration outweigh the risks of tumor proliferation and how such determination may shift through the course of treatment. Some researchers and clinicians have also suggested administration of transketolase inhibitors as a complementary tactic in treating some oncology patients. Thus, the evidence supports a flexible strategy involving phased restriction of thiamine intake during chemotherapy, followed by compensatory dietary enhancement and/or thiamine supplementation as a reasonable conservative approach, with the particulars of such implementation ultimately dependent on the prior history, emerging needs, and evolving response of the individual patient.

Intercurrent thiamine supplementation may be clinically appropriate for some patients at critical stages in their therapeutic regimen if thiamine depletion presents an overriding concern for patient survival and well-being. Implementation of such an approach to integrative personalized care requires active collaboration by health care professionals trained and experienced in both conventional pharmacology and nutritional therapeutics. When tumor-bearing patients receive thiamine-containing supplements, it would seem prudent to use RDA levels of thiamine (1-2 mg/day) and avoid higher doses (10-100 or more mg/day) of thiamine, unless the patient has cardiac, neurological, or musculoskeletal symptoms consistent with severe thiamine deficiency and promptly ameliorated by a therapeutic trial of higher-dose thiamine administration. Once corrected, a return to RDA-level supplementation and encouraging dietary intake of thiamine-rich foods, such as brewer's/nutritional yeast, would seem appropriate in view of the data on thiamine's potential to enhance tumor growth. In patients with recurrent or metastatic malignant disease, even with no evidence of tumor on scans and physical examination after treatment, micrometastatic disease is probable, and in the absence of a life-threatening deficiency syndrome, it would seem prudent to avoid high levels of thiamine administration (as well as niacin/niacinamide, shown to support growth of new blood vessels—angiogenesis—on which tumor growth and metastasis depend).

Furosemide and Related Loop Diuretics

Evidence: Furosemide (Lasix).
Extrapolated, based on similar properties: Bumetanide (Bumex), ethacrynic acid (Edecrin), torsemide (Demadex).

Interaction Type and Significance

≈≈≈ Drug-Induced Nutrient Depletion, Supplementation Therapeutic, Not Requiring Professional Management
☼ Prevention or Reduction of Drug Adverse Effect
◇ Adverse Drug Effect on Nutritional Therapeutics, Strategic Concern

Probability:	Evidence Base:
1. Certain	● Consensus

Effect and Mechanism of Action

Several studies have suggested that loop diuretics, especially furosemide (Lasix), can cause thiamine depletion due to increased urinary excretion, contributing to cardiac insufficiency in patients with CHF.[16-21] Further research has indicated that the compromised thiamine status of individuals with CHF may be caused by altered metabolism, rather than simple deficiency, of thiamine. In a study of the diuretic effects of single IV doses of furosemide on six healthy volunteers,

Rieck et al.[22] observed a doubling of thiamine excretion rate, along with the expected increased urine volume and sodium excretion. Another study examined cardiac function and status of select nutrients in 30 patients with idiopathic dilated cardiomyopathy using diuretics, compared with a similar number of healthy control individuals. Measuring the activity of erythrocytic transketolase and the effect of TPP, da Cunha et al.[22a] determined the presence of thiamine deficiency in 33% of the patients with heart disease (vs. 10% of controls).

Even though all loop diuretics work by inhibiting sodium and chloride reabsorption in the thick ascending limb of Henle's loop, no conclusive research on the effects of other loop diuretics on thiamine has been published. However, CHF is characteristic of wet beriberi, caused by thiamine deficiency. Patients receiving furosemide are likely to have compromised kidney function, decreased metabolic function associated with aging, malnourishment, alcoholism and other lifestyle factors, and other variables aggravating thiamine depletion, deficiency, and dysregulation.[17,19,23]

Research

As noted earlier, numerous studies have determined that thiamine depletion is a common phenomenon among patients undergoing loop diuretic therapy. For example, an investigation of 38 sequential patients in a cardiology clinic assessed thiamine status by in vitro erythrocyte transketolase activity assay and dietary intake of thiamine. Thiamine deficiency was found in 21% of the patients and evidence of risk for dietary thiamine inadequacy in 25%.[19]

A small pilot study in 1991 examined the effects of long-term furosemide therapy (80-240 mg for 3-14 months) in hospitalized patients with CHF to determine the occurrence of clinically significant thiamine deficiency caused by urinary loss.[17] Elevated levels of thiamine pyrophosphate effect (TPPE), indicating thiamine deficiency, were found in 21 of 23 furosemide-treated patients and in 2 of 16 age-matched controls. Biochemical evidence of thiamine deficiency tended to be more common among patients with poor left ventricular ejection fractions (LVEF). A 7-day course of IV thiamine, 100 mg twice daily, lowered TPPE levels to normal in six of the subjects, indicating normal thiamine utilization capacity, and improved LVEF in four of five patients, as demonstrated by echocardiography. These preliminary findings suggest that long-term furosemide therapy may be associated with clinically significant thiamine deficiency, presumed to result from urinary loss, and contribute to impaired cardiac performance in patients with CHF. Further, this apparent drug-induced depletion pattern responded to appropriate thiamine administration within an inpatient setting.

In 1995 the same research team conducted a double-blind, placebo-controlled trial in which they initially randomized 30 subjects to 1 week of either IV thiamine (200 mg/day) or placebo within inpatient care.[18] In the second phase, all individuals were discharged and given oral thiamine (200 mg/day) for 6 weeks. After the initial IV thiamine, thiamine status normalized, and LVEF increased significantly in those who received IV thiamine, in contrast to no measurable response in thiamine status among those given IV placebo. After the 7-week intervention, the 27 remaining subjects showed 22% improvement in LVEF. The researchers concluded that cardiac function in CHF patients may be exacerbated by thiamine depletion attributable to long-term furosemide therapy; thiamine supplementation or systematic dietary enhancement may avert or correct this adverse effect and its probable sequelae in patients with moderate to severe CHF.

Although there is consensus on an association between loop diuretic therapy and compromised thiamine status, conclusive evidence is lacking to confirm a consistent causal relationship. Using high-pressure liquid chromatography (HPLC) to assess blood thiamine and thiamine ester concentrations in erythrocytes of 41 elderly patients with CHF treated with furosemide (and a control group), a Swedish team found reduced thiamine diphosphate (TPP), the storage form of thiamine, but not thiamine phosphate (TP). The researchers concluded that the observed change in CHF patients taking furosemide was most likely not an expression of a thiamine deficiency, but rather of altered thiamine metabolism not yet explained.[24]

Zenuk et al.[25] investigated the thiamine status of 32 patients with CHF who received either 40 to 80 mg or 80 mg or more of furosemide daily. Using erythrocyte transketolase enzyme activity and the degree of TPPE, these researchers found that 96% (24 of 25) of those receiving the higher diuretic dose demonstrated biochemical evidence of severe thiamine deficiency, as did 57% (4 of 7) of patients taking 40 mg furosemide daily. No other clinical variables showed a significant association with thiamine status.

Thus, collectively, the body of evidence suggests that thiamine deficiency occurs in a substantial proportion of CHF patients being treated with furosemide.

Nutritional Therapeutics, Clinical Concerns, and Adaptations

Long-term diuretic administration remains a central pharmacological therapy of heart insufficiency and hypertension in conventional practice. However, loop diuretics can aggravate the high-risk status inherent to many conditions for which these medications are prescribed, especially among hospitalized or chronic care elderly patients. Thiamine supplements should be considered in patients undergoing sustained diuresis, particularly when dietary deficiency may be present. Investigating the risk posed by diuretic use for subclinical thiamine deficiency in elderly patients, Swiss researchers suggested that low-dose thiamine supplementation may help prevent the development of subclinical wet beriberi in such patients.[20] Pending conclusive evidence to the contrary, patients taking furosemide, and possibly other loop diuretics, would most likely benefit from thiamine support of 100 mg per day, orally.

Nortriptyline and Related Tricyclic Antidepressants

Evidence: Nortriptyline (Aventyl, Pamelor).
Extrapolated, based on similar properties: Amitriptyline (Elavil); combination drug: amitriptyline and perphenazine (Triavil, Etrafon, Triptazine); amoxapine (Asendin), clomipramine (Anafranil), desipramine (Norpramin, Pertofrane), doxepin (Adapin, Sinequan), imipramine (Janimine, Tofranil), nortriptyline (Aventyl, Pamelor), protriptyline (Vivactil), trimipramine (Surmontil).

Interaction Type and Significance

≈≈≈ **Drug-Induced Nutrient Depletion, Supplementation Therapeutic, Not Requiring Professional Management**
⊕⊕⊕ **Beneficial or Supportive Interaction, Not Requiring Professional Management**

Probability:	Evidence Base:
3. Possible	○ **Preliminary**

Effect and Mechanism of Action

The mechanism of action involved in the proposed interactions between nortriptyline and thiamine, or more exactly B-vitamin complex, is uncertain at this time, and various explanations are available. Interference with nutrient metabolism of other drug-induced depletion effects may be corrected by supplementation. A synergistic interaction between the antidepressant and the nutrient(s) may also be contributing to improved outcome measures.[26] Further research to determine the mechanism(s) of action could clarify the physiological processes and help refine integrative therapies to enhance clinical outcomes.

Research

A 1992 study involving 14 institutionalized geriatric patients with impaired cognitive function undergoing treatment for depression is the primary evidence for augmentation of nortriptyline therapy using supplemental B-vitamin complex. In this 4-week, randomized, placebo-controlled, double-blind trial, the elderly inpatients were administered open tricyclic antidepressant (TCA) treatment (nortriptyline titrated to doses yielding blood levels of 50-150 ng/mL) along with vitamins B₁, B₂, and B₆ (each 10 mg/day). The researchers reported that "the active vitamin group demonstrated significantly better B₂ and B₆ status on enzyme activity coefficients and trends toward greater improvement in scores on ratings of depression and cognitive function, as well as in serum nortriptyline levels compared with placebo-treated subjects."[27]

Nutritional Therapeutics, Clinical Concerns, and Adaptations

The coadministration of thiamine, as part of a B-vitamin complex formula at customary dosage levels, offers reasonable potential for enhancing treatment of depression (especially with cognitive dysfunction) with nortriptyline, or other TCAs, particularly in elderly of other patients who have restricted mobility or who are living in institutionalized care settings, at increased risk of inadequate and inconsistent nutrient intake.

Oral Contraceptives: Monophasic, Biphasic, and Triphasic Estrogen Preparations (Synthetic Estrogen and Progesterone Analogs)

Ethinyl estradiol and desogestrel (Desogen, Ortho-TriCyclen).
Ethinyl estradiol and ethynodiol (Demulen 1/35, Demulen 1/50, Nelulen 1/25, Nelulen 1/50, Zovia).
Ethinyl estradiol and levonorgestrel (Alesse, Levlen, Levlite, Levora 0.15/30, Nordette, Tri-Levlen, Triphasil, Trivora).
Ethinyl estradiol and norethindrone/norethisterone (Brevicon, Estrostep, Genora 1/35, GenCep. 1/35, Jenest-28, Loestrin 1.5/30, Loestrin 1/20, Modicon, Necon 1/25, Necon 10/11, Necon 0.5/30, Necon 1/50, Nelova 1/35, Nelova 10/11, Norinyl 1/35, Norlestin 1/50, Ortho Novum 1/35, Ortho Novum 10/11, Ortho Novum 7/7/7, Ovcon-35, Ovcon-50, Tri-Norinyl, Trinovum).
Ethinyl estradiol and norgestrel (Lo/Ovral, Ovral).
Mestranol and norethindrone (Genora 1/50, Nelova 1/50, Norethin 1/50, Ortho-Novum 1/50).
Related, internal application: Etonogestrel/ethinyl estradiol vaginal ring (Nuvaring).

Interaction Type and Significance

≈≈≈ **Drug-Induced Nutrient Depletion, Supplementation Therapeutic, Not Requiring Professional Management**
☼ **Prevention or Reduction of Drug Adverse Effect**

Probability:	Evidence Base:
2. Probable	◉ **Emerging**

Effect and Mechanism of Action

The use of oral contraceptives (OCs) may be associated with altered metabolism of many nutrients and increased susceptibility to depletion in some women, particularly vitamins B_1, B_2, B_3, B_6, B_{12}, and C, as well as folic acid, manganese, magnesium, and zinc.[28]

Research

Researchers have observed slight to moderate decreases in thiamine levels in some women taking OCs.[29-32] Evidence is still insufficient to confirm consistent patterns of nutritional deficiencies resulting from OC.[33,34] Although thiamine levels have not been consistently lower in women taking OCs compared with controls, urinary thiamine levels are higher in women using OCs who also take supplemental thiamine.[35]

Nutritional Therapeutics, Clinical Concerns, and Adaptations

The clinical implications of this probable interaction are uncertain at this time. Further research focusing on variable susceptibility to thiamine depletion, particularly such factors as pharmacogenomic variables, dietary intake, age, and concomitant medications and health conditions, could further define conditions of increased risk and elucidate approaches for optimal correction with nutritional therapies. Pending such evidence, coadministration with customary supplemental daily doses of thiamine, particularly in a B-complex formulation to address parallel depletion effects, would safely and effectively reduce risks of adverse effects.

Phenytoin and Related Anticonvulsant Medications

Evidence: Phenytoin (diphenylhydantoin; Dilantin, Phenytek). Extrapolated, based on similar properties: Carbamazepine (Carbatrol, Tegretol), clonazepam (Klonopin), clorazepate (Tranxene), divalproex semisodium, divalproex sodium (Depakote), ethosuximide (Zarontin), ethotoin (Peganone), felbamate (Felbatol), fosphenytoin (Cerebyx, Mesantoin), levetiracetam (Keppra), mephenytoin, mephobarbital (Mebaral), methsuximide (Celontin), oxcarbazepine (GP 47680, oxycarbamazepine; Trileptal), phenobarbital (phenobarbitone; Luminal, Solfoton), piracetam (Nootropyl), primidone (Mysoline), sodium valproate (Depacon), topiramate (Topamax), trimethadione (Tridione), valproate semisodium, valproic acid (Depakene, Depakene Syrup), vigabatrin (Sabril), zonisamide (Zonegran).

Interaction Type and Significance

≈≈≈ **Drug-Induced Nutrient Depletion, Supplementation Therapeutic, Not Requiring Professional Management**

☼ **Prevention or Reduction of Drug Adverse Effect**

Probability:	Evidence Base:
1. Certain	●●● Consensus

Effect and Mechanism of Action

In their study of phenytoin's effects on the in vivo kinetics of thiamine in rat nervous tissues, Patrini et al.[36] reported that phenytoin appeared to interfere mainly with thiamine and thiamine monophosphate (TMP) uptake, thiamine pyrophosphate (TPP) dephosphorylation to TMP, and TPP turnover times, and that these effects were particularly prominent in the cerebellum and brainstem of chronically treated animals.

Research

The research team led by M.I. Botez in Montreal has contributed significantly to our understanding of the effects of phenytoin on thiamine in humans. In a 1982 study, Botez et al.[37] determined by microbiological assay a statistically significant difference between whole-blood thiamine and cerebrospinal fluid (CSF) thiamine levels in comparing samples from 23 control subjects and 11 phenytoin-treated epileptic patients. Similar studies of 157 epileptic patients observed low levels of folate and thiamine in the blood and CSF, associated with phenytoin therapy.[38] In a subsequent clinical trial this research team conducted a clinical trial investigating the effects of thiamine and folate on verbal and nonverbal intelligence quotient (IQ) testing in 72 epileptic patients receiving phenytoin alone or in combination with phenobarbital for more than 4 years. They noted that 31% had subnormal blood thiamine levels and 30% had low folate at baseline assessment, and that such vitamin deficiencies were independent phenomena. After a 6-month, randomized, double blind trial, they found that thiamine (50 mg/day) improved neuropsychological functions in both verbal and nonverbal IQ testing. In particular, higher scores were recorded on the block design, digit symbol, similarities, and digit span subtests. The researchers concluded that, in epileptic patients chronically treated with phenytoin, thiamine supplementation improves neuropsychological functions, such as visuospatial analysis, visuomotor speed, and verbal abstracting ability.[39]

Nutritional Therapeutics, Clinical Concerns, and Adaptations

Individuals undergoing anticonvulsant therapy, particularly using phenytoin, will most likely benefit from coadministration of 50 to 100 mg of oral thiamine daily. Such corrective nutrient therapy seems prudent, especially given that vitamin B_1 has no known toxicity. All currently available evidence indicates that such coadministration is safe and can be undertaken without close supervision or specific monitoring. Nevertheless, individuals using any anticonvulsant medication should consult with their prescribing physician and a health care professional experienced in nutritional therapeutics before introducing any significant levels of supplementation into their therapeutic regimen.

Scopolamine

Scopolamine

Interaction Type and Significance

⊕⊕ **Beneficial or Supportive Interaction, with Professional Management**

☼ **Prevention or Reduction of Drug Adverse Effect**

Probability:	Evidence Base:
2. Probable	○ Preliminary

Effect and Mechanism of Action

Thiamine is involved in the presynaptic release of acetylcholine and exerts a cholinomimetic effect in the central nervous system. Thiamine binds to nicotinic receptors and may exhibit anticholinesterase activity. Scopolamine exerts an anticholinergic effect.[40]

Research

A small human study investigated the effects of pharmacological doses of thiamine on the cognitive deficits typically associated with scopolamine therapy. In this randomized, double-blind, placebo-controlled, double-crossover clinical trial with 13 healthy subjects, the group receiving 5 g thiamine orally (with scopolamine, 0.007 mg/kg IM) demonstrated significantly reduced adverse effects of scopolamine compared with the placebo group. Improvements were measured in P3 latency, spectral components of electroencephalography, and memory recall.[40]

Nutritional Therapeutics, Clinical Concerns, and Adaptations

Patients undergoing scopolamine therapy will most likely benefit from oral thiamine coadministration, generally 2 to 4 g/day. Such supportive nutrient therapy probably will have significant clinical benefit and generally is considered to present negligible risk. The available research has been conducted with higher doses and close supervision (in a research setting with healthy patients). Pending further research into specific doses and response patterns with patient populations prescribed scopolamine for typical medical conditions, close supervision and regular monitoring are advisable, preferably within an integrative care setting providing for collaboration between the prescribing physician and a health care professional experienced in nutritional therapeutics.

Stavudine and Related Reverse-Transcriptase Inhibitor (Nucleoside) Antiretroviral Agents

Evidence: Stavudine (d4T, Zerit).
Extrapolated, based on similar properties: Abacavir (Ziagen), didanosine (ddI, dideoxyinosine; Videx); dideoxycytidine (ddC, zalcitabine; Hivid), lamivudine (3TC, Epivir), stavudine (D4T; Zerit), tenofovir (Viread), zidovudine (azidothymidine, AZT, ZDV, zidothymidine; Retrovir); combination drugs: zidovudine and lamivudine (Combivir); abacavir, lamivudine, and zidovudine (Trizivir).

Interaction Type and Significance

≈≈≈ **Drug-Induced Nutrient Depletion, Supplementation Therapeutic, Not Requiring Professional Management**
☼ **Prevention or Reduction of Drug Adverse Effect**

Probability: Evidence Base:
3. Possible   **○ Preliminary**

Effect and Mechanism of Action

With expanded use of stavudine and similar medications, often with highly active antiretroviral therapy (HAART) protocols, severe lactic acidosis has been increasingly reported as a severe and potentially fatal complication of HIV treatment.[41-45] Defects in the gene on the X chromosome encoding the E1 peptide of the E1 subunit (pyruvate decarboxylase), which binds TPP, can contribute to increased susceptibility to lethal lactic acidosis.[46]

Reports

Two case reports provide the evidence supporting thiamine therapy to reduce risk of or respond to adverse effects of stavudine. Schramm et al.[47] reported the case of a 30-year-old woman with AIDS and nucleoside analog–induced lactic acidosis that exacerbated shortly after introducing total parenteral nutrition and reversed within hours after treatment with IV thiamine. A 2001 paper described an asymptomatic HIV-infected woman treated with HAART (stavudine, lamivudine, and indinavir) for 1 year who demonstrated an "impressively rapid response (within a few hours)" to 100 mg IV thiamine.[48]

Preexisting vitamin deficiency appears to be an important cofactor in the susceptibility to this unpredictable adverse reaction to therapy in patients with HIV infection.

Nutritional Therapeutics, Clinical Concerns, and Adaptations

Lactic acidosis induced by stavudine or similar nucleoside analog medications for HIV infection is a serious and often life-threatening condition, and such patients are usually already hospitalized or under close supervision by their prescribing physician. The available reports involved critical care and physician administration of high-dose thiamine to address both the lactic acidosis and the patient's presumed background vitamin deficiency status. The clinicians submitting these reports recommended that physicians prescribing stavudine therapy take note of the rapid response to thiamine administration, suggest that high-dose B vitamins should be given to any patient presenting with lactic acidosis under nucleoside analog treatment, and advise thiamine infusion for critical care of this potentially life-threatening complication of HIV therapy.

Supplementation with customary oral doses of a B-vitamin complex may be self-administered as a prophylactic measure by patients undergoing stavudine or other antiretroviral therapy, particularly when nutrient intake has been compromised by an inadequate or imbalanced diet. Pending further research into preventive and reactive doses of thiamine with respective modes of administration, for coadministration with stavudine or similar nucleoside analog medications, close supervision and regular monitoring are advisable when lactic acidosis is present or threatening, preferably within an integrative care setting providing for collaboration between the prescribing physician and a health care professional experienced in nutritional therapeutics.

Tetracycline and Related Tetracycline Antibiotics

Evidence: Tetracycline (Achromycin, Actisite, Apo-Tetra, Economycin, Novo-Tetra, Nu-Tetra, Sumycin, Tetrachel, Tetracyn).
Extrapolated, based on similar properties: Demeclocycline (Declomycin), doxycycline (Atridox, Doryx, Doxy, Monodox, Periostat, Vibramycin, Vibra-Tabs), minocycline (Dynacin, Minocin, Vectrin), oxytetracycline (Terramycin), tetracycline combination drugs: chlortetracycline, demeclocycline, and tetracycline (Deteclo); bismuth, metronidazole, and tetracycline (Helidac).

Interaction Type and Significance

◇◇ **Impaired Drug Absorption and Bioavailability, Precautions Appropriate**

Probability: Evidence Base:
3. Possible   **○ Preliminary**

Effect and Mechanism of Action

Nutrient formulations containing B vitamins, including thiamine (B₁), may interfere with tetracycline pharmacokinetics.

Research

In an investigation of the effects of various nutrients on the pharmacokinetics of tetracycline hydrochloride in healthy subjects, researchers observed a significant impairment of drug bioavailability associated with concomitant oral administration of a B-complex vitamin formulation.[49]

Clinical Implications and Adaptations

Physicians prescribing tetracycline or related antibiotic medications should advise patients regularly supplementing with thiamine, alone or within a B-complex vitamin formulation, to take the nutrient(s) and the medication at least 4 hours apart from each other.

NUTRIENT-NUTRIENT INTERACTIONS

Thiaminases

Thiaminases are thiamine antagonists found in a few plants and some raw seafood. When these enzymes are ingested, in coffee, black tea, certain vegetables, and the raw flesh and viscera of certain fish and shellfish, especially carp, they can destroy dietary or supplemental thiamine. Such type I thiaminases render thiamine biologically inactive by displacing its pyrimidine methylene group with a nitrogenous base or SH-compound to eliminate the thiazole ring. Once the thiamine molecule is cleaved by a thiaminase, the body is incapable of restoring it. Thus, the ingestion of significant amounts of thiaminases can induce thiamine deficiency, even when dietary intake of thiamine may be otherwise adequate. The level of raw fish consumption by humans is rarely sufficient, even among frequent sushi eaters, to constitute a significant probability of clinically significant thiamine depletion. Thiaminases are denatured by heat, so cooking or other forms of heat treatment will render them inactive.

Chlorinated Water and Chlorogenic Acid

Chlorinated water tends to destroy thiamine, especially when heated in the cooking of grains. Chlorogenic acid, found both in decaffeinated and caffeinated coffee, also destroys thiamine.

B Vitamins and Other Synergistic Nutrients

Thiamine works synergistically with vitamin B₂ and vitamin B₃.

Ames et al.[50] suggest that combination therapy with thiamine, alpha lipoic acid, riboflavin, nicotinamide, and adequate potassium may be optimal for the initial treatment of patients with maple syrup urine disease, a rare, autosomal recessive disorder of branched-chain amino acid metabolism.

HERB-NUTRIENT INTERACTION

Horsetail

Horsetail *(Equisetum arvense)*

Equisetum arvense (horsetail) may impair thiamine absorption. This particular form of thiaminase poisoning occurs most often among farm animals where hay has been contaminated by horsetail. No cases have been reported of humans consuming *Equisetum* medicinally and experiencing clinically significant thiamine depletion or deficiency.

The 51 citations for this monograph, as well as additional reference literature, are located under Vitamin B₁ (Thiamine) on the CD at the back of the book.

Vitamin B₂ (Riboflavin)

Nutrient Name: Vitamin B₂, riboflavin.
Synonyms: 7,8-dimethyl-10-(11-ᴅ-ribityl)isoalloxazine, 7,8-dimethyl-10-(ᴅ-ribo-
2,3,4,5-tetrahydroxypentyl)isoalloxazine, flavin, flavine, hepatoflavin, lactoflavin,
lyochrome, ovoflavin, riboflavine, uroflavin, vitamin B₂, vitamin G.
Trade Names Include: Aqua-Flave, Beflavin, Beflavina, Béflavine, Beflavit, Berivine,
Dolo-Neurotrat, Flavaxin, Ribobis, Ribobutin, Ribipea.
Related Substance: Riboflavin-5-phosphate: Alloxazine mononucleotide, coflavinase,
cytoflav, flavine mononucleotide, FMN, riboflavin phosphate.

Summary

Drug/Class Interaction Type	Mechanism and Significance	Management
Anticonvulsant medications Barbiturates ≈≈/☼/◇≈≈	Anticonvulsant medications, especially those that induce cytochrome P450, may alter riboflavin metabolism and interfere with activity of riboflavin-related coenzymes and deplete riboflavin. Riboflavin is essential to the function of folate, MTHFR, and pyridoxine. Coadministration can mitigate adverse effects. Further research needed.	Riboflavin (and folate) coadministration may be beneficial, but interaction can vary depending on medication. Requires clinical management.
Antimalarial drugs ✗/◇◇/⊕✗/⊕	Strong evidence indicates that low riboflavin status is protective against malaria and advantageous in reducing the severity of malarial symptoms. Several antimalarial medications appear to act as riboflavin antagonists. Riboflavin intake is generally contraindicated in both prevention and treatment. However, limited research indicates that high doses of riboflavin may exert activity against *Plasmodium falciparum*. Further research needed.	Avoid concomitant riboflavin intake, as well as vitamin E, iron, and folate, except as indicated by extraordinary circumstances and then only under medical supervision.
Antiretroviral agents Nucleoside (analog) reverse-transcriptase inhibitors (NRTIs) ☼/≈≈/◇≈≈	Drug-induced mitochondrial toxicity associated with riboflavin deficiency contributes to lactic acidosis in patients treated with NRTIs. Riboflavin coadministration can prevent or reverse these and other adverse effects. Further research warranted to confirm consistent but limited evidence.	Coadministration, preferably with thiamine, can be beneficial. Supervise closely and monitor regularly.
Boric acid, borate, and boron ≈≈≈/☼	Boron, in various forms, tends to complex with riboflavin and thereby reduce absorption and increase urinary excretion. Effects are rapid, and continued use may cause riboflavin deficiency. Separation of intake can reduce gut absorption interference. Conversely, riboflavin may be used to treat acute boric acid poisoning.	Separate intake of boron/boric acid and riboflavin unless binding is intentional.
Chlorpromazine Phenothiazine antipsychotics ◇≈≈/≈≈/◇◇	Chlorpromazine and other phenothiazines can inhibit hepatic flavokinase and conversion of riboflavin to FMN and FAD. Binding and increased excretion may also occur; thus, simultaneous intake might impair activity of both agents. Interrelationships reported linking unipolar depression, low thyroxine status, deficiency of riboflavin, and folate. Riboflavin (or FAD) may protect against chlorpromazine-induced arrhythmia and mitochondrial dysfunction.	Consider coadministration of riboflavin (and folic acid), especially in unipolar depression. Separate intake. Evaluate and monitor riboflavin, FAD, and thyroxine status.
Doxorubicin Anthracyclines ◇≈≈/≈≈/☼/◇◇	Doxorubicin can inhibit the conversion to FMN and FAD but coadministration of riboflavin may not adequately counteract resulting toxic effects. Binding and increased excretion may also occur; thus, simultaneous intake might impair activity of both agents. Sunlight exposure in the presence of riboflavin may deactivate doxorubicin. Further research needed.	Coadministration, especially with coenzyme Q10, can be beneficial but may not be adequate. Separate intake. Sunlight avoidance may be prudent with coadministration. Supervise closely and monitor regularly.
Oral contraceptives (OCs) ◇≈≈/≈≈/☼	Mixed OCs may reduce levels of riboflavin (as well as B₆, folate, and B₁₂). Evidence mixed as to clinical significance of effects, but risk appears higher with high-dose hormones, high metabolic demands, poor nutritional status, and during initial months. Nutritional support may prevent or reverse adverse effects on riboflavin and related nutrients. Continued research necessary for conclusive determination of effects and susceptibility and effective clinical response.	Coadministration of a B-complex formulation can be beneficial. No adverse effects probable.
Probenecid ≈≈/≈≈≈	Probenecid can adversely affect riboflavin through several mechanisms, including impaired absorption in gastrointestinal tract, inhibited renal tubular secretion, and decreased urinary excretion. Evidence limited but generally accepted as plausible. Probable that riboflavin administration can prevent or reverse adverse drug-induced effects.	Coadminister riboflavin, especially with nutritionally compromised patients and with long-term therapy. Monitor for signs of deficiency.
Propantheline ✗/◇◇	Propantheline appears to elevate riboflavin levels by decreasing salivary flow and decreasing rate of gastric emptying and gastrointestinal motility. Minimal evidence, but low probability of significant risk due to minimal toxicity of riboflavin. Substantive research necessary for conclusive determination of effects and appropriate clinical response.	No response necessary. Patients need not avoid riboflavin in multivitamin.

Continued

Summary		
Drug/Class Interaction Type	Mechanism and Significance	Management
Tetracycline antibiotics Other antibiotics ✗✗/◇◇	Simultaneous intake of riboflavin and other B vitamins with tetracycline-class antibiotics can reduce absorption and bioavailability of both/all agents. Antibacterial effect on intestinal flora and gut ecology can produce secondary adverse effects on B-vitamin status and inflammatory processes.	Separate intake if concurrent administration indicated or necessary. Probiotic flora beneficial after antibiotic therapy.
Thyroid hormones ⊕⊕	Hypothyroidism and riboflavin deficiency share many characteristics. Triiodothyronine (T₃) enhances biosynthesis of FMN through the expression of riboflavin kinase. Thyroid status appears to influence activity of riboflavin (and folate) and response to tricyclic antidepressants and phenothiazines.	Coadministration may be beneficial, except with malaria susceptibility or treatment.
Tricyclic antidepressants (TCAs) ⊕⊕/◇≈≈/≈≈	TCAs can adversely affect riboflavin activity (and increase requirements) by impairing absorption and inhibiting synthesis of FMN and FAD. Coadministration may prevent or reverse depletion as well as augment clinical response to TCAs through an additive or synergistic effect. Continued research warranted. Coadministration potentially beneficial in migraine.	Coadministration of riboflavin can be protective and may enhance clinical response, especially with deficiency. Consider B₁, B₆, B₁₂, and folic acid. Check thyroxine status. Supervise closely and monitor regularly.

MTHFR, 5,10-Methylenetetrahydrofolate reductase; *FMN,* flavin mononucleotide; *FAD,* flavin adenine dinucleotide.

NUTRIENT DESCRIPTION
Chemistry and Forms

Riboflavin names: 7,8-dimethyl-10-(11-D-ribityl)isoalloxazine, 7,8-dimethyl-10-(D-ribo-2,3,4,5-tetrahydroxypentyl)isoalloxazine, and 7,8-dimethyl-10-ribitylisoalloxazine.
Formula: $C_{17}H_{20}N_4O_6$.
Molecular weight: 376.4 daltons.
Riboflavin is stable to heat, oxidation, and acid; it is destroyed by alkali and light, especially fluorescent light. Riboflavin is partially soluble in water.
Riboflavin is a water-soluble member of the B-vitamin family. The originally termed "yellow enzyme," which became known as "flavin mononucleotide" or "riboflavin phosphate," was initially synthesized in 1935. The name "riboflavine" was initially chosen because it contained the pentose side chain ribitol, and *flavius* is Latin for "yellow," in recognition of the deep color of the crystals formed from the pure vitamin and the deep-yellow color it imparts to urine. The final "e" was later dropped on learning that it really was not an amine. In 1952 the Commission on Biochemical Nomenclature formally adopted the name *riboflavin.* At this time, riboflavin is the Approved Name for use on pharmaceutical labels in Britain.

Physiology and Function

Riboflavin plays a critical role as a component of several key metabolic substances involved in oxidation of glucose, fatty acids, and certain amino acids; reactions with several intermediaries of the Krebs cycle; activation of pyridoxine phosphate (B₆) to form pyridoxal phosphate, its biologically active form; conversion of folate to its coenzymes; conversion of tryptophan to niacin; and support of antioxidant activity through *flavin adenine dinucleotide* (FAD) and reduced glutathione. Riboflavin exerts minimal direct or intrinsic metabolic activity, and only a small portion of the total flavin pool in the human body remains as riboflavin, primarily stored in the liver. Most is converted into coenzyme derivatives *flavin mononucleotide* (FMN) and its product, the more predominant FAD, before these flavins form complexes with numerous flavoprotein dehydrogenases and oxidases. Notably, *flavokinase,* the enzyme required for the production of FAD and FMN, is regulated by thyroxin so that thyroid hormones increase the synthesis of flavin cofactors.

As flavocoenzymes, FMN and FAD participate in oxidation-reduction reactions in metabolic pathways and in energy production through the respiratory chain. The isoalloxazine ring system of riboflavin serves as the functional moiety in both FAD and FMN by acting as a two-electron acceptor in enzymatic biochemical reductions. This property enables FMN and FAD to act as cofactors for flavoproteins, the enzymes involved in oxidation-reduction reactions of organic substrates and in intermediary metabolism. FAD and FMN serve as intermediate hydrogen carriers in the mitochondrial electron transport chain, accepting hydrogen ions and transferring electrons to the cytochrome system as part of the metabolism of carbohydrates to produce adenosine triphosphate (ATP). Riboflavin aids in beta oxidation in lipid metabolism and is involved, as a coenzyme component of the dehydrogenases, in the first step in glucose metabolism.

Xanthine oxidase, nicotinamide-adenine dinucleotide phosphate (NADP)–cytochrome *c* reductase, and D- and L-amino acid oxidase are among the key riboflavin-dependent flavoenzymes. Succinic dehydrogenase, monoamine oxidase (MAO), and other flavoenzymes have FAD covalently bound to them. As a component of these flavin coenzymes, riboflavin serves as a cofactor in numerous respiratory enzymes, including glutaryl coenzyme A dehydrogenase, erythrocyte glutathione reductase, sarcosine dehydrogenase, NADH dehydrogenase, electron-transferring flavoprotein, and ETF dehydrogenase. Flavocoenzymes are also involved in the biosynthesis of niacin-containing coenzymes from tryptophan (via FAD-dependent kynurenine hydroxylase), the FMN-dependent conversion of the 5'-phosphates of vitamin B₆ to pyridoxal 5'-phosphate, the FAD-dependent dehydrogenation of 5,10-methylenetetrahydrofolate to the 5'-methyl product, and the vitamin B₁₂–dependent formation of methionine and sulfur amino metabolism.

Riboflavin participates in other self-regulatory and protective processes, particularly by facilitating destruction of reactive oxygen species and prevention of cellular oxidative injury in a range of tissues. Glutathione reductase is a FAD-containing enzyme that generates reduced glutathione, which acts as a cofactor in the formation of glutathione peroxidases, major selenium-containing antioxidant enzymes central to the regulation of lipid peroxidation. The availability of riboflavin is also essential to maintaining the mitochondrial pool of reduced glutathione necessary to the activities of the flavoenzymes reduced nicotinamide-adenine dinucleotide phosphate (NADPH)–cytochrome P450 (CYP450) reductase and NADPH–cytochrome *b* reductase. Riboflavin may also play a role in maintaining the integrity of erythrocytes and nerve tissue. *Flavin reductase*, also known as methemoglobin reductase, is an NADPH-dependent enzyme that appears to provide protection against oxidative forms of hemeproteins, such as those involved in reperfusion injury. In this process, riboflavin acts as an antioxidant through its conversion to dihydroriboflavin, with methemoglobin reduced while riboflavin is oxidized. The dihydroriboflavin not only maintains the hemeproteins in their lower oxidation states, but also rapidly reduces higher oxidation states of hemeproteins and prevents peroxidative damage to the heme and protein groups. Moreover, because the 5,10-methylenetetrahydrofolate reductase gene product (MTHFR) is a riboflavin/FAD-dependent enzyme, riboflavin status modifies the metabolic effect of the MTHFR 677C→T polymorphism, a critical factor in regulation of plasma concentrations of total homocysteine (tHcy), coronary artery disease, and colon cancer risk. For individuals who carry the 677C→T polymorphism, improving both riboflavin and folate nutriture is protective.

Riboflavin is also required for gluconeogenesis, erythropoiesis, thyroid enzyme regulation, and the production of corticosteroids. Riboflavin is also important in deoxyribonucleic acid (DNA) and ribonucleic acid (RNA) metabolism and can be found in high concentration in the retina.

In normal physiological settings, riboflavin is readily absorbed in the upper gastrointestinal tract, principally in the duodenum, through a saturable active transport system. The presence of food can increase absorption fourfold when riboflavin is ingested with meals rather than taken separately. The gastric environment is important because acid is responsible for releasing B₂ from noncovalent bonding in foods so that it may be absorbed. Hepatitis, cirrhosis, or biliary obstruction can also significantly impair its absorption. Riboflavin absorption is increased in hypothyroidism and decreased in hyperthyroidism. Riboflavin and a number of other water-soluble vitamins can be synthesized by the microflora that should normally populate the large intestine. Circulating riboflavin can complex with a variety of proteins, including plasma albumin. Conversion of riboflavin to its coenzymes forms (e.g., FAD) predominantly takes place in the liver, heart, and kidneys, but also to some degree in most tissues. In the body tissue, riboflavin is predominantly present as the coenzyme FAD. Riboflavin is stored in the liver to a limited extent, but hepatic reserves will only reduce to 50% of maximum storage when availability is low. Riboflavin is excreted primarily in the urine, predominantly as metabolites, with a typical half-life elimination of 66 to 84 minutes. Excess riboflavin, approximately 9%, is excreted unchanged, imparting the well-known yellow color to urine. Riboflavin crosses the placenta readily and is also excreted in breast milk.

NUTRIENT IN CLINICAL PRACTICE
Known or Potential Therapeutic Uses

Treatment of *ariboflavinosis* (riboflavin deficiency) is the primary application of riboflavin recognized in conventional medical practice. An emerging body of evidence supporting the efficacy of riboflavin for the prevention of migraine and ocular cataract is becoming more widely recognized but is still generally viewed as mixed. Nevertheless, clinical experience and a close review of the literature reveal a solid basis for further research through well-designed and high-powered clinical trials aimed at developing guidelines for therapeutic application. The use of riboflavin in conjunction with antiviral regimens, especially nucleoside analog reverse-transcriptase inhibitors (NNRTIs), is well established, particularly for treatment and prevention of lactic acidosis.

Riboflavin is most often administered in conjunction with other nutrients, especially B vitamins, because its physiological functions and activities as well as its depletion patterns tend to cluster, and their coadministration produces a synergistic effect.

Historical/Ethnomedicine Precedent

Vitamin B₂ (riboflavin) has not been used historically as an isolated nutrient.

Possible Uses

Anemia, anorexia, aphthous ulcers, ariboflavinosis (riboflavin deficiency), bulimia, burn recovery, burning feet syndrome, carpal tunnel syndrome, cataracts, depression, esophageal cancer (risk reduction and treatment), ethylmalonic encephalopathy, fatigue, glaucoma, human immunodeficiency virus (HIV) support, hyperhomocysteinemia, involuntary eye movement, ischemia-reperfusion injury, malaria, methemoglobinemia (congenital), migraine headache (prophylaxis), mitochondrial encephalomyopathy (MEM), multiple acyl-coenzyme A dehydrogenase deficiency, neonatal jaundice (with phototherapy), Parkinson's disease, posttransplant headache, preeclampsia, red blood cell aplasia, sickle cell anemia, sports performance enhancement, thyroid disorders.

Deficiency Symptoms

Cheilosis, glossitis, and angular stomatitis (cracking at lip corners) are classic deficiency symptoms, but both hyporiboflavinosis and ariboflavinosis can also manifest as lethargy, depression, generalized weakness, hyperemia, edema of the pharyngeal and oral mucous membranes, dermatitis (particularly seborrheic dermatitis affecting the scrotum or labia majora and nasolabial folds), photosensitivity, burning and itching of the eyes, corneal vascularization, and normochromic normocytic anemia, leukopenia, and thrombocytopenia, sometimes associated with pure erythrocyte cytoplasia of the bone marrow. These clinical signs of deficiency in humans may appear at intakes less than 0.5 to 0.6 mg per day. Isolated riboflavin deficiency is rare and usually occurs in conjunction with broader nutritional deficiency patterns, particularly involving other B vitamins and contexts associated with increased vulnerability. Symptoms of niacin and vitamin B₆ deficiency may also appear because riboflavin is necessary to their metabolic activity.

The U.S. recommended dietary (daily) allowance (RDA) for riboflavin (vitamin B₂), as revised in 1998, was established based on dosage level necessary to prevent the pathophysiological changes associated with riboflavin deficiency, not to maintain normal enzyme function, promote optimal health, or treat specific conditions.

The most common cause of insufficient riboflavin status is unbalanced, nutritionally deficient diets, particularly affecting infants and children, elderly persons, low-income populations, and those in areas characterized by deprivation. Individuals in particular groups tend to be especially at risk for riboflavin deficiency, including chronic heavy alcohol use, people with chronic illnesses (especially chronic liver disease), patients with severe burns or sickle cell anemia, patients receiving total parenteral nutrition (TPN) with inadequate riboflavin, and gastric bypass bariatric surgery patients, if they neglect to take high-potency B-complex supplements. Impaired absorption and reduced assimilation of riboflavin can result from abnormal digestion caused by various conditions, including gastrointestinal (GI) infections or parasites, infectious enteritis, GI and biliary obstructions, chronic diarrhea, decreased GI passage time, celiac disease, tropical sprue, malignancy, and resection of the small intestine, as in management of patients with Crohn's enteritis. Infants receiving phototherapy for neonatal jaundice are also at risk for riboflavin deficiency. Inadequate thyroid hormone and cataract formation can also be associated with impaired riboflavin status. Inborn errors of metabolism affecting the formation of a flavoprotein, such as acyl-coenzyme A dehydrogenases, can cause deficiency in relatively rare cases. Children may be at increased risk of deficiency during phases of rapid growth. Riboflavin deficiency is relatively common in children with cardiac disease, especially congestive heart failure. Low milk consumption and lactose intolerance can also contribute to decreased riboflavin intake. Vegetarians tend to have depressed riboflavin levels, and vegans are considered at increased risk of riboflavin deficiency, although nutritional yeast is an excellent source for vegans. Individuals engaged in strenuous athletic activities tend to have increased riboflavin requirements and may be more susceptible to deficiency. Women using oral contraceptives tend to lower levels of riboflavin and other B vitamins. In many women, riboflavin levels tend to be lower during periods of exercise and calorie-restrictive dieting.

Dietary Sources

Even though all plant and animal cells contain riboflavin and it is widely distributed in foodstuffs, few foods provide abundant sources of this essential nutrient. The richest dietary sources of riboflavin are calf liver and other organ meats, torula (nutritional) yeast, brewer's yeast, and mushrooms. Milk products (especially yogurt), spinach, asparagus, broccoli and other leafy green vegetables, egg whites, fish roe, almonds and other nuts, legumes, sunflower seeds, whole grains (especially wild rice), wheat germ, and fortified grains can also contain significant amounts of vitamin B₂. Regular daily intake of riboflavin is important because, as with other B vitamins, vitamin B₂ is not stored in appreciable amounts. Healthy subjects restricted to a riboflavin-free diet may demonstrate symptoms of riboflavin deficiency within 7 days.[1] The requirement for riboflavin appears to be related more to nitrogen balance than to caloric intake.

The availability and stability of riboflavin vary with different food sources. Riboflavin from animal sources is better absorbed and thus exhibits higher bioavailability than from vegetable sources. Vegetarians, and vegans in particular, therefore are more susceptible to inadequate riboflavin intake. The milling and processing of grains usually result in substantial loss of riboflavin because the vitamin is concentrated in the germ and bran. Furthermore, being water soluble, the riboflavin in grains and vegetables is often leached away during cooking, unless those fluids are reused as soups and sauces. The riboflavin in milk is relatively abundant and generally stable, although it was often degraded by light exposure when distributed in clear-glass bottles.

Nutrient Preparations Available

Riboflavin and riboflavin 5'-monophosphate are the most common forms of riboflavin available in supplements. Riboflavin is rarely administered as a monotherapy or dispensed as an individual nutrient; it is almost always part of a multinutrient formulation, particularly as a component of a B-vitamin complex. In general, such coadministration is superior because vitamin B₂ is most effective in combination with vitamins B₁, B₃, and B₆.

Dosage Forms Available

Oral: Capsule, soft elastic capsule, tablet, enteric-coated tablet, extended-release tablet.

Injection: Injectable riboflavin sodium phosphate is available by prescription. Riboflavin is moderately unstable in glucose–amino acid solutions but is stabilized with addition of a lipid, typically a 3:1 mixture, in TPN admixtures.

Dosage Range

Adult

Dietary: 5 to 30 mg per day. However, a survey conducted by the U.S. Department of Agriculture estimated that daily riboflavin intake less than the RDA occurs in about a third of Americans. In the United Kingdom the average adult daily diet for men provides 2.24 mg and 1.98 mg for women.

Supplemental/Maintenance: The ideal level of riboflavin intake has not been established, but the 25 to 50 mg typically contained in nutritional supplements is generally considered more than adequate for most individuals.

In the United States the Food and Nutrition Board of the Institute of Medicine of the National Academy of Sciences recommends the following dietary reference intakes (DRIs) for riboflavin:

Men (> 18 years): 1.3 mg
Women (> 18 years): 1.1 mg
Pregnant women (any age): 1.4 mg
Lactating women (any age): 1.6 mg

Pharmacological/Therapeutic: 10 to 100 mg/day, although 400 mg/day is often administered for migraine prophylaxis.

Toxic: None established. The evidence on adverse effects has been deemed insufficient to set a tolerable upper intake level (UL) for riboflavin.

Pediatric (< 18 Years)

Dietary: 2.5 to 10 mg/day.
Infants, birth to 6 months: 0.3 mg/day (AI, adequate intake)
Infants, 7 to 12 months: 0.4 mg/day (AI)
Children, 1 to 3 years: 0.5 mg/day (RDA)
Children, 4 to 8 years: 0.6 mg/day (RDA)
Children, 9 to 13 years: 0.9 mg/day (RDA)
Adolescents, 14 to 18 years: 1.0 mg/day for females; 1.3 mg/day for males (RDA)
Supplemental/Maintenance: 0.4 to 1.8 mg/day.
Pharmacological/Therapeutic: Riboflavin is generally not administered in pharmacological doses to infants or children. Riboflavin at levels five times that in formulas for term infants is often provided in augmented preterm infant formulas (PIFs) administered enterally to very-low-birth-weight (VLBW)

infants; 5 mg three times daily has been used during photo-therapy for neonatal jaundice.

Toxic: Not established.

Laboratory Values

Erythrocyte riboflavin: This test is generally not considered to provide a sensitive index. Levels below 15 µg/dL of red blood cells indicate deficiency.

Red blood cell FAD and FMN: Because these forms constitute more than 90% of riboflavin, these levels (obtained after modest hydrolysis from FAD) have been used as indicators of the cellular concentration of riboflavin in its form as coenzyme.

Urinary riboflavin: Urinary excretion of riboflavin reflects an excess of current intake beyond tissue requirements. A normal adult excretes 120 µg or more in 24 hours. Excretion of less than 100 µg daily indicates deficiency.

Erythrocyte glutathione reductase (EGR) activity coefficients: Stimulation of FAD-dependent EGR in vitro, which relies on an associated oxidation of NADPH, can be readily monitored spectrophotometrically and expressed as an activity coefficient (AC) indicating the ratio of activities in the presence and absence of added FAD. Assessment of this riboflavin-dependent enzyme provides a reliable indicator of functional riboflavin status but has known limitations, particularly in individuals with glucose-6-phosphate dehydrogenase (G6PD) deficiency.

An activity coefficient less than 1.2 is defined as "acceptable," 1.2 to 1.4 as indicating low riboflavin status, and greater than 1.4 indicating deficiency.

Capillary electrophoresis with laser-induced fluorescence detection: This test may provide an effective tool for accurate assessment of riboflavin status by allowing detection of all riboflavin vitamers below physiological concentrations.

Urinary riboflavin levels are often measured to assess compliance with medication regimens, particularly with patients being treated for alcohol dependence, mental disorders, and other conditions.

High intake levels of riboflavin are known to interfere with the accuracy of many laboratory tests, including urinalysis based on spectrometry, drugs of abuse assays, and fluorometric determinations of catecholamines and urobilinogen.

SAFETY PROFILE
Overview

Riboflavin (vitamin B$_2$) is generally considered to be nontoxic at typical supplemental and dietary dosage levels. Its limited intestinal absorption and water solubility make riboflavin toxicity highly improbable.

Nutrient Adverse Effects

General Adverse Effects

Beyond flavinuria, the yellow discoloration of urine, with high doses and extremely rare instances of allergic reactions, riboflavin toxicity in humans is unknown. Although indications of serious adverse effects are lacking, very high doses have reportedly caused itching, numbness, and burning or prickling sensations. Only two minor, nonspecific adverse events (diarrhea and polyuria) were reported during the 4-month course of a clinical trial involving 400 mg per day for migraine prophylaxis.[2] A potential risk from the photosensitizing properties of riboflavin

has been raised, but no substantial evidence is available to confirm such a concern as clinically significant.

Mutagenicity. None has been found on testing or has otherwise been proposed or suspected.

Pregnancy and Nursing

Riboflavin is excreted in breast milk but is generally considered safe during pregnancy and lactation at usual dosage levels.

Teratogenicity. None has been reported.

Infants and Children

No pediatric adverse effects from vitamin B$_2$ have been established.

Contraindications

No contradictions have been established for riboflavin.

Precautions and Warnings

No warnings or precautions have been established for vitamin B$_2$, other than known allergy to constituents of the formulation.

INTERACTIONS REVIEW
Strategic Considerations

The administration of riboflavin as a monotherapy is atypical in conventional practice and nutritionally oriented therapeutics; its use in migraine prophylaxis represents its most well-known monotherapeutic application. Supplementation is usually unnecessary for individuals with a balanced diet and healthy lifestyle, although requirements can be increased with stresses such as poor nutritional intake (of riboflavin and other B vitamins), chronic illness, malabsorption disorders, alcohol consumption, hemodialysis, chemotherapy, or even vigorous athletic activity. The diagnosis of riboflavin deficiency is usually based on the symptoms and evidence of general undernutrition. Angular stomatitis is the most readily observable sign of emerging deficiency but frequently goes unrecognized at early stages. Diagnostic tests to confirm riboflavin deficiency are not readily available or particularly sensitive to functional depletion. In cases of frank riboflavin deficiency, high doses are typically administered orally until symptoms resolve. Impairment and deficiencies involving B vitamins are highly interdependent, and these nutrients are usually most effective when administered concomitantly. Riboflavin is generally considered to be nontoxic at typical supplemental and dietary dosage levels, with flavinuria (yellow-colored urine) being the primary side effect.

Although evidence from focused clinical trials is limited, adverse effects from coadministration appears to be improbable with most medications, given basic intake timing precautions. The major exception is individuals at high risk for malaria or being treated with antimalarial medications. Coadministration of riboflavin is particularly indicated with the several pharmaceuticals that impair riboflavin absorption and the many that inhibit conversion of riboflavin to its active coenzymes, FAD and FMN. The concomitant use of riboflavin and thiamine with the nucleoside analog reverse-transcriptase inhibitors used in HIV pharmacotherapy can prevent or reverse the uncommon but usually irreversible lactic acidosis caused by drug-induced mitochondrial toxicity and riboflavin deficiency. Coadministration with tricyclic antidepressants appears not only to counter drug-induced adverse effects but also to enhance therapeutic response, especially in depressed patients with low folate levels, defective methylation functions, and low thyroxine levels. Less dramatically, riboflavin's lack of toxicity suggests that it can be broadly prescribed to prevent or reverse drug-induced depletion effects, even in the absence of deficiency signs, as with oral contraceptives and CYP450-inducing antiseizure medications. Riboflavin appears to be safe even in the case of the anticholinergic agent propantheline, which can elevate riboflavin levels. Concomitant administration of other B vitamins is often indicated for full effectiveness of vitamin B₂.

Tetracycline-class antibiotics, chlorpromazine and related phenothiazine antipsychotics, and boric acid are prominent among the drugs with notable pharmacokinetic interactions with riboflavin, typically involving binding that impairs absorption of both substances. Chlorpromazine and boric acid and its derivatives promote renal excretion of riboflavin. Preliminary evidence suggests that riboflavin could theoretically impair the therapeutic activity of doxorubicin, selegiline, and some sulfa drugs in individuals exposed to sunlight or other bright light.

The role of riboflavin in cardiovascular function is emerging as an area of significant scientific research, providing new data on interactions involving related medications. Research involving patients with migraine demonstrated a decreased mitochondrial phosphorylation potential between migraine attacks and suggests that decreased brain mitochondrial energy reserve between attacks is related to the activity of flavoenzymes, particularly FMN and FAD, in the electron transport chain and the production of cellular energy. The pivotal role of riboflavin in FAD, which is the cofactor for the MTHFR enzyme, as well as the role of MTHFR in the regulation of homocysteine, may bring riboflavin into equal prominence with folic acid, vitamins B₆ and B₁₂, and possibly thiamine as a key agent in remethylation processes and modulation of risks associated with hyperhomocysteinemia. The antioxidant activity of vitamin B₂ and its clinical implications have yet to be fully elucidated but are derived from its role as a component of FAD and the role of this cofactor in the production of the antioxidant peptide reduced glutathione, as well as from its conversion to dihydroriboflavin. By affecting the mitochondrial pool of reduced glutathione, riboflavin deficiency in turn affects the activities of the flavoenzymes NADPH-CYP450 reductase, NADPH–cytochrome *b* reductase, and NADPH-dependent methemoglobin reductase (i.e., flavin reductase).

Oxidative forms of hemeproteins have been implicated in reperfusion injury, and elevated riboflavin levels have been reported to provide protection against such altered hemeproteins and reperfusion injury.[3-6] Continued research into these activities and functions will provide new insight into the importance of riboflavin nutriture, suggest expanded therapeutic uses for riboflavin administration, and present new challenges for understanding both beneficial and harmful interactions with conventional medications.

NUTRIENT-DRUG INTERACTIONS

Anticonvulsant Medications and Related Barbiturates

Evidence: Carbamazepine (Carbatrol, Tegretol), divalproex semisodium, divalproex sodium (Depakote), fosphenytoin (Cerebyx, Mesantoin), mephenytoin, oxcarbazepine (GP 47680, oxycarbamazepine; Trileptal), phenobarbital (phenobarbitone; Luminol, Solfoton), phenytoin (diphenylhydantoin; Dilantin, Phenytek), primidone (Mysoline), sodium valproate (Depacon), valproate semisodium, valproic acid (Depakene, Depakote).

Similar properties but evidence lacking for extrapolation: Amobarbital (Amytal), aprobarbital (Alurate), butabarbital (Butisol), butalbital (Fiorinal, Fioricet), clonazepam (Klonopin), clorazepate (Gen-Xene, Tranxene), diazepam (Valium), ethosuximide (Zarontin), ethotoin (Peganone), felbamate (Felbatol), gabapentin (Neurontin), lamotrigine (Lamictal), levetiracetam (Keppra), mephobarbital (Mebaral), methohexital (Brevital), methsuximide (Celontin), pheneturide (ethylphenacemide), pentobarbital (Nembutal), secobarbital (Seconal), thiopental (Pentothal), thiopentone (Thiopental), tiagabine (Gabitril), topiramate (Topamax), trimethadione (Tridione), zonisamide (Zonegran); combination drugs: acetylsalicylic acid, codeine, butalbital, and caffeine (Fiorinal); acetaminophen, butalbital, and caffeine (Fioricet). See also Folic Acid monograph.

Interaction Type and Significance

≈≈   **Drug-Induced Nutrient Depletion, Supplementation Therapeutic, with Professional Management**

☼   **Prevention or Reduction of Drug Adverse Effect**

◇≈≈   **Drug-Induced Adverse Effect on Nutrient Function, Coadministration Therapeutic, with Professional Management**

Probability:	Evidence Base:
4. Plausible to	○ **Preliminary** and
3. Possible	● **Consensus**

Effect and Mechanism of Action

Anticonvulsant medications may alter riboflavin metabolism, which could interfere with the activity of riboflavin-related coenzymes and deplete riboflavin. For example, by inducing CYP450 phenobarbital (and other enzyme-inducing antiepileptic drugs [AEDs], e.g., carbamazepine or phenytoin, and/or primidone) may increase destruction of riboflavin and thereby increase the risk of deficiency.[7] Riboflavin is the precursor for FAD, the cofactor for MTHFR, which catalyzes the formation of 5-methyltetrahydrofolate, which in turn acts as a methyl donor for homocysteine remethylation. Riboflavin is also necessary for activating vitamin B₆ to pyridoxal 5′-phosphate (PLP). Thus, the recycling of folate cofactors depends on vitamin B₆ and riboflavin.

Concurrent riboflavin administration appears to prevent or reverse these adverse effects.

Research

Although the evidence regarding the adverse impact of AEDs on folate and B₆ is abundant and consensus has emerged as to the character and significance of these interactions, the evidence regarding riboflavin has often been more indirect, associative, and inferential.

Numerous studies, primarily from the 1970s and 1980s, indicate that children undergoing anticonvulsant therapy with phenytoin (diphenylhydantoin) and related medications have exhibited subnormal riboflavin urinary excretion levels. Lewis et al.[8] found a wide range of variability in creatinine excretion of children treated with anticonvulsant drugs compared with normal, phenylketonuric and galactosemic children, 300% to 500% over 24 hours. In particular, they noted that "creatinine excretion rates were significantly more variable for children treated with anticonvulsant drugs than for normal children," and that "riboflavin-creatinine ratios determined on individual voidings were variable but adequate although total riboflavin was low."

Riboflavin, folate, and vitamin B$_6$ status influence the tendency toward elevated plasma total homocysteine (tHcy) concentrations often observed in patients taking AEDs. The effects of AEDs on riboflavin and other B vitamins appear to play a major role in the elevated tHcy concentrations.[9-16] In a 2003 study involving 101 patients with symptomatic, cryptogenic, or primary generalized epilepsy and 101 controls, Apeland et al.[16] investigated fasting and postmethionine loading concentrations of homocysteine (Hcy), vitamin B$_2$, and vitamin B$_6$ in patients taking AEDs. Patients receiving inducer AEDs (carbamazepine or phenytoin, phenobarbital, and/or primidone) had high plasma flavin nucleotide/riboflavin concentration ratios associated with low riboflavin concentrations, typically indicating a functional deficiency. Notably, riboflavin concentrations were positively correlated with serum folate and PLP concentrations, as well as weakly correlated with tHcy concentrations. The authors concluded that "it therefore seems reasonable to ensure an adequate intake of riboflavin in patients on inducer AEDs."[16]

In a cross-sectional design that included 423 healthy blood donors, age 19 to 69 years, Hustad et al.[17] determined that "plasma riboflavin is an independent determinant of plasma tHcy," but that the riboflavin-tHcy relationship was modified by MTHFR C677T genotype and "was essentially confined to subjects with the C677T transition of the MTHFR gene." Other data, derived from the Framingham Offspring cohort, suggest that "riboflavin status may affect homocysteine metabolism, but only in a small segment of the population who have both low folate status and are homozygotes for the MTHFR C677T mutation."[18] Subsequently, Moat et al.[19] studied B-vitamin status and plasma tHcy in 126 healthy individuals, 20 to 63 years of age (42 CC, 42 CT, and 42 TT MTHFR genotypes), at baseline and after three interventions lasting 4 months. At baseline and after nutritional intervention, lower riboflavin status was associated with increased plasma tHcy concentrations, with the mean plasma tHcy 2.6 μmol/L higher in the lowest quartile of plasma riboflavin levels compared with the highest quartile. This effect was not restricted to those with the T allele. Notably, folic acid given as a 400-μg/day supplement appeared to exacerbate a tendency toward riboflavin deficiency, as suggested by an increase in the proportion of individuals with erythrocyte glutathione reductase activation coefficient (EGRAC) of 1.4 or greater, from 52% to 65% after supplementation. These authors concluded that "folate and riboflavin interact to lower plasma tHcy, possibly by maximizing the catalytic activity of MTHFR," and that this observed effect "may be unrelated to MTHFR genotype."[19] Further research is warranted to elucidate these various factors and their clinical implications.

Overall, the limited evidence currently available is consistent with earlier findings, but research is still in preliminary phases. Nevertheless, adequately powered and well-designed clinical trials more specifically focusing on riboflavin are warranted. Pending such conclusive findings, the probability of such effects can be considered substantial given the established activity of these drugs on folate and related nutrients and the inherent interdependencies among these nutrients.

Nutritional Therapeutics, Clinical Concerns, and Adaptations
Physicians prescribing anticonvulsant medications (including barbiturates) are advised to consider nutritional support, including riboflavin, in patients undergoing long-term therapy.

Such concomitant nutrient administration is more likely to be important in children, patients with compromised nutritional status, those receiving AED polypharmacy, and patients with genetic polymorphisms adversely influencing methionine metabolism and Hcy levels, such as the C677T MTHFR mutation. Pending conclusive research, coadministration of folic acid and vitamins B$_{12}$ and B$_6$ is also prudent in most cases. Close supervision and regular monitoring of both medication and Hcy levels are essential to responsible and effective clinical management of such patients.

Antimalarial Drugs

Chloroquine (Aralen, Aralen HCl), hydroxychloroquine (Plaquenil), mefloquine (Lariam), quinacrine (Atabrine, Mepacrine); combination drug: atovaquone and proguanil (Malarone).

Interaction Type and Significance

✗   **Potential or Theoretical Adverse Interaction of Uncertain Severity**

◇◇   **Drug-Induced Effect on Nutrient Function, Supplementation Contraindicated, Professional Management Appropriate**

⊕✗   **Bimodal or Variable Interaction, with Professional Management**

⊕   **Potential or Theoretical Beneficial or Supportive Interaction, with Professional Management**

Probability:
3. Possible or
2. Probable

Evidence Base:
∇ **Mixed** or
○ **Preliminary**

Effect and Mechanism of Action
Scientific information on the interrelationships among riboflavin, malaria, and antimalarial drugs is complex, paradoxical, and inconclusive. Low dietary intake of riboflavin, especially to the level of deficiency, appears to be protective against malaria and advantageous in reducing the severity of malarial symptoms. Several antimalarial medications appear to act as riboflavin antagonists, which may play a significant role in their therapeutic efficacy. Quinacrine and related antimalarials impair riboflavin utilization by inhibiting the conversion of riboflavin to FMN and FAD, its active coenzyme derivatives.[20,21] The resultant diminished availability of glutathione reductase and reduced glutathione may render intraerythrocytic malaria parasite more vulnerable to oxidative stress.[22,23] Several antimalarial drugs appear to bind with and increase urinary excretion of riboflavin. Stereospecific complexes with riboflavin-binding protein (RBP) do not appear to form.[24] For example, the phenothiazine ring of chlorpromazine and the isoalloxazine ring of riboflavin exhibit a number of shared structural characteristics.[25] These similarities contribute to the tendency to bind the nutrient and promote riboflavinuria.

Conversely, and paradoxically, high doses of riboflavin may exert activity against the human malaria parasite *Plasmodium falciparum* through its action as a reducing agent and its effects on methemoglobin.[26]

Research
Research findings from animal and human studies indicate that deficient riboflavin nutriture can greatly decrease malarial parasitemia, inhibit the growth of *Plasmodium,* and mitigate the severity of malarial symptoms.[27-31] Dutta et al.,[32] who

conducted many experiments in this area, offered two hypotheses to explain this phenomenon:

It is therefore likely that the conditions which riboflavin deficiency produce have a common biochemical mechanism for their antimalarial activity—namely, they compromise the composition and integrity of membrane phospholipids. Alternatively, it is conceivable that riboflavin deficiency may selectively affect glutathione metabolism in the parasitised red blood cells, since glutathione reductase is an FAD-requiring enzyme.

More recently Akompong et al.[26] investigated the in vitro activity of riboflavin against the *P. falciparum* parasite. The human malaria parasite digests hemoglobin and polymerizes the released free heme into hemozoin, and high doses of riboflavin are used clinically to treat congenital methemoglobinemia without any adverse effects. First, the authors found that the acidic environment of food vacuoles is essential for survival of the parasite in erythrocytes, and such an environment also enhances the auto-oxidation of hemoglobin. They then released parasites from their host cells and separately analyzed hemoglobin ingested by the parasites from that remaining in the erythrocytes; isolated parasites contained elevated amounts of oxidized hemoglobin (methemoglobin) compared with levels found in normal, uninfected erythrocytes. Finally, they treated infected cells with riboflavin, as a reducing agent, for 24 hours, which decreased the parasite methemoglobin level by 55%; hemozoin production was inhibited by 50%, and the average size of the food vacuole decreased by 47%. Administration of riboflavin for 48 hours resulted in a 65% decrease in food vacuole size and inhibited asexual parasite growth in cultures. Based on these findings, the authors concluded that riboflavin is "attractive as a safe and inexpensive drug for treating malaria caused by *P. falciparum*."[26]

The exact mechanism by which riboflavin status influences malaria parasitemia has yet to be fully elucidated. Quinacrine and several drugs with known antimalarial properties, including chlorpromazine, imipramine, and amitriptyline, inhibit biosynthesis of FMN and FAD from riboflavin, most likely because of their structural similarity to riboflavin (e.g., phenothiazine ring of chlorpromazine and isoalloxazine ring of riboflavin), and increase urinary excretion of riboflavin.[20,25,32] Related in vitro research, however, indicates that quinacrine, chlorpromazine, and daunomycin do not form stereospecific complexes with RBP.[24] Furthermore, malaria parasites are known to be highly susceptible to activated oxygen species because of very limited activities of catalase and superoxide dismutase and because their plasma membranes, composed of very high amounts of phospholipids containing unsaturated fatty acids, apparently render them susceptible to the damaging effects of lipid peroxidation.[22,23,33] Thus, given the importance of riboflavin availability to glutathione reductase activity and redox capacity, the parasites may have a higher requirement for riboflavin than do host erythrocytes, and thus they may be more vulnerable to riboflavin deficiency, whether dietary or induced by competition. Consequently, in a review of these conflicting and unresolved findings, Rivlin and Dutta[34] note that "under certain circumstances, specific nutrient deficiencies, such as deprivation of vitamin E, iron, riboflavin, and folate, may prove to be beneficial for the treatment of malaria," and caution that "the indiscriminate use of vitamin supplementation, while well intended, may prove to be potentially harmful."

All the investigators who have conducted research in this area have emphasized the need for further research, through well-designed clinical trials of sufficient power, into the implications of riboflavin availability and activity for drug design and therapeutic strategy, especially given the wide prevalence of resistance to conventional antimalarial drug therapy.

Nutritional Therapeutics, Clinical Concerns, and Adaptations

Physicians treating patients infected with malaria are advised to query patients about any nutritional supplement use and to advise that they avoid concurrent intake of riboflavin, as well as vitamin E, iron, and folate, except as indicated by some extraordinary circumstances and then only under medical supervision. Pending more conclusive research, the potential benefit from high-dose riboflavin administration deserves consideration, but pending actual clinical trials of such an intervention in malaria patients, implementation could pose a significant risk of aggravating the condition, particularly in terms of inhibiting efficacy of standard antimalarial drugs.

Antiretroviral Agents, Nucleoside (Analog) Reverse-Transcriptase Inhibitors (NRTIs or NNRTIs)

Evidence: Didanosine (ddI, dideoxyinosine; Videx), lamivudine (3TC, Epivir), stavudine (D4T, Zerit), zidovudine (azidothymidine, AZT, ZDV, zidothymidine; Retrovir). **Extrapolated, based on similar properties:** Abacavir (Ziagen), dideoxycytidine (ddC, zalcitabine; Hivid), tenofovir (Viread), zidovudine combination drugs: zidovudine and lamivudine (Combivir); abacavir, lamivudine, and zidovudine (Trizivir).

Interaction Type and Significance

☼   **Prevention or Reduction of Drug Adverse Effect**

≈≈   **Drug-Induced Nutrient Depletion, Supplementation Therapeutic, with Professional Management**

◇≈≈ **Drug-Induced Adverse Effect on Nutrient Function, Coadministration Therapeutic, with Professional Management**

Probability:	Evidence Base:
3. Possible or	◉ **Emerging** or
2. Probable	● **Consensus**

Effect and Mechanism of Action

Riboflavin deficiency, even at mild levels, appears to increase the risk of nonischemic (type B) lactic acidosis, which infrequently occurs in patients treated with reverse-transcriptase anti-HIV agents. Several adverse effects associated with nucleoside reverse-transcriptase inhibitors (NRTIs) appear to derive from drug-induced mitochondrial toxicity.[35-42] Didanosine/ ddI, stavudine, zidovudine/AZT, and other drugs in this class can inhibit DNA polymerase and critical DNA-related riboflavin activity, resulting in impaired mitochondrial DNA synthesis; such adverse effects may be mitigated by riboflavin coadministration.[43] Further, NRTI-induced lactic acidosis is not readily reversible after discontinuation of NRTI and is often fatal because of progressive lactic acidosis and hypotension.[44] Hepatic steatosis and fatty liver are other serious mitochondrial-related complications observed in HIV patients undergoing antiretroviral therapy.[45] These adverse effects have been reversed with riboflavin administration, with concurrent thiamine in some patients.

Research/Reports

Mild to moderate riboflavin deficiency is common among HIV-infected individuals because of compromised nutritional status, lifestyle stressors, pregnancy, and drug-induced depletion or interference.[46] In 1998, Fouty et al.[43] achieved a major breakthrough in the pathophysiology of this NRTI-associated disorder in the cases of three patients with riboflavin deficiency who were exhibiting lactic acidosis and hepatic steatosis during antiviral treatment and responded well on restoration of normal riboflavin concentrations. In the most striking example, a 46-year-old woman with AIDS who had been on triple-antiretroviral therapy (stavudine, lamivudine, and indinavir) for 4 months was admitted with lactic acidosis, low blood urea nitrogen (BUN), and marked hepatic steatosis. The treating physicians observed that she was taking amitriptyline and suspected an actual or functional deficiency of riboflavin, which was confirmed on testing her enzyme EGRAC. The patient recovered rapidly after receiving 50 mg of riboflavin daily. Subsequently, two other HIV-infected patients on similar triple-drug therapy who had fatty liver on abdominal computed tomography (CT) and (less severe) lactic acidosis demonstrated normalization of serum lactate levels after administration of riboflavin.

In 1999, on the basis of Fouty's report, Luzzati et al.[47] treated a 35-year-old HIV-infected pregnant woman with 50 mg oral riboflavin daily after she presented with severe lactic acidosis. Blood lactate levels returned to normal within 4 days of initiating riboflavin. That patient had been undergoing antiviral therapy with stavudine and lamivudine over the previous 12 months (after previous treatment with zidovudine and zalcitabine). The authors also noted the work of Vir et al.[36] in suspecting increased risk of riboflavin deficiency with pregnancy. Later in 1999, Schramm et al.[48] described a 30-year-old female with AIDS and nucleoside analog–induced lactic acidosis that exacerbated shortly after introducing total parenteral nutrition. She demonstrated a therapeutic recovery within hours after administration of high dose thiamine.

Dalton and Rahimi[49] describe a case of type B lactic acidosis in a 51-year-old HIV-positive woman receiving three nucleotide analogs. She presented with nausea, vomiting, abdominal pain, and hepatic steatosis. Serum riboflavin levels documented a deficiency, and signs of mitochondrial toxicity were demonstrated by diffuse myopathy and pancreatitis. Immediately after treatment with 50 mg of riboflavin daily, serum BUN level, lactic acid levels, and arterial blood pH all returned to normal values, and her signs of mitochondrial toxicity improved. These authors concluded that it is "impossible to predict which patients are predisposed to the development of this syndrome," and suggested that "it may be important to screen and treat riboflavin deficiency in patients on nucleoside analogues."

Vasseur et al.[50] reported the case of a 47-year-old woman with HIV and end-stage renal disease on hemodialysis, treated with combination antiretroviral drug therapy, who developed an acute, severe lactic acidosis 24 hours after surgery for endocarditis. This patient fully recovered after administration of riboflavin, discontinuation of antiretroviral medication, and other supportive measures, including hemodialysis. The authors suggest that the timing of this complication and previous reports imply that open-heart surgery may be a risk factor for nonischemic (type B) lactic acidosis in patients taking NRTIs.

Nutritional Therapeutics, Clinical Concerns, and Adaptations

Physicians treating patients with HIV infection are advised to test for riboflavin deficiency and initiate nutritional support with riboflavin, thiamine, and possibly other B vitamins before beginning treatment with NRTIs. Such a course of action seems warranted given the nontoxic character and low cost of the vitamin therapy and the relative severity of the potential adverse effects. Although the anecdotal case literature provides repeated examples of using a 50-mg dose, no parameters have been established for prophylactic dosage levels.

Even though the body of available evidence is limited and reliant on case reports, the pattern of deficiency-related susceptibility, drug-induced toxicity, and favorable response provides a consistent clinical reference and pharmacologically plausible rationale for preventive intervention, pending conclusive research. Well-designed trials are clearly warranted to confirm the efficacy of riboflavin for preventing and treating this serious adverse effect.

Boric Acid, Borate, and Boron

Interaction Type and Significance

≈≈≈ **Drug-Induced Nutrient Depletion, Supplementation Therapeutic, Not Requiring Professional Management**

☼ **Prevention or Reduction of Drug Adverse Effect**

Probability:
3. Possible or
    2. Probable

Evidence Base:
☐ Inadequate or
○ Preliminary
    (presumed
    ● Consensus)

Effect and Mechanism of Action

Most administered forms of boron are readily converted to boric acid. Boric acid and borate can bind riboflavin, by complexing with its polyhydroxyl ribitol side chain, and displace it from plasma-binding sites. By thus increasing water solubility and urinary excretion of riboflavin, high intake levels of boric acid can potentially cause a deficiency of the nutrient, particularly in the first 24 to 48 hours after ingestion.[25]

Conversely, riboflavin increases urinary excretion of boric acid and can be used to treat boric acid poisoning.

Research

In a review of drugs that promote renal excretion of riboflavin, Pinto and Rivlin[25] discuss the mechanism involved and conclude that boric acid or borate, as typically found in nutritional supplements, eye products, and mouthwashes, can bind riboflavin and significantly impair its bioavailability. Such activity would inherently involve the binding and reduced therapeutic activity of the boric acid or related substance.

Nutritional Therapeutics, Clinical Concerns, and Adaptations

Physicians prescribing boric acid or its derivatives, or treating a patient who is self-administering such agents, are advised to consider coadministration of riboflavin. The probability of this interaction occurring is relatively high given the known mechanisms, but the probability of a clinically significant drug-induced depletion depends on the individual's initial nutritional status, drug dosage and duration, and other factors of susceptibility or individual variability. Prudence suggests that concurrent administration of riboflavin alone or within a B-complex vitamin formulation is warranted during continued administration of boric acid or high-dose boron, with intake separated by at least 4 hours. The exact dose level at which such an effect occurs, and how it changes proportionately, has yet to be determined, especially for any given individual.

Chlorpromazine and Related Phenothiazine Antipsychotics

Evidence: Chlorpromazine (Largactil, Thorazine).
Similar properties but evidence lacking for extrapolation: Acetophenazine (Tindal), fluphenazine (Modecate, Permitil, Prolixin, Prolixin Decanoate, Prolixin Enanthate), mesoridazine (Serentil), methotrimeprazine (levomepromazine; Nozinan), pericyazine (Neuleptil), perphenazine (Trilafon); combination drug: perphenazine and amitriptyline (Etrafon, Triavil, Triptazine); prochlorperazine (Compazine, Stemetil), promazine (Sparine), promethazine (Phenergan, Promacot, Promethegan), propiomazine (Largon), thioproperazine (Majeptil), thioridazine (Mellaril), trifluoperazine (Stelazine), triflupromazine (Vesprin).

Interaction Type and Significance

◇≈≈ **Drug-Induced Adverse Effect on Nutrient Function, Coadministration Therapeutic, with Professional Management**
≈≈ **Drug-Induced Nutrient Depletion, Supplementation Therapeutic, with Professional Management**
◇◇ **Impaired Drug Absorption and Bioavailability, Precautions Appropriate**

Probability: Evidence Base:
2. Probable   ○ Preliminary

Effect and Mechanism of Action

Chlorpromazine, a phenothiazine derivative, impairs riboflavin utilization by inhibiting the activity of hepatic flavokinase and thus the conversion of riboflavin to FMN and FAD, its active coenzyme derivatives.[20,21] The phenothiazine ring of chlorpromazine and the isoalloxazine ring of riboflavin exhibit a number of shared structural characteristics.[25] Consequently, chlorpromazine tends to bind with and increase urinary excretion of riboflavin, although stereospecific complexes with RBP do not appear to form.[24] This similarity contributes to the tendency to bind the nutrient and promote riboflavinuria. Such a mechanism of action would imply the binding and reduced therapeutic activity of the chlorpromazine or related phenothiazine drugs.

Research

Using a rat model, Pinto et al.[20] demonstrated that chlorpromazine, as well as imipramine and amitriptyline, "inhibited the incorporation of [14C]riboflavin into [14C]FAD in liver, cerebrum, cerebellum, and heart." They found that in vitro these drugs inhibited hepatic flavokinase, the first of two enzymes in the conversion of riboflavin to FAD. After 3 or 7 weeks, the effects of chlorpromazine administration, at doses comparable on a weight basis to those used clinically, impaired conversion of riboflavin to its coenzyme derivatives and interfere with riboflavin metabolism and utilization "in the animal as a whole" to a significant degree, as indicated by several standard indices of riboflavin status. The EGRAC, an FAD-containing enzyme, was elevated, indicating a riboflavin deficiency state. The urinary excretion of riboflavin was more than twice that of age- and gender-matched pair-fed control rats. Tissue levels of FMN and FAD in test animals were significantly lower than those of pair-fed controls after administration of chlorpromazine for 7 weeks, despite consumption of a diet estimated to contain 30 times the RDA. Thus the authors concluded that low doses of chlorpromazine in rats fed abundant riboflavin increase urinary riboflavin excretion and reduce hepatic flavin stores.[20] In a

follow-up study, this research team confirmed that low doses of chlorpromazine increased urinary riboflavin excretion and greatly depleted FAD levels in liver, kidney, and heart, both in animals fed a normal diet and in animals fed a riboflavin-deficient diet. Notably, "brain levels of FAD by contrast were relatively resistant to both dietary riboflavin withdrawal and treatment with chlorpromazine."[51] Subsequent studies showed that urinary riboflavin excretion began to increase within 6 hours of administration of chlorpromazine.

In related research, animal studies have found that administration of riboflavin or FAD can protect against chlorpromazine-induced arrhythmia and mitochondrial dysfunction, particularly when used with coenzyme Q10.[52,53]

In a study involving 52 male and female acute psychiatric inpatients (see Tricyclic Antidepressants), Bell and colleagues[112] investigated the relationship between FAD, which is "reportedly sensitive to thyroid status and to phenothiazine and tricyclic drug exposure," and folate-dependent methylation pathways that "may play a role in the etiology and treatment of such mental disorders as major depression." Nine subjects (17%) demonstrated riboflavin deficiency on a functional red blood cell enzyme assay, thus indicating insufficient FAD activity, with only one riboflavin-deficient subject exhibiting deficiency in another B-complex vitamin, folate. Notably, all patients demonstrating riboflavin deficiency were women, who were characterized by being significantly younger than the rest of the sample, having significantly lower thyroxine levels (even when controlling for gender and covarying for age), and exhibiting "a nonsignificant trend toward more unipolar depression (44% vs 14%), but not toward bipolar or schizophrenic disorders." Moreover, "drug exposure did not show a relationship to riboflavin deficiency in this sample." The authors concluded that these "findings suggest that B₂ (FAD) activity may serve as a sensitive marker of thyroxine status in certain female psychiatric inpatients and that B₂ deficiency may play an etiological role in defects of the methylation pathways in a subset of mentally ill individuals."

Nutritional Therapeutics, Clinical Concerns, and Adaptations

Physicians prescribing chlorpromazine or related phenothiazines to individuals for unipolar depression, schizophrenia, anxiety, porphyria, or nausea are advised to evaluate riboflavin, FAD, and thyroxine status and to consider coadministration of a B-complex formulation containing riboflavin and folate. Such nutrient supplementation may address fundamental susceptibilities in these patients while preventing drug-induced nutrient depletion patterns. Given the available information regarding potential binding of riboflavin and chlorpromazine, it would be prudent to separate intake of the nutrients and other medications by 4 hours or more.

Doxorubicin and Related Anthracycline Chemotherapy

Evidence: Doxorubicin (Adriamycin, Rubex).
Extrapolated, based on similar properties: Daunorubicin (Cerubidine, DaunoXome), epirubicin (Ellence, Pharmorubicin), idarubicin (Idamycin, Zavedos), mitoxantrone (Novantrone, Onkotrone).
Similar properties but evidence lacking for extrapolation: Doxorubicin, pegylated liposomal (Caelyx, Doxil, Myocet).

Interaction Type and Significance

◇≈≈ **Drug-Induced Adverse Effect on Nutrient Function, Coadministration Therapeutic, with Professional Management**

≈≈   **Drug-Induced Nutrient Depletion, Supplementation Therapeutic, with Professional Management**
☼   **Prevention or Reduction of Drug Adverse Effect**
◇◇   **Impaired Drug Absorption and Bioavailability, Precautions Appropriate**

Probability: Evidence Base:
4. Plausible to   ○ **Preliminary** to
  2. Probable   ◉ **Emerging**

Effect and Mechanism of Action

Doxorubicin has been shown to form a 1:1 stoichiometric complex with riboflavin, increasing urinary excretion, and competing for binding to tissue proteins.[25,54-57] Such a pharmacokinetic interaction would impair activity of both agents.

Doxorubicin can interfere with the normal metabolism and function of riboflavin by inhibiting the conversion to FMN and FAD.

Riboflavin 2',3',4',5'-tetrabutyrate (B₂-butyrate) may be effective in reducing lipid peroxidation and other toxic effects associated doxorubicin therapy.[58-60]

Riboflavin may deactivate doxorubicin (ADR) in the presence of daylight. "The inactivation of the drug results from its direct oxidation by the excited triplet riboflavin in a type I photosensitization reaction, and 3-methoxysalicyclic acid is an ADR breakdown product."[61,62]

Research

Animal models and clinical reviews indicate that Adriamycin/doxorubicin can cause riboflavin deficiency, even when dietary sources of riboflavin have been sufficient, and that such drug-induced depletion plays a role in drug toxicity and adverse effects. Pinto et al.[54,63] demonstrated that the increased levels in aldosterone associated with doxorubicin are the result of the drug's inhibition of flavin coenzyme biosynthesis. Based on findings using a rat model, these researchers concluded that flavins play a decisive role in regulating the levels of aldosterone and suggested that a doxorubicin-induced increase in serum aldosterone may play a significant role in the pathogenetic mechanisms of cardiovascular toxicity and overall muscular weakness. In related experiments, this research team found that Adriamycin intensifies depletion of reduced glutathione by riboflavin deficiency in rat lens.[63,64]

The findings indicating that the effects of light exposure on riboflavin may impair the activity of doxorubicin are preliminary and of uncertain clinical significance. Ramu et al.[62] investigated the enhancement of doxorubicin inactivation through light-excited riboflavin by histidine and other imidazole analogs. The rate of bleaching of doxorubicin by light-excited riboflavin was enhanced in the presence of histidine in a concentration-dependent manner. These researchers concluded that "in contrast to singlet oxygen, the trans-annular peroxide, formed by the interaction of histidine and the singlet oxygen produced by photoexcited riboflavin, is an efficient oxidizer" of doxorubicin. Based on these findings, they noted that the "presence of urocanic acid in the skin suggests that significant degradation of ADR could occur in the presence of biologically relevant concentrations of riboflavin if patients treated with ADR are exposed to sunlight."[62]

Nutritional Therapeutics, Clinical Concerns, and Adaptations

Physicians administering doxorubicin are advised to coadminister riboflavin to prevent or reverse adverse effects of the agent on riboflavin and its coenzymes. Administration of riboflavin before, during, and after chemotherapy with anthracyclines, particularly doxorubicin, is supported by the body of scientific evidence and experienced clinicians. A daily dosage of 20 to 25 mg of riboflavin, the amounts found in many multivitamin supplements, is most likely sufficient to compensate for doxorubicin-induced deficiency; intake should be separated by 4 hours to minimize risk of binding. Riboflavin is nontoxic, even in high doses, and evidence of any interference by the nutrient on the therapeutic effect of the chemotherapy is lacking and generally considered as unlikely, apart from risk of mutual interference with absorption. Patients might be instructed to avoid significant exposure to sunlight or other sources of major light exposure. All cases inherently require close supervision and regular monitoring. Notably, riboflavin administration may not adequately counteract the toxic effects of doxorubicin related to interference with biosynthesis of FAD and FMN. Concurrent administration of coenzyme Q10 may mitigate doxorubicin cardiotoxicity and myopathy (see Coenzyme Q10 monograph).

Physicians and other health care professionals may consider reviewing the potential for such synergistic therapies with appropriate patients and provide referral information to centers specializing in such integrative approaches. Further research with large, well-designed clinical trials is needed.

Oral Contraceptives: Monophasic, Biphasic, and Triphasic Estrogen Preparations (Synthetic Estrogen and Progesterone Analogs)

Ethinyl estradiol and desogestrel (Desogen, Ortho-TriCyclen). Ethinyl estradiol and ethynodiol (Demulen 1/35, Demulen 1/50, Nelulen 1/25, Nelulen 1/50, Zovia). Ethinyl estradiol and levonorgestrel (Alesse, Levlen, Levlite, Levora 0.15/30, Nordette, Tri-Levlen, Triphasil, Trivora). Ethinyl estradiol and norethindrone/norethisterone (Brevicon, Estrostep, Genora 1/35, GenCep 1/35, Jenest-28, Loestrin 1.5/30, Loestrin1/20, Modicon, Necon 1/25, Necon 10/11, Necon 0.5/30, Necon 1/50, Nelova 1/35, Nelova 10/11, Norinyl 1/35, Norlestin 1/50, Ortho Novum 1/35, Ortho Novum 10/11, Ortho Novum 7/7/7, Ovcon-35, Ovcon-50, Tri-Norinyl, Trinovum). Ethinyl estradiol and norgestrel (Lo/Ovral, Ovral). Mestranol and norethindrone (Genora 1/50, Nelova 1/50, Norethin 1/50, Ortho-Novum 1/50). Related, internal application: Etonogestrel/ethinyl estradiol vaginal ring (Nuvaring).

Interaction Type and Significance

◇≈≈   **Drug-Induced Adverse Effect on Nutrient Function, Coadministration Therapeutic, with Professional Management**
≈≈   **Drug-Induced Nutrient Depletion, Supplementation Therapeutic, with Professional Management**
☼   **Prevention or Reduction of Drug Adverse Effect**

Probability: Evidence Base:
4. Plausible to **3. Possible**   ◉ **Emerging**

Effect and Mechanism of Action

Oral contraceptives (OCs), particularly in high doses in women with compromised nutriture, tend to alter levels of several nutrients, lowering some, elevating others, and producing ambiguous effects in a few. The mechanisms of such effects have yet to

Nutrient-Drug Interactions and Drug-Induced Nutrient Depletions

be fully elucidated but almost certainly involve the physiological interrelationships among vitamin B$_6$, vitamin B$_1$, riboflavin, folate, and tryptophan, such that a deficiency in one nutrient induces alterations in the activity of others.[65] Concurrent administration of riboflavin and related nutrients appears to prevent or compensate for these adverse effects.

Research

Beginning in the mid-1970s, a series of studies and reviews reported an association between OCs and alterations in physiological levels of several nutrients, most notably depressing serum levels of vitamin B$_6$, but also B$_{12}$ and riboflavin.[65-69] In a 1974 letter regarding a study by Sanpitak and Chayutimonkul[70] on OCs and riboflavin nutriture, Briggs[71] noted that the data showed "striking decreases in women taking oral contraceptives in all the water-soluble vitamins (C, B$_{12}$, riboflavine, B$_6$), no change in vitamin E, but an increase in plasma-retinol." As Wynn[66] summarized in 1975: "Biochemical evidence of co-enzyme deficiency has been reported for vitamin B$_2$, vitamin B$_6$, and folic acid." Webb[69] noted that "OC users need more pyridoxine and riboflavin is needed to oxidize pyridoxine phosphate to pyridoxal phosphate." Generally, however, summary remarks echoed this theme: "The clinical significance of these alterations is unknown." However, given the apparent need for enhanced nutriture, consumption of multivitamins was often the ensuing, tentative recommendation.

Ahmed et al.[68] investigated the effects of OCs on nutrient status through a series of animal and human studies. In 1975 they compared biochemical parameters used for assessing vitamin nutritional status in a group of women who had used low-estrogen combination OCs for 6 to 12 months with those of another group of nontreated women, initially and at one or more times in the 6 months. Among several changes relating to nutrient levels and activity, they noted a "fall in erythrocyte riboflavin concentration associated with a decrease in erythrocyte glutathione reductase activity and increase in vitro stimulation with FAD." Notably, "most of these changes were observed during the first few cycles of oral contraceptive treatment."[68]

In a 1979 cross-sectional and follow-up study, Vir and Love[72] found "no significant adverse effect" of OCs on riboflavin nutriture in 65 "young healthy women." Biochemical deficiency of riboflavin manifested in 3 of 33 women in the cross-sectional group, whereas in the follow-up group, only one developed biochemical deficiency after 3 months. Notably, "biochemical riboflavin status did not correlate with OC use," with no correlation observed "between riboflavin intake and activity coefficient of erythrocyte glutathione reductase activity (EGR)." "Most of the subjects had adequate riboflavin intake," and the authors suggested that for women "in developing countries it is possible that the combined effects of poor dietary riboflavin nutrition and OCs contribute to the further deterioration of dietary riboflavin nutrition."[72]

In 1980, Lewis and King[72a] published findings from a small clinical trial indicating that women taking OCs were responsive to riboflavin and thiamin supplementation at relatively low levels, even though deficiencies were not detectable by standard laboratory assessment. In this experiment involving 13 young women, age 19 to 25, thiamin, riboflavin, and pantothenic acid status were determined at the beginning and end of a 12-day confined study. The subjects were fed a constant formula diet containing 2.0 mg thiamin, 3.0 mg riboflavin, and 10 mg pantothenic acid on entering the metabolic unit during the first week of their menstrual cycle. The activity of erythrocyte transketolase or erythrocyte glutathione reductase (EGR) was responsive to the levels of thiamin and riboflavin fed during the study, even though use of OCs did not appear to influence the activity of these enzymes or their response to in vitro stimulation by their cofactors. In the group receiving OCs, erythrocyte transketolase and EGR stimulation by their cofactors was significantly decreased by day 12.

These studies suggest that coadministration of riboflavin may provide support against potential effects of OCs by reversing or preventing nutritional deficits, particularly in those with inadequate intake or preexisting depletion patterns.

Inconsistent findings in various reports have been attributed to differences of OC formulation or riboflavin intake, but more recent research indicates that the women, their biochemical individuality, and variable demands on their systems may play significant roles in determining the effects of OCs. Roe et al.[73] compared the riboflavin requirements of eight healthy OC users and 10 nonusers on diets prepared in a metabolic unit using a single daily menu and meal pattern. On measurement, "erythrocyte glutathione reductase assay values and urinary riboflavin excretion showed intersubject and interperiod differences but no significant group differences (OC versus non-OC)." These authors concluded that "when dietary intake is controlled, OC do not significantly influence riboflavin status," but that "riboflavin needs were related to energy requirements of the subjects." In related research not involving OCs, Belko et al.[74] investigated the riboflavin requirement of young women during periods of sedentary living and exercise determined during a 12-week metabolic study. After examining intake of calories and riboflavin, exercise effects, and EGRAC, they concluded that "healthy young women require more riboflavin to achieve biochemical normality" than the 1980 RDAs, and that "exercise increases riboflavin requirements."

Overall, the body of available evidence indicates that OC effects on riboflavin status, as with other nutrients, are significantly influenced by interindividual variability in diet, nutritional status, energy requirements, and response to OCs. Given adequate nutrient intake relative to activity levels, OCs, particularly at the lower estrogen dose levels more typical in recent years, are not likely to exert a significant adverse effect on riboflavin status in most women. In some women, levels of riboflavin and other nutrients may be adversely affected during the initial months of use, but such effects tend to diminish after the initial 3 to 6 months relative to other factors, although long-term use of estrogen-containing OCs can induce folic acid and B-vitamin deficiency. As always, individual variations in tolerance and susceptibility to adverse effects are probable. Further research is warranted through well-designed and adequately powered clinical trials.

Nutritional Therapeutics, Clinical Concerns, and Adaptations

The supplemental dose of riboflavin, 20 to 25 mg, found in most multivitamins is probably adequate to compensate for any potential deficiency resulting from OC use, although requirements can increase with significant changes in dietary intake or activity level. Coadministration of vitamin B$_6$, folic acid, and B$_{12}$ is usually appropriate when nutritional support is indicated. Enhanced nutrient intake is most important in women with compromised nutritional status, lifestyle factors, or medical conditions impairing vitamin nutriture, or taking medications that tend to deplete riboflavin or interrelated nutrients.

Probenecid

Probenecid (*p*-(di-*n*-propylsulfamyl)-benzoic acid; Benemid, Parbenem, Probalan).
Related: Sulfinpyrazone (Anturane).

Interaction Type and Significance

≈≈ **Drug-Induced Adverse Effect on Nutrient Function, Coadministration Therapeutic, Not Requiring Professional Management**

≈≈≈ **Drug-Induced Nutrient Depletion, Supplementation Therapeutic, Not Requiring Professional Management**

Probability:	Evidence Base:
4. Plausible	○ Preliminary

Effect and Mechanism of Action

Probenecid may decrease the absorption of riboflavin from the GI tract, but it can also inhibit renal tubular secretion of riboflavin and decrease riboflavin excretion in the urine.[75-79]

Research

Although widely discussed as a probable interaction, the research findings regarding the effects of probenecid on riboflavin absorption and function are preliminary and limited in scope.

Using an in vitro cellular model system, Said et al.[80] found that uptake of riboflavin by colonic epithelial cells was not inhibited in a competitive manner by probenecid, although it was inhibited by the membrane transport inhibitor amiloride (used clinically as a potassium-sparing diuretic).

Nutritional Therapeutics, Clinical Concerns, and Adaptations

Physicians prescribing probenecid are advised to administer riboflavin concurrently because requirements for riboflavin may be increased by the drug's action. Risk is likely to be higher with nutritionally compromised patients and long-term therapy. Physicians should monitor closely for any signs of deficiency.

Propantheline Bromide (Pro-Banthine)

Propantheline bromide (Pro-Banthine)

Interaction Type and Significance

✗ **Potential or Theoretical Adverse Interaction of Uncertain Severity**

◇◇ **Drug-Induced Effect on Nutrient Function, Supplementation Contraindicated, Professional Management Appropriate**

Probability:	Evidence Base:
4. Plausible or	○ Preliminary but
6. Unknown	● Consensus

Effect and Mechanism of Action

Propantheline is an antimuscarinic (anticholinergic) agent that can significantly increase riboflavin absorption by decreasing salivary flow, rate of gastric emptying, and GI motility.[81-85]

Research

The available research investigating the effects of propantheline on riboflavin absorption lacks evidence from clinical trials, but its conclusions are generally accepted as consensus in the pharmacological literature. Nevertheless, even though this effect is apparently "probable to certain" in occurrence, its clinical significance is minimal because the capacity to absorb riboflavin from the GI tract by humans is limited, and riboflavin is generally considered nontoxic at known doses.[86-88] In most cases the effect would be minimal, and it could be beneficial in patients with compromised riboflavin nutriture. Further research would be required to determine whether this pharmacokinetic effect might diminish over time and to assess more accurately any subtle physiological effects of long-term propantheline therapy on riboflavin metabolism and its relationships with coenzymes, related nutrients, and their activities.

Nutritional Therapeutics, Clinical Concerns, and Adaptations

Physicians prescribing propantheline can better understand the drug's actions by analyzing its effects on riboflavin. Derivative literature typically cautions patients taking propantheline to "seek medical advice." In most cases, however, no changes in clinical management are necessary as a result of these highly probable effects. In particular, avoidance of multivitamins containing typical doses of riboflavin is generally unnecessary.

Tetracyclines and Other Antibiotics

Demeclocycline (Declomycin), doxycycline (Atridox, Doryx, Doxy, Monodox, Periostat, Vibramycin, Vibra-Tabs), minocycline (Dynacin, Minocin, Vectrin), oxytetracycline (Terramycin), tetracycline (Achromycin, Actisite, Apo-Tetra, Economycin, Novo-Tetra, Nu-Tetra, Sumycin, Tetrachel, Tetracyn); combination drugs: chlortetracycline, demeclocycline, and tetracycline (Deteclo); bismuth, metronidazole, and tetracycline (Helidac).
Related: Antibiotics, all classes.

Interaction Type and Significance

✗✗ **Minimal to Mild Adverse Interaction—Vigilance Necessary**

◇◇ **Impaired Drug Absorption and Bioavailability, Precautions Appropriate**

Probability:	Evidence Base:
2. Probable	○ Preliminary

Effect and Mechanism of Action

B vitamins, including riboflavin, may interfere with tetracycline pharmacokinetics, impairing absorption and bioavailability. Such an interaction would also impair bioavailability of the vitamins. Thus, tetracyclines can increase urinary riboflavin excretion. More broadly, riboflavin can impair the antibiotic activity of tetracyclines (as well as streptomycin, erythromycin, tyrothricin, and carbomycin) but generally does not inhibit the activity of chloramphenicol, penicillin, or neomycin.[88-90]

Extended use of tetracycline antibiotics could adversely affect bioavailability and function of riboflavin and other B-complex nutrients, both directly and indirectly. Apart from the two-way pharmacokinetic issues, the destructive impact of antimicrobial agents on gut microflora can impair production of B vitamins (as well as folate and vitamin K) and could contribute to systemic inflammatory processes and depressed immune system function.[91-100]

Research

Experiments have demonstrated inactivation of tetracycline solutions by riboflavin in vitro.[89,101] Omray and Varma[102] demonstrated that oral administration of a vitamin C and vitamin B complex could impair absorption and reduce bio-availability of tetracycline hydrochloride through pharmacokinetic interference.

Clinical Implications and Adaptations

Physicians prescribing tetracycline or related antibiotic medications should advise patients regularly supplementing with riboflavin, alone or within a B-complex vitamin formulation, to take the nutrient(s) and the medication at least 4 hours apart from each other.

Patients treated with tetracyclines or other broad-spectrum antibiotics for an extended period or with high doses will usually benefit from a course of probiotic flora for an equivalent duration to restore intestinal microbiota. Short-term use of tetracyclines is unlikely to lead to clinically significant alterations in the GI ecology. A diet rich in leafy green vegetables and whole grains would typically provide sufficient compensation for any drug-induced decrease in nutrient intake or synthesis, although a multivitamin (taken separate from the medication) may be appropriate in patients with compromised nutritional status undergoing extended tetracycline therapy.

Thyroid Hormones

L-triiodothyronine (T₃): Cytomel, liothyronine sodium, liothyronine sodium (synthetic T₃), Triostat (injection).
Levothyroxine (T₄): Eltroxin, Levo-T, Levothroid, levothyroxine (synthetic), levoxin, Levoxyl, Synthroid, thyroxine, Unithroid.
L-Thyroxine and L-triiodothyronine (T₄ + T₃): Animal levothyroxine/liothyronine, Armour Thyroid, desiccated thyroid, Westhroid.
L-Thyroxine and L-triiodothyronine (synthetic T₄ + T₃): Euthroid, Euthyral, liotrix, Thyar, Thyrolar.
Dextrothyroxine (Choloxin).
See also Antimalarial Drugs and Tricyclic Antidepressants.

Interaction Type and Significance

⊕⊕ **Beneficial or Supportive Interaction, with Professional Management**

Probability:	Evidence Base:
4. Plausible or	○ Preliminary to
3. Possible	◉ Emerging

Effect and Mechanism of Action

Thyroid hormone regulates the enzymatic conversion of riboflavin to FMN and FAD, its active coenzyme forms.[103] Specifically, triiodothyronine (T₃) plays a key role in the conversion of riboflavin into FMN by enhancing biosynthesis through the expression of riboflavin kinase.[104,105]

Riboflavin is necessary for thyroxine synthesis, as are niacin, pyridoxine, and iodine. Inadequate riboflavin intake can also contribute to diminished thyroid function.

Research

Although a significant body of scientific research explores the physiological functions and the relationships involving riboflavin, its coenzymes, and thyroid hormones, evidence from clinical trials directly investigating coadministration and therapeutic strategies is limited.

Using a rat model, Lee and McCormick[104] reported a "correspondence of flavokinase activity with the amount of a high-affinity flavin-binding protein quantitated immunologically in hypo-, eu-, and hyperthyroid rats [which] indicated

that the thyroid response is caused by an increased amount of enzyme; moreover, the concomitant decrease in a low-affinity flavin-binding protein suggests an inactive precursor form of flavokinase." Furthermore, "FAD synthetase activity showed a similar but less pronounced trend than flavokinase."

In 1968, Rivlin et al.[106] observed that hypothyroidism has biochemical similarities to riboflavin deficiency, including lowered FAD biosynthesis, depressed basal EGR activity, and elevated EGRAC. In 1969, Rivlin and Wolf[107] reported diminished responsiveness to thyroid hormone in riboflavin-deficient rats. Croxson and Ibbertson[108] reported low serum T₃ and hypothyroidism in patients with anorexia nervosa. They noted that "a probable decrease of peripheral T₄ to T₃ conversion leads to low serum T₃ concentrations." In a clinical trail involving six hypothyroid human adults, Cimino et al.[105] demonstrated that the activity of EGR, an accessible FAD-containing enzyme, is decreased to levels comparable to those found in riboflavin deficiency, and thyroxine therapy resulted in normal EGR levels while the subjects were on a controlled dietary regimen. Subsequently, in a clinical trial of 17 adolescent girls diagnosed with anorexia nervosa, Capochichi et al.[109] found that "triiodothyronine concentrations were low and negatively correlated with plasma riboflavin concentrations." They concluded that the "low triiodothyronine concentrations observed in anorexia nervosa could alter the extent of riboflavin conversion into cofactors, thus leading to high erythrocyte riboflavin concentrations, low plasma flavin adenine dinucleotide concentrations, and high rates of ethylmalonic acid and isovalerylglycine excretion."

Notably, as discussed in reviewing interactions between riboflavin and antimalarial drugs, hypothyroidism is known to be associated with decreased susceptibility to parasitemia.[110]

Some secondary sources have suggested that synthetic thyroid medication (T₄) tends to decrease riboflavin absorption, but evidence is lacking to support this hypothesis.

Nutritional Therapeutics, Clinical Concerns, and Adaptations

Physicians treating patients diagnosed with hypothyroidism are advised to consider concurrent nutritional support that includes riboflavin, as well as iodine, niacin, and vitamins B₆ and C, as appropriate to the patient's particular characteristics and needs. Patients receiving Synthroid or equivalent exogenous T₄ may particularly benefit from enhanced riboflavin nutriture. Further research using well-designed clinical trials is warranted to explore these potential therapeutic synergies.

Tricyclic Antidepressants (TCAs)

Evidence: Amitriptyline (Elavil), imipramine (Janimine, Tofranil), nortriptyline (Aventyl, Pamelor).
Similar properties but evidence lacking for extrapolation: Amitriptyline combination drug: amitriptyline and perphenazine (Etrafon, Triavil, Triptazine); amoxapine (Asendin), clomipramine (Anafranil), desipramine (Norpramin, Pertofrane), doxepin (Adapin, Sinequan), protriptyline (Vivactil), trimipramine (Surmontil).

Interaction Type and Significance

⊕⊕ **Beneficial or Supportive Interaction, with Professional Management**
◇≈≈ **Drug-Induced Adverse Effect on Nutrient Function, Coadministration Therapeutic, with Professional Management**

≈≈   **Drug-Induced Nutrient Depletion, Supplementation Therapeutic, with Professional Management**

Nutrient Depletion
Probability: Evidence Base:
3. Possible or 2. Probable   ● Emerging

Coadministration Benefit
Probability: Evidence Base:
4. Plausible to 2. Probable ○ Preliminary

Effect and Mechanism of Action

Tricyclic antidepressants (TCAs) can decrease riboflavin absorption and inhibit the incorporation of riboflavin into FMN and FAD.[20] Consequently, the potential for riboflavin depletion and impairment of physiological functions can increase riboflavin requirements during extended therapy using these medications. Moreover, coadministration of riboflavin and other B vitamins may elevate levels of these nutrients and their metabolites and augment the therapeutic activity of TCAs and clinical outcomes from such therapy.

Research

A review of the scientific literature reveals a significant trend suggesting a probable additive or synergistic effect with TCA/riboflavin coadministration, the occurrence and degree of which are influenced by the patient's nutritional status and other individual variables.

In two clinical trials in 1992, Bell et al.[111,112] demonstrated the potential clinical advantages of coadministering riboflavin and TCAs to influence intermediates in the folate-dependent methylation pathways. In a 4-week, randomized, placebo-controlled, double-blind study involving 14 geriatric inpatients diagnosed with depression, they investigated augmentation of open TCA treatment with 10 mg each of vitamins B₁, B₂, and B₆. The "active vitamin group demonstrated significantly better B₂ and B₆ status on enzyme activity coefficients and trends toward greater improvement in scores on ratings of depression and cognitive function, as well as in serum nortriptyline levels compared with placebo-treated subjects."[111] In the second study, starting with a sample of 52 male and female acute psychiatric inpatients, they found that nine women (17% of total) exhibited "B₂ deficiency (i.e., insufficient FAD activity) on a functional red blood cell enzyme assay, but only one B₂-deficient individual showed deficiency in another B-complex vitamin (folate)." Notably, the "B₂-deficient women had significantly lower thyroxine levels, even when controlling for sex and covarying for age" and "exhibited a nonsignificant trend toward more unipolar depression (44% vs 14%), but not toward bipolar or schizophrenic disorders." Furthermore, as in the parallel trial, "drug exposure did not show a relationship to riboflavin deficiency in this sample." These researchers concluded that their "findings suggest that B₂ (FAD) activity may serve as a sensitive marker of thyroxine status in certain female psychiatric inpatients and that B₂ deficiency may play an etiological role in defects of the methylation pathways in a subset of mentally ill individuals."[112] (See also Chlorpromazine and Related Phenothiazine Antipsychotics.)

The TCAs, particularly amitriptyline, and riboflavin are both used clinically for migraine prophylaxis. Research into potential synergy is suggested by the available data on their mutual effects and the ability of riboflavin to counter possible adverse effects of the drug.

Note: Riboflavin is often used to monitor drug compliance with a range of medications, including TCA therapy. Riboflavin is coadministered with the medication because it is simple to assess riboflavin in urine (e.g., bright-yellow flavinuria).[113-115] Thus, a patient's noncompliance is easily detected because their urine will not exhibit riboflavin (unless the patient is taking vitamins that contain riboflavin, which would confound results). This use is not intended to function as an interaction and is mentioned only to clarify potential confusion regarding such coadministration.

Nutritional Therapeutics, Clinical Concerns, and Adaptations

Physicians prescribing TCAs, particularly for unipolar depression, are advised to coadminister riboflavin to prevent or reverse adverse effects on nutrient bioavailability and activity and to consider further adjunctive therapy with thiamine and cyanocobalamin (B₁ and B₁₂). The aim is to achieve pharmacological synergy and enhanced therapeutic outcomes through the supportive interaction of these nutrients with riboflavin and TCAs. Although riboflavin and thiamine are considered relatively nontoxic, the coadministration of a TCA and pyridoxine (B₆) amplifies the usual admonition that close supervision and regular monitoring are warranted. Because PLP-dependent enzymes play a role in serotonin synthesis, concomitant pyridoxine may prevent or reverse depletion as well as augment clinical response to TCAs through an additive or synergistic effect. See the Vitamin B₆ monograph for further discussion.

THEORETICAL, SPECULATIVE, AND PRELIMINARY INTERACTIONS RESEARCH, INCLUDING OVERSTATED INTERACTIONS CLAIMS

Acetylsalicylic Acid

Acetylsalicylic acid (acetosal, acetyl salicylic acid, ASA, salicylsalicylic acid; Arthritis Foundation Pain Reliever, Ascriptin, Aspergum, Asprimox, Bayer Aspirin, Bayer Buffered Aspirin, Bayer Low Adult Strength, Bufferin, Buffex, Cama Arthritis Pain Reliever, Easprin, Ecotrin, Ecotrin Low Adult Strength, Empirin, Extra Strength Adprin-B, Extra Strength Bayer Enteric 500 Aspirin, Extra Strength Bayer Plus, Halfprin 81, Heartline, Regular Strength Bayer Enteric 500 Aspirin, St. Joseph Adult Chewable Aspirin, ZORprin); combination drugs: ASA and caffeine (Anacin); ASA, caffeine, and propoxyphene (Darvon Compound); ASA and carisoprodol (Soma Compound); ASA, codeine, and carisoprodol (Soma Compound with Codeine); ASA and codeine (Empirin with Codeine); ASA, codeine, butalbital, and caffeine (Fiorinal); ASA and extended-release dipyridamole (Aggrenox, Asasantin).

Concurrent intake of aspirin and riboflavin has been reported to cause gastric intolerance in some patients. In a migraine prophylaxis pilot study involving 49 individuals administered 400 mg riboflavin and 75 mg aspirin daily, one subject withdrew from the trial after 2 weeks because of gastric intolerance.[46] Both the relatively high dose of riboflavin and the lack of corroborating evidence from other clinical trials or qualified case reports render this isolated report preliminary and speculative. No mechanism of action has been documented, and given the known adverse effects of aspirin, the role of riboflavin as the predominant aggravating factor is doubtful.

Beta-1-Adrenoreceptor Antagonists (Beta-Adrenergic Blocking Agents)

Oral forms (systemic).
Evidence: Bisoprolol (Zebeta), metoprolol (Lopressor, Toprol XL).

Extrapolated, based on similar properties: Acebutolol (Sectra), atenolol (Tenormin); combination drugs: atenolol and chlortalidone (Co-Tendione, Tenoretic); atenolol and nifedipine (Beta-Adalat, Tenif); betaxolol (Kerlone), carteolol (Cartrol), esmolol (Brevibloc), labetalol (Normodyne, Trandate); metoprolol combination drug: metoprolol and hydrochlorothiazide (Lopressor HCT); nadolol (Corgard), nebivolol (Nebilet), oxprenolol (Trasicor), penbutolol (Levatol), pindolol (Visken), propranolol (Betachron, Inderal LA, Innopran XL, Inderal); combination drug: propranolol and bendrofluazide (Inderex); sotalol (Betapace, Betapace AF, Sorine), timolol (Blocadren).

Through distinct but complementary mechanisms, coadministration of riboflavin and a beta blocker could theoretically enhance migraine prevention effects without introducing adverse effects.

Sándor et al.[116] investigated the effects of riboflavin and beta blockers on migraineurs, specifically focusing on intensity dependence of auditory-evoked cortical potentials, in 26 patients before and after 4 months of prophylaxis with metoprolol or bisoprolol (all with migraine without aura) or riboflavin (13 with migraine without aura, 2 with migraine with aura). The intensity dependence of the auditory-evoked cortical potentials was significantly decreased after the treatment with beta blockers, and this decrease correlated significantly with clinical improvement. In contrast, although most patients treated with riboflavin showed clinical improvement, they demonstrated no change in intensity dependence. Based on these findings, the authors concluded that "beta-blockers and riboflavin act on two distinct pathophysiological mechanisms" and suggested that coadministration for migraine prophylaxis "might enhance their efficacy without increasing central nervous system side effects."[116]

Bile Acid Sequestrants

Cholestyramine (Locholest, Prevalite, Questran), colesevelam (Welchol), colestipol (Colestid).

Concomitant intake of riboflavin and a bile acid sequestrant may decrease the absorption of riboflavin by binding riboflavin (and many other nutrients). The tendency of these drugs to adsorb nutrients is well established with regard to fat-soluble vitamins, although controversy remains as to the frequency, extent, and clinical significance of this probable drug-induced nutrient depletion pattern.

This interaction is cited in many reviews and derivative sources as being a known effect of hypocholesterolemic resins on riboflavin absorption.[117] Although plausible and consistent with established principles of pharmacological activity, a conclusive set of evidence derived from well-designed clinical trials and qualified case reports to confirm this possibility is not readily discoverable through standard search methodologies.

Physicians prescribing bile acid sequestrants are advised to consider coadministration of riboflavin, as well as folic acid, vitamins B₁₂ and B₆, mixed tocopherols and tocotrienols, vitamin D, coenzyme Q10, magnesium, and other synergistic nutrients, within a comprehensive and individualized strategy of integrative therapeutics to prevent and treat cardiovascular disease. The relationship between riboflavin and homocysteine may be sufficient to justify increased intake of riboflavin and these complementary nutrients in patients with known cardiovascular disease or factors indicating high risk. The probable interference with absorption and bioavailability of riboflavin and other relevant nutrients by these hypocholesteremic resins further heightens the imperative for enhanced nutritional support, particularly in patients with compromised nutriture.

Daily administration of a high-potency multivitamin/mineral formulation will replace the nutrients impeded by the drug, thus serving as prudent prophylaxis against potential depletion. Riboflavin (as well as other nutrients and medications) should be taken 1 hour before or 4 to 6 hours after bile acid sequestrants to reduce impairment of absorption and obtain optimal bioavailability.

Imidazole Antibiotics

Clotrimazole (Mycelex) and related imidazole antibiotics.

Flavohemoglobins metabolize nitric oxide (NO) to nitrate and protect bacteria and fungi from NO-mediated damage, growth inhibition, and attack by NO-releasing immune cells. Imidazole antibiotics inhibit the NO dioxygenase function of microbial flavohemoglobin and disruption of the riboflavin pathways.[118,119] Consequently, riboflavin supplementation theoretically could impair the antimicrobial activity of imidazole antibiotics or similar agents that rely on the greater sensitivity to riboflavin depletion in the pathogen than in the host.

Physicians prescribing imidazole antibiotics may consider it prudent to query patients about vitamin intake and to suggest temporary discontinuation of riboflavin intake during treatment. Although speculative, the mechanism of action is plausible and consistent with known pharmacological principles. Further research may be warranted to determine the occurrence and probability of this potential interaction and the circumstances under which it might be clinically significant.

Methotrexate

Methotrexate (Folex, Maxtrex, Rheumatrex).

Numerous derivative articles mention that methotrexate interferes with riboflavin absorption and may inhibit the activities of riboflavin. A few others caution that high-dose riboflavin may impair the therapeutic efficacy of methotrexate. However, evidence from the scientific literature is lacking other than a brief discussion in a 1973 review on riboflavin and cancer by Rivlin[120] and the 1990 review of nutritional deficiencies associated with chemotherapy by Dreizen et al.[57] More substantive evidence from well-designed clinical trials is necessary to establish a clear pattern of interaction between riboflavin and methotrexate and determine its probability, severity, and characteristics.

In a case report, Svahn et al.[121] describe severe lactic acidosis caused by thiamine deficiency in an 11-month-old girl with B-cell leukemia/lymphoma on total parenteral nutrition during high-dose methotrexate therapy. "Treatment with a vitamin cocktail (OH-cobalamin, pyridoxine, thiamine, riboflavine, biotin, carnitine) at pharmacologic doses rapidly improved the child's clinical and laboratory status." Such adverse effects resulting from imbalanced parenteral supplementation are widely recognized and highlight the need for appropriate nutritional support as an integral component of treatment for severe conditions, especially with medications that have a narrow therapeutic index.

Metoclopramide

Metoclopramide (Reglan).

Increased GI motility is associated with a decrease in the rate of absorption for riboflavin. Metoclopramide, a 5HT3-receptor antagonist and a dopamine antagonist, has been effective in increasing underactive GI motility toward normal and thereby treating gastric stasis, which often accompanies migraine attacks. However, by altering the rate of gastric emptying, metoclopramide tends to decrease the absorption of riboflavin.[82]

Given this observed pattern, the concurrent administration of riboflavin with metoclopramide in patients being treated for migraine appears potentially beneficial as a means of ensuring riboflavin sufficiency and providing its possible therapeutic activity.

Selegiline

Selegiline (deprenyl, L-deprenil, L-deprenyl; Atapryl, Carbex, Eldepryl, Jumex, Movergan, Selpak).

Some secondary reviews of interactions involving riboflavin mention that riboflavin may deactivate selegiline in the presence of daylight. Based on in vitro research into sensitized photodegradation of selegiline in the presence of riboflavin and light, Takacs et al.[122] asserted that such "experiments proved that in the presence of riboflavin, both daylight and the light of daylight-lamps are sufficient to significantly decompose selegiline." However, evidence is lacking to confirm such activity with coadministration in a clinical setting, based on human trials or qualified case reports. Nevertheless, pending conclusive research, prudence suggests that patients being treated with selegiline be advised to avoid riboflavin supplementation or exposure to direct sunlight or other bright lights if they use both agents concurrently. Further research may be warranted.

Thiazide Diuretics

Bendroflumethiazide (bendrofluazide; Naturetin), combination drug: bendrofluazide and propranolol (Inderex); benzthiazide (Exna), chlorothiazide (Diuril), chlorthalidone (Hygroton), cyclopenthiazide (Navidrex); combination drug: cyclopenthiazide and oxprenolol hydrochloride (Trasidrex); hydrochlorothiazide (Aquazide, Esidrix, Ezide, Hydrocot, HydroDiuril, Microzide, Oretic); combination drugs: hydrochlorothiazide and amiloride (Moduretic); hydrochlorothiazide and captopril (Acezide, Capto-Co, Captozide, Co-Zidocapt); hydrochlorothiazide and enalapril (Vaseretic); hydrochlorothiazide and lisinopril (Prinzide, Zestoretic); hydrochlorothiazide and losartan (Hyzaar); hydrochlorothiazide and metoprolol (Lopressor HCT); hydrochlorothiazide and spironolactone (Aldactazide); hydrochlorothiazide and triamterene (Dyazide, Maxzide), hydroflumethiazide (Diucardin); methyclothiazide (Enduron), metolazone (Zaroxolyn, Mykrox), polythiazide (Renese), quinethazone (Hydromox), trichlormethiazide (Naqua).

Hydrochlorothiazide and related thiazide diuretics may increase the loss of riboflavin in the urine and could contribute to a cumulative depletion over time, especially in patients with poor nutritional status. Such an adverse effect is highly plausible given general knowledge of thiazide-induced depletion affecting many nutrients. However, specific evidence from clinical trials or qualified case reports is lacking. Further research is warranted. Pending such conclusive findings, coadministration of a multivitamin may be appropriate, particularly in patients with compromised dietary intake. Supervision and monitoring are appropriate.

Trimethoprim and Trimethoprim-Sulfamethoxazole

Trimethoprim (Proloprim, Trimpex); combination drug: trimethoprim and sulfamethoxazole (cotrimoxazole, co-trimoxazole, SXT, TMP-SMX, TMP-sulfa; Bactrim, Bactrim DS, Cotrim, Septra, Septra DS, Sulfatrim, Uroplus).

Interference with the therapeutic activity of sulfa drugs by riboflavin is widely reported in derivative literature. However, specific evidence from clinical trials or qualified case reports is lacking. Conversely, long-term use of sulfa-based antibiotics

may deplete riboflavin and other B vitamins, primarily through their adverse effect on the GI environment and its microbiota. See Tetracycline and Other Antibiotics for discussion and citations regarding this effect.

Note: Sulfamethazine is photodegraded in the presence of fluorescent light and FMN. This effect is not related to coadministration but does have implications for accurate laboratory assessment. Procedures for quantitating sulfa drugs and their metabolites need to be performed in subdued lighting and using amber or low-actinic vessels to prevent losses from photochemical reactions.[123]

NUTRIENT-NUTRIENT INTERACTIONS

Boron

See Boric Acid, Borate, and Boron.

Calcium

Calcium

Calcium absorption is impaired in riboflavin deficiency. Dairy products are rich sources of both nutrients.

Folate (Folic Acid)

Folate (Folic Acid)

The activities of folate and riboflavin are interdependent. Riboflavin is a cofactor for MTHFR, the FAD-dependent enzyme responsible for maintaining the specific folate coenzyme required to form methionine from homocysteine. The recycling of folate cofactors depends on riboflavin and vitamin B₆, whereas riboflavin is required for activating vitamin B₆ to PLP.[16] Thus, the regulation of homocysteine metabolism represents an activity of clinical significance dependent on the presence and activity of both nutrients.

Bates and Fuller[124] reported that the "effects of acute riboflavin deficiency on fetal development have similarities with effects of folate deficiency, possibly mediated by effects of flavins on folate metabolism." Weanling rats fed a riboflavin-deficient diet exhibited a marked reduction in activity of hepatic MTHFR.

In general, B vitamins can be most effective when administered together because of their interrelationships and interdependencies and the consequent cascade effect of functions or deficits.

Iron

Iron

Iron absorption and metabolism are impaired in riboflavin deficiency through multiple mechanisms not fully elucidated. Riboflavin deficiency may impair iron absorption, increase intestinal loss of iron, and impair iron utilization in hemoglobin synthesis. Powers[125] reported that coadministration of riboflavin and iron to individuals who are deficient in both nutrients enhances the therapeutic response to iron in iron deficiency anemia.

Psyllium, Fiber, and Related Laxatives

Methylcellulose (e.g., Citrucel), polycarbophil (e.g., FiberCon), psyllium (e.g., Metamucil).

Concomitant intake of psyllium may decrease the absorption of riboflavin.[126] Separating oral intake by at least 2 hours will usually minimize any such interference.

Vitamin B₃ (Niacin)

Vitamin B₃ (Niacin)

Kynurenine mono-oxygenase, an FAD-dependent enzyme, is necessary for the synthesis of NAD and NADP, niacin-containing coenzymes, from tryptophan. Therefore, in the presence of a low-niacin diet, riboflavin sufficiency would be necessary for endogenous synthesis of niacin from tryptophan.

Vitamin B₆ (Pyridoxine)

Vitamin B₆ (Pyridoxine)

Riboflavin and pyridoxine are intimately related, both physiologically and clinically. The clinical signs of riboflavin deficiency and pyridoxine deficiency are similar, and significant interactions between indicators of their nutritional status have been documented, notably in two studies involving elderly patients.[127,128] Riboflavin is a cofactor in the activation of vitamin B₆. Pyridoxine 5′-phosphate oxidase (PPO), an FMN-dependent enzyme, is necessary for the conversion of most naturally available vitamin B₆ (i.e., pyridoxamine phosphate and pyridoxine phosphate), to pyridoxal 5′-phosphate (PLP), its coenzyme form.[129] Correcting a riboflavin deficiency can restore normal activity to that enzyme (PPO). In general, B vitamins can be most effective when administered together because of their interrelationships and interdependencies.

Vitamin B₁₂

Vitamin B₁₂

The numerous interactions between riboflavin and B₁₂ are critical to normal function in many physiological processes. For example, methionine synthase, the enzyme that converts homocysteine to methionine, depends on both 5-methyltetrahydrofolate (as a methyl donor) and vitamin B₁₂, as methylcobalamin.[130] Conversely, biosynthesis of methylcobalamin depends on flavoproteins. Riboflavin deficiency interferes with the metabolism of other nutrients, especially the other B vitamins. Nevertheless, evidence is lacking to confirm that riboflavin deficiency leads to a functional deficiency of vitamin B₁₂. In general, B vitamins can be most effective when administered together because of their interrelationships and interdependencies and the consequent cascade effect of functions or deficits.

Vitamin E

Vitamin E

Riboflavin deficiency has been associated with increased oxidative stress. Both vitamin E and riboflavin can act as antioxidants. Concomitant intake may produce a synergistic effect that potentiates this antioxidant effect. In particular, glutathione reductase requires FAD to regenerate reduced glutathione from oxidized glutathione. Thus, riboflavin may protect vitamin E from lipid peroxidation while facilitating regeneration of oxidized vitamin E through its role in production of reduced glutathione.

Zinc

Zinc

Zinc absorption is impaired in riboflavin deficiency.

The 131 citations for this monograph, as well as additional reference literature, are located under Vitamin B₂ (Riboflavin) on the CD at the back of the book.

Vitamin B₃ (Niacin)

Nutrient Names: Vitamin B3, niacin, niacinamide.
Synonyms: Niacin: Nicotinic acid, nicotinate.
  Niacinamide: Nicotinamide, nicotinic acid amide, nicotinic amide.
Related Substances: Hexaniacin, inositol hexaniacinate, inositol hexanicotinate, inositol nicotinate.
Other Synonyms: 3-Pyridine carboxamide, anti-blacktongue factor, antipellagra factor, benicot, nicamid, nicosedine, nicotylamidum, pellagra-preventing factor, vitamin G.
Trade Names Include: Efacin, Endur-Acin, Enduramide, Hexopal, Niaca, Niacor, Niasafe, Niaspan, Nicalex, Nicamin, Nico-400, Nicobid, Nicolar, Nicotinex, Nico-Span, Papulex, Slo-Niacin, Tega-Span, Tri-B3, Wampocap.

Summary

Drug/Class Interaction Type	Mechanism and Significance	Management
Acetylsalicylic acid (ASA, aspirin) Acetaminophen Nonsteroidal anti-inflammatory drugs (NSAIDs) ☼/⊕✗/✗✗✗	Anti-inflammatory agents, particularly aspirin, are often administered to moderate superficial adverse effects associated with niacin (e.g., flushing, pruritus) due to effect of competitive inhibition on nicotinuric acid conjugation pathway. Coadministration may also enhance benefits on cardiovascular risk.	Coadministration of aspirin or NSAID may increase tolerance of, and enhance compliance with, niacin therapy. Consider lower-dose niacin. Monitor liver enzymes.
Anticonvulsant medications ✗✗✗/⊕✗/⊕	Concurrent niacinamide may potentiate action of anticonvulsants (particularly primidone and carbamazepine) by decreasing drug clearance. Niacinamide may also decrease conversion of primidone to phenobarbital. Further research warranted.	Niacinamide coadministration may be beneficial, but interaction can vary depending on medication. Requires clinical management.
Bile acid sequestrants ⊕⊕/⊕✗/◇◇/◇	Concurrent use of niacin and bile acid sequestrants may produce an "additive effect" on hypolipidemic activity, particularly lipoprotein B levels, by separate, well-established mechanisms. However, simultaneous intake may interfere with absorption and bioavailability of both agents and reduce their effectiveness. Combining colestipol and niacin may reduce thyroxine-binding globulin and total serum thyroxine (T₄) levels and increase triiodothyronine (T₃) uptake ratios. Further research warranted, including use of inositol hexaniacinate.	Coadministration of niacin and bile acid sequestrant can enhance efficacy of hypolipidemic strategy. Separate intake. Monitor liver enzymes. Supplement fat-soluble nutrients and coenzyme Q10 with resin therapy. Support healthy dietary and lifestyle changes.
Gemfibrozil Fibrates ⊕⊕/⊕✗/✗	Niacin and fibrates can elevate high-density lipoprotein cholesterol (HDL-C) levels and provide secondary beneficial effects of shifting low-density lipoprotein (LDL) particle size and lowering triglycerides. Niacin appears to exert more effect on HDL-C and fibrates on triglycerides. Thus coadministration can provide complementary cardioprotective effects and reduce risk of vascular events. Both agents, however, can cause hyperhomocysteinemia, with gemfibrozil the exception.	Coadministration can be beneficial, particularly in patients for whom low HDL-C represents the primary lipid disturbance. Coadminister B₆, B₁₂, and folic acid. Monitor liver enzyme and homocysteine levels. Support healthy dietary and lifestyle changes.
HMG-CoA reductase inhibitors (statins) ⊕⊕/⊕✗/✗✗	Coadministration of niacin and statin therapy has been widely researched and subsumed within conventional treatment of hyperlipidemia and atherosclerosis. Although exerting a broadly additive effect, niacin exerts greater influence on HDL-C levels, whereas statins primarily reduce levels of LDL-C. Combined effect also increases risk of hepatotoxicity, myositis, and other adverse effects. Niacin also depletes methyl donors and contributes to hyperhomocysteinemia and hypocysteinemia, whereas statins interfere with biosynthesis of coenzyme Q10.	Coadministration can be particularly appropriate in patients for whom low HDL-C represents the primary lipid disturbance. Coadminister B₆, B₁₂, and folic acid. Coadminister coenzyme Q10 and consider SAMe or other methyl donors to reduce adverse effects. Monitor liver enzyme and homocysteine levels. Support healthy dietary and lifestyle changes.
Insulin, biguanides, meglitinide analogs Oral hypoglycemic agents ⊕⊕/⊕✗/✗	Niacinamide supports pancreatic beta cells, enhances insulin secretion, and increases insulin sensitivity, potentially delaying onset or reducing symptoms of type 1 diabetes mellitus. Niacin influences glucose tolerance but may elevate glucose levels; most relevant with metabolic syndrome and dyslipidemia. Thus high-dose niacin may disrupt glycemic control, whereas niacinamide is unlikely to interfere with activity of insulin or oral hypoglycemic medications. Evidence of effects of niacin and niacinamide on glucose function and dysglycemia is mixed and inadequate; further research needed.	Coadministration of either niacinamide or low-dose niacin may be appropriate in some patients. Careful evaluation, close supervision, and regular monitoring essential. Monitor liver enzymes with niacin. Promote appropriate diet and exercise.
Isoniazid, rifampin Antitubercular agents ≈≈/☼	Isoniazid is well known for depleting niacin, primarily by interfering with the functions of vitamin B₆ and tryptophan, but also through competition in NAD. Adverse effects more severe in nutrient-	Coadminister niacin and B₆, especially with nutritionally compromised patients, and always with long-term therapy. Monitor closely for any signs of deficiency.

Continued

Summary

Drug/Class Interaction Type	Mechanism and Significance	Management
	depleted patients, especially with long-term use, but often subtle and pervasive. Coadministration of niacin and vitamin B₆ may prevent or reverse deficiency pattern without compromising therapeutic activity.	
Mercaptopurine, azathioprine, and thioguanine Thiopurines ≈≈/☼	Niacin depletion, to stage of pellagra, is a well-known effect associated with thiopurine therapy. Adverse effects are more severe in nutrient-depleted patients, especially with long-term use. Coadministration of niacin may prevent or reverse deficiency pattern without compromising therapeutic activity.	Coadminister niacin, especially with nutritionally compromised patients, and always with long-term therapy. Monitor closely for any signs of deficiency.
Tetracycline antibiotics ⊕⊕/⊕ X/◇ ◇/≈≈	Simultaneous intake of B₃ and other B vitamins with tetracycline antibiotics can reduce absorption and bioavailability of both/all agents. Coadministration of niacinamide with tetracycline or minocycline often effective against inflammatory skin conditions. Antibacterial effect on intestinal flora and gut ecology can produce secondary adverse effects on B vitamin status and inflammatory processes.	Separate intake if concurrent administration indicated or necessary. Administer probiotic flora after antibiotics.
Thioridazine ⊕⊕	Concomitant administration of niacin and thioridazine may cause increased therapeutic effect, through uncertain mechanism(s), possibly involving stimulation of GABA receptors by niacin. Limited but positive evidence from clinical trials.	Consider coadministration. Close supervision and regular monitoring appropriate.
Tricyclic antidepressants (TCAs) ⊕⊕/⊕ X/X X	Coadministration of niacinamide may support the serotonergic effects of L-tryptophan and its potentiation of therapeutic activity of TCAs. Preliminary evidence mixed; rationale plausible. Research indicates narrow therapeutic range and importance of titrating tryptophan dose, particularly in unipolar patients.	Consider coadministration of niacinamide and L-tryptophan. Effect can be very dose-dependent. Close supervision and regular monitoring critical.
Ursodeoxycholic acid Chenodeoxycholic acid X X	These anticholelithogenic agents increase cholesterol saturation of bile and thus may reduce antihyperlipidemic activity of niacin. Evidence limited but treated as consensus.	Concurrent use contraindicated as incompatible.

HMG-CoA, 3-Hydroxy-3-methylglutaryl–coenzyme A; *NAD*, nicotinamide adenine dinucleotide; *SAMe*, S-adenosylmethionine; *GABA*, gamma-aminobutyric acid.

NUTRIENT DESCRIPTION

Chemistry and Forms

Niacin and niacinamide are the two principal forms of the water-soluble B-complex vitamin, B₃. Nicotinic acid and nicotinamide are alternate names for niacin and niacinamide, respectively. Niacin was initially isolated from rice bran in 1911. Later, in 1934, Warburg and Christian isolated niacinamide, the amide of niacin, when coenzyme II (NADP) was extracted from equine erythrocytes. The structure of niacinamide consists of a pyridine ring with an amide group in position three. Inositol hexaniacinate is the hexanicotinic acid ester of meso-inositol; it also called inositol hexanicotinate or inositol nicotinate.

Niacin is extremely stable to heat, light, acid, alkali, and oxidation.

Physiology and Function

Although niacin and niacinamide have divergent pharmacological activities, they share the fundamental function that identifies them as B₃, the vitamin activity that prevents pellagra. However, niacin does not meet the criteria for being defined as a vitamin in the strictest sense because it can be derived from tryptophan. However, at a 60:1 ratio for biosynthesis, this process is highly inefficient and depends on vitamins B₁, B₂, and B₆ as essential cofactors.

Niacin, as either nicotinamide or nicotinic acid, is rapidly absorbed in the proximal small intestine by facilitated diffusion (at low concentrations) and by passive diffusion (at high concentrations). A small proportion of niacinamide is metabolized to niacin, primarily through the activity of enteric flora.

The pharmacokinetics of niacinamide vary significantly depending on dose, species, gender, and route of administration. In humans, peak serum concentrations of niacinamide are attained within 1 hour of oral ingestion because it is rapidly cleared from circulation and distributed. Niacin is primarily eliminated via the urine, but also appears in breast milk.

Nicotinamide adenine dinucleotide (NAD+, coenzyme I) and nicotinamide adenine dinucleotide phosphate (NADP+, coenzyme II) are the active forms of nicotinamide. The nicotinamide component of NAD and NADP plays a key role in hydrogen transfer reactions by acting as a hydride ion acceptor or donor in numerous intracellular oxidation-reduction (redox) reactions. Thus, they are required for the activity of more than 200 enzymes participating in a broad range of metabolic processes, including glycolysis, tissue respiration, and lipid, amino acid, and purine metabolism. Notably, NAD is required for the redox reactions in glycolysis and in Krebs cycle during oxidative phosphorylation, through which biological systems derive most of their energy from carbohydrates. NADPH is also involved in fatty acid and steroid synthesis as well as the pentose phosphate shunt pathway, one pathway by which ribose is synthesized. Consequently, niacin is essential to biosynthesis of hormones such as estrogen, progesterone, testosterone, and insulin, along with stress-related hormones in the adrenals. Niacinamide is known to stimulate gamma-aminobutyric acid (GABA) receptors, without binding to the receptor sites, an effect likened to that of benzodiazepines. Both NAD+ and NADP+ function as cofactors for numerous dehydrogenase enzymes (e.g., lactate and malate dehydrogenases) responsible for innumerable biochemical reactions in the body, including detoxifying alcohol and utilizing carbohydrates, fats, and proteins. Niacin is a precursor of glucose tolerance factor, and niacinamide facilitates beta-cell regeneration in vivo and in vitro.

Nicotinamide adenine dinucleotide is the substrate for mono–adenosine diphosphate (ADP)–ribosyltransferases and poly-ADP-ribose polymerase (PARPs), two classes of enzymes that separate the niacin moiety from NAD and transfer ADP-ribose units from NAD to acceptor proteins. Although their functions are not yet well understood, PARPs also appear to play an important role in DNA replication and repair, as well as cell differentiation. Niacinamide inhibits free-radical formation and acts as an antioxidant, at least in part by preventing NAD depletion during DNA repair by inhibiting PARP. In particular, niacinamide protects pancreatic islet cell lysis (e.g., after exposure to oxygen free radicals and nitric oxide) and suppresses cytokine-mediated induction of nitric oxide synthase. Through its inhibition of PARP, niacinamide also modulates major histocompatibility complex (MHC) class II expression and exerts an anti-inflammatory action affecting neutrophil chemotaxis.

NUTRIENT IN CLINICAL PRACTICE
Known or Potential Therapeutic Uses

Within conventional medical practice, vitamin B₃ usage, typically as niacinamide, is primarily framed in terms of prophylaxis and treatment of frank vitamin B₃ deficiency states, particularly pellagra. However, the most common clinical application of niacin is treatment of primary hyperlipidemia, specifically type IIa/IIb, III, IV, or V hyperlipoproteinemia, where it is a first-line therapy, often in combination with an HMG-CoA reductase inhibitor, for reducing low-density lipoprotein cholesterol (LDL-C) concentrations and triglycerides and increasing high-density lipoprotein cholesterol (HDL-C) concentrations.

Supplementation with vitamin B₃ can play an essential role in treatment of individuals with malabsorption syndromes associated with pancreatic insufficiency and diseases of the small intestine, such as celiac and tropical sprue. Diabetes mellitus, hyperthyroidism, malignant carcinoid syndrome, and other pathophysiological states can increase metabolic requirements for B₃ and carry a significant risk for B₃ deficiency. Hartnup's disease is a rare autosomal recessive tryptophan metabolism disorder wherein inborn errors of metabolism cause tryptophan absorption and transport to be impaired and tryptophan to be diverted to form 5-hydroxytryptamine, thereby impairing conversion of tryptophan to niacin and increasing risk of niacin deficiency and the need for niacin (and tryptophan) intake.

Historical/Ethnomedicine Precedent

The use of lime or other alkalinating agents in the diets and cooking practices of many traditional cultures represents an institutionalized application of the empirical observation that bound niacin in many food sources, especially maize, needs to be liberated to supply adequate dietary intake of niacin.

Possible Uses
General
Burns, human immunodeficiency virus (HIV) support, postpartum support, pregnancy, schizophrenia, skin cancer.

Niacin
Anxiety, atherosclerosis, Bell's palsy, diabetes mellitus, dysmenorrhea, Hartnup's disease, high hypercholesterolemia, hyperlipidemia, hyperlipoproteinemia (type IIa/IIb, III, IV, V), hypertriglyceridemia, hypothyroidism, intermittent claudication, hypothyroidism, migraines, multiple sclerosis, myocardial infarction (recurrence), photosensitivity, Raynaud's disease, smoking cessation, tardive dyskinesia.

Niacinamide
Acne (topical), alcohol withdrawal support, anxiety, bursitis, cataracts, dermatitis herpetiformis (with tetracycline), diabetes mellitus (type 1; prevention), Hartnup's disease, hypoglycemia, osteoarthritis, pellagra, photosensitivity, Raynaud's disease, tardive dyskinesia.

Inositol Hexaniacinate
Hypercholesterolemia, intermittent claudication, peripheral vascular disease, Raynaud's disease.

Deficiency Symptoms

Niacin deficiency manifests pervasively, affecting every cell in the body. Symptoms of mild niacin deficiency include indigestion, fatigue, canker sores, vomiting, and depression. In its classic presentation as pellagra, severe niacin deficiency is characterized by cutaneous, mucous membrane, central nervous system (CNS), and gastrointestinal (GI) symptoms, alone or in combination; a pattern commonly described as the "four Ds": dermatitis, diarrhea, dementia, and death. Nutritionally based pellagra usually involves a simultaneous tryptophan deficiency. The dermatitis caused by a niacin deficiency is characterized by cracked, thick, scaly skin forming a symmetrical, darkly pigmented rash and exacerbated by sun exposure, a phenomenon known as "mal del sol." This condition is often complicated by other B-vitamin deficiencies. Scarlet glossitis and stomatitis are characteristic of acute deficiency. The tongue and mouth become inflamed, painful with a burning sensation, and take on a bright, beefy red appearance. Diarrhea results from decreased hydrochloric acid secretion accompanied by inflammation of the GI tract. Dementia caused by a lack of niacin begins with irritability, headaches, and insomnia, followed by mental confusion, amnesia, hallucinations, and severe depression. If untreated, pellagra is ultimately fatal.

The most common causes of niacin deficiency are alcoholism and inadequate intake of niacin (and tryptophan) with sufficient bioavailability; genetic, pathophysiological, and iatrogenic factors also constitute significant risks. High dietary intake of cereals (e.g., sorghum, corn) not processed with lime, to increase tryptophan bioavailability, is a common cause of niacin deficiency in settings of poverty and poor diet. However, a broad nutritional deficit is usually required, especially involving protein, tryptophan and/or thiamine, riboflavin, and pyridoxine. Excessive leucine intake (e.g, with high millet intake, as common in India) can lead to a niacin deficiency even with normal intake because leucine blocks NAD synthesis. Diarrhea, cirrhosis, and inadequate or imbalanced nutrient infusions during postoperative recovery are common causes of secondary niacin deficiency.

Dietary Sources

Liver, poultry, meat, fish, eggs, peanuts, brewer's yeast, torula yeast, rice bran, rice polishings, and wheat bran are rich dietary sources of vitamin B₃. Legumes, mushrooms, nuts, sunflower seeds, and wheat germ can also serve as significant nutrient sources. In general, however, although whole grains and cereal products may contain some vitamin B₃, fortification of white flour is the primary means of ensuring that commonly consumed grain products provide adequate niacin nutriture. Niacin tends to be bound to glycosides in mature cereal grains, such as corn and wheat, which significantly decreases its bioavailability. Alkali treatment of grains, such as with alkaline-cooking process using lime, may result in release of the bound niacin and increase its bioavailability; however, this has been disputed. Dietary tryptophan can be converted to niacin and can enhance available supplies, but evidence indicates that the 60:1 conversion ratio may be overly optimistic.[1]

Food sources of B₃ often also contain thiamine, riboflavin, pantothenic acid, pyridoxine, cyanocobalamin, and folic acid. B-complex vitamins (especially B₁, B₂, and B₆), vitamin C, magnesium, zinc, protein, and essential fatty acids enhance absorption of vitamin B₃, whereas alcohol, coffee, excess sugar, antibiotics, and steroids reduce niacin absorption.

Nutrient Preparations Available

Vitamin B₃ as a nutritional supplement is primarily available as niacinamide (nicotinamide) or niacin (nicotinic acid). Multivitamin formulations typically contain some form of B₃. Nicotinamide is the form of niacin most often used in nutritional supplements and in food fortification. Nicotinate and inositol hexaniacinate (the hexanicotinic acid ester of meso-inositol) are also available as nonprescription forms. Timed-release supplemental niacin (OTC) can produce fewer superficial adverse effects (e.g., flushing) but can also be more hepatotoxic. Nicotinic acid in a shorter-acting, timed-release preparation, sometimes referred to as "intermediate release" or "extended release," is available by prescription. Limited but relatively consistent evidence indicates that inositol hexaniacinate may be the best-tolerated form of niacin, with minimal incidence of skin flushing, nausea, vomiting, agitation, and hepatotoxicity.[2-4]

Within conventional medical practice the crystalline, immediate-release form (usually taken two to four times daily) and the extended-release form (once daily) are the two prescription formulations of niacin approved for treatment of dyslipidemia. The American Heart Association advises against using OTC supplemental niacin.[5]

Note: Niacin dosage values for requirements and foods are described in niacin equivalents (NE), which are calculated by combining nicotinic acid and niacinamide intake and adding an estimate for tryptophan conversion.

$$\begin{aligned} \text{Niacin (mg equivalents)} = {}& \text{Nicotinic acid (mg)} \\ &+ \text{Nicotinamide (mg)} \\ &+ \text{Tryptophan (mg)}/60 \end{aligned}$$

Dosage Forms Available

Capsule, liquid, powder, tablet, effervescent tablet. Injectable forms are sometimes administered by health care professionals.

Source Materials for Nutrient Preparations

All B vitamins are predominantly synthesized, except for the "food form," in which synthesized B vitamins are added to nutrient broth for yeast, which (supposedly) incorporates higher amounts of them into the cells, which are then dried and tableted.

Dosage Range

Adult

Dietary: The U.S. dietary reference intake (DRI) for niacin is 16 mg niacin equivalents per day for men and 14 mg equivalents daily for women.[6] Pregnant or lactating women: 18 mg daily.

Supplemental/Maintenance: 100 mg daily, combined forms.

Pharmacological/Therapeutic: 500 mg three times daily.

Toxic: U.S. tolerable upper limit (UL) established for nicotinic acid in adults is 35 mg per day; this level was selected to avoid the adverse effect of flushing in the general population, even though flushing and other adverse effects from nicotinamide are significantly less common. No separate tolerable UL has been established for nicotinamide. Reports of nicotinamide overdosage are not present in the literature.

Nicotinic acid/niacin: Transient acute flushing symptoms can occur at 100 to 200 mg niacin. Elevated liver enzymes, jaundice, and other signs of hepatotoxicity have been observed at nicotinic acid intakes as low as 750 mg/day for less than 3 months. Timed-release nicotinic acid has been associated with chemical hepatitis at levels as low as 500 mg/day for 2 months, although most cases have involved significantly higher doses and longer periods of intake,

Nicotinamide/niacinamide: Low toxicity generally characterizes the safety profile of nicotinamide. Intake of 3 g/day of nicotinamide for longer than 3 months has been associated with adverse effects such as nausea, vomiting, elevated liver enzymes, and jaundice. However, rare occurrences of liver toxicity have been reported at doses in excess of 1000 mg/day.

Pediatric (<18 Years)

Dietary:

Infants, birth to 6 months: 2 mg/day (AI, adequate intake)
Infants, 7 to 12 months: 4 mg/day (AI)
Children, 1 to 3 years: 6 mg/day (RDA)
Children, 4 to 8 years: 8 mg/day (RDA)
Children, 9 to 13 years: 12 mg/day (RDA)
Adolescents, 14 to 18 years: 14 mg (females) or 16 mg (males) daily (RDA)

Supplemental/Maintenance: Usually not recommended for children under 12 years of age. Avoid extended-release forms.

Pharmacological/Therapeutic: Usually not recommended for children under 12 years of age. Niacinamide has been administered in research and clinical settings involving prevention of type 1 diabetes mellitus in "high-risk" individuals at daily doses of 150 to 300 mg per year of the child's age, or 25 mg per kilogram body weight daily. Avoid extended-release forms.

Toxic: No tolerable UL for niacin in infants has been proposed. The U.S. tolerable UL established for niacin in children age 1 to 8 years is 10 to 15 mg daily and 20 mg daily for children 9 to 13 years; for adolescents (14-18 years) it is 30 mg daily. These levels were selected to avoid the adverse effect of flushing in the general population; flushing from nicotinamide is unreported and not considered an associated effect.

Laboratory Values

Cellular NAD and NADP content: Some clinicians and researchers suggest this test may provide the most clinically relevant indicators of niacin nutritional status.[7]

Erythrocyte nicotinamide adenine nucleotide (NAD): This test can provide a sensitive indicator of niacin status.
Red blood cell (RBC) NAD/NADP ratio: A ratio of RBC NAD to RBC nicotinamide nucleotide phosphate (NADP) less than 1.0 may indicate deficiency.
Urinary 1-N-methyl-nicotinamide (NMN) and 2-N-pyridone (2-N-P): Excretion of less than 0.8 mg NMN per day and/or less than 1.0 mg 2-N-P per day indicates niacin deficiency. Although this measurement of excretion levels of major niacin metabolites can provide relatively accurate indices of niacin status, the results are often not conclusive.
Whole-blood niacin: Reference range 1.2 to 2.9 µg/mL.
Abnormal liver function studies: All individuals taking pharmacological doses of niacin should be monitored for liver function and enzyme levels; elevations in AST (SGOT) and ALT (SGPT) are common.
Lymphocytic growth response.

Niacin or nicotinic acid administration can alter findings from several laboratory tests.

Urinary catecholamine concentration measurements by fluorimetric methods may be falsely elevated by niacin.
Urine glucose determination using Benedict's reagent (cupric sulfate) may produce false-positive reactions. However, nicotinic acid may elevate blood glucose levels.
Nicotinic acid may falsely elevate blood growth hormone levels.
High-dose nicotinic acid may elevate blood uric acid levels.
Niacin may falsely elevate homocysteine (Hcy) levels (by interference with the assay). It can also truly elevate Hcy levels by consuming methyl donor nutrients in its metabolism.
Niacin may decrease high-sensitivity C-reactive protein (hsCRP).

SAFETY PROFILE
Overview

The safety profile for pharmacological preparations of vitamin B₃ varies significantly for different forms of the nutrient and exhibits a major differentiation between short-term, non-threatening but uncomfortable adverse effects and longer-term toxicity. Evaluation of vitamin B₃ toxicity is further complicated by over 50 years of research findings and clinical observations that use varied preparations and poor methodology or that are inadequately powered, rendering contradictory and inconsistent conclusions, and that are often simply obsolete or clinically irrelevant.

Generally, adverse effects (predominantly flushing and itching) are significantly more likely with nicotinic acid than with nicotinamide, and, conversely, nicotinamide is better tolerated than nicotinic acid. Moreover, adverse reactions to niacinamide, at doses less than 1000 mg/day, are rare (and possibly linked to impure materials), and as such the nutrient is generally considered safe in most situations.[8-11] However, the possibility exists that adverse effects of niacinamide have not been adequately documented because significantly fewer clinical trials have involved niacinamide and the lack of data simply reflects a study bias. No adverse effects are associated with intake of niacin from food sources in typically consumed forms.[6] Adverse effects ranging from minor discomfort to severe toxicity are possible with nicotinic acid. Close supervision and regular monitoring are warranted when administering doses of niacin greater than 1000 mg/day.

Nutrient Adverse Effects
General Adverse Effects

Niacin often causes skin flushing with burning and tingling sensations, especially in the face, at levels more than 100 mg, although some sensitive individuals can experience flushing with as low a dose as 10 to 20 mg. These symptoms are of rapid onset and limited duration and may be accompanied by stomach distress, itching, and headache. The vasodilatory response involved constitutes a significant mechanism of action in the therapeutic action of niacin and is considered beneficial by many who self-administer niacin. However, many patients who discontinue or refuse niacin do so to avoid this unpleasant effect. These niacin-induced adverse effects typically resolve with discontinuation. Tachyphalaxis also develops with continued daily use, although tolerance may disappear with breaks of just a few days, but is usually quickly reestablished shortly after daily intake is resumed.

Nausea and GI upset are usually the first signs of toxicity with both niacin and niacinamide. Niacin is excreted as methylated pyridones, the formation of which uses S-adenosylmethionine (SAMe), the primary physiological methyl donor. The resulting niacin-induced interference with methionine metabolism and depletion of SAMe impairs detoxification processes and contributes to many of niacin's adverse effects, including decreased levels of vitamin B₆ and increased plasma homocysteine concentrations. Changes in hepatic transaminase enzyme levels, indicating liver inflammation, are often the second detectable sign of niacin toxicity. Prudence warrants that aspartate transaminase (AST, SGOT) and alanine transaminase (ALT, SGPT) be monitored regularly during therapy with any form of niacin. Elevated liver enzymes, jaundice, and other signs of hepatotoxicity have been observed at nicotinic acid intakes as low as 500 mg/day for less than 3 months, although doses of 1500 to 3000 mg/day are more typically associated with clinically significant adverse effects. A significant body of evidence indicates that slow-release or extended-release forms of niacin are more likely to cause adverse effects and hepatic toxicity reactions. Niacin administration needs to be discontinued or the dose significantly reduced at first indication of adverse effects on liver function. When initiating pharmacological doses of time-release niacin, beginning with 500 mg and increasing by 500 mg each month up to the target dose (usually 1.5-3.0 g) improves tolerance to the therapy.

Other symptoms rarely or infrequently associated with niacin intake include headache, dizziness, anxiety, panic attacks, hypothyroidism, abnormal cardiac rhythms, heart palpitations, difficult breathing, lactic acidosis, myopathy, elevated creatine kinase levels, tooth or gum pain, macular swelling, blurred vision, and toxic amblyopia.

In a multicenter randomized, placebo-controlled trial, Garg et al.[12] found that niacin therapy, at 1000 mg or more per day, can substantially increase plasma homocysteine levels.

Niacinamide, at high dosage levels, has been associated with nausea, heartburn, vomiting, flatulence, and diarrhea. Parenteral administration of niacinamide has been reported to cause mild headaches and dizziness.

Rare occurrences of anaphylactic shock have been reported following intravenous or oral niacin therapy.

Adverse Effects Among Specific Populations

Individual characteristics that increase susceptibility to adverse effects from excess nicotinic acid intake include abnormal liver function or a history of liver disease, active peptic ulcer disease, alcohol abuse, diabetes, hypoglycemia, gout, cardiac arrhythmias, severe hypotension, inflammatory bowel disease, and migraine headaches.

Pregnancy and Nursing

Use of niacin supplementation during pregnancy or breastfeeding is not recommended because research on safety and effectiveness is insufficient. No problems have been reported.

Children

Use of niacin supplementation in children is not recommended because of insufficient research on safety and effectiveness and diminished hepatic detoxification capacity. No problems have been reported.

Contraindications

Vitamin B₃ is contraindicated in persons with hypersensitivity or allergy to niacin or niacin-containing substances and in children under 12 years of age, especially time-release forms.

Precautions and Warnings

Niacin should be avoided, or used only under close supervision and with appropriate monitoring, in patients with liver disease or compromised hepatic function, especially time-release forms.

Concomitant use of niacin and HMG-CoA reductase inhibitors (statins) significantly increases the risk of adverse effects, ranging from mild and reversible to severe and potentially fatal, especially in patients with compromised renal or hepatic function (see later discussion).

For decades, warnings have been voiced regarding potential risks for individuals with diabetes or hypoglycemia. Nicotinic acid can induce elevation in blood glucose and depletion of glycogen stores. Recent clinical trials found that niacin does not appear to raise blood glucose levels in patients with type 2 diabetes.[13,14] Thus, although niacin may cause significant alterations in blood sugar levels and insulin, such effects warrant clinical management rather than avoidance. (See Nutrient-Drug Interactions.)

Niacin can increase uric acid production and elevate blood uric acid concentrations. Individuals with gout, or predisposition to gout, should be administered niacin only under close supervision, preferably within the context of a comprehensive approach to dietary change and risk reduction. This adverse effect is primarily theoretical and evidence preliminary or inconsistent.

Niacin may elevate plasma homocysteine levels and should only be used under close supervision and with appropriate monitoring by patients with hyperhomocysteinemia or elevated risk of stroke or heart disease.

High-dose niacin intake can aggravate peptic ulcer and should be avoided in these patients except under close supervision and with appropriate monitoring.

Rare occurrences of leukopenia and slightly increased blood eosinophils have been reported in individuals taking niacin. Caution is advised in patients with bleeding disorders or undergoing anticoagulant therapy.

INTERACTIONS REVIEW

Strategic Considerations

With its long-standing role within standard practice of cardiovascular care, niacin is a nutrient that belies the labels of "alternative" and "conventional" and demonstrates the importance of an integrative approach to risk reduction and therapeutic intervention based on scientific evidence and clinical outcomes. The use of niacin with statins, resins, and fibrates is well established in conventional medicine. As such, niacin confirms the need for a multidisciplinary and collaborative model in both the benefits it conveys and the risks it amplifies when coadministered with various drug regimens and in the ways in which a strategic approach employing multiple nutrients can reduce adverse effects, optimize efficacy, and expand benefits.

Vitamin B₃ is among the most frequently researched nutrients in conventional medicine. However, a review of the available evidence illustrates that the combination of widespread usage and scientific research of limited character and narrow focus has resulted in an incomplete and unevenly distributed set of data characterized by many more speculative, ill-founded, or inadequately investigated "interactions" than thoroughly researched and well-documented ones.

Niacin can play an important role in a comprehensive strategy for reducing dyslipidemia and the risk of coronary disease, but low doses may be safer and just as effective as high doses. Also, there is an even greater need to coadminister vitamins B₆ and B₁₂ and folate, as well as methyl donor support through nutrients such as SAMe and betaine, to counter the tendencies to hepatoxicity and hyperhomocysteinemia, especially if statins are also employed. The issue of how antioxidants, singly or as networks, may interact with niacin to impair some of its therapeutic activity deserves focused research.

Two primary issues consistently arise regarding clinical application of niacin: toxicity and glucose control. The issue of *toxicity* is inherent to the nature of niacin and manifests primarily in adverse effects on the liver and interference with B₆-tryptophan-methionine metabolism, leading to elevation of homocysteine (Hcy). The use of low-dose niacin or the alternative administration of nontoxic inositol hexaniacinate may adequately address the former. Coadministration of B₂, B₆, B₁₂, folic acid, SAMe, and possibly betaine may diffuse the adverse effect on methyl donor supply and Hcy regulation.

The issue of interference with *glucose control,* particularly the often-asserted possibility of interference with oral hypoglycemic medications, may have been resolved with recent evidence indicating a lack of clinically significant interaction; nevertheless, continued research into potential benefits, drawbacks, and clinical implementation of coadministration is needed. Regular monitoring of liver enzyme levels, specifically AST and ALT, as well as plasma Hcy, is critical whenever administering niacin, especially in conjunction with statins.

The multiple concerns with niacin-induced toxicity highlight the need for further research into the efficacy of inositol hexaniacinate, or low-dose niacin, for treatment of dyslipidemias.

Likewise, the role of niacinamide in relation to insulin sensitivity, glucose tolerance, and dysglycemia suggests the need for integrative strategies that can both prevent the progression of dysfunction to disease and evolve within a multidisciplinary treatment strategy that responds flexibly to improvement or decline in the patient's condition.

In almost all its uses, vitamin B₃ exemplifies several fundamental principles operative in the clinical practice of integrative medicine. Less may do more, or enough, for any given agent. Static monotherapy using any agent is often less effective than flexible, personalized, and synergistic polypharmacy/polynutrient strategies crafted to the individual patient and evolving with their changing condition. Moreover, the spectrum of clinical applications for niacin and niacinamide and these agents' interactions with various drugs emphasize the importance of the guiding principles in the management of most clinically significant interactions: the centrality of physician-patient trust and dialogue, the importance of collaboration among health care professionals bringing together various perspectives and expertises, the continuum of dosage from nutrient support to pharmacological intervention, the opportunities to emphasize therapeutic actions or mitigate adverse effects through combinations and dosage manipulation, and the essential need for ongoing supervision, monitoring, and titration.

NUTRIENT-DRUG INTERACTIONS

Acetylsalicylic Acid, Acetaminophen, and Related Nonsteroidal Anti-Inflammatory Drugs (NSAIDs)

Evidence: Acetylsalicylic acid (acetosal, acetyl salicylic acid, ASA, salicylsalicylic acid; Arthritis Foundation Pain Reliever, Ascriptin, Aspergum, Asprimox, Bayer Aspirin, Bayer Buffered Aspirin, Bayer Low Adult Strength, Bufferin, Buffex, Cama Arthritis Pain Reliever, Easprin, Ecotrin, Ecotrin Low Adult Strength, Empirin, Extra Strength Adprin-B, Extra Strength Bayer Enteric 500 Aspirin, Extra Strength Bayer Plus, Halfprin 81, Heartline, Regular Strength Bayer Enteric 500 Aspirin, St. Joseph Adult Chewable Aspirin, ZORprin).
Extrapolated, based on similar properties:
ASA combination drugs: ASA and caffeine (Anacin); ASA, caffeine, and propoxyphene (Darvon Compound); ASA and carisoprodol (Soma Compound); ASA, codeine, and carisoprodol (Soma Compound with Codeine); ASA and codeine (Empirin with Codeine); ASA, codeine, butalbital, and caffeine (Fiorinal); ASA and extended-release dipyridamole (Aggrenox, Asasantin).
Acetaminophen (APAP, Paracetamol, Tylenol).
COX-1 inhibitors: Diclofenac (Cataflam, Voltaren), diclofenac and misoprostol (Arthrotec), diflunisal (Dolobid), etodolac (Lodine), fenoprofen (Dalfon), furbiprofen (Ansaid), ibuprofen (Advil, Excedrin IB, Motrin, Motrin IB, Nuprin, Pedia Care Fever Drops, Provel, Rufen); combination drug: hydrocodone and ibuprofen (Reprexain, Vicoprofen); indomethacin (indometacin; Indocin, Indocin-SR), ketoprofen (Orudis, Oruvail), ketorolac (Acular ophthalmic, Toradol), meclofenamate (Meclomen), mefenamic acid (Ponstel), meloxicam (Mobic), nabumetone (Relafen), naproxen (Anaprox, Naprosyn), oxaprozin (Daypro), piroxicam (Feldene), salsalate (salicylic acid; Amigesic, Disalcid, Marthritic, Mono Gesic, Salflex, Salsitab), sulindac (Clinoril), tolmetin (Tolectin)
COX-2 inhibitor: Celecoxib (Celebrex).

Interaction Type and Significance

☼   **Prevention or Reduction of Nutrient Adverse Effect**
⊕✗   **Bimodal or Variable Interaction, with Professional Management**
✗✗✗**Potentially Harmful or Serious Adverse Interaction—Avoid**

Adverse Interaction
Probability:
4. Plausible

Evidence Base:
○ Preliminary

Adverse Effect Reduction
Probability:
2. Probable

Evidence Base:
● Consensus

Effect and Mechanism of Action

Aspirin or other anti-inflammatory agents can be administered to reduce cutaneous flushing and other unwanted reactions associated with niacin intake. Both nicotinic acid and salicylic acid agents undergo glycine conjugation. Competitive inhibition with coadministration may reduce total nicotinic acid clearance and thereby cause saturation (and effective elimination) of the nicotinuric acid conjugation pathway.[15]

Theoretically, concomitant use of niacin and aspirin may increase the risk of bleeding.

Research

The use of aspirin or other anti-inflammatory agents to moderate niacin-induced effects is a well-known, empirically based practice among health care professionals experienced in nutritional therapeutics and self-medicating individuals. Several clinical trials have investigated and confirmed the efficacy of concomitant aspirin to relieve the adverse effects of niacin (nicotinic acid), such as flushing, headache, pruritus, tingling, and heat. As of 1992, the National Cholesterol Education Program recommended pretreatment with aspirin or another NSAID before niacin therapy as a means of enhancing compliance with niacin-based treatment of hyperlipidemia.

Ding et al.[15] conducted a pharmacokinetic study of the interaction between nicotinic acid and salicylic acid by investigating the impact of aspirin administration on nicotinic acid steady-state levels and total clearance in six healthy subjects. Nicotinic acid solutions were infused at constant rates (0.075-0.100 mg/kg/min) for 6 hours to establish steady-state concentrations. Two hours after the nicotinic acid infusion began, they orally administered 1 g aspirin. By analyzing nicotinic acid, nicotinuric acid, and salicylic acid in plasma samples, they observed an immediate marked decrease of nicotinuric acid levels and an increase in nicotinic acid concentrations after aspirin administration. The authors hypothesized that "salicylic acid causes a concentration-dependent decrease of total nicotinic acid clearance that results in the saturation (and effective elimination) of the nicotinuric acid conjugation pathway."

Whelan et al.[16] conducted the first randomized, double-blind, placebo-controlled trial to evaluate the efficacy of aspirin in reducing cutaneous reactions caused by niacin. They administered four different treatment regimens to 31 healthy subjects who had been randomized into four groups. They found that 325 mg of aspirin decreased intolerability to niacin significantly better than 80 mg aspirin. Aspirin reduced the incidence of warmth and flushing associated with niacin, but not the itching and tingling. Subsequently, in a randomized, double-blind, placebo-controlled, crossover study, Jungnickel et al.[17] compared the effects of pretreatment with two aspirin regimens and placebo on niacin-induced cutaneous reactions in 42 healthy adult subjects. Subjects received 325 mg aspirin, 650 mg aspirin, and placebo for 4 consecutive days and also ingested 500 mg immediate-release niacin 30 minutes after taking aspirin or placebo on the fourth day. They concluded that an aspirin regimen of 325 mg effectively suppressed niacin-induced cutaneous reactions, with no additional benefit derived from increasing the aspirin dose to 650 mg.[17]

Nutritional Therapeutics, Clinical Concerns, and Adaptations

The use of aspirin or other anti-inflammatory agents to reduce the discomfort of cutaneous reactions to niacin represents a viable option to offer patients during niacin therapy. A daily dose of 325 mg aspirin per day has proved effective and is generally assumed to be safe for most patients. Close supervision may be warranted for patients at risk for bleeding given the theoretical possibility of an additive interaction between these two agents. In general, time-release niacin should generally be avoided unless supervised by an experienced health care professional.

Anticonvulsant Medications, Including Phenobarbital, Phenytoin, and Valproic Acid

Evidence: Carbamazepine (Carbatrol, Tegretol), diazepam (Valium), divalproex semisodium, divalproex sodium (Depakote), primidone (Mysoline), sodium valproate (Depacon), valproate semisodium, valproic acid (Depakene, Depakene Syrup).

Extrapolated, based on similar properties: Clonazepam (Klonopin), clorazepate (Tranxene), ethosuximide (Zarontin), ethotoin (Peganone), felbamate (Felbatol), fosphenytoin (Cerebyx, Mesantoin), levetiracetam (Keppra), mephenytoin, mephobarbital (Mebaral), methsuximide (Celontin), phenobarbital (phenobarbitone; Luminol, Solfoton), phenytoin (diphenylhydantoin, Dilantin, Dilantin-125, Dilantin Infatabs, Dilantin Kapseals, Phenytek), tiagabine (Gabitril), topiramate (Topamax), trimethadione (Tridione), zonisamide (Zonegran). Similar properties but evidence lacking for extrapolation: Gabapentin (Neurontin), lamotrigine (Lamictal), oxcarbazepine (GP 47680, oxycarbazepine; Trileptal), pheneturide (ethylphenacemide).

Interaction Type and Significance

✗✗✗ Potentially Harmful or Serious Adverse Interaction—Avoid

⊕✗ Bimodal or Variable Interaction, with Professional Management

⊕ Potential or Theoretical Beneficial or Supportive Interaction, with Professional Management

Probability:	Evidence Base:
4. Plausible	○ Preliminary

Effect and Mechanism of Action

Concomitant use of niacinamide with antiepileptic drugs (AEDs) may decrease drug clearance of AEDs, specifically carbamazepine, diazepam, and sodium valproate, through inhibition of cytochrome P450 (CYP450) and thereby potentiate the anticonvulsant action of these drugs.[18,19] Nicotinamide (niacinamide) may also decrease the conversion of primidone to phenobarbital.[18]

Research

Bourgeois et al.[18] conducted related experiments examining the effect of nicotinamide on the conversion of primidone to phenobarbital in mice and in three epileptic patients. They observed that in mice "200 mg per kilogram of nicotinamide increased the half-life of primidone by 47.6%, and the conversion to phenobarbital and phenylethylmalonamide was decreased by 32.4% and 14.5%, respectively." Similarly, nicotinamide also decreased the conversion of primidone to phenobarbital in the human patients in a dose-dependent manner. They also reported increased carbamazepine levels in two patients coadministered nicotinamide. These researchers proposed that the observed nicotinamide-induced inhibition of primidone and carbamazepine metabolism in humans "probably occurs by inhibition of cytochrome P-450 by nicotinamide."

Subsequently, Kryzhanovskii and Shandra[19] studied the effects of nicotinamide (250 mg/kg), pyridoxal 5-phosphate (B₆; 10 mg/kg), and alpha-tocopherol (100 mg/kg) with diazepam, carbamazepine, sodium valproate, and their combinations on epileptic activity in acute experiments on mice with corazole-induced seizures. This nutrient formulation "potentiated anticonvulsive action" of the AEDs studied, specifically improving their effects on "convulsive intensity and lethality." The authors concluded that their findings provided "new evidence of the advisability of using vitamins in combination with synthetic anticonvulsive drugs."

Nutritional Therapeutics, Clinical Concerns, and Adaptations

The available research findings suggest that physicians prescribing anticonvulsant medications might consider the possible therapeutic benefit of coadministering vitamin B₃, specifically as niacinamide, along with other nutrients as a means of enhancing drug activity and potentially enabling use of these drugs at reduced dosage levels. The preliminary nature of the data reviewed indicates that further research through well-designed clinical trials is warranted to determine the efficacy, safety, and clinical management of concomitant nutrient support, including niacinamide, during AED therapy. Pending conclusive research-based evidence, close supervision and regular monitoring are prudent during coadministration of niacinamide with AED therapy to ensure that the vitamin does not significantly potentiate excessive drug activity and to adjust drug doses accordingly. When nicotinamide is started or stopped, AED drug levels should be determined, and adjusted as necessary.

Bile Acid Sequestrants

Evidence: Cholestyramine (Locholest, Prevalite, Questran), colestipol (Colestid).

Extrapolated, based on similar properties: Colesevelam (Welchol).

See also Gemfibrozil and Related Fibrates, as well as HMG-CoA Reductase Inhibitors (Statins).

Interaction Type and Significance

⊕⊕ Beneficial or Supportive Interaction, with Professional Management

⊕✗ Bimodal or Variable Interaction, with Professional Management

◇◇ Impaired Drug Absorption and Bioavailability, Precautions Appropriate

◇ Adverse Drug Effect on Nutritional Therapeutics, Strategic Concern

Probability:	Evidence Base:
2. Probable	◉ Emerging to ● Consensus

Effect and Mechanism of Action

Niacin and bile acid sequestrants reduce cholesterol levels by separate, well-established mechanisms that produce an additive effect. The action of cholesterol-lowering resins is largely derived from their interference with lipid absorption, as are their primary adverse effects on bioavailability of numerous nutrients. In particular, niacin and resin agents can bind in the digestive tract and mutually interfere with absorption and bioavailability when ingested close to each other. Furthermore, by an unknown mechanism, combined colestipol and niacin can reduce thyroxine-binding globulin (TBG) and total serum thyroxine (T$_4$) levels and increase triiodothyronine (T$_3$) uptake ratios.[20]

Research

A narrow but significant and consistent body of evidence spanning many years provides a solid base of research data supporting the coadministration of niacin and bile acid sequestrants. Starting in 1983, an evolving research team, including Blankenhorn, Nessim, Cashin-Hemphill, Azen, Hodis, and others, conducted extensive research and published numerous studies documenting the beneficial effects of combined colestipol-niacin therapy in the treatment of patients with hyperlipidemia, coronary atherosclerosis, femoral atherosclerosis, and coronary venous bypass grafts.[21-31] In a 1990 review of this body of work, Blankenhorn et al.[32] presented this overview:

> The evaluation of the results of Cholesterol Lowering Atherosclerosis Study has shown that some triglyceride-rich lipoproteins play an important role in the progression of atherosclerosis. The combined niacin-colestipol treatment resulted in a forty to fifty per cent decrease in the levels of cholesterol-rich lipoprotein B but had no effect on triglyceride-rich lipoproteins. Patients who had increased levels of [the] latter lipoproteins ... showed progression of atherosclerotic lesions [despite niacin-colestipol therapy]. On the other hand, in the Helsinki Heart Study, despite minimal reduction in the levels of LDL-cholesterol, patients with phenotypes IIB and IV had higher reduction rates in coronary end points than patients with phenotype IIA.

Furthermore, these researchers have extensively investigated, refined, and documented techniques for assessing atherosclerosis, evaluating efficacy and predicting outcomes of these and related antihyperlipidemic interventions, including innovative use of computer- and human-derived coronary angiographic endpoint measures.[23,32-34]

In a serial blood-lipid-lowering study, during routine thyroid function monitoring, these researchers unexpectedly observed that after 1 year of combined colestipol and niacin therapy, previously euthyroid patients demonstrated reduced total serum T$_4$ levels and increased T$_3$ uptake ratios, apparently as a result of reduced TBG levels.[20]

Nutritional Therapeutics, Clinical Concerns, and Adaptations

Bile acid sequestrants and niacin constitute two of the many conventional therapies used alone or in various combinations for treating hyperlipidemia, atherosclerosis, and interrelated conditions. The body of evidence strongly supports beneficial interaction on hyperlipidemia, atherosclerosis, and mortality from coronary heart disease from concomitant administration of niacin and cholesterol-lowering resins, particularly on coronary and femoral atherosclerosis, where continued regression can continue for several years. However, bile acid sequestrants and niacin may interfere with the absorption of each other if the two agents are ingested at the same time; therefore, separation of oral intake should be separated by 4 to 6 hours to avoid diminished bioavailability and obtain more effective therapeutic response.

Supervision and regular monitoring, not only of lipid levels, but more critically of liver enzymes, is essential given the known risks associated with niacin therapy. Monitoring of thyroid hormone levels is also judicious because the combined action of these two agents has been associated with adverse changes in total serum T$_4$ levels, T$_3$ uptake ratios, and TBG levels. Complementary thyroid support may be warranted.

Furthermore, bile acid sequestrants can reduce absorption and bioavailability of fat-soluble nutrients (e.g., vitamins A, D, E, and K), as well as coenzyme Q10 and omega-3 fats, which are essential to healthy cardiovascular function and reducing cardiovascular risk, particularly mortality from coronary heart disease. Enhanced nutrient intake, through foods and supplements, is recommended, with intake being separated from the resin agent by at least 2 hours before and 4 hours after the medication.

The use of niacin in a less toxic form, inositol hexaniacinate, may provide a prudent option within such an integrative lipid management strategy. However, further research with well-designed, adequately powered clinical trials will be necessary to confirm efficacy and safety and establish clinical guidelines. Pending conclusive evidence, such an approach may be preferable because no available evidence indicates diminished therapeutic activity or increased probability of adverse effects compared with the use of nicotinic acid.

Gemfibrozil and Related Fibrates

Evidence: Gemfibrozil (Apo-Gemfibrozil, Lopid, Novo-Gemfibrozil).
Extrapolated, based on similar properties: Bezafibrate (Bezalip), ciprofibrate (Modalim), clofibrate (Atromid-S), fenofibrate (Lofibra, Tricor, Triglide).
See also Bile Acid Sequestrants and HMG-CoA Reductase Inhibitors (Statins).

Interaction Type and Significance

⊕⊕ **Beneficial or Supportive Interaction, with Professional Management**
⊕✗ **Bimodal or Variable Interaction, with Professional Management**
✗ **Potential or Theoretical Adverse Interaction of Uncertain Severity**

Probability:	Evidence Base:
3. Possible or	○ Preliminary to
2. Probable	◉ Emerging

Effect and Mechanism of Action

Achieving and maintaining increased plasma concentrations of high-density lipoprotein cholesterol (HDL-C) produces a cardioprotective effect that is increasingly being recognized as complementary to and equally important as reducing low-density lipoprotein cholesterol (LDL-C) in reducing risk of heart attack and stroke. Central to the function and activity of HDL-C is its influence and impact on reverse cholesterol transport. Among its many beneficial functions, HDL also exerts anti-inflammatory effects, reduces oxidation of LDL, and promotes fibrinolysis. Niacin is currently the most effective agent for increasing low HDL-C levels. Fibrates represent the other main class of HDL-elevating drugs. Both agents can also shift small, dense LDL particles toward larger, more buoyant particles and lower elevated triglyceride levels, thereby reducing atherogenic tendencies.[35,36]

Gemfibrozil, fenofibrate, and other fibrates are well known for their triglyceride-lowering effects, but they also raise HDL-C levels by 10% to 15%. Fibrates are classified as peroxisome proliferator-activated receptor (PPAR) agonists, even though their mechanism of action is also complex and not fully understood. Whereas PPAR agonists are located throughout the body, fibrates are known particularly to stimulate hepatic PPAR-alpha and thereby increase apolipoprotein AI and AII synthesis, decrease triglyceride synthesis, and enhance catabolism of triglyceride-rich particles. Alone, and apparently more so together, fibrates and niacin can reduce the risk for the combined endpoint of myocardial infarction or death from coronary artery disease (CAD) in patients with CAD for whom low HDL cholesterol represents the primary lipid disturbance.

Research

Spencer et al.[37] conducted a retrospective review of 161 patients who were prescribed a combination of gemfibrozil (1200 mg/day) and niacin (1229 mg/day) for 6 to 12 months to determine the effect of the combination therapy on lipid profile. In conjunction with dietary instruction, coadministration of niacin and gemfibrozil produced marked and significant changes in lipid levels: total cholesterol and LDL decreased by 14%, HDL increased by 24%, total/HDL cholesterolratio decreased by 30%, and triglycerides decreased by 52%. This beneficial effect was most marked in patients with initial levels of HDL less than 40 mg/dL, triglycerides greater than 250 mg/dL, and LDL greater than 160 mg/dL. The authors reported no episodes of ALT elevation or symptomatic myositis.

In a placebo-controlled, angiographic regression trial involving subjects with normal or modestly elevated LDL-C and low levels of HDL-C, Andrews et al.[38] found that 30 months of treatment with gemfibrozil and (if necessary) niacin and/or cholestyramine raised HDL by 25% and lowered LDL to less than 110 mg/dL. However, despite these significant improvements in lipid profile, the treatment group exhibited no significant difference from the controls in flow-mediated dilation or nitroglycerin-induced dilation. Furthermore, subjects with a history of systemic hypertension demonstrated greatly impaired flow-mediated dilation that was not significantly improved with treatment.

In a randomized, open-label, crossover study, Zema[39] investigated the effects of nicotinic acid, gemfibrozil, and combination therapy on the lipid profile of 23 subjects with clinically well-defined atherosclerosis and isolated hypoalphalipoproteinemia (low HDL-C alone). In the 14 subjects "able to tolerate all forms of pharmacotherapy," HDL-C increased by 15% (34.5 to 39.7 mg/dL) with gemfibrozil (1200 mg/day); by 35% (to 46.5 mg/dL) with nicotinic acid (mean dose, 2250 mg/day); and by 45% (to 50.0 ± 7.5 mg/dL) with combination therapy of gemfibrozil and nicotinic acid. The authors reported statistically significant favorable alterations with LDL-C, LDL-C/HDL-C, non–HDL-C/HDL-C, apolipoprotein (apo) B and apo B/apo A-I. The author concluded that coadministration of gemfibrozil and nicotinic acid is both "feasible" and "effective" in raising HDL-C levels in "the majority of patients with clinical atherosclerotic disease and isolated hypoalphalipoproteinemia."[39]

Sakai et al.[40] found that niacin, but not gemfibrozil, selectively increases apo A-I, a cardioprotective subfraction of HDL, in patients with low HDL-C.

Whitney et al.[41] conducted a randomized, double-blind, placebo-controlled trial, involving 143 military retirees under 76 years of age with low HDL-C levels and angiographically evident coronary disease, to determine if increasing HDL-C levels would produce beneficial effects on progression of coronary heart disease and clinical events. They found that the group administered a combination of gemfibrozil, niacin and cholestyramine, along "with aggressive dietary and lifestyle intervention" involving regular exercise and low-fat diets, experienced a 20% decrease in total cholesterol level, 36% increase in HDL-C level, 26% decrease in LDL-C level,

and 50% reduction in triglyceride levels, compared with placebo. Focal coronary stenosis decreased by 0.8% in the treated group, but increased by 1.4% in the placebo group. A composite cardiovascular event endpoint was reached in 26% of patients in the placebo group and 13% of those in the treated group. Notably, the treated group reported a higher incidence of adverse effects, particularly flushing and GI intolerance, but these rarely led to withdrawal from the study. These findings are limited by the small size and use of a composite clinical outcome. Furthermore, it is unknown whether the observed improvements in angiographic findings resulted from reductions in LDL-C or increases in HDL-C, or both.[41]

Most fibrates elevate plasma levels of the atherogenic amino acid homocysteine (Hcy), a known cardiovascular risk factor, at least in part through an alteration of creatine-creatinine metabolism and changes in methyl transfer. For example, fenofibrate and bezafibrate lead to a 20% to 40% elevation of plasma Hcy levels. In contrast, gemfibrozil does not increase Hcy. Niacin use has also been associated with elevations in plasma Hcy levels. Concurrent administration of folic acid and vitamins B₁₂ and B₆ is often warranted to modulate plasma Hcy and prevent the fibrate and/or niacin from counteracting the desired cardiovascular protection.[42] The causal effects of Hcy are unconfirmed by single, large-scale, prospective clinical intervention trials, but the association between hyperhomocysteinemia and a range of pathophysiological processes is widely recognized, and a 2006 meta-analysis reached the conclusion that lowering Hcy levels reduces the risk of vascular events.[43]

Fibrates, particularly gemfibrozil, are known to interact with statins to increase the risk of myositis, myopathy, and rhabdomyolysis (as is niacin).[44,45] Whether such an adverse interaction is possible with concomitant use of fibrates and niacin has yet to be investigated. Further research through well-designed clinical trials is warranted to establish efficacy and safety.

Nutritional Therapeutics, Clinical Concerns, and Adaptations

Physicians treating individuals with dyslipidemia are advised to consider the combination of niacin and a fibrate agent in patients for whom the elevation of HDL-C constitutes a principal therapeutic goal. Along with periodic evaluation of lipid levels, assessment of liver function and plasma Hcy levels may also be appropriate given the adverse effects of both agents. Concomitant folic acid and vitamins B₁₂ and B₆ play an important role in a comprehensive strategy, especially when administering fenofibrate or bezafibrate. Repletion of SAMe, especially with betaine, may also moderate the hepatotoxic effects of these agents on methionine metabolism, methyl group availability, and Hcy levels. Coadministration of coenzyme Q10 may also be appropriate in enhancing cardiovascular health and reducing risk.

HMG-CoA Reductase Inhibitors (Statins)

Evidence: Atorvastatin (Lipitor), fluvastatin (Lescol, Lescol XL), lovastatin (Altocor, Altoprev, Mevacor); combination drug: lovastatin and niacin (Advicor); pravastatin (Pravachol), simvastatin (Zocor); combination drug: simvastatin and extended-release nicotinic acid (Niaspan).

Extrapolated, based on similar properties: Rosuvastatin (Crestor).

See also Insulin, Biguanides, Meglitinide Analogs, and Related Oral Hypoglycemic Agents.

See also Antioxidants in Nutrient-Nutrient Interactions.

Interaction Type and Significance

⊕⊕ **Beneficial or Supportive Interaction, with Professional Management**

⊕✗ **Bimodal or Variable Interaction, with Professional Management**

✗✗ **Minimal to Mild Adverse Interaction—Vigilance Necessary**

Probability:

2. Probable to
1. Certain

Evidence Base:

● **Consensus** but also
◉ **Emerging**

Effect and Mechanism of Action

Concomitant administration of niacin and HMG-CoA reductase inhibitors (statins) may produce additive effects that enhance the reduction of serum cholesterol levels but also increase the risk of adverse effects. As indicated by their collective name, statins limit synthesis of LDL-C by interfering with the normal cholesterol-synthesizing activity of the enzyme 3-hydroxy-3-methylglutaryl–coenzyme A (HMG-CoA) reductase in the liver. Niacin can elevate levels of HDL-C by 15% to 30% while also preferentially increasing HDL2 and LpA-I particles and slightly to moderately reducing LDL-C. Niacin's mechanisms of action are broad and complex and include selectively increasing the antiatherogenic HDL subfraction, lipoprotein (Lp) A-I (without apolipoprotein A-II), while inhibiting triglyceride synthesis, lipolysis in adipose tissue, and apo A-I catabolism. Collectively, these objectives are central to reducing hypercholesterolemia, limiting atherogenic processes and supporting cardiovascular health.[5,46-50]

All statin drugs are metabolized by the CYP450 isoform 3A4. Consequently, many drugs and other substances that share this metabolic pathway can elevate plasma levels of a statin and thereby increase the risk of myopathy and other adverse effects.

Statin drugs are associated with adverse symptoms that are typically considered insignificant but potentially severe, including elevated liver enzymes (SGOT/AST and SGPT/ALT), myositis, myopathy, and rhabdomyolysis, as well as impairment of coenzyme Q10 synthesis.[51-53] For example, HMG-CoA reductase inhibitors occasionally cause myopathy, which is manifested as muscle pain and weakness and accompanied by grossly elevated creatine kinase (>10 times ULN). Rhabdomyolysis is a relatively uncommon condition in which muscle cells are broken down, releasing myoglobin, muscle enzymes, and electrolytes into the blood, sometimes resulting in kidney failure. The risk of statin-induced myopathy and other adverse effects appears to be increased by high levels of HMG-CoA reductase inhibitory activity in plasma. The severity and probability of such reactions vary considerably among individuals and may be based on genetic factors influencing hepatic function and statin metabolism, such as CYP3A genotype.[54] The reported incidence of elevated hepatic transaminases and myopathy with lovastatin use over 4 years is 1.3% and 0.1% of cases, respectively; however, safety at 5 years appears predominant, but long-term data (≥20 years) on adverse effects is still not available.[53,55-57]

Niacin is also associated with adverse effects on the liver, including elevating hepatic transaminases, depleting methyl donors and increasing homocysteine levels. Niacin can lower plasma levels of vitamin B6 and interfere with the metabolism of methionine, leading to hyperhomocysteinemia and hypocysteinemia with attendant increase of cardiovascular risks.[58-60] Specifically, elevated levels of niacin (e.g., >1 g/day) can deplete SAMe because niacin is excreted as methylated pyridones, the formation of which uses SAMe as the methyl donor. SAMe is formed by the adenylation of methionine via S-adenosylmethionine synthase and acts as the methyl donor in virtually all known biological methylations. Thus, depletion of SAMe impairs detoxification processes and may account for many of niacin's adverse effects. The concomitant use of niacin and a statin drug increases the risk of many adverse effects, including development of toxicity symptoms, such as myopathy and rhabdomyolysis, in patients previously stable when treated with a single agent.

Research

The therapeutic benefits of coadministering niacin with statin agents, generally, have been well documented, as have the potential risks. The body of scientific literature demonstrating this interaction and its clinical implications is sufficiently well known to establish it as a standard therapy within the armamentarium of conventional medical practice. Consequently, rather than provide an exhaustive review of pertinent literature, this section focuses on landmark research as well as studies that illustrate issues of particular clinical significance, suggest parameters of therapeutic application, or raise questions of safety and patient variability. Furthermore, although the research beginning with Altschul et al. and continuing through the Coronary Drug Project on the efficacy of niacin therapy in the treatment of hyperlipidemia, especially with low HDL-C, deserves mention, a review and analysis of the research on niacin monotherapy is beyond the scope of this section. However, broadly viewed, the available evidence from clinical trials more consistently supports the use of niacin in conjunction with statins, resins, or other antihyperlipidemic agents, rather than as niacin monotherapy, for decreasing cholesterol levels and slowing the progression of atherosclerotic plaque formation in individuals being treated for atherosclerosis. Lastly, the limited duration of many studies restricts use of the resultant data in conclusively assessing adverse effects associated with usage over years or decades on a diverse patient population.

Efficacy. Malloy et al.[61] conducted an open sequential study involving 22 patients with clinical characteristics of familial hypercholesterolemia to compare serum lipoprotein responses to three interventions: diet alone, colestipol and niacin with diet, and colestipol, niacin, and lovastatin with diet. The respective characteristics of the treatment components were diet: less than 200 mg/day of cholesterol and less than 8% of total calories from saturated fat; colestipol: 30 g/day; lovastatin: 40 to 60 mg/day; and niacin: 1.5 to 7.5 g/day. These researchers reported significantly improved responses, as measured by lower mean total serum cholesterol and LDL-C levels and elevated HDL-C levels, with the multiple intervention than with any binary combination. They concluded that "colestipol, lovastatin, and niacin are mutually complementary in treating hypercholesterolemia" and noted that "this regimen produces reductions in serum cholesterol levels similar to those associated with regression of atheromatous plaques in animal studies." Adverse effects were not reported among the study participants.[61]

In 1994, Davignon et al.[62] conducted a study comparing the effects of placebo, nicotinic acid extended-release capsules (0.5-1.0 g twice daily), pravastatin (40 mg at bedtime), or the combination for 8 weeks in 158 patients with type IIa or IIb primary hypercholesterolemia. They observed greater declines in LDL-C levels and increases in HDL-C levels, relative to baseline, with the niacin and pravastatin combination than

Nutrient-Drug Interactions and Drug-Induced Nutrient Depletions

with either agent alone; all three treatments were significantly more effective than placebo.

Jacobson et al.[63] conducted a randomized, double-blind trial involving 74 hypercholesterolemic patients to investigate gender differences in efficacy of fluvastatin and niacin in the treatment of hypercholesterolemia. After an initial 6 weeks in which subjects received fluvastatin or placebo, open-label niacin, to a maximum of 3 g daily, was added to each treatment for the next 9 weeks. In the initial phase of 3 to 6 weeks of treatment, the reduction in LDL-C was significantly greater with fluvastatin (20.8%) compared with placebo. At the end of 12 to 15 weeks, the addition of niacin potentiated the response to 43.7% in those administered the fluvastatin and niacin combination and to 26.5% in those receiving placebo plus niacin. Notably, these researchers reported significant gender differences in the LDL-C response to the fluvastatin and niacin combination. Women demonstrated LDL-C reductions of 54.6%, whereas men exhibited LDL-C reductions of 38.2%. Female subjects also tended to experience greater LDL-C reductions with the placebo plus niacin combination than did male subjects. At the end of 12 to 15 weeks, HDL-C increased by 33.1%, whereas triglyceride levels declined by 32.3%.[63] These variable responses based on gender deserve further research, as do other factors that shape interindividual variability in clinical response, adverse effects, lifestyle influences, compliance, and other relevant characteristics.

In a randomized trial involving 65 patients with low HDL levels and hypertriglyceridemia, O'Keefe et al.[64] (1995) compared pravastatin in combination with niacin, magnesium, and placebo. They found that, after 18 weeks, subjects in the pravastatin plus niacin group had a −41% change in the total cholesterol/HDL-C ratio, whereas those in the pravastatin plus magnesium and pravastatin plus placebo arms demonstrated −13% and −16% changes, respectively. Furthermore, the HDL2 and HDL3 subfractions, as well as the apolipoprotein A-I levels, were increased significantly and postprandial lipemia diminished significantly (−32% change in the remnant particle triglyceride concentration and decreased very-low-density lipoprotein (VLDL) remnant levels) only in the pravastatin/niacin arm. Additionally, the levels of small dense LDL3 cholesterol were decreased to a greater extent in the pravastatin plus niacin group than in the other groups. The authors concluded that the pravastatin and niacin combination produced significant and more numerous benefits than those produced by a pravastatin-magnesium combination (or placebo), and that such effects were clinically important in "patients with clustered risk factors."[64]

In a randomized, open-label trial, Jokubaitis[65] administered fluvastatin (20 mg/day) or placebo for six weeks and noted that fluvastatin produced a 20.8% reduction in LDL-C levels from baseline. Then, starting at six weeks, open-label niacin was administered to all patients and titrated to a final dose of 3 g/day. Subjects treated with both niacin and fluvastatin exhibited a 43.7% reduction in LDL-C levels at the week 15 endpoint, in contrast to a 26.5% reduction seen with niacin monotherapy. The author concluded by recommending that "use of combination therapies may result in optimal management of patients with moderately severe hypercholesterolaemia and mixed dyslipidaemic profiles."

In a 14-week, prospective, open-label trial involving 16 diabetic patients with LDL-C concentrations of at least 150 mg/dL after dietary therapy, Gardner et al.[66] found that coadministration of niacin (titrated to a maximum of 500 mg three times daily) and "low-dose" pravastatin (20 mg/day) produced favorable results on lipid profiles, including

significant lowering of LDL cholesterol, compared with pravastatin monotherapy. Notably, only five of these diabetic subjects required minor alterations (three increased, two decreased) in their hypoglycemic regimens to maintain glycemic control; most were treated without compromising glycemic control.

Guyton et al.[67] conducted a multicenter, open-label study involving 269 hypercholesterolemic adult subjects to determine the long-term safety and efficacy of an extended-release once-a-night niacin preparation, Niaspan, in the treatment of hypercholesterolemia. After 48 weeks of treatment, the extended-release niacin alone (median dose, 2000 mg) reduced LDL cholesterol (18%), apolipoprotein (apo) B (15%), total cholesterol (11%), triglycerides (24%), and lipoprotein Lp(a) (36%), and increased HDL-C (29%). However, the extended-release niacin plus a statin lowered LDL-C (32%), apo B (26%), total cholesterol (23%), triglycerides (30%), and lipoprotein Lp(a) (19%), and increased HDL cholesterol (26%). Notably, 2.6% of patients exhibited reversible elevations of aspartate aminotransferase or alanine aminotransferase more than twice the normal range. A pair of trials conducted by Goldberg and associates arrived at similar conclusions.[68,69]

McKenney et al.[70] conducted a multicenter, randomized, open-label, parallel-design study to assess the effect of niacin and atorvastatin on lipoprotein subclasses in patients with atherogenic dyslipidemia. At baseline, all subjects demonstrated total cholesterol greater than 200 mg/dL, triglycerides between 200 and 800 mg/dL, and apo B greater than 110 mg/dL, as measured by nuclear magnetic resonance spectroscopy. After a low-fat diet stabilization period, subjects were randomly assigned to atorvastatin (10 mg) or immediate-release niacin (3000 mg) daily for 12 weeks. The authors reported that both atorvastatin and niacin significantly reduced the concentrations of VLDL particles (−31% and −29%, respectively) and small LDL particles (−44% and −35%). Niacin increased the concentration of large LDL (+75%), "shifted the LDL subclass distribution toward the larger particles, more effectively converted patients from LDL phenotype B to phenotype A, and increased levels of the larger and perhaps more cardioprotective high-density lipoprotein particles." In contrast, atorvastatin reduced the number of LDL particles more than niacin (31% vs. 14%), "preferentially lowered the concentration of small LDL particles without increasing levels of large LDL, and more effectively, reduced LDL particle numbers." Thus, these two agents exhibited their strengths and respective contributions to potential synergistic use with atorvastatin showing a preferred LDL effect and niacin a preferred HDL effect.[70]

In a three-year, randomized, controlled, double-blind trial involving 160 patients with documented coronary heart disease (CHD), low HDL-C levels, and normal LDL-C levels, Brown, Zhao, et al.[71] found that a combination of simvastatin and niacin increased HDL2 levels, inhibited the progression of coronary artery stenosis, and decreased the frequency of occurrence of a first cardiovascular event, such as myocardial infarction, stroke, death, or revascularization. Other findings from this study, indicating that protective increase in HDL2 with simvastatin plus niacin was attenuated by concurrent therapy with antioxidants, were widely interpreted as indicating a negative interaction between antioxidants and statins.[72] However, a closer analysis more likely shows a blunting effect of the antioxidants on the rise of HDL cholesterol, more associated with niacin, rather than a direct effect on the statin therapy.

In a 52-week, multicenter, open-label study involving a total of 814 men and women (mean age, 59 years) with dyslipidemia, Kashyap et al.[73] administered niacin-lovastatin combination in four escalating doses: 500 mg niacin plus 10 mg lovastatin for the first month, 1000 mg niacin plus 20 mg lovastatin for the second, 1500 mg niacin plus 30 mg lovastatin for the third, and 2000 mg niacin plus 40 mg lovastatin for the fourth month through week 52. They observed dose-dependent effects for all major lipid parameters. At week 16, mean LDL-C and triglycerides were reduced by 47% and 41%, respectively, and LDL/HDL cholesterol and total/HDL cholesterol ratios were also decreased by 58% and 48%, respectively; these effects persisted through week 52. Mean HDL cholesterol was increased by 30% by the sixteenth week but slowed to attain an increase to 41% at the end of 1 year. Lipoprotein Lp(a) and C-reactive protein also decreased in a dose-related manner by 25% and 24%, respectively, at 2000 mg niacin plus 40 mg lovastatin.[73] In a randomized, double-blind trial involving 39 patients undergoing stable statin therapy, published that same month (March 2002), Wink et al.[74] demonstrated that coadministration of very-low-dose niacin (50 mg orally twice daily) for 3 months increased the mean HDL-C by 2.1 mg/dL, compared with statin therapy and placebo, while avoiding the adverse effects (and dropout rates) associated with niacin therapy at higher dosage levels.

Taylor et al.[75] have conducted various phases of the Arterial Biology for the Investigation of the Treatment Effects of Reducing Cholesterol (ARBITER) study over an extended period. In the ARBITER 2 study, these researchers found that statins alone are not enough to halt the progression of atherosclerosis, as measured by carotid intima media thickness (CIMT), even when the LDL-C target is achieved. In that study, investigators demonstrated that the combination extended-release nicotinic acid 1000 mg daily (Niaspan) and a statin (usually simvastatin 40 mg daily) halted the progression of atherosclerosis while the atherosclerotic process continued in patients treated with statin alone.[76] At the Scientific Sessions of the American Heart Association (2005), Taylor et al.[77] presented findings from the ARBITER 3 study, involving 148 patients, demonstrating that a further 12 months of treatment with prolonged-release nicotinic acid 1000 mg daily (Niaspan) and a statin (usually simvastatin 40 mg daily) achieved regression of atherosclerosis, including among patients with diabetes mellitus or the metabolic syndrome. This significant reduction in CIMT was associated with a 23.7% increase in HDL-C, leading to a reduction of approximately 5% in atherosclerotic plaque in the carotid arteries of patients.

In related research, a retrospective analysis of 44,351 patients with a mean follow-up of 30 ± 12 months found that raising HDL-C, in addition to lowering LDL-C and triglycerides, significantly improves outcomes in a wide spectrum of patients. After categorizing patients by primary or secondary prevention, gender, and the presence or absence of diabetes mellitus, Stanek and associates observed that achieving optimal lipid values for HDL-C in addition to LDL-C and triglycerides resulted in a significant 30% reduction in cardiovascular event risk, overall and across all subgroups.[78] Research comparing a Niaspan-simvastatin combination versus simvastatin alone is continuing through the Atherothrombosis Intervention in Metabolic Syndrome with Low HDL-C/High Triglyceride and Impact on Global Health Outcomes (AIM-HIGH) studies.

Safety. In a rat model, Basu and Mann[58] found that niacin administration can lower plasma levels of vitamin B₆ and interfere with the metabolism of methionine, leading to hyperhomocysteinemia and hypocysteinemia.

Coadministration of B₆ normalized Hcy levels without compromising niacin's therapeutic effects on dyslipidemia.

Subsequent to the reports of myotoxicity in individuals treated with lovastatin and niacin concomitantly, other researchers investigated the potential for increased adverse effects with other statin agents.[79,80] Davignon et al.[62] reported no significant differences regarding adverse events or laboratory parameters in both placebo and pravastatin groups at 8 and 88 weeks. However, compared with placebo, treatment with nicotinic acid resulted in significant increases in aspartate and alanine transaminase (ALT). Thus the adverse effects associated with niacin alone or niacin-pravastatin together were both greater than with niacin alone. Jokubaitis[65] studied the coadministration of niacin with fluvastatin to examine the possibility of similar adverse effect from this alternative combination. He reported that fluvastatin (20 mg/day) with niacin (titrated to final dosage of 3 g/day) was "well tolerated, with no reports of myopathy or of significant elevations in creatine kinase or liver transaminase levels," over 6 weeks. Guyton et al.[67] found that adverse hepatic effects from the combination of a statin and an extended-release, once-a-night niacin preparation (0.5-3.0 g/day) were "minor and occurred at rates similar to those reported for statin therapy." In the study previously mentioned, Kashyap et al.[73] noted that treatment with escalating doses of a niacin-lovastatin combination was "generally well tolerated" and that "drug-induced myopathy did not occur in any patient." Flushing was the most common adverse event, causing 10% of subjects to withdraw, while the "incidence of elevated liver enzymes to >3 times the upper limit of normal was 0.5%." Secondary compendiums consistently state that increased adverse effects have not been reported with the combination of niacin and pravastatin.

In a retrospective case-control study, Wilke et al.[54] found that CYP3A genotype was associated with increased severity of atorvastatin-induced muscle damage, but not an increased risk for development of such adverse effects, as indicated by elevated serum creatine kinase (CK) levels. Thus, individuals who were homozygous for CYP3A5*3 demonstrated greater serum CK levels than patients heterozygous for CYP3A5*3, when concomitant lipid-lowering agents (gemfibrozil with or without niacin) were sequentially removed from the analysis. Consequently, individuals who have a genetic problem with metabolizing statins might have a larger depletion of coenzyme Q10 (due to a higher level of the statin drug) and thus a greater incidence of adverse effects; conversely, individuals who tolerate statins better may be metabolizing them more rapidly and thus depleting coenzyme Q10 to lesser degree.[81]

Reports

Reaven and Witztum[79] reported the case of a patient on lovastatin therapy who developed rhabdomyolysis subsequent to the introduction of nicotinic acid, 2.5 g daily, and briefly discussed a case of myositis in another patient concurrently taking lovastatin and nicotinic acid. Even though such events are consistent with known pharmacological effects of both agents, Stockley[82] commented on these data: "These adverse reports are therefore isolated and it is by no means certain that the addition of nicotinic acid was responsible for what happened."

Nutritional Therapeutics, Clinical Concerns, and Adaptations

The coordinated administration of niacin with statin drugs represents a constructive application of drug-nutrient interactions that has been fully integrated into conventional medical practice. Niacin therapy has generally been found to be most effective in patients with the highest total cholesterol levels and is particularly indicated in patients with low HDL-C levels. However, the National Cholesterol Education Program (NCEP) guidelines suggest combination niacin/statin therapy only when diet and single-drug therapy are not effective. The importance of this broad approach cannot be emphasized enough in educating patients to adopt a proactive and comprehensive approach to enhancing cardiovascular health rather than just reducing risk by focusing on any single indicator of pathophysiological processes. Thus, pharmacotherapy, even when complemented by coordinated use of niacin and synergistic nutrients within an integrative strategy, can never take the place of patient initiative in adopting healthy dietary habits, maintaining a consistent exercise regimen, minimizing stress, and cultivating a supportive social network.

The clinical efficacy, potential for beneficial interaction, and risk of adverse reactions from coadministration of niacin vary among the statin agents. A wide range of substances and conditions alter the pharmacokinetics of and clinical response to statin therapy, and the various HMG-CoA reductase inhibitors have different potentials for interactions. Hepatic dysfunction may influence the pharmacokinetics of pravastatin; all HMG-CoA reductase inhibitors are contraindicated in patients with liver disease or unexplained elevations in serum transaminases. The pharmacokinetics of pravastatin, simvastatin, and fluvastatin are only minimally altered by renal dysfunction, but modification of lovastatin dosage may be necessary in patients with severe renal insufficiency; nevertheless, caution is warranted in all such patients. This interindividual variability and the broad range of factors influencing cardiovascular health and risk highlight the importance of individualized and flexible prescribing practices characterized by close monitoring and attention to signs of clinical response to the medication program.

Both statins and niacin possess problematic safety profiles, and their concomitant use can increase the risk of adverse effects just as it offers increased potency for therapeutic benefit. Close supervision and regular monitoring of hepatic transaminases (AST, ALT) and CK (for myositis) are appropriate, in addition to standard lipid profiles. Patients need to be educated about potential adverse effects of antihyperlipidemic pharmacotherapy and advised to observe for unexplained muscle pain, tenderness, weakness, cramps, or stiffness and immediately report any such untoward developments. Particular caution is warranted if the patient is being treated with another agent that can affect CYP3A4 metabolism.

A range of nutritional therapies can play important roles within an integrative strategy of comprehensive medical care for individuals with hyperlipidemia. The use of niacin in a less toxic form (inositol hexaniacinate) may provide a prudent option within such an integrative lipid management strategy. However, further research with well-designed, adequately powered clinical trials will be necessary to confirm efficacy and safety and establish clinical guidelines. Pending such conclusive evidence, such an approach may be preferable because no available evidence indicates diminished therapeutic activity or increased probability of adverse effects compared with the use of nicotinic acid. Additionally, coadministration of coenzyme Q10 (100 mg three times daily) and methyl donors may mitigate some adverse effects of statins and niacin, respectively, while supporting the strategic goals of reducing cardiovascular risk and enhancing cardiovascular, specifically myocardial, function. In particular, repletion of SAMe, especially with

vitamin B₆ and betaine, may also moderate the hepatotoxic effects of these agents on methionine metabolism, methyl group availability, and Hcy levels. As discussed later, supplemental chromium can enhance the activity of niacin in lipid management (thereby allowing lower niacin dosage levels) as well as directly decrease triglycerides and total cholesterol and increase HDL-C. More broadly, folic acid and vitamin B₁₂ can complement this nutrient support by helping to moderate tendencies to hyperhomocysteinemia and reducing the risk of vascular events.

Insulin, Biguanides, Meglitinide Analog Oral Hypoglycemics

Insulin: Animal-source insulin (Iletin); human analog insulin (Humalog); human insulin (Humulin, Novolin, NovoRapid, Oralin).

Biguanides: Buformin (Andromaco Gliporal, Buformina), metformin (Dianben, Glucophage, Glucophage XR), phenformin (Debeone, Fenformin).

Sulfonylureas: Acetohexamide (Dymelor), chlorpropamide (Diabinese), glimepiride (Amaryl), glyburide (glibenclamide; Diabeta, Glynase Prestab, Glynase, Micronase, Pres Tab), glipizide (Glucotrol; Glucotrol XL), tolazamide (Tolinase), tolbutamide (Orinase; Tol-Tab).

Combination drugs: Glipizide and metformin (Metaglip), glyburide and metformin (Glucovance).

Extrapolated, based on similar properties:

Alpha-glucosidase inhibitors: Acarbose (Glucobay, Precose).

Meglitinide analogs: Nateglinide (Starlix), repaglinide (Prandin).

Thiazolidinediones (Glitazones): Pioglitazone (Actos), rosiglitazone (Avandia).

See also Chromium monograph.

Interaction Type and Significance

⊕⊕ **Beneficial or Supportive Interaction, with Professional Management**

✗⊕ **Bimodal or Variable Interaction, with Professional Management**

✗ **Potential or Theoretical Adverse Interaction of Uncertain Severity**

Probability: Evidence Base:
4. Plausible or   ▽ **Mixed** and/or
  3. Possible   ◉ **Emerging**

Effect and Mechanism of Action

The activity and mechanisms (as well as use and interactions) of niacin and niacinamide are distinct in regard to the effects of vitamin B₃ on glycemic control.

Agents in the meglitinide class of antidiabetic drugs work by stimulating the beta cells to produce and release insulin in the presence of glucose postprandially.

Acute use of nicotinic acid (niacin) inhibits lipolysis in adipose tissue and thus suppresses circulating nonesterfied fatty acid (NEFA) levels. However, NEFA levels increase above baseline once the niacin effect abates.[83] With this increased NEFA availability, NEFA oxidation occurs at the expense of glucose oxidation, and according to the Randle cycle hypothesis, the resultant reduction in glucose uptake by skeletal muscle is associated with an increase in blood glucose levels.[84] Niacin administration, in large doses, could interfere with the therapeutic activity of medications designed to lower blood glucose levels. Thus, theoretically, hyperglycemia may occur with concomitant intake of niacin and sulfonylureas. However, niacin has also been identified as a constituent of the glucose tolerance factor in yeast that enhances insulin response.

Chronic administration of nicotinic acid can disrupt glycemic control in diabetic patients being treated with insulin or hypoglycemic medications.

Niacinamide may enhance insulin secretion and increase insulin sensitivity, at least in part by protecting and preserving pancreatic beta–islet cell function. The activation of poly-ADP-ribose polymerase (PARP), as an adaptive response to minimize oxidative damage to DNA, appears to deplete cellular NAD+ and cause beta–islet cell death.[85] Therefore, repletion of cellular NAD+ levels through administration of niacinamide, would prevent cell death and preserve beta–islet cell function and sustain insulin response and may be beneficial in the prevention and delay of type 1 diabetes mellitus. Niacinamide has been shown to have no effect on insulin secretion or glucose kinetics and is generally considered unlikely that concomitant niacinamide, at typical dosages, would interfere with the activity of insulin or oral hypoglycemic medications.

Research

Niacinamide (Nicotinamide). Treatment with high-dose niacinamide, at doses ranging from 200 mg to 3 g per day, appears to exert protective effects on beta-cell function in animals and humans, particularly patients with newly diagnosed diabetes mellitus (type 1) and children at high risk.[86-91] Subsequently, a recent meta-analysis of 10 randomized, controlled trials involving 158 niacinamide-treated and 129 control patients with recent-onset type 1 diabetes revealed significantly better preservation of basal C-peptide secretion (a stable indicator of insulin secretion) in the niacinamide-receiving cohort after 1 year. Subanalysis of the five placebo-controlled trials yielded the same result.

Elliott and Chase[92] conducted a controlled but nonrandomized and unblinded trial involving 22 high-risk children (<16 years of age) to investigate the efficacy of oral nicotinamide in preventing the onset of diabetes mellitus. They concluded that "all of eight untreated control subjects have developed diabetes, whereas only one of fourteen treated children has diabetes to date." Likewise, in an experiment involving nine adult volunteers, Paul et al.[93] reported that niacinamide, at a dose of 1.2 g/m² for 7 days, caused no significant differences from baseline in insulin sensitivity, glucose disappearance rate, or acute insulin response to glucose.

Conversely, the findings from one large, well-designed and adequately powered trial and a small case series strongly suggest the limitations of niacinamide in effectively preventing type 1 diabetes.[94,95]

Greenbaum et al.[95a] investigated the effects of short-term administration of nicotinamide on glucose metabolism in subjects at high risk of developing insulin-dependent diabetes mellitus (IDDM), specifically to determine if such intake might cause insulin resistance in such subjects. They observed a 23.6% decrease in insulin sensitivity after administering nicotinamide (2 g/day) to eight islet cell antibody–positive (ICA+) relatives of IDDM patients for 2 weeks.

Thus, overall, niacinamide monotherapy, outside the context of dietary changes and complementary pharmacological support (pharmaceutical, nutritional, or botanical) is unlikely to forestall the onset of type 1 diabetes in most individuals, especially in those with strong genetic susceptibility, or to provide effective treatment for such patients once the disease process has progressed. However, the research directed toward investigating the interactions between niacinamide and antidiabetic therapies suggests that the pharmacological activity of this nutrient can be beneficial for some patients given appropriate dosage levels and proper monitoring and supervision.

Bingley et al.[96] performed intravenous tolerance tests in 10 healthy adult subjects before and after 14 days of treatment with nicotinamide (25 mg/kg/day) and concluded that "nicotinamide does not affect insulin secretion and glucose kinetics in normal subjects."

Polo et al.[97] conducted a 6-month, single-blind study involving 18 patients with "non-insulin-dependent (type 2) diabetes mellitus of normal body weight without signs of autoimmunity, i.e., negative for islet cell antibodies, with secondary failure of sulphonylureas, defined as persistent hyperglycaemia in spite of maximal doses of sulphonylureas." The subjects were randomly assigned to one of three treatments: (1) insulin plus nicotinamide (0.5 g three times daily), (2) insulin plus placebo (three times daily), or (3) current sulphonylureas plus nicotinamide (0.5 g three times daily). At baseline and after 6 months, all subjects were evaluated for C-peptide release under basal conditions and 6 minutes after intravenous glucagon, for glycosylated hemoglobin (HbA₁c), and for fasting and mean daily blood glucose levels. Compared with insulin plus placebo group, C-peptide release increased in both groups receiving nicotinamide, and HbA₁c, fasting, and mean daily blood glucose levels improved in the three groups to the same extent. Applying multiple-regression analysis, they determined that "nicotinamide administration was the only significant factor for the improvement of C-peptide release." The authors concluded that "nicotinamide improves C-peptide release in type 2 diabetic patients with secondary failure of sulphonylureas, leading to a metabolic control similar to patients treated with insulin."[97]

Niacin (Nicotinic Acid). Many secondary sources, reviews, and derivative reference works have stated, with varying degrees of certainty, that niacin administration could impair insulin activity, significantly elevate blood glucose concentrations, and cause glucose intolerance and insulin resistance, and that such effects could produce adverse effects on glycemic control in patients receiving insulin or oral hypoglycemic agents. Many studies have produced findings that support, or have been interpreted as supporting, such a conclusion, particularly in the context of dyslipidemia.[68,69,98-114] Consequently, standard treatment guidelines for years recommended against the use of niacin in patients with diabetes. Over time these preliminary cautionary notes have failed to achieve confirmation through well-designed clinical trials, and countervailing evidence has emerged. However, even if confirmed, this potentially beneficial effect of niacin intake would more accurately be characterized as a convergence of patient communication, case management, and drug titration issues rather simply than as an adverse effect or interaction. At this time, the trend in the evidence supports the position that coadministration of niacin, at low to moderate doses and with proper medical supervision, does not interfere with the therapeutic efficacy of oral hypoglycemic therapy and may provide strategic benefit in individuals with dyslipidemia, especially proportionately low HDL-C concentrations.

Elam et al.[114a] conducted a prospective, randomized, placebo-controlled clinical trial involving 468 participants, including 125 with diabetes, who had diagnosed peripheral arterial disease, to investigate the efficacy and safety of relatively high, lipid-modifying dosages of niacin in diabetic patients. After an active run-in period, subjects were randomly assigned to receive immediate-release niacin (crystalline nicotinic acid), 3000 mg/day (or maximum tolerated dosage), or placebo for up to 60 weeks (including 48-week double-blind phase). Glucose levels were modestly increased by niacin, 8.7 and 6.3mg/dL, in participants with and without diabetes,respectively. Furthermore, niacin use significantly increased HDL-C by 29% and 29%, decreased triglycerides by 23% and 28%, and reduced LDL-C by 8% and 9%, respectively, in subjects with and without diabetes. There were "no significant differences in niacin discontinuation, niacin dosage, or hypoglycemic therapy in participants with diabetes assigned to niacin vs placebo." The authors concluded that their "study suggests that lipid-modifying dosages of niacin can be safely used in patients with diabetes and that niacin therapy may be considered as an alternative to statin drugs or fibrates for patients with diabetes in whom these agents are not tolerated or fail to sufficiently correct hypertriglyceridemia or low HDL-C levels."[114a]

In a 16-week, double-blind, placebo-controlled trial, Grundy et al.[115] evaluated the efficacy and safety of 1000-mg or 1500-mg, once-daily extended-release (ER) niacin in 148 patients with diabetic dyslipidemia. Sixty-nine patients (47%) were also receiving concomitant therapy with statins. In addition to dose-dependent increases in HDL-C levels for both niacin doses (vs. placebo) and reductions in triglyceride levels for the 1500-mg ER niacin (vs. placebo), baseline and week 16 values for glycosylated hemoglobin levels were 7.13% and 7.11%, respectively, in the placebo group; 7.28% and 7.35%, respectively, in the 1000-mg ER niacin group (vs. placebo); and 7.2% and 7.5%, respectively, in the 1500-mg ER niacin group. Four subjects discontinued participation because of inadequate glucose control, whereas four others (including one given placebo) quit because of flushing. No significant adverse effects were observed, including myopathy or hepatoxic effects. Thus, low doses of ER niacin (1000 or 1500 mg/day) provide "a treatment option for dyslipidemia in patients with type 2 diabetes" that is unlikely to produce significant adverse effects or disrupt glycemic control in most patients.[115]

Nutritional Therapeutics, Clinical Concerns, and Adaptations

Physicians prescribing oral hypoglycemic agents, especially an initial course of treatment or change in medication dosage, are advised to ask the patient about vitamin B₃ intake, in all forms, including within multivitamin formulations. Niacinamide may enhance insulin secretion and increase insulin sensitivity, whereas niacin may alter the action of insulin and levels of blood glucose in some individuals.

Whether prescribed or self-administered, the potential effect of either nutrient must be factored into dosing and monitoring schedules. Coadministration of niacin or niacinamide in patients on insulin therapy may warrant reduced insulin dose in those with type 1 diabetes or reduced oral hypoglycemic dose in those with type 2 diabetes, respectively. In particular, dosage may need to be adjusted when high-dose niacin (nicotinic acid) appears to antagonize the medication's antidiabetic activity. Similar cautions may be appropriate in patients with hypoglycemia or metabolic syndrome.

The concomitant administration of niacin and such medications may provide a significant beneficial synergistic effect, especially in patients with comorbid dyslipidemia and type 2 diabetes or metabolic syndrome. Monitoring of liver enzymes becomes more critical in such patients, especially with concurrent statin therapy.

Thus, although the balance of the available evidence indicates that concomitant use of niacin or niacinamide with insulin or oral hypoglycemic agents may not result in an adverse interaction, such coadministration requires an open and trusting therapeutic relationship, patient awareness, and professional supervision and regular monitoring if clinically beneficial outcomes are to be obtained. In some patients, if niacinamide therapy is particularly effective, insulin requirements will either decline or it may no longer be required.

Isoniazid, Rifampin, and Related Antitubercular Agents

Isoniazid (isonicotinic acid hydrazide; INH, Laniazid, Nydrazid), rifampicin (Rifadin, Rifadin IV).
Extrapolated, based on similar properties: Ethambutol (Myambutol), pyrazinamide (PZA); combination drugs: isoniazid and rifampicin (Rifamate, Rimactane); isoniazid, pyrazinamide, and rifampicin (Rifater).

Interaction Type and Significance

≈≈ **Drug-Induced Nutrient Depletion, Supplementation Therapeutic, with Professional Management**
☼ **Prevention or Reduction of Drug Adverse Effect**

Probability:	Evidence Base:
3. Possible or 2. Probable	● Consensus

Effect and Mechanism of Action

Pellagra and peripheral neuropathy are recognized complications of isoniazid therapy, especially with long-term treatment. This important antitubercular drug is a hydrazide derivative of isonicotinic acid that acts as a niacin and pyridoxine antagonist. The mechanisms of this interaction are complex and have yet to be fully elucidated. Isoniazid significantly inhibits the activity of kynurenine aminotransferase in the conversion of tryptophan to niacin. However, it appears that this direct interference is the prime factor in isoniazid-induced depletion of niacin.[116,117] Isoniazid's well-established interference with vitamin B₆ appears to be the more significant cause of impaired conversion of tryptophan to niacin. Moreover, as a form of isonicotinic acid, isoniazid replaces niacinamide in nicotinamide adenine dinucleotide (NAD). Consequently, isoniazid may deplete levels of niacin and cause a niacin deficiency, particularly in poorly nourished patients. Enhanced intake of vitamin B₆ may reduce this adverse effect, but dose levels need to reach an adequate threshold.[118,119] Niacin administration can prevent or reverse this drug-induced deficiency pattern.

Research

Isoniazid-induced vitamin B₃ deficiency has been recognized within the pharmacological literature since 1967.[120,121]

Shibata et al.[117] used rats fed a niacin-free diet to investigate in vivo inhibition of kynurenine aminotransferase activity by isoniazid. A diet containing INH and an injection of INH significantly inhibited kynurenine aminotransferase activity, and this inhibition was sufficient to reduce the urinary excretion of xanthurenic acid, the side-reaction product of the conversion pathway of tryptophan to niacin, to a level "below the limit of detection." However, the conversion ratio of tryptophan to niacin was "no different between the control and INH groups."

Reports

Bjornstad[122] and Harrington[123] have also reported cases of pellagra induced by isoniazid therapy in 1972 and 1977, respectively.

Comaish et al.[124] reported a case in which topical administration of niacinamide produced a positive response in a patient with tuberculous meningitis who had developed a pellagra-like skin eruption after treatment with isoniazid. In addition to the "almost complete resolution of the rash..., there was noticeable improvement in the patient's depression and apathy" subsequent to the "percutaneous absorption of niacinamide."

Ishii and Nishihara[116] investigated 106 necropsy cases of tuberculosis and diagnosed eight cases of pellagra, on the grounds of neuropathological findings and retrospective study of clinical data. None of these patients had been diagnosed as niacin deficient, even though pellagra symptoms had developed during isoniazid therapy in every case. These patients died 4 to 16 weeks after manifesting pellagra symptoms. The authors concluded: "Pellagra should be suspected whenever tuberculous patients under treatment with isoniazid develop mental, neurological or gastrointestinal symptoms, even in the absence of typical pellagra dermatitis."

Darvay et al.[119] reported a case of isoniazid-induced pellagra that occurred despite pyridoxine (10 mg daily) supplementation. Drug withdrawal and administration of niacin "led to a rapid and sustained clinical improvement."

Nutritional Therapeutics, Clinical Concerns, and Adaptations

Although coadministration of pyridoxine with INH has become routine, niacin coadministration is also recommended during long-term treatment of tuberculosis with isoniazid. A daily dosage of 200 mg niacin is typical in most cases. Depletion of vitamin B₃, even to the level of frank deficiency manifested as pellagra, is a well-known adverse effect of isoniazid therapy. In some individuals such depletion is of limited significance, especially with short-term use in well-nourished populations. However, the diagnosis of vitamin B₃ deficiency is often overlooked or delayed, even with overt dermatological, mental, neurological, and gastrointestinal (GI) symptoms. In particular, pellagra lacking skin lesions may develop in patients with minimal sun exposure (e.g., bedridden); thus the condition known as *pelle sine pelle agra* (i.e., pellagra psychosis without skin lesions) can develop with significant GI symptoms, neurological pathology, and even psychosis without obvious signs of typical pellagra-induced dermatitis. Close monitoring and attention to the broad spectrum of the clinical presentation of niacin depletion is critical to clinical management of patients undergoing isoniazid therapy.

Mercaptopurine, Azathioprine, and Thioguanine (Thiopurines)

Mercaptopurine (6-Mercaptopurine, 6-MP, NSC 755; Purinethol), azathioprine (asathioprine; Azamun, Imuran, Thioprine), thioguanine (6-thioguanine, 6-TG, 2-amino-6-mercaptopurine; Lanvis, Tabloid).

Interaction Type and Significance

≈≈ **Drug-Induced Nutrient Depletion, Supplementation Therapeutic, with Professional Management**
☼ **Prevention or Reduction of Drug Adverse Effect**

Probability:	Evidence Base:
3. Possible or 2. Probable	● Consensus

Effect and Mechanism of Action

Mercaptopurine, azathioprine, and thioguanine are cytotoxic antimetabolites used in the treatment of irritable bowel syndrome, leukemia, and some cancers. The mechanisms involved in their therapeutic activity have not been fully elucidated. Thiopurine *S*-methyltransferase (TPMT) catalyzes the *S*-methylation of all three drugs. Mercaptopurine requires intracellular anabolism by hypoxanthine guanine phosphoribosyl transferase (HGPTPT or HGPRT) to become cytotoxic. Likewise, azathioprine is an immunosuppressive prodrug, the *S*-imidazole precursor of 6-MP, converted to 6-mercaptopurine in the liver by TPMT. Intracellular activation of thioguanine, a 6-thiopurine analog of the naturally occurring purine

bases hypoxanthine and guanine, results in incorporation into DNA as a false purine base.

Pellagra is a recognized adverse effect of treatment with mercaptopurine, azathioprine, and thioguanine. Coadministration of vitamin B₃ can prevent or reverse this drug-induced deficiency pattern.

Research

Thiopurine-induced vitamin B₃ deficiency has been recognized within the pharmacological literature.

Reports

In a case report, Jarrett et al.[125] described two patients who developed pellagra during treatment with azathioprine for inflammatory bowel disease.

Nutritional Therapeutics, Clinical Concerns, and Adaptations

Niacin coadministration is recommended during treatment with thiopurines. Depletion of vitamin B₃, even to the level of frank deficiency manifested as pellagra, is a well-known adverse effect of thiopurine therapy. In some individuals such depletion is of limited significance, especially with short-term use in well-nourished populations. Concomitant folic acid is also usually warranted to prevent or reverse depletion. Close monitoring and attention to the clinical presentation of niacin depletion is critical to clinical management of patients undergoing thiopurine therapy.

Tetracycline Antibiotics

Demeclocycline (Declomycin), doxycycline (Atridox, Doryx, Doxy, Monodox, Periostat, Vibramycin, Vibra-Tabs), minocycline (Dynacin, Minocin, Vectrin), oxytetracycline (Terramycin), tetracycline (Achromycin, Actisite, Apo-Tetra, Economycin, Novo-Tetra, Nu-Tetra, Sumycin, Tetrachel, Tetracyn); combination drugs: chlortetracycline, demeclocycline, and tetracycline (Deteclo); bismuth, metronidazole, and tetracycline (Helidac).

Interaction Type and Significance

⊕⊕ **Beneficial or Supportive Interaction, with Professional Management**
⊕✗ **Bimodal or Variable Interaction, with Professional Management**
◇◇ **Impaired Drug Absorption and Bioavailability, Precautions Appropriate**
≈≈ **Drug-Induced Nutrient Depletion, Supplementation Therapeutic, with Professional Management**

Probability:	Evidence Base:
2. Probable	◉ Emerging to ● Consensus

Effect and Mechanism of Action

B-vitamin supplements, including B₃, may interfere with tetracycline pharmacokinetics, impairing absorption and bioavailability; such an interaction would also impair bioavailability of the vitamin. Separation of intake timing can mitigate this possible unintended effect.

Extended use of tetracycline antibiotics could adversely affect bioavailability and function of vitamin B₃ and other B-complex nutrients, both directly and indirectly. Apart from the two-way pharmacokinetic issues, the destructive impact of antimicrobial agents on gut microflora can impair production of B vitamins (as well as vitamin K) and potentially contribute to systemic inflammatory processes and depressed immune system function.[126-135]

High doses of niacinamide can exert significant anti-inflammatory effects. The coadministration of niacinamide with tetracycline or minocycline may be effective against several types of dermatological pathologies, particularly blistering skin diseases such as bullous pemphigoid and dermatitis herpetiformis.[136]

Research

In an investigation of the effects of various nutrients on the pharmacokinetics of tetracycline hydrochloride in healthy subjects, researchers observed a significant impairment of drug bioavailability associated with concomitant oral administration of a B-complex vitamin supplement.[137]

Some small studies and a number of cases have been published in which the combination of niacinamide and tetracycline or minocycline has found to be efficacious in the treatment of bullous pemphigoid, cicatricial pemphigoid, pemphigus vegetans, dermatitis herpetiformis, and similar dermatoses.[138-148]

Clinical Implications and Adaptations

Physicians prescribing tetracycline or related antibiotic medications should advise patients regularly supplementing with B₃, alone or within a B-complex vitamin formulation, to take the nutrient(s) and the medication at least 4 hours apart.

Concomitant use of niacinamide and a tetracycline-class antibacterial may be effective in the treatment of dermatological conditions, whether infectious or autoimmune, under proper medical supervision.

Prudence suggests that individuals treated with oral tetracyclines or other broad-spectrum antibiotics for an extended time be administered a course of probiotic flora for an equivalent duration to restore intestinal microbiota. Short-term use of tetracyclines is unlikely to lead to clinically significant alterations in the GI ecology, as is use of topical preparations.

Thioridazine and Related Phenothiazines

Evidence: Thioridazine (Mellaril).
Extrapolated, based on similar properties: Acetophenazine (Tindal), chlorpromazine (Largactil, Thorazine), fluphenazine (Modecate, Permitil, Prolixin, Prolixin Decanoate, Prolixin Enanthate), mesoridazine (Serentil), methotrimeprazine (levomepromazine; Nozinan), pericyazine (Neuleptil), perphenazine (Trilafon); combination drug: perphenazine and amitriptyline (Etrafon, Triavil, Triptazine); prochlorperazine (Compazine, Stemetil), promazine (Sparine), promethazine (Phenergan, Promacot, Promethegan), propiomazine (Largon), thiethylperazine (Torecan), thioproperazine (Majeptil), trifluoperazine (Stelazine), triflupromazine (Vesprin).
See also Antipsychotics in Theoretical, Speculative, and Preliminary Interactions Research.

Interaction Type and Significance

⊕⊕ **Beneficial or Supportive Interaction, with Professional Management**

Probability: Evidence Base:
4. Plausible   ○ **Preliminary**

Effect and Mechanism of Action

The concurrent administration of niacin and thioridazine appears to exert an additive or synergistic beneficial effect based on one or more unknown mechanisms.

Niacinamide appears to stimulate gamma-aminobutyric acid (GABA) receptors without binding to receptor sites.[149,150]

Research

In a much-cited study, Mohler et al.[150] found that niacinamide exerts benzodiazepine-like actions capable of producing an anxiolytic effect equivalent to a potent benzodiazepine.

Saxena, Lehmann, and colleagues investigated the coadministration of niacin and thioridazine in a series of clinical trials involving geriatric patients conducted during the early 1970s.[151,152] In one controlled trial, addition of niacin (300-1500 mg/day) to the thioridazine (and fluoxymesterone) regimen of elderly patients being treated for psychosis produced higher levels of cooperation and decreased tendency to withdraw from other people.[153]

Nutritional Therapeutics, Clinical Concerns, and Adaptations

Physicians prescribing thioridazine or related phenothiazine antipsychotic agents might consider the potential benefits of concomitant niacin, as suggested by this preliminary research. Prudence and close supervision are warranted given the limited scope and size of the available evidence. Further research may be warranted.

Tricyclic Antidepressants (TCAs)

Evidence: Imipramine (Janimine, Tofranil).
Extrapolated, based on similar properties: Clomipramine (Anafranil).
Similar properties but evidence lacking for extrapolation: Amitriptyline (Elavil); combination drug: amitriptyline and perphenazine (Etrafon, Triavil, Triptazine), amoxapine (Asendin), desipramine (Norpramin, Pertofrane), doxepin (Adapin, Sinequan), nortriptyline (Aventyl, Pamelor), protriptyline (Vivactil), trimipramine (Surmontil).

Interaction Type and Significance

⊕⊕ **Beneficial or Supportive Interaction, with Professional Management**
⊕✗ **Bimodal or Variable Interaction, with Professional Management**
✗✗ **Minimal to Mild Adverse Interaction—Vigilance Necessary**

Probability: Evidence Base:
4. Plausible   ○ **Preliminary**

Effect and Mechanism of Action

L-Tryptophan supplementation can potentiate the action of tricyclic antidepressants (TCAs) through its serotonergic effects. The coadministration of niacinamide appears to support this synergistic interaction by reducing peripheral breakdown of tryptophan.[154]

Research

In a 4-week, double-blind, controlled study, Chouinard et al.[154] randomly assigned 25 newly admitted, severely depressed patients to receive tryptophan-nicotinamide, imipramine, or tryptophan-nicotinamide-imipramine combination. They observed that "there were no substantial differences between the three treatments," but that the efficacy of tryptophan-nicotinamide combination tended to decline after 2 weeks when the nutrient doses were increased: tryptophan from 4 to 6 g per day and nicotinamide from 1.0 to 1.5 g per day. Notably, the "therapeutic response of patients treated with tryptophan-nicotinamide was significantly correlated with the rise in plasma tryptophan." In contrast, the therapeutic response and rise in plasma tryptophan were negatively correlated within the tryptophan-nicotinamide-imipramine group, "implying that tryptophan levels were too high in some patients." The authors concluded that their findings "suggest that tryptophan-nicotinamide may be as effective as imipramine in unipolar patients providing the dose is kept within the therapeutic window, and that at low doses it could also potentiate the action of tricyclic antidepressants." They also noted that "bipolar patients seem to require higher doses of tryptophan than unipolar patients."[154]

Subsequent research investigated the pivotal role of tryptophan in potentiating the antidepressant action of TCAs and confirmed that the dose level of tryptophan was critical to obtaining a beneficial outcome.[155,156] However, other research into the interaction between L-tryptophan and TCAs failed to produce findings of efficacy.[155,157]

Nutritional Therapeutics, Clinical Concerns, and Adaptations

Physicians treating individuals diagnosed with depressive disorders using TCAs can reasonably consider the potential benefits of coadministering L-tryptophan and niacinamide within the context of an integrative therapeutic strategy. The ability of such nutrients to potentiate TCAs is notably dose dependent and requires close supervision and regular monitoring. Pretreatment tryptophan depletion status and carefully calibrated dosages of L-tryptophan (typically 4 g/day) and niacinamide (1.0 g/day) appear to be primary factors in determining probability of an optimal effect. Once stabilization occurs, reduction of antidepressant medication levels can be considered if consistent with the expressed patient treatment goals, particularly in patients with a history of adverse effects attributable to the antidepressant medication. Evolving personalized treatment protocols coordinated by health care professionals trained and experienced in both nutritional therapeutics and conventional psychopharmacology offer opportunities for deriving clinical benefits greater than what might be achieved by conventional antidepressant medications alone.

Ursodeoxycholic Acid and Chenodeoxycholic Acid

Chenodeoxycholic acid (CDCA, chenodiol; Chenix).
Ursodeoxycholic acid (UDCA, ursodiol; Actigall, Destolit, Urdox, Urso, Ursofalk, Ursogal).

Interaction Type and Significance

✗✗ **Minimal to Mild Adverse Interaction—Vigilance Necessary**

Probability:
4. Plausible to
2. Probable

Evidence Base:
● Consensus but
□ Inadequate

Effect and Mechanism of Action

Cholesterol makes up only 5% of bile, but approximately 75% of the gallstones found in the U.S. population are formed from cholesterol. Ursodiol and chenodiol are anticholelithogenic agents that contain bile acids and are sometimes used for dissolution of cholesterol-based stones less than 1.5 cm in diameter. Chenodiol and ursodiol are considered equally effective as cholesterol gallstone solubilizing agents. Both ursodeoxycholic acid (ursodiol) and chenodeoxycholic acid (chenodiol) undergo 7-dehydroxylation to form lithocholic acid, with chenodiol being more efficiently 7-dehydroxylated than ursodiol. However, ursodiol is generally preferred over chenodiol because of its lower incidence of diarrhea and hepatotoxicity. Some portion of ursodeoxycholic acid is epimerized to chenodeoxycholic acid via a 7-oxo intermediate.

Among conventional pharmacologic agents administered in the treatment of cholelithiasis, only niacin and the statins do not contribute to the formation of gallstones.

Because of their tendency to increase cholesterol saturation of bile, concomitant use of ursodiol or chenodiol may reduce the antihyperlipidemic activity of niacin.[158,159]

Research

The information on these interactions is derived from literature distributed by the manufacturers of proprietary products. Specific research derived from clinical trials or animal research may be extant but was not accessible to multiple searches conducted using standard resources.

Nutritional Therapeutics, Clinical Concerns, and Adaptations

The concomitant use of ursodeoxycholic acid (ursodiol) or chenodeoxycholic acid (chenodiol) with niacin appears to be incompatible and inappropriate as complementary therapies within a strategy for treatment of hyperlipidemia. Coadministration is generally not recommended unless otherwise indicated and then only under close supervision.

Associated Therapies

Radiotherapy

Administration of niacinamide may enhance the efficacy of radiotherapy in the treatment of cancer. Using a rat model, Agote et al. observed that concomitant nicotinamide with radioactive iodine treatment enhanced the radiosensitivity of normal and goitrous thyroid in the rat and increased effectiveness of radiation at lower doses.[160] In a 1997 review of preclinical and clinical studies, Denekamp and Fowler[161] found that niacinamide increased tissue sensitivity to radiation in cancer therapy.

Physicians and other health care professionals may consider reviewing the potential for such synergistic therapies with appropriate patients and provide referral information to centers specializing in such integrative approaches. Further research is warranted.

THEORETICAL, SPECULATIVE, AND PRELIMINARY INTERACTIONS RESEARCH, INCLUDING OVERSTATED INTERACTIONS CLAIMS

Adrenoreceptor Antagonists (Systemic)

Alpha-1-adrenoreceptor antagonists (alpha-1-adrenergic blocking agents): Doxazosin (Cardura), guanabenz (Wytensin), prazosin (Minipress).
Beta-1-adrenergic antagonists (beta-1-adrenergic blocking agents): Oral forms (systemic): Acebutolol (Sectral), atenolol (Tenormin); combination drugs: atenolol and chlortalidone (Co-Tendione, Tenoretic); atenolol and nifedipine (Beta-Adalat, Tenif); betaxolol (Kerlone), bisoprolol (Zebeta), carteolol (Cartrol), esmolol (Brevibloc), labetalol (Normodyne, Trandate), metoprolol (Lopressor, Toprol XL); combination drug: metoprolol and hydrochlorothiazide (Lopressor HCT); nadolol (Corgard), nebivolol (Nebilet), oxprenolol (Trasicor), penbutolol (Levatol), pindolol (Visken), propranolol (Betachron, Inderal LA, Innopran XL, Inderal); combination drug: propranolol and bendrofluazide (Inderex); sotalol (Betapace, Betapace AF, Sorine), timolol (Blocadren).

Related but evidence against extrapolation: **Beta-adrenergic blocking eyedrops (ophthalmic forms):** Betaxolol (Betoptic), carteolol (Cartrol, Ocupress), levobunolol (AKBeta, Betagan), metipranolol (OptiPranolol), timolol (Timoptic).

Both niacin and adrenergic blocking agents can produce vasodilation and lower blood pressure; the concomitant use of such agents could theoretically induce an additive effect resulting in postural hypotension. Even though the pharmacological principles of this potential interaction appear plausible, if not self-evident, substantive evidence from well-designed controlled trials is lacking. Pending such research, physicians prescribing these medications should ask patients about any prescribed or self-administered use of niacin, advise patients to be watchful for such effects, and closely monitor for excessive changes in blood pressure.

Atypical Antipsychotics

Aripiprazole (Abilify, Abilitat), clozapine (Clozaril), olanzapine (Symbyax, Zyprexa), quetiapine (Seroquel), risperidone (Risperdal), ziprasidone (Geodon).
Extrapolated, based on similar properties: Haloperidol (Haldol).
See also Thioridazine and Related Phenothiazines and Benztropine sections.

Since the 1940s, Hoffer and others have investigated the management of schizophrenia and related psychiatric disorders using orthomolecular therapy emphasizing megadose niacin and niacinamide as means of elevating levels of NAD, their biologically active form. In early double-blind trials, a doubling of the recovery rate, a 50% reduction in hospitalization rates, and dramatic reductions in suicide rates were reported with treatment using 3 g of niacin daily. Based on years of clinical practice and research involving more than 1000 patients treated with either niacinamide or niacin (1.5-6.0 g/day) for 3 months to 5 years, Hoffer and others have concluded that B₃ monotherapy is most efficacious with early and acute schizophrenia. However, they have cautioned that B₃ monotherapy is usually relatively ineffective in the treatment of individuals with chronic schizophrenia, although multinutrient megadose therapy is reported to be beneficial in some chronic cases.[8,149,162-165]

Green[166] and others have suggested that some of the reported success with individuals diagnosed as schizophrenic may be the result of misdiagnosis and that such patients were actually suffering from subclinical pellagra. Thus, the perceptual changes, neurasthenia, and other characteristic deficiency symptoms would be expected to respond significantly to high doses of B₃ in any form.

This controversial research has been debated for decades, and evidence from double-blind clinical trials is mixed and generally limited by study size, duration, and design. In some studies, patients were also being treated with psychoactive medications, potentially limiting therapeutic response and confounding findings.[167-171]

Nevertheless, such usage suggests the possibility of an additive or synergistic interaction with coadministration of niacin or niacinamide and an antipsychotic medication. No clinical trials have applied coadministration to investigate this plausible interaction directly, nor has any substantive evidence emerged to suggest any pattern for an adverse or beneficial outcome. Pending conclusive research, physicians prescribing benzodiazepines are advised to query patients about vitamin intake and closely supervise and regularly monitor patients initiating or making any changes in therapeutic regimen, particularly involving megadose intake of vitamins.

Benzodiazepines

Alprazolam (Xanax), bromazepam (Lexotan), chlordiazepoxide (Librium), clonazepam (Klonopin, Rivotril), clorazepate (Gen-Xene, Tranxene), diazepam (Valium), estazolam (ProSom), flurazepam (Dalmane), lorazepam (Ativan), medazepam (Nobrium), midazolam (Hypnovel, Versed), oxazepam (Serax), prazepam (Centrax), quazepam (Doral), temazepam (Restoril), triazolam (Halcion).

The therapeutic activity of benzodiazepines derives from their potentiating the activity of GABA. Specifically, benzodiazepines bind to a receptor on the GABA A receptor complex, which facilitates the binding of GABA to its specific receptor site. This binding by benzodiazepines causes increased frequency of opening of the chloride channel complexed with the GABA A receptor. Such opening of the chloride channel results in membrane hyperpolarization and subsequent inhibition of cellular excitation.

Mohler et al.[150] found that niacinamide exerts benzodiazepine-like actions capable of producing an anxiolytic effect equivalent to a potent benzodiazepine.

Niacinamide appears to stimulate GABA receptors without binding to receptor sites.[149,150] Thus, the concomitant administration of niacinamide and a benzodiazepine could theoretically produce an additive effect with potential for an excessive sedative-hypnotic response. Furthermore, because benzodiazepines are metabolized predominantly in the liver by oxidation and conjugation, any adverse effects on the liver caused by vitamin B₃ could theoretically impair drug metabolism and elevate blood levels.

Substantive evidence from well-designed clinical trials or qualified case reports is lacking to confirm these hypothetical interactions and to suggest any pattern for an adverse or beneficial outcome. Pending such research, physicians prescribing benzodiazepines are advised to query patients about vitamin intake and closely supervise and regularly monitor patients initiating or making any changes in therapeutic regimen, particularly involving megadose intake of vitamins.

Benztropine

Benztropine (Cogentin).

Benztropine is used to treat Parkinson's disease and to mitigate akathisia and other adverse reactions to neuroleptics and other antipsychotic drugs. Kramer et al.[172] reported in a letter that coadministration of 4000 mg of L-tryptophan and 25 mg niacin per day taken with benztropine enhances the treatment of akathisia. Further research in such potentially beneficial interactions is warranted.

Carbidopa and Related Antiparkinsonian Agents

Carbidopa (Lodosyn), levodopa (L-dopa; Dopar, Larodopa); combination drugs: levodopa and benserazide (co-beneldopa; Madopar); levodopa and carbidopa (Atamet, Parcopa, Sinemet, Sinemet CR); levodopa, carbidopa, and entacapone (Stalevo).

In animal models, Bender and Smith[173] found that benserazide, carbidopa, and other aromatic hydrazine derivatives can induce subclinical iatrogenic niacin deficiency by inhibiting kynurenine hydrolase, an enzyme involved in niacin synthesis. Subsequently, Bender et al.[174] reported niacin depletion in parkinsonian patients treated with L-dopa, benserazide, and carbidopa.

These preliminary findings suggest the need for close monitoring of vitamin B₃ status in patients using antiparkinsonian medications, looking for indications of depletion rather than waiting for signs of frank deficiency. Moreover, well-designed clinical trials are warranted to determine potential benefits and risks of B_3 coadministration.

Fluorouracil (5-FU)

Fluorouracil (5-FU; Adrucil, Efudex, Efudix, Fluoroplex).

Pellagra has been reported in patients with long-term administration of 5-FU.[175-178] Monitoring of vitamin B_3 and general nutrient status is always important during chemotherapy. Concurrent administration of appropriate nutrient support may be appropriate and is usually best provided within the context of coordinated care by health care professionals trained and experienced in both conventional oncology and nutritional therapeutics.

Ganglionic Blocking Agents

Mecamylamine hydrochloride (Inversine), trimethaphan camsylate (Arfonad).

Some derivative publications have proposed a potential adverse interaction between niacin and ganglionic blocking agents based on the known direct vasodilator action of these medications and the possibility of an additive interaction potentiating hypotensive effects. Although theoretically plausible, such assertions may be overstated given the lack of substantive evidence from well-designed clinical trials or qualified case reports, and of minimal relevance given that these drugs are not currently in clinical use because of toxicity and the difficulty of titrating their hypotensive effects. Nevertheless, pending such research, physicians administering these drugs are advised to query patients about vitamin intake and closely supervise and regularly monitor patients initiating or making any changes in therapeutic regimen, particularly involving intake of niacin in pharmacological doses.

Griseofulvin

Griseofulvin (Fulvicin, Grifulvin, Gris-PEG, Grisactin, Gristatin).

Rasool et al.[179] conducted in vitro research that indicates griseofulvin solubility increases in a nonlinear fashion as a function of nicotinamide concentration. They studied two aliphatic analogs of nicotinamide (nipecotamide and N,N-dimethylacetamide) as ligands with griseofulvin and found that they increased the solubilities of the drug in a linear fashion.

Thus, theoretically, the simultaneous administration of niacinamide and griseofulvin could result in increased levels of the drug, a potentially adverse reaction of clinical significance if induced unintentionally. However, use of nicotinamide might enable use of lower dosages of griseofulvin to achieve the same level of therapeutic effect while reducing effects from the drug. Physicians prescribing griseofulvin are advised to query patients regarding vitamin intake and to consider potential benefits of coadministration under supervision. Further research is warranted into parameters of effects and, on confirmation, as a basis for developing guidelines for enhancing benefits and minimizing risk of adverse effects.

Guanethidine

Guanethidine (Apo-guanethidine; Ismelin).

Guanethidine lowers blood pressure by blocking norepinephrine release from adrenergic synapses; in the process it can deplete norepinephrine over time. Niacin may theoretically increase guanethidine effect, but a clear mechanism has not been established, nor has substantive clinical research been published. Pursuit of such research is improbable given the minimal use of guanethidine in clinical practice.

Neomycin

Neomycin (Mycifradin, Myciguent, Neo-Fradin, NeoTab, Nivemycin).

Niacin and neomycin have both been shown to reduce serum lipoprotein Lp(a) levels in patients with hyperlipidemia. Thus, for example, in an experiment involving 14 type II hyperlipoproteinemic subjects, Gurakar et al.[180] observed that concomitant treatment with neomycin (2 g/day) and niacin (3 g/day) "induced a 48% decline in low density lipoprotein cholesterol levels and a 45% reduction in the concentration of lipoprotein Lp(a)." However, the primary value of such findings is not in their direct clinical application; rather, such observations elucidate the ways in which "lipoprotein Lp(a) concentrations can be altered pharmacologically and that the progression of cardiovascular disease may be altered through changes in lipoprotein (a) levels."

Thus, although such an interactive effect might be interpreted to suggest that coadministration of neomycin with niacin might enhance the cholesterol-lowering effects of niacin, such use is inadvisable because of the numerous adverse effects of extended neomycin administration, especially the well-documented depletion of numerous key nutrients. Pharmacologic dose niacin is also well documented to lower Lp(a) levels by itself, but it is unclear whether or not this effect is enhanced by coadministration of neomycin.

Nicotine Transdermal Patches

Nicotine (Habitrol, NicoDerm CQ, Nicotrol).

The relationship between nicotine and niacin is often confused in secondary literature, especially when using the nicotinic acid nomenclature. Fundamentally, niacin is a vasodilator, whereas nicotine is a vasoconstrictor. Nicotine clearly binds to and stimulates nicotinic acetylcholine receptors, which are divided into two types: nicotinic and muscarinic.

Using a rat model, Turenne et al.[181] observed that "neither acute (0.25mg/kg) or chronic (0.5mg/kg/day for 14 days) administration of nicotine... had any significant effect" on the normal vasodilatory response to ingestion of nicotinic acid.

Notably, tobacco can decrease vitamin B3 absorption.

In a letter published in *The Lancet* (1980), Clarkes[182] suggested an intriguing approach to the relationship between niacin and nicotine in the context of tobacco addiction, as follows:

> Morphine works by tricking the endorphin receptors— might not nicotine similarly dupe the niacin (vitamin B_3) receptors of the CNS?... Is it not possible, then, that nicotine fills niacin receptor sites and creates a deficiency of a nutrient required by the CNS? Perhaps this is why some say they need a cigarette to "calm their nerves."
>
> If this hypothesis is valid, it might be possible to wean some smokers off their nicotine addiction by administering nicotinic acid (niacin).[182]

Subsequently, a few letters in professional publications have discussed the possibility that the concomitant use of supplemental niacin and transdermal nicotine could result in increased adverse effects associated with the vitamin, particularly flushing.[183,184] Since then, several secondary articles and lay publications have reiterated these concerns as if they had been proved. In the absence of well-designed clinical trials or qualified case reports, this purported interaction may simply be an example of overuse of inadequately examined citations.

Overall, a clinically significant effect on blood pressure is improbable from concurrent use of transdermal nicotine (or tobacco smoking) and oral niacin given limited available knowledge of this interaction. Further research using well-designed clinical trials may be appropriate to determine the probability and characterization of a clinically significant interaction.

Oral Contraceptives: Monophasic, Biphasic, and Triphasic Estrogen Preparations (Synthetic Estrogen and Progesterone Analogs)

Ethinyl estradiol and desogestrel (Desogen, Ortho-TriCyclen).
Ethinyl estradiol and ethynodiol (Demulen 1/35, Demulen 1/50, Nelulen 1/25, Nelulen 1/50, Zovia).
Ethinyl estradiol and levonorgestrel (Alesse, Levlen, Levlite, Levora 0.15/30, Nordette, Tri-Levlen, Triphasil, Trivora).
Ethinyl estradiol and norethindrone/norethisterone (Brevicon, Estrostep, Genora 1/35, GenCep 1/35, Jenest-28, Loestrin 1.5/30, Loestrin1/20, Modicon, Necon 1/25, Necon 10/11, Necon 0.5/30, Necon 1/50, Nelova 1/35, Nelova 10/11, Norinyl 1/35, Norlestin 1/50, Ortho Novum 1/35, Ortho Novum 10/11, Ortho Novum 7/7/7, Ovcon-35, Ovcon-50, Tri-Norinyl, Trinovum).
Ethinyl estradiol and norgestrel (Lo/Ovral, Ovral).
Mestranol and norethindrone (Genora 1/50, Nelova 1/50, Norethin 1/50, Ortho-Novum 1/50).
Related, internal application: Etonogestrel/ethinyl estradiol vaginal ring (Nuvaring).

Norethindrone Enanthate

Norethindrone, injectable (NET EN; Noristerat).
Related progestin injectable: Medroxyprogesterone (depot medroxyprogesterone acetate, DMPA; Depo-Provera, Depo-subQ Provera 104).
Related progestin and estrogen injectable: Estradiol cypionate and medroxyprogesterone acetate (Cyclofem, Lunelle); norethisterone enanthate and estradiol valerate (Mesigyna).
See also Vitamin B₆ monograph.

The use of oral contraceptives (OCs) has been associated with both elevated and decreased levels of vitamin B₃. Pyroxidine, as the coenzyme pyridoxal phosphate, is involved in conversion of tryptophan to niacin, and tryptophan load tests have shown that certain metabolites of B₆ have increased secretion when OCs are used, with compromised B₆ status a frequent outcome.[185-194] Resulting deficiencies of vitamin B₆ caused by OC use could lead to a subsequent decrease in the formation of niacin from tryptophan and an increased risk of niacin deficiency. Furthermore, OC formulations with a high progestin/progestogen content can induce tryptophan pyrrolase, thereby diverting pyridoxine for niacin synthesis to the detriment of 5-hydroxytryptamine (serotonin) formation and contributing to tendencies to premenstrual syndrome and depression. In such patients, supplementation with vitamin B₆ (pyridoxine), at levels of 25 mg two or three times daily, may mitigate such adverse effects. Conversely, with estrogen-containing formulations (and/or in different individuals), OC use might decrease the need for niacin intake by increasing the efficiency of niacin synthesis from tryptophan.[195]

The clinical implications of this potential interaction are uncertain at this time and are likely to vary depending on patient characteristics as well as specific medication and dosage. Further research with well-designed clinical trials of adequate power are warranted to clarify these outstanding issues and to provide guidelines for understanding the variable influences of diverse OC formulations on individuals of differing genetic and metabolic constitutions as well as dietary, lifestyle, and economic characteristics.

In a related study of a long-acting, low-dose injectable OC, norethisterone enanthate (20 mg monthly), Bamji et al.[196] reported a peculiar aberration in the tryptophan-niacin pathway, as indicated by increased kynurenic acid excretion after tryptophan load was observed.

Nutritional counseling should be an ongoing part of any comprehensive patient education program. Health care professionals prescribing OCs are advised to encourage patients to adopt healthy dietary patterns and an increased understanding of how eating well directly influences both their feeling of well-being and their long-term health. The levels of niacin, 10 to 25 mg, found in most B-complex or multivitamin formulations are probably adequate to compensate for any potential deficiency caused by OC use, particularly in women from high-risk groups. In general, increased intake of the entire B-vitamin complex appears warranted in women taking hormonal OCs.

Pargyline

Pargyline (Eutonyl).
Pargyline (hydrochloride) is a selective monoamine oxidase inhibitor. The concomitant use of pargyline and niacin could theoretically cause an excessive drop in blood pressure. Substantive evidence of such interaction-induced hypotension is lacking, but caution and medical supervision are advisable when introducing a new agent or changing dosages in an ongoing therapeutic regimen.

Pyrazinamide

Pyrazinamide (PZA; Tebrazid); combination drug: isoniazid, pyrazinamide, and rifampicin (Rifater).
Using a rat model, Shibata et al.[197] observed that pyrazinamide, an antituberculosis agent, may elevate niacin levels by altering the metabolism of tryptophan to niacin and of tryptophan to serotonin. Substantive evidence of this potential interaction occurring in humans is lacking.

Notably, both niacin and pyrazinamide are known to cause hyperuricemia and increase the risk for gout. Prudence suggests the avoidance of any concurrent use outside the context of close supervision and regular monitoring by a qualified health care professional.

Selective Serotonin Reuptake Inhibitor and Serotonin-Norepinephrine Reuptake Inhibitor (SSRI and SSRI/SNRI) Antidepressants

Citalopram (Celexa), duloxetine (Cymbalta), escitalopram (S-citalopram; Lexapro), fluoxetine (Prozac, Sarafem), fluvoxamine (Faurin, Luvox), paroxetine (Aropax, Deroxat, Paxil, Seroxat), sertraline (Zoloft), venlafaxine (Effexor).

Vitamin B₃ saturation might theoretically encourage diversion of tryptophan to serotonin synthesis and provoke excessive serotonin levels in individuals being treated with serotonin reuptake inhibitors. However, evidence is lacking to confirm such a phenomenon. Should this interaction be confirmed by well-designed clinical trials, such an effect could be characterized as a "potential synergistic opportunity" or a "potential adverse effect," depending primarily on communication, coordination, and clinical management.

Sulfinpyrazone and Probenecid

Sulfinpyrazone (Anturane), probenecid (Benemid, Parbenem, Probalan).
The use of niacin at higher dosage levels could potentially interfere with the uricosuric effects of sulfinpyrazone or probenecid by impairing uric acid excretion and thereby elevating uric acid levels. Although the mechanism of this

potential interaction is plausible, substantive evidence of its occurrence in humans and well-defined characterization of its clinical significance are lacking. Nevertheless, individuals diagnosed with gout should avoid supplementing with niacin outside the context of close supervision and regular monitoring by a qualified health care professional.

Warfarin and Other Anticoagulants

Primary: Warfarin (Coumadin, Dicumarol, Marevan).

Related medications: Anisindione (Miradon), dicumarol, ethyl biscoumacetate (Tromexan), nicoumalone (acenocoumarol; Acitrom, Sintrom), phenindione (Dindevan), phenprocoumon (Jarsin, Marcumar).

Similar properties but evidence lacking for extrapolation: Antiplatelet thromboprophylactics: Acetylsalicylic acid, cilostazol (Pletal), clopidogrel (Plavix), dipyridamole (Permole, Persantine), ticlopidine (Ticlid); combination drug: ASA and extended-release dipyridamole (Aggrenox, Asasantin); heparin (Calciparine, Hepalean, Heparin Leo, Minihep Calcium, Minihep, Monoparin Calcium, Monoparin, Multiparin, Pump-Hep, Unihep, Uniparin Calcium, Uniparin Forte).

The derivative literature frequently asserts that niacin may increase the risk of bleeding when used concurrently with anticoagulants or antiplatelet drugs. Evidence from clinical trials or well-qualified case reports is lacking to substantiate claims of probable risk of clinically significant adverse effects from concomitant use in typical doses under proper medical supervision.

Coagulopathy is a well-known complication of severe niacin-induced hepatotoxic reactions, primarily associated with sustained-release niacin preparations. Based on the available case reports, such effects are possible even in patients with minimal transaminase level elevations; however, the frequency of such events appears to be rare. "Deficiency in protein synthesis, including coagulation factors, and coagulopathy are unrecognized complications of sustained-release niacin therapy." In the cases described, "protein deficiency, coagulopathy, and aminotransferase level elevation resolved promptly after withdrawal of niacin therapy."[198,199]

Notably, niacin improves prothrombotic tendencies by reducing plasminogen activator inhibitor-1 (PAI-1), fibrinogen, and alpha-2 antiplasmin. Coagulation parameters are altered in peripheral arterial disease (PAD), and altered coagulation may play a critical role in the susceptibility to cardiovascular complications in PAD. In a randomized trial, Philipp et al.[200] found that niacin decreases plasma fibrinogen and LDL cholesterol in patients with PAD. They observed that changes in fibrinogen levels were "highly correlated with changes in low-density lipoprotein cholesterol in subjects taking niacin." Likewise, in a multicenter, randomized, placebo-controlled trial, Chesney et al.[201] found that niacin "favorably modifies fibrinogen and plasma F1.2." Such a decrease in F1.2 suggests that niacin reduces the production of thrombin from prothrombin, although the mechanism and parameters of occurrence of such a phenomenon have yet to be fully elucidated. This beneficial effect on abnormal procoagulation factors indicates the possibility of a strategic "interaction" of clinical significance given proper dosing, medical supervision, and regular monitoring.

The probability of a clinically significant interaction between niacin and anticoagulants appears to be low, based on presently available evidence. Although niacin and such agents can both affect related metabolic functions, a direct interaction would be considered as "confirmed" only if niacin altered prothrombin times in patients previously stabilized on warfarin. In general, it is prudent to monitor the international normalized ratio (INR) when altering any pharmacological treatment given with oral anticoagulants, especially warfarin. Furthermore, periodic monitoring of liver enzymes in patients being treated with niacin is advisable, especially sustained-release forms. Moreover, the previous cases indicate the need to measure prothrombin times routinely in patients who develop even mild transaminase level elevation while receiving niacin therapy. The niacin should be discontinued if such abnormalities develop.

NUTRIENT-NUTRIENT INTERACTIONS

Antioxidants

Antioxidants

Odetti et al.[202] found that concomitant administration of niacin and retinol, along with tocopherols, produced more marked effects on plasma cholesterol levels did than niacin alone. Likewise, serial coronary angiographic evidence developed by Hodis et al.[203] demonstrated that the combination of niacin, colestipol, and vitamin E reduces progression of coronary atherosclerotic lesions.

However, recent evidence emerging in the context of the interaction between vitamin E and other antioxidants and niacin-statin combinations has raised serious questions about the efficacy of antioxidants supplements in preventing cardiovascular disease, especially in patients being treated with conventional hypolipidemic agents. In particular, antioxidants may blunt the therapeutic activity of niacin on cholesterol levels, possibly by interfering with niacin's effects on proteins involved with the formation of high-density lipoproteins (HDLs).[204] As part of the HDL Atherosclerosis Treatment Study (HATS), Brown, Cheung, and associates investigated the respective and collective roles of statins, niacin, and antioxidants (vitamins E and C, beta-carotene, and selenium) in cardiovascular protection in patients with coronary artery disease and low HDL cholesterol. They found that simvastatin-niacin substantially improved HDL parameters, but that these favorable responses were blunted by the antioxidants, especially with regard to Lp(A-I).[205] In an accompanying paper, focusing on coronary atherosclerotic plaques and the occurrence of a first cardiovascular event, the niacin-simvastatin combination was significantly superior to placebo with regard to average stenosis progression (0.4% and 3.6%, respectively), but in participants also receiving antioxidants, this benefit was reduced to 0.7% average stenosis progression, a finding interpreted as possible interference by antioxidants.[71] When surrogate markers of cholesterol absorption and synthesis were later measured in a subset of HATS participants, at 24 months (on treatment) and 38 months (off treatment), treatment with simvastatin-niacin continued to be associated with favorable changes in cholesterol metabolism and stenosis.[206] These findings were subsequently interpreted in many quarters as suggesting that antioxidant supplementation was contraindicated in the treatment of hyperlipidemia and prevention of cardiovascular disease.[72,207]

A more critical analysis of the data suggests that the primary observed adverse interaction is between niacin and antioxidants, not statins and antioxidants. The affected HDL increases that occurred were probably attributable to the niacin therapy because low-dose simvastatin monotherapy has only limited effects in raising the levels of HDL cholesterol and apolipoprotein (apo) A-I. Thus, one or more of the antioxidants might be interfering with niacin's ability to alter the expression of proteins responsible for the formation of HDL.

Further, the findings derived from the population studied may have limited general relevance to individuals who have only elevated LDL cholesterol levels (and normal HDL levels) and to women, who made up only 13% of the cohort. Also, with regard to HDL status, there was no detriment to the antioxidants alone (i.e., given to a group without simvastatin/niacin), and actually a slight benefit, which, if involving thousands of patients as with the previous statin and the thrombolytic trials, might have become a trend, or even statistically significant. Lastly, the composition of the antioxidant nutrient formulation used has been questioned. Given that niacin depletes the liver of methyl donors, thereby raising homocysteine levels and contributing significantly to the vitamin's hepatotoxicity, researchers might have obtained different results if they had included methyl donor–relevant nutrients with the antioxidants, such as folic acid, choline/betaine, and possibly coenzyme Q10, the synthesis of which is inhibited by statins.

Betaine

Betaine

The hepatotoxicity of niacin reflects, to a significant degree, the high demand for methyl groups imposed by niacin catabolism, leading to a reduction in hepatic levels of S-adenosylmethionine (SAMe). Such depletion of SAMe by niacin is likely to play a major role in the elevation of plasma homocysteine and other adverse effects associated with high-dose niacin intake.[60] Coadministration of equimolar doses of betaine may alleviate the hepatotoxic risk associated with niacin therapy.[208] Well-designed and adequately powered clinical trials are warranted to determine the efficacy of such coadministration.

Chromium

Chromium

A potential interaction between niacin and chromium has been discussed, but only preliminary evidence is available as to its clinical implications. Niacin plays an essential role in the physiological activity of chromium, particularly glucose regulation.[209-214] Therefore, many chromium formulations contain niacin, most directly as chromium polynicotinate, a niacin-bound form of chromium, but also as glucose tolerance factor (GTF), a complex of chromium and nicotinic acid believed to facilitate insulin binding.[210] Concomitant intake may improve glucose tolerance, particularly in individuals whose diet provides inadequate levels of dietary nicotinic acid and chromium.

Urberg and Zemel[209] investigated the possibility that inconsistent response to chromium might result from inadequate levels of dietary nicotinic acid to serve as substrate for GTF synthesis. They randomly divided 16 healthy elderly volunteers into three groups and administered 200 μg chromium, 100 mg nicotinic acid, or 200 μg chromium plus 100 mg nicotinic acid daily for 28 days, with evaluation at onset and on day 28. Fasting glucose and glucose tolerance were unaffected by either chromium or nicotinic acid alone, but the group receiving the chromium–nicotinic acid combination demonstrated a 15% decrease in a glucose area integrated total (AUC) and a 7% decrease in fasting glucose. Notably, none of the treatments exerted any effect on fasting or 1-hour insulin levels. The authors interpreted their findings as suggesting that "the inability to respond to chromium supplementation may result from suboptimal levels of dietary nicotinic acid."[209] In contrast, in a double-blind crossover study involving 14 healthy adults and five adults with non-insulin-dependent diabetes mellitus (NIDDM), Thomas

and Gropper[215] found that daily supplemental chromium (200 μg) complexed with 1.8 mg nicotinic acid produced no statistically significant effects on plasma insulin, glucose, or lipid concentrations. However, chromium–nicotinic acid administration slightly lowered fasting plasma total and LDL cholesterol, triglyceride, and glucose concentrations and 90-minute postprandial glucose concentrations in individuals with NIDDM.

A variety of sources indicate that the synergistic effect from coadministration of niacin and chromium may be most significant in individuals with insulin resistance and a predisposition for type 2 diabetes mellitus.[216,217] Such coadministration also can produce an enhanced effect in reducing triglycerides and elevating HDL cholesterol, often allowing for efficacy of niacin at a reduced dose.[200] Moreover, low-dose niacin can be effective in reducing plasma fibrinogen levels (elevated levels being associated with thrombotic risk) in subjects with peripheral vascular disease.[200,201]

Individuals who do not respond to administration of chromium may have inadequate levels of vitamin B₃. Coadministration may be beneficial. However, inadvertent, excessive, or unsupervised coadministration might theoretically induce a hypoglycemic state in patients taking prescription diabetes medications. This largely unexplored territory is further confounded by the possibility that niacin in larger doses may contribute to insulin resistance. Patient caution, and possibly supervision by a health care professional experienced in nutritional therapeutics, may be appropriate in the unlikely event (in the absence of prescription antidiabetic medication) that such supplementation induces hypoglycemia.

Phytosterols

Phytosterols

Yeganeh et al.[218] investigated the effects on lipid profile and atherosclerosis of combining dietary phytosterols with niacin or fenofibrate in apolipoprotein E–knockout mice. In contrast to fenofibrate, "niacin caused an increase of 150% in HDL-cholesterol concentrations and a decrease of 22% in total cholesterol levels which were associated with significant reductions in atherosclerotic lesion size as compared to controls."

Policosanol

Policosanol

Policosanol, a mixture of long-chain (13- to 24-carbon) fatty alcohols derived from sugarcane, brown rice, or beeswax, may exert many of the same therapeutic effects as statin drugs without the associated risks, especially the known adverse effect on coenzyme Q10 synthesis.[219-223] Research on policosanol as a monotherapy has thus far not lived up to earlier claims.[224] Well-designed and adequately powered clinical trials of extended duration are warranted to determine whether coadministration of policosanol and low-dose niacin or inositol hexaniacinate might produce the effects on intermittent claudication, dyslipidemias, coronary disease, and cardiovascular mortality demonstrated by statins, with or without niacin.

S-Adenosylmethionine (SAMe)

S-Adenosylmethionine (SAMe)

The hepatotoxicity of niacin reflects, to a significant degree, the high demand for methyl groups imposed by niacin catabolism, leading to a reduction in hepatic levels of SAMe. The depletion of the hepatic SAMe pool plays a role in decreased detoxification activity and is similar to hepatotoxic effects of ethanol, methotrexate, and niacinamide. Such depletion of SAMe by niacin is likely to play a major role in the elevation of plasma homocysteine and other adverse effects associated with high-dose niacin intake.[60] Coadministration of SAMe may decrease adverse effects associated with niacin. Well-designed and adequately powered clinical trials are warranted to determine the efficacy of such a therapeutic approach.

Vitamin B₆ (Pyridoxine)

Vitamin B₆ (Pyridoxine)

Pharmacological doses of niacin can interfere with the metabolism of methionine, leading to hyperhomocysteinemia and hypocysteinemia. Coadministration of vitamin B₆ with niacin could reasonably be expected to mitigate such effects. Basu and Mann[58] found that vitamin B₆ can normalize the homocysteine-altered sulfur amino acid status of rats fed diets containing pharmacological levels of niacin, without reducing niacin's hypolipidemic effects.

For several decades a number of clinicians have reported that vitamin B₆ and niacin have been effective in managing patients diagnosed with schizophrenia and related psychiatric conditions; research findings, however, have been mixed. Such use has led to suggestions that coadministration of vitamin B₆ and niacin might produce a beneficial additive or synergistic effect that could enhance therapeutic outcomes.[225,226] In a 48-week study, conducted as part of the Canadian Mental Health Association Collaborative Study, Petrie et al.[227] found that coadministration of both nicotinic acid and pyridoxine with conventional neuroleptic treatment did not produce the significant therapeutic changes that resulted from coadministration of either nutrient (nicotinic acid or pyridoxine).

Zinc

Zinc

Enhanced zinc intake appears to cause activation of niacin metabolism and increase the excretion of niacin metabolites N′methylnicotinamide (N′MN) and N′methyl-2-pyridone-5-carboxamide (2-PYR), especially in a context of nutrient depletion. In a series of experiments involving niacin-depleted rats and then human subjects with alcoholic pellagra, Vannucchi et al.[228,229] found that zinc interacts with niacin metabolism through a probable mediation by vitamin B₆.

The 231 citations for this monograph, as well as additional reference literature, are located under Vitamin B₃ (Niacin) on the CD at the back of the book.

Vitamin B₆

Nutrient Name: Vitamin B$_6$.
Synonyms: Adermine hydrochloride, pyridoxal (PL), pyridoxine (PN), pyridoxamine (PM), and their phosphate derivatives: pyridoxal 5′-phosphate (PLP or P5P), pyridoxine 5′-phosphate (PNP), pyridoxamine, pyridoxamine 5′-phospate (PNP), pyridoxine hydrochloride.
Related Substance: Pyritinol.

Summary

Drug/Class Interaction Type	Mechanism and Significance	Management
Amiodarone ☼/⊕✗/✗	Amiodarone typically causes cutaneous photosensitivity with increased risk of sunburn. This effect, which usually is slow to resolve even after drug discontinuation, is most likely due to drug-induced oxidative stress on erythrocyte membranes. Coadministration of B$_6$ may ameliorate this adverse effect without impairing therapeutic activity of amiodarone.	Pyridoxine may be beneficial in preventing or reversing inflammatory reaction due to amiodarone.
Anticonvulsant medications Barbiturates ✗✗/✗✗✗/⊕✗/⊕ ⊕/☼/ ◇≈≈/◇	Anticonvulsant medications, especially carbamazepine and valproic acid, may displace pyridoxal 5′-phosphate (PLP), interfere with activity of pyridoxine-related coenzymes, and deplete these B$_6$ and interdependent nutrients. However, phenobarbital and phenytoin may elevate levels of B$_6$ (and B$_{12}$). Anticonvulsants can cause or aggravate hyperhomocysteinemia. Coadministration can mitigate adverse effects and may enhance therapeutic effect (e.g., valproic acid, phenobarbital). Potential for accelerated drug metabolism (and decreased circulating levels), but substantive and consistent evidence lacking, and probably only with high-dose pyridoxine. Vitamin B$_6$ is a known anticonvulsant. Further research needed.	Low-dose coadministration of pyridoxine (with B$_{12}$, riboflavin, and folate) may be beneficial, but interaction can vary depending on medication; anticonvulsant polytherapy known for greater adverse effects. Assess homocysteine and consider testing for MTHFR SNPs. Coadministration requires clinical management with regular monitoring.
Chemotherapy ☼/⊕✗/✗	Vitamin B$_6$ may mitigate certain drug-induced adverse effects but can impair therapeutic activity of some agents. Pyridoxine coadministration can reduce or reverse palmar-plantar erythrodysesthesia (hand-foot) syndrome associated with 5-fluorouracil, docetaxel, and doxorubicin HCl liposome injection without impairing drug activity. However, while B$_6$ may significantly reduce altretamine-associated neurotoxicity, it may also adversely affect response duration in a cisplatin (CDDP)—hexamethylmelamine regimen. Limited data suggest that further research warranted.	Coadministration can be beneficial but may impair drug activity of some agents. Watch for drug-induced adverse effects. Supervise closely and monitor regularly. Use with altretamine generally contraindicated.
Doxylamine ⊕⊕	Vitamin B$_6$ is effective for many women with nausea and vomiting of pregnancy and is generally considered safe. Combination of doxylamine and pyridoxine is effective in reducing the severity of such symptoms. Claims of adverse effects largely disproved. Available by prescription in some countries; Diclectin in Canada.	Consider doxylamine prescription for women with nausea and vomiting of pregnancy. Supportive dialogue and informed decision making especially important. Monitor as always during pregnancy. Ginger may also be beneficial.
Erythropoiesis-stimulating agents ≈≈/◇⊕ ⊕/☼/⊕ ⊕	EPO therapy increases hemoglobin synthesis, which can decrease erythrocyte pyridoxine status and increase nutritional requirements. Further, vitamin B$_6$ deficiency is common in patients with chronic renal failure, during dialysis, and with furosemide. Even absent signs of deficiency, administration of B$_6$ can prevent or reverse adverse effects, as well as sequelae of accompanying hemodialysis, such as peripheral polyneuropathy. Nutrient support is unlikely to impair EPO efficacy. Continued research warranted.	Coadministration of low-dose to moderate-dose vitamin B$_6$ can be beneficial, especially with folic acid. Supervise closely and monitor regularly, especially with renal failure.
Furosemide Loop diuretics ≈≈/☼	Furosemide acutely increases urinary excretion of B$_6$ (as well as vitamin C) in chronic renal failure; accompanying excretion of oxalic acid may mitigate tendency to accumulate oxalic acid.	Coadministration can be beneficial, especially with renal failure and/or dialysis. Monitor levels of vitamins B$_6$ and C. Supervise closely.
Gentamicin Aminoglycoside antibiotics ☼/◇≈≈/≈≈/⊕≈	Gentamicin and PLP tend to complex. This can interfere with B$_6$ metabolism, particularly renal PLP, and contribute to B$_6$ depletion. Concomitant B$_6$ appears to prevent gentamicin-induced adverse effects, particularly nephrotoxicity, without reducing drug efficacy. However, even though administration of PLP may reduce severity of symptoms, it may not prevent nephrotoxicity. Clinical trials needed to confirm limited but consistent findings from animal experiments.	Coadministration of vitamin B$_6$ may be beneficial and, at low dose, safe. No adverse effects probable.
Haloperidol Neuroleptic agents ◇≈≈/☼	Haloperidol and related neuroleptics can cause tardive dyskinesia, dystonia and other parkinsonian symptoms, most likely due to oxidative stress and lipid peroxidation. Concomitant B$_6$ can prevent or reduce such drug-induced extrapyramidal symptoms, even in the absence of deficiency signs, but may not enhance therapeutic outcomes. Nutrient support is not likely to impair drug efficacy. Further research warranted.	Coadminister pyridoxine, especially with long-term therapy. High-dose B$_6$ may be necessary and will require close supervision. Monitor for signs of deficiency or excess; standard assays may not reveal CNS levels.
Hydralazine ≈≈/◇≈≈/⊕✗/◇◇	Hydralazine and B$_6$ can bind to form inactive complex excreted in urine. This pharmacokinetic interaction may decrease hydralazine availability, deplete pyridoxine, and impair B$_6$-related functions. Preliminary evidence suggests	Coadministration of vitamin B$_6$ may be beneficial, but moderate-level doses warrant supervision and regular monitoring. Separate intake. Impairment of drug efficacy improbable.

Summary

Drug/Class Interaction Type	Mechanism and Significance	Management
	that pyridoxine-deficiency neuropathy and other well-known hydralazine-induced adverse effects are caused by its action as a B_6 antagonist, but evidence is lacking to prove benefits of B_6 coadministration. Clinical trials needed to confirm limited but consistent findings from animal experiments.	
Isoniazid, rifampin Antitubercular agents ◇≈≈/≈≈/☼/⊕✗/✗	Isoniazid and cycloserine are pyridoxine antagonists that produce a functional vitamin B_6 deficiency. Thus, antitubercular drugs can cause adverse effects, such as anemia or peripheral neuropathies, which may be prevented or reduced by B_6 (as well as B_3 and folic acid). Further, B_6 depletion is common among at-risk populations, and disease process of tuberculosis may aggravate deficiency. In some cases, pyridoxine has been inadequate to reverse toxic drug effects such as seizures. Routine coadministration of B_6 remains controversial despite a history of effective clinical application, evidence of benefit, and lack of evidence demonstrating adverse effects.	Coadministration of vitamin B_6 (and niacin and folic acid) may be beneficial. Separate intake. Low risk of adverse effects from B_6 at typical doses. Impairment of drug efficacy improbable. High-dose pyridoxine, often intravenously, may be necessary in severe cases. Supervise closely and monitor regularly. Discontinue medication if signs of hepatotoxicity.
Levodopa, carbidopa, benserazide Antiparkinsonian medications ✗✗/◇≈≈/☼	PLP acts as a cofactor in conversion of levodopa to dopamine. Thus, high levels of pyridoxine intake can accelerate peripheral metabolism of levodopa to dopamine, reduce the availability of dopa for conversion to dopamine, and impair the therapeutic activity of levodopa. A dopa-decarboxylase inhibitor (DDI; e.g., carbidopa, benserazide) can reduce excessive metabolism of levodopa and increase amounts available to the CNS. Conversely, as a B_6 antagonist, levodopa can increase metabolic requirements for pyridoxine. Concomitant low-dose B_6, in the presence of a DDI, can prevent or reverse nutrient depletion and adverse sequelae.	Avoid supplemental intake of vitamin B with levodopa monotherapy. No contraindication with carbidopa or benserazide. Coadministration of vitamin B_6 may prevent or reduce B_6 deficiency. Supervise closely and monitor regularly.
Methotrexate ◇≈≈	Methotrexate is known to elevate homocysteine levels by interfering with B_6- and folate-dependent reactions and may thereby increase risks of vascular disease. Vitamin B_6 is depleted by inflammation and tends to be particularly depleted in individuals with rheumatoid arthritis. Concomitant B_6 may reduce adverse effects without impairing drug activity in treatment of rheumatoid arthritis. Further research warranted, especially with regard to genomic variability.	Coadministration of vitamin B_6 and folic acid may be beneficial. Impairment of drug efficacy improbable at low to moderate doses and in nononcological settings. Consider genomic assessment. Supervise and monitor.
Neomycin ≈≈≈☼	Neomycin may interfere with activity of B_6, directly and through its effects on interdependent nutrients. Evidence is limited and dated but suggests that neomycin for longer than 2 weeks may have adverse effects on B_6 status, particularly in the presence of compromised nutritional status, other medications, and comorbid conditions. Further research warranted.	Coadministration of vitamin B_6 and broad range of nutrients, plus probiotics, may be beneficial, especially with extended neomycin therapy.
Oral contraceptives (OCs) ☼/⊕⊕⊕	OCs can impair 5-hydroxytryptophan decarboxylase in the tryptophan to niacinamide pathway and thus decrease serotonin levels. Higher estrogen doses may aggravate symptoms in some cases. Vitamin B_6 may reduce OC-related adverse effects, especially in women with compromised nutritional status, but often also in those with no measurable B_6 deficiency. Evidence is mixed but appears inadequate to confirm the necessity of routine nutrient support. Further research warranted.	Coadministration of vitamin B_6, preferably with folic acid, may prevent or reduce adverse effects. No adverse effects probable at typical doses, but higher doses may be indicated, and monitoring would be appropriate.
Penicillamine ◇◇/≈≈/☼	Penicillamine is a pyridoxine antagonist that reacts with PLP to form a metabolically inactive thiazolidine. Vitamin B_6 activity can be impaired and, over time, a deficiency may develop. Concomitant vitamin B_6 may counteract potential adverse effects such as anemia and peripheral neuritis. Separating intake can avoid any decrease in either agent's activity.	Coadministration of vitamin B_6 may be beneficial. Separate intake. Low risk of adverse effects from B_6 at typical doses. Impairment of drug efficacy improbable.
Phenelzine Monoamine oxidase-B inhibitors ◇◇/⊕✗/≈≈/☼	Phenelzine may act as pyridoxine antagonist by reacting with PLP to form metabolically inactive hydrazone compound and could reduce blood levels of vitamin B_6. Administration of B_6 reported to reverse drug-induced effects such as neuropathy. Separating intake would reduce risk of any decrease in either agent's activity. Evidence limited but consistent with accepted pharmacological knowledge.	Coadministration of vitamin B_6 may be prevent depletion and reverse adverse drug effects. Separate intake. Low risk of adverse effects from B_6 at typical doses. Supervise and monitor.
Tetracycline antibiotics ⊕⊕/⊕✗/◇◇/≈≈	Simultaneous intake of pyridoxine and other B vitamins with tetracycline-class antibiotics can reduce absorption and bioavailability of both/all agents. Antibacterial effect on intestinal flora and gut ecology can produce secondary adverse effects on B-vitamin status and inflammatory processes. Evidence limited but consistent with accepted pharmacological knowledge.	Separate intake if concurrent administration indicated or necessary. Probiotic flora beneficial after high-dose and/or extended antibiotics.
Theophylline, aminophylline ◇≈≈/≈≈/☼/⊕	Theophylline can cause seizures, hand tremor, and other adverse effects by acting as potent, noncompetitive inhibitor of pyridoxal kinase and by inducing pyridoxal kinase activity. Consequently, circulating PLP concentrations may be depressed and body stores of pyridoxine depleted, but circulating pyridoxal levels may remain unchanged. Vitamin B_6 administration can counter increased intake requirements and may reduce drug-	Coadministration of vitamin B_6 may prevent depletion and reverse adverse drug effects. Low risk of adverse effects from B_6 at typical doses. Supervise and monitor.

Continued

Summary

Drug/Class Interaction Type	Mechanism and Significance	Management
	induced adverse effects without impairing the therapeutic activity of theophylline.	
Tricyclic antidepressants (TCAs) ⊕⊕	PLP-dependent enzymes play a role in serotonin synthesis. Deficiency of vitamin B$_6$ more common in depressed individuals than in general population. Coadministration may prevent or reverse depletion as well as augment clinical response to TCAs through an additive or synergistic effect. Evidence is consistent but limited; continued research warranted.	Coadministration of B$_6$ can be supportive and may enhance clinical response, especially with deficiency. Consider B$_1$, B$_2$, B$_{12}$, and folic acid. Supervise closely and monitor regularly. Counsel exercise and healthier dietary choices.

NUTRIENT DESCRIPTION

Chemistry and Forms

Vitamin B$_6$ is a water-soluble vitamin that was first isolated in the 1930s by Paul Gyorgy. Catalyzed by pyridoxal kinase, an adenosine triphosphate (ATP)–dependent enzyme, pyridoxal, pyridoxamine, and pyridoxine are converted to pyridoxal 5′-phosphate, the active coenzyme form, which plays the most significant role in human metabolism. Thus, "vitamin B$_6$" is a generic term used to collectively describe the six related compounds that exhibit the biological activity of pyridoxine: pyridoxal (PL), pyridoxine (PN), pyridoxamine (PM), and their phosphate derivatives: pyridoxal 5′-phosphate (PLP or P5P), pyridoxine 5′-phosphate (PNP), and pyridoxamine 5′-phospate (PNP).

In addition to being water soluble, pyridoxine is stable in heat, especially in acid media, but unstable in alkaline solutions and very unstable to light.

Physiology and Function

Humans cannot synthesize vitamin B$_6$, so dietary intake is necessary. Pyridoxine and its vitamers are absorbed in the upper small intestine by simple diffusion. The more acidic the environment, the greater is the absorption. After being transported to the liver, pyridoxine and pyridoxal (oxidized by pyridoxine oxidase) are phosphorylated by pyridoxal kinase to form pyridoxine 5′-phosphate and pyridoxal 5′-phosphate (PLP, the active coenzyme), which is then exported from the liver bound to albumin. Tissue uptake is through extracellular dephosphorylation, followed by metabolic trapping intracellularly as PLP.

Through a variety of reactions involving transamination, deamination, desulfuration, decarboxylation, side-chain cleavage, and one-carbon metabolism, pyridoxine and approximately 100 PLP-dependent enzymes are involved in amino acid metabolism; glycogen release and blood glucose regulation; hemoglobin synthesis and oxygen transport; synthesis of niacin and a variety of lipids, hormones, and neurotransmitters; cysteine metabolism and homocysteine regulation; and formation of alpha-aminolevulinic acid, sphingolipids, and intrinsic factor.

Vitamin B$_6$ plays a central role in the metabolism of amino acids through the transfer of NH$_2$ to form keto acids and enable oxidation (i.e., transamination) and the removal of amino groups from certain amino acids (i.e., deamination), both reactions enabling their use as sources for energy. Similarly, transfer of the sulfhydryl group from methionine to serine (i.e., desulfuration or trans-sulfuration) enables the formation of cysteine and regulation of homocysteine. The removal of COOH groups from certain amino acids to yield amines (i.e., decarboxylation) is central to the synthesis of neurotransmitters such as serotonin, norepinephrine, and histamine from tryptophan, tyrosine, and histidine,

respectively, and the conversion of phosphatidylserine to phosphatidylethanolamine in phospholipid synthesis. Relatedly, PLP is a coenzyme in the synthesis of niacin from tryptophan, thereby supplementing niacin intake from the diet. Dopamine and gamma-aminobutyric acid (GABA) are likewise depen-dent on B$_6$ coenzymes, as is the formation of sphingolipids involved in the development of the myelin sheath surrounding nerve cells. Notably, PLP can be highly concentrated in the brain even when blood levels are low, and dementia may be associated with reduced transport. Pyridoxal 5′-phosphate–dependent enzymes catalyze these and many other essential metabolic transformations.

Equally important is the role of B$_6$, as well as folic acid, B$_{12}$, and B$_2$, as the source of coenzymes which participate in one-carbon metabolism. Thus, the freely reversible interconversion of serine and glycine is catalyzed by serine hydroxymethyltransferase (SHMT), a reaction that is both folate dependent and PLP dependent. This mobilization of folate-linked single-carbon functional groups enables the biosynthesis of purines and 2′-deoxythymidine 5′-monophosphate and the remethylation of homocysteine to methionine.

A significant portion of the PLP in the human body is bound to glycogen phosphorylase in muscle tissue and in the liver. PLP functions as a coenzyme in the phosphorolytic cleavage of glycogen as glucose-1-phosphate; it also serves as a coenzyme in gluconeogenesis, where amino acids are used to produce glucose. Vitamin B$_6$ nutriture may have a beneficial effect on glucose tolerance by activating apokynureninase or kynureninase that has been inactivated by undergoing transamination, particularly under the influence of elevated estrogen levels.

Pyridoxal 5′-phosphate functions as a coenzyme in the formation of alpha-aminolevulinic acid, which is a precursor of heme. Heme is a component of hemoglobin and thus is critical to the formation of erythrocytes and function of transport oxygen. Both pyridoxal and PLP are able to bind to the hemoglobin molecule.

Vitamin B$_6$ plays a role in modulating the activities of several major hormones. PLP can bind to steroid hormone receptors and decrease the effects of estrogen, testosterone, and other steroid receptors through competitive inhibition. Notably, exogenous estrogens (i.e., oral contraceptives) may deplete vitamin B$_6$ levels, possibly through inhibition of kynureninase by estrogen metabolites and induction of tryptophan oxidase, causing increased oxidative metabolism of tryptophan.

NUTRIENT IN CLINICAL PRACTICE

Known or Potential Therapeutic Uses

The role of vitamin B$_6$ in conventional medicine is controversial but evolving. Other than prevention and treatment of vitamin B_6 deficiency, standard practice primarily limits the application of B_6 to intravenous administration for pyridoxine-dependent seizures in infants and adjunctive treatment of acute toxicity from cycloserine, hydralazine, or isoniazid overdose. Furthermore, warnings of potential adverse effects from supplemental use of pyridoxine appear abundantly within conventional medical literature and press releases. Nevertheless, for decades practitioners of nutritional therapeutics have reported significant efficacy in the treatment of individuals with premenstrual syndrome, estrogen overload, adverse effects of oral contraceptives, nausea and vomiting in pregnancy, depression, carpal tunnel syndrome, and asthma. Enhancement of cognitive function and immune system activity, as well as prevention of kidney stones, have also been proposed by numerous researchers and clinicians. The role of B_6, independently or in conjunction with folate, riboflavin, and vitamin B_{12}, in regulating hyperhomocysteinemia and reducing the risk of and improving outcomes in vascular disease and heart attacks remains inconclusive. Well-designed, long-term clinical trials investigating both primary and secondary prevention and integrative therapeutics are warranted.

Low circulating vitamin B_6 is associated with elevation of the inflammation marker C-reactive protein independently of plasma homocysteine levels. Furthermore, inflammation appears to induce a tissue-specific depletion of vitamin B_6 as vitamin B_6 coenzymes are used to meet the higher demands of certain tissues during inflammation and the circulating concentration of PLP declines.

Historical/Ethnomedicine Precedent

Vitamn B_6 has not been used historically as an isolated nutrient.

Possible Uses

Acne, age-related cognitive decline, alcohol withdrawal support, Alzheimer's disease, amenorrhea, anemia (if deficient, and for genetic vitamin B_6–responsive anemia), aphthous ulcers, asthma, atherosclerosis, attention deficit disorder, autism, bulimia, burns, carpal tunnel syndrome, celiac disease, childhood intelligence (for deficiency), colorectal cancer (risk reduction), coronary artery disease (risk reduction), dementia, depression, diabetic neuropathy, fibrocystic breast disease, gestational diabetes, human immunodeficiency virus (HIV) support, hyperhomocysteinemia, hypoglycemia, immune response enhancement (critically ill patients), infant seizures (inborn error in B_6 metabolism), iron-resistant anemia, low back pain, monosodium glutamate (MSG) sensitivity or poisoning, myocardial infarction, nausea and vomiting of pregnancy, nephrolithiasis, Osgood-Schlatter disease, Parkinson's disease, photosensitivity, presurgery and postsurgery support, preeclampsia, pregnancy and postpartum support, premenstrual syndrome, retinopathy, rheumatoid arthritis, schizophrenia, seborrheic dermatitis, sickle cell anemia, sideroblastic anemia, stroke prevention, tardive dyskinesia, toxemia of pregnancy, vertigo.

Deficiency Symptoms

Vitamin B_6 deficiency can manifest as impaired immunity, irritability, depression, confusion, skin lesions, inflammation of the tongue, sores or ulcers of the mouth, and ulcers of the skin at the corners of the mouth. Inflammation appears to induce a tissue-specific depletion of vitamin B_6. Adults given

deoxypyridoxine, a B_6 antagonist, developed depression, nausea, vomiting, mucous membrane lesions, seborrheic dermatitis, peripheral neuritis, and a range of neurological effects, including ataxia, hyperacusis, hyperirritability, altered mobility and alertness, abnormal head movements, and convulsions.

Although frank deficiencies are considered rare, marginal vitamin B_6 status may be relatively common.[1] Deficiencies of vitamin B_6 are usually related to an overall deficiency of all the B vitamins. The risk of B_6 deficiency or insufficiency is greatest in alcoholics, women using oral contraceptives, individuals suffering from depression, and patients with chronic fatigue syndrome and kidney failure. However, several surveys have found that daily intake of B_6 is less than the recommended dietary allowance (RDA) for a significant proportion of the population. In the United States, 90% of women and 71% of men reportedly have diets deficient in B_6, with dietary intake of vitamin B_6 averaging approximately 1.5 mg and 2 mg daily for women and men, respectively.[2] In industrialized societies, children and the elderly experience B_6 deficiency more than any other B vitamin, with men and women over 60 years of age consuming an average of approximately 1.2 mg/day and 1.0 mg/day, respectively.[3,4] The milling of grain, which removes 40% to 90 % of naturally occurring B_6, and exposure to medications and environmental pollutants that act as B_6 antagonists constitute the greatest causes of vitamin B_6 deficiency or increased metabolic requirement; food fortification may mitigate some of these losses. Other factors associated with increased risk of deficiency or insufficiency and increased metabolic need include life stages characterized by rapid growth, such as pregnancy and lactation, childhood, and adolescence; increased dietary protein intake; high alcohol and coffee intake; institutionalization; tobacco smoking; chronic digestive and malabsorption disorders, including irritable bowel syndrome, diarrhea, liver disease; and chronic diseases, including asthma, diabetes, heart disease, and rheumatoid arthritis. Some individuals on a very restricted vegetarian diet may be at increased risk of insufficient B_6 intake.

Dietary Sources

Calf liver, turkey, tuna, spinach, banana, lentils, and potatoes are among the dietary sources relatively rich in vitamin B_6. Other foods containing B_6 include organ meats, pork, poultry, milk, egg yolks, fish, corn, legumes, seeds, grains, wheat, wheat germ, wheat bran, brewer's yeast, green leafy vegetables, green beans, avocados, cantaloupe, cabbage, green peppers, carrots, soybeans, blackstrap molasses, walnuts, peanuts, and pecans.

Vitamin B_6 in food sources appears as pyridoxine, pyridoxal, and pyridoxamine. Not all forms of dietary B_6 are equally bioavailable. In a mixed diet, approximately 75% of vitamin B_6 present is bioavailable. Pyridoxine glucoside, found in certain plant foods, exhibits only 50% the bioavailability as vitamin B_6 from other food sources or supplements. Furthermore, cooking and food processing can destroy a significant portion of vitamin B_6 originally present in foods. Freezing of vegetables decreases B_6 content by 20%, canning by 54%, and processing of grains by 40% to 90%.

The dietary requirement for vitamin B_6 is proportional to the level of protein consumption, ranging from 1.4 to 2.0 mg daily for a normal adult. The requirement for vitamin B_6 during pregnancy and lactation increases approximately by 0.6 mg daily.

Nutrient Preparations Available

Pyridoxine hydrochloride and pyridoxal 5′-phosphate (PLP) are the more commonly available forms, with pyridoxal and pyridoxamine also being available as supplements. Pyridoxine hydrochloride is the form most widely used in conventional medicine and typical supplements and has the advantage of efficient transport through cell membranes and the ability to cross the blood-brain barrier. However, many practitioners experienced in nutritional therapeutics frequently administer PLP because it is the activated form and is particularly important in patients with conditions characterized by impaired conversion of pyridoxine hydrochloride to PLP, such as liver disease and zinc or magnesium deficiency. Some sources maintain that PLP is better absorbed, but these claims are contentious.

Dosage Forms Available

Capsules, liquids, liposomal sprays, lozenges, softgels, tablets, effervescent tablets, and enteric-coated tablets. Vitamin B$_6$ is usually contained in multivitamins or B-complex formulations, including chewable tablets and liquid drops for children.

Supplemental B$_6$ is best taken between or with meals, preferably with doses divided throughout the day. Individuals who experience alterations in sleep patterns with B$_6$ may benefit from emphasizing morning intake.

Dosage Range

Adult
Dietary:
   Men and women: 1.3 to 1.7 mg/day, increasing with age
   Pregnant women: 1.9 mg/day
   Lactating women: 2.0 mg/day

Note: Vitamin B$_6$ requirements rise with increased dietary protein intake. Before 1998 the U.S. RDA for vitamin B$_6$ was expressed in terms of protein intake. However, when the Food and Nutrition Board (FNB) of the Institute of Medicine revised the RDA for vitamin B$_6$ in 1998, they factored in protein intake but established fixed RDA levels.

Supplemental/Maintenance: 10 to 40 mg/day.
Optimal daily intake: Women: 50 mg/day; men: 35 mg/day.
Pharmacological/Therapeutic: 50 to 200 mg/day, occasionally as high as 500 mg daily; typically safe at levels of 200 to 300 mg daily; even so, individuals using more than 100 to 200 mg daily for more than 2 months should be supervised by a nutritionally trained health care professional.

Toxic: According to the U.S. Institute of Medicine, conservative practice recommends that adults not consume more than 100 mg of pyridoxine daily, the tolerable upper intake level (UL) for adults.[5] However, no studies have produced evidence of sensory nerve damage, as confirmed by objective neurological examination, at intakes of pyridoxine below 200 mg/day. Intakes up to 200 mg/day are usually safe in adults. Regardless, a daily dose of 500 mg should never be exceeded, even under physician supervision. Most cases of toxicity, particularly sensory neuropathy, have developed in individuals who have ingested doses of pyridoxine in excess of 1000 mg/day for extended periods.[6]

Pregnant and lactating women should avoid daily doses of vitamin B$_6$ greater than 100 mg daily. Vitamin B$_6$ crosses the placenta. However, available evidence suggests safe use during pregnancy.

Pediatric (<18 Years)
Dietary:
   Infants, birth to 6 months: 0.1 mg/(AI, adequate intake)
   Infants, 7 to 12 months: 0.3 mg/day (AI)
   Children, 1 to 3 years: 0.5 mg/day (RDA)
   Children 4 to 8 years: 0.6 mg/day (RDA)
   Children 9 to 13 years: 1.0 mg/day (RDA)
   Adolescents, 14 to 18 years: 1.2 mg/day for females; 1.3 mg/day for males (RDA)

Supplemental/Maintenance

Vitamin B$_6$ is usually not recommended for children under 12 years of age.

Pharmacological/Therapeutic

Viatmin B$_6$ is usually not recommended for children under 12 years of age, except intravenous administration for pyridoxine-dependent seizures in infants.
   Toxic: Tolerable upper intake level (UL) for vitamin B$_6$:
Infants, birth to 12 months: Not possible to establish.
   Children, 1 to 3 years: 30 mg/day
   Children, 4 to 8 years: 40 mg/day
   Children, 9 to 13 years: 60 mg/day
   Adolescents, 14 to 18 years: 80 mg/day

Laboratory Values

At present, there is no generally accepted test for assessing vitamin B$_6$ status.
   Plasma pyridoxal 5′-phosphate (P5P, PLP; active form of B$_6$): Levels less than 30 nmol/L indicate deficiency.
   Plasma total vitamin B$_6$: Levels less than 40 nmol/L indicate deficiency.
   Urinary 4-pyridoxic acid: Levels less than 3.0 μmol/day indicate deficiency; 4-pyridoxic acid is the major urinary metabolite of B$_6$.
   Erythrocyte glutamic-pyruvic (alanine) transaminase index (EGPT): A ratio greater than 1.25 (or 1.5) indicates deficiency, depending on the amount of PLP added and the method of testing.
   Enzymatic assays run before and after addition of PLP can be used to generate an activity coefficient ratio for this PLP-dependent enzyme. This represents the functional availability of erythrocyte vitamin B$_6$ in its coenzyme form. The value increases with vitamin B$_6$ deficiency.
   Erythrocyte glutamic-oxaloacetic (aspartate) transaminase index (EGOT): This dual enzymic assay is effective to detect and measure human deficiencies of both PLP and activity of this PLP-dependent enzyme.
   Serum glutamic-oxaloacetic transaminase (SGOT) reactivation: Although primarily used to diagnose and monitor the course of liver disease, decreased levels in this standard measure of aspartate transaminase (AST) can indicate pyridoxine deficiency.
   Serum B$_6$: Radioimmunoassay (RIA) of serum pyridoxal phosphate can be used to detect both vitamin B$_6$ deficiency and vitamin B$_6$ toxicity.
   Reference range: 18 to 175 nmol/L.
Tryptophan load test (tryptophan challenge): Urinary xanthurenic acid excretion greater than 65 μmol/L indicates deficiency.
Tryptophan catabolism is PLP dependent. Thus, an oral tryptophan dose (50 mg/kg for children and up to 2 g/kg for

adults) is administered and xanthurenic acid measured to provide a functional assessment of vitamin B_6 status.

SAFETY PROFILE
Overview

Although water soluble and efficiently excreted, vitamin B_6 occupies the unenviable position of being the only B vitamin for which toxicity is a reasonable concern. Although typical dosage levels in most available supplements are unlikely to produce adverse effects in most healthy individuals, concern surrounds this nutrient, as codified by regulatory agencies worldwide.

Sensory neuropathy is the primary adverse effect caused by chronic pyridoxine overdose. Other effects reported, but without established frequency, include nausea, headache, seizures (after very large intravenous doses), insomnia, suppressed lactation, increased AST levels, decreased serum folic acid levels, and miscellaneous allergic reactions.

Nutrient Adverse Effects

Peripheral neuropathy characterized by loss of reflexes and paresthesias and pain in the extremities constitutes the primary toxic effect associated with vitamin B_6 administration. Such adverse effects are almost exclusively associated with high-dose intake, in excess of 1000 mg daily, for an extended period. However, several case reports describe individuals exhibiting sensory neuropathies at dosage levels of less than 500 mg daily over several months.

Parry and Bredesen[7] described sensory neuropathy in 16 patients associated with pyridoxine abuse, defining "low-dose pyridoxine" intake as "0.2 to 5g"/day. They noted that "duration of consumption before symptoms was inversely proportional to the daily intake." Furthermore, they observed that for "all patients with adequate follow-up, improvement followed discontinuation of pyridoxine."[7]

Subsequently, Dalton and Dalton[8] published a paper from a controlled trial describing a "newly recognised neurotoxic syndrome due to pyridoxine (B_6) overdose." They reported an elevated serum B_6 level in 172 women, "of whom 60% had neurological symptoms, which disappeared when B_6 was withdrawn and reappeared in 4 cases when B_6 was restarted." They observed that the "mean dose of B_6 in the 103 women with neurological symptoms was 117 ± 92 mgs, compared with 116.2 ± 66 mgs in the control group" and noted "a significant difference (P less than 0.01) in the average duration of ingestion of B_6 in the neurotoxic group of 2.9 ± 1.9 years compared with 1.6 ± 2.1 years in controls." Finally, the documented symptoms included "paraesthesia, hyperaesthesia, bone pains, muscle weakness, numbness and fasciculation, most marked on the extremities and predominantly bilateral unless there was a history of previous trauma to the limb."[8]

Very high doses of B_6 have also been reported to produce exacerbation of acne, breast tenderness, or increased milk production (when administered while lactating). However, in reviewing all available data, the FNB concluded: "The data fail to demonstrate a causal association between pyridoxine intake and other endpoints (e.g., dermatological lesions and vitamin B_6 dependency in newborns)."[5] Large doses may theoretically result in increased urinary excretion of other B vitamins, leading to imbalances.

The adverse effects observed have been attributed to intake levels that exceed the liver's capacity to convert pyridoxine to PLP. Consequently, administration of PLP may be advantageous (compared with pyridoxine) when high doses are required for therapeutic efficacy, although this concept has not been evaluated in clinical trials, and monitoring for neurotoxicity would still be prudent.

Adverse Effects Among Specific Populations

Pregnancy and Nursing. Pregnant and lactating women should avoid daily doses of vitamin B_6 greater than 100 mg. Confirmed reports of teratogenicity are lacking.

Infants and Children. Vitamin B_6 is generally not indicated for children under 12 years of age.

Contraindications

Major contraindication is hypersensitivity to vitamin B_6 or any component of a B_6-containing preparation. A yeast-free form is advisable for individuals who are sensitive to yeast.

Precautions and Warnings

A variety of drugs can interact with vitamin B_6, and in some cases, B_6 may significantly reduce the therapeutic activity of the medication.

INTERACTIONS REVIEW
Strategic Considerations

Vitamin B_6 represents a substance that, as a dietary constituent, is widely recommended as beneficial for its physiological function and preventive effects but, as a nutritional supplement or therapeutic agent, is obscured by controversy, prejudice, and partial information. The continuing controversy over the causal role or coincident occurrence and consequent clinical significance of hyperhomocysteinemia in cerebrovascular and cardiovascular disease, and the value of folate, B_6, B_{12}, and B_2 in reducing such risks, has kept this key nutrient in the medical news for several years. However, its broader uses by health care professionals remain largely ignored by conventional practitioners and academic researchers.

Coadministration of vitamin B_6 may counter the pyridoxine-depleting effects of medications such as chemotherapy, methotrexate, theophylline, furosemide and related loop diuretics, isoniazid, cycloserine and other antitubercular agents, and thiosemicarbazide, but especially in individuals and patient populations with high incidences of compromised nutritional status, dysfunctional pharmacogenomic variations, preexisting insufficiency or deficiency, and exacerbating comedication. In most typical situations, coadministration of B_6 usually mitigates adverse effects, with or without marked deficiency, and without impairing drug efficacy.

High-dose oral contraceptives, gentamicin, neomycin, and other aminoglycoside antibiotics can both interfere with the physiological functions of B_6 and deplete available levels. Nevertheless, it appears that administration of pyridoxal 5'-phosphate (PLP, the activated form of vitamin B_6) may not prevent gentamicin-induced nephrotoxicity, even though it may reduce severity of symptoms. Likewise, with haloperidol and related neuroleptic agents, concomitant B_6 can prevent or reduce adverse effects, including drug-induced extrapyramidal symptoms, even in the absence of deficiency signs, but may not enhance therapeutic outcomes.

The situation of antiparkinsonian medications is more complicated because high levels of pyridoxine intake can accelerate peripheral metabolism of levodopa to dopamine, reducing the availability of dopa for central nervous system (CNS) conversion to dopamine, and impair the therapeutic activity of levodopa. The clinical significance of this effect is usually absent or minimal given the predominant use of low-dose B₆ and the standard practice of combining levodopa with a dopa-decarboxylase inhibitor (DDI), such as carbidopa or benserazide, to reduce excessive peripheral metabolism of levodopa and increase amounts available to the CNS. However, because levodopa acts as a vitamin B₆ antagonist, it can increase the metabolic requirements for pyridoxine. Consequently, coadministration of low-dose vitamin B₆, in the presence of a DDI, can prevent or reverse nutrient depletion and adverse sequelae.

In the case of anticonvulsant medications and related barbiturates, amiodarone, erythropoietin and other erythropoiesis-stimulating agents, or tricyclic antidepressants, the coadministration of B₆ may prevent or mitigate adverse effects and, in some cases, may potentially enhance clinical outcomes. Here the conventional use of vitamin B₆ with antitubercular medications, particularly isoniazid, represents a widely accepted example of integrative principles in action through the dual activity of reducing adverse drug-induced effects and enhancing clinical outcomes.

Although vitamin B₆ is considered an effective preventive or treatment for nausea and vomiting of pregnancy in some women, the combination of doxylamine and pyridoxine may enhance these benefits and is widely used in Canada.

In regard to pharmacokinetic interactions, substances such as tetracycline antibiotics, hydralazine, and penicillamine can bind with vitamin B₆ to form an inactive complex, which is usually excreted in the urine. These interactions tend to decrease drug availability, deplete pyridoxine, and impair B₆-related functions, athough not always to a clinically significant degree.

Somewhat similarly, phenelzine can react with PLP to form a metabolically inactive hydrazone compound and thereby reduce vitamin B₆ levels. Conversely, B₆ coadministration may reverse drug-induced effects such as neuropathy.

The broad, diverse, and profound implications of the adverse effects of antibiotics, in general, on symbiotic intestinal microflora are only beginning to receive the attention of researchers. The secondary adverse effects of such changes on B-vitamin status and inflammatory processes will undoubtedly become the subject of deeper investigation.

The primary adverse effects and risks of vitamin B₆ relate to its classic and well-described overdose symptoms, particularly neuropathies. Although frequently emphasized in the medical literature as a cause for concern, and subsequently restricted as an over-the-counter nutritional supplement in the United Kingdom, the occurrence of such adverse effects is minimal given the large number of self-prescribed users of vitamin B₆.

NUTRIENT-DRUG INTERACTIONS

Amiodarone

Amiodarone (Cordarone).

Interaction Type and Significance
☼ **Prevention or Reduction of Drug Adverse Effect**
⊕✗ **Bimodal or Variable Interaction, with Professional Management**
✗ **Potential or Theoretical Adverse Interaction of Uncertain Severity**

Probability: Evidence Base:
6. Unknown   ▽ Mixed

Effect and Mechanism of Action
Cutaneous photosensitivity, with subsequent increased tendency to sunburn, is one of the more common adverse effects associated with amiodarone, occurring in as many as 70% of patients. In rare cases, extended use of the drug ($\geq$12 months) can cause gradual onset of a slate-gray or violaceous discoloration of sun-exposed sites. Onset of photosensitivity primarily occurs during the second year of therapy, presumably from drug accumulation, and discontinuation of the medication usually leads to resolution of these effects within 2 years.[9-14] Early research by Ferguson et al.[15] indicated that amiodarone has a phototoxic potential against erythrocytes, suggesting a membrane-directed effect. Studying red blood cell hemolysis, Kahn and Fleischaker[16] reported that photo-oxidation of membrane proteins and photoperoxidation of unsaturated fatty acids of membrane lipids could be responsible for this amiodarone-induced damage. Using electron spin resonance (ESR) Guerciolini et al.[17] determined that the triggering mechanism is the creation of a long-lived excited state (triplet state) in the photosensitizer after the absorption of a photon.

Data on the effects of pyridoxine on the phototoxicity of amiodarone are mixed and inconclusive. Cozzani and Jori[18] observed inactivation of L-glutamate decarboxylase from *Escherichia coli*, sensitized by the coenzyme pyridoxal phosphate. Kaufmann[19] reported that coadministration of pyridoxine can "suppress the photosensitivity" of patients with amiodarone-induced photosensitivity. He suggested that amiodarone inhibits melanin formation in the skin via a "hypothetical anti-vitamin-B₆ effect, and that after a latent period of several months, it causes hypersensitivity to solar irradiation."[19] In response, Guerciolini et al.[17] cited the work of Cozzani and Jori, as well as other findings, and proposed that pyridoxine can enhance the phototoxicity of amiodarone, although they specifically declared that this "does not rule out a protective effect of pyridoxine *in vivo*."

Research
In a randomized controlled trial, Mulrow et al.[20] indicated that pyridoxine may exacerbate amiodarone-induced photosensitivity. However, no subsequent research or reports have corroborated this preliminary findings, and the predominant trend in the available data suggests that a protective effect is probable.

Reports
In a letter, Kaufmann[19] described successful amelioration of photosensitivity with coadministration of oral pyridoxine in three patients who had experienced "a marked tendency to sunburn, caused by amiodarone." These patients were able to continue amiodarone treatment, with initial pyridoxine doses ranging from 40 to 300 mg, and maintain good tolerance of solar irradiation with 20 to 40 mg daily doses. He noted that the vitamin B₆ "in no way impaired the desired pharmacological effects of amiodarone" and concluded that the "minimum effective daily dose of pyridoxine remains to be established."[19]

In related research, Ross and Moss[21] reported two cases of erythropoietic protoporphyria in which use of pyridoxine was associated with a marked reduction in photosensitivity without evidence of adverse effects. These patients had been only moderately responsive to beta-carotene and sunscreens.

Nutritional Therapeutics, Clinical Concerns, and Adaptations
Physicians prescribing amiodarone for extended use as an antiarrhythmic and coronary vasodilator are advised to be watchful for cutaneous toxicity symptoms and consider coadministration of pyridoxine as a preventive or in response to such effects.

Despite the suggestion of potential adverse effects from concomitant intake of amiodarone and vitamin B₆ based on preliminary research, no clinical research or qualified case reports have confirmed such concerns. An initial trial dose of 100 to 200 mg pyridoxine daily for 3 months followed by 20 to 40 mg daily would usually be appropriate. However, both the scientific literature and clinical experience show that the effective dosage levels to prevent or reverse adverse effects of amiodarone vary considerably among individual patients, and that initial dosage levels are typically larger than maintenance doses. Close supervision is warranted during initial higher dose levels because of the possible, but improbable, risk of B₆-induced neuropathy.

Short-term use of amiodarone prophylaxis with major cardiac surgery is unlikely to result in drug accumulation, although administration of vitamin B₆ (as well as folic acid, B₂, and B₁₂) may be indicated in the strategic approach to cardiovascular care in such individuals, at least in relationship to hyperhomocysteinemia.

Anticonvulsant Medications and Related Barbiturates

Evidence: Carbamazepine (Carbatrol, Tegretol), divalproex semisodium, divalproex sodium (Depakote Delayed Release; Depakote ER), fosphenytoin (Cerebyx, Mesantoin), gabapentin (Neurontin), mephenytoin, phenobarbital (phenobarbitone; Luminal, Solfoton), phenytoin (diphenylhydantoin; Dilantin, Phenytek), primidone (Mysoline), valproate sodium (Depacon), valproic acid (Depakene Syrup, Depakene)

Similar properties but evidence lacking for extrapolation: Acetazolamide (Diamox, Diamox Sequels), amobarbital (Amytal), aprobarbital (Alurate), butabarbital (Butisol), butalbital (Fiorinal, Fioricet), clonazepam (Klonopin), clorazepate (Gen-Xene, Tranxene), diazepam (Valium), ethosuximide (Zarontin), ethotoin (Peganone), felbamate (Felbatol), levetiracetam (Keppra), mephobarbital (Mebaral), methohexital (Brevital), methsuximide (Celontin), oxcarbazepine (GP 47680, oxycarbamazepine; Trileptal), pheneturide (ethylphenacemide), pentobarbital (Nembutal), secobarbital (Seconal), thiopental (Pentothal), tiagabine (Gabitril), topiramate (Topamax), trimethadione (Tridione), zonisamide (Zonegran).

Related but evidence against extrapolation: Lamotrigine (Lamictal).

See also Folic Acid monograph.

Interaction Type and Significance

✗✗　　Minimal to Mild Adverse Interaction—Vigilance Necessary

✗✗✗　Potentially Harmful or Serious Adverse Interaction—Avoid

⊕✗　　Bimodal or Variable Interaction, with Professional Management

⊕⊕　　Beneficial or Supportive Interaction, with Professional Management

☼　　　Prevention or Reduction of Drug Adverse Effect

◇≈≈　Drug-Induced Adverse Effect on Nutrient Function, Coadministration Therapeutic, with Professional Management

◇　　　Adverse Drug Effect on Nutritional Therapeutics, Strategic Concern

Probability:
4. Plausible

Evidence Base:
▽ Preliminary and
▽ Mixed

Nutrient Depletion
Probability:
4. Improbable or
3. Possible

Evidence Base:
◉◉ Emerging and
▽ Mixed

Coadministration Benefit
Probability:
3. Possible or 2. Probable

Evidence Base:
◉◉ Emerging

Effect and Mechanism of Action

High doses of pyridoxine can increase metabolism and decrease serum levels of certain anticonvulsants and barbiturates, specifically phenytoin and phenobarbitone, in some individuals, although not in others. Pyridoxine may accelerate hepatic metabolism of antiepileptic drugs (AEDs) by increasing enzyme activity.[22] However, no mechanism for this reported activity has been confirmed.

Chronic anticonvulsant therapy can exert differing effects on vitamin B₆ metabolism and levels, which may vary for different individuals or different agents or act through diverse mechanisms. Plasma pyridoxal 5′-phosphate (PLP) levels can be significantly decreased with chronic use of carbamazepine and valproic acid, especially in children. Both valproic acid and PLP are strongly protein bound, and valproic acid tends to displace PLP from protective protein-binding sites and induce a deficit in PLP.[23] Conversely, prolonged phenobarbitone and phenytoin (diphenylhydantoin) therapy is associated with fine structural changes in hepatocytes and significantly elevated serum levels of vitamins B₆ and B₁₂.[24]

Pyridoxine-dependent seizures result from an increased genetically derived requirement for the nutrient within the CNS. Researchers have reported that, in some but not all patients, the "binding affinity of glutamate decarboxylase (GAD) to the active form of pyridoxine is low in cases of pyridoxine-dependent seizures (PDS) and that a quantitative imbalance between excitatory (i.e. glutamate) and inhibitory (i.e. gamma-aminobutyric acid, GABA) neurotransmitters could cause refractory seizures."[25] Continued administration of vitamin B₆ in pharmacological doses has contributed to a marked reduction in infantile seizures in some cases. The combination of B₆ and valproic acid or phenobarbital may work synergistically in these patients, even in patients lacking typical indicators of B₆ deficiency.[26]

The reported effect of AEDs on vitamin B₆ levels may be causal to or exacerbating of the elevated levels of homocysteine (Hcy) found in some individuals with seizure disorders using anticonvulsant medications or barbiturates.[27-33] Although Hcy has been used as an experimental convulsant, this hyperhomocysteinemia may be attributable to the underlying disease process, the medication, or both. Enzyme-inducing AEDs, including phenytoin, phenobarbital, and primidone, are associated with numerous adverse effects on B vitamins and Hcy regulation, including low PLP concentrations, decreased folate absorption, decreased plasma folate concentrations, low riboflavin concentrations, and elevated total Hcy concentrations in adults and in children. These effects vary among individuals, with genetic variables, with monotherapy or polytherapy, and with drug mechanisms of action. Coadministration of B₆, folate, and related nutrients, at low to moderate doses, may normalize Hcy levels, particularly in patients receiving AED monotherapy.

Research and Reports

Over more than three decades, researchers have reported numerous possible and proven interactions between vitamin B₆ and related nutrients in individuals undergoing therapy with anticonvulsants and barbiturates. Evidence indicates the probability of interactions that might adversely affect drug activity and nutrient levels and function, but other research suggests that coadministration under medical supervision may be beneficial in certain patients by mitigating drug-induced hyperhomocysteinemia or enhancing therapeutic response.

Effect on Drug Activity. A study conducted by Hansson and Sillanpaa[22] constitutes the primary, if not singular, published paper mentioned in most accounts of the interactions between vitamin B$_6$ and the broad range of medications commonly clustered together as antiepileptic drugs. In many instances the details of the report have been misrepresented, exaggerated, or overextended. In this short letter the authors reported marked drops in serum concentrations of phenytoin or phenobarbitone in a small number of patients receiving "long-term multiple antiepileptic medications," most of whom were significantly compromised with "non-progressive brain-damage syndromes in addition to mental retardation and epilepsy." Doses of pyridoxine of 200 or 400 mg daily for 4 weeks elicited the most frequent changes in drug levels, up to 50% in some cases. However, in "several other cases, pyridoxine added to the anticonvulsant treatment did not alter the phenytoin or phenobarbitone concentrations." The most extreme case of decreased serum phenytoin concentrations following administration of 200 mg and then 400 mg per day of pyridoxine involved a 6-year-old girl "during subacute intoxication." The authors noted that the "doses used were arbitrarily chosen," and no attempt was made to determine the "real amount needed per day." Levels of PLP were not assessed. While offering no supportive evidence, the authors suggested that the addition of the pyridoxine may have "increased activity of pyridoxal-phosphate-dependent enzymes involved in the biotransformation (hydroxylation?) of the drugs."[22] Such alterations in drug concentrations could theoretically trigger seizures, but these authors did not relate any such occurrences in their small study. Subsequent research from controlled trials is lacking to confirm these preliminary findings and establish their clinical implications.

Effects on Nutrients and Homocysteine. A broad range of sources present as "incontrovertible" that anticonvulsants decrease the levels and impair the function of numerous key nutrients, including vitamin B$_6$. Notably, seizures are a known effect of vitamin B$_6$ deficiency, and certain seizure disorders are specifically pyridoxine dependent. Furthermore, decreased levels of B$_6$ and related nutrients (folate, B$_2$, B$_{12}$) are also strongly associated with elevations in plasma Hcy. Nevertheless, the body of evidence available at this time, although highly suggestive, is mixed and inadequate to confirm or disprove the hypothesis that AEDs promote clinically significant B$_6$ deficiency or that AED-induced hyperhomocysteinemia inherently results in increased adverse outcomes, or to determine which drugs are more likely to induce such changes and what patient characteristics are associated with increased vulnerability to Hcy elevations and subsequent adverse events. Moreover, some studies have found that serum levels of vitamin B$_6$ (and/or B$_{12}$) are elevated in some patients treated with AEDs.

Anticonvulsant medications appear capable of either lowering or elevating levels of vitamin B$_6$. In a study involving patients with epilepsy on long-term antiepileptic treatment Hagberg et al.[34] found that plasma PLP concentrations were normal in single determinations using tryptophan load tests. However, in patients followed before and during therapy using antiepileptic medication with hydantoin and succinimide (ethosuximide), Reinken[35] observed significant repeated decreases in serum concentrations of PLP. Subsequent research by Reinken[36] suggested an association between anticonvulsant therapy and possible depletion of vitamin B$_6$ in children.

Haust et al.[23] reported "increased levels of erythrocyte protoporphyrin (EP)" and a "progressive fall in plasma pyridoxal 5'-phosphate (B6-P)" as well as decreased levels of 5-aminolevulinic acid dehydratase (ALA-D) and uroporphyrinogen I synthetase (URO-S) in an epileptic boy undergoing long-term treatment with valproic acid (VPA, 1.3 g/day), CBMZP (0.9 g/day), and folic acid (7.5 mg/day). They administered "pyridoxine HCl (B6-HCl), 87.5 mg/d followed by administration of both B6-HCl and preformed B6-P (50 mg/d each)" and were subsequently able to achieve "the eventual withdrawal of VPA and a net reduction of CBMZP to 450 mg/d." They obtained increases in ALA-D and URO-S before any reduction of CBMZP with pyridoxine hydrochloride alone and then normalization of enzyme levels after "administration of both B6-HCl and B6-P and withdrawal of VPA. During stepwise reduction of VPA, EP remained elevated to values as high as 2.48 µmol/L (upper reference limit, 1.33 µmol/L). Only after permanent withdrawal of VPA did concentrations of EP fall to normal levels." The authors interpreted these findings to suggest "that VPA displaced B6-P from protective protein binding sites" because "both VPA and B6-P are strongly proteinbound," and "that the resulting deficit in B6-P (rather than CBMZP) reduced ALA-D and URO-S activities via primary reduction of ALA-synthetase activity."[23]

In contrast, other researchers have observed apparent elevations of vitamin B$_6$ levels in individuals being treated with AEDs. Dastur and Dave[24] observed that contrasting pattern when they studied the effects of prolonged anticonvulsant medication in 27 epileptic patients, primarily from low socioeconomic groups, age 15 to 54 years. These subjects had received phenobarbitone (90 mg/day phenobarbital) and diphenylhydantion (300 mg/day phenytoin) regularly for 3 to 32 years and had no history of B-vitamin supplementation. "Besides reduced serum and cerebrospinal fluid (CSF) folate levels, significantly increased levels of total vitamin B$_6$ in CSF and serum and of vitamin B$_{12}$ in serum were found in patients as compared with normal healthy subjects." Furthermore, despite a lack of "clinical hepatic involvement, liver biopsy performed in nine of twenty-seven patients revealed fine structural changes in hepatocytes suggestive of varying degrees of drug-induced changes. A ramifying network of short, smooth, endoplasmic cisternae with depleted rough endoplasmic reticulum (RER), distended sinusoids with Kupffer cells, dark shrunken hepatocytes with reduced mitochondria, and increased lipofuscin were observed." The authors suggested that these elevations in serum vitamin levels, along with "significant elevation of serum triglycerides and/or cholesterol," might be the result of hepatic damage, specifically "an adaptive response of the liver, a reversible change."[24]

The recycling of folate cofactors depends on vitamin B$_6$ and riboflavin, and riboflavin is necessary for activating vitamin B$_6$ to PLP. Plasma Hcy levels tend to be elevated in individuals undergoing long-term AED therapy and may play a role in the increased incidence of atherosclerosis, vascular disease, and stroke observed in this patient population. Although controversial, numerous epidemiological data indicate that chronic

AED administration is associated with various occlusive vascular disease.[37-40]

Numerous researchers have demonstrated that treatment with phenytoin, phenobarbital, and primidone and other enzyme-inducing AEDs is associated with elevated total homocysteine (tHcy) concentrations or decreased plasma folate concentrations in adults and in children.[27,28,41-45] For example, Schwaninger et al.[29] conducted a controlled trial involving 51 consecutive outpatients in an epilepsy clinic receiving stable, individually adjusted AED treatment and 51 gender- and age-matched controls. Assessing plasma concentrations of tHcy and vitamin B$_6$ and serum levels of vitamin B$_{12}$ and folate in fasted subjects, they observed that "patients and controls differed significantly in concentrations of folate (13.5 ± 1.0 vs. 17.4 ± 0.8 nM) and vitamin B$_6$ (39.7 ± 3.4 vs. 66.2 ± 7.5 nM), whereas serum concentrations of vitamin B$_{12}$ were similar." Furthermore, they found that plasma Hcy concentration was "significantly increased to 14.7 ± 3.0 microM in patients compared with controls" and that "number of patients with concentrations of >15 microM was significantly higher in the patient group than among controls." The authors noted that these patterns were present with both AED polytherapy and with carbamazepine monotherapy. However, they also cautioned that the observed elevations in homocysteine might be "associated with the disease and not the treatment."[29]

Verrotti et al.[30] evaluated hyperhomocysteinemia in 60 epileptic children (29 females, 31 males), age 14.2 to 17.9 years, receiving sodium valproate (VPA) and carbamazepine (CBZ), monotherapy. They observed "no significant differences in fasting and post-methionine Hcy, plasma PLP, serum folate, erythrocyte folate and serum vitamin B$_{12}$ values between the control group and the two groups of epileptic children" before the initiation of therapy. However, "patients treated with VPA and CBZ showed a significant increase of the plasma concentrations of Hcy when compared to baseline data and controls values" and demonstrated "a significant decrease of serum folate and plasma PLP" after 1 year of therapy. Notably, "serum vitamin B$_{12}$ and erythrocyte folate levels remained in the normal range." The authors suggested two possible interpretations for the increased plasma concentrations of Hcy with prolonged VPA or CBZ treatment. They proposed that remethylation of Hcy to methionine uses 5-methyltetrahydrofolate as a methyl donor and vitamin B$_{12}$ as a cofactor, or "Hcy may conjugate with serine to form cystathionine in a reaction which requires pyridoxal 5'-phosphate ... as a cofactor."[30] Thus, significantly decreased levels of PLP (P5P) or folate in presence of increased Hcy levels might be predicted with carbamazepine, a potent enzyme inducer, whereas only a small reduction of folate values might be associated with valproate, an AED with less enzyme-inducing activity.[46,47]

Yoo and Hong[41] (1999) and Ono et al.[32] (2002) suggested that a drug-gene interaction involving the C677T variant of the 5,10-methylenetetrahydrofolate reductase (MTHFR) gene might be related to AED-mediated decrease in plasma folate concentrations and an independent predictor of hyperhomocysteinemia in patients receiving AED therapy. Nevertheless, Apeland et al.[48] (2003) reported that patients receiving enzyme-inducing AEDs (carbamazepine monotherapy; phenytoin, phenobarbital, and/or primidone) had low PLP concentrations that were negatively correlated with plasma Hcy concentrations as well as high plasma flavin nucleotide/riboflavin concentration ratios with low riboflavin concentrations.

Notably, these patients had higher plasma tHcy concentrations (fasting and after methionine loading) than controls, but such changes in tHcy were not observed in patients who received valproate.

However, more recent research indicates that elevated Hcy levels may not be clinically significant in AED-treated epileptic patients with adequate folate intake. Tamura et al.[31] measured blood concentrations of Hcy, folate, vitamin B$_{12}$, and PLP and determined MTHFR genotypes in sixty-two patients receiving AED monotherapy (phenytoin, lamotrigine, carbamazepine, or valproate). They reported hyperhomocysteinemia in only 7 (11.4%) of 62 patients overall and 3 (15.0%) of the 20 patients receiving phenytoin. Notably, more than 55% of the patients overall exhibited PLP concentrations below the normal range. In contrast, serum vitamin B$_{12}$ concentrations were elevated in patients treated with valproate. The authors concluded that "hyperhomocysteinemia is not a serious clinical concern in AED-treated epileptic patients" with adequate folate nutriture. However, only "three patients had the homozygous thermolabile genotype of MTHFR; therefore, meaningful statistical analysis [of that particular factor] was not possible in this study."[31] Five years later, Gidal, Tamura, et al.[33] found that 32 weeks of treatment with lamotrigine (mean daily dose, 250 mg) had "no significant effect on concentrations of plasma total homocysteine (tHcy), plasma and red-cell folate and plasma vitamin B$_{12}$" but that "2070 mg of valproate resulted in a 57% increase in plasma vitamin B$_{12}$ concentrations over the baseline value and a 27% decline in plasma tHcy concentrations." The authors concluded that the data indicated "hyperhomocysteinemia may not be a serious clinical problem" among patients with epilepsy treated with either lamotrigine or valproate.[33] Thus, despite minimal data, it appears that newer AEDs, such as lamotrigine, which lack hepatic enzyme-inducing activity, are less likely to be associated with altered folate concentrations or Hcy metabolism.

Coadministration Benefits. Pyridoxine, alone and in concert with conventional AEDs, has been efficacious in the treatment of certain forms of seizure disorders. Some seizures are pyridoxine dependent, including inborn errors of metabolism, and require an increased intake of the nutrient. Furthermore, low vitamin B$_6$ is associated with a lowered seizure threshold.[49,50]

In a trial involving 20 patients with infantile spasms, Ito et al.[26] studied the effects of "high doses of vitamin B$_6$," valproic acid, or both and concluded that the combination of vitamin B$_6$ and valproic acid was effective and safe in the treatment of infantile spasms (i.e., seizures). Their research found that although vitamin B$_6$ alone provided some benefit, patients who were given a combination of vitamin B$_6$ and valproic acid had significantly fewer seizures and better electroencephalogram findings than did the group treated initially with vitamin B$_6$ alone. However, "vitamin B$_6$ therapy alone was continued in a single patient who remained seizure-free during the 15-month follow-up period."[26] Pietz et al.[50a] found that 300 mg/kg/day of vitamin B$_6$ (pyridoxine HCl orally) reduced infantile spasms in 5 of 17 children within the first 2 weeks of treatment, and within 4 weeks, all five patients were free of seizures. "Two patients developed other seizures (partial seizures, etiologically unclear blinking attacks), but no relapse of infantile spasms was observed among the five responders to vitamin B$_6$." Notably, "no serious adverse reactions were noted," with gastrointestinal symptoms, reversible after dosage reduction, being the primary adverse effects reported. Noting "the life-threatening side effects of treatment with ACTH/corticosteroids or valproate," the authors concluded by recommending a controlled clinical trial with "high-dose vitamin B₆" to either prove or disprove efficacy.[50a] In a controlled study, Walter-Sack and Klotz[51] found that coadministration of vitamin B₆, 200 mg daily for 4 weeks, resulted in a 45% reduction in phenobarbital blood levels.

Subsequently, Goto et al.[25] investigated binding affinity of glutamate decarboxylase (GAD) in relation to cerebrospinal fluid (CSF) glutamate/GABA concentrations to determine the etiology of pyridoxine-dependent seizures (PDS) and the mechanisms of pyridoxine action in seizure control. They described a patient with PDS whose generalized seizures terminated after intravenous pyridoxine phosphate. This patient's condition had been refractory to conventional antiepileptic medicines and was not accompanied by an elevated CSF glutamate concentration. "No seizure occurred once oral pyridoxine (13.5 mg/Kg per day) was started in combination with phenobarbital sodium (PB, 3.7 mg/Kg per day). The electroencephalogram (EEG) normalized approximately 8 months after pyridoxine was started." Based on these observations, they suggested that pyridoxine-dependent seizure "is not a discrete disease of single etiology in that insufficient activation of GAD may not account for seizure susceptibility in all cases and (2) mechanism(s) of anti-convulsive effect of pyridoxine, at least in some cases, may be independent of GAD activation."[25]

In a rat model, Reyes-Garcia et al.[52] found that B vitamins can enhance the antiallodynic effect of gabapentin (Neurontin). These researchers induced neuropathic pain and measured paw withdrawal in Wistar rats. Tactile allodynia was determined after oral administration of gabapentin (30-300 mg/kg), B vitamins (75-600 mg/kg), or a combination of gabapentin and B vitamins. Their findings "indicate that systemic administration of gabapentin and B vitamins can interact synergistically to reduce neuropathic pain in the rat and suggest the use of this combination to relieve neuropathy in humans."[52]

Nutritional Therapeutics, Clinical Concerns, and Adaptations

Physicians prescribing AEDs and related barbiturates are advised to be aware that these medications can decrease circulating levels of vitamin B₆ or its activated form, pyridoxal 5′phosphate (PLP), and may cause elevations in plasma homocysteine, with attendant risks. The probability of such adverse effects appears to be significantly greater with enzyme-inducing AEDs (carbamazepine monotherapy; phenytoin, phenobarbital, and/or primidone) than in those receiving valproate or lamotrigine monotherapy; in general, AED polytherapy carries greater risks for this and other adverse effects than does AED monotherapy with any agent. Furthermore, pharmacogenomic variability in metabolism of AEDs and genetic variants affecting folate metabolism, particularly MTHFR polymorphism C677T, can significantly influence drug efficacy and toxicity.

Coadministration of vitamin B₆, usually in combination with folate, vitamin B₁₂, and riboflavin, may be warranted to mitigate adverse effects of these medications on nutrient metabolism as well as increased risks of teratogenicity, hyperhomocysteinemia, and other well-known toxic effects. Moreover, within the context of appropriate clinical management by experienced health care professionals, vitamin B₆ may be indicated as a component of an integrative approach to treatment of seizure disorders, and coadministration with AEDs may enhance the therapeutic response.

Close supervision and regular monitoring is warranted with concomitant use, particularly B₆ doses greater than 200 mg/day. It is particularly important to regularly evaluate serum concentrations of phenytoin and phenobarbital and

clinical response in patients receiving concomitant pyridoxine at doses of 200 mg/day or greater. Evidence is lacking to suggest that the small dose levels of vitamin B₆ in typical multivitamins and B-complex formulations might interfere with effective drug dose and therapeutic response.

Chemotherapy

Evidence: Altretamine (hexamethylmelamine, HMM; Hexalen), cisplatin (*cis*-diaminedichloroplatinum, CDDP; Platinol, Platinol-AQ), docetaxel (taxotere), doxorubicin, pegylated liposomal (Caelyx, Doxil, Myocet), fluorouracil (5-FU, Adrucil, Efudex, Efudix, Fluoroplex).
Extrapolated: Other chemotherapeutic agents and combinations.

Interaction Type and Significance

☼   **Prevention or Reduction of Drug Adverse Effect**
⊕✗   **Bimodal or Variable Interaction, with Professional Management**
✗   **Potential or Theoretical Adverse Interaction of Uncertain Severity**

Coadministration Benefit Probability:	Evidence Base:
4. Plausible to **2. Probable**	○ Preliminary to ◉◉ Emerging

Drug Interference Probability:	Evidence Base:
4. Plausible to **2. Probable**	○ Preliminary

Effect and Mechanism of Action

Vitamin B₆ may reduce the severity of certain adverse effects associated with several chemotherapeutic agents but may also diminish the therapeutic efficacy of some medications. Palmar-plantar erythrodysesthesia (PPE) syndrome is an adverse effect often associated with antineoplastic treatment using 5-fluorouracil, docetaxel, and doxorubicin HCl liposome injection. This painful condition often constitutes the limiting toxicity of such therapies.[53] Pyridoxine has been shown to mitigate this painful cutaneous toxicity, but the mechanisms of these activities have yet to be elucidated.[54-57] Pyridoxine can reduce altretamine-associated neurotoxicity but may diminish the therapeutic activity of altretamine (hexamethylmelamine) when used in combination with cisplatin.[58] Again, the mechanisms for these effects are as yet unknown.

Research and Reports

Molina, Fabian, et al.[54,56] published two papers on the coadministration of pyridoxine therapy for palmar-plantar erythrodysesthesia associated with low dose continuous infusion 5-fluorouracil (200-300 mg/m²/day). Their preliminary report (1987) described reversal of PPE, without impairment of therapeutic efficacy, in colon cancer patients receiving 200 mg/m²/day continuous 5-FU following coadministration of 100 mg/day of pyridoxine.[54] Three years later they published their complete findings showing that concomitant pyridoxine therapy can reverse 5-FU–induced PPE without any adverse effects or interruption of chemotherapy. "Five previously untreated patients who developed PPE received 50 or 150 mg of pyridoxine/day when moderate PPE changes were noted. Reversal of PPE without interruption of the 5-FU was seen in 4/5 patients. Four of these patients who received pyridoxine had responded to 5-FU treatment. No adverse affect of pyridoxine on clinical response was noted."[56]

Vukelja et al.[59] reported two cases in which symptoms of PPE began to resolve within 12 to 24 hours after initiation of pyridoxine, 50 mg three times daily, and continued to improve for several weeks.

In a randomized, double-blind clinical trial involving 41 dogs with non-Hodgkin's lymphoma, Vail et al.[57] compared concomitant pyridoxine therapy to placebo in preventing the development of PPE (PPES) during chemotherapy using Doxil, a doxorubicin-containing pegylated (Stealth) liposome. They observed that the "likelihood of developing serious PPES and having to decrease or discontinue Doxil therapy was 4.2 times (relative risk) greater in placebo group dogs than in pyridoxine group dogs." Although pyridoxine "did not completely abrogate PPES, it occurred later and less dramatically than in placebo-treated dogs and resulted in fewer treatment delays or discontinuations, allowing a higher cumulative dose of Doxil to be received." Furthermore, "no difference was observed in remission rates (71.4 versus 75%) achieved between groups" and a "trend (P = 0.084) toward prolongation of remission length was observed in dogs receiving pyridoxine, which was likely attributable to their ability to receive more Doxil without delay or discontinuation." The authors concluded "that pyridoxine is effective in delaying the onset and severity of PPES in this canine model."[57]

Altretamine, also known as hexamethylmelamine (HMM), is a synthetic cytotoxic antineoplastic s-triazine derivative associated with a small but significant occurrence of neurological toxicity. Fabian et al.[60] administered prophylactic pyridoxine or the drug alone in a Phase II trial of hexamethylmelamine (HEX) involving 98 patients with metastatic breast cancer, heavily pretreated with other agents. They reported "a 2% response rate in 89 partially or fully evaluable patients. Seven percent of these patients developed neurologic toxicity which occurred in the HEX-alone group only."[60] Subsequently, Wiernik et al.[58] conducted a trial involving a total of 248 analyzable patients with stages III-IV ovarian epithelial cancer (114 with and 134 without prior chemotherapy) who were randomized to one of four cisplatin (DDP)–hexamethylmelamine (HMM) regimens. Pyridoxine was coadministered at a dose of 300 mg/m² orally to evaluate its ability to reduce the neurotoxicity of HMM. Applying multivariate analysis, they identified prior chemotherapy, pyridoxine administration, recent diagnosis, and large tumor size as factors adversely affecting response duration. They concluded: "Although pyridoxine administration significantly reduced neurotoxicity, its adverse effect on response duration suggests that the agent should not be administered with DDP or HMM." The authors recommended further investigation of the "mechanism by which pyridoxine may unfavorably affect response duration."[58]

Nutritional Therapeutics, Clinical Concerns, and Adaptations

Pyridoxine coadministration represents a valuable option for adjunctive use with certain forms of chemotherapy (e.g., 5-fluorouracil, docetaxel, doxorubicin HCl liposome injection) as a means of preventing or reducing specific adverse effects, particularly PPE syndrome and neurotoxicity. In contrast, administration of pyridoxine during chemotherapy using altretamine (HMM), especially in conjunction with cisplatin, while potentially beneficial, warrants caution and should be considered as contraindicated in most cases. Safe and effective implementation of any therapeutic strategy combining chemotherapy and pyridoxine requires clinical management within the context of integrative care involving health care professionals trained and experienced in both conventional pharmacology and nutritional therapeutics.

The usual dosage of vitamin B₆ ranges from 50 to 100 mg, three times daily orally, and inherently requires close supervision and regular monitoring given the increased risk for pyridoxine toxicity in compromised patients and potential interference with therapeutic efficacy of the concomitant antineoplastic therapy. Physicians and other health care professionals may consider reviewing the potential for such synergistic strategies with appropriate patients and provide referral information to centers specializing in such integrative approaches. The available evidence is limited but suggestive of a broader pattern deserving further research with large, well-designed clinical trials.

Doxylamine

Doxylamine and pyridoxine, combination drug (Bendectin, Diclectin).

Interaction Type and Significance:

⊕⊕ **Beneficial or Supportive Interaction, with Professional Management**

Probability: Evidence Base:
2. Probable   ●●● **Consensus**

Effect and Mechanism of Action

Bendectin was introduced in the United States in 1956 by Merrell Dow as medication specifically for nausea and vomiting of pregnancy (NVP). Originally it was formulated as a combination of "doxylamine succinate, an antihistamine with antiemetic properties, dicyclomine hydrochloride, an antispasmodic agent, and pyridoxine hydrochloride (vitamin B₆) to prevent possible deficits during pregnancy and to synergize the antinauseant activity."[61] Based on results of randomized control trials comparing each component alone and in combination versus placebo, dicyclomine hydrochloride was dropped from the formulation in 1976. The standard formulation of Diclectin as of 2003 was 10 mg vitamin B₆ and 10 mg doxylamine per tablet.

Research

Beginning in 1969, allegations and lawsuits appeared, based on single case incidents, claiming possible teratogenic effects of Bendectin resulting in congenital limb deformities. These legal claims were based on limited evidence and failed in court. Several clinical trials and a meta-analysis of 20 studies, including review of Bendectin use by 200,000 patients, failed to demonstrate any causal relationship between Bendectin and congenital malformations.[62-66] Nevertheless, Merrell Dow withdrew Bendectin from the U.S. market and ceased worldwide production in 1983 because of business rather than medical factors, specifically adverse publicity, rising legal costs, and insurance premiums, despite winning their legal battles and continued evidence of safety and efficacy. Diclectin is the only prescription medication recommended for the treatment of NVP available in Canada and is considered the drug of choice.

Physicians have continued to prescribe doxylamine-pyridoxine, and further research has investigated its therapeutic application in subsequent years even as the legal and market history of the medication are cited as a striking example of poorly founded litigation interfering with rational, safe, and effective therapeutics.[67-69] According to a review by Bishai et al.,[70] the "efficacy of the delayed-release combination of doxylamine and pyridoxine (Bendectin, Diclectin) has been shown in several randomized, controlled trials." Nevertheless, a significant discrepancy appears to exist between the reported rate of taking Diclectin and physicians' self-reported prescribing practices for Diclectin.[71] Thus, in 1999, 90% of physicians reported prescribing Diclectin to their pregnant women with NVP, but only 66% of respondents in a study were actually taking the medication.[72]

In a population-based case-control study, Boneva et al.[73] investigated nausea during pregnancy and congenital heart defects. They found that, overall, early nausea and use of antinausea medication, particularly Bendectin "was associated with a lower risk for congenital heart defects compared with: 1) absence of nausea..., and 2) nausea without medication use." These researchers concluded that these "results suggest that pregnancy hormones and factors or, alternatively, a component of Bendectin (most probably pyridoxine) may be important for normal heart development" and proposed that their "findings outline potential areas for future research on and prevention of congenital heart defects."[73]

Fear of litigation, cautious prescribing, and inadequate communication have all contributed to a pattern of suboptimal dosing in patients treated with doxylamine-pyridoxine. In an observational, prospective study, Atanackovic et al.[74] determined the incidence of adverse maternal and fetal effects and pregnancy outcome in 225 women taking doxylamine-pyridoxine for NVP at the recommended or higher-than-recommended doses. They reported "two pregnancies with major malformation, a finding that is consistent with the rates of birth defects in the general population." They concluded that "the higher than standard dose of Diclectin, when calculated per kg of body weight, does not affect either the incidence of maternal adverse effects or pregnancy outcome." The authors recommended that "if needed, Diclectin can be given at doses higher than four tablets per day to normalize for body weight or optimize efficacy."[74] Likewise, in a clinical trial involving 68 women with moderate to severe NVP, Boskovic et al.[74a] found that "most women (50/68) were receiving 2 tablets a day of Diclectin instead of the recommended dose of 4 tablets a day."

An innovative study suggests that compliance in use of medications such as doxylamine-pyridoxine is influenced by many factors and that cultivation of a strong physician-patient relationship might deserve greater attention. Using survey data from interviews with 59 women recruited from the Motherisk Nausea and Vomiting Helpline, Baggley et al.[72] investigated factors that influence women's decision making on whether to treat NVP pharmacologically. Although all participants were informed that Diclectin was considered safe for use during pregnancy, investigators found that at "a follow-up telephone call, 34% were not using any pharmacologic treatment, and of those who were taking the drug, 26% were using less than the recommended dose." These researchers learned that the rationale offered "for not using the medication were insufficient safety data, preference for non-pharmacologic methods, and being made to feel uncomfortable by the physician." Notably, "of the women who did use Diclectin, the most convincing reassuring information that it was safe to use came from friends and family."[72] Moreover, in a survey conducted by Hollyer et al.,[75] women suffering from NVP expressed significant fear of using "drugs" during pregnancy and stated that they were more comfortable using "natural" and "alternative" therapies to treat NVP and engaged in such self-care with little or no supervision by their medical or naturopathic physicians.

Nutritional Therapeutics, Clinical Concerns, and Adaptations

The combination of doxylamine and pyridoxine represents a poignant example of the promises and hazards of drug-nutrient interactions as both therapeutic synergy and medicolegal

challenge. The body of evidence indicates that this medication can safely and effectively reduce NVP when used at recommended doses, which at four tablets per day provides 40 mg each of pyridoxine and doxylamine. As mentioned, one study found that the inclusion of vitamin B₆ might actually enhance fetal development and reduce the risk of congenital heart malformations. Most importantly, the tortured history of this innovative medication suggests that the cultivation of a frank, honest, and trusting therapeutic relationship may play a greater role in patient decision making and compliance than any claims of safety or efficacy and attendant scientific "evidence." Further research is warranted, as might be investigation of concomitant use of ginger (*Zingiber officinale*), which has also been shown to be safe and effective in NVP, with doxylamine and pyridoxine.[76-78]

Erythropoiesis-Stimulating Agents

Epoetin alpha (EPO, epoetin alfa, recombinant erythropoietin; Epogen, Eprex, Procrit), epoetin beta (NeoRecormon), darbepoetin alpha (darbepoetin alfa; Aranesp).
See also Furosemide and Related Loop Diuretics.

Interaction Type and Significance

≈≈   **Drug-Induced Nutrient Depletion, Supplementation Therapeutic, with Professional Management**
◇⊕⊕ **Drug-Induced Adverse Effect on Nutrient Function, Coadministration Therapeutic, with Professional Management**
☼   **Prevention or Reduction of Drug Adverse Effect**
⊕⊕   **Beneficial or Supportive Interaction, with Professional Management**

Probability: Evidence Base:
2. Probable   ◉◉ **Emerging,**
                                           ○ **Mixed**

Effect and Mechanism of Action

Erythropoietin (EPO) therapy increases hemoglobin synthesis, which can decrease erythrocyte pyridoxine status and increase nutritional requirements.

The water-soluble nature and small-to-medium molecular size of vitamin B₆, as well as folic acid and vitamin B₁₂, renders B₆ particularly susceptible to being lost in the dialysate in patients undergoing either peritoneal dialysis or hemodialysis, especially with high-flux dialysis.

Research

It is well known that vitamin B₆ deficiency, from many causes, develops in the majority of patients with chronic renal failure and in patients during various forms of renal replacement therapy. Mydlik, Derzsiova, and Zemberova[79-81] have conducted a series of studies investigating erythrocyte levels of various B vitamins in kidney disease as well as the influence of water, furosemide, and sodium diuresis on the metabolism and urinary excretion of vitamin B₆, oxalic acid, and vitamin C in patients with chronic renal failure. Their most important finding was that erythrocyte vitamin B₆ is consumed by the stimulated hemoglobin synthesis at an increased rate during EPO treatment in hemodialysis patients. In a 1993 study involving 26 patients undergoing regular dialysis treatment (RDT), they investigated the influence of recombinant human erythropoietin (r-HuEPO) on erythrocyte vitamins B₁, B₂, and B₆ by comparing vitamin erythrocyte levels with and without EPO. The non-EPO group received oral pyridoxine 5 mg daily for

9 months while the EPO-treated group received oral pyridoxine 5 mg daily for the first 6 months and 20 mg daily during the following 3 months. They observed a significant elevation in erythrocyte vitamin B_2 levels and a significant decrease in erythrocyte vitamin B_6. However, after administration of the higher doses of pyridoxine (20 mg daily), subjects exhibited "a significant increase in vitamin B_6 and at the end of the 9 months, the values of vitamin B_6 were within the normal range."[79] Further, after establishing that intravenous administration of furosemide (20 mg) leads to an increase of urinary excretion and fraction excretion of vitamin B_6 in patients with chronic renal failure, this research team found that a "daily oral dose of pyridoxine 6 mg was optimal for the patients without erythropoietin (EPO) treatment during the period of 12 months of CAPD." Using pyridoxal 5-phosphate (PLP) as an indirect method of determining erythrocyte vitamin B_6, they concluded that for "prevention of vitamin B_6 deficiency in hemodialysis and CAPD patients we recommend the following doses of pyridoxine: for patients without EPO treatment 5 mg/day, and with EPO treatment 20 mg/day." They also noted that a "favorable effect of pyridoxine 50 mg/day has also been found on several parameters of cellular immunity in hemodialysis patients."[80] Subsequently, they published the results of a 15-month study investigating the influence of erythropoietin on the biochemical parameters of several nutrients. Among these they demonstrated that "erythrocyte vitamin B_6 and folic acid significantly decreased due to erythropoietin treatment." In response, they found that oral administration of vitamin B_6 (20 mg/day) and folic acid (5 mg/week) during the last 3 months positively "influenced the deficiency of erythrocyte vitamin B_6 and folic acid."[81]

In related research, Kasama et al.[82] found the "average *in vivo* PLP clearance for six patients on standard hemodialysis increased by more than 50%... at average blood flows of 375 mL/min" and that levels of "PLP decreased from a baseline of 50 ± 13.8 ng/mL to 24 ± 9.7 ng/mL ... after 3 months of HF/HE [high-flux/high-efficiency] treatments; the levels returned to 45 ± 6.4 ng/mL on resumption of standard dialysis treatments." They concluded that HF/HE dialysis "treatments can have a dramatic impact on vitamin B_6 homeostasis." The authors also noted that the use of different types of dialysis membranes and reprocessing in dialysis significantly affected PLP clearance to varying degrees.[82]

In a 1999 review of comprehensive approaches to patients being treated with EPO, Horl[83] summarized the available research regarding pyridoxine and concluded: "Vitamin B_6 requirements are increased during epoetin therapy, and supplementation at a dose of 100-150 mg/week is recommended."

Peripheral polyneuropathy (PPN) is a known adverse effect of nutrient depletion from high-flux hemodialysis. Okada et al.[84] found that vitamin B_6 coadministration can improve PPN in patients with chronic renal failure on high-flux hemodialysis (HD) and r-HuEPO. Their study included 36 patients undergoing chronic high-flux HD and receiving r-HuEPO, 26 of whom suffered from PPN. After determining initial predialysis serum pyridoxal 5'-phosphate (P5P) levels and ranking PPN symptoms in these patients, they administered vitamin B_6 (60 mg/day) prescribed to 14, randomly assigned, and vitamin B_{12} (500 μg/day) to the others. Notably, "predialysis serum P5P levels of HD patients with PPN were not significantly lower than those of matched HD patients without PPN." However, they demonstrated that "supplementation with vitamin B_6 for 4 weeks significantly increased the predialysis level of P5P and dramatically attenuated PPN symptoms compared with initial symptoms." In contrast, no

improvement was observed in response to administration of vitamin B_{12}. Thus, coadministration of B_6 was beneficial to HD patients on EPO therapy even though indications of B_6 deficiency, as ascertained by serum levels, were absent.[84]

Nutritional Therapeutics, Clinical Concerns, and Adaptations
Physicians administering EPO therapy, particularly in the context of hemodialysis, are advised to consider coadministration of vitamin B_6, 20 to 50 mg/day orally, as well as folic acid, 1 mg/day orally, to prevent or reverse adverse effects on these nutrients and their physiological functions. The body of available evidence strongly suggests that such nutritional support is often appropriate in the absence of overt signs or standard laboratory indications of deficiency. Vitamin B_6 intake at these levels is generally considered safe, although regular monitoring would be judicious in compromised patients, such as those with chronic renal failure. Folic acid is safe at all relevant levels of intake, although care should be taken to rule out concurrent B_{12} deficiency states.

Furosemide and Related Loop Diuretics

Evidence: Furosemide (Lasix).
Extrapolated, based on similar properties: Bumetanide (Bumex), ethacrynic acid (Edecrin), torsemide (Demadex).
See also Erythropoiesis-Stimulating Agents.

Interaction Type and Significance
≈≈ **Drug-Induced Nutrient Depletion, Coadministration Therapeutic, with Professional Management**
☼ **Prevention or Reduction of Drug Adverse Effect**

Probability:	Evidence Base:
4. Plausible	○ Preliminary

Effect and Mechanism of Action
Furosemide acutely increases urinary excretion of oxalic acid and vitamin B_6 (as well as vitamin C) in individuals with chronic renal failure. This effect could reverse the tendency in uremic patients toward accumulation of oxalic acid, which can result in elevated plasma levels.

Research
Several preliminary human trials have reported increased excretion of vitamin B_6 in individuals administered furosemide and investigated the influence of the nutrient on hyperoxalemia and increased oxalic acid excretion with furosemide.

In a small trial involving eight chronic hemodialysis patients with secondary hyperoxalemia, Balcke et al.[85] observed that pyridoxine administration decreased mean plasma oxalic acid concentration from 149.5 to 99.0 μmol/L within 2 weeks and to 93.8 μmol/L after 4 weeks, with a 46% mean reduction. Notably, the "decrease in plasma oxalic acid levels was most pronounced in patients with the highest pretreatment values." Furthermore, the "two patients who received pyridoxine therapy prior to the beginning of the study had low initial values of plasma oxalic acid concentrations and showed no further decline."[85]

Subsequently, Mydlik et al.[86,87] conducted a series of investigations of the effect of furosemide on urinary excretion of oxalic acid, vitamin C, and vitamin B_6 in patients with chronic renal failure (CRF). In one controlled clinical trial (1998), they observed an increased urinary excretion of oxalic acid, vitamin C, and vitamin B_6 during the first 3 hours after a single intravenous (IV) dose of 20 mg furosemide in a control group and in CRF patients without dialyzation treatment. They noted that this effect persisted for 6 hours in CRF patients without dialysis. "The authors described a new hitherto unknown positive side-effect of furosemide, i.e. enhanced urinary oxalic acid excretion in the control group and in patients with chronic renal failure without dialyzation treatment and a negative side-effect of furosemide, i.e. increased urinary vitamin B6 excretion in both examined groups." In conclusion, based on these findings, they recommended monitoring of vitamin C and of "vitamin B₆ in plasma during long-term administration of large doses of furosemide to patients with chronic renal failure as deficiency of these vitamins could develop."[86] A year later these researchers published results of another trial in which they compared urinary excretion of vitamin B₆, oxalic acid, and vitamin C in three groups: 15 healthy subjects during maximal water diuresis, 12 patients in polyuric stage of CRF without dialysis treatment receiving a diet high in sodium chloride (15 g/day), and 15 patients in polyuric stage of CRF without dialysis treatment after IV administration of 20 mg furosemide. "Urinary excretion of vitamin B₆, oxalic acid and vitamin C significantly increased during maximal water diuresis while during high intake of sodium chloride the urinary excretions of these substances were not affected." The authors interpreted these results to suggest that "urinary excretion of vitamin B₆, oxalic acid and vitamin C depends on the urinary excretion of water" and to confirm their earlier findings that IV furosemide (20 mg) increases urinary excretion of vitamin B₆, as well as oxalic acid and vitamin C, in patients with CRF.[87]

Nutritional Therapeutics, Clinical Concerns, and Adaptations

Physicians prescribing furosemide or related loop diuretics are advised to monitor levels of vitamin B₆ and other nutrients and to supplement as indicated, particularly in patients with CRF and on dialysis. Because furosemide also depletes thiamine (vitamin B₁), it is probably best to supplement a B-complex preparation with adequate amounts of B₁ and B₆. Close supervision is warranted with these patients, especially after introducing a new medication or nutrient or changing the dose or combination of any agents.

Gentamicin and Related Aminoglycoside Antibiotics

Evidence: Gentamicin (G-mycin, Garamycin, Jenamicin).
Extrapolated, based on similar properties: Amikacin (Amikin), kanamycin (Kantrex), neomycin (Mycifradin, Myciguent, Neo-Fradin, NeoTab, Nivemycin), netilmicin (Netromycin), paromomycin (monomycin; Humatin), streptomycin, tobramycin (AKTob, Nebcin, TOBI, TOBI Solution, TobraDex, Tobrex).

Interaction Type and Significance

☼ **Prevention or Reduction of Drug Adverse Effect**
◇≈≈ **Drug-Induced Adverse Effect on Nutrient Function, Coadministration Therapeutic, with Professional Management**
≈≈ **Drug-Induced Nutrient Depletion, Supplementation Therapeutic, with Professional Management**
⊕✗ **Bimodal or Variable Interaction, with Professional Management**

Probability: Evidence Base:
2. Plausible   ○ Preliminary

Effect and Mechanism of Action

Pyridoxal 5'-phosphate (PLP), the active form of vitamin B₆, readily forms complexes with gentamicin, as well as a wide variety of other potentially toxic substances. This pharmacodynamic interaction interferes with vitamin B₆ metabolism, specifically resulting in a reduction of renal PLP, and has been associated with B₆ depletion. Concomitant vitamin B₆ appears to prevent adverse effects associated with gentamicin, particularly nephrotoxicity, without reducing the drug's efficacy.

Research

A number of animal studies, many conducted by Enriquez, Keniston, Weir, and associates, have documented the adverse effects of gentamicin on vitamin B₆ metabolism and plasma concentrations and the potential benefit of B₆ coadministration. Using a rat model, Keniston et al.[88] found that "PLP protected against GM-induced neuromuscular paralysis and death." Kacew[89] observed that coadministration of PLP for 4 days lowered gentamicin levels in the kidneys and restored renal concentration of PLP to normal levels, but 14 days of PLP administration was required to inhibit gentamicin-induced nephrotoxicity in the rat. Similarly, Weir et al.[90] reported gentamicin administration in rabbits led to a 47% drop in plasma PLP levels. Their findings also suggested that "gentamicin interferes with vitamin B₆ metabolism, but that vitamin B₆ status does not affect levels of gentamicin." Subsequently, these researchers demonstrated that vitamin B₆ can protect against the nephrotoxicity of gentamicin in rabbits, particularly acute tubular necrosis. They did note, however, the possibility of interstitial nephritis with intramuscular injection of high doses of vitamin B₆ based on the reaction of one rabbit.[91] In other research using a rat model, Smetana et al.[92] determined that a "specific concentration of pyridoxal-5-phosphate may be necessary to provide protection against all manifestations of aminoglycoside-induced renal damage." Ali and Bashir[93] found that although PLP, at the doses used, "reduced significantly the severity of some of the manifestations of nephrotoxicity,... [it] was ineffective in completely preventing the development of nephrotoxicity."

Nutritional Therapeutics, Clinical Concerns, and Adaptations

Physicians prescribing gentamicin or other aminoglycoside antibiotics are advised to consider the potential benefit of coadministering vitamin B₆ to mitigate adverse effects, particularly aminoglycoside-induced nephrotoxicity. The available evidence is consistent in its findings but limited by the exclusive presence of animal studies. The research reviewed suggests that such concomitant intake is unlikely to impair the therapeutic efficacy of the medication. Clinical trials are warranted to investigate patterns of adverse effects and interactions and to determine guidelines for a safe and effective clinical response.

Haloperidol and Other Neuroleptic Agents

Evidence: Haloperidol (Haldol).
Extrapolated, based on similar properties: Chlorpromazine (Largactil, Thorazine), clozapine (Clozaril), fluphenazine (Modecate, Permitil, Prolixin, Prolixin Decanoate, Prolixin Enanthate), prochlorperazine (Compazine, Stemetil).
Similar properties but evidence lacking for extrapolation: Atypical antipsychotics: Aripiprazole (Abilify, Abilitat), clozapine (Clozaril), olanzapine (Symbyax, Zyprexa), quetiapine (Seroquel), risperidone (Risperdal), ziprasidone (Geodon).

Interaction Type and Significance

◇≈≈ **Drug-Induced Adverse Effect on Nutrient Function, Coadministration Therapeutic, with Professional Management**
☼ **Prevention or Reduction of Drug Adverse Effect**

See also Risperidone in Theoretical, Speculative, and Preliminary Interactions Research.
See also Vitamin E monograph.

Reduction of Adverse Drug Effects
Probability:
2. Probable

Evidence Base:
●●● Consensus

Enhancement of Therapeutic Outcomes
Probability:
4. Plausible or
2. Improbable

Evidence Base:
▽ Mixed

Effect and Mechanism of Action
Tardive dyskinesia and parkinsonian symptoms, especially dystonia, are adverse effects typically associated with haloperidol and other psychotropic medications. Neuroleptic agents are known to induce oxidative stress, and lipid peroxidation appears to play a central role in the development of tardive dyskinesia.[94]

Vitamin B$_6$ plays a key role in the synthesis of serotonin, dopamine, norepinephrine, and gamma-aminobutyric acid (GABA) and other neurotransmitters, all of which have been proposed to be involved in the development of tardive dyskinesia. Concomitant administration of vitamin B$_6$ can prevent or reduce drug-induced tardive dyskinesia and related extrapyramidal symptoms but may not enhance therapeutic outcomes in the management of psychotic symptoms in schizophrenic and schizoaffective patients.[95]

Research
Miodownik, Lerner, Kotler, and colleagues have conducted a series of small trials investigating the use of vitamin B$_6$ in the treatment of neuroleptic-induced tardive dyskinesia (TD). They have consistently found that coadministration or addition of vitamin B$_6$ (100-500 mg/day) produced "clinically significant (greater than 30%) improvement on measures of involuntary movement" using the Abnormal Involuntary Movement Scale (AIMS), Barnes Akathisia Rating Scale (BARS), the Simpson-Angus Scale (SAS), and the Extrapyramidal Symptom Rating Scale (ESRS). In some cases, they also measured "clinically significant improvement" on the Brief Psychiatric Rating Scale (BPRS).[95,96] Subsequently, they reported "significant improvement in tardive dyskinesia and parkinsonian symptoms" in a double-blind crossover trial lasting 9 weeks involving 15 patients, suffering from schizophrenia and schizoaffective disorder with positive psychotic symptoms and TD, who received up to 400 mg vitamin B$_6$ daily. However, their findings in this study "did not show any therapeutic effect on psychotic symptoms from vitamin B$_6$ added to antipsychotic agents," which patients received on a constant basis.[97] None of the patients in these trials experienced adverse effects attributable to vitamin B$_6$. The emerging pattern in these studies strongly suggested that continued research is warranted to clarify the relationship between vitamin B$_6$ and TD.

These investigators examined whether basal levels of vitamin B$_6$ might serve as a predictive marker to distinguish which patients might be more vulnerable to such adverse reactions. In one paper they reported that, "although patients in the TD group were exposed to neuroleptic drugs for significantly longer periods of time, there were no differences" in serum PLP levels between the treated group and controls. Based on these findings, they concluded that "reports of the effectiveness of vitamin B$_6$ supplementation in the treatment of

TD could therefore be explained by the assumption that central nervous system or intracellular vitamin B$_6$ levels, which are involved in the pathogenesis of TD, are not the same as vitamin B$_6$ peripheral serum levels."[98] Likewise, in a subsequent paper, these researchers noted that there was "no direct correlation between pathological symptoms and the serum baseline level of vitamin B$_6$ nor its level during the treatment."[97] Thus, the available evidence has yet to reach a level of clarity to confirm that these medications consistently deplete functional levels of vitamin B$_6$ or to clarify the mechanisms involved in the adverse effects or their mitigation.

In a review of research on the treatment of TD and tardive dystonia, Simpson[99] wrote: "Tardive dyskinesia not only may be painful and disfiguring, but it also predicts poor outcome in patients with schizophrenia .... The best treatment for tardive dyskinesia and dystonia is prevention, which is a function of medication choice."

Nutritional Therapeutics, Clinical Concerns, and Adaptations
Physicians prescribing neuroleptic drugs known to cause TD and related adverse extrapyramidal effects are advised to coadminister vitamin B$_6$ to prevent or reduce the occurrence and severity of such reactions. The pyridoxine levels, 200 to 400 mg daily, indicated in such situations are potentially capable of causing adverse neurological effects (primarily peripheral neuropathy) and require close supervision and regular monitoring.

Hydralazine

Hydralazine (hydralazine hydrochloride, 1-hydrazinophthalazine monohydrochloride; Apresoline); combination drugs: hydralazine and hydrochlorothiazide (Apresazide); hydralazine and isosorbide dinitrate (BiDil).

Interaction Type and Significance
≈≈   **Drug-Induced Nutrient Depletion, Supplementation Therapeutic, with Professional Management**
◇≈≈   **Drug-Induced Adverse Effect on Nutrient Function, Coadministration Therapeutic, with Professional Management**
⊕✗   **Bimodal or Variable Interaction, with Professional Management**
◇◇   **Impaired Drug Absorption and Bioavailability, Precautions Appropriate**

See also Levodopa, Carbidopa, Benserazide, and Related Antiparkinsonian Medications.

Nutrient Depletion
Probability:
4. Plausible to
2. Probable

Evidence Base:
○ Preliminary

Drug Interference
Probability:
4. Plausible to
2. Probable

Evidence Base:
○ Preliminary

Effect and Mechanism of Action
Hydralazine and vitamin B$_6$ can bind to form a complex that is excreted in the urine, potentially decreasing available levels of hydralazine, depleting pyridoxine, and impairing B$_6$-related functions.[100] Thus, hydralazine acts as pyridoxine antagonist, inhibits a number of enzymes requiring pyridoxal as a cofactor, and may increase vitamin B$_6$ requirements and/or cause

anemia, peripheral neuritis, or other B$_6$-deficiency neuropathies.[101] Conversely, such pharmacokinetic interaction with vitamin B$_6$ may decrease the therapeutic effectiveness of hydralazine.[102]

Reports and Research

Pyridoxine-deficiency neuropathy and other B$_6$-related adverse effects due to hydralazine have been well known for decades, beginning with a case report published in 1965 by Raskin and Fishman.[101] Rumsby and Shepherd[100] elaborated on the effect of hydralazine (as well as penicillamine and phenelzine) on the function of PLP. Subsequently, Vidrio[102] investigated the potential role of hydralazine's interaction with pyridoxal as the basis for its hypotensive effect. He noted that the "drug interacts with pyridoxal and can produce B$_6$ deficiency; it also inhibits a number of enzymes requiring pyridoxal as a cofactor, but there is no apparent relation between its enzymatic and blood pressure effects." Using a rat model, he found that "responses to hydralazine were diminished by pyridoxine and [that the] inhibitory effect of pyridoxine was absent when rats were pretreated with the calcium antagonists verapamil or cinnarizine. Hydralazine hypotension in anesthetized rats was also reduced by pyridoxal pretreatment." The author concluded that these findings "suggest that at least part of hydralazine-induced hypotension may be related to interaction with pyridoxal, possibly through interference with an effect of the vitamer on calcium and/or sodium transport into vascular smooth muscle," a "vitamer" being one or more related chemical substances that fulfill the same specific vitamin function.[102]

Nutritional Therapeutics, Clinical Concerns, and Adaptations

Physicians prescribing hydralazine, alone or as a combination drug, are advised to consider potential benefits of vitamin B$_6$ coadministration. Such concomitant pyridoxine therapy may prevent or reverse adverse effects due to the known actions of the medication. Furthermore, an integrative approach combining these agents may be potentially valuable strategically (preventing hyperhomocysteinemia and potentially reducing the risk of vascular disease, stroke, and dementia). Nevertheless, evidence from well-designed and adequately powered human trials is lacking to confirm need for and benefit of vitamin B$_6$ coadministration or increased pyridoxine intake. Further research is warranted, although it may be a low priority because of the substantially decreased clinical usage of this agent over the past few decades.

In cases where pyridoxine is indicated, certain precautions are recommended. A daily dose of 50 to 100 mg vitamin B$_6$ would be typical in such usage. At such levels the probability of adverse effects from the nutrient are low, but extended use could theoretically cause toxicity symptoms in some individuals. Attention to the potential for adverse effects is judicious within the usual schedule of supervision and monitoring for individuals being treated for hypertension. Caution patients to separate intake of hydralazine and vitamin B$_6$ by at least 2 hours to minimize the risk of any diminished bioavailability of either agent due to complex formation.

Isoniazid, Rifampin, and Related Antitubercular Agents

Cycloserine (Seromycin), ethambutol (Myambutol), ethionamide (2-ethylthioisonicotinamide; Trecator SC), isoniazid (isonicotinic acid hydrazide; INH, Laniazid, Nydrazid), pyrazinamide (PZA; Tebrazid), rifampicin (Rifadin, Rifadin IV); combination drugs: isoniazid and rifampicin (Rifamate, Rimactane); isoniazid, pyrazinamide and rifampicin (Rifater).

Interaction Type and Significance

◇≈≈ **Drug-Induced Adverse Effect on Nutrient Function, Coadministration Therapeutic, with Professional Management**

≈≈ **Drug-Induced Nutrient Depletion, Supplementation Therapeutic, with Professional Management**

☼ **Prevention or Reduction of Drug Adverse Effect**

⊕✗ **Bimodal or Variable Interaction, with Professional Management**

✗ **Potential or Theoretical Adverse Interaction of Uncertain Severity**

See also Folic Acid monograph.

Nutrient Interference Probability:	Evidence Base:
3. Possible	◉◉ Emerging

Coadministration Benefit Probability:	Evidence Base:
3. Possible or 1. Certain	▽ Mixed or ●●● Consensus

Drug Interference Probability:	Evidence Base:
4. Plausible	☐ Inadequate

Effect and Mechanism of Action

A number of antitubercular drugs exert significant adverse effects on normal metabolism and function of vitamin B$_6$, as well as folate and niacin/niacinamide. These medications are occasionally used as single agents but are more often administered in multidrug regimens for the treatment of tuberculosis (TB), especially in patients co-infected with HIV.

Isoniazid is a hydrazine derivative and pyridoxine antagonist that reacts with PLP to form a metabolically inactive hydrazone, inactivating PLP, and thereby producing a functional vitamin B$_6$ deficiency. Thus, isoniazid can interfere with the normal activity of pyridoxine through competitive inhibition, usually in a dose-dependent manner.[103] These effects may lead to anemia or peripheral neuropathies.[104-108] Further, the ingestion of toxic amounts of isoniazid, as little as 1.5 g in adults, can cause increasingly severe adverse effects, with refractory seizures, profound metabolic acidosis, coma, and occasionally death at doses larger than 30 mg/kg.[109] Intravenous pyridoxine is considered the specific antidote for acute isoniazid neurotoxicity and is often used before or along with hemodialysis.[110,111]

Cycloserine acts as a pyridoxine antagonist by forming a metabolically inactive oxime. The resulting impairment of vitamin B$_6$ availability reduces blood levels of pyridoxine and may lead to anemia or peripheral neuropathies.[112,113] However, seizures, which may accompany cycloserine administration, may result from pyridoxine depletion associated with the underlying tubercular infection rather from a direct pyridoxine antagonism by the drug.[114]

Both isoniazid and cycloserine inhibit human erythrocyte pyridoxal kinase using pyridoxal, but not pyridoxamine, as substrate and can react with pyridoxal or PLP to form covalent complexes. Kinetic studies suggest that the observed pyridoxal kinase inhibition resulted from these formed complexes.[115]

Ethionamide, an antileprosy drug sometimes used in combination with other agents for treating multidrug-resistant tuberculosis, may also increase vitamin B$_6$ requirements.[106]

Research

The action of isoniazid and related antitubercular drugs as pyridoxine antagonists is generally agreed on, and the efficacy of pyridoxine in countering the toxic effects of isoniazid is well established.[107,113] Nevertheless, the issue of whether all patients are vulnerable to clinically significant adverse effects with typical clinical practice involving antitubercular drugs has been contentious, and the benefits of routine vitamin B_6 coadministration have been the subject of long-standing controversy.

The relationship between the toxic effects of isoniazid and other anti-TB drugs and their interference with vitamin B_6 has been developed over many years and is regarded as consensus.[107,112,113,116] Several early studies by Polish researchers focused on the effects of isoniazid and ethionamide on pyridoxine metabolism in children and the use of the tryptophan test as an assay for determining pyridoxine levels.[106,117,118] However, an investigation of the effect of cycloserine on pyridoxine-dependent metabolism in TB by Nair et al.[114] indicated that the pathological processes of TB itself contributed significantly to B_6 depletion. Measuring urinary tryptophan metabolites, they observed an "abnormally high level of xanthurenic acid excretion in untreated patients," which they interpreted to suggest "a decreased availability of pyridoxal phosphate related to the disease process. Although plasma cycloserine levels were kept high once therapy began, xanthurenic acid excretion before and after tryptophan load became progressively more normal as symptoms diminished." The authors noted that "throughout the study, no significant changes in 5-hydroxyindoleacetic acid excretion were observed" and suggested that "the convulsions which may sometimes accompany cycloserine administration are not due to a direct pyridoxine antagonism by the drug."[114]

In a 1980 review of the scientific literature on pyridoxine administration during isoniazid therapy, Snider[103] reported on the frequency of INH-induced neuropathy in various studies and identified population groups at relatively high risk of developing this often-serious complication. He reported that pyridoxine administration "during isoniazid (INH) therapy is necessary in some patients to prevent the development of peripheral neuropathy" and concluded that the "routine use of pyridoxine supplementation to prevent peripheral neuropathy in high risk populations is recommended."[103] Subsequently, Mbala et al.[119] conducted a prospective, single-blind, placebo-controlled, randomized trial involving 85 children with TB in Zaire. These researchers observed no occurrences of "neurological or neuropsychiatric disorder ... in the two groups during the 6 months of the treatment and 3 months after the treatment" and interpreted their findings to "suggest that the vitamin B_6 supplementation of isoniazid therapy is unnecessary in childhood TB."[119] However, in a review article on recognition and management of isoniazid overdose, also published in 1998, Romero and Kuczler[109] cautioned that "physicians must be aware of its potentially fatal effects." They concluded: "Given in gram-per-gram amounts of the isoniazid ingested, pyridoxine (vitamin B_6) usually eliminates seizure activity and helps to correct the patient's metabolic acidosis. Isoniazid toxicity should be suspected in any patient who presents with refractory seizures and metabolic acidosis." Overall, the consensus within the scientific literature indicates that patient characteristics are more significant than drug toxicity alone in determining the need for nutrient coadministration, but that pyridoxine is effective in the prevention and treatment of isoniazid toxicity.[120]

The coadministration of isoniazid (INH) and pyridoxine has frequently been used in the treatment of HIV-infected individuals at risk for or diagnosed with TB. Chaisson[121] and Gordin et al.[122] reported the findings of two independent clinical trials that compared combinations of isoniazid with pyridoxine or rifampin and pyrazinamide (PZA) in the treatment of patients with HIV and latent TB infections and prevention of active TB development. INH/pyridoxine given for 6 to 12 months was effective in preventing TB in dually infected adults. However, treatment with rifampin and pyrazinamide, dosed either daily or twice weekly, required only 2 months of treatment to prevent TB effectively in such patients.

In 1957, McCune et al.[123] conducted in vivo animal studies suggesting that administration of high doses of vitamin B_6 can interfere with the effect of isoniazid and indicating that the appearance of this isoniazid antagonism might be delayed. Evidence from human trials is lacking to confirm this proposed interaction or to determine its clinical significance and frequency.

Reports

Haden[105] described a case of pyridoxine-responsive sideroblastic anemia due to antitubercular drugs.

Brent et al.[111] reported "three cases of obtundation secondary to isoniazid overdose that was immediately reversed by intravenous pyridoxine." Status epilepticus seizures were stopped by IV pyridoxine administration in two of these cases; although the patients remained comatose for prolonged periods, the comas were immediately reversed by the administration of additional pyridoxine. In the third case, isoniazid-induced lethargy was treated by IV pyridoxine on presentation, and the patient responded with immediate reversal of lethargy. The authors concluded that pyridoxine is "effective in treating not only isoniazid-induced seizures, but also the mental status changes associated with this overdose" and noted that the "dose required to induce awakening may be higher than that required to control seizures."[111]

Chan[124] described a case in which administration of 10 mg/day of pyridoxine was ineffective in reversing isoniazid-induced psychosis. This dose is relatively low, and the author suggested that a larger dose, such as 50 mg/day, might have been necessary.

Nutritional Therapeutics, Clinical Concerns, and Adaptations

Physicians treating individuals with latent or active TB are advised to consider coadministration of vitamin B_6 (as well as folic acid and niacinamde) to prevent or counter potential adverse drug effects, particularly development of nutrient deficiency and peripheral neuropathy, associated with isoniazid and related antitubercular drugs. Assessment of risk for nutrient deficiency at the initiation of treatment and testing of nutrient levels during therapy may be warranted in certain cases.

Although almost certain to occur to some degree, clinically significant adverse effects on vitamin B_6 levels and related functions are generally considered improbable in most healthy, well-nourished patients with typical dosage levels, such as isoniazid (INH) 5 mg/kg. However, these medications can pose significant risks in major segments of the populations at greatest risk of exposure to TB, latent TB infection, or active TB: impoverished, malnourished, or homeless persons; IV drug users; HIV-positive individuals; institutionalized elderly persons; and those with severe illness or compromised health. Risks of adverse drug effects are also heightened in patients who are pregnant, have underlying seizure disorders, or are at significant risk for the development of peripheral neuropathy due to comorbid conditions such as malnutrition, diabetes, HIV infection, alcoholism, or uremia.

In cases where pyridoxine is indicated certain precautions are recommended. Although no recommended dosage level has been established, a daily dose of 50 mg vitamin B_6 is typical in such cases. At such low levels, the probability of adverse effects from the nutrient are low. Monitoring for potential adverse effects from pyridoxine is nevertheless recommended as judicious because extended use, especially with 'higher doses,' could theoretically cause toxicity in some individuals. However, the intercurrent development of peripheral neuropathy while receiving antitubercular treatment could also reflect inadequate pyridoxine status, so there may be a role for laboratory evaluation in such cases.

The general toxicity, and hepatotoxicity in particular, associated with antitubercular medications remains a significant clinical concern in all patients. In particular, isoniazid, pyrazinamide, and rifampin are not recommended for patients with a history of liver toxicity related to any antitubercular medication or underlying liver disease and should be used with caution in patients being treated with other potentially hepatotoxic drugs. Close supervision and regular monitoring are recommended, beginning with complete blood count, platelet levels, and hepatic functioning at the initiation of treatment, then monthly in patients being treated with single-drug therapy (INH or rifampin) and at 2, 4, 6, and 8 weeks for those receiving both rifampin and pyrazinamide for 2 months. Clinical monitoring consists of a detailed review for possible signs and symptoms of drug-induced hepatitis or other adverse effects, including rash, fever, fatigue, nausea, vomiting, jaundice, right upper quadrant abdominal pain, and paresthesias. Refractory seizures and metabolic acidosis are hallmarks of toxicity and demand urgent intervention with parenteral pyridoxine. "Isoniazid should be discontinued in symptomatic patients whose serum aminotransferases are more than three times normal and in asymptomatic patients whose aminotransferases are more than five times normal."[125]

Levodopa, Carbidopa, Benserazide, and Related Antiparkinsonian Medications

Carbidopa (Lodosyn), levodopa (L-dopa; Dopar, Larodopa); combination drugs: levodopa and benserazide (co-beneldopa; Madopar); levodopa and carbidopa (Atamet, Parcopa, Sinemet, Sinemet CR); levodopa, carbidopa, and entacapone (Stalevo).
Levodopa Monotherapy

Interaction Type and Significance

✗ ✗   Minimal to Mild Adverse Interaction—Vigilance Necessary

◇≈≈   Drug-Induced Nutrient Depletion, Supplementation Contraindicated, Professional Management Appropriate

Probability: Evidence Base:
3. Possible to   ● Consensus
  2. Probable
Levodopa with a Peripheral Dopa-Decarboxylase Inhibitor (DDI)

Interaction Type and Significance
☼ Prevention or Reduction of Drug Adverse Effect

Probability: Evidence Base:
5. Improbable   ● Consensus

Effect and Mechanism of Action

Pyridoxal 5'-phosphate (PLP) acts as a cofactor in the conversion of levodopa to dopamine. Levodopa acts as a vitamin B_6 antagonist, and increased levels can increase the metabolic requirements for pyridoxine. Concomitant low-dose vitamin B_6 can prevent or reverse nutrient depletion and adverse sequelae. Conversely, excessive levels of pyridoxine can accelerate peripheral metabolism of levodopa to dopamine (in the gastrointestinal tract). Because levodopa can cross the blood-brain barrier, but dopamine cannot, this reduces the levodopa normally available to the central nervous system (CNS).[126-128] Pyridoxine may also alter levodopa metabolism by Schiff-base formation.[129] Consequently, high levels of pyridoxine intake can reduce the availability of dopa for conversion to dopamine and impair the therapeutic activity of levodopa administered in the treatment of Parkinson's disease. However, combining a DDI such as carbidopa or benserazide with levodopa reduces excessive metabolism of levodopa and increases amounts available to the CNS. Under such conditions, pyridoxine, even at high concentrations, is usually unlikely to affect peripheral metabolism, diminish serum levels of levodopa, or impair drug activity.[130]

Reports and Research

Stockley[129] characterizes the interaction between pyridoxine and levodopa as "clinically important, well documented and well established." Beginning in 1969, a series of reports described and studies consistently demonstrated a pattern of predictable interaction between these two agents. Barham Carter[131] noted that in "the treatment of parkinsonism with levodopa it is often necessary to prescribe drugs to combat the nausea which occasionally occurs," and thus vitamin B_6 had been recommended or self-prescribed based on its potential benefit in alleviating nausea and vomiting. In a much-cited paper, Duvoisin et al.[132] delineated the basic pattern of the antagonism of the effects of levodopa by pyridoxine. They reported that high-dose pyridoxine, 750 to 1000 mg daily, produced a noticeable reduction in the effects of levodopa within 24 hours, and that the effects of the medication were completely abolished within 3 to 4 days. Further, the effects of levodopa were reduced or abolished with daily doses of 50 to 100 mg per day. Notably, daily intake of 5 to 10 mg pyridoxine was associated with an increase in the signs and symptoms of parkinsonism in eight of ten patients. Leon et al.[133] observed a 66% reduction in plasma levodopa levels and exacerbation of Parkinson's disease symptoms in three of four patients administered 50 mg pyridoxine daily concomitantly. A number of other reports and trials confirmed these findings, and a consensus was established by the early 1970s.[126,134-139]

Yahr and Duvoisin[140] determined that a pyridoxine-deficient diet is probably unnecessary to achieve avoidance of B_6-induced impairment of levodopa therapy and might result in pyridoxine deficiency and subsequent adverse effects.

A DDI such as carbidopa or benserazide can neutralize the interactions between pyridoxine and levodopa but may also deplete vitamin B_6. In 1972, Papavasiliou et al.[130] demonstrated the lack of adverse effect from pyridoxine when carbidopa was coadministered with levodopa in a paper describing the "potentiation of central effects with a peripheral inhibitor." In a small study involving six patients on chronic levodopa treatment for Parkinson's disease, Mars[141] reported that mean levodopa plasma levels dropped by from 356 to 109 ng/mL (70%), when 50 mg pyridoxine was coadministered with 250 mg levodopa. In contrast, with levodopa-carbidopa, their mean plasma levels of levodopa increased to 845 ng/mL, almost threefold. Moreover, with 50 mg pyridoxine, mean plasma levels of levodopa rose slightly higher, to 891 ng/mL, although the plasma-integrated area was 22% less than that observed with levodopa-carbidopa. However, in a series of in vitro, animal, and preliminary human studies, Bender et al.[142-145] suggested that benserazide and carbidopa may cause vitamin B₆ depletion by forming hydrazones, inhibiting enzymes in the oxidative pathway of tryptophan metabolism and of nicotinamide nucleotide synthesis, and depleting niacin. Overall, most researchers and reviewers concur that use of a DDI with levodopa functionally eliminates the probability of a clinically significant impairment of levodopa's activity and therapeutic efficacy from vitamin B₆ at typical dosage levels. Thus, Stockley's review concludes that "even in the presence of large amounts of pyridoxine, the peripheral metabolism remains unaffected and the serum levels of levodopa are virtually unaffected."[129] Research is lacking to substantiate the suggestion that either carbidopa or benserazide may deplete vitamin B₆ levels to a greater degree than levodopa alone.

Nutritional Therapeutics, Clinical Concerns, and Adaptations

Physicians prescribing levodopa as monotherapy need to caution patients to avoid unplanned consumption of vitamin B₆ above typical dietary levels, such as greater than 5 mg per day, particularly in the form of B₆ supplements or multivitamins containing pyridoxine. Such contraindications are generally considered moot for individuals administered levodopa combined with a DDI such as carbidopa or benserazide, as is currently the standard of care in Parkinson's disease management.

Concomitant administration of low-dose vitamin B₆, 5 to 10 mg per day, may be appropriate to prevent drug-induced pyridoxine deficiency and attendant adverse effects from levodopa or benserazide and carbidopa. Vitamin B₆ may also be indicated in certain patients for prevention of dietary deficiencies, reduction of known health risks, and treatment of comorbid conditions. Close supervision and regular monitoring for decreased effects of levodopa are necessary in individuals for whom vitamin B₆ is indicated during levodopa therapy (without a DDI), particularly since the dose required to counter nutrient depletion overlaps with the lowest dose observed to reduce the therapeutic effect of non-DDI protected levodopa. Limited pyridoxine intake may also be prudent in patients being treated with levodopa-carbidopa (Sinemet) or levodopa-benserazide (Madopar) because these agents may deplete B₆, but high doses of pyridoxine might potentially overwhelm the protective effect of the DDI. In general, any vitamin B₆ intake should be accompanied by food, a meal, or a light snack at bedtime, and separated from levodopa by at least 2 hours. Patients should be advised that increased parkinsonian symptoms would be the typical warning sign of diminished drug activity.

Methotrexate

Methotrexate (Folex, Maxtrex, Rheumatrex)
See also Folic Acid monograph.

Interaction Type and Significance

◇≈≈ **Drug-Induced Adverse Effect on Nutrient Function, Coadministration Therapeutic, with Professional Management**

Nutrient Depletion
Probability: Evidence Base:
3. Possible or   ●●● Consensus
  2. Probable

Coadministration Benefit
Probability: Evidence Base:
4. Plausible or   ▽ Mixed
  3. Possible

Effect and Mechanism of Action

Because inflammation causes tissue-specific depletion of vitamin B₆, individuals with rheumatoid arthritis (RA) more likely tend be to be vitamin B₆ depleted, and abnormal vitamin B₆ status is associated with severity of symptoms in patients with RA.[146-149]

Homocysteine (Hcy) can be metabolized by various pathways, requiring various enzymes, such as methylenetetrahydrofolate reductase and cystathionine beta-synthase, involving reactions that require vitamin B₆ and folate as cofactors. Specifically, vitamin B₆ is involved in the formation of cystathionine from Hcy and is critical to the formation of 5,10-methylenetetrahydrofolate from tetrahydrofolate. Folate and vitamin B₁₂ are involved in the remethylation of Hcy to methionine via a B₁₂-dependent reaction. Elevated plasma total homocysteine (tHcy) has been established as an independent risk factor for cerebrovascular disease, coronary atherosclerosis, peripheral vascular disease, and thrombosis, although the preventive and therapeutic benefit of nutritional therapies to lower Hcy remains to be conclusively demonstrated.

Methotrexate interferes with folate and Hcy metabolism. Both methotrexate and decreased vitamin B₆ (and folate) status can contribute to increased Hcy levels and attendant risks. Coadministration of vitamin B₆, usually with folic acid or activated folic acid, may lower Hcy levels and reduce related pathogenic processes and risks.

Research

A series of studies by Chiang, Selhub, Roubenoff, and colleagues have focused on the relationship between inflammatory processes, RA, and vitamin B₆ status. They reported that plasma pyridoxal 5′-phosphate (PLP) concentration is correlated with functional vitamin B₆ indices in patients with RA and marginal vitamin B₆ status.[150] Furthermore, they have documented strong and consistent associations between vitamin B₆ status and several indicators of inflammation in patients with RA and observed an inverse correlation between circulating vitamin B₆ levels and clinical indicators, including the disability score, length of morning stiffness, degree of pain, and biochemical markers, including erythrocyte sedimentation rate and C-reactive protein levels.[146,148] Based on these findings, they have suggested that "such strong associations imply that impaired vitamin B₆ status in these patients results from inflammation."[149] Subsequently, they conducted a cross-sectional, case-controlled, human clinical trial in parallel with experiments in an animal model of inflammation to investigate whether inflammation directly alters vitamin B₆ tissue contents and its excretion in vivo. Human subjects with RA had low plasma PLP levels compared with healthy control subjects, but normal erythrocyte PLP and urinary 4-pyridoxic acid excretion. Adjuvant arthritis induced in rats did not affect 4-pyridoxic acid excretion or muscle storage of PLP, but did result in significantly lower PLP levels in circulation and in liver during inflammation. Based on these findings, they concluded that the "low plasma pyridoxal 5′-phosphate levels seen in inflammation are unlikely to be due to insufficient intake or excessive vitamin B₆ excretion," but that instead, "inflammation induced a tissue-specific depletion of vitamin B₆" as vitamin B₆ coenzymes are removed from the circulation to meet the higher demands of certain tissues during inflammation.[149]

Although the issue of methotrexate's adverse effect on the role of vitamin B_6 in regulating Hcy is largely agreed on, the clinical significance of Hcy, and its possible elevation by methotrexate, remains contentious. In a 12-month, randomized double-blind trial involving 62 patients with RA and elevated Hcy (≥ 12 μmol/L), Yxfeldt et al.[151] investigated the effects of administering a combination of vitamins B_6, B_{12}, and folic acid on Hcy levels and analyzed the relationship between Hcy levels and inflammatory variables, and/or methotrexate (MTX) treatment. The Hcy level decreased significantly in the subjects treated with B vitamins compared with those given placebo. Furthermore, in a "multiple regression model there was an association between the alteration in Hcy level over 0-12 months and MTX treatment, as well as the alteration in CRP, adjusted for B-vitamin treatment." The authors concluded that Hcy levels in patients with RA can be reduced by treatment with B vitamins, and that Hcy levels were related to markers of inflammation and MTX treatment.[151] However, in a pilot study involving 17 juvenile idiopathic arthritis patients and 17 age-matched and gender-matched healthy children, Huemer et al.[152] found that hyperhomocysteinemia in children with juvenile idiopathic arthritis is not influenced by MTX treatment and folic acid supplementation.

Further research is warranted to determine the degree to which methotrexate adversely influences levels and functions of vitamin B_6, as well as factors influencing interpatient variability, alterations in Hcy status, the influence of B-vitamin supplementation on clinical outcomes, and appropriate nutrient support levels when administration is indicated.

No sources reviewed cited any evidence to suggest that concurrent administration of vitamin B_6, alone or in a multivitamin formulation, might impair the therapeutic efficacy of methotrexate in the treatment of RA or other nononcological applications.

Nutritional Therapeutics, Clinical Concerns, and Adaptations

Physicians administering methotrexate for the treatment of rheumatoid arthritis are advised to consider coadministration of vitamin B_6 (50-100 mg/day) with folic acid, possibly in an activated form, such as folinic acid or 5-L-methyl folate. Such concurrent nutrient support may be effective in countering adverse effects of methotrexate on the physiological activities of vitamin B_6, particularly in the regulation of Hcy, and thereby may reduce related risks of vascular disease. More broadly, individuals with RA are more likely to be nutritionally compromised and benefit from enhanced intake of all key nutrients. Similarly, evaluation of patients for genetic polymorphisms, such as MTHFR 677 C→T, are potentially at greater risk for adverse effects from medications that impair folate metabolism or deplete folate levels.

Neomycin

Neomycin (Mycifradin, Myciguent, Neo-Fradin, NeoTab, Nivemycin).

Interaction Type and Significance

≈≈≈ **Drug-Induced Nutrient Depletion, Supplementation Therapeutic, Not Requiring Professional Management**

☼ **Prevention or Reduction of Drug Adverse Effect**

Probability:
5. **Improbable** or
2. **Probable** (depending on duration)

Evidence Base:
○ **Preliminary** (though generally regarded as
●●● **Consensus**)

Effect and Mechanism of Action

Neomycin may impair the activity of vitamin B_6.[153] Furthermore, oral neomycin can decrease absorption or increase elimination of folic acid and other nutrients, including beta-carotene, calcium, carbohydrates, fats, iron, magnesium, potassium, sodium, vitamin A, vitamin B_{12}, vitamin D, and vitamin K.[116,154] The effects on folic acid and vitamin B_{12}, in particular, can adversely effect vitamin B_6 activity. These effects increase with time in long-term neomycin therapy and can be most significant in the elderly population.[155]

Research

Faloon et al.[156] (1966) documented the adverse effects of neomycin on intestinal absorption of nutrients. Hardison and Rosenberg[157] further elucidated the effect of neomycin on bile salt metabolism and fat digestion in humans. Subsequently, the adverse effects of neomycin on nutrient status were explored extensively in the pioneering work of Daphne A. Roe, MD (1923-1993), of Cornell University, Division of Nutritional Sciences, through publications such as "Drug-Induced Nutritional Deficiencies" (1976). As such, this interaction has largely passed into the "consensus" of the literature documenting adverse drug effects and drug-induced nutrient depletions, without passing through the stages of published case reports, human trials, reviews, etc., which constitute the emerging standard within the scientific literature of drug-nutrient interactions. Further research may be warranted.

Nutritional Therapeutics, Clinical Concerns, and Adaptations

Physicians prescribing a course of oral neomycin lasting more than a few days are advised to coadminister a multivitamin-mineral supplement containing vitamin B_6. Depletion is improbable with short-term use of oral neomycin associated with surgery or perioperative care. A course of probiotic flora is also appropriate following broad-spectrum antibiotics to restore normal gut ecology.

Oral Contraceptives: Monophasic, Biphasic, and Triphasic Estrogen Preparations (Synthetic Estrogen and Progesterone Analogs)

Ethinyl estradiol and desogestrel (Desogen, Ortho-TriCyclen).
Ethinyl estradiol and ethynodiol (Demulen 1/35, Demulen 1/50, Nelulen 1/25, Nelulen 1/50, Zovia).
Ethinyl estradiol and levonorgestrel (Alesse, Levlen, Levlite, Levora 0.15/30, Nordette, Tri-Levlen, Triphasil, Trivora).
Ethinyl estradiol and norethindrone/norethisterone (Brevicon, Estrostep, Genora 1/35, GenCept 1/35, Jenest-28, Loestrin 1.5/30, Loestrin 1/20, Modicon, Necon 1/25, Necon 10/11, Necon 0.5/30, Necon 1/50, Nelova 1/35, Nelova 10/11, Norinyl 1/35, Norlestin 1/50, Ortho Novum 1/35, Ortho Novum 10/11, Ortho Novum 7/7/7, Ovcon-35, Ovcon-50, Tri-Norinyl, Trinovum).
Ethinyl estradiol and norgestrel (Lo/Ovral, Ovral).
Mestranol and norethindrone (Genora 1/50, Nelova 1/50, Norethin 1/50, Ortho-Novum 1/50).
Related, internal application: Etonogestrel/ethinyl estradiol vaginal ring (Nuvaring).

Interaction Type and Significance

☼ **Prevention or Reduction of Drug Adverse Effect**
⊕⊕⊕ **Beneficial or Supportive Interaction, Not Requiring Professional Management**

Nutrient Depletion
Probability: Evidence Base:
5. Improbable   ▽ Mixed

Coadministration Benefit
Probability: Evidence Base:
3. Possible or **2. Probable** ◉◉ Emerging

Effect and Mechanism of Action

Oral contraceptives (OCs) are associated with many symptoms suggestive of a drug-induced vitamin B₆ deficiency and in many ways parallel to postpartum depression or gestational diabetes mellitus. However, these iatrogenic elevations of exogenous estrogen and progestins may contribute to adverse effects such as depression, premenstrual syndrome, and dysglycemia by altering the metabolism and functions of vitamin B₆ more than by directly affecting vitamin B₆ status or causing B₆ deficiency.

Oral contraceptives can interfere in the role that vitamin B₆ plays in facilitating the tryptophan conversion to niacinamide pathway. PLP-dependent enzymes are required in the conversion of L-tryptophan to 5-hydroxytryptamine and L-tyrosine to norepinephrine, as well as synthesis of dopamine, norepinephrine, and gamma-aminobutyric acid (GABA). OCs appear to impair 5-hydroxytryptamine (5-HT, serotonin) formation through interference with 5-hydroxytryptophan decarboxylase and thus contribute to depression due to resulting decreased brain levels of serotonin. Tryptophan dioxygenase is a glucocorticoid-induced enzyme. Elevating concentrations of pyridoxal phosphate by administering pyridoxine reduces synthesis and activity of this enzyme and attenuates the response to glucocorticoid hormones. The resulting reduction in the oxidative metabolism of tryptophan increases the amount of tryptophan available for CNS synthesis of serotonin. OCs with higher estrogen dose increase levels of estrogen metabolites that inhibit kynureninase. The resulting increased tissue and blood concentrations of xanthurenic acid tend to complex with insulin to form a relatively inactive complex and thus impair glucose tolerance.[158,159] Furthermore, abnormal metabolism of tryptophan results not only from induced hepatic tryptophan oxygenase, but also from specific changes in the activity of enzymes beyond kynurenine in the pathway of tryptophan metabolism.[160-162] Additionally, abnormally elevated excretion of tryptophan metabolites could potentially cause some degree of true vitamin B₆ deficiency.[163-165]

Coadministration of vitamin B₆ may ameliorate symptoms associated with OCs, especially when exacerbated in women with compromised nutritional status or other susceptibility factors.[158,166-169] Concomitant pyridoxine support during OC use appears to enable a direct effect of pyridoxal phosphate in inducing tryptophan oxidase and thereby corrects the effects of OCs on tryptophan metabolism, even in the absence of preexisting deficiency.[6,164,170-178] Vitamin B₆ can also enhance glucose tolerance by activating apokynureninase or kynureninase that has been inactivated by undergoing transamination.[179] The dosage of estrogen in the OC formulation appears to influence the probability of adverse effects, at least in some women.

In regard to adverse cardiovascular effects of OCs and other exogenous estrogens, it is noteworthy that pyridoxal 5-phosphate is essential for the metabolism of the atherogenic amino acid homocysteine.

Nutritional requirements for riboflavin may also be higher in OC users because this nutrient is needed to oxidize pyridoxine phosphate to pyridoxal phosphate. Conversely, niacin requirements may be reduced due to alterations in tryptophan metabolism.

Research

A large body of scientific literature indicates that OCs can cause a number of adverse effects in some women, but the issue of whether vitamin B₆ is necessary and should be routinely coadministered to prevent such outcomes remains contentious and unresolved.

Several studies have documented that vitamin B₆ deficiency is relatively common in the U.S. and U.K. population, and numerous papers have reported that reduced levels of vitamin B₆ in women using OCs compared with the general population.[2-4,180-184]

The impact of OCs on vitamin B₆ itself and its functions and the clinical benefit of concurrent pyridoxine administration have been the subject of debate for decades. Variations in the choice of subjects, characteristics of controls, composition and dosage levels of the OCs tested, measures of B₆ status used, adverse effects assessed, and duration of the trials have all contributed to inconsistencies in findings and mixed conclusions.

Over more than a decade the research team of Adams, Rose, Wynn, and colleagues conducted a series of investigations into the relationship between OCs and vitamin B₆. In 1972 they reported that 80% of women taking OCs had abnormal tryptophan metabolism and about 20% demonstrated evidence for absolute deficiency of the nutrient.[185] Reviewing the scientific literature on the subject in early 1973, they wrote that "the altered excretion of tryptophan metabolites observed in women on o.c. is similar to that found in nutritional vitamin-B₆ deficiency, and is corrected by the administration of vitamin B₆. Vitamin B₆ requirements may be further increased by the effect of oestrogen conjugates competitively inhibiting pyridoxal phosphate."[158,160,186-188] Then, in a double-blind, crossover trial involving 22 women "whose depression was thought on clinical grounds to be due to o.c. administration," these researchers observed positive clinical responses on depression with coadministration of B₆ (20 mg twice daily), but notably only in that half of subjects with "absolute vitamin-B₆ deficiency." They suggested that other factors needed to be considered for depression in the other half of depressed women and mentioned insufficient substrate due to tryptophan deficiency as a possible factor.[161] Their continued investigation into the effects of excretion of metabolites after oral loading doses of L-kynurenine led them to conclude that OC use "does not generally change the requirement for vitamin B₆ but rather produces a specific change in activity of enzymes beyond kynurenine in the pathway of tryptophan metabolism."[162] Bennink and Schreurs[181] reported that "vitamin B₆ blood concentration was not affected" in 50 women using combined OCs but also observed that "OCs increased XA [xanthurenic acid] excretion after tryptophan administration in 80% of the users." Amatayakul et al.[159] reported no significant adverse effects on B₆ status but also noted that "urinary xanthurenic acid excretion ... [was] significantly increased by OC treatment, although this excessive XA excretion was adequately corrected with 18 mg of daily vitamin B-6 supplementation." In a 6-month trial, van der Vange et al.[189] investigated the effect of seven low-dose OC preparations, containing equivalent amounts of ethinyl estradiol but different amounts and types of progestagen, on vitamin B₆ status in 55 women. They observed increases in erythrocyte glutamic-oxaloacetic transaminase (EGOT) activity, a pyridoxal phosphate–dependent enzyme, and the calculated total EGOT activity after 6 months' treatment, but no changes were observed in the degree of in vitro stimulation, considered a more reliable parameter. Plasma PLP levels initially decreased during the first 3 months of treatment, but levels returned to normal after 6 months. Based on these findings, the authors concluded that "the low-dose preparations investigated in this study have no any adverse effects on vitamin B$_6$ status."[189] Notably, several studies used women with intrauterine devices (IUDs) as controls; a questionable proposition given the emerging understanding of the impact of inflammation on B$_6$ status.

Massé et al.[190] investigated the effects of a low-dose triphasic OC preparation (30 μg estrogen) in 14 young female subjects (and nine matched controls). They found that short-term OC use did not demonstrably alter PLP levels in plasma and erythrocytes in the majority of women with adequate dietary intake. Although by employing two methods of assessment, "only one case (7%) of deficiency due to OC was evidenced, ... a disturbance in vitamin B$_6$ metabolism was detected. PL levels in both blood components have increased steadily and did not subside to pretreatment values at the end of the experiment." They concluded by suggesting that "the single use of the PLP vitamer can be misleading as demonstrated by other investigators" and suggested the need to explore B$_6$ status further by evaluating "the other aldehydic form of vitamin B$_6$, to fully establish and comprehend hormone-induced adverse effects on this metabolism, particularly those of progesterone/progestin that have not yet been explored."[190] In a double blind, placebo-controlled trial, involving women taking low-dose OCs, Villegas-Salas et al.[191] reported no significant benefit in the prevention of adverse effects, such as nausea, vomiting, dizziness, depression, and irritability, from coadministration of up to 150 mg of pyridoxine daily.

In overview, the trend in the scientific literature indicates that OCs, especially in lower dose forms, usually do not directly deplete vitamin B$_6$ in most women, but may increase such risk or may be more likely to contribute to related adverse effects in those with higher B$_6$ requirements or compromised nutritional intake. However, most but not all researchers have found that OCs present a significant risk of altering several normal physiological pathways that involve B$_6$-dependent enzymes, and that in many cases, coadministration of pyridoxine, even in low doses, can prevent or reverse adverse effects related to hyperestrogenism, such as depression, dysglycemia, and premenstrual syndrome. Evidence is lacking at this time to support routine supplementation because of the inconsistencies in methodology and limited nature of the available research. Further investigation through well-designed and adequately powered long-term clinical trials is warranted to evaluate which patients are at greatest risk for adverse effects and most likely to benefit from nutrient support, as well as clinical parameters for determining dosage levels and concomitant nutrients indicated for optimal intervention.

The issue of whether or not concomitant vitamin B$_6$ supplementation might be beneficial or necessary in women taking OCs remains unresolved, but the discussion of adverse effects from such coadministration has usually not extended beyond the usual medical caution regarding dose-related pyridoxine toxicity. However, in 1973, Adams et al.[161] suggested that women with low daily protein consumption might be at increased risk for adverse effects with pyridoxine supplementation due to an increase in amino acid catabolism as a result of excess pyridoxine relative to protein intake. Throughout the

lengthy but limited history of human research on this issue, the absence of incidents of actual adverse effects attributable to excess pyridoxine intake is notable, especially given the loud warnings so often voiced regarding the potential risk of nutrient-induced toxicity.

Nutritional Therapeutics, Clinical Concerns, and Adaptations

Physicians prescribing OCs are advised to assess the patient's individual physiological characteristics, medical history, and nutritional status to determine the probability of an adverse reaction to the treatment. Based on such evaluation, or in response to a patient's expressed concern, it would then be appropriate to consider whether vitamin B$_6$ coadministration might reduce the risk and severity of potential adverse effects of the exogenous hormones, including effects on pyridoxine levels and function and increased incidence and severity of depression, dysglycemia, premenstrual syndrome, and disorders associated with elevated estrogen levels. Although the typical supplemental dose for pyridoxine in such situations is 10 to 75 mg per day, higher levels in the range of 100 to 400 mg per day may be indicated for short periods in cases where individual preventive and therapeutic requirements may be greater. Adverse effects from pyridoxine are improbable at lower doses, but such higher doses of vitamin B$_6$ may have significant risk of causing adverse effects and require caution, professional supervision, and regular monitoring, even for short periods. In cases where broader nutritional deficits are apparent, the administration of a multivitamin-mineral formulation may be more appropriate than a narrower pyridoxine prescription.

The tryptophan load test may provide a functional assessment of vitamin B$_6$ status and its influence upon tryptophan metabolism. With depression, as with any complex condition, the presence of OCs is unlikely to constitute the sole cause, or even be the decisive factor. Nevertheless, in certain cases, OCs may be inappropriate because of adverse effects.

Experienced practitioners of natural therapies frequently coadminister a range of agents to women who seek care for presumed adverse effects from OCs. Botanical preparations such chasteberry (*Vitex agnus castus*), dandelion root (*Taraxacum officinale*), fringetree root and bark (*Chionanthus virginicus*), dong quai (*Angelica sinensis*), burdock root (*Arctium lappa*), and wild yam root (*Dioscorea villosa*) have an extensive history of traditional usage and are administered clinically to enhance hepatic conjugation of estrogen, facilitate hormonal self-regulatory systems, and mitigate hyperestrogenism. Calcium, magnesium, evening primrose oil, riboflavin, folic acid, ascorbic acid, vitamin B$_{12}$, and vitamin E may also be beneficial for some women, particularly with preexisting insufficiency or drug-induced deficiency. Individualized assessment and an evolving therapeutic response involving collaboration of health care professionals trained and experienced in the various therapeutic modalities applied are usually essential to successful clinical outcomes.

Penicillamine

Penicillamine (D-Penicillamine; Cuprimine, Depen).

Interaction Type and Significance

◇◇ **Impaired Drug Absorption and Bioavailability, Precautions Appropriate**

≈≈ **Drug-Induced Nutrient Depletion, Supplementation Therapeutic, with Professional Management**

☼ **Prevention or Reduction of Drug Adverse Effect**

Probability:

5. **Improbable** or
   3. **Probable**

Evidence Base:

◉ **Emerging**

Effect and Mechanism of Action

Penicillamine can act as a pyridoxine antagonist by reacting with pyridoxal 5′-phosphate (PLP) to form a metabolically inactive thiazolidine. This pharmacokinetic interaction can increase vitamin B₆ excretion, reduce its physiological activity, and over time, increase the risk for a functional pyridoxine deficiency.[100,192,193] Vitamin B₆ may be coadministered to counteract potential adverse effects, such as anemia and peripheral neuritis.[194]

The formation of a metabolically inactive chelate could also potentially interfere with penicillamine to impair its therapeutic action to a clinically significant degree.

Separating the intake of two substances that tend to bind by several hours usually minimizes such interaction in the gastrointestinal tract.

Research

The long-term use of penicillamine may increase pyridoxine requirements. Pyridoxine administration can prevent or reverse pyridoxine deficiency as a result of this interaction.

Vitamin B₆ can act as an anticonvulsant. Conversely, seizures have been induced by DL-penicillamine and other vitamin B₆ antagonists, such as hydrazine and thiosemicarbazide. Using a mouse model, Abe and Matsuda observed that "the onset of convulsions induced by these convulsants coincides with the fall in GABA [gamma-aminobutyric acid] content and GAD [glutamic acid decarboxylase] activity in the mesencephalon area, and in contrast, the cessation of the convulsions by PN [pyridoxine] supplement coincides with the recovery in both the parameters."[195,196]

Researchers have noted an interrelationship between zinc and magnesium depletion and pyridoxine inactivation in autoimmune complications and other adverse effects associated with D-penicillamine.[197,198] In a trial involving 144 rheumatoid arthritis patients treated with penicillamine (125-1000 mg/day), Rumsby and Shepherd[199] found that 17% developed vitamin B₆ deficiency. However, clinical signs of deficiency were absent, using in vitro measurement of percentage stimulation of erythrocyte alanine aminotransferase (ALT) on addition of an excess of PLP to the blood sample. The investigators observed significantly higher unstimulated activity of PLP, a PLP-dependent apoenzyme, in penicillamine-treated subjects than in controls, as expected if ALT were deficient in its PLP coenzyme. Furthermore, they reported less marked in vitro ALT stimulation by PLP at intermediate penicillamine dosage levels, compared to controls. Such a pattern suggests that a pyridoxine deficiency is more likely in the early stages of penicillamine therapy, after which some degree of recovery might occur, and that lasting or recurrent deficiency is more likely in individuals later administered higher doses of the drug. These findings suggest that, barring clinical signs of pyridoxine deficiency, most patients are unlikely to require pyridoxine coadministration, unless they have a history of poor nutritional intake or other compromising factors.[199] Nevertheless, Rothschild[194] and other investigators have suggested that coadministration of vitamin B₆, in daily doses as high as 50 mg, may be indicated. Other methods of assessing B₆ deficiency might also be sensitive, such as measuring urinary xanthurenic acid excretion following an oral tryptophan load test.

Nutritional Therapeutics, Clinical Concerns, and Adaptations

Physicians prescribing penicillamine are advised that coadministration of vitamin B₆ may be prudent. Substantive evidence is lacking to confirm the need for and benefit of routine B₆ coadministration, and further research with well-designed and adequately powered clinical trials may be warranted. Nevertheless, the available evidence is adequately consistent from both pharmacological and clinical perspectives to warrant preventive measures, especially since they carry minimal risk. Monitoring of pyridoxine status may be warranted with chronic penicillamine therapy.

Certain patients are at higher risk for adverse reactions to penicillamine and risk of complications from pyridoxine deficiency. In particular, because of their dietary restrictions, individuals with Wilson's disease and cystinuria being treated with penicillamine would benefit from 25 mg of pyridoxine daily during therapy. Likewise, a daily supplement of pyridoxine is also indicated for patients with rheumatoid arthritis whose nutrition is impaired. In general, individuals taking penicillamine for any reason should supplement with the relatively small dose of 5 to 20 mg of vitamin B₆ daily. However, given the potential for binding, oral intake should be separated by at least 2 hours.

Phenelzine and Related Monoamine Oxidase (MAO) Inhibitors

Evidence: Phenelzine (Nardil), tranylcypromine (Parnate).
Extrapolated, based on similar properties, as MAO-A inhibitors: Isocarboxazid (Marplan), procarbazine (Matulane). Similar properties but evidence indicating no or reduced interaction effects: Poclobemide (Aurorix, Manerix), pargyline (Eutonyl).
Not supported by extrapolation from evidence (MAO-B inhibitors): selegiline (deprenyl, L-deprenil, L-deprenyl; Atapryl, Carbex, Eldepryl, Jumex, Movergan, Selpak).
See also Selegiline in Theoretical, Speculative, and Preliminary Interactions Research.

Interaction Type and Significance

◇◇ **Impaired Drug Absorption and Bioavailability, Precautions Appropriate**

⊕✗ **Bimodal or Variable Interaction, with Professional Management**

≈≈ **Drug-Induced Nutrient Depletion, Supplementation Therapeutic, with Professional Management**

☼ **Prevention or Reduction of Drug Adverse Effect**

Probability:

2. **Probable** or
   3. **Possible**

Evidence Base:

○ **Preliminary**

Effect and Mechanism of Action

The conversion of tryptophan to serotonin (5-hydroxytryptamine) is catalyzed by a PLP-dependent enzyme. Dopamine, norepinephrine, and gamma-aminobutyric acid (GABA) are other neurotransmitters synthesized using PLP-dependent enzymes. CNS serotonin is metabolized by monoamine oxidase (MAO) to 5-hydroxyindoleacetic acid (5-HIAA). MAO inhibitors elevate serotonin concentrations (along with other monoamine neurotransmitters, e.g., dopamine) by inhibiting such metabolic breakdown of the monoamine neurotransmitters.

Phenelzine can act as a pyridoxine antagonist by reacting with PLP to form a metabolically inactive hydrazone compound and reduce blood levels of vitamin B_6. Isoniazid and hydralazine, agents with chemical structures similar to phenelzine, are known to cause vitamin B_6 deficiency.[107,108,178] Thus, these drugs can decrease pyridoxine status and induce peripheral neuropathy, carpal tunnel syndrome, and other conditions associated with pyridoxine deficiency.

Reports and Research

There have been numerous reports of vitamin B_6 deficiency and subsequent adverse effects associated with long-term MAO inhibitor therapy. Despite the well-documented adverse effects of similar substances, there has been no definitive confirmation of the consistent but anecdotal and preliminary evidence involving phenelzine and related agents. Likewise, substantive evidence is lacking to prove benefit from nutrient coadministration. Research through well-designed and adequately powered clinical trials is warranted.

Harrison et al.[200] published a case report of carpal tunnel syndrome associated with tranylcypromine in 1983. That same year, Heller and Friedman[201] reported a case of pyridoxine deficiency and peripheral neuropathy associated with long-term phenelzine therapy. In 1984, Demers et al.[202] reported pyridoxine deficiency in two young men treated with phenelzine. "Alleviation of symptoms possibly associated with this deficiency and correction of subnormal serum B_6 levels occurred with the administration of pyridoxine." Several years later, Goodheart et al.[203] described the cases of two patients in whom clinical and electrophysiological findings confirmed sensorimotor peripheral neuropathy associated with phenelzine therapy. "Symptoms were predominantly sensory, and improvement occurred after withdrawal of phenelzine. Electrophysiologic findings were consistent with an axonal process."

Nutritional Therapeutics, Clinical Concerns, and Adaptations

Physicians prescribing phenelzine or related MAO inhibitors need to be alert to the possibility of this potential adverse interaction and instruct patients to eat a diet providing adequate amounts of vitamin B_6. Preventive coadministration of vitamin B_6 supplements may be warranted, especially in patients with compromised nutritional intake or comorbid conditions or medications that might also impair B_6 status. Many providers trained and experienced in nutritional therapeutics routinely advise patients treated with these medications to supplement with vitamin B_6, usually at moderate levels, such as 25 to 50 mg per day. Alternately, nutrient support can be initiated if untoward reactions occur during phenelzine treatment suggestive of B_6 deficiency. Monitoring of pyridoxine status may be warranted with chronic MAO inhibitor therapy. Although the MAO inhibitors are much less frequently used in the modern era of psychopharmacology, because of their well-known and dangerous interactions with medications such as meperidine, propoxyphene, and dextromethorphan, as well as food components such as tyramine, they remain important agents for certain patients with bipolar or unipolar depression who respond to none of the other classes of agents.

Tetracycline Antibiotics

Demeclocycline (Declomycin), doxycycline (Atridox, Doryx, Doxy, Monodox, Periostat, Vibramycin, Vibra-Tabs), minocycline (Dynacin, Minocin, Vectrin), oxytetracycline (Terramycin), tetracycline (Achromycin, Actisite, Sumycin, Topicycline; combination drugs: Detereclo, Helidac).

Interaction Type and Significance

⊕⊕   **Beneficial or Supportive Interaction, with Professional Management**

⊕✗   **Bimodal or Variable Interaction, with Professional Management**

◇◇   **Impaired Drug Absorption and Bioavailability, Precautions Appropriate**

≈≈   **Drug-Induced Nutrient Depletion, Supplementation Therapeutic, with Professional Management**

Probability:	Evidence Base:
4. Plausible	⊙ **Emerging**

Effect and Mechanism of Action

Oral B vitamin intake, including pyridoxine, may interfere with tetracycline pharmacokinetics, impairing absorption and bioavailability. Such an interaction would also impair bioavailability of the nutrient(s). Tetracyclines can also increase vitamin B_6 urinary excretion.

Research

Omray and Varma[204] demonstrated that oral administration of a formulation containing vitamin B complex and vitamin C could impair absorption and reduce bioavailability of tetracycline through pharmacokinetic interference.

Nutritional Therapeutics, Clinical Concerns, and Adaptations

Physicians prescribing tetracycline or related antibiotic medications can prudently advise patients regularly supplementing with vitamin B_6, alone or within a B-complex vitamin formulation, to take such supplements and the medication at least 4 hours apart. Although depletion of vitamin B_6 (from simultaneous intake and binding) may not have clinical significance with short-term use of tetracycline, individuals using the drug longer than 2 weeks may benefit from supplementation. A moderate supplemental dose of pyridoxine is usually in the range of 20 to 25 mg per day, easily obtained through most multivitamin formulas. Sustained use of higher doses of B_6 can potentially result in adverse effects and warrants supervision. Significant dietary sources of vitamin B_6 include bananas, lentils, potatoes, raisin bran, turkey, and tuna.

Prudence suggests that individuals treated with tetracyclines or other broad-spectrum antibiotics for an extended time be administered a course of probiotic flora for an equivalent duration to restore intestinal microbiota. Short-term use of tetracyclines may not lead to clinically significant alterations in the gastrointestinal ecology.

Theophylline/Aminophylline

Theophylline/aminophylline (Phyllocontin, Slo-Bid, Slo-Phyllin, Theo-24, Theo-Bid, Theocron, Theo-Dur, Theolair, Truphylline, Uni-Dur, Uniphyl); combination drug: ephedrine, guaifenesin, and theophylline (Primatene Dual Action).

Similar properties but evidence lacking for extrapolation: Dyphylline (Dilor, Lufyllin), oxytriphylline (Choledyl).

Interaction Type and Significance

◇≈≈   **Drug-Induced Adverse Effect on Nutrient Function, Coadministration Therapeutic, with Professional Management**

≈≈   **Drug-Induced Nutrient Depletion, Supplementation Therapeutic, with Professional Management**

☼ **Prevention or Reduction of Drug Adverse Effect**
⊕ **Potential or Theoretical Beneficial or Supportive**
   Interaction, with Professional Management

Nutrient Depletion
Probability: Evidence Base:
1. Certain   ●●● Consensus

Coadministration Benefit
Probability: Evidence Base:
2. Probable   ◉◉ Emerging or
                                ●●● Consensus

Effect and Mechanism of Action

Theophylline is a potent noncompetitive inhibitor of pyridoxal kinase, the enzyme needed to convert vitamin B₆ to its active form, pyridoxal 5′-phosphate (PLP) and therefore is a pyridoxine antagonist.[115,205] Theophylline also, paradoxically, induces pyridoxal kinase synthesis, thus speeding up pyridoxine metabolism, depending on the balance of these two opposing actions, and sometimes may result in depressed circulating PLP concentrations and body stores of pyridoxine, even though circulating pyridoxal levels may remain unchanged.[90,206-210] The resultant deficit of PLP results in multiple decreased B₆-dependent enzyme activities, including GABA synthesis, and can increase the risk of seizures, hand tremor, and other adverse CNS effects of theophylline.[209] Thus, theophylline may increase intake requirements for vitamin B₆, whereas concomitant pyridoxine or pyridoxal administration may normalize B₆ levels and reduce many theophylline-induced adverse effects without impairing the therapeutic activity of theophylline.[211,212] This beneficial effect may result, at least in part, from the modulating effect of pyridoxine and that of theophylline on catecholamine release.[213,214] Moreover, pyridoxine levels tend to be low in many asthmatic individuals, and its administration may play an important role in the treatment of asthma.

Research

A large number of animal experiments and human trials consistently demonstrate an adverse effect of theophylline on vitamin B₆ levels and functions that can be clinically significant, a high probability of benefit from administration of B₆ in some form, and a lack of adverse effects from concurrent intake.

Delport, Ubbink, Bartel, and colleagues at the University of Pretoria researched the interaction between theophylline and vitamin B₆ in many studies over several years.[215] In a 1988 study they reported that plasma PLP concentrations were significantly lower in a group of 28 asthmatic women, compared to 33 controls, although plasma pyridoxal levels were not different between the two groups. When they administered theophylline to 17 volunteers, they observed "large reductions in plasma pyridoxal-5′-phosphate levels, while plasma pyridoxal levels and urinary 4-pyridoxic acid excretion were unaffected by theophylline therapy."[205] The following year, in a 4-week placebo-controlled, double-blind trial involving apparently healthy young men, they demonstrated that theophylline greatly reduced serum vitamin B₆ levels and erythrocyte PLP levels through noncompetitive inhibition of erythrocyte pyridoxal kinase, and that both plasma PLP levels and the tryptophan load test normalized after 1 week of pyridoxine vitamin B₆ (10 mg/day).[206] Subsequently, they "demonstrated a significant correlation...between drug plasma levels and erythrocyte pyridoxal kinase activities"

and showed that vitamin B₆ coadministration produced "a four-fold increase in circulating pyridoxal 5′-phosphate levels."[211]

Other researchers have also reported depression of vitamin B₆ levels due to theophylline. Using a rabbit model, Weir et al.[90] observed that administration of "theophylline preparations intraperitoneally (aminophylline) or orally (sustained release anhydrous theophylline) resulted in a 47% depression of plasma pyridoxal 5′-phosphate (PLP) levels. The 87% increase in PLP with pyridoxine administration was only 18% when aminophylline was also given." They described the mechanism of the theophylline-B₆ interaction as "obscure" but noted that the "ethylenediamine in some theophylline preparations binds directly to PLP, potentially increasing the less direct theophylline effect." Furthermore, they cautioned that "pyridoxine supplementation resulted in higher average PLP levels but did not prevent death in animals with profoundly low PLP levels."[90] In a study of 26 asthmatic children, Shimizu et al.[216] found a depression of serum PLP levels existed in asthmatic children treated with theophylline compared with those not receiving theophylline; thus a "significant negative correlation between the serum levels of PLP and theophylline was demonstrated in the subjects." Oral administration of 200 mg of theophylline (Theo-Dur) to five children with asthma significantly depressed serum PLP levels 4 hours after the drug intake, whereas theophylline did not affect serum pyridoxal levels. Subsequently, this team of researchers studied 23 asthmatic children, 7 to 15 years old, including 16 patients who were treated with slow-release theophylline and seven patients not receiving any theophylline preparation. They evaluated steady-state serum theophylline and vitamin A, B₁, B₂, B₆, B₁₂, and C levels and demonstrated a "significant negative correlation between theophylline and circulating levels of vitamin B₆," with serum vitamin B₆ levels lowered by 40% in the children treated with slow-release theophylline for more than a year.[217] Likewise, Tanaka et al.[209] investigated the effect of sustained-release theophylline preparations on circulating vitamin B₆ concentrations in 26 children with asthma and determined that "serum PL and PLP concentrations in children within theophylline therapeutic ranges (5 to 15 micrograms/mL) were significantly lower than those with theophylline concentrations of less than 5 micrograms/mL." Martinez de Haas et al.[218] studied 141 adults and found that both geriatric and nongeriatric patients with chronic obstructive pulmonary disease being treated with theophylline exhibited markedly higher prevalence of subnormal vitamin B₆ status, as measured by PLP in whole blood, than did those not being treated with theophylline. Notably, 70% of the 40 chronic obstructive pulmonary disease (COPD) patients not treated with theophylline and 56% of the 84 geriatric non-COPD patients also had a subnormal vitamin B₆ status, suggesting a rather high baseline B₆ deficiency rate in the geriatric population.

The adverse effects of theophylline on the nervous system are well documented, with theophylline-induced seizures, in particular, being widely recognized for their significant morbidity and mortality given their recalcitrance to treatment. Glenn et al.[208] investigated the relationship between depressed plasma PLP levels and decreased GABA synthesis with theophylline treatment and the occurrence of seizures in experiments involving mice and rabbits. They observed that pyridoxine administration significantly decreased rates of seizure and death, and that "serum theophylline levels and plasma PLP levels showed significant negative correlation prior to pyridoxine infusion." They noted that "all six rabbits developed abnormal EEGs during theophylline infusion and all six rabbit EEG patterns returned to baseline during treatment with pyridoxine."[208] In a randomized, double-blind, placebo-controlled, crossover study, the South African researchers previously discussed administered theophylline to 15 young, healthy adults daily for 4 weeks, at a dosage level adjusted to produce plasma levels of 10 mg/L (10 µg/mL), combined with either placebo or 15 mg pyridoxal hydrochloride. Theophylline-induced tremor was greatly reduced with vitamin B₆ administration "after a single dose of theophylline and a similar but nonsignificant trend was observed with repeated doses." Subjects treated with pyridoxine also reported lessening of faint feeling, trembling, irritability, and other adverse effects on nervous system function associated with theophylline. Nevertheless, a variety of psychomotor and electrophysiological tests and self-report questionnaires failed to confirm any significant response differences within these parameters.[219] More recently, Seto et al.[210] measured serum pyridoxal (PAL) levels in children with bronchial asthma treated with theophylline to study whether a theophylline-related seizure is caused by a decrease in serum vitamin B₆. They determined that the serum PAL levels of 31 asthmatic children treated with theophylline were significantly lower than those of 21 control subjects. Moreover, three of the four subjects who experienced a seizure, with or without fever, exhibited low PAL levels within 24 hours.

None of the studies reviewed reported an adverse interaction with concurrent intake of pyridoxal and theophylline.

Nutritional Therapeutics, Clinical Concerns, and Adaptations

Physicians prescribing theophylline or related medications for extended periods are advised to coadminister vitamin B₆, 10 to 25 mg per day, to prevent or reverse adverse effects of the medication. The probability of drug-induced adverse effects is relatively high, especially at higher doses, given for extended periods, and in patients at higher risk for compromised nutritional status (e.g., children, elderly, chronically ill), and the safety profile of vitamin B6 at these conservative dosage levels is quite strong. Supervision and monitoring are appropriate, particularly in unstable patients or those undergoing a change in medication or dosage.

Tricyclic Antidepressants (TCAs)

Evidence: Nortriptyline (Aventyl, Pamelor).

Similar properties but evidence lacking for extrapolation: Amitriptyline (Elavil), combination drug: amitriptyline and perphenazine (Etrafon, Triavil, Triptazine), amoxapine (Asendin), clomipramine (Anafranil), desipramine (Norpramin, Pertofrane), doxepin (Adapin, Sinequan), imipramine (Janimine, Tofranil), protriptyline (Vivactil), trimipramine (Surmontil).

Interaction Type and Significance

⊕⊕ **Beneficial or Supportive Interaction, with Professional Management**

Probability: Evidence Base:
4. **Plausible** or 3. **Possible**   O **Preliminary**

Effect and Mechanism of Action

The conversion of tryptophan to serotonin (5-hydroxytryptamine) is catalyzed by a PLP-dependent enzyme. Dopamine, norepinephrine, and GABA are other neurotransmitters synthesized using PLP-dependent enzymes.

Research

Vitamin B₆ deficiency may be more common in individuals diagnosed with depression than in the general population. In a small study, Russ et al.[220] found that four of seven patients suffering from depression had subnormal plasma concentrations of PLP, the active form of vitamin B₆. Likewise, Stewart et al.[221] observed that among a group of 101 depressed outpatients, 21% of those assessed had low plasma levels of pyridoxine.

In a small clinical trial involving 14 institutionalized geriatric patients diagnosed as depressed, Bell et al.[222] reported improved cognitive functioning and depression ratings with coadministration of vitamins B₁, B₂, and B₆ (10 mg each) at the start of tricyclic antidepressant (TCA) therapy using nortriptyline.

Well-designed and adequately powered clinical trials are warranted to further investigate this possible synergy and determine the parameters of its clinical application.

Nutritional Therapeutics, Clinical Concerns, and Adaptations

Physicians prescribing nortriptyline or related TCA medications are advised to evaluate the patient's nutritional status, especially B vitamins and vitamin D. Nutrient coadministration may be prudent, pending more conclusive evidence from qualified case reports and substantive clinical trials, given the potential for benefit. A low dose of vitamin B₆ (e.g., 10-25 mg/day) may be adequate, especially when used in combination with thiamine and cyanocobalamin (B₁ and B₁₂); other nutrients such as vitamin D warrant significantly higher dose levels (e.g., 800-2000 IU/day). No available research suggests significant risk of adverse effects or interference with the therapeutic efficacy of TCA therapy with recommended doses.

Health care providers are advised to educate patients about the therapeutic benefits of a balanced healthy diet, supportive social engagement, regular exercise, and exposure to sunlight and fresh air and strongly encourage such building of these synergistic lifestyle practices.

THEORETICAL, SPECULATIVE, AND PRELIMINARY INTERACTIONS RESEARCH, INCLUDING OVERSTATED INTERACTIONS CLAIMS

Amphetamines, Mixed

Amphetamine aspartate monohydrate, amphetamine sulfate, dextroamphetamine saccharate, dextroamphetamine sulfate; D-amphetamine, Dexedrine.

Methylphenidate (Metadate, Methylin, Ritalin, Ritalin-SR; Concerta).

Combination drug: Mixed amphetamines: Amphetamine and dextroamphetamine (Adderall; dexamphetamine).

Compulsive behavior and anxiety develop in some patients treated with amphetamines, even after the medication is discontinued. Frye and Arnold[223] described the case of an 8-year-old boy in whom anxiety and persistent dextroamphetamine-induced compulsive rituals declined significantly within 3 weeks after initiation of pyridoxine (200 mg) daily for 1 week, followed by by a reduced dose of 100 mg daily. The positive response manifested after a few months of concomitant treatment, with elimination of the drug-induced adverse effects.

Bhagavan and Brin[193] studied serotonin and pyridoxal phosphate (PLP) levels in the blood of 11 hyperactive children and 11 controls and noted significantly lower levels of serotonin in the hyperactive patients than in controls. They found no differences in PLP content of blood between the two groups.

However, when four children who had displayed low serotonin levels were administered oral doses of pyridoxine, these investigators observed an appreciable increase in the serotonin content and a very large increase in the PLP content of blood in the hyperactive patients. These preliminary and indirect research findings suggest that pyridoxine intake, especially relative to tryptophan intake, can alter serotonin levels. However, the clinical significance of these data to vitamin B₆ supplementation in human patients being treated with mixed amphetamines has yet to be thoroughly and systematically researched.

Clinical trials investigating coadministration of pyridoxine/B vitamins along with stimulant medications prescribed for attention-deficit disorder (ADD) may be warranted.

Beta-Adrenoreceptor Antagonists and Calcium Channel Blockers

Beta-1-adrenoreceptor antagonists (beta-1 blocking agents)
   Oral forms (systemic)
   Evidence: Bisoprolol (Zebeta), metoprolol (Lopressor, Toprol XL).

Extrapolated, based on similar properties: Acebutolol (Sectral), atenolol (Tenormin); combination drugs: atenolol and chlortalidone (Co-Tendione, Tenoretic); atenolol and nifedipine (Beta-Adalat, Tenif), betaxolol (Kerlone); carteolol (Cartrol), esmolol (Brevibloc), labetalol (Normodyne, Trandate); metoprolol combination drug: metoprolol and hydrochlorothiazide (Lopressor HCT); nadolol (Corgard), nebivolol (Nebilet), oxprenolol (Trasicor), penbutolol (Levatol), pindolol (Visken), propranolol (Betachron, Inderal LA, Innopran XL, Inderal); combination drug: propranolol and bendrofluazide (Inderex); sotalol (Betapace, Betapace AF, Sorine), timolol (Blocadren).
Calcium channel blockers
   Amlodipine (Norvasc); combination drug: amlodipine and benazepril (Lotrel); bepridil (Bapadin, Vascor), diltiazem (Cardizem, Cardizem CD, Cardizem SR, Cartia XT, Dilacor XR, Diltia XT, Tiamate, Tiazac), felodipine (Plendil); combination drugs: felodipine and enalapril (Lexxel); felodipine and ramipril (Triapin); gallopamil (D600), isradipine (DynaCirc, DynaCirc CR), lercanidipine (Zanidip), nicardipine (Cardene, Cardene I.V., Cardene SR), nifedipine (Adalat, Adalat CC, Nifedical XL, Procardia, Procardia XL); combination drug: nifedipine and atenolol (Beta-Adalat, Tenif); nimodipine (Nimotop), nisoldipine (Sular), nitrendipine (Cardif, Nitrepin), verapamil (Calan, Calan SR, Covera-HS, Isoptin, Isoptin SR, Verelan, Verelan PM); combination drug: verapamil and trandolapril (Tarka).

Evidence of direct pharmacological interactions between vitamin B₆ and either calcium channel blockers or beta blockers is lacking, but there is a broader strategic interaction in terms of cardiovascular risk factors and comprehensive therapeutic strategies related to pyridoxine's role in homocysteine (Hcy) metabolism.

The biochemical conversion of homocysteine to cysteine depends on two consecutive, vitamin B₆–dependent reactions. Homocysteine is strongly associated with atherosclerosis, coronary artery disease, thromboembolism, and vascular endothelial cell injury. There is strong evidence that the prothrombotic and endothelial vascular dysfunction produced by Hcy may result from oxidative stress and subsequent endothelial cell damage. Furthermore, inflammation causes tissue-specific depletion of vitamin B₆. The pathogenic effects of Hcy, inflammation, and cholesterol are additive. Hyperhomocysteinemia is associated with numerous conditions, including coronary disease, stroke, peripheral vascular disease (carotid artery and cerebrovascular atherosclerosis), venous thrombosis, renal disease, diabetes mellitus, and organ transplant.

Ubbink et al.[224] performed oral methionine load tests on 22 vitamin B₆–deficient asthma patients treated with theophylline (a B₆ antagonist) and 24 age-matched and gender-matched controls with normal vitamin B₆ status. Both groups had normal circulating vitamin B₁₂ and folate concentrations. Methionine loading resulted in significantly higher increases in circulating total homocysteine (tHcy) and cystathionine concentrations in B₆-deficient subjects compared with controls. However, 6 weeks of vitamin B₆ administration (20 mg/day) significantly reduced post–methionine load increases in circulating tHcy concentrations in deficient subjects, but had no significant effect on the increase in tHcy concentrations in controls. These investigators concluded that a vitamin B₆ deficiency may contribute to metabolic changes associated with premature vascular disease.

Physicians prescribing beta blockers or calcium channel blockers are advised to consider a comprehensive cardiovascular care strategy incorporating vitamin B₆ along with vitamins B₂, B₁₂, omega-3 fatty acids (fish oils), magnesium, and coenzyme Q10. Typical therapeutic dosages of B₆ are in the range of 50 to 200 mg per day, with higher dosages warranting monitoring due to potential adverse effects associated with higher dosages for an extended period.

Corticosteroids, Oral

Betamethasone (Celestone), cortisone (Cortone), dexamethasone (Decadron), fludrocortisone (Florinef), hydrocortisone (Cortef), methylprednisolone (Medrol) prednisolone (Delta-Cortef, Orapred, Pediapred, Prelone), prednisone (Deltasone, Liquid Pred, Meticorten, Orasone), triamcinolone (Aristocort).

Similar properties but evidence indicating no or reduced interaction effects: Inhaled or topical corticosteroids.

Many review articles suggest that prednisone and related oral corticosteroid drugs can contribute to depletion of vitamin B₆. However, in a double-blind, placebo-controlled trial, Sur et al.[207] found that concomitant therapy with inhaled steroids and pyridoxine (300 mg/day) produced no significant differences (vs. placebo in place of pyridoxine) in the treatment of 31 patients with steroid-dependent asthma for 9 weeks.

Physicians prescribing oral corticosteroids for longer than 2 weeks are advised to evaluate the potential need to coadminister vitamin B₆ to counter the depleting effects of the medication. The limited available evidence suggests that coadministration of vitamin B₆ at low dose levels (e.g., 25-50 mg/day) may be sufficient to prevent drug-induced deficiency, and that larger doses may not provide any additional benefit. However, patients also being treated with theophylline may have greater vitamin B₆ requirement because that agent acts as a B₆ antagonist.

Diclofenac, Ketorolac, and Related Nonsteroidal Anti-Inflammatory Drugs (NSAIDs)

Diclofenac potassium (Cataflam), diclofenac sodium (Voltaren).

Using a rat model, Rocha-Gonzalez et al.[225] investigated a possible synergistic interaction between oral diclofenac and B vitamins (100:100:1 of vitamin B₁, B₆, and B₁₂, respectively) in increasing the analgesic effect of diclofenac and reducing inflammatory pain. "Diclofenac (0.31-316 mg/Kg), B-vitamins (32-178 mg/Kg), or a combination of B-vitamins and diclofenac was administered orally and the antinociceptive effect was determined" in the rat formalin test. During second phase of the test, they found that diclofenac, B vitamins, and "fixed-ratio B-vitamins–diclofenac combinations dose-dependently reduced flinching behavior." These researchers concluded that their findings "indicate that oral diclofenac and B-vitamins can interact synergistically to reduce inflammatory pain in the formalin test and suggest the use of those combinations to relief this kind of pain in humans."[225]

Medina-Santillan et al.[226] reported that B vitamins can increase the analgesic effect of ketorolac in the formalin test in the rat. "Ketorolac (0.32-10 mg/Kg, po), B-vitamins (56-316 mg/Kg), or a combination of B-vitamins (either 100:100:1 or 100:100:5 proportion of vitamin B_1, B_6 and B_{12}, respectively) and ketorolac was administered orally and the antinociceptive effect was determined." During second phase of the test, they found that ketorolac, B vitamins, and "fixed-ratio B-vitamins–ketorolac combinations dose-dependently reduced flinching behavior." These researchers concluded that their findings "indicate that oral ketorolac and B-vitamins can interact synergistically to reduce inflammatory pain in the formalin test and suggest the use of those combinations to relief this kind of pain in humans."[226]

These preliminary findings suggest that further research appears warranted, particularly given other emerging data elucidating the relationship between inflammation and depletion of vitamin B_6.[148,149]

Erythromycin and Related Macrolide Antibiotics (Oral)

Erythromycin oral (EES, EryPed, Ery-Tab, PCE Dispertab, Pediazole), troleandomycin (Tao).
Extrapolated, based on similar properties: Azithromycin (Zithromax), clarithromycin (Biaxin), dirithromycin (Dynabac).
Related but evidence against extrapolation: Erythromycin topical (A/T/S, Akne-Mycin, Erygel, Erycette, Eryderm, Erygel).

Oral erythromycin therapy, especially with long-term administration, may interfere with the absorption and activity of vitamin B_6, and other B vitamins, as well as minerals such as calcium and magnesium. Simple preventive action through coadministration of a multivitamin-mineral formulation is prudent when antibiotics are used for more than 2 weeks or repeatedly. Evidence is lacking, and claims of drug impairment are absent, regarding potential pharmacokinetic interference that might occur if these agents were ingested simultaneously; separation of oral intake by at least 2 hours would be judicious, pending substantive research findings.

Broad-spectrum antimicrobial agents tend to damage the ecology of the gastrointestinal tract by eliminating probiotic flora. Synthesis of B vitamins is among the many important functions performed by intestinal microbiota, and their restoration through oral intake of probiotic flora is recommended after use of any significant course of antibiotic medications. Nevertheless, the evidence pertaining to the effects of macrolide antibiotics specifically on vitamin B_6 is suggestive but remains preliminary or inconclusive. The burgeoning body of research underway into the critical role of gut microflora in the normal functioning of the digestive tract, immune system, neurotransmitter synthesis, and other central physiological processes portends a significantly greater knowledge and deeper understanding of this fundamental symbiotic relationship.

Fenofibrate, Bezafibrate, and Related Fibrates

Bezafibrate (Bezalip), ciprofibrate (Modalim), clofibrate (Atromid-S), gemfibrozil (Apo-Gemfibrozil, Lopid, Novo-Gemfibrozil), fenofibrate (Lofibra, Tricor, Triglide).

See also Folic Acid monograph.

Fenofibrate and other fibrates can greatly increase plasma homocysteine levels. Vitamin B_6, along with folic acid, B_{12}, and riboflavin, plays a key role in Hcy metabolism and increasing nutrient intake can lower plasma Hcy concentration. However, circulating levels of these vitamins are not typically lower with fibrates. Although the benefits of folic acid coadministration have been investigated and confirmed, evidence from human research focusing on the interaction between fibrates and vitamin B_6 is lacking. Clinical trials investigating the potential benefits of pyridoxine coadministration during fibrate therapy is warranted. Pending conclusive findings, physicians prescribing fibrates are advised to consider coadministration of vitamins B_6, B_{12}, riboflavin, and folic acid as prudent. In addition to regular exercise and prudent dietary habits, enhanced intake of magnesium, omega-3 fatty acids, L-carnitine, pantethine, and fiber, as well as coenzyme Q10 therapy, may also be beneficial in these cases.

Hormone Replacement Therapy (HRT): Estrogen-Containing and Synthetic Estrogen and Progesterone Analog Medications

HRT, estrogens: Chlorotrianisene (Tace); conjugated equine estrogens (Premarin); conjugated synthetic estrogens (Cenestin); dienestrol (Ortho Dienestrol); esterified estrogens (Estratab, Menest, Neo-Estrone); estradiol, topical/transdermal/ring (Alora Transdermal, Climara Transdermal, Estrace, Estradot, Estring FemPatch, Vivelle-Dot, Vivelle Transdermal); estradiol cypionate (Dep-Gynogen, Depo-Estradiol, Depogen, Dura-Estrin, Estra-D, Estro-Cyp, Estroject-LA, Estronol-LA); estradiol hemihydrate (Estreva, Vagifem); estradiol valerate (Delestrogen, Estra-L 40, Gynogen L.A. 20, Progynova, Valergen 20); estrone (Aquest, Estragyn 5, Estro-A, Estrone '5', Kestrone-5); estropipate (Ogen, Ortho-Est); ethinyl estradiol (Estinyl, Gynodiol, Lynoral).
HRT, estrogen/progestin combinations: Conjugated equine estrogens and medroxyprogesterone (Premelle cycle 5, Prempro); conjugated equine estrogens and norgestrel (Prempak-C); estradiol and dydrogesterone (Femoston); estradiol and norethindrone, patch (CombiPatch); estradiol and norethindrone/norethisterone, oral (Activella, Climagest, Climesse, FemHRT, Trisequens); estradiol valerate and cyproterone acetate (Climens); estradiol valerate and norgestrel (Progyluton); estradiol and norgestimate (Ortho-Prefest).
HRT, estrogen/testosterone combinations: Esterified estrogens and methyltestosterone (Estratest, Estratest HS).
See also Oral Contraceptives.

The potential adverse effects of exogenous estrogen (with or without progestins) on the levels and functions of vitamin B_6 remain an area of controversy and discovery. Research into the interactions between OCs and vitamin B_6 has demonstrated an adverse effect on B_6-dependent enzymes along the tryptophan-niacin pathway and revealed the breadth, complexity, and nuances of these issues, particularly with regard to hormone formulations and interindividual variability in drug response.

Conjugated estrogens may be associated with compromised vitamin B_6 status or deficiency. In a small, preliminary trial, Haspels et al.[227] observed a "relative pyridoxine deficiency ... in all of 12 women using conjugated estrogens unopposed by progestagens." They attributed this effect to "disturbed tryptophan metabolism, expressed in increased xanthurenic acid (XA) excretion (greater than or equal to 60 μmol/8 h) during 8 h following oral administration of 2 g L-tryptophan." This finding parallels the results from a number of studies focusing on OCs and potentially extrapolates to such patterns of interaction involving HRT in postmenopausal women. The authors found that this "disturbance is clear after 1 yr of oestrogen treatment," and that "xanthurenic acid excretion was only slightly increased in 3 women who used progestagens in high dosages at the same time." Based on these findings, the authors suggested that "biochemical changes induced could easily be corrected by administration of vitamin B₆" and concluded by noting that their "cyclic treatment regimen now consists of 25 days of oestrogens per month," after which "a 250 mg tablet per day of vitamin B₆ is prescribed."[227] Further research through well-designed and adequately powered clinical trials is warranted to confirm this adverse interaction, delineate patterns of susceptibility, and develop clinical guidelines for individualized hormone prescription and nutrient coadministration.

Hydroxychloroquine

Hydroxychloroquine (Plaquenil).

In 1991, McCarty[228] reported a case of complete reversal of rheumatoid nodulosis in a woman with a history of seropositive rheumatoid arthritis (RA) of 12 years' duration (with attacks of palindromic rheumatism for 3 years) after treatment with D-penicillamine, pyridoxine, and hydroxychloroquine. The author noted that "this is the first instance of complete resolution of all nodules in a patient with RA with the nodulosis variant." The specific role of vitamin B₆ in this clinical response remains uncertain, as does its generalizability to other patients with RA or similar autoimmune conditions. Further research through well-designed clinical trials may be appropriate.

Ketorolac

Ketorolac (Toradol).

See Diclofenac, Ketorolac, and Related Nonsteroidal Anti-Inflammatory Drugs (NSAIDs).

Nitrofurantoin

Nitrofurantoin (Furadantin, Macrobid, Macrodantin).

Lacerna and Chien[229] described the case of an elderly female patient who developed paresthesias after concomitant intake of nitrofurantoin and vitamin B₆ for an extended period. Corroborative evidence of such an interaction is lacking, as is research specifically investigating the mechanisms of action involved and parameters of clinical significance. The concerns previously discussed regarding the potential adverse effect on vitamin B₆ status due to the antimicrobial activity against probiotic flora in the gastrointestinal tract can be reasonably extrapolated to nitrofurantoin. However, specific human research is lacking to confirm this interaction or any potential benefit of supplementing probiotic flora, vitamin B₆, or other relevant nutrients during or after nitrofurantoin therapy.

Risperidone

Risperidone (Risperdal).

Dursun et al.[230] described the case of a 74-year-old woman who developed neuroleptic malignant syndrome while being treated for schizoaffective disorder with risperidone. Administration of "high-dose vitamin E plus vitamin B₆" effectively alleviated this known adverse drug reaction.

Evidence from further qualified case reports and/or research findings from clinical trials is lacking to confirm whether coadministration of vitamin E and vitamin B₆ might help prevent this condition in patients treated with risperidone and, if so, what dose would be appropriate.

Selegiline

Selegiline (deprenyl, L-deprenil, L-deprenyl; Atapryl, Carbex, Eldepryl, Jumex, Movergan, Selpak).

Selegiline is a highly potent and selective, irreversible inhibitor of B-type monoamine oxidase (MAO), a predominantly glial enzyme in the brain.

Several case reports have described individuals exhibiting the characteristic clinical picture of an extrapyramidal movement disorder due to aromatic L-amino acid decarboxylase (AADC) deficiency, which results in in an impaired synthesis of catecholamines and serotonin and manifests as oculogyric crises and vegetative symptoms. Many of these patients have demonstrated significant clinical improvement when treated with a combination of pyridoxine (an AADC cofactor), selegiline, and bromocriptine, especially when treatment is initiated during the first year of life.[231]

Selective Serotonin Reuptake Inhibitor and Serotonin-Norepinephrine Reuptake Inhibitor (SSRI and SSRI/SNRI) Antidepressants

Citalopram (Celexa), duloxetine (Cymbalta), escitalopram (S-citalopram; Lexapro), fluoxetine (Prozac, Sarafem), fluvoxamine (Faurin, Luvox), paroxetine (Aropax, Deroxat, Paxil, Seroxat), sertraline (Zoloft), venlafaxine (Effexor).

The conversion of tryptophan to serotonin (5-hydroxytryptamine) is catalyzed by a PLP-dependent enzyme. Dopamine, norepinephrine, and GABA are other neurotransmitters synthesized using PLP-dependent enzymes.

Vitamin B₆ deficiency may be more common in individuals diagnosed with depression than in the general population. In a small study, Russ et al.[220] found that four of seven patients suffering from depression had subnormal plasma concentrations of PLP, the active form of vitamin B₆. Likewise, Stewart et al.[221] observed that among a group of 101 depressed outpatients, 21% of those assessed had low plasma levels of pyridoxine.

Several animal and human studies have reported an interaction between pyridoxine intake and tryptophan or histidine affecting brain serotonin and histamine metabolism. Using a rat model and applying different levels of pyridoxine, Lee et al.[232] observed that "when dietary tryptophan was fed at the requirement level, excess pyridoxine caused essentially no changes in hypothalamic serotonin and 5HIAA ... [but that with] elevated tryptophan intake, excess pyridoxine significantly increased serotonin and 5HIAA (+32%, +20%) in the hypothalamus." They interpreted these findings to "indicate a clear interaction between substrate and coenzyme precursor which influences brain metabolism of histamine and serotonin." Ten years later (1998), Schaeffer et al.[233] fed seven female rats (vs. one control) "10, 100, 175 or 250x the National Research Council recommended level of pyridoxine HCl (7 mg/kg) for 10 wk and measured serum amino acids, amino acids and neurotransmitters in brain regions and the binding properties of serotonin receptors in the cerebral cortex using a ketanserin binding assay." They found that "excess dietary pyridoxine affected brain and serum concentrations of some amino acids and binding properties of cortical serotonin receptors in a biphasic pattern over the range of concentrations fed in this study." Bhagavan and Brin[193] studied serotonin and pyridoxal phosphate (PLP) levels in the blood of 11 hyperactive children and 11 controls and noted significantly lower levels of serotonin in the hyperactive patients compared with controls. They found no differences in PLP content of blood between the two groups. However, when four children who had displayed low serotonin levels were administered oral doses of pyridoxine, these investigators observed an appreciable increase in the serotonin content and a very large increase in the PLP content of blood in the hyperactive patients. These preliminary and indirect research findings suggest that pyridoxine intake, especially relative to tryptophan intake, can alter serotonin levels. However, the clinical significance of these data to vitamin B₆ supplementation in human patients being treated with serotonin reuptake inhibitors has yet to be thoroughly and systematically researched.

Physicians treating individuals diagnosed with depression or other conditions using serotonin reuptake inhibitors are advised to assess vitamin B₆ status and consider coadministration of vitamin B₆, or possibly a B-complex formulation. However, close supervision, regular monitoring, and dose titration are warranted given the theoretical potential for excessive serotonin buildup with suppression of reuptake. Patients stabilized on antidepressants should be advised to avoid sudden changes in dose levels of pyridoxine or other B vitamins, including abrupt termination of supplementation. Further research through well-designed and adequately powered clinical trials is recommended to determine the safety and efficacy of such concomitant therapy and, on confirmation, clinical guidelines for synergistic support. Research into the concomitant application of vitamin B₆ and an SSRI for the management of premenstrual syndrome also deserves consideration.

Health care providers are advised to educate patients as to the therapeutic benefits of a balanced healthy diet, supportive social engagement, regular exercise, and exposure to sunlight and fresh air and strongly encourage building these synergistic lifestyle practices.

Sulfamethoxazole, Trimethoprim-Sulfamethoxazole, and Related Sulfonamides Antibiotics

Sodium sulfacetamide (AK-Sulf, Bleph-10, Sodium Sulamyd), sulfamethoxazole (Gantanol), sulfanilamide (AVC), sulfasalazine (Salazosulfapyridine, salicylazosulfapyridine, suphasalazine; Apo-Sulfasalazine, Azulfidine, Azulfidine EN-Tabs, PMS-Sulfasalazine, Salazopyrin, Salazopyrin EN-Tabs, SAS), sulfisoxazole (Gantrisin); combination drug: sulfamethoxazole and trimethoprim (cotrimoxazole, co-trimoxazole, SXT, TMP-SMX, TMP-sulfa; Bactrim, Bactrim DS, Cotrim, Septra, Septra DS, Sulfatrim, Uroplus); triple sulfa (Sultrin Triple Sulfa).

Sulfamethoxazole and other sulfonamides may interfere with the activity of vitamin B₆, as well as that of folic acid and vitamin K. However, the limited data available suggest that the risk of a clinically significance adverse effect on the physiological functions of vitamin B₆ evidence is low in most individuals treated with sulfamethoxazole for 2 weeks or less. Furthermore, evidence is lacking to indicate that this interaction might occur with trimethoprim alone, apart from combination with sulfamethoxazole.

Physicians prescribing sulfamethoxazole or trimethoprim-sulfamethoxazole for longer than 2 weeks are advised to consider coadministration of vitamin B₆ and other nutrients that may be depleted. Monitoring of nutrient levels may be warranted, especially in individuals with compromised nutritional intake or immune status. Patients may generally benefit from systematic intake of probiotic bacterial flora for several weeks to months after any substantial antibiotic therapy, because 6 months of supplementation with at least 10 billion organisms daily is considered necessary to ensure full restoration of the symbiotic gut flora.

NUTRIENT-NUTRIENT INTERACTIONS

Coenzyme Q10

Coenzyme Q10: CoQ10

Coenzyme Q10 and vitamin B₆ exhibit a synergistic relationship both physiologically and clinically. "The endogenous biosynthesis of the quinone nucleus of coenzyme Q10 (CoQ10) from tyrosine is dependent on adequate vitamin B₆ nutriture."[234] Blood levels of both nutrients tend to decline with age and are associated with many pathological conditions more prevalent among the elderly population.

Coenzyme Q10 and vitamin B₆ have been widely applied in nutritional therapeutics to support healthy cardiovascular function and for the treatment of cardiovascular disease. However, other researchers have focused on the functions and therapeutics of these nutrients in relation to neurological conditions and immune function, some of which are also associated with elevated homocysteine levels.

Folkers et al.[235] observed that blood levels of both CoQ10 and immunoglobulin G (IgG) increased when CoQ10 and pyridoxine were administered together, and when CoQ10 was administered alone, to three groups of human subjects. Likewise, the blood levels of T4 lymphocytes and the ratio of T4/T8 lymphocytes increased when CoQ10 and pyridoxine were administered together and separately. The authors concluded that "these increases in IgG and T4-lymphocytes with CoQ10 and vitamin B₆ are clinically important for trials on AIDS, other infectious diseases, and on cancer." Willis et al.[234] collected blood samples from 29 patients who were not currently taking either CoQ10 or vitamin B₆ as nutritional supplements. They found that "means for all parameters were within normal ranges," but that a "strong positive correlation was found between CoQ10 and the specific activity of EGOT … and between CoQ10 and the percent saturation of EGOT with PLP." These authors suggested that it would be "prudent to recommend that patients receiving supplemental CoQ10 be concurrently supplemented with vitamin B₆ to provide for better endogenous synthesis of CoQ10 along with the exogenous CoQ10."

In a preliminary study involving 27 patients with Alzheimer's disease, Imagawa[236] demonstrated considerable effectiveness of mitochondrial activation therapy with CoQ10, iron, and vitamin B₆. Subsequently, in a published letter, Imagawa et al.[237] reported that progression of genetically confirmed familial Alzheimer's disease had been halted for 18 to 24 months in a subset of these patients, two sisters, treated with a daily combination of CoQ10 (60 mg), vitamin B₆ (180 mg), and iron (sodium ferrous citrate, 150 mg). Both patients exhibited improved mental status. The younger sister, 49 years old, who had "had a 1-year history of progressive memory impairment," showed marked improvement, such that her "mental state improved to almost normal after 6 months of therapy." The authors concluded that, in contrast to the rapid progression typical in such familial Alzheimer's disease patients, they "consider that treatment prevented the progression of dementia for 1.5-2 years."[237]

Folic Acid (Folate)

Folic Acid (Folate)

Vitamin B₆ and folate work together in a wide range of physiological processes, including the regulation of homocysteine. Their coadministration, often in conjunction with folic acid and riboflavin, can favorably alter methionine and cysteine metabolism and reduce plasma Hcy levels. In a controlled trial involving healthy individuals, Mansoor et al.[238] found that concomitant administration of folic acid (0.3 mg) and of pyridoxine hydrochloride (120 mg) for 5 weeks produced a greater plasma tHcy response than did either nutrient alone. Furthermore, these authors noted that long-term oral administration of vitamin B₆ alone might reduce concentrations of serum folate. Consequently, it would be prudent to "combine low to medium divided doses" of folic acid with vitamin B₆ routinely, particularly in individuals with known or significant risk for hyperhomocysteinemia.

Iron

Iron

See final paragraph of previous Coenzyme Q10 section for Imagawa's Alzheimer's disease study.[236,237]

Magnesium

Magnesium

Magnesium Magnesium and vitamin B₆ exhibit an interdependent relationship both physiologically and clinically. Concomitant vitamin B₆ can increase bioavailability of oral magnesium by facilitating active transport across cell membranes and significantly elevate mean plasma and red blood cell (RBC) magnesium levels.[197] Conversely, magnesium deficiency can impair conversion of pyridoxine hydrochloride to PLP; consequently, PLP may be more effective with patients experiencing magnesium (or zinc) deficiency or liver disease. Pyridoxine, magnesium, and zinc are all required for the action of delta-6 desaturase, the initial step in the conversion of essential fatty acids to prostaglandins and related regulatory compounds.[239] Concurrent administration of magnesium may prevent insomnia reportedly associated with high-dose intake of vitamin B₆. These two nutrients have been used in combination with zinc and manganese in the treatment of Osgood-Schlatter disease. Likewise, some clinicians have suggested the combination of vitamin B₆ and magnesium for treating social, communication, and behavioral responses of children and adults with autism; research findings have been mixed and inconclusive.[240]

Vitamin B₂ (Riboflavin)

Vitamin B₂ (Riboflavin)

Vitamin B₆ and riboflavin work together in a wide range of physiological processes, including the regulation of homocysteine. Their coadministration, often in conjunction with folic acid and vitamin B₁₂, can favorably alter methionine and cysteine metabolism and reduce plasma Hcy levels.

Vitamin B₁₂

Vitamin B₁₂

Vitamin B₆ and B₁₂ work together in a wide range of physiological processes, including the regulation of homocysteine. Their coadministration, often in conjunction with folic acid

and riboflavin, can favorably alter methionine and cysteine metabolism and reduce plasma Hcy levels.

Zinc

Zinc

Zinc is involved in the activation of pyridoxine. Pyridoxal kinase, in particular, requires a zinc-ATP complex as a substrate and a zinc-metallothioneine is necessary for the formation of that zinc-ATP complex.[241] Pyridoxine, zinc, and magnesium are all required for the action of delta-6 desaturase, the initial step in the conversion of essential fatty acids to prostaglandins and related regulatory compounds.[239]

In a rat model, Evans[242] found that vitamin B₆ enhances the absorption of zinc. In contrast, in a study involving 40 lactating women, Moser-Veillon and Reynolds[243] observed that B₆ intake significantly increased plasma total vitamin B₆, plasma pyridoxal phosphate (PLP), and milk total vitamin B₆ but exhibited no effect on plasma, erythrocyte, or milk zinc concentrations. However, zinc deficiency can impair conversion of pyridoxine hydrochloride to PLP; consequently, PLP may be more effective with patients experiencing zinc (or magnesium) deficiency or liver disease.

These two nutrients have been used in combination with magnesium and manganese in the treatment of Osgood-Schlatter disease. Likewise, some clinicians have suggested the combination of vitamin B₆ and zinc for treating mental illness, but such approaches remain controversial and unsupported by substantive evidence from well-designed and adequately powered clinical trials.[244,245]

HERB-NUTRIENT INTERACTIONS

Ginger

Ginger (Zingiber officinale)

According to most, but not all, researchers and clinicians, vitamin B₆ and ginger (Zingiber officinale) can safely and effectively relieve the severity of nausea and vomiting in early pregnancy in many cases.[76-78,246-249] Their concomitant use is common in clinical practice but has not been the subject of high-quality clinical trials; such research is warranted.

The 251 citations for this monograph, as well as additional reference literature, are located under Vitamin B₆ on the CD at the back of the book.

Nutrient-Drug Interactions and Drug-Induced Nutrient Depletions

Vitamin B₁₂

Nutrient Name: Vitamin B$_{12}$.
Synonyms: Cobalamin, cyanocobalamin.
Chemistry and Forms: Adenosylcobalamin, cobalamin, cyanocobalamin, hydroxocobalamin, hydroxycyanocobalamin, methylcobalamin.

Summary

Drug/Class Interaction Type	Mechanism and Significance	Management
Aminoglycoside antibiotics ≈≈≈/☼	Aminoglycosides decrease B$_{12}$ absorption and biosynthesis, interfere with B$_{12}$ metabolism, and increase elimination; also adversely impact bowel flora. Possible significant adverse effects with extended aminoglycoside administration. Methylcobalamin can reduce drug-induced ototoxicity.	Intramuscular (IM) methylcobalamin or oral B$_{12}$ during extended aminoglycoside therapy.
Anticonvulsant medications ⊕≈≈/☼/≈≈≈	Anticonvulsants may decrease absorption of cobalamin. Anemia common due to drug-induced folic acid and B$_{12}$ deficiency. Significant effect plausible; evidence inconclusive.	Supplement B$_{12}$ during extended anticonvulsant therapy. Monitor cobalamin status.
Antidepressants ⊕⊕	Low B$_{12}$ associated with increased susceptibility to depression. Low B$_{12}$ (and folate) status may result in elevated levels of homocysteine and lead to excitotoxic reactions within the CNS. Healthy B$_{12}$ levels may enhance response to antidepressant therapy through multiple mechanisms, including role in biosynthesis of serotonin and dopamine, and S-Adenosylmethionine (SAMe). Certain antidepressants may deplete and/or antagonize B$_{12}$. Significant effect probable; evidence preliminary.	Coadminister vitamin B$_{12}$, with folic acid, both for depression and for synergy with pharmacotherapy. Supervision and monitor as nutrients may elevate medication levels.
Bile acid sequestrants ≈≈≈	Bile acid sequestrants may reduce absorption of many nutrients, including B$_{12}$. Intrinsic factor (IF)-cyanocobalamin complex appears to be strongly adsorbed by cholestyramine and colestipol, but cyanocobalamin itself may not be adsorbed. Mechanisms plausible but evidence minimal and clinical significance uncertain.	Consider multivitamin-multimineral during extended resin therapy; separate intake. Monitor status of B$_{12}$ and other nutrients (particularly fat-soluble nutrients).
Chloramphenicol ≈≈≈/◇≈≈/☼	Chloramphenicol may reduce B$_{12}$ absorption and can oppose the erythropoieitic activity of B$_{12}$ (or iron) in treatment of anemia; bone marrow depression possible. Evidence suggests that B$_{12}$ coadministration (with B$_6$) may reduce or reverse adverse effects associated with chloramphenicol, including optic neuritis.	Lower-dose chloramphenicol may reduce risk of bone marrow suppression. Supplement B$_{12}$ and/or multivitamin-multimineral during extended chloramphenicol. Monitor B$_{12}$ and iron status. High-dose cyanocobalamin and pyridoxine neccessary for reversing severe adverse effects.
Clofibrate ☼/≈≈≈	Clofibrate can impair B$_{12}$ absorption; fenofibrate or other fibrates may also. Fenofibrate and bezafibrate (but not gemfibrozil) can cause hyperhomocysteinemia by binding and activating peroxisome-proliferator activated receptors (PPAR) alpha. Clinical significance unclear. Coadministration of folic acid or a vitamin combination with fenofibrate can reduce Hcy elevation; no evidence indicating interference with drug activity.	Coadministration of B$_{12}$, folic acid, and/or B$_6$ is advisable with most fibrates, particularly if Hcy elevated. Consider change to gemfibrozil and support healthy lifestyle practices.
Colchicine ≈≈≈	Colchicine may interfere with B$_{12}$ absorption and interfere with B$_{12}$ metabolism by reducing IF-B$_{12}$ receptors. Colchicine-induced neuropathies may be related to B$_{12}$ depletion or another unknown mechanism. Evidence preliminary and clinical significance uncertain.	Coadminister B$_{12}$ as protective, particularly with higher deficiency risk. Separate intake. IM injection may be required if any indications of neuropathy. Monitor B$_{12}$; urinary methylmalonic acid may be necessary.
Histamine (H$_2$) receptor antagonists ≈≈≈	H$_2$ receptor antagonists (H$_2$RAs) decrease secretion of gastric acid and pepsin, as well as IF, and thus can impair absorption of dietary cobalamin. Possible clinically significant B$_{12}$ depletion, especially in compromised patients.	Supplement B$_{12}$ during extended H$_2$RA therapy. Monitor cobalamin status.
Metformin Biguanides ≈≈≈/◇≈≈/☼	Biguanides, especially metformin, reduce B$_{12}$ absorption and lower serum B$_{12}$ and holotranscobalamin by depressing IF secretion and interfering with B$_{12}$/IF uptake at ileal membrane. Possible decrease of folate and increase Hcy.	Supplement B$_{12}$, folic acid, and calcium. Monitor folate and cobalamin status.
Methotrexate ≈≈≈/◇≈≈/ ☼/⊕	Methotrexate interferes with folate metabolism and increases risk of B$_{12}$ deficiency, leading to risk of elevated Hcy. Risk is uncertain but probably significant for nutrient adverse effects. B$_{12}$ is not contraindicated, although prolonged use of therapeutic doses in cancer patients may be problematic, but folic acid is generally contraindicated in cancer treatment (except for folinic acid "rescue" after high-dose methotrexate).	Supplement B$_{12}$. Coadminister folic acid with rheumatoid arthritis and psoriasis; avoid with cancer. Monitor folate and cobalamin status.
Nitrous oxide (N$_2$O) ≈≈≈/☼	N$_2$O inactivates B$_{12}$, methionine synthase. Chronic N$_2$O exposure may lead to B$_{12}$ deficiency, decreased folate activity, and possibly elevated Hcy levels. Clinical significance controversial; evidence mixed.	B$_{12}$ supplementation may be prudent with long-term daily exposure. Monitor cobalamin and folate status.
Oral contraceptives (OCs) ≈≈≈/☼	Decreased B$_{12}$ levels associated with OC use. B$_{12}$ supplementation may reduce adverse effects associated with OC use (e.g., elevated Hcy). Clinical significance controversial; evidence strong but mixed.	B$_{12}$ supplementation may be beneficial. Monitor cobalamin, folate, and Hcy.
Pemetrexed ☼/⊕⊕	Pemetrexed inhibits several folate-dependent enzymes and may cause serious adverse effects, including elevated Hcy. Folic acid and B$_{12}$ can reduce Hcy, enhance drug safety profile, and reduce drug toxicity, without reducing efficacy or survival time.	Concomitant B$_{12}$ and folic acid, with supervision. Closely monitor cobalamin, folate, and Hcy.
Proton pump inhibitors (PPIs) ≈≈≈/☼	PPIs decrease secretion of gastric acid and thus can impair absorption of dietary B$_{12}$. Possible clinically significant B$_{12}$ depletion, especially in compromised patients, CYP2C19 polymorphism, Zollinger-Ellison syndrome, and atrophic gastritis.	Oral or IM cobalamin recommended. Monitor cobalamin and folate status.

Summary

Drug/Class Interaction Type	Mechanism and Significance	Management
Zidovudine/AZT Reverse-transcriptase inhibitor (nucleoside) antiretroviral agents ≈≈≈	Individuals with HIV/AIDS tend to exhibit low levels of vitamin B_{12} and suffer from B_{12} malabsorption. B_{12} deficiency and its sequelae are often aggravated by antiretroviral agents. Both trends are amplified at more advanced stages. However, coadministration of vitamin B_{12} and folinic acid does not appear to prevent or significantly reduce AZT-induced bone marrow suppression.	Regularly monitor nutritional status and blood counts of HIV-infected patients. Consider concomitant B_{12} and folate; increased dose with anemia or granulocytopenia.

NUTRIENT DESCRIPTION

Physiology and Function

Vitamin B_{12} is the generic term for the group of compounds, collectively known as *cobalamins*, that exhibit the biological activity of cyanocobalamin. Vitamin B_{12} was isolated from liver extract in 1948 and was shown to control pernicious anemia; its structure was elucidated in 1955, and cobalamin was first synthesized in 1973. Cobalamin is the precursor to methylcobalamin and adenosylcobalamin, the bioactive cofactor forms of cobalamin. This water-soluble, crystalline substance derives its red color from the heavy metal cobalt molecule it contains. It is susceptible to degradation by dilute acid, alkali, light, and oxidizing or reducing agents; 30% is typically destroyed by cooking.

Vitamin B_{12} from foods is released from the protein complex that it comes from via the action of hydrochloric acid and proteases. The absorption of cobalamin is highly dependent on *intrinsic factor*, a protein produced by the parietal cells, without which less than 1% of vitamin B_{12} would be absorbed. The secreted intrinsic factor binds to the B_{12}, enabling transfer of compound across the intestinal mucosa, and the resulting complex travels down to the ileum, where it is absorbed from the terminal aspect in the presence of calcium. Vitamin B_{12} is normally actively transported into the blood via protein binding to transcobalamin II and carried to the liver, its major storage site for up to 3 years, and to the kidneys and adrenals. It is distributed throughout the body, where it is converted in tissues to active coenzymes, methylcobalamin and deoxyadenosylcobalamin, and plays a vital role in the metabolism of all cells, especially those of the gastrointestinal tract, bone marrow, and nervous tissue. Excretion is through the urine.

Vitamin B_{12} acts as a coenzyme for various metabolic functions, including fat and carbohydrate metabolism and protein synthesis, and is used in cell replication and hematopoiesis. Its key functions include activation of folate to its active form (tetrahydrofolate, THF); conversion of homocysteine to methionine; fat and carbohydrate metabolism; synthesis of DNA and myelin; and antioxidant (maintains reduced glutathione).

Cobalamin is involved as a cofactor in the transfer of methyl groups in the synthesis of methionine and in folic acid metabolism. In particular, it is needed to remove the methyl group from methyltetrahydrofolate (MTHF) so that THF can be used for reducing RNA in the synthesis of DNA. Vitamin B_{12} is necessary for the maturation of red blood cells (RBCs) as well. Thus, in the absence of B_{12}, DNA is severely compromised, and RBCs grow without dividing, becoming megaloblasts, thus the term *megaloblastic anemia*, which occurs with deficiencies of either folate or B_{12}.

Vitamin B_{12} and folic acid work together to regulate homocysteine (Hcy) levels. Methyl-B_{12} is used to transfer the methyl group onto Hcy to form methionine. Methionine is an essential sulfur-containing amino acid that is converted in the liver into *S*-adenosylmethionine (SAMe), considered the activated form of methionine. Methionine is important in methyl transfers and is necessary for the synthesis of myelin sheaths, among numerous other vital functions. Methionine synthase (5-MTHF–homocysteine S–methyltransferase) catalyzes the cobalamin-dependent methylation of Hcy, using 5-MTHF as the methyl donor. Defects in methionine synthase result in hyperhomocysteinemia and are implicated as the lesion in the cblG complementation group of disorders in cobalamin metabolism. Lower Hcy levels are associated with decreased risk of cardiovascular disease; high Hcy levels may also be associated with Alzheimer's disease, osteoporosis, and strokes. Methionine synthase reductase (MSR) is responsible for the reductive methylation and reactivation of methionine synthase with SAMe as a methyl donor. MSR is a member of the ferredoxin-NADP reductase family of electron transferases, containing the FMN, FAD, and NADPH binding sites necessary to maintain methionine synthase in its functional state.[1] SAMe plays an important role in detoxification processes, the synthesis of antioxidants, and the regulation of emotional states.

Vitamin B_{12} is also involved in carbohydrate metabolism, plays a key role in nerve cell activity, and is required for the synthesis of myelin. Lactic acid and pyruvate production can increase from 50% to 100% during B_{12} deficiency. Neurological problems often occur when there is a B_{12} deficiency because the nervous system relies on carbohydrates as its main source of fuel.

NUTRIENT IN CLINICAL PRACTICE

Known or Potential Therapeutic Uses

Vitamin B_{12} deficiency is a common but underrecognized, yet easily treatable disorder in older adults. Although several causes exist, food-cobalamin malabsorption is considered the most common etiology. Therapeutic administration of vitamin B_{12} is used primarily to prevent or treat a deficiency state or counter depletion. Although oral intake can serve some supportive function, intramuscular injection was considered the primary therapeutic mode of administration for many years. More recently, it has been shown that large oral doses (1-2 mg/day) are equally effective in treating even the severe B_{12} deficiency associated with pernicious anemia. Concomitant folic acid therapy is also necessary in many circumstances.

Possible Uses

Acquired immunodeficiency syndrome and human immunodeficiency virus (AIDS/HIV) support, age-related cognitive decline (with vitamin B_{12} deficiency), age-related hearing dysfunction, allergies, Alzheimer's disease, anemia (for thalassemia if deficient), anemia (if deficient), anemia of pregnancy, asthma, atherosclerosis, atopic dermatitis, Bell's palsy, bipolar disorder, bursitis, canker sores (for deficiency only), cardiac events and death (risk reduction after first stroke), chronic fatigue syndrome, contact dermatitis, Crohn's disease, cyanide poisoning (hydroxycobalamin form only), cystic fibrosis (with vitamin B_{12} deficiency), depression (with vitamin B_{12} deficiency), dermatitis herpetiformis (with vitamin B_{12} deficiency), diabetes mellitus, diabetic neuropathies, diabetic retinopathy, Down's syndrome, heart attack, hepatitis, herpes zoster, hives, hypercholesterolemia, hyperhomocysteinemia, immune function, inherited cobalamin disorders, insomnia, low back pain, lung cancer (risk reduction), male infertility, methionine synthase reductase (MSR) deficiency (genetic), methionine synthase apoenzyme deficiency (genetic), methylmalonic aciduria (genetic), multiple sclerosis, neural tube defects (risk reduction), neuralgias, neuropathy, osteoporosis (with hyperhomocysteinemia), pain, pernicious anemia, phenylketonuria (with vitamin B_{12} deficiency), presurgery and postsurgery support, postherpetic neuralgia, preclampsia, pregnancy support, restless leg syndrome, retinopathy (associated with childhood diabetes), schizophrenia, sciatica, seasonal affective disorder, seborrheic dermatitis, sickle cell anemia (with B_{12} deficiency), stroke and second stroke (risk reduction), thyrotoxicosis, tinnitus, vitamin B_{12} deficiency, vitiligo.

Deficiency Symptoms

Increased risk of vitamin B_{12} deficiency is associated with deficiency of intrinsic factor and pernicious anemia; achlorhydria; atrophic gastritis; gastric carcinoma; gastrectomy, especially of the cardia or fundus; pregnancy and lactation; malnourished children; the elderly, especially those physically disabled and with urinary incontinence, tinnitus, or hearing loss; HIV-infected individuals; psychiatric disorders; liver disease or cancer; *Helicobacter pylori* infection; intestinal diseases, especially involving malabsorption, such as celiac disease, Crohn's disease, colitis, chronic diarrhea (e.g., in AIDS), pancreatic disease, and tapeworms; vegan diets, especially over an extended period; chronic heavy cigarette smoking and/or alcohol use; excessive or prolonged use of medications such as antibiotics, anticonvulsants, cholestyramine, colchicine, gentamicin, metformin, neomycin, and para-aminosalicylic acid (PAS); protracted intake of megadoses of vitamin C and copper.

Genetic

Deficiency of methylmalonyl-CoA mutase, leading to methylmalonic aciduria.

Elevated adenosylcobalamin, most likely due to a perturbation in cofactor binding.

Defects in methionine synthase result in hyperhomocysteinemia and are implicated as the lesion in the cblG complementation group of disorders in cobalamin metabolism.

Genetic mutations in the cobalamin-binding domain of methyltransferase.

Methionine synthase reductase (MSR) deficiency, such as mutation(s) in cblE complementation group.

Signs and Symptoms of B₁₂ Deficiency

Depression, irritability, agitation, bone loss, confusion and memory loss (especially in elderly), fatigue, psychosis, classic pernicious anemia due to lack of intrinsic factor, macrocytic anemia, decreased phagocyte and polymorphonucleocyte response, impaired lymphocyte response, poor blood clotting and easy bruising, progressive peripheral neuropathy, spinal degeneration, unstable gait, decreased coordination, paresthesias, loss of appetite, nausea, vomiting, glossitis, tongue and mouth irregularities, achlorhydria, dermatitis and skin sensitivity.

Complications associated with long-term depletion of this nutrient can take years to develop, and frank vitamin B_{12} deficiency is considered rare. Years of deficiency are usually required before hematological and neurological signs and symptoms become evident. Vitamin B_{12} deficiencies manifest primarily as anemia and neurological changes. Pernicious anemia is usually the first symptom of B_{12} deficiency and results from either inadequate intake or inhibited absorption associated with reduced gastric secretion of intrinsic factor. Vitamin B_{12} deficiency, and subsequent impairment of cell replication in atrophy and inflammation of mucus membranes in the mouth and throughout the digestive tract, not only results in reduced absorption of nutrients, gastric atrophy, anorexia, and weight loss, but also creates a gastric environment of increased susceptibility to imbalance and infection. Thus, numerous studies have observed a strong association between *Helicobacter pylori* and B_{12} deficiency, even in the absence of gastric atrophy,[2-11] with infection detected in 56% of individuals diagnosed with pernicious anemia in one trial.[12] Likewise, inhibited DNA synthesis associated with B_{12} deficiency can lead to megaloblastic anemia and manifest as weakness, decreased ability to concentrate, and shortness of breath. Cobalamin-deficiency polyneuropathy is considered particularly difficult to diagnose, and deficiency for longer than 3 months can result in irreversible degenerative central nervous system (CNS) lesions. Low B_{12} levels may also be associated with an increased risk of brain disorders, birth defects, colon cancer, and heart disease. Vitamin B_{12} deficiency can mask signs of polycythemia vera.

In a clinical trial, Eussen et al.[13] found that the lowest dose of oral cyanocobalamin required to normalize mild vitamin B_{12} deficiency is more than 200 times greater than the recommended dietary allowance (RDA).

Dietary Sources

Liver, meat, salt-water fish, oysters, milk, eggs, aged cheese such as Roquefort, fortified brewer's yeast. All foods of animal origin, especially organ meats, provide vitamin B_{12} because it is produced by microbial synthesis in the digestive tract of animals. It does not occur in fruits, vegetables, grain, or legumes. A few foods of vegetable origin, specifically seaweed and microalgae (including nori, chlorella, and spirulina) and tempeh, can provide small but inconsistent amounts.[14,15]

Nutrient Preparations Available

Hydroxycobalamin and cyanocobalamin are synthetic forms of vitamin B_{12}. Methylcobalamin and 5-deoxyadenosylcobalamin are the two forms of vitamin B_{12} that occur naturally in foods.

Hydroxycobalamin, cyanocobalamin, and adenosylcobalamin are the principal forms used in conventional clinical practice. Methylcobalamin is also used but is very expensive.

Absorption of large doses of B_{12} in the form of oral supplements is relatively poor. Sublingual forms are available but may not offer significant absorption advantages. Intramuscular or deep subcutaneous injection, usually as hydroxycobalamin, is the most effective route of B_{12} administration, especially for the elderly or those suffering from chronic depletion. However, some research indicates that oral doses may be as effective, even in the elderly.[13] Large doses (e.g., 1 mg), whether sublingual or oral, completely overcome the need for intrinsic factor.

Dosage Forms Available

Capsules, effervescent tablets, gels, injectable (prescription only), intranasal sprays, liposomal sprays, liquids, lozenges, powder, sublingual lozenges, tablets.

Dosage Range

Adult

Dietary: 1 to 3 μg daily.

Supplemental/Maintenance: 100 μg daily. Vegans (individuals who avoid all foods of animal origin) will generally benefit from a daily dose of 2 to 3 μg or more of vitamin B$_{12}$. Individuals who include animal products in their regular diet usually do not need to supplement with B$_{12}$. However, several studies show that B$_{12}$ absorption declines with increasing age and suggest that the elderly may generally benefit from regular supplementation with 10 to 25 μg per day of vitamin B$_{12}$.[16-19]

Pharmacological/Therapeutic: Pharmacological dosages in the scientific literature range from 100 to 3000 μg. For example, long-term supplementation might involve 30 μg/day for 5 to 10 days initially, followed by 100 to 200 μg per month. A daily dose of 250 μg is often used to treat deficiency, and daily doses as high as 2000 μg have been used in chronic renal insufficiency. Therapy for pernicious anemia usually involves vitamin B$_{12}$ injections, but oral administration of 1000 μg/day may be effective for some individuals.[20-25] Some evidence indicates that individuals, particularly elderly, whose serum cobalamin concentration is less than 300 pg/mL should receive replacement parenteral therapy. Nonspecific neurological signs and symptoms, particularly in the elderly, including fatigue, appear to respond to B$_{12}$ supplementation, despite low-normal serum levels. Ralph Carmel, a hematologist, has researched and published extensively on this issue.

Gel, intranasal (Nascobal): 500 μg/0.1 mL (5 mL)

Injection: 100 μg/mL (1 mL, 10 mL, 30 mL); 1000 μg/mL (1 mL, 10 mL, 30 mL)

Tablet [OTC]: 50 μg, 100 μg, 250 μg, 500 μg, 1000 μg.

Dibencozide is a supplemental form of deoxyadenosylcobalamine that has been widely used by athletes and bodybuilders.

Toxic: Few adverse effects and no reports of toxicity have been associated with B$_{12}$ therapy, even at unusually high oral doses such as 5000 μg/day.

Pediatric (<18 years)

Dietary:

Infants, birth to 6 months: 0.4 μg/day (AI, adequate intake)
Infants, 7 to 12 months: 0.5 μg/day (AI)
Children, 1 to 3 years: 0.9 μg/day (RDA)
Children, 4 to 8 years: 1.2 μg/day (RDA)
Children, 9 to 13 years: 1.8 μg/day (RDA)
Adolescents, 14 to 18 years: 2.4 μg/day (RDA)

Pharmacologic/Therapeutic: 1 to 5 mg given in single doses of 100 μg over 2 or more weeks, followed by 30 to 50 μg per month.

Laboratory Values

Elevated levels of urinary methylmalonic acid (MMA) is the most reliable sign of a need for increased intake of B$_{12}$, regardless of the serum level of the vitamin.

Serum Vitamin B$_{12}$

Normal range: 150 to 750 pg/mL; this represents 0.1% of total body content.

Levels less than 150 pmol/L indicate clear deficiency.

Serum levels may be normal even when anemia or neurological symptoms due to vitamin B$_{12}$ deficiency are present.

Urinary Methylmalonic Acid

Levels greater than 5 μg/mg creatinine indicate deficiency.

Urinary MMA is a more sensitive index of B$_{12}$ status than serum levels of the vitamin.

Hypersegmentation Index of Nuclei of Neutrophils

The ratio of neutrophils with five lobes or more to those with four lobes or less; values greater than 30% indicate deficiency.

Note: These findings can also result from folate deficiency and are not reliable during pregnancy.

Note: Antibiotics may interfere with microbiological assay for serum and erythrocyte vitamin B$_{12}$ (false low results).

Methotrexate, pyrimethamine, and most antibiotics invalidate folic acid and vitamin B$_{12}$ diagnostic microbiological blood assays.

SAFETY PROFILE

Overview

Vitamin B$_{12}$ is nontoxic in recommended dosages.

Nutrient Adverse Effects

No toxicities have been reported or suspected as being associated with vitamin B$_{12}$ in healthy adults, even at very high oral doses (>10 mg/day). However, no studies have specifically confirmed long-term safety in individuals with severe hepatic or renal disease.

General Adverse Effects

Adults: Infrequent diarrhea, urticaria, itching skin, peripheral vascular thrombosis. Megadoses of B$_{12}$ may cause or exacerbate acne symptoms.[26-28]

Hydroxycobalamin is usually administered as an injectable. Some evidence indicates that the cyano part of cobalamin may be toxic to cells (related to cyanide) and rarely may provoke significant or even severe reactions.[29,30] Most, but not all, injectable vitamin B$_{12}$ products contain preservatives; some may contain benzoyl alcohol. An intradermal test dose should be performed for hypersensitivity. Avoid use of preparations containing benzoyl alcohol in premature infants.

Reactions to intramuscular injections of cyanocobalamin:

Less than 10%: Weakness (1%-4%), anxiety, pain, nervousness, hypoesthesia, dizziness, paresthesia, abnormal gait, headache (2%-11%), sore throat, dyspnea, rhinitis, nausea and vomiting, dyspepsia, diarrhea, back pain, arthritis, myalgia, urticaria.

Less than 1%: Peripheral vascular thrombosis, urticaria, anaphylaxis, congestive heart failure (CHF), pulmonary edema.

Adverse Effects Among Specific Populations

Studies specifically confirming long-term safety in individuals with severe hepatic or renal disease are lacking.

Pregnancy and Nursing

No significant safety issues have been demonstrated regarding the use of vitamin B$_{12}$ by pregnant or lactating women. B$_{12}$ enters breast milk; compatible.

Infants and Children

No significant safety issues have been demonstrated regarding the use of vitamin B$_{12}$ by infants or children. Supplementation can be important for children on a vegetarian, especially vegan, diet.

Contraindications

Hypersensitivity to cyanocobalamin or any component of the formulation, cobalt; patients with hereditary optic neuropathy (Leber's disease).

Precautions and Warnings

Apparent vitamin B$_{12}$ deficiency should not be treated with vitamin B$_{12}$ alone until a definitive diagnosis has been established; that is, folate deficiency has been ruled out.

Treatment of vitamin B$_{12}$–related megaloblastic anemia may result in severe hypokalemia, sometimes fatal, when anemia corrects, due to cellular potassium requirements. Because of the rapid DNA synthesis, with resulting rapid cell division in bone marrow, when a severe B$_{12}$ deficiency is corrected, it is prudent to supplement folate (1 mg/day) and ensure high dietary/supplemental (prescription) potassium intake. Conversely, because of vitamin B$_{12}$'s role in DNA synthesis, high doses of B$_{12}$ and folic acid should generally be avoided in oncology patients with known tumors.

INTERACTIONS REVIEW
Strategic Considerations

Vitamin B$_{12}$ deficiency inhibits DNA synthesis, which systemically affects the growth, function and repair of all cells and tissues. Other than the expected epidemiological patterns among individuals exclusively under a long-term vegan diet, the elderly, malnourished, heavily medicated, and institutionalized populations are particularly at risk for developing deficiency or subclinical depletion patterns. Healthy gastric pH and gut ecology play a critical role in B$_{12}$ absorption and metabolism. Some reviewers have explored whether the association between *Helicobacter pylori* infection and coronary heart disease might be related to reduced cobalamin absorption and cobalamin status and, consequently, elevated homocysteine levels, but no conclusions have been ventured.[9] Scientific knowledge of the diverse roles and profound implications of enteric flora and healthy gut ecology has begun to emerge and is contributing to a fundamental reconceptualization of our understanding of assimilation and nutriture, immune function, neurotransmitter metabolism, and other core aspects of human physiology.[31-35]

The primary commonly accepted drugs that deplete vitamin B$_{12}$ include AZT, cholestyramine, colchicine, and metformin. Histamine (H$_2$) blockers and proton pump inhibitors impair B$_{12}$ absorption from food but do not appear to interfere significantly with B$_{12}$ absorption from supplemental sources. Medications that reduce folate absorption or interfere with its metabolism, such as methotrexate, oral contraceptives, and anticonvulsants, also contribute to B$_{12}$ depletion and decreased function. Generally, avoiding high doses of B$_{12}$ and folate with oncology patients is prudent, pending careful clinical study of the issue, because of vitamin B$_{12}$'s role in DNA synthesis and because large doses of B$_{12}$/folate might stimulate tumor growth.

Vitamin B$_{12}$ deficiency is more common than suspected and can be difficult to recognize because of its often subtle and pervasive symptomatology at early and middle stages. Serum levels may be normal even when significant deficiency has been present for an extended period; urinary MMA provides a more sensitive assessment of B$_{12}$ status. There is some evidence that supplementation can improve symptoms of diabetic neuropathy and delay the progress of dementia related to vitamin B$_{12}$ deficiency. Health care providers are advised to elicit risk factors and discuss susceptibility, consequences, and preventive steps with patients at risk for B$_{12}$ deficiency or depletion. Hydroxycobalamin and adenosylcobalamin are the preferred forms of injectable B$_{12}$; bioactive methylcobalamin tablets are the preferred sublingual form.

It appears that generous quantities of B$_{12}$ may be critical to effectiveness much more often than previously thought, especially in the elderly. Generally, nutritional education has framed B$_{12}$ dosing in single-digit micrograms, and folate dosing in hundreds of micrograms, because of the difference in quantity that prevent serious deficiency states. However, a pivotal clinical trial by Eussen et al.[13] showed that once deficient (by MMA levels), it takes 500 to 600 µg of oral vitamin B$_{12}$, at minimum, to correct an established pattern of "mild" depletion. Moreover, it is advisable always to give equivalent amounts of B$_{12}$ with folate. The primary caution generally voiced against folic acid administration is the oft-repeated warning that vitamin B$_{12}$ deficiency, especially severe deficiencies such as those associated with pernicious anemia, might be masked. This caution, however, seems misplaced or at least uninformed, since almost all folic acid products on the market are formulated with vitamin B$_{12}$, at the least, or a comprehensive range of synergistic nutrients, as in a multivitamin or B-complex formulation. All health care providers trained and experienced in nutritional therapeutics would routinely coadminister folic acid and vitamin B$_{12}$ as a matter of safety, synergy, and efficacy.

Homocysteine (Hcy) regulation appears as a recurrent theme in reviewing the strategic significance of drug interactions with dietary sources and supplemental forms of vitamin B$_{12}$. The pervasive and destructive effects of elevated Hcy levels are well documented and widely known. Methionine synthase, the enzyme that metabolizes Hcy to methionine, uses 5-methyltetrahydrofolate and vitamin B$_{12}$ as cofactors. Folic acid may have antiatherogenic mechanisms independent of lowering Hcy levels. Apart from effects on the vascular system, plasma total homocysteine (tHcy) level (and low serum folate concentrations) is an independent risk factor for dementia, as well as low bone mineral density, particularly among women.[36-42]

The evolving debate as to whether Hcy represents a causal or coincident factor in heart disease, stroke, and related conditions shifted to a new level with publication of the Vitamin Intervention for Stroke Prevention (VISP) trial. When the VISP trial's intention-to-treat analysis failed to show efficacy of combined-vitamin therapy for recurrent vascular events in patients with nondisabling stroke, Spence et al.[43] conducted an "efficacy analysis limited to patients most likely to benefit from the treatment, based on hypotheses arising from evidence developed since VISP was initiated." They cited many reasons for the lack of observed efficacy, including "folate fortification of grain products, inclusion of the recommended daily intake for B$_{12}$ in the low-dose arm, treatment with parenteral B$_{12}$ in patients with low B$_{12}$ levels in both study arms, a dose of B$_{12}$ too low for patients with malabsorption, supplementation with nonstudy vitamins, and failure of patients with significant renal impairment to respond to vitamin therapy." Consequently, they "excluded patients with low and very high B$_{12}$ levels at baseline (< 250 and > 637 pmol/L, representing the 25th and 95th percentiles), to exclude those likely to have B$_{12}$ malabsorption or to be taking B$_{12}$ supplements outside the study and patients with significant renal impairment." On analyzing data for this subgroup of 2155 patients (37% female, mean age of 66 ± 10.7 years), "there was a 21% reduction in the risk of events in the high-dose group compared with the low-dose group." They also noted that "patients with a baseline B$_{12}$ level at the median or higher randomized to high-dose vitamin had the best overall outcome, and those with B$_{12}$ less than the median assigned to low-dose vitamin had the worst." They concluded: "In the era of folate fortification, B$_{12}$ plays a key role in vitamin therapy for total homocysteine. Higher doses of B$_{12}$, and other treatments to lower total homocysteine may be needed for some patients."[43]

Subsequently, the NORVIT and HOPE-2 trials supported the conclusions of a consistent body of scientific research demonstrating that these nutrients help lower Hcy levels, but failed to support the hypothesis that lowering Hcy levels alone will provide protection against a future cardiovascular event in high-risk patients with established cardiovascular disease. For example, in the Norwegian study of post–myocardial infarction (MI) patients randomized to a folate/B$_{12}$/B$_6$ formulation or placebo, Bønaa et al.[44,45] observed a pattern of increased risk of a second MI in the intervention group, despite a lowering of Hcy. Although relevant to certain patient populations, the findings from these trials suggest that such a study of secondary prevention (patients with previous MI) has limited applicability to primary prevention (individuals without previous vascular events) in healthy individuals and in those with elevated risk. Notably, the HOPE-2 study demonstrated a statistically significant, 25% reduction in nonfatal strokes.[46]

Nevertheless, the current data are confounded because all patients were taking standard post-MI medications, such as beta blockers, angiotensin-converting enzyme (ACE) inhibitors, and aspirin, and investigators did not monitor drug levels to see if the B vitamins were depleted by the medications or, conversely, if the medications were impaired or levels lowered by the nutrients, as is possible if they induce the pregnane X receptor (PXR), as occurs, for example, with vitamin E.[47,48] Such potentially significant variables, which were not assessed or factored in, might explain the unexpected "increased risk" associated with the B vitamins, which would actually be analogous to poor compliance with medication. Research into PXR is in preliminary stages, and a focus on its relevance to B vitamins may be warranted and could shed some light on these and other findings. More broadly, such findings do not detract from other potential benefits derived from lowering Hcy levels, or at least reversing processes associated with elevated Hcy.

The causes of hyperhomocysteinemia are broadly categorized as "inherited" and "acquired"; many involve vitamin B$_{12}$ (and folate) nutriture, metabolism, and function. The inherited causes include MTHFR deficiency or defect, methionine synthase defect, vitamin B$_{12}$ transport defect, vitamin B$_{12}$ coenzyme synthesis defect, and cystathionine beta-synthase deficiency. The acquired cause can be grouped as vitamin deficiencies, chronic diseases, and medication effects. Nutritional deficits of vitamin B$_{12}$, folic acid, and vitamin B$_6$ can usually be remedied by ensuring adequate dietary sources and administering supplements providing these synergistic nutrients. As with folate, medications that adversely affect B$_{12}$ status and function constitute one of the primary risk factors for

hyperhomocysteinemia. Fortunately, this last factor may be the most amenable to clinician intervention—with this monograph being a tool in providing safe and effective medical management by employing an evidence-based, integrative approach to health care delivery.

NUTRIENT-DRUG INTERACTIONS

Aminoglycoside Antibiotics

Evidence, supportive interaction: Gentamicin (G-mycin, Garamycin, Jenamicin).

Evidence, nutrient depletion: Neomycin (Mycifradin, Myciguent, Neo-Fradin, NeoTab, Nivemycin).

Extrapolated, based on similar properties: Amikacin (Amikin), kanamycin (Kantrex), netilmicin (Netromycin), paromomycin (monomycin; Humatin), streptomycin, tobramycin (AKTob, Nebcin, TOBI, Tobrex).

Interaction Type and Significance

≈≈≈ Drug-Induced Nutrient Depletion, Supplementation Therapeutic, Not Requiring Professional Management

☼ Prevention or Reduction of Drug Adverse Effect

Nutrient Depletion
Probability:
2. Probable

Evidence Base:
● Consensus

Coadministration Benefit
Probability:
2. Probable

Evidence Base:
○ Preliminary

Effect and Mechanism of Action

Aminoglycosides, particularly neomycin, are typically recognized to decrease absorption, reduce endogenous synthesis, interfere with metabolic functions, and increase elimination of vitamin B$_{12}$ and many other nutrients.[49,50] Eradication of healthy intestinal bacterial flora and disruption of gut ecology by antimicrobials can reduce or eliminate the endogenous synthesis of B$_{12}$ by intestinal microbiota.[51,52]

Ototoxicity, a common adverse effect of medication in this class, can be greatly reduced by simultaneous administration of methylcobalamin. Methylcobalamin's inhibition of the ototoxic effect of gentamicin may derive from the vitamin's inherent nutritive effect on nerve cells. Although recent research indicates that free-radical formation may be pivotal in aminoglycoside-induced ototoxicity, the mechanism of this probable protective interaction remains unclear. Nevertheless, cobalamin plays a fundamental role in the synthesis of methionine and glutathione peroxidase, both of which appear to provide significant antioxidant and neuroprotective activity.

Research

Elevated aminoglycoside blood levels have demonstrated a strong tendency to induce hearing loss and impair equilibrium (eighth cranial nerve disease), often permanently.[53-55] Moore et al.[56] reported that 22% of patients receiving aminoglycosides experienced hearing loss, and the incidence of ototoxicity may be as high as 75% in patients undergoing streptomycin therapy for more than 60 days. Familial susceptibility to aminoglycoside ototoxicity has been discussed in several studies[57-59] and appears to result from the A1555G mutation in the mitochondrial DNA.[60] Oxidative damage appears to be central to the kidney damage often associated with gentamicin and other aminoglycosides.[61] Furthermore, patients with kidney disease may have increased aminoglycoside blood levels and increased susceptibility to these and other adverse effects. Interestingly, in the physiological model of classical Chinese medicine, the functions of the inner ear are traditionally associated with the kidneys; embryologically, the two tissues originate from the same cells. Aminoglycosides are also known to cause muscular problems, resulting in further muscle weakness in patients with myasthenia gravis, Parkinson's disease, or similar conditions.

Aminoglycosides have been shown to activate and increase the rate of production of oxygen metabolites in the cochlea of mature and developing rats.[62] In vitro experiments indicate that scavengers of such reactive oxygen species, particularly D-methionine, can exert a neuroprotective effect on vestibular sensory cells in relation to gentamicin ototoxicity when combined with either a neurotrophin or a calpain inhibitor.[63] Animal research in aminoglycoside ototoxicity has demonstrated significantly decreased levels of superoxide dismutase, catalase, glutathione peroxidase, glutathione-S-transferase, glutathione reductase activities, and malondialdehyde in cochlear samples from albino guinea pigs administered 200 mg/kg/day amikacin for 28 days. This study showed that differences in cochlear antioxidant enzyme activity between treated and control groups inversely correlated significantly with the change in auditory brainstem response thresholds, with the greatest correlation for the high frequencies, which are most affected by aminoglycosides.[64] Subsequently, Jin and Sheng[65] found that simultaneous administration of methylcobalamin greatly reduced the ototoxic effect of gentamicin on the inner ear of guinea pigs.

The potential relevance to vitamin B₁₂ nutriture to inner ear lesions is suggested by the findings of Shemesh et al.,[66] who reported a 47% incidence of vitamin B₁₂ deficiency in patients with chronic tinnitus and noise-induced hearing loss. The emerging picture of aminoglycoside-induced oxidative stress and observed benefits conferred by cobalamin in reducing the severity of resulting ototoxicity strongly suggest that concomitant administration of vitamin B₁₂ may provide more than protection against drug-induced depletion. Further research involving well-designed clinical trials are clearly warranted to investigate the potential of this nutrient in integrative care strategies in those cases where gentamicin, tobramycin, amikacin, and other aminoglycosides are indicated as therapeutically appropriate.

Nutritional Therapeutics, Clinical Concerns, and Adaptations

When used appropriately, aminoglycosides can play a critical role in the treatment of many life-threatening infections. These potent systemic antibacterial and antimycobacterial agents are typically administered in an inpatient setting intravenously, by inhalation, or by irrigation, and their adverse effects are well documented and generally recognized. Short-term use of aminoglycosides, such as administration of oral neomycin in preparation for surgery, is unlikely to lead to clinically significant B₁₂ deficiencies, because people with normal B₁₂ absorption store at least a 3-year supply in the liver. However, the high safety profile of B₁₂ and the lack of evidence indicating that B₁₂ interferes with the antimicrobial properties of aminoglycosides, along with the significant potential risk associated with these medications, suggest that physicians prescribing aminoglycoside therapy for more than a few days might find it prudent to coadminister vitamin B₁₂, preferably by intramuscular injection or possibly within a multivitamin-mineral supplement, with extended outpatient care. Research indicates that

alpha-tocopherol may also provide a protective effect against gentamicin-induced otovestibular toxicity.[67] Further research is warranted to determine if concomitant use of these two nutrients might provide a synergistic beneficial effect in conjunction with aminoglycoside therapy, possibly through their activity against oxidative stress and free-radical–induced damage. Restoration of intestinal microbiota through oral intake of probiotic flora is also essential after use of any significant course of antibiotic medications and can be especially important to normalization of B₁₂ status.

Anticonvulsant Medications, Including Phenobarbital, Phenytoin, and Valproic Acid

Evidence: Carbamazepine (Carbatrol, Tegretol), divalproex semisodium, divalproex sodium (Depakote), phenobarbital (phenobarbitone; Luminal, Solfoton), phenytoin (diphenylhydantoin; Dilantin, Phenytek), sodium valproate (Depacon), valproate semisodium, valproic acid (Depakene, Depakene Syrup).

Extrapolated, based on similar properties: Clorazepate (Tranxene), ethosuximide (Zarontin), ethotoin (Peganone), felbamate (Felbatol), fosphenytoin (Cerebyx, Mesantoin), levetiracetam (Keppra), mephenytoin, methsuximide (Celontin), oxcarbazepine (GP 47680, oxycarbamazepine; Trileptal), piracetam (Nootropyl), primidone (Mysoline), topiramate (Topamax), trimethadione (Tridione), vigabatrin (Sabril), zonisamide (Zonegran).

Interaction Type and Significance

$\oplus \approx \approx$ **Drug-Induced Nutrient Depletion, Supplementation Therapeutic, Not Requiring Professional Management**

☼   **Prevention or Reduction of Drug Adverse Effect**

$\approx \approx \approx$ **Drug-Induced Nutrient Depletion, Supplementation Therapeutic, Not Requiring Professional Management**

Probability:	Evidence Base:
4. Plausible	⊙ Emerging, ▽ Mixed

Effect and Mechanism of Action

In general, anticonvulsants may cause vitamin B₁₂ depletion or deficiency, at least in part from decreased absorption of cobalamin.[68] Anemia in individuals undergoing long-term antiepileptic therapy appears usually to derive from drug-induced folic acid and B₁₂ deficiency. In vitro experiments with human promyelocytic leukemia cell line, HL60, suggest that one mechanism underlying some undesirable effects of long-term therapy with phenytoin may be a drug-related impairment of both folate and vitamin B₁₂ uptake by certain cells, including hemopoietic and neural cells.[69] Homocysteine (Hcy) is a known convulsant agent and has been used experimentally to induce seizures. Antiepileptic drugs (AEDs, and possibly seizure disorders themselves) are also known to contribute to elevated plasma tHcy levels in many individuals, and drug-induced depletion of vitamin B₁₂ and folic acid plays a significant role in that process.[70-73] Interactions between anticonvulsants and folic acid are well documented,[74-76] and drug-induced folic acid deficiency contributes to vitamin B₁₂ deficiency.

Research

Findings from human trials investigating the potential for anticonvulsant medications to cause clinically significant vitamin B₁₂ depletion and deficiency are mixed and, thus far, suggestive but inconclusive. Frenkel et al.[77] found that, even in the absence of laboratory confirmation of anemia, individuals on long-term anticonvulsant therapy demonstrated significantly lower levels of vitamin B$_{12}$ in their cerebrospinal fluid (CSF) compared with controls. A majority of symptomatic individuals demonstrated improved mental status and nerve function after several days of supplemental vitamin B$_{12}$, 30 µg daily. Subsequently, in a trial with 51 patients receiving treatment at an outpatient epilepsy clinic, Schwaninger et al.[78] found that long-term AED therapy, using carbamazepine (Tegretol), phenytoin (Dilantin), or phenobarbital, was associated with elevated plasma Hcy concentrations but had no measurable effect on serum levels of vitamin B$_{12}$ compared with controls. In a study comparing 16 healthy children and 16 children with epilepsy who had been receiving carbamazepine for 1 to 4.5 years, Deda et al.[79] found lower mean serum level folic acid in the medicated group, although within normal limits, but no statistically significant difference in serum vitamin B$_{12}$. This same research team later published a paper showing no significant differences in serum vitamin B$_{12}$ and folic acid concentrations in 26 children with epilepsy who had been receiving long-term valproate therapy, compared to 28 healthy children.[79] Although these findings may initially appear contradictory, such variance may be attributable to research design, the medications used, their dosage and duration, B$_{12}$ assay methods, or other ancillary factors, including patient age and health status. Overall, the available evidence indicates that long-term therapy with the most commonly used AEDs (carbamazepine, phenytoin, phenobarbital, valproate) does not inherently induce significant declines in serum concentrations of vitamin B$_{12}$.

Early-onset cobalamin (Cbl) C/D deficiency is an inborn error of intracellular Cbl metabolism characterized by high plasma levels of methylmalonic acid (MMA), homocystine, and homocysteine. Biancheri et al.[80] studied 10 children with early-onset cobalamin C/D deficiency and reported epilepsy and electroencephalogram (EEG) abnormalities as prominent features associated with the early-onset type of combined methylmalonic aciduria and homocystinuria, possibly related to the pathologically and persistently high Hcy levels. Furthermore, within the emerging field of toxicogenomics, phenobarbital and other enzyme inducers are associated with distinct gene-expression profiles that influence how different medications affect individuals in divergent ways,[81] most likely including their adverse effects and impact on vitamin B$_{12}$ and other nutrients.

Nutritional Therapeutics, Clinical Concerns, and Adaptations

The research available at this time indicates that anticonvulsant medications as a class do not consistently cause clinically significant patterns of vitamin B$_{12}$ depletion, at least as indicated by the assay methods (usually serum levels) applied and the medications studied. Further research indicated in this important but until recently somewhat neglected area, especially given increased knowledge of the impact of B$_{12}$ deficiency on neurological and psychiatric conditions and the elusive nature of detecting depletion patterns before the onset of overt pathological changes. Physicians prescribing anticonvulsant therapy may consider it judicious to measure urinary MMA levels, and/or recommend supplemental vitamin B$_{12}$ to counter potential effects of drug-induced depletion patterns, despite the lack of strong evidence of regular occurrence, given the subtle and long-term implications of such a deficiency and the lack of toxicity or interference with the antiepileptic treatment associated with the nutrient. Furthermore, some nutritionally oriented health care professionals generally supplement with vitamin

B$_{12}$, vitamin B$_6$, and folate in patients undergoing long-term anticonvulsant therapy as a preventive measure against increased Hcy plasma concentrations associated with seizure disorders, their treatment, and other sources of deficiencies of these nutrients. Periodic monitoring of fasting plasma Hcy levels in this patient population would also be prudent.

Antidepressants

Evidence: Amitriptyline (Elavil); combination drug: amitriptyline and perphenazine (Etrafon, Triavil, Triptazine); amoxapine (Asendin), citalopram (Celexa), clomipramine (Anafranil), desipramine (Norpramin, Pertofrane), doxepin (Adapin, Sinequan), fluoxetine (Prozac, Sarafem), imipramine (Janimine, Tofranil), nortriptyline (Aventyl, Pamelor), paroxetine (Aropax, Deroxat, Paxil, Seroxat), protriptyline (Vivactil), trimipramine (Surmontil).
Extrapolated, based on similar properties:
   Selective serotonin reuptake inhibitor (SSRI) antidepressants: Escitalopram (S-citalopram; Lexapro), fluvoxamine (Faurin, Luvox), sertraline (Zoloft).
   SSRI/SNRI antidepressants: Duloxetine (Cymbalta), venlafaxine (Effexor).

Interaction Type and Significance

⊕⊕ **Beneficial or Supportive Interaction, with Professional Management**

Probability:	Evidence Base:
2. Probable	◉ Preliminary

Effect and Mechanism of Action

Although scientific understanding is incomplete and conclusive evidence is lacking, numerous mechanisms may account for research findings suggesting that adequate or high vitamin B$_{12}$ levels may decrease susceptibility to depression and enhance response to antidepressant therapy through multiple mechanisms. Of first order is the intimate relationship between B$_{12}$ and folate and the numerous linkages between these nutrients and neurotransmitters, emotional state, and general well-being. Low vitamin B$_{12}$ (and folate) status may result in elevated Hcy levels and lead to exitotoxic reactions in the CNS that may enhance depression. Vitamin B$_{12}$ is also necessary for endogenous formation of S-adenosylmethionine (SAMe), which has a known antidepressant action. Vitamin B$_{12}$ may also play an important role in alleviating depression through its involvement in the synthesis of monoamine neurotransmitters such as serotonin and dopamine. Notably, some antidepressants invoke a mechanism of action involving inhibition of monamine metabolism. In a broader contextual perspective, the nutrient status of individuals with depression may be compromised by their life situations or as part of their depressive behavior. Lastly, the potential for B$_{12}$ depletion/antagonism by some antidepressants also deserves consideration and further investigation.

Research

Individuals with depressive disorders have been characterized as more likely to have low levels of vitamin B$_{12}$ and folate,[82-85] with a doubled risk of depression in elderly, physically disabled women with significant B$_{12}$ deficiency. Tiemeier et al.[86] found that B$_{12}$ deficiency, but not folate deficiency, is independently associated with depressive disorders.[86] However, Bjelland et al.[87] found no significant correlation between low plasma folate or B$_{12}$ levels and depression without comorbid anxiety disorder in the general population.

Researchers have noted that individuals with low folate levels demonstrate a poor response to antidepressant therapy.[85,88,89] In a 4-week, randomized, placebo-controlled, double-blind clinical trial involving 14 elderly patients under treatment for major depression with cognitive dysfunction, Bell et al.[90] reported that subjects receiving small doses of vitamins B$_1$, B$_2$, and B$_6$ (10 mg each daily) demonstrated significantly better B$_2$ and B$_6$ status on enzyme activity coefficients and trends toward greater improvement in scores on ratings of depression and cognitive function, along with increased vitamin B$_{12}$ levels and serum nortriptyline levels. Those receiving placebo (i.e., no B complex) also exhibited reduced B$_{12}$ levels. Hintikka et al.[91] conducted a 6-month, "naturalistic prospective follow-up study" involving 115 outpatients (45 male and 70 female outpatients) being treated for depression using a range of antidepressive medications (citalopram, fluoxetine, paroxetine, tricyclics), most with some degree of active concomitant therapeutic relationship. No patients had a low vitamin B$_{12}$ status at baseline (and 12% exhibited elevated initial B$_{12}$ levels), and there was no correlation between severity of depression and baseline B$_{12}$. However, the participants who fully responded to treatment had the highest serum vitamin B$_{12}$ levels at the beginning and end of the study, with that significance remaining after factoring out smoking, drinking habits, type of treatment, and family history.

Nutritional Therapeutics, Clinical Concerns, and Adaptations
Further epidemiological studies and larger, well-designed clinical trials are warranted to clarify the role of vitamin B$_{12}$ (and folate) in depressive disorders. Pending such conclusive investigation, physicians prescribing antidepressant medications are advised to consider concomitant supplementation of vitamin B$_{12}$, preferably with folic acid, as a potential adjunctive therapy for the depression itself and as a possible means of enhancing therapeutic response to the pharmacological therapy. Close supervision and regular monitoring are warranted because nutrient supplementation has been observed to elevate medication levels in certain cases.

Bile Acid Sequestrants

Evidence: Cholestyramine (Locholest, Prevalite, Questran), colestipol (Colestid).
Extrapolated: Colesevelam hydrochloride (WelChol).

Interaction Type and Significance
≈≈≈ Drug-Induced Nutrient Depletion, Supplementation Therapeutic, Not Requiring Professional Management

Probability:
4. Plausible

Evidence Base:
○ Preliminary

Effect and Mechanism of Action
Bile acid sequestrants, such as cholestyramine, decrease lipid digestion and absorption, as well as absorption of the fat-soluble vitamins and other nutrients, including vitamin B$_{12}$.[50,92-94] In particular, the intrinsic factor–cyanocobalamin complex appears to be strongly adsorbed by cholestyramine and colestipol, while cyanocobalamin itself may not be adsorbed by these antihypercholesterolemic resins.[95]

Research
Intrinsic factor–mediated binding of cyanocobalamin by bile acid sequestrants can occur but may not be clinically significant. In 1973, Coronato and Glass[92] reported depression of the intestinal uptake of radiovitamin B$_{12}$ in the presence of cholestyramine. In a clinical trial involving 18 children with familial hypercholesterolemia, West and Lloyd[96] observed that prolonged treatment with cholestyramine was associated with a fall in mean serum folate concentration, as well as decreased mean serum concentrations of vitamins A and E and of inorganic phosphorus, but no significant changes in concentrations of serum iron, vitamin B$_{12}$, plasma calcium, or protein. In an in vitro investigation of cholestyramine and colestipol, Leonard et al.[97] found that both resins bound, to a high extent, vitamin B$_{12}$–intrinsic factor complex, folic acid, and iron citrate. In a related in vitro experiment, Teo et al.[98] found that dihydroxy bile acids (deoxycholic, glycodeoxycholic, taurodeoxycholic, glycochenodeoxycholic, and taurochenodeoxycholic), at concentrations found in duodenal juice, inhibit the binding of intrinsic factor to vitamin B$_{12}$, suggesting that vitamin B$_{12}$ absorption might be reduced. These collective data suggest that bile acid sequestrants may inhibit B$_{12}$ absorption, but that such effects are not usually measurable through serum B$_{12}$ levels. Further human research is warranted using more sensitive measures of B$_{12}$ status, such as urinary MMA, to determine how frequently clinically significant inhibition of absorption occurs, which patient populations are most susceptible to drug-induced depletion, and what compensatory measures, if any, might be appropriate.

Nutritional Therapeutics, Clinical Concerns, and Adaptations
Given the limitations of the available evidence, monitoring of vitamin B$_{12}$ status, using a sensitive index, is prudent for patients using bile acid sequestrants, especially in "at-risk" populations. Supplementation with a multivitamin-mineral formulation may be judicious in preventing drug-induced depletion of B$_{12}$ and other nutrients susceptible to decreased absorption; no adverse effects or interactions would be expected from such nutritional support.

Chloramphenicol

Interaction Type and Significance
≈≈≈ Drug-Induced Nutrient Depletion, Supplementation Therapeutic, Not Requiring Professional Management
◇≈≈ Drug-Induced Adverse Effect on Nutrient Function, Coadministration Therapeutic, with Professional Management
☼ Prevention or Reduction of Drug Adverse Effect

Probable:
2. Probable

Evidence Base:
○ Preliminary

Effect and Mechanism of Action
Chloramphenicol may reduce the absorption of vitamin B$_{12}$. It can also oppose the erythropoieitic activity of B$_{12}$ or iron in the treatment of anemia. Vitamin B$_{12}$ may reduce or reverse adverse effects associated with chloramphenicol.

Research
Chloramphenicol may cause bone marrow depression and can oppose the erythropoieitic activity of B$_{12}$ or iron in the treatment of anemia.[99-101] Saidi et al.[100] reported that four patients receiving B$_{12}$ therapy for pernicious anemia were all similarly refractory to treatment until chloramphenicol was withdrawn. "Very high daily doses" of pyridoxine and cyanocobalamin appear capable of reversing chloramphenicol-induced optic neuritis.[102]

Nutritional Therapeutics, Clinical Concerns, and Adaptations

Physicians prescribing chloramphenicol therapy for an extended period are advised to monitor vitamin B$_{12}$ (and iron) status, using a sensitive index, especially in at-risk populations. Prescribing moderate dosage levels of chloramphenicol (e.g., 25-30 mg/kg) can usually obtain efficacious effects against infections without introducing the risk of marrow depression, which usually does not occur unless serum levels rise to 25 μg/mL or higher[103]; alternative antibacterial agents could also be considered. Thus, chloramphenicol is rarely used in the United States at this time because of its rare but devastating complication of aplastic anemia. It is still used often in other countries, such as Mexico. Its use in the United States is almost always in the hands of infectious disease specialists in treatment of rare and highly antibiotic-resistant infections.

Supplementation with a multivitamin-mineral formulation may be judicious in preventing chloramphenicol-induced depletion of B$_{12}$. No adverse effects or interactions would be expected from such nutritional support. In the event that chloramphenicol causes optic neuritis, health care professionals trained and experienced in both conventional pharmacology and nutritional therapeutics can institute a collaborative response using high doses of pyridoxine and cyanocobalamin to reverse the condition.

Clofibrate and Related Fibrates

Evidence: Clofibrate (Atromid-S), fenofibrate (Lofibra, Tricor, Triglide).
Related but evidence against extrapolation: Bezafibrate (Bezalip), ciprofibrate (Modalim), gemfibrozil (Apo-Gemfibrozil, Lopid, Novo-Gemfibrozil).

Interaction Type and Significance

☼   **Prevention or Reduction of Drug Adverse Effect**
≈≈≈ **Drug-Induced Nutrient Depletion,**
      Supplementation Therapeutic, Not Requiring Professional Management

Probability:	Evidence Base:
2. Probable	○ Preliminary

Effect and Mechanism of Action

Clofibrate impairs absorption of vitamin B$_{12}$.[104] Fenofibrate or other fibrates may have similar activity. Fenofibrate and bezafibrate are known causes of iatrogenic hyperhomocysteinemia. Gemfibrozil does not influence plasma Hcy in the same way because, unlike other fibrates, it does not bind and activate the peroxisome proliferator-activated receptors alpha (PPAR-α), which downregulate the renal cyclooxygenase-2 (COX-2) enzyme system.

Research

Concern has been raised that inhibition of vitamin B$_{12}$ absorption by fibrates might contribute to hyperhomocysteinemia associated with these medications. Dierkes et al.[105] reported that serum Hcy significantly increases after therapy with fenofibrate or bezafibrate; no corresponding changes in folate and cobalamin concentrations were observed, although there was a slight but significant lowering of vitamin B$_6$ with fenofibrate. These authors postulated that this effect resulted from fenofibrate effects on renal function. Two years later, they published a second paper showing that in a crossover study with 22 hypertriglyceridemic patients, Hcy, creatinine, and cystatin-C were raised by fenofibrate but not by gemfibrozil, another fibrate, which does not affect

renal function.[106] Thus, these medications may disrupt absorption of B$_{12}$ and other nutrients, but it appears that nutrient depletion may not be the direct mechanism underlying fenofibrate-induced elevations in Hcy blood levels. Nevertheless, these studies demonstrate that coadministration of folic acid or a vitamin combination with fenofibrate can prevent most of the Hcy increase associated with fenofibrate. Further research is warranted to determine whether coadministration of vitamin B$_{12}$, folic acid and vitamin B$_6$ might lower Hcy in individuals taking gemfibrozil, clofibrate, or other fibrates.

Nutritional Therapeutics, Clinical Concerns, and Adaptations

Gemfibrozil is the only fibrate still in wide clinical use, and it is generally associated with fewer interactions and adverse effects than other fibrates. Although the interference of B$_{12}$ absorption by clofibrate and possibly other fibrates appears undisputed, its impact on physiological levels and any consequent clinical implications remain unclear. However, the iatrogenic hyperhomocysteinemia associated with fenofibrate and bezafibrate aggravates the risk of atherosclerosis and cardiovascular risk in general, and as such, these medications present a strategic contradiction. Supplementation with vitamin B$_{12}$, folic acid, and vitamin B$_6$ is generally appropriate in individuals prescribed fibrates, except possibly gemfibrozil, particularly if Hcy levels are elevated.[107] No adverse effects or interference with the medications would be expected at usual dosages of these nutrients. Alternatively, treatment could be changed to gemfibrozil, an effective cardioprotective agent in patients with hypertriglyceridemia or low HDL (high-density lipoprotein) cholesterol, or both,[108] which does not increase plasma Hcy levels, or to an integrative approach to treatment of dyslipidemia incorporating regular exercise and restricted intake of high-glycemic carbohydrates, as well as nutritional support, including fiber, fish oil (EPA/DHA), pantethine, vitamin B$_3$ (niacin or inositol hexaniacinate), garlic, and beta-glucan.

Colchicine

Interaction Type and Significance

≈≈≈ **Drug-Induced Nutrient Depletion,**
      Supplementation Therapeutic, Not Requiring Professional Management

Probability:	Evidence Base:
2. Probable	○ Preliminary, ▽ Mixed

Effect and Mechanism of Action

Colchicine interferes with vitamin B$_{12}$ metabolism by reducing intrinsic factor–B$_{12}$ receptors.[109-113] Neuropathies are a known adverse effect associated with colchicine use; research findings remain mixed and inconclusive as to whether such phenomena result from drug-induced B$_{12}$ depletion or another, unknown mechanism.[109,113-116]

Research

The research findings on the clinical significance of colchicine's effect on the absorption of vitamin B$_{12}$ is mixed, as is that pertaining to the mechanisms of colchicine-related neuropathies and their potential relationship to drug-induced B$_{12}$ depletion. Variations in methods applied for assessing B$_{12}$ status may play an important role in the respective findings of the various studies. For example, Ehrenfeld et al.[114] found no difference in serum B$_{12}$ levels after long-term colchicine therapy in patients with recurrent polyserositis (familial Mediterranean fever).

Nutritional Therapeutics, Clinical Concerns, and Adaptations

Despite uncertainty about the exact relationship between colchicine and vitamin B$_{12}$ with regard to neuropathies, caution is indicated in elderly individuals taking colchicine and experiencing neurological symptoms. Pending well-designed clinical trials aimed at clarifying these questions, physicians prescribing colchicine are advised to coadminister vitamin B$_{12}$ to counter the known drug-induced interference with absorption, particularly in patients at higher risk for B$_{12}$ deficiency for other reasons, and even more so if any indications of neuropathy emerge; intramuscular (IM) injection may be necessary. Serum levels of B$_{12}$ may still be normal during the initial phase of the onset of B$_{12}$-deficiency neuropathies; a more sensitive test, such as urinary MMA, may be necessary to detect a deficiency of gradual onset. In any event, the nontoxic nature of the nutrient presents a low-risk prophylactic option for the prudent physician to discuss with patients.

Histamine (H$_2$) Receptor Antagonists

Evidence: Cimetidine (Tagamet; Tagamet HB), famotidine (Pepcid RPD, Pepcid, Pepcid AC), ranitidine (Zantac).
Similar properties but evidence lacking for extrapolation: Nizatidine (Axid, Axid AR), ranitidine bismuth citrate (Tritec).

Interaction Type and Significance

≈≈≈ **Drug-Induced Nutrient Depletion, Supplementation Therapeutic, Not Requiring Professional Management**

Probability:	Evidence Base:
3. Possible	● Consensus

Effect and Mechanism of Action

Histamine (H$_2$) receptor antagonists (H$_2$RAs) decrease secretion of gastric acid and pepsin by gastric parietal cells. Gastric acid and pepsin are required for the cleavage of vitamin B$_{12}$ from animal protein-bound dietary sources. Thus, cimetidine, ranitidine, and related medications significantly impair liberation of dietary B$_{12}$ from its protein binder during digestion. Further, intrinsic factor (IF), also produced by gastric parietal cells, is required for vitamin B$_{12}$ absorption from the gastrointestinal (GI) tract.[117-119]

Research

Comparing the effect of cimetidine on the absorption of orally administered crystalline or food (egg yolk–bound) vitamin B$_{12}$ in 13 patients, Salom et al.[117] observed that whereas absorption of crystalline B$_{12}$ was normal and not significantly changed by cimetidine, the uptake of food-bound B$_{12}$ decreased by a mean of 53% in all patients. These authors further noted that their findings indicated that cimetidine-induced B$_{12}$ malabsorption would not be detected by the standard Schilling test.[117] Nevertheless, Walan and Strom[120] investigated the effect of continuous treatment with cimetidine (400 mg at night or twice daily) for 3 years and found no significant difference on plasma vitamin B$_{12}$, as well as weight, hemoglobin, plasma iron, plasma folate, and albumin; a slight decrease of plasma calcium was observed. They concluded that moderate and inconstant reduction of acidity over 24 hours, typical of twice-daily administration of those H$_2$ antagonists available in 1985, was unlikely to result in metabolic consequences. Later, in a randomized controlled prospective study, Thorens et al.[121] investigated the incidence of gastric and duodenal bacterial overgrowth in 47 outpatients with peptic disease being treated with omeprazole or cimetidine. After a 4-week treatment regimen, they found higher basal gastric pH and a significantly higher level of bacterial overgrowth in patients receiving omeprazole than in those receiving cimetidine. However, even with this significant disruption of the digestive tract's environment, serum concentrations of vitamin B$_{12}$, beta-carotene, and albumin were similar before and after treatment with both drugs.[121]

Kirch et al.[122] reported that ranitidine (300 mg daily) distinctly reduced protein-bound cobalamin absorption from a mean of 7.66% before ranitidine administration to 0.84% during treatment with ranitidine.

Overall, a consensus emerged starting in the 1980s that H$_2$RAs interfered with absorption of vitamin B$_{12}$ from food sources, more so than from supplemental sources, and that consistent long-term use in at-risk populations posed a significant potential for clinically significant nutrient depletion. Short-term or intermittent use has generally been considered to have an inconsequential effect on nutrient absorption.[123,124] In particular, Aymard et al.[123] noted that hematological adverse effects attributable to H$_2$RAs are relatively uncommon, usually involving cimetidine, and that the inhibition of gastric secretion by the H$_2$RAs may theoretically contribute to the occurrence of cobalamin (or iron) malabsorption and deficiency anemia with long-term use.

The interaction of H$_2$RAs and other medications may also affect B$_{12}$ status. For example, metformin decreases absorption of vitamin B$_{12}$ and folic acid, and cimetidine decreases the elimination of metformin; therefore a reduced metformin dosage is usually recommended when these agents are combined.[125] The clinical implications of such multiple interactions have yet to be studied in any systematic manner in well-designed human trials, even though patients taking multiple pharmaceuticals may constitute the norm more than the exception among affected populations.

Report

In a case report, Ruscin et al.[126] described vitamin B$_{12}$ deficiency in a 78-year-old nonvegetarian woman with symptomatic gastroesophageal reflux after long-term use (~4.5 years) use of H$_2$RAs, starting with cimetidine, and a proton-pump inhibitor. They noted a moderate decline in serum vitamin B$_{12}$ concentration, from an initial normal serum level of 413 pg/mL to a low-normal level of 256 pg/mL after almost 2 years. However, on the latter occasion, MMA and Hcy, clinically important biochemical markers of B$_{12}$-dependent enzyme activity, were significantly elevated. These researchers then observed that MMA and Hcy concentrations decreased dramatically when oral replacement of vitamin B$_{12}$ (1000 μg daily) was instituted. This response not only confirmed vitamin B$_{12}$ deficiency, but also demonstrated that the woman was able to adequately absorb nonprotein-bound vitamin B$_{12}$ from the GI tract, suggesting that her deficiency was a result of food-cobalamin malabsorption, and that the accumulation of MMA and Hcy was not a consequence of renal dysfunction.

Nutritional Therapeutics, Clinical Concerns, and Adaptations

Although H$_2$RAs have not conclusively been shown to decrease IF secretion, studies have demonstrated a significant reduction in protein-bound vitamin B$_{12}$ absorption secondary to decreased gastric acid and pepsin secretion in patients taking these drugs. Although this interaction probably lacks clinical importance during the short term, continuous use of these medications for more than 2 years could cause or contribute to vitamin B$_{12}$ deficiency, including anemia, especially in patients with a history of poor nutrition and other causes of inadequate stores of vitamin B$_{12}$. Such impairment of vitamin

B$_{12}$ absorption could be amplified for individuals also using antacids on a regular basis along with the H$_2$RAs. Further research is warranted into the effect of these medications on the function of gastric acid and pepsin in the initial step of the B$_{12}$ absorption process and the clinical implications of any resulting impaired release of cobalamin from food protein.

Physicians prescribing H$_2$RAs are advised to monitor cobalamin status, preferably using a sensitive test, such as urinary MMA, and to coadminister supplemental vitamin B$_{12}$ in individuals on H$_2$RA and/or proton pump inhibitor (PPI) therapy for an extended period, especially when other risk factors for deficiency are present. In the event that supplementation is determined to be necessary, a typical adult dose of 10 to 25 µg per day would be appropriate, a level commonly found in a B-complex vitamin or in many multivitamins. Given the likely mechanism of action involved, patients taking H$_2$RAs who are prone to or have developed a vitamin B$_{12}$ deficiency will generally respond to oral supplementation, which does not require stomach acid to be absorbed.

Metformin and Related Biguanides

Evidence: Metformin (Dianben, Glucophage, Glucophage XR).
Extrapolated: Buformin, metformin combination drugs: glipizide and metformin (Metaglip), glyburide and metformin (Glucovance).

Interaction Type and Significance

≈≈≈ Drug-Induced Nutrient Depletion, Coadministration Therapeutic, Not Requiring Professional Management

◇≈≈ Drug-Induced Adverse Effect on Nutrient Function, Coadministration Therapeutic, with Professional Management

☼ Prevention or Reduction of Drug Adverse Effect

Probability:
2. Probable

Evidence Base:
● Consensus

See Folic Acid monograph for further discussion.

Effect and Mechanism of Action

Biguanide therapy, particularly metformin, causes reduced vitamin B$_{12}$ absorption and low serum total vitamin B$_{12}$ and holotranscobalamin (B$_{12}$-TCII) levels by depressing intrinsic factor (IF) secretion[127] and through a calcium-dependent ileal membrane antagonism affecting B$_{12}$-IF complex uptake.[128] B$_{12}$-IF complex uptake by ileal cell surface receptors depends on calcium availability, and metformin specifically affects calcium-dependent membrane action; this effect can be reversed by supplemental calcium.

Research

Of patients who are prescribed metformin, conservatively 10% to 30% have evidence of reduced vitamin B$_{12}$ absorption, accompanied by a decline in folic acid status and elevation of Hcy. An early study by Carpentier et al.[129] involving diabetic individuals determined that whereas biguanides depleted vitamin B$_{12}$, folic acid was not similarly affected. In a subsequent study involving nondiabetic male patients with coronary heart disease, Carlsen et al.[130] observed that metformin increases total serum Hcy levels and depletes vitamin B$_{12}$ and sometimes folic acid. More recently, in a randomized, placebo-controlled trial involving 390 patients with type 2 diabetes, Wulffele et al.[131] found that 16 weeks of treatment with metformin reduces serum levels of vitamin B$_{12}$ and folate, resulting in a modest increase in Hcy.[131] This pattern has been confirmed by Ting et al.,[132] who found "an increased risk of vitamin B$_{12}$ deficiency associated with current dose and duration of metformin use despite adjustment for many potential confounders."

Caspary et al.[133] initially noted that the vitamin B$_{12}$ malabsorption, pathological Schilling tests, and elevated fecal bile acid excretion observed with biguanides, particularly metformin, improved when the medication was discontinued or antibiotics were administered. They interpreted these findings to suggest that small intestinal bacterial overgrowth, leading to binding of the IF-B$_{12}$ complex to bacteria, was responsible for the B$_{12}$ depletion observed in diabetic patients receiving biguanide therapy. Subsequently, Adams et al.[127] surveyed 46 randomly selected diabetic patients on biguanide therapy and found that 30% demonstrated malabsorption of vitamin B$_{12}$, apparently by two different mechanisms. On withdrawal of the drug, normal absorption returned in only half of those with malabsorption. Using absorption tests with exogenous IF, these researchers further determined that biguanide-induced depression of IF secretion mediated the persistent malabsorption in most individuals of the latter group.[127] Finally, Bauman et al.[128] performed a comparative study in which type 2 diabetic patients who had been receiving sulfonylurea therapy were switched to metformin for 3 months, after which oral calcium supplementation was administered. Monthly serial measurements of serum total vitamin B$_{12}$ and B$_{12}$-TCII revealed parallel declines in those taking metformin compared with controls. The observed depression of B$_{12}$-TCII was reversed by the introduction of oral calcium supplementation.

Nutritional Therapeutics, Clinical Concerns, and Adaptations

Physicians prescribing metformin or other biguanides are advised to supplement vitamin B$_{12}$, folic acid, and calcium and regularly monitor folic acid and vitamin B$_{12}$ levels.

Methotrexate

Methotrexate (Folex, Maxtrex, Rheumatrex)
See also Antifolates section in Folic Acid monograph.

Interaction Type and Significance

≈≈≈ Drug-Induced Nutrient Depletion, Supplementation Therapeutic, Not Requiring Professional Management

◇≈≈ Drug-Induced Adverse Effect on Nutrient Function, Coadministration Therapeutic, with Professional Management

☼ Prevention or Reduction of Drug Adverse Effect

⊕ Potential or Theoretical Beneficial or Supportive Interaction, with Professional Management

Probability:
1. Certain

Evidence Base:
◉ Emerging

Effect and Mechanism of Action

Given methotrexate's intentional interference with normal functioning of folic acid metabolism, problems with vitamin B$_{12}$ deficiency can be expected. Further, vitamin B$_{12}$ and folic acid work together to control homocysteine (Hcy) levels and prolonged methotrexate therapy may contribute to elevated Hcy levels.

Research

Investigators have found that patients taking methotrexate have lower B_{12} levels within RBCs than in controls, but that serum levels of B_{12} were not different. They concluded that folate depletion may be related to B_{12} deficiency in RBCs.[134]

Further, in an experiment using mice with mammary adenocarcinoma, Miasishcheva et al.[135] measured the effect of methylcobalamin on 3H-methotrexate uptake by tumor and normal tissues. They found a dose-related response in which methylcobalamin stimulated the rate of 3H-methotrexate influx into the tumor and small intestine, but did not change its influx into the spleen.

Nutritional Therapeutics, Clinical Concerns, and Adaptations

In no circumstances is methotrexate-induced vitamin B_{12} deficiency considered important to the drug's therapeutic efficacy. However, because folate deficiency inherently results from methotrexate use, some support to counterbalance the unintentional adverse effects on vitamin B_{12} levels would appear valuable. Supplementation with vitamin B_{12} is harmless and indicated. Physicians prescribing methotrexate are advised to coadminister vitamin B_{12}. In such cases, supplementation is often up to or greater than 1000 µg of cobalamin per day orally or by IM injections. In cancer patients with known tumors, however, caution is warranted because malignant tumors are known to be avid for B_{12} and folate, which are rate-limiting nutrients for DNA synthesis. Although not an issue for noncancer applications of methotrexate, caution with use of B_{12} and folate at above RDA/DV levels in cancer patients is warranted, pending careful clinical trial investigation of this issue.

Well-designed human trials are warranted to investigate the extent and implications of B_{12} depletion by methotrexate, as well as therapeutic guidelines for compensatory supplementation, and to explore potential concomitant administration of methylcobalamin to enhance the activity of methotrexate, and possibly enable reduction of the medication's dosage and amelioration of associated adverse effects.

Nitrous Oxide

Nitrous Oxide (N_2O)

Interaction Type and Significance

≈≈≈ **Drug-Induced Nutrient Depletion, Supplementation Therapeutic, Not Requiring Professional Management**

☼ **Prevention or Reduction of Drug Adverse Effect**

Probability: Evidence Base:
2. Possible   ● **Consensus**

Effect and Mechanism of Action

Repeated or prolonged nitrous oxide (N_2O) anesthesia can inactivate vitamin B_{12} and thereby interferes with the activity of folic acid, particularly in susceptible individuals; Hcy levels in turn can become elevated.[136-139] In particular, research has shown that N_2O induces inactivation of methionine synthase.[140] Among many potential sequelae, N_2O's interference with normal B_{12} activity can also lead to megaloblastic hematopoiesis.[141,142]

It is worth noting that in the research design of many investigations, such as on the effects of methotrexate, N_2O is used to inactivate cobalamin.[135,143]

Research

A broad consensus exists as to the nature of the interaction between N_2O and vitamin B_{12}. However, opinions appear mixed and the evidence is seemingly inconsistent as to the clinical significance, frequency, and severity of this interaction and the variable potential for such occurrence in patients and health care providers. In an animal experiment, O'Leary et al.[144] observed a synergistic interaction between vitamin B_{12} deficiency and N_2O exposure when they compared the bone marrow cells of rats raised on a B_{12}-deficient or B_{12}-sufficient diet and then exposed or not exposed to N_2O for 3 hours. In a study of urinary excretion of formic acid and forminoglutamic acid (FIGLU) in surgical patients exposed to isoflurane alone or combined with N_2O, Koblin et al.[140] observed only a small, transient increase in the FIGLU-to-creatinine ratio in some patients that peaked at the end of anesthetic exposure and returned toward control levels by the first day after anesthesia and surgery. These authors concluded that "although an occasional patient may prove highly susceptible to and develop signs of severe vitamin B_{12} and folic acid deficiency after exposure to N_2O, our findings suggest that this is a rare event." Ermens et al.[138] reported measurable changes in Hcy and folate plasma and urine levels indicative of cobalamin inactivation during N_2O anesthesia. In a review article, Flippo and Holder[139] noted a pattern of neurological degeneration associated with N_2O anesthesia in patients with vitamin B_{12} deficiency.

However, Salo et al.[141] gathered peripheral blood samples from eight anesthetists and seven internists in a survey of potential occupational health hazard to operating theater personnel chronically exposed to trace N_2O concentrations. They reported that no evidence of definite signs of B_{12}-N_2O interaction could be observed in peripheral blood counts and films, serum vitamin B_{12}, and plasma and erythrocyte folate concentrations.[141] The issue of how this interaction might affect individuals abusing N_2O has not been addressed in a systematic or direct manner and deserves consideration as a potential area of concern.

Reports

Both Amos et al.[145] and Nunn et al.[142] reported cases of individuals in whom N_2O anesthesia induced B_{12}-related adverse effects, including megaloblastic bone marrow changes, which were reversed by administration of folic acid or folinic acid.

Nutritional Therapeutics, Clinical Concerns, and Adaptations

Although the mechanism of nitrous oxide's effect on vitamin B_{12} activity is generally recognized and agreed on, the research on the topic has come to differing conclusions as to the probability of clinically significant adverse effects. Nevertheless, an analysis of these findings reveals a clear and consistent pattern indicating that short-term or occasional administration of N_2O, or even repeated minimal exposure over an extended period in the case of medical personnel, is unlikely to present a significant risk of substantive adverse effects on B_{12} (and folic acid) levels or activity. Overall, the incidence of severe adverse reactions appears to be rare. However, repeated or prolonged exposure to N_2O anesthesia in individuals with preexisting B_{12} (or folate) deficiency, significantly compromised general health status, pharmacogenomic limitations in detoxification functions, or other risk factors can create a situation of meaningful risk for a moderate to severe adverse reaction of a transient or cascading nature.

Evidence is lacking to support a recommendation for routine supplementation by medical or dental staff regularly exposed to N$_2$O. However, the need for B$_{12}$ and folate administration should be considered for individuals who have a recent history of, or are known to be currently engaged in, the habitual use of N$_2$O as a recreational drug. Urinary MMA level determination would be a useful monitoring test in both situations.

Normally, most patients with normal vitamin B$_{12}$ levels who undergo short-duration N$_2$O anesthesia (<2 hours) do not require supplementation. Nevertheless, prophylactic supplementation with vitamin B$_{12}$ and folate can provide a relatively certain preventive measure, with little or no risk of (additional) adverse effects, for patients who will undergo N$_2$O anesthesia for several hours, especially if these individuals are in poor health, have indications of compromised B$_{12}$ status, or demonstrate other cause for elevated risk.[145] Some health care professionals trained and experienced in nutritional therapies within an integrative context recommend 100 µg of vitamin B$_{12}$ and 1000 µg folic acid, starting 1 week before and continuing for 1 week after prolonged N$_2$O exposure.

Oral Contraceptives: Monophasic, Biphasic, and Triphasic Estrogen Preparations (Synthetic Estrogen and Progesterone Analogs)

Ethinyl estradiol and desogestrel (Desogen, Ortho-TriCyclen).
Ethinyl estradiol and ethynodiol (Demulen 1/35, Demulen 1/50, Nelulen 1/25, Nelulen 1/50, Zovia).
Ethinyl estradiol and levonorgestrel (Alesse, Levlen, Levlite, Levora 0.15/30, Nordette, Tri-Levlen, Triphasil, Trivora).
Ethinyl estradiol and norethindrone/norethisterone (Brevicon, Estrostep, Genora 1/35, GenCep. 1/35, Jenest-28, Loestrin 1.5/30, Loestrin1/20, Modicon, Necon 1/25, Necon 10/11, Necon 0.5/30, Necon 1/50, Nelova 1/35, Nelova 10/11, Norinyl 1/35, Norlestin 1/50, Ortho Novum 1/35, Ortho Novum 10/11, Ortho Novum 7/7/7, Ovcon-35, Ovcon-50, Tri-Norinyl, Trinovum).
Ethinyl estradiol and norgestrel (Lo/Ovral, Ovral).
Mestranol and norethindrone (Genora 1/50, Nelova 1/50, Norethin 1/50, Ortho-Novum 1/50)
Related, internal application: Etonogestrel/ethinyl estradiol vaginal ring (Nuvaring).

Interaction Type and Significance

≈≈≈ **Drug-Induced Nutrient Depletion, Supplementation Therapeutic, Not Requiring Professional Management**
☼ **Prevention or Reduction of Drug Adverse Effect**

Probability:	Evidence Base:
3. Possible	● **Consensus**

Effect and Mechanism of Action
The use of oral contraceptives (OCs), especially those with higher estrogen content, has been consistently associated with decreased levels of vitamin B$_{12}$.[146-148]

Research
Several decades of evidence indicate, and a broad consensus of researchers and reviewers recognize and agree, that OCs can cause a biochemical deficiency of vitamin B$_{12}$ and other nutrients.[109,148-151] The clinical implications of this probable interaction are uncertain at this time, but the conventional judgment expressed in the literature postulates that direct adverse effects of clinical significance are unlikely in most cases. Nevertheless, in a 1975 letter, Briggs[152] stated that requirements for riboflavin, thiamine, B$_{12}$, B$_6$, and tocopherols

may be increased by the use of OCs, whereas niacin and possibly vitamin A requirements may be reduced, and that normalization in nutrient status "can be effected fairly quickly by use of a daily multivitamin," which he recommended as a "routine prophylactic prescription." He further noted that "clinical signs of hypovitaminosis include depression, susceptibility to infections, and skin signs, all of which were found in users of oral contraceptives in an epidemiological survey of 46,000 women in Great Britain."[152] Megaloblastic anemia has been linked to OC use, although this has been infrequently observed and reported.

Wertalik et al.[146] compared B$_{12}$-binding proteins and serum folate concentration in 20 women who had been taking OCs for 2 to 60 months, 26 women in the third trimester of pregnancy, and 23 control women. They found that mean serum vitamin B$_{12}$ levels were 221 pg/mL in OC users (vs. 372 pg/mL in controls, i.e., 40% lower), and that half these women had serum B$_{12}$ levels below normal limits (i.e., <200 pg/mL). Generally, women in the OC group demonstrated normal B$_{12}$-binding protein capacity and RBC levels of vitamin B$_{12}$. The mean for serum folic acid was within normal range among OC users, but 30% had levels below normal (4 ng/mL). Evidence of anemia or hypersegmentation was lacking in any of these women.

However, in regard to adverse cardiovascular effects of OCs, it is also important to note that vitamin B$_{12}$ is essential for the metabolism of the atherogenic amino acid homocysteine. Well-designed clinical trials are warranted to investigate this deeper pattern of relationship between exogenous estrogen and cardiovascular risk that may be mediated by Hcy, or reflected in Hcy levels, and may be selectively detrimental to certain individual possessing as-yet unknown pharmaco/toxicogenomic characteristics involving estrogen conjugation and influenced by nutrient depletion.

Nutritional Therapeutics, Clinical Concerns, and Adaptations
Women taking OCs could reduce potential adverse effects on their cobalamin levels through supplementation with vitamin B$_{12}$. Although supplemental use of vitamin B$_{12}$ is not usually considered necessary for most of the population, the suggested dose of cobalamin in vegans is 2 to 3 µg per day, and higher levels in the range of 50 to 200 µg per day may be indicated for OC users. Supplementation with vitamin B$_{12}$ (and folate) may also reduce tendencies toward or the degree of hyperhomocysteinemia, particularly in women with compromised liver function, symptoms of an estrogen-dominance pattern, or genomic susceptibility. Physicians prescribing OCs are advised to discuss potential benefits from vitamin B$_{12}$ (and folic acid) supplementation with their patients.

Para-Aminosalicylic Acid

Para-Aminosalicylic Acid (4-aminosalicylic acid, 4-ASA, aminosalicylic acid, p-aminosalicylic acid, PAS; Paser).

Para-aminosalicylic acid (PAS) is a medication used in the treatment of tuberculosis, but it is rarely prescribed anymore, except for some of the multidrug-resistant strains. PAS is known to cause vitamin B$_{12}$ malabsorption and depletion.[153] When PAS is used clinically, it would be prudent to coadminister B$_{12}$, monitoring urinary MMA to determine sufficiency of nutrient support.

Pemetrexed

Pemetrexed (Alimta); combination drug: pemetrexed and cisplatin.
See also Antifolates section in Folic Acid monograph.

Interaction Type and Significance

☼   **Prevention or Reduction of Drug Adverse Effect**

⊕⊕   **Beneficial or Supportive Interaction, with Professional Management**

Probability:	Evidence Base:
2. Probable	◉ Emerging, possibly
	● Consensus

Effect and Mechanism of Action

Pemetrexed is a multitargeted antifolate/antimetabolite chemotherapeutic agent that inhibits several folate-dependent enzymes, including thymidylate synthase, dihydrofolate reductase, and glycinamide ribonucleotide transformylase, and causes elevation of plasma total homocysteine (tHcy) levels. Sporadic, severe myelosuppression, with GI toxicity, is a life-threatening and predictable, if infrequent, adverse effect associated with antifolates as a class.

Research

Pretreatment plasma tHcy and, to a lesser extent, MMA can be used as vitamin deficiency markers to predict nutrient depletion and severe toxicity, such as severe thrombocytopenia and neutropenia, from pemetrexed-based therapy.[154] Niyikiza et al.[155] report that concomitant folic acid and vitamin B₁₂ can reduce plasma tHcy levels and improve the safety profile for pemetrexed, without reducing and possibly increasing its efficacy.

Vogelzang and associates[156] conducted a clinical trial involving 456 chemotherapy-naive patients with malignant pleural mesothelioma, which also studied the use of concomitant folate and vitamin B₁₂ as part of a Phase III study of pemetrexed in combination with cisplatin versus cisplatin alone. After an initial 117 patients had enrolled, folic acid and vitamin B₁₂ were added to reduce toxicity, resulting in a significant reduction in toxicities in the pemetrexed/cisplatin arm. Folic acid was administered orally (350-1000 μg daily) beginning 1 to 3 weeks before the initial chemotherapy treatment and continued throughout the study. Vitamin B₁₂ (1000 μg) was administered intramuscularly starting 1 to 3 weeks before the first dose of chemotherapy and repeated every 9 weeks while each patient was receiving the study therapy. Coadministration of folate and vitamin B₁₂ with pemetrexed plus cisplatin treatment resulted in superior survival time, time to progression, and response rates compared with treatment with cisplatin alone. These researchers concluded that the addition of folic acid and vitamin B₁₂ to the chemotherapeutic regimen significantly reduced toxicity without adversely affecting treatment efficacy and survival time.[156]

Nutritional Therapeutics, Clinical Concerns, and Adaptations

Physicians prescribing pemetrexed, or related antifolates, alone or in combination with cisplatin, are advised to identify patients at risk of toxicity before initiating treatment, by measuring plasma tHcy and administering concomitant folic acid and vitamin B₁₂, as indicated, to decrease Hcy levels through vitamin supplementation, enhance the drug safety profile, reduce drug toxicity, and possibly improve efficacy.

Proton Pump Inhibitors (PPIs)

Evidence: Omeprazole (Losec, Prilosec).
Extrapolated, based on similar properties: Esomeprazole (Nexium), lansoprazole (Prevacid, Zoton), pantoprazole (Protium, Protonix, Somac), rabeprazole (AcipHex, Pariet).

Interaction Type and Significance

≈≈≈   **Drug-Induced Nutrient Depletion, Supplementation Therapeutic, Not Requiring Professional Management**

☼   **Prevention or Reduction of Drug Adverse Effect**

Probability:	Evidence Base:
3. Possible	● Consensus

Effect and Mechanism of Action

Omeprazole binds in its active form in the parietal cells of the gastric mucosa with H⁺,K⁺-ATPase. This enzyme is responsible for the pumping of protons into the gastric lumen in exchange for potassium ions ("proton pump"). By design, omeprazole leads to a dose-dependent inhibition of gastric acid secretion. This in turn will interfere with cleavage of vitamin B₁₂ from dietary proteins and will decrease protein absorption. Consequently, concern has been raised that prolonged omeprazole therapy could be responsible for a cobalamin deficiency from malabsorption of protein-bound dietary vitamin B₁₂.[157,158] Absorption of protein-bound cobalamin is further impaired in patients being treated for Zollinger-Ellison syndrome and individuals with atrophic gastritis, often associated with omeprazole therapy, especially in patients with *Helicobacter pylori* infections.[159,160]

Research

Reduced serum vitamin B₁₂ levels have been documented occasionally in relation to long-term treatment with a proton pump inhibitor (PPI) in selected groups of patients. Several studies have found that omeprazole interferes with the absorption of vitamin B₁₂ from food sources. Long-term omeprazole treatment leads to significant decreases in serum vitamin B₁₂ but not folate levels.[120,161-163] These results suggest patients treated with H⁺, K⁺-ATPase inhibitors such as omeprazole should have vitamin B₁₂ levels monitored regularly, via serum levels or as urinary MMA. The Schilling test will not detect malabsorption of food-bound cobalamin. However, other researchers, such as Koop,[164] have come to different conclusions. In general, the available evidence indicates that PPIs do not promote the development of pernicious anemia.

Schenk et al.[159] evaluated serum cobalamin levels and performed histopathological scoring of corpus biopsy specimens in 49 *H. pylori*–positive patients before and after omeprazole treatment for gastroesophageal reflux disease (GERD). Although none had signs of atrophic gastritis at inclusion, 15 patients (33%) had developed atrophic gastritis, nine of whom had moderate to severe atrophy at follow-up. Although no change was observed in the median serum cobalamin level in the 34 patients without atrophy, a decrease in cobalamin was seen from 340 at baseline to 285 at follow-up in the 15 patients who developed atrophy. These findings confirmed the hypothesis that development of atrophic gastritis during omeprazole treatment in *H. pylori*–positive GERD patients is associated with a decrease of serum vitamin B₁₂ levels.[159] Subsequently, Shuval-Sudai and Granot[11] surveyed 133 supposedly healthy, non–vitamin B₁₂–deficient adults and found that the prevalence of *H. pylori* seropositivity was significantly higher among subjects with borderline (>145-180 pg/mL) or low-normal (>180-250 pg/mL) serum vitamin B₁₂ levels than among those with vitamin B₁₂ greater than 250 pg/mL.

As it alters the gastric environment, acid suppression also increases the risk of intragastric overgrowth of non–*H. pylori* bacterial species and formation of *N*-nitrosamines.[121,165] In chronic atrophic gastritis, atrophy of the stomach glands leads to intrinsic factor deficit, with consequent failure to absorb vitamin B$_{12}$ and gastric achylia, which predisposes to *Giardia* infection, which in itself leads to further depletion of vitamin B$_{12}$.[166]

Sagar et al.[167] investigated the role of *S*-mephenytoin hydroxylase, a polymorphic cytochrome P450 (CYP) enzyme, identified as CYP2C19, which catalyzes the metabolism of omeprazole and some other drugs in the effect on serum vitamin B$_{12}$ levels during long-term treatment with omeprazole. No difference in B$_{12}$ levels was found between heterozygous (wt/mut) and homozygous (wt/wt) in 111 patients after receiving one dose of 20 mg omeprazole. However, they found that the CYP2C19 polymorphism significantly affected serum vitamin B$_{12}$ levels in patients on omeprazole therapy for more than 1 year.[167] Such findings strongly suggest that genotyping of CYP2C19 may be appropriate for patients in need of long-term treatment with omeprazole or other PPIs. Use of PPIs that do not depend primarily on 2C19 for metabolic clearance would be preferable in those patients found to have mutations in the gene encoding the 2C19 phase I hepatic enzyme, so as to avoid potentially excessive drug levels.

Reports

Bellou et al.[168] reported a case of cobalamin deficiency with megaloblastic anemia in a patient who received omeprazole (40-60 mg daily) for 4 years as treatment for a gastroesophageal reflux (GER) complicated by peptic esophagitis. Even though the Schilling test was normal (13%) with crystalline cobalamin, it was at 0% with cobalamin-labeled trout meat, and serum vitamin B$_{12}$ was dramatically decreased at 80 pmol/L. Intramuscular treatment with cobalamin restored normal hematological status of B$_{12}$.

In a case report, Ruscin et al.[126] described vitamin B$_{12}$ deficiency in a 78-year-old nonvegetarian woman with symptomatic GER after long-term use (~4.5 years) of histamine (H$_2$) receptor antagonists, starting with cimetidine, and a PPI. They noted a moderate decline in serum vitamin B$_{12}$ concentration, from an initial normal serum of 413 pg/mL to a low-normal level of 256 pg/mL after almost 2 years. However, on the latter occasion, MMA and Hcy, clinically important biochemical markers of B$_{12}$-dependent enzyme activity, were significantly elevated. These researchers then observed that MMA and Hcy concentrations decreased dramatically when oral replacement of vitamin B$_{12}$ (1000 µg daily) was instituted. This response not only confirmed vitamin B$_{12}$ deficiency, but also demonstrated that the woman was able to adequately absorb nonprotein-bound vitamin B$_{12}$ from the GI tract, suggesting that her deficiency was a result of food-cobalamin malabsorption, and that the accumulation of MMA and Hcy was not a consequence of renal dysfunction.

Nutritional Therapeutics, Clinical Concerns, and Adaptations

Physicians prescribing omeprazole or other PPIs are advised to monitor their patient's B$_{12}$ status regularly and, as indicated, administer concomitant vitamin B$_{12}$ supplementation (10-50 µg/day orally) or IM injection. Supplemental forms of B$_{12}$ do not require stomach acid to achieve proper absorption and protect against drug-induced vitamin depletion. Large oral doses (at least 1 mg daily) also bypass the need for intrinsic factor to be absorbed adequately to correct a B$_{12}$ deficiency.

Well-designed clinical trials are warranted to evaluate the effect of omeprazole and related PPIs on B$_{12}$ absorption over an extended follow-up period to determine the clinical significance of omeprazole-associated vitamin B$_{12}$ deficiency and possibly identify patients at increased risk for deficiency. Physicians prescribing PPIs are advised to consider the possibility of dietary vitamin B$_{12}$ malabsorption in patients receiving long-term PPI treatment and presenting with signs and symptoms of deficiency. Monitoring of B$_{12}$ status using a sensitive index, such as urinary MMA, is critical in preventing the potential clinical complications of PPI-associated vitamin B$_{12}$ deficiency. Individuals with the CYP2C19 polymorphism (poor metabolizers of omeprazole), elderly patients with poor dietary intake of vitamin B$_{12}$, individuals with impaired vitamin B$_{12}$ stores, and those with certain GI disorders are at increased risk of adverse drug effects and in greater need of nutrient support. Since omeprazole became available without a prescription, there is a greater need for careful history taking of over-the-counter (OTC) medication use, as well as awareness of this potentially devastating complication in the at-risk population by all health care practitioners.

Zidovudine (AZT) and Related Antiretroviral Agents, Reverse-Transcriptase Inhibitor (Nucleoside)

Evidence: Zidovudine (azidothymidine, AZT, ZDV, zidothymidine; Retrovir).
Extrapolated, based on similar properties: Abacavir (Ziagen), didanosine (ddI, dideoxyinosine; Videx); dideoxycytidine (ddC, zalcitabine; Hivid), lamivudine (3TC, Epivir), stavudine (D4T, Zerit), tenofovir (Viread); zidovudine combination drugs: zidovudine and lamivudine (Combivir); abacavir, lamivudine, and zidovudine (Trizivir).

Interaction Type and Significance

≈≈≈ **Drug-Induced Nutrient Depletion, Supplementation Therapeutic, Not Requiring Professional Management**

Probability:	Evidence Base:
2. Probable—Situational	○ **Preliminary**

Effect and Mechanism of Action

Individuals infected with HIV tend to be at greater risk of compromised vitamin B$_{12}$ status, and these medications may be associated with decreased B$_{12}$ levels.

Research

Subnormal serum B$_{12}$ levels appear to be common among individuals infected with HIV, even at early asymptomatic stages,[169] but particularly among those in advanced stages of AIDS. Furthermore, in several placebo-controlled studies, macrocytosis, anemia, and granulocytopenia were the most significant adverse effects associated with zidovudine use, especially among patients with advanced, symptomatic HIV disease. Significant anemia most often occurred after 4 to 6 weeks of therapy and in many cases required dose adjustment, discontinuation of zidovudine, and/or blood transfusions.

In an early study of azidothymidine (AZT) toxicity, Richman et al.[170] found that HIV-infected individuals with low vitamin B$_{12}$ levels were more likely to develop anemia and other blood-related adverse effects after taking AZT.[170] In 1993, Snower and Weil[171] studied 100 consecutive inpatients in a large metropolitan urban hospital with macrocytosis and found that 44% were patients with AIDS being treated with zidovudine. In a descriptive cross-sectional survey involving 200 HIV-infected individuals, Paltiel et al.[172] found subnormal serum B$_{12}$ levels in 61 subjects (30.5%) and observed that malabsorption of vitamin B_{12}, as evidenced by abnormal Schilling tests, was more likely among patients with more advanced HIV disease or GI symptoms, but was not necessarily associated with low B_{12} levels. In a 1995 prospective, randomized study, Falguera et al.[173] determined that concomitant administration of vitamin B_{12} and folinic acid did not significantly prevent or reduce AZT-induced bone marrow suppression in most treated individuals.

Nutritional Therapeutics, Clinical Concerns, and Adaptations

Physicians prescribing AZT or related retroviral therapy are advised to monitor the nutritional status of HIV-infected patients and discuss potential benefit from supplementation with vitamin B_{12} and folate. Regular monitoring of nutritional status and frequent blood counts are strongly recommended in patients with symptomatic HIV disease taking zidovudine. For asymptomatic HIV-infected individuals and patients with early HIV disease, most of whom have better marrow reserve, blood counts may be obtained less frequently, depending on the patient's overall status. If anemia or granulocytopenia develops, dosage adjustments may be necessary. In the event that supplementation is determined to be necessary, a typical adult dose of 10 to 25 µg daily, or 1000 to 1500 µg monthly, might be beneficial.

THEORETICAL, SPECULATIVE, AND PRELIMINARY INTERACTIONS RESEARCH, INCLUDING OVERSTATED INTERACTIONS CLAIMS

Aminosalicylates

Mesalazine (5-aminosalicylic acid, 5-ASA, mesalamine; Azacol, Canasa, Ipocal, Pentasa, Rowasa, Salofalk), para-aminosalicylic acid (4-aminosalicylic acid, 4-ASA, aminosalicylic acid, p-aminosalicyclic acid, PAS; Paser).
Aminosalicylates may reduce absorption of vitamin B_{12}.[174]
See also Para-aminosalicylic Acid.

Antibiotics, Particularly Cycloserine and Erythromycin

Cycloserine (Seromycin), erythromycin oral (EES, EryPed, Ery-Tab, PCE Dispertab, Pediazole).

The effects of antibiotics on vitamin B_{12} metabolism and function constitute an area of interactions research that has often been alluded to but rarely investigated in a direct and systematic manner. Many antibiotics are recognized to decrease absorption, reduce endogenous synthesis, and increase elimination of vitamin B_{12} and many other nutrients.[50,175,176] Some antibiotics rely on mechanisms of action that interfere with B_{12} metabolism (e.g., membrane transport) within bacterial cells.[177] Eradication of healthy intestinal bacterial flora and disruption of gut ecology by antimicrobials can reduce or eliminate the endogenous synthesis of B_{12} by symbiotic intestinal microbiota.[51,52] Restoration of intestinal microbiota through oral intake of probiotic flora is essential after use of any significant course of antibiotic medications and can be especially important to normalization of B_{12} status. Conversely, in some infections characterized by severe mucosal lesions and subsequent malabsorption, antibiotic therapy can help restore healthy B_{12} absorption.[178] Likewise, Crohn's disease patients who either have involvement or have had resection of the terminal ileum are at high risk of developing B_{12} deficiency because this is the site of absorption of the B_{12}–intrinsic factor complex.

Further research into the effects of antibiotics on vitamin B_{12} is warranted to clarify the particular mechanisms and outcomes of such interactions and enable formulation of guidelines for clinical practice. However, this potential for drug-induced deficiency may be more of an issue for vitamin K than for B_{12}, given the 3-year stores (or longer) of B_{12}, the 3 to 6 µg per day requirement, and the ubiquity of the vitamin in nonvegan diets.

Methyldopa

Methyldopa (Aldomet); combination drugs: methyldopa and chlorothiazide (Aldoclor), methyldopa and hydrochlorothiazide (Aldoril).

Methyldopa use can reduce vitamin B_{12} levels, potentially leading to a vitamin B_{12} deficiency, and may interfere with B_{12} metabolism.[179] Supplementation of vitamin B_{12} at moderate levels of 10 to 25 µg per day can counteract this tendency to depletion with no significant risk of adverse effects. The clinical implications of this potential interaction may be considered negligible/improbable, because methyldopa is rarely used anymore as an antihypertensive medication, being primarily employed in the treatment of pregnant women with hypertension, since it appears to be one of the safest antihypertensives for use in pregnancy.

Simvastatin

Simvastatin (Zocot).

In a preliminary clinical trial the coadministration of simvastatin (80 mg/day) and a combination of folic acid (2 mg/day) and vitamin B_{12} (0.8 mg/day) produced both serum lipid changes (with reductions in low-density lipoprotein cholesterol) and reductions in homocysteine. The combination group and simvastatin-alone group experienced similar serum lipid changes, and the combination group and vitamins-alone group experienced similar homocysteine reductions. Furthermore, no detectable antagonistic effect was observed when simvastatin and folic acid/vitamin B_{12} were administered concomitantly.[180] Further research with well-designed clinical trials is warranted for this novel approach to the multiple needs of prevention and treatment of cardiovascular disease using integrative approaches combining conventional pharmacology and nutritional therapeutics.

NUTRIENT-NUTRIENT INTERACTIONS

Alcohol

Excessive alcohol intake may reduce absorption of vitamin B_{12}.

Calcium

As previously discussed, increased intake of calcium can reverse vitamin B_{12} malabsorption induced by metformin.[128]

Folic Acid

Vitamin B_{12}, folic acid, and vitamin B_6 work together in a broad range of physiological functions, including controlling homocysteine levels. Supplementation with folic acid may mask a deficiency of vitamin B_{12}. Testing of B_{12} status by a physician is appropriate whenever anemia is suspected, and the combined supplementation of folic acid and B_{12} is usually advisable.

Folic acid deficiency, drug-induced or otherwise, can induce a deficiency of vitamin B_{12}. However, large doses of folic acid, given continuously, may reduce blood levels of vitamin B_{12}.

Potassium Chloride, Sustained/Controlled-Release Medications

Potassium administration can alter the amount of acid in the stomach and thereby inhibit the absorption of vitamin B_{12}.[181] Physicians prescribing slow-release potassium chloride may find it judicious to supplement these patients with vitamin B$_{12}$, with separaton of intake.

Vitamin B$_6$

Vitamin B$_{12}$ functions in concert with vitamin B$_6$ and folic acid in a broad range of physiological functions, including controlling homocysteine levels.

Vitamin C

Some sources suggest that vitamin C may damage or diminish the effectiveness of vitamin B$_{12}$ if taken together. This interaction may be prevented by not taking large doses of vitamin C within 1 hour of oral vitamin B$_{12}$ intake.

Vitamin D

A synergistic interaction between mecobalamin (B$_{12}$) and vitamin D appears to be involved in reducing the risk of hip fracture among stroke patients, with homocysteine as a predictive factor.[182,183]

The 183 citations for this monograph, as well as additional reference literature, are located under Vitamin B$_{12}$ on the CD at the back of the book.

Nutrient-Drug Interactions and Drug-Induced Nutrient Depletions

The quality of mercy is not strained.

Vitamin C (Ascorbic Acid)

Nutrient Names: Vitamin C, ascorbic acid.
Synonyms: Antiscorbutic vitamin, ascorbate, ascorbic acid, ascorbyl palmitate, calcium ascorbate, cevitamic acid, chromium ascorbate, dehydroascorbic acid (DHA), isoascorbic acid, magnesium ascorbate, manganese ascorbate, molybdenum ascorbate, potassium ascorbate, sodium ascorbate, zinc ascorbate; Ester-C.
Related Substances: Acerola, rose hips.

Nutrient-Drug Interactions and Drug-Induced Nutrient Depletions

Summary

Drug/Class Interaction Type	Mechanism and Significance	Management
Acetaminophen ⊕⊕/⊕✗/✗	Concomitant intake of vitamin C can competitively inhibit the conjugation of acetaminophen with sulfate and increase the apparent biological half-life of acetaminophen, thus potentially increasing risk of acetaminophen-induced hepatotoxicity. Conversely, esters of ascorbic acid may reduce reactive intermediate back to parent compound such that hepatic ascorbate can protect against acetaminophen-induced hepatotoxicity. L-Ascorbic acid esters may reduce hepatic glutathione (GSH) depletion and facilitate regeneration. Not fully understood or adequately researched, but supervised coadministration of vitamin C with acetaminophen may enable reduced drug dosages and help protect against hepatotoxicity.	Consider vitamin C during acetaminophen therapy. Monitor liver enzymes with chronic acetaminophen use.
Acetylsalicylic acid (ASA, aspirin) Salsalate ☼/≈≈≈/⊕✗/✗	Aspirin and salicylic acid can increase urinary excretion of vitamin C, lower leukocyte ascorbic acid levels, and decrease its metabolic availability. Gastric mucosa stores ascorbic acid, which is important in protecting epithelial cells, particularly against gastric erosion and hemorrhage. Compromised nutritional status can increase risk of adverse drug effects. Vitamin C may reduce gastric mucosal damage and gastric toxicity induced by ASA-generated free radicals. However, research findings have been mixed, and further study is warranted. Coadministration of vitamin C and other antioxidants may also potentiate aspirin's antiaggregative effects.	Watch for nutritional deficiencies in patients on long-term aspirin therapy and promote nutrient-rich diet. Consider ascorbic acid coadministration especially with potential ascorbic acid depletion.
Antihypertensive medications ⊕⊕	Enhanced levels of ascorbic acid may play a protective role against reactive oxygen species associated with essential hypertension and endothelial dysfunction. Concomitant intake of hypertensive medications and vitamin C may be beneficial in blood pressure management. Strong evidence is lacking and more research is needed. However, coadministration is unlikely to introduce any significant risks and may reduce cardiovascular risk and support therapeutic outcomes.	Consider vitamin C during antihypertensive therapy. Monitor regularly. Promote patient self-management of blood pressure and diet high in nutrient-rich vegetables and fruits.
Chemotherapy Radiotherapy ✗✗✗/⊕✗/✗✗/☼/≈≈	Coadministration of vitamin C, as with other antioxidants, may enhance the therapeutic effects of chemotherapy but, particularly if unsupervised and poorly timed, may interfere with radiotherapy and some forms of chemotherapy, particularly when free radicals are primary mechanism of action. Concomitant ascorbic acid beyond nutritional levels is controversial and, if indicated, demands close management by experienced clinicians. Direct research is limited and findings have been mixed. Generalized conclusions are inherently inadequate given the diversity of patients, pathologies, and medications. Further study through well-designed trials is warranted.	Unsupervised coadministration of high-dose vitamin C generally contraindicated. Coordinated care using high doses of intravenous ascorbic acid may be beneficial with experienced clinicians.
Cimetidine Histamine (H₂) receptor antagonists (H₂RAs) ☼	Cimetidine can cause decrease in serum hydrocortisone concentrations by binding to cytochrome P450, covering active heme group, and impairing hydroxylation reactions involved in human steroidogenesis. Preliminary evidence indicates that ascorbic acid, by an unknown mechanism, can prevent such a cimetidine-induced decrease in CYP450 activity and may normalize serum hydrocortisone concentration.	Coadministration of ascorbic acid before or with abdominal surgery may help mitigate adverse effects of cimetidine on cortisone levels.
Corticosteroids, oral ⊕⊕/≈≈/◇≈≈/☼	Ascorbic acid is essential in biosynthesis and metabolic regulation of certain steroid hormones, and its administration can increase serum hydrocortisone concentrations, particularly when steroidogenesis is inhibited. However, exogenous hydrocortisone can inhibit cellular uptake of ascorbic acid, impair its normal accumulation in adrenal tissues, and increase urinary excretion. Coadministration of ascorbic acid with glucocorticoids may enhance their therapeutic activity and reduce adverse effects of extended use, including vitamin C depletion. Research is limited but further study is warranted. Adverse effects are unlikely with clinical management.	Consider coadministration of ascorbic acid with long-term glucocorticoid therapy.
Cyclosporine ☼/≈≈/⊕✗/✗	Coadministration of vitamin C, and possibly other antioxidants, with cyclosporine may reduce adverse effects without decreasing therapeutic efficacy. However, drug dose needs to monitored closely and possibly reduced because vitamin C could enhance bioavailability and decrease the clearance and steady-state	Consider concomitant ascorbic acid. Supervise closely and monitor drug levels regularly.

356

Summary

Drug/Class Interaction Type	Mechanism and Significance	Management
	volume of drug's distribution. Further research warranted given limited knowledge of mechanisms involved and clinical implications.	
Desferoxamine Chelating agents ⊕✗/⊕⊕	Vitamin C can enhance absorption of nonheme iron, so concomitant intake of iron and vitamin C could theoretically increase risk of iron overload in certain predisposed individuals. Ascorbic acid modulates iron transport and storage, but increased iron levels can reduce blood levels of ascorbic acid through oxidation. Coadministration of vitamin C with deferoxamine can enhance iron excretion. However, rare complications have been reported due to exacerbation of toxic drug effects; although increased oxidation is suspected, no mechanism has been confirmed in humans. Research limited and further study needed.	Intravenous vitamin C may increase iron excretion by deferoxamine. Close supervision and monitoring are warranted, particularly in patients with cardiac disease.
Disulfiram ☼/⊕	Vitamin C may prevent (orally) or reduce severity (intravenously) of acetaldehyde toxicity associated with disulfiram-alcohol reactions. Coadministration can enhance therapeutic efficacy by reducing adverse effects and supporting drug compliance.	Use of vitamin C and related nutrients established in critical care of disulfiram toxicity; proper training required. Preventive use may be beneficial.
Erythropoiesis-stimulating agents ⊕⊕/⊕✗/✗✗/✗	Resistance to recombinant human erythropoietin (rHuEpo) is common in hemodialysis patients with functional iron deficiency, as is ascorbic acid deficiency. Adequate levels of available iron are necessary, but parenteral iron can produce iron overload with significant risks. Intravenous ascorbic acid improves anemia in iron-overloaded, EPO-hyporesponsive hemodialysis patients and facilitates elimination of iron from stores without reducing functional iron levels. Most but not all evidence is positive, and further research is warranted to further determine safety, efficacy, and indications.	Intravenous vitamin C may be appropriate in some patients resistant to EPO and at risk of iron overload. Close supervision and regular monitoring are warranted, particularly in dialysis patients.
Furosemide Loop diuretics ⊕/≈≈/☼	Ascorbic acid coadministration appears to significantly increase bioavailability of furosemide and enhance its diuretic and natriuretic effects. Several mechanisms are involved, with reduced gastric first-pass metabolism of furosemide the most important influence. Furosemide acutely increases urinary excretion of oxalic acid and vitamin C in individuals with chronic renal failure and may protect uremic patients against accumulation of oxalic acid. Limited evidence indicates absence of adverse effects and suggests further research warranted.	Coadminister vitamin C, as well as B vitamins, to optimize therapeutic effects and prevent depletion. Monitor for depletion of vitamins C and B_6, especially with renal failure and dialysis.
HMG-CoA reductase inhibitors (statins) ✗/✗✗/⊕✗/⊕	Relationship of statin drugs to oxidative stress is unclear and of potentially major significance as an adverse effect. Concomitant vitamin C may improve some lipid parameters (particularly LDL and triglycerides), promote glutathione, protect and regenerate vitamin E, and inhibit lipid peroxidation, all of which may contribute to reducing cardiovascular risk. However, the interaction between statins and antioxidants is controversial, and evidence suggests potential impairment of HDL-ogenic effects of niacin by antioxidants. Well-designed long-term trials are necessary to conclusively clarify mixed findings.	Consider coadministration of multiple antioxidants, including ascorbic acid, as well as fish oil and coenzyme Q10, to reduce adverse effects of statins and enhance therapeutic outcomes. Avoid combination in some cases. Monitor drug levels and liver enzymes regularly.
Indinavir Protease inhibitors ◇◇/◇◇◇	Concomitant high-dose ascorbic acid can reduce steady-state plasma concentrations of indinavir. However, while findings suggest possibility of subtherapeutic concentrations, limited evidence has not confirmed clinical significance. Further research needed, especially given high rate of self-medication among patient population.	Review inventory of nutrient and herb intake and caution against unsupervised intake of vitamin C and other agents in pharmacological doses. If nutrients indicated, monitor drug levels.
Lansoprazole-amoxicillin-metronidazole (LAM) triple therapy ⊕⊕/⊕✗/✗✗	Ascorbic acid secretion in the stomach is impaired with increased occurrence of *Helicobacter pylori*. LAM triple therapy enhances gastric vitamin C levels and recovery from gastritis, but eradication of *H. pylori* is not enhanced and may be impaired by simultaneous administration of vitamin C (and E). Evidence limited and research warranted.	Prudence suggests that patients be advised to avoid concomitant high-dose vitamin C during LAM triple therapy. Otherwise, advise diet rich in vitamin C in preventing gastric disease or reducing effects of *H. pylori* infection.
Levodopa, carbidopa Antiparkinsonian medications ⊕⊕/☼/◇≈≈/⊕✗/✗✗	Oxidative stress may contribute to Parkinson's disease and may be aggravated by levodopa monotherapy. Dopamine agonists and vitamin C both exert neuroprotective effects through antioxidant mechanisms, thus slowing neuron degeneration in the substantia nigra and preventing levodopa-induced neurotoxicity. Concomitant ascorbic acid can improve levodopa absorption, particularly in elderly patients, and possibly enable reduction of levodopa dosage without diminishing its effectiveness. Coadministration with levodopa-carbidopa can enhance functionality and symptom reduction in some but not all individuals. High-dose vitamin C contraindicated in certain patients, who may experience an exacerbation of dyskinesia; pretreatment screening is critical.	Administration of vitamin C (and E) may slow disease progression in Parkinson's patients. Coadministration of moderate-dose ascorbic acid (and B_6 and coenzyme Q10) with levodopa-carbidopa may be beneficial but needs to be gradually introduced, closely supervised, and regularly monitored.
Methotrexate ☼	Minimal case report data suggest that vitamin C might mitigate adverse effects associated with methotrexate therapy, particularly nausea. The particular case involved multiple medications, but signs of adverse effects or decreased drug efficacy from 1-3 g ascorbic acid were absent. Limited character of available evidence suggests caution in extrapolating to broader clinical implications. Use of antioxidants during chemotherapy is generally contraindicated outside context of medical care by trained and experienced clinicians.	Consider coadministration of vitamin C in moderate to high dose to alleviate nausea from methotrexate. However, caution, structured protocols, and close monitoring required during chemotherapy.
Nitroglycerin Nitrates ☼	Coadministration of vitamin C during nitrate therapy may prevent or reduce development of tolerance, at least in part, by mitigating free-radical formation. In particular, stabilization of mitochondrial aldehyde dehydrogenase involved in	Oral vitamin C may be used to prevent onset of nitrate tolerance, but intravenous ascorbic acid may be indicated in acute situations.

Continued

Nutrient-Drug Interactions and Drug-Induced Nutrient Depletions

Summary

Drug/Class Interaction Type	Mechanism and Significance	Management
	bioconversion of organic nitrates by ascorbic acid may also contribute to reduction of tolerance. Further research warranted, especially toward establishing patient predictors of risk and efficacy.	Requires close supervision and regular monitoring by experienced clinicians.
Oral contraceptives (OCs) ≈≈≈/✗	Oral contraceptives may cause increased ascorbic acid turnover in tissues and reduce plasma, leukocyte, and platelet ascorbic acid levels. Conversely, high-dose ascorbic acid may impair conversion of ethinyl estradiol to its sulfates and elevate plasma levels of ethinyl estradiol although without interfering with ethinyl estradiol pharmacokinetics. Unqualified case reports of contraceptive failure or breakthrough bleeding following vitamin C use have not been confirmed by research. Evidence generally limited with inconsistencies and qualifications although findings generally suggest minimal adverse effect of either agent upon the other. Further research through well-designed trials warranted.	Monitor for adverse effects of oral contraceptives especially in women with compromised nutritional status. Consider coadministration of vitamins C, B_{12} and B_6, as well as folate and magnesium, in women demonstrating or at risk of adverse effects from exogenous estrogens.
Propranolol Beta-1-adrenoceptor antagonists ✗ ✗	Vitamin C may decrease the absorption and first-pass metabolism of propranolol, but this interaction appears to be of minimal clinical significance.	Separate oral intake of vitamin C if indicated during beta-blocker therapy. Monitor.
Tetracycline antibiotics ⊕⊕⊕/☼/≈≈≈	Concomitant intake of vitamin C can enhance bioavailability and elevate blood levels of tetracycline. It may also protect against adverse effect of tetracyclines, including dental and oral discoloration and hepatic and renal toxicity. Chronic tetracycline may reduce blood levels of and interfere with the activity of ascorbic acid, particularly in compromised individuals. Preliminary data promising and consistent but limited; further research is warranted.	Consider concomitant vitamin C with long-term tetracycline therapy to enhance therapeutic effects, reduce adverse effects, and prevent depletion, especially with compromised nutritional status.

NUTRIENT DESCRIPTION

Chemistry and Forms

The generic term *vitamin C* is used to describe the various compounds that exhibit the biological activity of ascorbic acid. Albert Szent-Györgyi first isolated ascorbic acid in 1928 from porcine adrenal glands. Originally called "hexuronic acid," *ascorbic acid* (Latin *a*, "not"; *scorbutus*, "scurvy") became the official nomenclature in 1933 after the correct structural formula was determined and it was successfully synthesized.

In nature, vitamin C appears in both its reduced form (L-ascorbic acid) and its oxidized form (L-dehydroascorbic acid), which interconvert in a reversible equilibrium. L-Ascorbic acid is the most active form, but both possess antiscorbutic activity. Vitamin C is water soluble and easily oxidized in solution and with heat.

Physiology and Function

Unlike many species that are able to synthesize vitamin C, humans require intake as a nutrient. Vitamin C is readily absorbed, predominantly in the distal portion of the small intestine (jejunum) and to a lesser degree in the mouth, stomach and proximal small intestine, through active transport mechanisms as well as passive diffusion. The pharmacokinetic profile of vitamin C is significant for decreased nonlinear absorption and increased nonlinear elimination with increasing oral doses. Intake of 400 mg per day (or 75 mg/dL) is required to saturate serum. Thus, although 70% to 90% of the dietary intake is absorbed, absorption falls to 50% with a dose of 1.5 grams (g). Once maximum serum level (> 1.4 mg/dL) has been attained, intake of greater than 400 mg/day results in increased tissue levels of vitamin C. It is transported in the free form with higher concentrations in leukocytes and platelets than red blood cells (RBCs) and plasma. RBCs reach saturation with 60 mg/day. Once in circulation, vitamin C is readily taken up and concentrated in a wide range of body tissues, with the adrenal glands containing the highest concentration, and other glandular tissues (e.g., pituitary, thymus, corpus luteum) also holding relatively higher concentrations. Whole-body stores are typically about 1.5 g. Vitamin C crosses the placenta and is excreted in breast milk. It is primarily eliminated through urine, but only a small proportion is excreted unchanged (unless plasma concentration > 1.4 mg/dL).

Vitamin C plays a central role in the biosynthesis and function of many key physiological substances. Given its high concentration in the adrenals (50 times that of serum), it is not surprising that vitamin C is required for the synthesis of adrenaline/epinephrine, noradrenaline/norepinephrine, cortisol, and histamine, all of which are involved in stress response. Moreover, adrenocorticotropic hormone (ACTH) stimulation induces significant loss of ascorbic acid from the adrenal cortex as part of glucocorticoid mobilization. Vitamin C is necessary for the synthesis of carnitine and thus essential to metabolism of fat as an energy source. It is also essential in the metabolism of folic acid, histamine, phenylalanine, tryptophan, and tyrosine and the optimal activity of several enzymes, specifically enabling the conversion of folacin to tetrahydrofolic acid, dopamine to epinephrine, and tryptophan to 5-hydroxytryptophan and eventually 5-hydroxytryptamine (serotonin). Vitamin C also enhances the bioavailability of iron, as well as aiding the reduction of ferric iron to ferrous iron and limiting the degradation of ferritin to hemosiderin.

Vitamin C is a powerful protective agent within the antioxidant, detoxification, and immune systems. Its activity as an antioxidant *par excellence* is well established and widely recognized. As a water-soluble substance with universal access to cells throughout the body, vitamin C acts as a powerful reducing agent in its own right, neutralizing free radicals by donating hydrogen atoms from its two hydroxyl (OH) positions. Furthermore, it functions synergistically with other antioxidants, particularly glutathione, the other major hydrophilic antioxidant, and vitamin E, a major lipophilic antioxidant, which it can regenerate. Moreover, unlike other antioxidants that exhibit the potential of converting to pro-oxidant activity under conditions of high oxidative stress (or during in vitro experiments involving free metal ions), evidence from well-designed and physiologically relevant research is lacking to substantiate suggestions that oral vitamin C intake promotes oxidative damage in humans under physiological conditions.[1] Vitamin C protects cholesterol from oxidative damage by free radicals, lowers elevated low-density lipoprotein (LDL) cholesterol, and increases high-density lipoprotein (HDL) cholesterol. It decreases total cholesterol by facilitating the formation of bile, aiding cholesterol degradation/metabolism, and participating in its conversion to bile acids for excretion. It also decreases levels of lipoprotein(a) or Lp(a), which forms atherosclerotic plaques and helps dissolve such plaques, by reacting with insoluble calcium-phospholipid-cholesterol plaque to form soluble sodium-phospholipid-cholesterol and calcium ascorbate; it may also reverse dysfunction of endothelial cells lining the blood vessels.

Vitamin C is essential for the optimal activity of many important detoxification systems, particularly the hepatic cytochrome P450 (CYP450) mixed-function oxidase system and other enzymes responsible for metabolizing toxic substances, including heavy metals (e.g., mercury, lead, arsenic, cadmium, nickel) and many pharmaceuticals. Vitamin C inhibits hyaluronidase (the enzyme that degrades hyaluronic acid, a high-molecular-weight compound that functions as an intercellular matrix) and prevents formation of nitrosamines, carcinogenic compounds formed from dietary nitrate/nitrite compounds in the digestive tract. The numerous and profound roles of vitamin C in facilitating and regulating immune function include increasing levels of macrophage activity, lymphocyte production (neutrophils, lymphocytes, natural killer cells), and antibodies (IgA, IgG, IgM). It also elevates interferon production, modulates prostaglandin synthesis, and exerts antihistamine effects.

The activity of vitamin C is fundamental to the structural integrity, strength, and elasticity of the human body through its central role in the synthesis of collagen and elastin. These organic materials are essential to the formation, activity, and maintenance of skin, tendons, cartilage, muscles, intercellular connective tissue matrix, blood vessels, bone matrix, and tooth dentin. Specifically, the hydroxylysine cross-links in collagen require the activity of prolylhydroxylase and lysyl hydroxylase, enzymes that hydroxylate lysine and proline, and for which ascorbic acid acts as a reducing agent and coenzyme. Overall, collagen comprises 25% to 30% of total body protein, making it the most abundant protein in the body. Thus, vitamin C and its allied nutrients inherently play an important role in the healing and rebuilding of damaged tissues, such as strains, sprains, burns, scars, and fractures.

NUTRIENT IN CLINICAL PRACTICE
Known or Potential Therapeutic Uses

Vitamin C surpasses almost every other nutrient in the range of claims made for its use in promoting health and treating disease and in the popularity of its use as a supplement. Nevertheless, after more than half a century of controversy, evidence from controlled clinical trials and epidemiological studies remains limited and often speculative. Many groups within the general population, such as children, the elderly, and smokers, exhibit significant risk of vitamin C deficiency due to inadequate and inconsistent intake of vitamin C–rich foods and depletion due to medications and stressors. Nevertheless, observational studies largely indicate that populations with a higher dietary intake of vitamin C exhibit a lower incidence of cataracts, macular degeneration, cardiovascular disease, osteoarthritis, and some cancers.

Assertions of vitamin C's efficacy in the prevention of the common cold and cancer, in particular, have been focal points in a contentious and often unsubstantiated war of words, citations, and incongruous sets of assumptions, methods, and goals among divergent schools of medicine. For example, evidence for the protective effects of vitamin C against cancer is mixed, depending on study design, size and duration, nutrient source, dose, mode of administration, and the form of cancer involved, with cancers of the mouth, throat and vocal chords, lungs, esophagus, stomach, colon-rectum, and breast demonstrating inverse correlations, broadly or in select populations, in at least some studies. The application of "megadose" vitamin C as part of nutritional therapies in cancer care is even more controversial, and substantive dialogue between advocates and critics has rarely produced meaningful data or mutually satisfactory research. Review of numerous studies indicates beneficial effects of regular vitamin C, at moderate to high doses, in modestly reducing the duration of the common cold and respiratory infections and possibly the severity of symptoms. Research findings are more mixed regarding reductions in the frequency of infection. The weight of evidence in research within conventional medicine suggests a lack of benefit from long-term daily supplementation in preventing colds, except in individuals with low dietary intake, marathon athletes, or other populations with unusual circumstances.

Nevertheless, issues such as dosing strategies and delivery techniques, possible differences in physiological potency of supplemental forms from different sources, and concomitant nutrient synergies continue to separate the divergent therapeutic approaches. For example, in conventional discourse (and most human trials) a daily dose of 200 mg orally is often termed as "megadose vitamin C," and 2000 mg is considered a tolerable daily upper limit. However, among physicians specializing in nutritional therapeutics, such descriptors would be reserved for doses starting at 4 g (4000 mg) daily, and therapeutic intervention can involve intravenous (IV) administration. Consequently, the parties in this long-standing debate too often operate from such divergent views of clinical application, research methodology, and outcomes interpretation, so fundamental questions often go unanswered, the most meaningful issues remain go unresolved, and opportunities for effective collaboration can be lost.

Although findings from well-designed and adequately powered clinical trials have rarely attained the dramatic level of benefit asserted by pioneers and proponents, clinicians experienced in nutritional therapeutics have regularly been able to offer substantive critiques of conventional research methodology and suggest limited relevance of many trials to actual clinical application. As with nutritional research to this point in many areas, mixed findings may result more from variations in intervention (forms used, dose levels, methods of administration), trial characteristics (duration, patient populations, methods of assessing outcomes), and other variables than from the actual effects of the "vitamin C." Here the issues of dietary versus "supplemental" sources, as well as the multitude of supplemental forms, constitute fundamental factors in parsing evidence and extrapolating research findings. Overall, the use of oral doses may be appropriate for maintaining or restoring tissue levels, whereas IV administration of pharmacological doses is significantly more effective at obtaining greatly elevated plasma levels for short periods. Likewise, the benefits of multiple interdependent and synergistic nutrients in food sources and many prescribing strategies using nutrients as cotherapies render distinguishing the effects of any single component virtually impossible and contrasts sharply with the more decontextualized, single-agent investigational methodology modeled on studies designed for pharmacological interventions and pathological conditions. Meaningful and enduring conclusions and an operative consensus within the broader medical community will require development of an expansive set of in-depth research from controlled clinical trials integrating insights from the full range of therapeutic perspectives.

Historical/Ethnomedicine Precedent

The discovery of scurvy prevention through citrus intake among British sailors resulted from what is generally considered the first example of a controlled experiment comparing results in two populations administered different diets. It implicitly revealed a connection between the diets of disparate cultures and their respective ecological settings and traditional diets and the impact of their deficits on human health and disease.

Possible Uses

Acute anterior uveitis, aging or sun-damaged skin, alcohol withdrawal, allergies, anti-inflammatory, asthma, atherosclerosis, autism, bedsores, bronchitis, bruising (easy, excessive), cancer (risk reduction), cancer treatment, candidiasis, capillary fragility, cataract, cervical dysplasia, chronic obstructive pulmonary disease (COPD), common cold, Crohn's disease, dermatitis, diabetes mellitus, dysbiosis, eczema, fatigue, gallbladder disease, gallstone prevention, gastritis, gingivitis, glaucoma, gout, hay fever, heart disease prevention, heavy metal detoxification, hepatitis, *Helicobacter pylori* infection, herpes simplex infection, herpes zoster infection, human immunodeficiency virus and acquired immunodeficiency syndrome (HIV/AIDS) support, hives, hypercholesterolemia, hypertension, hypertriglyceridemia, hypoglycemia, immune function enhancement, influenza, insomnia, intervertebral disc inflammation, iron deficiency anemia, low back pain, macular degeneration, male infertility (sperm agglutination, low sperm count), menopausal symptoms, menorrhagia, mitral valve prolapse, multiple sclerosis, muscle soreness recovery (postexercise), nausea of pregnancy, nitrate tolerance, oral premalignant lesions (risk reduction), osteoarthritis, otitis media (recurrent), Parkinson's disease, peptic ulcers, periodontal disease, peripheral vascular disease, photosensitivity, platelet adhesiveness, postherpetic neuralgia, preeclampsia (prevention), premature placental rupture, reflex sympathetic dystrophy (RSD) prevention, retinopathy, rheumatoid arthritis, schizophrenia, scurvy, sinusitis, skin ulcers, sports injuries, stress, sunburn (prevention), tardive dyskinesia, urinary tract infection, vascular dementia prevention, viral or bacterial infections, vitiligo, wound healing.

Deficiency Symptoms

Scurvy is the fundamental and defining picture of severe vitamin C deficiency and its description as the first identified nutritional deficiency disease constituted a landmark development in nutritional medicine. Frank scurvy is rare in the United States (U.S.) and Europe, but subclinical deficiencies are common. Symptoms of advanced vitamin C deficiency derive primarily from defective collagen synthesis and degenerative changes in capillaries, bone, and connective tissue, and include listlessness, fatigue, weakness, fever, shortness of breath, anorexia, erupted teeth with bleeding gums, ecchymoses, hemorrhage, anemia, edema, hypotension, convulsions, personality changes, hypertrophy of the cornea, icterus, perifollicular hyperkeratotic papules, dry skin, muscle cramps, aching bones, joints, and muscles, and secondary infections. Scurvy, uncorrected, is eventually fatal. Children can experience abnormal development of bones, teeth, and blood vessels and disturbances of growth. Capillary fragility, bleeding gums, easy bruising, poor wound healing, diminished antioxidant protection, increased susceptibility to infection, and fatigue are among the indicators of possible subclinical vitamin C deficiency.

Smokers are foremost among groups at risk of vitamin C deficiency, but the elderly, institutionalized persons, hospital patients, and diabetics are also highly susceptible. The Third National Health and Nutrition Examination Survey also identified those who did not use supplements and non-Hispanic black males as having elevated risks of vitamin C deficiency and depletion in the U.S.[2] Other groups characterized by specific metabolic stresses may need greater levels of vitamin C intake for proper physical activity and protective functions, including individuals with high alcohol intake, those with increased oxidative stress (e.g., exposure to chemicals, heavy metals, radiation), those in life phases of rapid growth (pregnancy, lactation, childhood, adolescence), and individuals with chronic illnesses (e.g., rheumatoid arthritis, diabetes, hyperthyroidism, chronic kidney failure). As discussed later, numerous medications can deplete vitamin C or interfere with its normal activities. Increased risk of developing cataracts and heart disease can result from degenerative processes associated with chronic vitamin C deficiency.

Other than humans and other primates (specifically gorillas, chimpanzees, and monkeys), guinea pigs and a rare species of bat are the only mammals that lack the ability to synthesize ascorbic acid from glucose.

Dietary Sources

Public education is necessary to correct the widely held misconception, founded more in marketing and advertising than in nutritional science, that fruits, especially citrus, are exceptionally rich sources of vitamin C. In fact, vegetables are richer dietary sources. Vitamin C can be lost through oxidation during storage and cooking, and boiling can cause leaching of the nutrient into the water (unless recovered by use, such as in gravy or soup).

Almost all fresh vegetables and fruits are potential sources of vitamin C. Foods particularly rich in vitamin C include broccoli, cauliflower, red bell peppers, red chili peppers, black currants, Brussels sprouts, cantaloupe, kale, parsley, turnip greens, collard, rose hips, citrus fruits, strawberries, apples, persimmons, papaya, guava, acerola cherries, potatoes, cabbage, tomatoes, and green bell peppers.

Nutrient Preparations Available

Vitamin C is present in most multivitamin preparations. Intravenous ascorbate solutions (sodium ascorbate, or ascorbic acid buffered to a pH > 5.5) are only administered by drip; IV push is contraindicated because of venous irritation. Osmalality of IV ascorbate solutions up to 1200 mOsm/L are well tolerated if the patient can take adequate fluids by mouth.

Scientific evidence is lacking to demonstrate superior bio-availability of any single form of orally administered vitamin C (L-ascorbic acid) compared with any other form. Although vitamin C from naturally occurring sources is favored by advocates of vitamin C therapy, naturally derived and synthesized forms of L-ascorbic acid are chemically identical, and limited human research has thus far demonstrated no significant differences in their respective biological activities or bioavailability, using standard assay methods and parameters of physiological effect. When formulated as a mineral salt, ascorbic acid is buffered (i.e., less acidic) and thus theoretically less irritating than simple ascorbic acid to the gastrointestinal (GI) tract. A wide range of mineral ascorbates are available, with sodium ascorbate (131 mg sodium per 1000 mg ascorbic acid) and calcium ascorbate (114 mg calcium per 1000 mg ascorbic acid) being the most common. The addition of small amounts of dehydroascorbate (oxidized ascorbic acid), calcium threonate, and trace levels of xylonate and lyxonate, all metabolites of vitamin C, to a base of calcium ascorbate, marketed as Ester-C, is purported to provide for enhanced bioavailability, but supportive evidence is lacking, although Ester-C does appear to be "much better tolerated" than "regular ascorbic acid," as indicated by "fewer epigastric adverse effects."[3] Similarly, although bioflavonoids and vitamin C often occur together in many fruits and vegetables, claims that combining them in supplements provides superior activity have yet to be substantiated. Vitamin C is normally water soluble, but a fat-soluble form, known as *ascorbyl palmitate,* has been synthesized for use in topical applications by esterifying vitamin C to palmitic acid, a saturated fatty acid; an oral form would be unlikely to escape breakdown through hydrolyzation before being absorbed in the digestive tract. Erythorbic acid is an isomer of ascorbic acid but may lack the primary antiscorbutic activity of ascorbic acid; it is used in the U.S. as a food additive, but not as a nutritional supplement.

Based on the finding that some tumors accumulate high levels of vitamin C, concern has been raised that vitamin C might make cancer treatment less effective.[4] However, there is virtually no evidence from clinical trials that vitamin C interferes with any type of cancer therapy. In contrast, multiple animal and clinical studies suggest that vitamin C may enhance cancer therapy, possibly by acting as a pro-oxidant when accumulated in large intracellular stores by tumors, then exposed to chemotherapy or radiation.[5-7,7a] (See Chemotherapy for further discussion.)

The tissue levels of ascorbic acid concentration obtained through IV administration are significantly greater than those associated with oral intake. Intravenous administration of vitamin C at 18 g/day can produce plasma concentrations 25 times those resulting from oral administration of the same dose. Recent pharmacokinetics models indicates that with oral administration, even large frequent doses of vitamin C, will increase plasma concentrations only modestly, from 70 mmol/L to a maximum of 220 mmol/L, whereas IV administration increases concentrations as high as 14,000 mmol/L. Plasma concentrations of 1000 to 5000 mmol/L are selectively cytotoxic to tumor cells in vitro, and emerging evidence indicates that vitamin C at concentrations achieved only by IV administration may function as a prodrug for hydrogen peroxide (H_2O_2) delivery to tumor tissues.[8-15] Such observations may account for the inconsistent findings and divergent conclusions in studies using oral versus IV modes of delivery. Rigidly imposing a preconceived model of the beneficial or adverse effects of pro-oxidant effects of nutrients is not likely to lead to clinically useful conclusions.

Dosage Forms Available

Capsules, liposomal spray, powders, tablets, chewable tablets, effervescent tablets.

Source Materials for Nutrient Preparation

Commercial vitamin C is synthesized from glucose by two primary methods. The Reichstein process, developed in the 1930s, applies a single prefermentation, followed by a purely chemical route. The two-step fermentation process, introduced in China in the 1960s, replaces the later chemical stages with further fermentation. The yield from either process is approximately 60% ascorbic acid from the glucose feed, usually derived from corn.

Sago palm–derived ascorbic acid has been developed for individuals with putative corn sensitivity.

Camu camu *(Myrciaria dubia),* a bioflavanoid-rich berry from the Amazon rain forest, is an innovative source of vitamin C emerging in the marketplace

Dosage Range

Adult

Dietary: Vitamin C intake of 10 mg per day can prevent scurvy. The U.S. recommended dietary allowance (RDA) for vitamin C, or the daily dose required to prevent deficiency disease, is 90 mg/day for men and 75 mg/day for women; it was recently revised upward from 60 mg daily and had been 45 mg until 1974. The new, higher RDA takes into account for the first time the vitamin's role as an antioxidant as well as protection from deficiency. A special RDA has been established for adult smokers: 125 mg/day for men and 110 mg/day for women; Ames[16] has recommended that smokers need to consume two to three times more vitamin C than nonsmokers. The mean dietary intakes of vitamin C for adults in the United Kingdom (U.K.) and Germany were 87 and 76 mg daily and 75 and 72 mg daily for adult men and women, respectively.[17,18] Among elderly men and women in the U.K., vitamin C intakes of 72 and 68 mg daily, respectively, have been reported.[19] The National Health and Nutrition Examination Survey found that the median consumption of vitamin C from foods during the years 1988 to 1991 was 73 and 84 mg daily for men and women in the U.S., respectively.[20] All these studies have demonstrated a wide variation in vitamin C intake, with 25% to 30% of the U.S. population consuming less than 2.5 servings of fruit and vegetables daily. Dietary intake levels in other areas, such as Latin America, Africa, and Asia, are typically lower. Based on a review of the scientific literature, the Linus Pauling Institute recommends "that the RDA for vitamin C should be 120 mg/day for optimum risk reduction of heart disease, stroke, and cancer in healthy individuals. Special populations, such as older adults and individuals with disease, may require substantially larger amounts of vitamin C to achieve optimum body levels and derive therapeutic benefits."[21] Consuming at least five servings of fruits and vegetables daily may provide about 200 mg of vitamin C.[22]

Supplemental/Maintenance:
   60 to 1000 mg/day.
      Optimal daily intake: 0.5 to 3 g/day, depending on the individual.

Some research suggests that blood levels reach saturation at an oral intake of approximately 200 mg daily in healthy individuals, and assuming tissues are saturated, any intake above that amount may be excreted. However, the Linus Pauling

Institute recommends a vitamin C intake of at least 400 mg daily; this amount has been found to fully saturate plasma and circulating cells with vitamin C in young, healthy nonsmokers.[12,22] Individual variability can alter the metabolic effects of supplemental vitamin C, including nutrigenomic response variability, body weight, depletion status, and degree of tissue saturation based on recent patterns of intake.

Pharmacological/Therapeutic:

300 to 1000 mg/day typical for adults treated for scurvy.

500 mg/day to 20 g/day reported in scientific literature.

Up to 70 g/day used therapeutically and in research settings.

Dosing to bowel tolerance is typically applied clinically as a practical (as well as variable and evolving) parameter in therapeutic administration of vitamin C. The laxation effects of large oral doses of vitamin C are likely because of the osmotic effects of unabsorbed ascorbate. The common clinical observation that the bowel tolerance of vitamin C increases substantially during acute viral illnesses suggests that more ascorbate is absorbed from the GI tract during such episodes.

Toxic: Although toxicity is rare, the tolerable upper intake level (UL) established by the Food and Nutrition Board (FNB) of the Institute of Medicine for vitamin C in adults was set at 2000 mg. Notably, this advisory body established the "no adverse effect level" (NOAEL) for vitamin C arbitrarily out of necessity because they were mandated to do so, even though their review of the scientific literature failed to find any "solid data" to support a toxic dose for vitamin C.[23] As stated by Johnston[24] in 1999: "The available data indicate that very high intakes of vitamin C (2 to 4 grams per day) are well tolerated biologically in healthy mammalian systems. Currently, strong scientific evidence to define and defend a UL for vitamin C is not available." Thus, this level is based on the potential for discomfort from possible diarrhea and GI disturbances (i.e., temporary and easily reversible responses) rather than actual toxicity in most individuals and is derived from uncontrolled case reports.[23]

Pediatric (<18 years)

Dietary:

Neonates to 6 months: 40 mg/day (AI, adequate intake)

6 to 12 months: 50 mg/day (AI)

1 to 3 years: 15 mg/day (RDA)

4 to 8 years: 25 mg/day (RDA)

9 to 13 years: 45 mg/day (RDA)

Adolescents, 14 to 18 years: 65 mg for females; 75 mg for males (RDA)

Supplemental/Maintenance: Usually not recommended for children under 12 years of age.

Pharmacological/Therapeutic: The treatment of scurvy in children typically requires 100 to 300 mg per day orally in divided doses for 2 weeks. Otherwise, vitamin C is generally not administered in pharmacological doses to infants or children.

Toxic: UL levels (oral):

0 to 12 months: none established

1 to 3 years old: 400 mg/day

4 to 8 years old: 650 mg/day

9 to 13 years old: 1200 mg/day

Adolescents, 14 to 18 years old, including pregnant or breast-feeding females: 1800 mg/day

Toxicity is rare.

Laboratory Values

Physicians usually do not test vitamin C status, except for rare occasions of suspected scurvy. Most methods of laboratory assessment are generally considered neither sensitive nor precise in determining functional deficiency or systemic depletion. Further, high intake of vitamin C can interfere with some of the more frequently used laboratory tests.

Assessment of deficiency or depletion status.

Leukocyte ascorbate:

Normal range: not established.

Levels less than 114 mmol/108 cells (buffy coat) indicate deficiency.

Leukocyte concentrations may provide a good index of tissue stores of vitamin C.

Plasma ascorbate:

Normal range: not established.

Levels less than 2.6 mg/L (15 μmol/L) may indicate deficiency, but consistency in standards is lacking.

Plasma levels indicate metabolic turnover status of vitamin C. However, "extreme individual variability" has been documented with an identical vitamin C repletion dose in different individuals producing different plasma ascorbate levels based on body weight, prior depletion, and prior repletion.[25]

Urinary ascorbate:

Normal range: not established.

Excretion of less than 10 mg/day indicates severe deficiency.

Urinary ascorbate is generally considered an insensitive index of status except in severe deficiency.

Ascorbate loading test: An oral dose of 0.5 to 2.0 g ascorbic acid is administered over 4 days, and then urinary ascorbate is measured; excretion of less than 60% of dose indicates depletion of tissue ascorbate.

Lingual ascorbic acid test (LAAT): In this physician-administered test, a drop (from 25-gauge needle) of blue dye (2,6-dichloroindophenol sodium salt solution) is put on the tip of the tongue. Vitamin C status is indicated by the time required for the dye to disappear. Less than 20 seconds indicates normal levels; 20 to 25 seconds, marginal levels; and longer than 25 seconds, depletion of vitamin C levels. This is a functional test of the oxidation-reduction (redox) status of saliva and tissue, which is influenced by ascorbate status, but not specific for it.

As a strong reducing agent, ascorbic acid (>1 g daily) can interfere with some diagnostic tests, particularly those based on redox reactions. Evidence for some of these effects is mixed.

False-negative results on stool occult blood (guaiac assay) have been attributed to "high-dose" vitamin C intake within preceding 48 to 72 hours. False-negative results on urine acetaminophen tests have also been reported.

Vitamin C intake may produce false increases in levels in these serum tests: bilirubin, carbamazepine, creatinine, aspartate transaminase (AST; glutamic-oxaloacetic transaminase [SGOT]), uric acid.

Vitamin C intake may produce false decreases in levels in these serum tests: lactate dehydrogenase (LDH), theophylline.

Inaccurate readings on urinary glucose tests have been observed, with false negatives using glucose oxidase and false positives using cupric sulfate as the reagent test. Vitamin C–induced interference with blood glucose tests has been reported in the scientific literature but disputed.

Several unqualified case reports from the 1970s suggested that high-dose vitamin C could lower prothrombin time (PT) and cause increased clotting. Vigilance is appropriate whenever employing anticoagulant therapy, but evidence is too weak and inconsistent to represent this potential effect as highly probable or predictable, as discussed later.

SAFETY PROFILE
Overview

Vitamin C is safe across a broad range of intakes for most adults, according to a review and editorial by a team of eminent nutritional researchers.[26] Scientific evidence is lacking to demonstrate that even very large amounts of vitamin C are toxic or exert adverse health effects. Regular intake of dose levels well above the RDAs has been common in large numbers of individuals for decades. Adverse effects have been lacking in individuals, including Linus Pauling, who have consumed 10 g or more daily for extended periods. Systemic toxicity is improbable in healthy individuals because the primary effects of excess intake are mainly caused by large amounts of unabsorbed ascorbic acid in the intestine and, as such, typically do not alter circulating levels, are easily excreted, and respond rapidly to a decrease in intake. Thus, the Linus Pauling Institute, Oregon State University, concluded "that there is currently no consistent and compelling data for serious adverse effects of vitamin C in humans, and a UL can therefore not be established."[21]

Nutrient Adverse Effects
General Adverse Effects

Gastrointestinal (GI) discomfort, abdominal bloating, flatulence, dysuria, increased urinary frequency, skin rashes, loose stools, and diarrhea, resulting from the osmotic effects of unabsorbed vitamin C in the intestine, constitute the primary adverse effects in most individuals. Although providing the basis for the UL in the U.S., these responses are all dose related, resolve rapidly with decreased intake, and present no serious risk. Tolerance typically develops over time with gradual increase in dose. Diarrhea usually occurs with doses of 6 to 10 g daily but has been reported to afflict some individuals after only a single 1-g dose. Lowering the dosage to the highest level that does not provoke diarrhea (i.e., to "bowel tolerance") is a common method of determining maximal dosage for therapeutic effect.

Adverse Effects Among Specific Populations

Because of the importance of excretion as a regulatory process, individuals with compromised renal function may experience impaired elimination, excess accumulation, and increased lithogenicity.

Individuals with inadequate levels of glucose-6-phosphate dehydrogenase (G6PD) are at increased risk of a potentially severe adverse reaction, including possible hemolysis, after intake of certain oxidizing substances, such as high doses of vitamin C, orally or intravenously, suggesting that ascorbate might function as a pro-oxidant under certain conditions.[27] Genetic or G6PD enzyme activity testing is appropriate, particularly when IV ascorbic acid administration is contemplated.

In the general (U.S.) population, researchers have found "no association between serum ascorbic acid level and prevalence of kidney stones in women or men."[28] Nevertheless, certain individuals may theoretically exhibit increased risk of calcium oxalate stones with high-dose vitamin C intake becasue of potentially increased oxalate levels.[29] Vitamin C (ascorbic acid) is metabolized to dehydroascorbic acid, which in turn is metabolized to oxalic acid. In general, individuals who consume large amounts of vitamin C have shown either no change or a decreased risk of kidney stone formation in large-scale observational studies.[28,30,31] However, one of every 400 individuals possesses a defect in oxalate metabolism,

resulting in idiopathic hypercalciuria, that could put them at increased risk of stone formation due to elevated urinary oxalic acid levels when administered high dose vitamin C (4-10 g orally). In a trial investigating the effect of calcium citrate supplementation on urinary calcium oxalate saturation in female stone-formers, Levine et al.[32] and associates found that "calcium citrate supplementation did not increase the lithogenicity." However, 2 years later in a study of vitamin C pharmacokinetics in healthy volunteers, these researchers reported that some individuals can experience an elevation in urinary oxalate levels after consuming 1000 mg of vitamin C per day, even in the absence of a history of kidney stones.[11] Auer et al.[33] expressed concern in reporting a small trial in which they observed sharp increases in excretion of urinary oxalate and sudden onset of hematuria due to formation of kidney stones in a single male subject who had consumed "large doses of ascorbic acid" for 8 days. Notably, in the paper describing the trial as a whole, these same authors "concluded that ingestion of large doses of ascorbic acid does not affect the principal risk factors associated with calcium oxalate kidney stone formation."[34]

In an interesting line of research, several small trials and a decade of clinical experience have consistently demonstrated the efficacy of lemonade in improving urinary citrate levels and reducing the occurrence of hypocitraturic calcium nephrolithiasis, in a manner similar to that of potassium citrate.[35-37]

Oxalate formation is saturable, and most of the population is unlikely to experience this complication. Hoffer[38,39] and other senior vitamin C researchers consider this kidney stone risk as exaggerated and inadequately demonstrated, possibly an artifact resulting from failure to acidify urine samples during collection. Some physicians experienced in nutritional therapies suggest that this risk may be mitigated by vitamin C's tendency to bind calcium, causing it to be excreted in urine, and rendering it unavailable for forming calcium oxalate stones. Likewise, Ester-C may be less likely than other forms of vitamin C to cause this rise in oxalate. Research is lacking to validate either of these propositions conclusively. Vitamin B$_6$ decreases oxalate production and may mitigate this risk.[31] Thiamine can also inhibit oxalate formation, as can correction of magnesium deficiency.[40] Nevertheless, health care professionals treating individuals at risk are advised to exercise extra caution in administering doses greater than 300 mg/day on a regular basis and to consider measuring urinary oxalate levels before and after beginning ascorbate supplementation.

Pregnancy and Nursing

Vitamin C is not known to cause mutations or birth defects in healthy individuals.[23] However, in one randomized, placebo-controlled trial involving 722 pregnant women at risk for pre-eclampsia, researchers observed a slightly elevated incidence of small-for-gestational-age neonates among women administered vitamin C (1000 mg) and vitamin E (RRR alpha-tocopherol, 400 IU) versus placebo.[41] A larger trial would be necessary to determine if this is a statistically significant and etiological effect, or if these events occurred by chance.

Infants and Children

The risk of "rebound scurvy" has been reiterated in innumerable secondary sources for decades, even though substantive scientific evidence is lacking. Theoretically, rebound scurvy could potentially occur in infants if the mother takes megadoses of vitamin C during gestation. This assertion is largely based on one poorly controlled study done by Cochrane in 1965 involving two infants whose mothers who had consumed 400 mg of supplemental vitamin C during pregnancy. The vitamin C was discontinued abruptly after the births. These infants were receiving formula, and it was presumed that the formula had adequate levels of vitamin C. However, there was no analysis of the vitamin C content in the formula, nor was any attention given to the storage, preparation, or administration of the formula.[42] Thus, considering the number of women who have taken vitamin C during pregnancy, this small study occurring more than 30 years ago, and no similar cases documented, the risk is likely to be extremely low, if existent at all. The FNB Panel on Dietary Antioxidants and Related Compounds concluded that vitamin C does not cause "rebound scurvy" in healthy individuals.[23]

Contraindications

Cystinuria.

Glucose-6-phosphate dehydrogenase (G6PD) deficiency.

Individuals with a history of hemosiderosis, hemochromatosis, or other forms of iron overload.

Individuals with a history of recurrent nephrolithiasis, especially oxalate stone-formers, should avoid daily doses of 1000 mg or more outside the context of close supervision by an appropriately trained and experienced health care professional.

Megadoses (> 4 g/day) in individuals with a history of renal failure outside the context of supervision by an appropriately trained and experienced health care professional, particularly on initiation of intake or significant change in dose.

Pregnant women should avoid daily doses above 500 mg without close medical supervision.

Use of doses greater than 1000 mg/day is generally contraindicated during forms of chemotherapy and radiation in which free-radical formation is an intentional part of the therapeutic mechanism. As discussed later, vitamin C and other antioxidants should be administered only in the context of direct supervision and close monitoring because of their potential inhibition of oxidation.

Precautions and Warnings

Patients with renal impairment or on chronic hemodialysis. Doses of vitamin C should not exceed 100 to 200 mg daily in individuals with renal failure.

Caution and close supervision are appropriate in administering vitamin C to individuals diagnosed with sickle cell anemia, sideroblastic anemia, or thalassemia.

Patients preparing for major surgery, particularly those at increased risk of hemorrhage, should not exceed 400 mg daily in the week before the procedure except under the supervision of an experienced health care professional.[43]

Individuals with sensitivities to corn may react to commercially available forms of vitamin C because most are derived from corn. Ascorbates derived from sago palm have been produced for extremely corn-sensitive individuals.

Long-term intake of high doses of vitamin C may induce copper deficiency.

INTERACTIONS REVIEW

Strategic Considerations

Whether in cardiovascular health, immune function, oncology, or preventing the common cold, vitamin C, or perhaps more accurately "the view of vitamin C," may constitute the most contentious and misunderstood topic, and thus probably the greatest single test of scientific discovery and clinical pragmatism, in integrative therapeutics and patient self-care. For decades, vitamin C has been the subject of intense controversy in medicine, the virtual bogeyman of medicine's Cold War era, and with its central physiological roles and its pervasive therapeutic potential, it presents a central opportunity for transdisciplinary collaboration and the emerging model of integrative therapeutics. Leading scientists and experienced clinicians, and throngs of self-administering patients, have voiced strong support for the preventive and therapeutic value of ascorbic acid ever since it was taken up by Linus Pauling and the clinicians proposing "orthomolecular medicine." On the side of the status quo, researchers and the institutions of conventional medicine have consistently voiced skepticism, disinterest, and often disdain for the exuberance of what they have seen as overamplified extrapolations of questionable anecdote. Nevertheless, the paradigm and treatment protocols of the pioneers and their successors have rarely been studied or applied intact by the conventional researchers who have investigated vitamin C. Richards,[44] Segerstråle,[45] and others have described a systematic pattern of bias against vitamin C therapeutics, particularly in contrast to conventional agents such as 5-fluorouracil and interferon. Hemilä[46] has suggested that "Pauling's conclusions were dismissed because of the fundamental divergence with the traditional notion that the only purpose of vitamin C is to prevent scurvy and not because of experimental findings." He also cited the work of Goodwin and Tangum[47] as providing "several examples to support the conclusion that there has been systematic bias against the concept that vitamins might be beneficial in levels higher than the minimum required to avoid classic deficiency diseases."[46]

In the absence of a theoretically clear and clinically operative model of integrative medicine, a strident attitude and lack of respect on both sides have contributed to the absence of a substantive scientific debate, to the detriment of both scientific knowledge and patients. Fortunately, scientific knowledge of vitamin C has grown progressively, as has a deeper appreciation of nutritional therapies in general. Moreover, new "discoveries" have become possible with the greater openness in scientific research to incorporating the therapeutic models of natural medicine, and thus more accurately resembling its clinical practice. These changes within the broader world of medical practice, education, and research have opened the doorway for a more systematic and comprehensive study of vitamin C, its essential role in human health, possibilities for therapeutic application, and the operative considerations for beneficial and adverse interactions within a clinical context encompassing conventional pharmacology. Considering the widespread use of vitamin C by all sectors of the patient population, self-administered or prescribed by nonconventional health care professionals, the sparsity of substantive clinical research data is striking and the basis for any sweeping generalizations about benefits, dangers, or interactions woefully inadequate.

It is useful to divide the clinical investigation of vitamin C into its physiological (coenzyme and antioxidant) functions (up to intakes of 400 mg/day, at which point tissue levels become saturated) and its pharmacological dosage range (multigram doses orally, up to 100 g intravenously). Evidence suggests that high-dose, particularly parenteral, ascorbic acid functions as a redox potential–modulating agent rather than a vitamin or antioxidant. Confusion between these two distinct roles of ascorbic acid may be the source of conflicting data in this field.

Under certain conditions, ascorbic acid, whether from natural or synthetic sources, can interact with numerous pharmacological agents, beneficially, adversely, or bimodally, depending on clinical management. In particular, through its antioxidant activity and influence on drug-metabolizing enzymes, vitamin C may amplify or mitigate adverse effects (sometimes intended effects) of numerous pharmacological agents or, in some cases, potentially impair the desired therapeutic activity of such agents. Here the issue of ascorbic acid coadministration with chemotherapy or statin drugs has been the most contentious. In both regards, theoretical concerns about the antioxidant or pro-oxidant effects of vitamin C in conjunction with conventional therapies have been based all too often on questionable assumptions and limited research. Many conclusions have been made absent substantive evidence from large, lengthy, and well-designed trials focusing on the specific proposed interactions involving vitamin C. Health care professionals of all schools of thought and therapeutic approaches share these concerns, but those experienced in their application in clinical settings regularly point out that most cited research is preliminary and of only limited similarity to actual clinical practice. The paramount need is for well-designed and adequately powered trials that will critically assess the therapeutic use of vitamin C in these clinical contexts; determine the frequency, character, and clinical significance of any substantive interactions; and offer guidelines for shaping the clinical adaptations necessary for ensuring safety and optimizing outcomes. Moreover, in such investigations, particular attention must focus the form, dosage, and mode of vitamin C administration, concomitant conditions and treatments, and individual pharmacogenomic, lifestyle, and personal history factors characterizing the subject population, so as to discern specific influential variables and customize therapeutic responses accordingly.

Distinguishing use of vitamin C as nutritional supplement and patient self-care practice from high-dose ascorbic acid administration, orally or intravenously, by trained and experienced health care professionals applying coherent multidisciplinary strategies constitutes a critical first step to any meaningful scientific dialogue and productive research agenda. For example, approaches such as alternating administration but avoiding simultaneous intake, as practiced in many integrative oncology clinics, and purposeful selection of IV or oral administration represent significant clarifications that could benefit research design. Thus, in most observed interactions, doses less than 1 g/day are generally much less likely to precipitate adverse interactions, particularly given adequate separation of intake when indicated. High versus low dosage levels and IV versus oral administration almost always need to be considered as distinct from each other.

Likewise, few conclusive judgments can be made (or even hypothesized) as to the efficacy or risks of vitamin C within oncological treatment programs until further research is conducted into the contentious but largely unexplored issue of whether vitamin C always acts as an antioxidant or whether and when it may shift to pro-oxidant activity, as well as the corollary questions as to under what certain conditions this might occur and how that might affect interactions, effects, and outcomes. Further, the question of whether vitamin C can and should be investigated as an isolated nutrient or as a component of a broader nutrient-based interventions needs to be recognized, addressed, and sorted, especially with regard to such key issues as the preventive and therapeutic use of antioxidants and the respective emphasis on dietary versus supplement versus pharmacological forms. The important concepts embodied in the work of Bruce Ames and his collaborators regarding the importance of nutrients to genetic stability and

exemplified by the extended SU.VI.MAX study in France provide useful models for the further development of research methodology that can deliver clinically relevant findings.

A wide range of drugs and drug classes can cause adverse effects or induce harmful reactions by interfering with the normal physiological activities of vitamin C and depleting functional levels in diverse tissues. As with most patterns of nutrient depletion or physiological impairment, patient susceptibility to clinically significant adverse effects from drug-induced vitamin C depletion depends largely on the nutritional status, concomitant medical conditions, and drug intake and other patient-specific factors, as well as the dosage level and treatment duration of the medication(s) involved. In some situations, coadministration of vitamin C, usually with synergistic nutrients, may only be appropriate for individuals with compromised nutritional status resulting from diet, disease, genetics, or medications, and then primarily in relation to intensive or prolonged drug regimens. In other situations, where concomitant ascorbic acid presents no significant risk of adverse effects or interactions, routine prophylactic administration may be judicious.

NUTRIENT-DRUG INTERACTIONS

Acetaminophen

Acetaminophen (APAP, paracetamol; Tylenol); combination drugs: acetaminophen and codeine (Capital and Codeine; Phenaphen with Codeine; Tylenol with Codeine); acetaminophen and hydrocodone (Anexsia, Anodynos-DHC, Co-Gesic, Dolacet, DuoCet, Hydrocet, Hydrogesic, Hy-Phen, Lorcet 10/650, Lorcet-HD, Lorcet Plus, Lortab, Margesic H, Medipain 5, Norco, Stagesic, T-Gesic, Vicodin, Vicodin ES, Vicodin HP, Zydone); acetaminophen and oxycodone (Endocet, Percocet 2.5/325, Percocet 5/325, Percocet 7.5/500, Percocet 10/650, Roxicet 5/500, Roxilox, Tylox); acetaminophen and pentazocine (Talacen); acetaminophen and propoxyphene (Darvocet-N, Darvocet-N 100, Pronap-100, Propacet 100, Propoxacet-N, Wygesic); acetaminophen, butalbital and caffeine (Fioricet).

Interaction Type and Significance
⊕⊕ **Beneficial or Supportive Interaction, with Professional Management**
⊕✗ **Bimodal or Variable Interaction, with Professional Management**
✗ **Potential or Theoretical Adverse Interaction of Uncertain Severity**

See also Indomethacin and related Nonsteroidal Anti-inflammatory Drugs (NSAIDs) in Theoretical, Speculative, and Preliminary Interactions Research.

Probability: Evidence Base:
4. Plausible   ○ **Preliminary**

Effect and Mechanism of Action
Both acetaminophen and ascorbic acid are metabolized and excreted in part by conjugation to sulfate. Their competition for available sulfate in the body can inhibit the conjugation of acetaminophen with sulfate. This can significantly decrease the fraction of a dose of acetaminophen excreted as acetaminophen sulfate and increase the fraction excreted as acetaminophen glucuronide. Thus, by decreasing the excretion rate of acetaminophen sulfate, ascorbic acid can increase the apparent biological half-life of acetaminophen.[48] Such effects may

increase therapeutic activity but can also elevate risks associated with excess acetaminophen, particularly hepatotoxicity (caused by depletion of hepatic glutathione). However, esters of ascorbic acid, such as ascorbyl stearate or ascorbyl palmitate, may also be capable of reducing the reactive intermediate back to the parent compound, and thus hepatic ascorbate can provide enhanced protection against acetaminophen-induced hepatotoxicity, as indicated by reductions in biochemical markers of hepatotoxicity, such as serum transaminase and serum isocitrate dehydrogenase (SICD) activities. Furthermore, L-ascorbic acid esters appear to facilitate hepatic glutathione (GSH) regeneration after coadministration of a hepatotoxic dose of acetaminophen.[49,50]

Research

Acetaminophen remains one of the most common toxic exposures and causes significant morbidity and mortality. Acetaminophen-induced acute hepatic failure, usually by intentional overdose but sometimes inadvertent, represents a major risk in conventional medical practice.[51-53]

In a clinical experiment involving five healthy adult volunteers, Houston and Levy[48] administered an oral dose of ascorbic acid (3 g) 1.5 hours after an oral dose of 1 g acetaminophen. They observed a "rapid and pronounced decrease in the excretion rate of acetaminophen sulfate" with a "significant increase in the fractions of the dose of acetaminophen excreted as acetaminophen glucuronide" and a "decrease in the fraction excreted as acetaminophen sulfate." Thus, competitive inhibition of acetaminophen's conjugation with sulfate by the ascorbic acid produced an increase in the "apparent biological half-life of acetaminophen from 2.3 ± 0.2 (mean $\pm$ SD) to 3.1 ± 0.5 hr." Notably, concomitant administration of sodium sulfate prevented these effects; thus confirming the pivotal role of sulfate conjugation.

Mitra et al.[49] conducted two investigations exploring the effect of ascorbic acid esters on acetaminophen-induced hepatotoxicity in mice. In the first, they administered a hepatotoxic dose of acetaminophen alone and with ascorbyl stearate or ascorbyl palmitate at 600 mg/kg for each substance and observed that coadministration of the ascorbate esters with acetaminophen "prevented an increase in liver weight/body weight ratios and hepatic glutathione depletion... by reducing the reactive intermediate back to the parent compound." Further, the combined acetaminophen–ascorbyl stearate treatment demonstrated enhanced antipyretic effect, compared to acetaminophen alone or with ascorbyl palmitate, as evidenced in significantly greater reductions in rectal temperature at 15- to 30-minute postdosing periods. Subsequently, Mitra et al.[50] examined the effects of acetaminophen alone and with each of the same ascorbic acid esters on the activities of serum transaminases (glutamic-pyruvate transaminase [SGPT, ALT], glutamic-oxaloacetic transaminase [SGOT, AST]) and SICD. They observed significant reductions in serum transaminase and SICD activities in the animals treated with either acetaminophen–ascorbate ester combination, compared with acetaminophen-positive controls. Although oral coadministration of acetaminophen with ascorbate ester did not prevent the initial hepatic GSH depletion (15 minutes to 4 hours after dosing), they reported that hepatic GSH content began to rise in the animals treated with either acetaminophen–ascorbate ester combination at 4 hours and reached control values within 12 hours after dosing. Further, urinary mercapturate conjugates measured over a 60-minute postdosing period were significantly lower and plasma sulfobromophthalein (BSP) retention was approximately eight times higher in the animals treated with acetaminophen alone versus either acetaminophen–ascorbate ester combination. These findings indicate "maintenance of hepatic excretory functions" in the presence of ascorbyl stearate or ascorbyl palmitate and the "possible role of L-ascorbic acid esters in GSH regeneration."[50] Although limited in their extrapolation to humans, these studies using a rodent model provide potential value in understanding the mechanisms of vitamin C in mitigating the adverse effects of acetaminophen in hepatoxicity.

Emerging research indicates that "profuse and dysregulated production of cytokines, growth factors, and/or other endogenous substances during viral/bacterial infections and inflammation states play a role in the development of drug-induced liver injury," particularly in relation to "administration of drugs or hepatotoxicity associated with administration of therapeutic doses of acetaminophen in some genetically predisposed subjects."[54] The relevance of therapeutic administration of vitamin C and nutrients with similar activity within a comprehensive and individualized strategic approach to inflammation and infection (and avoidance of hepatotoxicity) deserves further investigation.

Nutritional Therapeutics, Clinical Concerns, and Adaptations

The collective findings from these initial studies indicate a complex, and as-yet incompletely understood, relationship between acetaminophen and vitamin C. The potential for elevated circulating levels of acetaminophen in the presence of vitamin C suggests the opportunity for equivalent therapeutic effects with a lowered drug dose. Given the well-established toxicity of acetaminophen, such a potentially beneficial interaction deserves further exploration through well-designed, adequately powered clinical trials. However, this potential value is complicated by the significant likelihood of patients self-administering both agents during acute infections and is therefore worthy of frank inquiry and educational overtures. Although such effects are unlikely to constitute a major risk with short-term acetaminophen use for pain or fever in most individuals, acute acetaminophen toxicity in previously healthy individuals has been documented. Moreover, such risks are significantly greater in individuals with compromised hepatic or renal function, and any use of acetaminophen is contraindicated, with or apart from vitamin C, in such individuals except under the supervision of a medical professional.

Acetylsalicylic Acid (Aspirin) and Salsalate

Acetylsalicylic acid (acetosal, acetyl salicylic acid, ASA, salicylsalicylic acid; Arthritis Foundation Pain Reliever, Ascriptin, Aspergum, Asprimox, Bayer Aspirin, Bayer Buffered Aspirin, Bayer Low Adult Strength, Bufferin, Buffex, Cama Arthritis Pain Reliever, Easprin, Ecotrin, Ecotrin Low Adult Strength, Empirin, Extra Strength Adprin-B, Extra Strength Bayer Enteric 500 Aspirin, Extra Strength Bayer Plus, Halfprin 81, Heartline, Regular Strength Bayer Enteric 500 Aspirin, St. Joseph Adult Chewable Aspirin, ZORprin); combination drugs: ASA and caffeine (Anacin); ASA, caffeine, and propoxyphene (Darvon Compound); ASA and carisoprodol (Soma Compound); ASA, codeine, and carisoprodol (Soma Compound with Codeine); ASA and codeine (Empirin with Codeine), ASA, codeine, butalbital, and caffeine (Fiorinal); ASA and extended-release dipyridamole (Aggrenox, Asasantin).

Salsalate (salicylic acid; Amigesic, Disalcid, Marthritic, Mono Gesic, Salflex, Salsitab).

See also Indomethacin and Related Nonsteroidal Anti-Inflammatory Drugs (NSAIDs) in Theoretical, Speculative, and Preliminary Interactions Research.

Interaction Type and Significance

☼　**Prevention or Reduction of Drug Adverse Effect**

≈≈≈　**Drug-Induced Nutrient Depletion, Supplementation Therapeutic, Not Requiring Professional Management**

⊕✗　**Bimodal or Variable Interaction, with Professional Management**

✗　**Potential or Theoretical Adverse Interaction of Uncertain Severity**

Nutrient Depletion
Probability:
3. **Possible** or
2. **Probable**

Evidence Base:
○ Preliminary
◉ Emerging

Coadministration Benefit
Probability:
3. **Possible** or
2. **Probable**

Evidence Base:
● Consensus

Coadministration Risk
Probability:
4. **Plausible** or
3. **Possible**

Evidence Base:
▽ Mixed
○ Preliminary

Effect and Mechanism of Action

Vitamin C has been shown to reduce gastric mucosal damage and gastric toxicity induced by ASA-generated reactive oxygen metabolites.[55,56] After ingestion, both aspirin and salsalate are rapidly converted to salicylic acid. Aspirin and salicylic acid can increase urinary excretion of vitamin C, lower leukocyte ascorbic acid levels (by 50%), and decrease its metabolic availability.[57-60]

The gastric mucosa is the largest depot of ascorbic acid in the human body, with ascorbic acid concentrations 25 times higher than in plasma.[61] Some data suggest that aspirin may protect endothelial cells from oxidant damage via the nitric oxide (NO)–cyclic guanosine monophosphate (cGMP) pathway.[62,63] However, gastric epithelial cells require vitamin C to translate inducible heme oxygenase (HO-1) mRNA "into active protein, which then may exert gastroprotection by its antioxidant and vasodilative properties.... Induction of HO-1 is considered to be an adaptive cellular mechanism in response to oxidative stress."[64] Thus, a significant body of data shows that the oxidative damage caused by aspirin can induce exfoliation of gastric epithelial cells, formation of gastric erosions, and GI hemorrhage. In particular, the gastric mucosa of individuals deficient in vitamin C (and possibly other, synergistic nutrients) might be less able to increase the rate of cell production and therefore susceptible to increased bleeding after aspirin ingestion.

Vitamins A, E, and C and bioflavonoids may enhance the "antiaggregative effect of aspirin, prolongate its activity, [and] increase hypocoaguloemia due to reduced releasing of thrombocytic factors 3 and 4 into plasma."[65]

Research

Russell, Goldberg, et al.[57,66] published two related studies in *The Lancet* in 1968 that examined the relationships between leukocyte ascorbic acid levels (L.A.A.) and GI hemorrhage in humans and aspirin and gastric mucosa in vitamin C–depleted guinea pigs. On measuring leukocyte–ascorbic acid levels in 60 patients with GI hemorrhage, they found that the mean value of 14.2 μg/10^8 white blood cells (WBCs) was "significantly lower than that found in a matched peptic ulcer control group (17.6) and in a healthy control group (23.7)." They determined that ascorbic acid levels were "significantly lower in patients in whom aspirin or alcohol might have precipitated bleeding than in those in whom no precipitating factor was present," and that "the association of low L.A.A. levels with aspirin or alcohol ingestion was present whatever the causation of haemorrhage." they concluded: "Subclinical scurvy may be an additional factor in maintaining haemorrhage initially precipitated by aspirin or alcohol, and poor dietary intake of vitamin C seems the most probable explanation for the low L.A.A. levels observed." This susceptibility to bleeding from acute gastric lesions (erosions) appears greater in elderly individuals.[57] In the animal experiment they observed:

> "Guineapigs on the scorbutogenic diet bled from the gastric mucosa significantly more often than those on a normal diet. The addition of aspirin to a scorbutogenic diet significantly increased the likelihood of gastric mucosal bleeding." These findings led them to conclude that aspirin "thus seems to precipitate gastric mucosal haemorrhage more readily when guineapigs are in a subclinical scorbutic condition." Thus, based on both studies they interpreted their results to "suggest that aspirin is more likely to cause significant gastric mucosal haemorrhage when subclinical scurvy is present."[66] In a subsequent letter, Croft[67] reviewed several studies regarding the impact of malnourishment on compromised gastric mucosa and aspirin-induced loss of epithelial cells and proposed that an "explanation of their findings could be that a low turnover of gastric epithelial cells renders the mucosa particularly susceptible to aspirin."

Sahud and Cohen[68] compared platelet and plasma levels of ascorbic acid and the effect of aspirin ingestion in 48 healthy individuals and 34 patients with rheumatoid arthritis. They observed that plasma ascorbic acid levels were "abnormally low in all rheumatoid subjects except those taking supplemental vitamin C." Moreover, looking at platelet levels of ascorbic acid, which more accurately reflect tissue stores than plasma levels, they found "significantly low platelet levels of ascorbic acid... only in those rheumatoid patients receiving high doses of aspirin—i.e., 12 or more tablets per day." Based on these findings, they concluded that "a high dosage of aspirin in patients with rheumatoid arthritis is associated with tissue ascorbic acid depletion" and recommended that "administration of supplemental ascorbic acid to rheumatoid patients receiving a high dosage of aspirin as primary therapy seems warranted."[68]

Loh et al.[58] examined the effect of aspirin on uptake of ascorbic acid into leukocytes in both in vitro and human studies. First, they compared the uptake of ascorbic acid into leukocytes incubated in a buffered medium of ascorbic acid with that in a medium also containing aspirin and observed that the aspirin completely inhibited absorption of the ascorbic acid. In normal adults, they observed a significant increase in plasma and leukocyte ascorbic acid during the 2 hours after administration of 500 mg ascorbic acid but found that simultaneous administration of 600 mg aspirin "further increased plasma ascorbic acid concentrations but completely arrested uptake of ascorbic acid into the leukocytes." Likewise, administration of ascorbic acid every 6 hours increased urinary excretion of ascorbic acid and produced a concomitant increase in leukocyte ascorbic acid. In contrast, the "simultaneous administration of aspirin with the ascorbic acid resulted in a further significant increase in excretion of ascorbic acid and a simultaneous fall in leukocyte ascorbic acid." Further, administration of aspirin every 6 hours for 7 days "resulted in diminished plasma and leukocyte ascorbic acid concentrations within four days. Thereafter, reduced ascorbic acid levels just in excess of those associated with production of scorbutic symptoms were maintained." The authors concluded that "supplementary ascorbic acid should be administered to individuals receiving aspirin therapy."[58]

Not all researchers have demonstrated this adverse effect of aspirin on vitamin C levels; at least not in healthy populations. Johansson and Akesson[69] conducted a clinical trial in which healthy adults were given four different diets for 1 week: "low ascorbic acid diet, low ascorbic acid diet plus acetylsalicylic acid" (3 g/day), "high ascorbic acid diet" (1 g/day), and high ascorbic acid diet plus acetylsalicylic acid. They observed that "at low ascorbic acid intake, acetylsalicylic acid increased urinary ascorbic acid, but at high ascorbic acid intake, acetylsalicylic acid instead decreased urinary ascorbic acid." They hypothesized that the latter effect resulted from inhibited intestinal absorption of ascorbic acid, and the former effect from "decreased protein binding and tissue uptake of ascorbic acid caused by acetylsalicylic acid." Overall, they reported that in "no instance" did the acetylsalicylic acid affect plasma ascorbic acid levels.

In a double-blind, randomized, crossover study involving 14 healthy volunteers, McAlindon et al.[56] administered aspirin 900 mg twice daily and either placebo, vitamin C 1 g twice daily, allopurinol 100 mg twice daily, or sulphasalazine 1 g twice daily for 3 days. They demonstrated that aspirin induced gastric injury, as assessed endoscopically and by quantifying mucosal reactive oxygen metabolite release by measuring chemiluminescence, but reported that no drug reduced any parameter of gastric injury. However, they found that vitamin C reduced duodenal injury, as assessed by Lanza score.

In two studies involving healthy subjects, Dammann et al.[70] and Schulz et al.[61] investigated the effects of the interaction between aspirin and ascorbic acid on gastric mucosa and plasma ascorbic acid concentrations. In the first, a randomized, four-fold crossover study, they performed serial esophago-gastro-duodenoscopy on 17 healthy subjects before and after each course of 4-day dosing and collected gastric aspirates to detect microbleeding. They observed that subjects administered the combination of buffered acetylsalicylic acid and ascorbic acid "yielded the lowest Lanza score, the lowest increase in the number of mucosal petechiae and the lowest increase in the amount of gastric microbleeding." In contrast, those subjects receiving "acetylsalicylic acid plus paracetamol plus caffeine showed the highest Lanza score of all treatments, and a considerably greater sum of petechiae in the oesophagus, stomach and duodenum compared with those receiving buffered acetylsalicylic acid plus ascorbic acid." The authors concluded that this "trial confirms that buffering of acetylsalicylic acid improves local gastric tolerability."[70] In a related prospective, randomized, double-blind, parallel-group study involving three groups of 15 subjects each, these researchers compared concentrations of ascorbic acid in "gastric mucosa, gastric juice, urine and plasma in healthy subjects under steady state and fasted conditions" after 6 days of ascorbic acid (0.48 g/day) with and without concomitant administration of acetylsalicylic acid (0.8 g/day). Treatments were switched without any washout, resulting in a 14-day study period overall. Initially, they found that ascorbic acid concentrations were highest in the gastric mucosa, followed by gastric juice, plasma, and urine. Subsequently, on day 7, ascorbic acid concentrations in gastric

mucosa, plasma, and urine had increased to a statistically significant degree in those groups receiving ascorbic acid and decreased significantly in the group receiving aspirin only. During this period, differences in ascorbic acid concentrations in gastric juice, between the treatment groups, were not statistically significant. Thus, in healthy subjects, "clinically relevant doses" of aspirin reduced ascorbic acid concentrations in gastric mucosa "by about 10% within six days resulting from antioxidative defense mechanisms." The authors concluded by recommending, as beneficial, a "protective adjunct administration" of vitamin C, particularly in "patients with long-term ASA treatment or conditions with additional risks such as elderly subjects with unfavorable dietary conditions and impaired antioxidative protection."[61]

Animal experiments by Byshchevskil et al.[65] indicate that concomitant administration of aspirin with antioxidants, specifically, vitamins A, E, and C and bioflavonoids, "in balanced diet in doses adequate to therapeutic ones" may potentiate aspirin's antiaggregative effect. They recommended more research and suggested that "administration of [the] vitamin combination studied is likely to diminish thrombocyte aggregative activity to a level needed using lower aspirin doses." More recently, Fiebich et al.[71] reported "synergistic inhibitory effect of ascorbic acid and acetylsalicylic acid on prostaglandin E_2 release in primary rat microglia."

The effects of vitamin C on renal clearance of aspirin suggest another potential interaction from coadministration, although bimodal in its clinical implications. In a review on drug-nutrient interactions among elderly patients, Schumann[72] noted that "high doses of vitamin C" can further reduce renal clearance of acetylsalicylic acid and other acidic drugs among elderly patients, in whom renal clearance is often impaired. As suggested by the author, and concurrent with the findings of several studies previously discussed, this possible pattern of interaction indicates an influence of vitamin C on the risk of toxicity inherent to aspirin that is neither inherently adverse nor beneficial. Professional supervision and reasonable monitoring are warranted, with titration of aspirin dose being an advantageous possibility. Such situations can represent risks or opportunities, depending on the characteristics of the patient and the rationale for aspirin administration, and reiterate the preeminent need for inquiry about patient use of supplemental nutrients and comprehensive and coordinated clinical management of the intake of drugs and nutrients among geriatric patients, which is numerous and complex in most cases.

Nutritional Therapeutics, Clinical Concerns, and Adaptations

Aspirin and vitamin C may be the most frequently self-prescribed medicinal substances in modern culture, and as a result, many individuals forget that adverse effects are a possibility with any agent. Health care professionals treating patients regularly taking aspirin are advised to educate them regarding the inherent risks of aspirin intake, particularly damage to the GI mucosa and microhemorrhage. In this context, it may also be prudent to suggest the potential protective value of supplementing with 200 to 500 mg vitamin C per day, as typically found in multivitamins. Although not conclusive, the body of available evidence indicates that vitamin C may moderate several of the adverse effects associated with aspirin intake and may provide some synergistic influence. Further, the populations more likely to use aspirin regularly are also more likely to be elderly, to have aspirin-induced gastric mucosal damage and bleeding, and to be on a nutrient-compromised diet, all of which increase the adverse effects of aspirin on vitamin C status and general health. Professional supervision and periodic monitoring are warranted in such patients, as well as in those with compromised renal function, to avoid adverse effects of aspirin and any potential added risk that might theoretically derive from coadministration of vitamin C. Although not yet the direct subject of scientific research, the known supportive influence of vitamin C on absorption of nonheme iron might be of benefit in countering the tendency to anemia in those using aspirin on a regular basis. Lastly, chronic use of aspirin, other than as cardiovascular prophylaxis, suggests the need for a more fundamental therapeutic strategy aimed at analyzing and resolving the causes of pain and inflammation.

Antihypertensive Medications (Generally)

See also Propanolol and Related Beta-1-Adrenoceptor Antagonists (Beta-Adrenergic Blocking Agents).

Interaction Type and Significance
⊕⊕ **Beneficial or Supportive Interaction, with Professional Management**

Probability:
3. Possible

Evidence Base:
○ **Preliminary**

Effect and Mechanism of Action
The antioxidant activity of vitamin C may play a protective role against the increased production of reactive oxygen species associated with essential hypertension.[73] High-dose intra-arterial ascorbic acid levels may ameliorate endothelial dysfunction in individuals with hypertension.[74]

Research
In a small, randomized, double-blind, placebo-controlled trial, Duffy et al.[75] investigated the effect of ascorbic acid treatment on blood pressure in 45 patients with hypertension who continued conventional antihypertensive medications. Systolic, diastolic, and mean blood pressures in the treatment and placebo groups were similar at baseline and after acute treatment. They observed that 1 month of ascorbic acid treatment (500 mg/day) significantly decreased systolic blood pressure, in contrast to placebo, which had no effect. Likewise, after 1 month, ascorbic acid decreased mean blood pressure from 110 (12) to 100 (8) mm Hg, an effect significantly different from placebo. However, whereas 1 month of ascorbic acid decreased diastolic blood pressure, this response was not significant compared with placebo. Based on these findings, the researchers concluded that "the present study suggests that 500 mg of ascorbic acid daily is useful for blood pressure control in patients with hypertension" and suggested continued research with larger and longer clinical trials. They also noted: "Epidemiological studies show that dietary intake of ascorbic acid correlate inversely with hypertension and its clinical sequelae."[75]

Another study on the progression of hypertension produced potentially important findings related to vitamin C usage, but not directly related to an interaction between vitamin C and conventional antihypertensive drugs. Kim et al.[76] conducted a double-blind, randomized, controlled trial comparing the effects of 50 or 500 mg daily for 5 years on blood pressure in 224 Japanese subjects in a region with high gastric cancer and stroke mortality levels. Before supplementation, neither systolic nor diastolic blood pressure was significantly related with the serum vitamin C concentration. They found that vitamin C administration failed to produce any significant decrease in systolic or diastolic blood pressure. After 5 years, systolic blood pressure significantly increased in groups, regardless of vitamin C dose, compared with baseline, with the increase in low-dose and moderate-dose groups quite similar. Notably, study subjects were slightly less likely to smoke than the general population, but had all been serologically diagnosed with atrophic gastritis.

Nutritional Therapeutics, Clinical Concerns, and Adaptations
Further research into the potential interaction between antihypertensive medications and vitamin C is warranted. Pending substantive findings, physicians might find it prudent to prescribe vitamin C, at a modest dose level, to patients undergoing treatment for hypertension. Proper monitoring at home and during periodic examinations is appropriate, but no substantive research data indicate a significant risk for such individuals with vitamin C administration over an extended period. The importance of a diet emphasizing vegetables and fruits (i.e., rich in nutrients such as vitamin C) is fundamental and should be vigorously conveyed to patients.[77]

Chemotherapy and Radiotherapy

Including cisplatin (*cis*-diaminedichloroplatinum, CDDP; Platinol, Platinol-AQ), cyclophosphamide (Cytoxan, Endoxana, Neosar, Procytox), docetaxel (Taxotere), doxorubicin (Adriamycin, Rubex), etoposide (Eposin, Etophos, VePesid, VP-16), fluorouracil (5-FU; Adrucil, Efudex, Efudix, Fluoroplex), gemcitabine (Gemzar), rinotecan (camptothecin-11, CPT-11; Campto, Camptosar), methotrexate (Folex, Maxtrex, Rheumatrex), paclitaxel (Paxene, Taxol).
See also specific agents: Fluorouracil and Methotrexate.

Interaction Type and Significance
✗✗✗ **Potentially Harmful or Serious Adverse Interaction—Avoid**
⊕✗ **Bimodal or Variable Interaction, with Professional Management**
✗✗ **Beneficial or Supportive Interaction, with Professional Management**
☼ **Prevention or Reduction of Drug Adverse Effect**
≈≈ **Drug-Induced Nutrient Depletion, Supplementation Therapeutic, with Professional Management**

Probability:
4. Plausible and/or
2. Probable

Evidence Base:
▽ **Mixed** or
○ **Preliminary**

Effect and Mechanism of Action
Oxygen radicals can act as highly toxic stressors contributing to oncogenesis and other pathological processes. Higher intake of vitamin C and related nutrients through dietary sources is generally associated with reduced risk for many forms of cancer. In particular, vitamin C is known for direct activity as a free-radical scavenger, its central role in supporting intracellular glutathione (GSH) stores, and its synergistic relationship with other antioxidant nutrients and *N*-acetylcysteine (NAC).[78] Emerging research indicates that pharmacological ascorbic acid concentrations, as attainable through IV administration, selectively kill cancer cells in vitro and act as a prodrug to deliver hydrogen peroxide to tissues.[14]

In most cases the interaction between vitamin C and antineoplastic agents may be characterized most accurately as bimodal in nature. Chemotherapeutic agents and vitamin C and other antioxidants, dietary or administered, may interact in a synergistic manner to reduce drug toxicity and enhance therapeutic efficacy. Conversely, many antineoplastic agents, as well as radiotherapy, rely on a mechanism of action employing focused exposure to intensified levels of free radicals, which may contribute to destruction of tumor cells, although many mechanisms are believed to be involved. The simultaneous administration of vitamin C with chemotherapeutic agents or radiotherapy could theoretically diminish the therapeutic action of these interventions, to the degree that free-radical generation is central to the tumoricidal mechanism, and to the degree that ascorbic acid can quench the free radicals generated. Dietary sources of vitamin C and associated antioxidant nutrients are theoretically capable of exerting a similar activity. Such a judgment, however, assumes that the vitamin C or other nutrient is acting in its antioxidant mode and has not shifted to a pro-oxidant effect, and that such influence is inherently problematic. Moreover, nutrient form, dose, and mode of administration and clinical management, particularly timing and coordination of interventions (concurrent or alternating), can be decisive factors influencing effects and outcomes.

In two review papers, Prasad et al.[7] and Simone et al.[79] summarized the mechanisms that contribute to the effects of vitamin C and other antioxidants in the treatment of neoplastic diseases. First, "individual antioxidants such as vitamin A (retinoids), vitamin E (primarily alpha-tocopheryl succinate), vitamin C (primarily sodium ascorbate) and carotenoids (primarily polar carotenoids) induce cell differentiation and growth inhibition to various degrees in rodent and human cancer cells by complex mechanisms."[7] The proposed mechanisms for these effects in limiting carcinogenic processes include blocking destruction imposed by free radicals (thus protecting healthy tissue from damage), inhibiting protein kinase C activity (thus restraining tumor cell division and proliferation), inducing transforming growth factor-beta (TGF-β) and p21 genes, and inhibiting oncogene expression, prostaglandin E_1–stimulated adenylate cyclase activity, expression of c-myc, H-ras, and E2F, a transcription factor.[7,79] "Furthermore, antioxidant vitamins individually or in combination enhance the growth-inhibitory effects of x-irradiation, chemotherapeutic agents, hyperthermia, and biological response modifiers on tumor cells, primarily *in vitro*. These vitamins, individually, also reduce the toxicity of several standard tumor therapeutic agents on normal cells."[7] Notably, these papers and most research by experts in the field emphasize administration of multiple antioxidant nutrients concomitantly.

In reference to cisplatin, Weijl et al.[80] also proposed that "cisplatin-combination chemotherapy induces a fall in plasma antioxidant levels that may reflect a failure of the antioxidant defense mechanism against oxidative damage induced by commonly used anticancer drugs."

Vitamin C may aggravate cardiac toxicity of doxorubicin and related anthracyclines by mobilizing iron from storage sites and thus increasing levels of iron-catalyzed free radicals. Such adverse effects are less probable with liposome-encapsulated anthracyclines, which appear to have significantly less cardiac toxicity.

Research

The complex issue of concurrent administration of vitamin C and other antioxidants, whether as nutrients, herbs, or foods, during conventional therapy with antineoplastic agents in their various forms, as both monotherapy and polytherapy, has been the subject of protracted controversy and heated debate but minimal specific and substantive clinical research. Numerous surveys have found that the use of natural medicine and

alternative therapies tends to be more widespread among individuals with cancer than in any other patient population, and that such use is more often self-prescribed or "nonintegrative," that is, lacking in coordination among the health care professionals and their respective therapeutic models.[81-90] Nevertheless, despite decades of attentions and a broad range of papers, offering mostly extrapolation, belief, opinion, and polemic, there have still been essentially no well-designed randomized trials of antioxidants versus placebo during the same chemotherapy or radiotherapy of adequate power to elucidate the fundamental clinical questions at hand or confirm any pattern of interaction that might be applied in a clinically consistent manner. Further, generalizations and extrapolations have especially limited value given the wide range of cancers among patients receiving oncological care and the diverse combinations of cancer drugs and radiotherapy employed in such interventions. Moreover, and perhaps most significantly in terms of developing a definitive research-based body of scientific evidence, any meaningful clinical trial would require that the diet of subjects be controlled for its antioxidant content. Adequately accounting for such confounding factors renders development of substantive clinical evidence extremely complicated, difficult, and expensive. The pervasive issue of patient disclosure of concurrent treatments and the need to cultivate a trusting therapeutic relationship further convolute professional collaboration, clinical decisions, and outcomes assessment. The following discussion of the key permutations of themes underlying possible and proven interactions between vitamin C and various forms of conventional chemotherapy (and radiotherapy) provides a clinical review of the available evidence, although some agents are discussed separately in other sections of this monograph.

Definitive research findings from large-scale, well-controlled, randomized clinical trials are lacking to demonstrate the long-term effects of combining chemotherapeutic agents and vitamin C or other oral antioxidants. The scattered evidence from in vitro and animal experiments and clinical reports of varying degrees of quality suggests, as concluded in a much-cited 1999 paper by Labriola and Livingston,[91] that "there is sufficient understanding of the mechanisms of action of both chemotherapeutic agents and antioxidants to predict the obvious interactions and to suggest where caution should be exercised with respect to both clinical decisions and study interpretation." However, in reviewing the data, it appears that the highly variable quality of available evidence and the wide range of agents involved render any consistent characterization and broad conclusions impossible, or at least premature. Instead, an overview and synthesis of the scientific evidence and clinical insight of professionals experienced in applying nutritional therapies in oncological care suggest that safe and effective therapeutic models are possible in certain cases and that flexible protocols are emerging, but that risks from mismanagement are real and continued research is critical.[7,7a,79,92-105] In such a comprehensive approach, each intervention constitutes a viable tactic in a comprehensive strategy employing integrative principles to craft individualized and evolving interventions based on the condition(s) being treated, agents being administered, and the characteristics and needs of the particular patient. This approach requires ongoing research and a posture of open-minded discovery, critical analysis, and flexible response in which all elements, whether conventional or nonconventional, chemotherapy or nutrient, are subject to rigorous standards of scientific evidence and equally vigorous clinical assessments of safety, tolerance, and outcomes.

Chemotherapy of many types (and all radiotherapy) leads to an increase in levels of reactive oxygen species, which stress the antioxidant defense system. Oxygen radicals are highly toxic, produce a variety of pathological changes through lipid peroxidation and DNA damage, and have been implicated in various disease processes, including carcinogenesis and aging.[106] For example, the cardiotoxicity of doxorubicin can be of rapid onset and endure for decades, often without cardiac complaints. In a longitudinal assessment of cardiac function in 22 patients treated with anthracycline for osteogenic sarcoma or malignant fibrous histiocytoma, Brouwer et al.[107] found systolic dysfunction in more than a quarter of the patients and diastolic dysfunction in almost half after two decades (22 years median). Moreover, cardiac dysfunction was progressive as measured at 9, 14, and 22 years.[107]

Many forms of chemotherapy release free radicals as a means of inducing irreversible tissue injury, and thereby reduce circulating levels of antioxidants. Weijl et al.[80] demonstrated that cisplatin combination chemotherapy induces a fall in plasma antioxidants of oncology patients with vitamin C, vitamin E, uric acid, and ceruloplasmin levels falling significantly; these levels returned to baseline levels before the start of the next chemotherapy cycle. Thus, although oxidative stress represents a significant causal or contributing factor in the development of tumors, its focused use in the form of chemotherapy and radiotherapy also provides a powerful tool in attacking cancer cells. These effects constitute one of the primary causes of adverse effects and toxicity associated with conventional antineoplastic therapy.

A variety of in vitro experiments, animal studies, and human trials have found that coadministration of vitamin C, usually in combination with other antioxidant nutrients, may enhance the therapeutic activity of chemotherapy in certain types of cancer and may reduce the adverse effects associated with such interventions.[7a,96,108-119] Ray et al.[120] observed that ascorbic acid could suppress cyclophosphamide-induced lipid peroxidation in vitro to a significant extent, as indicated by tissue levels of malondialdehyde, 4-hydroxy-2-nonenal, reduced glutathione, and nitric oxide. In animal experiments using mice and guinea pigs, Umezawa, Fujita, and associates found that vitamin C was associated with reduced severity of doxorubicin-induced cardiotoxicity and significantly increased life expectancy of mice and guinea pigs without interfering with the drug's antineoplastic activity.[121,122] Likewise, in an experiment using fibrosarcoma-bearing rats, Muralikrishnan et al.[123] found that coadministration of vitamin C mitigated lipid abnormalities typically associated with combined application of cyclophosphamide, methotrexate, and 5-fluorouracil (CMF), as applied in the treatment of breast cancer.[123]

In a prospective, placebo-controlled, randomized, double-blind pilot study involving 13 patients receiving "high-dose" chemotherapy and 12 patients receiving radiotherapy, Wagdi et al.[124] found that an antioxidant combination consisting of vitamin C, vitamin E, and N-acetylcysteine (NAC) protected against heart damage induced by chemotherapy without reducing the drug's effectiveness. For example, 46% patients in the placebo-chemotherapy group and 66% in the radiotherapy-placebo group showed a reduction in left ventricular ejection fraction (LVEF) of 10% or greater; in contrast, no patient in either antioxidant group group, plus chemotherapy or plus radiation, showed a fall greater than 10%, and most demonstrated significantly smaller change, if any. While cautioning that the "small number of patients in the study precludes a definitive statement," the authors concluded that these preliminary results "suggest efficient cardioprotection by this nontoxic and inexpensive antioxidant combination, so larger studies are warranted for confirmation."

Babu et al.[125] reported a "salubrious effect of vitamin C and vitamin E" on tamoxifen-induced hypertriglyceridemia in postmenopausal women with breast cancer. They coadministered vitamin C (500 mg) and vitamin E (400 mg) for 90 days along with tamoxifen (10 mg twice daily). Among the "tamoxifen-treated patients, total cholesterol (TC), free cholesterol (FC), phospholipids (PL), free fatty acids (FFA), low density lipoprotein cholesterol (LDL) levels were decreased and the triglycerides (TG), ester cholesterol (EC), high density lipoprotein cholesterol (HDL) and very low density lipoprotein cholesterol (VLDL) levels were increased." However, subjects treated with combination therapy exhibited a reduction in total cholesterol levels, VLDL, and LDL, whereas "TG levels were significantly decreased and HDL, EC levels were significantly increased."[125]

Pediatric oncologists Kennedy et al.[126] performed a 6-month observational study of 103 children with acute lymphoblastic leukemia in which they demonstrated that low dietary antioxidant vitamin intakes are associated with increases in adverse effects of chemotherapy. Among their findings was the observation that greater vitamin C intakes at 6 months were "associated with fewer therapy delays, less toxicity, and fewer days spent in the hospital."

In a phase II study involving the combination of "antioxidants, both in the diet and supplemented, pharmaco-nutritional support, progestagen, and anti-cyclooxygenase-2," Mantovani et al.[127] demonstrated "efficacy and safety" in 44 patients with "cancer-related anorexia/cachexia and oxidative stress." They evaluated data on four variables (clinical, nutritional, laboratory, quality of life) in 39 "advanced" cancer patients, with "cancer-related anorexia/cachexia and oxidative stress," who completed 4 months of an integrative treatment regimen consisting of "diet with high polyphenols content (400 mg), antioxidant treatment (300 mg/d alpha-lipoic acid + 2.7 g/d carbocysteine lysine salt + 400 mg/d vitamin E + 30,000 IU/d vitamin A + 500 mg/d vitamin C), and pharmaconutritional support enriched with 2 cans per day (n-3)-PUFA (eicosapentaenoic acid and docosahexaenoic acid), 500 mg/d medroxyprogesterone acetate, and 200 mg/d selective cyclooxygenase-2 inhibitor celecoxib." They reported significant increases from baseline of body weight, lean body mass (LBM), and appetite; "important decrease of proinflammatory cytokines interleukin-6 (IL-6) and tumor necrosis factor-alpha, and a negative relationship worthy of note was only found between LBM and IL-6 changes"; and "a marked improvement" in quality of life, as assessed using several standard scoring systems. Of the 39 patients, 22 were determined to be "responders" or "high responders" at the end of the study. The authors concluded that "the treatment was effective and more importantly was shown to be safe," and that "therefore, a randomized phase III study is warranted."[127]

As to the general issue of coadministering antioxidant agents during chemotherapy, it is noteworthy that several pharmacological agents are used within conventional care specifically for the protective effects of their antioxidant activity. Mesna (Mitexan, sodium 2-mercaptoethane-sulfonate) protects the urinary tract from the urotoxic effects of oxazaphosphorine cytostatics (ifosfamide, cyclophosphamide, sufosfamide, and trofosfamide) by forming a nontoxic additive compound with acrolein, a chemotherapy metabolite, which is spontaneously formed in the urine from the primary metabolites eliminated through the kidneys.[128,129] Dexrazoxane (Zinecard), a cyclic derivative of EDTA, has been prescribed as a cardioprotective agent based on its role in modulating free-radical production by chelating free iron in doxorubicin-induced cardiomyopathy; coadministration permits significantly greater doses of doxorubicin to be administered to patients with greater tolerance and safety.[130-140] Amifostine (Ethyol) is a phosphorylated prodrug with antioxidant effects analogous to those of glutathione. It is selectively dephosphorylated by normal cells, which express much higher levels of the cleaving phosphatase enzyme than do malignant cells. Dephosphorlyation allows the drug to move intracellularly, thus selectively protecting normal cells from chemotherapy and radiation. Amifostine was initially approved to protect against renal injury by cisplatin in ovarian cancer patients, and approval was then extended to decrease the loss of salivary function from radiotherapy in head and neck cancer, although some oncologists use it in a broader context for chemoprotection and radioprotection.[141-146]

Birdsall et al.[147] and Cancer Treatment Centers of America conducted an exploratory trial to investigate effect of concomitant naturopathic therapies on clinical tumor response to external-beam radiation therapy for early-stage prostate cancer (tumor stages 1b through 2, N0M0). External-beam radiation therapy of up to 72 Gy was given to 22 patients on a conventional 8-week treatment regimen; the 13 patients in the naturopathic group received at least one antioxidant supplement, with antioxidant naturopathic treatments most frequently including green tea extract, melatonin, and a high-potency multivitamin, vitamin C, or vitamin E. "All patients were monitored for at least 12 months (range 12-42) and no patient received concomitant hormonal therapy." The investigators reported that in the patients "who did not receive naturopathic [antioxidant] treatments, the median pretreatment PSA level was 5.4 ng/mL, the median PSA nadir was 0.66 ng/mL, and the median time to PSA nadir was 16.0 months," whereas in the "patients who did receive naturopathic treatments, the corresponding values were 5.8 ng/mL; 0.59 ng/mL; and 16.0 months" (PSA, prostate-specific antigen). One tumor treatment failure occurred in the nonnaturopathic group "based on PSA elevation > 2 ng from nadir which occurred at 14 months"; there were no treatment failures in the patients who received concomitant naturopathic regimens. The authors noted as "also significant that 9/9 patients in the non-CAM group were considered to be low risk (based on pretreatment PSA levels of 4-10 ng) whereas 3 patients in the CAM group were classified as intermediate risk (PSA >10-20 ng) and 1 patient as high risk (PSA > 20 ng)" (CAM, complementary and alternative medicine). Thus, the authors concluded that "concomitant naturopathic treatment does not appear to inhibit the capacity of external beam radiation therapy to control localized prostate cancer, and does not interfere with either the magnitude of the response, the velocity of the response, or its durability for at least 1 year." They added that these "results provide definitive evidence that antioxidant-based CAM modalities, designed to improve patient tolerance, quality of life, and possibly improve survival, do not inhibit tumor responses that depend on oxidative [tumor] killing mechanisms elicited by external beam radiation therapy."[147] Although encouraging, this small, retrospective study did not have sufficient power to draw any statistically significant conclusions. Similar studies involving much larger groups of patients receiving radiotherapy are warranted.

Nutritional Therapeutics, Clinical Concerns, and Adaptations

Further research with large, well-designed clinical trials is essential, but vitamin C therapy is already playing a role in many cancer treatment protocols, employing multiple therapeutic modalities within an integrative clinical strategy. Physicians and other health care professionals may consider reviewing the potential for such synergistic therapies with appropriate patients and provide referral information to centers specializing in such integrative approaches. Self-administration of vitamin C by patients during conventional chemotherapy is not advised, and health care providers should caution patients against initiating this outside the context of close supervision and regular monitoring by health care professionals trained and experienced in these practices.

In clinical practice, health care professionals specializing in multidisciplinary oncological care often consider "pulse therapy" as a safe and effective means of administering vitamin C, antioxidants, and other nutritional support with conventional antineoplastic treatment. As discussed at numerous professional conferences, this technique typically involves cessation of nutrient administration just before delivery of a large chemotherapeutic bolus or radiation treatments, followed by reintroduction of high-dose antioxidants (e.g. IV ascorbate, NAC). This alternating dosing approach allows maximum cytotoxic effect on tumor cells (without potential interference by simultaneous pharmacological-dose nutrient input) while enabling patients to benefit from the protective and restorative effects of the nutrient support at appropriate intervals.[148,149] Juices made from foods rich in antioxidants may also be administered during the nutrient therapy phase, and conversely, prudence suggests their avoidance during nutrient-withdrawal phases.

Cimetidine and Related Histamine (H₂) Antagonists

Evidence: Cimetidine (Tagamet; Tagamet HB).
Extrapolated: Famotidine (Pepcid RPD, Pepcid, Pepcid AC), nizatidine (Axid, Axid AR), ranitidine bismuth citrate (Tritec), ranitidine (Zantac).
Similar properties but evidence lacking for extrapolation: Proton pump inhibitors: Esomeprazole (Nexium), lansoprazole (Prevacid, Zoton), omeprazole (Losec, Prilosec), pantoprazole (Protium, Protonix, Somac), rabeprazole (AcipHex, Pariet).

Interaction Type and Significance

☼ **Prevention or Reduction of Drug Adverse Effect**

Probability:	Evidence Base:
2. Probable	○ Preliminary

Effect and Mechanism of Action

Cimetidine can bind to cytochrome P450 covering the active heme group. The cytochrome proves to be vital to hydroxylation reactions in human steroidogenesis. Serum hydrocortisone concentrations will decrease when CYP450 becomes blocked.[150] Ascorbic acid can prevent cimetidine-induced decrease of human serum hydrocortisone concentrations. Researchers, however, have not elucidated the mechanisms for this observed phenomenon.

Research

In a blinded, parallel, prospective, clinical trial, Boidin et al.[150] compared the effect of IV ascorbic acid on cimetidine-induced decreases in concentrations of serum hydrocortisone in 16 male adults undergoing major abdominal vascular surgery. Cimetidine is administered to surgical patients under anesthesia and is known to inhibit steroidogenesis. In contrast to patients receiving a placebo, in whom serum hydrocortisone concentrations decreased, patients receiving ascorbic acid exhibited a significant increase in serum hydrocortisone concentration.

Nutritional Therapeutics, Clinical Concerns, and Adaptations

The available evidence suggests that surgeons consider the potential benefits of coadministering vitamin C, when using cimetidine in conjunction with major abdominal surgery, to reduce undesirable effects of cimetidine on cortisone levels and attendant implications for inflammation and recovery. Adverse effects from such concomitant application have neither been reported nor would be expected based on established scientific evidence available at this time. Further research and more conclusive findings from adequately powered clinical trials are warranted to determine the efficacy of this observed interaction. Moreover, since cimetidine is clinically used less often than newer H_2 blockers, investigation into whether this effect and interaction occur with other histamine (H_2) antagonists appears worthy of consideration.

Corticosteroids, Oral and Topical, Including Prednisone

Evidence: Corticosteroids, oral: Betamethasone (Celestone), cortisone (Cortone), dexamethasone (Decadron), fludrocortisone (Florinef), hydrocortisone (Cortef), methylprednisolone (Medrol) prednisolone (Delta-Cortef, Orapred, Pediapred, Prelone), prednisone (Deltasone, Liquid Pred, Meticorten, Orasone), triamcinolone (Aristocort); corticosteroids, topical: cortisone eyedrops.

Extrapolated, based on similar properties: Other topical corticosteroids.

Similar properties but evidence lacking for extrapolation: Inhaled corticosteroids.

See also Cimetidine and related Histamine (H_2) Antagonists

Interaction Type and Significance

$\oplus\oplus$ **Beneficial or Supportive Interaction, with Professional Management**

$\approx\approx$ **Drug-Induced Nutrient Depletion, Supplementation Therapeutic, with Professional Management**

$\diamondsuit\approx\approx$ **Drug-Induced Adverse Effect on Nutrient Function, Coadministration Therapeutic, Not Requiring Professional Management**

$\diamondsuit$ **Prevention or Reduction of Drug Adverse Effect**

Probability: Evidence Base:
4. Plausible to   ○ Preliminary
   2. Probable

Effect and Mechanism of Action

Ascorbic acid is an important cofactor for both adrenal cortex and adrenal medulla and essential in the biosynthesis and metabolic regulation of certain steroid hormones.[151,152] However, exogenous hydrocortisone can inhibit cellular uptake of ascorbic acid as well as the normal accumulation of ascorbic acid by adrenal chromaffin cells.[153,154]

Ascorbic acid administration can increase serum hydrocortisone concentrations, particularly when steroidogenesis is inhibited by exogenous agents such as cimetidine.[150]

Exogenous glucocorticoids, in the form of oral corticosteroids, can increase urinary loss of vitamin C, as well as related nutrients such as vitamin K, selenium, and zinc.[155]

Research

Chowdhury and Kapil[156] found that administration of two doses of dexamethasone caused a "sharp decline" in testicular

ascorbic acid and cholesterol levels in prepubertal rat tissues. This adverse effect was reversible by administration of DHEA (dehydroepiandrosterone), 80 μg, but not by lower doses (20 μg).

Mehra et al.[153] confirmed that cortisone eyedrops reduced the concentration of ascorbic acid in the aqueous humor and lens. They also found that simultaneous administration of vitamin A drops "neutralized" this adverse effect and mitigated the risk of drug-induced glaucoma or cataract.

Kodama et al.[157] have conducted extensive research into the relationships between vitamin C and the pituitary and adrenal glands, particularly in the context of immune function and chronic fatigue syndrome (CFS). In one series of four experiments using a healthy male volunteer, they investigated the "relation between ACTH, cortisol and vitamin C in plasma in the course of vitamin C infusion or injection treatment with and without the use of methyl-prednisolone annex, a suppressor of the homeostatic mechanism of the pituitary ACTH." First, they noted a three-phase response pattern in which a steroid-free vitamin C infusion treatment induced "distinct depletion of both cortisol and vitamin C from the circulation at the initial to moderate stages of the experiment,...a small surge of plasma cortisol at the middle stage, and...skyrocket-like rises of ACTH and cortisol of plasma at the terminal stage." Second, the "use of methylprednisolone annex in the vitamin C infusion set completely suppressed the emergence of the plasma ACTH/cortisol surges of the terminal stage, but not the small surge of plasma cortisol. The synthetic steroid also suppressed the depletion of vitamin C and cortisol of the initial to moderate stages." In a subsequent 9-month pilot trial, the authors compared the effects of a "dehydroepiandrosterone-annexed vitamin C infusion set" and an "annex-free vitamin C infusion set," with and without the oral intake of erythromycin and chloramphenicol, in the treatment of a male patient with CFS characterized by persistent pneumonia signs and dermatomyositis. They reported that the "megadose" vitamin C–antibiotic combination produced improvement for 3 months, followed by a return of symptoms. However, the DHEA–vitamin C "infusion treatments together with the long-term antibiotics treatment, as conducted in the 3rd stage...led to substantial extinction of pneumonia signs (leucocytosis, tachycardia, etc.)." They also observed that the DHEA-C-antibiotic "treatment markedly increased the excretion of both 17-ketosteroids and 17-hydroxycorticosteroids in the urine" and suggested that the DHEA administered "was converted to testosterone, which in turn made a contribution to the control of CFS." These authors concluded that the results "could be taken as evidence to indicate that the new vitamin C infusion treatment effectuates the clinical control of CFS by fortifying the endogenous activities of both cortisol and testosterone."[157]

Kodama et al.[158,159] have continued their research with several studies of this vitamin C–DHEA infusion method, usually with antibiotic therapy, in the treatment of many patients in Nagoya, Japan, with CFS characterized by interstitial pneumonia and autoimmune processes. In overview, they stated that the "merit of our treatment system is to create a new hormonal environment to improve the state of immunodeficiency by use of a non-steroid substance—vitamin C—which encounters little resistance from the feedback mechanism of steroid metabolism in the in vivo system."

Report

Masugi et al.[160] published a case report describing the beneficial effects of combining ascorbic acid and methylprednisolone pulse (mp) therapy in the treatment of a patient with idiopathic thrombocytopenic purpura who had not responded adequately to treatment with methylprednisolone alone. They concluded that the "effect of this combination therapy seems to be better than MP therapy alone" and suggested that such coadministration is worth further examination as another therapeutic choice due to its fewer secondary effects than the usual regimen of corticosteroids, splenectomy, and other immunosuppressive drugs."

Nutritional Therapeutics, Clinical Concerns, and Adaptations

Physicians prescribing oral corticosteroids, especially for extended periods of therapy, are advised to consider the potential depleting effects of these medications on the status of vitamin C (and other vital nutrients) and resultant adverse effects on immune and adrenal function. Although conclusive evidence from adequately powered human trials is lacking, the available data indicate that such coadministration of vitamin C may mitigate certain adverse drug effects, particularly impaired healing response, and could enhance treatment efficacy and tolerance. A daily dose of 500 to 1500 mg vitamin C constitutes a typical level of nutrient support and would generally be considered safe in most patients. Ascorbic acid infusions may be appropriate in some cases but require specialized training and monitoring. Further clinical trials focused on reducing adverse effects and enhancing therapeutic outcomes, as well as safety and protocols for determining the appropriateness of such coadministration, are warranted.

Cyclosporine

Cyclosporine (Ciclosporin, cyclosporin A, CsA; Neoral, Sandimmune, SangCya).

Interaction Type and Significance

☼   **Prevention or Reduction of Drug Adverse Effect**
≈≈   **Drug-Induced Nutrient Depletion, Supplementation Therapeutic, with Professional Management**
⊕✗   **Bimodal or Variable Interaction, with Professional Management**
✗   **Potential or Theoretical Adverse Interaction of Uncertain Severity**

Probability:
4. Plausible or
2. Probable

Evidence Base:
○ Preliminary or
◉◉ Emerging

Effect and Mechanism of Action

The use of cyclosporine as an immunosuppressive agent in the treatment of allograft patients presents with a significant incidence of adverse effects, particularly nephrotoxicity. The risk of such events is heightened because the drug is poorly bioavailable (~30%). Some individuals are unable to achieve or maintain therapeutic cyclosporine blood levels. Further, the antioxidant activity of vitamin C may provide protective support against the reactive oxygen species induced by the drug's action and the lipid peroxidation products suspect in its toxic effects within the kidneys. Concomitant administration of vitamin C during cyclosporine therapy may enhance bioavailability and decrease the clearance and steady-state volume of distribution of the drug, as well as enabling a reduction in adverse effects and cost. Such a supportive interaction could potentially allow for decreased dosage levels of the medication. Vitamins C and E have also been used as adjunctive therapy in the context of transplants on the basis that they might slow progression of transplant-associated arteriosclerosis.

Research

Parra Cid et al.[161] reported that antioxidant nutrients, including vitamin E, may protect against cyclosporine A nephrotoxicity.

In a retrospective study of data on 22 consecutive heart transplant patients, reduced trough levels of cyclosporine were observed in those who took twice-daily doses of 500 mg vitamin C and 400 IU vitamin E, compared with other patients. Although no other interactions were found between the antioxidants and cyclosporine, cyclosporine trough levels decreased from 136 to 103 ng/mL in the first 2 weeks after antioxidants were administered. The decrease in trough concentrations averaged 25% but was as high as 60% in some patients. The researchers concluded: "We also don't know what the mechanism of this interaction is, so that should be studied in a more detailed analysis."[162]

On a practical level, many substances interact with cyclosporine, and because of its erratic pharmacokinetics, drug levels are routinely used to determine doses. With proper monitoring, any such interactions can be readily corrected by titration of the drug doses. Cyclosporine is a classic CYP3A4 intestinal enzyme substrate; some physicians routinely administer cyclosporine with grapefruit juice (which contains a CYP3A4 enzyme inhibitor) to reduce drug costs because a smaller dose of the drug will produce a higher blood level from a reduction in the first-pass drug metabolism by intestinal CYP3A4 enzyme. Vitamin C, or the combination of vitamins C and E, may have various effects on cyclosporine pharmacokinetics, but more research is needed to establish this.

Nutritional Therapeutics, Clinical Concerns, and Adaptations

Individuals undergoing immunosuppressive therapy with cyclosporine may benefit from coadministration of vitamin C and possibly other antioxidants such as vitamin E. Such adjunctive therapy may reduce adverse effects but would require vigilant drug level monitoring and drug dosage adjustment as necessary. Effective care of these patients will require active collaboration among physicians trained and experienced in both conventional pharmacology and nutritional therapeutics within an integrative therapeutic strategy. Given that vitamin C and allied nutrients might alter cyclosporine absorption and pharmacokinetics and that a wide range in individual responses has been reported, drug levels should be checked regularly, perhaps more frequently than customary, starting at 2 weeks. Among vitamin C–rich foods, unsupervised intake of grapefruit juice in particular is strongly contraindicated in patients taking cyclosporine because of effects on pharmacokinetics and drug levels.

Desferoxamine and Related Chelating Agents

Desferoxamine (Desferrioxamine mesilate, desferoxamine mesylate; Desferal).
Similar properties but evidence lacking for extrapolation: Deferasirox (Exjade); EDTA, ethylenediaminetetraacetic acid.

Interaction Type and Significance

⊕✗   **Bimodal or Variable Interaction, with Professional Management**
⊕⊕   **Beneficial or Supportive Interaction, with Professional Management**

Coadministration Benefit
Probability:
2. Probable

Evidence Base:
○ Preliminary

Coadministration Risk
Probability:
4. Plausible

Evidence Base:
○ **Preliminary** to
◉ **Emerging**

Effect and Mechanism of Action

In general, vitamin C can slightly to moderately increase absorption of nonheme iron; it also modulates iron transport and storage in the body. Iron overload may theoretically result from coadministration of iron and vitamin C in patients genetically (hemochromotosis) or medically (frequent RBC transfusions) predisposed to it. Conversely, high iron levels or iron administration can reduce blood levels of ascorbic acid, a water-soluble antioxidant as well as a reducing agent, through oxidation. Administration of vitamin C can enhance the activity of deferoxamine in excreting iron, even at low levels such as 200 mg daily, but with dose-dependent enhancement particularly in the 750 to 2000 mg dose range.[163]

Ascorbic acid is reported to enhance the toxic effects of deferoxamine, but no mechanism of action has been confirmed. Ascorbate has been proposed to induce cytotoxicity from iron-catalyzed oxidation, even in iron-deficient medium, but these in vitro findings of a pro-oxidant action of ascorbate in the context of free metal ions do not correlate with generally accepted observations under physiological conditions in humans.[164-166] Complications involving left ventricular dysfunction are reported to be of particular concern, and its occurrence is purported to be rapid in onset and severe.

Research

Hussain et al.[163] investigated the effect of dose, time, and ascorbate on iron excretion after subcutaneous desferrioxamine in a series of experiments involving 13 patients with beta-thalassemia major and one with congenital sideroblastic anemia, all of whom were receiving regular blood transfusions. After establishing that midlevel doses (1500 or 2000 mg) of desferrioxamine were more effective than lower doses (750 mg), with higher doses (4000 mg) showing a variable response, these researchers found that concomitant ascorbic acid therapy was invariably associated with increased iron excretion after subcutaneous desferrioxamine (D.F.). "In twelve studies at different dose levels of D.F., ascorbate therapy was associated with increased iron excretion ranging from 24 to 245%." They concluded that "in most patients with transfusional iron overload subcutaneous D.F over a 12 h period, at a dose ranging from 2 to 4 g daily with ascorbic-acid saturation, is at present the most satisfactory method of removing excess iron."

Coadministration of ascorbic acid is reported to enhance the toxic effects of desferoxamine, but evidence from large human trials is lacking to confirm any deleterious effect of vitamin C on iron status in patients with iron overload being treated with desferrioxamine. However, published reports have described a few incidents of clinically important, transient deterioration of left ventricular function in patients receiving 500 mg/day of ascorbic acid concurrent with iron chelation therapy. Henry et al.[167] have documented echocardiographic abnormalities in the majority of patients with transfusion-dependent anemia and secondary myocardial iron deposition. Nevertheless, the authors reported that they subsequently "observed a reduction in ejection fraction in several of the patients at National Institutes of Health following the addition of ascorbic acid to a program of iron chelation with intramuscular desferrioxamine." Also, "discontinuation of the ascorbic acid has been followed by a return to normal left ventricular function in all but one patient."[167]

Nutritional Therapeutics, Clinical Concerns, and Adaptations

The coadministration of vitamin C with parenteral agents, especially desferoxamine, may enhance therapeutic efficacy by increasing iron excretion, but rarely may also increase risks of left ventricular dysfunction or other significant adverse effects.

Many clinicians experienced in iron chelation therapy of iron overload states administer 500 mg of vitamin C an hour before beginning each desferal infusion to mobilize iron from storage sites and render it more available for chelation and subsequent excretion. Clinicians should monitor for cardiac decompensation, particularly in patients with preexisting cardiac disease. Administration of vitamin C after desferal injection may increase toxicity.

The limited state of the evidence and the mixed outcomes suggest the need for continued research through well-designed clinical trials. Particularly because deferasirox is orally active and a more potent iron chelator than parenteral desferoxamine, clinical studies of potential interactions, both positive and negative, between deferasirox and ascorbate should be performed.

Disulfiram

Disulfiram (Antabuse and Antabus; tetraethylthiuram disulfide.)

Interaction Type and Significance

☼ **Prevention or Reduction of Drug Adverse Effect**
⊕ **Potential or Theoretical Beneficial or Supportive Interaction, with Professional Management**

Probability:
2. Plausible to
1. Certain

Evidence Base:
● **Consensus**

Effect and Mechanism of Action

Ethyl alcohol (ethanol) is metabolized through the activity of alcohol dehydrogenase, which is the primary enzyme involved in its oxidation, and the microsomal ethanol-oxidizing system (MEOS), a key metabolic pathway, and manifests its toxic effects throughout the body, but most profoundly in the central nervous system (CNS).[168] Disulfiram is frequently used in the treatment of alcoholism but has a high level of noncompliance and dropout because of adverse effects, especially those attributable to acetaldehyde toxicity.[169]

Administration of vitamin C, alone or in combination with nutrients such as L-cysteine, and vitamin B₁ may provide a period of almost complete protection against acetaldehyde lethality, although it may not completely abrogate acetaldehyde toxicity.[170] Moreover, IV vitamin C (typically 1 g) is among the supportive measures possibly indicated to restore blood pressure and treat shock in severe disulfiram reactions.[168,171,172]

Vitamin C and other antioxidants (e.g., NAC) can inhibit the cytotoxic effect associated with disulfiram. Chronic administration of disulfiram appears to cause axonal degeneration and neurotoxicity, "at least in part, due to the cytotoxic effect of the disulfiram-Cu(2+) complex formed endogenously." The "disulfiram-Cu(2+) complex induces apoptosis and perhaps necrosis at a late stage mediated by oxidative stress followed by sequential activation of JNK, caspase-3 and poly (ADP-ribose) polymerase degradation" in a time-dependent manner. This "death-signaling pathway" involves "decreased mitochondrial membrane potential, increased free radical production, and depletion of non-protein-thiols (glutathione)."[173]

Both disulfiram and vitamin C can support abstinence in a supervised alcohol abuse program. Gamma-glutamyl transpeptidase (GGT) can fall with disulfiram but rise with vitamin C.[169]

Research

Vitamin C has been studied and used clinically for more than 50 years in the prophylaxis and treatment of disulfiram-alcohol reactions.[171,172] In 1975, Sprince et al.[170] published a paper discussing the protective action of vitamin C and other nutrients against acetaldehyde toxicity caused by heavy drinking, but also associated with heavy smoking. Using a rat model, they found that ascorbic acid, L-cysteine, and thiamine (in paired combinations) provided the greatest degree of protection against acetaldehyde lethality, although no combination completely prevented acetaldehyde toxicity. These researchers proposed that these particular nutrients acted synergistically and recommended coadministration to "enhance their individual activity in the body."

In a randomized, partially blind, 6-month follow-up study involving 126 patients, Chick et al.[169] compared the efficacy of supervised disulfiram (200 mg) and vitamin C (100 mg) as an adjunct to outpatient treatment of alcoholics. "In the opinion of the (blinded) independent assessor, patients on disulfiram increased average total abstinent days by 100 and patients on vitamin C by 69, thus enhancing by one-third this measure of treatment outcome. Mean weekly alcohol consumption was reduced by 162 units with disulfiram, compared with 105 units with vitamin C, and the disulfiram patients reduced their total six-month alcohol consumption by 2572 units compared with an average reduction of 1448 units in the vitamin C group." The researchers also observed that serum GGT "showed a mean fall of 21 IU/l in patients on disulfiram but rose by a mean of 13 IU/l with vitamin C." Although there were "no medically serious adverse reactions," seven patients in the disulfiram group reduced their dose due to "unwanted" adverse effects and four withdrew from treatment; one subject receiving vitamin C withdrew. Nevertheless, two thirds of the patients receiving disulfiram asked to continue the treatment at the conclusion of the study period. Such findings suggest that clinical trials investigating coadministration of these agents is warranted as a potential means of enhancing therapeutic outcomes while preventing or reducing adverse effects.

Clinical Implications and Adaptations

Clinicians using disulfiram in the treatment of alcohol addiction are advised to investigate the administration of vitamin C for application in situations of complications caused by Antabuse. Research into vitamin C coadministration in a preventive and synergistic role may be warranted.

Erythropoiesis-Stimulating Agents

Epoietin alpha (EPO, recombinant erythropoietin alfa; Epogen, Eprex, Procrit), epoietin beta (NeoRecormon), darbepoietin alpha darbepoietin alfa; (Aranesp).

Interaction Type and Significance

⊕⊕ **Beneficial or Supportive Interaction, with Professional Management**

⊕✗ **Bimodal or Variable Interaction, with Professional Management**

✗✗ **Minimal to Mild Adverse Interaction—Vigilance Necessary**

✗ **Potential or Theoretical Adverse Interaction of Uncertain Severity**

Coadministration Benefit
Probability:
2. Probable

Evidence Base:
◉ **Emerging** but
▽ **Mixed**

Coadministration Risk
Probability:
5. **Improbable** to
4. **Plausible**

Evidence Base:
☐ **Inadequate** and
▽ **Mixed**

Effect and Mechanism of Action

Resistance to recombinant human erythropoietin (rHuEpo) is common in hemodialysis patients with functional iron deficiency. Adequate levels of available iron are necessary for optimal response to rHuEpo, but in some cases, parenteral iron can produce iron overload, thereby increasing morbidity and mortality rates. Functional iron deficiency is a condition in which iron supply is reduced to meet the demands for increased erythropoiesis. Consequently, rHuEpo hyporesponsiveness can occur patients who are iron-overloaded (ferritin level of 500-800 μg/L) but also in those with normal iron status.[174-177]

Intravenous ascorbic acid improves anemia in iron-overloaded, erythropoietin (rEPO)–hyporesponsive hemodialysis patients. Vitamin C participates in many aspects of iron metabolism, including uptake, transport, regulation, mobilization, utilization, and sequestration.[178-183] Patients undergoing hemodialysis tend to develop ascorbic acid deficiency resulting from lack of dietary intake, increased vitamin oxidation catalyzed by iron, and nutrient depletion during dialysis. Although administration of iron can exacerbate hemosiderosis, ascorbic acid can beneficially alter hemosiderin metabolism and effect hemosiderin deposits. Hemosiderin is a pathological deposition of iron in tissues, including the spleen, small intestine, and bone marrow. Ascorbic acid can potentiate the mobilization of ferritin stores from inert tissue stores and facilitate the incorporation of iron into protoporphyrin in iron-overloaded hemodialysis patients being treated with rHuEpo.[183-188]

Thus, ascorbic acid administration, usually IV, not only improves the therapeutic response to rHuEpo but also facilitates elimination of iron from stores without reducing functional iron levels, including risk of rapid decline after discontinuing parenteral maintenance iron.[189]

Vitamin C is generally thought to reduce oxidative stress generated by iron administration, particularly in compromised patients. However, concerns have been raised that high-dose (usually IV) ascorbic acid might act as a pro-oxidant.[190]

Research

Over several decades, researchers have investigated the relationships between vitamin C and iron with regard to erythropoiesis and hemosiderin metabolism. Ascorbic acid intake augments the absorption of nonheme iron from dietary sources and reduces ferric iron (Fe^{3+}) to ferrous iron (Fe^{2+}) by mobilizing iron from the ferritin crystal core.[180,181] Since the 1950s, scientists have recognized that ascorbic acid facilitates heme synthesis by incorporation of iron into protoporphyrin. Bothwell et al.[184] noted in 1964 that individuals with scurvy often present with excessive iron deposits in the tissues. Nevertheless, evidence from well-controlled studies evaluating hemosiderosis and IV ascorbic acid is lacking. In the 1990s, researchers determined that ascorbic acid enhances iron-induced ferritin mRNA translation by promoting the conversion of the iron regulatory protein (IRP) RNA-binding form to aconitase. Ponka and Kuhlback[185] reported a high incidence of ascorbic acid deficiency in hemodialysis patients caused by limited dietary intake and its removal during dialysis. Further, in studying individuals with iron overload, particularly hereditary hemochromatosis, Young et al.[186] observed generally low plasma levels of ascorbic acid, possibly as a result of increased iron-induced oxidation.

Using a rodent model, Srigiridhar and Nair[191] demonstrated that administration of alpha-tocopherol or a combination of ascorbic acid and alpha-tocopherol protects the GI tract of iron-deficient rats against iron-induced oxidative damage during iron repletion.

A number of studies of varying size and quality have investigated the efficacy and safety of ascorbic acid during EPO therapy, and most have found that such coadministration can promote increased iron utilization and counter anemia by facilitating iron release from inert depots and circumventing the defective iron utilization in chronic hemodialysis (HD) patients who are treated with rHuEPO. In a trial involving four iron-overloaded HD patients who had developed relative resistance to erythropoietin (and three of whom exhibited features of "functional iron deficiency") Gastaldello et al.[174] found that resistance to erythropoietin in iron-overloaded HD patients can be overcome by IV ascorbic acid (500 mg after hemodialysis, one to three times per week).

Tarng, Huang, and associates conducted a series of trials over several years investigating the efficacy of IV ascorbic acid for erythropoietin-hyporesponsive anemia in HD patients with iron overload. In a parallel, comparative study in 1998, Tarng and Huang[175] compared the effects of IV iron versus IV ascorbic acid for erythropoietin-hyporesponsive anemia in 50 HD patients with iron overload and hyperferritinemia. Patients in both the IV iron group and the IV ascorbic acid group were hyporesponsive to erythropoietin and functionally iron deficient. They administered IV ferric saccharate (100 mg) post-HD on five consecutive dialysis sessions in the first 2 weeks to the IV iron group, and IV ascorbic acid (300 mg) three times weekly for 8 weeks to the ascorbic acid group. After 8 weeks of ascorbate therapy, mean hematocrit significantly increased $(25.8 \pm 0.5\%$ to $30.6 \pm 0.6\%)$, with a concomitant reduction of 20% in erythropoietin dose. Furthermore, a rise in transferrin saturation $(27 \pm 3\%$ to $48 \pm 6\%)$ and serum iron $(70 \pm 11$ $\mu g/dL$ to 107 ± 19 $\mu g/dL)$ paralleled the enhanced erythropoiesis. Although lacking statistical significance, serum ferritin fell modestly. In contrast, "intravenous iron therapy neither improved erythropoiesis nor reduced erythropoietin dose" during 12 weeks. Notably, after significant increases in indices of iron metabolism at 2 and 6 weeks, they decreased at 12 weeks and returned to the baselines. Thus, these findings demonstrated that IV ascorbic acid, but not IV iron, can effectively circumvent the functional iron-deficient erythropoiesis associated with iron overload in HD patients. The authors concluded: "Intravenous administration of ascorbic acid not only facilitates iron release from storage sites, but also increases iron utilization in the erythron."[175]

In a prospective trial involving 65 HD patients with iron overload (serum ferritin levels >500 μg/L) in 1999, Tarng et al.[192] investigated inadequate iron mobilization and defective iron utilization to determine criteria for prediction of a response to ascorbic acid treatment and establish guidelines for adjuvant therapy. They reported that 18 patients exhibited a "dramatic response" to IV ascorbic acid with a "significant

increase in their hemoglobin and reticulocyte index and a concomitant 24% reduction in rEPO dose after eight weeks," as well as "a significant rise" in serum iron and transferrin saturation and a fall in erythrocyte zinc protoporphyrin (which accumulates when hemoglobin synthesis is impeded) and serum ferritin. In contrast to responders, controls and nonresponders showed no significant changes in mean values of hemoglobin, rEPO dose, iron metabolism parameters, and erythrocyte zinc protoporphyrin. Furthermore, by analyzing data from 18 responders and 19 nonresponders, the authors determined that erythrocyte zinc protoporphyrin at a cutoff level of more than 105 μmol/mol heme and transferrin saturation at a level of less than 25% were "more specific to confirm the status of functional iron deficiency in iron-overloaded patients" and served as the "two criterion values [that] had the highest accuracy to predict a response to treatment."[192]

Subsequently, in 2004, Tarng et al.[193] investigated the effects of IV ascorbic acid "on serum concentrations of soluble transferrin receptors (TfR) on the basis of the hypothesis that an increase of labile iron in the cytosol will lead to inhibition of TfR expression." First, applying a stepwise multivariate analysis to evaluate the interrelation between serum TfR and iron status in 138 HD patients, they confirmed that serum EPO and transferrin saturation were the two independent predictors for serum TfR in HD patients (high TfR levels are indicative of iron deficiency, functional or absolute). They also noted that the lower the serum EPO and the higher the transferrin saturation, "the lower the serum TfR in HD patients who are on maintenance rHuEPO treatment." Then, in a controlled study, 36 HD patients were randomly administered IV ascorbic acid (total dose of 2000 mg) or placebo (normal saline). Neither serum EPO nor ferritin levels changed significantly in either group. However, compared with presupplemental values, serum TfR levels significantly declined, and transferrin saturation rose within 7 days in ascorbic acid–treated patients before any apparent alteration in hematocrit values; in contrast, no such changes were observed in the placebo group. Notably, the trend of decreased serum TfR and increased transferrin saturation was similar among ascorbic acid–treated subjects with ferritin less than or greater than 500 μg/L. They concluded that "ascorbic acid status can significantly decrease serum TfR concentrations and increase percentage of TSAT, probably through alterations in intracellular iron metabolism."[193]

In a 6-month, randomized, double-blind, crossover trial involving 27 HD patients, Giancaspro et al.[194] investigated the effects of IV ascorbic acid on functional iron deficiency and whether this results in a better correction of anemia in patients with stable hemoglobin concentration and functional iron deficiency. During the treatment phase, subjects in each group received vitamin C, 500 mg intravenously three times a week for 3 months, with treatment discontinued during the other 3 months as control. Hemoglobin concentration rose in one group but dropped slightly in the other group. However, percentage transferrin saturation significantly increased, and ferritin fell significantly in both groups during their respective treatment phase. The rHuEpo dose was kept unchanged throughout the study. These investigators concluded that IV ascorbic acid "may partially correct" functional iron deficiency and consequently help rHuEPO-hyporesponsive anemia.

Similarly, in a trial involving 36 patients whose ferritin levels were higher than 500 μg/L and who needed more than 100 U/kg/week of rHuEPO, Sezer et al.[195] found that IV ascorbic acid "effectively overrides rHuEpo resistance in iron-overloaded hemodialysis patients." Using a two-phase structure, they administered 500 mg IV ascorbic acid twice weekly to all the patients for 8 weeks during an initial phase and then, during an 8-week maintenance phase, separated the patients into groups, one of which received 500 mg ascorbic acid once weekly while the other group received no therapy. These researchers noted that the therapeutic response "remained stable in patient groups during the maintenance phase" and that in the six nonresponders, the hypochromic RBCs were less than 10%.

In a subsequent 12-month, prospective, randomized, double-blind, crossover study involving 63 subjects, Keven et al.[177] compared hemoglobin levels, weekly EPO dose, and ratio of EPO to hemoglobin (an index of EPO need) in patients treated with IV vitamin C, 500 mg three times a week, or with placebo over two consecutive 6-month periods. Subjects in both treatment groups, 20 patients (66.7%) in one group and 18 patients in the other group (64.3%), demonstrated positive response to vitamin C. Likewise, in both groups, vitamin C resulted in a significant increase in hemoglobin levels, a significant decrease in EPO-hemoglobin ratio, and increased transferrin saturation. In contrast, subjects in both groups exhibited no change in these parameters during their placebo phase. Although concluding that vitamin C "can be used as an effective adjuvant therapy to EPO in hemodialysis patients," including those with normal iron status, these authors added that "further studies are needed to determine possible predictors of hematologic response to vitamin C."

Lin et al.[196] have investigated the effects of low-dose IV ascorbic acid in diabetic ESRD patients with hyperferritinemia. In one trial they studied 22 chronic HD patients with type 2 diabetes in a single dialysis unit by comparing responses to different sequential treatment phases, including control period and post–IV ascorbic acid periods. The subjects received IV ascorbic acid, 100 mg three times per week for 8 weeks of treatment and 4 months of posttreatment follow-up. Hemoglobin and hematocrit increased significantly in the post–ascorbic acid period after 3 months compared with the control period, whereas mean corpuscular volume (MCV; red cell size, which is reduced in both absolute and functional iron deficiency) did not increase significantly. Also, serum ferritin significantly decreased at study completion and transferring saturation significantly increased at 1 month and further at 3 months. These researchers concluded that their findings demonstrated that short-term low-dose IV ascorbic acid therapy "can facilitate iron release from reticuloendothelial system but also increase iron utilization in diabetic hemodialysis patients with iron overload" and recommended that IV ascorbic acid be considered as "a potential adjuvant therapy to treat erythropoeitin-hyporesponsive anemia in iron-overloaded patients."[196]

Ogi et al.[196a] conducted a small trial contrasting the effects of IV ascorbic acid versus IV iron on functional iron deficiency in EPO-treated HD patients. Thirteen patients on chronic HD with functional iron deficiency (serum ferritin levels >300 ng/mL, serum iron levels <50 μg/dL) received IV injections of ascorbic acid, 100 mg three times a week, after HD until serum ferritin decreased to below 300 ng/mL (maximum, 3 months). The iron group (seven subjects) received more than 10 IV injections of saccharated ferric oxide (40 mg/dose) after HD. The seven patients of the control group received no iron preparation during the 3 months. Hemoglobin did not change in the ascorbic acid group during the 3-month period, but "serum iron increased significantly," from 37 to 49 ± 4 μg/dL, after 1 month ($p < 0.01$) and remained elevated until the end of the 3 months, and serum ferritin decreased

significantly after 3 months. In contrast, hemoglobin and serum iron increased significantly in the iron group from the respective pretreatment levels during the 2-month period, and serum ferritin rose significantly after 2 months. Notably, recombinant erythropoietin dose remained stable for 3 months in all three groups. "These results suggest that in hemodialysis patients with a functional iron deficiency, treatment with intravenous ascorbic acid can prevent iron overload due to treatment with intravenous iron, and provide a useful adjuvant means of maintaining hemoglobin and serum iron levels."

A few studies found limited benefit and increased risk from ascorbic acid therapy in iron-overloaded, erythropoietin (rEPO)–hyporesponsive HD patients. In one trial involving 61 "unselected" HD patients, Taji et al.[197] found that patients who received 100 mg IV ascorbic acid after each dialysis session demonstrated no significant improvements in erythropoiesis or various measures of quality of life and "significantly higher adverse events" compared with controls. These researchers interpreted their findings as suggesting that ascorbic acid treatment would most likely provide no significant benefit to "unselected" HD patients (i.e., not selected based on predictive factors).

The safety and efficacy of oral ascorbic acid in patients receiving HD has also been discussed and remains controversial. Some reviewers of the scientific literature on vitamin replacement therapy in renal failure patients, such as Makoff,[198] have proposed that supplemental vitamin C intake be limited to 60 mg/day, derived from the RDA, based on the supposition that "inappropriately high supplementation of vitamin C may cause toxicities which exacerbate existing pathologies."[198] In an 8-week, open-label randomized parallel study, Chan et al.[199] compared the efficacy and safety of 250 mg oral ascorbic acid with 250 mg IV ascorbic acid, three times weekly, on hemoglobin (Hb), ferritin, and rEPO dose in 21 iron-overloaded HD patients. These researchers also examined the effect of 3 months of 500 mg oral ascorbic acid three times weekly compared with no treatment on Hb, ferritin, and rEPO dose in 153 HD patients. They noted that all patients had "severe" ascorbic acid deficiency (mean, 2.2 mg/L; normal range, 4.0-14.0), and that with treatment, the plasma ascorbic acid level "increased, but was not significantly different between the groups." Further, they found that there was no change in Hb, iron availability, and rEPO dose with either form of ascorbic acid, even in a subgroup of 30 subjects with anemia taking the oral form for a longer duration. Notably, although there was a significant increase in serum oxalate, there were no accompanying significant changes in left ventricular function or renal calculi formation. Despite this lack of improvement with either form in the smaller iron-overloaded group or the larger group of HD patients, the authors suggested that ascorbic acid (AA) "administration may still be warranted in view of severe AA deficiency in haemodialysis patients."[199]

In view of the positive studies of IV ascorbate previously discussed, it would seem that a careful search for a dose-response effect in such nonresponsive patients would be warranted, with careful monitoring for potential adverse effects, given the possibility of pro-oxidant effects of higher doses of ascorbate, and because HD patients are known to have high baseline levels of oxidative stress. Combining IV ascorbate with oral antioxidant administration of a broad spectrum of antioxidants, such as alpha-lipoic acid, tocopherols and tocotrienols, OPCs, anthocyanins and other plant-derived antioxidant polyphenols, astaxanthin, and other antioxidant carotenoids (providing an extensive network of diet-derived antioxidant compounds that cover both lipid and aqueous physiological compartments), would seem a promising research avenue for this patient population.

Researchers and clinicians have expressed concern regarding the risk of iron overload after parenteral iron administration and the potential need to discontinue such therapy. Deira et al.[189] conducted a 6-month, prospective, randomized trial comparing IV ascorbic acid (AA, 200 mg three times weekly) versus low-dose desferroxamine (DFO, 1 mg/kg/week) in 27 HD patients with hyperferritinemia (>800 ng/mL) who had previously received parenteral iron (Ferlecit). "When Ferlecit was discontinued, functional iron did not vary and the epoetin resistance index (rhuEPO dose/Hb) was reduced by 21% in the i.v. AA group. In the DFO and control groups, functional iron levels fell. In the DFO group the epoetin resistance index increased by 20%, with no modifications in the control group." Overall, they observed no significant differences in iron loss or mobilization from dialysis, as well as a positive correlation between serum transaminases and ferritin, indicative of the hepatotoxicity associated with iron overload.

Other researchers have suggested that excessive dosing of ascorbic acid in HD patients with iron overload might "raise the risk of increasing free radical generation" and adversely influence serum ferritin levels because of a hypothetical pro-oxidant effect of ascorbic acid. Thus, in an experiment involving six healthy subjects and 29 HD patients, Chen et al.[190] studied the effect of IV ascorbic acid on oxidative stress parameters in blood samples. They reported that ascorbic acid presented "a strong antioxidant effect in DPPH chemical reaction," an index of free-radical scavenging activity. However, they also observed a "pro-oxidant effect when mixed with plasma or whole blood of healthy subjects and hemodialysis patients." This "pro-oxidant effect of ascorbic acid detected by LucCL [lucigenin chemiluminescence, which detects in vitro free-radical generation] was attenuated by various iron chelators and superoxide dismutase," and there was "no significant correlation between the responses of LucCL intensity to ascorbic acid administration and transferrin saturation." The changes of LucCL intensity were significantly higher in the ascorbic acid–treated group of HD patients than those in the control group. The ascorbic acid therapy produced significantly higher LucCL intensity in HD patients with elevated ferritin (≥600 ng/mL) than in those with ferritins less than 600 ng/mL. Although the "changes of LucCL intensity were positively correlated with serum ferritin level...," there was no significant correlation between the responses of LucCL intensity to ascorbic acid administration and transferrin saturation." These results are strongly suggestive that the presence of excess iron stores (as reflected by serum ferritin level) is a key factor in catalyzing oxidative stress (in vitro) in the presence of higher levels of serum ascorbate. The authors noted that the presence of iron-chelator-suppressible chemiluminescence in persons with higher ascorbic acid levels in the blood or plasma are "suggestive of free radical formation." However, they qualified this potential interpretation by adding that their data neither conclusively answered the question of "whether the findings occur *in vivo*" nor proved "that the free radicals generated *in vitro* lead to toxicity in patients." Overall, they concluded that their "results suggest that either lower parenteral dose or lower infusion rate of ascorbic acid may be more appropriate for adjuvant therapy in iron-overloaded uremic patients."[190]

The generally positive findings in these many experiments and preliminary studies have led researchers to recommend large-scale, prospective, and controlled trails to determine the long-term safety and efficacy of IV ascorbic acid therapy in iron-overloaded and functionally iron-deficient HD patients receiving epoetin alpha. The emerging trend in the research indicates that the need for determining patient characteristics predictive of iron-overloaded EPO hyporesponders most likely to achieve a beneficial response from ascorbic acid coadministration is of paramount importance. Based on their investigation into early prediction of response to intravenous iron medications in hemodialysis patients receiving rHuEPO, Chuang, Tarng, et al.[199a] suggested that changes in reticulocyte hemoglobin content (CHr) and reticulocytes in a high-fluorescence intensity region (HFR) at either 2 or 4 weeks "are superior to the conventional erythrocyte and iron metabolism indices and may serve as reliable parameters to detect iron-deficient erythropoiesis in HD patients undergoing rHuEpo therapy." As for predictors of response to coadministration of vitamin C, depleted nutrient status, elevated erythrocyte zinc protoporphyrin, elevated ferritin, and decreased transferrin saturation are generally considered the most important indicators.

Nutritional Therapeutics, Clinical Concerns, and Adaptations

Physicians treating hemodialysis or other patients undergoing EPO therapy are advised to evaluate patients for possible predictors of iron-overload risk (generally from repeated RBC transfusions) and inadequate therapeutic response (usually either from absolute or functional iron deficiency). In such cases the coadministration of ascorbic acid, typically parenteral but possibly oral administration, may enhance the response to EPO therapy and reduce adverse effects of iron administration. Identification of iron-overloaded EPO hyporesponders before treatment or at the earliest possible stage provides the most effective means of determining whether ascorbate therapy is appropriate to any given patient, so as to reduce the probability of long-term adverse reactions to iron therapy, minimize risk of anemia, and enhance erythropoeitic response. Further studies are needed to determine possible predictors of hematological response to vitamin C.

Furosemide and Related Loop Diuretics

Evidence: Furosemide (Lasix).
Extrapolated, based on similar properties: Bumetanide (Bumex), ethacrynic acid (Edecrin), torsemide (Demadex).

Interaction Type and Significance

⊕ **Potential or Theoretical Beneficial or Supportive Interaction, with Professional Management**
≈≈ **Drug-Induced Nutrient Depletion, Supplementation Therapeutic, with Professional Management**
☼ **Prevention or Reduction of Drug Adverse Effect**

Probability:
4. Plausible

Evidence Base:
○ **Preliminary**

Effect and Mechanism of Action

Ascorbic acid may amplify the bioavailability and activity of furosemide through several possible mechanisms. Vitamin C appears to enhance the GI absorption of furosemide, inhibit metabolism of furosemide at the gut wall, enhance the reabsorption of furosemide from the renal tubules, and increase the unionized fraction of furosemide at the receptor sites. Of these effects, reduced gastric first-pass metabolism of furosemide with coadministration of ascorbic acid is most likely to contribute to the significant increase in the oral bioavailability.[200]

Furosemide acutely increases urinary excretion of oxalic acid and vitamin C (as well as vitamin B_6) in individuals with chronic renal failure. This effect could reverse the tendency in uremic patients toward accumulation of oxalic acid resulting in elevated plasma levels.[201]

Research

Using animal models, Lee and Chiou[200] observed that the combination of furosemide and vitamin C produced significant increases in oral bioavailability of orally administered furosemide as well as its diuretic and natriuretic effects. They observed increases in both urine output and excretion of unchanged furosemide after coadministering furosemide (20 mg intravenously or 40 mg orally) and ascorbic acid (150 or 500 mg orally) to dogs. They attributed this effect to reduced gastric first-pass metabolism of furosemide rather than increased furosemide absorption. They subsequently administered furosemide (6 mg orally) and ascorbic acid (up to 100 mg orally) to rats and reported that "amounts of furosemide remaining per gram of stomach after 30-min incubations of 50 micrograms of furosemide with 9000g supernatant fractions of stomach homogenates were increased significantly (48.5 vs. 42.4 micrograms) by the addition of 100 micrograms of ascorbic acid." In contrast, the percentages of the oral doses of furosemide recovered from the GI tract 8 hours after oral administration were similar without and with ascorbic acid coadministration. These and related findings led the authors to suggest that the "significant increases in the diuretic and natriuretic effects of furosemide with ascorbic acid could be the result of increases in the reabsorption of furosemide from renal tubules and increases in the unionized fraction of furosemide at the renal tubular receptor sites."[200]

Mydlik et al.[202,203] conducted a series of investigations of the effect of furosemide on urinary excretion of oxalic acid, vitamin C, and vitamin B_6 in patients with chronic renal failure (CRF). In one controlled clinical trial (1998), they observed an increased urinary excretion of oxalic acid, vitamin C, and vitamin B_6 during the first 3 hours after a single IV dose of 20 mg furosemide in a control group and in patients with CRF without dialysis treatment. This effect persisted for 6 hours in CRF patients without dialysis. The authors described a new positive side effect of furosemide—enhanced urinary oxalic acid excretion in the control group and in CRF patients without dialysis treatment—and a negative side effect of furosemide: increased urinary vitamin B_6 excretion in both groups. They recommended monitoring of vitamin C and vitamin B_6 in plasma "during long-term administration of large doses of furosemide to patients with chronic renal failure as deficiency of these vitamins could develop."[202] A year later these researchers published results of another trial in which they compared urinary excretion of vitamin B_6, oxalic acid, and vitamin C in three groups: 15 healthy subjects during maximal water diuresis, 12 patients in polyuric stage of CRF without dialysis treatment receiving a diet high in sodium chloride (15 g/day), and 15 patients in polyuric stage of CRF without dialysis treatment after IV administration of 20 mg furosemide. "Urinary excretion of vitamin B_6, oxalic acid and vitamin C significantly increased during maximal water diuresis while during high intake of sodium chloride the urinary excretions of these substances were not affected." The authors interpreted these results to suggest that "urinary excretion of vitamin B_6,

oxalic acid and vitamin C depends on the urinary excretion of water" and to confirm their earlier findings that IV furosemide (20 mg) increases urinary excretion of vitamin B_6, as well as oxalic acid and vitamin C, in patients with CRF.[203]

Nutritional Therapeutics, Clinical Concerns, and Adaptations

Physicians prescribing furosemide or related loop diuretics are advised to monitor levels of vitamin C and other nutrients and to supplement as indicated, particularly in patients with CRF and on dialysis. The evidence is limited but indicates that individuals prescribed furosemide might demonstrate greater efficacy from their medication with the simultaneous use of vitamin C. Further, these preliminary findings do not provide adequate guidelines for determining the appropriate dosage in a range of patients using furosemide. However, in most cases, a dosage of 1000 to 2000 mg of vitamin C two to three times daily could provide benefit without causing significant risk. If diarrhea results from ingestion of excessive vitamin C, the dose can simply be lowered to bowel tolerance.

Regular monitoring is warranted after introducing a new medication or nutrient or changing the dose or combination of any agents, and close supervision is especially critical in patients with compromised renal function. It may also be prudent to increase dietary intake of or to supplement the B-complex vitamins in patients taking furosemide because the drug increases excretion of vitamins B_1 and B_6.

HMG-CoA Reductase Inhibitors (Statins)

Evidence: Atorvastatin (Lipitor), lovastatin (Altocor, Altoprev, Mevacor), pravastatin (Pravachol), simvastatin (Zocor); combination drugs: Niacin and lovastatin (Advicor); simvastatin and extended-release nicotinic acid (Niaspan).
Extrapolated, based on similar properties: Fluvastatin (Lescol, Lescol XL), rosuvastatin (Crestor).
See also Vitamin B_3 (Niacin), Vitamin E, Coenzyme Q10, and Omega-3 Fatty Acids monographs.

Interaction Type and Significance

✗ **Potential or Theoretical Adverse Interaction of Uncertain Severity**
✗✗ **Minimal to Mild Adverse Interaction—Vigilance Necessary**
⊕✗ **Bimodal or Variable Interaction, with Professional Management**
⊕ **Potential or Theoretical Beneficial or Supportive Interaction, with Professional Management**

Probability:	Evidence Base:
4. Plausible or	▽ **Mixed** and
3. Possible	○ **Preliminary**

Effect and Mechanism of Action

Vitamin C, along with vitamin E and coenzyme Q10, plays a critical role in endogenous antioxidant activity, synthesis of glutathione, and inhibition of lipid peroxidation. Vitamin C is also protective of and participates in the regeneration of vitamin E. Conversely, statin drugs appear to exert an adverse impact on oxidative stress.

Concomitant intake of vitamin C and other antioxidants with conventional lipid-lowering agents may improve some lipid parameters, particularly low-density lipoprotein (LDL) cholesterol and triglycerides.[204]

Antioxidants, including vitamin C, may interfere with the high-density lipoprotein (HDL)–elevating activity of statin-niacin combinations, although the specific role of ascorbic acid in such potential interference, including possible mechanisms of action, have not been elucidated. Presumably, nutrient-rich foods could also impair the activity of such agents, if the hypothesis were to bear out under further investigation.

Research

The mixed evidence from clinical trials investigating the use of antioxidant nutrients during statin therapy indicates that scientific knowledge of the mechanisms of action and diverse effects of this common lipid management intervention, as well as its interaction with vitamin C and other nutrients, is incomplete. As part of the HDL Atherosclerosis Treatment Study (HATS), Brown, Cheung, and associates reported that coadministration of 1000 mg vitamin C, 800 IU alpha-tocopherol, 100 μg selenium, and 25 mg beta-carotene daily diminished the therapeutic activity of a simvastatin-niacin combination. In particular, this antioxidant combination appeared to interfere with the HDL-elevating activity of the statin-niacin combinations, especially with regard to Lp(A-I), even though statins alone generally lower HDL as well as LDL (with possible exception of atorvastatin).[205] In an accompanying paper focusing on coronary atherosclerotic plaques and the occurrence of a first cardiovascular event, the niacin-simvastatin combination was significantly superior to placebo with regard to average stenosis progression, although in participants also receiving antioxidants, this benefit was significantly attenuated, a finding interpreted as possible interference by antioxidants.[206] Notably, the specific role of vitamin C in such potential interference, including possible mechanisms of action, have not been presented in a precise and substantiated form. Moreover, the HDL increases were probably attributable to the niacin therapy because low-dose simvastatin monotherapy has only limited effects in raising the levels of HDL cholesterol and apolipoprotein (apo) A-I. Thus, one or more of the antioxidants might be interfering with niacin's ability to alter the expression of proteins responsible for the formation of HDL. Further, the findings derived from the population studied may have limited general relevance to individuals who have only elevated LDL cholesterol levels (and normal HDL levels) and to women, who made up only 13% of the cohort. Also, with regard to HDL status, there was no detriment to the antioxidants alone (i.e., given to a group without simvistatin/niacin) and actually a slight benefit, which, if involving thousands of patients as in the previous statin and the thrombolytic trials, might have become a trend or even statistically significant. Also of note is that statins block endogenous synthesis of ubiquinone (coenzyme Q10), and thus far no trials in this area have included coadministration of this important mitochondrial-protective antioxidant, with or without other antioxidants.

Subsequently, in a much larger, randomized, controlled trial involving more than 20,000 men and women with coronary artery disease (CAD) or diabetes, Collins et al.[207] found that the administration of an antioxidant combination (250 mg vitamin C, 600 mg vitamin E, and 20 mg beta-carotene daily) in conjunction with simvastatin did not impair the cholesterol-lowering effects of simvastatin over a 5-year period.

Arad et al.[204] conducted a double-blind, placebo-controlled, randomized clinical trial investigating whether coadministration of conventional lipid-lowering therapy and antioxidants could retard the progression of coronary calcification (as assessed by CT-determined calcium score) and prevent atherosclerotic cardiovascular disease (ASCVD) events. They administered atorvastatin (20 mg daily), vitamin C (1 g daily), and vitamin E (alpha-tocopherol, 1000 U daily), versus matching placebos, to 1005 asymptomatic, apparently healthy men and women age 50 to 70 with coronary calcium scores at or above the 80th percentile for age and gender. Notably, all subjects received concomitant aspirin (81 mg daily). The authors halted the trial prematurely, after more than 4 years, because no statistically significant effect was observed on progression of coronary calcium score. They concluded that the combined treatment "induced substantial and sustained reductions in LDL cholesterol and triglycerides but failed to achieve conventional levels of statistical significance in the reduction of either all ASCVD events or CAD events."

Nutritional Therapeutics, Clinical Concerns, and Adaptations

Physicians prescribing statin therapy for dyslipidemia are advised to ask patients about their intake of vitamin C and other antioxidant nutrients. Monitoring for any adverse impact from high levels of antioxidant intake, including nutrient-rich foods, may be judicious in the event that a niacin-based formulation is used. No scientifically based and clinically useful conclusions have emerged to address the paradox of whether patients should be similarly advised of a potential "risk" from eating fruits and vegetables rich in vitamin C (as well as E and other antioxidants) as part of supporting cardiovascular health. Further research through well-designed, adequately powered, and clinically relevant trials are necessary to investigate these issues more conclusively. In such research the confounding factors of nutrient dose, source, and combination, as well as controlling for and focusing on food sources of antioxidant nutrients, need to be adequately accounted for to produce substantial findings with clinically relevant implications.

Indinavir and Related Protease Inhibitors

Evidence: Indinavir (Crixivan).
Related: Amprenavir (Agenerase), atazanavir (Reyataz), brecanavir, darunavir (Prezista), fosamprenavir (Lexiva), nelfinavir (Viracept), ritonavir (Norvir), saquinavir (Fortovase, Invirase), tipranavir (Aptivus); combination drugs: lopinavir and ritonavir (Aluvia, Kaletra), saquinavir and ritonavir (SQV/RTV).

Interaction Type and Significance

◇◇ **Impaired Drug Absorption and Bioavailability, Precautions Appropriate**
◇◇◇ **Impaired Drug Absorption and Bioavailability, Avoidance Recommended**

Probability:	Evidence Base:
4. Plausible	○ **Preliminary**

Effect and Mechanism of Action

Concomitant administration of ascorbic acid at doses of 1000 mg per day can reduce steady-state plasma concentrations of indinavir.[208]

Research

In a small, prospective, open-label, longitudinal, two-period time series involving seven healthy volunteers, Slain et al.[208] found that daily "high-dose" vitamin C (1000 mg/day) can reduce steady-state plasma concentrations of indinavir. They observed that mean steady-state peak concentration (C_{max}) of indinavir was significantly reduced (20%) after 7 days of vitamin C administration, and that the corresponding mean area under the curve (AUC 0-8 hours) was also significantly decreased

(14%). The mean minimum concentration (C_{min}) of indinavir was 32% lower in the presence of vitamin C, although not to a statistically significant degree. Oral clearance and half-life of indinavir were not significantly different. Notably, with regard to evolving standards of trial design, all "subjects were given a vitamin C content-controlled diet for 1 week before the study began and throughout the study period." Such levels of vitamin C intake are common in the HIV/AIDS patient population based on presumed enhancement of immune function. The authors noted that "subtherapeutic concentrations of antiretroviral agents have been associated with viral resistance and regimen failure" but cautioned that "the clinical significance of our findings remains to be established."[208] No data are yet available regarding lower intakes of ascorbic acid concurrently with indinavir or other protease inhibitors.

Nutritional Therapeutics, Clinical Concerns, and Adaptations

These findings emphasize the need for physicians prescribing antiretroviral drugs to interview patients about treatments from other practitioners, as well as self-prescribed supplements and dietary programs, and to maintain an ongoing inventory of such concomitant factors. Although the research is limited in size, duration, and subject characteristics, its findings suggest that vitamin C used at pharmacological doses can reduce drug concentrations and potentially impair therapeutic efficacy. In cases where continued administration of vitamin C is deemed clinically appropriate or is the established choice of the patient, regular monitoring and dose titration of antiretroviral medications are essential. Well-designed and adequately powered clinical trials are warranted to investigate the potential risks and benefits of such coadministration, as well as compensatory integrative protocols.

Lansoprazole-Amoxicillin-Metronidazole (LAM) Triple-Therapy Regimen

Lansoprazole (Prevacid, Zoton); amoxicillin (Amoxicot, Amoxil, Moxilin, Trimox, Wymox); metronidazole (Dirozyl, Flagyl).

Related: HeliMet (Wyeth; discontinued in United Kingdom August 2005): Lansoprazole (Zoton), clarithromycin (Klaricid), metronidazole.

Interaction Type and Significance

⊕⊕ **Beneficial or Supportive Interaction, with Professional Management**

⊕✗ **Bimodal or Variable Interaction, with Professional Management**

✗✗ **Minimal to Mild Adverse Interaction—Vigilance Necessary**

Probability:
2. Probable

Evidence Base:
◉ Emerging or
○ Preliminary

Effect and Mechanism of Action

Helicobacter pylori infection is recognized as a risk factor for peptic ulcers and gastric lymphoma/adenocarcinoma and an opportunistic pathogen in a compromised gastric environment. Ascorbic acid, the reduced form of vitamin C, is secreted by the normal stomach, supports a healthy gastric environment, including greater resistance to *H. pylori*, and may protect against gastric cancer. Ascorbic acid secretion in the stomach is impaired with increased occurrence of *H. pylori*, particularly as associated with chronic/atrophic gastritis.[209,210] Increased oxidation and a decreased secretion of ascorbic acid have been proposed as mechanisms for *H. pylori* infection and low ascorbic acid levels in gastric juice.[211]

Eradication of *H. pylori* using the lansoprazole-amoxicillin-metronidazole (LAM) triple therapy regimen enhances gastric vitamin C levels and recovery from gastritis.[209,211,212]

However, administration of ascorbic acid alone does not appear to eradicate *H. pylori* effectively or reduce gastric inflammation and may impair the therapeutic efficacy of triple therapy if coadministered, particularly against a metronidazole-susceptible strain of infection.[213]

Research

Several studies have found that successful treatment of *H. pylori* using LAM triple therapy correlates with restoration of normal ascorbic acid levels in gastric juice. Sobala et al.[209] investigated gastric juice ascorbic acid concentrations in patients participating in trials of *H. pylori* eradication for duodenal ulcer disease and intestinal metaplasia before and up to 15 months after attempted eradication. In 12 patients in whom *H. pylori* was successfully eradicated, they found that gastric juice ascorbate and total vitamin C concentrations and the ratio of gastric secretion to plasma vitamin C increased after treatment, with the increase greatest in subjects with high final plasma vitamin C concentrations. In contrast, in 22 subjects in whom *H. pylori* eradication failed, there were "no significant changes in juice or plasma concentrations after treatment." The authors concluded that "successful eradication of *H. pylori* improves secretion of vitamin C into gastric juice" and suggested that such an environment in the stomach enhanced protection against gastric cancer.

Subsequently, in a study involving 70 patients with *H. pylori*–associated gastritis before and after therapy, Ruiz et al.[211] reported that among patients who experienced reduction of gastric pH, "gastric juice ascorbic acid increased significantly after *H. pylori* clearance." They also observed that such benefical changes paralleled "improvement of the compromise of the gastric epithelium, reduction of the proportion of vitamin C composed by dehydroascorbic acid, and increase of the gastric juice/plasma vitamin C concentration gradient." Notably, in a manner consistent with an influential role of oxidative stress, they observed that "smokers had lower vitamin C concentrations in plasma and gastric juice before and after *H. pylori* clearance than nonsmokers."

Rokkas et al.[212] investigated gastric juice and plasma vitamin C levels in 88 dyspeptic patients, 58 of whom were *H. pylori* positive, before and after attempted eradication with LAM triple therapy. Before intervention, they observed that gastric juice vitamin C levels were statistically lower in *H. pylori*–positive patients than in the *H. pylori*–negative patients. Gastric juice vitamin C levels increased significantly in the 45 patients (77.6%) for whom triple therapy achieved eradication of *H. pylori*, reaching levels comparable to those among the 30 *H. pylori*–negative subjects. Moreover, these patients demonstrated a "significant... improvement of gastritis after eradication, which paralleled the elevation of gastric juice vitamin C levels." In contrast, they observed "no difference... in plasma vitamin C levels between *H. pylori*–negative and –positive patients or in the latter before and after *H. pylori* treatment." Thus, effective elimination of *H. pylori* using LAM triple therapy facilitated the restoration of normal levels of vitamin C secretion as part of successful treatment of dyspepsia and gastric pathology.

No research has been conducted to determine if increased intake and elevated blood levels of vitamin C might prevent initial *H. pylori* infection, which often occurs during childhood, and reduce risk of peptic ulcers and stomach cancer. Nevertheless, using data from a random sample of almost 7000 American adults collected during the first phase of the Third National Health and Nutrition Examination Survey (NHANES-III), researchers have found that, after accounting for age, ethnicity, weight, and other factors, among white participants, those with the highest serum levels of ascorbic acid had a 25% lower prevalence of infection.[214] Thus, individuals with higher levels of vitamin C may have greater advantage in preventing *H. pylori* infection, peptic ulcers, and stomach cancer.

Although eradication of *H. pylori* using LAM triple therapy or other medications may enhance gastric vitamin C status and healthy stomach function, the concomitant administration of vitamin C may detract from therapeutic efficacy in recovery from *H. pylori* infection. In a trial involving 210 *H. pylori*–positive patients, Kockar et al.[215] compared the effect of several treatment regimes alone and in various combinations over 14 days in seven treatment groups (each with 30 patients). Of those receiving the standard treatment (lansaprasol 30 mg twice daily, clarithromycin 500 mg twice daily, amoxicillin 1 g twice daily), 20 (66%) achieved eradication. In contrast, 15 (50%) of those receiving ascorbic acid (1000 mg/day) in addition to the standard treatment achieved eradication, and only three (10%) did so among subjects treated only with ascorbic acid (1000 mg/day). The following year, in a randomized trial involving a total of 104 *H. pylori*–infected patients, Chuang et al.[213] compared the effects of LAM twice daily for 1 week versus LAM plus vitamin C (250 mg) and vitamin E (200 mg) twice daily for 1 week, followed immediately by vitamin C and E once daily for 6 consecutive weeks. Eight weeks after the completion of triple therapy, they assessed the patients for the effectiveness of *H. pylori* eradication and the histological severity of gastric inflammation. Intention-to-treat and per-protocol eradication rates in the LAM-plus-vitamin group were significantly lower (40% and 44%, respectively) than in the triple-only group (59.1% and 64.4%, respectively). Among patients infected with metronidazole-susceptible isolates, the LAM-only group had a higher intention-to-treat eradication rate than those in the LAM-plus-vitamin group (80% vs. 53.1%). However, the intention-to-treat eradication rates between the two groups were no different for the metronidazole resistance isolates. No significant differences in gastric inflammation were observed. The authors concluded that combining vitamin C and E with triple therapy failed to improve the *H. pylori* eradication rate and gastric inflammation and apparently reduced the eradication rate of triple therapy in patients with metronidazole-susceptible strain infection.

Nutritional Therapeutics, Clinical Concerns, and Adaptations

Physicians are advised to recommend that individuals increase their consumption of vitamin C–rich foods as a means of reducing risk of *H. pylori* infection and as a possible means of mitigating the effects of infection in those with gastric disease who test positive for *H. pylori*. However, patients should be further advised to eliminate high-dose vitamin C intake while being treated with LAM triple therapy, to avoid any potential interference with the efficacy of the medication. It is known that low gastric pH is protective of *H. pylori*, which is why proton pump inhibitors to achieve neutral gastric pH are combined with antibiotics. From this preliminary research, prudence would suggest that ascorbic acid (and perhaps other organic acids capable of lowering intragastric pH) should be avoided during anti–*H. pylori* therapy. Related research indicates that coadministration of probiotic flora to restore gut ecology can enhance clinical outcomes.[216]

Carbidopa (Lodosyn), levodopa (L-dopa; Dopar, Larodopa); combination drugs: levodopa and benserazide (co-beneldopa; Madopar); levodopa and carbidopa (Atamet, Parcopa, Sinemet, Sinemet CR); levodopa, carbidopa, and entacapone (Stalevo).

Interaction Type and Significance

⊕⊕　**Beneficial or Supportive Interaction, with Professional Management**

☼　**Prevention or Reduction of Drug Adverse Effect**

◇≈≈　**Drug-Induced Adverse Effect on Nutrient Function, Coadministration Therapeutic, with Professional Management**

⊕✗　**Bimodal or Variable Interaction, with Professional Management**

✗✗　**Minimal to Mild Adverse Interaction—Vigilance Necessary**

Probability:	Evidence Base:
3. Possible or	⊙ **Emerging**
2. Probable	

Effect and Mechanism of Action

Oxidative stress appears to play a significant role in the pathogenesis of Parkinson's disease (PD), and levodopa monotherapy may aggravate that stressor.[217-219] Individuals with PD tend to exhibit elevated levels of oxidative stress. However, L-dopa undergoes autoxidation (as does dopamine), thus generating reactive oxygen species and decreasing plasma antioxidants, and thereby contributes to levodopa-induced neurotoxicity.[220-222] In contrast, dopamine agonists act through several antioxidant mechanisms that confer neuroprotective effects, including slowing dopamine neuron degeneration and their influence on the nigrostriatal synthesis and release and turnover of dopamine.[223] Vitamin C and deprenyl are both effective in preventing the levodopa-induced inhibition of complex I activity, one of the enzymatic units of the mitochondrial respiratory chain, as demonstrated in different tissues from patients with PD.[224]

Ascorbic acid is a cofactor required in both adrenal steroidogenesis and catecholamine biosynthesis for conversion of dopamine to norepinephrine by dopamine beta-hydroxylase.[152,225] Vitamin C does not cross the blood-brain barrier but does enter the cerebrospinal fluid and can be found there in concentrations proportional to dietary intake.[226-228] Vitamin C is a highly effective antioxidant and, as such, has a particular affinity for hydroxyl radicals. Because hydroxyl radicals are considered especially significant in destruction of dopamine-producing cells in the substantia nigra, vitamin C may play an especially important role in preventing and slowing the progression of PD.

Most patients with PD are elderly and may experience difficulty with levodopa absorption because of the adverse effects of aging on the drug absorption processes. However, ascorbic acid can improve levodopa absorption, particularly in elderly PD patients with poor levodopa bioavailability. Consequently, coadministration of ascorbic acid with levodopa can enable reduction of levodopa dosage without diminishing its effectiveness.[229]

Research

Fahn[218,218a] found that Parkinson's disease patients administered "high-dosage" vitamin C and synthetic alpha-tocopherol

(3000 mg and 3200 IU daily, respectively) delayed the progression of their disease to the point where they needed L-dopa 2½ years later than subjects without nutrient support.

In an unblinded, uncontrolled clinical trial, Linazasoro and Gorospe[230] prescribed a solution of levodopa-carbidopa and ascorbic acid to 21 parkinsonian patients with motor complications. "Eight patients continued the treatment for a mean period of 16.8 months, experiencing substantial increases in the number of hours with good functional capacity." In particular, troublesome symptoms "such as dystonia and akathisia in 'off' periods disappeared in all cases in which they had been present," and the combined treatment was tolerated (i.e., in six of eight subjects who continued in the study and in four who ceased treatment late in the study). Furthermore, subjects reported substantial increases in the number of hours with good functional capacity and a reduction in "intake of other anti-Parkinsonian drugs." However, 13 patients (62%) "abandoned the study, citing exacerbation of biphasic dyskinesia as the main reason." These investigators concluded that the combination of levodopa-carbidopa and ascorbic acid "is a useful therapy in some Parkinsonian patients whose motor complications are not managed with conventional drug treatment" but cautioned that pretreatment screening "is probably of utmost importance" to ensure that this approach is not administered to patients with "intense biphasic dyskinesia."[230]

Buhmann et al.[223] studied markers of systemic oxidative stress and levels of hydrophilic and lipophilic antioxidants in plasma and cerebrospinal fluid (CSF) and investigated the influence of levodopa and dopamine agonist therapy on the oxidative status in patients with PD. When they compared samples from PD patients, patients with other neurological diseases (OND), and healthy controls they observed "increased oxidative stress, seen as higher levels of lipoprotein oxidation in plasma and CSF, decrease of plasma levels of protein sulfhydryl (SH) groups and lower CSF levels of alpha-tocopherol in PD patients compared to OND patients and controls." Furthermore, they found that, although levodopa treatment did not significantly change the plasma lipoprotein oxidation, levodopa "monotherapy tended to result in an increase of autooxidation and in a decrease of plasma antioxidants with significance for ubiquinol-10" (coenzyme Q10). In contrast, dopamine agonist therapy monotherapy was "significantly associated with higher alpha-tocopherol levels," and patients with dopamine agonist monotherapy or comedication with dopamine agonist exhibited "a trend to lower lipoprotein oxidation." Overall, these researchers concluded that their data supported "the concept of oxidative stress as a factor in the pathogenesis" of PD and "might be an indicator of a potential prooxidative role" of levodopa and a "possible antioxidative effect of dopamine agonists" in the treatment of PD.[223]

In a clinical trial involving sixty-seven elderly patients with PD, Nagayama et al.[229] compared various pharmokinetic parameters in plasma drug concentrations following ingestion of a tablet containing 100 mg levodopa (LD) and 10 mg carbidopa, with and without concomitant ascorbic acid (200 mg). They observed "significant increases" in AUC and C_{max} and a "significant reduction" in time to c_{max} (T_{max}) with addition of ascorbic acid in 25 patients with baseline AUC of 2500 ng/hour/mL or greater. The authors concluded that ascorbic acid "can improve LD absorption in elderly PD patients with poor LD bioavailability," and that levodopa therapy in combination with ascorbic acid "may be one of the strategies for PD treatment."

These emerging findings suggest that continued research through well-designed and adequately powered clinical trials is warranted to determine safety, efficacy, and predictors of patient suitability, as well as the benefits of combined application of coenzyme Q10, glutathione (parenteral), alpha-lipoic acid, tocopherols/tocotrienols, and other potentially synergistic antioxidant nutrients.

Reports

Numerous unqualified case reports have suggested that high-dose ascorbic acid may reduce adverse effects of levodopa therapy, including nausea or malcoordination. In a letter (1975), Sacks and Simpson[231] described a patient, previously unable to tolerate L-dopa because of severe nausea, whose condition greatly improved when ascorbic acid was coadministered. Subsequently, his condition rapidly deteriorated each time he received a placebo instead of vitamin C.

Nutritional Therapeutics, Clinical Concerns, and Adaptations

Physicians prescribing antiparkinsonian drugs can reasonably consider the potential benefits of ascorbic acid coadministration as part of their therapeutic strategy. Advising patients to increase their intake of vitamin C and related antioxidants, in nutrient-rich foods or as combination nutrient formulations, may reduce risk or delay onset of Parkinson's disease, although conclusive evidence is still lacking. Limited evidence indicates that certain individuals may benefit from combining vitamin C at moderate doses (200-400 mg/day orally), along with coenzyme Q10 and vitamin B6, with levodopa-carbidopa therapy. The effects of such nutrient support include improved drug absorption and reductions in nausea, malcoordination, and other common adverse effects associated with antiparkinsonian drugs. Such an integrative approach may be particularly indicated in patients whose motor symptoms are recalcitrant to standard drug therapy. However, careful evaluation of patient suitability and close supervision are warranted because certain individuals may experience exacerbation of biphasic ("on/off" phenomena) dyskinesia. Notably, ascorbic acid is sometimes used clinically in the treatment of levodopa toxicity.

Methotrexate

Methotrexate (Folex, Maxtrex, Rheumatrex).
See also Chemotherapy and Radiotherapy.

Interaction Type and Significance

☼ **Prevention or Reduction of Drug Adverse Effect**

Probability:	Evidence Base:
4. Plausible	○ Preliminary

Effect and Mechanism of Action

See Chemotherapy section.

Reports

Sketris et al.[232] reported the case of a female patient being treated for breast cancer with methotrexate and cyclophosphamide, but also taking propranolol, amitriptyline, perphenazine, and prochlorperazine. The patient experienced relief from the nausea caused by the cytotoxic therapy with the concurrent ingestion of 1 to 3 g of vitamin C daily. The authors noted that this nutrient coadministration produced little effect on the urinary excretion of methotrexate.

Nutritional Therapeutics, Clinical Concerns, and Adaptations

Coadministration of vitamin C with methotrexate (and cyclophosphamide) may potentially moderate adverse effects of this chemotherapeutic agent without diminishing its therapeutic activity. However, the limited character of the available data on this specific interaction and the complexity of the broader interactions between antioxidants and chemotherapy render a generalized conclusion premature.

Nitroglycerin and Related Nitrates

Nitroglycerin (glyceryl trinitrate, GTN; Deponit, Minitran, Nitrek, Nitro-Bid, Nitro-Dur, Nitro-Time, Nitrodisc, Nitrogard, Nitroglyn, Nitrolingual, Nitrol, Nitrostat, Transderm-Nitro, Tridil), Isosorbide Dinitrate (ISDN, Isordil, Sorbitrate); combination drug: hydralazine and isosorbide dinitrate (BiDil); isosorbide mononitrate (Imdur, ISMN, ISMO, Isotrate, Monoket).

Interaction Type and Significance
☼ **Beneficial or Supportive Interaction, with Professional Management**

Probability: Evidence Base:
2. Probable   ◉ Emerging

Effect and Mechanism of Action
Organic nitrates have been used widely in conventional practice for the treatment of both coronary artery disease (CAD) and congestive heart failure (CHF), but the tendency of many individuals to build up tolerance to nitrates is an important factor limiting their clinical effectiveness. Nitroglycerin and the other organic nitrates are prodrugs that appear to undergo a biotransformation process to yield nitric oxide (NO) or some NO adjunct as their vasoactive metabolite. While providing clear benefits in acute care, nitrate tolerance develops, and these medications rapidly lose some of their hemodynamic activity and clinical effectiveness when applied as sustained therapy. Numerous investigations and ongoing debate have produced no conclusive knowledge of the mechanism(s) underlying nitrate tolerance. However, coadministration of vitamin C with nitroglycerin can help maintain the nitroglycerin-induced dilation response and changes in the orthostatic blood pressure by one or more possible mechanisms.

Increased formation of superoxide radicals may play a significant role in the development of nitrate tolerance in certain patients. Coadministration of vitamin C may help reduce or eliminate vascular tolerance and help maintain the nitroglycerin-induced changes in the orthostatic blood pressure during long-term nitrate therapy. Some evidence indicates that antioxidant activity and free-radical scavenging produces this beneficial effect, but other data suggest that oxidative stress is not a critical contributor to nitrate tolerance and that tolerance reduction by vitamin C may be caused by "a stabilizing effect on enzymes involved in the bioconversion" of glyceryl trinitrate (GTN) to NO.[233-236] Other research indicates GTN tolerance is "a metabolic syndrome characterized by mitochondrial dysfunction," based on evidence that "nitrate tolerance is mediated, at least in significant part, by inhibition of vascular ALDH-2 [aldehyde dehydrogenase] and that mitochondrial ROS [reactive oxygen species] contribute to this inhibition."[237]

Research
Using continuous IV infusion in a canine model in 1996, Bassenge and Fink[233] administered nitroglycerin (GTN 1.5 μg/kg/min), alone or in combination with ascorbate (55 μg/kg/min), as an antioxidant, for 5 days while monitoring hemodynamic parameters and measuring ex vivo platelet function. With GTN alone, they observed both an initial maximal coronary dilator response and a fall of left ventricular end-diastolic pressure (LVEDP), which "declined progressively and disappeared during the infusion period," and "a progressive, unexpected upregulation of platelet activity demonstrated by enhanced thrombin-stimulated intracellular Ca^{++} levels and increases in the microviscosity of platelet membranes (indicating enhanced receptor expression) associated with a progressive impairment in basal, unstimulated cGMP levels." In contrast, with the combination of GTN and ascorbate as antioxidant, "the dilator responses were maintained fully throughout the infusion period," and adverse changes in platelet activity and microviscosity of platelet membranes were "prevented completely." Based on these findings, the authors concluded that "vascular tolerance is closely reflected by simultaneous changes in platelet function and further, that both can be prevented completely by appropriate antioxidants such as ascorbate."

In 1998, Bassenge et al.[234] conducted an experiment in which they monitored hemodynamic effects and tolerance development in nine healthy subjects randomly administered transdermal GTN (0.4 mg/hour), oral vitamin C (500 mg), or the combination, three times daily for 3 days. With GTN alone, they observed "an immediate rise in arterial conductivity (a/b ratio of dicrotic pulse), but within 2 d of initiating GTN, the a/b ratio progressively decreased and reached basal levels," followed by "a progressive loss of the orthostatic decrease in blood pressure." In contrast, "coadministration of Vit-C and GTN fully maintained the GTN-induced changes in the orthostatic blood pressure, and the rise of a/b ratio was augmented by 310% for the duration of the test period." Furthermore, changes in "vascular tolerance in GTN-treated subjects were paralleled by upregulation of the activity of isolated platelets, which was also reversed by Vit-C administration." The authors concluded that these findings demonstrate that coadministration of vitamin C "eliminates vascular tolerance and concomitant upregulation of ex vivo-washed platelet activity during long-term nonintermittent administration of GTN in humans."[234]

Subsequently, Watanabe et al.[235] reported similar findings in two small trials focused on patients with established cardiovascular disease. They found that coadministration of oral vitamin C (2 g three times daily) with nitroglycerin prevented attenuation of development of nitrate tolerance in a randomized, double-blind, placebo-controlled trial involving 24 healthy volunteers and equal number of patients with ischemic heart disease.[238] They also demonstrated the preventive effect of ascorbate on the nitrate tolerance in another randomized, double-blind, placebo-controlled study involving 20 patients with CHF.

An in vitro experiment conducted by Hinz and Schroder,[236] however, suggests that the ability of vitamin C to attenuate nitrate tolerance occurs, at least in part, independently of its antioxidant effects. First, using LLC-PK1 kidney epithelial cells, they observed that a 5-hour "pretreatment with glyceryl trinitrate (GTN) resulted in substantial desensitization of the intracellular cyclic GMP response to a subsequent 10-min challenge with GTN (1 microM)." They noted that "GTN-tolerant cells were fully sensitive to the spontaneous nitric oxide (NO) donor spermine NONOate, which does not require enzymatic bioactivation." In contrast, cyclic GMP stimulation by GTN was "up to 3.1-fold higher when vitamin C (1-10 mM) was present during the pretreatment period." However, they also noted that "other oxygen radical scavengers such as tiron or dimethylsulfoxide and the NO scavenger PTIO left tolerance induction unaltered." The authors concluded that these collective data "suggest that reactive oxygen species or NO do not contribute to the development of nitrate tolerance" and proposed that reduction of nitrate tolerance by vitamin C "may be due to a stabilizing effect on enzymes involved in the bioconversion of GTN to NO."

Subsequently, however, other research data have suggested, and evidence from an experiment using an in vivo model of nitrate tolerance supports the hypothesis, that the denitrification of organic nitrates is mediated by mitochondrial aldehyde dehydrogenase (ALDH) and that dysfunction of this enzyme is an important cause of tolerance. In particular, using a rat model, Sydow et al.[237] have observed that GTN infusions "were accompanied by decreases in vascular ALDH-2 activity, GTN biotransformation, and cGMP-dependent kinase (cGK-I) activity." In a related in vitro experiment using cultured endothelial cells, they demonstrated that "GTN increased the production of reactive oxygen species (ROS) by mitochondria,... these increases were associated with impaired relaxation to acetylcholine, [and] antioxidants/reductants decreased mitochondrial ROS production and restored ALDH-2 activity." Based on these multiple findings, the authors suggested that "nitrate tolerance is mediated, at least in significant part, by inhibition of vascular ALDH-2 and that mitochondrial ROS contribute to this inhibition," and therefore, "GTN tolerance may be viewed as a metabolic syndrome characterized by mitochondrial dysfunction," which ascorbate is capable of preventing. Certain other compounds with antioxidant activity appear not to be able to do this, although as yet there has been no comprehensive evaluation of the important nutritional antioxidants. There are some hints of mechanisms involved in ascorbate's GTN tolerance prevention, but this remains somewhat unclear.

Nutritional Therapeutics, Clinical Concerns, and Adaptations

Physicians prescribing organic nitrates for more than acute therapy are advised to consider coadministration of ascorbic acid at a clinically effective dose, such as 400 to 800 mg three times daily or more, as a means of enhancing the therapeutic effectiveness of nitrate therapy by preventing nitrate tolerance, as well as providing other potential benefits in reducing cardiovascular risk, such as prevention of platelet activation by chronic nitrate administration. In acute situations, IV ascorbic acid may be indicated to optimize nitrate intervention and prevent the onset of nitrate tolerance; close monitoring and supervision by clinicians experienced in such interventions are essential to safety and therapeutic efficacy.

Despite limitations and apparent contradictions in scientific knowledge of the mechanisms involved in nitrate tolerance and vitamin C's ability to attenuate such developments, the available scientific literature tentatively supports the use of vitamin C during nitrate therapy as a means of attenuating such problematic developments. Moreover, although data showing possible or probable benefits are preliminary in many respects, no evidence yet suggests any adverse effects or impairment of drug activity from such concomitant therapy.

In patients requiring nitrate therapy for a sustained period, a comprehensive, evolving, and individualized therapeutic strategy is essential. Physicians prescribing long-acting nitroglycerin often advise patients to refrain from nitroglycerin for 10 to 12 hours each day as a means of reducing the tendency to nitrate tolerance. Furthermore, coadministration of L-arginine (substrate for nitric oxide synthase) and folic acid may also inhibit development of nitrate tolerance, although preliminary clinical trial evidence suggesting worse outcomes in post–

myocardial infarction (MI) patients with L-arginine would argue against its use in this setting, pending larger and longer randomized clinical trials. The appropriateness of antioxidants in such an integrative strategy is controversial because the role of oxidative stress in cardiovascular disease in general and nitrate tolerance in particular remains unclear and the clinical application of antioxidants contentious. Further research through well-designed and adequately powered clinical trials is clearly warranted and strongly recommended.

Oral Contraceptives: Monophasic, Biphasic, and Triphasic Estrogen Preparations (Synthetic Estrogen and Progesterone Analogs)

Ethinyl estradiol and desogestrel (Desogen, Ortho-TriCyclen).
Ethinyl estradiol and ethynodiol (Demulen 1/35, Demulen 1/50, Nelulen 1/25, Nelulen 1/50, Zovia).
Ethinyl estradiol and levonorgestrel (Alesse, Levlen, Levlite, Levora 0.15/30, Nordette, Tri-Levlen, Triphasil, Trivora).
Ethinyl estradiol and norethindrone/norethisterone (Brevicon, Estrostep, Genora 1/35, GenCep. 1/35, Jenest-28, Loestrin 1.5/30, Loestrin1/20, Modicon, Necon 1/25, Necon 10/11, Necon 0.5/30, Necon 1/50, Nelova 1/35, Nelova 10/11, Norinyl 1/35, Norlestin 1/50, Ortho Novum 1/35, Ortho Novum 10/11, Ortho Novum 7/7/7, Ovcon-35, Ovcon-50, Tri-Norinyl, Trinovum).
Ethinyl estradiol and norgestrel (Lo/Ovral, Ovral).
Mestranol and norethindrone (Genora 1/50, Nelova 1/50, Norethin 1/50, Ortho-Novum 1/50).
Related, internal application: Etonogestrel/ethinyl estradiol vaginal ring (Nuvaring).

Interaction Type and Significance

≈≈≈ **Drug-Induced Nutrient Depletion, Supplementation Therapeutic, Not Requiring Professional Management**

✗ **Potential or Theoretical Adverse Interaction of Uncertain Severity**

Nutrient Depletion Probability:	Evidence Base:
3. Possible	▽ Mixed
	○ Emerging

Nutrient Interference Probability:	Evidence Base:
4. Plausible,	▽ Mixed,
5. Improbable	○ Emerging

Effect and Mechanism of Action

In a review of this possible interaction, Stockley[239] concludes that no mechanism has been established. Nevertheless, numerous hypotheses have been proposed over the past 30 years. Oral contraceptives (OCs) may cause increased ascorbic acid turnover in tissues and reduce plasma, leukocyte, and platelet ascorbic acid levels.[240-242] Conversely, ascorbic acid (in gram doses) may elevate plasma levels of ethinyl estradiol by interfering with the conjugation of ethinyl estradiol to its sulfate for excretion, but other evidence indicates that high-dose vitamin C does not interfere with the pharmacokinetics of ethinyl estradiol.[243-245] Paradoxically, multivitamins, including vitamin C, may play a role in incidents of contraceptive failure or breakthrough bleeding.[243,246,247] In such instances, ascorbic acid could theoretically cause elevated blood concentrations of ethinyl estradiol resulting from competition for sulfation; in contrast, "progestogens are only metabolised in the liver and have no significant enterohepatic recirculation."[248]

Research

The scientific data concerning interactions between OCs and vitamin C are limited, diverse, inconsistent and contentious. Overall, OCs may lower vitamin C levels in plasma and white blood cells (WBCs), whereas ascorbic acid may (or may not) elevate serum ethinyl estradiol levels.[239] However, changes in OC formulations over the past several decades, the use of vitamin C in conjunction with other nutrients, and the diverse characteristics of the patient populations render much of the available information obsolete or inappropriate for deriving valid generalizations. Moreover, the preponderance of unqualified case reports, the small size of the few relevant clinical trials, and the lack of any substantive evidence as to mechanisms involved collectively fail to provide a coherent body of findings of adequate quality to enable anything other than a cursory review of the scientific literature.

Numerous studies conducted in the mid-1970s produced findings indicating that OCs can adversely affect levels and functions of several key nutrients, including vitamin C. These original papers led to an extended reiteration of such conclusions in numerous editorials and reviews. In particular, researchers described lowered levels of ascorbic acid in plasma, leukocytes, and platelets in women using estrogen-containing OCs.[240-242,249-254]

Oral contraceptives can increase requirements of several key nutrients, including vitamin C, and may induce nutrient depletions in certain women, especially those with compromised nutrient intake or metabolic stressors. Based on research of OC effects on ascorbic acid metabolism in rhesus monkeys, Weininger and King[242] proposed that the observed reduction could be caused by increased ascorbic acid turnover in tissues. In a study involving 10 healthy young women who had taken OCs of the combined type for several cycles, Briggs and Briggs[255] initially observed "plasma concentrations of ascorbic acid and vitamin B_{12} below the range seen in a matched group of untreated women," whereas red blood cell (RBC) aspartate transaminase (AST) and glutathione reductase (GTR) "were less saturated by their essential co-factors." However, daily administration of "a high-potency vitamin B complex with vitamin C... restored all four biochemical indices of vitamin nutrition to the normal ranges." In a 1974 letter regarding a study by Sanpitak and Chayutimonkul[256] on OCs and riboflavin nutriture, Briggs[257] noted that the data showed "striking decreases in women taking oral contraceptives in all the water-soluble vitamins (C, B_{12}, riboflavine, B_6), no change in vitamin E, but an increase in plasma-retinol." In a subsequent prospective trial involving five lactating women, Cummings[258] found "little change in plasma ascorbic acid but a slight, nonsignificant, decrease in [breast] milk ascorbic acid levels," which was "promptly" corrected on initiation of supplementation with ascorbic acid.

In contrast, other researchers have produced findings indicating a lack of adverse effect of OCs on vitamin C, although in many cases, depletion of or adverse effects on other nutrients were confirmed. Prasad et al.[259] reported that plasma ascorbate levels were not affected by OC use. Subsequently, Mooij et al.[260] observed a similar pattern of depletion when they investigated the effects of OCs containing 30 μg of ethinyl estradiol on concentrations of several nutrients in serum and RBCs of 59 nonpregnant female volunteers, 28 of whom were taking OCs, for four cycles. Although "vitamin A levels were significantly higher and vitamin B_{12} levels were significantly lower in the group using OC,...comparison of the baseline values of vitamin total B_2, FAD, C, serum and red blood cell folate as determined on days 3 and 23 of the first cycle of the two groups compared revealed no significant differences." However, whereas "multivitamin and folic acid supplementation did not affect the concentrations of vitamin A and vitamin B_{12} with either group,... all other vitamins increased significantly" in both OC and control groups.

Effects inherently vary based on a woman's dietary intake, nutrigenomic makeup, and metabolic stressors, including nutrient depletion due to diet, lifestyle, and concomitant drug therapies. Thus, for example, Veninga[261] reported, "Among patients who are well nourished and nonsmokers, OC use does not appear to jeopardize vitamin C levels." As with other vitamins affected by OCs, biochemical deficiencies caused by the exogenous hormones may not manifest in any form easily ascertained by standard clinical parameters. In such cases, repletion of nutrient status through supplementation or enhanced dietary intake may produce beneficial effects even in the absence of overt clinical deficiency symptoms, as can occur with vitamin B_6. Nevertheless, opinions in clinical trials, editorials, and reviews range in their conclusions from recommendations for universal prophylactic multinutrient treatment with OC use to warnings that such nutritional support is unjustified or even potentially dangerous.[247,262]

Preliminary data suggesting a potential adverse effect on bioavailability of OCs has not borne up to deeper investigation. For example, Morris et al.[243] reported that oral intake of 1 g ascorbic acid substantially raised serum ethinyl estradiol levels (48% elevation at 24 hours) in women using OCs. However, in a definitive study of the influence of vitamin C on pharmacokinetics of ethinyl estradiol, Zamah et al.[244] found no effect of high vitamin C dosage on the systemic availability of ethinyl estradiol in women using a combination OC. In a blinded, randomized trial, 37 women using a combination monophasic OC (30 μg EE2 and 150 μg levonorgestrel) were administered concomitant daily doses of 1 g ascorbic acid, taken ½ hour before OC intake, during the first or second cycle of OC use, for two consecutive cycles. Using blood samples drawn 11 times over 12 hours on the first and fifteenth day of OC intake, they measured levels and calculated C_{max} and AUC (0-12 hours) of ascorbic acid, free and sulfated ethinyl estradiol, and a number of other parameters. Only 6-hour postintake samples were obtained on pill days 10 and 21. "No effect of ascorbic acid was observed" when "C_{max} and AUC values for EE2 and EE2-sulfate in cycles with and without ascorbic acid were evaluated statistically for days one and fifteen and the ratios of day 15/day 1 for each of the substances." They noted that only on day 15 "was there a significantly lower AUC for EE2-sulfate in the presence of ascorbic acid intake." These researchers interpreted the findings as demonstrating that "competition between ascorbic acid and EE2 for sulfation does not lead to an increased systemic availability of EE2 and is, therefore, unlikely to be of any clinical importance." They concluded: "Ascorbic acid can, therefore, be removed from the list of drugs interfering with the pharmacokinetics of ethinyl estradiol."[244]

Subsequently, in a study involving American women, Kuhnz, Zamah, et al.[245] reported the absence of an effect of high oral doses of vitamin C on the systemic availability of ethinyl estradiol in women using a levonorgestrel-containing (LNG) combination OC. They reported that "no effect of vitamin C was observed for any of the parameters investigated," concluding that "repeated oral administration of gram quantities of vitamin C does not impair the sulfation of hydroxylated metabolites of LNG." Furthermore, they noted "no observable effect on the serum protein binding of LNG and the concentrations" of sex hormone–binding globulin (SHBG) and corticosteroid-binding globulin (CBG) in the serum. In a review, Shenfield[248] proposed that differences in the way OC formulations interact with diverse agents derives from ethinyl estradiol being "sulphated in the gut wall, hydroxylated and glucuronidated in the liver, and undergoes enterohepatic recirculation" while the "progestogens are only metabolised in the liver and have no significant enterohepatic recirculation."

For many years, clinicians, researchers, and patients have sought to determine whether the occurrence of cervical dysplasia might be associated with exogenous estrogens, particularly OCs, and nutrient intake, including vitamin C. In a case-control study involving 257 women with confirmed cervical dysplasia and 133 controls, Liu et al.[263] assessed dietary intake of various nutrients and risk factors. They found no significant correlation with OC use or other presumed risk factors, even after adjusting for their potential confounding effects. However, along with vitamin A, folate, and riboflavin, they did observe an increased risk for lower intakes of vitamin C compared with the highest intake level.

In unrelated but potentially relevant research, Huang et al.[264] found that low concentrations of 17β-estradiol, close to physiological levels, reduced oxidative modification of LDLs in the presence of vitamin C and vitamin E in vitro. In contrast to this activity of protecting LDLs from oxidation, 17β-estradiol monotherapy demonstrated no antioxidant effect.

Reports

Numerous contradictory and unqualified case reports present a range of potential interactions so broad and diverse as to suggest that the given outcome in any single case is highly individual and strongly influenced by numerous factors, such as diet, drug dose and formulation, health status, lifestyle factors, genetics, and concomitant drug and nutrient intake. No single conclusions can reasonably be drawn from these data.

Some reports suggest that vitamin C may impair the efficacy of OC steroids, leading to breakthrough bleeding and pregnancy. Morris et al.[243] published an unqualified report describing the case of one women taking the triphasic OC Logynon who reported heavy breakthrough bleeding within 2 to 3 days of ceasing her self-prescribed, 1-g daily dose of ascorbic acid. DeSano and Hurley[246] cited multivitamins, including vitamin C, as a contributing factor in contraceptive failure, although no mechanism was proposed or demonstrated.

Nutritional Therapeutics, Clinical Concerns, and Adaptations

Physicians prescribing OCs are advised to consider possible adverse effects associated with such treatment and discuss these potential risks and means of preventing or reversing them with the patient. The available evidence indicates several possible interactions, with permutations ranging from depletion of several key nutrients, including vitamin C, to improbable occurrence of reduced drug efficacy. Dietary intake, tissue nutriture status, metabolic stressors, individual pharmacogenomic variability, and numerous other factors influence the probability and character of any potential interaction. In many cases, an actual interaction may not manifest any clinically significant changes, or such changes may be subclinical, subtle, or simply slow to exhibit obvious effects.

Prophylactic nutritional support may be appropriate for certain individuals, while monitoring over time may elucidate the need for supplementation based on clinical response to OCs. In many patients, nutritional support may relieve symptoms associated with OC use, even though no objective signs of nutrient depletion are evident. In such cases, ascorbic acid in the range of 200 to 500 mg twice daily, along with folic acid,

vitamin B6, and magnesium, can be beneficial in preventing or reversing adverse effects of OCs. More comprehensive clinical assessment is appropriate in individuals who develop premenstrual syndrome or other signs of estrogen accumulation, for whom stronger support of hepatic estrogen conjugation functions may be necessary. Although most evidence indicates that vitamin C supplementation is unlikely to interfere with the intended activity of OCs, it is always prudent to be watchful for any indications that vitamin supplementation might be impairing OC activity.

Propranolol and Related Beta-1-Adrenoceptor Antagonists (Beta-Adrenergic Blocking Agents)

Oral forms (systemic)
Evidence: Propranolol (Betachron, Inderal LA, Innopran XL, Inderal)
Extrapolated: Acebutolol (Sectral), atenolol (Tenormin); combination drugs: atenolol and chlortalidone (Co-Tendione, Tenoretic); atenolol and nifedipine (Beta-Adalat, Tenif); betaxolol (Kerlone), bisoprolol (Zebeta), carteolol (Cartrol), esmolol (Brevibloc), labetalol (Normodyne, Trandate), metoprolol (Lopressor, Toprol XL); combination drug: metoprolol and hydrochlorothiazide (Lopressor HCT); nadolol (Corgard), nebivolol (Nebilet), oxprenolol (Trasicor), penbutolol (Levatol), pindolol (Visken); propranolol combination drug: propranolol and bendrofluazide (Inderex); sotalol (Betapace, Betapace AF, Sorine), timolol (Blocadren).

Interaction Type and Significance

✗✗   **Minimal to Mild Adverse Interaction—Vigilance Necessary**

Probability:	Evidence Base:
4. Plausible and	○ **Preliminary**
5. Improbable	

Effect and Mechanism of Action

Vitamin C may decrease the absorption and first-pass metabolism of propranolol to a minimal degree.

Research

In an experiment involving five healthy subjects, Gonzalez et al.[265] measured plasma concentrations and urinary excretion of propranolol and its metabolites following oral administration of a single 80-mg dose of propranolol with or without ascorbic acid pretreatment (2 g). Compared with controls, they observed that subjects treated concurrently with vitamin C exhibited decreases in maximum plasma concentration (C_{max}) of propranolol (28%), area under the propranolol concentration-time curve (from 0 to 24 hours; 37%), and the total amount of drug recovered in urine (66%). Furthermore, the time to reach C_{max} of propranolol was increased (from 1.9 to 2.7 hours). However, "no change in elimination rate was observed, indicating that ascorbic acid had affected both the absorption process and the first pass metabolism." The heart rate "decreased less when propranolol was administered with ascorbic acid" than in control subjects, but this was considered of "little biological importance." The authors proposed that ascorbic acid impaired both absorption and the metabolic conjugation of the propranolol. Overall, this interaction appears to be of minimal clinical significance.

Clinical Implications and Adaptations

Prudence suggests that physicians prescribing propranolol or related beta-adrenergic blocking agents caution patients to separate oral intake of vitamin C from intake of the medication by at least 2 hours. The available evidence is limited and indicates that any effect that might occur would probably be of minimal clinical significance.

Tetracycline Antibiotics

Demeclocycline (Declomycin), doxycycline (Atridox, Doryx, Doxy, Monodox, Periostat, Vibramycin, Vibra-Tabs), minocycline (Dynacin, Minocin, Vectrin), oxytetracycline (Terramycin), tetracycline (Achromycin, Actisite, Apo-Tetra, Economycin, Novo-Tetra, Nu-Tetra, Sumycin, Tetrachel, Tetracyn); combination drugs: chlortetracycline, demeclocycline, and tetracycline (Deteclo); bismuth, metronidazole, and tetracycline (Helidac).
See also Ampicillin and Related Beta-Lactam Antibiotics in Theoretical, Speculative, and Preliminary Interactions Research.

Interaction Type and Significance

⊕⊕⊕   **Beneficial or Supportive Interaction, Not Requiring Professional Management**
☼   **Prevention or Reduction of Drug Adverse Effect**
≈≈≈   **Drug-Induced Nutrient Depletion, Supplementation Therapeutic, Not Requiring Professional Management**

Probability:	Evidence Base:
4. Plausible	○ Preliminary

Effect and Mechanism of Action

Concomitant intake of vitamin C can enhance bioavailability and elevate blood levels of tetracycline.[266,267]

Prolonged use of tetracycline may reduce blood levels of ascorbic acid and can interfere with the activity of vitamin C as well as folic acid, potassium, and vitamins B_2, B_6, B_{12}, and K, particularly in individuals with digestive pathologies or otherwise compromised health or nutritional status.[268]

Vitamin C may also protect against hepatic and renal toxicity occasionally associated with tetracycline therapy, as well as the much more common adverse effect of dental and oral discoloration.[269-271]

Research

As early as 1957, Freinberg and Lite[266] found that coadministration of 500 mg vitamin C with tetracycline increased blood levels of tetracycline. Similarly, Omray and Varma[267] reported that coadministration of vitamin C (100 mg/day) increased the bioavailability of tetracycline in experiments evaluating the pharmacokinetic parameters of tetracycline hydrochloride in healthy subjects.

Polec et al.[269] observed that ascorbic acid could exert a protective effect against tetracycline-induced nephrotoxicity. Naseer and Alam[270] subsequently reported a similar protective effect of ascorbic acid against nephrotoxicity and hepatotoxicity induced by oxytetracycline.

Nutritional Therapeutics, Clinical Concerns, and Adaptations

Limited evidence suggests that physicians prescribing tetracycline-class antibiotics consider the potential benefits of ascorbic acid coadministration, particularly with extended periods of administration and in patients with compromised nutritional status and hepatic or renal function. Nothing in the available data has been interpreted to suggest a significant probability of any adverse effect with coadministration, whereas the general trend in the literature suggests a supportive and possibly protective effect from concomitant vitamin C. In particular,

prudence suggests that the possible protective effect against the discoloration of children's teeth by tetracycline (a relative contraindication for pediatric use) deserves consideration.

Although controversial, most advocates of vitamin C usage would further, and more fundamentally, recommend high-dose vitamin C for its direct effects on bacterial infection and the immune system. A supplemental (or moderate therapeutic) dose of vitamin C is usually in the range of 2000 to 4000 mg per day, in divided doses, although higher-dosage ascorbic acid therapy is relatively common.

Further research into the safety and efficacy of such purposeful coadministration is warranted, especially given the high incidence of self-prescribed vitamin C dosing during acute illnesses and the associated high probability of unsupervised self-administration.

THEORETICAL, SPECULATIVE, AND PRELIMINARY INTERACTIONS RESEARCH, INCLUDING OVERSTATED INTERACTIONS CLAIMS

Aluminum Hydroxide and Related Aluminum-Containing Antacids

Evidence: Aluminum hydroxide (Alternagel, Amphojel).
Related: Aluminum carbonate gel (Basajel), aluminum magnesium hydroxide sulfate; combination drugs: aluminum hydroxide, magnesium carbonate, alginic acid, and sodium bicarbonate (Gaviscon Extra Strength Tablets, Gaviscon Regular Strength Liquid, Gaviscon Extra Strength Liquid); aluminum hydroxide and magnesium hydroxide (Advanced Formula Di-Gel Tablets, Co-Magaldrox, Di-Gel, Gelusil, Maalox, Maalox Plus, Mylanta, Wingel); aluminum hydroxide, magnesium trisilicate, alginic acid, and sodium bicarbonate (Alenic Alka, Gaviscon Regular Strength Tablets).
See also Cimetidine and Related Histamine (H_2) Antagonists.

A consensus within the scientific literature recognizes that citrate, particularly from citrus juice or calcium citrate, can greatly enhance gastrointestinal (GI) absorption of aluminum from both dietary sources and aluminum-containing antacids, can elevate blood aluminum concentrations, and may lead to retention and increased aluminum concentrations in the liver, brain, and bones.[272-280] The pattern of increased aluminum toxicity from this well-documented interaction with citrate is particularly of concern in patients with renal failure. Notably, calcium citrate without aluminum antacids does not cause aluminum retention in patients with functioning kidneys.[281,282]

Although broadly observed in both humans and experimental animals, the mechanism of this effect of citrate is not well understood, and its extrapolation to ascorbic acid is supported by only limited clinical evidence. The formation of a highly soluble aluminium-citrate complex has been proposed. Nevertheless, there are no functional correlations between ascorbic acid and citric acid, the only two common traits being their presence in citrus fruits and status as organic acids.

In regard to the interaction between ascorbic acid and aluminum hydroxide, the evidence is more limited. In particular, the series of animal and human studies conducted by Domingo, Gomez, et al.[283-285] found that coadministration of vitamin C and aluminum hydroxide can lead to increased aluminum absorption and excretion. In two experiments using a rat model, they observed that among a range of eight acid compounds commonly found as dietary constituents, all eight substances "significantly increased the aluminum concentrations [from drinking water] in most of the tissues [liver, spleen, kidney, brain and bone], with ascorbic and citric acids showing the highest rate of aluminum accumulation."[283] Their primary conclusion was that because of "the wide presence and consumption of the above dietary constituents, in order to prevent aluminum accumulation and toxicity we suggest a drastic limitation of human exposure to aluminum."[284] They also recommended: "Meanwhile, the diet of uremic patients should be carefully monitored."[283] More directly, in an experiment involving 13 healthy volunteers, they observed that oral administration of aluminum hydroxide (900 mg three times daily) along with ascorbic acid (2 g daily) for 3 days produced "a significant increase in urine aluminum excretion, presumably because of enhanced gastrointestinal absorption." Based on these findings, they cautioned against administration of ascorbic acid in patients with renal failure who are taking aluminum-containing antacids.[285]

Evidence thus far suggests that administration of ascorbic acid, possibly even at dietary levels, is inappropriate with the simultaneous use of aluminum-containing antacids and is particularly incompatible in patients with compromised renal function, especially those on dialysis, although probably not as dangerous as citrate. Further human research is warranted to determine parameters of risk in terms of dose of each substance, timing, and patient susceptibility characteristics in this potentially significant interaction. Pending further evidence from well-designed trials, health care professionals should advise healthy individuals to avoid aluminum-based antacids within 2 to 3 hours of food and drink that contain citrates, ascorbic acid, and other organic acids, as in soft drinks. However, the entire question of the necessity and safety of aluminum-containing antacids deserves scrutiny, because their inherent toxicity is ultimately more responsible for the risk in this possible interaction than is the vitamin C (or citrate), whether in food or supplemental form, or its effects on aluminum metabolism. In the meantime, with patients who need antacid therapy, calcium-based or magnesium-based antacids offer safer options within the conventional pharmaceutical repertoire. Notably, aluminum hydroxide has been used in renal failure patients as a phosphate binder but is less effective than calcium carbonate and is associated with aluminum retention, particularly in children and young adults with chronic renal disease, and can lead to aluminum bone disease.

Amphetamines, Mixed

Amphetamine (amphetamine aspartate monohydrate, amphetamine sulfate), dextroamphetamine (dextroamphetamine saccharate, dextroamphetamine sulfate, D-amphetamine; Dexedrine); combination drug, mixed amphetamines: amphetamine and dextroamphetamine (Adderall; dexamphetamine).

Extraploated, based on similar properties: Methylphenidate (Metadate, Methylin, Ritalin, Ritalin-SR; Concerta); modafinil (Provigil), pemoline (Cylert).

The absorption of amphetamines in the gut can be increased by the acidification of the contents in the GI tract. Certain forms of ascorbic acid could theoretically alter the pH in the intestines and increase bioavailability, thus producing elevated drug levels.[286]

Pending substantive research findings, physicians prescribing mixed amphetamines may find it prudent to caution against unsupervised high-dose ascorbic acid intake, and advise patients to ingest vitamin C in supplemental form, and presumably acidic foods, at least 1 hour before or 2 hours after the medication.

Ampicillin, Related Beta-Lactam and Other Antibiotics

Evidence: Ampicillin (Amficot, Omnipen, Principen, Totacillin), aztreonam (Azactam injection), benzyl and procaine penicillin combination (Seclopen), cefotaxime (Claforan), gentamicin (G-mycin, Garamycin, Jenamicin); combination drug: sulfamethoxazole and trimethoprim (cotrimoxazole, co-trimoxazole, SXT, TMP-SMX, TMP-sulfa; Bactrim, Bactrim DS, Cotrim, Septra, Septra DS, Sulfatrim, Uroplus); streptomycin.

Similar properties but evidence indicating no or reduced interaction effects: Chloramphenicol (Chloromycetin).

Cephalosporins: Cefaclor (Ceclor), cefadroxil (Duricef), Cefamandole (Mandol), cefazolin (Ancef, Kefzol), cefdinir (Omnicef), cefepime (Maxipime), cefixime (Suprax), cefoperazone (Cefobid), cefotetan (Cefotan), cefoxitin (Mefoxin), cefpodoxime (Vantin), cefprozil (Cefzil), ceftazidime (Ceptaz, Fortaz, Tazicef, Tazidime), ceftibuten (Cedax), ceftizoxime (Cefizox), ceftriaxone (Rocephin), cefuroxime (Ceftin, Kefurox injection, Zinacef), cephalexin (Keflex, Keftab), cephapirin (Cefadyl), cephradine (Anspor, Velocef), loracarbef (Lorabid), meropenem (Merrem I.V.).

Clindamycin (Cleocin) and related lincosamide-class antibiotics.

Penicillins: Amoxicillin (Amoxil, Trimox); combination drugs: amoxicillin and clavulanate (Augmentin, Augmentin XR, Clavulin, Nuclav); ampicillin combination drug: ampicillin and sulbactam (Betamp, Unasyn), bacampicillin (Spectrobid); carbenicillin (Geocillin), combination drug: clavulanic acid and ticarcillin (Timentin); cloxacillin (Cloxapen), dicloxacillin (Dynapen, Dycill); imipenem combination drug: imipenem and cilastatin (Primaxin I.M., Primaxin I.V.); mezlocillin (Mezlin), nafcillin (Unipen), oxacillin (Bactocill), penicillin G (Bicillin C-R, Bicillin L-A, Pfizerpen), penicillin V (Beepen-VK, Veetids), piperacillin (Pipracil), piperacillin and tazobactam (Zosyn), ticarcillin (Ticar), ticarcillin and clavulanate (Timentin).

See also Tetracycline Antibiotics.

Alabi et al.[287] conducted in vitro experiments showing that a number of antibacterial agents may significantly reduce plasma levels of ascorbic acid: ampicillin, chloramphenicol, cefotaxime, gentamicin, benzyl and procaine penicillin combination (seclopen), co-trimoxazole, and streptomycin, in descending magnitude of effect.

Concomitant use of vitamin C could theoretically enhance antimicrobial activity and support immune response, but research is limited and findings have been preliminary. For example, Shoeb et al.[288] observed that "*Enterobacter cloacae* ATCC 13047 showed increasing susceptibility to ampicillin when incubated anaerobically in the presence of increasing concentrations of ascorbic acid." Under anaerobic growth conditions, "ascorbic acid abrogated the induction of the enzyme [beta-lactamase] completely. On the other hand, the constitutive enzymatic activity was markedly decreased as the bacterium was grown anaerobically."

A series of negative interactions were found by Belicova et al.,[288a] who conducted a series of in vitro experiments investigating effects of ascorbic acid on the antibacterial activity of selected antibiotics and synthetic chemotherapeutic agents by means of spectrophotometric measurements. They found that "ofloxacine, N-succinimidylofloxacine, fleroxacine, tetracycline, 6-thiatetracycline, and doxycycline reacted with ascorbic acid with the development of the superoxide radical (O_2^-)." Further, using Heatley's method, they demonstrated "that in the presence of ascorbic acid the antibacterial effect of substances was decreased by 9.6 to 40.7% and 10.1 to 45.1% in *Staphylococcus aureus* and *Escherichia coli,* respectively." In particular, they noted that "the kinetics of the process of the survival of cells within twenty-four hours demonstrated that a combination of ofloxacine as well as tetracycline with ascorbic acid produced a statistically significant increase in log10 of CFU/ml in *S. aureus* as well as *E. coli*."

In contrast, Cursino et al.[289] subsequently documented a pattern of synergistic interaction between ascorbic acid (AA) and six antibiotics, in vitro, against 12 multidrug-resistant *Pseudomonas aeruginosa* isolates. They observed "synergic activity" with ascorbic acid and chloramphenicol, kanamycin, streptomycin, and tetracycline. "Indifference was observed to any antibiotics and antagonism only for chloramphenicol." The authors concluded that their findings "indicated that multiresistant *P. aeruginosa* was affected by combination of AA and antibiotics" and that continued "research on ascorbic acid–antimicrobial interactions may find new methods to control strains of multiresistant *P. aeruginosa*." The preliminary character and mixed findings of the available data indicate that further research is required before any well-founded conclusions can be made and clinical responses formulated.

Although specific survey data are unavailable, it seems highly probable that self-administration of vitamin C by patients undergoing treatment with antibiotics prescribed by physicians is relatively common practice in the United States, Europe, and elsewhere. The need for well-designed and adequately powered clinical trials investigating the safety and efficacy of such interactions and their permutations is imperative given such unsupervised coadministration. The uncertainties inherent in applying in vitro phenomena to in vivo clinical situations also suggest that placebo-controlled clinical trials involving patients with similar infections treated by the same antibiotics, informed by laboratory observations, would be necessary to formulate any clinically useful conclusions.

Governmental regulatory bodies, such as the U.K. Committee on Safety of Medicines (CSM), recommend that beta-lactam antibiotics be specifically reserved for treatment of verified bacterial infections associated with amoxicillin-resistant beta-lactamase–producing strains, and that treatment normally be limited to 14 days.

Anticonvulsant Medications, Including Phenytoin and Valproic Acid

Evidence: Carbamazepine (Carbatrol, Tegretol), divalproex semisodium, divalproex sodium (Depakote), primidone (Mysoline), sodium valproate (Depacon), valproate semisodium, valproic acid (Depakene, Depakene Syrup).
Extrapolated, based on similar properties: Clonazepam (Klonopin), clorazepate dipotassium (Tranxene), diazepam (Valium), ethosuximide (Zarontin), ethotoin (Peganone), felbamate (Felbatol), fosphenytoin (Cerebyx, Mesantoin), lamotrigine (Lamictal), levetiracetam (Keppra), mephenytoin, methsuximide (Celontin), oxcarbazepine (GP 47680, oxycarbamazepine; Trileptal), phenobarbital (phenobarbitone; Luminol, Solfoton), phensuximide (Milontin), phenytoin (diphenylhydantoin; Dilantin, Phenytek), piracetam (Nootropyl), tiagabine (Gabitril), topiramate (Topamax), trimethadione (Tridione), vigabatrin (Sabril), zonisamide (Zonegran).

Primidone and other antiepileptic drugs (AEDs) may increase urinary excretion of ascorbic acid. Furthermore, the depleting effects of anticonvulsants on folate status could in turn adversely affect vitamin C status because ascorbic acid facilitates the conversion of folic acid to folinic acid, its active form.

Jurima-Romet et al.[290] conducted in vitro experiments demonstrating that vitamin C and vitamin E exerted a cytoprotective effect against 4-ene valproic acid–induced cytotoxicity in glutathione-depleted rat hepatocytes.

Secondary literature occasionally cites research indicating that concomitant use of barbiturates or primidone may increase urinary excretion of ascorbic acid, but substantive human research findings are lacking.[291]

Further research into the potential interaction between anticonvulsant medications and vitamin C is warranted. Pending substantive findings, physicians might find it prudent to prescribe vitamin C, at a modest dose level and with proper monitoring, to patients undergoing AED therapy.

The importance of folic acid during pregnancy is widely known, but equally important is the maintenance of sufficient levels of ascorbic acid and other antioxidant nutrients to prevent DNA damage. Such support is especially critical in women being treated with anticonvulsant therapy because of the drug-induced effects (e.g., reduction in plasma ascorbic acid, retinol, and beta-carotene levels) observed in nonsupplemented women on long-term AED therapy.

Clozapine and Related Atypical Antipsychotics

Clozapine (Chozaril).
Related but evidence lacking for extrapolation: Aripiprazole (Abilify, Abilitat), olanzapine (Symbyax, Zyprexa), quetiapine (Seroquel), risperidone (Risperdal), ziprasidone (Geodon).

Bioactivation of clozapine, a dibenzodiazepine antipsychotic, occurs in several tissues, including the liver, where it is catalyzed by the cytochrome (CYP) P450 enzymes, which results in the formation of both stable and protein-reactive metabolites. During hepatic metabolism of the piperazine ring, *N*-demethylation appears to be performed by CYP1A2, whereas *N*-oxidation and formation of chemically reactive metabolites depend on multiple forms of the CYP450 system.[292]

Agranulocytosis and hepatotoxicity are among the adverse effects uniquely associated with clozapine therapy. The unstable protein-reactive drug metabolites formed through bioactivation, particularly a nitrenium intermediate, have been implicated in this toxicity pattern. In the presence of a full hepatic enzyme-metabolizing system, both clozapine and demethylclozapine, a stable product, exhibit cytotoxicity toward polymorphonuclear leukocytes (PMNs) and mononuclear leukocytes. In contrast, clozapine *N*-oxide is not cytotoxic but is readily reduced (enzymatically) back to clozapine in the presence of NADPH; however, this conversion can be inhibited by ascorbic acid, probably by inhibiting the (unknown) reducing enzyme.[292,293] Further, fractions of the drug undergo covalent binding to microsomes and to protein in neutrophils and myeloid cells (drug-protein adducts).[294] Consequently, the action of these cytotoxic metabolites can inhibit the formation of neutrophils and stem cells, induce agranulocytosis, and cause abnormalities in the normal antioxidant defense system.[295]

Vitamin C (as well as glutathione and *N*-acetylcysteine) may block the adverse effects of these oxidative compounds and limit their damage to immune cells, most likely through their free-radical–scavenging activity. Further, because vitamin C can restore normal glutathione peroxidase levels, its presence can further enhance antioxidant protection. Intracellular reduced glutathione (GSH) is depleted with bioactivation of clozapine and demethylclozapine, but not clozapine *N*-oxide. In the presence of glutathione, clozapine glutathionyl adducts are formed as additional metabolites.[292] Thus, coadministration of ascorbic acid with clozapine may, directly and indirectly, reduce oxidative stress and prevent protein adduct formation.[293,296] However, the clinical implications of these in vitro findings have yet to be established.

In a cross-sectional pilot study, Linday et al.[295] found that patients with clozapine-induced agranulocytosis exhibited lower levels of glutathione peroxidase, compared with controls, as well as evidence of free-radical–scavenging enzyme activity and levels of related trace metals. Levels of selenium, another important antioxidant, were lower in both groups of patients treated with clozapine, with and without agranulocytosis, than those of controls.

The mechanisms involved in adverse effects associated with bioactivation of clozapine have yet to be fully elucidated. Significant knowledge has emerged indicating the interrelated roles and implications of oxidation, free radicals, various clozapine metabolites and their respective effects, and the reversibility or irreversibility of reduction processes. However, these probable pathways have yet to be confirmed in humans. Further research through well-designed and adequately powered clinical trials are warranted to determine whether coadministration of vitamin C, alone or in combination with glutathione (most effective parenterally) and/or N-acetylcysteine (orally), can prevent, mitigate, or reverse adverse protein adduct formation, toxicity, and agranulocytosis. The low incidence of stark adverse effects of this nature suggests that genetic variability significantly influences the occurrence of a toxic response, and that assessment of pharmacogenomic risk factors may provide a useful tool for determining which patients are at higher risk and thus might be more likely to benefit from antioxidant support. The second- and third-generation atypical antipsychotics have different and milder adverse effect profiles than clozapine. Research such as that with clozapine is warranted with the other agents of this class.

Epinephrine

Epinephrine (Adrenaline, Epi; Adrenalin, Ana-Gard, AsthmaHaler, Asthma-Nefrin, Bronchaid, Bronkaid Mist, Brontin Mist, Epifin, Epinal, EpiPen, Epitrate, Eppy/N, Medihaler-Epi, Primatene Mist, S-2, Sus-Phrine; injectable: Adrenalin Chloride Solution, EpiPen Auto-Injector).

In an experiment involving healthy subjects, Cox et al.[297] observed that intravenous (IV) administration of epinephrine reduced plasma concentrations of vitamin C. The clinical implications of these findings for patients being treated with epinephrine are unknown at this time.

Further research through well-designed clinical trials may be warranted. Pending substantive findings, increased intake of vitamin C and related nutrients appears judicious in individuals using epinephrine on a regular or repeated basis.

Fenofibrate

Fenofibrate (Lofibra, Tricor, Triglide).
In one controlled human trial, Eberlein-Konig et al.[298] found that the combination of two grams of ascorbic acid and 1000 IU of d-alpha-tocopherol before ultraviolet exposure dramatically blocked ultraviolet phototoxic lysis of erythrocytes associated with fenofibrate. Pending further controlled human trials, these preliminary findings suggest that coadministration of ascorbic acid and vitamin E, preferably as naturally occurring tocopherols, might provide potential support to individuals undergoing fenofibrate therapy with minimal risk.

Haloperidol and Other Neuroleptic Agents

Haloperidol (Haldol)
Similar properties: Chlorpromazine (Largactil, Thorazine), clozapine (Clozaril), fluphenazine (Modecate, Permitil, Prolixin, Prolixin Decanoate, Prolixin Enanthate), olanzapine (Symbyax, Zyprexa), prochlorperazine (Compazine, Stemetil), quetiapine (Seroquel), risperidone (Risperdal).

See also Clozapine.
In relatively high systemic doses, ascorbate may exert an antidopaminergic action on striatal function, which mimics the pharmacology of haloperidol.[299,300]

Using a rodent model, Rebec et al.[301] observed that ascorbic acid (1000 mg/kg) alone failed to exert significant behavioral effects, but it "enhanced the antiamphetamine and cataleptogenic effects of haloperidol" (0.1 or 0.5 mg/kg), compared with saline. Subsequently, Pierce, Rebec, et al.[299] found that the combination of ascorbate (100 or 500 mg/kg) over 21 days can potentiate the effects of chronic haloperidol (0.5 mg/kg) on behavioral supersensitivity to apomorphine, but did not affect striatal dopamine (D$_2$) receptor binding. These researchers concluded that "these findings indicate that although chronic ascorbate produces behavioral supersensitivity to apomorphine through central mechanisms, they appear to differ from those induced by chronic haloperidol." In a related experiment, they found that "repeated treatment with ascorbate or haloperidol, but not clozapine, elevates extracellular ascorbate in the neostriatum of freely moving rats."[302] Finally, Gulley and Rebec[300] demonstrated a modulatory effect of ascorbate (100 and 1000 mg/kg intraperitoneally), alone or with haloperidol (0.01 and 0.05 mg/kg subcutaneously), on a lever-release conditioned avoidance response task in male rats. They interpreted the observed contrast between increase in avoidance latency and the lack of effect on conditioned avoidance response when the two agents were coadministered as indicating "an antidopaminergic action of ascorbate on striatal function, but suggest that this effect requires relatively high systemic doses."

However, in a 2-week open trial, Straw et al.[303] administered oral doses of ascorbic acid, 4.5 g daily, to eight male inpatients diagnosed with chronic schizophrenia and stabilized on a fixed dose of haloperidol. They reported no significant clinical change in psychopathology in these subjects, nor any apparent pharmacokinetic interaction with haloperidol, associated with the addition of ascorbic acid.

Although lacking evidence from adequately powered clinical trials, these collective findings suggest a potential dose-dependent synergistic interaction between ascorbate and haloperidol. Further research may be warranted. In the meantime, patients should be advised to avoid such concomitant usage without first discussing such practices with their prescribing physician. Monitoring and supervision are appropriate in individuals using both agents.

Heparin, Unfractionated; Low-Molecular-Weight Heparin

Heparin, unfractionated (UFH): Heparin (Calciparine, Hepalean, Heparin Leo, Minihep Calcium, Minihep, Monoparin Calcium, Monoparin, Multiparin, Pump-Hep, Unihep, Uniparin Calcium, Uniparin Forte).
Low-molecular-weight heparin (LMWH): Ardeparin (Normiflo), certoparin (Mono-Embolex), enoxaparin (Clexane, Lovenox), dalteparin (Fragmin), nadroparin (Fraxiparine), tinzaparin (Innohep).
Similar properties but evidence lacking for extrapolation: Argatroban, bivalirudin (Angiomax), dabigatran etexilate (Rendix; investigational), danaparoid (Orgaran), desirudin (Iprivask, Revasc), fondparinux (Arixtra), hirudin, lepirudin (Refludan).

The preliminary discussion of potential heparin–ascorbic acid antagonism by Owen et al.[304] in 1970 never lead to substantive research.

The integrity of heparin, in both forms (UFH, LMWH), can be adversely affected by oxidative stress, such as that resulting from iron, copper, peroxidases, and other sources of free radicals, although LMWH may be less susceptible than UFH because of its uniform shorter chain length and the significantly less nonspecific binding required to inactivate it.[305-307] Consequently, coadministration of antioxidant nutrients including vitamin C may protect heparin and enable it to maintain its therapeutic activity. In several studies, Deepa and Varalakshmi[308-313] have investigated the cytoprotective activity and beneficial effect of LMWH on cardiac, hepatic, and renal lipid peroxidation and collapse of antioxidant defenses resulting from gentamicin-induced glomerulotoxicity, adriamycin-induced cardiac and hepatic toxicity, atherogenic diet, oxalate-mediated lithogenesis, and other stressors.[314] These and related findings indicate that further investigation into the clinical implications of potential synergy among heparin, ascorbic acid, and other antioxidant nutrients is warranted.

Indomethacin and Related Nonsteroidal Anti-Inflammatory Drugs (NSAIDs)

Evidence: Indomethacin (indometacin; Indocin, Indocin-SR). Similar properties but evidence lacking for extrapolation
COX-1 inhibitors: Diclofenac (Cataflam, Voltaren); combination drug: diclofenac and misoprostol (Arthrotec); diflunisal (Dolobid), etodolac (Lodine), fenoprofen (Dalfon), furbiprofen (Ansaid), ibuprofen (Advil, Excedrin IB, Motrin, Motrin IB, Nuprin, Pedia Care Fever Drops, Provel, Rufen; combination drug: hydrocodone and ibuprofen (Reprexain, Vicoprofen), ketoprofen (Orudis, Oruvail), ketorolac (Acular ophthalmic, Toradol), meclofenamate (Meclomen), mefenamic acid (Ponstel), meloxicam (Mobic), nabumetone (Relafen), naproxen (Anaprox, Naprosyn), oxaprozin (Daypro), piroxicam (Feldene), salsalate (salicylic acid; Amigesic, Disalcid, Marthritic, Mono Gesic, Salflex, Salsitab), sulindac (Clinoril), tolmetin (Tolectin).
COX-2 inhibitors: Celecoxib (Celebrex).
See also Acetaminophen and Acetylsalicylic Acid (Aspirin) and Salsalate sections.

Several small and preliminary studies directly and indirectly indicate patterns of interaction between vitamin C and specific NSAID drugs. However, evidence is lacking from in-depth and focused research on particular interactions and their clinical implications. Potential issues involve synergistic or additive anti-inflammatory activity, impairment of normal nutrient physiological activity, and drug-induced nutrient depletion. The limited evidence available does not suggest a significant risk of impairment of drug therapeutic activity by vitamin C, although any conclusions, especially generalizations for the drug class as a whole, would be speculative.

In a small study on airway tone in the basal state in six healthy, nonsmoking male adults, Ogilvy et al.[314a] investigated the effects of ascorbic acid and indomethacin. Neither ascorbic acid (1.0 g orally) nor indomethacin (50 mg orally) alone produced a significant change in measurements assessing basal tone. However, the researchers noted that "both the duration and intensity of the bronchoconstriction induced by methacholine aerosol (10 mg/mL for 30 sec) were significantly reduced by prior administration of ascorbic acid," but that this "ameliorating action of ascorbic acid was blocked by ingestion of indomethacin." They interpreted their primary findings as suggesting that "ascorbic acid exerts its effects by altering the production of a bronchodilator prostaglandin."

In a double-blind, randomized, crossover study involving 14 healthy volunteers, McAlindon et al.[56] administered aspirin (900 mg twice daily) and placebo, allopurinol (100 mg twice daily), sulfasalazine (1 g twice daily), or vitamin C (1 g twice daily) for 3 days to assess gastric mucosal reactive oxygen metabolite release and gastroduodenal injury. They found that no agent "reduced any parameter of gastric injury but vitamin C reduced duodenal injury assessed by Lanza score," and concluded that vitamin C had demonstrated a previously unrecognized protective effect against aspirin-induced duodenal injury.

The limited data available regarding interactions between NSAIDs and vitamin C suggest that further research is warranted, especially given the high incidence of use, prescribed and self-administered, of these agents.

Isoniazid and Related Antitubercular Agents

Evidence: Isoniazid (isonicotinic acid hydrazide; INH, Laniazid, Nydrazid).
Related but evidence lacking for extrapolation: Cycloserine (Seromycin), ethambutol (Myambutol), ethionamide (2-ethylthioisonicotinamide; Ethide, Ethiocid, Ethomid, Etomide, Mycotuf, Myobid, Trecator SC), pyrazinamide (PZA; Tebrazid), rifampicin (Rifadin, Rifadin IV); combination drugs: isoniazid and rifampicin (Rifamate, Rimactane); isoniazid, pyrazinamide, and rifampicin (Rifater).

Isoniazid (INH) and its metabolites, particularly hydrazine, are known to cause formation of the free-radical intermediates and are thus suspected as the source of INH-induced hepatic injury. The hydrazyl radical alpha-(4-pyridyl-1-oxide)-N-tert-butylnitrone (4-POBN), one of these toxic intermediates, appears to be formed by the CYP450-dependent microsome systems. The antioxidant activity of ascorbic acid may mitigate such oxidative damage.

In an in vitro experiment using electron spin resonance (ESR) spectroscopy and spin-trapping technique, Matsuki et al.[314b] generated findings indicating that hydrazine (Hy) was "most intensive" among the free-radical intermediates formed by isoniazid (INAH) and its metabolites and likely to be a "potent intermediate" involved in INAH-induced hepatic injury. "In the presence of ascorbic acid (AA), the free radical formation of Hy, INAH and acetyl hydrazine was significantly inhibited, suggesting that AA may affect the INAH-hepatitis." They confirmed that "the radical is formed by the cytochrome P-450 dependent microsome systems" when they observed a decrease in the generation of the radical from hydrazine on the addition of CYP450 inhibitors.

These preliminary findings suggest that coadministration of vitamin C, preferably as part of a multinutrient-antioxidant network, might prevent or reduce drug toxicity effects resulting from free-radical damage associated with isoniazid and other antituberculotic medications. Further research into potential protective effects of concomitant antioxidant support, particularly compatibility, dosage, and timing, may be warranted.

Mexiletine

Mexiletine (Mexitil).
Doses of ascorbic acid greater than 1 g daily have been reported to accelerate the excretion of the antiarrhythmic drug mexiletine. The clinical significance of this is unclear.

Mexiletine has also been found to possess antioxidant activity in brain membranes, although at millimolar concentration, significantly less potent than vitamin C and most antioxidant nutrients.[315]

Pending substantive research findings, physicians prescribing mexiletine for ventricular arrhythmias should caution patients to use vitamin C in supplemental form at levels of 1 g daily or higher only with medical supervision and appropriate monitoring.

Phenothiazines

Evidence: Fluphenazine (Modecate, Permitil, Prolixin, Prolixin Decanoate, Prolixin Enanthate), perphenazine (Trilafon), thioridazine (Mellaril).

Extrapolated: Acetophenazine (Tindal), chlorpromazine (Largactil, Thorazine), mesoridazine (Serentil), methotrimeprazine (levomepromazine; Nozinan), pericyazine (Neuleptil); perphenazine combination drug: perphenazine and amitriptyline (Etrafon, Triavil, Triptazine); prochlorperazine (Compazine, Stemetil), promazine (Sparine), promethazine (Phenergan, Promacot, Promethegan), propiomazine (Largon), thiethylperazine (Torecan), thioproperazine (Majeptil), trifluoperazine (Stelazine), triflupromazine (Vesprin).

Hoffer, VanderKamp, Smythies, and others have discussed metabolic abnormalities involving ascorbic acid as potential contributors in the etiology of schizophrenia and other forms of mental illness. Such assertions remain contentious within conventional medicine, with no agreement on mechanisms of action and a lack of evidence from well-designed and adequately powered clinical trials.

Beauclair et al.[316] stated that 8 of 10 schizophrenic subjects in an uncontrolled trial reported decreases in disorganized thoughts, hallucinations, and paranoia when ascorbic acid (8 g/day) was added to their standard drug therapy.

Dysken et al.[316a] described a male patient with a history of manic behavior whose serum fluphenazine levels decreased by 25% (from 0.93 to 0.705 ng/mL) and whose clinical condition greatly deteriorated over 13 days during which 500 mg ascorbic acid was taken twice daily.

Amenorrhea occurs in many female patients undergoing treatment with phenothiazines. In one clinical anecdote, Kanofsky et al.[317] described a 45-year-old woman taking thioridazine who resumed menstruating after initiating daily intake of 6 g of ascorbic acid.

No substantive body of qualified evidence or clear pattern of interaction is present in these inconsistent data. Consequently, the question of whether a clinically significant interaction occurs with known probability cannot be answered at this time. Given the absence of a predictable generalized pattern of interaction, the medical condition of a given patient, their pharmacognomic individuality, concomitant medication regimen, and nutritional status all play potentially significant roles. Caution, close supervision, and regular monitoring are essential if acscorbic acid, in pharmacological doses, and a phenothiazine drug are used concomitantly. Controlled clinical trials may be warranted to determine the safety and efficacy of coadministration of vitamin C and neuroleptic agents.

Probenecid

Probenicid (Benemid, Probalan).

Probenecid increases excretion of uric acid and is used to treat patients with gout. Vitamin C can also increase uric acid excretion and has been administered in graduated doses to treat gout. However, concerns have been voiced that high ascorbate intake might precipitate an acute gouty episode in some individuals, based on possible changes in uric acid solubility within joint spaces. The concomitant administration of probenecid and ascorbic acid, under professional supervision, could theoretically enhance the therapeutic efficacy of gout therapy, but substantive evidence from human research is lacking. Controlled trials may be warranted.

Selective Serotonin Reuptake Inhibitor (SSRI) Antidepressants

Evidence: Fluvoxamine (Faurin, Luvox); paroxetine (Aropax, Deroxat, Paxil, Seroxat).

Extrapolated, based on similar properties: Citalopram (Celexa), escitalopram (S-citalopram; Lexapro), fluoxetine (Prozac, Seraphim), sertraline (Zoloft).

Limited data from a published case report suggest that vitamin C might reduce bleeding associated with paroxetine and fluvoxamine.[318]

Tacrine

Tacrine (Tetrahydroaminoacridine, THA; Cognex).

Hepatotoxicity resulting in irreversible liver damage is a known adverse effect associated with tacrine. Research indicates that, in the course of bioactivation, tacrine undergoes "extensive oxidative metabolism to a variety of mono- and dihydroxylated metabolites in animals and humans."[319] Limited evidence from in vitro experiments using human and rat liver microsomes suggests that concomitant intake of ascorbic acid might inhibit the formation of cytotoxic metabolites from tacrine. In particular, researchers found that reduced glutathione (500 µM) "completely blocked NADPH-dependent cytotoxicity and inhibited protein-reactive metabolite formation by 60%," and "ascorbic acid (500 µM) inhibited the generation of cytotoxic and protein-reactive metabolites" by 75% and 35%, respectively.[319]

Clinical trials may be warranted to investigate potential hepatoprotective activity from coadminsitration of ascorbic acid during tacrine therapy.

Warfarin and Related Oral Vitamin K Antagonist Anticoagulants

Warfarin (Coumadin, Marevan, Warfilone).

Extrapolated, based on similar properties: Anisindione (Miradon), dicumarol, ethyl biscoumacetate (Tromexan), nicoumalone (acenocoumarol; Acitrom, Sintrom), phenindione (Dindevan), phenprocoumon (Jarsin, Marcumar).

Data from some, but not all, animal experiments and rare, unqualified case reports indicates that vitamin C, in high doses, might decrease functional levels and therapeutic activity of warfarin, but the cumulative body of evidence fails to support a well-founded, consistent, and generalizable conclusion.[320-325] Reports of lowered prothrombin time (PT) in individuals taking large doses of vitamin C, outside of professional supervision, have not lead to confirmation of clinically significant complications (e.g., increased clotting), nor has awareness of such potential resulted in substantial reports of any broader patterns or frequency of occurrence. The actual occurrence and clinical implications of a potential interaction remain controversial, and most probably derive from individual patient characteristics, warfarin tolerance and other pharmacogenomic variability, dose factors and regularity of drug-nutrient intake, dietary factors, concomitant medications, and comorbid pathologies.

No generally agreed-on or well-supported mechanism of action has emerged to confirm or explain an interaction between vitamin C and warfarin or related anticoagulants. After declaring the mechanism involved as "not understood," Stockley[239] suggests that decreased warfarin bioavailability resulting from diarrhea induced by high-dose ascorbic acid may be a factor in reported but inconsistent and unpredictable alterations in warfarin levels and therapeutic activity.

Isolated case reports involving uncoordinated ascorbic acid self-administration from the early 1970s form the foundation of speculative claims that ascorbic acid can adversely affect warfarin kinetics and impair therapeutic activity.[325] In a published letter, Rosenthal[326] described the case of a woman, stabilized on 7.5 mg warfarin daily, in whom initiation of regular intake of ascorbic acid (at an unstated dose) was associated with a steady decline in PT from 23 seconds to 19, 17, and then 14 seconds; further, the patient failed to respond to an increase in the dosage of warfarin to 10, 25, and eventually 20 mg per day. This patient returned to PT of 28 seconds within 2 days of halting ascorbic acid supplementation. Smith et al.[327] reported the case of a female patient who exhibited warfarin resistance while taking self-prescribed vitamin C at 16 g/day. A significant increase in PT was obtained after increasing her warfarin dose to 25 mg/day.

Findings from the four controlled trials involving large numbers of subjects indicate a lack of clinically significant interaction between warfarin and ascorbic acid, even at doses as high as 10 g vitamin C per day. Hume et al.[328] observed no significant alterations in anticoagulant effects in five warfarin-treated patients administered 1 g ascorbic acid daily for a 2-week period. Similarly in a trial involving 84 patients on chronic anticoagulant therapy, Dedichen[329] reported no observable effects after administration of an unstated amount of ascorbic acid for 10 weeks. In a study involving 19 patients administered ascorbic acid at doses up to 5 to 10 g daily for 1 or 2 weeks, Feetam et al.[330] observed a mean fall of 17.5% in total plasma warfarin concentrations but reported no "clinically important interaction," as demonstrated by changes in medication effects. Likewise, Blakely[331] reported an absence of clinically significant alteration in warfarin activity in 11 patients administered up to 4 g ascorbic acid daily for 2 weeks.

Physicians prescribing warfarin or related anticoagulant medications are advised to obtain an inventory of both regularly and occasionally used supplements and caution patients against initiating or abruptly changing dosage levels of vitamin C or other nutrients (or herbs) without proper professional supervision and increased monitoring of INR and other relevant hematological parameters. Even with cautious acknowledgment of the available reports, tentative and inconsistent as they are, it is improbable that a clinically significant interaction might occur, in most individuals, at doses less than 1 g daily. Thus, Stockley[239] concluded: "There is no good reason for avoiding the concurrent use." Nevertheless, as always, regular monitoring and repeated inquiry, as well as concern for warfarin resistance, are essential in managing patients undergoing anticoagulant therapy.

NUTRIENT-NUTRIENT INTERACTIONS

Alpha-Lipoic Acid

Alpha-lipoic acid and vitamin C both possess significant antioxidant properties and, as such, demonstrate synergistic activities against free radicals. In general, antioxidant agents function most effectively, and with the least risk of shifting into pro-oxidant activity, when used in clusters to create the effect of an antioxidant network.[332,333] Although widespread and growing scientific research into the physiological activities and therapeutic implications of antioxidants remains largely preliminary, with the well-designed, large, long-term French SU.VI.MAX (Supplementation en Vitamines et Mineraux Antioxydants) prospective study being the significant exception.[334] Diabetic neuropathies and ocular diseases are among the most prominent of numerous areas of clinical importance,

which are the subjects of ongoing and anticipated research into potential synergies between vitamin C and alpha-lipoic acid.[335,336]

The interdependent relationships and biochemical interactions among vitamin C, alpha-lipoic acid, and other antioxidants, particularly vitamin E, demonstrate important aspects of the model of antioxidant networks, their physiological activities, and clinical implications. Alpha-lipoic acid demonstrates significant antioxidant activities by deactivation of reactive oxygen and nitrogen species, both in vivo and in vitro. Furthermore, dihydrolipoic acid may act as a "strong direct chain-breaking antioxidant" and enhance the antioxidant potency of ascorbate and vitamin E. In 1992, Kagan et al.[337] found that dihydrolipoic acid (but not thioctic acid, its oxidized form) "reduced ascorbyl radicals (and dehydroascorbate) generated in the course of ascorbate oxidation by chromanoxyl radicals. This interaction resulted in ascorbate-mediated dihydrolipoic acid–dependent reduction of the vitamin E chromanoxyl radicals, i.e. vitamin E recycling." Casciari et al.[13] found that "ascorbate increased the percentage of apoptotic cells in SW620 hollow fibre tumours" and that coadministration of lipoic acid "synergistically enhanced [this] ascorbate cytotoxicity." Furthermore, lipoic acid, "unlike ascorbate, was equally effective against proliferating and non-proliferating cells." Lu and Liu[338] investigated the synergistic interaction of lipoic acid with other endogenous and exogenous antioxidants. They found that vitamin C, as well as Trolox (a water-soluble derivative of alpha-tocopherol) and hydroxycinnamic acid derivatives, were able to "recycle lipoic acid by donating electrons to lipoic acid radical cations, thereby increasing the antioxidant capacity of lipoic acid in vivo and in vitro."

Bioflavonoids

Bioflavonoids and vitamin C often function synergistically, as might be expected from their frequent presence together in many foods. Simultaneous oral intake with bioflavonoids can enhance bioavailability of vitamin C.[339] Bioflavonoids perform antioxidant functions in concert, and ascorbic acid can protect flavonoids from oxidative degradation.[340]

Copper

Limited evidence suggests that vitamin C intake, at greater than 1 g/day, may reduce copper retention and contribute to copper depletion. Copper absorption may theoretically be impaired by concomitant high ascorbic acid intake, possibly resulting in lowered ceruloplasmin levels, but conclusive evidence is lacking to confirm a pattern of clinically significant interaction.

Finley and Cerklewski[341] investigated the influence of ascorbic acid supplementation on copper status in an experiment involving young adult men consuming self-selected diets and administered 500 mg of ascorbic acid with each meal (1500 mg/day) for 64 days. "Each subject thus served as his own control." They observed that serum ceruloplasmin activity was "significantly reduced...at every data point throughout the ascorbic acid supplementation period," and that a "similar but nonsignificant trend was observed for serum copper. Furthermore there was a significant increase...in serum copper concentration 20 days after the supplementation period." Although these observed effects "occurred within physiological ranges of normal values, this study confirms that a high ascorbic acid intake is antagonistic to copper status of men, as has been demonstrated in laboratory animals." Subsequently, Jacob et al.[342] conducted a study of intestinal copper absorption and blood measures of copper status in healthy young men receiving varying intakes of ascorbic acid over 14 weeks using a live-in nutrition suite. Using "both enzymatic and immunochemical methods," they observed that copper "absorption, copper retention, total serum copper and the serum level of ceruloplasmin protein were not affected significantly by the changes" in ascorbic acid (AA) intake, but that the "oxidase activity of serum ceruloplasmin was decreased an average of 21% during the high (605 mg/d)" AA intake phase. The authors interpreted their findings as suggesting that "in adult men moderate supplemental intakes of AA reduce ceruloplasmin oxidase activity specifically but do not depress intestinal copper absorption or overall body copper status." Notably, the levels of ascorbic acid administered in this latter study were about one-third those used in the former study.

Folic Acid

Vitamin C appears to play an important role in the activation of folic acid to form folinic acid, possibly by acting as a reducing agent. Well-founded conclusions are as yet premature because data from primary scientific literature are inconclusive, and secondary discussions are conflicting in their interpretations.

Glutathione (GSH)

Unlike most mammals, which are able to synthesize ascorbic acid in the liver, humans and guinea pigs possess no ability to synthesize ascorbate de novo. In particular, hepatic glutathione plays an essential role in regeneration of vitamin C. During in vitro experiments using serum albumin from rats, Vethanayagam et al.[343] observed that albumin "acts as an antioxidant and exerts a significant glutathione-dependent DHAA-reductase activity that may be important in the physiologic recycling of ascorbic acid" from dehydroascorbate (DHAA), its oxidized byproduct. Likewise, using cultured liver-derived cells from humans (HepG2 cells) and rats (H4IIE cells) Li, May, et al.[344] confirmed that GSH is required to recycle ascorbic acid. They noted that in "both cell types, DHA [dehydroascorbic acid] reduction lowered glutathione (GSH) concentrations and was inhibited by prior depletion of GSH" and concluded that "both cell types rely largely on GSH- or NADPH-dependent mechanisms for ascorbate recycling from DHA." These researchers also found that GSH is required for recycling of ascorbic acid in endothelial cells.[345] Subsequently, using a mouse model, Gao et al.[346] demonstrated "enhancement of glutathione cardioprotection by ascorbic acid in myocardial reperfusion injury."

Consistent with the antioxidant network model, coadministration of these two antioxidants can be reasonably expected to synergistically enhance the activity of both agents. Glutathione levels can be positively influenced by parenteral glutathione (prepared by compounding pharmacies), oral liposomal glutathione, oral supplements of N-acetylcysteine, and whey-derived cysteine peptide supplementation.

Grape Seed Extract

In a randomized, double-blind, placebo-controlled trial, Ward et al.[347] investigated the effects of coadministration of vitamin C and grape seed polyphenols in 69 individuals being treated for hypertension. The participants received 500 mg/day vitamin C, 1000 mg/day grape seed polyphenols, both vitamin C and polyphenols, or neither for 6 weeks. Vitamin C alone reduced systolic blood pressure (BP, vs. placebo), whereas no effect was observed with polyphenols. However, these investigators reported a "significant interaction between grape-seed and vitamin C treatments" in which systolic BP and diastolic BP increased 4.8 ± 0.9 mm Hg and 2.7 ± 0.6 mm Hg, respectively (vs. placebo). Notably, "endothelium-dependent and independent vasodilation, and markers of oxidative damage were not significantly altered." The authors added that, although the mechanism underlying these phenomena "remains to be elucidated," these results "suggest caution for hypertensive subjects taking supplements containing combinations of vitamin C and polyphenols." Further research appears warranted to confirm and determine the frequency, characteristics, and clinical significance of this possible interaction.

Iron

Vitamin C, in supplements or vitamin C–rich foods, can strongly enhance the absorption of nonheme iron in the GI tract by reducing dietary ferric iron (Fe^{3+}) to ferrous iron (Fe^{2+}), forming a highly absorbable iron–ascorbic acid complex, and increasing bioavailability of the iron twofold to threefold.[239,348-352] Levine et al.[12] reported that concomitant intake of vitamin C at 200 mg/30 mg elemental iron increases iron absorption, especially ferric iron.[12] This effect, however, apparently is influenced by gastric pH, bile function, and other dietary constituents; is highly dose dependent; and is relatively minor at ascorbic acid doses under 200 mg, even in individuals with low iron stores.[349,353,354]

However, ascorbic acid can prevent the dose-dependent inhibitory effects of polyphenols and phytates on nonheme-iron absorption.[355] Furthermore, ascorbate stabilizes the iron cores of ferritin in cells and retards ferritin degradation and autophagic uptake of ferritin clusters into lysosomes.[356]

Iron deficiency anemia affects one third to half of children in the developing world. Zlotkin et al.[357] found that adding "sprinkles" (ferrous fumarate and ascorbic acid microencapsulated in a thin, soy-based coat) to weaning foods can be an effective tool in reducing rates of anemia in susceptible children.

The two primary risks potentially attributed to the combined influence of iron and ascorbic acid are iron overload and increased oxidative stress. (See earlier erythropoietin section for a discussion of these issues in that context.)

Overall, the probability of iron overload from concomitant intake of iron and vitamin C is extremely low in individuals without transfusion or IV iron–produced iron overload or genetic hemochromotosis. However, the risk of an adverse interaction is significant in individuals with genetic hematochromatosis, which remains asymptomatic until late stages of iron overload, and iron intake should absolutely be restricted in such patients. A transferrin saturation of greater than 70% should trigger high suspicion of hemachromatosis and further investigation.

Limited in vitro evidence has suggested that concomitant iron and ascorbic acid might result in a paradoxical pro-oxidant effect within the context of high oxidative stress, but human trials have failed to confirm such findings. In a study involving 40 healthy female and male volunteers, Proteggente et al.[358] investigated the potential for a pro-oxidant interaction of iron and ascorbate by testing the effects of iron supplementation on oxidative damage to DNA. Subjects "with plasma ascorbate levels at the upper end of the normal range (mean plasma ascorbate approximately equal to 70 micromol/L)" were "supplemented with a daily dose of syrup (ferrous glycine sulphate equivalent to 12.5 mg iron)" over 6 weeks. After assessing a number of relevant parameters in serum and plasma samples, including serum ferritin, transferrin-bound iron, percent saturation of transferrin and plasma ascorbate, and measurement of oxidative damage to DNA bases from WBCs using gas chromatography/mass spectrometry, they determined that "iron supplementation did not affect any of the iron status parameters," and that there were "no detrimental effects, over the period under investigation, in terms of oxidative damage to DNA." The authors cautioned, however, that "the effects of larger doses or of longer supplementation periods should also be investigated."[358] A dose of 12.5 mg iron is below the daily value (DV) for most population groups and far below therapeutic doses used to correct iron deficiency states.

Lutein

The mutual occurrence of high levels of both lutein and vitamin C in some plants suggests a potential synergistic relationship between these two antioxidant nutrients. Carotenoids are lipophilic and hydrophobic, and absorption is enhanced by dietary fat. In an experiment involving nine young adults, however, Tanumihardjo et al.[359] found that simultaneous administration of ascorbic acid facilitated lutein absorption.

Selenium

The relationship between ascorbic acid and selenium is complex and only partially understood. The allied roles of these nutrients are well established, particularly with regard to the activity of glutathione peroxidase, and often relied on in clinical application of antioxidants. For example, among the numerous selenium-dependent enzymes, also known as *selenoproteins*, thioredoxin reductase maintains the antioxidant function of vitamin C by catalyzing its regeneration.[360] However, other evidence derived from short-term human experiments investigating the interaction between dietary ascorbic acid at extremes of intake and selenium (Se) in young adult males indicates that doses of vitamin C greater than 1 g may reduce the absorption of selenium. Nevertheless, the authors concluded that these "data and those previously obtained in subjects with more usual ascorbic acid intakes point to a possible important role for ascorbic acid in the maintenance of Se homeostasis."[361] Pending more conclusive evidence, prudence suggests that selenium be ingested 1 hour before or 20 minutes after taking vitamin C.

Taurine

In an animal experiment, Mochizuki et al.[362] reported an "amplifying effect of dietary taurine on the induction of cytochrome P-450 and on the urinary excretion of ascorbic acid in rats fed on phenobarbital-containing diets." Such observations suggest the potential for clinically significant implications involving both medications and xenobiotics metabolized by hepatic cytochrome P450 enzymes and thus indicate that further research is warranted.

Vitamin B₆

Urinary excretion of pyridoxine may be increased in individuals with vitamin C deficiency. Conversely, rare individuals may develop profound hyperoxaluria in response to supraphysiological intake of vitamin C, which could increase risk of renal oxalate calculi. In such individuals, pyridoxine in doses of 100 to 300 mg per day (often in conjunction with magnesium supplementation) has been shown to normalize the oxalate production and excretion.

Vitamin B₁₂

Some sources suggest that vitamin C may damage or diminish the effectiveness of vitamin B_{12} if taken together. This potential interaction may be prevented by not taking large doses of vitamin C within 1 hour of oral vitamin B_{12} intake.

Vitamin E

Vitamin C facilitates regeneration of vitamin E and restoration of its antioxidant activity, thus providing an excellent example of an effective antioxidant network. Their strong presence in diets rich in vegetables and fruits associated with reduced risk of cardiovascular disease and cancer suggests that coadministration may be beneficial. Regarding their role in secondary cardiovascular prevention, Gey[78] concluded that "vitamin E acts as first risk discriminator, vitamin C as second one; optimal health requires synchronously optimized vitamins C + E, A, carotenoids and vegetable conutrients."

Zandi et al.[363] examined data from the Cache County Study, a large, population-based investigation of the prevalence and incidence of Alzheimer's disease and other dementias, and determined that regular use of vitamin E in nutritional supplement doses, especially in combination with vitamin C, may protect the aging brain against pathological changes associated with Alzheimer's disease and reduce the risk of developing the condition. Further study with randomized prevention trials is needed before drawing firm conclusions about the protective effects of such coordinated antioxidant supplementation. If effective, the use of these (and possibly other) antioxidant nutrients may offer a safe and inexpensive strategy for reducing the risk of developing Alzheimer's dementia.

Bruno et al.[364,365] have conducted extensive research into the relationship between vitamin C and alpha-tocopherol, with a focus on the conditions of high oxidative stress found in smokers. First, they found that vitamin E disappearance "is accelerated in cigarette smokers due to their increased oxidative stress and is inversely correlated with plasma vitamin C concentrations."[364] Then, in a double-blind, placebo-controlled, randomized crossover trial, they demonstrated that ascorbic acid (500 mg twice daily for weeks) doubled "plasma ascorbic acid concentrations in both groups and attenuated smokers', but not nonsmokers', plasma alpha- and gamma-tocopherol...fractional disappearance rates by 25% and 45%, respectively. Likewise, smokers' plasma deuterium-labeled alpha- and gamma-tocopherol concentrations were significantly higher...at 72 h during ascorbic acid supplementation compared with placebo." They concluded that "cigarette smoking increased plasma alpha- and gamma-tocopherol fractional disappearance rates, suggesting that the oxidative stress from smoking oxidizes tocopherols, and that plasma ascorbic acid reduces alpha- and gamma-tocopherol radicals to nonoxidized forms, thereby decreasing vitamin E disappearance in humans."[365]

Vitamin K

In 1952, Merkel[366] found that coadministration of menadione bisulfite (vitamin K_3 sodium bisulfite, which lacks vitamin K activity until metabolized to menaquinone, also known as vitamin K_2) and ascorbate provided complete relief of symptoms within 3 days in 64 of 70 consecutive cases of nausea and vomiting of pregnancy. These findings have not been followed up.

Vitamin K_2 combined with IV ascorbate has shown recent promise as an oxidative therapy for cancer. Similar preliminary studies have involved use of K_3 in conjunction with IV and oral ascorbate. Vitamin K_3 is a more active free-radical generator than is K_2.[367-371]

HERB-NUTRIENT INTERACTION

Reishi Mushroom (Ganoderma lucidum)

Futrakul et al.[372] found that coadministration of vitamins C and E along with *Ganoderma lucidum* as a treatment for steroid-resistant nephrosis "helps to neutralize oxidative stress and suppress the toxic effect to the glomerular endothelial function."

The 380 citations for this monograph, as well as additional reference literature, are located under Vitamin C (Ascorbic Acid) on the CD at the back of the book.

Vitamin D (Calciferol)

Nutrient Names: Vitamin D, calciferol.
Synonyms: 1,25-Dihydroxyvitamin D, calciferol, calcipotriol, cholecalciferol (vitamin D_3), ergocalciferol (vitamin D_2), irradiated ergocalciferol, ergosterol (provitamin D_2), activated/irradiated ergosterol (vitamin D_2).
Related Substance: Calcitriol is also the name of a drug that is the active (1,25-dihydroxycholecalciferol) form of vitamin D.

Summary

Drug/Class Interaction Type	Mechanism and Significance	Management
Allopurinol ⊕⊕	Allopurinol may elevate serum concentrations of 1,25(OH)$_2$-vitamin D_3 by reducing uric acid's inhibition of 1-hydroxylase activity.	Assess vitamin D status. Allopurinol may increase 1,25(OH)$_2$D levels, especially with supplementation.
Androgen-deprivation therapy (ADT) ☼/⊕⊕	Concomitant vitamin D and calcium can counter skeletal impact of deficiency patterns associated with prostate cancer treatment, decreased sex hormone levels, and ADT, especially when used with bisphosphonates. Consensus of evidence is emerging for this clinically significant, supportive interaction, as are clinical guidelines.	Coadminister vitamin D and calcium and monitor bone and D status. Promote sunlight exposure and exercise.
Anticonvulsant medications ≈≈≈/◇/☼	Phenytoin and phenobarbital accelerate vitamin D metabolism in liver (CYP450 induction) and may reduce serum levels of 25(OH)D. Thus, anticonvulsants may impair mineralization, leading to increased risk of bone loss, osteoporosis, osteomalacia, rickets, and fractures. Coadministration of "high-dose" vitamin D can mitigate drug-induced vitamin D depletion and related bone loss.	Coadminister vitamin D and calcium. Monitor serum 25-OHD and bone status. Promote sunlight exposure and weight-bearing exercise.
Bisphosphonates ⊕⊕⊕	Synergistic interaction; vitamin D assists calcium absorption, and both enable bisphosphonates in maintaining bone mineralization, including with hormone replacement therapy (HRT).	Coadminister vitamin D; administer calcium but separate intake from bisphosphonates. Promote appropriate sunlight exposure and weight-bearing exercise.
Calcitriol Vitamin D analogs ✗✗/✗✗✗/◇◇	Additive effect from concurrent use would increase risk of vitamin D toxicity, especially since 1,25(OH)$_2$D and analogs bypass renal feedback controls.	Caution; generally avoid. Possible value in coadministration (e.g., renal disease) with monitoring.
Cholestyramine Colestipol Bile acid sequestrants ≈≈≈/◇	Bile acid sequestrants decrease lipid digestion and absorption and thereby reduce absorption of vitamin D and fat-soluble nutrients. Risk of deficiency and sequelae.	Supplement vitamin D. Promote sunlight exposure and weight-bearing exercise.
Cimetidine Histamine (H$_2$) receptor antagonists ≈≈≈/◇	Cimetidine may inhibit action of vitamin D hydroxylase and could reduce hepatic activation of vitamin D through hydroxylation. Possible risk of deficiency.	Monitor 25(OH)D. Compensatory supplementation may be appropriate.
Corticosteroids, oral ≈≈≈/◇≈≈/◇	Oral corticosteroids reduce calcium absorption and may increase excretion while decreasing vitamin D availability and lowering serum levels. Increased risk of bone loss, osteoporosis, and fractures with long-term oral steroid use.	Supplement vitamin D and calcium. Monitor bone and 25(OH)D status with steroid use > 1 month. Promote sunlight exposure and exercise.
Estrogens/progestins Hormone replacement therapy (HRT) ⊕⊕/✗✗	Synergistic interaction, especially with osteoporosis. Vitamin D assists calcium absorption, and both enable estrogen in inhibiting osteoclastic activity and bone resorption and maintaining bone mineralization. Progestins may counter benefit.	Coadminister vitamin D and calcium (separate intake), possibly bisphosphonates. Monitor bone, 25(OH)D, and HDL. Promote sunlight and exercise.
Heparin, unfractionated ◇≈≈/≈≈	Heparin therapy is associated with bone loss. Heparin may also inhibit formation of 1,25(OH)$_2$D by kidneys. Risks of bone loss and associated nutrient depletion with extended heparin use are significant. Limited evidence supporting protective effect of oral vitamin D.	Coadminister vitamin D and calcium, possibly as hydroxyapatite. Monitor bone and 1,25(OH)$_2$ status with heparin use > 1 month.
Isoniazid (INH) ≈≈	Isoniazid can lower levels of both activated vitamin D and calcium levels; can also inhibit hepatic mixed-function oxidase activity, hepatic 25-hydroxylase and renal 1α-hydroxylase and reduce corresponding vitamin D metabolites. Drug-induced vitamin D deficiency can produce hypocalcemia and elevate parathyroid hormone. Nutrient support unlikely to interfere with drug's therapeutic activity.	Supplement vitamin D and calcium when INH used for > 1 month. Promote sunlight exposure. Monitor 25(OH)D and bone status.
Ketoconazole ⊕✗	Ketoconazole inhibits P450 enzymes to block adrenal steroidogenesis; also inhibits both synthesis of activated vitamin D and its metabolism by 1 alpha-hydroxylase and 24-hydroxylase, thus maintaining 1,25(OH)$_2$-vitamin D levels if it is supplemented. Ketoconazole reduces calcium (and 1,25-D) in hypercalcemia and sarcoidosis.	Monitor for vitamin D deficiency with long-term use. Calcitriol may be necessary. Half-life of administered calcitriol prolonged in presence of ketoconazole.
Neomycin ≈≈≈/◇	Long-term use of neomycin decreases absorption and/or increases elimination of many nutrients, including vitamin D. Risk of deficiency and sequelae.	Supplement multivitamin-mineral with extended use.

Continued

Summary

Drug/Class Interaction Type	Mechanism and Significance	Management
Orlistat ≈≈≈	Orlistat binds fat to prevent absorption and can interfere with absorption of vitamin D and other fat-soluble nutrients. Possible risk of significant deficiency.	Supplement multivitamin with extended use. Separate intake timing.
Raloxifene ⊕⊕	Synergistic interaction; vitamin D assists calcium absorption, and both enable raloxifene in inhibiting bone resorption.	Coadminister D_3 plus calcium. Monitor 25(OH)D and bone status. Promote sunlight exposure and exercise.
Rifampin ≈≈/◇≈≈	Rifampin induces cytochrome P450, resulting in decreased plasma levels of 25-hydroxycholecalciferol (25-OHD). Risk of significant deficiency uncertain.	Supplement D_3 when rifampin > 1 month. Monitor 25(OH)D status.
Thiazide diuretics ◇◇/✗✗	Thiazides reduce calcium excretion and could potentially lead to hypercalcemia (rare) and changes in vitamin D metabolism. Significance of interaction uncertain.	Monitor serum calcium.
Thioridazine ✗✗✗	Cholecalciferol inhibits hepatic cytochrome P2D6 and may decrease the metabolism of thioridazine. Concurrent use might increase activity and adverse effects of drug.	Monitor vitamin D status; supplementation may be appropriate but only under close supervision. Consider alternatives to thioridazine.
Verapamil Calcium channel blockers ✗✗✗/◇◇◇/◇◇	Vitamin D can increase calcium availability, which opposes verapamil's activity as calcium antagonist. Excess vitamin D might theoretically contribute to hypercalcemia on rare occasions, which in turn might theoretically precipitate cardiac arrhythmia in patients taking verapamil. Minimal evidence and low probability but potentially severe.	Concurrent supplementation with vitamin D (and calcium) may be appropriate but only under close supervision. Consider bone support needs.

NUTRIENT DESCRIPTION

Chemistry and Forms

Vitamin D is the generic term for compounds that exhibit the biological activity of calciferol: vitamin D_2 (ergocalciferol), vitamin D_3 (cholecalciferol), $1\alpha(OH)D_3$ (alfacalcidol), $25(OH)D_3$ (calcifediol, calcidiol), $1,25(OH)_2D_3$ (calcitriol), and dihydrotachysterol.

Physiology and Function

Vitamin D functions as both a fat-soluble vitamin and a hormone. From dietary sources, vitamin D is absorbed from the small intestine in the presence of bile and is transported into the circulation via the lymph in chylomicrons (similar to vitamin A transport). Vitamin D can also be synthesized in the skin as a result of direct exposure to the ultraviolet light in sunlight (UVB radiation) through the conversion of 7-dehydrocholesterol to cholecalciferol (vitamin D_3). This ability of animals to produce vitamin D from a cholesterol derivative makes the nutrient a "conditionally essential" vitamin. On entering the circulation from either the diet or the skin, vitamin D_3 is bound to the vitamin D–binding protein and transported to the liver. Two successive hydroxylations of vitamin D, first in the liver (to 25-hydroxycholecalciferol) and then in the kidneys, produce the hormonally active form, calcitriol, or 1,25-dihydroxycholecalciferol (1,25-dihydroxyvitamin D_3), in coordination with the parathyroid glands and calcium-sensitive parathyroid hormone (PTH, parathormone) secretion.

Calcitriol binds to the *vitamin D receptor* (VDR), a nuclear transcription factor that regulates gene expression. When the calcitriol/VDR complex subsequently combines with the *retinoic acid X receptor* (RXR), the resulting VDR/RXR heterodimer can interact with the vitamin D–responsive elements (VDREs) within the DNA. This interaction between the VDR/RXR heterodimer and a VDRE alters the rate of transcription of a related gene and thereby regulates the activity of vitamin D–dependent calcium transporters in the small intestine, osteoblasts in bone, and the 1-hydroxylase enzyme in the kidneys. Defects in the vitamin D receptor lead to hypocalcemic vitamin D–resistant rickets, congenital total lipodystrophy, and persistent müllerian duct syndrome. Research suggests that bone may be more responsive to

exercise in some genotypes of VDR than in others,[1] and that gene-environment interactions such as leisure physical activity and VDR genotype may play a role in maintaining the bone mineral density (BMD) at the lumbar spine in active postmenopausal women, especially in older active women.[2]

The vitamin D endocrine system is responsible for maintaining tight regulation of serum calcium levels within the narrow range critical to bone metabolism and healthy functioning of the nervous system. Calcitriol mediates the intestinal absorption and blood levels of calcium and phosphorus. It facilitates mineral deposition into bone, modulates bone mineralization and demineralization, and enhances muscle strength and balance. Vitamin D is necessary to calcium absorption and increases the absorption of calcium from the intestine (by stimulating the synthesis of calcium-binding protein and the epithelial calcium channel) and maintains serum calcium levels in the normal range; thus increasing resorption of calcium from bone as well as facilitating calcium storage in the bones. Consequently, even though it initially causes bone resorption, the net effect is to increase calcium deposition in the bone. In addition to promoting calcium absorption, calcitriol mediates the intestinal absorption of phosphorus, possibly magnesium and zinc as well, and may promote renal tubule phosphate resorption. Vitamin D is stored in body fat.

Vitamin D also plays many important roles in hormonal regulation and immune function. It helps maintain adequate blood levels of insulin and may assist the metabolism of sugar. Vitamin D may also assist healthy thyroid function, and the active form of vitamin D_3 may have a mechanism of action similar to thyroid hormone. Vitamin D and VDRs participate in the regulation of cell growth and development, particularly white blood cells and epithelial cells. In particular, the presence of VDRs in T lymphocytes suggests that vitamin D facilitates the development, activity, and response of T cells against antigens (and in autoimmune disorders).

NUTRIENT IN CLINICAL PRACTICE

Known or Potential Therapeutic Uses

Vitamin D is used to prevent osteoporosis and osteoporotic fractures, and intake is associated with reduced risk of breast cancer, colorectal cancer, prostate cancer, as well as cancers of the lung, skin (melanoma), colon, and bone. Administration of vitamin D in conjunction with bisphosphonate therapy (e.g., alendronate, risedronate, or etidronate) or exogenous hormone therapy (e.g., HRT) may enhance clinical outcomes in preventing and treating osteoporosis. A range of autoimmune diseases, particularly type 1 diabetes mellitus, rheumatoid arthritis, and multiple sclerosis, may be responsive to integrative therapeutics employing vitamin D, especially when they involve a VDR gene polymorphism. Calcitriol, the active metabolite of vitamin D, has been found to inhibit the growth of human prostate cancer cells in vitro; however, findings from preliminary human trials have been disappointing for its use (or that of analogs) as part of innovative protocols in the treatment of hormone-refractory prostate cancer.

Historical/Ethnomedicine Precedent

The physiological parameters of vitamin D may be premised on the ancient origins of humans in equatorial Africa. The high level of exposure to sun inherent to such an interaction with the environment may play a fundamental role in the high susceptibility for insufficiency or deficiency among modern humans less exposed to the sun, especially for dark-skinned individuals, because melanin acts as an ultraviolet absorber.

Possible Uses

Atherosclerosis, autoimmune diseases, breast cancer, burns, cancer prevention, celiac disease, digestive system cancers (oral, esophageal, stomach, pancreas, colorectal; risk reduction, especially in individuals with dark skin), Crohn's disease, depression (particularly seasonal affective disorder), diabetes mellitus, epilepsy, falls (prevention, especially in the elderly), fractures (especially in the elderly), hearing loss, hyperparathyroidism (secondary), hypertension, hypoparathyroidism, migraine headaches, multiple sclerosis, obesity, osteoarthritis, osteomalacia, osteoporosis, prevention of vitamin D deficiency, prostate cancer, psoriasis, rheumatoid arthritis (risk reduction), rickets, scleroderma, skin cancer (risk reduction), tuberculosis.

Deficiency Symptoms

Rickets, osteomalacia, osteoporosis, and fracture risk remain the most obvious and well-known outcomes associated with vitamin D deficiency. Researchers have increasingly expressed concern that the low levels of vitamin D found in a large percentage of Americans and Europeans may be associated with increased risk of a range of conditions, including cancer, heart disease, hypertension, diabetes, multiple sclerosis, and diminished immune status. The classic groups known for increased risk of deficiency are breast-fed infants, individuals on vegetarian diets, the elderly, individuals with fat malabsorption or chronic kidney disease, and individuals with compromised sun exposure due to lifestyle, climate, season, or cultural practices. Other significant etiologies include alcoholism, burns (and burn scarring), Crohn's disease, Cushing's disease, dark skin, decreased consumption of vitamin D, hypothyroidism, anticonvulsant drug therapy, kidney or liver disease, malabsorption (as in celiac disease or after intestinal surgery), ulcerative colitis, and vitamin D–resistant rickets. Vitamin D receptor polymorphic alleles have been linked to diabetes mellitus and colon cancer.[3,4] Low dietary calcium intake may enhance the phenotypic expression of VDR gene polymorphisms.[5]

Awareness of previously unrecognized vitamin D deficiency and its implications in long-term pathological processes has been growing in recent years.[6,7] Chapuy et al.[8] (1997) reported that one of seven adults may be deficient in vitamin D. Similarly, a study in 1998 by Thomas et al.[9] found that 37% of the total group surveyed were deficient in vitamin D, even though their reported diets should have provided the currently recommended levels of vitamin. This study also found that 42% of hospitalized patients under age 65 were deficient in vitamin D. Overall, vitamin D inadequacy has been reported in up to 57% of general medicine inpatients in the United States.[10] Spanish researchers found that healthy postmenopausal women in modern societies have an extremely high prevalence of vitamin D deficiency.[11] Likewise, young adults exhibit an unexpectedly high incidence of vitamin D insufficiency.[12] Vitamin D deficiencies may also raise the risk of prostate cancer by disrupting the relationship between androgens and VDR in prostate cells.[13]

Dietary Sources

Cod liver oil, oily cold-water fish (salmon, mackerel, herring), butter, egg yolks, vitamin D–fortified milk, and orange juice.

Most vitamin D in humans is derived from endogenous synthesis subsequent to sun exposure rather than from dietary sources. Vitamin D is found primarily in foods of animal origin, unless they are fortified. Cod liver oil is considered an excellent dietary source. Vegetables are usually low in vitamin D, although mushrooms, if irradiated, can be a significant source of vitamin D. Milk used to make cheese or yogurt is usually not fortified with vitamin D. Human milk contains the 25-hydroxycholecalciferol form of D, possibly to compensate for the limited ability of the liver in infants to achieve the first hydroxylation of cholecalciferol. The vitamin D content in human milk varies with maternal sun exposure and vitamin D intake.

Sunshine

With exposure to ultraviolet light, the skin synthesizes vitamin D. It is estimated that 20 minutes, with face and arms exposed, will stimulate about 600 to 1000 IU per day, during spring, summer, and fall in temperate regions, and year-round in tropical and subtropical regions. Enough sun or UVB exposure to produce minimal skin erythema (known as the *minimal erythemic dose*) can produce 10,000 to 20,000 IU in about an hour. Adequate amounts of vitamin D can theoretically be synthesized and stored in fat to carry an individual through the winter. In temperate latitudes, above 35° to 50°, a minimum of 15 minutes of sun exposure on the arms, face, and hands three times per week in the morning or late afternoon during the spring, summer, and fall is needed to avoid vitamin D deficiency at the end of winter. However, research indicates that, in actuality, many individuals in higher latitudes, especially with seasonal clothing, overcast climates, and minimal time outdoors, do not receive adequate sun exposure to avoid compromised vitamin D status. Sun exposure with sunscreen significantly prevents skin synthesis of vitamin D.

Dosage Forms Available

Capsules, injection (IM), liquid, tablets. Intramuscular (IM) form is not available in the United States.

Oral dosing (with meals) is preferred, but malabsorption associated with gastrointestinal, liver, or biliary disease may necessitate IM injection.

Nutrient Preparations Available

Cholecalciferol (vitamin D_3) is more potent and bioavailable than ergocalciferol (D_2).

Dosage Range

Adult

Dietary: The adequate intake of vitamin D (cholecalciferol, or vitamin D_3) is 5 µg (200 IU) per day for adults age 19 to 50 years, 10 µg (400 IU) for adults age 51 to 70 years, and 15 µg (600 IU) for adults 71 years and older.

Supplemental/Maintenance: 10 µg (400 IU) per day. However, in some cases this may be unnecessary, given consistent adequate direct exposure to the sun, usually 20 minutes per day. Supplement with cod liver oil if 25(OH)D levels are low (1 tsp per 50 pounds of body weight). One tablespoon of cod liver oil provides approximately 1200 IU (30 µg) of vitamin D_3.

A dose of 20 µg (800 IU) per day for individuals, especially the elderly, not adequately exposed to sunlight or living in farther northern or southern latitudes.

Pharmacological/Therapeutic: 800 to 2000 IU per day, including dietary sources, under supervision of a physician or health care professional experienced in nutritional therapeutics.[14,15] Dosages used in clinical studies range from 5 µg (200 IU) to 250 µg (10,000 IU) daily. Significantly higher doses are often used in the treatment of secondary hypoparathyroidism, vitamin D–resistant rickets, nutritional rickets and osteomalacia, and familial hypophosphatemia.

Toxic: The current official tolerable upper intake level (UL) is 50 µg (2000 IU) per day. However, many experts in the field strongly support raising the UL to at least 4000 IU, and 10,000 IU may be tolerable for most individuals, but such a daily dose should be medically monitored.

Adverse effects have been reported at concentrations ranging from 250 to 1250 µg (10,000-50,000 IU) per day.

Pediatric (<18 years)

Dietary: The adequate intake (AI) of vitamin D (cholecalciferol, or vitamin D_3) is 5 µg (200 IU) per day for infants and children up to 18 years.

Supplemental/Maintenance: One teaspoon of cod liver oil per 50 lb/wt. Sun exposure of 20 minutes daily is adequate and preferable. Do not give cod liver oil when sun exposure is being implemented.

Pharmacological/Therapeutic

> Premature infants: 10 to 20 µg (400-800 units) per day, up to 750 µg (30,000 IU) per day.
> Infants and healthy children: 10 µg (400 IU) per day.

Significantly higher doses are often used in the treatment of hypoparathyroidism, nutritional rickets and osteomalacia, vitamin D–resistant rickets, and familial hypophosphatemia. Vitamin D receptor defects, specifically tissue resistance to vitamin D, or vitamin D–dependent rickets (VDDR), are usually treated with 20 µg/day of the bioactive form, calcitriol, or 5 mg/day of the dietary form, vitamin D_2, plus oral calcium and phosphate.[16]

Toxic: UL for infants (0-12 months) is 25 µg (1000 IU) per day and for children (1-18 years) is 50 µg (2000 IU) per day.

Note: Requirements depend on the exposure of a person's skin to ultraviolet radiation. The intensity of exposure is also a factor. The latitude determines how much exposure to sunlight the person requires to synthesize adequate levels of vitamin D. Pollution, clouds, and skin color also affect an individual's ability to produce vitamin D. The darker the skin, the less vitamin D will be produced (up to 95% blocked). However, with longer exposure times, even with the darkest skin color, sufficient levels of vitamin D are produced. Glass and topical sunscreens block UV light.

Laboratory Values

Laboratory assessment of vitamin D status has been in a state of controversy and evolution in recent years, particularly since the effects of mild vitamin D deficiency or insufficiency have become more widely recognized.

Plasma 25(OH)-Vitamin D

This assay reflects body reserves. Plasma levels less than 25 nmol/L indicate deficiency.

However, results from laboratories doing 25-hydroxyvitamin D (25-OHD) tests vary widely.[17] Reference ranges from most labs are too low. Optimal serum levels of 25-OHD to avoid increases in PTH are at least 20 ng/mL,[18] but may actually be in the range of 45 to 55 ng/mL (115-140 nmol/L). Heaney et al.[19,20] suggest that the appropriate serum 25-OHD level is 32 ng/mL.[8] Concurrent parathyroid tests (PTH) may elucidate equivocal laboratory findings because one could expect a high PTH if there is a low vitamin D concentration in the blood.

Plasma 1,25(OH)$_2$-Vitamin D

This assay measures the active form of the vitamin. As 25-OHD levels drop, PTH secretion increases (secondary hyperparathyroidism), which maintains the 1,25(OH)$_2$-vitamin D level in the normal range. For this reason, measuring the 25-OHD level is necessary to diagnose vitamin D deficiency or insufficiency. Normal 1,25(OH)$_2$D levels are 48 to 100 pmol/L.

Also, measure serum calcium, blood urea nitrogen (BUN), and phosphorus every 1 to 2 weeks; and monitor bone density regularly until stabilized.

Serum calcium concentration times phosphorus concentration should not exceed 70 mg/dL to avoid ectopic calcification; ergocalciferol levels: 10 to 60 ng/mL; serum calcium: 9 to 10 mg/dL; phosphorus: 2.5 to 5.0 mg/dL.

SAFETY PROFILE

Overview

Vitamin D is generally well tolerated, and excessive doses from sunlight exposure or dietary source are considered highly improbable, if not impossible. Its UL of 50 µg (2000 IU) per day reflects that vitamin D has long been considered the most likely of all vitamin supplements to cause toxicity. Although a revised consensus has developed in recent years among researchers and some clinicians, regulatory and institutional guidelines are only gradually beginning to respond to and integrate the new data into their recommendations.

Adverse effects have been reported at concentrations ranging from 250 to 1250 µg/daily.[21] Hypervitaminosis D has generally been associated with intake of 625 to 1500 µg (25,000-60,000 IU) daily for 1 to 4 months, or several years of vitamin D supplementation at 250 to 1250 µg (10,000-50,000 IU) daily, and has never been associated with sun exposure. Published case reports of vitamin D toxicity with hypercalcemia, for which the 25(OH)D concentration and vitamin D dose are known, all involve intake of at least 1000 µg (40,000 IU) per day, and only one case occurred at a level of intake under 40,000 IU/day.[14]

However, emerging evidence and the opinions of many vitamin D researchers now suggest that the daily value (DV) of 400 IU for vitamin D, which was based on the amount necessary to prevent rickets in infants (initially given as 5 mL of cod liver oil 100 years ago) is an order of magnitude below the amount necessary for older adults, and those not exposed to sun without sunscreen on a regular basis, to achieve and maintain blood levels of vitamin D that are optimum for bone health and cancer prevention.[15,22-33] "Estimates of the population distribution of serum 25(OH)D values, coupled with available dose-response data, indicate that it would require input of an additional 2600 IU/d (65 mcg/d) of oral vitamin D_3 to ensure that 97.5% of older women have 25(OH)D values at or above desirable levels."[34] Absent lymphoma or granulomatous disease, which can cause vitamin D sensitivity, it appears that long-term ingestion of greater than 10,000 IU/day is necessary to cause vitamin D toxicity and hypercalcemia.

Nutrient Adverse Effects
General Adverse Effects

Excessive levels of vitamin D intake over an extended period can lead to headaches, kidney stones, and weight loss. Less common symptoms include diarrhea, increased thirst, increased urination, irritability, and failure to gain weight in children. More extreme consequences include blindness, deafness, and potentially death. Elevated vitamin D levels (as well as vitamin D deficiency) may be related to increased risk of prostate cancer.[35] Vitamin D intake increases both calcium and phosphorus absorption. Although the increased levels of calcium associated with enhanced vitamin D status may be an indicator of benefit for those at risk for bone loss, elevated blood levels of calcium may also be associated with increased risk of heart disease. Elevated serum calcium levels induced by hypervitaminosis D are responsible for many of its primary adverse effects.

Acute overdose is associated with increased urinary frequency, nausea, vomiting, loss of appetite, diarrhea, muscle weakness, dizziness, and calcification of heart, blood vessels, and lungs; symptoms reverse after overdosing is discontinued.

Adverse Effects Among Specific Populations

Individuals with sarcoidosis, other granulomatous diseases, and certain types of lymphoma may quickly develop elevated levels of $1,25(OH)_2$-vitamin D_3 (the activated form), if supplemented with cholecalciferol or other vitamin D precursor, because of autonomous conversion of 25-OHD to the active hormone, $1,25(OH)_2D$. Elevated levels of activated vitamin D significantly increase risk of hypercalcemia, which might require treatment with hydration, intravenous bisphosphonates, ketoconazole, hydroxychloroquine (Plaquenil), and corticosteroids, as well as avoidance of dietary sources of vitamins D_2 and D_3 and calcium.

Pregnancy and Nursing

Vitamin D enters breast milk and is considered compatible at usual dosage levels.

Infants and Children

Vitamin D intakes of 50 to 75 µg (2000-3000 IU) per day may cause toxicity symptoms in some children. Also, some hypersensitive infants have developed toxicity symptoms at 1000 IU/day.

Most cases of toxicity involve the intake of 625 to 1500 µg (25,000-60,000 IU) per day for 1 to 4 months.

Children taking 250 µg (10,000 IU) per day for 4 months can develop the following toxicity symptoms, related to hypercalcemia: headaches, weakness, nausea and vomiting, constipation, polyuria, polydipsia, diarrhea, and calcification of soft tissues, such as kidneys, lungs, tympanic membrane, or ears.

Contraindications

Hypercalcemia, hyperparathyroidism (primary), hypersensitivity to cholecalciferol or any component of the formulation, malabsorption syndrome, sarcoidosis, granulomatous disease, lymphoma; evidence of vitamin D toxicity. If vitamin D insufficiency or deficiency is documented in a patient with lymphoma, cautious supplementation of vitamin D_3 with monitoring of blood levels of both forms of vitamin D and calcium may be undertaken. Not all lymphomas will autonomously convert 25-OHD to its activated form, and no predictive tests yet exist for this capability. Successful treatment of the lymphoma with a complete response obviates the risk of vitamin D hyperconversion. Vitamin D sufficiency may decrease risk of relapse in treated lymphoma patients because vitamin D deficiency is associated with increased risk of developing the disease (along with several other cancers, including breast, colon, and prostate).

Precautions and Warnings

Administer with extreme caution in patients with impaired renal function, heart disease, renal stones, or arteriosclerosis.
Administer concomitant calcium supplementation.
Maintain adequate fluid intake.
Avoid hypercalcemia, although not likely in absence of $1,25(OH)_2$-vitamin D_3 excess.

Caution may be appropriate with renal function impairment with secondary hyperparathyroidism. However, impaired renal function is often associated with a need to administer prescription vitamin D as well as D_3 because second hydroxylation of the 25-OH form is lacking. Furthermore, secondary hyperparathyroidism is an indication for D_3 therapy.

INTERACTIONS REVIEW
Strategic Considerations

Several classes of common pharmacological agents interact with vitamin D and its metabolic processes. These interactions take on greater significance in light of the elevated probability of vitamin D deficiency in many of the patient populations likely to be prescribed the medications under consideration. More broadly, the occurrence of vitamin D deficiency has been recognized as being more widespread than previously believed, and in turn the implications of vitamin D insufficiency for health maintenance and disease prevention have become better understood. Thus, although conventional medical practice and governmental nutritional policies have focused on prevention of short-latency deficiency diseases, vitamin D represents a prime example of the growing awareness of the central role of nutritional factors in health maintenance and prevention of long-latency deficiency diseases. Factors such as lack of time outdoors with significant sunlight exposure, air pollution, cultural practices, and geographic population distribution all add to the subtle but profound significance of seasonal decrease in sunlight availability, even in areas generally considered as "sunny."[7,9,11,36,37] The combined effect of these many factors contributes to what some experts have described as an "epidemic" of vitamin D deficiency, affecting 20% to 60% of the population.

The issues of pervasive vitamin D deficiency status and underutilization of laboratory assessment for 25-hydroxyvitamin D levels influence and limit research design, interpretation, and clinical practice within conventional medicine. For example, in 2005, two randomized controlled trials of calcium carbonate and cholecalciferol (vitamin D$_3$) administration for prevention of fractures in primary care reported widely publicized conclusions that such nutrient supplementation provided no value in preventing fractures.[38,39] Such declarations were made despite disclosures that (1) vitamin D levels had been tested in only a small sample of the subjects in one of the studies; (2) vitamin D deficiency appeared to be common within the subject populations, as indicated by responses to vitamin D supplementation; (3) quality control of the supplements was very poor, and compliance was marginal and declined over time (e.g., 63%, or as low as 45%); and (4) the use of calcium carbonate in a population of older and often hypochlorhydric subjects would be considered suboptimal by many, if not most, experienced practitioners of nutritional therapeutics. Digestion of calcium carbonate relies on the integrity of gastric function and the bowel culture to produce the ionizing acids. Thus, gastrointestinal adverse effects, typical of calcium carbonate, were cited as a major factor in greater noncompliance with calcium intake.

In the study in which 1% of the subjects had their vitamin D levels actually measured, there was only a marginal increase after 1 year of supplementation with 800 IU of vitamin D per day (although some supplements, when analyzed, contained as little as 372 IU, mean value, per tablet). Average 25-OHD levels at beginning of the study (15 ng/mL) were in the range of severe deficiency and after 1 year improved only to 24 ng/mL, still well below what many vitamin D researchers consider to be adequate levels (30-40 ng/mL).[40]

Subsequently, in a trial involving 944 healthy Icelandic adults, Steingrimsdottir et al.[41] found that with 25-OHD levels below 10 ng/mL, maintaining calcium intake above 800 mg/day appeared to normalize calcium metabolism, as determined by the PTH level, but in individuals with higher 25-OHD levels, no benefit was observed from calcium intake above 800 mg/day. Likewise, Jackson et al.[42] found that the combination of 1000 mg elemental calcium (as calcium carbonate) and 400 IU vitamin D daily did not appreciably reduce risk of hip fracture over 7 years, except in those who took their nutrients regularly. Thus, among adherent women (i.e., those who followed the treatment protocol 80% of the time), the supplements reduced hip fractures by 29%. Nevertheless, the relatively low dose of vitamin D, the use of calcium carbonate (a less-than-optimal form in the opinion of many and one associated with reduced compliance), and the late start and relatively limited duration of supplementation suggest that the treatment protocol was less than adequate (unless consistently adhered to) and thus render these findings less than conclusive. Such studies also indicate the importance of nutrient support throughout adulthood, as opposed to beginning it past midlife. Clearly, further research on calcium and other minerals involved in bone metabolism needs to take into account, and preferably optimize, vitamin D status.

Notably, the main conventional pharmacological intervention against osteoporosis is *antiresorptive drugs,* such as

bisphosphonates, for which almost every clinical trial has included coadministration of calcium or vitamin D. Moreover, the decontextualization and narrow focus of these studies highlight the shortcomings of standard research methodology and clinical practice to account for the broad factors of aging, lifestyle, activity level, drug depletions, and poor nutritional status characteristic of the populations in question, as well as the complex nature of bone health and its reliance on interdependencies of multiple nutrients and tissues, rather than such a narrow focus on supplemental calcium and vitamin D. As public and practitioner attention on vitamin D grows, it may prove a pivotal issue in expanding perceptions and awareness, analysis, and intervention through a broad integrative model more accurately reflecting patient needs and scientifically comprehending the breadth and complexity of the processes involved.[14,24,28,37]

The well-known interactions between vitamin D and pharmaceutical medications cluster into several main groups. The use of calcium and vitamin D appears to enhance the bone-maintaining effectiveness of hormone replacement therapy (HRT) and bisphosphonates, especially for women who already have osteoporosis; this benefit appears greater for women supplementing with calcium citrate than for those using calcium carbonate. Anticonvulsants, particularly phenobarbital and phenytoin, may reduce serum levels of calcidiol (25-hydroxycholecalciferol, calcifediol) by altering hepatic metabolism of vitamin D. Notably, physicians prescribing agents that impair vitamin D function for extended periods (e.g., anticonvulsants, opioids, oral corticosteroids) usually do not advise or prescribe adequate countermeasures, whether vitamin D and calcium, bisphosphonates, or the combination, to effectively address the common occurrence of drug-induced decreases in bone mineral density and increased risk of fracture.[43,44] Numerous medications that alter fat absorption, such as cholestyramine, colestipol, mineral oil, orlistat, and olestra, can interfere with intestinal absorption of vitamin D. Ketoconazole can reduce serum levels of calcitriol. Conversely, excessive vitamin D intake may, in rare cases, induce hypercalcemia and could theoretically precipitate cardiac arrhythmia in patients receiving cardiovascular medications such as verapamil or digoxin. Moreover, cardiac glycosides could potentially increase toxicity. Thiazide diuretics may increase vitamin D effects. Finally, it is now recognized that cholecalciferol inhibits CYP2C8/9, 2C19, and 2D6, although the full implications of such activity and the potential effects on pharmaceuticals metabolized by these enzymes have yet to be fully investigated and documented.

Because vitamin D toxicity from supplemental sources is a real (though improbable) possibility, health care providers are reminded to counsel their patients to avoid taking more than the recommended amount of vitamin D, and to take it in conjunction with a calcium supplement and possibly a special diet. The encouragement of greater exposure to sunlight (outdoors) cannot be overemphasized. Although contrary to prevailing dogma of the past decade and as yet poorly studied, it is becoming increasingly evident that use of high-potency sunscreens that block UVB may significantly contribute to vitamin D deficit. Oral supplementation can be used to compensate for lack of adequate UV exposure from sunlight. However, significantly higher amounts of supplementation may be necessary than previously believed and currently available in most vitamin preparations. Titrating intake to blood level of 25-OHD is the most reliable way to ensure adequate intake.

Although some innovative therapeutic strategies are emerging using vitamin D analogs, most examples of such approaches are considered separately in a brief review later.

NUTRIENT-DRUG INTERACTIONS

Allopurinol

Allopurinol (Loporin, Zyloprim)

Interaction Type and Significance
⊕⊕ **Beneficial or Supportive Interaction, with Professional Management**

Probability:
2. Probable

Evidence Base:
○ **Preliminary**

Effect and Mechanism of Action
The uric acid–lowering agent allopurinol may elevate serum concentrations of 1,25-dihydroxycholecalciferol, the active form of vitamin D. Uric acid may directly decrease the serum concentration of $1,25(OH)_2$-vitamin D_3 in patients with gout by inhibiting 1-hydroxylase activity.

Research
Takahashi et al.[45] measured the serum concentrations of $1,25(OH)_2$-vitamin D_3, $25(OH)$-vitamin D_3, and parathyroid hormone (PTH) in 82 male patients with primary gout whose serum uric acid was significantly higher than that of 41 normal control male subjects. The patients with gout exhibited a significantly decreased serum concentration of $1,25(OH)_2$-vitamin D_3, which was corrected as uric acid levels dropped. These researchers reported that administration of allopurinol for 1 year caused a significant increase in their serum $1,25(OH)_2$-vitamin D_3 concentration (along with a significant decrease in their serum uric acid concentration). Notably, the serum concentrations of $25(OH)$-vitamin D_3 and PTH were not affected.

Nutritional Therapeutics, Clinical Concerns, and Adaptations
Individuals diagnosed with gout may have compromised vitamin D status and should be assessed for vitamin D deficiency. Coadministration of a uric acid–lowering agent such as allopurinol may elevate $1,25(OH)_2$-vitamin D_3 levels. Supplementation with vitamin D (5-10 µg/day) may be advisable and is unlikely to present any significant risk, particularly under reasonable supervision and regular monitoring.

Androgen-Deprivation Therapy

Antiandrogens: Bicalutamide (Casodex), cyproterone (Androcur, Cyprostat, Cyproteron, Cyprone, Cyprohexal, Ciproterona, Cyproteronum, Neoproxil, Procur, Siterone), flutamide (Chimax, Drogenil, Euflex, Eulexin), nilutamide (Anandron, Nilandron).
Gonadotropin-releasing hormone (GnRH) agonists/analogs: Goserelin (Zoladex), leuprolide (Eligard, Lupron, Lupron Depot, Viadur), triptorelin (De-capeptyl Trelstar, Trelstar LA).

Interaction Type and Significance
☼ **Prevention and Reduction of Drug Adverse Effect**
⊕⊕ **Beneficial or Supportive Interaction, with Professional Management**

Probability:
2. Probable

Evidence Base:
● **Consensus**

Effect and Mechanism of Action
Decreased levels of sex hormones are generally associated with increased risk of diminished bone mineral density (BMD) and osteoporosis. Supplementation of vitamin D can optimize and preserve bone mass, which tends to be adversely affected by androgen-deprivation therapy (ADT) and is associated with increased risk of osteoporosis and fractures.

Research
Research directly investigating prevention and treatment of osteoporosis caused by ADT is limited. Normally, the incidence of osteoporotic fractures usually increases a decade later in men than in women. Osteoporosis in men with gonadal steroid deficiency can derive from a variety of causes. Gonadotropin-releasing hormone agonists (which, after causing an initial surge in testosterone, result in castrate levels that are maintained as long as the drug is administered) hasten this process and increase bone loss, increasing the risk of osteoporosis and fractures, which have been widely documented in men prescribed ADT for the treatment of prostate carcinoma.[46-53] Four retrospective studies have shown a significant association between ADT and elevated fracture risk in men with prostate cancer.[48,54-56] In particular, with GnRH agonists, men with fractures had lower BMD and higher biochemical markers of bone resorption than men without fractures.[55] Collectively, the available studies indicate that the first year of ADT results in a 5% to 10% decrease in BMD in men with prostate cancer, an effect greater than that associated with menopause.[57] Furthermore, in a cross-sectional study of hormone-naive men with prostate cancer, Smith et al.[58] observed vitamin D deficiency and inadequate dietary intake of calcium in 17% and 59%, respectively.

Smith et al.[59] also found that concurrent treatment with calcium, vitamin D, and pamidronate (a bisphosphonate drug) during ADT increases serum concentrations of both 25-hydroxyvitamin D and 1,25-dihydroxyvitamin D. Bisphosphonates have come to play an important role in supporting bone mass.[59-62] Coadministration of vitamin D (and calcium), particularly with bisphosphonates, is generally accepted.[51] The rationale and supporting research are further discussed in the Bisphosphonates section.

Nutritional Therapeutics, Clinical Concerns, and Adaptations
As with postmenopausal women and HRT, concomitant calcium and vitamin D enable and enhance the fundamental preventive support provided by diet and regular weight-bearing exercise in maintaining (or restoring) bone health, particularly bone mass and BMD. Smoking cessation, moderate alcohol consumption, and other supportive lifestyle modification should be also encouraged. The administration of bisphosphonates constitutes a further intervention as part of conventional care. Clinical management should evolve in response to the results of urinary assessment of bone breakdown (e.g., deoxypyridinium metabolites) and radiographic, DXA (dual-energy x-ray absorptiometry), ultrasound, or other techniques for BMD assessment. Oral intake of the bisphosphonate and calcium should be separated by at least 2 hours.

Anticonvulsant Medications, Including Phenobarbital, Phenytoin, and Valproic Acid

Evidence: Divalproex semisodium, divalproex sodium (Depakote), gabapentin (Neurontin), phenobarbital (phenobarbitone; Luminal, Solfoton), phenytoin (diphenylhydantoin; Dilantin, Phenytek), sodium valproate (Depacon), valproate semisodium, valproic acid (Depakene, Depakene Syrup).
Extrapolated, based on similar properties: Carbamazepine (Carbatrol, Tegretol), clonazepam (Klonopin), clorazepate (Tranxene), diazepam (Valium), ethosuximide (Zarontin),

ethotoin (Peganone), felbamate (Felbatol), fosphenytoin (Cerebyx, Mesantoin), lamotrigine (Lamictal), levetiracetam (Keppra), mephenytoin, mephobarbital (Mebaral), methsuximide (Celontin), oxcarbazepine (GP 47680, oxycarbamazepine; Trileptal), piracetam (Nootropyl), primidone (Mysoline), topiramate (Topamax), trimethadione (Tridione), vigabatrin (Sabril), zonisamide (Zonegran).

Interaction Type and Significance

≈≈≈ **Drug-Induced Nutrient Depletion, Supplementation Therapeutic, Not Requiring Professional Management**

◇ **Adverse Drug Effect on Nutritional Therapeutics, Strategic Concern**

☼ **Prevention or Reduction of Drug Adverse Effect**

Probability: Evidence Base:
2. Probable   ● **Consensus**

Effect and Mechanism of Action

Phenobarbital and related anticonvulsants are inducers of cytochrome P450 and the mixed-function oxidase system. Phenobarbital impairs bioavailability of vitamin D. Phenytoin and phenobarbital may reduce serum levels of 25(OH)D (calcidiol) by altering hepatic metabolism of vitamin D, at least in part by accelerating its metabolism.[63, 64] Antiepileptic drugs (AEDs) that induce the enzyme CYP3A4 are of particular concern because 3A4 degrades vitamin D, which can create effects consistent with secondary hyperparathyroidism; AEDs that induce 3A4 include phenytoin, phenobarbital, carbamazepine, oxcarbazepine, and felbamate. Vitamin D therapy does not appear to alter serum phenytoin levels, but phenytoin may limit the ability of some individuals to respond to vitamin D therapy or may require larger doses of vitamin D to maintain optimal blood levels of 25-OHD. Thus, anticonvulsants impair mineralization, leading to increased risk of osteomalacia and osteoporosis.

High-dose vitamin D therapy can significantly counter vitamin D depletion and improve BMD and prevent bone loss associated with anticonvulsant treatment.

Research

Long-term therapy with phenytoin and other anticonvulsants can disturb vitamin D and calcium metabolism and result in osteomalacia. Both epilepsy and anticonvulsant medications are independent risk factors for low BMD, regardless of vitamin D levels. Long-term anticonvulsant treatment can cause excessive metabolism and deficiency of vitamin D and is believed to be associated with decreased BMD and bone loss.

In a 1982 study of 30 adult epileptic patients, Zerwekh et al.[65] reported decreased serum 24,25-dihydroxyvitamin D concentration during long-term anticonvulsant therapy (with phenytoin, phenobarbital, or carbamazepine), with phenobarbital-treated patients exhibiting a significant decrease in serum 25(OH)D. They noted that various anticonvulsant agents appear to exert different effects on vitamin D metabolism.

After finding no pattern of low serum levels of vitamin D (25[OH]D) or radiological evidence of osteomalacia or rickets in more than 400 individuals using anticonvulsants in Florida, Williams et al.[66] concluded that the climate provided adequate exposure to sunshine and thereby prevented the development of anticonvulsant-induced osteomalacia or rickets. "In contrast to reports from northern climates, we found minimal evidence of anticonvulsant-induced bone disease." Subsequently, in a controlled trial, Riancho et al.[67] studied 17 ambulatory epileptic children taking anticonvulsants for two seasons with high

and low levels of solar radiation and observed that although serum 25-OHD concentrations were normal among medicated subjects during the summer, their levels were significantly lower than those of controls during the winter months.

In initiating a prospective 3-year study, Hunt et al.[68] found that, of 144 children and young adults who required anticonvulsant therapy, 52 were found to have serum alkaline phosphatase (ALP) levels elevated more than two standard deviations (SDs) above normal, and half of these showed signs of rickets or osteomalacia. After slow and gradual but varying rates of response to calcitriol, all patients showed significant lowering of serum ALP levels by 30 months of follow-up. In a later controlled study, Jekovec-Vrhovsek et al.[69] determined that bone strength improved (specifically, BMD increased) in 13 institutionalized children under long-term anticonvulsant therapy who were supplemented for 9 months with 0.25 µg daily 1,25-dihydroxycholecalciferol vitamin D, the activated form of vitamin D, and 500 mg daily calcium.[69]

Telci et al.[70] compared bone turnover in 52 epileptic patients receiving chronic anticonvulsant therapy with 39 healthy volunteers as matched controls and found that the resorption phase of bone turnover is affected during chronic anticonvulsant therapy. Total serum ALP levels (a marker of bone formation) were significantly increased in patients from both genders compared with those of controls. Among male epileptic patients, urinary deoxypyridinoline levels (a marker of bone resorption) were significantly increased and 25-OHD levels significantly reduced compared with controls.[70]

Farhat et al.[71] compared the effects of various AEDs on bone density in 71 adults and children over at least 6 months. More than half the adults and children/adolescents had low serum 25-OHD levels. Although this finding did not correlate with their BMD, AEDs were strongly associated with decreased BMD in the adults, particularly at skeletal sites enriched in cortical bone. Furthermore, lower BMD was more consistently associated with enzyme-inducing agents (e.g., phenytoin, phenobarbital, carbamazepine, primidone) than with medications that did not induce enzymes (e.g., valproic acid, lamotrigine, clonazepam, gabapentin, topamirate, ethosuximide). These researchers concluded: "Generalised seizures, duration of epilepsy, and polypharmacy were significant determinants of bone mineral density."[71]

Although it has been generally established that certain AEDs constituted a risk factor for osteoporosis and fractures in postmenopausal women, data regarding men have largely been lacking. In findings presented at the First North American Regional Epilepsy Congress, Jetter et al.[72] found that "enzyme-inducing AEDs do significantly affect vitamin D, calcium, and parathyroid hormone levels." In this study, researchers focused on phenytoin, phenobarbital, carbamazepine, oxcarbazepine, and felbamate as enzyme 3A4–inducing AEDs. Because 3A4 degrades vitamin D, they set out to determine whether levels of 25-hydroxyvitamin D_3 (25-OH-D_3), PTH, or calcium differed between men taking 3A4 enzyme–inducing AEDs and those taking other types of AEDs. The researchers obtained 25-OH-D_3, intact PTH, and calcium levels in 210 male veterans, age 20 to 89 (average, 58), who had been treated with AEDs for an average of 20.3 years. On analysis, they found that the 126 patients treated with at least one enzyme-inducing AED for at least the past 6 months exhibited an average 25-OH-D_3 level of 19.2 ng/mL, compared with 23.8 ng/mL in those taking non–enzyme-inducing AEDs ($p = .005$). The patients taking enzyme-inducing AEDs had a blood calcium level of 8.83 mg/dL, whereas the 64 treated with only non–enzyme-inducing AEDs for that period exhibited levels of 9.16 mg/dL ($p = .00009$). The intact PTH levels averaged 52.5 pg/mL for patients on enzyme-inducing AEDs and 38.2 pg/mL for patients on non-enzyme-inducing AEDs ($p = .0002$). The 20 patients treated with divalproex sodium were analyzed separately. The authors concluded that the "findings suggest that a secondary hyperparathyroidism is associated with the use of these drugs and that dietary supplementation of vitamin D may be necessary to prevent osteoporosis." Furthermore, the investigators emphasized that neurologists need to monitor BMD in men treated with these medications, parallel to recommendations regarding female patients.[72]

In 2001, Valmadrid et al.[73] published a survey of practice patterns of neurologists. They found that only 41% of pediatric and 28% of adult neurologists performed routine evaluation of patients taking AEDs for either bone or mineral disease. Further, among those physicians who detected bone disease through such diagnostic testing, 40% of pediatric and 37% of adult neurologists prescribed either calcium or vitamin D. However, only 9% of pediatric and 7% of adult neurologists prescribed prophylactic calcium or vitamin D for patients receiving AED therapy.

In two parallel, randomized, controlled trials involving 72 adults (18-54 years old) and 78 children and adolescents (10-18 years), Mikati, Fuleihan, et al.[74] investigated the effects of two doses of vitamin D given over 1 year on BMD in ambulatory patients on long-term AED therapy. Adult subjects received either "low-dose vitamin D" (400 IU/day) or "high-dose vitamin D" (4000 IU/day), and children and adolescents received 400 or 2000 IU/day. At baseline, 34% of the adults were in the deficient range of vitamin D levels, and 46% were in the insufficient range; the parallel levels for children were 18% and 44%, respectively. Likewise, using DXA, baseline BMD in adults was lower than that of age-matched and gender-matched controls versus either a Western or an ethnically identical population. After treatment, none of the adults and only a few of the children in the high-dose group still exhibited vitamin D deficiency, and relatively few had vitamin D insufficiency. Furthermore, the authors demonstrated that "significant increases in BMD at all skeletal sites compared to baseline" after 1 year in the high-dose, but not in the low-dose, vitamin D group. Nevertheless, BMD at 1 year remained below normal. Notably, baseline BMD was normal in children (compared with age- and gender-matched controls), and both treatment groups "showed significant and comparable increases" in BMD. The authors concluded that in "ambulatory adults on antiepileptic drugs, high-dose vitamin D therapy substantially increased bone mineral density at several skeletal sites," and that "both doses resulted in comparable increases in bone mass" in children. These findings represent the first clinical trials demonstrating that high-dose vitamin D therapy significantly improves BMD in patients receiving AED therapy.[74]

Report

Duus[75] reported a case of several severe fractures in a patient following epileptic seizures. The patient had epileptic osteomalacia and responded well to vitamin D treatment.

Nutritional Therapeutics, Clinical Concerns, and Adaptations

Many individuals with epilepsy, especially children, lead restricted lifestyles and are often institutionalized or under other forms of full-time care. Such individuals not only experience the effects of the pathophysiology on vitamin D metabolism, but also tend to have compromised nutritional status and restricted time outdoors in the sun, especially during winter months. Thus, sunlight represents an effective and low-risk method of supporting vitamin D status. Oral supplementation can also be recommended. A moderate dose of 400 to 1500 IU/day of vitamin D could exert a protective function for individuals using phenobarbital or phenytoin who are concerned about potential drug-induced rickets, osteomalacia, or osteoporosis. Pretreatment and posttreatment monitoring of serum 25-OHD and 1,25-$(OH)_2$D levels would also identify individuals at risk of treatment-induced and nutritional/sunlight-related deficiencies of vitamin D. Available evidence indicates that such supplementation does not represent a significant risk of interfering with the therapeutic activity of standard anticonvulsant agents. However, as previously suggested, regular exposure to sunlight represents an effective and low-risk method of supporting vitamin D status by providing adequate stimulation of endogenous synthesis of necessary levels of vitamin D. Others have advocated a proactive approach toward the risks of bone loss while voicing caution that given the increased risk of osteomalacia, osteoporosis, and rickets among those taking anticonvulsants, withdrawal from such drugs carries potential for increased risk of seizure-related fractures. Monitoring of bone status is often appropriate.

Bisphosphonates

Evidence: Alendronate (Fosamax), etidronate (Didronel). Extrapolated, based on similar properties: Clodronate (Bonefos, Ostac), ibandronate (Bondronat, Boniva), risedronate (Actonel), tiludronate (Skelid), zoledronic acid (Zometa). Similar properties but evidence lacking for extrapolation: Pamidronate (Aredia).

Interaction Type and Significance

⊕⊕⊕ **Beneficial or Supportive Interaction, Not Requiring Professional Management**

Probability	Evidence Base
2. Probable or	◉ **Emerging** or
1. Certain	● **Consensus**

Effect and Mechanism of Action

The ability of bisphosphonates to inhibit osteoclastic activity and bone resorption, maintain healthy bone mineralization, and produce substantial gains in bone mass depends on the presence of adequate vitamin D and other nutrients (e.g., protein, calcium, phosphorus).[76,77] Calcium, the principal element in bone, can be absorbed in the brush border of the intestinal mucosa only when vitamin D is present. Notably, bisphosphonates have been used effectively to treat the more resistant cases of vitamin D–induced hypercalcemia.

Research

All currently approved, bone-active pharmacological agents have been studied only in conjunction with supplemental calcium, and newer anabolic agents increase mineral demand in skeletal tissue and will thus require even higher levels of calcium repletion.[78] The consensus underlying the fundamental importance of vitamin D and calcium nutriture is underscored by the observation that when Greenspan et al.[79] investigated the relative efficacy of HRT (conjugated estrogen with or without medroxyprogesterone) plus alendronate, HRT alone, alendronate alone, or placebo on spine and hip BMD in 373 osteopenic elderly women, all subjects received calcium and vitamin D supplements. After 3 years, DXA scans showed that participants taking combination therapy had greater improvement in BMD at the hip and spine than those taking HRT or alendronate alone or taking placebo, all with calcium and vitamin D.

In an uncontrolled clinical trial involving osteoporosis patients with a poor response to bisphosphonate therapy, Heckman et al.[80] found that the addition of 25 µg (1000 IU) per day of vitamin D to the bisphosphonate regimen resulted in significantly increased BMD of the lumbar spine after 1 year. In a randomized, double-blind trial involving 48 osteopenic and osteoporotic women, Brazier et al.[81] compared one group who received 10 mg alendronate once daily along with 500 mg elemental calcium daily and 10 µg (400 IU) cholecalciferol (vitamin D_3) twice daily for 3 months and a second group who received the same dosage of alendronate and calcium but placebo instead of the vitamin D. All subjects had low BMD, serum 25-hydroxyvitamin D_3 (25-OHD, calcifediol) less than 12 µg/L, and dietary calcium intake less than 1 g/day. Although markers of bone remodeling, such as serum and urinary CTX and urinary NTX (C- and N-terminal telopeptides of type I collagen), were dramatically and significantly decreased after as little as 15 days of treatment and remained decreased throughout the course of treatment in both groups, the group also receiving the vitamin D demonstrated a more pronounced effect, particularly after 1 month, for the bone resorption markers serum CTX and urinary NTX. These researchers concluded that coadministration of calcium and vitamin D is appropriate in elderly women with calcium and vitamin D insufficiencies receiving alendronate, to achieve rapid reduction of bone loss.[81]

In a randomized trial involving 154 patients with Crohn's disease, Siffledeen et al.[82] investigated the efficacy of etidronate plus calcium and vitamin D for treatment of low BMD. The subjects, most of whom had T scores in the osteopenic range (−1.5 to −2.5), were administered etidronate (400 mg orally) or placebo for 14 days, and then both groups were given daily calcium (500 mg) and vitamin D (400 IU) for 76 days, in a treatment cycle repeated every 3 months for 2 years. After 24 months, BMD at the lumbar spine, ultradistal radius, and trochanter sites, but not the total hip, increased steadily, significantly, and similarly in both treatment arms. The findings demonstrate that in patients with low BMD on absorptiometry, treatment with calcium and vitamin D alone will increase BMD by about 4% per year, and that adding etidronate to the treatment program does not appear to enhance the effects of calcium and vitamin D.[82] In an accompanying editorial on the preeminence of calcium and vitamin D in limiting fracture risk in Crohn's disease, Bernstein[83] commented that this study provides reassurance that bisphosphonates are "rarely needed in IBD [inflammatory bowel disease] patients, most of whom have T scores greater than −2.5, and many of whom are using corticosteroids to some extent."

Some patients with prostate carcinoma and a diffuse metastatic invasion of the skeleton exhibit indirect biochemical and histologic indications of osteomalacia. Bisphosphonates are known to cause symptomatic hypocalcemia in prostate cancer patients with diffuse skeletal metastases. Bisphosphonate administration can aggravate osteomalacia and give the appearance of symptomatic hypocalcemia because of the transient, striking prevalence of osteoblastic activity over bone resorption by osteoclasts, which are inhibited by bisphosphonate drugs. Calcium supplementation is often considered as contraindicated in individuals with prostate cancer. However, concomitant use of calcium with bisphosphonates has been proposed as a means of inhibiting the osteoclastic activation that often precedes the abnormal osteoblastic bone formation within metastases.

In regard to men with nonmetastatic prostate cancer, findings from a small, randomized, double-blind, controlled trial conducted by Nelson et al.[84] showed that treatment with alendronate, 70 mg weekly, plus daily calcium and vitamin D, reversed bone loss in 56 men receiving antiandrogen therapy. In contrast, the 56 subjects taking placebo, calcium, and vitamin D lost bone density during the same period. Notably, among these 112 men, with an average age of 71, only 9% had normal bone mass, whereas 52% had low bone mass and 39% developed osteoporosis after an average 2 years of ADT.

Nutritional Therapeutics, Clinical Concerns, and Adaptations

Calcium and vitamin D are essential for maintaining bone mass and density and imperative to the success of drug therapies for inducing bone augmentation.[77] Deficiencies of both nutrients are common in the patient populations at highest risk for osteoporosis. The importance of exercise and sound nutrition (including adequate protein, calcium, and phosphorus intake) as foundational cannot be overemphasized and is supported by growing evidence. Calcium has a clearly demonstrated effect of enhancing estrogen's effects on bone metabolism. Further, most research indicates that consistent exposure to sunlight (excluding winter in northern latitudes) provides a safe and effective, as well as otherwise beneficial, method of elevating vitamin D levels. Doses of 1500 mg calcium and 800 IU vitamin D daily provide prudent nutritional support for osteoporosis prevention and treatment, or more exactly, 30 to 40 mmol calcium with sufficient intake vitamin D daily to maintain serum 25(OH)D levels above 80 nmol/L (∼30 µg/ L).[78]

Thus, a synergistic combination of oral calcium and vitamin D, within the context of an active lifestyle, constitutes the core proactive intervention within integrative therapeutics for all individuals at high risk for osteoporosis, or a foundational treatment for diagnosed bone loss. Notably, low serum vitamin D levels have been associated with the incidence of falls in older women,[85] and vitamin D has been found to be helpful in reducing the incidence of falls, a major factor in fracture risk, by improving muscle strength, walking distance, and functional ability.[86] Also, hormone supplementation or replacement regimens (conventional HRT, bio-identical estrogens/progesterone, herbal hormone precursors/modulators) should be considered if indicated in women.

In addition to these primary and secondary therapies, a bisphosphonate can provide a potent intervention in reversing bone loss and supporting healthy bone mass. Whereas oral calcium preparations need to be taken at least 2 hours before or after the bisphosphonate to avoid pharmacokinetic interference, such timing of oral vitamin D intake is unnecessary because no evidence has indicated potential pharmacological interference with bisphosphonates or other components of the treatment. It is generally recommended that alendronate or etidronate be taken with a full glass (6-8 ounces) of plain water on an empty stomach, avoiding the recumbent position for at least 30 minutes to prevent the potential for severe esophageal irritation associated with incomplete transfer of the tablet to the stomach.

Calcitriol and Vitamin D Analogs

Alfacalcidol, calcitriol, dihydrotachysterol.
See also later discussion for therapeutics involving vitamin D analogs and other agents.

Interaction Type and Significance

✗✗   Minimal to Mild Adverse Interaction—Vigilance
       Necessary
✗✗✗   Potentially Harmful or Serious Adverse
       Interaction—Avoid
◇◇   Drug-Induced Effect on Nutrient Function,
       Supplementation Contraindicated, Professional
       Management Appropriate

Probability: Evidence Base:
1. Certain   ● Consensus

Effect and Mechanism of Action

The simultaneous use of supplemental vitamin D and vitamin D analogs, such as calcitriol, inherently produces an additive effect. The potential for vitamin D toxicity is particularly increased because calcitriol [$1,25(OH)_2D_3$] and its drug formulations bypass physiological feedback mechanisms and control systems that normally limit its production in the kidneys. The clinical significance and severity of the interaction primarily depend on the respective dosages involved and duration of intake, although individual variability based on VDR genotype, diet, and other factors may modify the intensity and character of the response.

Research

Research into coordinated administration of supplemental vitamin D and vitamin D analogs represents a viable approach to integrative therapeutics that has yet to be conducted in a systemic manner.

The use of calcitriol and other vitamin D analogs in combination with other pharmaceutical agents represents an emerging area of therapeutic synergy. Even though these agents are drugs and not nutrients per se, their action is derived from their relationship to vitamin D, and their therapeutic application is discussed briefly later.

Reports

Reports of vitamin D toxicity resulting from simultaneous intake of vitamin D and pharmaceutical analogs are lacking.

Clinical Implications and Adaptations

Coadministration of vitamin D and analogs such as calcitriol may be appropriate in some circumstances, as in renal disease, but only under close medical supervision. Unintentional concomitant use of vitamin D and its pharmacological analogs should be avoided through direct inquiry by health care providers of patients initiating therapy and routine implementation of a thorough inventory of vitamin and other supplement intake.

Cholestyramine, Colestipol, and Related Bile Acid Sequestrants

Evidence: Cholestyramine (Locholest, Prevalite, Questran), colestipol (Colestid).
Extrapolated, based on similar properties: Colesevelam (WelChol).

Interaction Type and Significance

≈≈≈   Drug-Induced Nutrient Depletion,
       Supplementation Therapeutic, Not Requiring
       Professional Management
◇   Adverse Drug Effect on Nutritional
       Therapeutics, Strategic Concern

Probability: Evidence Base:
4. Plausible   ○ Preliminary

Effect and Mechanism of Action

Absorption of dietary sources of vitamin D requires bile. Bile acid sequestrants, such as cholestyramine and colestipol, decrease lipid digestion and absorption. In the process, they also reduce absorption of the fat-soluble vitamins, such as vitamin D, and other nutrients.[87-89]

Research

Tonstad et al.[90] conducted a study of 37 boys and 29 girls age 10 to 16 years with familial hypercholesterolemia, first in an 8-week, double-blind, placebo-controlled protocol, then in open treatment for 44 to 52 weeks. After 1 year of colestipol, those who took 80% or more of the prescribed dose had a greater decrease in serum 25-OHD levels than those who took less than 80%. They also found that levels of serum folate, vitamin E, and carotenoids were reduced in the colestipol group.[90]

In a rodent model, Watkins et al.[91] found that cholestyramine may deplete calcium (and zinc), an effect that could adversely impact the function of vitamin D, especially in regard to bone health.

Nutritional Therapeutics, Clinical Concerns, and Adaptations

Fat-soluble vitamins, and vitamin D nutriture in particular, can play a valuable role in the prevention and treatment of many conditions involving the cardiovascular system and lipid metabolism (including atherosclerosis, heart disease, obesity, hypertension, and diabetes), such that interference with its absorption could be counterproductive in relation to the broad therapeutic strategy and clinical outcomes. Modest supplementation with vitamin D (10-20 μg or 400-800 IU daily) may be advisable for many individuals, particularly those at high risk for deficiency sequelae, but consistent exposure to sunlight (without sunscreen) may be sufficient to maintain healthy vitamin D levels and can be combined with the exercise usually critical to those prescribed bile acid sequestrants. Exposure to sunlight in the winter months of higher latitudes, however, is likely to be insufficient to maintain adequate vitamin D levels, making dietary use of supplements or a rich natural source of vitamin D (e.g., cod liver oil) necessary, separated from the bile acid sequestrant by at least 2 hours.

Cimetidine

Cimetidine (Tagamet)

Interaction Type and Significance

≈≈≈   Drug-Induced Nutrient Depletion,
       Supplementation Therapeutic, Not Requiring
       Professional Management
◇   Adverse Drug Effect on Nutritional
       Therapeutics, Strategic Concern

Probability: Evidence Base:
4. Plausible   ○ Preliminary

Effect and Mechanism of Action

Cimetidine inhibits vitamin D hydroxylase (a hepatic mixed-function oxidase) and may reduce hepatic activation of vitamin D through hydroxylation.[92]

Research

In limited animal and human research, cimetidine has been found to decrease the synthesis of vitamin D and adversely affect serum levels of 25-OHD.

In a small, uncontrolled trial, Odes et al.[93] treated nine adult subjects with 400 mg cimetidine orally twice daily during a period from winter to summer, as the daily duration of sunlight was increasing. They measured serum levels of 25-OHD, 24,25(OH)$_2$D, and 1,25(OH)$_2$D before treatment, after 4 weeks of treatment, and 1 month after cessation of treatment. The normal seasonal increase in the level of 25-OHD was not observed during treatment. However, 25-OHD did rise significantly after the cimetidine was withdrawn. These researchers concluded that their findings "suggest that short-term treatment with cimetidine could potentially perturb vitamin D metabolism in man."

Further clinical trials would be necessary confirm these preliminary findings and to determine whether other H$_2$ receptor antagonists might similarly affect vitamin D metabolism in humans.

Nutritional Therapeutics, Clinical Concerns, and Adaptations

Laboratory tests can determine blood levels of 25-hydroxycholecalciferol, the form of vitamin D after it has been hydroxylated in the liver. Low levels require prescription of an activated form of vitamin D (e.g., calcitriol) because activation of a regular vitamin D supplement (or even cholecalciferol derived from sunlight exposure) would be vulnerable to blockage by the cimetidine. In this case it would be prudent to monitor the serum level of 1,25-dihydroxyvitamin D to be certain that replacement is adequate but not excessive.

Corticosteroids, Oral, Including Prednisone

Betamethasone (Celestone), cortisone (Cortone), dexamethasone (Decadron), fludrocortisone (Florinef), hydrocortisone (Cortef), methylprednisolone (Medrol) prednisolone (Delta-Cortef, Orapred, Pediapred, Prelone), prednisone (Deltasone, Liquid Pred, Meticorten, Orasone), triamcinolone (Aristocort).

Similar properties but evidence indicating no or reduced interaction effects: Inhaled or topical corticosteroids.

Interaction Type and Significance

≈≈≈ **Drug-Induced Nutrient Depletion, Supplementation Therapeutic, Not Requiring Professional Management**

◇≈≈ **Drug-Induced Adverse Effect on Nutrient Function, Coadministration Therapeutic, with Professional Management**

◇ **Adverse Drug Effect on Nutritional Therapeutics, Strategic Concern**

Probability: Evidence Base:
2. Probable, 3. Possible   ○ **Emerging**

Effect and Mechanism of Action

Oral corticosteroids are associated with osteoporosis. The mechanism is multifactorial, including reduced calcium absorption, decreased vitamin D availability, lowered serum 25-hydroxycalciferol levels, and interference with vitamin D activation and metabolism, all increasing risk of bone loss.[94-99] Corticosteroids also contribute to osteoporosis through increased renal calcium excretion and decreased bone formation by osteoblasts and serum levels of sex hormones. Administration of cortisone impairs net calcium absorption through two mechanisms: depressed vitamin D–dependent calcium absorption and increased vitamin D–independent calcium backflux.[100]

Research

It is generally recognized that long-term use of corticosteroids can lead to loss of bone mineral density (BMD) and higher risk for fractures. Of patients using corticosteroids for long periods, 25% develop at least one fracture. Although the usefulness of calcium and vitamin D supplements in the treatment and the prevention of steroid-induced osteoporosis may seem self-evident, research into the effectiveness of such nutritional therapies has been slow to evolve. Nevertheless, it now appears that the adverse effects of glucoactive corticosteroids on intestinal calcium transport and bone turnover can usually be counteracted by the combined administration of supplemental doses of calcium and physiological doses of 25-OHD$_3$.

In 1977, Hahn et al.[101] observed no significant serum 25-OHD concentrations in 21 adults receiving chronic, moderate-dose corticosteroid therapy and who demonstrated radiological osteopenia (vs. controls). However, in 1978, Chesney et al.[98] found a reduction of serum 1,25(OH)$_2$D in children receiving long-term glucocorticoid treatment for various glomerular diseases (vs. children with chronic glomerulonephritis but not treated with glucocorticoids). They further observed that this reduction in serum 1,25(OH)$_2$D$_3$ concentration correlated with the dose of steroid administered as well as with the severity of reduction in forearm bone mineral content.

By administering 20 mg/day of prednisone to 12 normal adults for 14 days, Hahn et al.[94] confirmed that glucocorticoids suppress intestinal calcium absorption (by 31%), but not by decreasing circulating concentrations of biologically active vitamin D metabolites, since mean serum concentrations of 25-OHD and 24,25(OH)$_2$D did not change significantly from initial values; serum 1,25(OH)$_2$D concentration was even slightly increased.

In a 2-year, randomized, double-blind, placebo-controlled trial, Buckley et al.[102] administered 500 IU of vitamin D$_3$ and 1000 mg of calcium carbonate daily to 65 rheumatoid arthritis patients being treated with low amounts of prednisone (mean dosage, 5.6 mg daily). They found that those who received the nutrients maintained or gained BMD in the lumbar spine and trochanter, whereas those receiving prednisone therapy but were given placebo (i.e., no supplements) lost BMD in the same areas during the course of the study. In a subsequent study (1998), Lems et al.[103] reported that low-dose (10 mg/day) prednisone (LDP) treatment led to a decrease in osteocalcin, P1CP, and alkaline phosphatase and an increase in urinary excretion of calcium. They concluded that LDP has a negative effect on bone metabolism because bone formation decreased while bone resorption remained unchanged or decreased slightly. They also found parathyroid hormone (PTH) increased (insignificantly) during LDP (+19%) and LDP plus calcium (+14%), but decreased during coadministration of with calcitriol (−16%) and calcium/calcitriol (−44%). The increase in PTH during LDP could be prevented by calcitriol combined with calcium supplementation.

Wissing et al.[104] conducted a 1-year controlled trial investigating the effect of low-dose corticosteroids on post–renal transplant bone loss and the ability of cholecalciferol to further decrease bone loss. They administered either 400 mg oral calcium or 400 mg oral calcium daily in association with a monthly dose of 25,000 IU vitamin D$_3$ to 90 patients admitted for renal transplantation and scheduled to be treated with low doses of prednisolone. All subjects experienced a "moderate but significant" loss of lumbar spine BMD, but no bone loss at the femoral neck and shaft during the first posttransplant year. Subjects in the calcium/D$_3$ group had significantly higher 25-OHD but not 1,25(OH)$_2$D levels and exhibited slightly higher bone loss, but the difference did not reach statistical significance. The researchers also reported "a highly significant negative correlation between 25(OH) vitamin D and intact parathyroid hormone (iPTH) serum levels." They concluded that "cholecalciferol supplementation did not prevent posttransplant bone loss but contributed to the normalization of iPTH levels after renal transplantation."[104] Notably, the dose administered, 25,000 IU of D_3 once a month, is less than the 1000 IU per day recommended by experts as the minimum for those not exposed to adequate sunlight, and it is not well timed for an agent with a half-life of 2 weeks.

A meta-analysis of well-designed clinical trials by Amin et al.[105] concluded that supplementation with vitamin D and calcium was more effective than placebo or calcium alone in providing a "moderate" protective effect against corticosteroid-induced osteoporosis, using change in lumbar spine BMD as the primary outcome measure. However, bisphosphonates and fluoride were more effective than vitamin D in some trials.

In contrast, numerous studies and several reviews of inhalant and nasal corticosteroids have consistently concluded that such medications, in and of themselves, do not generally pose a significant risk of inducing bone loss in children or adults.[106] For example, Elmstahl et al.[107] reported no difference in BMD in a group of subjects taking inhaled corticosteroids and unexposed control subjects, nor was any dose-response relationship observed between inhalant steroid therapy and BMD. Likewise, Suissa et al.[108] conducted a case-control study nested within a population-based cohort of all Quebec patients at least 65 years of age who were given respiratory medications and followed for at least 4 years. The rate of fracture for current inhaled corticosteroid use was not increased, and the rate of upper extremity fracture increased by 12% (RR 1.12) with every 1000-μg increase in the daily dose of inhaled corticosteroids. No such increase was observed for hip fracture. Among a subgroup of subjects followed more than 8 years, "only the use of more than 2000 μg of inhaled corticosteroids per day for an average of 6 years was associated with an elevated risk of fracture." No increase in the rate of fractures was observed at any dose of nasal corticosteroids.

Nutritional Therapeutics, Clinical Concerns, and Adaptations

Physicians prescribing corticosteroids, possibly for only 1 month but especially for longer periods, are advised to discuss the potential adverse metabolic implications of such medications with patients and compensatory options. In 1998, Lems et al.[109] noted that "in spite of guidelines according to which patients protractedly using corticosteroids should take sufficient calcium and cholecalciferol, only about one-tenth of them takes any form of medication to prevent osteoporosis." Most research indicates that calcium intakes from dietary and supplemental sources totaling 1000 to 1500 mg of calcium per day in conjunction with 10 to 20 μg (400-800 IU) of vitamin D are required to prevent adverse effects, although much higher doses may be necessary in the context of a preexisting 25OHD deficiency.[40] Monitoring serum levels of both 25-OHD and 1,25(OH)$_2$D (activated form of vitamin D) is appropriate, and supplementation (or possibly a prescription of calcitriol) is often necessary if a deficiency is indicated. If 25-OHD levels are low (< 50 nmol/L), correction with up to 7000 IU vitamin D_3 per day, or 50,000 IU vitamin D_2 per week, for 1 to 2 months will correct the 1,25(OH)$_2$D level in patients with normal renal function. Often the 1,25(OH)$_2$D (dihydroxycholecalciferol) level is maintained, even in the face of a 25-OHD deficiency, due to increased secretion of PTH, which speeds up renal conversion of 25-OHD to the active form. Thus, measuring intact PTH, as well as both forms of vitamin D, provides the most complete picture of vitamin D status.[40] It is also prudent to monitor for

hypercalciuria and hypercalcemia when supplementing with both calcium and vitamin D, although the occurrence of hypercalcemia is rare.

Physicians prescribing steroids for longer than 2 weeks should encourage all patients to modify their lifestyles, including smoking cessation and limitation of alcohol consumption. The importance of mild to moderate weight-bearing exercise cannot be overemphasized; 30 minutes to 1 hour every day, particularly with sunlight exposure, should be strongly encouraged, if feasible. However, individuals with known or potential bone loss should be advised to develop an exercise program under the supervision of a physician or other health care professional familiar with the increased risks of fracture associated with long-term use of steroids.

Some physicians may consider it necessary and appropriate to prescribe calcitriol in individual cases. Concomitant use of bisphosphonates and estrogen/progesterone support may also be appropriate for some individuals using oral steroids longer than 3 months, especially if low BMD is evident or likely.

Hormone Replacement Therapy (HRT): Estrogen-Containing and Synthetic Estrogen and Progesterone Analog Medications

Evidence: HRT, estrogens: Chlorotrianisene (Tace); conjugated equine estrogens (Premarin); conjugated synthetic estrogens (Cenestin); dienestrol (Ortho Dienestrol); esterified estrogens (Estratab, Menest, Neo-Estrone); estradiol, topical/transdermal/ring (Alora Transdermal, Climara Transdermal, Estrace, Estradot, Estring FemPatch, Vivelle-Dot, Vivelle Transdermal); eestradiol cypionate (Dep-Gynogen, Depo-Estradiol, Depogen, Dura-Estrin, Estra-D, Estro-Cyp, Estroject-LA, Estronol-LA); estradiol hemihydrate (Estreva, Vagifem); estradiol valerate (Delestrogen, Estra-L 40, Gynogen L.A. 20, Progynova, Valergen 20); estrone (Aquest, Estragyn 5, Estro-A, Estrone '5', Kestrone-5); estropipate (Ogen, Ortho-Est); ethinyl estradiol (Estinyl, Gynodiol, Lynoral).

HRT, estrogen/progestin combinations: Conjugated equine estrogens and medroxyprogesterone (Premelle cycle 5, Prempro); conjugated equine estrogens and norgestrel (Prempak-C); estradiol and dydrogesterone (Femoston); estradiol and norethindrone, patch (CombiPatch); estradiol and norethindrone/norethisterone, oral (Activella, Climagest, Climesse, FemHRT, Trisequens); estradiol valerate and cyproterone acetate (Climens); estradiol valerate and norgestrel (Progyluton); estradiol and norgestimate (Ortho-Prefest).

Related but evidence lacking for extrapolation: HRT, estrogen/testosterone combinations: Esterified estrogens and methyltestosterone (Estratest, Estratest HS).

HRT, progestins: Dydrogesterone (Duphaston), intrauterine L-norgestrel system (Mirena), medroxyprogesterone acetate (Provera), norethisterone (norethindrone; Micronor).

HRT, progesterone: Micronized progesterone (Prometrium, Utrogestan).

Medroxyprogesterone: Conjugated equine estrogens and medroxyprogesterone (Premelle cycle 5, Prempro); medroxyprogesterone, oral (Cycrin, Provera); medroxyprogesterone, injection (depot medroxyprogesterone acetate, DMPA; Depo-Provera, Depo-subQ Provera 104); progestin and estrogen injectable: estradiol cypionate and medroxyprogesterone acetate (Cyclofem, Lunelle).

Interaction Type and Significance

⊕⊕   **Beneficial or Supportive Interaction, with Professional Management**

✗✗   **Minimal to Mild Adverse Interaction—Vigilance Necessary**

Probability:
3. Possible or
  2. Probable

Evidence Base:
○ Emerging

Effect and Mechanism of Action

The combination of vitamin D and estrogen replacement therapy (ERT, in the context of calcium supplementation) increases bone mass more than ERT alone, especially in osteoporotic women. The ability of exogenous female hormones, particularly forms of estrogen, to effectively inhibit osteoclastic activity and bone resorption, maintain healthy bone mineralization, and support bone mass is inherently dependent on the presence of vitamin D and other nutrients (e.g., protein, calcium, phosphorus).[76,77] Calcium, the principal element in bone, can be absorbed in the brush border of the intestinal mucosa only when vitamin D is present. Estrogen appears to have a beneficial effect on vitamin D (and calcium) metabolism, although progestins may diminish that benefit. Estrogen also inhibits osteoclastic action, which would represent an additive interaction with vitamin D.

Research

The negative calcium balance usually associated with aging is accentuated in osteoporotic women who have decreased calcium absorption and decreased serum levels of $1,25(OH)_2D$. In a controlled trial involving 17 women with surgically induced menopause, Lobo et al.[110] (1985) observed that serum levels of $1,25(OH)_2D$ increased and urinary calcium loss decreased after 2 months of conjugated estrogens (0.625 mg daily).[110] Subsequently, several studies have investigated various aspects of the question of whether such elevated vitamin D levels might correspond with increased bone strength and reduced risk of fractures and how this effect might vary given initial BMD status, for different individuals, under different HRT regimens, or with different forms of calcium.

Several studies have examined the role of HRT in improving vitamin D activity and calcium balance in women with postmenopausal osteoporosis. In an early study of postmenopausal women by Bikle et al.,[111] treatment with 17β-estradiol alone increased serum $1,25(OH)_2D$, but the addition of medroxyprogesterone, a progestin, lowered vitamin D levels such that total and free $1,25(OH)_2D$ returned toward baseline and thus appeared to antagonize part of the beneficial effects on calcium homeostasis attributable to estrogen. In the first prospective trial confirming the beneficial effect of HRT on prevention of peripheral fractures in nonosteoporotic postmenopausal women and subsequent controlled studies, Komulainen et al.[112-114] determined that supplementation with 300 IU/day of vitamin D_3 (cholecalciferol) does not prevent bone loss in healthy, nonosteoporotic, early-postmenopausal women, nor does such low-dose vitamin D_3 provide significant benefit beyond that attributable solely to combined estradiol and progestin. However, in a 4-year, prospective, partly randomized study of 60 osteoporotic women, Tuppurainen et al.[115] found that vitamin D_3 (cholecalciferol, 300 IU/day, no intake during June–August) together with a combination of 2 mg estradiol valerate and 1 mg of a progestin (cyproterone acetate) daily resulted in greater improvement in BMD compared with estradiol/progestin alone (as well as with baseline or placebo). The osteoporotic women in both HRT groups demonstrated a significant increase in lumbar BMD, but there were no statistically significant differences in either lumbar or femoral BMD changes between these two HRT groups. Furthermore, the combination of HRT and vitamin D_3 was associated with a greater increase in femoral neck BMD than with HRT alone.

In a randomized, double-blind, placebo-controlled trial involving 128 healthy Caucasian women over age 65 with low spinal BMD, Recker et al.[116] compared parameters of BMD and bone loss under continuous low-dose HRT (conjugated equine estrogen, 0.3 mg/day, and medroxyprogesterone, 2.5 mg/day) in conjunction with calcium and vitamin D supplementation versus placebo. Subjects in both groups were administered sufficient calcium supplementation to bring all calcium intakes above 1000 mg/day and oral 25-OHD sufficient to maintain serum 25-OHD levels of at least 75 nmol/L. Through the course of 3.5 years of observation, significant increases were seen in spinal BMD as well as in total-body and forearm bone density, particularly among patients with greater than 90% adherence to therapy. Meanwhile, breast tenderness, spotting, pelvic discomfort, mood changes, and other symptoms typically associated with HRT were mild and short-lived under this relatively low-dose regimen. These authors concluded that "continuous low-dose HRT with conjugated equine estrogen and oral medroxyprogesterone combined with adequate calcium and vitamin D provides a bone-sparing effect that is similar or superior to that provided by other, higher-dose HRT regimens in elderly women" and is well tolerated by most patients.[116]

In a 6-month, placebo-controlled clinical trial involving 21 postmenopausal women with osteoporosis, Gallagher et al.[117] observed that conjugated equine estrogen increased both calcium absorption and serum vitamin D levels [$1,25(OH)_2D$]. Subsequently, these researchers investigated the roles of estrogen deficiency and declining calcium absorption from reduced activated vitamin D (calcitriol) levels or intestinal resistance to calcitriol as central factors in age-related bone loss. In a randomized, double-blind, placebo-controlled trial involving 485 elderly women (66-77 years old) with normal BMD for their age, Gallagher et al.[118] compared the effects of ERT (0.625 mg conjugated estrogens daily for women without a uterus) and HRT (ERT plus 2.5 mg medroxyprogesterone acetate daily for those women with a uterus) with or without calcitriol (1,25-OHD) versus placebo. Hormone therapy alone and in combination with calcitriol were both highly effective in reducing bone resorption and increasing BMD at the hip and other key sites. In particular, calcitriol was effective in increasing BMD in the femoral neck and spine. The combination of ERT/HRT and calcitriol increased BMD in the total hip and trochanter significantly more than did ERT or HRT alone, particularly in women adherent to treatment. Thus, the concomitant use of vitamin D, calcium, and conventional forms of HRT appear generally to raise vitamin D levels but especially to enhance BMD in women who demonstrate osteoporosis, that is, those for whom BMD is most critical. Furthermore, such nutritional support may also allow for reduced HRT dosages and corresponding decrease in risk of attendant adverse effects and sequelae.

The form of calcium used for supplementation presents a potential confounding factor that has not been considered by most researchers but that would be a central concern to most practitioners of nutritional therapeutics. By examining data from a trial involving 25 postmenopausal women, Heller et al.[119] (2002) found that variable results of reported calcium supplementation studies may be caused by the effects of estrogen treatment or vitamin D status on the bioavailability of calcium citrate versus calcium carbonate. Using data derived from a prior trial in 25 postmenopausal women, the authors found that change in area under the curve (ΔAUC) of serum calcium after subtraction of placebo was significantly higher after calcium citrate than after calcium carbonate in non-estrogen-treated patients. Estrogen-treated patients showed no evident difference in the bioavailability of calcium between the two calcium formulations. Bioavailability was also significantly higher with the citrate salt for the subgroups with lower serum 25-OHD and higher serum $1,25(OH)_2D$ concentrations. Thus, bioavailability of calcium from calcium carbonate was more dependent on estrogen treatment and vitamin D status than that of calcium citrate.

Preliminary research into polymorphisms of the estrogen receptor (ER), vitamin D receptor (VDR), and their interactions may help clarify individual genetic variations in the influence of hormone therapies, exercise, ethnic background, and other factors on bone mineral density (BMD) and peak bone mass. In a population-based, 3-year, longitudinal study of BMD, Willing et al.[120] found that two genetic ER polymorphisms were significantly predictive of both lumbar spine and total-body BMD level, but not change in BMD during the study. A genetic VDR variant was not associated with baseline BMD, change in BMD over time, or any of the bone-related serum and body composition measurements in the 372 women in whom it was evaluated. Further, no other polymorphic markers were identified as being significantly associated with BMD measurements. However, these researchers did identify a significant impact on BMD levels associated with an interaction of two ER polymorphisms and two VDR genotypes. Subjects who had the $(-/-)$ PvuII ER and bb VDR genotype combination had a very high average BMD, whereas women with the $(-/-)$ PvuII ER and BB VDR genotype had significantly lower BMD levels. Differences in serum levels of osteocalcin, PTH, $1,25(OH)_2D$, or $25(OH)_2D$ did not explain this contrast. These authors concluded that their findings "suggest that genetic variation at the ER locus, singly and in relation to the vitamin D receptor gene, influences attainment and maintenance of peak bone mass in younger women, which in turn may render some individuals more susceptible to osteoporosis than others."[120]

Subsequently, in a study involving 108 postmenopausal Caucasian women, Deng et al.[121] found that VDR and ER genotypes may have different effects on BMD at different sites and on total-body bone mineral content (tbBMC). They assessed associations of BMD with VDR BsmI genotypes and ER XbaI (ERX) and PvuII (ERP) polymorphisms with spine, femoral neck, and distal radius BMD and with tbBMC. In this sample, researchers did not detect a significant association for ER genotypes with spine and radius BMD, or for VDR genotypes with femoral neck and radius BMD and tbBMC, or find a significant interaction between VDR and ER genotypes. However, they did note significant associations between (1) VDR genotypes and spine BMD variation, (2) both ERX and ERP genotypes and femoral neck BMD variation, and (3) ERX genotypes and tbBMC variation. Based on these observations, these researchers concluded that "if significant factors influencing bone are not appropriately controlled, true significant associations can easily be missed."[121] Related research suggests that bone may be more responsive to exercise in some genotypes of VDR than in others,[1] and that gene-environment interactions such as leisure physical activity and VDR genotype may play a role in maintaining the BMD at the lumbar spine in active postmenopausal women, especially older women.[2]

The importance of individual genotypes as important factors in determining changes in bone mass in the elderly, with and without HRT, as well as other factors, such as vitamin D and mineral nutriture and exercise, is becoming increasingly clear and will undoubtedly receive greater consideration in shaping individualized therapeutic strategies to optimize and preserve bone mass.

Myrup et al.[122] cautioned against a possible limiting effect of cholecalciferol on the lipid benefits of HRT, along with potential risk of hypercalcemia. In a double-blind, randomized trial involving 74 postmenopausal women, they investigated the effect of cholecalciferol and estrogen-norethindrone treatment for 1 year on total cholesterol level, high-density lipoprotein (HDL) cholesterol level, blood pressure, and body mass index. A similar decrease in serum cholesterol level was demonstrated in subjects receiving estrogen-norethindrone (11%) and those receiving hormones combined with cholecalciferol (13%); this hypocholesterolemic effect was most pronounced in lean women. However, the HDL cholesterol/total cholesterol ratio increased only 25% in women administered both estrogen-norethindrone and cholecalciferol, versus an increase of 45% with estrogen-norethindrone treatment alone.[122] Subsequently, in a in a population-based, prospective, 3-year study involving 464 women, Heikkinen et al.[123] arrived at similar conclusions. They found that serum concentrations of HDL cholesterol did not change significantly in the group receiving HRT (sequential combination of 2 mg estradiol valerate and 1 mg cyproterone acetate) alone, but decreased in the groups receiving vitamin D_3, HRT plus vitamin D_3, or placebo.

Nutritional Therapeutics, Clinical Concerns, and Adaptations

Hormone support, calcium, and vitamin D act in concert to enhance the primary activities of nutrition and exercise in healthy bone metabolism. HRT has been the mainstay of osteoporosis prevention but is limited because of dose-related risks, adverse effects, and patient acceptance. Furthermore, because estrogen alone can be safely used only in women without a uterus, due to an unacceptably high incidence of uterine cancer with unopposed estrogen, all postmenopausal women with an intact uterus receiving hormonal therapy must be treated with some combination of estrogen and progestins or their analogs, even though estrogen's effect on bone appears potentiated by calcium and vitamin D, and progestins may work against it. Calcium and vitamin D are essential for maintaining bone mass and density and imperative to the success of drug therapies for inducing bone augmentation.[77] Deficiencies of both nutrients are common in the patient populations at highest risk for osteoporosis. The importance of exercise and sound nutrition (including adequate protein and phosphorus intake) as foundational cannot be overemphasized and is supported by growing evidence.[2,124,125]

Calcium and estrogen have a clearly demonstrated synergistic effect of enhancing each other's effects on bone metabolism. Further, most research indicates that consistent exposure to sunlight provides a safe and effective, as well as otherwise beneficial, method of elevating vitamin D levels. Nevertheless, prudent nutritional support for osteoporosis prevention and treatment can be provided through diet or supplementation including 1500 mg/day of calcium and 800 IU (20 μg) vitamin D, or more exactly, sufficient intake vitamin D per day to maintain serum $25(OH)D$ levels above 80 nmol/L.[78]

Thus, a synergistic combination of oral calcium and vitamin D, within the context of an active lifestyle, constitutes the core proactive intervention within integrative therapeutics for all individuals at high risk for osteoporosis, or a base treatment for diagnosed bone loss. Additionally, hormone supplementation or replacement regimens (conventional HRT, bio-identical estrogens/progesterone, isoflavones, herbal hormone precursors/modulators) may produce the same effects, but conclusive evidence is lacking. Further research through well-designed clinical trials is warranted.

Although exogenous hormone therapy (and possibly understudied/untested "natural" alternatives) appears to enhance vitamin D metabolism, the importance of consuming adequate levels of vitamin D through diet and supplements cannot be overstated while taking hormones. As indicated by some of the research reviewed, total cholesterol, low-density lipoprotein (LDL) cholesterol, and HDL cholesterol ratios deserve monitoring in the event that vitamin D supplementation might exert a dyslipidemic effect. Again, exercise might be indicated as playing a fundamental role in the comprehensive therapeutic approach. Notably, low serum vitamin D levels have been associated with the incidence of falls in older women,[85] and vitamin D has been found to be helpful in reducing the incidence of falls, a major factor in fracture risk, by improving muscle strength, walking distance, and functional ability.[86] Overall, further research is needed to determine the character and full implications of the interaction(s) between supplemental vitamin D and exogenous hormone therapy and their relationship to the many factors influencing bone health and the risks of osteoporosis and fractures.

Heparin, Unfractionated

Heparin, unfractionated (Calciparine, Hepalean, Heparin Leo, Minihep Calcium, Minihep, Monoparin Calcium, Monoparin, Multiparin, Pump-Hep, Unihep, Uniparin Calcium, Uniparin Forte).

Interaction Type and Significance

◇≈≈ Drug-Induced Adverse Effect on Nutrient Function, Coadministration Therapeutic, with Professional Management

≈≈ Drug-Induced Nutrient Depletion, Supplementation Therapeutic, with Professional Management

Probability:	Evidence Base:
2. Probable	● Consensus

Effect and Mechanism of Action

Over time, heparin causes bone loss, especially in the spine, hips, pelvis, and legs. This effect is more pronounced with standard (unfractionated) heparin (UFH) than with low-molecular-weight heparin (LMWH). At least one mechanism of the negative effect of UFH on bone is nonspecific binding of the longer polysaccharide chains to bone, with inhibition of osteoblastic function. Heparin may also inhibit formation of 1,25-dihydroxyvitamin D by the kidneys.[126]

Research

Majerus et al.[127] reported that use of heparin, at high doses, for several months causes osteoporosis. Likewise, both Wise and Hall[128] and later Haram et al.[129] found that women who received heparin therapy during pregnancy experienced decreased bone density (i.e., osteopenia). On the other hand, in one study, nine women on heparin treatment received 6.46 g daily of a special calcium preparation, ossein-hydroxyapatite compound (OHC) for 6 months and were compared to 11 women not receiving the bone-protective treatment. In the OHC group, good compliance was observed, with no side effects and reduced back pain. Those taking the calcium preparation did not demonstrate the expected decrease in bone mass, and bone mass decreased significantly in the controls.[130]

Nutritional Therapeutics, Clinical Concerns, and Adaptations

Although the adverse effects of heparin on vitamin D and bone metabolism are well documented, research confirming the benefits of supplementing vitamin D and calcium in individuals on heparin therapy for any extended period is limited. However, in the meantime, such nutritional support would most likely be beneficial and is not contraindicated. Physicians prescribing UFH may find it prudent to coadminister with calcium and vitamin D supplementation. With chronic use, the vitamin D metabolite that should be measured to determine vitamin D status is 25(OH)D (25-hydroxyvitamin D), which is the major circulating form of vitamin D, circulating at 1000 times the concentration of 1,25(OH)$_2$D (1,25-dihydroxyvitamin D) and having a half-life of 2 weeks; after D$_3$ repletion has been initiated, monitoring 1,25(OH)$_2$D may be adequate. In some cases, if low, calcitriol may be necessary and appropriate to restore normal activated vitamin D levels; calcitriol is usually required (or appropriate) only in those patients unable to convert 25(OH)D to calcitriol. With long-term heparin therapy, assessment and monitoring of BMD may also be indicated.

Isoniazid and Related Antitubercular Agents

Isoniazid (isonicotinic acid hydrazide, INH; Laniazid, Nydrazid); combination drugs: isoniazid and rifampicin (Rifamate, Rimactane); isoniazid, pyrazinamide, and rifampicin (Rifater). Extrapolated, based on similar properties: Cycloserine (Seromycin), ethambutol (Myambutol), ethionamide (2-ethylthioisonicotinamide; Ethide, Ethiocid, Ethomid, Etomide, Mycotuf, Myobid, Trecator SC), pyrazinamide (PZA; Tebrazid).

See also Rifampin.

Interaction Type and Significance

≈≈ Drug-Induced Nutrient Depletion, Supplementation Therapeutic, with Professional Management

Probability:	Evidence Base:
2. Probable	◉ Emerging

Effect and Mechanism of Action

Research indicates that antituberculous drugs, including isoniazid (INH), induce vitamin D deficiency. Vitamin D levels have been found to be lowered in children with tuberculosis (TB), both in untreated children and in those taking isoniazid. Observed declines in activated vitamin D (1α,25-dihydroxyvitamin D) can produce relative hypocalcemia and induce elevation in PTH levels. Isoniazid can inhibit hepatic mixed-function oxidase activity, as evidenced by a reduction in antipyrine and cortisol oxidation, as well as hepatic 25-hydroxylase and renal 1α-hydroxylase; thereby causing such a reduction in the corresponding vitamin D metabolites.[131,132]

Research

Brodie et al.[131] investigated the effect of isoniazid on vitamin D metabolism, serum calcium and phosphate levels, and hepatic monooxygenase activity by administering isoniazid, 300 mg daily, to eight healthy subjects for 14 days. They observed several responses, including a 47% drop in the concentration of 1α,25(OH)$_2$D (the most active metabolite of vitamin D) after a single dose of isoniazid, with lowered levels continuing throughout the study; declines in levels of 25OHD (the major circulating form of the vitamin) in all subjects and to below normal range in six; and a 36% elevation in PTH levels in response to the relative hypocalcemia produced. In a study involving 46 children with asymptomatic TB, Toppet et al.[133] found that children administered isoniazid for 3 months demonstrated a decrease in blood levels of 1,25(OH)$_2$D. Isoniazid appears to interfere similarly with the activity of many other nutrients, including magnesium.

Specific evidence is lacking to determine if isoniazid or related agents actually cause symptoms of vitamin D deficiency and calcium depletion, especially with long-term therapy. Clinical trials are warranted to investigate the clinical significance of any depletion pattern and efficacy of prophylactic intervention. Such research is particularly important in children undergoing long-term therapy, in whom potential adverse effects may significantly impair the calcium economy during this critical life stage, when maximum bone density is being attained and will be relied on for life.

Nutritional Therapeutics, Clinical Concerns, and Adaptations

Physicians prescribing isoniazid or related antitubercular therapy, especially for longer than 1 month, are advised to recommend coadministration of vitamin D and calcium, preferably as part of a multivitamin and mineral formulation (at least 50 mg vitamin B$_6$ daily is indicated with INH as well); this prudent measure is unlikely to interfere with the efficacy of the medication(s). Vitamin D supplementation may be of great value in addition to antituberculous drugs in the treatment of tuberculous children, and its use is highly recommended.[134] Exposure to sunlight is the simplest and most natural way to provide activated vitamin D; sunshine and mountain air were characteristic of the great TB sanitoriums in the pre–anti-TB drug era. However, when vitamin D is to be supplemented orally, the typical dosage would be in the range of 5 to 10 μg (200-400 IU) per day, depending on size and body weight. Concurrent calcium supplementation in the range of 100 to 250 mg three times daily would be appropriate, but research is lacking to confirm specific effective dosage levels.

Granulomatous lesions, such as those present in extensive TB infection, often contain active 1-hydroxylase enzymes that activate 25-OH-cholecalciferol and are independent of the feedback mechanisms that regulate the renal 1-hydroxylase enzymes. Regular monitoring of serum calcium would reveal early vitamin D toxicity in this setting. Research findings emphasize the need for regular monitoring of 25(OH)D and bone status in this population, even if no sign of rickets is observed in these patients.

Ketoconazole

Ketoconazole (Nizoral).

Interaction Type and Significance

⊕✗ **Bimodal or Variable Interaction, with Professional Management**

Probability:
2. Probable

Evidence Base:
◉ **Emerging**

Effect and Mechanism of Action

Ketoconazole blocks adrenal steroidogenesis by inhibiting P450 enzymes involved in steroid hormone synthesis. In so doing, however, ketoconazole also inhibits 1α-hydroxylase and 24-hydroxylase, the P450 enzymes that metabolize vitamin D; inhibits renal 1,25(OH)$_2$D synthesis; and reduces serum levels of calcitriol.[135,136]

This activity enables ketoconazole to serve as a second-line ADT in the treatment of prostate cancer. The ability of vitamin D to inhibit growth of prostate cancer cells depends on levels of the active metabolite, 1,25(OH)$_2$D (calcitriol). Because 24-hydroxylase converts calcitriol to less active products, its inhibition by ketoconazole maintains the magnitude and duration of response to calcitriol.[137]

Research

Adams et al.[138] reported that ketoconazole decreases the serum 1,25(OH)$_2$D and calcium concentration in sarcoidosis-associated hypercalcemia. In several studies, Glass et al.[139-141] found that ketoconazole reduced previously elevated serum 1,25(OH)$_2$D and total serum calcium in hypercalcemic patients, particularly those with sarcoidosis. In a study of 19 patients with well-characterized absorptive hypercalciuria, Breslau et al.[142] found they could separate subjects into those who responded to ketoconazole and those who were nonresponders. Responders demonstrated reduced serum 1,25(OH)$_2$D, decreased intestinal calcium absorption, and decreased 24-hour urinary calcium excretion.

Nutritional Therapeutics, Clinical Concerns, and Adaptations

Physicians prescribing ketoconazole for extended periods, including use in conjunction with calcitriol for the treatment of prostate cancer, are advised to closely supervise and regularly monitor for drug-induced vitamin D deficiency. Given the nature of ketoconazole's action, simple oral vitamin D supplementation may not provide adequate protection, and calcitriol might need to be prescribed to avoid adverse effects of vitamin D deficiency. Monitoring is essential because the half-life of administered calcitriol tends to be prolonged in presence of ketoconazole.

Neomycin

Neomycin (Mycifradin, Myciguent, Neo-Fradin, NeoTab, Nivemycin); combination drugs: Adcortyl with Graneodin, Betnovate-N, Dermovate-NN, Gregoderm, Synalar N, Tri-Adcortyl, Trimovate.

Interaction Type and Significance

≈≈≈ **Drug-Induced Nutrient Depletion, Supplementation Therapeutic, Not Requiring Professional Management**

◇ **Adverse Drug Effect on Nutritional Therapeutics, Strategic Concern**

Probability:
2. Probable

Evidence Base:
● **Consensus**

Effect and Mechanism of Action

It is widely accepted that extended use of neomycin can significantly decrease absorption or increase elimination of vitamin D as well as many other nutrients, including beta-carotene, folic acid, vitamin A, vitamin B$_{12}$, vitamin K, calcium, iron, magnesium, potassium, and sodium.[89]

Research

No specific evidence is cited because the literature treats this interaction as axiomatic.

Nutritional Therapeutics, Clinical Concerns, and Adaptations

Physicians prescribing extended courses of neomycin are advised to coadminister a multivitamin and mineral supplement as a prudent measure to avoid potential drug-induced deficiencies. Separation of oral intake by at least 2 hours will reduce the risk of intrerference with absorption of either preparation.

Orlistat

Orlistat (alli, Xenical).

Interaction Type and Significance

≈≈≈ **Drug-Induced Nutrient Depletion, Supplementation Therapeutic, Not Requiring Professional Management**

Probability:
2. Probable

Evidence Base:
○ Preliminary

Effect and Mechanism of Action

Orlistat is a gastrointestinal lipase inhibitor that binds dietary fat and prevents its absorption. Such activity can interfere with the absorption of vitamin D and other fat-soluble nutrients and potentially induce deficiency patterns.

Research

In a 52-week, double-blind, randomized, parallel-group, placebo-controlled multicenter study, preceded by a 4-week, single-blind, placebo run-in period, James et al.[143] observed that vitamin D (and beta-carotene) concentrations decreased in patients treated with 120 mg orlistat three times daily, compared with those receiving placebo (even though fat-soluble vitamin levels remained within the normal range in the treatment group). Van Gaal et al.[144] conducted a 6-month, multicenter, randomized, double-blind, parallel-group clinical trial involving 676 obese men and women. Most subjects demonstrated reduced blood levels of vitamins D and A, but these remained within the clinical reference ranges, and only few individuals developed nutrient deficiency patterns that required supplementation. However, in a clinical trial involving 17 obese African-American and Caucasian adolescents receiving orlistat, 120 mg three times daily, McDuffie et al.[145] observed several significant nutrient depletion patterns despite coadministration of a daily multivitamin supplement containing vitamin A (5000 IU), vitamin D (400 IU), vitamin E (300 IU), and vitamin K (25 µg). In particular, mean serum levels of vitamin D were significantly reduced compared with baseline after 1 month of orlistat, despite multivitamin supplementation.

Nutritional Therapeutics, Clinical Concerns, and Adaptations

Predictably, in view of its known pharmacological effects, orlistat interferes with absorption of fat-soluble nutrients, including vitamin D. The question of whether, and for which individuals, the probable decline in vitamin D blood level reaches a threshold of clinical significance remains unclear and worthy of further clinical trials. Pending conclusive research findings, physicians prescribing orlistat for 6 months or longer are advised to err on the side of prudence and coadminister supplemental vitamin D (and possibly vitamin A), potentially in the form of a moderate-dosage multivitamin combination. Separating intake of orlistat and supplemental nutrients by 2 or more hours may reduce adverse effects on absorption. Notably, the U.S. Food and Drug Administration (FDA) requires that food products containing olestra, which also inhibits fat absorption, include vitamin D and other fat-soluble vitamins (i.e., vitamins A, E, and K).

Raloxifene

Raloxifene (Evista).

Interaction Type and Significance

⊕⊕ **Beneficial or Supportive Interaction, with Professional Management**

Probability:
2. Probable

Evidence Base:
○ Preliminary

Effect and Mechanism of Action

The ability of raloxifene, a selective estrogen receptor modifier (SERM) that is an analog of tamoxifen, to inhibit bone resorption and maintain or increase BMD depends on calcium nutriture and vitamin D's role in enabling calcium absorption and bone metabolism. Vitamin D can increase effectiveness of the drug.

Research

Boivin et al.[146] found that the coadministration of calcium (500 mg) and vitamin D_3 (400-600 IU) with raloxifene increased the degree of mineralization of bone in postmenopausal women, as demonstrated by iliac crest biopsies. All currently approved bone-active pharmacological agents have been studied only in conjunction with supplemental calcium, and newer anabolic agents increase mineral demand in skeletal tissue and will thus require even higher levels of calcium repletion.[78]

Nutritional Therapeutics, Clinical Concerns, and Adaptations

Calcium and vitamin D are essential for maintaining bone mass and density and imperative to the success of drug therapies for inducing bone augmentation.[77] Deficiencies of both nutrients are common in the patient populations at highest risk for osteoporosis. The importance of exercise and sound nutrition (including adequate protein and phosphorus intake) as foundational cannot be overemphasized and is supported by growing evidence. Calcium has a clearly demonstrated effect of enhancing estrogen's effects on bone metabolism. Further, most research indicates that consistent exposure to sunlight provides a safe and effective, as well as otherwise beneficial, method of elevating vitamin D levels. Doses of 1500 mg calcium and 800 IU vitamin D daily provide prudent nutritional support for osteoporosis prevention and treatment.

Thus, a synergistic combination of oral calcium and vitamin D, within the context of an active lifestyle, constitutes the core proactive intervention within integrative therapeutics for all individuals at high risk for osteoporosis, or a foundational treatment for diagnosed bone loss. Notably, low serum vitamin D levels have been associated with the incidence of falls in older women,[85] and vitamin D has been found to be helpful in reducing the incidence of falls, a major factor in fracture risk, by improving muscle strength, walking distance, and functional ability.[86] Also, hormone supplementation or replacement regimens (conventional HRT, bio-identical estrogens/progesterone, herbal hormone precursors/modulators) should be considered if indicated in women.

In addition to these primary and secondary therapies, the use of raloxifene in postmenopausal women can provide a potent intervention in reversing bone loss and supporting healthy bone mass, although it does tend to increase, rather than decrease, menopausal symptoms. Raloxifene may also be useful in reducing the risk of breast cancer in this population.

Rifampin

Rifampin (Rifadin, Rifadin IV); combination drugs: isoniazid and rifampicin (Rifamate, Rimactane); isoniazid, pyrazinamide, and rifampicin (Rifater).
See also Isoniazid section.

Interaction Type and Significance

≈≈   **Drug-Induced Nutrient Depletion, Coadministration Therapeutic, with Professional Management**

◇≈≈   **Drug-Induced Adverse Effect on Nutrient Function, Coadministration Therapeutic, with Professional Management**

Probability: Evidence Base:
2. Probable   ○ Preliminary

Effect and Mechanism of Action

Pharmacokinetic interaction occurs because rifampin is a potent inducer of hepatic drug metabolism, specifically (cytochrome P450) 2C9, 2C19, and 3A4. Rifampin inhibits CYP1A2 and increases oxidation of antipyrine and 6β-hydroxycortisol, potentially causing decreased plasma levels of 25-hydroxycholecalciferol (25-OHD), which represents the body stores of active vitamin D precursor.[147]

Research

In a small study with eight male subjects, Brodie et al.[147] found that a 2-week course of rifampicin (600 mg/day orally) produced a consistent fall in plasma 25-OHD levels of approximately 70%. Within the time frame of the study, plasma levels of 1,25-dihydroxycholecalciferol, PTH, and calcitonin were not significantly altered.

Nutritional Therapeutics, Clinical Concerns, and Adaptations

Physicians prescribing rifampicin for extended periods would be prudent to coadminister supplemental vitamin D at a dosage level appropriate to the patient's age, weight, sun exposure, and other characteristics and needs. Regular monitoring of 25-OHD would be appropriate.

Thiazide Diuretics

Bendroflumethiazide (bendrofluazide; Naturetin); combination drug: bendrofluazide and propranolol (Inderex); benzthiazide (Exna), chlorothiazide (Diuril), chlorthalidone (Hygroton), cyclopenthiazide (Navidrex); combination drug: cyclopenthiazide and oxprenolol hydrochloride (Trasidrex); hydrochlorothiazide (Aquazide, Esidrix, Ezide, Hydrocot, HydroDiuril, Microzide, Oretic); combination drugs: hydrochlorothiazide and amiloride (Moduretic); hydrochlorothiazide and captopril (Acezide, Capto-Co, Captozide, Co-Zidocapt); hydrochlorothiazide and enalapril (Vaseretic); hydrochlorothiazide and lisinopril (Prinzide, Zestoretic); hydrochlorothiazide and losartan (Hyzaar); hydrochlorothiazide and metoprolol (Lopressor HCT); hydrochlorothiazide and spironolactone (Aldactazide); hydrochlorothiazide and triamterene (Dyazide, Maxzide), hydroflumethiazide (Diucardin), methyclothiazide (Enduron), metolazone (Zaroxolyn, Mykrox), polythiazide (Renese), quinethazone (Hydromox), trichlormethiazide (Naqua).

Interaction Type and Significance

◇◇   **Drug-Induced Effect on Nutrient Function, Supplementation Contraindicated, Professional Management Appropriate**

✗✗   **Minimal to Mild Adverse Interaction—Vigilance Necessary**

Probability: Evidence Base:
5. Improbable   ☐ Inadequate

Effect and Mechanism of Action

Thiazide diuretics induce changes in renal tubules that reduce calcium excretion and could potentially lead to hypercalcemia in rare instances and changes in vitamin D metabolism (particularly increases in serum levels of 24,25-dihydroxycholecalciferol).

Research

Riis and Christiansen[148] studied the actions of bendroflumethiazide (5 mg/day), along with 500 mg/day calcium, on vitamin D metabolism in a 12-month, placebo-controlled clinical trial in 19 healthy, early-postmenopausal women. Subjects in the thiazide group demonstrated a significant elevation in the serum concentration of 24,25-dihydroxycholecalciferol and a tendency toward decreased serum 1,25-dihydroxycholecalciferol, although mean serum 25-hydroxycholecalciferol remained unchanged.

Nutritional Therapeutics, Clinical Concerns, and Adaptations

Given the uncertain implications of such findings, physicians are advised to closely supervise and regularly monitor serum calcium levels when prescribing thiazide diuretics. Special testing before initiating or increasing any vitamin D supplementation is probably unnecessary.

Thioridazine

Thioridazine (Mellaril).

Interaction Type and Significance

✗✗✗   **Potentially Harmful or Serious Adverse Interaction—Avoid**

Probability: Evidence Base:
2. Probable   ● Consensus

Effect and Mechanism of Action

Cholecalciferol (vitamin D_3), as a cytochrome P2D6 inhibitor, may decrease the metabolism of thioridazine via CYP isoenzymes.

Research

In a double-blind, randomized-order, crossover study of thioridazine pharmacodynamics, Hartigan-Go et al.[149] used debrisoquin, an agent presumed to be extensively metabolized by CYP2D6, to determine the hydroxylation status of thioridazine. They also found that thioridazine can prolong QTc intervals in a dose-dependent manner in normal subjects.[149] Furthermore, a manufacturer of thioridazine determined that the peak concentration (C_{max}) of thioridazine (single oral dose of 25 mg) is highly variable, and that some individuals are "slow hydroxylators" and others are "rapid hydroxylators." In regard to the effects of CYP2D6 inhibition, compared with placebo, thioridazine increased QTc intervals by 9 msec and 23 msec with 10-mg and 50-mg doses, respectively.[150]

Clinical Implications and Adaptations

Concomitant use of thioridazine and agents that inhibit CYP2D6 isoenzymes such as cholecalciferol is contraindicated and should be avoided. Evidence is lacking to suggest that supplementation with forms of vitamin D other than cholecalciferol (vitamin D_3) is problematic, and vitamin D support is often important in patients being treated with thioridazine.

Alternatives to thioridazine may need to be considered when supplementation with vitamin D_3 is critical to a patient's medical needs and central to the therapeutic strategy for their comprehensive care. Regardless, an alternate drug choice may be necessary because this phenothiazine antipsychotic has been withdrawn from the market in many jurisdictions.

Verapamil and Related Calcium Channel Blockers

Evidence: Verapamil (Calan, Calan SR, Covera-HS, Isoptin, Isoptin SR, Verelan, Verelan PM).

Extrapolated, based on similar properties: Amlodipine (Norvasc); combination drug: amlodipine and benazepril (Lotrel); bepridil (Bapadin, Vascor), diltiazem (Cardizem, Cardizem CD, Cardizem SR, Cartia XT, Dilacor XR, Diltia XT, Tiamate, Tiazac), felodipine (Plendil); combination drugs: felodipine and enalapril (Lexxel); felodipine and ramipril (Triapin); gallopamil (D600), isradipine (DynaCirc, DynaCirc CR), lercanidipine (Zanidip), nicardipine (Cardene, Cardene I.V., Cardene SR), nifedipine (Adalat, Adalat CC, Nifedical XL, Procardia, Procardia XL); combination drug: nifedipine and atenolol (Beta-Adalat, Tenif); nimodipine (Nimotop), nisoldipine (Sular), nitrendipine (Cardif, Nitrepin), verapamil combination drug: Verapamil and trandolapril (Tarka).

Interaction Type and Significance

✗ ✗ ✗   **Potentially Harmful or Serious Adverse Interaction—Avoid**

◇ ◇ ◇   **Impaired Drug Absorption and Bioavailability, Avoidance Recommended**

◇ ◇   **Drug-Induced Effect on Nutrient Function, Supplementation Contraindicated, Professional Management Appropriate**

Probability: Evidence Base:
5. Improbable   ○ Preliminary

Effect and Mechanism of Action

Verapamil is a calcium antagonist, whereas vitamin D facilitates calcium absorption and metabolism. An interaction involving supplemental vitamin D, due to pharmacodynamic antagonism, is theoretically plausible but considered improbable. Vitamin D (or calcium) supplementation could potentially interfere with the primary activity of verapamil, and thus its therapeutic effectiveness, by increasing calcium availability. Further, hypercalcemia induced by toxic levels of vitamin D may precipitate cardiac arrhythmia in patients taking verapamil, although this is extremely rare, if it ever occurs. Conversely, verapamil may decrease endogenous production of vitamin D. Verapamil may also induce target-organ parathyroid hormone (PTH) resistance.

Research

The evidence for this interaction is minimal, but it is often considered self-evident. In a 1982 in vitro study, Lerner and Gustafson[151] reported that verapamil inhibited 1α-hydroxyvitamin D_3–stimulated bone resorption in tissue culture. In an animal model using rats fed a high-calcium diet, Fox and Della-Santina[152] found that chronic oral verapamil administration decreased 1,25-dihydroxyvitamin D_3 [$1,25(OH)_2D_3$] levels (by reducing production) and increased plasma immunoreactive PTH (most likely by inducing target-organ PTH resistance). In contrast, verapamil produced no significant effect on $1,25(OH)_2D_3$ levels in rats fed a low-calcium diet.

Reports

Bar-Or and Gasiel[153] reported that calcium adipate and calciferol antagonized the heart rate–limiting effect of verapamil in a patient being treated for atrial fibrillation.

Clinical Implications and Adaptations

Physicians prescribing verapamil or other calcium channel blockers are advised to exercise caution regarding the concomitant use of vitamin D. This possible interaction can present strategic concerns because many patients receiving verapamil may also have or be at risk for osteoporosis, such that calcium and vitamin D support is an important concomitant need. For example, Holick[154] suggests that such patients typically need vitamin D support. Close supervision and regular monitoring, preferably within the context of integrative care involving health care professionals trained and experienced in both conventional pharmacology and nutritional therapeutics, are essential in cases where concurrent use of verapamil and vitamin D is clinically appropriate. In cases of overdose with verapamil or other calcium channel blockers, intravenous calcium chloride or gluconate is the treatment of choice.

Related Discussion

Calcitriol and Vitamin D Analogs

Alfacalcidol, calcitriol, dihydrotachysterol.

Investigations into the pharmacology and clinical application of $1,25(OH)_2D_3$, the hormonal active form of vitamin D, have proceeded far beyond those of the nutrient itself. In many situations, including adverse drug-induced effects on vitamin D metabolism, calcitriol has been administered to increase effective activated vitamin D levels. In some recent research and emerging clinical protocols, calcitriol has been used as a central component of the pharmacological repertoire, that is, as a drug and not as a nutrient.

Stio et al.[155] demonstrated synergistic immunoregulatory properties and inhibitory effect of cyclosporine A and vitamin D derivatives on T-lymphocyte proliferation in T lymphocytes prepared from ulcerative colitis patients. Such an alternative therapeutic approach in these patients could reduce the dose, and consequently the toxicity, of cyclosporine A. In an animal model using mice with breast tumor xenografts, Sundaram et al.[156] found that treatment with a vitamin D_3 analog, EB 1089, before ionizing radiation reduces tumor growth and induces apoptosis, without inducing hypercalcemia. In another in vitro experiment, Dunlap et al.[157] reported that treating human prostate cancer cells with calcitriol and its analog, 19-nor-1α,25(OH)$_2$D$_2$, may potentiate the effects of ionizing radiation and make these cells more susceptible to the effects of radiotherapy.

In a phase II clinical trial, Beer et al.[158] demonstrated that coadministration of high-dose calcitriol to weekly treatment with the chemotherapy agent docetaxel (Taxotere) appears to improve the therapeutic response in men with hormone-refractory prostate cancer without compromising safety, with the combination providing as much as twice the efficacy as docetaxel alone, as measured by prostate-specific antigen (PSA) response rate. Subjects received oral calcitriol, 0.5 µg/kg, on the first day of the treatment cycle, followed by an infusion of docetaxel, 36 mg/m², on the following day. This sequence was repeated weekly for 6 weeks of an 8-week cycle until there was evidence of disease progression or unacceptable toxicity, or until the patient requested to be withdrawn from the study. The phase III, randomized clinical trials following from this study evaluate the use of weekly docetaxel versus weekly docetaxel plus calcitriol in hormone-refractory prostate cancer.

THEORETICAL, SPECULATIVE, AND PRELIMINARY INTERACTIONS RESEARCH, INCLUDING OVERSTATED INTERACTIONS CLAIMS

Antacids, Especially Magnesium-Containing Antacids

Aluminum carbonate gel (Basajel), aluminum hydroxide (Alternagel, Amphojel); combination drugs: aluminum hydroxide, magnesium carbonate, alginic acid, and sodium bicarbonate (Gaviscon Extra Strength Tablets, Gaviscon Regular Strength Liquid, Gaviscon Extra Strength Liquid); aluminum hydroxide and magnesium hydroxide (Advanced Formula Di-Gel Tablets, co-magaldrox, Di-Gel, Gelusil, Maalox, Maalox Plus, Mylanta, Wingel); aluminum hydroxide, magnesium trisilicate, alginic acid, and sodium bicarbonate (Alenic Alka, Gaviscon Regular Strength Tablets); calcium carbonate (Titralac, Tums), magnesium hydroxide (Phillips' Milk of Magnesia MOM); combination drugs: magnesium hydroxide and calcium carbonate (Calcium Rich Rolaids); magnesium hydroxide, aluminum hydroxide, calcium carbonate, and simethicone (Tempo Tablets); magnesium trisilicate and aluminum hydroxide (Adcomag trisil, Foamicon); magnesium trisilicate, alginic acid, and sodium bicarbonate (Alenic Alka, Gaviscon Regular Strength Tablets); combination drug: sodium bicarbonate, aspirin, and citric acid (Alka-Seltzer).

Chronic use of some antacids may alter availability, levels, and metabolism of vitamin D. Evidence is lacking to confirm this potential interaction or determine its patterns of clinical significance.

Calcitonin

Calcitonin

The effect of calcitonin (clinically used primarily for treatment of hypercalcemia, but also osteoporosis and painful bone metastases, especially of multiple myeloma) may be antagonized by supplemental vitamin D.

Digoxin

Digoxin (Digitek, Lanoxin, Lanoxicaps, purgoxin).

Vitamin D enhances calcium absorption and elevated calcium levels may potentiate the effects of digoxin and contribute to increased risk of digoxin toxicity, potentially precipitating cardiac arrhythmia. At toxic levels, vitamin D could aggravate hypercalcemia and increase adverse effects of digoxin. Conversely, digoxin can potentiate the arrhythmogenic effects of hypercalcemia, leading to a symptomatic rhythm disorder.[159]

Although pharmacologically plausible, evidence from clinical studies regarding a direct interaction between digoxin and supplemental vitamin D is lacking. The risks associated with elevated or unstable calcium levels in patients receiving digoxin therapy are well known.

Most cases of hypercalcemia are unrelated to vitamin D intake. Vitamin D toxicity from supplemental sources is uncommon, if not rare, and would usually require an extended period of excessive vitamin D intake. However, even though rare, hypercalcemia would be a characteristic of hypervitaminosis D and would carry a significant probability of clinical significance in an individual undergoing digoxin therapy.

The combined use of vitamin D and digoxin may be therapeutically appropriate but involves judicious prescribing, cautious scrutiny, and careful follow-up. In particular, close supervision and regular monitoring of calcium levels are appropriate and prudent when prescribing digoxin therapy, especially in conjunction with any agents that might alter calcium status. The probability of an adverse reaction is generally quite low, but the consequences of such an event could potentially be severe and rapid in onset once a critical mass (hypervitaminosis D, hypercalcemia) had been reached. Physicians and other health care practitioners are advised to discuss use of and create an inventory of herbs and nutritional supplements with their patients in a respectful yet frank dialogue. Vitamin D excess to the degree that could cause hypercalcemia through sun exposure is generally considered impossible.

Doxorubicin

Doxorubicm (Adriamycin, Rubex).

Supplemental vitamin D may enhance the effects of doxorubicin. Given the positive trend in the findings from studies investigating the coadministration of calcitriol with a range of conventional cancer therapies, this potential supportive interaction warrants clinical trials. In an in vitro experiment, Ravid et al.[160] found that $1,25(OH)_2D_3$ may enhance the susceptibility of breast cancer cells to doxorubicin-induced oxidative damage.

Flurbiprofen

Flurbiprofen (Ansaid).

Through its primary mechanism of prostaglandin synthetase inhibition or possibly through other activities, flurbiprofen appears to reduce calcium and vitamin D levels in individuals with hypercalcemia. Buck et al.[161] found that flurbiprofen reduced circulating $1,25(OH)_2D$ in patients with recurrent calcium lithiasis. In a double-blind study, Brown et al.[162] reported on an individual with sarcoidosis in whom flubiprofen reduced plasma calcium levels and urinary hydroxyproline excretion to normal, while plasma $1,25(OH)_2D_3$ remained high. Clinical trials are warranted to determine whether flurbiprofen might influence calcium and vitamin D levels in healthy subjects or individuals with conditions involving other calcium and vitamin D metabolic disorders.

Hydroxychloroquine

Hydroxychloroquine (Plaquenil).

In a case report, Barré et al.[163] stated that 24 weeks of treatment with hydroxychloroquine reversed hypercalcemia and returned calcium and $1,25(OH)_2D$ levels to normal in a 45-year-old woman with sarcoidosis undergoing hemodialysis. The authors noted that these findings demonstrated the capacity of hydroxychloroquine to inhibit the conversion of $25(OH)D$ to $1,25(OH)_2D$ and suggested "the efficacy of hydroxychloroquine as an alternate to corticosteroids in the treatment of hypercalcemia of granulomatous disease." Controlled clinical trials are warranted to follow up on this report and also to determine whether hydroxychloroquine might beneficially influence calcium and vitamin D levels in healthy subjects or individuals with conditions other than sarcoidosis. Pending clarification by such research, physicians prescribing hydroxychloroquine are advised to discuss the potential effects of calcium and vitamin D supplementation with patients and closely supervise and regularly monitor calcium and vitamin D status in individuals for whom such supplementation may be appropriate for comorbid conditions.

Indapamide

Indapamide (Lozol).

Indapamide is a thiazide-like diuretic, but evidence is lacking as to whether it might enhance the activity of vitamin D in the manner of thiazide diuretics and whether such interaction might rise to the level of clinical significance. Pending clarification by controlled clinical trials, physicians prescribing indapamide are advised to discuss the potential effects of vitamin D supplementation with patients and closely supervise and

Nutrient-Drug Interactions and Drug-Induced Nutrient Depletions

regularly monitor calcium and vitamin D status in individuals for whom such supplementation may be appropriate for comorbid conditions.

Mineral Oil

Mineral Oil (Agoral, Kondremul Plain, Liquid Parafin, Milkinol, Neo-Cultol, Petrogalar Plain).

Mineral oil, as a lipid solvent, interferes with normal absorption of vitamin D (and other nutrients) and increases its elimination from the body. Some disagreement surrounds the degree of clinical significance, particularly with regard to vitamin D in particular, but most research has found that mineral oil interferes with the absorption of many nutrients, including beta-carotene, calcium, phosphorus, potassium, and vitamins A, D, K, and E. Chronic use of mineral oil can cause a deficiency of vitamins A, D, E, and K.[164]

If mineral oil is used for any extended period, concomitant administration of a multivitamin and mineral supplement would be generally be advisable. Malabsorption of fat-soluble vitamins due to ingestion of mineral oil can be minimized by administering mineral oil on an empty stomach or consuming vitamin or mineral supplements at least 2 hours before or after the mineral oil. In general, it is advisable to limit the internal use of mineral oil to less than 1 week.

Sodium Fluoride

Sodium Fluoride (Fluorigard, Fluorinse, Fluoritab, Fluorodex, Flura-Drops, Flura-Tab, Karidium, Luride, Pediaflor, PreviDent).

In an in vitro experiment using serum-free cultures of human marrow, stromal osteoblast-like cells, Kassem et al.[165] found that $1,25(OH)_2D_3$ potentiated fluoride-enhanced type I collagen production in a dose-dependent way (as well as production of ALP and osteocalcin), compared with sodium fluoride alone, which did not increase type I collagen production. Controlled clinical trials would be necessary to determine if coadministration of $1,25(OH)_2$-cholecalciferol and sodium fluoride might promote beneficial collagen growth.

Sucralfate

Sucralfate (Carafate).

In a multiclinical and randomized study involving 100 patients with chronic gastric ulcer, Patty et al.[166] reported that sucralfate may reduce intestinal absorption of vitamin D. However, in a clinical trial of 30 patients with chronic renal failure on intermittent hemodialysis, Vucelic et al.[167] found that sucralfate intake was associated with slight increases in serum calcium levels. Physicians prescribing sucralfate are advised to discuss the possible implications of vitamin D (and calcium) supplementation with patients for whom such nutriture is important to strategic clinical goals and to monitor vitamin D and calcium levels regularly should supplementation be deemed appropriate.

Warfarin

Warfarin (Coumadin, Marevan, Warfilone).

Based on a single letter published in *JAMA* (1975), concern has been raised about a possible adverse interaction between vitamin D and anticoagulant medicines such as warfarin.[168] The potential for increased activity of anticoagulants due to vitamin D has not been confirmed by other case reports or any substantial clinical research. Physicians prescribing warfarin should be aware of rumors arising from recurring reference to this warning of theoretical risk of enhanced drug activity from vitamin D supplementation. Even though the occurrence of this interaction would seem to be widespread if it represented a significant risk, given the widespread use of vitamin D, health care professionals are advised to discuss this theoretical concern, and the lack of evidence supporting it, with patients before initiating supplementation with vitamin D in doses greater than 10 µg (400 IU) daily. Nevertheless, in conventional practice, vitamin D supplementation at usual dosages is not considered contraindicated during anticoagulant therapy. In general, because warfarin interacts with such a wide variety of substances, it is wise to monitor the prothrombin time (PT) twice weekly when new medications or nutrients that are to be administered for more than a few days are added to the patient's regimen. Only in recent years have the profound interactions between warfarin and acetaminophen and between warfarin and cranberry juice been identified. There are likely many such interactions that are yet unrecognized. Frequent monitoring of the PT/INR when diet, medication, or nutrient regimens are changed is the best protection against untoward clinical events occurring from such as-yet unrecognized interactions, especially those that may occur only in patients with certain genetic polymorphisms.

NUTRIENT-NUTRIENT INTERACTIONS

Boron

Boron appears to play a significant role in converting vitamin D from 25-OHD to its active form [$1,25(OH)_2D$], thus facilitating calcium absorption. This observation is clinically relevant because it supports the practice of using supplemental vitamin D_3 with boron, rather than calcitriol, thereby avoiding the high costs of calcitriol.

After examining animal nutrition models, Hunt[169] concluded that that dietary boron alleviates perturbations in mineral metabolism characteristic of vitamin D_3 deficiency. Hunt et al.[170] found that dietary boron modifies the effects of vitamin D_3 nutrition on indices of energy substrate utilization and mineral metabolism in the chick. For example, chicks fed a diet containing insufficient vitamin D for 26 days exhibited decreased food consumption and plasma calcium concentrations, as well as increased plasma concentrations of glucose, β-hydroxybutyrate, triglycerides, triiodothyronine (T_3), cholesterol, and alkaline phosphatase (ALP) activity. After administration of boron, plasma glucose and triglycerides returned to concentrations exhibited by chicks that had been fed a diet adequate in vitamin D. Such findings support the coadministration of boron and vitamin D_3 as a potentially useful strategy in diabetes management. Likewise, boron elevated the numbers of osteoclasts and alleviated malformation of the marrow sprouts of the proximal tibial epiphysial plate in rachitic (vitamin D–deficient) chicks, thus correcting a distortion characteristic of vitamin D_3 deficiency.[171] In an experiment investigating the effects of dietary boron in rats fed a vitamin D–deficient diet, Dupre et al.[172] observed that introduction of boron into the diet resulted in higher apparent-balance values of calcium, magnesium, and phosphorus.

In a study involving male subjects over 45 years of age and postmenopausal women fed a low-magnesium and low-copper diet, Nielsen et al.[173] showed that administration of 3.25 mg of boron daily increased levels of plasma vitamin D_2.

Caffeine

Rapuri et al.[174] found that elderly women with high caffeine intakes had significantly higher rates of bone loss at the spine than those with low intakes, and that caffeine intake interacts with vitamin D receptor (VDR) genotypes. Nevertheless, the role of caffeine as a risk factor for bone loss remains controversial.

Calcium

Coadministration of vitamin D and calcium, along with weight-bearing exercise and sunlight exposure, are generally considered the foundational approaches to calcium nourishment, attainment, and maintenance of bone mineral density (BMD) and prevention of bone loss.[175-177] A normal physiological function of vitamin D is to facilitate intestinal calcium absorption.

Although findings have varied, often significantly influenced by methodology (especially in meta-analyses), most research indicates that concomitant intake of vitamin D and calcium reduces risk of fractures and enhances bone health, particularly for individuals with a preexisting insufficiency and with consistent patient compliance. In general, according to Heaney and Weaver,[78] prudent nutritional support for osteoporosis prevention and treatment consists of 30 to 40 mmol calcium per day together with sufficient vitamin D to maintain serum 25(OH)D levels above 80 nmol/L ($\sim$25 µg or 1000 IU vitamin D daily).[78] In a Cochrane Library review of 38 randomized or quasirandomized trials, Avenell and Handoll[178] found that the risk of fractures of the hip and other nonspinal bones was reduced slightly in elderly people who are frail and at risk for bone fractures, particularly those who live in nursing homes or other institutions, if vitamin D and calcium were given. Nevertheless, the risk of spinal fractures did not appear to be reduced.

In a trial involving 944 healthy Icelandic adults, Steingrimsdottir et al.[41] found that with 25-OHD levels below 10 ng/mL (i.e., significant vitamin D deficiency), maintaining calcium intake above 800 mg/day appeared to normalize calcium metabolism, as determined by the PTH level, but in individuals with higher 25-OHD levels, no benefit was observed from calcium intake greater than 800 mg/day.

In 2005 and 2006, three major papers were published discussing the relationship between calcium, vitamin D, and osteoporotic fracture risk. Findings from the RECORD study (*The Lancet*, 2005) suggested a lack of benefit from concomitant calcium and vitamin D in the prevention of fractures in menopausal women.[39] Subsequently, Jackson et al.[42] (2006) used data from the Women's Health Initiative that questioned the assumption that calcium and vitamin D can prevent osteoporosis-related hip fractures. They randomly assigned 36,000 postmenopausal women to receive elemental calcium, as calcium carbonate (500 mg twice daily), plus vitamin D (200 IU twice daily) or a placebo for an average of 7 years. Notably, the average calcium consumption in both groups was approximately 1150 mg/day, close to the appropriate recommended intake level. After 7 years, subjects in the treatment group exhibited 12% fewer hip fractures than those in the placebo group, a finding that was not statistically significant. However, a deeper analysis of the data reveals that more significant differences appear when considering compliance and initial calcium intake levels. For example, on excluding women who were not adhering to the program, the reduction in fractures was greater, with 29% fewer fractures in the treatment group than in the placebo group, a statistically significant difference. Likewise, hip fracture risk decreased by about 22% in treated subjects whose initial calcium intake was low or moderate.[42] Overall, in both trials, compliance was only about 40% and 50%.

In contrast, Boonen et al.[179] conducted a multifaceted meta-analysis of major randomized, placebo-controlled trials that analyzed the effects of vitamin D alone or in combination with calcium. In one analysis they found that randomized clinical trials comparing vitamin D alone to placebo showed no effect. Likewise, a subsidiary analysis showed that low doses of vitamin D (<800 units/day) exerted no effect. However, they demonstrated a statistically significant 21% reduction in risk of fracture, compared with placebo, among subjects receiving 800 IU vitamin D and more than 1000 mg calcium daily. The authors concluded that vitamin D exerts its beneficial effect on bone predominantly by increasing absorption of calcium.

In some individuals and with certain medical conditions, supplementation with vitamin D, particularly at excessive levels, can induce an excessive increase in the absorption of calcium and increase the risk of hypercalcemia and kidney stone formation.[42] The risk of such adverse effects may be influenced by the form of calcium used, as well as other, individual patient variables.

Phosphorus

Vitamin D may cause an increase in the absorption of phosphorus. The clinical implications of this potential pattern of interaction have yet to be fully investigated in controlled human trials.

Sodium

In a small clinical trial involving 11 normal subjects and two patients with postsurgical hypoparathyroidism, Breslau et al.[180] found that in normal subjects, sodium-induced renal hypercalciuria is accompanied by increased $1,25(OH)_2D$ synthesis and enhanced intestinal calcium absorption. Since this adaptive mechanism did not occur in two patients with hypoparathyroidism, the authors suggested that mediation of this effect by parathyroid hormone was possible.

Vitamin A

Vitamin A antagonizes some of the activity of vitamin D. High doses of vitamin A, given concurrently with vitamin D, tend to reduce the toxic effects of vitamin D.[181,182] Vitamin A toxicity, such as hepatotoxicity, must also be considered in such contexts.

The 182 citations for this monograph, as well as additional reference literature, are located under Vitamin D (Calciferol) on the CD at the back of the book.

Vitamin E

Nutrient Name: Vitamin E.
Synonyms: Vitamin E; d-alpha-tocopherol.
Related Compounds: d-beta-tocopherol, d-gamma-tocopherol, d-delta-tocopherol; tocopheryl acetate, tocopheryl succinate.
Trade Names: Aqua Gem E, Aquasol E, E-Gems, Key-E, Key-E Kaps.

Summary

Drug/Class Interaction Type	Mechanism and Significance	Management
Acetylsalicylic acid (ASA, aspirin) ⊕⊕/✗	Concomitant use of aspirin and vitamin E may provide an additive effect in reducing platelet aggregation and otherwise reducing cerebrovascular risk. Evidence mixed but suggesting positive trend for clinically significant supportive interaction; use of antioxidant could clarify findings and enhance preventive effect.	Coadminister aspirin with multiple antioxidants, including mixed tocopherols and coenzyme Q10.
Anthralin ☼	Combining topical application of vitamin E with anthralin can provide antioxidant protection against drug-induced lipid peroxidation and inflammation. Narrow but strong evidence indicating clinically significant supportive interaction.	Compound and coadminister.
Bile acid sequestrants ≈≈≈/◇	Bile acid sequestrants may interfere with absorption of vitamin E, as well as of folic acid and other fat-soluble nutrients. Despite mixed evidence, reasonable probability of clinically significant adverse effect on status of nutrients relevant to cardiovascular health, particularly in at-risk individuals.	Supplement with vitamin E and other affected nutrients away from medication.
Chemotherapy and radiotherapy ✗✗✗/⊕✗/◇≈≈/◇◇/⊕⊕/≈◇◇ Associated oral mucositis ☼	Vitamin E and other antioxidants may provide protective activity against lipid peroxidation and other damaging forms of oxidative stress induced by conventional oncological therapies and may exert synergistic therapeutic activity when coadministered in a systematic and clinically appropriate manner. However, inappropriate or ill-timed usage may interfere with therapies relying on action of free radicals for therapeutic effect. Evidence of interference is lacking while evidence of synergy is mixed. Research into strategic coadministration and clinical guidelines is preliminary and evolving. Blanket declarations of risk, efficacy, or clinical significance are premature and unsupported.	Avoid concomitant use outside appropriate care. Concurrent or alternating administration can be appropriate in certain clinical situations under close supervision and regular monitoring.
Cisplatin, oxaliplatin Platinum chemotherapy ☼/≈≈/⊕⊕	Coadministration of vitamin E may reduce the adverse effects of platinum-based chemotherapy due to free-radical damage, particularly neuropathies and nephrotoxicity, while compensating for nutrient depletion and potentially enhancing therapeutic efficacy. Growing body of evidence suggests a supportive interaction of clinical significance with appropriate clinical management.	Avoid concomitant use outside appropriate care. Concurrent or alternating administration can be appropriate in certain clinical situations under close supervision and regular monitoring.
Cyclosporine ⊕⊕/☼/✗	Vitamin E coadministration may reduce nephrotoxicity and other adverse effects of cyclosporine while enhancing its bioavailability and decreasing its clearance and steady-state volume of distribution.	Coadministration may be beneficial unless otherwise indicated. Supervise and monitor.
Dapsone ☼	The strong oxidative action of dapsone can cause hemolysis by damaging red cell membranes. Coadministration of vitamin E may partially protect against dapsone-induced hemolysis. Evidence supportive but mixed and inconclusive.	Coadminister vitamin E, preferably as mixed tocopherols; effect may be enhanced by other antioxidants.
Doxorubicin Anthracycline Chemotherapy ☼	Oxidative damage contributes to the cardiomyopathy typical of anthracycline chemotherapy. Vitamin E coadministration may mitigate such adverse effects through its antioxidant activity and enhance tolerance of adverse effects; synergistic effects also possible. Evidence of benefit inadequate; possibility of interference with drug activity contentious but unproven.	Coadministration of vitamin E, preferably as mixed tocopherols, may help prevent or treat cardiotoxicity. Consider coenzyme Q10 and other antioxidants, as well as L-carnitine, L-taurine, ginkgo, and fish oils. Concurrent or alternating administration can be appropriate in certain clinical situations under close supervision and regular monitoring.
Gemfibrozil ≈≈≈/◇≈≈	Gemfibrozil may reduce serum levels of alpha- and gamma-tocopherol, and other antioxidants. Evidence mixed and contradictory. Clinical significance uncertain.	Patients with or at risk for cardiovascular disease likely to benefit from a diet rich in vitamin E and other antioxidant nutrients; role of supplementation contentious.
Glyburide ⊕⊕	Vitamin E can reduce lipid peroxidation and may enhance glycemic control and improve insulin action. Evidence supportive but preliminary.	Diet rich in vitamin E and allied nutrients and emphasizing low glycemic index advisable. Supplementation, preferably as mixed tocopherols, may be appropriate. Regular monitoring of blood glucose levels essential.
Haloperidol ≈≈/☼/◇≈≈	Free radical production and oxidative damage caused by haloperidol contribute to tardive dyskinesia and other adverse effects, and	Coadminister vitamin E, preferably as mixed tocopherols; effect may be enhanced by other antioxidants. Supervise and monitor.

Summary

Drug/Class Interaction Type	Mechanism and Significance	Management
	may be due, to some degree, to drug-induced vitamin E depletion. Research indicates that vitamin E coadministration may reduce adverse effects in certain patient subgroups with minimal risk of significant adverse effects or interference with drug activity.	
HMG-CoA reductase inhibitors (statins) ✗/◇≈≈/⊕⊕	Vitamin E may support therapeutic action of statin agents and reduce their adverse effects, particularly on oxidative status; however, vitamin E may interfere with therapeutic action of statins, but concerns remain unclear and unsubstantiated. Antioxidant combinations, including vitamin E, may interfere with the HDL-elevating activity of statin-niacin combinations, most likely through their interaction with niacin. Vitamin E may also enhance clearance of statins by promoting detoxification processes. Coadministration may enhance antihyperlipidemic therapy and reduce cardiovascular risk. Evidence is preliminary but emerging. Efficacy controversial and clinical significance unclear.	Statins (without niacin) may be compatible with administration of multiple antioxidant combinations emphasizing mixed tocopherols and coenzyme Q10. Supervise and monitor within an integrative strategy.
Omeprazole Proton pump inhibitors ⊕⊕⊕	Antioxidant activity of vitamin E may reduce esophagitis and support omeprazole therapy by increasing the mucosal resistance to oxidative damage from gastroesophageal reflux. Preliminary evidence indicates reasonable probability of clinically significant beneficial interaction from coadministration.	Coadminister. Drug dose may be reduced.
Orlistat ≈≈≈/☼/◇	Orlistat may decrease absorption of vitamin E and other fat-soluble nutrients. Preliminary evidence indicates vitamin E depletion pattern with reasonable probability of clinical significance over extended period.	Supplement with vitamin E and other nutrients preventively or if indication of deficiency with extended orlistat therapy.
Warfarin Oral vitamin K antagonist anticoagulants ✗✗/⊕✗/⊕⊕	Research involving individuals not taking anticoagulants as well as warfarin-related case reports indicate that high-dose vitamin E may enhance effect of coumadin-derivative anticoagulants by decreasing vitamin K levels and activity, reflected by PIVKA-II, an underactive form of prothrombin produced in presence of vitamin K insufficiency. Further research is warranted to determine nutrient interaction between vitamins K and E in patients using oral anticoagulants and appropriate clinical responses to coadministration.	Closely monitor and titrate if coadministration is appropriate.

NUTRIENT DESCRIPTION

Chemistry and Forms

Alpha-tocopherol is either d-alpha (RRR) or dl- (all-racemic) alpha tocopherol.

Naturallly ocurring forms of vitamin E include tocopherols (d-alpha-tocopherol, d-beta-tocopherol, d-gamma-tocopherol, d-delta-tocopherol) and tocotrienols (alpha-tocotrienol, d-beta-tocotrienol, d-gamma-tocotrienol, d-delta-tocotrienol).

Physiology and Function

Vitamin E was discovered in the 1920s, but our comprehension of the full implications of this nutrient in health, dysfunction, and disease is only beginning to emerge. Alpha-tocopherol is the only recognized form of the lipid-soluble vitamin E in animal tissues and plasma. However, vitamin E antioxidants are a group of eight tocopherol and tocotrienol compounds, including four tocopherols and four additional tocotrienol (alpha, beta, gamma, delta), which occur naturally in foods. Research over the past decade has focused on this nutrient's role in antioxidant functions, but important discoveries have also emerged concerning the direct role of vitamin E in control of cell division, inflammatory processes, xenobiotic detoxification, blood cell regulation, and connective tissue growth.

Vitamin E absorption depends on the presence of bile and decreases as dosage increases. At normal levels of intake, about 50% of dietary vitamin E is absorbed. A diet high in unsaturated fat increases vitamin E requirements. Vitamin E is distributed to all body tissues but has a particular affinity for adipose tissue. Adipose tissue slowly accumulates vitamin E and then in time slowly releases it while the liver just briefly stores vitamin E, and does so continuously. *Alpha-tocopherol transfer protein* (TTP), present in the liver and cerebellum, is the lipophilic vitamin-binding protein responsible for the incorporation of alpha-tocopherol into lipoproteins and for the transport of alpha-tocopherol between membranes. Dietary intake of vitamin E is metabolized in the liver to CEHCs, which are then glucuronidated and excreted via the urine.

Vitamin E's principal physiological role is to act as an antioxidant to prevent free-radical damage (lipid peroxidation) and protect the stability and integrity of cellular tissues and membranes. Vitamin E's role in stabilizing cell membranes is especially important in the lungs and red blood cells (RBCs), which are particularly susceptible to oxidative damage because of their high oxygen tension. As a fat-soluble nutrient, this antioxidant activity occurs particularly in lipid media and protects fatty acids against oxidative damage caused by various pollutants, peroxides, and free radicals formed during metabolic processes. It also reduces formation of *lipofuscin,* an oxidized fat that has been implicated in the aging process. If insufficient vitamin E is present, polyunsaturated fatty acids (PUFAs) may become oxidized in the body, creating toxins that may lead to chromosomal damage and carcinogenesis. Alpha-tocopherol has been shown to inhibit platelet aggregation, enhance vasodilation, affect the expression and activity of immune and inflammatory cells, and inhibit the activity of protein kinase C, an important cell-signaling molecule. Researchers have recently determined that vitamin E, especially as d-alpha-tocopherol, can act as a ligand for, and thereby increase the metabolic activity of, *pregnane X receptor* (PXR), which regulates a constellation of genes involved in detoxification of xenobiotics.[1] Vitamin E also plays an important role in preventing neurological abnormalities such as peripheral neuropathies.

NUTRIENT IN CLINICAL PRACTICE

Known or Potential Therapeutic Uses

Research into the role of vitamin E in health and disease has yet to mature and remains the subject of controversy and discovery. Within the conventional perspective on nutrition, the metabolic function of vitamin E is usually considered as still unidentified, although its major function as a nonspecific chain-breaking antioxidant is acknowledged and emphasized. In contrast, since the 1940s, health care professionals practicing nutritional therapeutics have often presented vitamin E as a primary component of health optimization, disease prevention, and therapeutic intervention. Although conventional medicine usually disclaims the value of antioxidant therapy via nutritional supplements in the primary prevention of cardiovascular disease and cancer, the lack of cohesive understanding of the role of vitamin E and other antioxidants in secondary prevention is also acknowledged. Clinical trials have typically investigated individual antioxidants, such as vitamin E, without considering that most health care professionals practicing nutritional therapeutics employ antioxidant formulations aimed at achieving synergistic action from multiple ingredients. Such factors may account for many of the recent inconsistencies and disappointments in outcomes of studies examining the efficacy of vitamin E supplementation for heart disease and other conditions. Further, research employing vitamin E, as with most other studies involving nutritional supplements, have often been designed without regard to the particular form of the nutrient(s) employed, dosage levels typical of informed clinical practice, or the underlying pathophysiological mechanisms.

This subject exemplifies the need for well-designed clinical trials focused on clearly defined health care goals and informed by an integrative approach utilizing the knowledge and experience of clinicians and researchers from a diverse range of perspectives. Furthermore, the conclusions of reviews and meta-analyses of vitamin E studies require a careful parsing of trial data based on form of the nutrient involved, design and time frame, concomitant therapies, and patient population characteristics if they are to be accurate and clinically useful. Fortunately, in the meantime, a broad consensus supports the primary value of a balanced and diverse diet rich in antioxidants as the foundation of health optimization and disease prevention.

Possible Uses

Acne, allergies, Alzheimer's disease, amyotrophic lateral sclerosis (risk reduction), anemia (sickle cell anemia and other types of hemolytic anemia), angina, anti-inflammatory, antioxidant, ataxia with isolated vitamin E deficiency (AVED), atherosclerosis, bronchitis, burns, cardiovascular effects, cataracts, cold sores, cystic fibrosis, dermatitis herpetiformis, diabetes mellitus, diabetic retinopathy (prevention), Down syndrome, Dupuytren's contracture, dysmenorrhea, epilepsy (pediatric), fibrocystic breast disease, fibromyalgia, hemolytic anemia (deficiency), hepatitis, herpetic lesions and postherpetic neuralgia, high-altitude exercise performance, human immunodeficiency virus and acquired immunodeficiency syndrome (HIV/AIDS) support, hypercholesterolemia, mild hypertension, hypoglycemia, immune support (especially for elderly), infertility, inflammatory thrombophlebitis, intermittent claudication, leukoplakia, lung cancer (risk reduction), macular degeneration, menopause (including hot flashes and atrophic vaginitis), menorrhagia (heavy menstruation), muscular dystrophy, myocardial infarction, nocturnal cramping, Osgood-Schlatter disease, osteoarthritis, pancreatic insufficiency, peripheral neuropathy (due to deficiency), photosensitivity, preeclampsia (risk reduction), premature infants, premenstrual syndrome, prostate cancer (risk reduction), psoriasis, Raynaud's syndrome, restless legs syndrome, retinopathy, retrolental fibroplasia, rheumatoid arthritis, scar tissue, seborrheic dermatitis, scleroderma, skin ulcers, spinocerebellar ataxia (due to deficiency), spontaneous abortion, sudden infant death syndrome (SIDS), sunburn, systemic lupus erythematosus (SLE), tardive dyskinesia, vaginal atrophy, vaginitis, wound healing, yellow nail syndrome.

Deficiency Symptoms

Frank vitamin E deficiency is rare in humans, but dietary intake in developed countries is often compromised by heavy reliance on processed foods. Very little vitamin E is transferred across the placenta, so premature infants, who are not breast-fed or supplemented, are susceptible to deficiency and subsequent damage of the retina (retrolental fibroplasia) if exposed to high oxygen tension from oxygen supplementation. Individuals with a genetic defect in alpha-tocopherol transfer protein (TTP) have an especially significant susceptibility to a severe vitamin E deficiency, characterized by low blood and tissue levels of vitamin E and progressive nerve abnormalities. Deficiency of vitamin E can cause a peripheral neuropathy, in which sensory neurons are particularly affected, such that the large-caliber axons die, ultimately resulting in a spinocerebellar ataxia.

Possible signs and symptoms of vitamin E deficiency include decreased integrity of RBC membranes, hemolytic anemia (with consequent elevated indirect bilirubin), peripheral neuropathy, spinocerebellar ataxia, elevated heavy metal levels, cataracts, cystic fibrosis, cholestatic liver disease, various lipid malabsorption syndromes, atrophy of reproductive organs, infertility, premenstrual syndrome, hot flashes, fibrocystic disease, benign prostatic hypertrophy, dry skin, eczema, psoriasis, poor wound healing, atrophy and weakness in skeletal and smooth muscles, and Osgood-Schlatter disease (also associated with selenium deficiency), as well as increased risk of cancer, atherosclerosis, rheumatoid arthritis, major depression, and preeclampsia. Sickle cell anemia and beta-thalassemia predispose to vitamin E insufficiency.

Dietary Sources

Unrefined, cold-pressed vegetable oils, particularly wheat germ oil, sunflower seed oil, and olive oil and all whole, raw, or sprouted seeds, nuts, and grains (especially whole wheat) are considered the best dietary sources of vitamin E. Asparagus, avocados, brussels sprouts, egg yolks, legumes, shrimp, spinach, sweet potatoes, and leafy green vegetables, generally, can be good sources. Although wheat germ can be an excellent source, it must be absolutely fresh (less than a week old) because the oil oxidizes rapidly, and rancid wheat germ does not contain active vitamin E.

Food sources can provide the recommended dietary allowance (RDA) level of 15 mg alpha-tocopherol per day, an appropriate intake for many conditions, while offering a rich diversity of gamma-tocopherol and other tocopherols. However, clinical research indicates that the maintenance dosage levels and especially the higher range of therapeutic dosage levels, typically hundreds of units per day, required for some conditions may be difficult to obtain through diet alone. This is particularly true for individuals who reduce their intake of dietary fats, because vitamin E tends be more abundant in diets richer in fats. Moreover, recent research on vitamin E bioavailability shows that absorption of vitamin E is higher if it is part of or closely associated with the digestion of a food that contains fat. For example, grain cereal fortified with vitamin E raised plasma levels of new vitamin E more consistently and to higher levels proportionally than did vitamin E as a supplement only, with liquids on an empty stomach, or even taken with milk.[2] On a broader level, there is a growing body of evidence that large doses of vitamin E, especially if used without an accompanying diverse antioxidant network, may be deleterious for some individuals.

Tocopherols are oily yellow liquids that are water insoluble, heat and acid stable, and deteriorate with exposure to alkali, light, oxygen, iron, or lead. Frying of foods as well as freezing also decreases the potency of vitamin E. In contrast, tocopheryl esters, which are most often found in fortified foods (particularly breakfast cereals), tend to be fairly resistant to both frying and freezing (as well as highly bioavailable).

Nutrient Preparations Available

Although alpha-tocopherol has long been the standard of vitamin E supplementation, research is evolving to a greater understanding of the importance of naturally occurring forms and the advantages of mixed tocopherols. RRR-alpha-tocopherol, more commonly known as d-alpha-tocopherol, is the only form of alpha-tocopherol that occurs naturally in foods, whereas synthetic dl-alpha-tocopherol (all-racemic alpha-tocopherol) is composed of equal amounts of all stereoisomers. The establishment of d-alpha as the "active" isomer was based on the rat fetus resorption assay developed in the 1940s, in which only the d-alpha isomer is active; in pregnant rats made vitamin E deficient, the fetuses die and are resorbed, which is prevented only by d-alpha-tocopherol. The other isomers may have superior in vivo biological antioxidant activity, and gamma appears to have greater prostate cancer–preventive activity than alpha. The tocotrienols are much superior in cellular membrane protection because of a greater ability to move within membrane structures. Naturally occurring d-alpha-tocopherol is significantly more bioavailable, perhaps 200%, and exerts greater physiological activity than synthetic dl–alpha-tocopherol.[3] Some clinicians have reported that water-soluble forms of vitamin E can be better absorbed and more effective with individuals experiencing fat malabsorption problems, especially middle-age and menopausal women. Vitamin E is sold in both esterified and nonesterified forms but is usually manufactured as acetate or succinate esters because pure vitamin E compounds are easily oxidized. A tocopherol form is appropriate in topical use; tocopheryl forms require an enzyme to split the vitamin E from the acid moiety to which it is attached by an ester linkage.

Dosage Forms Available

Capsule, gel capsule; emulsified liquid drops, mycelized liquid drops; injection; liquid; ointment; powder; solution, oral drops; spray; suppository; tablet; topical.

Equivalencies:
1 mg d-alpha-tocopheryl acetate = 1.49 IU
1 IU all-racemic alpha-tocopherol = 0.45 mg
The current RDA is given in milligrams of alpha-tocopherol.

Dosage Range
Adult
Dietary: RDA based on RRR-alpha-tocopherol (d-alpha-tocopherol):

Adults, 19 years and older: 15 mg (22.5 IU)/day
Pregnancy (all ages): 15 mg (22.5 IU)/day
Breastfeeding (all ages): 19 mg (28.5 IU)/day

Supplemental/Maintenance: 15 mg/day, higher doses may not be more efficacious.[4,5]
Pharmacologic/Therapeutic: 400 to 2500 IU/day (excluding pregnant or lactating women) in clinical practice; 100 to 1000 IU/day in the scientific literature.
Toxic: The safe upper intake level (UL) of vitamin E for adults as d-alpha-tocopheryl acetate is 1500 IU/day (1000 mg), or 1100 IU/day dl-alpha.

Pediatric (<18 years)
Dietary: RDA based on RRR-alpha-tocopherol (d-alpha-tocopherol)

Infants, birth to 6 months: 4 mg (6 IU)/day
Infants, 7 to 12 months: 5 mg (7.5 IU)/day
Children, 1 to 3 years: 6 mg (9 IU)/day
Children, 4 to 8 years: 7 mg (10.5 IU)/day
Children, 9 to 13 years: 11 mg (16.5 IU)/day
Adolescents, 14 to 18 years: 15 mg (22.5 IU)/day

Supplemental/Maintenance: Not established.

Laboratory Values
Plasma vitamin E: Less than 11.6 μmol/L indicates deficiency. Plasma alpha-tocopherol (μmol/L)/plasma cholesterol (mmol/L): Ratio less than 2.2 indicates deficiency. Accurate measurement of vitamin E status inherently includes the ratio of vitamin E/total cholesterol because vitamin E level in the blood is directly correlated with the blood lipid level.
Plasma tocopherol: Less than 10 μmol/L generally indicates deficiency.

Note: Alpha-tocopherol normally constitutes more than 90% of total plasma vitamin E.

There is no correlation between plasma levels and vitamin E stores. A serum peroxide value can give an indirect status.

SAFETY PROFILE
Overview

Vitamin E supplements are widely considered to be safe and unlikely to cause adverse side effects in most individuals at typical dosage levels. At common therapeutic doses intended for long-term use, 800 IU per day, vitamin E, in its various forms, is considered nontoxic in most individuals. Daily doses of 2000 to 3500 IU have been used in clinical setting for extended periods without adverse effects. Nevertheless, there has been a recent trend in the scientific literature suggesting potential adverse effects of dosages significantly higher than the recently revised RDA. Warnings against use of dosage levels greater than 200 IU/day usually derive from trials using vitamin E as an isolated antioxidant, synthetic dl-alpha-tocopherol, and patients with pathologies, behaviors, diet, or other factors characterized by high oxidative stress. Meta-analyses and reviews encompassing such studies are limited by their failure to emphasize the clinical implications of such study factors and attendant mixing of findings from trials employing essentially different substances (e.g., natural vs. synthetic forms, multiple vs. single nutrient). Thus, a potentially dangerous pro-oxidant effect can be created when one or two antioxidants, especially in synthetic forms, are given in high dosages to individuals who are chronically antioxidant deficient and under increased oxidative stress. Even so, "higher circulating concentrations of alpha-tocopherol within the normal range are associated with significantly lower total and cause-specific mortality in older male smokers."[6] Unfortunately, the mainstream of scientific research and medical practice has yet to consider, let alone investigate this concept.

Nutrient Adverse Effects
General Adverse Effects

The rare occasions of adverse effects from supplemental forms of vitamin E, typically in high dosages for extended durations, have been characterized by fatigue, headache, hemorrhage, double vision, nausea, flatulence, diarrhea, gastrointestinal distress, and muscular weakness. One study, published in 2005 and widely publicized in the popular press when initially released online in late 2004, was a meta-analysis suggesting that high dosages of vitamin E were associated with a small increase in risk for all-cause mortality at doses above 400 IU daily among individuals being treated for various health conditions, and this dose-dependent increase began to be seen above doses of 150 IU/day. These researchers also found that the meta-analysis of the vitamin E studies involving low doses (i.e., < 200 IU/day) indicated a small decrease in all-cause mortality, although it did not reach statistical significance. These conclusions were based on meta-analysis from 19 randomized, placebo-controlled trials involving d-alpha-tocopherol and dl-alpha-tocopherol (synthetic form) in diverse populations, including high proportions of the elderly and high-risk individuals with chronic pathologies.[7] None of these studies included any of the other naturally occurring tocopherol or tocotrienol isomers of the vitamin E complex.

Pregnancy and Nursing

Note: With pregnant women, monitor plasma tocopherol concentrations (normal range, 6-14 μg/mL).

In one randomized, placebo-controlled trial involving 722 pregnant women at risk for preeclampsia, researchers observed a slightly elevated incidence of small-for-gestational-age neonates among women administered vitamin C (1000 mg) and vitamin E (RRR-alpha-tocopherol, 400 IU) versus placebo.[8]

Infants and Children

Reports of infant deaths from vasculocentric hepatotoxicity in 1983 due to parenteral administration of vitamin E were found to be related to the solubilizing agent polysorbate instead of vitamin E.[9] This compound, E-Ferol, was subsequently banned. In a 1989 review article, Mino[10] summarized a cautious perspective: "In the course of therapy with elevated dosages of vitamin E, administered either orally, intramuscularly, or intravenously, many problems arose in the infants, such as unexpected death, increased frequency of necrotizing enterocolitis (NEC) and sepsis, and the development of unusual symptoms including hepatic injuries."

Toxicity: Vitamin E toxicity is generally considered to be very rare. Increased risk of hemorrhage may result from vitamin E toxicity. A dose of 1800 IU/day has been shown to cause a prolonged bleeding time (an in vivo test of platelet function).

Contraindications

Chronic rheumatic heart disease: Avoid initial use of high doses; increase gradually.

Hypertension.

Congestive heart failure (CHF): Large doses of a single antioxidant supplement, such as vitamin E, in patients likely to be under oxidative stress who do not consume a diet rich in antioxidants, may contribute to further oxidative stress.

Precautions and Warnings

Hypersensitivity to vitamin E, source material, or any component of the formulation; intravenous (IV) route.

INTERACTIONS REVIEW
Strategic Considerations

Vitamin E deficiency resulting from inadequate dietary intake is relatively uncommon in the developed world, but it may occur within certain populations, such as elderly persons and institutionalized individuals. Further, a wide range of common drugs deplete key nutrients, including vitamin E and other antioxidants, and the risk of drug-induced deficiency of vitamin E and consequent adverse effects is considered to be substantial.

Conversely, supplementation with naturally occurring forms of vitamin E may prevent or reverse adverse effects of many medications. However, controversy continues as to whether coadministration of vitamin E with drugs that deplete it offers superior therapeutic outcomes, or whether such polypharmacy simply obscures the outcome or even interferes with intended drug actions.

The role of vitamin E in conventional medicine has undergone many sharp turns, particularly at the start of the twenty-first century, as a number of interventional clinical trials, as well as several meta-analysis studies, were published. Perhaps most importantly, the issue of single versus multiple isomers of vitamin E, as well as natural versus synthetic sources, reveals deep divisions within the medical and scientific community as to nutritional therapeutics and underlying assumptions. This pivotal factor in clinical practice, research design, and scientific discourse was further exacerbated by the recent redefinition of "vitamin E" away from the previous functional definition based on physiological action to a narrower, more pharmaceutic definition exclusively specifying d-alpha-tocopherol.

Any discussion of "vitamin E" first requires a common understanding of meaning and context and should begin with questions as to forms and sources being applied. Thus, studies referring to "vitamin E" could indicate alpha-tocopherol more exactly (although often failing to differentiate isomer and source), supplements containing multiple tocopherol isomers, supplements containing multiple forms of naturally occurring vitamin E (i.e., mixed tocopherols and tocotrienols), or food sources. Many controversies and much confusion would be rapidly resolved if discourse was founded on such clear communication and consistent nomenclature. The clinical significance of such discriminations becomes apparent in the treatment of conditions such as congestive heart failure, in which the interaction between different forms of "vitamin E" may constitute one of the more significant physiological factors. The exclusive reliance on alpha-tocopherol in almost all clinical trials of vitamin E fails to acknowledge the inherent balance and synergistic interplay among alpha-, beta-, gamma-, and delta-tocopherol and thus limits both the immediate applicability of any resultant findings and their extrapolation.

Over the past 40 years the role of vitamin E in preventing heart disease has been the subject of often acrimonious debate and collegial miscommunication. The ongoing controversy regarding the role of vitamin E in the prevention and treatment of cardiovascular disease reveals a deep schism in the often opposing world views of the linear reductionistic philosophy that permeates much of conventional medicine, and the more holistic empirical approaches of "natural" medicine. This dynamic suggests an emerging paradigm that might offer novel approaches to research, prevention, and therapeutics that can transcend and yet be inclusive of previously conflicting viewpoints. *Oxidative stress* plays a central role in the physio-pathology underlying many chronic degenerative diseases, particularly cardiovascular disease, but its clinical implications are not understood in a consistent and comprehensive way. The underlying assumption in the field was that if the antioxidant effect of vitamin E conclusively proved to be clinically significant, vitamin E would logically be confirmed as playing an integral role in the prevention and treatment of heart disease. The role of antioxidant nutrients has evolved through a cycle of ill-founded enthusiasm and premature expectations that verge on regarding them as a panacea, into a body of research using single antioxidants in high doses (and often synthetic forms), with mostly negative results, and toward an emerging reconceptualization of nutrients' physiological nature and function, clinical uses, and effects. The interactions between antioxidants and statin drugs provide an important illustration of this dialogue and suggest ways in which both research and clinical practice can mature.

Thus, over the past two decades, the attitude toward vitamin E has gone from acceptance and often enthusiasm in some quarters, especially in relation to heart disease, to near-condemnation in more recent papers. However, the limitations of the research thus far clearly point to the need for further research into the differences between pharmaceutical and food sources of vitamin E, the physiological functions of and interplay among the various forms of naturally occurring tocopherol isomers, and the implications of such findings in formulating preparations for research and clinical practice. Furthermore, the emerging knowledge of physiological detoxification systems, such as hepatic phase I, II, and III enzyme systems, and the operative mechanisms of nuclear receptors, such as pregnane X receptor (PXR), offers significant prospects for understanding the clinical significance of drug metabolism and its stimulation by vitamin E and other nutrients. Further research, education, and communication will also be necessary to clarify the importance of using naturally occurring forms of vitamin E, preferably mixed tocopherols and tocotrienols, within the context of a comprehensive antioxidant strategy and with a respect for the particular needs and vulnerabilities of specific patient populations.

Some aspects of this controversy may derive from differences in the research questions being asked, trial design, observational studies versus randomized controlled clinical trials versus meta-analyses, characteristics of subject populations, nutrient forms and dosages, dietary sources versus supplemental intake, concomitant dietary and lifestyle factors, polypharmacy, and outcome measures. From early research into the possible beneficial nature of the interaction between the two, the ground shifted dramatically to claims that antioxidants diminish the effectiveness of statins, and finally to frank warnings that key antioxidants such as beta-carotene and alpha-tocopherol might actually increase risk of coronary artery disease and heart failure.[11,12] Conversely, the unresolved concerns regarding the safety and ultimate efficacy of statin drugs increasingly suggest that the dominant paradigm of scientific knowledge of their nature and action (i.e., lowering of cholesterol) may provide an inadequate explanation of their preventive and therapeutic effects as observed in a wide range of conditions. Ultimately the key to resolving such apparent conflicts may reside in greater individualization of care, with reference to the emerging tools of pharmaco-/nutrigenomics, through titration of drug doses to effect and/or blood levels and close monitoring within a flexible, responsive, and evolving integrative approach.

Many of the issues that arise in clinical research regarding vitamin E reflect clinical experience with vitamin E in particular and nutritional therapies in general, and the role such interventions play in defining clinical options and shaping therapeutic strategy. For example, the HATS study published in fall 2001 (discussed later) was widely interpreted as a negative interaction between antioxidants and statins, but on closer analysis more likely shows a blunting effect of the antioxidants on the rise of high-density lipoprotein (HDL) cholesterol, more associated with niacin, rather than a direct effect on the statin therapy. Most statins have minimal if any positive effects on HDL, and often actually reduce HDL, along with low-density lipoprotein (LDL), which is why the statin-niacin combination has become widely used since that study. Even so, the accepted fact that simvastatin is metabolized by cytochrome P450 3A4 (CYP3A4) may be a potentially significant observation given the findings of a single in vitro experiment showing that alpha-tocopherol could theoretically stimulate drug metabolism, particularly through its effect on PXR, with subsequent increased expression of the CYP3A4 enzyme. Nevertheless, failure to include coenzyme Q10 and methyl donors in the nutrient mix may also have represented a significant limitation in the trial design. Such modification would have addressed underlying mechanisms at issue: the inhibitory activity of statins on endogenous synthesis of coenzyme Q10 and niacin's depletion of methyl donors, particularly in the liver. Correction of these two drug-nutrient interactions with supplementation might have led to a very different outcome.

Lastly, an important aspect of antioxidant function rarely factored into the design of clinical trials is a recognition of the pro-oxidant potential of antioxidants. One or two antioxidants, especially synthetic ones (e.g., all-*trans* beta carotene), given in high doses to individuals under high oxidative stress, who consume diets low in antioxidants (e.g., male Finnish smokers, alcohol/tobacco users), can create a situation in which the antioxidants are forced to act as pro-oxidants. The resultant deficit in the antioxidant network causes the carotene and/or tocopherol and/or ascorbate radicals to persist without being quenched, and thereby increase free-radical damage. The increased incidence of heart failure among high-risk individuals taking 400 mg/day of vitamin E (with ramipril), observed in the HOPE study, appears to reveal such an adverse effect of increased oxidative stress when a comprehensive antioxidant network is not available.[13] Subsequent meta-analyses will be limited by their indiscriminate inclusion of trials using varied agents in isolation with diverse populations. Similarly, the related findings of HOPE and HOPE-TOO trials emphasized the limitations and potential adverse response to use of vitamin E as a single antioxidant in individuals characterized by a state of oxidative stress. These researchers reported that natural-source vitamin E (400 IU alpha-tocopherol daily) failed to significantly reduce risk of cancer or cardiovascular events, the primary focus of the study, and appeared to be associated with an increased risk of heart failure. It is noteworthy that the subject group comprised older patients (average age, >70 years) with a history of heart disease, stroke, or diabetes, most of whom demonstrated very strong risk factors and were taking numerous medications. Furthermore, the authors of this study, as well as most commentators, do not appear to have considered the established relationship between alpha-tocopherol and gamma-tocopherol and its implications in such a patient population. High doses of alpha-tocopherol are known to deplete gamma-tocopherol, not only disrupting the natural balance among the various forms, but particularly influencing the production of natriuretic hormone, which plays a central role in regulating fluid and salt balance and for which gamma-tocopherol is a precursor. Any gamma-tocopherol deficiency induced by alpha-tocopherol could further stress the heart in this already-compromised population and thus contributed to an increased risk of heart failure. The authors conceded that the "unexpected" results "cannot be confirmed at this time by other trials" and "could be due to chance."[11] Such findings reveal an emerging pattern, approaching consensus, confirming the lack of efficacy of an exclusively pharmacological approach to vitamin E therapeutics, narrowly defined as alpha-tocopherol, in achieving the successes attributed to "vitamin E," particularly in individuals with heart disease, diabetes, or similarly compromised conditions. The findings point strongly toward the appropriate use of nutrient-rich food sources, or at least their closest approximation in the form of supplements, providing coordinated, multiple antioxidants, particularly mixed tocopherols and tocotrienols (which are up to 50 times more potent antioxidants than the tocopherols).

As knowledge of interactive complexity at molecular and cellular levels unfolds, so do prospects for more appropriately designed clinical trials. The French SuViMax study, which coadministered five antioxidants, showed a cancer prevention effect in likely dietarily antioxidant-deficient males. This exemplifies the hypothesis that the larger the number of antioxidant nutrients combined, that act in both aqueous and lipidic compartments, the better the clinical results should be. As collective knowledge of the mechanisms and nuances of integrative therapeutics matures, so do prospects for increasingly relevant, large-scale, well-designed clinical trials focusing on clinical outcomes. In the meantime, the role of vitamin E as a key antioxidant is undergoing a reassessment as clinicians and researchers obtain greater knowledge and deeper insight into antioxidant networks, the influences of dietary and supplemental sources, and their roles in health promotion, disease prevention, and therapeutic intervention.

NUTRIENT-DRUG INTERACTIONS

Acetylsalicylic Acid (ASA, aspirin)

Acetylsalicylic acid (acetosal, acetyl salicylic acid, ASA, salicylsalicylic acid; Arthritis Foundation Pain Reliever, Ascriptin, Aspergum, Asprimox, Bayer Aspirin, Bayer Buffered Aspirin, Bayer Low Adult Strength, Bufferin, Buffex, Cama Arthritis Pain Reliever, Easprin, Ecotrin, Ecotrin Low Adult Strength, Empirin, Extra Strength Adprin-B, Extra Strength Bayer Enteric 500 Aspirin, Extra Strength Bayer Plus, Halfprin 81, Heartline, Regular Strength Bayer Enteric 500 Aspirin, St. Joseph Adult Chewable Aspirin, ZORprin); combination drugs: ASA and caffeine (Anacin); ASA, caffeine, and propoxyphene (Darvon Compound); ASA and carisoprodol (Soma Compound); ASA, codeine, and carisoprodol (Soma Compound with Codeine); ASA and codeine (Empirin with Codeine); ASA, codeine, butalbital, and caffeine (Fiorinal); ASA and extended-release dipyridamole (Aggrenox, Asasantin).

Interaction Type and Significance

⊕⊕ **Beneficial or Supportive Interaction, with Professional Management**
✗ **Potential or Theoretical Adverse Interaction of Uncertain Severity**

Probability:	Evidence Base:
2. Probable	◉ **Emerging**

Effect and Mechanism of Action

Given a perception of aspirin and vitamin E as both acting as blood thinners (e.g., reducing platelet aggregations), an additive effect from coadministration of these substances has been proposed.

Research

The emerging body of human research into the potential interaction between vitamin E and aspirin has yet to reach the plateau of evolution and clarity necessary to understanding the apparent inconsistencies between clinical practice and the scientific literature. Steiner et al.[14] conducted a double-blind, randomized clinical trial investigating the antiaggregating agent containing vitamin E in 100 patients at risk for transient ischemic attacks (TIAs). Over 2 years, subjects were administered either aspirin (325 mg) or aspirin plus vitamin E (400 IU/day). Comparing two randomized subgroups from both sets of subjects, those receiving the combination medication demonstrated a significant reduction in ischemic events and platelet adhesiveness. There was no significant difference in the incidence of hemorrhagic stroke, although both individuals who developed it were taking vitamin E. The authors noted that the coadministration of vitamin E and aspirin appears to be safe and concluded that "combination of vitamin E and a platelet antiaggregating agent (e.g., aspirin) significantly enhances the efficacy of the preventive treatment regimen in patients with transient ischemic attacks and other ischemic cerebrovascular problems."[14]

In a double-blind clinical trial into the related issue of vitamin E's impact in patients undergoing chronic warfarin therapy, Kim and White[15] found that none of the subjects who received vitamin E had a significant change in the international normalized ratio (INR). Looking at the controversial topic of antioxidant use by smokers, Liede et al.[16] performed an endpoint examination of a random sample of 409 male smokers, age 55 to 74 years, who had participated in a larger, controlled, double-blind clinical trial. They reported a statistically significant increase in gingival bleeding among subjects taking the combination of acetylsalicylic acid (ASA) and alpha-tocopherol (50 mg/day) compared with those taking aspirin alone (33.4% vs. 25.8%); ASA alone increased bleeding only slightly. These authors concluded that alpha-tocopherol supplementation, particularly when combined with aspirin, might increase the risk of bleeding gums and other clinically important hemorrhage.

Subsequently, in an in vitro study, Celestini et al.[17] investigated the capacity of vitamin E to enhance the antiplatelet effect of aspirin by assessing the dose-response curves of platelet aggregation, dense body secretion, phospholipase C activation, and calcium mobilization in aspirin-treated platelets incubated with and without added vitamin E (50 and 100 mg daily). They also looked at the important issue of vitamin E's role in reducing platelet adhesion to collagen. These researchers demonstrated significant induction of maximal platelet aggregation and calcium mobilization compared with controls and concluded that vitamin E can potentiate the antiplatelet activity of aspirin by inhibiting the early events of platelet activation pathways induced by collagen.

The clear direction of this research, collectively, supports further research into the combined use of vitamin E, preferably naturally occurring tocopherols, together with aspirin, in the prevention of undesirable platelet aggregation, particularly thrombotic complications in atherosclerotic patients.[17]

Nutritional Therapeutics, Clinical Concerns, and Adaptations

For decades, clinicians and patients have been exposed to research and subjected to debate on the potential benefits of both aspirin and vitamin E in the prevention of cardiovascular disease.[18-24] Unfortunately, the certainty of the evidence and its penetration into common knowledge have been delayed and obscured by the often contradictory and hyperbolic nature of the claims and counterclaims. At the time of this review, the evolving body of evidence suggests that the probable additive effect from coadministration of aspirin and vitamin E could enhance valuable antiplatelet activity or produce undesirable effects on hemorrhagic tendencies, depending on characteristics of the patient population, respective dosage and forms employed, and coordination of attending health care providers. Given the high likelihood that conscientious patients could be using both vitamin E and aspirin as daily preventive measures, it would seem critical that the nature and implications of this potentially beneficial interaction be clarified and guidelines for integrative practice management be developed and implemented. Innovative approaches, similar to the "polypill" proposed by Wald and Law,[25] incorporating tocopherols deserve further investigation as the clinical implications of vitamin E and antioxidants in relation to aspirin, statin therapy, and other conventional approaches reveal their nuances to well-designed clinical trials, especially if clinicians experienced in the dosage and forms of the nutrients involved are integrated into the research process. In particular, therapeutic use of both vitamin E and aspirin might benefit from a fresh view that expands beyond the long-held conception of their beneficial action deriving solely, or even primarily, from their effects on coagulability and opens into supportive and even nutritive effects. Through development of such integrative approaches to polypharmacy, especially toward preventive effects, clinicians of all therapeutic schools would do well to disown their historical prejudices for or against pharmaceuticals and natural products per se and focus instead on our shared avowed dedication to the health and well-being of those who entrust us with their care.

Pending further research, combined use of aspirin and vitamin E, particularly as d-alpha-tocopherol or other naturally-occurring forms, presents a potentially valuable asset in the emerging repertoire of pharmacological and behavioral tools for the prevention of excess coagulation and reduction of the incidence of hemorrhagic stroke, especially among individuals at increased at risk for TIAs. Nevertheless, there is a critical need to remain cognizant of the potentially dangerous increased tendency to bleed, which may represent a manifestation of vitamin E toxicity in some cases. Although individual needs must be assessed within the clinical context of each patient's genetic susceptibility, lifestyle risks, medical history, and other factors, 100 IU tocopherol, mixed or d-alpha, and 80 mg aspirin per day may provide a conservative starting point for such integrative care.

Anthralin

Anthralin (Anthra-Derm, Dithranol, Drithocreme, Micanol Cream).

Interaction Type and Significance

☼ **Prevention or Reduction of Drug Adverse Effect**

Probability:
2. Probable

Evidence Base:
◉ Emerging

Effect and Mechanism of Action

Anthralin causes skin inflammation as a result of free-radical formation, through lipid peroxidation and production of inflammatory endoperoxides or by a more direct mechanism.

Research

In a clinical trial, Finnen et al.[26] determined that topical application of the tocopherol form of vitamin E inhibited inflammation of forearm skin by scavenging free radicals of the oxygen species.

Nutritional Therapeutics, Clinical Concerns, and Adaptations

Physicians prescribing anthralin as a topical antipsoriatic might reduce the risk of adverse effects by requesting that the pharmacist compound alpha-tocopherol into the preparation.

Bile Acid Sequestrants

Evidence: Cholestyramine (Locholest, Prevalite, Questran), colestipol (Colestid).
Extrapolated, based on similar properties: Colesevelam (Welchol).

Interaction Type and Significance

≈≈≈ **Drug-Induced Nutrient Depletion, Supplementation Therapeutic, Not Requiring Professional Management**
◇ **Adverse Drug Effect on Nutritional Therapeutics, Strategic Concern**

Probability:
2. Probable

Evidence Base:
▽ Mixed

Effect and Mechanism of Action

Through their intended effect of limiting absorption and assimilation of dietary lipids, bile acid sequestrants may prevent absorption of vitamin E, as well as of folic acid and other fat-soluble vitamins (A, D, K, carotenoids, and coenzyme Q10).[27-31]

Research

Researchers have investigated both supportive and depleting interactions between vitamin E and bile acid sequestrants, especially colestipol. Hodis et al.[32] found that the combination of colestipol, vitamin E (100 IU/day) and niacin was associated with added benefits on progression of coronary atherosclerotic lesions, as demonstrated in serial coronary angiographic studies. Schwarz et al.[33] observed that during 24 months of colestipol therapy plus diet, serum vitamin A and E concentrations did decrease in the five patients with good drug adherence, but deemed the resultant concentrations as within normal limits and hence insignificant. In monitoring plasma levels of fat-soluble vitamins, including vitamin E, and several other nutrients in young patients with familial hypercholesterolemia after 5 years of colestipol therapy, Schlierf et al.[34] observed no adverse drug effects with respect to the previous parameters and noted that plasma levels of carotenoids and vitamin E were elevated in the patients according to elevated concentrations of lipoproteins. Tonstad et al.[35] conducted a study of 37 boys and 29 girls age 10 to 16 years with familial hypercholesterolemia, first in an 8-week, double blind, placebo-controlled protocol, then in open treatment for 44 to 52 weeks. They found that levels of serum folate, vitamin E, and carotenoids were reduced in the colestipol group.

Nutritional Therapeutics, Clinical Concerns, and Adaptations

Although bile acid sequestrants inherently reduce absorption of fat-soluble nutrients such as vitamin E and alter their availability and functionality within the body, evidence is lacking as to whether and when this impingement on normal physiological processes results in clinically significant effects and deleterious outcomes. Depletion due to unintended effects on absorption of fat-soluble nutrients, including vitamin E, may not be adequate to adversely affect many segments of the population to a clinically significant degree, or at least one discernible using standard research methodology. Importantly, plasma levels of fat-soluble vitamins, especially vitamin E, are typically elevated along with the elevated concentrations of lipoproteins that are carriers of nutrients. Further, any such impact may be potentially problematic in susceptible individuals most at risk for deficiency patterns and increased risk of cardiovascular dysfunction and disease, especially through extended courses of treatment. If vitamin E is being taken as part of an explicit strategy to reduce oxidative stress, thereby possibly reducing risk of cardiovascular disease, and support healthy lipid metabolism, the potential interference from these agents needs to be considered in establishing dosage, timing, and form of any concomitant therapy using vitamin E. Water-soluble forms of d-alpha-tocopherol provides one readily available means of circumventing this potential adverse interference with normal assimilation of nutrients in individuals for whom vitamin E plays an essential role in clinical care strategy, whether for cardiovascular effects or other preventive or therapeutic effects. Otherwise, regular use of a high-potency multivitamin/mineral formulation will replace the nutrients depleted by the drug. Individuals taking vitamin E, or other nutritional supplements and some drugs, may reduce interference of absorption by cholestyramine, colestipol, or other bile acid sequestrants by allowing an interval of 1 hour before or 4 to 6 hours after the medication.

Chemotherapy (Various Agents)

Including cisplatin (cis-diaminedichloroplatinum, CDDP; Platinol, Platinol-AQ), cyclophosphamide (Cytoxan, Endoxana, Neosar, Procytox), docetaxel (Taxotere), doxorubicin (Adriamycin, Rubex), etoposide (Eposin, Etophos, VePesid, VP-16), fluorouracil (5-FU; Adrucil, Efudex, Efudix, Fluoroplex), gemcitabine (Gemzar), irinotecan (camptothecin-11, CPT-11; Campto, Camptosar), methotrexate (Folex, Maxtrex,

Rheumatrex), mitomycin (Mutamycin), paclitaxel (Paxene, Taxol), vinblastine (AlkabanAQ, Velban, Velsar), vincristine (Leurocristine, Oncovin, VincasarPFS), vinorelbine (Navelbine).

Antioxidants with Chemotherapy and Radiotherapy

Interaction Type and Significance

✗✗✗   **Potentially Harmful or Serious Adverse Interaction—Avoid**

⊕✗   **Bimodal or Variable Interaction, with Professional Management**

◇≈≈   **Drug-Induced Adverse Effect on Nutrient Function, Coadministration Therapeutic, with Professional Management**

◇◇   **Drug-Induced Effect on Nutrient Function, Supplementation Contraindicated, Professional Management Appropriate**

⊕⊕   **Beneficial or Supportive Interaction, with Professional Management**

≈◇◇   **Drug-Induced Nutrient Depletion, Supplementation Contraindicated, Professional Management Appropriate**

Probability:	Evidence Base:
3. Probable	▽ Mixed

Effect and Mechanism of Action

Oxygen radicals have increasingly come under investigation as highly toxic stressors contributing to the causes of many diseases, including many forms of cancer. Vitamins E, C, and A are well known antioxidant agents. N-acetylcysteine (NAC) is a free-radical scavenger and might access the endothelial cell, thus increasing intracellular glutathione (GSH) stores. Even so, some concerns have been raised that antioxidants might be contraindicated during chemotherapy because one way in which chemotherapeutic agents attack cancer cells is by causing oxidative damage.[36,37]

Research

A variety of test tube–based and animal studies have found vitamin A, C, and E to increase the effectiveness of chemotherapy in several types of cancer.[36,38-44] In a double-blind study, Wagdi et al.[45] found that an antioxidant combination consisting of vitamin C, vitamin E, and NAC provided protection against heart damage induced by chemotherapy without reducing its effectiveness. NAC therapy may be useful therapy in advanced cervical cancers, especially squamous cell carcinomas. Several researchers have offered the seemingly paradoxical conclusion that the appropriate administration of antioxidant inhibitors and/or free-radical–generating compounds may be a useful strategy in the treatment of solid tumors. After performing a comprehensive review of the relationship between chemotherapy and antioxidants, Weijl et al.[46] rebuffed warnings that antioxidants need to be avoided during chemotherapy, but also determined that definitive evidence was lacking to support the use of antioxidants to provide relief from the adverse side effects of chemotherapy. Subsequently, however, conference reports (unpublished proceedings) by Salignik and Zeisel at a 1999 American Society of Cell Biology meeting suggest that vitamin A–deficient and vitamin E–deficient mice were less susceptible to brain tumor progression than non–vitamin-deficient control animals. Salignik et al.[47] suggested suppression of free radicals by the antioxidant vitamins may suppress apoptosis (programmed cell death).

In a randomized, double-blind, placebo-controlled trial among 540 head and neck cancer patients treated with radiation therapy, Bairati et al.[48] found that coadministration of alpha-tocopherol (400 IU/day) and beta-carotene (30 mg/day) administered during radiation therapy and for 3 years thereafter resulted in "less severe acute adverse effects during radiation therapy" (vs. placebo), with that reduction being "statistically significant... for adverse effects to the larynx... and overall at any site." However, "quality of life was not improved" by the nutrient coadministration. Moreover, the "rate of local recurrence of the head and neck tumor tended to be higher in the supplement arm of the trial." Notably, "beta-carotene was discontinued because of ethical concerns" during trial. The authors concluded that concomitant treatment "with high doses of alpha-tocopherol and beta-carotene during radiation therapy could reduce the severity of treatment adverse effects," but they cautioned that their data suggest that "use of high doses of antioxidants as adjuvant therapy might compromise radiation treatment efficacy."[48]

Kennedy et al.[49] conducted a 6-month observational study of 103 children with acute lymphoblastic leukemia (ALL) being treated with chemotherapy. They reported that a large percentage of children undergoing ALL treatment have inadequate intakes of antioxidants and vitamin A, and that lower intakes of antioxidants are associated with increases in the adverse side effects of chemotherapy. In particular, greater vitamin E intake at 3 months was associated with a lower incidence of infections.

Birdsall et al.[50] and Cancer Treatment Centers of America conducted an exploratory trial to investigate effect of concomitant naturopathic therapies on clinical tumor response to radiation for early-stage prostate cancer (tumor stages 1b through 2, N0,M0). External-beam radiation therapy of up to 72 Gy was given to 22 patients on a conventional 8-week treatment regimen, whereas the 13 patients in the naturopathic group received at least one antioxidant supplement, with the most frequent antioxidant naturopathic treatments including green tea extract, melatonin, and a high-potency multivitamin, vitamin C, or vitamin E. "All patients were monitored for at least 12 months (range 12-42) and no patient received concomitant hormonal therapy." The investigators reported that in the patients "who did not receive naturopathic [antioxidant] treatments, the median pretreatment PSA level was 5.4 ng/mL, the median PSA nadir was 0.66 ng/mL, and the median time to PSA nadir was 16.0 months," and in the "patients who did receive naturopathic treatments, the corresponding values were 5.8 ng/mL; 0.59 ng/mL; and 16.0 months." One tumor treatment failure occurred in the nonnaturopathic group "based on PSA elevation > 2 ng from nadir which occurred at 14 months," but there were no treatment failures in the patients who received concomitant naturopathic regimens. The authors noted as "also significant that 9/9 patients in the non-CAM group were considered to be low risk (based on pretreatment PSA levels of 4-10 ng) whereas 3 patients in the CAM group were classified as intermediate risk (PSA > 10-20 ng) and 1 patient as high risk (PSA > 20 ng)" (PSA, prostate-specific antigen; CAM, complementary and alternative medicine). Thus, the authors concluded that "concomitant naturopathic treatment does not appear to inhibit the capacity of external beam radiation therapy to control localized prostate cancer, and does not interfere with either the magnitude of the response, the velocity of the response, or its durability for at least 1 year." They added that these "results provide definitive evidence that antioxidant-based CAM modalities, designed to improve patient tolerance, quality of life, and possibly improve survival, do not inhibit

tumor responses that depend on oxidative [tumor] killing mechanisms elicited by external beam radiation therapy."[50] Although encouraging, this small, retrospective study did not have sufficient power to draw any statistically significant conclusions. Similar studies involving much larger groups of patients receiving radiotherapy are warranted.

Clinical Implications and Adaptations

Some oncologists have raised reasonable concerns that supplementation with antioxidants might interfere with or limit the effectiveness of chemotherapeutic agents and radiation therapy. However, no substantial prospective, randomized, controlled clinical research has emerged to support this speculation or to warrant considering antioxidants as contraindicated during chemotherapy or radiotherapy, and emerging evidence indicates that effects of coadministration (particularly during radiotherapy) are more likely to be beneficial or negligible than harmful.[50a] Many nutritionally oriented health care professionals consider the oxidative damage caused by chemotherapy to be a particularly troublesome adverse effect given that evidence increasingly points to oxidative damage as being a contributing factor in the causation of many cancers. Individuals receiving chemotherapy should consult their treating physician and a nutritionally trained health care professional about the potential value of adding antioxidants to their regimen before starting such concomitant use. Well-designed clinical trials addressing this issue are sorely needed, but are moving into the necessary state of refinement. Such trials are particularly difficult to perform because the potential antioxidant contribution from diet, and its extreme variability among cancer patients during treatment, can seriously confound the effects of adjunctive antioxidant intake. For studies to be meaningful, diet needs to be standardized, which is logistically difficult. Studies that use a small number of antioxidants (i.e, fewer than four agents) concurrently with high oxidative stress inducers, such as chemotherapy and radiation, in patients consuming an antioxidant-poor diet, also are likely seeing the oxidant effects of the "antioxidant" compounds, because the antioxidant network necessary to recycle oxidized antioxidants is severely compromised.

Oral Mucositis

Interaction Type and Significance
☼   **Prevention or Reduction of Drug Adverse Effect**

Probability: Evidence Base:
2. Probable   ◉ **Emerging**

Effect and Mechanism of Action
Acute reductions in plasma concentrations of essential nutrients, including alpha-tocopherol, have been associated with impaired immune responses in some clinical settings. In particular, oral mucositis, inflammation of mucous membranes, represents one of the most frequent complications during conventional cancer therapy using chemotherapy or radiotherapy. Topical vitamin E has been proposed as a preventive agent based on effects on inflammation and lipid peroxidation.

Research
In a randomized, double-blind, placebo-controlled study involving 18 patients, Wadleigh et al.[51] used topical vitamin E in the treatment of oral mucositis in patients receiving chemotherapy. They found that six of nine patients receiving vitamin E had complete resolution of their oral lesions, whereas lesions did not

resolve completely in eight of nine patients who received placebo. Lopez et al.[52] conducted further studies examining the efficacy of topical vitamin E for the treatment of this condition and found that although topical vitamin E applied once daily was beneficial to some subjects, others did not experience relief from their symptoms.

In 1998, Mills[53] demonstrated the beneficial modifying effect of beta-carotene on oral mucositis caused by radiation and chemotherapy. Subsequently, in a preliminary study, topical application of honey also proved to be of benefit against radiation-induced mucositis.[54] More recently, Ferreira et al.[55] conducted a randomized, placebo-controlled clinical trial involving 54 patients receiving radiotherapy as the only treatment for cancers of the mouth and oropharynx. Subjects were administered an oil solution containing 400 IU vitamin E twice daily or a placebo (presumed to be nonactive) containing 500 mg evening primrose oil twice daily, before every conventional fraction of 2 Gy (200 rad) and again 8 to 12 hours later during the 5 to 7 weeks of radiotherapy. Participants were instructed to dissolve each capsule and hold the oil in their mouth for 5 minute before swallowing. At the conclusion of the study, the occurrence of painful mucositis events was significantly less (21.6% vs. 33.5%) among subjects who had received vitamin E than those receiving placebo. Likewise, pain and eating restrictions were significantly less in participants receiving vitamin E compared with the placebo group. These findings demonstrate that vitamin E can be useful in preventing and reducing the severity of mucositis in patients receiving radiotherapy for head and neck cancer. The equivalent survival statistics between the two groups would argue against any interference by vitamin E's antioxidant activity with efficacy of the radiotherapy.

Nutritional Therapeutics, Clinical Concerns, and Adaptations

The research reviewed might be considered weak or unreliable because of its limited scale, but the collective conclusions indicate that topical vitamin E represents a potentially effective approach to the prevention of mouth sores typically associated with chemotherapy and radiation. The trend revealed in the extant research recommends that well-designed, placebo-controlled trials are warranted. In the meantime, conservative principles of care, with a preventive orientation and integrative repertoire, suggest that vitamin E may provide a safe and inexpensive remedy to a highly probable adverse effect. In such cases, topical application of alpha-tocopherol twice daily would be the form most likely to be effective; with alpha-tocopheryl being the less preferred form. Formulations combining vitamin E and selenomethionine might also be considered, especially as a radioprotective agent.

Cisplatin and Oxaliplatin

Cisplatin (*cis*-diaminedichloroplatinum, CDDP; Platinol, Platinol-AQ); oxaliplatin (Eloxatin).
See also previous section on mucositis.

Interaction Type and Significance

☼　**Prevention or Reduction of Drug Adverse Effect**
≈≈　**Drug-Induced Nutrient Depletion,**
　　　Supplementation Therapeutic, with
　　　Professional Management
⊕⊕　**Beneficial or Supportive Interaction, with**
　　　Professional Management

Probability:　　　　　　Evidence Base:
2. Probable　　　　　◉ **Emerging**

Effect and Mechanism of Action

Cisplatin is one of the most active antineoplastic agents for the treatment of various malignant tumors. However, platinum-based chemotherapy regimens are often associated with a wide range of adverse effects and often irreversible damage, including nephrotoxicity, peripheral neuropathy, ototoxicity, gastrointestinal dysfunction, and myelosuppression. In particular, cisplatin therapy reduces antioxidant levels in the blood at the same time that it increases levels of free radicals and lipid peroxidation. Peripheral neuropathy is a particularly common adverse effect, especially affecting the hands and feet. Dorsal root ganglia are key sites in cisplatin-induced neurotoxicity because these are the neural tissue with the highest degree of platinum accumulation[56]; these ganglia also are the most vulnerable neural structures in vitamin E deficiency neuropathies.[57] Cisplatin neurotoxicity has been attributed to demyelinization of the sensitive axons of the peripheral nerve sheaths, gangliar cell loss of the dorsal root ganglion and neural body, and axonal degeneration of the posterior horns of the spinal cord, paralleling the neurotoxic damage induced by chronic alpha-tocopherol deficiency.[58] Oxaliplatin is a novel, third-generation, platinum-based anticancer agent, recently approved and now widely used to treat colorectal cancer, and it appears to be even more neurotoxic than cisplatin. Vitamin E supplementation apparently enhances antioxidant activity and prevents or limits free-radical damage.

Research

The neuropathy induced by cisplatin is characterized by symptoms of peripheral sensory neuropathy, with ataxia and areflexia, similar to that observed in alpha-tocopherol deficiency syndromes. McCarron et al.[59] observed that alpha-tocopherol deficiency determines a peripheral neuropathy and spinocerebellar ataxia caused by retrograde degeneration of the large-caliber axons in the peripheral nerves and degeneration of the posterior columns in the spinal cord.

Pathak et al.[60] reported potentiation of the effect of paclitaxel and carboplatin on a human lung squamous carcinoma cell line after pretreatment with an antioxidant mixture containing vitamin C, vitamin E, and beta-carotene.

A team of Italian researchers investigating the issue of cisplatin-induced neurotoxicity and potential benefits of vitamin E administration published two important papers in 2003. An animal study, with accompanying in vitro research, demonstrated that alpha-tocopherol supplementation provided for decreased severity of adverse effects, particularly protection from drug-induced lipid peroxidation and toxic sequelae, without compromising therapeutic effect, thus contributing to enhanced survival.[58] In their human trial, the team randomly assigned 27 individuals, age 28 to 74, with a wide range of cancers to receive cisplatin chemotherapy alone or cisplatin chemotherapy combined with alpha-tocopherol, 300 IU daily. Supplementation began 3 days before onset of cisplatin therapy and concluded after 3 months, with both objective and subjective assessments at the beginning, midpoint, and conclusion of the therapeutic trial. Subjects receiving both vitamin E and cisplatin reported significantly lower neurotoxicity scores at the conclusion of their treatment (2.1), compared with participants who been given cisplatin alone (4.7). Only 31% of the group receiving alpha-tocopherol developed nerve damage, whereas such adverse reactions occurred in more than 85% of those receiving cisplatin alone. The severity of nerve damage was significantly different, with only mild to moderate effects among the nutrient-supplemented group, whereas two members of the drug-only group experienced severe neuropathies.[61]

In a randomized, open-label, controlled trial, Argyriou et al.[62] investigated the effects of oral vitamin E (600 mg/day) on chemotherapy-induced peripheral neuropathy in 40 patients who underwent six courses of cumulative cisplatin, paclitaxel, or a combination regimen. Treatment was administered during chemotherapy and for 3 months after treatment cessation. Thirty-one patients completed the study; 4 of 16 patients in the vitamin E group demonstrated neurotoxicity versus 11 of 15 patients in the control group. One vitamin E patient and three controls experienced mild neurotoxicity. Moderate toxicity occurred in three vitamin E patients and five controls. Three controls developed severe neurotoxicity. The researchers concluded that the "relative risk (RR) of developing neurotoxicity was significantly higher in the control group than in the treatment group, RR = 0.34," and recommended a large, randomized placebo-controlled trial.[62]

Nutritional Therapeutics, Clinical Concerns, and Adaptations

The evolution of research into the interaction of vitamin E and cisplatin is clearly heading in a promising direction. Although the studies thus far are limited in scale and inherently preliminary in nature, they indicate that vitamin E coadministration, preferably with naturally occurring tocopherol(s), not only can compensate for nutrient depletion pattern and mitigate adverse drug effects, but also can offer the potential for employing higher concentrations of cisplatin, thus improving the antitumor agent's therapeutic index. Research with oxaliplatin may also reveal similar potential for coadministration. Strategic integrative protocols, adapted to the particular characteristics and needs of the individual patient, offer expanded possibilities for enhanced care and improved outcomes within the context of collaborative care involving health care professionals trained and experienced in both conventional oncology and nutritional therapeutics.

Cyclosporine

Cyclosporine (Ciclosporin, cyclosporin A, CsA; Neoral, Sandimmune, SangCya)

Interaction Type and Significance

⊕⊕　**Beneficial or Supportive Interaction, with Professional Management**

☼　**Prevention or Reduction of Drug Adverse Effect**

✗　**Potential or Theoretical Adverse Interaction of Uncertain Severity**

Probability:	Evidence Base:
3. Possible	◉ **Emerging**

Effect and Mechanism of Action

The use of cyclosporine as an immunosuppressive agent in the treatment of allograft patients presents with a significant incidence of adverse effects, particularly nephrotoxicity. The risk of such events is heightened because the drug is poorly bioavailable (~30%). Some individuals are unable to achieve or maintain therapeutic cyclosporine blood levels. Further, the antioxidant activity of vitamin E may provide protective support against the reactive oxygen species (ROS) induced by the drug's action and the lipid peroxidation products suspected in its toxic effects within the kidneys. Concomitant administration of vitamin E during cyclosporine therapy may enhance bioavailability and decrease clearance and steady-state volume of distribution of the drug, as well as reduce adverse effects and cost. Such a supportive interaction could potentially allow for decreased dosage levels of

the medication. Vitamins E and C have also been used as adjunctive therapy in transplant patients on the basis that they might slow progression of transplant-associated arteriosclerosis.

Research

In a small study published in 1996, Chang et al.[63] investigated the effect of water-soluble vitamin E (d-alpha-tocopheryl polyethylene glycol 1000 succinate) on the oral pharmacokinetics of cyclosporine in 10 healthy volunteers. In those individuals who randomly received the vitamin E after two doses of cyclosporine (10 mg/kg orally), cyclosporine clearance and steady-state volume of distribution for the drug were significantly decreased, and an increased area under the curve (AUC) for cyclosporine was observed. In a human trial, using the same water-soluble vitamin E at 6.25 IU/kg twice daily, Pan et al.[64] determined that cyclosporine blood levels during the early posttransplant period were significantly improved in 26 liver transplant patients (both adults and children) previously unable to achieve or maintain therapeutic levels. In contrast, in a different application of cyclosporine, a subsequent in vitro study using a P-glycoprotein–expressing human lung cancer cell line suggested that alpha-tocopherol could antagonize the multidrug-resistance–reversal activity of cyclosporine A and other chemosensitizing agents.[65] Elsewhere, Parra Cid et al.[66] reported that antioxidant nutrients, including vitamin E, protect against cyclosporine A nephrotoxicity.

In a recent retrospective study of data on 22 consecutive heart transplant patients, reduced trough levels of cyclosporine were observed in those who took twice-daily doses of 400 IU vitamin E and 500 mg vitamin C, as compared to other patients. These researchers found no other interactions between the antioxidants and cyclosporine, but cyclosporine trough levels decreased from 136 to 103 ng/mL in the first 2 weeks after antioxidants were administered. The average decrease in trough concentrations was 25% but in some patients was as high as 60%. The authors concluded: "We also don't know what the mechanism of this interaction is, so that should be studied in a more detailed analysis."[67]

On a practical level, many substances interact with cyclosporine, and because of its erratic pharmacokinetics, drug levels are routinely used to determine doses. With such monitoring, any undesirable interaction effects can be readily corrected. Cyclosporine is a classic CYP3A4 intestinal enzyme substrate; some physicians routinely administer cyclosporine with grapefruit juice (which contains a CYP3A4 enzyme inhibitor) to reduce drug costs, since a smaller dose of the drug will produce a higher blood level due to a reduction in the first-pass drug metabolism by intestinal CYP3A4 enzyme. Vitamin E, or the combination of vitamins E and C, may have various effects on cyclosporine pharmacokinetics, but more research is needed to establish this.

Nutritional Therapeutics, Clinical Concerns, and Adaptations

Individuals undergoing immunosuppressive therapy with cyclosporine may benefit from concomitant administration of vitamin E, and possibly other antioxidants such as vitamin C. Such adjunctive therapy may reduce adverse effects and enable lower drug dosage levels while maintaining therapeutic efficacy. Effective care of these patients will require active collaboration among physicians trained and experienced in both conventional pharmacology and nutritional therapeutics within an integrative therapeutic strategy. Given that vitamin E and allied nutrients might alter cyclosporine absorption and pharmacokinetics and that a wide range in individual responses has been reported, drug levels need to be checked regularly, perhaps more frequently than usual, starting at 2 weeks.

Dapsone

Dapsone (4,4′ diaminodiphenyl-Sulphone)

Interaction Type and Significance

☼ **Prevention or Reduction of Drug Adverse Effect**

Probability:
4. Plausible

Evidence Base:
○ **Preliminary**

Effect and Mechanism of Action

Dapsone is strongly oxidative in a way that damages the membranes of RBCs and can result in hemolysis.

Research

In several trials, individuals with leprosy or dermatitis herpetiformis taking dapsone were given 800 IU of vitamin E for periods ranging from 4 weeks to 3 months. Kelly et al.[68] found that dl-alpha-tocopherol acetate, 800 mg/day for up to 3 months, did not substantially ameliorate the hemolytic effect of dapsone at 100 mg/day. In another study of patients with dermatitis herpetiformis, vitamin E therapy was followed by vitamin C therapy, and then combined therapy with vitamins E and C. This study concluded that the vitamin C had exerted no beneficial effect, but that oral administration of 800 units of vitamin E daily for 4 weeks confers partial protective effect against dapsone-induced hemolysis in patients with dermatitis herpetiformis.[69] Subsequently, Lardo et al.[70] studied patients with leprosy and concluded that oral vitamin E, 800 IU/day, conferred partial protective effect but did not correct the hemolysis parameters produced by dapsone treatment, 100 mg/day, except for methemoglobin levels, which were a more sensitive indicator of the oxidant damage.

Nutritional Therapeutics, Clinical Concerns, and Adaptations

Preliminary clinical evidence suggests that vitamin E may counter the adverse effects of dapsone but remains somewhat inconclusive. However, supplementation of 800 IU daily could provide many other potential benefits for such individuals beyond the antioxidant effect against dapsone-induced hemolysis indicated in these studies. Furthermore, clinicians are advised to consider recommending a strict gluten-free diet for certain patients. Dermatitis herpetiformis is often secondary to an unrecognized gluten sensitivity (celiac sprue); such an approach over time may make dapsone treatment unnecessary in these cases.

Doxorubicin and Related Anthracycline Chemotherapy

Evidence: Doxorubicin (Adriamycin, Rubex).
Extrapolated, based on similar properties: Daunorubicin (Cerubidine), epirubicin (Ellence, Pharmorubicin), idarubicin (Idamycin, Zavedos), mitoxantrone (Novantrone, Onkotrone). Similar properties but evidence lacking for extrapolation: Daunorubicin, liposomal (DaunoXome); doxorubicin, pegylated liposomal (Caelyx, Doxil, Myocet).

Interaction Type and Significance

☼ **Prevention or Reduction of Drug Adverse Effect**

Probability:
4. Plausible

Evidence Base:
○ **Preliminary**

Effect and Mechanism of Action

Doxorubicin is a highly effective antineoplastic agent, but cardiotoxicity, acute and chronic, is an adverse effect occurring in up to one third of the patients treated after a cumulative dose of 300 mg/m^2, and increasing sharply beyond a cumulative dose of 360 mg/m^2. Consequently, it is often used in less-than-optimal doses in an attempt to mitigate resultant irreversible and dose-dependent cardiomyopathy. As an antioxidant with a particular affinity for cardiac tissue, vitamin E has been investigated as a potential tool in mitigating such adverse effect and enabling treatment with higher dosage levels of doxorubicin.[71]

The cardiotoxicity of anthracycline chemotherapy agents can be of rapid onset and persist for decades, often absent cardiac complaints. The cardiotoxicity is multifactorial and involves oxidative stress, in part mediated by an iron-catalyzed Fenton reaction; iron-chelating agents have been shown to decrease doxorubicin cardiac toxicity. Two conditions of cardiotoxicity have been recognized. The first is a dose-independent idiosyncratic phenomenon appearing immediately after anthracycline administration and is based on a pericarditis-myocarditis syndrome in patients without previous cardiac disease. The second condition is dose related and characterized by progressive decline of left ventricular systolic function, as assessed by the ejection fraction on nuclear medicine and echocardiographic studies, which may lead to congestive heart failure (CHF). Diastolic dysfunction may also lead to CHF, with or without concomitant compromise of left ventricular ejection fraction. On pathological examination, progressive anthracycline-related cardiac damage may include restrictive endomyocardial disease, characterized by fibrous thickening of the endomyocardium, and dilated cardiomyopathy, as a result of myocardial fibrosis and hypertrophy of surviving myocytes. Symptoms can appear many years after completion of chemotherapy, although sequential assessment of left ventricular systolic and diastolic function will show compromise long before symptomatic CHF ensues. Risk of anthracycline-induced CHF is increased by radiotherapy fields that involve all or part of the heart.[72-74] In a longitudinal assessment of cardiac function in the 22 patients treated with anthracycline for osteogenic sarcoma or malignant fibrous histiocytoma, Brouwer et al.[75] found systolic dysfunction in more than a quarter of the patients and diastolic dysfunction in almost half after two decades (median, 22 years). Moreover, cardiac dysfunction was progressive, as measured at 9, 14, and 22 years.

Hair loss is another adverse effect typically associated with doxorubicin.

Cardiac Toxicity for Anthracycline Class of Antineoplastic Agents. Cardiac toxicity is similar between equipotent doses of doxorubicin and daunorubicin, slightly lower for epirubicin, and only one-sixth that of doxorubicin for equipotent doses of mitoxantrone. Doxil and DaunoXome (liposomal doxorubicin and daunorubicin, respectively) have negligible cardiotoxicity, presumably because of negligible cardiac exposure to the active drug with the pharmacokinetics of the liposome-encapsulated preparation.

Research

Initial studies using rodents found that vitamin E exerted a protective effect against doxorubicin-induced cardiotoxicity.[76,77] In 1979, Krivit[78] proposed that alpha-tocopherol might ameliorate or prevent cardiac dysfunction without impairing the drug's antitumor effectiveness. Subsequently, a study by Legha et al.[79] showed that use of the vitamin did not compromise the drug's antitumor activity but also failed to demonstrate substantial protection against doxorubicin-induced cardiac toxicity.

Wood[80] reported the severity of hair loss typically associated with doxorubicin therapy might be ameliorated by administration of tocopherol at 1600 IU/day, a relatively high dosage. These findings were supported by a subsequent study using doxorubicin-treated rabbits that showed evidence of protection against doxorubicin-dependent inhibition of new hair growth after being fed a alpha-tocopherol–supplemented diet;[81] human trials have not been published confirming such potential efficacy.

Other investigations have focused on possible synergistic relationships between vitamin E and doxorubicin. In vitro research with human prostatic carcinoma cells by Ripoll et al.[82] found that vitamin E enhanced the medication's chemotherapeutic effects.

Review teams led by Weijl[46] and Quiles[71] noted that antioxidant activity can protect against chemotherapy-induced cellular oxidative damage and suggested that the body of evidence indicates that vitamin E coadministration might enable tolerance of higher doxorubicin dose levels, but concluded that evidence from human trials of the nutrient's ability to attenuate the drug's cardiotoxicity remained inadequate.

Nutritional Therapeutics, Clinical Concerns, and Adaptations
Pending further positive research findings, no substantive evidence exists to support the use of alpha-tocopherol as a method of reducing cardiac toxicity caused by doxorubicin. In the meantime, clinicians seeking to integrate such nutritional support into their treatment protocols might consider ubiquinone (coenzyme Q10, L-taurine, L-caritine, fish oils, and/or ginkgo), for which there is more substantial evidence of cardiac protection from doxorubicin.

Gemfibrozil
Gemfibrozil (Apo-Gemfibrozil, Lopid, Novo-Gemfibrozil).

Interaction Type and Significance
≈≈≈ **Drug-Induced Nutrient Depletion, Supplementation Therapeutic, Not Requiring Professional Management**
◇≈≈ **Drug-Induced Adverse Effect on Nutrient Function, Coadministration Therapeutic, with Professional Management**

Probability: Evidence Base:
4. Plausible   ▽ Mixed

Effect and Mechanism of Action
Gemfibrozil may reduce serum antioxidant levels (coenzyme Q10, alpha-tocopherol, gamma-tocopherol) in a manner paralleling changes in lipid levels, but through mechanisms as yet unclear.[83]

Research
The evidence provides an incomplete understanding of the interaction between gemfibrozil and vitamin E. In a randomized, placebo-controlled, crossover trial of 21 men with combined hyperlipidemia, 10 to 12 weeks of gemfibrozil therapy reduced alpha- and gamma-tocopherol serum levels to the levels comparable to those of normolipemic control subjects.[83] Other researchers, also in 1998, reported an antioxidant activity attributable to gemfibrozil that resulted in significantly decreased LDL lipid peroxides and an increased LDL vitamin E/lipid peroxide ratio, with no observable effect on vitamin E status.[84]

Nutritional Therapeutics, Clinical Concerns, and Adaptations
The contradictory and incomplete evidence concerning the interaction(s) between gemfibrozil and vitamin E could be interpreted to suggest a depletion pattern. Clarification of this potential adverse interaction may require a larger study sample and a longer time. However, these seemingly contradictory findings may simply reflect individual pharmacogenomic variability and a normal physiological response to a reduction in serum cholesterol levels. Further, the context of the entire discussion is to some degree held in abeyance, pending further developments in the ongoing controversy regarding the respective roles of antihyperlipidemic drugs and antioxidants in promoting cardiovascular health and treating lipid disorders.

Glyburide
Glyburide (Glibenclamide; Diabeta, Glynase, Glynase Prestab, Micronase, Pres Tab).

Interaction Type and Significance
⊕⊕ **Beneficial or Supportive Interaction, with Professional Management**

Probability: Evidence Base:
4. Plausible   Preliminary

Effect and Mechanism of Action
Glyburide is a sulfonylurea drug used in the treatment of type 2 (non-insulin-dependent) diabetes mellitus (NIDDM) and as such is designed to lower blood glucose levels. The nutritive status and physiological status of vitamin E have often been considered factors of potentially major significance in dysglycemia and development of type 2 diabetes mellitus. This long-standing hypothesis has grown more complex and subtle with the increased knowledge of the interplay between glycemic control and oxidative stress in health and disease. Thus, in addition to normalization of lipid peroxidation, vitamin E might stimulate pancreatic insulin-producing function. Both actions could improve blood glucose control in many individuals with type 2 diabetes and alter the appropriate dose levels of hypoglycemic medications. Notably, oxidative damage plays a central role in many of the pathological changes associated with diabetes, particularly peripheral neuropathies and diabetic retinopathy.

Research
Paolisso et al.[85,86] published two relevant papers in 1993. In a double-blind human trial with 10 healthy control subjects and 15 NIDDM subjects, they observed reduced oxidative stress and improved insulin action in response to 900 mg vitamin E per day for 4 months, compared to placebo.[85] After a randomized clinical trial with 25 type 2 diabetic subjects, they concluded that d-alpha-tocopherol (900 mg/day) for 3 months "seems to produce a minimal but significant improvement in metabolic control but not insulin secretion in elderly type 2 diabetic patients."[86] Subsequently, Balabolkin et al.[86a] prescribed vitamin E in daily doses 600 and 1200 mg to 41 type 2 diabetic patients, who were then divided into four treatment groups: "(1) diets, (2) predian, (3) glyburide, and (4) sugar-reducing drugs and insulin". The authors concluded that while receiving vitamin E, all groups demonstrated enhanced pancreatic insulin production and normalization of lipid peroxidation.[85] Sharma et al.[87] subsequently investigated the role of vitamin E in reducing levels of oxidative stress in

diabetic patients, in the uncontrolled diabetic state or under good glycemic control. They found that maintenance of glycemic control only partially reduced oxidative stress and that oxidant injury continued despite optimal control of the diabetes. After administering supplemental vitamin E for 4 weeks, they reevaluated these patients and observed a further reduction in the oxidative stress, suggesting that vitamin E supplementation might be helpful in reducing free-radical–induced oxidant injury in diabetic patients. These collective findings could be interpreted as supporting the hypothesis that vitamin E may promote blood glucose stabilization and prevent the oxidative damage typically resulting from dysglycemia and likely contributing to the cascading sequelae common among diabetic individuals.

Nutritional Therapeutics, Clinical Concerns, and Adaptations

Enhanced vitamin E intake, through dietary or supplemental sources, may modulate blood glucose levels and reduce oxidative stress resulting from dysglycemic states. Individual genetic susceptibility, diet, lifestyle and contextual stress (or supportive) factors, and pharmacogenomic variability in response to nutrients and medications all significantly influence vitamin E status and the impact of vitamin E supplementation in diabetic individuals taking glyburide or other oral sulfonylurea hypoglycemic agents. Individuals taking any medication for blood glucose and insulin control need to be especially attentive with self-monitoring whenever any of these variables is altered. In particular, changes that enhance glycemic control increase the risk of an unforeseen hypoglycemic reaction.

Haloperidol

Haloperidol (Haldol).

Interaction Type and Significance

≈≈   **Drug-Induced Nutrient Depletion, Supplementation Therapeutic, with Professional Management**

☼   **Prevention or Reduction of Drug Adverse Effect**

◇≈≈   **Drug-Induced Adverse Effect on Nutrient Function, Coadministration Therapeutic, with Professional Management**

Probability: Evidence Base:
4. Plausible   ▽ **Mixed**

Effect and Mechanism of Action

Haloperidol may deplete vitamin E levels and produce adverse effects similar to those of vitamin E deficiency and characteristic of conditions responsive to vitamin E therapy, particularly tardive dyskinesia. Treatment with conventional antipsychotic medications increases free-radical production and oxidative damage, which exerts neurotoxic effects and appears to contribute to the development of dyskinetic phenomena.

Research

Tardive dyskinesia is a common adverse effect of long-term therapy using haloperidol and related neuroleptic drugs and also occurs outside the context of drug reactions, for which some clinicians have found vitamin E to be an effective therapy. An animal study compared the effects of haloperidol on rats fed a normal or a vitamin E–deficient diet and found depleted vitamin E levels in the deprived group.[88] In 1993, Gattaz et al.[89] examined the issue of tardive dyskinesia as part of an investigation of vitamin E's ability to attenuate the development of haloperidol-induced dopaminergic hypersensitivity in rats.

In a series of short-term, controlled trials, Adler et al.[90,91] investigated the therapeutic efficacy of alpha-tocopherol in the treatment of tardive dyskinesia, with generally positive findings, culminating in the 1998 publication of a 36-week study involving 40 subjects who received d-alpha vitamin E (1600 IU/day) or placebo, which confirmed and extended the earlier results.[92] However, shortly thereafter the same research group published a larger, prospective, randomized, nine-site trial of up to 2 years that showed no significant advantage from a similar treatment protocol.[93] A 1998 meta-analysis of studies focusing on vitamin E and tardive dyskinesia published since 1987 noted that the collective findings indicated that a significant subgroup (28.3%) of patients with neuroleptic-induced tardive dyskinesia who were treated with vitamin E showed a modest improvement, and that the supplementation was well tolerated, with only rare and clinically insignificant adverse effects.[94]

Nutritional Therapeutics, Clinical Concerns, and Adaptations

The role of increased oxidative damage in cases of tardive dyskinesia resulting from antipsychotic medications has become increasingly clear. However, as clinical studies have evolved, the weight of the evidence continues to shift away from exclusive use of tocopherol toward a greater appreciation of broader antioxidant approaches for prevention of neurotoxic effects and treatment of long-standing tardive dyskinesia.[95] The increasing use of atypical antipsychotics as effective treatments may also reduce the prevalence and incidence of drug-induced tardive dyskinesia. The emerging tools of pharmacogenomic assessment offer the potential for prescribing medications more precisely suited to a given patient, and thus less likely to produce adverse effects, and for sorting potential antioxidant nutrients or combinations to prevent oxidative damage and ameliorate drug-induced neurotoxicity. Pending further clinical trials with modified supportive protocols and drug-nutrient combinations, physicians prescribing haloperidol can present coadministration of vitamin E, preferably as naturally occurring tocopherols and possibly within a broader antioxidant formulation, as a potentially beneficial means of moderating adverse drug effects, with no known risk of interfering with the haloperidol's therapeutic action.

HMG-CoA Reductase Inhibitors (Statins)

Atorvastatin (Lipitor), fluvastatin (Lescol, Lescol XL), lovastatin (Altocor, Altoprev, Mevacor); combination drug: lovastatin and niacin (Advicor); pravastatin (Pravachol), rosuvastatin (Crestor), simvastatin (Zocor); combination drug: simvastatin and extended-release nicotinic acid (Niaspan).

Interaction Type and Significance

✗   **Potential or Theoretical Adverse Interaction of Uncertain Severity**

◇≈≈   **Drug-Induced Adverse Effect on Nutrient Function, Coadministration Therapeutic, with Professional Management**

⊕⊕   **Beneficial or Supportive Interaction, with Professional Management**

Probability: Evidence Base:
2. Probable (but   ○ **Preliminary** and
contradictory)   ▽ **Mixed**

Effect and Mechanism of Action

Vitamin E has long been presented as preventing the oxidative damage to LDL cholesterol that is generally considered a major component of heart disease. Vitamin E appears to support the therapeutic action of 3-hydroxy-3-methylglutaryl–coenzyme A (HMG-CoA) reductase inhibitors (statins) and reduce their adverse effects, in the prevention and treatment of cardiovascular disease, particularly hyperlipidemia and atherosclerosis. In the critical area of endogenous antioxidant activity and inhibition of lipid peroxidation, statin drugs appear to exert an adverse impact on oxidative status, and statin therapy may enhance oxidizability of alpha-tocopherol and ubiquinol (coenzyme Q10). More recently, concerns have been raised that antioxidants, including vitamin E, may interfere with the HDL-elevating activity of statin-niacin combinations, even though statins alone generally lower HDL as well as LDL (with possible exception of atorvastatin). Vitamin E's specific role in such potential interference, including possible mechanisms of action, has not been presented in a precise and substantiated form. Nevertheless, simvastatin is metabolized by CYP3A4,[96] an important observation given the hypothesis that alpha-tocopherol may stimulate drug metabolism, particularly through its effect on PXR.[97]

Concomitant intake of vitamin E and other antioxidants with conventional lipid-lowering agents may improve some lipid parameters, particularly LDL cholesterol and triglycerides.[98]

Research

Over the past decade, emerging trends in both pathophysiologic and therapeutic research have expanded beyond the earlier emphasis on cholesterol to a deepening appreciation of the fundamental role of inflammation in cardiovascular risk and outcomes, as well as other disease processes.[99] Within this context, previous conceptions of both statin therapies and vitamin E, as an antioxidant and beyond, have yet to form a comprehensive model encompassing healthy function and prevention, therapeutics, and mechanisms of action.

The issue of cholesterol's contribution to heart disease, especially coronary artery disease (CAD), has often focused on the particular risks associated with oxidative damage to LDL cholesterol. Coronary endothelial function has been shown to improve under lipid-lowering and antioxidant therapy. Chen et al.[100] conducted initial research into the antiatherosclerotic effects of vitamin E, through preservation of endogenous antioxidant activity and inhibition of lipid peroxidation, when used with lovastatin and amlodipine (a calcium channel blocker). Palomaki et al.[101,102] showed that lovastatin treatment enhanced oxidizability of alpha-tocopherol and ubiquinol (coenzyme Q10). A subsequent randomized, double-masked, crossover clinical trial involving 28 men with coronary heart disease and hypercholesterolemia determined that alpha-tocopherol supplementation (450 IU daily) significantly increased the antioxidative capacity of LDL when measured ex vivo, which was partially abolished by concomitant lovastatin therapy.[103] In a small study of seven patients with hypercholesterolemia, Neunteufl et al.[104] found that coadministration of simvastatin (20 mg) and vitamin E (300 IU) improved markers of blood vessel elasticity, reduced total cholesterol and LDL cholesterol, and augmented alpha-tocopherol levels (normalized to LDL) more than simvastatin monotherapy.

Recent studies suggest that antioxidant nutrients, including vitamin E, may interfere with the therapeutic action of combination statin-niacin medications, which have become an innovative and increasingly respected form of statin therapy because of the synergistic interaction of the drug and vitamin. This combination has been shown to be effective in lowering LDL cholesterol and raising HDL cholesterol levels in high-risk individuals with hyperlipidemia, particularly in the context of personal history of cardiac events, malignant family history of heart disease, elevated inflammatory index markers (IIMs), or other high-risk factors.[105,106] As part of the HDL Atherosclerosis Treatment Study (HATS), researchers investigated the respective and collective roles of statins, niacin, and antioxidants (vitamins E and C, beta-carotene, selenium) in cardiovascular protection in patients with CAD and low HDL cholesterol. Cheung et al.[107] found that simvastatin-niacin substantially improved HDL parameters, but that these favorable responses were blunted by the antioxidants, especially with regard to Lp(A-I). In an accompanying paper, focusing on coronary atherosclerotic plaques and the occurrence of a first cardiovascular event, Brown et al.[108] found that the niacin-simvastatin combination was significantly superior to placebo with regard to average stenosis progression, but in participants also receiving antioxidants, this benefit was reduced to 0.7%, a finding interpreted as possible interference by antioxidants. When surrogate markers of cholesterol absorption and synthesis were later measured in a subset of HATS participants, at 24 months (on treatment) and at 38 months (off treatment), treatment with simvastatin-niacin continued to be associated with favorable changes in cholesterol metabolism and stenosis.[109] These findings were subsequently interpreted in many quarters as suggesting that adjuvant antioxidant administration was contraindicated in the treatment of hyperlipidemia and prevention of cardiovascular disease.[110,111]

A more critical analysis of the data suggests that the primary observed adverse interaction is between niacin and antioxidants, not statins and antioxidants. The HDL increases that occurred were probably attributable to the niacin therapy because low-dose simvastatin monotherapy has only limited effects in raising the levels of HDL cholesterol and apolipoprotein (apo) A-I. Thus, one or more of the antioxidants might be interfering with niacin's ability to alter the expression of proteins responsible for the formation of HDL. Further, the findings derived from the population studied may have limited general relevance to individuals who have only elevated LDL cholesterol levels (and normal HDL levels) and to women (who made up only 13% of the cohort). Also, with regard to HDL status, there was no detriment to the antioxidants alone (i.e., given to a group without simvastatin/niacin), and actually a slight benefit, which if involving thousands of patients as in the previous statin and thrombolytic trials, might have become a trend, or even statistically significant. Lastly, the composition of the antioxidant nutrient formulation used has been questioned. Given that niacin depletes the liver of methyl donors, thereby raising homocysteine levels and contributing significantly to the vitamin's hepatotoxicity, researchers might have obtained different results if they had included methyl donor–relevant nutrients with the antioxidants (e.g., folic acid, choline/betaine, and possibly coenzyme Q10, the synthesis of which is inhibited by statins). The principles of nutritional therapeutics also suggest that nutrient therapies might gain potency by looking beyond single-nutrient supplementation to multi-constituent formulations analogous to the antioxidant composition of fruits and vegetables, which involve complex mixtures of many antioxidant compounds rather than single entities.

Nevertheless, evidence from other quarters suggests that some forms of vitamin E may enhance clearance of statin drugs, as well as other hepatotoxic compounds. In particular, alpha-tocopherol can stimulate the activity of pregnane X receptor (PXR), which regulates a constellation of genes involved in detoxification of xenobiotics and upregulates phase I, II, and III enzymes, especially CYP3A.[97] Given that simvastatin appears to be metabolized by CYP3A,[96] a valid case might be made that alpha-tocopherol, although not gamma-tocopherol,[1] may be facilitating liver clearance of the statin drug in a manner consistent with its protective function in xenobiotic detoxification. Significantly, especially when looking at integrative therapeutic options, fluvastatin and pravastatin are the two statins that are not metabolized by the cytochrome P450 3A4 system; they are also the two statins that have exhibited very low propensities to elicit myopathy when combined with other agents.[112] Apart from the necessary continuing research to confirm and elaborate these emerging findings, there remain unanswered fundamental strategic concerns arising from the adverse effects of any therapeutic agent(s) that obstruct and potentially damage normal liver function.

A broadening of the approach to prevention and therapeutics of CAD is coinciding with a growing understanding that the action of statins on cholesterol is not their exclusive or even primary therapeutic mechanism. The emerging emphasis on the role of inflammation in the pathogenesis of cardiovascular disease may provide a clearer understanding of the respective roles of both vitamin E and statins, as well as opening the discussion into further considerations of the potential therapeutic roles of natural thrombolytic agents, such as nattokinase and urokinase, proteolytic enzymes, and natural anti-inflammatory agents such as green tea, omega-3 fatty acids, garlic, and curcumin. The broad incidence and life-threatening implications of CAD and other forms of cardiovascular disease make further research into these complex questions imperative and indicate that building refinement and personalization into study design might open pathways to more definite conclusions and effective interventions better than would premature declarations and prohibitions.

In a related piece of innovative research, Hecht and Harman[113] used electron-beam tomography to assess the relationship of aggressiveness of lipid-lowering treatment to changes in calcified plaque burden in patients with subclinical atherosclerosis. They found that calcified coronary plaque progression appears to be unaffected by the degree of lipid lowering achieved by statin therapy. This study suggests that simply focusing on lowering LDL cholesterol levels may not produce the clinical outcomes presumed by manipulation of isolated pathophysiological phenomenon, as least with regard to slowing progression of subclinical disease in asymptomatic patients. Subsequently, Arad et al.[98] conducted a double-blind, placebo-controlled, randomized clinical trial investigating whether coadministration of conventional lipid-lowering therapy and antioxidants could retard the progression of coronary calcification and prevent atherosclerotic cardiovascular disease (ASCVD) events. They administered atorvastatin (20 mg daily), vitamin C (1 g daily), and vitamin E (alpha-tocopherol, 1000 U daily), versus matching placebos, to 1005 asymptomatic, apparently healthy men and women age 50 to 70 with coronary calcium scores at or above the 80th percentile for age and gender. Notably, all subjects received concomitant aspirin (81 mg daily). The authors halted the trial prematurely, after more than 4 years, because no statistically significant effect was observed on progression of coronary calcium score. They concluded that the combined treatment "induced substantial and sustained reductions in LDL cholesterol and triglycerides but

failed to achieve conventional levels of statistical significance in the reduction of either all ASCVD events or CAD events, though statistically significant reduction of CAD events was found in analysis of the subgroup with a baseline calcium score of > 400."[98] The lack of a group taking atorvastatin and aspirin with placebo antioxidant vitamins also makes the study uninterpretable in regard to the contribution, if any, of vitamins C and E.

Although these preliminary studies are important, the most definitive studies will be large, well-designed, randomized, double-blind trials of these therapies with clinical endpoints, such as cardiac events and survival, rather than the myriad of shorter-term surrogate endpoints, which have not been firmly established and universally accepted as "clinically relevant." Such studies are expensive, however, and tend not to involve natural products, which carry no patent protection and therefore (presumably) cannot subsequently be marketed profitably enough to recoup the considerable clinical research costs. Such studies will of necessity be funded by public institutions, which have the public health as their foremost concern.

Nutritional Therapeutics, Clinical Concerns, and Adaptations

Given the unresolved state of current knowledge, the collective evidence warns against overstated conclusions and generic clinical guidelines. Coadministration of vitamin E may reduce adverse effects and enhance efficacy of simple statin therapy (i.e., without niacin). However, the introduction of niacin into antihyperlipidemic therapy complicates the issue. In addition, individual variations in liver function and lipid metabolism, as well as pharmacogenomic variability in clinical response to conventional interventions, further confound any generic statin drug protocol that fails to account for each patient's characteristics and needs and a willingness to modify periodically the course of treatment in a flexible manner based on regular monitoring and patient preferences.

Integrative Medicine Approaches to Lipid Management. In clinical practice, it may be reasonable to add nutraceuticals to the standard diet and exercise phase of lipid management, then add a statin if the lipid profile is not brought into what is currently considered an acceptable risk profile. Likewise, future clinical trials investigating hypercholesterolemia and cardiovascular health might incorporate and extend the principle of reflecting healthy dietary intake by including not only the previously mentioned nutrients but also magnesium, vitamin B6, copper, zinc, and chromium and liver-supporting agents such as silymarin, apha-lipoic acid, L-carnitine, and flavonoids. For example, the emergence of policosanol also offers a potential natural alternative to statin therapy in some patients; it has been shown, in some but not all studies, to reduce serum cholesterol levels with a more favorable adverse effect profile than the statins. Furthermore, genetic factors influence individual variations in cardiovascular risk factors, lipid metabolism, and pharmacogenomic response to conventional antihyperlipidemic drugs. Thus, Zambon et al.[114] showed that in middle-aged men with established CAD and dyslipidemia, the hepatic lipase (HL) gene −514 C→T polymorphism significantly predicts changes in coronary stenosis with lipid-lowering treatment that appear to involve an HL-associated effect on LDL metabolism. Subjects with the C:C genotype had the greatest decrease in HL activity and the most improvement in LDL density and HDL(2)-C with therapy, as well as the greatest angiographic improvement, compared with the other genotypes studied.

Omeprazole

Omeprazole (Losec, Prilosec).

Interaction Type and Significance

⊕⊕⊕ **Beneficial or Supportive Interaction, Not Requiring Professional Management**

Probability: Evidence Base:
2. Probable   ○ Preliminary

Effect and Mechanism of Action

Mucosal damage in erosive esophagitis is mediated primarily by free radicals. The antioxidant properties of vitamin E can increase the mucosal resistance in gastroesophageal reflux.

Research

Mirmomen et al.[115] conducted a preliminary double-blind, placebo-controlled clinical trial involving 58 individuals with moderate to severe erosive esophagitis; 29 received omeprazole 20 mg every other day plus vitamin E 800 mg daily, and 29 received omeprazole 20 mg every other day along with a daily placebo. At entry, all patients had been cured of endoscopically confirmed esophagitis by antisecretory therapy. All patients underwent endoscopic control to assess relapse rates at 24 and 48 weeks, or when they presented with symptoms. At 24 weeks, 82.8% of patients in the vitamin E group were still in remission compared with only 58.6% in the placebo group. Later, at 48 weeks, 79.3% and 55.2%, respectively, were in remission. Further, 68.9% of patients in the vitamin E group were symptom free versus 48.2% in the placebo group. The authors concluded that the combination of low-dose omeprazole and vitamin E is more effective than omeprazole alone for maintenance of moderate to severe esophagitis.[115]

Nutritional Therapeutics, Clinical Concerns, and Adaptations

The concomitant administration of omeprazole and vitamin E may provide an effective tool to physicians treating patients with recurrent esophagitis. In addition to expanding and extending proton pump inhibitor therapy by addressing underlying oxidative stress and inflammation and supporting restoration of healthy tissue and function, this integrative treatment option might also allow a lower dose of omeprazole. Further clinical trials involving a larger subject population are warranted.

Orlistat

Orlistat (alli, Xenical).

Interaction Type and Significance

≈≈≈ **Drug-Induced Nutrient Depletion, Supplementation Therapeutic, Not Requiring Professional Management**
☼ **Prevention or Reduction of Drug Adverse Effect**
◇ **Adverse Drug Effect on Nutritional Therapeutics, Strategic Concern**

Probability: Evidence Base:
2. Probable   ◉ Emerging

Effect and Mechanism of Action

Orlistat inhibits gastric and pancreatic lipases in the lumen of the gastrointestinal (GI) tract to decrease systemic absorption of dietary fat, along with fat-soluble nutrients.

Research

Clinical trials and observational data indicate that orlistat may reduce absorption of vitamin E, and that in some individuals, this effect may be dramatic enough to result in deficiency symptoms.[116-118] In one trial involving 12 healthy volunteers who were administered a single oral dose of 400 IU vitamin E, pharmacokinetic assessment revealed that orlistat significantly reduced the absorption of vitamin E (~43% according to maximum concentration, and ~60% according to area under concentration-time curve), but not that of vitamin A. In a clinical trial involving 17 obese African-American and Caucasian adolescents receiving orlistat, 120 mg three times daily, McDuffie et al.[119] observed several significant nutrient depletion patterns despite coadministration of a daily multivitamin supplement containing vitamin A (5000 IU), vitamin D (400 IU), vitamin E (300 IU), and vitamin K (25 µg). In particular, during 3 to 6 months of orlistat treatment, acute absorption of alpha-tocopherol was significantly reduced compared with baseline levels ($p < 0.001$), but serum levels of alpha-tocopherol did not change significantly.

Nutritional Therapeutics, Clinical Concerns, and Adaptations

A vitamin E supplementation strategy is advised in the event vitamin deficiency occurs in patients undergoing orlistat therapy.[120] More proactively, individuals taking orlistat for extended periods would benefit from prophylactic vitamin E supplementation,[118,121] 400 IU daily of naturally occurring tocopherols. Alternatively, employing a water-soluble form of the nutrient could bypass this interference, if nutritional treatment using vitamin E supplementation is part of a broader therapeutic strategy including orlistat.

Warfarin and Related Oral Vitamin K Antagonist Anticoagulants

Primary: Warfarin (Coumadin, Marevan, Warfilone).
Extrapolated, based on similar properties: Nicoumalone (acenocoumarol; Acitrom, Sintrom), phenindione (Dindevan), phenprocoumon (Jarsin, Marcumar).

Interaction Type and Significance

✗✗ **Minimal to Mild Adverse Interaction—Vigilance Necessary**
⊕✗ **Biomodal or Variable Interaction, with Professional Management**
⊕⊕ **Beneficial or Supportive Interaction, with Professional Management**

Probability: Evidence Base:
4. Plausible   ▽ Mixed or
                                ○ Preliminary

Effect and Mechanism of Action

Vitamin E may indirectly enhance the anticoagulant effect of warfarin by altering production of vitamin K–dependent coagulation factors, specifically at the vitamin K–dependent step of carboxylation at the gamma position of precursor prothrombin (factor II), as well as the other three vitamin K–dependent coagulation cascade enzymes, thus potentiating the warfarin-induced functional vitamin K insufficiency. Although no mechanism for vitamin E's action in these situations had been known until 2004, reductions in fully gamma-carboxylated vitamin K–dependent coagulation factors (II, VII, IX, and X) have previously been observed in subjects taking supplemental vitamin E.

Research

Corrigan and Ulfers[122] administered vitamin E (100 or 400 IU/day) orally for 4 weeks to 12 individuals receiving warfarin. The subjects showed no significant change in the prothrombin time (PT), factor II coagulant activity, or factor II antigen (which measures the amount of prothrombin present, but not its activity). However, a significant reduction was observed compared with pretreatment ratios on using a ratio of factor II activity to factor II antigen, as measured by the immunoreactive protein technique, suggesting that vitamin E influences the final activation step (gamma carboxylation) of prothrombin production, which is mediated by vitamin K. Further research by Corrigan[123] has supported the hypothesis that coagulation characteristics in normal individuals (i.e., those without vitamin K deficiency) are unaffected by vitamin E and that doses significantly higher than 400 IU/day are generally necessary to induce adverse effects in susceptible individuals.

In two independent, randomized clinical trials, Booth et al.[124] investigated the effect of 12 weeks of supplementation with RRR-alpha-tocopherol (1000 IU/day) on vitamin K status, as represented by several biochemical indicators, in 38 men and women with rheumatoid arthritis (study A) and in 32 healthy men (study B), none of whom were taking oral anticoagulants. Plasma phylloquinone (vitamin K_1) concentrations and the percentage of undercarboxylated osteocalcin (a marker of vitamin K insufficiency unrelated to coagulation proteins) did not change significantly in response to the vitamin E. However, the degree of mean PIVKA-II increased from 1.7 to 11.9 ng/mL in study A and from 1.8 to 5.3 ng/mL in study B after the 12 weeks of vitamin E supplementation, which represent highly significant increases. PIVKA-II is an abbreviation for the underactive form of prothrombin produced in the presence of either vitamin K deficiency due to dietary or endogenous production defects, or to the presence of a vitamin K antagonist such as Coumadin (warfarin). This significant increase in PIVKA-II, indicative of poor vitamin K status in adults not receiving oral anticoagulant therapy, strongly suggests that high doses of vitamin E may functionally antagonize vitamin K's activity in catalyzing gamma-carboxylation (activation) of at least factor II, and possibly also of factors VII, IX, and X. Insufficient levels of any one of these four vitamin K–dependent coagulation factors will prolong the PT/INR, although lowering of all four factors to a therapeutic level is necessary for full protection from inappropriate clot formation in the thrombophilic patient.

Reports

Cases of enhanced anticoagulant effect in response to high-dose vitamin E supplementation have been reported among patients taking oral anticoagulants. A single case report from 1974 led to a long-standing perception of risk from simultaneous use of warfarin and vitamin E and repeated warnings of contraindication. In this event, a vitamin K–deficient patient on warfarin therapy began to exhibit a range of adverse effects, including bleeding, ecchymoses, and prolonged PT, suggesting excessive anticoagulation within 2 months of beginning consumption of up to 1200 IU/day of vitamin E. Nevertheless, although decreased serum concentrations of blood-clotting factors were reported, warfarin serum concentrations were not altered, suggesting an enhancement of the warfarin effect on vitamin K–dependent coagulation factor synthesis. The patient's coagulation status normalized within 1 week of discontinuing the vitamin E supplementation.[125] Subsequently, Kim and White[15] investigated the pharmacological effect of concomitant warfarin and vitamin E in a randomized, double-blind clinical trial with

21 subjects receiving chronic warfarin therapy and found no significant changes in warfarin activity or INR in those who received vitamin E at doses up to 1200 IU/day. Within the context of integrative clinical management, the patient in the case report likely could have continued the vitamin E and reduced the dose of warfarin until the PT was again in the therapeutic range.

Clinical Implications and Adaptations

For many years, warnings have been voiced regarding potential adverse effects from use of vitamin E supplementation by individuals undergoing warfarin therapy, but only recently is the evidence beginning to suggest a possible basis for such contraindications. Continued research is warranted to determine whether the effects of this nutrient interaction are beneficial or adverse in and of themselves, whether they might be reversed by concomitant supplementation with vitamin K, and how they might affect oral anticoagulant therapy. Nevertheless, prudence supports operating under the assumption that the intended effect of warfarin therapy to cause functional vitamin K insufficiency, as reflected by a therapeutically prolonged PT and INR, may be enhanced by vitamin E coadministration, at least in some individuals undergoing long-term anticoagulant therapy. Furthermore, certain individuals with pharmacogenomic variations in vitamin K and warfarin metabolism, particularly in the context of vitamin K deficiency, may experience differing degrees of alteration in coagulation status in response to vitamin E supplementation. High doses of vitamin E for sustained periods may also mildly inhibit platelet activation. In the event of clinically significant changes in anticoagulant effects from concomitant use of warfarin and vitamin E, such effects would most likely be delayed in onset and of moderate severity. Physicians prescribing anticoagulant therapy are advised to monitor INR levels more frequently in patients who are beginning or increasing the dosage levels of vitamin E therapy, especially if those doses exceed 1000 IU/day, as well as in patients who significantly reduce their intake of vitamin E after sustained periods of supplementation.

THEORETICAL, SPECULATIVE, AND PRELIMINARY INTERACTIONS RESEARCH, INCLUDING OVERSTATED INTERACTIONS CLAIMS

Amiodarone

Amiodarone (Cordarone, Pacerone).

Research using human pulmonary artery endothelial cells, in vitro, suggests that alpha-tocopherol may reduce lung toxicity associated with amiodarone.[126] Establishing efficacy of and clinical protocols for this potentially protective interaction warrants further research.

Benzamycin and Benzoyl Peroxide

Benzamycin, benzoyl peroxide.

Benzoyl peroxide (BPO), one of the two components in Benzamycin (and also widely used in OTC acne preparations), is well known for promoting carcinogenesis in animals. An in vitro study, using a human keratinocyte cell line, found that human skin cells exposed to vitamin E were more resistant to cytotoxicity caused by BPO.[127] A subsequent human trial determined that alpha-tocotrienol supplementation significantly counteracted BPO-induced lipid peroxidation, although it did not significantly mitigate drug-induced barrier perturbation in the stratum corneum and increased transepidermal water loss.[128] Whether these medications cause similar adverse effects in humans, and whether any countervailing effect is exerted by vitamin E, have yet to be researched in controlled human trials. Physicians prescribing such agents might suggest to their patients that supplemental vitamin E could potentially provide a means of reducing adverse effects associated with BPO and minimizing risk of further complications.

Cationic Amphiphilic Drugs

Chloroquine, Chlorpromazine, Desipramine, and Propranolol.

Cationic amphiphilic drugs (CADs) represent a wide range of therapeutic classes of medications used in the treatment of arrhythmias, depression, and seizure disorders and are well known for adverse effects on lysosomal phospholipid (PL) storage. Scuntaro et al.[129] conducted an in vitro study investigating the mechanisms of alpha-tocopherol action on drug kinetics and PL storage using a model of human cultured fibroblasts exposed to single and repetitive doses of desipramine and other CADs. They found that although alpha-tocopherol did not influence the initial, pH-dependent, rapid phase of drug uptake, it did inhibit, in a dose-dependent manner, the slow and cumulative phases of drug uptake and the accumulation of cellular phospholipids. The researchers hypothesized that this activity was caused by competition between alpha-tocopherol and CADs for PL complex formation and noted that the influence of alpha-tocopherol on drug uptake varies among different CADs. Although these findings suggest that alpha-tocopherol may counteract many adverse effects of CAD exposure on lysosomal PL storage and appear to restore normal membrane recycling, further research is necessary to determine if such benefits would be obtained in human subjects, and whether such activity would interfere with the effectiveness of the medications. Knowledge of the clinical implications of this apparent supportive interaction is too preliminary to suggest implementation in a clinical setting.

Clofibrate

Clofibrate (Aromid-S).

The issue of an interaction between vitamin E and clofibrate has been raised in two primary forms. A small, randomized, double-blind clinical trial investigated the effect of tocopherol on serum cholesterol and triglycerides in hyperlipidemic patients treated with diet and clofibrate and found no significant effect.[130] Others have voiced concern that clofibrate may impair absorption of vitamin E.[131] The severity of any resulting depletion, the frequency with which it occurs, and its clinical implications have yet to be determined in any conclusive form. However, because this is no longer a widely used lipid-lowering agent, further work in this area seems unlikely.

Cyclophosphamide

Cyclophosphamide (Cytoxan, Endoxana, Neosar, Procytox).

Oxidation in the liver is required for activation of cyclophosphamide. Vitamin E and other antioxidant nutrients could theoretically interfere with this process and reduce the agent's antitumor activity. However, separate animal studies have found that both vitamin A and vitamin C supplementation potentiated the antineoplastic activity of cyclophosphamide, particularly in the context of nutrient deficiency, without introducing any adverse effects.[38,132] In another animal study, combined cyclophosphamide treatment and vitamin E administration increased level of key enzymes (LDH, SGPT, SGOT, acid phosphatase, alkaline phosphatase) and produced greater efficacy in the treatment of fibrosarcoma in rats.[133] Furthermore, in a preliminary human trial, researchers reported increased survival among patients with small cell lung cancer (SCLC) whose treatment with cyclophosphamide and

radiation was supplemented with a combination of beta-carotene, vitamin A, and vitamin E, compared with most published chemoradiation treatment regimens alone.[134] Because the current standard of care for SCLC involves platinum and etoposide with concurrent radiation treatment, however, it is difficult to extrapolate from the cyclophosphamide/radiation/vitamin E study. No research, human or otherwise, has been published investigating the occurrence or clinical implications of such a potential interaction specifically involving vitamin E. Well-designed clinical trials are warranted to determine the beneficial or detrimental nature of this potential interaction and to develop clinical protocols to optimize outcomes based on such emergent understanding. As noted previously, well-designed randomized clinical trials of cancer treatment, with and without antioxidant supplements, that carefully standardize the antioxidant contribution of diet are sorely needed.

Cytochrome P450 3A4 Substrates

Recent findings indicate that d-alpha-tocopherol interacts with the pregnane X receptor (PXR) and increases its activity.[135] PXR is a promiscuous nuclear receptor that is expressed in the liver and intestine and is activated by a broad array of endogenous and exogenous toxic compounds, especially lipophilic xenobiotics, including prescription drugs, herbs, pesticides, endocrine disruptors, and other environmental contaminants. On activation, PXR coordinately regulates a number of genes involved in drug clearance via the liver (cytochrome P450s) and intestine (P-glycoprotein) and thus upregulates phase I, II, and III enzymes.[136] This activity can provide a protective effect, especially in relation to xenobiotic clearance, but it also strongly suggests a potential for drug interactions, particularly involving medications metabolized by the CYP3A phase I enzymes. No work documenting actual drug interactions of clinical significance has been published at this time. However, more than 50% of the most frequently used prescription medications are metabolized by members of the CYP3A group.[97] Vitamin E acting as a PXR ligand could alter these PXR-mediated reactions. Unfortunately, the extent to which pharmacological doses of vitamin E modulate these pathways in vivo has not been determined. Although PXR regulation of hepatic alpha-tocopherol metabolism appears to be of central importance, other hepatic systems, such as P-glycoprotein (MDR2), participate in vitamin E trafficking and excretion.[1] If patients are taking vitamin E when they start a drug, and this drug is titrated to either effect (e.g., blood pressure) or blood level (e.g., cyclosporine), it most likely would be of no consequence, as long as they continued to take vitamin E. Starting or stopping vitamin E supplementation, however, while stable on a medication metabolized by those enzymes, could potentially be problematic, especially outside the context of professional supervision. Further research into this metabolic activity and related pharmacovigilance are warranted.

Fenofibrate

Fenofibrate (Lofibra, Tricor, Triglide).

In one controlled human trial, researchers found that the combination of 1000 IU d-alpha-tocopherol and 2 g ascorbic acid and prior to ultraviolet (UV) exposure dramatically blocked UV phototoxic lysis of erythrocytes associated with fenofibrate.[137] An animal study found that alpha-tocopherol content was decreased by 51% in the livers of fenofibrate-treated mice.[138] In another animal study, Chaput et al.[139] observed that coadministration of alpha-tocopherol and fenofibrate produced a synergistic effect in which fenofibrate's lag phase was prolonged and its lipoprotein oxidation parameters were improved. Pending further controlled human trials, these preliminary findings suggest that coadministration of vitamin E, preferably as naturally occurring mixed tocopherols, might provide potential support to individuals undergoing fenofibrate therapy with minimal risk.

Gentamicin

Gentamicin (G-Mycin, Garamycin, Jenamicin).

Animal research indicates that alpha-tocopherol interferes with gentamicin-induced free-radical formation and suggests that this drug may be useful in preventing aminoglycoside oto-vestibulo-toxicity.[140] Vitamin B_{12} may provide a complementary protective effect.[141] Familial susceptibility to aminoglycoside ototoxicity has been discussed in several studies[142-144] and appears to be caused by the A1555G mutation in the mitochondrial DNA.[145]

Griseofulvin

Griseofulvin (Fulvicin, Grifulvin, Gris-PEG, Grisactin, Gristatin).

Research involving children and guinea pigs indicates that vitamin E coadministration can elevate blood levels of this antifungal medication and thus allow for reduced dosage levels of griseofulvin, well known for its adverse effects.[146,147] It appears that elevated alpha-tocopherol levels can reduce activity of the cytochrome P450 system enzymes that metabolize griseofulvin, thereby slowing the rate of griseofulvin biotransformation, which in turn allows for significantly sustained elevation of blood and skin concentrations of the medication. Even though these findings are still at a preliminary stage, physicians prescribing griseofulvin may want to discuss the option of concomitant vitamin E, 100 IU daily, with their patients as a safe and potentially effective means of reducing griseofulvin dosage levels and attendant adverse effects, without compromising efficacy. Conversely, the unsupervised concomitant use of griseofulvin and vitamin E, at significant dosages, could potentially increase severity of the drug's adverse effects due to CYP450 inhibition and subsequent elevation of blood and skin levels.

Hormone Replacement Therapy (HRT): Estrogen-Containing and Synthetic Estrogen and Progesterone Analog Medications

HRT, estrogens: Chlorotrianisene (Tace); conjugated equine estrogens (Premarin); conjugated synthetic estrogens (Cenestin); dienestrol (Ortho Dienestrol); esterified estrogens (Estratab, Menest, Neo-Estrone); estradiol, topical/transdermal/ring (Alora Transdermal, Climara Transdermal, Estrace, Estradot, Estring FemPatch, Vivelle-Dot, Vivelle Transdermal); estradiol cypionate (Dep-Gynogen, Depo-Estradiol, Depogen, Dura-Estrin, Estra-D, Estro-Cyp, Estroject-LA, Estronol-LA); estradiol hemihydrate (Estreva, Vagifem); estradiol valerate (Delestrogen, Estra-L 40, Gynogen L.A. 20, Progynova, Valergen 20); estrone (Aquest, Estragyn 5, Estro-A, Estrone '5', Kestrone-5); estropipate (Ogen, Ortho-Est); ethinyl estradiol (Estinyl, Gynodiol, Lynoral).
HRT, estrogen/progestin combinations: Conjugated equine estrogens and medroxyprogesterone (Premelle cycle 5, Prempro); conjugated equine estrogens and norgestrel (Prempak-C); estradiol and dydrogesterone (Femoston); estradiol and norethindrone, patch (CombiPatch); estradiol and norethindrone/norethisterone, oral (Activella, Climagest, Climesse, FemHRT, Trisequens); estradiol valerate and

cyproterone acetate (Climens); estradiol valerate and norgestrel (Progyluton); estradiol and norgestimate (Ortho-Prefest). Extrapolated, based on similar properties: HRT, estrogen/testosterone combinations: Esterified estrogens and methyltestosterone (Estratest, Estratest HS).
Over 6 months, Clemente et al.[148] treated 15 postmenopausal women with climacteric symptoms using 50 µg/24 hours estradiol transdermally applied twice a week for 21 days and a daily dose of 10 mg oral medroxyprogesterone acetate, which was added for 12 days in each treatment cycle. Their preliminary findings suggest that HRT can preserve the content of alpha-tocopherol and beta-carotene in LDL particles and keep the LDL in a reduced antioxidant state. In a randomized study involving 66 postmenopausal women, Inal et al.[149] found that concomitant administration of transdermal estradiol and vitamin E (600 mg/day, orally) improved LDL, HDL, and total cholesterol status, compared to pretreatment levels. However, within the Women's Angiographic Vitamin and Estrogen (WAVE) Trial, all-cause mortality increased in postmenopausal women, with at least one coronary stenosis at baseline coronary angiography, who were administered 400 IU vitamin E plus 500 mg vitamin C, both twice daily, eversus placebo.[150] These apparently contradictory findings strongly suggest further research into hormone metabolism and variable responses to exogenous administration of estrogen compounds, particularly in the presence of nutritional supplementation.

Women appear to clear CYP3A substrates more efficiently than men[151] and may possess additional alternative vitamin E–metabolizing systems, perhaps under the regulation of estrogen. Estrogen is metabolized by CYP3A4[152] (phase II), and some CYP3As may be regulated by estrogen. Alpha-tocopherol appears to induce the metabolic activity of PXR, a known regulator of steroid hormone and sterol homeostasis,[153] and thereby upregulate CYP3A4, resulting in stimulation of drug metabolism. Consequently, estrogen and alpha-tocopherol may interact through nuclear receptors, particularly nuclear estrogen receptor (ER) and PXR. The clinical implications of these potential interactions remain unclear, particularly given the evolving evidence concerning HRT's effect on cardiovascular risk and the emerging state of knowledge regarding estrogen conjugation and related detoxification systems.

Insulin

Animal-source insulin (Iletin); human analog insulin (Humanlog); human insulin (Humulin, Novolin, NovoRapid, Oralin).

Clinical experience and some human trials have suggested possible efficacy of vitamin E in improving glucose tolerance in individuals with diabetes. If such findings are confirmed by well-designed clinical trials, the central issue of an interaction between insulin and vitamin E must be the avoidance of hypoglycemic states. In such cases, clinical management within an integrative strategy characterized by collaboration among health care professionals experienced in conventional pharmacology and nutritional therapeutics becomes imperative. However, to further complicate the always-complex and individual issue of dysglycemia and physiological compensations, a trial by Skrha et al.[153a] reported that 3 months of vitamin E (600 mg daily) was associated with a deterioration in insulin action and fibrinolysis in obese type 2 diabetic patients. Such seemingly contradictory findings remind us that further research is necessary to establish a clear understanding of the complex interrelationships among insulin resistance, glucose regulation, oxidative stress, and obesity. Pending such discoveries, caution is warranted regarding self-prescribing of high doses of supplemental vitamin E by diabetic individuals; conservative practice would especially caution against rapid escalation of dosage levels among obese diabetic patients. As with any introduction of changes intended to alter metabolism significantly and affect a disease process, a moderate pace of change, close observation, and collaboration among health care professionals trained in both conventional pharmacology and nutritional therapeutics are central to safe and effective application of integrative therapeutics.

Isoniazid

Isoniazid (isonicotinic acid hydrazide, INH; Laniazid, Nydrazid); combination drugs: isoniazid and rifampicin (Rifamate, Rimactane); isoniazid, pyrazinamide, and rifampicin (Rifater).

Isoniazid may interfere with the activity of vitamin E and many other nutrients. Pending further evidence from well-designed clinical trials looking at drug-induced nutrient depletion patterns and compensatory interventions, physicians prescribing isoniazid may want to present patients with the option of using a daily multivitamin/multimineral supplement.

Isotretinoin and Related Retinoids

Acitretin (Soriatane), bexarotene (Targretin), etretinate (Tegison), isotretinoin (13-*cis* retinoic acid; Accutane), tretinoin (all-*trans* retinoic acid, ATRA; Atragen, Avita, Renova, Retin-A, Vesanoid, Vitinoin).

Several potent retinoids deplete vitamin E levels in the skin, which increases the skin toxicity (e.g., cheilosis, drying, The chapping) of these agents. The results of a phase I trial indicate that alpha-tocopherol substantially reduces the initial toxicity of high-dose 13-*cis* retinoic acid (isotretinoin) without compromising drug efficacy.[154] A daily dose of 800 IU alpha-tocopherol has been suggested to reduce retinoid toxicity.[155] In another direction of emerging integrative therapeutics, some clinicians and researchers have been investigating coadministration of 13-*cis* retinoic acid and alpha-tocopherol, often in conjunction with other agents, in the treatment of various cancers recalcitrant to conventional chemotherapy. Several other potent retinoids have also become standard treatments for certain malignancies, such as all-*trans* retinoic acid (etretinate) in acute promyelocytic leukemia, acitretin, and bexarotene for cutaneous T-cell lymphoma (mycosis fungoides), although bexarotene does not have prominent skin toxicity, other than as a photosensitizer. Many clinicians have found that co-prescribing vitamin E (800-1000 IU daily) with these agents reduces their skin toxicity significantly. Large, randomized trials are needed to ensure that there is also no interference with therapeutic efficacy.

Lindane

Lindane (Kwell Shampoo).

Lindane use is associated with a wide range of often significant adverse effects, including promotion of tumor formation.[156] In particular, in vitro studies have found that vitamin E protects human leukocytes against toxic effects of lindane.[157] At this time, evidence is lacking to confirm such protective effects from concomitant use of vitamin E during lindane therapy. However, given that the nutrient is generally considered nontoxic, supplementation at moderate levels during treatment might be judicious.

Mineral Oil

Mineral Oil (Agoral, Kondremul Plain, Liquid Parafin, Milkinol, Neo-Cultol, Petrogalar Plain).

Mineral oil, as a lipid solvent, may also absorb many substances and interfere with normal absorption of alpha-tocopherol and other nutrients.[158] Some disagree, but most researchers have found that mineral oil interferes with the absorption of many nutrients, including beta-carotene, calcium, phosphorus, potassium, and vitamins A, D, K, and E.[159,160] Chronic use of mineral oil may cause a deficiency of these nutrients, the clinical significance of which is as yet undetermined. Individuals taking mineral oil for any extended period may benefit from regular use of a multivitamin supplement that includes all the fat-soluble vitamins. Malabsorption of fat-soluble vitamins from ingestion of mineral oil can also be minimized by administering mineral oil on an empty stomach or consuming vitamin or mineral supplements at least 2 hours before or after the mineral oil. In general, it is advisable to limit the internal use of mineral oil to periods of less than 1 week.

Oral Contraceptives: Monophasic, Biphasic, and Triphasic Estrogen Preparations (Synthetic Estrogen and Progesterone Analogs)

Ethinyl estradiol and desogestrel (Desogen, Ortho-TriCyclen).
Ethinyl estradiol and ethynodiol (Demulen 1/35, Demulen 1/50, Nelulen 1/25, Nelulen 1/50, Zovia).
Ethinyl estradiol and levonorgestrel (Alesse, Levlen, Levlite, Levora 0.15/30, Nordette, Tri-Levlen, Triphasil, Trivora).
Ethinyl estradiol and norethindrone/norethisterone (Brevicon, Estrostep, Genora 1/35, GenCept 1/35, Jenest-28, Loestrin 1.5/30, Loestrin1/20, Modicon, Necon 1/25, Necon 10/11, Necon 0.5/30, Necon 1/50, Nelova 1/35, Nelova 10/11, Norinyl 1/35, Norlestin 1/50, Ortho Novum 1/35, Ortho Novum 10/11, Ortho Novum 7/7/7, Ovcon-35, Ovcon-50, Tri-Norinyl, Trinovum).
Ethinyl estradiol and norgestrel (Lo/Ovral, Ovral).
Mestranol and norethindrone (Genora 1/50, Nelova 1/50, Norethin 1/50, Ortho-Novum 1/50).
Related, internal application: Etonogestrel/ethinyl estradiol vaginal ring (Nuvaring).

Use of oral contraceptives (OCs) is associated with increased risk of thrombosis in women, at least in part because of their adverse effects on vitamins and enzymes involved in the oxidative defense system; this risk is known to be significantly elevated by smoking.[161] Susceptibility to lipid peroxidation is greater when antioxidant status is impaired, which may further increase the risk of thrombosis.[162] Supplementation with vitamin E may mitigate some of these adverse effects and elevated risks, although large clinical trials would be necessary to confirm this.

See also Hormone Replacement Therapy.

Paclitaxel

Paclitaxel (Paxene, Taxol).

Paclitaxel monotherapy is not generally associated with significant cardiotoxicity, but it can dramatically increase the cardiac toxicity of anthracyclines such as doxorubicin. In a double-blind pilot study involving 13 cancer patients receiving chemotherapy and 12 patients receiving radiotherapy, Japanese researchers found that an antioxidant regimen (vitamin E, vitamin C, and *N*-acetylcysteine) protected against chemotherapy-induced heart damage without interfering with the action of the primary therapies.[45] Although these preliminary results suggest efficient cardioprotection by this nontoxic and inexpensive adjunctive supplementation, the study's small size precludes a definitive conclusion. Larger, well-designed clinical trials are warranted for confirmation.

Pentoxifylline

Pentoxifylline (Pentoxil, Trental).

In a clinical trial of 43 patients, presenting with 50 symptomatic radiation-induced fibrosis (RIF) areas involving the skin and underlying tissues, were treated with a combination of pentoxifylline (800 mg/day) and tocopherol (1000 IU/day). Dramatic regression of chronic radiotherapy damage was demonstrated, with all assessable injuries exhibiting continuous clinical regression and functional improvement.[163] Based on these preliminary findings of reversal of human chronic radiotherapy damage, and because no other treatment is presently available for RIF, the researchers concluded that coordinated use of these two agents in a supportive interaction should be considered a therapeutic measure. Further research with larger, well-designed trials is warranted to confirm these findings and develop therapeutic protocols.

Phenobarbital, Phenytoin, Valproic Acid, and Related Anticonvulsant Medications

Carbamazepine (Carbatrol, Tegretol), clonazepam (Klonopin), clorazepate (Tranxene), divalproex semisodium, divalproex sodium (Depakote), ethosuximide (Zarontin), ethotoin (Peganone), felbamate (Felbatol), fosphenytoin (Cerebyx, Mesantoin), levetiracetam (Keppra), mephenytoin, methsuximide (Celontin), oxcarbazepine (GP 47680, oxycarbazepine; Trileptal), phenobarbital (Luminal, Phenobarbitone, Solfoton), phenytoin (Dilantin, Phenytek), piracetam (Nootropyl), primidone (Mysoline), sodium valproate (Depacon), topiramate (Topamax), trimethadione (Tridione), valproate semisodium, valproic acid (Depakene, Depakene Syrup), vigabatrin (Sabril), zonisamide (Zonegran).

Two studies conducted by a Japanese research team found lower serum vitamin E levels in individuals taking phenobarbital and phenytoin compared with those who received no anticonvulsant medications for seizures. In the first study, 10 patients undergoing anticonvulsant therapy who had demonstrated low vitamin E levels were then administered dl-alpha-tocopherol acetate, 100 mg/day; after 1 month, both their serum vitamin E levels and hemolysis tests returned to normal, having been abnormal before supplementation.[164] These researchers recommended coadministration with vitamin E for some patients undergoing anticonvulsant therapy. These findings indicate that long-term use of anticonvulsants, particularly phenytoin and phenobarbital, can result in a deficiency of vitamin E, as well as of zinc, which may produce several problems, especially in children.[165] The full clinical implications of this nutrient depletion pattern have yet to be investigated in a large trial, but physicians prescribing anticonvulsant therapy, especially for children, are advised to present the option of supplementing with 100 to 200 IU of vitamin E daily, preferably in a naturally occurring tocopherol form, as prophylaxis against deficiency and its sequelae.

Ramipril and Other Angiotensin-Converting Enzyme (ACE) Inhibitors

Benazepril (Lotensin), captopril (Capoten), cilazapril (Inhibace), enalapril (Vasotec), fosinopril (Monopril), lisinopril (Prinivil, Zestril), moexipril (Univasc), perindopril (Aceon), quinapril (Accupril), ramipril (Altace), trandolapril (Mavik); combination drugs: benazepril and amlodipine (Lotrel); enalapril and felodipine (Lexxel); enalapril and hydrochlorothiazide (Vaseretic); lisinopril and hydrochlorothiazide (Prinzide, Zestoretic).

Long-term data from the Heart Outcomes Prevention Evaluation (HOPE) study might be interpreted to suggest a potential interaction between vitamin E and ramipril (and possibly other ACE inhibitors).[13] In high-risk individuals with diabetes or heart disease undergoing ramipril therapy, concomitant use of vitamin E appears to be associated with increased risk of heart failure. The observed pattern more likely is simply an effect of using large doses of a single antioxidant supplement in patients likely to have high oxidative stress, rather than a true interaction. Until more is known, concomitant use of ACE inhibitors and any single antioxidant nutrient preparation in high doses should be avoided.

Rifampicin

Rifampicin (Rifadin, Rifadin IV); combination drugs: isoniazid and rifampicin (Rifamate, Rimactane); isoniazid, pyrazinamide, and rifampicin (Rifater).

In an in vitro experiment, both vitamin E and rifampicin activated PXR, an orphan nuclear receptor central to xenobiotic metabolism. Production of vitamin E metabolites increased when hepatocytes were incubated with rifampicin and vitamin E (all-racemic alpha-tocopherol). This observation suggests that a CYP3A-type cytochrome initiates tocopherol metabolism by omega oxidation.[166] The clinical implications of this potential interaction are unknown at this time.

Risperidone

Risperidone (Risperdal).

In a case report of a 74-year-old woman being treated for schizoaffective disorder with risperidone, coadministration of vitamins E and B_6 was efficacious in reversing neuroleptic malignant syndrome (NMS), an adverse effect associated with the medication.[167] Although encouraging, further research with well-designed clinical trials into the general effectiveness of adjunctive vitamins E and B_6 to treat (or prevent) NMS in individuals taking risperidone is necessary to confirm these observations and develop therapeutic recommendations.

Verapamil

Verapamil (Calan, Calan SR, Covera-HS, Isoptin, Isoptin SR, Verelan, Verelan PM); combination drug: trandolapril and verapamil (Tarka).

P-glycoprotein (P-gp) mediates resistance of cancer cells to chemotherapy agents that are, or are derived from, natural products. In an in vitro experiment, using a P-gp–expressing human small cell lung cancer line, the inclusion of alpha-tocopherol antagonized the multidrug-resistance (MDR)–modifying ability of verapamil, as well as other chemosensitizing agents, and prevented restoration of sensitivity to both doxorubicin and vinblastine.[65] The clinical implications of such observations in humans are untested and unknown.

Zidovudine (AZT)

Zidovudine (azidothymidine, AZT, ZDV, zidothymidine; Retrovir); combination drugs: zidovudine and lamivudine (Combivir); abacavir, lamivudine, and zidovudine (Trizivir).

In vitro and animal studies indicate that coadministration of AZT and vitamin E (as d-alpha-tocopherol acid succinate) enhanced antiviral activity and therapeutic efficacy, compared with AZT alone.[168] Further research found that this form of vitamin E increased erythroid colony-forming unit (CFU-E)–derived colonies and provided protection against

AZT-induced toxicity to bone marrow at a level equivalent to recombinant human erythropoietin (rhEpo).[169] The clinical significance of such findings has yet to be explored in human trials.

NUTRIENT-NUTRIENT INTERACTIONS

Antioxidants

Vitamin E works synergistically with other antioxidant nutrients to "quench" free radicals, peroxides, and other potentially harmful substances. Antioxidants function best as a network to quench high levels of free radicals safely and effectively. Vitamin E can spare other antioxidants, and vice versa. When given singly, especially at higher dosage levels, antioxidant agents can induce variable antioxidant or pro-oxidant effects in different physiological settings.

Large doses of vitamin E in patients likely to be under oxidative stress (based on their pathology and lifestyle, e.g., smoking, alcohol, recreational drugs) who do not consume a diet rich in antioxidants may contribute to further oxidative stress. In general, individuals with established cardiovascular disease and diabetes represent populations particularly characterized by high oxidative stress. Consequently, long-term daily use of even 400 mg of d-alpha-tocopherol, outside the context of other antioxidant support, by such patients can carry a significant risk that they will produce tocopherol radicals in excess of their ability to quench them. A parallel phenomenon has also been reported with beta-carotene in smokers. This susceptibility applies to all antioxidants, with the possible exception of oligomeric proanthocyanadins (OPCs), and other complex mixtures of flavonoids, such as anthocyanins and anthocyanidin, which contain a variety of compounds with differing redox potentials, and thus have some intrinsic network characteristics. Vitamin E is particularly cardiotrophic and may therefore exert special stress on cardiac tissue. Ultimately, somewhere in the network, a compound is needed that can decompose harmlessly after accepting the electron that has been passed around. A single chemical entity, such as tocopherol or a carotenoid (especially synthetic), usually cannot perform this critical function adequately. Thus, antioxidants are best utilized in a form that maximizes their network effect and minimizes the risk of a paradoxical pro-oxidative effect. At least five antioxidant supplements should be combined, preferably more (e.g., tocopherol, coenzyme Q10, ascorbate, mixed carotenes, vitamin A, selenium, flavonoids). Foods with high ORAC (oxygen radical–absorbing capacity) should always be encouraged in the diet as well.

Chitosan

Chitosan, a supplement proposed to promote weight loss, decreases dietary absorption of fats and therefore also of vitamin E and other fat-soluble nutrients, as shown in an animal model.[170] The clinical significance of this probable pharmacokinetic interaction has yet to be investigated in clinical trials. However, separating intake of therapeutic nutrients such as vitamin E by at least 2 hours before or 4 hours after taking chitosan can avert nutrient depletion in susceptible individuals undergoing long-term use of this nutraceutical.

Iron

Vitamin E can counteract the pro-oxidant activity of iron by, for example, attenuating oxidative stress induced by intravenous iron in patients on hemodialysis.[171] Nevertheless, the mineral can bind and inactivate vitamin E. Vitamin E can also decrease the hematological response to iron salts to a degree that may be clinically significant, particularly in anemic children.[172] Monitoring is warranted.

Polyunsaturated Fatty Acids; Omega-3 and Omega-6 Fatty Acids

High dietary intake of polyunsaturated fatty acids (PUFAs) can induce decreased vitamin E levels.[173] Such long-term dietary patterns require increased vitamin E intake, possibly through supplementation.

Selenium

Selenium potentiates the antioxidant activity of vitamin E. Selenium and vitamin E act synergistically and are more effective when taken together. Among other activities, glutathione peroxidase, the enzyme that recycles oxidized glutathione to its reduced (active) form, is selenium dependent.

Vitamin A

High levels of vitamin E intake may interfere with the absorption of vitamin A.

Vitamin C

Vitamin C facilitates regeneration of vitamin E and restoration of its antioxidant activity, an example of how an antioxidant network functions. Zandi et al.[174] examined data from the Cache County Study, a large, population-based investigation of the prevalence and incidence of Alzheimer's disease and other dementias. They determined that regular use of vitamin E in nutritional supplement doses, especially in combination with vitamin C, may protect the aging brain against pathological changes associated with Alzheimer's disease and reduce the risk of developing the condition. Further study with randomized prevention trials is needed before drawing firm conclusions about the protective effects of such coordinated antioxidant supplementation. If effective, the use of these (and possibly other) antioxidant nutrients may play an important role in a safe and inexpensive strategy for the prevention of Alzheimer's disease.

Bruno et al.[175] have conducted extensive research into the relationship between vitamin C and alpha-tocopherol, with a focus on the conditions of high oxidative stress found in smokers. First, they found that vitamin E "disappearance is accelerated in cigarette smokers due to their increased oxidative stress and is inversely correlated with plasma vitamin C concentrations." Then, in a double-blind, placebo-controlled, randomized crossover trial, Bruno et al.[176] demonstrated that ascorbic acid (500 mg twice daily for weeks) doubled "plasma ascorbic acid concentrations in both groups and attenuated smokers', but not nonsmokers', plasma alpha- and gamma-tocopherol... fractional disappearance rates by 25% and 45%, respectively. Likewise, smokers' plasma deuterium-labeled alpha- and gamma-tocopherol concentrations were significantly higher... at 72 h during ascorbic acid supplementation compared with placebo." Based on these findings, they concluded that "cigarette smoking increased plasma alpha- and gamma-tocopherol fractional disappearance rates, suggesting that the oxidative stress from smoking oxidizes tocopherols and that plasma ascorbic acid reduces alpha- and gamma-tocopheroxyl radicals to nonoxidized forms, thereby decreasing vitamin E disappearance in humans."[176] Therefore, these investigators confirmed faster plasma vitamin E disappearance in smokers and its normalization with vitamin C administration.

Vitamin K

Vitamin E in high doses may interfere with the absorption and utilization of vitamin K and induce vitamin K deficiency.[124] This potential pattern might be playing a role in cases in which enhanced anticoagulant effect has been reported among patients taking oral anticoagulants following high-dose vitamin E administration. Vitamin E, at levels greater than 1000 IU per day, may alter the activity of vitamin K–dependent clotting factor production and thus coagulation status, possibly increasing the risk of an excessive hypoprothrombinemic response in some individuals on warfarin therapy. (See Warfarin for further discussion.)

The 179 citations for this monograph, as well as additional reference literature, are located under Vitamin E on the CD at the back of the book.

Vitamin K

Nutrient Name: Vitamin K.
Synonyms: Phylloquinone, phytonadione.
Related Substances: Phylloquinone, phytomenadione or phytonadione (K_1),
menaquinone (K_2), menadione (K_3).

Summary

Drug/Class Interaction Type	Mechanism and Significance	Management
Antibiotics ≈≈/≈≈≈/◇/☼	Antibacterial agents can inhibit or eliminate beneficial intestinal flora, thus disrupting gut ecology and interfering with endogenous vitamin K_2 synthesis. Cephalosporins also disrupt synthesis of active clotting factors by inhibiting hepatic vitamin K epoxide reductase. Clinical significance varies with vitamin K status and length of treatment; can be rapid and severe, especially with patients on warfarin therapy.	Administer vitamin K and follow with probiotics. Monitor INR and prothrombin and titrate anticoagulants, if indicated, especially with long-term or repeated antibiotics. Vitamin K administration for excess coumadin effect should be done only by practitioners experienced in this maneuver.
Bile acid sequestrants Cholestyramine, colestipol ≈≈≈	Bile acid sequestrants interfere with absorption of vitamin K and other fat-soluble nutrients. Consensus on mechanism; clinical significance variable, but more important for those with higher cardiovascular risk.	Supplement vitamin K, as well as mixed tocopherols, coenzyme Q10 and other fat-soluble nutrients important for cardiovascular health.
Corticosteroids, oral Prednisone ☼/≈≈≈	Oral corticosteroids can cause increased urinary loss of vitamin K as well as depletion of other key nutrients. Long-term oral steroid use may lead to clinically significant depletion, particularly affecting bone mass; may be prevented or reversed with vitamin K administration, especially in conjunction with synergistic nutrients.	Coadminister vitamin K (may require menatetrenone, a form of K_2), and monitor for bone loss, especially BMD, with extended steroid therapy.
Phenytoin, phenobarbital Anticonvulsant medications ≈≈≈/◇◇	Many anticonvulsants increase breakdown of vitamin K by inducing hepatic microsomal oxidase enzymes. Clinical significance unclear; greatest in pregnancy.	Coadminister vitamin K (possibly IM), especially during pregnancy.
Mineral oil ≈≈≈	Mineral oil may interfere with absorption of vitamin K and other nutrients. Evidence minimal but effect probable, though of variable clinical significance. Malabsorption of vitamin K can increase anticoagulant activity of warfarin.	Supplement with vitamin K–containing multivitamin; seperate intake. Avoid extended intake of mineral oil. Monitor and titrate with concomitant warfarin.
Warfarin Oral vitamin K antagonist anticoagulants ◇◇/⊕✗/◇◇	Warfarin and indandione anticoagulants act by inhibiting conversion of the vitamin K epoxide back to vitamin K. Excessive vitamin K intake, directly or within foods or herbs, will interfere with therapeutic action unless closely monitored, dose-titrated, and properly managed within comprehensive therapeutic strategy. Adverse effects can be rapid and serious. Close management, multidisciplinary collaboration, and active patient dialogue essential.	Limit and tightly regulate vitamin K intake. Closely monitor INR and titrate anticoagulant at close intervals when administering herbs, nutrients, or foods with substantial K content.

INR, International normalized ratio; *IM*, intramuscularly; *BMD*, bone mineral density.

NUTRIENT DESCRIPTION

Chemistry and Forms

Vitamin K refers to a family of compounds exhibiting the activity of phytomenadione. Phylloquinone (or phytomenadione) is the K_1 form naturally occurring in plants and fish. Bacteria synthesize menaquinone (K_2), a fat-soluble form. Menadione (K_3), the water-soluble parent compound, does not occur naturally.

Physiology and Function

Vitamin K serves as a coenzyme during the synthesis of many proteins involved in blood clotting and bone metabolism. Vitamin K_1 is fat soluble and requires bile salts for absorption in the upper gastrointestinal tract. Vitamin K acts as a cofactor in the final synthesis of proteins with a modified amino acid residue. This modified glutamic acid residue is found in the blood and along vessel walls, along with platelet-derived phospholipid, where it binds and facilitates the action of calcium, and is an integral part of the clotting process. It is also found in bone proteins and can bind onto calcium ions to cause calcification. This role in calcium transport is central to vitamin K's functions within healthy bone formation and blood clotting.

Vitamin K enables both coagulation and fibrinolysis. Vitamin K's central role in blood coagulation involves synthesis of coagulation components, such as prothrombin (factor II), as well as factors VII, IX, and X and proteins C, S, and Z in the liver. Proteins C and S promote fibrinolysis and anticoagulation. Thus, they are involved with reducing inflammation.

Osteocalcin, matrix Gla protein, and protein S are vitamin K–dependent structural and regulatory proteins in bone and vascular metabolism. Vitamin K plays the critical role of allowing calcium ions to bind, thus resulting in the calcification of bone. Osteocalcin metabolism has been implicated in the pathogenesis of osteoporosis through an unknown mechanism that may be linked to suboptimal vitamin K status, resulting in its undercarboxylation and presumed dysfunction.

Probiotic microflora in the intestines, when a healthy microecology is functioning, normally manufacture significant amounts of vitamin K, contributing up to half of daily requirements in some individuals.

NUTRIENT IN CLINICAL PRACTICE

Historical/Ethnomedicine Precedent

In most cultural traditions, herbs and green leafy vegetables have historically been used to enrich and tonify the blood and support its metabolic functions. Consumption of cultured foods can support vigorous probiotic flora population and healthy gut ecology.

Possible Uses

Acute myeloid leukemia (vitamin K_2 only), bone loss (risk reduction), calcium oxalate kidney stones (prevention), celiac disease (malabsorption-induced deficiency), coagulation disorders, cystic fibrosis, epistaxis, floaters (in eyes), fractures (risk reduction), gastric bypass with Roux-en-Y (bariatric surgery), hemorrhagic disease of the newborn, inflammatory conditions, myelodysplastic syndromes (vitamin K_2 only), nausea and vomiting of pregnancy, osteoporosis, phenylketonuria (if deficient), preterm infants (K_1 prophylaxis), pruritus, rheumatoid arthritis, stroke prevention; vitamin K malabsorption (e.g., with celiac disease or bariatric surgery), warfarin overanticoagulation.

When the clotting mechanism is disrupted by medications such as certain antibiotics, cephalosporin possessing an MTT side chain, or excessive doses of oral anticoagulants (warfarin), vitamin K can be administered to correct the situation.

Deficiency

Symptoms: Easy bruising, small amounts of blood in stool, prolonged bleeding; impaired bone remodeling, and mineralization.

Vitamin K deficiency is rare in the general population, but the risk is significantly greater in infants, especially premature infants and those who are exclusively breast-fed, for whom such a deficiency can be fatal (hemorrhagic disease of the newborn). Adults at increased risk of vitamin K deficiency include individuals with heavy alcohol intake, liver disease, fat malabsorption, or chronic digestive disorders, such as chronic diarrhea, celiac sprue, Crohn's disease or ulcerative colitis, and bariatric surgical procedures that bypass the duodenum.

In recent years, several published papers suggest that the dietary reference intakes (DRIs) for vitamin K are based solely on levels relevant to hepatic synthesis of clotting factors, and that much higher levels (10 mg/day) may be needed for optimal health of the skeletal and vascular systems. Vascular calcification may be related to chronic insufficiency of vitamin K intake. Patients receiving chronic warfarin, essentially an induced vitamin K deficiency, have a higher incidence of vascular calcification.

Dietary Sources

Leafy green vegetables are the single best dietary source of vitamin K because of their high chlorophyll content; the vitamin K content is proportionate to the degree to which the plant parts are green. Kale, green tea, and turnip greens are the most abundant food sources. Spinach, broccoli, lettuce, and cabbage are also rich sources. Other food sources include egg yolk, cow's milk, and liver, as well as soybean oil, olive oil, cottonseed oil, and canola oil.

The probiotic flora inhabiting intestines with a healthy ecology normally manufacture vitamin K_2, or *menaquinone*. Menaquinones (MK-*n*, with the *n* determined by the number of prenyl side chains) can also be found in the diet; MK-4 is in meat, and MK-7, -8, and -9 are found in fermented food products such as cheese. The Japanese fermented soy product *natto* is a rich source of MK-7. Some sources have said that MK-4, also known as *menatetrenone*, is synthetic vitamin K_2, but this is not accurate. However, MK-4 is distinct from other MKs because it is not produced in significant amounts by gut microflora, but it can be derived from vitamin

K_1 in vivo. Hydrogenation of plant oils appears to decrease the absorption and biological effect of vitamin K in bone, possibly as an effect of *trans*-fatty acids.

Nutrient Preparations Available

Phylloquinone (K_1) is the usual form of supplemental vitamin K. Vitamin K_2 is also used therapeutically, often parenterally. Mixed K_1 and K_2 formulations are increasingly available. The natural, long-chain menaquinone-7 (MK-7), derived from natto, exhibits a "very long half-life time,...resulting in much more stable serum levels and accumulation of MK-7 to higher levels (7-8 fold) during prolonged intake,"[1] compared to synthetic vitamin K_1. The MK-7 preparation can also induce "more complete carboxylation of osteocalcin," and thereby also increase activity against vitamin K antagonists.[1]

Dosage Forms Available

Capsule, tablet; injectable (prescription only).

Dosage Range

Adult
Supplemental/Maintenance: 30 to 100 µg per day.
Pharmacological/Therapeutic: 45 to 500 µg per day.
Toxic: None reported or suspected.

Pediatric (<18 years)
Supplemental/Maintenance
    Infants, birth to 6 months: 5 µg/day
    Infants, 7 to 12 months: 10 µg/day
    Children, 1 to 3 years: 15 µg/day
    Children, 4 to 6 years: 20 µg/day
    Children, 7 to 10 years: 30 µg/day
Pharmacological/Therapeutic: 45 to 150 µg per day.
Toxic: None reported or suspected.

Laboratory Values

Plasma vitamin K: Osteocalcin level is sometimes used as a surrogate test for vitamin K status.

Prothrombin time (PT) and clotting factors (X, IX, VII, and protein C) may also be used as reference values, but PT is not considered a reliable test for vitamin K status. Vitamin K deficiency will prolong PT, but so does hepatic insufficiency (which also results in inadequate levels of clotting factors).

SAFETY PROFILE

Overview

Supplemental vitamin K is generally considered safe when used in accordance with proper dosing guidelines. No adverse effects associated with vitamin K consumption from food or supplements have been reported in humans or animals. This does not mean, however, that no potential exists for adverse effects resulting from high intakes beyond normal dietary or supplemental levels. Because data on the adverse effects of vitamin K are limited, caution may be warranted.

Patients undergoing anticoagulant therapy should monitor vitamin K intake and avoid significant inconsistencies in intake levels. Regular monitoring of coagulation parameters (INR) and dose titration is essential.

Nutrient Adverse Effects

General Adverse Effects

Naturally occurring vitamin K_1 (phylloquinone) is generally considered nontoxic, whereas menadione (K_3), the synthetic derivative, has been associated with potentially severe toxicity reactions at high doses, particularly in infants and other highly vulnerable populations. Flushing and perspiration are the most common, although infrequent, adverse effects reported. Other potential toxicity symptoms include difficulty breathing, tightness in throat or chest, chest pain, hives, rash, or itchy or swollen skin. Rare cases of hemolytic anemia have been reported.

The primary risk associated with vitamin K has been limited to rare reports of cutaneous allergic reaction to intramuscular (IM) vitamin K_1.

Less than 1%: Abnormal taste, anaphylaxis, cyanosis, diaphoresis, dizziness (rarely), dyspnea, gastrointestinal upset (oral), hemolysis in neonates and in patients with glucose-6-phosphate dehydrogenase (G6PD) deficiency, hypersensitivity reactions, hypotension (rarely), pain, tenderness at injection site, transient flushing reaction.

More recently, discussions have arisen concerning potential risk of cirrhosis associated with supplemental intake of vitamin K, but not with food sources, in the treatment of osteoporosis.

Toxicity

Phylloquinone (vitamin K_1) is not toxic at 500 times the recommended dietary allowance (RDA, 0.5 mg/kg/day). No toxicities have been reported or suspected as being associated with natural vitamin K at any dose in humans when given orally. Intravenous (IV) administration of vitamin K at doses of 2 to 8 mg/kg has been found to be lethal in horses.

Menadione (vitamin K_3) has a finite toxicity resulting from its reaction with sulfhydryl groups. Large doses of menadione may produce hemolytic anemia, hyperbilirubinemia, and kernicterus in the infant. Other signs of synthetic vitamin K toxicity include flushing, sweating, and chest constriction. Most toxicity is associated with IV use and may be related to allergies to various preservatives or excipients.

Adverse Effects Among Specific Populations

Patients receiving anticoagulant therapy should monitor vitamin K intake. Possible risk of aggravation exists among individuals prone to form kidney stones.

Pregnancy and Nursing

No extant reports of adverse effects have been related to fetal development during pregnancy. This fat-soluble vitamin crosses the placenta and is excreted into breast milk.

Infants and Children

Vitamin K can cause a fatal form of jaundice in infants. No adverse effects have been reported among breast-fed infants.

Contraindications

Patients undergoing anti–vitamin K anticoagulant therapy, except within the context of appropriate professional supervision; some premature infants.

INTERACTIONS REVIEW

Strategic Considerations

The primary interactions of clinical significance involving vitamin K and pharmaceutical agents derive from interference of vitamin K with the therapeutic action of certain anticoagulant medications and the adverse effect of antimicrobial medications on normal vitamin K synthesis by gut bacterial flora. Although vitamin K's role in coagulation receives attention regularly, its influence on fibrinolysis also needs to be considered. The critical issue with anticoagulants is monitoring and managing the proportionate effects of the medication and dietary or supplemental sources of vitamin K. Strategic administration of probiotic flora and restoration of a healthy gut ecology can compensate for the tactical use of antimicrobial agents in the suppression of infectious bacteria. The interactions involving vitamin K provide challenging opportunities for reframing the constituent elements of medical intervention within the context of a dynamic and evolving individualized process emphasizing strategic goals and comprehensive clinical outcomes, such as improved function, decreased risk, and enhanced quality of life.

Oral Anticoagulant Overdose

Clinical surveys have found that a substantial number of anticoagulation clinics underutilize oral phytonadione for patients with supratherapeutic international normalized ratio (INR) values. These data indicate that such clinics do not comply with the guidelines for vitamin K use developed at the American College of Chest Physicians (ACCP) Fifth Consensus Conference on Antithrombotic Therapy, as published in 1998.

NUTRIENT-DRUG INTERACTIONS

Antibiotics/Antimicrobial Agents (Systemic)

Aminoglycoside Antibiotics: Amikacin (Amikin), gentamicin (G-mycin, Garamycin, Jenamicin), kanamycin (Kantrex), neomycin (Mycifradin, Myciguent, Neo-Fradin, NeoTab, Nivemycin), netilmicin (Netromycin), paromomycin (monomycin; Humatin), streptomycin, tobramycin (AKTob, Nebcin, TOBI, TOBI Solution, TobraDex, Tobrex).

Beta-Lactam Antibiotics: Methicillin (Staphcillin); aztreonam (Azactam injection); carbapenem antibiotics: meropenem (Merrem I.V.); combination drug: imipenem and cilastatin (Primaxin I.M., Primaxin I.V.); penicillin antibiotics: amoxicillin (Amoxicot, Amoxil, Moxilin, Trimox, Wymox); combination drug: amoxicillin and clavulanic acid (Augmentin, Augmentin XR, Clavulin); ampicillin (Amficot, Omnipen, Principen, Totacillin); combination drug: ampicillin and sulbactam (Unisyn); bacampicillin (Spectrobid), carbenicillin (Geocillin), cloxacillin (Cloxapen), dicloxacillin (Dynapen, Dycill), mezlocillin (Mezlin), nafcillin (Unipen), oxacillin (Bactocill), penicillin G (Bicillin C-R, Bicillin L-A, Pfizerpen, Truxcillin), penicillin V (Beepen-VK, Betapen-VK, Ledercillin VK, Pen-Vee K, Robicillin VK, Suspen, Truxcillin VK, V-Cillin K, Veetids), piperacillin (Pipracil); combination drug: piperacillin and tazobactam (Zosyn); ticarcillin (Ticar); combination drug: ticarcillin and clavulanate (Timentin).

Cephalosporin Antibiotics: Cefaclor (Ceclor), cefadroxil (Duricef), cefamandole (Mandol), cefazolin (Ancef, Kefzol), cefdinir (Omnicef), cefepime (Maxipime), cefixime (Suprax), cefoperazone (Cefobid), cefotaxime (Claforan), cefotetan (Cefotan), cefoxitin (Mefoxin), cefpodoxime (Vantin), cefprozil (Cefzil), ceftazidime (Ceptaz, Fortaz, Tazicef, Tazidime), ceftibuten (Cedax), ceftizoxime (Cefizox), ceftriaxone (Rocephin), cefuroxime (Ceftin, Kefurox, Zinacef), cephalexin (Keflex, Keftab), cephapirin (Cefadyl), cephradine (Anspor, Velocef); imipenem combination drug: imipenem and cilastatin (Primaxin I.M., Primaxin I.V.); loracarbef (Lorabid), meropenem (Merrem I.V.).

Fluoroquinolone (4-Quinolone) Antibiotics: Cinoxacin (Cinobac, Pulvules), ciprofloxacin (Ciloxan, Cipro), enoxacin (Penetrex), gatifloxacin (Tequin), levofloxacin (Levaquin), lomefloxacin (Maxaquin), moxifloxacin (Avelox), nalidixic acid (Neggram), norfloxacin (Noroxin), ofloxacin (Floxin, Ocuflox), sparfloxacin (Zagam), trovafloxacin (alatrofloxacin; Trovan).

Macrolide Antibiotics: Azithromycin (Zithromax), clarithromycin (Biaxin), dirithromycin (Dynabac), erythromycin, oral (EES, EryPed, Ery-Tab, PCE Dispertab, Pediazole), troleandomycin (Tao).

Sulfonamide Antibiotics: Sodium sulfacetamide (AK-Sulf, Bleph-10, Sodium Sulamyd), sulfamethoxazole (Gantanol), sulfanilamide (AVC), sulfasalazine (Salazosulfapyridine, salicylazosulfapyridine, suphasalazine; Apo-Sulfasalazine, Azulfidine, Azulfidine EN-Tabs, PMS-Sulfasalazine, Salazopyrin, Salazopyrin EN-Tabs, SAS), sulfisoxazole (Gantrisin); combination drug: sulfamethoxazole and trimethoprim (cotrimoxazole, co-trimoxazole, SXT, TMP-SMX, TMP-sulfa; Bactrim, Bactrim DS, Cotrim, Septra, Septra DS, Sulfatrim, Uroplus); triple sulfa (Sultrin Triple Sulfa).

Chemotherapy, Cytotoxic Antibiotics: Bleomycin (Blenoxane), dactinomycin (Actinomycin D, Cosmegen, Cosmegen Lyovac), mitomycin (Mutamycin), plicamycin (Mithracin).

Miscellaneous Antibiotics/Antimicrobials: Bacitracin (Caci-IM), chloramphenicol (Chloromycetin), chlorhexidine (Peridex), clindamycin, oral (Cleocin), colistimethate (Coly-Mycin M), dapsone (DDS, diaminodiphenylsulphone; Aczone Gel, Avlosulfon), furazolidone (Furoxone), lincomycin (Lincocin), linezolid (Zyvox), nitrofurantoin (Macrobid, Macrodantin), trimethoprim (Proloprim, Trimpex), vancomycin (Vancocin).

Interaction Type and Significance

≈≈   Drug-Induced Nutrient Depletion, Supplementation Therapeutic, with Professional Management, *or*

≈≈≈   Drug-Induced Nutrient Depletion, Supplementation Therapeutic, Not Requiring Professional Management

◇   Adverse Drug Effect on Nutritional Therapeutics, Strategic Concern

☼   Prevention or Reduction of Drug Adverse Effect

Probability: Evidence Base:
2. Probable   ◉ Emerging, possibly
                            ● Consensus

Effect and Mechanism of Action

Antimicrobial therapies, particularly chronic or recurrent courses of treatment, exert a detrimental and often devastating effect on beneficial bacterial flora naturally populating the human digestive tract. The diverse microorganisms comprising the gut microflora play a critical role in the synthesis of vitamin K, as well as synthesis of the B vitamins and the metabolism of bile acids, other sterols, and xenobiotics.[2,3] Broad-spectrum antibiotics reduce hepatic vitamin K_2 (menaquinone) stores, presumably by reducing its synthesis by gut microflora.[4-7] In relation to warfarin, the INR reflects the balance between the anticoagulant and vitamin K. When the intestinal flora are wiped out by antibiotics, their production of vitamin K diminishes, and the INR increases. Some antibiotics,

particularly trimethoprim/sulfamethoxazole (Bactrim, Septra), and fluoroquinolones to a slightly lesser degree, specifically increase warfarin effect independent of their effect on bacterial flora production of vitamin K, by displacing it from protein-binding sites and dramatically elevating the anticoagulant effect.

In particular, in addition to reducing bacterial vitamin K synthesis, cephalosporins containing an *N*-methylthiotetrazole (MTT) side chain can result in a clinically relevant coagulopathy, prolonged PT, and increased risk of bleeding complications because of a deficiency in active vitamin K–dependent clotting factors.[5,8-11] In particular, cephalosporins such as cefazolin, cefmetazole, cefoperazone, and cefotetan, which feature the MTT side chain, can cause vitamin K deficiency and hypoprothrombinemia, disrupting synthesis of active clotting factors by inhibiting hepatic vitamin K *epoxide reductase* (ER), an enzyme necessary to recycle vitamin K back to its active form.[12,13] Even so, in a study using dogs, Spurling et al.[9] found that cefuroxime, which lacks the MTT side chain, still appears to affect PT by reducing bacterial vitamin K synthesis. Other evidence indicates that antibiotics other than MTT–side chain cephalosporins may also act as weak inhibitors of the vitamin K epoxide cycle.

Research

During the past decade the scientific literature investigating probiotic intestinal flora has grown exponentially and with it a deeper appreciation of the clinical significance of these symbiotic microorganisms in healthy human physiology. The unintended adverse effects of antibiotics on gut flora will impact most individuals to some degree, but such actions pose a potentially significant risk to individuals living within tight parameters of vitamin K regulation via anticoagulant medications. Early animal studies led by Spurling, Shirakawa, and others found that deliberate destruction of intestinal flora induced a measurable decrease in vitamin K levels and amplified alterations in coagulation functions, including prolonged prothrombin time (PT) and activated partial thromboplastin time (aPTT).[4,9] A subsequent review by Lipsky[14] (1994) criticized some of the assertions used in previous studies and asserted that there was no definitive evidence that intestinal bacteria were an important source of vitamin K. Some later review articles, such as Covington, have claimed that antibiotic use infrequently causes significant disruption to gut flora and thus vitamin K. Although transient interference with flora vitamin K synthesis may not trigger clinically significant perturbations in plasma vitamin K levels, high doses of broad-spectrum antibiotics, especially in a repeated or chronic prescribing pattern, may fundamentally undermine the dynamic infrastructure of endogenous menaquinone synthesis.

Amid this controversy, an emerging body of reports and research have documented proposed, and discovered further, critical and irreplaceable functions of bacterial flora in the microecology of the digestive tract in relation to nutrient assimilation, transformation, and synthesis; immune function; infection resistance; detoxification; neurotransmitter function; hormonal regulation; and numerous other systemic functions. Along with the emergence of antibiotic-resistant bacterial strains, the often-indiscriminate and hasty overprescribing of antibiotics has contributed to systematic eradication of beneficial bacterial flora en masse, with no equally programmatic conventions for probiotic replacement. Further, growing research has demonstrated the importance of prebiotic substances that aim at stimulating the growth of such flora, thus modulating the composition of the natural ecosystem.

In recent years, increasing attention has focused on the possible beneficial effects of prebiotics, such as enhanced resistance to invading pathogens, improved bowel function, anti–colon cancer properties, lipid-lowering action, and improved calcium bioavailability.[15-20]

Thus, an emerging consensus of evidence indicates that these broad adverse effects are responsible for a disturbing pattern of apparent interactions between warfarin and antibiotics that do not seem to result from pharmacokinetics or other direct interaction, but rather from the destruction of gut flora and the ecosystem of which they are a part. Therefore, the initial dose of warfarin arrived at to bring the INR into the target therapeutic range always needs to be analyzed in the context of body stores, endogenous synthesis, and dietary intake of K_1 and synthesized K_2. If individuals have low stores and little endogenous synthesis, they will be "coumadin sensitive"; that is, a few milligrams will put them into therapeutic range. Conversely, only the change in the vitamin K status (or vitamin K ER function) creates an unstable INR situation. Thus, the state of an individual's intestinal ecology may not affect the ability to titrate to a stable INR, but someone with significant "dysbiosis" (i.e., disrupted gut ecology and attendant dysfunctions) may be started on 5 mg of coumadin and have an INR of 7 within a few days, potentially leading to an exaggerated or misunderstood perception of the overall situation by the physician.

Apart from consideration of general trends, the potential for disruption of vitamin K concentrations and coagulation functions subsequent to antibiotic administration warrants higher levels of monitoring and management than previously considered necessary in conventional practice. Olson[21] noted in 1999 that a reduction in prothrombin and other vitamin K–dependent factors can indicate a deficiency. In a comprehensive review (2000) of vitamin K and vitamin K antagonists Vermeer and Schurgers[22] further observed that severe vitamin K deficiency may be associated with detectable plasma levels of descarboxyprothrombin. The body of evidence suggests that any such decline in vitamin K status attributable to antibiotic effects on endogenous flora will carry a greater risk of contributing to a clinically significant disruption in coagulation stability in individuals with preexisting low vitamin K levels, suffering from renal failure, or recovering from organ transplant surgery.

Ofloxacin represents one notable, but partial, exception to the general concern regarding the action of antibiotics as a class in relation to interference with the vitamin K–dependent coagulation factors. In a small, preliminary study with seven healthy male subjects, Verho et al.[23] observed that ofloxacin, 200 mg once daily for 7 days, did not alter the anticoagulant response to phenprocoumon after a stabilization phase of 2 weeks. If subsequent research were to confirm this finding, individuals taking ofloxacin might not need to supplement vitamin K to protect against possible drug-induced depletion. Nevertheless, the indirect effect of ofloxacin on vitamin K synthesis by intestinal flora would remain an issue of concern and worthy of specific inquiry through clinical trials.

Reports

As clinicians and researchers have become increasingly aware of the multifaceted roles of intestinal microflora, there has been a steady rise in reports documenting interactions between anticoagulant medications, especially warfarin, and a range of antibiotic medications, which appear to be more widespread and deleterious than would be attributable to predictable pharmacokinetics and other direct mechanisms of interaction. In an innovative research methodology comparing postmortem liver tissue from 22 deceased patients, nine of whom had been given broad-spectrum antibiotics before death, Conly and Stein[7] observed a reduction in hepatic bacteria-produced menaquinone (K_2) concentration associated with the use of such antimicrobials; in contrast, there was a lack of significant difference in hepatic levels of dietary-derived phylloquinone between the two groups.[24] A 1996 case report by Bandrowsky et al.[25] documented significant postoperative bleeding caused by an amoxicillin-induced vitamin K deficiency, rather than a failure of the local tranexamic acid mouth rinse protocol being applied. In a review, Huilgol et al.[26] reported a case of antibiotic-induced vitamin K deficiency that resulted in hemobilia (bleeding into the biliary tract) complicating acalculous cholecystitis. Suzuki et al.[27] reported on an infant with intracranial hemorrhage, 2 days after the introduction of oral antibiotics, which was attributed to vitamin K deficiency despite K_2 prophylaxis. In 2002, Jones and Fugate[28] published four case reports demonstrating significant elevations in INR values during and up to 1 day after levofloxacin therapy in previously stable patients undergoing warfarin therapy. The authors attributed this unexpected interaction to displacement of warfarin from protein-binding sites, reduction in gut flora producing vitamin K, and decreased warfarin metabolism. In 2003, Davydov et al.[29] reported the case of a 58-year-old woman who developed an elevated INR and microscopic hematuria after taking amoxicillin/clavulanate potassium while on warfarin therapy. They concluded that a decrease in vitamin K–producing gut flora with resulting vitamin K deficiency was the most likely contributing factor.

Nutritional Therapeutics, Clinical Concerns, and Adaptations

Although the practice of regularly replacing probiotic flora after the use of antibiotics has been widespread in European and natural medicine for decades, integration of such prescribing practices has only recently entered mainstream practice of conventional medicine in the United States as the evidence of the importance of such flora and gut ecology has accumulated. A wide range of evidence demonstrates multifaceted benefits from recolonization of symbiotic microflora and reestablishment of a vigorous gut ecology after antibiotic therapy for the general population. The clinical significance of such replacement theraphy may be greater among individuals undergoing warfarin or other vitamin K–oriented anticoagulant therapy as a result of the antibiotic's adverse impact on normal intestinal microorganisms. Preventive supplementation is warranted, particularly in nutritionally deficient or otherwise compromised individuals, but the administration of probiotics would be especially appropriate for individuals with known or potential coagulation disorders manifesting hypoprothrombinemia, with internal and external hemorrhage or other signs and symptoms of deficiency. Among the agents discussed, cephalosporins are most likely associated with vitamin K deficiency. Quinolones and sulfonamides have further interactions complications of clinical significance in addition to the flora-depletion issues inherent to other antibiotic medications.

Conservative nutritional practice indicates the value of supplementing with vitamin K whenever an antibiotic medication is used. A daily dosage of 45 to 80 µg of vitamin K along with administration of diverse and vigorous cultures of probiotic flora, during and for a minimum of 2 weeks after the course of antibiotics, will generally be adequate to mitigate any disruptive effects on gut ecology and vitamin K synthesis. Although such combinations are available, most multivitamin formulations do not contain either vitamin K or probiotics. Further variables in the patient's clinical presentation, serum levels, age, gender, dietary habits, and medication regimen can be considered in crafting the therapeutic protocol to best support the broader strategic agenda. Regular monitoring and close clinical management are important during any vitamin K administration or recolonization of beneficial flora in patients taking vitamin K antagonist anticoagulants, such as warfarin. Just as production of vitamin K diminishes and the INR increases as the intestinal flora are damaged or eliminated by antibiotics, so, conversely, can their reintroduction shift the relationship between vitamin K and anticoagulant medications, especially warfarin. Until probiotic replacement can restore and maintain this balance, it is usually necessary to reduce the dose of warfarin during a course of antibiotics. During coadministration of probiotics and warfarin, the anticoagulant dose may need to be titrated, realizing that the effects of a dose adjustment on a given day will be seen in the INR 2 days later. Whenever possible, it can be beneficial for patients undergoing warfarin therapy to have a home monitor so that they can monitor their INR daily during such situations. As previously noted, different antibiotics appear to exert widely varying levels of effect on vitamin K activity, both directly and through effects on flora, so the urgency and scale of the clinical response can vary significantly based on the medication being administered as well as other factors relating to the individual characteristics of the patient. If hemorrhage occurs subsequent to antibiotic therapy, medical intervention is appropriate. In such cases, vitamin K should initially be administered by IM injection, or in urgent cases, a low dose of vitamin K_1, such as 0.5 mg, can be infused intravenously over 30 minutes.

Replacement therapy with exogenous probiotics subsequent to antimicrobial medications should be paced in individuals undergoing anticoagulant therapy, given the potential for increased endogenous production of vitamin K_2 by the resurgent ecology. Again, the effects of such administration are more likely to be significant with neonates and in individuals who have been nutritionally deficient in vitamin K. Even so, daily intake of vitamin K from a balanced and nutritious diet is usually greater than the levels produced by active flora. Additional research is warranted to better determine the particular dosages of vitamin K supplementation and probiotic replacement appropriate to respective antibiotic medications, particularly in the context of anticoagulant therapy. However, the availability of oral, direct thrombin inhibitors, such as Exanta (Astra-Zeneca), may soon reduce the risk of drug interactions and the need to restrict vitamin K intake, as well as provide a sufficiently predictable effect that monitoring is unnecessary.

Bile Acid Sequestrants

Cholestyramine (Locholest, Prevalite, Questran), colesevelam (WelChol), colestipol (Colestid).

Interaction Type and Significance

≈≈≈ **Drug-Induced Nutrient Depletion, Supplementation Therapeutic, Not Requiring Professional Management**

Probability:
3. Possible

Evidence Base:
● Consensus

Effect and Mechanism of Action

Bile acid sequestrants, such as cholestyramine and colestipol, are designed to prevent bile acids from being reabsorbed and recycled by the enterohepatic circulation, thus forcing the body to metabolize reserves of cholesterol into more bile acids. Because bile acids and their salts are used to solubilize and absorb many fat-soluble nutrients, as a direct consequence

such sequestrants may also interfere with absorption of vitamin K and other fat-soluble nutrients, including vitamins A, D, and E; carotenoids; essential fatty acids; and lipid-soluble antioxidants, such as coenzyme Q10.[30-36]

Research

Clinical studies and research reviews consistently acknowledge the high probability of vitamin K malabsorption resulting from bile acid sequestrants. Opinions have varied as to the clinical significance of such drug-induced depletion patterns; the general trend has been toward deeper appreciation of the importance of nutrients such as vitamin K and a growing awareness of the subtle and pervasive adverse effects resulting from such interference with normal nutritional intake and metabolism over time.

Nutritional Therapeutics, Clinical Concerns, and Adaptations

Vitamin K supplementation, as part of a multivitamin-mineral formulation, would probably be of benefit for individuals taking bile acid sequestrants. Taking such supplements daily, at least 1 hour before or 4 to 6 hours after the medication, will reduce the degree of interference with the intended nutriture.

Nevertheless, this interaction raises serious questions about continuity between tactical methods of specific interventions and strategic goals of improved health, reduced risk, and better outcomes, given the accumulating experimental, epidemiological, and clinical evidence of an association between nutrient intake and reduced risk of coronary heart disease.

Corticosteroids, Oral, Including Prednisone

Betamethasone (Celestone), cortisone (Cortone), dexamethasone (Decadron), fludrocortisone (Florinef), hydrocortisone (Cortef), methylprednisolone (Medrol) prednisolone (Delta-Cortef, Orapred, Pediapred, Prelone), prednisone (Deltasone, Liquid Pred, Meticorten, Orasone), triamcinolone (Aristocort).

Interaction Type and Significance

☼ **Prevention or Reduction of Drug Adverse Effect**
≈≈≈ **Drug-Induced Nutrient Depletion, Supplementation Therapeutic, Not Requiring Professional Management**

Probability:
3. Possible

Evidence Base:
● Consensus

Effect and Mechanism of Action

Vitamin K plays a key role in calcium transport and enhances bone formation. Oral corticosteroids can cause increased urinary loss of vitamin K, as well as of vitamin C, selenium, and zinc. Steroidal medications are also well known to enhance bone resorption and suppress bone formation, leading to loss of bone mineral density (BMD) and potentially to developmental problems and osteoporosis.

Research

Numerous studies examining the relationship between vitamin K status and osteoporosis have demonstrated the critical role played by the nutrient in maintaining and restoring bone health.[37] Other researchers have focused on the therapeutic benefits that vitamin K supplementation might provide to individuals whose bone health was likely to be compromised, particularly by iatrogenic loss of BMD. Yonemura et al.[38] conducted a small clinical trail investigating the short-term effect of vitamin K administration (as menatetrenone) on prednisolone-induced loss of BMD in 20 patients with chronic glomerulonephritis. Ten patients received prednisolone alone, and the other 10 patients received prednisolone plus 15 mg of menatetrenone three times daily. Their findings confirmed that prednisolone resulted in loss of BMD of the lumbar spine associated with suppression of both bone formation and enhancement of bone resorption, and that such prednisolone-induced reduction of BMD was prevented by menatetrenone administration.

Inoue et al.[39] conducted a prospective pilot study focusing on the important issue of adverse effects on skeletal development and bone health in children undergoing glucocorticoid therapy. Twenty children were divided in to two groups; one group received alfacalcidol (0.03 µg/kg/day) and the other alfacalcidol (0.03 µg/kg/day) plus menatetrenone (~2 mg/kg/day) for 24 weeks. Bone biochemical markers and BMD were measured at baseline and after treatment. The authors concluded that that menatetrenone effectively and safely increases lumbar BMD, probably through carboxylation of osteocalcin, in long-term prednisolone-treated children receiving alfacalcidol who have a high bone turnover; no adverse effects were observed.

Uncertainty remains as to the comprehensive processes and mechanisms of action involved in bone loss and protection against such unintended adverse effects, particularly the clinical significance of increased nutrient loss through urination resulting from steroids. Most likely, variables of age, gender, health status, and conditions being treated will all influence the degree to which urinary loss of vitamin K directly impacts BMD and increases risk of bone loss. These small, short-term studies suggest that large, well-designed, randomized, double-blind controlled trials focusing on different populations are warranted to understand better the physiological processes and risk factors involved and to develop responsive therapeutic protocols.

Nutritional Therapeutics, Clinical Concerns, and Adaptations

Individuals receiving oral corticosteroid therapy for extended periods will most likely benefit from increased vitamin K intake, whether supplemental or dietary. The studies cited and other research have involved physician-administered forms of vitamin K. Further research investigating food sources of vitamin K or oral forms of vitamin K suitable for self-care deserve attention because therapeutic levels of vitamin K are typically obtainable by such means. Given that this nutrient has small risk of adverse effects or toxicity, such supplementation could easily fit within the monitoring and supervision inherent to steroid therapy.

Topical and inhaled corticosteroids have generally been found to exert significantly lesser adverse effects on BMD. Therefore, patients receiving such therapy would be less likely to benefit from vitamin K supplementation.[40-42]

Mineral Oil

Mineral oil (Agoral, Kondremul Plain, Liquid Parafin, Milkinol, Neo-Cultol, Petrogalar Plain).

Interaction Type and Significance

≈≈≈ **Drug-Induced Nutrient Depletion, Supplementation Therapeutic, Not Requiring Professional Management**

Probability:
4. Plausible

Evidence Base:
○ **Preliminary,** possibly
◉ **Emerging**

Effect and Mechanism of Action

Mineral oil, as a lipid solvent, may absorb many substances and interfere with normal absorption of vitamin K and other nutrients. The sequelae of such effects can alter the activity of anticoagulant medications through reduced vitamin K levels.

Research

Although some disagree, most researchers have found that mineral oil interferes with the absorption of many fat-soluble nutrients, including beta-carotene, calcium, phosphorus, potassium, and vitamins A, D, K, and E.[43,44] Chronic use of mineral oil can cause a deficiency of vitamins A, D, E, and K, being fat soluble, because these vitamins are dissolved in the mineral oil, which is not absorbed from the intestine. This is especially problematic during pregnancy since the regular ingestion of mineral oil may reduce the assimilation of critical nutrients. The malabsorption of vitamin K can result in an increased anticoagulant activity by warfarin anticoagulants because of this adverse effect of mineral oil.

Nutritional Therapeutics, Clinical Concerns, and Adaptations

Individuals using mineral oil for any extended period will likely benefit from regular use of a multivitamin supplement containing more than 100 µg of vitamin K per daily dose. Malabsorption of fat-soluble vitamins caused by ingestion of mineral oil can be minimized by administering mineral oil on an empty stomach or consuming vitamin or mineral supplements at least 2 hours before or after the mineral oil. In general, it is advisable to limit the internal use of mineral oil to less than 1 week.

Phenytoin, Phenobarbital, and Other Anticonvulsant Medications

Carbamazepine (Carbatrol, Tegretol), clonazepam (Klonopin), clorazepate (Tranxene), divalproex semisodium, divalproex sodium (Depakote), ethosuximide (Zarontin), ethotoin (Peganone), felbamate (Felbatol), fosphenytoin (Cerebyx, Mesantoin), levetiracetam (Keppra), mephenytoin, mephobarbital (Mebaral), methsuximide (Celontin), oxcarbazepine (GP 47680, oxycarbazepine; Trileptal), phenobarbital (phenobarbitone; Luminal, Solfoton), phenytoin (diphenylhydantoin; Dilantin, Phenytek), piracetam (Nootropyl), primidone (Mysoline), sodium valproate (Depacon), topiramate (Topamax), trimethadione (Tridione), valproate semisodium, valproic acid (Depakene, Depakene Syrup), vigabatrin (Sabril), zonisamide (Zonegran).

Similar properties but evidence lacking for extrapolation: Acetazolamide (Diamox; Diamox Sequels).

Interaction Type and Significance

≈≈≈ **Drug-Induced Nutrient Depletion, Supplementation Therapeutic, Not Requiring Professional Management**

◇◇ **Drug-Induced Effect on Nutrient Function, Supplementation Contraindicated, Professional Management Appropriate**

Probability:
3. Possible

Evidence Base:
◉ **Emerging**

Effect and Mechanism of Action

Phenytoin, phenobarbital, primidone, and carbamazepine increase metabolic breakdown of vitamin K by inducing hepatic microsomal oxidase enzymes. The implications of drug exposure and iatrogenic vitamin K deficiency may pose particularly significant risks during and after pregnancy.

Research

Numerous researchers and clinicians have proposed that vitamin K deficiency due to anticonvulsant medications might pose significant risks for pregnant women. Vitamin K deficiency during fetal development has been known to result in facial bone abnormalities, specifically maxillonasal hypoplasia, known as Binder syndrome.[45,46] An elevated serum osteocalcin level indicates that the anticonvulsant drugs, particularly phenytoin and phenobarbital, are interfering with vitamin K metabolism.[47] The reduced levels of vitamin K–dependent clotting factors also increase the risk of bleeding problems during delivery. Such in utero exposure also results in increased risk for newborns because vitamin K–dependent hemostatic factors are present in reduced quantities at birth. Vitamin K administration during pregnancy offers preventive and therapeutic benefits, with little or no risk, for the general obstetric population. Nevertheless, although cases of increased bleeding and congenital abnormalities have been documented, evidence from clinical trials is lacking to validate the hypothesis that coadministration is particularly necessary and efficacious as a standard practice for women taking phenytoin and other hepatic enzyme-inducing antiepileptic drugs (AEDs) while pregnant.

For more than 60 years, public policy has recommended the prophylactic administration of vitamin K (1 mg intramuscularly) to infants at birth. Such clinical practice emerged before awareness of adverse effects of anticonvulsant medications and was largely derived from manufacturer recommendations aimed at general prevention of early, deficiency-related bleeding rather than specific concerns about maternal anticonvulsant use. Research into the frequency and severity of this risk suggests that previous studies and clinical concerns have overestimated the probability of significantly increased risk of excessive bleeding in newborns exposed to maternal enzyme-inducing anticonvulsants in utero. In 1993, Cornelissen et al.[48] published their findings from a multicenter observational case-control study comparing the incidence of vitamin K deficiency in mother-infant pairs exposed to anticonvulsant drugs, with 25 pregnant women receiving anticonvulsant therapy and 25 pregnant controls. Maternal vitamin K_1 concentrations were lower in women with epilepsy than in controls, but PIVKA-II (protein induced by vitamin K absence of factor II) was rarely present. Even though mothers were rarely vitamin K deficient, the incidence of vitamin K deficiency still was increased in neonates exposed to anticonvulsant drugs prenatally. In a 2002 paper, Kaaja et al.[49] prospectively followed 662 pregnancies in women with epilepsy who used a variety of enzyme-inducing AEDs and compared outcomes with 1324 nonepileptic pregnancies as controls. None of the mothers received vitamin K_1 during pregnancy, but all infants received 1 mg vitamin K_1 intramuscularly at birth. An analysis of bleeding outcomes revealed that factors other than maternal enzyme-inducing AED use were more likely to be associated with increased risk for bleeding in the offspring. Nevertheless, the authors advised that antenatal administration of vitamin K to mothers undergoing drug therapy may still be appropriate in selected cases.

Some literature reviewers considering formulation of preventive health care policy have criticized the practice of IM administration of vitamin K throughout the last third of pregnancy to all women receiving anticonvulsants as not supported by the available evidence.[50] Beyond the issue of maternal medications, the broader debate on vitamin K delivery for newborns has shifted, with multiple concerns arising about potential risks of injection and emerging research supporting the efficacy and safety of oral prophylaxis. In this area, as with many other concerns regarding therapies for at-risk pregnant women, the ability to adequately assess obstetric interventions is hampered by the limited number of interventional studies that included long-term outcome assessment. More research is warranted into the clinically important question as to whether maternal vitamin K oral administration reduces anticonvulsant-associated birth defects.

Nutritional Therapeutics, Clinical Concerns, and Adaptations

Women taking enzyme-inductive anticonvulsant medications may benefit, as may their infants, from vitamin K coadministration during pregnancy to prevent neonatal bleeding disorders and congenital facial bone abnormalities.

Warfarin and Related Oral Vitamin K Antagonist Anticoagulants

Evidence: Warfarin (Coumadin, Marevan, Warfilone).
Extrapolated, based on similar properties: Anisindione (Miradon), dicumarol, ethyl biscoumacetate (Tromexan), nicoumalone (acenocoumarol; Acitrom, Sintrom), phenindione (Dindevan), phenprocoumon (Jarsin, Marcumar).

Interaction Type and Significance

◇◇ **Drug-Induced Effect on Nutrient Function, Supplementation Contraindicated, Professional Management Appropriate**

⊕✗ **Bimodal or Variable Interaction, with Professional Management**

◇ **Adverse Drug Effect on Nutritional Therapeutics, Strategic Concern**

◇ **Adverse Drug Effect on Herbal Therapeutics, Strategic Concern**

◇≈≈ **Drug-Induced Adverse Effect on Nutrient Function, Coadministration Therapeutic, with Professional Management**

Probability: Evidence Base:
1. Certain   ● Consensus

Effect and Mechanism of Action

Coumarins are vitamin K antagonists that produce their anticoagulant effect by interfering with the cyclic interconversion of vitamin K and its 2,3-epoxide (vitamin K epoxide). Vitamin K is primarily located in hepatic microsomes, where the vitamin K–dependent gamma-carboxylation as the final step in synthesis of prothrombin and factors VII, IX, and X occurs. Gamma-carboxylation is linked to vitamin K metabolism, specifically the cyclic interconversion of vitamin K and vitamin K epoxide. The primary site of action of warfarin and indandione anticoagulants appears to be an inhibition of the conversion of epoxide to vitamin K in this cycle. Warfarin's anticoagulant effect is based on the the drug being structurally a vitamin K "mimic" that binds to the vitamin K–dependent enzymes more avidly than does vitamin K, but does not allow the enzyme its active form, thus preventing gamma-carboxylation of coagulation factors II, VII, IX, and X; paradoxically, warfarin can exert a procoagulant response by interfering with proteins C and S. Without the gamma-carboxylation step, the factors lack adequate activity in the coagulation cascade. This vitamin K–epoxide cycle occurs in extrahepatic tissues such as kidney, spleen, and lung and is inhibited by warfarin. Thus, vitamin K epoxide is an intermediary metabolite of vitamin K that accumulates when it cannot be utilized, and thus is a marker of warfarin effect. There is a correlation between the inhibition of prothrombin synthesis and the regeneration of vitamin K from the epoxide by anticoagulants.

Gamma-carboxylation of glutamyl residues, facilitated by vitamin K, not only activates clotting factors but also activates osteocalcin and other bone matrix proteins. By inhibiting this process, vitamin K antagonists such as warfarin impair bone metabolism and increase the risk of osteoporotic fractures.[51]

Research

The simple issue of whether or not vitamin K, alone or in plant materials, interacts with warfarin and similar anticoagulants appears inherent and formulaic, which it is to a major degree. However, the nuances and complexities of individual variations and competing therapeutic agendas reveal a wider range of hidden risks and clinical options than initially evident. Moreover, a review of the research literature indicates that a significant gap exists between the therapeutic guidelines and prevailing clinical practices regarding the use of vitamin K for treatment of warfarin-associated coagulopathy.

A long-term debate as to the safest and most effective form of vitamin K for stabilizing an excessively elevated INR has recently approached an evidence-based consensus.[52] A series of randomized controlled trials, particularly those by Crowther et al.[53,54] and Lubetsky et al.,[55] have determined that oral vitamin K (phytonadione) lowers the INR more rapidly than subcutaneous vitamin K. Moreover, in some compromised ill patients, subcutaneous absorption, due to shunting of blood away from the skin, may actually be even less effective. Oral delivery also carries a substantially reduced risk of adverse reactions. In particular, intravenous administration carries a risk of anaphylaxis, although this may be significantly reduced by infusing over 30 minutes.

Clinical surveys, including ongoing research by Libby and Garcia[56] at the University of New Mexico, have determined that despite published reports of its safety and efficacy and established clinical protocols, a substantial number of anticoagulation clinics underutilize oral phytonadione in treating patients taking warfarin whose INR values are above therapeutic levels. In a 2002 paper, 100 separate anticoagulation clinics in the southwestern United States were surveyed with respect to the implementation of the recommendations for phytonadione use from the ACCP Fifth Consensus Conference on Antithrombotic Therapy. Of 53 respondents, 13 (25%) indicated that their clinics never use oral phytonadione. Eighteen (34%) indicated that their clinics use subcutaneous phytonadione, despite the absence of a recommendation for this in the 1998 ACCP guidelines. Only 17 respondents (32%) provided all four answers consistent with the ACCP recommendations.[56] The reasons for and implications of this apparent pattern of practice warrant broader and more in-depth research, in addition to confirming whether the observed phenomenon is representative of other geographic regions.

Individual sensitivity to warfarin is not consistent or fixed and appears to be influenced by vitamin K status, drug protein binding, and warfarin metabolism, among other variables. Reduced dietary vitamin K_1 intake potentiates the effect of warfarin in sick patients treated with antibiotics and IV fluids without vitamin K coadministration and in states of fat malabsorption. Hepatic dysfunction potentiates the response to warfarin through impaired synthesis of coagulation factors. Hypermetabolic states produced by fever or hyperthyroidism increase warfarin responsiveness, probably by increasing the catabolism of vitamin K–dependent coagulation factors. Lubetsky et al.[57] followed 50 patients commencing warfarin and consuming their regular diets for 8 weeks and concluded that in 32% (16/50) of anticoagulated patients under usual dietary conditions, sensitivity to warfarin is decreased by vitamin K intake of 250 µg/day or greater. Similarly, Cushman

et al.[58] investigated the association of vitamin K status with warfarin sensitivity among 40 orthopedic patients beginning perioperative algorithm-dosed warfarin and found that dietary and biochemical measures of vitamin K status were associated with early warfarin sensitivity.

As Iqbal, Linder, and others have discussed, the pharmacodynamics of warfarin are subject to significant genetic and environmental variability.[59-62] Research by O'Reilly, Aggeler, et al.,[64-66] as well as by Alving et al.,[67] found that hereditary resistance to warfarin occurs in rats as well as humans. Individuals with genetic warfarin resistance require doses five-fold to 20-fold higher than average to achieve an anticoagulant effect. This pharmacogenomic pattern of response is attributed to altered affinity of the receptor for warfarin because the plasma warfarin levels required to achieve an anticoagulant effect are increased. Furthermore, Scordo et al.[68] evaluated the influence of CYP2C9 and CYP2C19 genetic polymorphisms on warfarin maintenance dose and metabolic clearance in 93 Italian outpatients receiving long-term warfarin anticoagulant therapy. They concluded that "CYP2C9 genetic polymorphisms markedly influence warfarin dose requirements and metabolic clearance of the S-warfarin enantiomer, although non-genetic factors may also contribute to their large interindividual variability."

Overall, a greater clinical understanding of, and development of experience with, the dynamic equilibrium between vitamin K intake and anticoagulant medications, with a heightened appreciation for and responsiveness to individual variability, physiological dynamics, and evolving health status, will enable safer and more effective utilization of anticoagulant therapy and reduce unrealistic assumptions of static physiological states.[69-71] Sconce, Kamali, et al.[72,73] have published a series of papers proposing an appraisal of current vitamin K–dosing algorithms for the reversal of overanticoagulation with warfarin, providing evidence to support vitamin K administration to "improve stability of anticoagulation for patients with unexplained variability in response to warfarin," and emphasizing the "need for a more tailored dosing regimen." Such an evolution of clinical practice will enable greater flexibility and reveal opportunities for support of a broader criterion for health than simple disease management as defined by INR levels, including integrative therapeutic strategies incorporating more robust dietary options and appropriate therapeutic application of herbal preparations, aimed at enhancing healthy function, reducing cardiovascular risk, and reducing reliance on anticoagulants over time.

Clinical Implications and Adaptations

By design, warfarin and similar anticoagulant medications achieve their therapeutic effect by interfering with vitamin K function and metabolism. Conversely, vitamin K therapy can be employed to antidote excessive effects of such anticoagulant therapies. Within the clinical practice of integrative medicine, warfarin therapy presents significant challenges to the implementation of botanical and nutritional therapeutics, let alone maintaining a simple healthy diet rich in nutritive plant foods. However, through communication, collaboration, and coordination, seemingly contraindicated therapies can be used together through high levels of vigilance, close monitoring, and responsive management within a context of integrative care bringing together medical practitioners trained and experienced in nutritional therapeutics, herbal medicine, and conventional pharmacology. As Jaffer and Bragg[74] judiciously pointed out in a 2003 review of warfarin dosing and monitoring: "There is no evidence that consuming less vitamin K is more beneficial in maintaining anticoagulation control than consuming more."

Although the actions of anticoagulant medications and supplements, herbs, or foods containing vitamin K may be antagonistic on a tactical level, achieving and maintaining stability of coagulation factors are more important than mere presence or intake levels. More fundamentally, the primary strategic goals of disease prevention and health optimization must always remain clear and central. Amid valid concerns for effective anticoagulant protection, many physicians who prescribe coumadin anticoagulation instruct their patients to avoid consuming anything high in vitamin K, a practice that deprives them of many health-promoting phytonutrients. Consequently, from whatever source of information, many patients have been misinformed or otherwise come to believe that substances rich in vitamin K should be avoided if they are taking warfarin. However, simply eliminating plant foods rich in vitamin K and prohibiting use of therapeutically beneficial herbal prescriptions will not necessarily guarantee normalized INR values or support long-term medical objectives. Foods, herbs, and nutritional supplements inherently contain variable amounts of vitamin K and need to be evaluated with a thorough dietary assessment; the phylloquinone content of a wide range of foodstuffs has been listed by Sadowski et al.[75] Green leafy vegetables, such as kale, Swiss chard, spinach, broccoli, and mustard and turnip greens, are the foods that contain the highest amount of vitamin K per serving and thus are most likely to cause fluctuations in the INR.[76] Furthermore, in warfarinized patients any sudden reduction in intake of vitamin K from any of these sources is contraindicated because it may induce increased anticoagulation and increase bleeding risk through enhanced unopposed action of the medication.

Ultimately, the fundamental clinical management concern is maintaining a dynamic balance between vitamin K intake and warfarin, as represented in the INR; as such, however, the INR itself is secondary, if not irrelevant, to clinical outcomes and patient health, whether the patient reaches a therapeutic INR with 3 mg of warfarin, or 5, or 10, or even 20 mg. Warfarin itself is inexpensive and, unlike many pharmacological agents of its therapeutic potency, has no inherent toxicity or dose-related adverse effects, apart from its effects on vitamin K–related functions. Maintaining fairly constant vitamin K levels from both endogenous and exogenous sources is the key to stable anticoagulation with vitamin K antagonist anticoagulants. Thus, therapeutic agents containing vitamin K, whose actions are desirable for other reasons, are not necessarily contraindicated and can be used in the presence of anticoagulant medications if the individual has been stable during coadministration of such substances and anticoagulants, or if gradual, staged introduction of such agents is closely supervised and regularly monitored. Trust, communication, and education, along with systematic monitoring and flexible responses, are pivotal in the safe and effective management of vitamin K intake and INR stability within the context of a healthy diet and therapeutic use of herbal and nutritional therapies.

Management of a proper equilibrium between vitamin K intake and warfarin levels can be a challenging balancing act for both health care providers and patients, given the clinical importance of effective anticoagulant therapy and warfarin's narrow therapeutic index. Excessive vitamin K consumption can promote increased production of the vitamin K clotting factors, decreasing the anticoagulant response to warfarin. On the other hand, decreased vitamin K consumption can increase the anticoagulant response to warfarin. Normally it is sufficient to inform individuals taking warfarin to maintain

a moderate and consistent level of vitamin K in their diet, to avoid binge eating of vitamin K–rich foods, and to report any significant changes in diet, supplement, or herbal intake to their anticoagulant management team. During the course of coadministration of vitamin K–rich herbs (or foods) and warfarin, the anticoagulant dose will need to be titrated, based on recognition that the effects of a dose adjustment on a given day will be seen in the INR 2 days later. In general, it would be reasonable to monitor the PT and INR more frequently when any dietary change, herbal therapy, or drug therapy is added or withdrawn from the regimen of a patient treated with an oral anticoagulant. Evidence from randomized controlled trials continues to support the use of less-intense warfarin treatment for many indications. For most patients, within an INR range of 2.0 to 3.0, the lower level generally is safer and equally effective. Whenever possible, it can be beneficial for patients undergoing warfarin therapy to have a home monitor so that they can monitor their INR daily during such transitional processes. However, the increasing availability of oral, direct thrombin inhibitors, such as Exanta, may soon reduce the risk of drug interactions and the need to restrict vitamin K intake, as well as provide a sufficiently predictable effect that high levels of monitoring become unnecessary.

Exercise is important in the elderly population and in individuals with cardiovascular disease. Clinical care needs to emphasize measures to counter the adverse effects of warfarin and other vitamin K antagonists on normal bone metabolism and subsequent elevation in the risk of osteoporotic fractures. Thus, particularly when prescribing anticoagulants to elderly individuals or others at high risk of falling, health care providers are advised to instruct patients to wear stable shoes, exercise regularly, maintain adequate intake of calcium and vitamin D, employ walking aids, and discontinue unnecessary and potentially complicating medications.

THEORETICAL, SPECULATIVE, AND PRELIMINARY INTERACTIONS RESEARCH, INCLUDING OVERSTATED INTERACTIONS CLAIMS

Acetylsalicylic Acid (Aspirin) and Salicylates

Acetylsalicylic Acid (acetosal, acetyl salicylic acid, ASA, salicylsalicylic acid; Arthritis Foundation Pain Reliever, Ascriptin, Aspergum, Asprimox, Bayer Aspirin, Bayer Buffered Aspirin, Bayer Low Adult Strength, Bufferin, Buffex, Cama Arthritis Pain Reliever, Easprin, Ecotrin, Ecotrin Low Adult Strength, Empirin, Extra Strength Adprin-B, Extra Strength Bayer Enteric 500 Aspirin, Extra Strength Bayer Plus, Halfprin 81, Heartline, Regular Strength Bayer Enteric 500 Aspirin, St. Joseph Adult Chewable Aspirin, ZORprin); combination drugs: ASA and caffeine (Anacin); ASA, caffeine, and propoxyphene (Darvon Compound); ASA and carisoprodol (Soma Compound); ASA, codeine, and carisoprodol (Soma Compound with Codeine); ASA and codeine (Empirin with Codeine); ASA, codeine, butalbital, and caffeine (Fiorinal); ASA and extended-release dipyridamole (Aggrenox, Asasantin).
Salsalate (salicylic acid; Amigesic, Disalcid, Marthritic, Mono Gesic, Salflex, Salsitab).
Related salicylates: Choline salicylate, magnesium salicylate, salsalate, diflunisal, sodium salicylate, sodium thiosalicylate.

The combination of vitamin K sources and aspirin or salicylates represents a possible bimodal interaction and as such could be beneficial or self-defeating, depending on intention, coordination, and implementation. Long-term use of aspirin is supported by a broad base of evidence for reducing cardiovascular risk but carries numerous adverse effects, including the possibility that it may increase the need for vitamin K. Aspirin and nonsteroidal anti-inflammatory drugs can produce gastric erosions that increase the risk of upper gastrointestinal bleeding. The resultant risk of clinically important bleeding is heightened when high doses of aspirin are taken in combination with high-intensity warfarin therapy (INR, 3.0-4.5). Conversely, vitamin K provides significant potential benefit in prevention of cardiovascular disease, but concern has been raised that increased intake may interfere with blood-thinning function of prophylactic aspirin. The mechanisms of such effect are uncertain and problematic because there is no well-known interaction between platelet function and vitamin K. Such concern may derive from a common misconception that because coumadin "thins blood," vitamin K in large amounts "thickens it" or creates a procoagulable state. Further research is warranted, and ultimately either a choice of therapeutic strategies may be required or protocols for innovative integrative options may prove effective in clinical trials.

Olestra

Olestra (Olean)

Olestra, the fat substitute composed of hexa-, hepta- and octa-esters of sucrose, may reduce the absorption of vitamin K and contribute to a deficiency.[77] Compensatory vitamin K supplementation may be advisable, espically on at-risk populations.

Orlistat

Orlistat (alli, Xenical)

Orlistat could theoretically reduce the absorption of vitamin K and other fat-soluble nutrients. Evidence of a significant depletion pattern is lacking. In a clinical trial involving 17 obese African-American and Caucasian adolescents receiving orlistat, 120 mg three times daily, McDuffie et al.[78] observed several significant nutrient depletion patterns, despite coadministration of a daily multivitamin containing vitamin A (5000 IU), vitamin D (400 IU), vitamin E (300 IU), and vitamin K (25 μg). However, during 3 to 6 months of orlistat treatment, the decrease in serum levels of vitamins K was not significant.[78]

NUTRIENT-NUTRIENT INTERACTIONS

Vitamin C

In 1952, Merkel[79] found that coadministration of menadione bisulfite and ascorbate provided complete relief of symptoms within 3 days in 64 of 70 consecutive cases of nausea and vomiting of pregnancy.

Vitamin K_2 combined with IV ascorbate has shown recent promise as an oxidative therapy for cancer. Similar preliminary studies have involved the use of vitamin K_3 in conjunction with IV ascorbate.[80-84] Vitamin K_3 is a more active free-radical generator than is K_2.

Vitamin E

Vitamin E in high doses may interfere with the absorption and utilization of vitamin K. In two independent, randomized clinical trials, Booth et al.[85] investigated the effect of 12 weeks of supplementation with RRR-alpha-tocopherol (1000 IU/day) on vitamin K status, as represented by several biochemical indicators, in 38 men and women with rheumatoid arthritis (study A) and in 32 healthy men (study B), none of whom were taking oral anticoagulants. Plasma phylloquinone concentrations and the percentage of undercarboxylated osteocalcin did not change significantly in response to the vitamin E. However, the degree of mean PIVKA-II (under-gamma-carboxylation of prothrombin; proteins induced by vitamin K absence—factor II), increased from 1.7 to 11.9 ng/mL in study A and from 1.8 to 5.3 ng/mL in study B after the 12 weeks of vitamin E supplementation. This pattern of potential interaction could play a role in cases of enhanced anticoagulant effect in response to high-dose vitamin E intake reported among patients taking oral anticoagulants.

Refer to the Warfarin section of the Vitamin E monograph for further discussion of these issues.

The 85 citations for this monograph, as well as additional reference literature, are located under Vitamin K on the CD at the back of the book.

Boron

Nutrient Name: Boron
Synonyms: Boron chelates—boron aspartate, boron citrate, and boron glycinate; sodium borate.
Elemental Symbol: B.
Related Substance: Borax, boric acid.

Summary

Drug/Class Interaction Type	Mechanism and Significance	Management
Hormone replacement therapy (HRT) Estrogens/progestins ✗/⊕✗/⊕⊕	Increased boron intake may contribute to elevated levels of estradiol (and testosterone). Coadministration of boron and estrogen enhancement therapies could provide synergistic benefit toward preventing bone demineralization, limiting bone loss, and treating osteoporosis. Concomitant use of exogenous female hormones and supplemental boron could theoretically increase risk of adverse effects of excess estrogen; however, available evidence suggests no association between high boron intake and elevated risk of breast cancer. Evidence from human research is limited. Well-designed long-term clinical trials are warranted.	Encourage increased dietary intake of boron-rich vegetables, fruits, and nuts as safe and efficacious, especially in conjunction with exercise and supplementation with calcium and vitamin D. Monitor when coadministration with supplemental boron indicated.

NUTRIENT DESCRIPTION

Chemistry and Form

Boron, the fifth chemical element, is a nonmetallic mineral present in the human body in trace amounts. In nature, boron is most prevalent as *borax*, which is a mixture of boron, sodium, and oxygen.

Physiology and Function

Boron is involved in the metabolic functions of many key nutrients, including calcium, copper, magnesium, phosphorus, potassium, and vitamin D. Although essential for plants, controversy remains unresolved as to whether boron is an essential nutrient for humans. Knowledge is incomplete as to the mechanism of absorption from the gastrointestinal tract, but it is known that dietary boron is rapidly absorbed. Boron is distributed throughout the body tissues, with the highest concentrations found in bones, dental enamel, spleen, and thyroid gland. Boron is primarily excreted in the urine, with bile, sweat, and breath serving as secondary routes of elimination.

The available streams of research have yet to coalesce into a comprehensive understanding of this nutrient's functions and relationships. Conventional research usually focuses on boron's particularly strong affinity for bone and joint tissue, where it influences composition, structure, and strength. However, a broader interpretation of the body of scientific evidence from animal and human studies indicates that boron acts as an essential ally of other substances in fine-tuning many human physiological interactions. Thus, boron exerts much of its influence by playing an integrative role in the areas of bone metabolism, joint health, mental acuity, wound healing, and proper functioning of the endocrine system.[1] Boron plays a major role in cell membrane functions, where it affects response to hormones (e.g., estrogen, vitamin D) that are involved in bone turnover and through its influence on transmembrane signaling or transmembrane movement of regulatory ions (e.g., calcium, magnesium). Boron participates in many aspects of the regulation of metabolism. For example, it lowers blood glucose levels in vitamin D deficiency states through its interaction with compounds having hydroxyl groups; it exhibits estrogen-mimetic activity; it appears to participate in regulating the respiratory burst of neutrophils; and it affects the activity of certain enzymes. Boron also plays an important but as-yet not fully elucidated role in cognitive and psychomotor functions.

The relationship between boron and calcium appears to be especially important, with increased boron levels associated with increased absorption of calcium, magnesium, and phosphorus and reduced urinary excretion of minerals, notably calcium. Boron facilitates metabolism of magnesium, copper, and potassium. It facilitates hydroxylation reactions to participate in the activation of vitamin D and to affect human steroid hormone levels and synthesis of estrogens and testosterone. Thus, increased boron intake may enhance both calcium absorption and serum levels of endogenous estradiol and testosterone. These multiple actions suggest that boron plays a key role in calcium and magnesium homeostasis, promotes bone mineralization, and mitigates bone loss, thus reducing the risk of osteoporosis. However, as with most nutrients, this effect is most significant in individuals with inadequate dietary intake of relevant minerals, with deficient magnesium intake being critical to variability in the activity of boron.

NUTRIENT IN CLINICAL PRACTICE

Known or Potential Therapeutic Uses

Consistent but limited evidence suggests that supplemental boron may be beneficial in supporting bone health and treating skeletal degeneration. In particular, preliminary evidence indicates that boron exerts beneficial effects on calcium metabolism and bone demineralization in postmenopausal women by reducing calcium loss (through excretion in the urine).[2,3] Findings from a double-blind, placebo-controlled pilot study involving 20 subjects with osteoarthritis demonstrated a significant favorable response to supplementation with 6 mg boron per day; 50% of subjects receiving the nutrient improved, compared with only 10% receiving placebo.[4] However, strong evidence is lacking from clinical trials to confirm boron's efficacy in preventing or treating osteoarthritis. Emerging epidemiological data and experimental research support the use of boron in prevention and treatment of prostate cancer.[1,5,6]

Some commentators have voiced the recommendation that food sources may be safer than supplements and therefore preferable. Nevertheless, health care professionals trained and experienced in nutritional therapies generally administer boron within the context of a comprehensive strategy including calcium, vitamin D, magnesium, and trace minerals such as zinc, copper, and manganese. Principles of judicious clinical management suggest that laboratory assessment of boron levels to elicit deficiency status may be valuable.

Historical/Ethnomedicine Precedent

Boron has not been used historically as an isolated nutrient.

Possible Uses

Osteoarthritis, osteoporosis, prostate cancer, rheumatoid arthritis.

Deficiency Symptoms

Consensus is lacking on specific signs and symptoms of boron deficiency. However, observed effects of boron depletion include increased urinary loss of calcium and magnesium and increased rate of bone demineralization. Epidemiological evidence from geographic areas with low soil boron reveals an inverse relationship between the dietary intake of boron and the incidence of arthritis. In areas of the world where daily boron intakes usually are 1.0 mg or less, the estimated incidence of arthritis ranges from 20% to 70%, whereas in areas of the world where boron intakes are usually 3 to 10 mg, the estimated incidence of arthritis ranges from 0% to 10%. Therefore, patients living in such areas should be especially informed regarding this factor, and the same approach applies to other elements, significantly influenced by locale, such as selenium and vitamin D.

Dietary Sources

Raisins, prunes, dates, almonds, hazelnuts, and peanuts are the richest sources of boron. Significant amounts are available in most leafy vegetables, noncitrus fruits, and legumes, as well as beer, wine, and cider. However, the actual amounts of boron in plant sources will vary widely, depending on boron levels in the soil in which the food is grown. Meat, fish, and poultry provide minimal amounts of boron.

Dosage Forms Available

Capsule, liquid, tablet.

Source Materials for Nutrient Preparations

Sodium borate is the simple sodium salt of boric acid. Chelates are produced by reacting boron compounds with various organic and amino acids.

Dosage Range

Adult

Dietary: No dietary or nutritional requirement for boron has been established. Average adult boron intake in the United States has been estimated at 1 mg per day.[7] Rainey and Nyquist[8] confirmed this in a six-nation comparison of dietary boron conducted during the 1990s for the World Health Organization. They found that U.S. adults consumed, on average, slightly more than 1 mg daily, approximately 7% to 10% less than average boron intake levels of individuals in Britain and Egypt and 32% to 41% less than Germans, Kenyans, and Mexicans. Individuals who eat healthy amounts of fruits and vegetables, nuts, and legumes will generally have a boron intake in the range of 2 to 6 mg per day.[9]

Supplemental/Maintenance: The optimal dose of boron for proper physiological function and prevention of osteoporosis appears to be 3 to 6 mg per day.

Pharmacological/Therapeutic: Pharmacological doses used in clinical studies range from less than 1 mg up to 12 mg per day. Administration of 3 mg three times daily constitutes a typical therapeutic dose in the treatment of arthritis. A trial period of 2 to 4 months is usually indicated. Individuals being treated for rheumatoid arthritis will generally report symptom amelioration within 4 weeks of beginning boron supplementation.[10]

Toxic: The potential lethal dose for adults is estimated at 15 to 20 g per day[11]; 150 mg per liter of water represents a toxic concentration of boron.

Pediatric (<18 Years)

Dietary: No minimal dietary requirement established specifically for infants and children.

Supplemental/Maintenance: Not currently recommended for children.

Pharmacological/Therapeutic: Reports based on clinical observations indicate that children with juvenile arthritis (Still's disease) may improve in 2 to 3 weeks with administration of 6 to 9 mg boron daily.[10]

Toxic: No toxic dosage level established specifically for infants and children.

Laboratory Values

Deoxypyridinoline (D-ppd), and to a lesser degree pyridinium (Pyd), can provide a noninvasive evaluation of the biochemical markers of bone loss and assessment of bone resorption, which may be affected by multiple factors, including boron status.

Blood levels and hair analysis may also provide useful data in establishing boron status.

SAFETY PROFILE
Overview

Boron is generally considered relatively nontoxic for most individuals at usual supplemental doses, which are approximately equivalent to typical dietary intake levels. Adverse effects such as nausea and vomiting are only associated with doses 50 times the upper level of the recommended range.

Nutrient Adverse Effects
General Adverse Effects

Accidental acute exposure to high levels of boron (e.g., oral doses >100 mg/day) can cause disturbances in appetite and digestion, nausea, vomiting, abdominal pain, diarrhea, dermatitis, convulsions, fatigue, and other symptoms; fatality is rare but has been reported.[12] The most frequently cited case involved a reported suicide where boric acid was ingested.[13]

Chronic exposures may be responsible for some toxic symptomatology. However, the daily dosage levels of 1 to 3 mg provided by most supplements containing boron have not been linked with toxicity in most reports. Areas with dietary boron intake of up to 41 mg/day have not produced associated patterns of adverse medical or health outcomes.

Adverse Effects Among Specific Populations

In one clinical trial, some menopausal women reported aggravations of hot flashes and night sweats with supplemental boron intake; others experienced amelioration of such symptoms.[14]

Pregnancy and Nursing

Qualified reports of adverse effects during pregnancy or nursing are lacking. However, the lack of clinical data from human trials or reports does not provide adequate evidence to confirm safety of boron during pregnancy and breastfeeding.

Infants and Children

Children exposed to boron-containing dusting powders and lotions, particularly containing borax or boric acid, constitute a high proportion of reports of toxicity. Irritation is common when such substances are applied to broken skin and mucous membranes. External boron-related preparations are generally best avoided.

Contraindications

Prudence suggests that supplemental boron be avoided during pregnancy because of potential effects on estrogen metabolism.

Precautions and Warnings

Newnham[10] has cautioned that individuals being treated for rheumatoid arthritis may experience an aggravation of symptoms (Herxheimer response) during the initial 1 to 3 weeks.

The increase in estrogen associated with elevated boron intake indicated by some preliminary research could theoretically increase the risk of several cancers. Nevertheless, no epidemiological evidence has confirmed an increased risk of cancer in areas of the world where dietary boron intake is high. Out of caution, some physicians have recommended that supplemental boron intake be limited to a maximum of 1 mg/day. Boron intake through regular consumption of fruits, vegetables, nuts, and legumes will generally exceed 1 mg/day and can provide a risk-free method for enhancing boron levels. Menopausal women experiencing increased hot flashes or night sweats might consider discontinuation of supplemental boron to determine whether the severity of their symptoms is reduced.

INTERACTIONS REVIEW
Strategic Considerations

The effects of boron on calcium metabolism and steroid hormone activity form the basis for the known and other potential therapeutic activity and related interactions. In particular, the probable interaction between boron and estrogen (as well as testosterone) may exemplify a bimodal interaction pattern. Boron's direct role in bone health and various effects on calcium, other minerals, and vitamin D provide its primary value (and common use) in preventing and treating osteoporosis and osteoarthritis.

Boron's potential ability to enhance estrogen (and possibly testosterone) could be therapeutically efficacious in supporting bone and joint health and preventing bone loss. However, concern has been raised as to potential risk of excessive estrogen response, especially in the context of hormone replacement therapy (HRT), which has already been associated with increased risk of breast and uterine cancer, as well as increased risk of dementia and thrombosis. Although long-term use of estrogen and progestin in combination does appear to lower a woman's overall risk for colon tumors, researchers say HRT users who do develop colon cancer are less likely to have it detected at an early stage, when it is most treatable. The coadministration of boron and estrogen support therapies could provide a valuable strategic synergy in the preventing bone loss and treating osteoporosis. Clinicians working to enhance

the effects of estrogen are advised to monitor any changes in hormone status related to coadministration of boron. Conversely, restriction of boron intake could conceivably play a supportive role in therapeutic strategies aimed at limiting or reducing estrogen levels, such as in the prevention or treatment of estrogen-sensitive breast cancer. Boron supplementation might also prove useful in situations of hormone blockade and chemotherapy-induced osteoporosis, common in treatment of breast and prostate cancer, although careful clinical trials would be necessary to ensure that any increase in hormone levels induced by boron would be adequately offset by boron's apparent chemoprevention properties.

Evidence from in vitro, animal, and human studies indicates that boron can inhibit enzymes such as serine proteases, notably prostate-specific antigen (PSA). In a prostate cancer mouse model employing the LNCaP human prostate cancer cell line, boric acid has been found to decrease PSA by 87%, reduce tumor size, and lower tumor expression of insulin-like growth factor-1 (IGF-1), a tumor trophic factor.[15-18] As previously noted, dietary boron intake is strongly associated with reduced risk of prostate cancer.[6,8,19] Strum[1] has cited boron's known ability to inhibit cyclooxygenase (COX) and lipoxygenase (LOX), key enzymes mediating the inflammatory cascade, and noted: "Such anti-inflammatory capabilities of boron are clearly pertinent to its anti-cancer effect, because the reduction of COX II and LOX enzymes leads to a decrease in prostaglandin E_2 (PGE_2) and other unfavorable eicosanoids such as leukotrienes."

No reports or studies documenting drug-induced depletion of boron were accessible for review.

NUTRIENT-DRUG INTERACTIONS

Hormone Replacement Therapy (HRT): Estrogen-Containing and Synthetic Estrogen and Progesterone Analog Medications

HRT, estrogens: Chlorotrianisene (Tace); conjugated equine estrogens (Premarin); conjugated synthetic estrogens (Cenestin); dienestrol (Ortho Dienestrol); esterified estrogens (Estratab, Menest, Neo-Estrone); estradiol, topical/transdermal/ring (Alora Transdermal, Climara Transdermal, Estrace, Estradot, Estring FemPatch, Vivelle-Dot, Vivelle Transdermal); estradiol cypionate (Dep-Gynogen, Depo-Estradiol, Depogen, Dura-Estrin, Estra-D, Estro-Cyp, Estroject-LA, Estronol-LA); estradiol hemihydrate (Estreva, Vagifem); estradiol valerate (Delestrogen, Estra-L 40, Gynogen L.A. 20, Progynova, Valergen 20); estrone (Aquest, Estragyn 5, Estro-A, Estrone '5', Kestrone-5); estropipate (Ogen, Ortho-Est); ethinyl estradiol (Estinyl, Gynodiol, Lynoral).

HRT, estrogen/progestin combinations: Conjugated equine estrogens and medroxyprogesterone (Premelle cycle 5, Prempro); conjugated equine estrogens and norgestrel (Prempak-C); estradiol and dydrogesterone (Femoston); estradiol and norethindrone, patch (CombiPatch); estradiol and norethindrone/norethisterone, oral (Activella, Climagest, Climesse, FemHRT, Trisequens); estradiol valerate and cyproterone acetate (Climens); estradiol valerate and norgestrel (Progyluton); estradiol and norgestimate (Ortho-Prefest).

HRT, estrogen/testosterone combinations: Esterified estrogens and methyltestosterone (Estratest, Estratest HS).

Interaction Type and Significance

✗   **Potential or Theoretical Adverse Interaction of Uncertain Severity**

⊕✗   **Bimodal or Variable Interaction, with
Professional Management**
⊕⊕   **Beneficial or Supportive Interaction, with
Professional Management**

Coadministration Benefit
Probability: Evidence Base:
2. Probable   ○ Preliminary or
                            ◉ Emerging

Coadministration Risk
Probability: Evidence Base:
4. Plausible   ○ Preliminary or
                            ▽ Mixed

Effect and Mechanism of Action

Boron may elevate estradiol and testosterone levels, especially in those with low dietary intake of boron and magnesium. The probable beneficial influence of boron in limiting calcium loss and supporting bone mineralization may be amplified by enhancement of steroid hormone status.

Research

Several small studies have shown an association between boron and increased estrogen levels, both in menopausal women not on estrogen replacement therapy (ERT) and healthy men and, more markedly, in women on ERT.

For many years a research team led by Nielsen, Hunt, and Penland in North Dakota has conducted numerous studies investigating boron, its activities, and therapeutic implications. In a 1987 clinical trial,[3] they observed marked changes in several indices of mineral metabolism in seven women consuming a low-magnesium diet and five women consuming a diet adequate in magnesium after administering a nutritional dose of boron (3 mg/day) for 48 days to these 12 women, age 48 to 82, not on ERT. Before the study, all subjects had consumed a conventional diet supplying about 0.25 mg boron daily for 119 days, that is, a diet essentially devoid of fruits and vegetables. Women receiving the boron demonstrated marked reductions in urinary excretion of calcium and magnesium and increased levels of plasma ionized calcium, especially in subjects receiving low dietary magnesium intake. Boron supplementation depressed the urinary excretion of phosphorus by the low-magnesium, but not by the adequate-magnesium, women. These researchers also reported marked elevations in serum concentrations of 17β-estradiol (the most potent of the naturally produced estrogens) and testosterone in response to the boron supplementation; again, the elevation was more pronounced in subjects on a low-magnesium diet. These findings "suggest that supplementation of a low-boron diet with an amount of boron commonly found in diets high in fruits and vegetables induces changes in postmenopausal women consistent with the prevention of calcium loss and bone demineralization."[3] Subsequently, Nielsen and Penland[14] reported elevated estrogen in several perimenopausal women administered 2.5 mg boron per day as well as other changes in boron metabolism and indices associated with macromineral metabolism, hormonal status, and immune function.

In a single-blind, placebo-controlled, crossover trial involving 18 healthy men, Naghii and Samman[20] reported that administration of boron at 10 mg/day for 4 weeks was associated with significantly increased plasma estradiol levels and a trend toward increased testosterone levels. These authors commented that the nutrient-induced elevation of endogenous estrogen suggests a protective role for boron in atherosclerosis.

Nutritional Therapeutics, Clinical Concerns, and Adaptations

The limited body of available evidence reveals a clear and emergent pattern indicating that health care professionals should encourage increased boron intake in individuals for whom elevated estrogen (and testosterone) levels will be beneficial, especially for preventing demineralization, limiting bone loss, and treating osteoporosis. Boron supplementation is especially important in postmenopausal women consuming a low-boron diet to prevent bone demineralization and osteoporosis; the importance of encouraging a varied diet rich in vegetables, fruits, and nuts cannot be overemphasized for general wellness and bone health in particular. A synergistic combination of oral calcium, vitamin D, boron, and magnesium, within the context of an active lifestyle, could reasonably be considered as a core proactive intervention within integrative therapeutics for all individuals at high risk for osteoporosis, or a foundational treatment for diagnosed bone loss. Additionally, hormone supplementation or replacement regimens (conventional HRT, bio-identical estrogens/progesterone, isoflavones, herbal hormone precursors/modulators) may achieve similar effects, but conclusive evidence is lacking; further research through clinical trials is warranted. Well-designed studies, published in peer-reviewed journals, have confirmed the benefits of ipriflavone and its amelioration of bone loss.

Dietary sources may be preferable, but evidence is lacking for claims of a significant adverse effects or increased risks attributable to boron supplementation at usual dosage levels of 1 to 3 mg/day. The consensus for increased dietary intake of foods rich in boron, especially nuts and fruits, receives at least nominal attention in conventional care and is strongly emphasized in health care providers trained and experienced in nutritional, preventive, and integrative approaches to healthy aging and bone-protective strategies. Some authors in secondary and derivative literature have voiced questionable, but often strong, cautions against use of supplemental boron as potentially risky because of possible elevated hormone levels. Such a concern for nutrient-induced adverse effects is curious, if not overstated, given the rising tide of research on adverse effects and limited efficacy of conventional estrogen-based HRT and momentous shift in health policy away from indiscriminate long-term HRT prescribing. Increased risks of breast and uterine cancer, as well as thromboembolism and dementia, may be related to artificial estrogen administration (and poor liver conjugation), but it is unreasonable to attribute such risks to boron. In fact, epidemiological evidence indicates that high boron intake from dietary sources does not affect breast cancer rates. Furthermore, the strong and growing trend of evidence supporting boron's role in reducing risk of prostate cancer (and potentially reversing pathological changes) dissuades against unfounded cautions regarding potential elevations in testosterone levels. Emerging evidence that boron functions as both a COX and LOX inhibitor may be related to its apparent activity as a candidate chemoprevention agent for both breast and prostate cancer. Clearly, the body of specific and general evidence from both the scientific literature and clinical experience supports increased boron intake as part of a comprehensive strategy for bone health.

THEORETICAL, SPECULATIVE, AND PRELIMINARY INTERACTIONS RESEARCH, INCLUDING OVERSTATED INTERACTIONS CLAIMS

Benign Prostatic Hypertrophy and Prostate Cancer Treatments

See Strategic Considerations.

NUTRIENT-NUTRIENT INTERACTIONS

Calcium

Boron exerts a favorable influence on calcium absorption, function, and excretion. In a 1987 clinical trial, Nielsen, Hunt, et al.[3] observed marked changes in several indices of mineral metabolism in seven women on a low-magnesium diet and five women on a diet adequate in magnesium, after a nutritional dose of boron (3 mg/day) for 48 days to these 12 women, age 48 to 82, not on ERT. Before the study, all subjects had consumed a conventional diet supplying about 0.25 mg boron daily for 119 days (i.e., a diet essentially devoid of fruits and vegetables). Women receiving the boron demonstrated marked reductions in urinary excretion of calcium and magnesium and increased levels of plasma ionized calcium, especially those receiving low dietary magnesium intake. Subsequent research by Nielsen et al.[21] indicated that 3 mg/day boron supplementation in men over age 45 and postmenopausal women on a low-magnesium diet contributed to several beneficial effects, including increased concentration of plasma ionized and total calcium, as well as reduced serum calcitonin concentration and urinary excretion of calcium. Later research by Nielsen[22] demonstrated that a low-boron diet elevated urinary calcium excretion.

Copper

Boron appears to increase serum levels of both copper and copper-dependent enzymes in humans. In a small trial involving five men over age 45, four postmenopausal women, and five postmenopausal women on estrogen therapy who had been fed a diet low in boron for 63 days, Nielsen et al.[21] demonstrated that boron (3 mg/day) administration resulted in higher erythrocyte superoxide dismutase (SOD), serum enzymatic ceruloplasmin, and plasma copper. Nielsen[22] confirmed these findings in a subsequent trial where the same variables were higher during boron repletion than while subjects were fed a diet low in boron. Higher SOD levels may be a mechanism of action for boron's improvement in degenerative joint disease. Some practitioners report using SOD in patients with outstanding results; SOD levels can be measured. The elevation in copper can be of concern because copper is a pro-angiogenesis element (in opposition to zinc).

Magnesium

Boron supports magnesium function and may assume some of its functions in states of magnesium deficiency. The interaction between boron and magnesium appears to be most significant when magnesium deprivation is severe enough to produce typical signs of deficiency.[23] Animal research by Hunt[24] indicated that a combined deficiency of boron and magnesium leads to detrimental alterations in the bones of animals. Introduction of additional boron elevated plasma magnesium concentrations and enhanced growth. Nielsen[2] and later Hunt et al.[25] found that boron's ability to reduce urinary loss of calcium disappeared when subjects were administered concomitant magnesium. Moseman[26] reported increased serum magnesium concentrations in female subjects after administration of supplemental boron. Meacham et al.[27] compared boron and magnesium in relation to exercise in women and found higher serum magnesium concentrations in sedentary females whose diets are supplemented with boron than in female athletes supplemented with boron while maintaining an exercise regimen.

Methionine and Arginine

In a series of nine experiments lasting 6 to 10 weeks using rats deprived of boron, Nielsen et al.[28] found that the severity of magnesium deprivation and the methionine status of the rat strongly influence the extent and nature of the interaction between magnesium and boron, as well as the response to boron deprivation. The beneficial impact of boron administration was consistently observed when the diet contained marginal methionine and luxuriant arginine. Depressed growth and bone magnesium concentration, as well as elevated spleen/body weight and kidney/body weight ratios, were among the signs exhibited by rats fed a diet marginal in methionine and magnesium. The authors interpreted their findings as indicating that the severity of such symptoms was alleviated with boron administration.

Phosphorus

Administration of boron appears to lower serum phosphorus concentrations. These effects have been observed in rats and in female subjects, age 20 to 27.[26,28] Exercise may diminish these effects as a result of increased loss of or elevated metabolic demand for boron.[26] Urinary excretion of phosphorus may be reduced when boron is administered in the context of low magnesium status, although not under conditions of adequate magnesium intake.

S-Adenosyl-L-Methionine (SAMe)

Ongoing studies are focusing on the naturally occurring molecules for which boron has an affinity, including S-adenosyl-L-methionine (S-adenosylmethionine, SAMe). Well-designed studies, published in peer-reviewed journals, have confirmed the benefits of SAMe in the treatment of osteoarthritis. Thus, given research demonstrating that boron may have a positive effect on osteoarthritis by helping to preserve bone, it may be reasonable to use boron in concert with SAMe to relieve painful arthritic symptoms.[29]

Vitamin B₂ (Riboflavin)

High doses of boron may increase excretion of riboflavin. Pinto et al.[30] showed that boric acid ingestion can induce urinary losses of riboflavin. Therefore, supplementation with B complex may be advised in patients with high boron intakes.

Vitamin D (Calciferol)

Boron appears to play a significant role in converting vitamin D to its more active form, thus facilitating calcium absorption. This observation is clinically relevant because it supports the practice of using vitamin D_3 with boron, rather than calcitriol, and thereby avoiding the high costs of calcitriol.

After examining animal nutrition models, Hunt[31] concluded that that dietary boron alleviates perturbations in mineral metabolism characteristic of vitamin D_3 deficiency. Hunt et al.[32] found that dietary boron modifies the effects of vitamin D_3 nutrition on indices of energy substrate utilization and mineral metabolism in the chick. For example, chicks fed a diet containing insufficient vitamin D for 26 days exhibited decreased food consumption and plasma calcium concentrations, as well as increased plasma concentrations of glucose, β-hydroxybutyrate, triglycerides, triiodothyronine, cholesterol, and alkaline phosphatase activity. Plasma glucose and triglycerides returned to concentrations exhibited by chicks fed a diet adequate in vitamin D after administration of boron. Such findings support the coadministration of boron and vitamin D_3 in diabetes management. Likewise, boron elevated the numbers of osteoclasts and alleviated malformation of the marrow sprouts of the proximal tibial epiphyseal plate in rachitic (vitamin D–deficient) chicks, thus correcting a distortion characteristic of vitamin D_3 deficiency.[24] In an experiment investigating the effects of dietary boron in rats fed a vitamin D–deficient diet, Dupre et al.[33] observed that introduction of boron into the diet resulted in higher apparent-balance values of calcium, magnesium, and phosphorus.

In a study involving male subjects over 45 years of age and postmenopausal women fed a low-magnesium and low-copper diet, Nielsen et al.[21] showed that administration of 3.25 mg of boron per day increased levels of plasma vitamin D_2.

The 33 citations for this monograph, as well as additional reference literature, are located under Boron on the CD at the back of the book.

Nutrient-Drug Interactions and Drug-Induced Nutrient Depletions

Calcium

Nutrient Name: Calcium.
Synonyms: Calcium ascorbate, calcium aspartate, calcium carbonate, calcium citrate, calcium gluconate, calcium lactate.
Elemental Symbol: Ca.
Related Substance: Microcrystalline hydroxyapatite (MCHC)

Nutrient-Drug Interactions and Drug-Induced Nutrient Depletions

Summary

Drug/Class Interaction Type	Mechanism and Significance	Management
Aminoglycoside antibiotics ≈≈/☼	Nephrotoxic effects of aminoglycosides can increase calcium excretion. Calcium coadministration may be protective but may potentiate adverse effects, especially of gentamicin, although such nephrotoxic synergy has only been demonstrated with parenteral, not oral, calcium coadministration.	Coadminister with extended use; closely monitor renal function and serum calcium, magnesium, and potassium.
Amphotericin B ≈≈≈/☼	Toxicity of amphotericin B associated with increased intracellular calcium concentration. This drug can deplete and disrupt calcium and other minerals. Well documented but not well understood.	Monitor electrolytes and coadminister minerals as indicated. Consider using less toxic liposomal formulation instead.
Antacids, aluminum- and magnesium-containing ✗✗✗/≈≈≈	Aluminum-based antacids may reduce calcium absorption and complex with phosphates to deplete calcium. Calcium citrate may increase aluminum absorption.	Avoid calcium citrate during therapy. Minimize use of aluminum-based antacids.
Anticonvulsant medications ≈≈≈/◇/☼	Antiepileptic drugs, particularly phenytoin and phenobarbital, can decrease calcium absorption, accelerate vitamin D metabolism in liver (CYP450 induction), and may reduce serum levels of 25(OH) vitamin D. Thus, anticonvulsants impair mineralization, leading to increased risk of bone loss, osteoporosis, and fractures. Mechanisms well established; clinical implications variable.	Coadminister calcium and vitamin D. Monitor serum 25(OH)D and bone status. Promote sunlight exposure and weight-bearing exercise.
Atenolol Beta-1-adrenoceptor antagonists ◇/◇/◇	Simultaneous intake may inhibit absorption and bioavailability of both agents, which over time may increase drug half-life and may cause accumulation.	Separate intake by 2 hours. Monitor blood pressure and heart rate as indices of beta-blocker levels.
Bisphosphonates ⊕⊕⊕/◇ ◇/◇	Synergistic interaction. Vitamin D assists calcium absorption, and both enable bisphosphonates in maintaining bone mineralization, including with HRT.	Coadminister calcium and vitamin D. Promote appropriate sunlight exposure and weight-bearing exercise.
Calcitonin ⊕⊕	Calcium intake may enhance bone-sparing effect of calcitonin in prevention or treatment of osteoporosis. Pharmacologically reasonable; emerging evidence.	Coadminister calcium (and vitamin D if needed).
Calcium acetate ✗✗✗	Possible adverse effect from concomitant administration due to additive effect. Generally accepted; direct evidence lacking.	Avoid concomitant calcium. Monitor for hypercalcemia with calcium acetate.
Cholestyramine, colestipol Bile acid sequestrants ≈≈≈/◇	Bile acid sequestrants can impair calcium absorption by binding calcium and by reducing absorption of vitamin D and fat-soluble nutrients as a result of decreasing lipid digestion and absorption. Risk of deficiency and sequelae with extended use.	Supplement calcium and vitamin D. Promote sunlight exposure and exercise.
Corticosteroids, oral ≈≈≈/◇/☼	Oral corticosteroids reduce calcium absorption and may increase excretion while decreasing vitamin D availability and lowering serum levels. Increased risk of bone loss, osteoporosis, and fractures with long-term oral steroid use.	Supplement additional calcium and monitor bone and 25(OH)D status with steroid use > 1 month. Promote sunlight exposure and exercise.
EDTA ≈≈/✗✗	EDTA binds to calcium; thereby increasing calcium excretion and increasing risk of hypocalcemia or negative calcium balance.	Assess levels of calcium and other affected nutrients before treatment. Coadminister minerals.
Estrogens/progestins Oral contraceptives (OCs) Hormone replacement therapy (HRT) ⊕⊕⊕/☼	Synergistic interaction, especially with osteoporosis. Calcium can protect bone mineral density (BMD) during attainment of maximal peak bone mass in adolescence and early adulthood (with which OCs can interfere) and minimize later bone loss. Vitamin D assists calcium absorption, and both enable estrogen to inhibit osteoclastic activity and bone resorption and maintain bone mineralization. Progestins may counter benefit.	Coadminister with calcium and vitamin D (separate intake), possibly bisphosphonates. Monitor bone, 25(OH)D and HDL. Promote sunlight, nutrient-rich diet, and weight-bearing exercise.
Fluoroquinolone/ quinolone antibiotics ◇◇/≈≈	Chelation between this class of antibiotics and calcium likely to impair absorption of both, as well as other minerals. Calcium depletion and effects of bone loss plausible with extended use but not established or probable.	Discontinue calcium or separate intake during short-term therapy. Mineral supplementation may be appropriate with extended therapy; intake separated by several hours.
Gastric acid—suppressive medications Cimetidine, Histamine (H₂) antagonists Omeprazole, Proton pump inhibitors ≈≈≈	Cimetidine can decrease calcium absorption and transport through effects on vitamin D hydroxylase and vitamin D and impairment of gastric acid environment. Omeprazole can decrease absorption by reducing gastric acid production and increasing gastric pH. Possible deficiency with extended use.	Supplement with calcium other than carbonate; take separate from meals. Monitor bone density and 25(OH)D with chronic use, especially postmenopausal women.
Heparin, unfractionated ◇≈≈/≈≈/◇	Heparin therapy is associated with bone loss. Heparin may also inhibit formation of 1,25-dihydroxyvitamin D by kidneys and thereby reduce calcium absorption. Significant risk of bone loss with extended heparin use and nutrient depletion. Limited evidence supporting protective effect of supplemental calcium (or vitamin D).	Coadminister calcium and vitamin D, possibly as hydroxyapatite, where indicated. Monitor bone and 1,25(OH)₂ status with heparin use > 1 month.

Summary

Drug/Class Interaction Type	Mechanism and Significance	Management
Isoniazid (INH) ≈≈/◇	Isoniazid can lower levels of both calcium and activated vitamin D levels; inhibit hepatic mixed-function oxidase activity, hepatic 25-hydroxylase and renal 1α-hydroxylase and reduce corresponding vitamin D metabolites. Drug-induced vitamin D deficiency can produce hypocalcemia and elevate parathyroid hormone (PTH). Nutrient support unlikely to interfere with therapeutic activity of medication.	Coadminister calcium and vitamin D when INH used for > 1 month. Promote sunlight exposure. Monitor 25(OH)D and bone status.
Levothyroxine Thyroid hormones ◇◇/≈≈≈/◇	Chelation between thyroid medications and calcium impairs absorption of both, particularly with calcium carbonate. Thyroid hormones increase urinary calcium excretion. Calcium depletion and effects of bone loss plausible with extended use, but not established or probable; risk greater in women with history of hyperthyroidism or thyrotoxicosis. Strong evidence for binding but evidence lacking for benefit from calcium coadministration.	Comorbid conditions may require both agents. Separate thyroid (morning) and calcium (bedtime). Monitor BMD with long-term use.
Metformin Biguanides ≈≈≈/◇≈≈/☼	Biguanides, especially metformin, reduce B_{12} absorption and lower serum B_{12} and holotranscobalamin by depressing intrinsic factor secretion and interfering with B_{12}/intrinsic factor uptake through calcium-dependent ileal membrane antagonism. Possible decrease of folate and increase of homocysteine.	Supplement B_{12}, folic acid, and calcium. Monitor folate and cobalamin status.
Sulfamethoxazole Sulfonamide antibiotics ≈≈≈	Sulfonamide can impair calcium absorption, as well as that of magnesium and vitamin B_{12}. Low probability of clinically significant effects on calcium balance with short-term therapy. Calcium depletion and effects of bone loss plausible with extended use, but not established or probable.	Intake separated by several hours. Additional calcium supplementation may be appropriate with extended therapy.
Tetracycline antibiotics ◇◇/≈≈≈/◇	Chelation between calcium and tetracycline antibiotics likely to impair absorption of both to clinically significant degree. Calcium intake, even small amounts, can significantly impair antimicrobial activity. Tetracycline also increases urinary calcium excretion. Calcium depletion and effects on calcium-dependent tissues (e.g., bones, teeth) probable, and adverse effect on bone formation or density possible with extended use; increased concern with adolescents and elderly.	Discontinue calcium (including dairy foods), or separate intake during short-term therapy. Calcium supplementation usually appropriate with extended therapy, with intake separated by several hours.
Thiazide diuretics ✗✗/◇◇/⊕✗/⊕⊕	Thiazide diuretics increase calcium retention by decreasing urinary calcium excretion; decreased calcium absorption, suppressed PTH secretion, and inhibited vitamin D synthesis also appear to be effects of thiazides. Concomitant use with supplemental calcium theoretically increases risk of hypercalcemia; low probability of occurrence. Not a substitute for increased calcium intake; benefits of increased calcium retention cease when thiazide discontinued. Evidence incomplete.	Monitor calcium levels before initiating and periodically during concomitant use of calcium or vitamin D.
Verapamil Calcium channel blockers ✗✗/⊕✗/⊕⊕/≈≈	Verapamil may decrease endogenous vitamin D synthesis and induce target-organ PTH resistance. Calcium administration can be used to reduce adverse effects of calcium channel blockers; concurrent use of verapamil and intravenous calcium salts, in particular, can be therapeutically efficacious (e.g., control cardiac tachyarrhythmias) yet avoid hypotensive effect of calcium channel blocker. Conversely, increased calcium availability may oppose verapamil's activity as calcium antagonist, particularly when antihypertensive effect desired. Theoretically, excess calcium (or vitamin D) might contribute to hypercalcemia, which in turn might precipitate cardiac arrhythmia in patients on verapamil. Minimal evidence; rare occurrence but potentially severe.	Concurrent supplementation with calcium (and vitamin D) may be appropriate, but only under close supervision. Consider bone support needs.

EDTA, Ethylenediaminetetraacetic acid; *HDL*, high-density lipoprotein; *INH*, international normalized ratio.

Nutrient-Drug Interactions and Drug-Induced Nutrient Depletions

NUTRIENT DESCRIPTION

Chemistry and Forms

Calcium ascorbate, calcium aspartate, calcium carbonate, calcium citrate, calcium citrate-malate (citramate), calcium gluconate, calcium lactate, calcium malate; microcrystalline hydroxyapatite (MCHC); calcium acetate; bonemeal, dolomite; calcium glycerophosphate, dicalcium phosphate, tricalcium phosphate; calcium phosphate (dairy calcium).

Physiology and Function

Calcium is the most abundant mineral in the human body, with 99% of it stored in bone and teeth. The remaining 1% of body calcium is found in the blood, extracellular fluid (ECF), and soft tissue. Normal physiological functioning requires that homeostatic systems in the intestines, bones, and kidneys, in concert with parathyroid hormone (PTH), calcitonin, vitamin D, and other hormones, maintain calcium levels in the blood and ECF within very narrow concentration parameters. Calcium absorption in the intestines will increase if blood levels decrease. Likewise, renal excretion can be reduced to maintain calcium levels. Ultimately, however, bone will be demineralized to maintain normal calcium parameters when intake is inadequate to sustain the physiological functions of calcium in bone and teeth, cellular structure, endocrine function, cell signaling, nerve transmission, blood clotting, blood pressure regulation, enzyme activation, and muscle contraction.

A dynamic and complex system involving calcium absorption, bone formation and resorption, renal reabsorption and excretion, and hormonal regulatory networks enables rapid and tight control of blood calcium levels. Calcium is absorbed in the duodenum, jejunum, and ileum by an active saturable process that involves vitamin D and PTH. Calcium exhibits threshold absorption that depends on the interplay among dietary intake, blood and tissue levels, gender, life stage and activity level, gastric pH, hormonal milieu, vitamin D receptor genotype, and numerous other factors. Except for dietary intake, the major factors influencing the efficiency of absorption are physiological requirements and age. Thus, in childhood, adolescence, pregnancy, and lactation, the intestinal calcium absorption process becomes more efficient; conversely, it is impaired in the elderly, especially with decreased physical activity levels. Calcium bioavailability depends to some extent on vitamin D status. PTH stimulates the conversion of vitamin D to calcitriol, its active form, primarily in the kidneys and to some degree in other tissues. Calcitriol increases the absorption of calcium from the small intestine. At high intakes, some calcium is absorbed by passive diffusion (independent of vitamin D). Some absorption can also occur from the colon. Together with PTH, calcitriol activates osteoclasts to stimulate the release of calcium from bone and increases renal tubular reabsorption to reduce excretion of calcium through the urine. On reaching normal blood calcium levels, the parathyroid glands suspend PTH secretion, and the kidneys resume excretion of any excess calcium through the urine. Unabsorbed and endogenously secreted calcium is eliminated through the feces. Perspiration and breast milk also act as pathways of calcium excretion.

Calcium ions play a major role in the structural aspect of physiology. Hydroxyapatite $[Ca_{10}(PO_4)_6(OH)_2]$, a crystalline calcium carbonate/calcium phosphate compound, is the form of calcium primarily responsible for providing rigidity and strength to bones and teeth. Positive calcium balance is maintained during development and growth until peak bone density is attained, becomes neutral as adults mature, and is often negative in the elderly. Thus, bone density increases during the first three decades of life until it reaches its peak at about age 30. Thereafter, bone density stabilizes before moving into a pattern of gradual decline. Both men and women experience diminishing bone density as they age, but women experience more significant and rapid decline after menopause. Calcium and vitamin D insufficiency during adolescence and young adulthood can significantly curtail peak bone density, dramatically increasing the risk of osteoporosis in later life.

Calcium facilitates muscle activity by aiding transport across cell membranes. Muscles require calcium for proper contractile function. Without calcium, the muscles tend to stay in the contracted state. The cell membranes of skeletal muscle cells, nerve cells, and other electrically excitable cells are characterized by voltage-dependent calcium channels that enable rapid changes in calcium concentrations. For example, the nerve impulse entering a muscle fiber to stimulate contraction triggers calcium channels in the cell membrane to allow influx of calcium ions into the muscle cell. Calcium ions are released from intracellular storage vesicles as these calcium ions bind to troponin-c and set in motion the process of muscle contraction. Meanwhile, the binding of calcium to calmodulin activates glycogenolysis in the muscle to provide energy necessary for contraction.

As with striated muscle throughout the body, the heart requires calcium for proper contractility. A sudden decrease of ionized serum calcium can cause tetany, leading to cardiac or respiratory failure. Likewise, calcium plays a role in mediating the constriction and relaxation of blood vessels (vasoconstriction and vasodilation).

An array of proteins and enzymes require calcium as a cofactor for optimal activity and stabilization. For example, activation of seven of the clotting factors in the coagulation cascade requires the binding of calcium ions. Ionized calcium initiates the formation of blood clotting by stimulating the release of thromboplastin from blood platelets. It is also a cofactor in the conversion of prothrombin to thrombin, which converts fibrinogen to fibrin, and then aids in its polymerization to form a stable clot.

Calcium also regulates membrane stabilization. Certain cells (e.g., mast cells) tend to rupture when calcium ions are depleted. In addition, neurotransmitters at synaptic junctions are regulated by calcium. This may have effects on such conditions such as anxiety, insomnia, and other stress-related conditions.

NUTRIENT IN CLINICAL PRACTICE
Known or Potential Therapeutic Uses

Calcium plays many essential roles in human physiology, but it primarily receives attention in conventional medicine and patient inquiries in regard to bone health, aging, and osteoporosis. Nevertheless, calcium has a proven influence on risk for numerous pathological patterns and needs to be emphasized as a critical nutrient beginning at an early age. Calcium intake during childhood and especially during adolescence is perhaps the most significant factor in establishing healthy bone mass and preventing osteoporosis, although exercise is an equally and possibly more important factor.[1] Calcium too often becomes a concern as aging progresses and the threat of bone loss is looming or initial signs of osteoporosis are already present. Unfortunately, when awareness of need develops during middle age and menopause, it is usually too late for optimal calcium nutriture to function in a preventive mode.[2-5]

Evidence for beneficial effects of calcium supplementation on *bone mineral density* (BMD), most often studied in women before and after menopause, is mixed, with slowing the pace of further bone loss becoming the realistic clinical objective in most cases. Inherently, the significance of variables such as calcium intake, beverage habits, hormone history and status, and lifestyle factors (e.g., exercise, smoking) all complicate the issues and confound analysis of the available data.[6,7] Thus, although the current dietary and calcium supplementation recommendations are almost always advisable, they are unlikely to reverse the process of age-related bone loss without a comprehensive and strategic approach utilizing multidisciplinary interventions.

The collective evidence indicates that a diet rich in calcium from plant sources deserves much more attention, and that the common advice to consume dairy products may be less well founded than generally presumed. Furthermore, the tendency of adolescents to displace milk consumption with carbonated beverages during the most critical life stage for peak bone mass development tips the calcium balance in a deleterious direction, given the calcium-depleting action of phosphates found in many soft drinks, as well as drawing on the skeletal mineral reserve to buffer the acid load imposed by habitual consumption of large quantities of these acidified carbonated drinks. Experts in clinical nutrition generally recommend that individuals obtain as much calcium as possible from a diverse, notrient-rich, and balanced diet. Foods that provide calcium usually contain other important nutrients, such as magnesium, manganese, copper, zinc, vitamin D, and vitamin K, that work synergistically with calcium. Moreover, intake of calcium levels above 800 mg (elemental calcium) per day is probably unnecessary for maintaining calcium metabolism in most individuals, provided that vitamin D status is adequate, except for pregnancy and lactation.[8]

Calcium absorption is variable, both between different individuals and also with differing forms of calcium. Individuals of Asian and African heritage absorb calcium more efficiently than do Caucasians.[9] Different forms of calcium are absorbed at different rates. The pH of the stomach often influences how well certain calcium salts will be absorbed. The more water-soluble forms of calcium, such as citrate and citrate-malate, tend to have a greater absorption rate, especially in people who are deficient in hydrochloric acid, such as the elderly, or those taking gastric acid–suppressive medications. Furthermore, vitamin D intake and blood levels, as well as vitamin D receptor genotype, can significantly influence calcium bioavailability and absorption.[10] Bran and high-fiber cereals are high in phytates, which can reduce calcium absorption, although this is probably not clinically significant for most individuals over time at typical levels of consumption.

Historical/Ethnomedicine Precedent

Dark-green leafy vegetables, hard cheeses, sesame seeds, seaweed, and other components of traditional indigenous diets have long been emphasized for their contributions to health and longevity. Dairy consumption has been part of some cultural traditions for long periods, although controversy continues as to whether it is always in association with a genetic capacity to digest, assimilate, and metabolize dairy foods.

Possible Uses

Amenorrhea (bone loss prevention), anxiety, arthritis, blood clotting, blood pressure regulation, cardiovascular disease, celiac disease (related deficiency), colon cancer (risk reduction), colorectal cancer, depression, dysmenorrhea, gestational hypertension, gingivitis, hyperactivity, hypercholesterolemia, hypertension, hypertriglyceridemia, hypoparathyroidism, insomnia, insulin resistance syndrome, kidney stones (calcium oxalate stone prevention), migraine, multiple sclerosis, obesity, osteoporosis, periodontal disease, postpartum support, preeclampsia (related deficiency), pregnancy support, premenstrual syndrome, restless legs syndrome, rickets, stroke.

Related Therapeutic Applications

Calcium carbonate is used as an antacid. Calcium carbonate and calcium acetate can be used as phosphate binders in renal failure. Calcium chloride and calcium gluconate are used intravenously in treating severe hypocalcemia.

Deficiency Symptoms

Simple calcium deficiency is not a recognized clinical disorder, and standard laboratory tests, except bone scans during middle age, offer little useful data to evaluate calcium status for individuals with suboptimal or even moderately compromised intake, development, and peak bone mass. Long-term calcium deficiency contributes to growth deficiency in children; poor tooth development is also characteristic. A lack of calcium in adults may cause osteoporosis and osteomalacia and result in bone deformities, bone pain, and fractures. Other symptoms related to a deficiency are tetany or other muscle spasms. These usually occur in the legs. However, they may also occur in the

blood vessels and may lead to hypertension. Other, typically more advanced, symptoms of calcium deficiency include nausea and vomiting, headaches, candidiasis, dry skin and nails, alopecia, neuromuscular irritability, muscular spasms and contracture, tetany, arrhythmias, convulsions, anxiety, depression, insomnia, and psychosis.

Calcium insufficiency, depletion, and deficiency can result from a wide range of factors and are usually gradual in onset and difficult to reverse once established. Decreased intake, inadequate weight-bearing exercise, blood loss (both internal and external), menorrhagia, lead toxicity, and malabsorption all can lead to calcium deficiency. Deficiencies in vitamin D and magnesium can contribute to calcium deficiency. A growing body of evidence indicates that vitamin D status is compromised in a large portion of the population, particularly adolescents and the elderly, because of inadequate intake and lack of exposure to sufficient sunlight. Magnesium deficiency results in decreased responsiveness of osteoclasts to PTH. Compromised calcium status during development will prevent the attainment of optimal peak bone mass. Once that opportune phase is passed, inadequate calcium intake may contribute to accelerated bone loss and ultimately the development of osteoporosis.

However, increased absorption of dietary calcium, rather than an increased intake or decreased excretion of calcium, appears to be the most influential factor in rapid acquisition of bone mineral during pubertal growth. Thus, the effects of dietary factors on calcium absorption efficiency are modulated by calcium status, genetic factors (e.g., specific vitamin D receptor gene polymorphisms), and height and body size.[10-14] Furthermore, malabsorption conditions (e.g., Crohn's disease, celiac disease, surgical intestinal resection), prolonged bed rest, excessive menstrual blood loss, and a range of pathologies and medical interventions can also contribute to calcium depletion and potential deficiency.

Dietary Sources

Hard cheese, almonds, sesame seeds, filberts, and dark-green leafy vegetables are considered *high* in calcium, with greater than 200 mg/100 g food.

Milk, yogurt, sunflower seeds, Brazil nuts, broccoli, parsley, and watercress are considered *medium* in calcium, with greater than 100 mg/100 g food.

Average dietary intakes of calcium in the United States (U.S.) are well below the adequate intake (AI) recommendation for every age and gender group, especially in females and most significantly in children 9 to 17 years old. Furthermore, surveys consistently find that up to 85% of postmenopausal women do not consume adequate calcium every day, and on average consume about 500 mg less than the U.S. recommended dietary allowance (RDA). "Despite increasing public awareness and patient education about the importance of calcium [intake], this analysis shows the average daily calcium intake has not improved since the landmark Study of Osteoporotic Fractures (SOF)," conducted from 1986 to 1988, which found that postmenopausal women's average daily calcium intake was 714 mg daily.[15]

The issue of calcium bioavailability from milk and dairy products remains a contentious issue, more often dominated by cultural habit and marketing than by nutritional science. In a systematic review of 58 clinical, longitudinal, retrospective, and cross-sectional studies on the relationship between milk, dairy products, or calcium intake and bone mineralization or fracture risk in children and young adults (1-25 years old), Lanou et al.[16]

concluded: "Scant evidence supports nutrition guidelines focused specifically on increasing milk or other dairy product intake for promoting child and adolescent bone mineralization." Furthermore, large segments of the populations may not have the genetic background for digestion and assimilation of cow's milk, or any milk, past infancy, with resulting food intolerances, lactase deficiency, and food allergies being increasingly recognized for their clinical import.

Consumption of cola-containing drinks, but not other carbonated beverages, appears to be associated with lower BMD in older women.[17]

Nutrient Preparations Available

The issue of which form of supplemental calcium is "best" belies the broader issues of biochemical individuality in general and gastrointestinal function in particular. Organically bound calcium, such as aspartate, citrate, gluconate, or chelated forms, generally demonstrates higher bioavailability than inorganic calcium, such as carbonate, phosphate, or sulfate; such bioavailability is particularly significant in individuals with insufficient gastric acid or poor bowel constitution and in the elderly. *Calcium carbonate* is the least expensive and most well-known form of calcium, but it frequently causes constipation and bloating and may not be well absorbed by individuals with reduced levels of stomach acid.[18] When calcium carbonate is taken with orange or other citrus juice, a significant amount of calcium citrate is formed, and absorption appears to be enhanced, even in subjects with low gastric acidity. Calcium citrate and heated oyster shell–seaweed calcium may be better absorbed than calcium carbonate; other evidence indicates no significant difference in bioavailability. Studies have shown a normally functioning bowel can ionize calcium carbonate and the lumen can absorb it well; after it is absorbed, it can be converted to aspartate, then an orotate, so that it can be absorbed into the cells.[19-21]

Calcium lactate and calcium gluconate are also more efficiently absorbed than calcium carbonate. Calcium citrate appears to be better tolerated in the elderly and by those with sensitive digestive systems and may offer superior efficacy in preventing the progression of osteoporosis. Calcium citrate-malate (citramate) is absorbed better and tolerated more consistently than calcium carbonate.[22] Many physicians and other health care professionals experienced in nutritional therapy have increasingly turned to calcium citramate as their preferred form of calcium. Some evidence suggests efficacy of microcrystalline hydroxyapatite (MCHC) in cases where osteoporosis is the greatest concern. This form of calcium is purported to have a special affinity for bone formation, but some have asserted that it may not be absorbed well.

Dosage Forms Available

Capsule, chewable tablet, functional foods (e.g., orange juice fortified with calcium citrate), liposomal spray, liquid, powder, tablet; injection (prescription only).

Source Materials for Nutrient Preparations

Oyster shells (calcium carbonate), dolomite, bonemeal (calcium hydroxyapatite); calcium ascorbate, calcium aspartate, calcium citrate, calcium citrate-malate, calcium gluconate, calcium glycerophosphate, calcium lactate, calcium malate, dicalcium phosphate, and tricalcium phosphate are calcium salts of the corresponding organic acid, produced by titrating the acid with calcium hydroxide or other basic form. Soluble forms of calcium phosphate along with other minerals present in milk have been extracted from milk and are being used to fortify other foodstuffs.

Most calcium supplements (85%) currently sold in the U.S. are made from calcium carbonate, which contains the greatest percentage of elemental calcium on a weight basis, but is also the least water-soluble calcium salt.

Note: Lead contamination has been observed in some forms of supplemental calcium, particularly dolomite, bonemeal, and oyster shell.[23-25] The U.S. federal limit for lead content is 7.5 micrograms (µg) per 1000 milligrams (mg) elemental calcium. Good manufacturing practice has established an industry standard of keeping the amount of lead in calcium supplements to less than 0.5 µg/1000 mg elemental calcium. A product survey published in 2000 reported measurable lead in 8 of 21 supplements, in amounts averaging 1 to 2 µg/1000 mg elemental calcium.[26] Calcium inhibits intestinal absorption of lead, and adequate calcium intake is protective against lead toxicity. Consequently, calcium deficiency could potentially present a greater risk of lead intake due to general lead exposure than associated with trace amounts in calcium supplements.

Dosage Range

No multivitamin/multimineral capsule or tablet contains 100% of the recommended daily dose of calcium because it would be too bulky and too large to swallow. For example, 1 g calcium carbonate contains 400 mg elemental calcium and 1 g calcium citrate contains 211 mg elemental calcium. Furthermore, because calcium exhibits an absorption threshold, absorption is maximized by limiting each dose to 500 mg elemental calcium.[27] Thus, supplemental calcium intake is most efficacious when the daily intake is divided into two or more doses, preferably with meals (and away from most medications). Concomitant vitamin D will enhance calcium absorption.

Adult

Dietary: In the United Kingdom, the average daily diet provides 961 mg for men and 764 mg for women.

Supplemental/Maintenance: 500 to 2500 mg per day.

For individuals age 19 to 50: 1000 mg/day (including diet)
For adults age 51 and older:
Women: 1500 mg/day (including diet)
Men: 1200 mg/day (including diet)
Pregnant and breastfeeding females under 19 years: 1300 mg/day (including diet)
Pregnant and breastfeeding females age 19 and older: 1000 mg/day (including diet)

Note: These recommendations do not incorporate research demonstrating that doses above 800 mg/day may be unnecessary with adequate vitamin D levels.

Pharmacological/Therapeutic: Calcium intake as high as 3000 mg/day, together with 10 to 50 µg/day vitamin D_3 (cholecalciferol), may be appropriate if plasma calcium and phosphate levels are stable and within normal range (e.g., in treatment of secondary hyperparathyroidism in uremia).[28]

Calcium deficits associated with vitamin D deficiency may warrant daily doses up to 6000 mg of calcium acetate or calcium carbonate.

Toxic: Total calcium intake, from combined dietary and supplemental sources, should not exceed 2500 mg/day for long-term use. Large, acute doses normally exhibit no toxic effects.

The tolerable upper intake level (UL) established by the U.S. Food and Nutrition Board (FNB), Institute of Medicine, for vitamin C in adults (≥ 19 years) is 2500 mg/day.

Pediatric (<18 years)
Dietary:

Infants, birth to 6 months: 210 mg/day; breast-feeding optimal
Infants, 7 months to 1 year: 270 mg/day
Children, 1 to 3 years: 500 mg/day
Children, 4 to 8 years: 800 mg/day

Supplemental/Maintenance: A daily intake of 1300 mg total calcium (diet plus supplements) is generally considered necessary to promote the attainment of maximal peak bone mass in children and adolescents.
Pharmacological/Therapeutic: 500 to 2500 mg/day.
Toxic: UL for calcium:

Infants, 0 to 12 months: Not established; dietary source only recommended
Children, 1 to 13 years: 2500 mg
Adolescents, 14 to 18 years: 2500 mg

Laboratoary Values
Serum Calcium
Normal levels: 2.2 to 2.6 mmol/L (8.4-10.2 mg/dL).

Serum calcium levels are maintained within tight parameters under most circumstances and do not provide accurate or sensitive markers for calcium status. Low blood calcium level usually implies abnormal parathyroid function and/or vitamin D deficiency, or low serum albumin. Elevated blood calcium levels are more likely to occur in response to higher absorption during calcium deficiency than with true excess. More often, elevated blood calcium occurs from hyperparathyroid states, vitamin D excess (usually in lymphoma, or sarcoid, or other granulomatous diseases where pathological tissues convert 25-OH vitamin D to calcitriol autonomously), or hypercalcemia of malignancy, which is usually caused by tumor-produced hormones that have PTH-like activity. Milk-alkali syndrome, as discussed later, is of historical interest only as a cause of hypercalcemia.

Ionized (Unbound) Serum Calcium
Normal levels: 1.17 to 1.29 mmol/L.
Low levels may indicate negative calcium balance.

Urinary Calcium
Normal levels:

Women: Approximately 150 to 250 mg/day
Men: Approximately 200 to 300 mg/day

SAFETY PROFILE
Overview
Calcium is generally considered safe at usual doses. Even in large doses, calcium absorption is limited, blood and tissue levels are tightly regulated, it is efficiently excreted, and toxicity rarely results. Some forms of calcium, notably calcium carbonate, may cause abdominal bloating, flatulence, and constipation in some individuals. Interference with absorption of other nutrients, particularly magnesium, iron, and zinc, as well as some medications, is the primary adverse effect associated

with large doses of calcium. However, concern has been raised in recent years about excessively high levels of lead in some forms of calcium, particularly those derived from bone-meal, dolomite, and oyster shell.

Nutrient Adverse Effects
General Adverse Effects
Hypercalcemia has been reported in association with calcium supplements and antacids but has never been attributed to dietary (i.e., food) sources of calcium. Ingestion of extremely large amounts of calcium (5000 mg/day, or >2000 mg/day over long period) can produce a toxic response. However, excess calcium levels are more likely to result from pathological processes such as hyperparathyroidism, certain types of cancer, kidney failure, breakdown of bone, or excessive levels of vitamin D.

Mild hypercalcemia is usually asymptomatic, but higher levels (>12 mg/dL) often result in symptoms that include loss of appetite, nausea, vomiting, constipation, abdominal pain, dry mouth, thirst, and frequent urination. More severe hypercalcemia may result in renal toxicity, cardiac arrhythmias, confusion, delirium, coma, and if not treated, death.

Milk-alkali syndrome, resulting from concomitant consumption of large quantities of milk, calcium carbonate (antacid), and sodium bicarbonate (absorbable alkali), represents the most well-known form of hypercalcemia. This obsolete treatment for peptic ulcers often involved calcium supplement levels from 1.5 to 16.5 g/day for 2 days to 30 years.

Increased excretion of calcium by the kidneys *(hypercalciuria)* constitutes a more significant risk factor for nephrolithiasis than does high calcium intake per se. In fact, most evidence indicates that enriched dietary calcium is associated with a decreased risk of oxalate kidney stones (which represent 80% of renal stones), presumably due to binding of dietary oxalate in the gut, thus decreasing its absorption. However, one large prospective study found that women taking supplemental calcium (of unspecified form) had a 20% higher risk of developing kidney stones than those who did not. These researchers also observed that women consuming low-calcium diets were at greater risk for stones than those with higher calcium intakes, perhaps, as they speculated, because of reciprocal hyperoxaluria.[29] Nevertheless, a diet low in animal protein and sodium, but with normal calcium levels, is more effective in preventing recurrence of calcium oxalate kidney stones than a diet low in calcium.[30] The form of calcium may be the differentiating factor deserving further investigations. Some clinicians have reported that calcium citrate can be beneficial in preventing or reversing kidney stones and bone spurs, and that calcium carbonate is more frequently associated with pathological calcification processes. As noted, higher levels of calcium from food may complex with dietary oxalates in the intestines and reduce their absorption; likewise, taking calcium supplements separate from food will significantly reduce their beneficial effect of decreasing intestinal oxalate absorption.

Adverse Effects Among Specific Populations
Risks from calcium supplementation are significantly greater in individuals with hyperparathyroidism, certain types of cancer, kidney failure, or other conditions that interfere with normal calcium regulation.

Pregnancy and Nursing
Evidence of adverse effects in pregnancy resulting from calcium supplementation is lacking. Calcium supplementation is

generally advised during pregnancy and lactation and can reduce risk of preeclampsia.

Infants and Children

Some sources have suggested that calcium supplements should be used under medical supervision in young children because of a risk of bowel perforation. Nondairy foods rich in calcium are preferred, with human breast milk being the superior food source for infants. Liquid forms are available when supplementation is appropriate. Children may also do well with some chewable forms, although some products contain sugar, which is not recommended.

Contraindications

Calcium supplementation is contraindicated in some individuals with hyperparathyroidism, chronic renal impairment or kidney disease, sarcoidosis or other granulomatous diseases, cancer patients with a history of hypercalcemia, or patients with a history of idiopathic calcium stones (except the common calcium oxalate stones, in which calcium supplementation with meals may reduce the risk of stone formation by binding dietary oxalate).

Precautions and Warnings

Caution is generally appropriate in conditions associated with hypercalcuria and hypercalcemia. Soft tissue calcification may occur with hyperparathyroidism, hyperphosphatemia, magnesium deficiency, or vitamin D overdoses. Calcium supplements should be used with caution and with medical supervision in hypertensive individuals because blood pressure control may be altered. As previously suggested, judicious selection of the form of calcium used may reduce or even reverse the risk factors involved with supplementation in individuals with these conditions.

High calcium intake, primarily from milk and dairy products, may increase prostate cancer risk by lowering concentrations of 1,25-dihydroxyvitamin D_3 [$1,25(OH)_2D_3$], a hormone thought to protect against prostate cancer. The epidemiological evidence, however, is mixed. Other evidence indicates that calcium supplementation is not associated with increased risk of prostate cancer.[31-36] Nevertheless, calcium supplementation is sometimes considered as contraindicated in men diagnosed with prostate cancer. If calcium were found to have such an adverse effect, concomitant supplementation with vitamin D might provide a safe, simple, and effective counterpoint.

INTERACTIONS REVIEW
Strategic Considerations

The many interactions involving calcium reveal several consistent patterns. Nevertheless, most of the available clinical research has inadequate specificity, depth, complexity, and duration and cannot capture many of the nuances that will enable clinicians to navigate their diverse implications. Calcium and many medications can interfere with each other in ways that are easily avoided or that require tactical choices within a strategic approach. On occasion, the adverse effects on calcium-rich tissue can be swift and permanent (e.g., tetracycline, sometimes corticosteroids). More often, medications interfere with calcium function or cause steady depletion that will increase risks of adverse effects over time. Notably, physicians prescribing such agents over extended periods (e.g., anticonvulsants, opioids and oral glucocorticoids) usually do not advise or prescribe adequate countermeasures, whether calcium and vitamin D, bisphosphonates, or the combination, to address effectively the common occurrence of drug-induced decreases in BMD and increased risk of fracture.[37,38] Conversely, the risk of hypercalcemia/hypercalciuria from calcium intake through supplements or dietary sources is improbable outside of metabolic pathologies influencing the calcium and vitamin D regulatory systems. Overall, calcium tends to follow the patterns of other dense aspects of nature and physiology, which come on gradually, move slowly, and can be difficult to reverse once established.

Calcium and many medications complex or otherwise bind to each other, thus reducing absorption of both agents. During short courses of treatment, this interaction may reduce drug absorption and activity to a clinically significant degree. In contrast, any short-term interference with calcium assimilation will not interfere with the intended therapeutic action in a strategically important degree, given that most uses of calcium are long term, preventive, or cumulative. In most situations, simple temporal separation of intake is adequate to avoid such interference; when not sufficient, however, the calcium may need to be temporarily discontinued, usually with minimal or no impact on therapeutic intentions. Importantly, calcium-fortified foods, such as orange juice, are often not thought of as "calcium supplements" and can significantly interfere with absorption of pharmaceutical medications that bind to calcium, when taken with such beverages.

Significant and often severe limitations in the ability to reach conclusions about interactions involving "calcium" occur because of the various calcium salts potentially involved. Too often, an easy but potentially misleading tendency is to generalize from research that often is not clear, especially in secondary sources and derivative literature, and particularly in abstract form. An even greater interpretive error is to extrapolate from findings involving parenteral calcium to the use of oral calcium supplements; the two situations are physiologically vastly different, and almost never comparable. Calcium carbonate and calcium phosphate are best taken with meals to optimize absorption.[21] Other calcium salts can be taken without regard to food intake or meals; this may make them preferable for hypochlorhydric individuals and patients prescribed H_2 antagonists or other medications that reduce gastric acidity, particularly proton pump inhibitors (PPIs).

The literature is further complicated by the presence of research and case reports involving calcium salts as antacids, particularly when observations regarding such substances are extrapolated to calcium supplements. Except for differences in the substances themselves, gastric acidity, achlorhydria, and acid suppression are all complicating issues of significant import. Likewise, some studies and many commentators fail to distinguish between calcium intake from calcium supplements and that from dietary intake of milk and dairy products.

Multiple variables (e.g., individual biochemical variability, gender, life stage, diet, vitamin D status) that influence how "calcium" will be absorbed and function in any given individual need to be further evaluated before considering the medications and conditions being treated.

The inadequacies of standard knowledge and clinical practice regarding the prevalence and assessment of vitamin D deficiency emerging in recent years will increasingly reveal deep implications for calcium balance, bone health, and much more. Many agents that deplete calcium or otherwise interfere with its metabolism do so indirectly through their adverse effects on vitamin D status. Although direct effects on calcium may also be present, the effects on vitamin D can significantly impair calcium absorption and activity. Conversely, elevated levels of vitamin D can cause an increased absorption of calcium.

Pervasive vitamin D deficiency status and underutilization of laboratory assessment for 25-hydroxyvitamin D [25(OH)D] levels influence and limit research design, interpretation, and clinical practice within conventional medicine. For example, in 2005, two randomized controlled trials of calcium carbonate and cholecalciferol (vitamin D_3) reported that administration for prevention of fractures in primary care produced widely publicized conclusions declaring that such nutrient supplementation provided no value in preventing fractures.[39,40] Such assertions were made despite disclosures that (1) vitamin D levels had been tested in only a small sample of the subjects in one of the studies; (2) vitamin D deficiency appeared to be common within the subject populations, as indicated by responses to vitamin D supplementation; (3) quality control of the supplements was very poor; (4) compliance was marginal and declined over time (e.g., 63%, or as low as 45%); and (5) the use of calcium carbonate in a population of older and often hypochlorhydric subjects would be considered suboptimal by many, if not most, experienced practitioners of nutritional therapeutics. Digestion of calcium carbonate relies on the integrity of gastric function and the bowel culture to produce the ionizing acids. Thus, gastrointestinal adverse effects, typical of calcium carbonate, were cited as a major factor in greater noncompliance with calcium intake.

In the study in which 1% of the subjects had their vitamin D levels actually measured, there was only a marginal increase after 1 year of supplementation with 800 IU of vitamin D per day (although when analyzed, some of the supplements contained as little as 372 IU, mean value, per tablet). Average 25(OH)D levels at beginning of the study (15 ng/mL) were in the range of severe deficiency, and after 1 year improved only to 24 ng/mL, still well below what many vitamin D researchers consider to be adequate levels (30-40 ng/mL).[41] Subsequently, in a trial involving 944 healthy Icelandic adults, Steingrimsdottir et al.[8] found that with 25(OH)D levels below 10 ng/mL, maintaining calcium intake above 800 mg/day appeared to normalize calcium metabolism, as determined by the PTH level, but in individuals with higher 25(OH)D levels, no benefit was observed from calcium intake above 800 mg/day. Clearly, further research on calcium and other minerals involved in bone metabolism need to take into account, and preferably optimize, vitamin D status.

Notably, in conventional practice, the main pharmacological intervention for the prevention of bone loss is antiresorptive drugs, such as bisphosphonates, for which almost every clinical trial has included coadministration of calcium or vitamin D. Moreover, the decontextualization and narrow focus of these studies highlight the shortcomings of standard research methodology and clinical practice to consider the broad factors of aging, lifestyle, activity level, drug depletions, and poor nutritional status characteristic of the populations in question, as well as the complex nature of bone health and its reliance on interdependencies of multiple nutrients and tissues, rather than using such a narrow focus on supplemental calcium and vitamin D. As public and practitioner attention on vitamin D grows, it may prove a pivotal issue in expanding perceptions and awareness, analysis, and intervention through a broad integrative model more accurately reflecting patient needs, with a scientific understanding of the breadth and complexity of the processes involved.

Ultimately, perhaps the most limiting aspects of the research findings generally available involve the questions asked, the assessment methods used, and the time frames considered. As noted in many sections, the markers of blood calcium levels and other short-term indices do not adequately address the issue of calcium depletion over time; the feedback systems of calcium homeostasis involve vitamin D synthesis and activation, calcium absorption, tubular reabsorption and urinary excretion, PTH production and secretion, and bone formation, catabolism, and resorption. Thus, as a drug interferes with calcium absorption and metabolism and induces a depletion pattern anywhere along the way, superficial parameters may remain within normal parameters, but the long-term state of bone density may be in steady decline. For this reason, it is often clinically useful to assess markers of bone breakdown, such as urinary pyridinium cross-links (pyridinium and deoxypyridinium), as a baseline, when starting a pharmaceutical intervention with the potential to impact calcium balance negatively. An increase in urinary markers of bone breakdown signifies the development of negative calcium balance, despite all other markers related to calcium appearing normal, because of intrinsic calcium homeostatic mechanisms. This can serve as an early warning sign and allow for nutritional interventions to correct negative calcium balance without waiting to find a decrease in bone density on a subsequent bone density scan.

See also Vitamin D in Nutrient-Nutrient Interactions.

NUTRIENT-DRUG INTERACTIONS

Aminoglycoside Antibiotics, Including Gentamicin and Neomycin

Evidence: Gentamicin (Garamycin), neomycin (Mycifradin, Myciguent, Neo-Fradin, NeoTab, Nivemycin).
Extrapolated, based on similar properties: Amikacin (Amikin), kanamycin (Kantrex), netilmicin (Netromycin), paromomycin (monomycin; Humatin), streptomycin, tobramycin (AKTob, Nebcin, TOBI, TOBI Solution, TobraDex, Tobrex).

Interaction Type and Significance

≈≈   **Drug-Induced Nutrient Depletion, Supplementation Therapeutic, with Professional Management**
☼   **Prevention or Reduction of Drug Adverse Effect**

Probability:	Evidence Base:
2. Probable	● **Consensus**

Effect and Mechanism of Action
Gentamicin exhibits a significant risk of nephrotoxic effects and can cause increased urinary calcium loss. Concomitant administration of calcium may have a protective effect but may also potentiate gentamicin-induced nephrotoxicity. Neurotoxic effects are also well known.

Neomycin impairs calcium absorption when taken orally.

Research
Animal studies indicate that renal tubular damage caused by aminoglycosides, such as gentamicin, can lead to hypocalcemia combined with hypokalemia, hypomagnesemia, and alkalosis.[42-44] In a retrospective study, Schneider et al.[45] found that coronary artery bypass graft (CABG) patients who received both a bypass prime with a high calcium concentration (6.25 mmol/L) and gentamicin perioperatively had a higher incidence of renal failure compared with those who received only the prime, gentamicin alone, or neither.

Reports

A 12-year-old boy developed renal wasting of magnesium, calcium, and potassium, with secondary hypomagnesemia, hypocalcemia, and hypokalemia (without hyperaldosteronism), after treatment with 14,400 mg gentamicin over 4 months.[46] Other case reports involving gentamicin have described similar adverse effects on electrolytes, particularly hypomagnesemia.[47-49]

Nutritional Therapeutics, Clinical Concerns, and Adaptations

Physicians administering extended courses of gentamicin or other aminoglycosides should monitor kidney function as well as plasma magnesium, calcium, and potassium levels during and after treatment. Magnesium levels in red blood cells (RBCs) can provide a more reliable picture of magnesium status than testing serum magnesium. Serum creatinine, blood urea nitrogen (BUN), and creatinine clearance should also be measured before initiating therapy and monitored throughout treatment. Nutritional support may be required to restore normal levels of calcium and other important minerals. Prolonged courses of gentamicin should be avoided if less nephrotoxic antibiotics are suitable. Oral neomycin in preparation for surgery is unlikely to produce clinically significant deficiencies.

Calcium coadministration in the range of 500 to 1000 mg per day may beneficial for individuals being treated with aminoglycosides for longer than 2 to 3 days. Slow-K and Micro-K are typical examples of the potassium suggested by most physicians. Patients can further enhance their potassium levels by eating several pieces of fresh fruit each day. However, increasing potassium intake by any means is usually contraindicated and often dangerous in patients with reduced kidney function. Coadministration of magnesium in the dosage range of 300 to 500 mg per day is usually appropriate but should be done in collaboration with a physician trained and experienced in nutritional therapies. Magnesium supplementation is risky in patients with renal insufficiency and is usually contraindicated in such cases. It is also important to note that magnesium is needed to maintain intracellular potassium due to magnesium dependence of the membrane Na^+, K^+-ATPase enzyme, as well as calcium, because parathyroid hormone (PTH) is a magnesium-requiring hormone. Intravenous (IV) magnesium replacement is preferred for correction of frank hypomagnesemia.

Amphotericin B

Amphotericin B (AMB; Fungizone).

Interaction Type and Significance

≈≈≈ **Drug-Induced Nutrient Depletion, Supplementation Therapeutic, Not Requiring Professional Management**

☼ **Prevention or Reduction of Drug Adverse Effect**

Probability:
2. Probable

Evidence Base:
● Consensus

Effect and Mechanism of Action

The ability of amphotericin B to increase intracellular calcium concentrations is associated with the toxicity of this antifungal agent. Calcium depletion is a generally accepted adverse effect of amphotericin B; sodium, potassium, and magnesium are similarly depleted. Hyperphosphatemia has also been observed. This medication exerts adverse effects on renal function, but details of possible metabolic pathways are not known.

Reports

Amphotericin B lipid complex (ABLC) is a liposomal formulation that is less nephrotoxic than conventional amphotericin B and can be given more safely to patients with preexisting renal impairment with no apparent loss of efficacy. Nevertheless, cases of severe hyperphosphatemia resulting from high-dose liposomal amphotericin have been reported.[50]

Nutritional Therapeutics, Clinical Concerns and Adaptations

Physicians administering amphotericin B are advised to monitor electrolyte status and consider supplementation with a multimineral formulation during extended treatment. Aberrations of serum electrolytes, including calcium, concomitant with amphotericin therapy may require parenteral management.

Antacids Containing Aluminum and Magnesium

Aluminum carbonate gel (Basajel), aluminum hydroxide (Alternagel, Amphojel), aluminum hydroxide and magnesium hydroxide (Advanced Formula Di-Gel Tablets, Co-Magaldrox, Di-Gel, Gelusil, Maalox, Maalox Plus, Mylanta, Wingel), aluminum hydroxide and magnesium trisilicate (Alenic Alka, Gaviscon Chewable); aluminum hydroxide, magnesium carbonate, alginic acid, and sodium bicarbonate (Gaviscon Extra Strength Tablets, Gaviscon Regular Strength Liquid, Gaviscon Extra Strength Liquid); aluminum hydroxide, magnesium hydroxide, calcium carbonate, and simethicone (Tempo Tablets); aluminum hydroxide, magnesium trisilicate, alginic acid, and sodium bicarbonate (Alenic Alka, Gaviscon Regular Strength Tablets); magnesium hydroxide (Phillips' Milk of Magnesia MOM), magnesium trisilicate (Adcomag trisil, Foamicon).
Similar properties but evidence indicating no or reduced interaction effects: calcium-containing combination drugs: aluminum hydroxide, calcium carbonate, magnesium hydroxide, and simethicone (Tempo Tablets); calcium carbonate and magnesium hydroxide (Calcium Rich Rolaids); magnesium hydroxide and calcium carbonate (Calcium Rich Rolaids).
See also Gastric Acid–Suppressive Medications.

Interaction Type and Significance

✗✗✗ **Potentially Harmful or Serious Adverse Interaction—Avoid**

≈≈≈ **Drug-Induced Nutrient Depletion, Supplementation Therapeutic, Not Requiring Professional Management**

Probability:
2. Probable

Evidence Base:
● Consensus

Effect and Mechanism of Action

Aluminum-based antacids may reduce calcium absorption and can complex with phosphates to cause a depletion of calcium stores. Aluminum hydroxide causes increased loss of calcium through urine and stool.

Calcium citrate has been found to act similar to citrus juice in significantly increasing aluminum absorption from antacids.

Research

Concomitant intake of calcium citrate can significantly increase aluminum absorption from both dietary sources and aluminum-containing antacids.[51-54] Weberg et al.[55] examined the mineral-metabolic effects of a 4-week course of a conventional low-dose aluminum-magnesium antacid in 10 healthy volunteers, who were given one antacid tablet after the three main meals and at bedtime (buffering capacity, 120 mmol/day). They observed significant changes from premedication state, including an increase in urinary excretion of magnesium, calcium, and aluminum; decrease in urinary excretion of phosphate; increase in maximal renal phosphate reabsorption; and increase in serum concentration of aluminum. All these parameters returned to normal levels within 3 to 4 days after cessation of antacids.[55] In a study involving eight male subjects, Coburn et al.[56] found that coadministration of 5 mL of aluminum hydroxide gel (2.4 g four times daily) and calcium citrate (950 mg four times daily) for 3 days "markedly enhances aluminum absorption from aluminum hydroxide" and increases urinary aluminum excretion. In a trial involving 30 healthy women, Nolan et al.[25] observed that calcium citrate (800 mg elemental calcium daily) significantly increased absorption of aluminum from dietary sources (i.e., with no additional exposure to aluminum in antacids) and resulted in significantly increased urinary aluminum excretion and plasma aluminum level. During monitoring, however, they noted no changes in urine or whole-blood lead levels. Further research is warranted to determine whether long-term use of calcium citrate contributes significantly to aluminum accumulation and toxicity and the relative role of antacids in such risk.

Antacids containing magnesium and aluminum can increase calcium elimination, particularly urinary and stool loss.[57]

Nutritional Therapeutics, Clinical Concerns, and Adaptations

Physicians prescribing antacids containing aluminum (and magnesium) should advise patients to avoid calcium supplements, particularly calcium citrate, during the course of treatment; citrus juice is also contraindicated. In general, use of aluminum-based antacids should be discouraged given the mineral's inherent toxicity. The risks of an adverse reaction between calcium citrate and aluminum-containing compounds are especially high for individuals with kidney failure, particularly those on dialysis. Consider alternative approaches to antacid therapy using calcium or magnesium compounds without aluminum content.

Anticonvulsant Medications

Carbamazepine (Carbatrol, Tegretol), clonazepam (Klonopin), clorazepate (Tranxene), divalproex semisodium, divalproex sodium (Depakote), ethosuximide (Zarontin), ethotoin (Peganone), felbamate (Felbatol), fosphenytoin (Cerebyx, Mesantoin), levetiracetam (Keppra), mephenytoin, methsuximide (Celontin), oxcarbazepine (GP 47680, oxycarbamazepine; Trileptal), phenobarbital (phenobarbitone; Luminal, Solfoton), phenytoin (Dilantin, Phenytek), piracetam (Nootropyl), primidone (Mysoline), sodium valproate (Depacon), topiramate (Topamax), trimethadione (Tridione), valproate semisodium, valproic acid (Depakene, Depakene Syrup), vigabatrin (Sabril), zonisamide (Zonegran).
Similar properties but evidence lacking for extrapolation: Acetazolamide (Diamox; Diamox Sequels).

Interaction Type and Signficance

≈≈≈ **Drug-Induced Nutrient Depletion, Supplementation Therapeutic, Not Requiring Professional Management**
◇ **Adverse Drug Effect on Nutritional Therapeutics, Strategic Concern**
☼ **Prevention or Reduction of Drug Adverse Effect**

Probability:　　　　　　Evidence Base:
2. Probable　　　　　◉ **Emerging**

Effect and Mechanism of Action

Many anticonvulsants, including phenobarbital, cause reduced calcium absorption with long-term use.[58] Some anticonvulsants, such as phenytoin and phenobarbital, adversely affect calcium metabolism by reducing serum levels of calcidiol and thereby altering hepatic metabolism of vitamin D, at least in part by accelerating its metabolism and increasing the excretion of its metabolites.[59,60] Thus, hypocalcemia and subsequent bone loss during anticonvulsant therapy may be the result of vitamin D deficiency. Consequently, by multiple possible mechanisms, anticonvulsant medications may reduce serum calcium levels.

Research

Long-term therapy with phenytoin and other anticonvulsants can disturb vitamin D and calcium metabolism and result in osteomalacia. Both epilepsy and anticonvulsant medications are independent risk factors for low bone density, regardless of vitamin D levels. Long-term anticonvulsant treatment can cause excessive metabolism and deficiency of vitamin D and is believed to be associated with decreased bone mineral density (BMD) and bone loss.

In vitro research involving rat bone culture by Somerman et al.[61] found that phenytoin reduced 1,25-dihydroxycholecalciferol and inhibited vitamin D–mediated bone resorption even after phenytoin treatment was discontinued. Several studies have found that patients on long-term anticonvulsant therapy exhibit reduced serum concentrations of 25-hydroxycholecalciferol.[62,63] Both forms of vitamin D are necessary for calcium absorption.[6,64]

In a 1982 study involving 30 adult epileptic patients, Zerwekh et al.[65] reported decreased serum 24,25-dihydroxyvitamin D concentration during long-term anticonvulsant therapy (with phenytoin, phenobarbital, or carbamazepine), with phenobarbital-treated patients exhibiting a significant decrease in serum 25-OHD. They noted that various anticonvulsant agents appear to exert different effects on vitamin D metabolism.

After finding no pattern of low serum levels of vitamin D (25-OHD) or radiological evidence of osteomalacia or rickets in more than 400 individuals using anticonvulsants in Florida, Williams et al.[66] concluded that the climate provided adequate exposure to sunshine and thereby prevented the development of anticonvulsant-induced osteomalacia or rickets. "In contrast to reports from northern climates, we found minimal evidence of anticonvulsant-induced bone disease." Subsequently, in a controlled trial, Riancho et al.[67] studied 17 ambulatory epileptic children taking anticonvulsants for two seasons with high and low levels of solar radiation and observed that although serum 25-OHD concentrations were normal among medicated subjects during the summer, their levels were significantly lower than those of controls during the winter months.

In initiating a prospective 3-year study, Hunt et al.[68] found that of 144 children and young adults who required anticonvulsant therapy, 52 were found to have serum alkaline phosphatase (ALP) levels elevated more than two standard deviations (SDs) above normal, and half these showed signs of rickets or osteomalacia. After slow and gradual but varying rates of response to calcitriol, all patients showed significant lowering of serum ALP levels by 30 months of follow-up. In a later controlled study, Jekovec-Vrhovsek et al.[69] determined that bone strength improved (specifically, BMD increased) in 13 institutionalized children undergoing long-term anticonvulsant therapy who were supplemented for 9 months with 0.25 µg daily 1,25-dihydroxycholecalciferol vitamin D, the activated form of vitamin D, and 500 mg daily calcium.

Telci et al.[70] compared bone turnover in 52 epileptic patients receiving chronic anticonvulsant therapy with 39 healthy volunteers as matched controls and found that the resorption phase of bone turnover is affected during chronic anticonvulsant therapy. Total serum ALP levels (a marker of bone formation) were significantly increased in patients from both genders compared with those of their controls. Among male epileptic patients, urinary deoxypyridinoline levels (a marker of bone resorption) were significantly increased while 25-OHD levels were significantly reduced compared with those of their controls.

Farhat et al.[71] compared the effects of various antiepileptic drugs (AEDs) on bone density in 71 adults and children anticonvulsant therapy for at least 6 months. More than half the adults and children/adolescents had low serum 25-OHD levels. Although this finding did not correlate with their BMD, the AEDs were strongly associated with decreased BMD in the adults, particularly at skeletal sites enriched in cortical bone. Furthermore, lower BMD was more consistently associated with enzyme-inducing agents (e.g., phenytoin, phenobarbital, carbamazepine, primidone) than with medications that did not induce enzymes (e.g., valproic acid, lamotrigine, clonazepam, gabapentin, topamirate, ethosuximide). These researchers concluded: "Generalised seizures, duration of epilepsy, and polypharmacy were significant determinants of bone mineral density."

In 2001, Valmadrid et al.[72] published a survey of practice patterns of neurologists. They found that only 41% of pediatric and 28% of adult neurologists performed routine evaluation of patients receiving AEDs for either bone or mineral disease. Further, among those physicians who detected bone disease through such diagnostic testing, 40% of pediatric and 37% of adult neurologists prescribed either calcium or vitamin D. However, only 9% of pediatric and 7% of adult neurologists prescribed prophylactic calcium or vitamin D for patients taking AED therapy.

Reports
Duus[73] reported a case of several severe fractures in a patient following epileptic seizures. The patient had epileptic osteomalacia and responded well to vitamin D treatment.

Nutritional Therapeutics, Clinical Concerns, and Adaptations
Physicians prescribing anticonvulsant medications are advised to coadminister calcium (200-400 mg three times daily) and vitamin D (200-400 IU twice daily) if the course of treatment is expected to last more than 1 month. Pretreatment and posttreatment monitoring of serum 25-OHD and 1,25-OH$_2$D levels would also identify individuals at risk of treatment-induced and nutritional/sunlight-related deficiencies of vitamin D. With regard to supplementation, calcium needs to be taken at least 2 hours before or 4 hours after the medication to avoid interfering with drug absorption; calcium carbonate should be avoided in favor of another form less likely to impair drug activity. Individuals in growth phases (children and adolescents) are most vulnerable to depletion patterns and resultant bone loss and other potential adverse effects. Furthermore, many individuals with epilepsy, especially children, lead restricted lifestyles and are often institutionalized or under other forms of full-time care. Such individuals not only experience the effects of the pathophysiology on vitamin D metabolism, but also tend to have compromised nutritional status and restricted time outdoors in the sun, especially

during winter months. Thus, sunlight represents an effective and low-risk method of supporting vitamin D status. Walking and other simple forms of weight-bearing exercise will also support bone health and increase the efficacy of nutrient enhancement through dietary and supplemental sources.

Concomitant calcium administration carries a low probability of adversely affecting the efficacy of anticonvulsant therapy. Further research is warranted to develop knowledge of this interaction pattern, factors influencing individual susceptibilities, and clinical options for appropriate therapeutic responses.

Atenolol and Related Beta-1-Adrenoceptor Antagonists (Beta-1-Adrenergic Blocking Agents)

Evidence: Atenolol (Tenormin), sotalol (Betapace, Betapace AF, Sorine).
Extrapolated, based on similar properties: Atenolol combination drugs: atenolol and chlorthalidone (Co-Tendione, Tenoretic); atenolol and nifedipine (Beta-Adalat, Tenif).
Similar properties but evidence lacking for extrapolation: Acebutolol (Sectral), betaxolol (Kerlone), bisoprolol (Zebeta), carteolol (Cartrol), esmolol (Brevibloc), labetalol (Normodyne, Trandate), metoprolol (Lopressor, Toprol XL); combination drug: metoprolol and hydrochlorothiazide (Lopressor HCT); nadolol (Corgard), nebivolol (Nebilet), oxprenolol (Trasicor), penbutolol (Levatol), pindolol (Visken), propranolol (Betachron, Inderal LA, Innopran XL, Inderal); combination drug: propranolol and bendrofluazide (Inderex); timolol (Blocadren).

Interaction Type and Significance
◇◇ **Impaired Drug Absorption and Bioavailability, Precautions Appropriate**
◇ **Adverse Drug Effect on Nutritional Therapeutics, Strategic Concern**

Probability:	Evidence Base:
4. Plausible	▽ Mixed

Effect and Mechanism of Action
Simultaneous intake of atenolol or other beta blockers along with calcium salts may inhibit absorption and bioavailability of both substances and reduce plasma concentrations of the medication.[74] Long-term coadministration may increase the drug half-life and lead to accumulation.

Research
In a clinical trial involving five healthy subjects, Kahela et al.[75] observed that administration of sotalol with a calcium gluconate solution substantially reduces the absorption and bioavailability of sotalol. In a similar experiment involving six healthy subjects, Kirch et al.[76] found that oral administration of 500 mg calcium salts (lactate, gluconate, and carbonate) with atenolol (100 mg) reduced plasma levels of atenolol by 51%, and elimination half-life increased to a mean of 11.0 hours (vs. 6.2 hours with atenolol alone). The prolongation of elimination half-life induced by calcium coadministration led to atenolol cumulation during a subsequent 6-day course. Furthermore, exercise tachycardia was lower 12 hours after atenolol and calcium than with atenolol alone. Gugler and Allgayer[53] reported that later pharmacokinetic research involving calcium antacids did not confirm an interaction with atenolol.

Direct evidence is lacking demonstrating any interaction between calcium and other systemic beta blockers.

Nutritional Therapeutics, Clinical Concerns, and Adaptations

Physicians prescribing atenolol or related beta blockers should advise patients to separate intake of the medication by at least 1 hour before or 2 hours after calcium supplements (or antacids). Prudence also suggests that physicians check the blood pressure of such patients before and after the initiation of calcium administration during beta-blocker therapy.

Well-designed clinical trials using specific forms of calcium are warranted to determine patterns of interaction, factors influencing clinical significance, and clinical responses to ensure efficacy of both beta blockers and calcium supplementation.

Bile Acid Sequestrants

See Cholestyramine, Colestipol, and Related Bile Acid Sequestrants.

Bisphosphonates

Evidence: Alendronate (Fosamax), etidronate (Didronel), risedronate (Actonel).
Extrapolated, based on similar properties: Clodronate (Bonefos, Ostac), ibandronate (Bondronat, Boniva), tiludronate (Skelid), zoledronic acid (Zometa).
Similar properties but evidence lacking for extrapolation: Pamidronate (Aredia).

Interaction Type and Significance

⊕⊕⊕   **Beneficial or Supportive Interaction, Not Requiring Professional Management**
◇◇   **Impaired Drug Absorption and Bioavailability, Precautions Appropriate**
◇   **Adverse Drug Effect on Nutritional Therapeutics, Strategic Concern**

Probability: Evidence Base:
2. Probable or   ◉ Emerging or
  1. Certain   ● Consensus

Effect and Mechanism of Action

The ability of bisphosphonates to effectively inhibit osteoclastic activity and bone resorption, maintain healthy bone mineralization, and produce substantial gains in bone mass depends on the presence of adequate vitamin D and other nutrients (e.g., protein, calcium, phosphorus).[77,78] Calcium, the principal element in bone, can only be absorbed in the brush border of the intestinal mucosa when vitamin D is present. Notably, bisphosphonates have been used effectively to treat the more resistant cases of vitamin D–induced hypercalcemia.

Research

All currently approved bone-active pharmacological agents have been studied only in conjunction with supplemental calcium; newer anabolic agents increase mineral demand in skeletal tissue and will thus require even higher levels of calcium repletion.[79] The consensus underlying the fundamental importance of vitamin D and calcium nutriture is underscored by the observation that when Greenspan et al.[80] investigated the relative efficacy of hormone replacement therapy (HRT, conjugated estrogen with or without medroxyprogesterone) plus alendronate, HRT alone, alendronate alone, or placebo on spine and hip BMD in 373 osteopenic elderly women, all subjects received calcium and vitamin D supplements. After 3 years, dual-energy x-ray absorptiometry (DXA) scans showed that participants taking combination therapy had greater improvements in BMD at the hip and spine than did those participants taking HRT or alendronate alone, or placebo, all with calcium and vitamin D.

In an uncontrolled clinical trial involving osteoporosis patients with a poor response to bisphosphonate therapy, Heckman et al.[81] found that the addition of 25 μg (1000 IU) vitamin D daily to the bisphosphonate regimen resulted in significantly increased BMD of the lumbar spine after 1 year.[81] In a randomized, double-blind trial involving 48 osteopenic and osteoporotic women, Brazier et al.[82] compared one group who received alendronate, 10 mg once daily, along with 500 mg elemental calcium daily and 10 μg (400 IU) cholecalciferol (vitamin D_3) twice daily for 3 months, and a second group who received the same dosage of alendronate and calcium but placebo instead of the vitamin D. All subjects had low BMD, serum 25-hydroxyvitamin D_3 (25-OHD, calcifediol) less than 12 μg/L, and dietary calcium intake less than 1 g/day. Although markers of bone remodeling such as serum and urinary CTX and urinary NTX (C- and N-terminal telopeptides of type I collagen) were dramatically and significantly decreased after as soon as 15 days of treatment and remained decreased throughout treatment in both groups, the group also receiving the vitamin D demonstrated a more pronounced effect, particularly after 1 month, for the bone resorption markers serum CTX and urinary NTX. These researchers concluded that coadministration of calcium and vitamin D could be appropriate in elderly women with calcium and vitamin D insufficiencies being treated with alendronate, to achieve rapid reduction of bone loss.[82]

Paget's disease is characterized by abnormal osteoclastic bone resorption, and bisphosphonates are powerful and selective inhibitors of osteoclastic bone resorption. In a randomized, placebo-controlled, double-blind study involving 15 patients with Paget's disease, O'Doherty et al.[83] observed that daily 1-hour infusions of alendronate caused small decreases in serum calcium, serum phosphate, and urinary calcium excretion.

Reasner et al.[84] observed acute changes in calcium homeostasis as a result of 7 days' treatment with risedronate. A decrease in serum calcium was accompanied by evidence of inhibition of bone resorption in patients with mild primary hyperparathyroidism, a condition typically characterized by hypercalcemia. Oral calcium partially suppressed serum hyperparathyroid hormone in both controls and subjects receiving risedronate. Although patients treated with risedronate had normal fasting serum calcium levels, serum calcium values in these normocalcemic patients were labile after oral calcium. After administration of 2 g calcium daily, serum calcium levels in risedronate-treated patients were similar to those in untreated patients with primary hyperparathyroidism. The authors interpreted these findings to suggest that serum calcium levels are likely to fluctuate in risedronate-treated patients with normal fasting serum calcium during postprandial periods. Further long-term research is warranted to determine whether the lability in serum calcium observed in the short term has clinical significance, how risedronate would influence serum calcium levels and BMD with extended use, and what clinical implications would be for concomitant calcium.

Some patients with prostate carcinoma and a diffuse metastatic invasion of the skeleton exhibit indirect biochemical and histological indications of osteomalacia. Bisphosphonates are known to cause symptomatic hypocalcemia in prostate cancer patients with diffuse skeletal metastases. Bisphosphonate administration can aggravate osteomalacia and give the appearance of symptomatic hypocalcemia because of the transient, striking prevalence of osteoblastic activity over bone resorption by osteoclasts, which are inhibited by bisphosphonate drugs. Calcium supplementation is often considered as contraindicated in individuals with prostate cancer. However, concomitant use with bisphosphonates has been proposed as a means of inhibiting osteoclastic activation that often precedes the abnormal osteoblastic bone formation within metastases. Thus, Adami[85] suggested that coadministration of high doses of calcium with alendronate therapy in prostate cancer patients with bone metastases (with evidence of osteomalacia) might contribute to improved clinical outcomes.

In regard to men with nonmetastatic prostate cancer, findings from a small, randomized, double-blind controlled trial conducted by Nelson et al.[86] showed that treatment with 70 mg alendronate weekly, plus daily calcium and vitamin D, reversed bone loss in men receiving antiandrogen therapy. In contrast, the 56 subjects taking placebo, calcium, and vitamin D lost BMD during the same period. Notably, among these 112 men, average age 71, only 9% had normal bone mass, whereas 52% had low bone mass and 39% developed osteoporosis after an average 2 years of androgen-deprivation therapy (ADT).[86]

In a nonblinded, randomized prospective trial examining BMD in 211 long-term adult renal transplant recipients, Jeffery et al.[87] compared calcitriol and alendronate and found that osteopenia or osteoporosis, which are experienced by the majority of such patients, can be effectively treated with calcium plus calcitriol or alendronate.

In a randomized trial involving 154 patients with Crohn's disease, Siffledeen et al.[88] investigated the efficacy of etidronate plus calcium and vitamin D for treatment of low BMD. The subjects, most of whom had T scores in the osteopenic range (−1.5 to −2.5), were administered etidronate (400 mg orally) or placebo for 14 days, and then both groups were given daily calcium (500 mg) and vitamin D (400 IU) for 76 days in a treatment cycle repeated every 3 months for 2 years. After 24 months, BMD at the lumbar spine, ultradistal radius, and trochanter sites, but not the total hip, increased steadily, significantly, and similarly in both treatment arms. The findings from this trial demonstrate that, in patients with low BMD on absorptiometry, treatment with calcium and vitamin D alone will increase bone density by about 4% per year and that adding etidronate to the treatment program does not appear to enhance the effects of calcium and vitamin D.[88] In an accompanying editorial on the preeminence of calcium and vitamin D in limiting fracture risk in Crohn's (inflammatory bowel) disease (IBD), Bernstein[89] commented that this study provides reassurance that bisphosphonates are "rarely needed in IBD patients most of whom have T scores greater than −2.5, and many of whom are using corticosteroids to some extent."

The National Osteoporosis Risk Assessment (NORA) Study, a longitudinal, observational study of osteoporosis among postmenopausal women in primary care practices across the U.S., reported in 2005 that 58% of women who might benefit from the osteoporosis treatment do not receive any of the standard medications, and when HRT is included, the number falls to 38%.[90]

Reports

In a review of 63 cases, Ruggiero et al.[91] described a pattern of osteonecrosis of the jaw (ONJ), an otherwise rare condition, in patients undergoing prolonged treatment with bisphosphonates. Fifty-six patients had received intravenous bisphosphonates for at least 1 year, and seven patients were receiving chronic oral bisphosphonate therapy. Fifty-five of these patients were being treated for various forms of cancer, one for osteoporosis. ONJ has occurred spontaneously in a significant number of patients. However, most cases have been associated with infections after dental surgeries, in patients on bisphosphonate therapy. The authors recommend that all patients on long-term bisphosphonate therapy have two or three preventive dental visits per year, and that physicians be watchful for any early signs of ONJ, such as tooth pain, swelling, numbness of the lip and chin, or pain in the jaw.

Nutritional Therapeutics, Clinical Concerns, and Adaptations

Calcium and vitamin D are essential for maintaining bone mass and density and imperative to the success of drug therapies for inducing bone augmentation.[78] Deficiencies of both nutrients are common in the patient populations at highest risk for bone loss. The importance of exercise and sound nutrition (including adequate protein, calcium, and phosphorus intake) as foundational cannot be overemphasized and is supported by growing evidence. Calcium has a clearly demonstrated effect of enhancing estrogen's effects on bone metabolism. Further, most research indicates that consistent exposure to sunlight (excluding winter in northern latitudes) provides a safe and effective, as well as otherwise beneficial, method of elevating vitamin D levels. Daily doses of 1500 mg calcium and 800 IU vitamin D provide prudent nutritional support for osteoporosis prevention and treatment, or more exactly, 30 to 40 mmol calcium with sufficient intake vitamin D daily, to maintain serum 25(OH)D levels above 80 nmol/L (∼ 30 µg/L).[79]

Thus, a synergistic combination of oral calcium and vitamin D, within the context of an active lifestyle and nutrient-rich diet, constitutes the core proactive intervention within integrative therapeutics for all individuals at high risk for osteoporosis, or a foundational treatment for diagnosed bone loss. Notably, low serum vitamin D levels have been associated with the incidence of falls in older women,[92] and vitamin D has been found to be helpful in reducing the incidence of falls, a major factor in fracture risk, by improving muscle strength, walking distance, and functional ability.[93] Also, hormone supplementation or replacement regimens (conventional HRT, bio-identical estrogens/progesterone, herbal hormone precursors/modulators) should be considered if indicated in women. In addition to these primary and secondary therapies, the use of a bisphosphonate can provide a potent intervention in reversing bone loss and supporting healthy bone mass.

Coadministration of bisphosphonates and calcium in patients with Paget's disease or prostate carcinoma requires close supervision and regular monitoring within the context of an integrative team of health care professionals trained and experienced in multidisciplinary therapeutics, including conventional pharmacology and nutritional therapeutics.

Oral calcium preparations need to be taken at least 2 hours before or after the bisphosphonate to avoid pharmacokinetic interference. However, the timing of oral vitamin D intake need not be managed because no evidence has indicated potential pharmacological interference with bisphosphonates or other components of the treatment. It is generally recommended to take alendronate or etidronate with a full glass (6-8 ounces) of plain water on an empty stomach and to avoid the recumbent position for at least 30 minutes to prevent potential severe esophageal irritation associated with incomplete transfer of the tablet to the stomach.

Calcitonin

Calcitonin (Calcimar, Miacalcin Nasal).

Interaction Type and Significance

⊕⊕ **Beneficial or Supportive Interaction, with Professional Management**

Probability:	Evidence Base:
2. Probable	◉ Emerging or
	● Consensus

Effect and Mechanism of Action

Calcitonin is a polypeptide hormone made by the thyroid gland that decreases bone resorption and reduces bone loss. Adequate calcium intake appears to enhance the bone-sparing benefit of calcitonin, particularly on the spine.

Research

Nieves et al.[94] reviewed six published clinical trials evaluating the effects of 200 IU intranasal salmon calcitonin in combination with calcium administration (total 1466 mg/day) as well as one using calcitonin alone. They observed that bone mass of the lumbar spine increased 2.1% with calcitonin and calcium, compared with −0.2% per year in those receiving calcitonin alone. These researchers concluded that the available data suggest that a high calcium intake potentiates the positive effect of calcitonin on bone mass of the spine. They also noted that these findings suggest that the dosage of nasal calcitonin used (200 IU) may be suboptimal.

Nutritional Therapeutics, Clinical Concerns, and Adaptations

Physicians prescribing intranasal calcitonin for prevention or treatment of osteoporosis are advised to coadminister calcium (400-500 mg three times daily).

Calcium Acetate

Calcium acetate (Phoslo).

Interaction Type and Significance

✗✗✗ **Potentially Harmful or Serious Adverse Interaction—Avoid**

Probability:	Evidence Base:
2. Probable	● Consensus

Effect and Mechanism of Action

Concomitant use of calcium supplements during calcium acetate administration can produce an additive effect that may be harmful in some individuals, especially in the context of renal failure.

Calcium acetate supplies an extremely bioavailable source of calcium because it ionizes readily and the acetate is quickly burned in the Krebs cycle, thereby providing a ready supply of calcium ions to complex with free phosphorus in renal patients with hyperphosphatemia. Care must be taken not to administer calcium if the serum calcium times phosphorus ($Ca \times PO_4$) product is greater than 70; calcium phosphate deposition in soft tissues is likely at this level. Aluminum salts were previously used for this purpose but were largely replaced by calcium acetate as the toxicity of aluminum became recognized.

Research

Although the additive interaction between these agents is considered formulaic and highly probable to result in clinically significant adverse effects, evidence from clinical trials focused directly on this interaction is lacking.

Clinical Implications and Adaptations

Physicians prescribing calcium acetate are advised to be watchful for indications of hypercalcemia (e.g., anorexia, depression, poor memory, muscle weakness), monitor serum calcium and phosphorus levels, and warn patients to avoid calcium supplementation. This interaction may be relevant only to the population with chronic renal insufficiency. It is not known whether it applies to those with normal renal function because clinical trials addressing this question are lacking. The probability of a clinically significant interaction involving hypercalcemia after concomitant intake of calcium acetate and other calcium supplements in normal individuals is low.

Cholestyramine, Colestipol, and Related Bile Acid Sequestrants

Evidence: Cholestyramine (Locholest, Prevalite, Questran), colestipol (Colestid).
Extrapolated, based on similar properties: Colesevelam (WelChol).

Interaction Type and Significance

≈≈≈ **Drug-Induced Nutrient Depletion, Supplementation Therapeutic, Not Requiring Professional Management**

◇ **Adverse Drug Effect on Nutritional Therapeutics, Strategic Concern**

Probability:	Evidence Base:
3. Possible	○ Preliminary or
	◉ Emerging

Effect and Mechanism of Action

The primary effect on calcium levels may be caused by lowered absorption of vitamin D under the influence of bile acid sequestrants. Medications in this class can bind calcium and thereby impair its absorption; they may also increase the loss of calcium in the urine.

Research

Diminished intestinal absorption of vitamin D, osteomalacia, and other metabolic alterations have been reported with long-term use of bile acid sequestrants. Colestipol lowers vitamin D absorption and thus adversely affects calcium metabolism. In vitro research indicates that cholestyramine causes appreciable binding of calcium (from calcium chloride) and thereby decreases absorption.[95] Animal studies suggest that cholestyramine may deplete calcium (and zinc). Watkins et al.[96] observed that rats fed cholestyramine for 1 month had a net negative balance for calcium, increased urinary excretion of calcium and magnesium, and a lower net positive balance for magnesium, iron, and zinc than the controls. They attributed these alterations in calcium, magnesium, and zinc metabolism to impaired vitamin D absorption from the intestine, followed by increased PTH secretion.

One study investigating possible malabsorption of minerals and vitamins in young patients with familial hypercholesterolemia after 5 years of colestipol therapy found no significant changes in plasma levels of calcium, PTH, and vitamin D, as well as other nutrients. However, changes in most of these parameters would not be predicted, and potential effects on bone mass were not assessed.[97] However, Tonstad et al.[98] conducted a study of 37 boys and 29 girls age 10 to 16 years with familial hypercholesterolemia, first in an 8-week, double-blind, placebo-controlled protocol, then in open treatment for 44 to 52 weeks. After 1 year of colestipol, those who took 80% or more of the prescribed dose had a greater decrease in serum 25-OHD levels than those who took less than 80%. Secondary effects on calcium metabolism and bone health were not investigated directly, but the observed adverse effect on vitamin D would be predicted to impair calcium absorption. Also, levels of serum folate, vitamin E, and carotenoids were reduced in the colestipol group.

Nutritional Therapeutics, Clinical Concerns, and Adaptations

Physicians prescribing bile acid sequestrants are advised to recommend supplementation with calcium (500 mg twice daily) along with vitamin D and other fat-soluble nutrients. Although modest supplementation with vitamin D (10-20 µg or 400-800 IU daily) may be advisable for many individuals, particularly those at high risk for deficiency sequelae, consistent exposure to sunlight (without sunscreen) may be sufficient to maintain healthy vitamin D levels and can be combined with the exercise usually critical to those being prescribed bile acid sequestrants. Exposure to sunlight in the winter months of northern latitudes, however, is likely to be insufficient to maintain adequate vitamin D levels, making it necessary to use dietary supplements or a rich natural source of vitamin D, such as cod liver oil, at least 2 hours before or after the bile sequestrant agents.

Corticosteroids, Oral, Including Prednisone

Betamethasone (Celestone), cortisone (Cortone), dexamethasone (Decadron), hydrocortisone (Cortef), methylprednisolone (Medrol) prednisolone (Delta-Cortef, Orapred, Pediapred, Prelone), prednisone (Deltasone, Liquid Pred, Meticorten, Orasone), triamcinolone (Aristocort).
Similar properties but evidence indicating no or reduced interaction effects: Inhaled or topical corticosteroids.

Interaction Type and Significance

≈≈≈ **Drug-Induced Nutrient Depletion, Supplementation Therapeutic, Not Requiring Professional Management**
◇ **Adverse Drug Effect on Nutritional Therapeutics, Strategic Concern**
☼ **Prevention or Reduction of Drug Adverse Effect**

Nutrient Depletion
Probability: Evidence Base:
2. Probable   ● **Consensus**

Drug Adverse Effect Reduction
Probability: Evidence Base:
2. Probable   ◉ **Emerging**

Effect and Mechanism of Action

Corticosteroids can impair calcium absorption and interfere with both calcium and vitamin D metabolism, thereby adversely affecting bone density and potentially other calcium-related functions. Several mechanisms have been implicated in these adverse effects. Corticosteroids interfere with the activation of vitamin D and thereby impair calcium absorption and contribute to secondary hyperparathyroidism. Decreases in tubular calcium reabsorption with increases in urinary excretion of calcium have also been demonstrated. Thus, increased bone resorption is caused by decreased calcium absorption and increased urinary calcium excretion, leading to secondary hyperparathyroidism. Furthermore, corticosteroids increase the risk for developing osteoporosis not only by

altering normal calcium metabolism, but also by reducing osteoblast activity. Also, steroids, even in low dose, can decrease osteocalcin, P1CP, and ALP.[99-112]

Research

Oral corticosteroids can adversely affect BMD and increase the risk of osteoporosis through their impact on both calcium and vitamin D. Numerous studies have demonstrated adverse effects on vitamin D and its functions due to steroid therapy; these are reviewed in the vitamin D monograph. Under active transport conditions, administration of corticosteroids produces a decrease of net calcium absorption by depressing vitamin D–dependent intestinal calcium absorption and increasing vitamin D–independent calcium backflux.[101,102,109,113]

Corticosteroids can adversely affect both bone formation and resorption. Serum osteocalcin, a sensitive marker of bone formation (and a vitamin K–dependent protein), is reduced with both short-term and chronic glucocorticoid treatment, corresponding to observed effects of reduced bone formation. In a double-blind placebo-controlled study involving 15 normal subjects, Nielsen et al.[106] found that oral prednisone at two dosage levels, 2.5 mg and 10 mg, proportionately inhibited serum osteocalcin levels within 3 to 4 hours and even reversed the normal nocturnal rise within the circadian rhythm of serum osteocalcin levels. In a 1998 study, Lems et al.[112] reported that low-dose (10 mg/day) prednisone (LDP) treatment led to a decrease in osteocalcin, P1CP, and ALP and an increase in urinary excretion of calcium. They concluded that LDP has a negative effect on bone metabolism because bone formation decreased and bone resorption remained unchanged or decreased slightly.

A strong trend in the cumulative research findings demonstrates that corticosteroids, especially long-term therapy or repeated use, can reduce bone density, cause development of corticosteroid-induced osteoporosis, and increase the risk of sustaining osteoporotic fractures.[110,114-118] By comparing asthmatic patients receiving long-term glucocorticoid therapy with a second group of age-matched and gender-matched asthmatic individuals not receiving these drugs, Reid et al.[115] measured a significant reduction in renal tubular calcium reabsorption in the glucocorticoid-treated patients. Tsugeno et al.[117] measured relative cortical volume (RCV) and other parameters in 86 postmenopausal asthmatic women taking high-dose oral steroid (> 10 g cumulative oral prednisolone) and 194 age-matched controls. Individuals treated with high doses of oral steroid demonstrated a significantly increased risk of fracture compared with control women after adjustment was made for years since menopause, body mass index, and RCV. In a study involving 117 patients taking oral corticosteroids for chronic lung disease, Walsh et al.[119] found that 58% had osteoporosis (a T score of less than −2.5) and 61% had a vertebral fracture, and that cumulative prednisolone dose was strongly associated with vertebral fracture. After analyzing the composite data, they concluded that "cumulative prednisolone dose is strongly related to fracture risk, and this effect is independent of its more modest impact on BMD." In a retrospective, cohort study, Steinbuch et al.[120] observed that oral glucocorticoid use is associated with an increased risk of fracture. Specifically, they found that dose dependence of fracture risk was observed for hip, vertebral, nonvertebral, and any fractures. Extended duration and continuous pattern of steroid use demonstrated a fivefold increase in risk of hip fracture and 5.9-fold increase in risk of vertebral fracture. Together, the combined effect of higher dose, longer duration, and continuous pattern further increased relative risk estimates to sevenfold for hip fractures and seventeenfold for vertebral fractures. Thus, a consensus has emerged confirming a strong association between oral corticosteroid therapy, especially chronic or repeated use, and adverse effects on calcium balance, BMD, and fracture susceptibility. Vitamin D deficiency is also associated with increased fracture risk as well as risk of falls. Overall, the degree of bone loss usually parallels the cumulative corticosteroid dose, and the highest rate of bone loss is observed in the first 3 to 6 months of therapy.

The adverse effects associated with inhaled corticosteroids (ICs) are generally considered as less common, less severe, and significantly less likely risk to contribute to fractures. For example, in a group of postmenopausal women, Elmstahl et al.[122] found no difference in BMD between the subset using ICs and unexposed control subjects, and no dose-response relationship between IC therapy and BMD.

The predominant weight of evidence suggests that coadministration of calcium and vitamin D can mitigate and possibly reverse loss of bone density and risk of osteoporosis associated with long-term oral corticosteroid therapy. In particular, the adverse effects of glucoactive corticosteroids on intestinal calcium transport and bone turnover can usually be counteracted by the combined administration of supplemental doses of calcium and physiologic doses of $25(OH)D_3$.[102,123,124] Reid and Ibbertson[125] studied the metabolic effects of administering 1 g of elemental calcium daily in 13 steroid-treated patients. After 2 months, they concluded that "calcium supplementation suppresses bone resorption without detectable suppression of indices of bone formation" and was therefore likely to result in increased bone mass. In a 2-year, randomized, double-blind, placebo-controlled trial involving 96 patients administered low-dose prednisone (mean dosage, 5.6 mg/day) for rheumatoid arthritis, Buckley et al.[113] found that subjects who received concomitant calcium carbonate (1000 mg) and vitamin D_3 (500 IU) daily maintained their bone density and gained BMD in the lumbar spine and trochanter. Subsequently, in a multiphase observational trial involving eight healthy, young male volunteers administered low-dose prednisone (10 mg/day), Lems et al.[126] found PTH (insignificantly) increased during prednisone (+19%) and prednisone plus 500 mg/day calcium (+14%), but decreased during supplementation with calcitriol (−16%) and calcium/calcitriol (−44%). The increase in PTH during prednisone could be prevented by coadministration of calcitriol and calcium.

Several recent reviews have come to somewhat divergent conclusions. Amin et al.[127] conducted a meta-analysis of all randomized controlled trials lasting at least 6 months (and reporting extractable results). They applied change in lumbar BMD as the primary outcome measure and observed that coadministration with the combination of calcium and vitamin D provided a "moderate beneficial effect," compared with placebo or calcium alone, in protecting against corticosteroid-induced osteoporosis. They concluded that "treatment with vitamin D plus calcium, as a minimum, should be recommended to patients receiving long-term corticosteroids." In contrast, in a review of the evidence on calcium supplementation for corticosteroid-induced bone loss during steroid therapy, also published in 1999, Adachi and Ioannidis[60] declared, "Calcium prophylaxis alone, when patients start corticosteroids, is associated with rapid rates of spinal bone loss and offers only partial protection from corticosteroid-induced spinal bone loss. Though calcium supplementation may have some benefit, it clearly cannot completely prevent corticosteroid-induced bone loss." Commenting on studies showing benefit from calcium supplementation, they also observed that

"caution should be taken when interpreting these results, since bone loss generally tapers or plateaus after the first 12 months of corticosteroid treatment; as such, any therapy might show benefit." They also questioned the methodology used in assessing bone density, particularly measurements at the radius rather than the spine. They also questioned the adequacy of calcium and vitamin D in counteracting the bone loss caused by corticosteroids and suggested the need for further support, including activated vitamin D.[60] In a 2000 Cochrane review, Homik et al.[128] evaluated five trials (totaling 247 patients) for lumbar and radial bone BMD after a minimum of 2 years supportive treatment. Their meta-analysis demonstrated "a clinically and statistically significant prevention of bone loss at the lumbar spine and forearm with vitamin D and calcium in corticosteroid treated patients." Noting the low cost and limited toxicity, they recommended that "all patients being started on corticosteroids should receive prophylactic therapy with calcium and vitamin D."

The issue of which forms of calcium and vitamin D provide the most effective protection with the least risk of adverse effects remains unresolved. Evidence is lacking from well-designed trials focusing on which of the of various forms of calcium, or combinations thereof, is most efficacious against steroid-induced bone loss, establishing appropriate dosage level, and determining possible variables in patient characteristics influencing efficacy. The question of safety and efficacy in selecting an appropriate form of vitamin D is similarly unresolved and remains contentious within conventional medicine. Numerous researchers and commentators have voiced concern over the risk of hypercalciuria and hypercalcemia when coadministering both calcium and vitamin D and noted experiences or cited reports of such.[111] Although the weight of evidence indicates that calcitriol ($1,25-OH_2D_3$), the most active form of vitamin D, may be the most effective, it also carries greater risk than calcifediol ($25-OHD$) or other forms of vitamin D.[129]

Nutritional Therapeutics, Clinical Concerns, and Adaptations

The primary concern regarding calcium in the context of corticosteroid therapy is bone loss through decreased absorption and increased urinary excretion. Corticosteroid-induced osteoporosis is a serious disorder that results in significant long-term morbidity. Optimal management strategies to prevent bone loss should include the use of the lowest efficacious dose of steroid medications and shortest duration of administration.

Prevention of adverse effects should include adequate calcium intakes from dietary and supplemental sources totaling 1000 to 1500 mg of calcium daily in conjunction with at least 500 IU of vitamin D daily, although much higher doses may be necessary in the context of a preexisting $25-OHD$ deficiency.[41] Monitoring serum levels of both $25-OHD$ and $1,25-OH_2D$ (activated form of vitamin D) is appropriate, and prescription of calcitriol may be necessary if a deficiency is indicated. If $25-OHD$ levels are low (< 50 nmol/L), correction with up to 7000 IU vitamin D_3 daily, or 50,000 IU vitamin D_2 weekly, for 1 to 2 months will correct the 1,25-dihydroxycholecalciferol level in patients with normal renal function. Often the $1,25-OH_2D$ level is maintained, even in the face of a $25-OHD$ deficiency, due to increased secretion of PTH, which speeds up renal conversion of $25-OHD$ to the active form. Thus, measuring intact PTH as well as both forms of vitamin D provides the most complete picture of vitamin D status.[41] It is also prudent to monitor for hypercalciuria and hypercalcemia when supplementing with both calcium and vitamin D. Physicians prescribing steroids for longer than 2 weeks should encourage all patients to modify their lifestyles, including smoking cessation and limitation of alcohol consumption. The importance of mild to moderate weight-bearing exercise cannot be overemphasized; 30 minutes to 1 hour every day, particularly with sunlight exposure, should be strongly encouraged, if feasible. However, individuals with known or potential bone loss should be advised to develop an exercise program under the supervision of a physician or other health care professional familiar with the increased risks of fracture associated with long-term use of steroids.

EDTA

EDTA (Ethylenediaminetetraacetic Acid)

Interaction Type and Significance

≈≈ **Drug-Induced Nutrient Depletion, Supplementation Therapeutic, with Professional Management**
✗✗ **Minimal to Mild Adverse Interaction—Vigilance Necessary**

Probability:
1. Certain

Evidence Base:
● Consensus

Effect and Mechanism of Action
EDTA binds to calcium and thereby increases calcium excretion.

Research
The chelation function of EDTA is central to its primary pharmacological action in therapeutic application.[130] As such, chelation with EDTA is considered among standard causes of hypocalcemia from increased loss of calcium, and EDTA is used experimentally to induce hypocalcemia.[131] However, in the presence of heavy metals, which bind more tightly to EDTA than calcium, the heavy metals will preferentially bind.

Experiments by Foreman and Trujillo[132] (1954) found that EDTA demonstrated 45% to 72% efficiency chelating Ca^{++} and that up to 3.2 mg/dL Ca^{++} is bound during infusion. Calcium excretion changed over time after chelation, with 28% excess Ca^{++} excreted during infusion, 60% excess Ca^{++} excreted 6 hours after infusion, and 12% excess Ca^{++} excreted 6 to 12 hours after infusion. Overall, serum ionized Ca^{++} was significantly reduced. Numerous responses to EDTA-induced hypocalcemia have been documented, including ionization of protein-bound and soft tissue Ca^{++}, induction of PTH secretion and vitamin D_3 synthesis, stimulation of bone resorption and osteoclast differentiation, and suppression of osteoblast differentiation.

Nutritional Therapeutics, Clinical Concerns, and Adaptations
Chelation with EDTA or other agents requires appropriate training and proper monitoring. Assessment of calcium levels is appropriate, and clinical responses will vary accordingly. When properly administered, EDTA chelation is considered unlikely to result in adverse reactions from hypocalcemia. Physicians who administer EDTA for chelation of heavy metals or other clinical applications routinely supplement their patients with minerals of nutritional importance.

ESTROGENS, PROGESTINS, AND ESTROGEN-PROGESTIN COMBINATIONS

Oral Contraceptives: Monophasic, Biphasic, and Triphasic Estrogen Preparations (Synthetic Estrogen and Progesterone Analogs)

Ethinyl estradiol and desogestrel (Desogen, Ortho-TriCyclen).

Ethinyl estradiol and ethynodiol (Demulen 1/35, Demulen 1/50, Nelulen 1/25, Nelulen 1/50, Zovia).
Ethinyl estradiol and levonorgestrel (Alesse, Levlen, Levlite, Levora 0.15/30, Nordette, Tri-Levlen, Triphasil, Trivora).
Ethinyl estradiol and norethindrone/norethisterone (Brevicon, Estrostep, Genora 1/35, GenCept 1/35, Jenest-28, Loestrin 1.5/30, Loestrin1/20, Modicon, Necon 1/25, Necon 10/11, Necon 0.5/30, Necon 1/50, Nelova 1/35, Nelova 10/11, Norinyl 1/35, Norlestin 1/50, Ortho Novum 1/35, Ortho Novum 10/11, Ortho Novum 7/7/7, Ovcon-35, Ovcon-50, Tri-Norinyl, Trinovum).
Ethinyl estradiol and norgestrel (Lo/Ovral, Ovral).
Mestranol and norethindrone (Genora 1/50, Nelova 1/50, Norethin 1/50, Ortho-Novum 1/50).
Related, internal application: Etonogestrel/ethinyl estradiol vaginal ring (Nuvaring).

Hormone Replacement Therapy (HRT): Estrogen-Containing and Synthetic Estrogen and Progesterone Analog Medications

HRT, estrogens: Chlorotrianisene (Tace); conjugated equine estrogens (Premarin); conjugated synthetic estrogens (Cenestin); dienestrol (Ortho Dienestrol); esterified estrogens (Estratab, Menest, Neo-Estrone); estradiol, topical/transdermal/ring (Alora Transdermal, Climara Transdermal, Estrace, Estradot, Estring FemPatch, Vivelle-Dot, Vivelle Transdermal); estradiol cypionate (Dep-Gynogen, Depo-Estradiol, Depogen, Dura-Estrin, Estra-D, Estro-Cyp, Estroject-LA, Estronol-LA); estradiol hemihydrate (Estreva, Vagifem); estradiol valerate (Delestrogen, Estra-L 40, Gynogen L.A. 20, Progynova, Valergen 20); estrone (Aquest, Estragyn 5, Estro-A, Estrone '5', Kestrone-5); estropipate (Ogen, Ortho-Est); ethinyl estradiol (Estinyl, Gynodiol, Lynoral).
HRT, estrogen/progestin combinations: Conjugated equine estrogens and medroxyprogesterone (Premelle cycle 5, Prempro); conjugated equine estrogens and norgestrel (Prempak-C); estradiol and dydrogesterone (Femoston); estradiol and norethindrone, patch (CombiPatch); estradiol and norethindrone/norethisterone, oral (Activella, Climagest, Climesse, FemHRT, Trisequens); estradiol valerate and cyproterone acetate (Climens); estradiol valerate and norgestrel (Progyluton); estradiol and norgestimate (Ortho-Prefest).
HRT, estrogen/testosterone combinations: Esterified estrogens and methyltestosterone (Estratest, Estratest HS).
See also Medroxyprogesterone.

Interaction Type and Significance

⊕⊕⊕ **Beneficial or Supportive Interaction, Not Requiring Professional Management**
☼ **Prevention or Reduction of Drug Adverse Effect**

Probability:
2. Probable

Evidence Base:
◉ Emerging

Effect and Mechanism of Action
Estrogen-containing medications can contribute to decreased BMD and increase the long-term risk of osteoporosis. Concomitant use of calcium (and vitamin D) supplements and exogenous estrogen may act synergistically to improve bone density and support the prevention and treatment of osteoporosis. Calcium, the principal element in bone, can only be absorbed in the brush border of the intestinal mucosa when vitamin D is present. Estrogen appears to enhance calcium absorption by increasing serum 1,25-dihydroxycholecalciferol [$1,25(OH)_2D$]. In contrast to the

beneficial effect on vitamin D (and calcium) metabolism exerted by estrogens, progestins may diminish that benefit. Estrogens may also contribute to an overall increase in calcium blood levels by decreasing urinary calcium loss. Overall, the ability of exogenous female hormones, particularly forms of estrogen, to effectively inhibit osteoclastic activity and bone resorption, maintain healthy bone mineralization, and support bone mass is inherently dependent on the presence of vitamin D, calcium, and other nutrients (e.g., protein, phosphorus).[77,78]

Research

In a randomized clinical trial, Teegarden et al.[133] studied the relationship between dietary calcium intake and BMD in 133 young women (18-30 years old) using oral contraceptives (OCs) who all were initially characterized by dietary calcium intake of less than 800 mg/day. The subjects were assigned to groups stratified by dietary intake: high calcium intake (1200-1300 mg/day), medium calcium intake (1000-1100 mg/day), and control (<800 mg/day). They found that higher levels of calcium intake, in the form of dairy products, positively impacted percent change of total-hip and total-body bone mineral density (BMD) and bone mineral content (BMC) and that such intake patterns "prevented a negative percent change in total hip and spine BMD" in women using OCs. They concluded: "Dairy product intake, at levels to achieve the recommended intakes of calcium, protected the total hip BMD and spine BMD from loss observed in young healthy women with low calcium intakes who were using [OCs]."[133]

The negative calcium balance usually associated with aging is accentuated in osteoporotic women who have decreased calcium absorption and decreased serum levels of $1,25(OH)_2D$. In a controlled trial involving 17 women with surgically induced menopause, Lobo et al.[134] (1985) observed that serum levels of $1,25(OH)_2D$ increased and urinary calcium loss decreased after 2 months of conjugated estrogens (0.625 mg daily).[134] Subsequently, several studies have investigated whether such elevated vitamin D levels might correspond with increased bone strength and reduced risk of fractures, and how such effect might vary given initial BMD status, for different individuals, under different HRT regimens, or with different forms of calcium.

Several studies have examined the role of estrogen in improving calcium balance in women with postmenopausal osteoporosis. In a randomized, double-blind, placebo-controlled trial involving 128 healthy Caucasian women over age 65 with low spinal BMD, Recker et al.[135] compared parameters of BMD and bone loss under continuous low-dose HRT (conjugated equine estrogen, 0.3 mg/day, and medroxyprogesterone, 2.5 mg/day) in conjunction with calcium and vitamin D versus placebo. Subjects in both groups were administered sufficient calcium to bring all calcium intakes above 1000 mg/day and oral 25-hydroxyvitamin D sufficient to maintain serum 25-OHD levels of at least 75 nmol/L. Through the course of 3.5 years of observation, significant increases were seen in spinal BMD as well as in total-body and forearm bone density, particularly among patients with greater than 90% adherence to therapy. Meanwhile, breast tenderness, spotting, pelvic discomfort, mood changes, and other symptoms typically associated with HRT were mild and short-lived under this relatively low-dose regimen. These authors concluded that "continuous low-dose HRT with conjugated equine estrogen and oral medroxyprogesterone combined with adequate calcium and vitamin D provides a bone-sparing effect

that is similar or superior to that provided by other, higher-dose HRT regimens in elderly women" and is well tolerated by most patients.[135]

In a 6-month placebo-controlled clinical trial involving 21 postmenopausal women with osteoporosis, Gallagher et al.[136] observed that conjugated equine estrogen increased both calcium absorption and serum vitamin D levels [1,25-$(OH)_2D$]. Subsequently, these researchers investigated the roles of estrogen deficiency and declining calcium absorption caused by reduced activated vitamin D (calcitriol) levels or intestinal resistance to calcitriol as central factors in age-related bone loss. In a randomized, double-blind, placebo-controlled trial involving 485 elderly women (age 66-77) with normal bone density for their age, they compared the effects of estrogen replacement therapy (ERT, 0.625 mg conjugated estrogens daily for women without a uterus) and HRT (ERT plus 2.5 mg medroxyprogesterone acetate daily for women with a uterus) with or without calcitriol (1,25-OHD) versus placebo. HRT alone and in combination with calcitriol were both highly effective in reducing bone resorption and increasing BMD at the hip and other key sites. In particular, calcitriol was effective in increasing BMD in the femoral neck and spine. In the adherent women, the combination of ERT/HRT and calcitriol increased BMD in the total hip and trochanter significantly more than did ERT or HRT alone, particularly in women who were adherent to treatment.[137]

Among several benefits observed in perimenopausal and postmenopausal women, calcium coadministration enhances the beneficial effect of exogenous estrogen on bone mass.[138,139] Nieves et al.[94] reviewed and analyzed 31 published clinical trials that measured bone mass of postmenopausal women from at least one skeletal site and determined that high calcium intake from diet or supplements potentiates the positive effect of estrogen on bone mass at all skeletal sites. In a retrospective study involving 315 women, Pines et al.[140] observed that early postmenopausal women taking calcium supplements with estradiol (or conjugated estrogens) demonstrate significantly greater gains in BMD than women taking HRT alone and concluded that calcium supplementation should be recommended in all postmenopausal women. In a placebo-controlled randomized trial involving 63 postmenopausal women, Ruml et al.[141] found that calcium citrate (400 mg twice daily) averted bone loss and stabilized BMD in the spine, femoral neck, and radial shaft in women relatively soon after menopause. They attributed this bone-sparing action to the inhibition of bone resorption from PTH suppression.

Nutritional Therapeutics, Clinical Concerns, and Adaptations

Calcium intake, along with vitamin D, remains the fundamental component supporting bone health at all ages and for both genders and is of particular importance in preventing bone loss in postmenopausal women. Requirements for healthy calcium intake begin at an early age because OC use may prevent attainment of maximal peak bone mass in young women. For women in postmenopausal years, HRT has been the mainstay of osteoporosis prevention but is limited because of dose-related risks, adverse effects, and patient acceptance. Estrogen may improve calcium absorption, vitamin D activity, and bone metabolism, but it remains important for women taking estrogen to maintain adequate calcium intake through diet and supplementation. Deficiencies of both nutrients are common in the patient populations at highest risk for osteoporosis. Calcium and estrogen have a clearly demonstrated synergistic effect of enhancing each other's effects on bone metabolism. Nevertheless, prudent nutritional support for osteoporosis prevention and treatment can be provided through diet or supplementation including 1500 mg/day of calcium and 800 IU (20 μg) vitamin D, or more exactly, sufficient intake vitamin D per day to maintain serum 25(OH)D levels above 80 nmol/L (30 ng/ml or μg/L).[79]

Thus, a synergistic combination of oral calcium and vitamin D, within the context of a calcium-rich diet and an active lifestyle, constitutes the core proactive intervention within integrative therapeutics for all women using exogenous estrogens, particularly individuals at high risk for osteoporosis, or a foundational treatment for diagnosed bone loss. Additionally, in the treatment of menopausal women, hormone supplementation or replacement regimens (conventional HRT, bio-identical estrogens/progesterone, isoflavones, herbal hormone precursors/modulators) may achieve similar effects, but conclusive evidence is lacking; further research through well-designed clinical trials is warranted. Bisphosphonates and calcitonin, as well as magnesium, boron, and other nutrients, may also play a role as options within a comprehensive approach to bone health through the later phases of the life cycle in both women and men.

The importance of exercise and sound nutrition as foundational cannot be overemphasized and is supported by growing evidence. Weight-bearing exercise is fundamental to maintaining BMD and reducing bone loss.[142-144] Vitamin D nutriture and adequate protein and phosphorus intake are also essential. Further, most research indicates that consistent, moderate exposure to sunlight provides a safe and effective, as well as otherwise beneficial, method of elevating vitamin D levels. Ultimately, prevention through exercise and calcium intake during the life stage of skeletal development is most important for establishing peak bone density. Patients should be educated and encouraged to make these lifelong habits.

Fluoroquinolone (4-Quinolone) Antibiotics

Cinoxacin (Cinobac, Pulvules), ciprofloxacin (Ciloxan, Cipro), enoxacin (Penetrex), gatifloxacin (Tequin), levofloxacin (Levaquin), lomefloxacin (Maxaquin), moxifloxacin (Avelox), nalidixic acid (Neggram), norfloxacin (Noroxin), ofloxacin (Floxin, Ocuflox), sparfloxacin (Zagam), trovafloxacin (Trovan).

Interaction Type and Significance

◇◇   **Impaired Drug Absorption and Bioavailability, Precautions Appropriate**

≈≈   **Drug-Induced Nutrient Depletion, Supplementation Therapeutic, with Professional Management**

Probability: Evidence Base:
1. Certain   ● **Consensus**

Effect and Mechanism of Action

The 3-carbonyl and 4-oxo functional groups on quinolone antibiotics form a chelate with calcium and other divalent metal cations, such as aluminum, copper, iron, magnesium, manganese, and zinc. This binding process can substantially interfere with the absorption, bioavailability, and activity of both the antimicrobials in this class and the supplemental calcium.

Research

The ability of multivalent cations to reduce the absorption and serum levels of oral quinolone antibiotics is well established.[145-156]

However, much research has involved mineral-based antacids rather than nutritional supplements; the limitations of extrapolating these data have not been analyzed. This interaction appears to have the greatest clinical significance with aluminum and magnesium ions, occurs to a lesser extent with bismuth and calcium ions, and is probably nonexistent with sodium ions. The observed reduction in quinolone absorption can significantly affect peak concentration (C_{max}) and percent bioavailability and in some circumstances will inhibit the therapeutic effectiveness of the antibiotic. Calcium intake appears to affect the rate, but not the extent, of moxifloxacin absorption.[157] Experimental data indicate that the degree of this interference is variable for different medications, with calcium-containing antacids reducing quinolone bioavailability to the following percentages: lomefloxacin (98%), levofloxacin (97%), ciprofloxacin (59%), and norfloxacin (37%).[150,152,154,158-162]

In studies with rats and human volunteers, Sanchez Navarro et al.[163] found that coadministration of 500 mg/L calcium carbonate ($CaCO_3$) to healthy volunteers significantly reduced the urinary excretion of 250 mg/L ciprofloxacin, although neither the fraction of absorbed dose nor the half-life was greatly affected. They concluded that calcium therefore shares the same propensity as other cations in impairing the absorption of ciprofloxacin. However, Lomaestro and Bailie[164] found that repeated doses of calcium carbonate, administered 2 hours before ciprofloxacin, did not significantly alter the relative bioavailability of ciprofloxacin. Pletz et al.[165] compared the effect different timing of calcium carbonate intake on the oral bioavailability of gemifloxacin. In an experiment involving 16 volunteers, gemifloxacin was administered alone, 2 hours before, simultaneously, or 2 hours after calcium carbonate. Only simultaneous coadministration of calcium carbonate reduced C_{max} (−17%) and AUC (−21%) significantly.

Calcium depletion resulting from chelation by this class of medications has not been studied per se. Although plausible, such an adverse effect on calcium balance is highly improbable given the normal physiological controls on blood calcium levels and the limited duration of standard drug use. Long-term quinolone therapy and simultaneous oral intake could theoretically contribute to bone loss.

Nutritional Therapeutics, Clinical Concerns, and Adaptations

Physicians treating patients for serious infections with quinolone antibiotics should advise them to refrain from ingesting calcium (and all other divalent mineral cation) supplements during therapy to avoid interfering with the absorption and thus the antimicrobial action of the medication. If this is not possible, administration of the medication 2 hours before or 6 hours after ingestion of an oral calcium supplement is suggested and can effectively minimize risk of an adverse interaction. This recommendation also applies to intake of calcium-containing antacids and calcium-rich or calcium-fortified foods. Monitor for decreased therapeutic effects of oral quinolones if inadvertently administered simultaneously with oral calcium supplements or calcium antacids.

GASTRIC ACID–SUPPRESSIVE MEDICATIONS

Cimetidine and Related Histamine (H₂) Receptor Antagonists

Evidence: Cimetidine (Tagamet; Tagamet HB).
Extrapolated, based on similar properties: Famotidine (Pepcid RPD, Pepcid, Pepcid AC), nizatidine (Axid, Axid AR), ranitidine bismuth citrate (Tritec), ranitidine (Zantac).

Omeprazole and Related Proton Pump Inhibitors

Evidence: Omeprazole (Losec, Prilosec).
Similar properties but evidence lacking for extrapolation: Esomeprazole (Nexium), lansoprazole (Prevacid, Zoton), pantoprazole (Protium, Protonix, Somac), rabeprazole (AcipHex, Pariet).

Interaction Type and Significance

≈≈≈ **Drug-Induced Nutrient Depletion, Supplementation Therapeutic, Not Requiring Professional Management**

Probability:	Evidence Base:
2. Probable or	◉ Emerging and
3. Possible	▽ Mixed

Effect and Mechanism of Action

Cimetidine may significantly decrease net calcium absorption and transport across the intestinal lumen to the mucosa, an action that may be secondary to its effect on the release of parathyroid hormone (PTH) or an effect on vitamin D metabolism.

Inhibition of gastric acid secretion by H_2 antagonists or proton pump inhibitors (PPIs), particularly at high doses, can impair calcium absorption and increase risk of fracture(s) since an acidic environment appears to enhance absorption of some forms of calcium. Furthermore, solubility of calcium is highly pH-dependent, particularly as seen in in vitro experiments. PPIs "also may reduce bone resorption through inhibition of osteoclastic vacuolar proton pumps."[166]

Research

Human studies have shown that cimetidine can lower the amount of calcium in the body, but the conditions, mechanisms, and clinical significance of this interaction pattern are not yet fully understood. Bo-Linn et al.[167] developed a method to measure gastrointestinal absorption of calcium after a single meal. Although a large dose of cimetidine significantly reduced gastric acid secretion, it had no effect on calcium absorption in normal subjects and in one patient with diagnosed achlorhydria. This pattern was observed for all the calcium sources investigated: milk, calcium carbonate ($CaCO_3$), and calcium citrate. Furthermore, calcium absorption from calcium carbonate was the same when intragastric contents were relatively acid (pH 3.0) and when acidity was relatively neutral (pH 7.4). A subsequent trial by Recker[18] found that calcium absorption from calcium carbonate was lower in patients with achlorhydria than in normal subjects. However, when calcium carbonate was taken with a meal, calcium absorption was normal, even in achlorhydric patients. In a review of studies on calcium bioavailability and stomach acid, Wood and Serfaty-Lacrosniere[168] concluded that the elderly, patients taking high doses of gastric acid–suppressive medications, and fasted individuals can most effectively absorb calcium carbonate ingested with a meal. Similarly, Heaney et al.[21] determined that bioavailability of calcium carbonate and calcium phosphate is enhanced when taken with meals.

Ghishan et al.[169] studied the effect of cimetidine on intestinal calcium transport in a rat model and observed a significant decrease in net intestinal calcium transport. In a double-blind, placebo-controlled crossover study, Fisken et al.[170] treated eight primary hyperparathyroid patients with cimetidine or placebo for 2 months and reported that serum calcium levels declined significantly in a single patient and that

PTH was affected in only one patient. In a clinical trial involving 16 patients with primary hyperparathyroidism treated with 1200 mg cimetidine daily, Caron et al.[171] proposed that the reduced calcium absorption observed with cimetidine may be secondary to the effects of the drug on vitamin D metabolism rather than inhibition of gastric acid secretion.

Kerzner, O'Connell, et al.[172] conducted a randomized, double-blind, placebo-controlled, crossover trial in which 18 women age 65 and older were administered omeprazole (20 mg daily) or placebo for 7 days, then after a 3-week washout period, switched over to the alternative treatment. On the morning of the seventh day of treatment after an overnight fast, subjects ingested radiolabeled calcium carbonate (500 mg elemental calcium), blood levels of which were measured in samples obtained at time zero and 5 hours later. Each woman also ingested a multivitamin containing 400 units of vitamin D daily throughout the study. The researchers observed that fractional calcium absorption was decreased from an average of 9.1% while treated with placebo to 3.5% with omeprazole. In confirming their hypothesis that omeprazole would alter calcium absorption, the authors added that further trials are needed to "determine whether the body could adapt to this decreased calcium absorption rate and to evaluate other solutions to overcome the omeprazole/proton pump inhibitor–calcium drug-drug interaction."[172] In a nested case-control study comparing users of PPI therapy and nonusers of acid suppression drugs who were over age 50, Yang et al.[166] found that "long-term PPI therapy, particularly at high doses, is associated with an increased risk of hip fracture." Furthermore, use of PPIs for longer than 1 year was associated with increased fracture risk by 44%, and long-term, high-dose users had 2.6 times greater risk than nonusers. However, they added that "short-term PPI use is unlikely to have a significant impact on fracture risk regardless of how high the daily dosage." The authors noted that PPIs "may interfere with calcium absorption through induction of hypochlorhydria but they also may reduce bone resorption through inhibition of osteoclastic vacuolar proton pumps."

Physicians experienced in nutritional therapeutics have often contended that gastric acid secretion declines with age in many individuals, and that this contributes to diminished calcium absorption, cumulative negative calcium balance, and eventually bone loss. In a cross-sectional study involving 248 white male and female volunteers age 65 or older, Hurwitz et al.[173] reported that "nearly 90% of elderly people in this study were able to acidify gastric contents, even in the basal, unstimulated state. Of those who were consistent hyposecretors of acid, most had serum markers of atrophic gastritis." Given the mixed evidence, long-term trials investigating this critical issue are warranted.

The relatively short duration of most trials and the utilization of serum calcium levels as a marker of calcium limit the strength of the available evidence in demonstrating a lack of effect on calcium balance over long periods (i.e., the scale of bone loss).

Report

Edwards et al.[174] reported the case of a 92-year-old woman with a normal serum calcium level who became severely hypocalcemic and exhibited tetany, seizures, and impaired mental status after receiving cimetidine postoperatively. Her condition responded to intravenous diazepam, phenytoin sodium, and parenteral calcium gluconate. Serum calcium levels were maintained by calcium infusions until the cimetidine treatment was stopped. The authors suggested that the effect of cimetidine on serum PTH level may have been responsible for the observed complications.

Nutritional Therapeutics, Clinical Concerns, and Adaptations
Physicians prescribing H$_2$ antagonists, PPIs, or other medications that reduce gastric acidity can advise patients to use calcium preparations other than calcium carbonate, which can be absorbed effectively when taken away from meals. Periodic assessment of calcium levels and BMD would be prudent in patients receiving chronic gastric acid–suppressive therapy, particularly postmenopausal women.

Heparin, Unfractionated

Heparin, unfractionated (Calciparine, Hepalean, Heparin Leo, Minihep Calcium, Minihep, Monoparin Calcium, Monoparin, Multiparin, Pump-Hep, Unihep, Uniparin Calcium, Uniparin Forte).

Interaction Type and Significance
◇ ≈≈ **Drug-Induced Adverse Effect on Nutrient Function, Coadministration Therapeutic, with Professional Management**
≈≈ **Drug-Induced Nutrient Depletion, Supplementation Therapeutic, with Professional Management**
◇ **Adverse Drug Effect on Nutritional Therapeutics, Strategic Concern**

Probability: Evidence Base:
4. Plausible or   ◉ Emerging or
2. Probable   ● Consensus

Effect and Mechanism of Action
Over time, heparin causes bone loss, especially in the spine, hips, pelvis, and legs. This effect is more pronounced with standard (unfractionated) heparin (UFH), than with low-molecular-weight heparin (LMWH). At least one mechanism of the negative effect of UFH on bone is nonspecific binding of the longer polysaccharide chains to bone, with inhibition of osteoblastic function. Heparin may also inhibit formation of 1,25-dihydroxyvitamin D by the kidneys.[175]

Research
Majerus et al.[176] reported that use of heparin, at full anticoagulation doses, for several months has been found to cause osteoporosis. Likewise, both Wise and Hall[177] and later Haram et al.,[178] found that women who received heparin therapy during pregnancy experienced decreased bone density, or osteopenia. On the other hand, in one study, nine women undergoing heparin treatment received 6.46 g daily of a special calcium preparation, ossein-hydroxyapatite compound (OHC), over 6 months and were compared to 11 women not receiving the bone-protective treatment. In the OHC-group, good compliance was observed, with no side effects and reduced back pain. Those taking the calcium preparation did not demonstrate the expected decreases in bone mass, whereas bone mass dropped significantly in the controls.[179]

Nutritional Therapeutics, Clinical Concerns, and Adaptations
Although the adverse effects of heparin on vitamin D, calcium, and bone metabolism are well documented, research confirming the benefits of coadministering calcium and vitamin D in individuals on heparin therapy for any extended period is limited. However, in the meantime, such nutritional support

would most likely be beneficial and is not contraindicated. Physicians prescribing UFH may find it prudent to coadminister calcium and vitamin D. With chronic use, the vitamin D metabolite that should be measured to determine vitamin D status is 25(OH)D, which is the major circulating form of vitamin D, circulating at 1000 times the concentration of 1,25(OH)$_2$D and having a half-life of 2 weeks; after D$_3$ repletion has been initiated, monitoring 1,25(OH)$_2$D may be adequate. With long-term heparin therapy, assessment of BMD may also be indicated.

Isoniazid

Isoniazid (isonicotinic acid hydrazide, INH; Laniazid, Nydrazid); combination drugs: isoniazid and rifampicin (Rifamate, Rimactane); isoniazid, pyrazinamide, and rifampicin (Rifater).

Interaction Type and Significance
≈≈ **Drug-Induced Nutrient Depletion, Supplementation Therapeutic, with Professional Management**
◇ **Adverse Drug Effect on Nutritional Therapeutics, Strategic Concern**

Probability: Evidence Base:
2. Probable   ◉ Emerging

Effect and Mechanism of Action
Isoniazid appears to decrease levels of both calcium and vitamin D and may interfere with the activity of both nutrients. Observed declines in activated vitamin D (1α,25-dihydroxyvitamin D) can produce relative hypocalcemia and induce elevation in PTH levels. Isoniazid can inhibit hepatic mixed-function oxidase activity, as evidenced by a reduction in antipyrine and cortisol oxidation, as well as hepatic 25-hydroxylase and renal 1α-hydroxylase; thereby causing such a reduction in the corresponding vitamin D metabolites.[180,181]

Research
Brodie et al.[180] investigated the effect of isoniazid on vitamin D metabolism, serum calcium and phosphate levels, and hepatic monooxygenase activity by administering isoniazid, 300 mg daily, to eight healthy subjects for 14 days. They observed several responses, including a 47% drop in the concentration of 1α,25(OH)$_2$D (most active metabolite of vitamin D) after a single dose of isoniazid, with lowered levels continuing throughout the study, declines in levels of 25(OH)D (major circulating form of the vitamin) in all subjects and to below normal range in six, and a 36% elevation in PTH levels in response to the relative hypocalcemia produced. In a study involving 46 children with asymptomatic tuberculosis (TB), Toppet et al.[182] found that children administered isoniazid for 3 months demonstrated a decrease in blood levels of 1,25(OH)$_2$D. Isoniazid appears to interfere similarly with the activity of many other nutrients, including magnesium.

Specific evidence is lacking to determine if isoniazid or related agents actually cause symptoms of vitamin D deficiency and calcium depletion, especially with long-term therapy. Clinical trials are warranted to investigate the clinical significance of any depletion pattern and efficacy of prophylactic intervention. Such research is particularly important in children undergoing long-term therapy, in whom potential adverse effects may significantly impair the calcium economy during the critical life stage when maximum bone density is being attained and will be relied on for a lifetime.

Nutritional Therapeutics, Clinical Concerns, and Adaptations

Physicians prescribing isoniazid or related antitubercular therapy, especially for greater than 1 month, are advised to recommend coadministration of calcium and vitamin D, preferably as part of a multivitamin-mineral formulation (at least 50 mg/day vitamin B_6 is indicated with INH as well), as a prudent measure, unlikely to interfere with the efficacy of the medication(s). Calcium in the range of 100 to 250 mg three times daily would be appropriate, but research is lacking to confirm specific effective dosage levels. Such nutrient support may be especially critical for children undergoing long-term therapy.

Concurrent vitamin D administration may be of great value in addition to antituberculous drugs in the treatment of tuberculous children, and its use is highly recommended.[183] Exposure to sunlight is the simplest and most natural way to provide activated vitamin D; sunshine and mountain air were characteristic of the great TB sanitoriums in the pre–anti-TB drug era. However, when vitamin D is to be administered orally, the typical dosage would be in the range of 5 to 10 µg (200-400 IU) per day, depending on size and body weight.

Granulomatous lesions, such as those present in extensive TB infection, often contain active 1-hydroxylase enzymes that activate 25-OH cholecalciferol and are independent of the feedback mechanisms that regulate the renal 1-hydroxylase enzymes. Regular monitoring of serum calcium would provide indication of early vitamin D toxicity in this setting. Research findings emphasize the need for regular monitoring of vitamin D status in this population, even if no sign of rickets is observed in these patients.

Levothyroxine and Related Thyroid Hormones

L-Triiodothyronine (T_3): Cytomel, liothyronine sodium, liothyronine sodium (synthetic T_3), Triostat (injection).
Levothyroxine (T_4): Eltroxin, Levo-T, Levothroid, levothyroxine (synthetic), levoxin, Levoxyl, Synthroid, thyroxine, Unithroid.
L-Thyroxine and L-triiodothyronine ($T_4 + T_3$): animal levothyroxine/liothyronine, Armour Thyroid, desiccated thyroid, Westhroid.
L-Thyroxine and L-triiodothyronine (synthetic $T_4 + T_3$): Euthroid, Euthyral, liotrix, Thyar, Thyrolar.
Dextrothyroxine (Choloxin).

Interaction Type and Significance

◇◇ **Impaired Drug Absorption and Bioavailability, Precautions Appropriate**
≈≈≈ **Drug-Induced Nutrient Depletion, Supplementation Therapeutic, Not Requiring Professional Management**
◇ **Adverse Drug Effect on Nutritional Therapeutics, Strategic Concern**

Probability: Evidence Base:
5. Improbable   ◉ **Emerging**

Effect and Mechanism of Action

Calcium compounds may form chelates with levothyroxine or related thyroid medications in the digestive tract, thereby reducing absorption, bioavailability, and efficacy of both agents. In particular, levothyroxine adsorbs to calcium carbonate in an acidic environment.[184] Thyroid hormone medications are known to increase calcium excretion. Most researchers agree that the complete mechanism of this interaction is unknown.

Research

Research on the clinical implications of the binding effect between calcium compounds and thyroid hormone medications is inconclusive, mixed, and contradictory. Several studies have found measurable changes in the bone density of women undergoing long-term treatment with thyroxine and other forms of thyroid medication at substitutive or suppressive doses. Controversy surrounds these findings' interpretation and their implications for bone metabolism. The results of studies examining the influence of T_4 therapy on bone mineral density (BMD) may produce conflicting findings, in part, as a reflection of the inclusion of patients with varying thyroid disorders. Apparently the impact of potential calcium depletion is greatest among women with a history of hyperthyroidism and thyrotoxicosis.

In 1988, Paul et al.[185] cautioned that women treated with L-T_4 for extended periods had a 12.8% lower BMD at the femoral neck and a 10.1% lower BMD at the femoral trochanter compared with matched controls. They suggested that excessive dosages of thyroid hormone might play a significant role in the occurrence of such patterns. In 1991, Adlin et al.[186] noted that long-term L-thyroxine therapy was associated with decreased density of the spine and hip. However, they concluded that because subclinical hyperthyroidism, decreased calcitonin responsiveness, and a history of hyperthyroidism were demonstrated in some or all of these patients, these factors must be considered as possible causes of the decreased BMD. Later in 1991, in a study involving 26 premenopausal women with Hashimoto's thyroiditis receiving long-term physiological doses of levothyroxine replacement therapy, Kung and Pun[187] observed that, compared with controls, women receiving the levothyroxine treatment had normal total-body BMD levels but had significantly lower BMD levels at the femoral neck (−5.7%), femoral trochanter (−7.0%), Ward's triangle (−10.6%), both arms (right, −7.8%; left, −8.9%), and pelvis (−4.9%). In contrast, lumbar spine BMD levels were similar in the two groups. These researchers concluded that patients receiving physiological doses of levothyroxine may have decreased BMD.

However, the findings of other investigators suggest that, under most circumstances, taking thyroid hormones may not be associated with reduced bone density. Franklyn et al.[188] compared case-control studies of patients on long-term T_4 therapy who had or had not previously received radioiodine treatment for thyrotoxicosis, as well as previously thyrotoxic patients who had not required T_4 replacement. After measuring BMD at several sites and comparing results among the three groups, they concluded that thyroxine therapy alone does not represent a significant risk factor for loss of BMD. However, they did note a risk of bone loss in postmenopausal (but not premenopausal) females with a previous history of thyrotoxicosis treated with radioiodine. Thyroid hormone use is much less common in men, who also have less osteoporosis. Schneider et al.[189] compared BMD at several sites in 33 men taking a mean thyroxine-equivalent dose of 130 µg daily, for an average of 15.5 years, with 653 nonusers; all 685 subjects were Caucasian men age 50 to 98. They found no significant differences in BMD at any site between users and nonusers, before or after controlling for age, body mass index, smoking, thiazide diuretics, and oral corticosteroid use. These authors concluded that long-term thyroid hormone use was not associated with adverse effects on BMD in men. Lopez Alvarez et al.[190] determined that histological type of thyroid neoplasia, doses of thyroid hormones, thyroid hormone levels, and duration of follow-up were not associated with changes in BMD.

No published findings among the research reviewed demonstrated the appropriateness or efficacy of calcium supplementation for individuals receiving long-term thyroid therapy.

Systematic research on the effect of calcium supplementation on the absorption of thyroid medication is still in preliminary stages. This probable interaction deserves continued investigation because concurrent treatment with both agents is quite common, particularly in peri- and postmenopausal women. Singh et al.[184] conducted an 8-month prospective cohort study, complemented by an in vitro investigation of T_4 binding to calcium carbonate ($CaCO_3$), and found that simultaneous ingestion of 1200 mg/day calcium carbonate and levothyroxine significantly reduced absorption of the thyroid hormone medication and increased serum thyrotropin levels. Mean levels of both free T_4 and total T_4 were significantly reduced during the calcium period and increased after calcium discontinuation. The in vitro experiment showed that adsorption of T_4 to calcium carbonate occurs at acidic pH levels.[184]

Reports

Schneyer[191] reported reduced levothyroxine effectiveness during simultaneous ingestion of calcium formulations in three women with thyroid cancer who were receiving levothyroxine to suppress serum thyroid-stimulating hormone (TSH) levels. In one case, TSH concentrations increased from 0.08 to 13.3 mU/L over a 5-month period during concomitant administration, and returned to normal after discontinuation of the calcium supplement. Separating the doses of levothyroxine (morning) and calcium carbonate (after lunch or dinner) was reported to minimize the effects of the interaction.

Nutritional Therapeutics, Clinical Concerns, and Adaptations

High calcium intake presents a high probability of interfering with the absorption and activity of thyroid hormone medications if taken simultaneously. Physicians prescribing thyroid therapy should advise patients to take the medication 2 hours before or 4 hours after ingestion of an oral calcium supplement (or calcium-rich foods) to effectively minimize risk of the nutrient interfering with the medication. Many patients find it easiest to take their thyroid medication in the morning and their calcium supplement before bedtime. Thyroid functions should be closely monitored in patients receiving long-term levothyroxine treatment.

No conclusive evidence demonstrates calcium depletion and decreased BMD attributable to thyroid hormone therapy, and no firm evidence supports the proposition that additional calcium supplementation is necessary for or even beneficial to individuals taking thyroid medication on a long-term basis. Even so, many health care providers trained in nutritional therapies have suggested the need for additional calcium supplementation by some patients using these drugs. The seemingly inconsistent findings may indicate that the effect of thyroid medications on calcium varies based on the individual's gender, history, condition, menstrual status, and other factors. Precisely because of this patient variability, many practitioners of nutritional medicine advocate the periodic testing of 24-hour urinary calcium levels for individuals using thyroid medication for more than a few months. Bone densitometry should be performed in patients at risk for osteoporosis. Physicians prescribing thyroid medication should discuss with patients their potential need for calcium supplementation beyond what would normally be recommended based on their age, gender, and menstrual status.

Metformin and Related Biguanides

Evidence: Metformin (Dianben, Glucophage, Glucophage XR).

Extrapolated: Buformin (Andromaco Gliporal, Buformina); metformin combination drugs: glipizide and metformin (Metaglip); glyburide and metformin (Glucovance); phenformin (Debeone, Fenformin).

Interaction Type and Significance

$\approx\approx\approx$ **Drug-Induced Nutrient Depletion, Supplementation Therapeutic, Not Requiring Professional Management**

$\diamondsuit\approx\approx$ **Drug-Induced Adverse Effect on Nutrient Function, Coadministration Therapeutic, with Professional Management**

☼ **Prevention or Reduction of Drug Adverse Effect**

Probability: Evidence Base:
2. Probable   ● **Consensus**

Effect and Mechanism of Action

Biguanide therapy, particularly metformin, causes reduced vitamin B_{12} absorption and low serum total vitamin B_{12} and holotranscobalamin (B_{12}-TCII) levels by depressing intrinsic factor secretion[192] and through a calcium-dependent ileal membrane antagonism affecting B_{12}–intrinsic factor complex uptake.[193] Vitamin B_{12}–intrinsic factor complex uptake by ileal cell surface receptors depends on calcium availability, and metformin specifically affects calcium-dependent membrane action; this effect can be reversed by concomitant calcium.

Research

Of patients prescribed metformin, conservatively 10% to 30% have evidence of reduced vitamin B_{12} absorption, accompanied by a decline in folic acid status and elevation of homocysteine (Hcy). An early study by Carpentier et al.[194] involving diabetic patients determined that whereas biguanides depleted vitamin B_{12}, folic acid was not similarly affected. In a subsequent study involving nondiabetic male patients with coronary heart disease, Carlsen et al.[195] observed that metformin increases total serum Hcy levels and depletes vitamin B_{12} and sometimes folic acid.[195] More recently, in a randomized, placebo-controlled trial involving 390 patients with type 2 diabetes, Wulffele et al.[196] found that 16 weeks of treatment with metformin reduces serum levels of vitamin B_{12} and folate, resulting in a modest increase in Hcy.

Caspary et al.[193] initially noted that the vitamin B_{12} malabsorption, pathological Schilling tests, and elevated fecal bile acid excretion observed with biguanides, particularly metformin, improved when the medication was discontinued or antibiotics were administered. They interpreted these findings to suggest that small intestinal bacterial overgrowth, leading to binding of the intrinsic factor–vitamin B_{12}-complex to bacteria, was responsible for the B_{12} depletion observed in diabetic patients on biguanide therapy. Subsequently, Adams et al.[192] surveyed 46 randomly selected diabetic patients on biguanide therapy and found that 30% demonstrated malabsorption of vitamin B_{12}, apparently by two different mechanisms. On withdrawal of the drug, normal absorption returned in only half of those with malabsorption. Using absorption tests with exogenous intrinsic factor, these researchers further determined that biguanide-induced depression of intrinsic factor secretion mediated the persistent malabsorption in most individuals of the latter group. Bauman et al.[197] performed a comparative study in which a group with type 2 diabetes who had been receiving sulfonylurea therapy was switched to metformin for 3 months, after which oral calcium was administered. Monthly serial measurements of serum total vitamin B_{12} and B_{12}-TCII revealed parallel declines in those taking metformin compared with controls. The observed depression of B_{12}-TCII was reversed by the introduction of oral calcium supplementation.

Nutritional Therapeutics, Clinical Concerns, and Adaptations

Physicians prescribing metformin or other biguanides are advised to supplement vitamin B_{12}, folic acid, and calcium and regularly monitor folic acid, vitamin B_{12}, and possibly Hcy levels.

Sulfamethoxazole and Related Sulfonamide Antibiotics

Sulfamethoxazole (Gantanol), combination drug: sulfamethoxazole and trimethoprim (cotrimoxazole, co-trimoxazole, SXT, TMP-SMX, TMP-sulfa; Bactrim, Bactrim DS, Cotrim, Septra, Septra DS, Sulfatrim, Uroplus).
Extrapolated, based on similar properties: Sodium sulfacetamide (AK-Sulf, Bleph-10, Sodium Sulamyd), sulfanilamide (AVC), sulfasalazine (salazosulfapyridine, salicylazosulfapyridine, suphasalazine; Apo-Sulfasalazine, Azulfidine, Azulfidine EN-Tabs, PMS-Sulfasalazine, Salazopyrin, Salazopyrin EN-Tabs, SAS), sulfisoxazole (Gantrisin), triple sulfa (Sultrin Triple Sulfa).

Interaction Type and Significance

≈≈≈ **Drug-Induced Nutrient Depletion, Supplementation Therapeutic, Not Requiring Professional Management**

Probability:	Evidence Base:
4. Plausible or	● Consensus
3. Possible	

Effect and Mechanism of Action

Sulfonamides, including sulfamethoxazole, can decrease absorption of calcium (as well as magnesium and vitamin B_{12}) and potentially lead to calcium depletion.

Research

This interaction is considered as well established, although specific evidence from well-designed clinical trials or qualified case reports is lacking.

Nutritional Therapeutics, Clinical Concerns, and Adaptations

The probability of adverse effects on calcium balance is low when medications in the sulfonamide family of antibiotics are used for 2 weeks or less. Physicians prescribing sulfamethoxazole or related medications, especially repeatedly or for longer than 2 weeks, are advised to monitor levels of calcium and other potentially affected nutrients and consider supplementation, such as coadministration of 1000 to 1500 mg calcium in divided doses, at least 2 hours before of after the medication.

Tetracycline Antibiotics

Demeclocycline (Declomycin), doxycycline (Atridox, Doryx, Doxy, Monodox, Periostat, Vibramycin, Vibra-Tabs), minocycline (Dynacin, Minocin, Vectrin), oxytetracycline (Terramycin), tetracycline (Achromycin, Actisite, Sumycin, Tetracyn; combination drugs: chlortetracycline,

demeclocycline, and tetracycline (Deteclo); bismuth, metronidazole, and tetracycline (Helidac).

Interaction Type and Significance

◇◇ **Impaired Drug Absorption and Bioavailability, Precautions Appropriate**
≈≈≈ **Drug-Induced Nutrient Depletion, Supplementation Therapeutic, Not Requiring Professional Management**
◇ **Adverse Drug Effect on Nutritional Therapeutics, Strategic Concern**

Probability:	Evidence Base:
2. Probable or	● Consensus
1. Certain	

Effect and Mechanism of Action

Tetracyclines form insoluble chelates with calcium and other polyvalent metal cations, including iron, magnesium, and zinc.[198,199] Thus, calcium and tetracycline-class antibiotics tend to bind with each other, and absorption of both agents is impaired.

Calcium may impair absorption of tetracycline antibiotics and therefore diminish their effectiveness. Tetracycline-class medications are primarily absorbed in the stomach and upper small intestine. Calcium, as well as dairy products and other foods containing high concentrations of calcium, may decrease the absorption of tetracyclines because of chelate formation in the gut.

Tetracyclines reduce absorption of calcium and can adversely affect calcium balance and mineralization of calcium-dependent tissues. The binding of the medication to calcium may also lead to growth retardation and pigmented teeth. Furthermore, tetracycline increases urinary calcium excretion. Thus, with prolonged use, tetracyclines contribute to calcium depletion and can adversely effect bone formation.

Research

Most of the findings leading to statements about this interaction involve calcium-based antacids and calcium-rich foods, but they are still reasonably applicable to calcium supplements. In a review of the effect of polyvalent metallic cations on absorption of tetracyclines, Neuvonen[198] noted that serum concentrations of these antibiotics generally remain within the therapeutic range. Nevertheless, he concluded that "the pharmacokinetic interactions in absorption of tetracyclines likely to be clinically significant in cases where the infecting pathogens are moderately resistant to tetracyclines and relatively high serum concentrations are needed for proper bacteriostasis." In a clinical trial (crossover design) involving 12 healthy volunteers, Jung et al.[200] observed that even a small volume of milk containing extremely small amounts of calcium can severely impair the absorption, and subsequent bioavailability, of tetracycline.

Long-term use of tetracycline antibiotics is highly likely to produce adverse effects on calcium and related tissues and developmental processes. Tetracyclines form a stable calcium complex in any bone-forming tissue. In particular, the interaction between tetracycline and calcium-rich foods (e.g., milk products) exerts adverse effects on bone and teeth that are well documented and widely recognized.[201,202] Unwanted pigmentation and other problems with tooth development caused by tetracycline are well known to dentists and the general public. The tetracyclines also tend to localize in tumors, necrotic or ischemic tissue, liver, and spleen and form tetracycline-calcium orthophosphate complexes at sites of new bone formation.

Tetracyclines are potent inhibitors of osteoclast function (i.e., antiresorptive). Vernillo and Rifkin[203] describe the processes by which tetracyclines can affect several parameters of osteoclast function and consequently inhibit bone resorption: (1) altering intracellular calcium concentration and interacting with the putative calcium receptor; (2) decreasing ruffled border area; (3) diminishing acid production; (4) diminishing the secretion of lysosomal cysteine proteinases (cathepsins); (5) inducing cell retraction by affecting podosomes; (6) inhibiting osteoclast gelatinase activity; (7) selectively inhibiting osteoclast ontogeny or development; and (8) inducing apoptosis, or programmed cell death, of osteoclasts. For example, a decrease in the fibula growth rate has been observed in premature infants receiving oral tetracycline in doses of 25 mg/kg every 6 hours. This reaction was shown to be reversible when the drug was discontinued.[204]

Nutritional Therapeutics, Clinical Concerns, and Adaptations
The mutual impairment of absorption characterizing the interaction between tetracyclines and calcium absorption is highly probable, usually clinically significant, and easily avoided through careful management and instruction. This effect on bone formation carries a significantly greater risk when growth and bone formation is most active, such as with infants and children. Avoiding this interaction is also particularly important in adolescents (e.g., being treated for acne) in the midst of the life stage where they need to attain maximum bone density.

Calcium in the form of antacids, milk products, and supplements should be avoided while using tetracycline-class antibiotics. When continued use of calcium supplements is deemed appropriate and necessary, the calcium supplement (as well as calcium-rich foods) should be taken at least 3 hours apart from ingestion of the medication. Properly managed, separation allows continued effective use of both calcium and the tetracycline antibiotic.

Thiazide Diuretics

Bendroflumethiazide (bendrofluazide; Naturetin); combination drug: bendrofluazide and propranolol (Inderex); benzthiazide (Exna), chlorothiazide (Diuril), chlorthalidone (Hygroton), cyclopenthiazide (Navidrex); combination drug: cyclopenthiazide and oxprenolol hydrochloride (Trasidrex); hydrochlorothiazide (Aquazide, Esidrix, Ezide, Hydrocot, HydroDiuril, Microzide, Oretic); combination drugs: hydrochlorothiazide and amiloride (Moduretic); hydrochlorothiazide and captopril (Acezide, Capto-Co, Captozide, Co-Zidocapt); hydrochlorothiazide and enalapril (Vaseretic); hydrochlorothiazide and lisinopril (Prinzide, Zestoretic); hydrochlorothiazide and losartan (Hyzaar); hydrochlorothiazide and metoprolol (Lopressor HCT); hydrochlorothiazide and spironolactone (Aldactazide); hydrochlorothiazide and triamterene (Dyazide, Maxzide); hydroflumethiazide (Diucardin), methyclothiazide (Enduron), metolazone (Zaroxolyn, Mykrox), polythiazide (Renese), quinethazone (Hydromox), trichlormethiazide (Naqua).

Interaction Type and Significance
✗ ✗   **Minimal to Mild Adverse Interaction—Vigilance Necessary**

◇ ◇   **Drug-Induced Effect on Nutrient Function, Supplementation Contraindicated, Professional Management Appropriate**

⊕✗   **Bimodal or Variable Interaction, with Professional Management**

⊕⊕   **Potential or Theoretical Beneficial or Supportive Interaction, with Professional Management**

Probability: Evidence Base:
4. Plausible   ◉ **Emerging** or
                                 ● **Consensus**

Effect and Mechanism of Action
Thiazide diuretics increase calcium retention by decreasing urinary calcium excretion through their effects on the cortical-diluting segment of the nephron, most likely from the peritubular side.[205-207] Decreased intestinal calcium absorption, suppressed PTH secretion, and inhibited vitamin D synthesis can also result as secondary compensations. Increased renal reabsorption of calcium induced by thiazide diuretics may increase the risk of developing hypercalcemia (and possibly metabolic alkalosis) as a result of concomitant administration of calcium supplements (and/or vitamin D).

Research
Consistent evidence indicates that thiazide-induced decrease in urinary calcium excretion can alter numerous parameters of calcium and vitamin D metabolism and increase risk of transient hypercalcemia, but research has not extended to investigation of potential long-term implications. Leppla et al.[208] conducted a small clinical trial involving seven patients with renal stones to investigate the potential therapeutic role of amiloride in calcium nephrolithiasis. They observed that two doses of amiloride (2.5 mg/day) reduced urinary calcium in two subjects with kidney stones. This decrease in urinary calcium was enhanced in five subjects when amiloride was coadministered with two doses of hydrochlorothiazide (25 mg/day). In a 6-month clinical trial involving six postmenopausal women with osteoporosis, Sakhaee et al.[209] demonstrated that coadministration of hydrochlorothiazide (50 mg/day) and vitamin D (50 µg/day) reduced urinary calcium excretion by 22% but also decreased gastrointestinal calcium absorption by 25%. Riis and Christiansen[206] studied the actions of bendroflumethiazide (5 mg/day), along with 500 mg/day calcium, on vitamin D metabolism in a 12-month placebo-controlled clinical trial in 19 healthy early-postmenopausal women. Subjects in the thiazide group demonstrated a significant elevation in the serum concentration of 24,25-dihydroxycholecalciferol and a tendency toward decreased serum 1,25-dihydroxycholecalciferol, although mean serum 25-hydroxycholecalciferol remained unchanged. The authors noted that all biochemical indices of calcium metabolism were unchanged in the thiazide group, except for a highly significant decrease in urinary calcium.

Some researchers and clinicians have proposed exploiting this interaction between thiazide diuretics and calcium as a potential therapeutic tool in reducing bone loss and preventing osteoporotic fractures. In a 1998 review article, Rejnmark et al.[210] reported that thiazide use is associated with higher BMD, reduced age-related bone loss, and a reduced risk of hip fractures and attributed it not only to decreased calcium excretion, but also possibly to a decrease in PTH-stimulated bone resorption and an associated reduction in the bone turnover rate. However, prudence suggests that such beneficial "side effects" do not provide adequate justification for prescribing this class of medications solely for that purpose, given the other risks associated with their use and the lack of evidence supporting efficacy. Furthermore, the most relevant evidence indicates that any beneficial effect on calcium in bone metabolism is transient. Thus, in the Rotterdam Study, a prospective population-based cohort study involving 7891 individuals 55 years of age and older, Schoofs et al.[211] reported 281 hip fractures and observed that current use of thiazides for more than 1 year was statistically significantly associated with a lower risk for hip fracture (with no clear dose dependency) compared with nonuse. However, this lower risk disappeared approximately 4 months after thiazide use was discontinued.

Reports

Concomitant use of thiazide diuretics and calcium supplements has been associated with numerous case reports describing hypercalcemia, as well as signs and symptoms of the milk-alkali syndrome, including dizziness, weakness, hypercalcemia, and metabolic alkalosis with respiratory compensation.[212-214] For example, Crowe et al.[215] described a case of symptomatic and reversible hypercalcemia in a 78-year-old female patient taking a combination diuretic (hydrochlorothiazide and amiloride) along with six to eight antacid tablets daily (each containing 680 mg calcium carbonate and 80 mg magnesium carbonate) for several years. Constipation, dehydration, and hypercalcemic alkalosis all resolved when the medications were discontinued during hospitalization. Gora et al.[216] published the case report of a 47-year-old man who was diagnosed with milk-alkali syndrome after being hospitalized with elevated serum calcium (6.8 mEq/L) and serum creatinine (7.2 mg/dL) as well as metabolic alkalosis. During the preceding 2 years he had been self-medicating for dyspepsia with 15 to 20 calcium carbonate tablets daily, each containing 500 mg, while also taking chlorothiazide. His condition improved shortly after this regimen was discontinued.

Nutritional Therapeutics, Clinical Concerns, and Adaptations

Physicians prescribing thiazide diuretics for treatment of hypertension frequently need to treat such patients concurrently for osteoporosis. In such situations, oral calcium supplements in common dosages do not usually influence blood calcium levels significantly and rarely would impact levels enough to cause clinically significant hypercalciuria.

Thiazides should not be used as a substitute for calcium (and vitamin D) supplementation in the prevention of bone loss and treatment of osteoporosis. Although individuals on long-term thiazide therapy could theoretically reduce calcium intake during such therapy, the available evidence indicates that such beneficial effects do not continue after the thiazide has been discontinued. Evidence is lacking and further research warranted to determine whether any rebound effects on calcium balance or bone loss occurs after thiazide use is suspended, as occurs with some medications.

Given the uncertain implications of the available evidence, physicians are advised to closely supervise and regularly monitor calcium levels when prescribing thiazide diuretics, particularly before initiating or increasing any vitamin D supplementation, and to instruct patients to watch for symptoms of hypercalcemia. In some cases, calcium intake may need to be reduced. When thiazides are indicated, supplementation with potassium and magnesium is usually appropriate to compensate for drug-induced nutrient depletion.

Verapamil and Related Calcium Channel Blockers

Evidence: Felodipine (Plendil), verapamil (Calan, Calan SR, Covera-HS, Isoptin, Isoptin SR, Verelan, Verelan PM).

Extrapolated, based on similar properties: Amlodipine (Norvasc); combination drug: amlodipine and benazepril (Lotrel); bepridil (Bapadin, Vascor), diltiazem (Cardizem, Cardizem CD, Cardizem SR, Cartia XT, Dilacor XR, Diltia XT, Tiamate, Tiazac); felodipine combination drugs: felodipine and enalapril (Lexxel); felodipine and ramipril (Triapin); gallopamil (D600), isradipine (DynaCirc, DynaCirc CR), lercanidipine (Zanidip), nicardipine (Cardene, Cardene I.V., Cardene SR), nifedipine (Adalat, Adalat CC, Nifedical XL, Procardia, Procardia XL); combination drug: nifedipine and atenolol (Beta-Adalat, Tenif); nimodipine (Nimotop), nisoldipine (Sular), nitrendipine (Cardif, Nitrepin); verapamil combination drug: trandolapril and verapamil (Tarka).

Interaction Type and Significance

✗✗   **Minimal to Mild Adverse Interaction—Vigilance Necessary**

⊕✗   **Bimodal or Variable Interaction, with Professional Management**

⊕⊕   **Beneficial or Supportive Interaction, with Professional Management**

≈≈   **Drug-Induced Nutrient Depletion, Supplementation Therapeutic, with Professional Management**

Probability:	Evidence Base:
2. Probable	◉ Emerging

Effect and Mechanism of Action

Enhanced renal vasoconstriction and renal tubular sodium reabsorption are calcium-dependent functions mediated by noradrenaline and angiotensin II (Ang II) that have been implicated in the pathogenesis of essential hypertension. Calcium supplements (especially in conjunction with high doses of vitamin D) may interfere with the hypotensive activity of and reduce the therapeutic response to verapamil and related calcium channel blockers by increasing calcium availability. Even though the primary activity of these medications involves calcium antagonism, the mechanism of these antagonistic effects on calcium has not yet been fully established. Felodipine use has been associated with increased calcium excretion, and calcium channel blockers may theoretically contribute to increased bone loss. Verapamil may decrease endogenous production of vitamin D and induce target-organ PTH resistance. Nevertheless, calcium administration may reduce adverse effects of calcium channel blockers, and concurrent use of verapamil and intravenous (IV) calcium salts, in particular, can be therapeutically efficacious.

Research

It has been reported that calcium salts may reverse the clinical effects and toxicities associated with verapamil.[217] Weiss et al.[218] found that calcium gluconate, when given as a pretreatment infusion, prevented the fall in blood pressure induced by verapamil, and when administered after verapamil, it restored blood pressure to control values. These researchers also noted that administration of calcium did not alter the antiarrhythmic effect of verapamil. Similarly, in a clinical trial conducted by Haft and Habbab,[219] pretreatment with IV calcium chloride in patients with supraventricular arrhythmias reduced the incidence of hypotensive side effects without compromising the antiarrhythmic effect of verapamil.

Calcium absorption depends on, and calcium function is intertwined with, vitamin D activity. In a 1982 in vitro study, Lerner and Gustafson[220] reported that verapamil inhibited $1\alpha(OH)_2D_3$-stimulated bone resorption in tissue culture. In an animal model using rats fed a high-calcium diet, Fox and Della-Santina[221] found that chronic oral verapamil administration decreased $1,25(OH)_2D_3$ levels (by reducing production) and increased plasma immunoreactive PTH (most likely by inducing target-organ PTH resistance). In contrast, verapamil produced no significant effect on $1,25(OH)_2D_3$ levels in rats fed a low-calcium diet. A study by Hulthen and Katzman[222] involving 10 patients with essential hypertension found that felodipine use was associated with increased calcium excretion.

Reports

In an isolated report, Bar-Or and Gasiel[223] described a case in which calcium adipate and calciferol antagonized the heart rate–limiting effect of verapamil in a patient being treated for atrial fibrillation.

Nutritional Therapeutics, Clinical Concerns, and Adaptations

Physicians prescribing verapamil or other calcium channel blockers are advised to exercise caution regarding the concomitant use of calcium (and vitamin D). Concurrent calcium administration in individuals undergoing treatment with calcium channel blockers may be problematic or beneficial, depending on the condition for which the drug has been prescribed, the dosage of calcium intake, and the characteristics of the individual patient being treated. Although of low probability, the potential for an adverse interaction can present strategic concerns because many patients treated with verapamil may also have or be at risk for osteoporosis, such that calcium and vitamin D support is an important concomitant need.

Patient self-administration of calcium should be avoided during treatment with a calcium channel blocker. However, some physicians routinely prescribe very low dosages of calcium, often in the range of 25 to 30 mg per day, for patients who have been diagnosed with angina pectoris or cardiac arrhythmias, but who have no history of hypertension, as a means of reducing excessive and unnecessary blood pressure–lowering activity by the medication. Close supervision and regular monitoring, preferably within the context of integrative care involving health care professionals trained and experienced in both conventional pharmacology and nutritional therapeutics, are essential in cases in which concurrent use of verapamil (or a related calcium channel blocker) and calcium (especially with vitamin D) is clinically appropriate. In particular, regular monitoring of blood pressure is required during any coadministration, especially before initiating or significantly changing the level of calcium intake. In cases of overdose with verapamil or other calcium channel blockers, IV calcium chloride or gluconate is the treatment of choice.

UNPROVEN, SPECULATIVE, AND OVERSTATED INTERACTIONS CLAIMS

Albuterol/Salbutamol and Related Beta-2-Adrenoceptor Agonists

Intramuscular (IM), intravenous (IV), and subcutaneous (SC) forms: Albuterol/salbutamol, rimiterol (Pulmadil).
Extrapolated: IM, IV, and SC forms: Fenoterol (Berotec), isoetharine (Arm-A-Med, Bronkosol, Bronkometer), pirbuterol (Exirel), salmeterol, tulobuterol (Brelomax).
Similar properties but evidence indicating no or reduced interaction effects: Inhalation forms: Albuterol (salbutamol; Albuterol Inhaled, Proventil, Ventolin); combination drug: albuterol and ipratropium bromide (Combivent);

isoproterenol (isoprenaline; Isuprel, Medihaler-Iso), levalbuterol (Xopenex), metaproterenol (Alupent), salmeterol (Serevent, combination drug: Advair), terbutaline (Brethaire, Brethine, Bricanyl).

Intravenous administration of salbutamol (albuterol) and rimiterol in therapeutic doses produced dose-related decreases in plasma levels of calcium, as well as magnesium, phosphate, and potassium, in four subjects.[224] These researchers advised caution in patients with abnormal glucose tolerance, potassium depletion, or predisposition to lactic acidosis and suggested rimiterol as preferable for infusion because of its short plasma half-life. Further research is warranted to determine if these beta-2-adrenoceptor agonists can induce such adverse effects to a clinically significant degree in individuals being treated for asthma and related conditions over an extended period.

Beclomethasone

Beclomethasone (Beclovent; Beconase; Beconase AQ; QVAR; Vancenase; Vancenase AQ; Vanceril).
Similar properties but evidence indicating no or reduced interaction effects: Other inhaled corticosteroids.

Adverse effects of inhaled corticosteroids are generally presumed to be significantly less than those from oral corticosteroids. However, investigators have reported that most of the beclomethasone from a metered-dose inhaler (MDI) is actually swallowed and can impair calcium absorption. In a 2-week randomized, double-blind, placebo-controlled, crossover trial involving 12 healthy subjects, Smith et al.[121] found that during the period in which they received oral doses of beclomethasone dipropionate (500-μg capsules twice daily), subjects demonstrated a 12% reduction in calcium absorption (measured by strontium absorption test) and a 23% reduction in 24-hour urinary cortisol excretion during the same week. These researchers concluded that decreased calcium absorption resulting from swallowed corticosteroids may contribute to adverse effects of inhaled steroids. Well-designed clinical trials of longer duration are warranted to investigate whether such effects may be a causative factor in long-term bone loss, and whether calcium supplementation or dietary calcium enrichment might be indicated.[225-228]

See also Corticosteroids, Oral.

Caffeine (and Coffee)

Caffeine (Cafcit, Caffedrine, Enerjets, NoDoz, Quick Pep, Snap Back, Stay Alert, Vivarin).
Combination drugs: Acetylsalicylic acid and caffeine (Anacin); acetylsalicylic acid, caffeine, and propoxyphene (Darvon Compound); ASA and carisoprodol (Soma Compound); acetylsalicylic acid, codeine, butalbital, and caffeine (Fiorinal); acetominophen, coffee (*Caffea arabica, Caffea canephora, Caffea robusta*), butalbital, and caffeine (Fioricet).

Caffeine is found in coffee, tea, soft drinks, chocolate, guaraná (*Paullinia cupana*), nonprescription over-the-counter (OTC) medications, and supplements containing caffeine or guaraná. For decades, caffeine in general and coffee in particular have been suspected of depleting calcium and contributing to bone loss. Although early studies suggested an epidemiological basis for this conclusion, the evolving picture from continued research has downsized the scope of clinical significance and clarified factors of susceptibility. Caffeine can lead to a small negative calcium balance because of a weak interference with calcium absorption efficiency, particularly in individuals with inadequate calcium intakes.[229] Caffeine can also induce a significant acute calcium diuresis,[224,230] but this renal effect is biphasic[231]; that is, an acute increase in calcium diuresis is followed by a fall in urinary calcium. Two human trials have found that coffee intake, rather than caffeine, was associated with a negative balance shift of 4 to 6 mg calcium daily for each 100 ml coffee consumed. Conversely, but consistent with the overall pattern, one observational study found accelerated bone loss in 205 healthy postmenopausal women who drank two to three cups of coffee daily and consumed less than 800 mg of calcium daily. Further research is warranted to determine the effects of caffeine in populations characterized by different levels and sources of calcium intake, gender, life stage, bone density, and other potentially influential factors and to compare the variable effects of different sources of caffeine, as well as decaffeinated coffee and differing methods of preparation.

Cisplatin

Cisplatin (cis-diaminedichloroplatinum, CDDP; Platinol, Platinol-AQ).

Cisplatin is nephrotoxic and may cause kidney damage, resulting in depletion of calcium, magnesium, potassium, and phosphate. Calcium supplementation may be appropriate but must be approached with caution and close monitoring, especially in patients with compromised renal function. Strategic integrative protocols, adapted to the particular characteristics and needs of the individual patient, offer expanded possibilities for enhanced care and improved outcomes within the context of collaborative care involving health care professionals trained and experienced in both conventional oncology and nutritional therapeutics.

Colchicine

Colchicine

An isolated case report published by Frayha et al.[232] describes acute colchicine poisoning resulting in symptomatic hypocalcemia in a young female with periodic polyserositis. Experimental data suggest that colchicine-induced hypocalcemia is secondary to colchicine inhibition of bone resorption. Findings from research using a rat model indicate that hypocalcemia may be mediated by interference with the regulatory mechanisms of bone cell calcium homeostasis, and that the destruction of microtubules may be closely related to the development of the hypocalcemia.[233]

Further research may be warranted to determine whether long-term colchicine therapy might contribute to bone loss or other calcium depletion effects, what circumstances or patient characteristics influence susceptibility to a clinically significant interaction, and what nutritional countermeasures might be safe and effective.

Cycloserine

Cycloserine (Seromycin).

Cycloserine may interfere with absorption of calcium and other nutrients, particularly minerals.[234,235] The clinical significance and therapeutic implications of this potential interaction are as yet not understood.

Diclofenac and Related Nonsteroidal Anti-Inflammatory Drugs (NSAIDs)

Diclofenac potassium (Cataflam), diclofenac sodium (Voltaren).

Related COX-1 inhibitors: Diclofenac combination drug: diclofenac and misoprostol (Arthrotec); diflunisal (Dolobid), etodolac (Lodine), fenoprofen (Dalfon), furbiprofen (Ansaid), ibuprofen (Advil, Excedrin IB, Motrin, Motrin IB, Nuprin, Pedia Care Fever Drops, Provel, Rufen); combination drug: hydrocodone and ibuprofen (Reprexain, Vicoprofen);

indomethacin (indometacin; Indocin, Indocin-SR), ketoprofen (Orudis, Oruvail), ketorolac (Acular ophthalmic, Toradol), meclofenamate (Meclomen), mefenamic acid (Ponstel), meloxicam (Mobic), nabumetone (Relafen), naproxen (Anaprox, Naprosyn), oxaprozin (Daypro), piroxicam (Feldene), salsalate (salicylic acid; Amigesic, Disalcid, Marthritic, Mono Gesic, Salflex, Salsitab), sulindac (Clinoril), tolmetin (Tolectin).

COX-2 inhibitor: Celecoxib (Celebrex).
See also Indomethacin.

Diclofenac can decrease the amount of urinary calcium excretion[236]; it may also inhibit bone resorption in postmenopausal women.[62] Thus, theoretically, coadministration could prevent bone loss in postmenopausal women. Further research is warranted.

Also, in a controlled clinical trial, Miceli-Richard et al.[237] demonstrated that acetaminophen (4 g/day) was not effective in treatment of symptomatic osteoarthritis of the knee.

Digoxin and Related Cardiac Glycosides

Digoxin (Digitek, Lanoxin, Lanoxicaps, purgoxin).
Deslanoside (cedilanin-D), digitoxin (Cystodigin), ouabain (g-strophanthin).

Calcium may interact with digoxin and related agents in two distinct ways. First, the two substances can interact in an additive or possibly synergistic manner. The inotropic action of cardiac glycosides appears to be associated, at least in part, with increased intracellular calcium availability. Chronotropic effects are also mediated by calcium. Thus, high calcium intake (especially by parenteral administration) can produce small increases in plasma calcium, thereby increasing the activity of digoxin and elevating the risk of arrhythmias and other aspects of digoxin toxicity. Second, digoxin also increases renal clearance and could lead to calcium depletion; hypocalcemia can negate the therapeutic activity of digoxin.

Evidence from clinical trials involving digoxin in human subjects, especially cardiac patients, is limited for obvious reasons given the high risk associated with any such experiments. In a 1965 paper, Kupfer and Kosovsky[238] reported that cardiac glycosides can interfere with calcium reabsorption and increase calcium excretion in a dog model through their effect on renal tubular transport of calcium. Although often cited, the clinical significance of this finding has never been established. Sonnenblick et al.[239] compared serum digoxin, calcium, potassium, and magnesium concentrations and arterial pH in 18 patients with gastrointestinal (GI) manifestations of digoxin toxicity with 19 patients with digoxin-induced cardiotoxicity, specifically automaticity. Patients with digoxin-induced GI symptoms had high serum concentrations of the drug. In contrast, those with drug-induced cardiotoxicity (automaticity) had therapeutic concentrations of digoxin but demonstrated higher calcium/potassium ratios and higher pH values.

The concern regarding this interaction dates back to a journal article published more than 70 years ago. In 1936, Bower and Mengle[240] published a "warning" in JAMA regarding two fatalities attributed to the "additive effects of calcium and digitalis." Although plausible and frequently cited for decades, no causal relationship was firmly established in these incidents. Techniques for laboratory assessment of digoxin serum levels were unavailable at that time, so it is more likely that the patients had digoxin toxicity and coincidentally were taking calcium. Other case reports describe cardiac arrhythmias associated with concomitant administration of cardiac glycosides and calcium preparations, primarily involving IV administration.[241]

In consideration of the drug's narrow therapeutic range, physicians prescribing digoxin and related cardioactive agents should advise patients to maintain stable calcium intake. Prudence suggests that blood calcium levels be monitored closely when significant or rapid changes in calcium status or intake are anticipated or undertaken. Calcium supplementation may be appropriate if deficiency is indicated, but any change in intake should be gradual and supervised closely. In most cases, checking serum calcium at onset of digoxin therapy is probably adequate. After that, monitoring digoxin level is probably the most important test. Hypocalcemia or hypercalcemia can clearly be problematic with digoxin therapy but generally is not caused by calcium supplements or their absence.

Although calcium status plays a significant role in the efficacy and safety of digoxin, supplemental or dietary calcium intake is unlikely to interact with digoxin to a clinically significant degree in most cases. Hypercalcemia increases digoxin toxicity, and hypocalcemia reduces digoxin's therapeutic effect. However, oral calcium supplements in common dosages do not usually influence blood levels of calcium levels to a significant degree and rarely would impact blood levels of calcium enough to cause a clinically significant interaction with digoxin. In absence of calcium deficiency, mimimal calcium is absorbed from the gut. In a deficiency state, calcium is mobilized from bone, through increased parathyroid hormone (PTH) secretion, to maintain the blood levels. Thus, under normal conditions, calcium homeostasis regulates blood calcium levels within a range unlikely to destabilize a patient taking digoxin.

Ionized calcium, normally tightly regulated by vitamin D, calcitonin, and PTH, would much more likely be problematic than calcium intake. Intravenous calcium carries a significant risk for an adverse interaction. Physicians administering parenteral or IV calcium to individuals undergoing digoxin therapy will presumably be closely monitoring such patients and working within a setting suitable to providing the necessary responses to unstable situations or unexpected developments. Low potassium and magnesium also increase digoxin toxicity.

Dobutamine

Dobutamine (Dobutrex).

Human research indicates that IV administration of calcium chloride may diminish the therapeutic effect of dobutamine, specifically its cardiac-stimulating properties.

In a clinical trial involving 22 patients administered dobutamine after coronary bypass surgery, Butterworth et al.[242] observed a 30% reduction in cardiac output with concomitant administration of calcium chloride by continuous infusion. These subjects had a normal cardiac output before calcium administration. In contrast, milrinone was not affected by the calcium administration. The authors could not demonstrate the mechanism involved in this interaction but suggested that calcium may interfere with signal transduction through the beta-adrenergic receptor complex.

Physicians administering dobutamine are advised to monitor for decreased cardiac output or other reduction of therapeutic effects if exogenous calcium is administered or the dose increased, especially intravenously. Evidence is lacking to support any extrapolation of this finding to oral calcium supplementation.

Erythromycin and Related Macrolide Antibiotics

Azithromycin (Zithromax), clarithromycin (Biaxin), dirithromycin (Dynabac), erythromycin, oral (EES, EryPed, Ery-Tab, PCE Dispertab, Pediazole), troleandomycin (Tao).

Erythromycin may interfere with the absorption and activity of calcium and other nutrients. Although not usually clinically significant with short-term administration, the increased risk of calcium depletion can become a concern with extended use. Further research is warranted to investigate potential adverse effects on calcium balance and bone metabolism with extended macrolide therapy.

Physicians prescribing erythromycin and related macrolide antibiotics internally for longer than 2 weeks are advised to supplement calcium (as well as folic acid, vitamins B_6 and B_2, and magnesium) as a preventive measure, with separation of oral intake. Any potential drug-induced adverse effect on bone formation would carry a significantly greater risk when growth and bone formation are most active, such as with infants and children. Avoiding such an interaction would also be particularly important in adolescents (e.g., being treated for acne) in the midst of the life stage where they need to attain maximum bone density.

Hydroxychloroquine and Chloroquine

Hydroxychloroquine (Plaquenil).
Related: Chloroquine (Aralen, Aralen HCl).

Preliminary data suggest that hydroxychloroquine might induce hypocalcemia or calcium depletion. An isolated case report described the use of hydroxychloroquine to block the formation of active vitamin D and normalize elevated blood levels of calcium in a 45-year-old woman with sarcoidosis.[243] Evidence is lacking to confirm or disprove such effects of hydroxychloroquine administration in individuals not presenting with sarcoidosis or elevated calcium. Pending further research with well-designed clinical trials, physicians prescribing hydroxychloroquine are advised to monitor vitamin 25(OH)D and calcium status.

Indapamide

Indapamide (Lozol).

As a thiazide-like diuretic, indapamide carries a high probability of interacting with nutrients in a manner similar to interactions observed with thiazide diuretics. Thus, preliminary data suggest that indapamide may cause slight elevation in blood calcium levels, and that concomitant administration of calcium supplements could potentially aggravate this risk.[244-247] Physicians prescribing indapamide should monitor blood calcium levels and consider whether calcium supplementation is contraindicated for the individual being treated.

Indomethacin

Indomethacin (Indometacin; Indocin, Indocin-SR).

Prostaglandins E_1 and E_2 (PGE_2) stimulate bone resorption. This has been proposed as a possible mechanism for hypercalcemia in malignancy (particularly renal cell carcinoma). Some in vitro and in vivo research has shown that indomethacin, a specific prostaglandin biosynthesis inhibitor, may reduce plasma calcium (and phosphate) levels. However, in a trial involving patients with breast cancer, Coombes et al.[248] found that indomethacin did not reduce serum calcium levels in patients with hypercalcemia, nor did it reduce skeletal destruction, as measured by the urinary hydroxyproline/creatinine ratio and urinary calcium in normocalcemic or hypercalcemic patients with osteolytic metastases. Similarly, in a study of PGE_2, parathormone (PTH), and response to indomethacin in patients with hypercalcemia of malignancy, Brenner et al.[249] found that PGE_2 and calcium fell to normal levels in 3 of 14 patients (breast, colon, renal carcinomas) after administration of indomethacin. In a rat model, Gomaa et al.[250] observed that indomethacin increased serum levels of calcium.

This potential interaction could be especially relevant in patients using indomethacin for joint pain and inflammation (e.g., osteoarthritis) or after orthopedic procedures. However, evidence is lacking to determine whether coadministration of nutrients might be appropriate or beneficial.

Laxatives, Stimulant

Laxatives, Stimulant

Stimulant laxatives may reduce absorption of calcium from dietary or supplemental sources.[251] With prolonged use, this action could result in adverse effects. Physicians are generally advised to inform patients to limit the duration of stimulant laxatives for many reasons, including potential for decreased absorption and potential depletion of key nutrients, including calcium.

Loop Diuretics

Bumetanide (Bumex), ethacrynic acid (Edecrin), furosemide (Lasix), torsemide (Demadex).

Loop diuretics act in the luminal side of the ascending part of the kidney's diluting segment and will increase the urinary excretion of calcium, subsequently increasing blood calcium levels.[252] This action could theoretically induce osteopenia; it may also increase the risk of calcium oxalate stones.

The available data from clinical research suggest that loop diuretics can alter calcium levels but are inadequate for determining whether and under what conditions such interaction may be clinically significant. In a trial involving 16 healthy volunteers treated with bumetanide, Davies et al.[253] found that the effects on calcium may be relatively less pronounced with this medication than with other drugs in this class; urinary calcium loss was initially elevated but was followed by retention at 24 hours (0.25-1.0 mg orally). Ogawa et al.[254] observed that furosemide (40 mg) caused marked calciuresis but also elevated serum calcium levels in an experiment involving five healthy male subjects. The authors noted that the effects of increased calcium excretion "may not extend to bone calcium remodeling at least in such a short-term experiment."

Fujita et al.[255] examined the effects of short-term administration of furosemide (4-7 days) on the response to exogenous parathyroid extract in six normal subjects. All six subjects demonstrated marked increases in urinary calcium excretion, reduced serum ionized calcium levels, and significant increase in urinary cyclic adenosine monophosphate (cAMP) from the control to the furosemide periods. Further research with well-designed clinical trials is warranted to clarify the clinical effects of loop diuretics on calcium metabolism and homeostasis and to determine guidelines for a safe, effective clinical response.

Physicians prescribing loop diuretics should advise patients to discuss their status, and/or consult with a health care professional trained and experienced in nutritional therapies, before initiating or increasing their level of calcium supplementation. Despite a lack of evidence establishing a general need for calcium support, increased calcium intake through diet or supplements may be appropriate during loop diuretic therapy in some individuals at high risk for bone loss. However, in patients taking both loop diuretics (especially furosemide) and calcium supplementation, testing of 24-hour urinary calcium levels may be prudent in patients with increased risk of calcium oxalate stones. Choosing which form of calcium to use may be significant in supporting bone density while minimizing risk of nephrolithiasis.

Medroxyprogesterone

Conjugated equine estrogens and medroxyprogesterone (Premelle cycle 5, Prempro); medroxyprogesterone, injection (Depo-Provera, Depo-subQ Provera 104); medroxyprogesterone, oral (Cycrin, Provera).

The evidence is mixed and preliminary, but the available data indicate that medroxyprogesterone administration probably increases bone loss, even with calcium coadministration. Hergenroeder et al.[256] conducted a randomized, controlled clinical trial involving 24 Caucasian women, age 14 to 28, with hypothalamic amenorrhea or oligomenorrhea, comparing the effects of treatment using oral contraceptives (OCs), medroxyprogesterone, or placebo over 12 months. Measuring bone mass at 6 and 12 months, they found that spine and total-body bone mineral measurements in amenorrheic subjects at 12 months were greater in the OC group than in the medroxyprogesterone and placebo groups, and that no detectable improvement in bone mineral associated with medroxyprogesterone use in oligomenorrheic subjects. There were no measurable differences in hip bone mineral calcium and bone mineral density (BMD) measurements at 12 months among the three groups. Merki-Feld et al.[257] conducted a 2-year prospective study on the effects of depot medroxyprogesterone acetate (DMPA) on bone mass response to estrogen and calcium therapy in women age 30 to 45. In particular, their investigation focused on the effects of estrogen or calcium substitution during the second year of follow-up in seven DMPA users with a high annual bone loss during the first year. The baseline cortical and trabecular bone mass (TBM) and the annual change was no different in DMPA users and controls. Over 24 months the researchers measured an increase in TBM of 0.6% and a decrease in cortical bone mass of 0.1% in exposed women. Some (but not all) DMPA users with bone loss during the first year could be successfully treated with estradiol or calcium. These authors concluded that no significantly accelerated bone loss was associated with DMPA use in women 30 to 45 years of age.

Berenson et al.[258] compared the effects of 24 months of DMPA on lumbar spine BMD compared with self-selected oral contraception (pills) and nonhormonal contraception (controls) in 191 women age 18 to 33. They observed that women using DMPA for 24 months demonstrated on average a 5.7% loss in BMD, with a 3.2% loss occurring between months 12 and 24. In contrast, users of desogestrel pills experienced an average 2.6% loss in BMD after 24 months. These authors concluded that DMPA appeared to be associated with linear pattern of decreased BMD during the first 2 years of use.

Calcium nutriture and weight-bearing exercise form the foundation of bone health in women during the menstrual years. Physicians prescribing medroxyprogesterone will want to remind patients of the basic preventive needs and suggest that consistency may be especially important given the potential for increased bone loss under the influence of this form of contraceptive.

Mineral Oil

Mineral Oil (Agoral, Kondremul Plain, Milkinol, Neo-Cultol, Petrogalar Plain).

Mineral oil, as a lipid solvent, may absorb many substances and interfere with normal absorption of calcium and other nutrients.[259] The effect of mineral oil on fat-soluble nutrients such as vitamin D, which is essential to calcium absorption, can further adversely influence calcium bioavailability. Although some research suggests that these interactions may be clinically significant, especially with long-term administration and simultaneous intake, the collective evidence is mixed and inconclusive.

Health care professionals advising patients using mineral oil for any extended time can recommend regular use of a multivitamin-mineral supplement as potentially beneficial. Administering mineral oil on an empty stomach or ingesting vitamin/mineral supplements at least 2 hours before or after the mineral oil can effectively minimize malabsorption of fat-soluble nutrients. However, in general, the internal use of mineral oil should be limited to less than 1 week.

Potassium-Sparing Diuretics

Amiloride (Midamor), spironolactone (Aldactone), triamterene (Dyrenium); combination drugs: amiloride and hydrochlorothiazide (Moduretic); spironolactone and hydrochlorothiazide (Aldactazide); triamterene and hydrochlorothiazide (Dyazide, Maxzide).

Potassium-sparing diuretics can increase calcium loss through urinary excretion, but evidence is lacking to determine whether and under what circumstances this effect might lead to a clinically significant pattern of calcium depletion.[260-262] Reduced calcium loss has also been posited, similar to that found with thiazide diuretics.

Leppla et al.[208] conducted a small clinical trial involving seven patients with renal stones to investigate the potential therapeutic role of amiloride in calcium nephrolithiasis. They observed that two doses of amiloride (2.5 mg/day) reduced urinary calcium in two subjects with kidney stones. This decrease in urinary calcium was enhanced in five subjects when amiloride was coadministered with two doses of hydrochlorothiazide (25 mg/day). The clinical implications of this observed effect on calcium metabolism are unclear at this time.

Triamterene may increase urinary calcium excretion. However, the clinical implications of this possible interaction are limited.

The evidence regarding this interaction is inconsistent and has yet to mature. Nevertheless, physicians prescribing potassium-sparing diuretics are advised to be aware of potential alterations in calcium status caused by these agents and to consider calcium supplementation or contraindication, as indicated by the individual patient's age, gender, medical history, BMD, and other relevant factors.

Retinoic Acid and Related Retinoids

Acitretin (Soriatane), bexarotene (Targretin), etretinate (Tegison), isotretinoin (13-*cis* retinoic acid; Accutane), tretinoin (All-Trans-Retinoic Acid, ATRA, Atragen, Avita, Renova, Retin-A, Vesanoid, Vitinoin).

Long-term or high-dose administration of vitamin A derivatives (retinoids) may produce a variety of skeletal adverse effects in humans. Kindmark et al.[263] investigated the early effects of oral isotretinoin therapy on bone turnover and calcium homeostasis in 11 consecutive patients with nodulocystic acne. They reported that markers of bone turnover and urine levels of calcium and hydroxyproline decreased significantly within 5 days of treatment. There was also a statistically significant decrease in serum calcium, with a minimum on day 5, and a marked increase in serum PTH. However, with continued treatment, the abnormal levels of these markers returned to baseline values within 14 days. Further research with well-designed clinical trials is warranted to investigate long-term

implications of retinoic acid therapy on calcium economy and bone health.

Physicians prescribing retinoic acid or related retinoid therapies internally for longer than 2 weeks are advised to supplement calcium (300 mg three times daily) as a preventive measure.

Salicylates

Acetylsalicylic acid (acetosal, acetyl salicylic acid, ASA, salicylsalicylic acid; Arthritis Foundation Pain Reliever, Ascriptin, Aspergum, Asprimox, Bayer Aspirin, Bayer Buffered Aspirin, Bayer Low Adult Strength, Bufferin, Buffex, Cama Arthritis Pain Reliever, Easprin, Ecotrin, Ecotrin Low Adult Strength, Empirin, Extra Strength Adprin-B, Extra Strength Bayer Enteric 500 Aspirin, Extra Strength Bayer Plus, Halfprin 81, Heartline, Regular Strength Bayer Enteric 500 Aspirin, St. Joseph Adult Chewable Aspirin, ZORprin); combination drugs: ASA and caffeine (Anacin); ASA, caffeine, and propoxyphene (Darvon Compound); ASA and carisoprodol (Soma Compound); ASA, codeine, and carisoprodol (Soma Compound with Codeine); ASA and codeine (Empirin with Codeine); ASA, codeine, butalbital, and caffeine (Fiorinal); ASA and extended-release dipyridamole (Aggrenox, Asasantin).

Salsalate (salicylic acid; Amigesic, Disalcid, Marthritic, Mono Gesic, Salflex, Salsitab).

Experimental data indicate that salicylic acid analogs with the carboxyl group adjacent to the hydroxyl group on the benzene ring can induce hypocalcemia. Kato et al.[264] found that orally administered aspirin and sodium salt of *o*-hydroxybenzoic acid (Na-salicylate), but not the sodium salt of *m*- and *p*-hydroxybenzoic acid (HBA), induced hypocalcemia; 2,5-dihydroxybenzoic acid (DHBA) and PAS sodium dihydrate (PAS-Na) caused hypocalcemia when administered intravenously but not orally. Related findings from IV injection of aspirin–dl-lysine (water-soluble aspirin) and SA–dl-lysine suggest that prostaglandins are not involved in the process of aspirin-induced hypocalcemia in the rat.[264]

Further research involving well-designed clinical trials is warranted to assess the short-term effects and long-term clinical implications of this potential interaction between salicylates and calcium, particularly in regard to long-term bone loss, joint pain, osteoarthritis, and analgesic use.

Sodium Fluoride

Sodium fluoride (Fluorigard, Fluorinse, Fluoritab, Fluorodex, Flura-Drops, Flura-Tab, Karidium, Luride, Pediaflor, PreviDent).

Calcium may reduce absorption of fluoride, and vice versa, when taken simultaneously.[265]

In a review article, Deal[266] reported that fluoride monotherapy can transfer calcium from leg bones to the spine, thus increasing the risk of stress fractures. However, coadministration of 1500 mg calcium daily and slow-release forms of fluoride increases the lumbar spine BMD without causing fractures.

Haguenauer et al.[267] conducted a meta-analysis of randomized controlled trials investigating efficacy of fluoride therapy on bone loss, vertebral and nonvertebral fractures, and adverse effects in postmenopausal women. Although fluoride therapy demonstrates an ability to increase lumbar spine BMD, it does not result in a reduction in vertebral fractures. Further, increasing fluoride dose raises the risk of nonvertebral fractures and incidence of GI adverse effects without providing any beneficial effect on the vertebral fracture rate. Health care professionals experienced in nutritional therapies report that sodium fluoride, when used as a treatment for osteoporosis, does harden bone, but it also renders bone less elastic and more brittle, and increases fracture risk. Further research is warranted to investigate this clinically important interaction and develop therapeutic guidelines integrating calcium supplementation and other nutritional interventions into a comprehensive strategy for treating osteoporosis that mitigates adverse effects and maximizes the therapeutic benefits of sodium fluoride therapy on bone quality.

Physicians prescribing fluoride to enhance bone mass are advised to coadminister calcium (400-500 mg three times daily) but to separate oral ingestion by at least 2 hours to reduce the risk of the two agents interfering with each other's absorption. Weight-bearing exercise, vitamin D, and sunlight exposure are also advisable to support bone health and reduce risk of bone loss.

Sucralfate

Sucralfate (Carafate).

Vucelic et al.[268] conducted a clinical trial investigating the effects of sucralfate on serum phosphorus, calcium, and alkaline phosphatase in 30 patients with chronic renal failure on intermittent hemodialysis. They reported an increase in serum calcium (as well as a significant reduction in serum phosphorus and alkaline phosphatase) after 14 days of treatment with sucralfate (1 g four times daily).

Calcium administration requires supervision during sucralfate therapy for hyperphosphatemia and secondary hyperparathyroidism in patients with chronic renal failure; avoidance of calcium may be appropriate in some cases. Physicians prescribing sucralfate should monitor patients for signs of hypercalcemia, which might be induced or aggravated by high calcium intake. Furthermore, serum phosphorus should be checked routinely in patients treated with sucralfate for peptic ulcer disease, although the risk of interference in calcium-phosphorus homeostasis is certainly much lower in patients with normal renal function. In the absence of clinical trial data, clinical vigilance is warranted.

Tamoxifen

Tamoxifen (Nolvadex).

Tamoxifen preserves BMD in postmenopausal women but may increase bone loss in premenopausal women.[269] Hypercalcemia is a rare adverse effect associated with tamoxifen therapy, the risk of which could theoretically be increased by calcium supplements. Hypercalcemia can occur in any advanced cancer in which the tumor cells make parathyroid-related protein (a peptide hormone), and in such tumors, concomitant calcium could aggravate the condition. However, the only time tamoxifen causes hypercalcemia is in breast cancer patients with bone metastases, who have a "tamoxifen tumor flare" in the first 2 to 3 weeks after initiating tamoxifen therapy; this is caused by the estrogen agonist activity of tamoxifen being asserted before the estrogen antagonist effect takes hold. Tumor flare is well known to be highly predictive of an ultimate therapeutic response in the breast cancer patient. Calcium intake during this brief window of tumor flare might exacerbate the hypercalcemia, but bone (rather than oral intake of calcium) is the primary source of the calcium in such cases. These patients respond to bisphosphonates, such as pamidronate and related drugs, which increase the binding of calcium to the bone matrix and shut down the function of osteoclasts, which are necessary to mobilize calcium from bone.

Calcium supplementation may be appropriate outside this volatile initial phase but must be approached with caution and close monitoring. In the longer term, physicians prescribing tamoxifen for prevention or treatment of breast cancer can enhance the bone health of these patients by recommending adequate calcium and vitamin D intake through dietary and supplemental sources (at appropriate phases in the therapeutic process), encouraging weight-bearing exercise and sunlight exposure and counseling about the relationship between smoking and alcohol and bone loss. Together these prudent recommendations will support overall health and may lessen bone loss and the risk of subsequent osteoporosis. BMD should be measured in women receiving chemotherapy of any type. Strategic integrative protocols, adapted to the characteristics and needs of the individual patient, offer expanded possibilities for enhanced care and improved outcomes within the context of collaborative care involving health care professionals trained and experienced in both conventional oncology and nutritional therapeutics.

NUTRIENT-NUTRIENT INTERACTIONS

Alcohol

Excessive alcohol intake may reduce calcium absorption.

Caffeine and Coffee

See Caffeine.

Essential Fatty Acids

Omega-6 fatty acids: Gamma-linolenic acid.
Omega-3 fatty acids: Alpha-linolenic acid (ALA), docosahexaenoic acid (DHA), eicosapentaenoic acid (EPA).

Animal studies and some evidence from human research indicate that essential fatty acids (EFAS) may enhance calcium absorption, at least in part, by enhancing the effects of vitamin D, to reduce urinary calcium excretion, to increase calcium deposition in bone and improve bone strength, and to enhance bone collagen synthesis.[270-272] Animals deficient in EFAs develop severe osteoporosis with increased renal and arterial calcification. In particular, these effects from the interaction between EFAs and calcium metabolism are associated with reduced ectopic calcification, specifically in the arteries and the kidneys, a major factor in mortality associated with osteoporosis.

In a randomized clinical trial involving 65 postmenopausal women taking a background diet low in calcium, Kruger et al.[272] observed that the coadministration of gamma-linolenic acid (omega-6 fatty acids from evening primrose oil) and eicosapentaenoic acid (omega-3 fatty acids from fish oil) with 600 mg/day calcium carbonate for 18 months was associated with improvements in markers of bone formation/degradation and bone mineral density (BMD), as well as a decreased incidence of fractures. In contrast, Bassey et al.[273] found no significant benefit in two randomized controlled trials comparing effects of calcium-EFA combination versus calcium alone on BMD in healthy premenopausal and postmenopausal women. The apparent inconsistency between these findings may reflect differences in the ages, general health status, diet, physical activity level, and other influential factors, which were significantly contrasting in the groups of women studied and need to be taken into account in any comparison between the studies and their results. In particular, long-term activity level and nutritional status, especially long-term dietary intake of calcium and EFAs, are known to affect calcium absorption and bone health.

Nutrient-Drug Interactions and Drug-Induced Nutrient Depletions

Both calcium and EFAs have beneficial effects on the population with or at risk for osteoporosis. However, further research is warranted to investigate the specific interaction(s) between calcium and EFAs, as well as the mechanisms of action, clinical significance, and therapeutic implications for bone health and other functions and conditions.

Iron

Concomitant administration of calcium and iron can decrease GI absorption of iron, particularly from nonheme sources.[274] Calcium supplements inhibit absorption of supplemental iron to a greater degree when taken with food.[275,276] Evidence, some extrapolated from research involving antacids, suggests that calcium can interfere with the absorption of iron and possibly other minerals by neutralizing stomach acid.[148,277] However, human research indicates that clinically significant effects on the status of either mineral are improbable, most likely because of compensatory changes in absorption rates.[278] Thus, it is unlikely that iron absorption is significantly reduced when iron and calcium are combined within a multimineral formulation. Nevertheless, when iron and calcium are being taken as separate supplements, separation of intake by 2 or more hours will avoid any impairment of absorption. Furthermore, taking calcium supplements away from meals appears to reduce adverse effects on absorption of iron and possibly other nutrients.

Lysine

Animal and human studies demonstrate that lysine can enhance intestinal calcium absorption and improve the renal conservation of the absorbed calcium, thus reducing urinary calcium excretion.[279,280] Coadministration of calcium and L-lysine supplements may provide a synergistic benefit for both preventive and therapeutic interventions in osteoporosis. Further research with well-designed, long-term clinical trials is warranted.

Magnesium

Magnesium intake from food and supplements is associated with BMD.[281] Concomitant administration of calcium and magnesium, particularly with high calcium intake, decreases GI absorption of magnesium. However, such competition does not appear to exert clinically significant effects on status of either mineral.[282-284]

Calcium supplementation, as well as cessation of magnesium administration, is typically used in treating hypermagnesemia.

Milk and Dairy Products

Cow's milk contains a different proportion of various mineral constituents than human milk. In particular, cow's milk, dairy products, and other foods that are high in phosphorus may reduce calcium absorption by forming insoluble complexes with calcium ions. Lactose does not enhance calcium availability in lactose-tolerant individuals.[285] Controversy continues as to whether calcium in many dairy products (1) may have limited bioavailability for individuals who do not properly digest dairy products because they lack sufficient lactase to digest the milk sugar or (2) may react to the characteristic proteins.

Phosphorus

Oral administration of calcium, as a divalent cation, may bind with oral phosphate and interfere with phosphorus absorption in the GI tract.[271,286] Most commentators portray the adverse impact of high phosphorus intake (e.g., in phosphoric acid—containing soft drinks, particularly in association with cola) on calcium function as the more clinically significant adverse effect of this interaction. Nevertheless, contentious debate and unresolved issues characterize the literature concerning the interactions, mechanisms, contextual influences, and clinical implications of high phosphorus intakes on calcium balance and bone health, as well as the impact of calcium on phosphorus balance.

Higher phosphorus intake has been associated with slightly lower levels of urinary calcium but also with slightly increased intestinal secretion of calcium, resulting in increased calcium loss in the feces.[287] Overall, the increase in endogenous fecal calcium from increasing phosphorus is generally about equal to the effect from decreasing urinary calcium. Diets high in phosphorus and low in calcium have been found to increase PTH secretion.

In terms of dietary consumption patterns, phosphorus intake tends to displace calcium intake. Animal protein, dairy products, and many carbonated beverages are especially high in phosphorus. The use of phosphorus-containing food additives contributes substantially to daily phosphorus intake for most people consuming a standard American diet, and their use is increasing, especially in processed foods. In particular, soft drinks often contain phosphoric acid as an acidulant to maintain carbonation, and the link between consumption of soft drinks and bone loss has been the subject of much discussion. Dietary intervention studies have shown that elevations in serum phosphorus resulting from high phosphorus intake may have physiological consequences that are harmful to both bone and kidney when sustained over time and particularly when calcium intake is low. Intake of foods rich in phosphorus (especially as additives) and low in calcium is associated with a persistent elevation in serum PTH levels but no increase in calcitriol (1,25-OH_2D, the active metabolite of vitamin D).[288] Such dietary patterns among children and adolescents do not bode well for long-term risk of osteoporosis in populations eating a standard American diet.[289]

One stream of research indicates that calcium intake, especially at relatively high levels, may adversely affect phosphorous balance. Thus, Heaney and Recker[225] concluded that no net association of different phosphorus intakes with calcium balance was likely because these two effects were opposite in direction. Twenty years later, Heaney and Nordin[290] led a team of researchers investigating the impact of high calcium intake on phosphorus absorption, metabolism, and function. They observed that phosphorus absorption falls and the risk of phosphorus insufficiency rises when calcium intake increases without a corresponding increase in phosphorus intake. In particular, they expressed a concern for dietary intakes with high Ca:P ratios that can occur with use of calcium supplements or food fortificants consisting of nonphosphate calcium salts. These researchers concluded that "older patients with osteoporosis treated with current generation bone active agents should receive at least some of their calcium co-therapy in the form of a calcium phosphate preparation."[290]

Health care professionals concerned with bone health and the unresolved complexities of the interaction between these two important nutrients can most benefit their patients by strongly advocating an active lifestyle supported by a diverse and balanced diet of fresh, nutrient-rich foods and minimal intake of processed foods and soft drinks throughout life, but especially during those life stages emphasizing attainment of maximal bone density and prevention of bone loss. Use of a multimineral formulations containing phosphorus has been recommended for individuals, especially the elderly, regularly taking high doses of calcium. In general, separating intake of supplemental phosphorus from calcium intake, either as calcium-rich foods or supplements, by at least 2 hours will minimize any impairment of absorption of either nutrient.

Protein

The effect of dietary protein on calcium balance is often treated as if it were a well-documented phenomenon, but it still remains contentious, seemingly paradoxical, and ultimately unresolved. Increases in dietary protein intake are directly associated with increased urinary calcium excretion and increased risk of bone loss over time. As the intake of dietary protein increases, the urinary excretion of calcium increases as a result of decreased fractional tubular reabsorption, such that doubling protein intake results in a 50% increase in urinary calcium excretion.[287] Using data from Zemel,[291] Weaver et al.[292] calculated that each additional gram of protein consumed results in an additional loss of 1.75 mg of calcium per day. Given an average absorption efficiency of 30% for dietary calcium, each 1-g increase in protein intake per day creates a requirement for an additional 5.8 mg of calcium per day to offset the protein-induced calcium loss.

Lifelong high intake of dietary animal protein correlates with increased risk of osteoporosis in most studies.[293] After sustaining an osteoporotic fracture, however, a 20-g/day supplement of protein reduced bone loss compared with similar patients not supplemented with protein.[294] Another randomized, double-blind trial showed that a supplement of soy protein powder providing 40 g protein and 90 mg soy isoflavones increased BMD at the spine in postmenopausal women.[295]

The effect of high protein on bone health remains unclear and controversial. The seemingly inconsistent findings could easily reflect differences in subject characteristics, medical conditions, materials tested, and dosage levels more than they reveal fundamental contradictions. Nevertheless, advising calcium supplementation along with increased dietary protein is probably reasonable. Diets simultaneously high in protein and inadequate in calcium especially may put people at risk for skeletal sequelae, particularly in later life. Furthermore, even though a large proportion of those consuming a standard American diet are more likely at risk of excess protein effects on calcium economy, those with insufficient protein intake are at perhaps greater risk of poor bone health. In particular, serum albumin levels (paralleling protein nutriture) are inversely related to hip fracture risk, and inadequate protein intakes have been associated with poor recovery from osteoporotic fractures.[289]

Sodium

The available evidence suggests that high sodium intake is associated with adverse effects on calcium and increased risk of bone loss. Increased sodium intake results in increased urinary calcium excretion, possibly because of competition between sodium and calcium for reabsorption in the kidney or through an effect of sodium on PTH secretion.[288,292,296] In a 2-year longitudinal study of the effect of sodium and calcium intakes on regional bone density in 124 postmenopausal women, Devine et al.[297] found that increased urinary sodium excretion (indicative of increased sodium intake) was associated with decreased BMD at the hip. Further research into this important interaction is clearly warranted, particularly given the strong association between diets high in sodium and decreased intake of foods rich in calcium and other beneficial nutrients.[289]

Soy

Phytic acid can interfere with the absorption of calcium. However, some research shows that soy products have relatively high calcium bioavailability, even though soybeans are rich in both oxalate and phytate.[292] Some health care professionals recommend a 2-hour separation between intake of calcium supplements and eating soya products.

Vitamin D

See also earlier Strategic Considerations discussion.

Coadministration of vitamin D and calcium, along with weight-bearing exercise and sunlight exposure, are generally considered the foundational approaches to calcium nourishment, attainment and maintenance of BMD, and prevention of bone loss.[298-300] A normal physiological function of vitamin D is to facilitate intestinal calcium absorption.

Although findings have varied, often significantly influenced by methodology (especially in meta-analyses), most research indicates that concomitant intake of calcium and vitamin D reduces risk of fractures and enhances bone health, particularly with individuals with a preexisting insufficiency and consistent patient compliance. In general, according to Heaney and Weaver,[79] prudent nutritional support for osteoporosis prevention and treatment consists of 30 to 40 mmol calcium daily with sufficient vitamin D to maintain serum 25(OH)D levels above 80 nmol/L (~25 µg [1000 IU] vitamin D/day). In a Cochrane Library review of 38 randomized or quasi-randomized trials, Avenell and Handoll[301] found that the risk of fractures of the hip and other nonspinal bones was reduced slightly in elderly people who are frail and at risk for bone fractures, particularly those who live in nursing homes or other institutions, if vitamin D and calcium were given. Nevertheless, the risk of spinal fractures did not appear to be reduced.

In a trial involving 944 healthy Icelandic adults, Steingrimsdottir et al.[8] found that with 25-OHD levels below 10 ng/mL (i.e., significant vitamin D deficiency), maintaining calcium intake above 800 mg/day appeared to normalize calcium metabolism, as determined by the PTH level, but in individuals with higher 25-OHD levels, no benefit was observed from calcium intake above 800 mg/day.

In 2005 and 2006, three major papers were published discussing the relationship between calcium, vitamin D, and osteoporotic fracture risk. Findings from the RECORD study, published in The Lancet (2005), suggested a lack of benefit from concomitant calcium and vitamin D in the prevention of fractures in menopausal women.[40] Subsequently, Jackson et al.[302] published a paper using data from the Women's Health Initiative that questioned the assumption that calcium and vitamin D can prevent osteoporosis-related hip fractures. They randomly assigned 36,000 postmenopausal women to receive elemental calcium, as calcium carbonate (500 mg twice daily), plus vitamin D (200 IU twice daily) or a placebo for an average of 7 years. Notably, the average calcium consumption in both groups was approximately 1150 mg/day, close to the appropriate recommended intake level. After 7 years, subjects in the treatment group exhibited 12% fewer hip fractures than did those in the placebo group, a finding that was not statistically significant. However, a deeper analysis of the data reveals that more significant differences appear when considering compliance and initial calcium intake levels. For example, after excluding women who were not adhering to the program, the reduction in fractures was greater, with 29% fewer fractures in the treatment group than in the placebo group, a statistically significant difference. Likewise, hip fracture risk decreased by about 22% in treated subjects whose initial calcium intake was low or moderate, but increased by 12% in treated women with high initial calcium intake (≥ 1200 mg/day).[302] Overall, in both trials compliance was only on the order of 40% and 50%.

In contrast, Boonen et al.[303] conducted a multifaceted meta-analysis of major randomized placebo-controlled trials that analyzed the effects of vitamin D alone or in combination with calcium. In one analysis they found that randomized clinical trials comparing vitamin D alone to placebo showed no effect. Likewise, a subsidiary analysis showed that low doses of vitamin D, less than 800 units/day, exerted no effect. However, they demonstrated a statistically significant 21% reduction in risk of fracture, compared to placebo, among subjects receiving 800 IU vitamin D and more than 1000 mg calcium daily. The authors concluded that vitamin D exerts its beneficial effect on bone predominantly by increasing absorption of calcium.

In some individuals and with certain medical conditions, supplementation with vitamin D, particularly at levels significantly in excess of those needed to overcome established deficiency, can induce an excessive increase in the absorption of calcium and increase the risk of hypercalcemia and kidney stone formation.[302] The risk of such adverse effects occurring may be influenced by the form of calcium used, as well as other, individual patient variables. Emerging evidence and the opinions of many vitamin D researchers now suggest, however, that the daily value (DV) of 400 IU for vitamin D, which was based on the amount necessary to prevent rickets in infants (initially

given as 5 mL of cod liver oil 100 years ago) is an order of magnitude below the amount necessary for older adults and those not regularly exposed to sun without sunscreen to achieve and maintain blood levels of vitamin D that are optimum for bone health and cancer prevention.[304-316] "Estimates of the population distribution of serum 25(OH)D values, coupled with available dose-response data, indicate that it would require input of an additional 2600 IU/d (65 mcg/d) of oral vitamin D_3 to ensure that 97.5% of older women have 25(OH)D values at or above desirable levels."[317] Absent lymphoma or granulomatous disease, which can cause vitamin D sensitivity, it appears that long-term ingestion of greater than 10,000 IU/day is necessary to cause vitamin D toxicity and hypercalcemia.

Zinc

Most available evidence from human studies indicates that simultaneous administration of calcium and zinc decreases GI absorption of zinc.[275,318-323] Research based on antacids suggests that calcium can interfere with the absorption of zinc (and possibly other minerals) by neutralizing stomach acid.[277] However, clinically adverse significant effects on bioavailability or status of either mineral are improbable. In particular, when ingested in the presence of meals, zinc levels appear to be unaffected by increases of either dietary or supplemental calcium.

The 323 citations for this monograph, as well as additional reference literature, are located under Calcium on the CD at the back of the book.

Chromium

Nutrient Name: Chromium.

Synonyms: Chromium 3, chromium acetate, chromium aspartate, chromium chloride, chromium histidine, chromium nicotinate, chromium picolinate, chromium polynicotinate, chromium sulfate, trivalent chromium; Cr(III), Cr^{+3}.

Elemental Symbol: Cr.

Related Substances: Brewer's yeast, high-chromium yeast; hexavalent chromium (VI; Cr^{+6}; toxic).

Summary

Drug/Class Interaction Type	Mechanism and Significance	Management
Beta-1-Adrenoceptor Antagonists ⊕⊕	Patients on beta-blocker therapy may derive improvements in lipid status, particularly elevations in HDL cholesterol, with concomitant chromium administration. Preliminary evidence primarily involved middle-aged men with hypertension, but findings may reasonably be extrapolated to other patient populations.	Coadminister. Standard monitoring usually adequate.
Corticosteroids, oral ≈≈/☼	Increased chromium excretion is associated with corticosteroid therapy and may play a role in steroid-induced diabetes. Coadministration can prevent drug-induced depletion and may reverse steroid-induced diabetes.	Coadminister. Standard monitoring usually adequate.
Insulin, glyburide, metformin Oral hypoglycemic agents ⊕⊕/⊕✗/✗	Compromised chromium status is quite common and may contribute to insulin resistance, dysglycemia, and onset of diabetes. Chromium potentiates insulin activity through multiple mechanisms, only some of which are well known, and is most active in those with chromium deficiency. Coadministration of chromium with exogenous insulin or oral hypoglycemic medications may provide therapeutic benefit by enhancing insulin activity and glucose control. However, inappropriate combining could induce hypoglycemic reaction.	Coadminister, especially with probable deficiency. Modify dosing of both agents gradually with titration. Monitor for hypoglycemia symptoms.
Sertraline Selective serotonin reuptake inhibitor (SSRI) antidepressants ⊕⊕	Disparate and indirect evidence indicates that chromium may benefit individuals with depression through effects on glucose control and potentiation of insulin. In particular, chromium picolinate appears to increase peripheral availability of tryptophan for brain serotonin (5-HT) synthesis and alter sensitivity of central 5-HT(2A) receptors. Clinical trials have reported increased efficacy (including efficacy in therapy-refractory patients) of standard antidepressant treatment, specifically sertraline, with coadministration. No evidence of adverse effects has been presented.	Coadministration judicious and considered safe, especially with probable deficiency. Standard monitoring usually adequate.

NUTRIENT DESCRIPTION

Chemistry and Forms

Chromium exists in several forms, with chrome-iron ore the predominant form in the planetary crust. The trivalent and hexavalent states constitute the most common valence states, with trivalent chromium being the stable and biologically active form found in most food sources and hexavalent chromium primarily associated with industrial exposure and toxicity.

Physiology and Function

Chromium is an essential trace mineral well known for its role in carbohydrate, lipid, and protein metabolism in general and insulin activity and glucose homeostasis in particular. Emerging knowledge indicates that chromium also plays an important role in nucleic acid synthesis and gene expression. Nevertheless, chromium, as an ultratrace element, is found in very low concentrations in the human body.

Dietary chromium is poorly absorbed (0.5% to 2.8% of intake), and almost all of an ingested dose is excreted in the feces. Absorption occurs in the small intestine by processes other than simple diffusion, the mechanisms of which are not yet fully understood. Chromium is subsequently transported in the serum or plasma bound to transferrin (named for its role in binding and transporting iron) primarily and albumin secondarily. Chromium is widely distributed throughout the human body, with highest concentrations in the bone, spleen, liver, and kidney into four different compartments that have rapid, medium, slow, and very slow turnover. Chromium that has been absorbed is excreted mainly in the urine. Small amounts are also lost in hair and sweat. Little excretion occurs via the biliary route.

Organic chromium increases insulin sensitivity, promotes glucose uptake, and potentiates the action of insulin by increasing insulin binding to cells, increasing the number of insulin receptors, and activating insulin receptor kinase. Trivalent chromium serves as the active component of a substance called *glucose tolerance factor* (GTF), along with nicotinic acid (a form of vitamin B_3) and amino acids in the form of a small oligopeptide known as *chromodulin*, or low-molecular-weight chromium-binding substance (LMWCr). Once activated by binding to chromium, chromodulin binds to insulin-activated insulin receptors in insulin-dependent cells and participates in auto-amplification of insulin signaling, thereby stimulating its tyrosine kinase activity and potentiating the activity of insulin. Chromium may also inhibit tyrosine phosphatase, which inactivates the insulin receptor. Such combined effects on insulin receptor kinase activity and tyrosine phosphatase would lead to increased phosphorylation of the insulin receptor and an associated increase in insulin sensitivity. Thus, through GTF, chromium acts as a cofactor to mediate the activity of insulin and facilitate glucose transport across cell membranes.

Chromium appears to possess hypocholesterolemic and antiatherogenic activities. Chromium can decrease levels of total cholesterol, low-density lipoprotein (LDL) cholesterol, and apolipoprotein B and may increase levels of high-density lipoprotein (HDL) cholesterol. The possible antiatherogenic activity of chromium is most likely derived from its glucose-regulatory activity. Chromium, like insulin, also increases uptake of amino acids into muscle, heart, and liver and enhances protein synthesis.

At this time, chromium remains the only essential transition metal whose mechanism of action has not been fully elucidated.

NUTRIENT IN CLINICAL PRACTICE
Known or Potential Therapeutic Uses

In 1957, researchers observed impaired glucose tolerance in chromium-deficient rats and discovered that administration of a chromium-containing compound extracted from pork kidney to diabetic rats maintained normal glucose tolerance and enabled more efficient use of insulin. They called this substance "glucose tolerance factor" (GTF). Later, other researchers reported an increased occurrence of glucose intolerance, weight loss, and peripheral neuropathy in patients receiving long-term total parenteral nutrition (TPN) without chromium. Intravenous administration of chromium chloride reversed these symptoms. Over the subsequent decades, chromium research has grown, with an emerging consensus confirming its therapeutic value in supporting insulin activity and glucose homeostasis. Wide-ranging and unresolved controversy surrounds its purported efficacy in weight loss, athletic training, dyslipidemia, depression, hyperactivity, and related conditions. Rigorous, blinded, and well-controlled studies of sufficient size and power are needed to assess fully the efficacy and mechanism of action of chromium administration and to establish clinical guidelines for its role within an integrative strategy for type 2 diabetes and impaired glucose tolerance.

Historical/Ethnomedicine Precedent

Based on familiarity with folk medicine traditions and empirical practice, naturopathic physicians and other practitioners of nutritional therapeutics have advocated the administration of brewer's yeast and foods rich in chromium for the prevention and treatment of hypoglycemia and diabetes for more than a century.

Possible Uses

Acne, atherosclerosis, athletic performance, atypical depression, depression, diabetes mellitus type 1, diabetes mellitus type 2, dysthymic disorder, gestational diabetes, glaucoma, hypercholesterolemia, hypertriglyceridemia, hypoglycemia, insulin resistance syndrome (metabolic syndrome/syndrome X), low HDL cholesterol, migraine, obesity, polycystic ovarian syndrome (PCOS), premenstrual syndrome (PMS), psoriasis, Turner's syndrome, weight loss.

Deficiency Symptoms

Suboptimal chromium intake is widespread, with as much as 90% of American diets low in chromium. Nevertheless, gross chromium deficiency is rare. Clinically, chromium deficiency was first characterized in three patients receiving long-term TPN lacking chromium. Compromised chromium status is most common in the elderly, individuals with diets high in simple carbohydrates and refined foods, pregnant women, and individuals experiencing extended periods of physiological stress, including those with chronic infections or those who regularly engage in strenuous exercise. Well-controlled studies have demonstrated chromium depletion in subjects with chromium intake level of 5 µg/1000 kcal. The primary sign of marginal chromium deficiency is impaired glucose tolerance, characterized by elevated levels of blood glucose and elevated circulating insulin concentration. Long-term deficiency results in elevated circulating cholesterol and triglyceride concentrations. Other observed effects include glycosuria, fasting hyperglycemia, hypoglycemia, decreased insulin binding, decreased insulin receptor number, impaired growth, central and peripheral neuropathy, and impaired humoral immune response. In many respects, chromium deficiency symptoms parallel those of diabetes. Low levels of chromium are also associated with increased risk of cardiovascular disease.

Dietary Sources

The amount of chromium in foods is variable because the actual chromium content in many foods can vary significantly in different batches of the same food. Brewer's yeast (particularly yeast grown in chromium-rich soil), lean meats (especially processed meats), oysters, liver and other organ meats, beer, and potatoes are relatively high in chromium. Seafood, whole grains, cheeses, chicken, bran, mushroom, oatmeal, prunes, nuts, broccoli, green beans, and asparagus are intermediate in chromium content. Most vegetables, fruit, refined grains, and processed foods (except for processed meats) contain low amounts of chromium. Notably, foods high in simple sugars, such as sucrose and fructose, not only are low in chromium content, but also are known to promote chromium loss.[1]

Note: Nutritional yeast and torula yeast do not contain significant amounts of chromium.

Nutrient Preparations Available

Several forms of trivalent chromium are available as stand-alone supplements or within combination nutrient formulations. Organic forms are preferable, including chromium aspartate, chromium histidine, chromium nicotinate, chromium picolinate, chromium polynicotinate; high-chromium yeast, and chromium-GTF. Chromium picolinate was considered the superior form for many years until chromium histidine was introduced by researchers from the U.S. Agricultural Research Service. Anderson et al.[2] found that men and women absorbed an average 3.1 µg of chromium from the chromium-histidine complex, compared with 1.8 µg from chromium picolinate, 0.4 µg from chromium chloride, and 0.2 µg from chromium polynicotinate. Typical maintenance doses of supplemental chromium range from 50 to 200 µg daily, expressed as elemental chromium. Chromium is best administered between meals, preferably in divided doses.

Dosage Forms Available

Capsule, tablet.

Source Materials for Nutrient Preparations

Trivalent chromium: Salt formed with picolinic acid, chloride, sulfate, nicotinic acid (niacin), or amino acid chelates, such as with histidine. Some forms of supplemental chromium are combined with GTF extracted from brewer's yeast.

Dosage Range

In recognition of the inadequacy of available data on chromium requirements the Food and Nutrition Board (FNB) of the U.S. Institute of Medicine proposed an adequate intake level (AI) based on the chromium content in normal diets rather than establish a recommended dietary allowance (RDA).

Adult

Dietary: Estimated average chromium intakes in the U.S. range from 23 to 29 µg per day for adult women and 39 to 54 µg per day for adult men.[3] The estimated safe and adequate daily dietary intake (ESADDI) for adults is 50 to 200 µg. Supplemental/Maintenance: 50 to 200 µg/day.

The AI for chromium in adult males is 30 to 35 µg per day and for females 20 to 25 µg per day (except while pregnant or lactating).
Pharmacological/Therapeutic: 200 to 3000 µg/day.

An individual's requirement for chromium parallels their degree of glucose intolerance.
Toxic: Some initial research indicated that doses as low as 300 µg per day were potentially toxic over extended periods. In the United States (U.S.), no tolerable upper level of intake (UL) has been set for chromium by the FNB. However, in the United Kingdom (U.K.) in 2004 the Food Standards Agency (FSA) established a maximum upper level of 10 mg (10,000 µg) elemental chromium from chromium picolinate per day.

Pediatric (< 18 Years)

Dietary: Breast-fed infants consume less than 1 µg/day.

Infants, 7 to 12 months: 5.5 µg/day (AI, adequate intake)
Children, 1 to 3 years: 11 µg/day (AI)
Children, 4 to 8 years: 15 µg/day (AI)

Supplemental/Maintenance: None established.
Pharmacologic/Therapeutic: 1 to 50 µg/day.
Toxic: None established.

Laboratory Values

No biomarker has established itself as the standard for assessing chromium status and distinguishing adequate or deficient chromium levels.

Serum chromium: Less than 2.0 nmol/L may indicate chromium deficiency, but this is a relatively insensitive indicator of tissue stores.
Whole-blood chromium: Normal range: 14 to 185 nmol/L.
Urinary chromium: Normal range: approximately 3 to 4 nmol/L; greater than 38 nmol/L indicates toxicity.

These tests have generally been considered to be of limited value in assessing status because of the extremely low concentrations of chromium present in biological tissues and fluids, and because these tests have only limited sensitivity in measuring response to chromium intake. Thus, they have primarily been used to measure overexposure to environmental chromium. Neutron activation analysis, mass spectrometry, and graphite furnace atomic absorption spectrometry represent the only analytical techniques with the required sensitivity to adequately provide clinically relevant measurements. However, these analytical methods are not widely available, are susceptible to interference from the sample matrix, and are too expensive to be clinically applicable. Additional investigation of urinary chromium in response to very low levels of intake has been suggested.

In a randomized, double-blind, crossover design involving 78 non-insulin-dependent diabetes mellitus patients, Bahijri and Mufti[4] (2002) found that both brewer's yeast and chromium chloride caused a significant increase in the mean values of urinary chromium (Cr) and a significant decrease in the means of glucose and fructosamine, concluding that "urinary Cr response to glucose load could be used as an indicator of Cr status."

SAFETY PROFILE

Overview

The limited safety data available suggest that chromium supplements are generally well tolerated at usual dosage levels. Both solubility and oxidation state affect the potential for toxicity. Furthermore, the type of complex may impact toxicity. There have been reports of toxic reactions to chromium picolinate at doses significantly higher than those typically used. No cause-effect relationship has been confirmed in human research. After several years of controversy regarding the potential toxicity of chromium, especially chromium picolinate, a consensus emerged in 2004 supporting the safety of chromium as a nutritional supplement.

Long-term daily intake of trivalent chromium (Cr^{+3}) and chromium in brewer's yeast in the range of 50 to 300 µg is generally considered safe. Supplementation with chromium picolinate at daily dosage levels of up to 1000 µg for as long as 64 months in adults has produced no adverse effects.[5-7] Even so, doses greater than 400 µg daily should generally not be taken for extended periods outside the context of care by a health care professional trained in nutritional therapies.

In contrast, chronic exposure to airborne or waterborne hexavalent chromium (Cr^{+6}), such as chromium dust in metalworking, printing, paint, textile, and other industrial settings, is associated with dermatitis and increased risk of lung and other cancers.

Nutrient Adverse Effects

General Adverse Effects

Self-administered chromium picolinate, at relatively high dosage levels, has been associated with adverse effects in a handful of case reports. Two case reports of renal failure, involving women consuming 600 and 1200 to 2400 µg chromium picolinate daily for 6 weeks and 5 months, respectively, have not been qualified to establish a causal link.[8,9] Toxic reactions to chromium picolinate have also been suspected in individual cases of interstitial nephritis, liver and kidney damage, thrombocytopenia, acute generalized exanthematous pustulosis, and rhabdomyolysis.[9-12] However, the dosage levels described in these unqualified reports are generally not recommended, especially outside the context of professional supervision.

Isolated in vitro evidence, mixed and still inconclusive, has suggested that chromium picolinate in high concentrations may be clastogenic. However, if proven, the picolinate component, rather than the chromium, might be the mutagenic factor because no reports have involved chromium chloride or chromium nicotinate. In vivo animal studies arrived at mixed conclusions. The significance of these results on humans taking the supplement for prolonged periods is unknown. In the U.K. the Committee on Mutagenicity commissioned by the FSA conducted a thorough genotoxicity review and, based on their recommendation, concluded that available evidence supported the safety of chromium at doses up to 10 mg per day. Nevertheless, judicious practice suggests that long-term intake of chromium picolinate, particularly at doses higher than 400 μg daily, are best undertaken under supervision of a health care professional trained and experienced in nutritional therapeutics. Continued study and postmarket surveillance is warranted.

Adverse Effects Among Specific Populations

The risk of chromium toxicity could theoretically be greater in individuals with preexisting liver or kidney disease.[3]

Pregnancy and Nursing

The maximum safe dosage levels of chromium for women who are pregnant or nursing have not been established. However, in a study involving 10 women administered 400 μg chromium picolinate daily, Kato et al.[13] found no evidence of increased oxidative damage to DNA, as measured by antibody titers to an oxidized DNA base of 5-hydroxymethyl uracil.

Chromium appears to be safe when used to improve glycemic control in gestational diabetes.[14] Furthermore, chromium appears safe in lactation when used orally; supplements do not appear to increase normal chromium concentration in human breast milk.[15]

Infants and Children

The maximum safe dosage levels of chromium for infants and children have not been established.

Contraindications

Chromium is contraindicated in those hypersensitive to any component of a chromium-containing formulation. Sensitivity to yeast warrants avoidance of yeast-derived or yeast-containing forms of chromium.

Precautions and Warnings

Pregnant women and nursing mothers should avoid doses of chromium greater than 50 μg per day.

Caution and professional supervision may be appropriate when introducing chromium to individuals with a history of hypoglycemia. Conversely, those with a history of hyperglycemia or type 2 diabetes mellitus who are taking prescription medications for blood sugar control should only initiate, use, or significantly change dosage levels of chromium supplements within the context of professional supervision and close monitoring.

Concern has been expressed that chromium picolinate might be contraindicated for individuals with depression, bipolar disease, or schizophrenia because picolinate can alter levels of neurotransmitters and chromium picolinate may decrease the sensitivity of 5-HT(2A) receptors by increasing the peripheral availability of tryptophan for brain serotonin (5-HT) synthesis.[16,17]

INTERACTIONS REVIEW

Strategic Considerations

For decades, chromium has played a central role in the prevention and treatment of hypoglycemia, insulin resistance, glucose intolerance, and diabetes mellitus within the clinical practice of nutritional therapeutics and natural medicine. Chromium is rarely, if ever, relied on as a monotherapy, or even a dominant intervention, within such a context. Exercise and lifestyle modification, balanced diet emphasizing low glycemic index/load foods, moderately high protein intake, and healthy fats and oils, along with individualized programs of nutrients and herbs, constitute the components of a more typical strategy.

Although often used in the treatment of dysglycemia in general, and hypoglycemic tendencies and insulin resistance in particular, chromium can also help prevent diabetes in susceptible individuals and play an adjunctive role in the treatment of diabetes. The dietary chromium intake of most individuals in the U.S. does not meet the level of 50 to 200 μg per day recommended by the U.S. National Academy of Science. Many clinicians and researchers have noted the parallels between suboptimal chromium levels, high intake of simple carbohydrates and sugars, and the escalating rates of insulin resistance and obesity, diabetes, and heart disease. An emerging pattern of evidence, but as yet not consistent, comprehensive, or conclusive, indicates that chromium may also improve lipid status by increasing HDL cholesterol and lowering total cholesterol. Furthermore, individuals with diabetes often have additional chromium depletion as a result of the disease process itself. Collectively, these findings suggest strongly that chromium may play a significant role in the prevention of heart disease through a variety of interconnected influences. Notably, chromium supplementation may also be of benefit in the treatment of individuals with Turner's syndrome through its effect on glucose tolerance. Preliminary research suggesting that chromium can reduce body fat, induce weight loss, and enhance lean muscle gain is intriguing and consistent with known activity, but has yet to be supported by a consistent and substantive body of evidence based on clinical trials of adequate size, strength, and design. At this point, the consistent theme in chromium research is that its therapeutic effect is greatest in individuals with diets low in chromium.

Chromium administration at typical dosage levels is generally unlikely to result in adverse effects or interactions with conventional medications. The available evidence regarding chromium interactions indicates that the use of supplemental chromium within the context of an integrative care model is likely to be safe and may provide added therapeutic benefits with reasonable administration and standard monitoring. In particular, concomitant use of chromium by diabetic patients introduces a high probability of enhanced insulin activity in response to the influence of the nutrient, especially in the context of suboptimal chromium intake and a diet high in refined carbohydrate foods, which contributes to both inadequate intake and increased urinary excretion. Thus, extra monitoring through stabilization may be required with chromium coadministration in patients being treated with conventional antidiabetic medications, such as insulin or oral hypoglycemic agents, because dosage requirements may be reduced as sensitivity of the insulin receptors to insulin increase.

Further research in all these areas is warranted. The findings likely to emerge over the coming decade will undoubtedly assist in clarifying knowledge, understanding, and effective clinical application of chromium in supporting healthy glucose regulation, preventing dysfunction of insulin and lipid metabolism, and treating resultant pathology.

NUTRIENT-DRUG INTERACTIONS

Beta-1-Adrenoceptor Antagonists (Beta-1-Adrenergic Blocking Agents)

Oral forms (Systemic): Acebutolol (Sectral), atenolol (Tenormin); combination drugs: atenolol and chlorthalidone (Co-Tendione, Tenoretic); atenolol and nifedipine (Beta-Adalat, Tenif); betaxolol (Kerlone), bisoprolol (Zebeta), carteolol (Cartrol), esmolol (Brevibloc), labetalol (Normodyne, Trandate), metoprolol (Lopressor, Toprol XL); combination drug: metoprolol and hydrochlorothiazide (Lopressor HCT); nadolol (Corgard), nebivolol (Nebilet), oxprenolol (Trasicor), penbutolol (Levatol), pindolol (Visken), propranolol (Betachron, Inderal LA, Innopran XL, Inderal); combination drug: propranolol and bendrofluazide (Inderex); sotalol (Betapace, Betapace AF, Sorine), timolol (Blocadren).

Interaction Type and Significance
⊕⊕   **Beneficial or Supportive Interaction, with Professional Management**

Probability: Evidence Base:
2. Probable   ○ Preliminary to
                                  ◉ Emerging

Effect and Mechanism of Action
Chromium supplementation may improve levels of HDL cholesterol through a mechanism that has not yet been fully elucidated.

Research
In a randomized, double-blind, placebo-controlled trial involving 63 men receiving beta-blocker therapy, primarily for hypertension, Roeback et al.[18] observed modest increases in HDL cholesterol levels after administration of 200 µg three times daily of "biologically active chromium" in the form of "glucose tolerance factor (GTF)–chromium" for 8 weeks.

Nutritional Therapeutics, Clinical Concerns, and Adaptations
Physicians prescribing beta blockers to individuals with hypertension can discuss with patients the potential benefits of adding chromium (e.g., 200 µg three times daily) to a comprehensive regimen for improving HDL cholesterol status as well as stabilizing glucose levels and generally reducing cardiovascular risk. Although not conclusive, these preliminary findings are promising in suggesting a potential role for chromium within an integrative strategy aimed at addressing the intertwining issues of dysglycemia, insulin resistance, hypertension, and cardiovascular risk. Furthermore, caution is appropriate in not summarily extrapolating from these findings based on men to presumed applicability to women. Further research through well-designed, long-term clinical trials is warranted to investigate the implications of this potential synergy and guide formulation of therapeutic options.

Corticosteroids, Oral

Betamethasone (Celestone), cortisone (Cortone), dexamethasone (Decadron), fludrocortisone (Florinef), hydrocortisone (Cortef), methylprednisolone (Medrol) prednisolone (Delta-Cortef, Orapred, Pediapred, Prelone), prednisone (Deltasone, Liquid Pred, Meticorten, Orasone), triamcinolone (Aristocort).

Interaction Type and Significance
≈≈   **Drug-Induced Nutrient Depletion, Supplementation Therapeutic, with Professional Management**
☼   **Prevention or Reduction of Drug Adverse Effect**

Probability: Evidence Base:
4. Plausible   ○ Preliminary

Effect and Mechanism of Action
Corticosteroid therapy increases chromium excretion; this effect may play a role in the development of corticosteroid-induced glucose intolerance and diabetes. Chromium coadministration may reverse steroid-induced diabetes.

Research
Ravina et al.[19] measured the effects of corticosteroid treatment on chromium losses in 13 patients 2 days before steroid administration and 3 days after treatment. They observed that urinary chromium losses after corticosteroid treatment increased significantly in the first 3 days following treatment. These researchers also reported that administration of 600 µg/day of chromium (as chromium picolinate) to three patients with steroid-induced diabetes "resulted in decreases in fasting blood glucose values from greater than 13.9 mmol/L (250 mg/dL) to less than 8.3 mmol/L (150 mg/dL)." Notably, hypoglycemic drugs were also "reduced 50% in all patients when given supplemental chromium."[19]

Nutritional Therapeutics, Clinical Concerns, and Adaptations
Physicians prescribing oral corticosteroids, especially for extended periods and at high dosage levels, are advised to coadminister chromium, 200 µg three times daily, to counter drug-induced chromium excretion, support glucose control and insulin sensitivity, and prevent corticosteroid-induced diabetes. Patients being treated with hypoglycemic agents will require supervision and monitoring because gradual decreases in medication levels will often be appropriate in response to the effects of chromium administration. Further research through well-designed, long-term clinical trials is warranted to investigate the implications of this potential synergy and guide formulation of therapeutic options.

Insulin, Glyburide, Metformin, and Related Oral Hypoglycemic Agents

Insulin: Animal-source insulin (Iletin); human analog insulin (Humanlog); human insulin (Humulin, Novolin, NovoRapid, Oralin).
Biguanides: Buformin (Andromaco Gliporal, Buformina), metformin (Dianben, Glucophage, Glucophage XR), phenformin (Debeone, Fenformin).
Sulfonylureas: Acetohexamide (Dymelor), chlorpropamide (Diabinese), glimepiride (Amaryl), glyburide (Diabeta, Glibenclamide, Glynase Prestab, Glynase, Micronase, Pres Tab), glipizide (Glucotrol; Glucotrol XL), tolazamide (Tolinase), tolbutamide (Orinase; Tol-Tab).
Combination drugs: Glipizide and metformin (Metaglip); glyburide and metformin (Glucovance).
Extrapolated, based on similar properties: **Alpha-glucosidase inhibitors:** Acarbose (Glucobay, Precose).

Meglitinide Analog Oral Hypoglycemics: Nateglinide (Starlix), repaglinide (Prandin).
Thiazolidinediones (glitazones): Pioglitazone (Actos), rosiglitazone (Avandia).

Interaction Type and Significance

⊕⊕ **Beneficial or Supportive Interaction, with Professional Management**
⊕✗ **Bimodal or Variable Interaction, with Professional Management**
✗ **Potential or Theoretical Adverse Interaction of Uncertain Severity**

Probability: Evidence Base:
2. Probable   ◉ Emerging

Effect and Mechanism of Action

In vitro, in vivo, and human studies indicate that chromium participates in glucose and lipid metabolism, influences circulating insulin levels, and potentiates the peripheral activity of insulin.[20-23] Chromium has been observed to improve insulin binding, insulin receptor number, insulin internalization, beta-cell sensitivity, and insulin receptor–related enzymes, with overall increases in insulin sensitivity. The proposed mechanism of action for chromium's effect is, at least in part, caused by enhanced intracellular tyrosine kinase activity that results from an interaction between chromium, chromodulin, and activated cell-surface insulin receptors.[24] Other research suggests that the potential in vivo mechanism of chromium (picolinate) on insulin action in human skeletal muscle may occur by increasing the activation of Akt phosphorylation.[25] This intracellular insulin-dependent protein facilitates the uptake of glucose into cells. Furthermore, by downregulating pancreatic islet beta-cell activity, chromium may increase glucagon secretion.[26] Nevertheless, at this time, knowledge of the biochemical basis underlying these reported and hypothesized effects remains conflicting and evolving.

Exogenous insulin therapy is designed to augment or replace endogenous insulin in individuals lacking sufficient synthesis capacity in the islets of Langerhans of the pancreas. Oral sulfonylureas (e.g., glyburide) act by stimulating the production and release of insulin (not sensitivity, or at least not primarily), and as such, these agents can only be used in patients with an intact pancreas with functioning islet cells. There are probably other activities of the oral drugs, but at one level, both insulin and oral hypoglycemic agents simply increase the amount of available insulin, one exogenously and the other endogenously. In most type 1 diabetic patients the islet cells have undergone autoimmune destruction, so the sulfonylurea-based agents are not useful. To the degree that type 1 diabetic individuals have chromium insufficiency and decreased insulin receptor sensitivity, increased dietary chromium may have benefit, but virtually all will require some exogenous insulin therapy.

Research

Numerous clinical trials, some well-designed, others less so, have demonstrated the ability of chromium to potentiate insulin and improve glucose control, especially in diabetic patients and individuals with less-than-optimal chromium intake. The nutritional biochemistry, physiological function, and therapeutic applications of chromium are gradually becoming elucidated. Consequently, studies on the effectiveness of chromium administration in patients with glucose intolerance and type 2 diabetes have produced findings that are inconsistent and evolving. These conflicting results are caused by many factors, including characteristics of subject population, concomitant medications and dietary influences, dose and form of chromium used, and duration of therapy.

Numerous studies have shown an association between chromium deficiency and impaired glucose regulation, onset of type 2 diabetes in susceptible individuals, and increased risk for lipid disorders and cardiovascular diseases.[27-34] The pathophysiology of diabetes itself may exacerbate chromium deficiency. For example, urinary loss of chromium is elevated in individuals with type 2 diabetes resulting, at least in part, from glycosuria. Thus, plasma chromium levels are about 40% lower in diabetic subjects compared with healthy individuals. In a symposium at the 59th annual scientific sessions of the American Diabetes Association (1999), Cefalu described an improvement in insulin sensitivity in obese people with prediabetic symptoms who received chromium picolinate. Conversely, excess chromium intake may result in tissue accumulation and subsequently could, at least theoretically, inhibit rather than enhance insulin activity. Findings from a rat study suggest that a chromium-induced increased in hepatic insulin clearance may offset the improvement in insulin sensitivity in some diabetic individuals, such that glycemic control might not improve appreciably.[35] Adequate and balanced chromium nutriture is clearly essential for normal insulin activity and glucose control. However, given the lack of human studies suggesting such effects of excess supplemental chromium intake and the low oral absorption of chromium compounds, it may be quite difficult to induce chromium excess with oral supplementation, especially in diabetic patients, with their tendency toward increased chromium excretion. These considerations are further supported by the safe upper limit of 10 mg daily established by the U.K. regulatory authorities.

Administration of chromium picolinate may help prevent or delay the need for antidiabetic medication and can often be used synergistically with such medications once they have been prescribed. The most relevant data indicate that chromium picolinate improves clinical results when used in combination with standard treatments, including insulin, sulfonylureas, or metformin alone and in combinations. Improvements have been observed in glucose tolerance tests in adult diabetic patients[36,37] and in glucose-intolerant men and women.[38-40] Uusitupa et al.[41] reported that administration of chromium produced a beneficial effect on insulin response at 1 hour but no improvement in glucose tolerance tests in non-insulin-requiring diabetics. However, researchers in three trials found no significant benefit of chromium with glucose tolerance, insulin levels, or blood lipid concentrations.[42-44]

Notably, in two of these studies, one used chromium chloride, which is poorly absorbed, and the other a low dose (200 µg/day) of chromium picolinate.

In a clinical trial involving 243 individuals with type 1 (105) and type 2 (138) diabetes, Ravina and Slezack[45] found that chromium supplementation (200 µg/day) decreased insulin, sulfonylurea drug, and metformin requirements in a significant number (115) of subjects. "The success rate was greater in those with NIDDM (57.2%) than in those with IDDM (33.6%). More women, of either type, reacted than men (62.5 vs. 50% in NIDDM and 37.6 vs. 28.6% in IDDM)." This trial exhibited major limitations; although frequently described as a controlled clinical trial, this study was largely open label in design with only 10 subjects enrolled in a double-blind protocol. In a subsequent placebo-controlled trial involving 48 patients with type 1 diabetes and 114 patients with type 2 diabetes, Ravina et al.[46] compared diets supplemented with chromium picolinate (200 μg/day) with placebo. They reported a reduced need for insulin or oral hypoglycemic medications in approximately 70% of patients coadministered chromium. Again, it is notable that trials using 1000 μg (1 mg) of chromium picolinate per day in diabetic patients show a strong positive trend.

Anderson et al.[6] conducted a promising but controversial randomized, placebo-controlled trial involving 180 Chinese men and women with type 2 diabetes, comparing the effects of 1000 μg chromium, 200 μg chromium, and placebo. The therapeutic response appeared to be dose related. The group receiving 1000 μg demonstrated significant improvements in lipids and hemoglobin A_{1c} (HbA$_{1c}$) values after 2 months; both groups receiving chromium showed such changes after 4 months. Fasting glucose was also lower in the higher dose (1000 μg) chromium group at 2 and 4 months, although no such change observed in the moderate (200 μg) chromium group. Serum insulin levels decreased significantly in both groups at 2 and 4 months.[6] The high dose used might be considered a strength of this trial because it is closer to the dosage levels found to be effective in clinical practice using monotherapy chromium in pharmacological doses. However, the characteristics of the Chinese patient population in this study may limit the applicability of its findings to patient populations in Europe and North America. Furthermore, the large number of subjects in this study has excluded it from some meta-analyses because it would overwhelm data from other, smaller trials.[47]

In a 4-month trial, Bahadori[48] and a team of Austrian researchers studied the effects of chromium picolinate (500 μg twice daily) in 16 obese patients with type 2 diabetes who were pretreated with, and continued to receive stable doses of, a sulfonylurea and metformin. These researchers reported that chromium picolinate appeared to enhance the effects of metformin and oral sulfonylureas. Chromium coadministration was associated with significant reductions in fasting insulin levels, without a detrimental effect on glucose control. Insulin resistance assessed by the insulin suppression test was not affected. They concluded that the positive effects seen in this clinical study could be associated with an effect of chromium picolinate on insulin clearance.

In a double-blind crossover trial involving 78 type 2 diabetic patients, Bahajri et al.[33] investigated the effects of brewer's yeast (23.3 μg Cr daily) and chromium chloride (200 μg Cr daily) sequentially with placebo in between, through four stages, each lasting 8 weeks. They found that both forms of chromium caused a significant decrease in the mean values of glucose (fasting and 2-hour post–glucose load), fructosamine, and triglycerides. The means of HDL cholesterol and serum and urinary chromium were all increased. Furthermore, the mean drug dosage decreased slightly (and significantly in an individual taking glibenclamide) after both supplements; some patients no longer required insulin. These researchers also noted that a higher percentage of subjects responded positively to brewer's yeast chromium.

In 2003, at the 18th International Diabetes Federation Congress, Cefalu et al.[25] presented the findings from a subsequently published double-blind, placebo-controlled trial involving two cohorts of patients with type 2 diabetes who were treated with either sulfonylureas or a diet program and randomized to receive either chromium picolinate (1000 μg/day) or placebo. Hyperinsulinemic, euglycemic clamp studies were used to measure insulin sensitivity and assess the efficacy of glucose uptake on all subjects before randomization and at the end of the study. Of the 16 subjects, those administered chromium picolinate demonstrated a mean increase in insulin

sensitivity of 8.9%, whereas those receiving placebo had a mean decrease of 3.6%. In addition, insulin-stimulated Akt activation was significantly increased at the end of the study compared with subjects on placebo. The authors stated that the enhanced activity of Akt phosphorylation associated with chromium administration in individuals with type 2 diabetes represents a possible mechanism to explain chromium picolinate's beneficial effect on insulin sensitivity.[25]

Rabinovitz et al.[49] conducted a controlled clinical trial involving 39 diabetic subjects, average age 73 years (18 males and 21 females), undergoing rehabilitation after stroke or hip fracture, who received 200 μg chromium twice a day for a 3-week period. Both the treated group and a control group of 39 diabetic patients continued their standard treatment for diabetes and received a diet of approximately 1500 kcal/day. At the end of the study, these researchers measured significant differences in the fasting blood level of glucose compared to the baseline (190 vs. 150 mg/dL, $p < 0.001$), improvements in HbA$_{1c}$ from 8.2% to 7.6% ($p < 0.01$), and reductions in total cholesterol from 235 to 213 mg/dL ($p < 0.02$). They also observed a trend toward lowered triglyceride levels. They concluded that, "in this population of elderly, diabetic patients undergoing rehabilitation, dietary supplementation with chromium is beneficial in moderating glucose intolerance."[49]

An overview of the most relevant literature shows that nine single-blind and double-blind trials over 10 years, involving 1349 total subjects, produced findings that are consistent. These studies concentrated on the effects of chromium picolinate on markers of blood glucose or on insulin regulation in subjects with type 2 diabetes or in individuals with induced diabetes. Overall, they found that chromium picolinate exerts a beneficial effect on fasting insulin values and on HbA$_{1c}$.[6,19,46,48,50-55] Cefalu et al.[52] and Morris et al.[56] have suggested that chromium picolinate increases insulin sensitivity and glucose utilization and maintains normal blood glucose concentrations. Many human studies have also reported that administration of chromium is associated with improvements in lipids, particularly triglycerides, LDL and HDL cholesterol,[57,58] and lipoprotein(a), as well as other benefits for coronary disease risk profiles that are important in both diabetic and nondiabetic populations. Nevertheless, in reviewing much of the same literature in a 2002 meta-analysis, Althuis et al.[47] concluded that "data from randomized clinical trials are sparse and inconclusive." Ultimately, everyone in the field agrees that further research emphasizing placebo-controlled, randomized clinical trials in well-characterized, at-risk populations is necessary to determine the effects of chromium, given in the more absorbable forms and in adequate amounts, on concentrations of glucose, insulin, and HbA$_{1c}$.

The controversy surrounding the efficacy of chromium in diverse populations continues; research has yet to deliver a consistent pattern of findings that might provide an evidence-based foundation for consensus. For example, two papers published in 2006 presented seemingly conflicting results with divergent implications. Following on the research previously mentioned, Martin, Cefalu, et al.[58a] conducted a trial involving 37 subjects with type 2 diabetes in which they first placed subjects, after baseline, on a sulfonylurea (glipizide, 5 mg/day) with placebo for 3 months. They then randomized subjects, in a double-blind fashion, to receive either the glipizide plus continued placebo or the glipizide plus 1000 μg chromium picolinate (CrPic) for 6 months. At the end of the trial period, they found that subjects administered glipizide and placebo, as opposed to those randomized to glipizide and chromium, exhibited a "significant increase" in body weight (2.2 kg), percent body fat (1.17%), and total abdominal fat (32.5 cm^2) from baseline. Conversely, those subjects receiving glipizide and chromium exhibited "significant improvements in insulin sensitivity corrected for fat-free mass" (28.8), HbA$_{1c}$ (glycosylated hemoglobin) (−1.16%), and free fatty acids (−0.2 mmol/L) "as opposed to sulfonylurea/placebo." The authors concluded that "this study demonstrates that CrPic supplementation in subjects with type 2 diabetes who are taking sulfonylurea agents significantly improves insulin sensitivity and glucose control," and that coadministration of chromium "significantly attenuated body weight gain and visceral fat accumulation compared with the placebo group." In contrast, in a 6-month, double-blind trial involving 53 subjects (46 of whom completed the study), Kleefstra et al.[59] found that, contrary to expectations, "high-dose chromium picolinate" (500 or 1000 μg) does not improve glycemic control or other parameters in "obese patients with poorly controlled, insulin-treated type 2 diabetes." The study participants had an HbA$_{1c}$ greater than 8% and insulin requirements of greater than 50 units per day. The investigators reported that among the three groups, receiving placebo or 500 or 1000 g chromium picolinate daily, the decrease in HbA$_{1c}$, the primary efficacy measure, was similar (−0.3%, −0.5%, and −0.3% for placebo, 500 μg, and 1000 μg, respectively). Secondary endpoints included changes in lipid profiles, body mass index (BMI), blood pressure, and insulin requirements. Likewise, no differences were observed in BMI, blood pressure, and insulin requirements; notably, however, a weak association was found between an increasing serum chromium concentration and improvement in the lipid profile. In light of the contrast between these results and earlier findings, the authors added: "Whether it is possible to select subgroups of patients with suitable certain phenotypes that may or may not benefit from chromium therapy also needs further attention."[59]

Nutritional Therapeutics, Clinical Concerns, and Adaptations

The ongoing epidemic of dysglycemia, insulin resistance, and diabetes, severe problems contributing to lipid disorders and cardiovascular morbidity, forcefully establishes the need to develop an integrative understanding of the therapeutic role of chromium. General agreement exists that chromium intake is inadequate for much of the population, and that compromised chromium nutriture status is common, even (or even more so) in developed countries with processed food–based diets. The body of literature suggests that individuals with diabetes may benefit from chromium administration in many ways, including more stable insulin levels and enhanced glucose control. Although inclusion of chromium in a comprehensive therapeutic strategy may contribute to these and many other potential benefits, the appropriate dosage levels and character of effects may vary among individuals and even change over time for a given patient. Furthermore, because the current data imply that some individuals respond better to chromium picolinate than do others (nonresponders), further research is needed to establish accurate and sensitive laboratory methods to identify the most suitable candidates for treatment with chromium picolinate or other well-absorbed forms, such as GTF or the histidine chelate. To date, the picolinate has been the best studied of the apparently efficacious forms of chromium.

Chromium's ability to enhance endogenous regulation of blood glucose levels, together with its potentiation of insulin's activity, make it a valuable option in stabilizing diabetic

physiology, potentially preventing diabetic complications, and eventually reducing dependence on medication. Health care professionals treating individuals with diabetes using conventional medications, natural therapies (e.g., acupuncture, herbs, other nutrients), and lifestyle changes (e.g., diet, exercise) will need to monitor such patients closely if chromium is introduced into the regimen. Thus, patients should be cautioned regarding the potential risks of inadvertent or unsupervised chromium administration in conjunction with conventional treatments, especially pharmaceutical treatments capable of inducing hypoglycemia. In particular, the prescribed dose of insulin or oral hypoglycemic medication may need to be reduced gradually to avoid a hypoglycemic reaction as the patient responds to the actions of chromium. Health care professionals trained and experienced in nutritional therapy typically prescribe chromium at a dosage of 200 μg, once or twice daily; higher dosage may be appropriate based on body surface area or failure to respond to lower doses. Chromium picolinate and chromium histidine are preferred forms.

Sertraline and Related Selective Serotonin Reuptake Inhibitor (SSRI) Antidepressants

Evidence: Sertraline (Zoloft).
Extrapolated, based on similar properties: Citalopram (Celexa), escitalopram (S-citalopram; Lexapro), fluoxetine (Prozac, Sarafem), fluvoxamine (Faurin, Luvox), paroxetine (Aropax, Deroxat, Paxil, Seroxat).

Interaction Type and Significance:

⊕⊕ **Beneficial or Supportive Interaction, with Professional Management**

Probability:	Evidence Base:
4. Plausible to	○ **Preliminary** to
2. Probable	◉ **Emerging**

Effect and Mechanism of Action

Dysglycemia can play an important role in the susceptibility of many individuals to depressive disorders. Chromium may have antidepressant activities in some individuals, at least in part by potentiating the action of insulin. Insulin, in turn, inhibits the reuptake of norepinephrine and enhances the blood-brain transport of tryptophan, a precursor of serotonin. Furthermore, picolinic acid (a component of chromium picolinate) can alter serotonin, dopamine, and norepinephrine metabolism in the central nervous system (CNS).[17]

Research

Following a patient's report of "dramatic response to the addition of chromium supplementation to sertraline pharmacotherapy" for dysthymic disorder, McLeod et al.[60] conducted a set of single-blind and open-label trials in which they substituted other nutritional supplements in each of the patients to test the specificity of response to chromium supplementation. They described significant improvements in mood and "remission of dysthymic symptoms" in five patients being treated for antidepressant-refractory dysthymic disorder with sertraline who were coadministered chromium picolinate or chromium polynicotinate at dosage levels of 200 to 400 μg per day. The authors suggested further study through controlled trials; such research appears warranted.

In more recent research, Attenburrow et al.[17] examined the relationship of chromium to serotonin, particularly chromium picolinate's apparent effect of increasing the peripheral availability of tryptophan for brain serotonin (5-hydroxytryptamine,

5-HT) synthesis and altering the sensitivity of central 5-HT(2A) receptors. They compared the effects of short-term chromium administration on plasma concentrations of tryptophan and other large, neutral amino acids in human and animal models and assessed brain serotonin function by measuring the corticosterone/cortisol response to 5-hydroxytryptophan (5-HTP), the 5-HT precursor, which is hypothesized to be mediated via indirect activation of 5-HT(2A) receptors. These researchers observed that administration of chromium lowered the cortisol response to challenge with 5-HTP in both rats and humans. Changes in peripheral tryptophan availability were not seen in humans, but chromium increased peripheral and central tryptophan availability and elevated brain 5-HT content in rats.

Clinical Implications and Adaptations

Physicians prescribing SSRI medications for treatment of individuals diagnosed with depressive disorders are advised to evaluate potential therapeutic benefit on serotonin levels with concomitant administration of chromium, 200 µg once or twice daily. Integrative therapy combining chromium and antidepressants could prove efficacious, especially in patients with a history of hypoglycemia/dysglycemia, insulin resistance, or diabetes. Close monitoring and periodic reevaluation are necessary because gradual decreases in medication levels may be appropriate. Further research through well-designed, long-term clinical trials is warranted to investigate the implications of this potential synergy and guide formulation of therapeutic options.

THEORETICAL, SPECULATIVE, AND PRELIMINARY INTERACTIONS RESEARCH, INCLUDING OVERSTATED INTERACTIONS CLAIMS

Antacids, Histamine (H₂) Receptor Antagonists, and Proton Pump Inhibitors

Antacids: Aluminum carbonate gel (Basajel), aluminum hydroxide (Alternagel, Amphojel); combination drugs: aluminum hydroxide, magnesium carbonate, alginic acid, and sodium bicarbonate (Gaviscon Extra Strength Tablets, Gaviscon Regular Strength Liquid, Gaviscon Extra Strength Liquid); aluminum hydroxide and magnesium hydroxide (Advanced Formula Di-Gel Tablets, co-magaldrox, Di-Gel, Gelusil, Maalox, Maalox Plus, Mylanta, Wingel); aluminum hydroxide, magnesium trisilicate, alginic acid, and sodium bicarbonate (Alenic Alka, Gaviscon Regular Strength Tablets); calcium carbonate (Titralac, Tums), magnesium hydroxide (Phillips' Milk of Magnesia MOM); combination drugs: magnesium hydroxide and calcium carbonate (Calcium Rich Rolaids); magnesium hydroxide, aluminum hydroxide, calcium carbonate, and simethicone (Tempo Tablets); magnesium trisilicate and aluminum hydroxide (Adcomag trisil, Foamicon); magnesium trisilicate, alginic acid, and sodium bicarbonate (Alenic Alka, Gaviscon Regular Strength Tablets); combination drug: sodium bicarbonate, aspirin, and citric acid (Alka-Seltzer).

Histamine (H₂) receptor antagonists: Cimetidine (Tagamet; Tagamet HB), famotidine (Pepcid RPD, Pepcid, Pepcid AC), nizatidine (Axid, Axid AR), ranitidine (Zantac); combination drug: ranitidine, bismuth, and citrate (Tritec).

Proton pump inhibitors:
Evidence: Omeprazole (Losec, Prilosec).
Related: Esomeprazole (Nexium), lansoprazole (Prevacid, Zoton), pantoprazole (Protium, Protonix, Somac), rabeprazole (AcipHex, Pariet).

Antacids, H₂ blockers, and proton pump inhibitors (PPIs) may inhibit chromium absorption and could contribute to chromium depletion, particularly in susceptible populations. The mechanism(s) underlying this apparent interaction include altered pH levels, formation of insoluble complexes, or some combination but remain unclear.

Concomitant intake of calcium carbonate can interfere with the absorption of chromium. Seaborn and Stocker[61] used an isotope of chromium in male rats to measure potential interaction between calcium and chromium. Their findings indicate that calcium carbonate may result in reduced absorption and tissue retention of chromium. Notably, this experiment employed chromium chloride, known for poor absorption compared to other forms. Subsequently, a related research team using female rats observed that administration of antacid (40 mg) by gastric intubation (0.5 mL), followed orally by 55 µg Cr 51 chromium chloride, resulted in decreased chromium absorption.[20]

Evidence is lacking to substantiate extension of these preliminary findings to humans. However, chromium status is marginal in a large segment of the population, increasing the probability of this possible interaction being clinically relevant in some individuals. Thus it is advisable to recommend that oral intake of chromium be separated from administration of any antacid (including calcium carbonate) by 2 to 3 hours to reduce the risk of interfering with absorption. Further research is warranted through well-designed clinical trials of sufficient size and power.

Antipsychotics

Aripiprazole (Abilify, Abilitat), chlorpromazine (Largactil, Thorazine), clozapine (Clozaril), fluphenazine (Permitil, Prolixin, Prolixin Decanoate, Prolixin Enanthate), haloperidol (Haldol), olanzapine (Zyprexa), prochlorperazine (Compazine, Stemetil), quetiapine (Seroquel), risperidone (Risperdal), ziprasidone (Geodon).

An interaction between chromium and antipsychotic medications is theoretically plausible, but no substantive evidence from case reports or clinical trials has emerged to confirm (or refute) this occurrence or articulate its clinical implications. Directly, and through its effects on insulin, chromium influences several neurotransmitters. Notably, insulin inhibits the reuptake of norepinephrine and enhances the blood-brain transport of tryptophan, a precursor of serotonin. Furthermore, picolinic acid, a component of chromium picolinate, is known to alter serotonin, dopamine, and norepinephrine metabolism in the CNS. Prudence suggests that, pending further research, the concomitant use of chromium preparations and antipsychotic medications should be avoided outside the context of supervision of health care professionals trained and experienced in both conventional psychopharmacology and nutritional therapeutics.

Lithium Carbonate

Lithium carbonate (Camcolit, Carbolith, Duralith, Eskalith, Li-Liquid, Liskonum, Litarex, Lithane, Lithobid, Lithonate, Lithotabs, PMS-Lithium, Priadel).

Lithium carbonate has been found to reduce blood glucose levels in diabetic individuals. Chromium potentiates the action of insulin. The combined effect of two substances with potential hypoglycemic action might present a significant risk for excessively low blood glucose levels.[62]

Chromium's ability to enhance endogenous regulation of blood glucose levels, together with its potentiation of insulin, make it a valuable tool in stabilizing diabetic physiology and eventually reducing dependence on insulin. Physicians prescribing lithium are advised to ask patients if they are taking or have been considering use of chromium supplementation. Such coadministration might be efficacious but requires close monitoring of blood glucose levels, especially in individuals with a history of hypoglycemia or in the presence of insulin/oral sulfonylurea therapy. Health care professionals experienced in nutritional therapeutics typically prescribe chromium at a dosage of 200 μg once or twice daily; chromium picolinate or histidine is the preferred form.

Meperidine

Meperidine (Demerol).

Tyramine intake may result in adverse effects in individuals taking meperidine (which has a lethal interaction with classic MAO inhibitor antidepressants). Brewer's yeast contains a significant amount of tyramine and thus should be considered a potentially harmful or serious adverse interaction.

It is highly improbable that the amount of tyramine contained in yeast-based chromium preparations is adequate to result in an adverse event, particularly at usual dosage levels. Nevertheless, physicians prescribing meperidine should advise patients to avoid significant intake of yeast, including chromium supplements containing yeast. Forms of chromium not derived from or containing yeast do not carry this potential risk.

Monoamine Oxidase (MAO) Inhibitors

MAO-A inhibitors: Isocarboxazid (Marplan), moclobemide (Aurorix, Manerix), phenelzine (Nardil), procarbazine (Matulane), tranylcypromine (Parnate).
MAO-B inhibitors: Selegiline (deprenyl, L-deprenil, L-deprenyl; Ataptyl, Carbex, Eldepryl, Jumex, Movergan, Selpak), pargyline (Eutonyl), rasagiline (Azilect).

Tyramine intake will often result in adverse effects in individuals taking MAO inhibitors. Brewer's yeast contains a significant amount of tyramine and thus should be considered as potentially harmful or serious adverse interaction.

It is highly improbable that the amount of tyramine contained in yeast-based chromium preparations is adequate to result in an adverse event, particularly at usual dosage levels. In a 1984 survey and critical review of the literature on the subject of diet and MAO inhibitors, Sullivan and Shulman[63] determined that "only four foods clearly warrant absolute prohibition: aged cheese, pickled fish (herring), concentrated yeast extracts and broad bean pods." Nevertheless, physicians prescribing MAO inhibitors should advise patients to avoid significant intake of yeast, including chromium supplements containing yeast. Forms of chromium not derived from or containing yeast do not carry this potential risk.

Nicotinic Acid (Vitamin B₃)

Nicotinic Acid (Vitamin B$_3$)

A potential interaction between chromium and nicotinic acid has been discussed, but only preliminary evidence is available as to its clinical implications. Nicotinic acid serves as substrate for synthesis of GTF, which is believed to facilitate insulin binding. Concomitant intake may improve glucose tolerance, particularly in individuals whose diet provides inadequate levels of dietary nicotinic acid. Consequently, inadvertent, excessive, or unsupervised coadministration might theoretically induce a hypoglycemic state. This largely unexplored territory is further confounded by the possibility that niacin may cause insulin resistance.

Urberg and Zemel[64] conducted an experiment in which 16 healthy elderly volunteers were divided into three groups and given either 200 μg chromium chloride, 100 mg nicotinic acid, or 200 μg chromium plus 100 mg nicotinic acid daily for 28 days, with evaluations on days 0 and 28. They observed the combined chromium–nicotinic acid supplement caused a 15% decrease in a glucose area integrated total and a 7% decrease in fasting glucose, whereas chromium or nicotinic acid alone did not affect fasting glucose or glucose tolerance. None of the interventions exerted any significant effect on fasting or 1-hour insulin levels. These researchers interpreted their findings to suggest that the inability to respond to chromium administration may result from suboptimal levels of dietary nicotinic acid. These findings also raise the question as to whether, as analogs, picolinate and nicotinate may share the same transport system for intestinal absorption, and if so, picolinate could then block nicotinate absorption, and vice versa.

Individuals who do not respond to administration of chromium may have inadequate levels of vitamin B$_3$. Coadministration may be beneficial. Patient caution, and possibly supervision by a health care professional trained and experienced in nutritional therapeutics, may be appropriate in the unlikely event (in the absence of prescription antidiabetic medication) that such intervention induces hypoglycemia.

Nonsteroidal Anti-Inflammatory Drugs (NSAIDs)

COX-1 inhibitors: Diclofenac (Cataflam, Voltaren); combination drug: diclofenac and misoprostol (Arthrotec); diflunisal (Dolobid), etodolac (Lodine), fenoprofen (Dalfon), furbiprofen (Ansaid), ibuprofen (Advil, Excedrin IB, Motrin, Motrin IB, Nuprin, Pedia Care Fever Drops, Provel, Rufen); combination drug: hydrocodone and ibuprofen (Reprexain, Vicoprofen); indomethacin (indometacin; Indocin, Indocin-SR), ketoprofen (Orudis, Oruvail), ketorolac (Acular ophthalmic, Toradol), meclofenamate (Meclomen), mefenamic acid (Ponstel), meloxicam (Mobic), nabumetone (Relafen), naproxen (Aleve, Anaprox, Naprosyn), oxaprozin (Daypro), piroxicam (Feldene), salsalate (salicylic acid; Amigesic, Disalcid, Marthritic, Mono Gesic, Salflex, Salsitab), sulindac (Clinoril), tolmetin (Tolectin).
COX-2 inhibitor: Celecoxib (Celebrex).

The NSAIDs may increase chromium levels in the body by enhancing chromium absorption from oral intake while also delaying or inhibiting chromium elimination. In a rat model, indomethacin and aspirin have been shown to increase chromium absorption.[61] Evidence is lacking to substantiate these proposed actions, and no case reports or clinical trials have documented clinically significant adverse effects.

NUTRIENT-NUTRIENT INTERACTIONS

Biotin

Chromium picolinate and biotin appear to work together to enhance glucose uptake in skeletal muscle cells and improve glucose disposal. Singer and Geohas[64a] conducted a placebo-controlled, double-blind, randomized trial investigating the effects on glycemic control of coadministering chromium and biotin in 43 type 2 diabetic subjects who were "poorly controlled" by oral antihyperglycemic agents. They coadministered chromium picolinate (600 μg) and biotin (2 mg) daily, in addition to their prestudy oral antihyperglycemic agent therapy. After 4 weeks, they observed "a significantly greater reduction in the total area under the curve for glucose" during the 2-hour oral glucose tolerance test for the treatment group compared with the placebo group, along with "significantly greater reductions" in fructosamine, triglycerides, and triglycerides/HDL cholesterol ratio in the treatment group. The authors concluded that coadministration of chromium picolinate and biotin "may represent an effective adjunctive nutritional therapy to people with poorly controlled diabetes with the potential for improving lipid metabolism." These findings indicate the need for continued research into the use of multiple nutritional interventions as complements to conventional pharmacological interventions within a broad and multifaceted, individualized and evolving strategic approach to dysglycemia and diabetes.

Calcium

The concomitant intake of calcium carbonate and chromium can interfere with the absorption of both agents and thus reduce the activity of chromium intake.[65] Optimal absorption can be maintained by separating intake of the two substances by at least 2 hours.

Further research is warranted to determine whether, and to what degree, the observed effect is caused by the antacid effect of calcium carbonate, or could be specific to calcium per se.

Carbohydrates

Excessive intake of sugars and other simple carbohydrates may increase the amount of chromium excreted through the urine.

In a 12-week trial, Kozlovsky et al.[66] compared chromium excretion in 37 subjects fed two diets containing equivalent chromium content, approximately 16 μg per 1000 calories. During the initial 6 weeks, the reference diet contained "optimal levels" of protein, fat, carbohydrate, and other nutrients, with 35% of total calories from complex carbohydrates and 15% from simple sugars. During the following 6 weeks, subjects consumed "high sugar diets" containing 15% complex carbohydrates and 35% simple sugars. During the high-sugar diets, subjects exhibited increased urinary chromium losses from 10% to 300% for 27 of 37 subjects, compared with the reference diets. The authors contextualized this significant stimulation of chromium loss associated with the high-sugar diet by further noting that "marginal intake of dietary Cr may lead to marginal Cr deficiency, which is associated with impaired glucose and lipid metabolism."

Using a mouse model, Seaborn and Stoecker[67] demonstrated that the source of carbohydrate can alter chromium absorption and retention. All animals were fed a diet in which 50% was composed of starch, sucrose, fructose, or glucose and compared with those fed a low-chromium diet and those administered 1 mg/kg chromium in the form of chromium chloride, a large dose. After 26 days they found that chromium concentrations were significantly higher in testes, spleen, kidney, and liver, as well as blood, epididymal fat pad, and femur, of animals given their carbohydrate load as starch than in animals fed sucrose, fructose, or glucose. Furthermore, elevated bone and kidney chromium concentrations and heart and muscle glycogen were associated with chromium administration.

In a small clinical trial, Anderson et al.[68] administered five different carbohydrate-based drinks to 20 subjects in amounts corresponding to body weight. They found that glucose plus fructose was the most insulinogenic, followed by glucose alone, starch plus fructose, starch alone, and water plus fructose.

Furthermore, they observed that subjects with the highest concentrations of circulating insulin displayed decreased ability to mobilize chromium on the basis of urinary chromium excretion. These researchers concluded that such urinary chromium losses parallel the insulinogenic properties of carbohydrates.

Urinary chromium excretion is greater in adults with diets high in simple sugars (e.g., sucrose) than in those with diets high in complex carbohydrates (e.g., whole grains). Increased insulin secretion in response to the consumption of simple sugars (vs. complex carbohydrates) appears to contribute significantly to this effect.[68-71] Decreased chromium intake and potentially compromised chromium status are also strongly associated with diets higher in simple carbohydrates and refined foods.

Chromium, 200 μg once or twice daily, may be beneficial in individuals with dietary intake high in sugars and simple carbohydrates. A dietary approach emphasizing lean meats, healthy fats and oils, carbohydrate sources low on the glycemic index (especially nutrient-rich fruits, vegetables, and whole grains), and a minimum of processed foods and refined carbohydrates will enhance the action and retention of dietary and supplemental chromium support for healthy insulin function and reduce the risk of dysglycemia, obesity, diabetes, and cardiovascular disease.[72]

Hydroxycitric Acid

See *Gymnema sylvestre*.

Iron

Chromium and iron compete for binding on transferrin, the iron transport protein. Thus, excessive levels of either mineral can interfere with transport of the other.

In an 8-week placebo-controlled study of younger men doing resistance training, Lukaski et al.[73] observed an insignificant decrease in transferrin saturation with iron after administration of 200 μg of chromium daily (3.3-3.5 μmol as chromium chloride or chromium picolinate). In a similar randomized, double-blind, placebo-controlled trial involving 18 older men (age 56-69) engaged in resistive training twice weekly, Campbell et al.[74] found that 925 μg of chromium picolinate daily for 12 weeks did not significantly affect hematologic indices, measures of iron metabolism, or iron status. Based on these and related findings, it has also been hypothesized that decreased chromium transport might contribute to the diabetes associated with hereditary hemochromatosis.

Well-designed long-term studies have yet to be published investigating this interaction more thoroughly.

Vanadium

Evidence from in vitro and in vivo research has been accumulating for more than 20 years showing that vanadyl and vanadate (i.e., vanadium salts) mimic insulin action in isolated cell systems and lower glucose levels in diabetic animals. Diabetic patients administered vanadium salts, containing 25 to 100 mg of elemental vanadium, daily for up to 6 weeks have demonstrated partial normalization of glucose metabolic irregularities.[75-78]

Human trials investigating the potential synergy between chromium and vanadium are warranted. Pending such clarification, professional supervision is appropriate for individuals with diabetes who choose to undertake such therapies, especially within the context of conventional therapy using insulin or oral hypoglycemic medications.

Vitamin C

Concomitant intake of vitamin C may increase chromium absorption. Animal research has shown that simultaneous intake of chromium and vitamin C enhances chromium uptake.[79] Seaborn et al.[80] studied the effects of chromium and ascorbate depletion in a guinea pig model and observed a synergistic relationship between ascorbic acid and chromium. They noted that their "findings suggest that dietary Cr may affect ascorbic acid metabolism and the metabolic response to stress."

A healthy intake of both chromium and vitamin C can play a role in the prevention and treatment of dysglycemia, lipid disorders, and cardiovascular disease.

Theoretically, an excess of chromium might result if a high intake was accompanied by high doses of vitamin C. The clinical significance of any potentially adverse effect is improbable, whereas the potential benefits of a synergistic interaction between these nutrients is plausible, even probable, at appropriate dosage levels in most individuals, particularly those with compromised dietary intake.

In vitro experiments have consistently found that the addition of ascorbic acid to plasma containing chromium(VI) leads to a dose-dependent reduction of chromium(VI) to chromium(III).

Zinc

Data from animal research indicate that coadministration of zinc and chromium may reduce intestinal content and absorption of zinc, particularly in the presence of zinc deficiency.[81] Pending further research, separating intake of these two minerals by at least several hours may be advisable to enhance absorption.

HERB-NUTRIENT INTERACTIONS

Gymnema sylvestre

Gymnema sylvestre, a plant native to the tropical forests of India, has played a role in the Ayurvedic treatment of diabetes for centuries. It has been postulated that *Gymnema* enhances the production of endogenous insulin. A typical dosage of *G. sylvestre* extract is 400 to 600 mg per day.

In a randomized, double-blind, placebo-controlled clinical trial, Preuss et al.[82] compared the effects of (-)-hydroxycitric acid alone and in combination with niacin-bound chromium and a standardized *G. sylvestre* extract in 60 moderately obese subjects over 8 weeks. Both groups receiving *Gymnema* demonstrated 5% to 6% reductions in body weight as well as significant reductions in food intake, total cholesterol, LDLs, triglycerides, and serum leptin levels, compared with those receiving placebo; HDL levels and excretion of urinary fat metabolites increased in both treated groups. The authors concluded that optimal doses of (−)-hydroxycitric acid and, to a greater degree, the combination of (−)-hydroxycitric acid, niacin-bound chromium, and *G. sylvestre* extract can serve as an effective and safe weight loss formula that can facilitate a reduction in excess body weight and BMI while promoting healthy blood lipid levels.

The 84 citations for this monograph, as well as additional reference literature, are located under Chromium on the CD at the back of the book.

Copper

Nutrient Name: Copper.
Synonyms: Copper carbonate, copper citrate, copper gluconate, copper glyconate, copper lysinate, copper sebacate, copper sulfate, cupric acetate, cupric oxide; cuprum.
Elemental Symbol: Cu.
Related Substance: Chlorophyllin.

Summary

Drug/Class Interaction Type	Mechanism and Significance	Management
Allopurinol ≈◇◇/☼	Allopurinol, a potent inhibitor of xanthine oxidase, forms a complex with copper that can reduce cardiac damage, which appears to be due to copper- and ascorbate-mediated DNA breakage, in patients undergoing cardiac bypass surgery. The mechanisms involved are not fully understood, but the resulting complex exhibits low redox activity.	Chelation of copper by allopurinol may help protect against cardiac damage during reperfusion of the heart. Avoid copper before bypass surgery.
Antacids ≈≈≈	Antacids can inhibit copper absorption and induce intestinal alkaline pH, which can precipitate dietary copper. Copper depletion and deficiency may result from excessive or extended use of antacids, especially with pyloric stenosis. Mechanism reasonable, but clinically significant adverse effects probably infrequent.	Coadminister with extended antacid use.
Cimetidine ✗✗/◇	Animal studies indicate cimetidine complexes with Cu(II) [and Fe(III)] ions and may elevate tissue copper concentrations, particularly in the liver. By binding copper (and iron), cimetidine may also act as a free-radical scavenger. Although the proposed mechanisms are plausible, evidence remains preliminary.	Coadminister if indicated. Separate intake by at least 2 hours.
Ciprofloxacin ◇◇	Copper and other minerals can bind to ciprofloxacin and reduce its absorption. Copper evidence preliminary, but parallel phenomenon with iron generally recognized. Drug efficacy could be impaired.	Separate intake by at least 2 hours.
Clofibrate fibrates ≈≈≈/⊕✗/◇◇/?	Clofibrate may enhance copper metabolism and elevate hepatic copper levels, and may reduce hypercholesterolemia, particularly with compromised copper status. Research is limited, with mixed findings and conclusions.	Coadminister, as appropriate; monitor.
Ethambutol ☼/◇≈≈/⊕⊕	Ethambutol forms chelate complexes with copper (and zinc), which may contribute to drug-induced optic neuropathy.	Coadminister and monitor visual function. Separate intake by at least 2 hours
Famotidine H₂ receptor antagonists (H₂RAs) ≈≈≈	Famotidine and H₂RAs interfere with the acidic gastric environment optimal for copper absorption. Such drug-induced changes can inhibit copper absorption and induce alkaline intestinal pH, which can precipitate dietary copper. Subsequent copper depletion and deficiency may result from excessive or extended gastric acid—suppressive therapy. Mechanism reasonable but frequency of clinically significant adverse effects unknown.	Coadminister with extended H₂RA use. Separate intake by at least 2 hours.
Nonsteroidal anti-inflammatory drugs (NSAIDs) ☼/⊕	Copper tends to complex with NSAIDs and might enhance their anti-inflammatory effects while reducing their ulcerogenic effects. Evidence preliminary and promising, but mixed; clinical implications likely significant.	Consider coadministration.
Oral contraceptives (OCs) Estrogens/progestins Hormone replacement therapy (HRT) ◇◇	Exogenous female hormones, especially progestins, may enhance copper absorption and elevate copper levels. Clinical significance may vary with age, specific medication, and other factors and could contribute to increased adverse drug effects, e.g., cardiovascular risk.	Avoid concomitant copper supplementation unless risk of depletion or other prevailing benefits.
Penicillamine, trientine, and tetrathiomolybdate Chelating agents ◇◇/≈◇◇	These chelating agents are designed to bind copper and limit its absorption and accumulation, particularly in treatment of mineral deposition disorders such as Wilson's disease and increasingly in antiangiogenic cancer therapy. Interaction is purposeful, and its clinical significance is generally recognized.	Limit dietary and avoid supplemental copper intake. Monitor for adverse drug effects.
Valproic acid Anticonvulsant medications ≈≈/◇≈≈	Valproic acid and related antiepileptics may induce copper deficiency and disrupt copper homeostasis by increasing excretion into bile. Preliminary evidence of depletion pattern; prevalence uncertain. Possible risk of clinical significance primarily with long-term anticonvulsant therapy.	Monitor copper (and zinc) status. Copper administrator warranted with deficiency indications or other risk factors.
Zidovudine (AZT) Reverse-transcriptase inhibitor (nucleoside) antiretroviral agents ≈≈/⊕/☼/◇	Coadministration of zinc with AZT can reduce adverse effects and enhance efficacy but extended therapy requires complement of copper to prevent adverse effects from zinc, thus providing a more comprehensive approach to supporting patients on AZT. Evidence preliminary, clinical significance unconfirmed.	Coadminister copper with extended zinc use.

NUTRIENT DESCRIPTION
Chemistry and Forms

Copper carbonate, copper citrate, copper gluconate, copper glycinate, copper lysinate, copper sebacate, copper sulfate; copper amino acid chelates; cupric acetate, cupric oxide.

Physiology and Function

Copper is an essential trace mineral that is present in all tissues and acts as a cofactor in several key enzyme systems. The average adult body contains about 80 to 120 milligrams of copper, most of which is stored in the liver. Copper stimulates iron absorption and is an important catalyst in hemoglobin synthesis and function. Copper is necessary to make adenosine triphosphate (ATP) and acts as an essential component of cytochrome oxidase, which is necessary for energy metabolism, cellular respiration, and myelin formation.

Copper is involved in the synthesis and breakdown of several hormones. Copper serves as a cofactor in dopamine–β-hydroxylase, which oxidizes ascorbic acid and synthesizes norepinephrine. It is also involved in the catabolism of estrogenic hormones. Copper may play a role in emotional regulation and cognitive function.

Copper is absorbed in the small intestine, where it is transferred across the gut wall by albumin, and carried on transcuprein and albumin to the liver, where it is incorporated into liver enzymes and secreted into the blood on the protein ceruloplasmin. Copper absorption has been found to be greater in women (71%) than in men (64%), age 20 to 59 years, but did not differ in men and women 60 to 83 years old. Copper elimination is primarily via bile, with small amounts eliminated in urine, sweat, and epidermal shedding.

Copper plays a central role in decreasing inflammation through both ceruloplasmin and the copper-containing form of superoxide dismutase (SOD). *Ceruloplasmin* is a weak, broad-specificity oxidase whose main functions include copper transport and extracellular scavenging of superoxide and other oxygen radicals. Adequate ceruloplasmin levels also minimize copper toxicity by limiting absorption of copper. Copper, along with zinc, as well as manganese, is found in cytostolic SOD. SOD is a primary quencher of superoxide radical, a prevalent and highly reactive free-radical form of oxygen produced during oxidative phosphorylation, which can be quite destructive if not rapidly quenched. SOD slows age-related deterioration, protects against chemical sensitivities (along with polyphenol oxidase), and enables the normal humoral immune response. There are also copper-containing amino acid chelates that have SOD activity. During inflammatory conditions, such as acute infections, serum copper levels, as ceruloplasmin, generally increase by 20% to 30%, whereas serum iron levels decline. Plasma copper, enzymatic ceruloplasmin, and immunoreactive (RID) ceruloplasmin have been observed to be significantly higher in women than in men, but SOD and in vitro ^{67}Cu uptake by red blood cells does not appear to differ between the genders.

Histaminase, which breaks down histamine to control allergies and inflammation, is another copper-dependent enzyme involved in regulating inflammatory processes. *Tyrosinase,* an enzyme that requires copper, plays a role in melanin synthesis, enabling skin pigmentation and hair coloration, as well as keratinization of hair.

Some researchers have proposed that copper deficiency is associated with elevated cholesterol and triglycerides, the development of atherosclerosis, and increased risk of cardiovascular disease.

Copper functions in the synthesis of collagen and repair of connective tissue, providing structural elasticity not only throughout the musculoskeletal system, but also in tissues of the lungs, blood vessels, and skin. Lysil oxidase, a copper-containing enzyme secreted by connective tissue cells, is necessary for the formation of the cross-links of collagen and elastin.

Copper is an essential element and its level in the body is strictly controlled. Under most conditions, excess copper is excreted in the urine and feces (via the bile). In cases of elevated copper, the adverse effects that develop are often caused less directly by copper toxicity than by its interference with the absorption and distribution of other mineral nutrients, such as iron and zinc.

Copper sulfate, cupric acetate, and alkaline copper carbonate are among the forms of copper best absorbed in the gut. Nevertheless, even though animal studies have demonstrated that it is poorly absorbed in the gut, *cupric oxide* (CuO) is the form of copper most often used in over-the-counter (OTC) preparations. *Chlorophyllin* is a relatively new, water-soluble copper complex of chlorophyll.

NUTRIENT IN CLINICAL PRACTICE
Known or Potential Therapeutic Uses

Copper has been proposed as offering therapeutic benefit in a wide range of conditions. Such therapeutic action has largely been premised on the hypothesis that administration will enhance or restore healthy function in the numerous enzyme systems where copper plays a critical role. Nevertheless, direct evidence confirming copper's efficacy in treating most of the diseases proposed is largely lacking, other than to prevent or treat those directly attributable to, or exacerbated by, copper deficiency or depletion.

Historical/Ethnomedicine Precedent: As the classical metal of Venus, copper was associated with the female reproductive system in ancient times.

Possible Uses

Anemia, aneurysms, atherosclerosis, athletic performance, benign prostatic hyperplasia, burns, cardiac arrhythmia, cardiovascular disease, decubitus ulcers, hypercholesterolemia, hypoglycemia, immune enhancement, Menkes' syndrome, muscle spasms, osteoporosis, peptic ulcer, peripheral vascular disease, rheumatoid arthritis, skin cancer (prevention), sprains and strains, stomach cancer (prevention), vitiligo, wound healing.

Deficiency Symptoms

Most research into copper deficiency has focused on acute, severe deficiency. Such frank clinical copper deficiency is relatively rare in humans and animals on typical, varied diets. However, marginal, chronic deficiency is not uncommon. Dietary surveys indicate that the average dietary intake of copper in the U.S. population is only half of the recently established recommended dietary allowance (RDA). Most cases of copper deficiency involve premature infants, infants suffering from malnutrition, or children with iron deficiency anemia, severe protein malnutrition, chronic diarrhea, or other malabsorption difficulties. Overt symptoms in adults are rare but may occur with inadequate or unbalanced dietary intake over an extended time or in those who consume zinc supplements chronically without counterbalancing copper. The determination of copper needs and marginal deficiency is obscured because copper deficiency may not manifest as decreased levels of copper-dependent enzymes, but it may still significantly lower their activity.

Because copper is required for a wide range of enzyme systems and metabolic processes, a deficiency can cause a variety of disorders. Laboratory animals fed copper-deficient diets tend to develop anemia, cardiac abnormalities and abnormal electrocardiograms, and elevated levels of serum cholesterol, triglycerides, and glucose. Symptoms of copper deficiency in humans include fatigue, hypotonia, hypothermia, growth retardation, reduced resistance to infection, various nervous system disorders, anemia, neutropenia, degeneration of vasculature, cardiac damage, hemolysis with potential liver and brain damage, various cardiovascular problems, impaired respiration, emphysema, elevated low-density lipoprotein (LDL) cholesterol and reduced high-density lipoprotein (HDL) cholesterol, impaired collagen formation, breakdown of connective tissue, bone demineralization, osteoporosis, depigmentation of skin, and changes in structure and appearance of hair.

Genetic Conditions Relating to Copper

Two primary genetic diseases involve copper metabolism: Menkes' syndrome and Wilson's disease.

Menkes' syndrome results from an X-linked mutation of genes encoding Cu-binding P-type adenosinetriphosphatase (ATPase) for the efflux of Cu, ATP7A. Apart from the distinctive kinky or steely hair, this syndrome is also characterized by stunted growth, abnormalities in cardiovascular and skeletal development, progressive cognitive decline, and premature death. This inborn error in metabolism limits absorption of copper in the intestines and uptake in the liver. Copper subsequently accumulates in the intestinal cells and produces symptoms resembling copper deficiency.

Wilson's disease, caused by the mutation of genes encoding Cu-binding ATPase for the efflux of Cu, ATP7B, is characterized by accumulation of copper in the liver, leading to severe hepatic damage; elevated copper levels subsequently affect the brain and result in neurological problems.

Dietary Sources

Oysters are the most abundant food source of copper. Other copper-containing foods include soy, peas, and other dried legumes; dark-green leafy vegetables; whole-grain breads and cereals; seafood, including crab and lobster; lamb, pork, and other meats, especially organ meats such as liver; nuts (almonds, pecans, walnuts); raisins, prunes, and pomegranates; and tea, coffee, and chocolate.

Foods rich in copper are generally also rich in iron.

Nutrient Preparations Available

Copper sulfate, cupric acetate, cupric oxide, and alkaline copper carbonate. As previously noted, CuO is the form most often used in OTC preparations, primarily because of its low cost. Chlorophyllin is a copper complex of chlorophyll.

Copper is usually found in multimineral or multivitamin/multimineral formulations.

Copper is often taken with, although preferably ingested apart from, long-term zinc administration to counteract the tendency to copper depletion associated with zinc intake without copper. Recommended Zn/Cu ratio in formulations is 10:1 to 15:1.

Dosage Forms Available

Capsule, tablet; cupric sulfate: injection (U.S.).

Dosage Range

Adult
Dietary: 1.0 to 1.5 mg/day
Supplemental/Maintenance: 1 to 2 mg/day
Pharmacological/Therapeutic: 2+ mg/day

Pharmacological doses of copper in scientific studies usually range from 2 to 4 mg per day. Copper dose is usually based on zinc intake. Many experts consider the optimal zinc/copper ratio as 10:1. Some practitioners of nutritional therapeutics use zinc at dosages up to 45 mg/day as part of therapeutic protocols. In such cases, LDL and HDL cholesterol levels need to be monitored. Zinc may need to be reduced or copper increased; even so, doses of copper greater than 3 mg/day are usually avoided.

Pediatric (<18 Years)
Supplemental/Maintenance: 0.5 to 1.0 mg/day
Pharmacological/Therapeutic: 1 to 2 mg/day

Laboratory Values

Serum ceruloplasmin concentrations and white blood cell (WBC) levels have been considered the most reliable methods of evaluation but often are insensitive to subtle changes in copper status. Copper-containing enzymes, such as Cu-Zn SOD, cytochrome-c oxidase, and diamine oxidase, may be more reliable, but evidence to date is not conclusive.[1] LDL and HDL cholesterol levels are sometimes used.

Serum, plasma, urinary, or hair copper concentrations are not considered particularly reliable because these monitoring parameters are subject to many variables and may not accurately demonstrate actual copper load; when used, such determinations are recommended monthly.

SAFETY PROFILE
Overview

Copper is generally considered safe when taken at customary dietary or typical supplemental dosage levels. Chronic copper toxicity from intentional intake in adults is rare. Long-term doses of 10 to 35 mg per day are considered safe. The tolerable upper limit (UL) of copper intake established by the U.S. National Institute of Medicine for adults is 10 mg per day, combining dietary and supplemental sources. However, research has suggested that the body cannot eliminate more than 3 mg/day, so in individuals who are copper replete or overloaded, greater than 3 mg/day dietary copper may contribute to further accumulation.

Nutrient Adverse Effects
General Adverse Effects

In adults, 10 mg of copper daily can induce nausea, and 60 mg may cause vomiting. Tissue elevations usually occur only when intake is 300 to 500 times above normal. The adverse effects on zinc metabolism represent the primary adverse effect of excessive copper levels.

Mutagenicity
No human data are available. Results from short-term tests on mutagenicity have been negative or inconclusive.

Adverse Effects Among Specific Populations
Copper intake exerts particular risk for individuals with Wilson's disease, a genetic disorder that causes a toxic accumulation of copper in the liver, kidneys, central nervous system (CNS), and cornea. Maximum safe daily dosages of copper intake for individuals with severe liver or kidney disease are of concern but have not been determined. Copper toxicity has occasionally been reported in individuals living in houses where copper from water pipes has leached into the drinking water.

Pregnancy and Nursing
Maximum safe daily dosages of copper intake for pregnant or nursing women have not been determined. There are no reports in the literature reviewed of teratogenicity or embryotoxicity in humans induced by excess copper intake. However, animal studies indicate that a deficiency or excess of copper in the body can cause significant harm to developing embryos.

Infants and Children
Maximum safe daily dosages of copper intake for infants and young children have not been determined. Copper can exert a lethal dose in children at levels as low as 3.5 g. The copper (and zinc) status of epileptic children taking valproate derivatives should be monitored.

Toxicity Signs and Symptoms
Symptoms of moderate copper toxicity include weakness, dizziness, fainting, headache (severe or continuing), burning sensation in the throat, gastrointestinal disturbances, loss of appetite, vomiting, excess salivation, metallic taste in mouth, dyspepsia, epigastric pain, painful urination, and low back pain. Severe cases can result in hemolytic anemia, hypertension, liver damage, jaundice, hemochromatosis, hemoglobinuria, hematuria, kidney failure, coma, and death. O'Donohue et al.[2] reported a case of adult chronic copper self-intoxication, after daily doses of 30 to 60 mg for 3 years, which resulted in severe liver cirrhosis necessitating orthotopic liver transplantation.

Contraindications

Biliary disease, cancer, heart bypass patients, liver disease, migraines, Wilson's disease. Copper is also contraindicated during the course of anticopper therapies. Some individuals may have a total body excess of copper resulting from a lifetime of drinking water from copper plumbing, and copper supplementation may not be desirable in such people.

Precautions and Warnings

Some individuals may become sensitized to copper sulfate and develop allergic contact dermatitis.

INTERACTIONS REVIEW
Strategic Considerations

Many medications may deplete copper or interfere with its metabolic functions, sometimes incidentally, but often intentionally. Copper supplementation may be appropriate to

correct drug-induced depletion patterns. In certain cases, however, such action is central to the therapeutic strategy, and supplementation is contraindicated, except in response to specific episodes of adverse effects of excessive copper deficiency caused by depletion. Conversely, in some situations, drugs such as allopurinol may provide benefit by reducing copper levels.

NUTRIENT-DRUG INTERACTIONS

Allopurinol

Allopurinol (Oxypurinol; Aloprim, Apo-Allopurinol, Lopurin, Purinol, Zyloprim).

Interaction Type and Significance
≈◇◇ **Drug-Induced Nutrient Depletion,**
           Supplementation Contraindicated,
           Professional Management Appropriate
☼   **Prevention or Reduction of Nutrient Adverse**
           Effect

Probability:	Evidence Base:
2. Probable	○ **Preliminary**

Effect and Mechanism of Action
Allopurinol, a potent inhibitor of xanthine oxidase, is known to protect the heart effectively against damage in patients undergoing cardiac bypass surgery. Nevertheless, the mechanism underlying the protective effect of allopurinol is unclear because of ambiguity concerning the presence of xanthine oxidase in the human heart. Allopurinol apparently chelates copper and reduces DNA breakage (see next).

Research
In 1993, Malkiel et al.[3] published a paper examining the possible role of the interaction between allopurinol and copper in myocardial protection. They found that allopurinol forms a one-to-one complex with Cu(II) ions in vitro, yielding a complex with low oxidation-reduction (redox) activity, and concluded that allopurinol substantially reduced copper-mediated and ascorbate-driven DNA breakage. Later research by Lapenna et al.[4] found that allopurinol, at therapeutically relevant concentrations (9-58 µM), significantly counteracted copper-catalyzed human non–HDL lipoprotein oxidation through metal complexation.

Nutritional Therapeutics, Clinical Concerns, and Adaptations
The ability of allopurinol to chelate copper may impart the protective effects against cardiac damage in bypass patients during reperfusion of the heart. These findings suggest that patients undergoing bypass surgery should avoid copper supplementation.

Antacids

Aluminum carbonate gel (Basajel), aluminum hydroxide (Alternagel, Amphojel); combination drugs: aluminum hydroxide, magnesium carbonate, alginic acid, and sodium bicarbonate (Gaviscon Extra Strength Tablets, Gaviscon Regular Strength Liquid, Gaviscon Extra Strength Liquid); aluminum hydroxide and magnesium hydroxide (Advanced Formula Di-Gel Tablets, co-magaldrox, Di-Gel, Gelusil, Maalox, Maalox Plus, Mylanta, Wingel); aluminum hydroxide, magnesium trisilicate, alginic acid, and sodium bicarbonate (Alenic Alka, Gaviscon Regular Strength Tablets); calcium carbonate (Titralac, Tums), magnesium hydroxide (Phillips' Milk of Magnesia MOM); combination drugs: magnesium hydroxide and calcium carbonate (Calcium Rich Rolaids); magnesium hydroxide, aluminum hydroxide, calcium carbonate, and simethicone (Tempo Tablets); magnesium trisilicate and aluminum hydroxide (Adcomag trisil, Foamicon); magnesium trisilicate, alginic acid, and sodium bicarbonate (Alenic Alka, Gaviscon Regular Strength Tablets); combination drug: sodium bicarbonate, aspirin, and citric acid (Alka-Seltzer). See also Cimetidine and Famotidine.

Interaction Type and Significance
≈≈≈ **Drug-Induced Nutrient Depletion, Supplementation Therapeutic, Not Requiring Professional Management**

Probability: Evidence Base:
3. Possible: ○ Preliminary

Effect and Mechanism of Action
The normally acidic environment of the stomach facilitates optimal absorption of copper and other nutrients. Antacids may induce a copper deficiency by inhibiting copper absorption and precipitating dietary copper through drug-induced alkaline pH in the intestines.

Reports
Roe, van Kalmthout, and other authors have reported cases where individuals have demonstrated the effects of copper deficiency subsequent to excessive use of antacids.[5-9] Such outcomes may appear to be more likely with extended use of antacids and the occurrence of pyloric stenosis.

Nutritional Therapeutics, Clinical Concerns, and Adaptations
Clinically significant adverse effects from antacids reducing copper absorption appear to occur infrequently. Nevertheless, individuals who take antacids for an extended period may benefit from 1 to 2 mg of copper supplementation daily, possibly in the form of a multivitamin/mineral formula.

Cimetidine

Cimetidine (Tagamet; Tagemet HB)

Interaction Type and Significance
✗✗ **Minimal to Mild Adverse Interaction—Vigilance Necessary**
◇ **Adverse Drug Effect on Nutritional Therapeutics, Strategic Concern**

Probability: Evidence Base:
4. Plausible   ○ Preliminary
See also Antacids and Famotidine.

Effect and Mechanism of Action
Cimetidine complexes with Cu(II) and Fe(III) ions and may elevate tissue copper concentrations.

Research
The considerations regarding this interaction derive from research involving rats. Naveh et al.[10] published a paper in 1987 that described elevated hepatic and plasma copper concentrations, mineral redistribution, and pathological changes in some tissues after intermediate to high doses of cimetidine (875-1750 mg/kg/day) administered intragastrically to young rats four times weekly for 5 weeks.

More recent research by Lambat et al.[11] and others has focused on the action of cimetidine as a free-radical scavenger and neuroprotective agent through its ability to bind to iron and copper, thus making them unavailable for free-radical production.

Nutritional Therapeutics, Clinical Concerns, and Adaptations
Given the consistent evidence of cimetidine's mineral-binding properties, individuals taking copper supplements are advised to allow at least a 2-hour interval after taking cimetidine to avoid diminished therapeutic effect from the nutrient. The therapeutically appropriate level copper supplementation would be in the range of 1 to 2 mg/day.

Ciprofloxacin

Ciprofloxacin (Ciloxan, Cipro)

Interaction Type and Significance
◇◇ **Impaired Drug Absorption and Bioavailability, Precautions Appropriate**

Probability: Evidence Base:
2. Probable   ◉ Emerging

Effect and Mechanism of Action
Minerals, including copper, can bind to ciprofloxacin, greatly reducing the absorption of the medication.

Research
The formation of a ferric ion–ciprofloxacin complex is a well-documented cause of the reduction in ciprofloxacin bioavailability in the presence of iron.[12-14] Complexation between Cu(II) and 4-quinolone antibacterials, including ciprofloxacin, has been studied in an aqueous medium.

Clinical Implications and Adaptations
Even though not as severe as with iron supplements, the tendency for copper and other minerals to bind ciprofloxacin suggests that individuals taking this and related antibacterial medications can reduce the risk of interfering with the drug's therapeutic effect by allowing at least a 2-hour interval after ingesting any copper or multimineral supplement.

Clofibrate and Related Fibrates

Evidence: Clofibrate (Atromid-S).
Extrapolated, based on similar properties: Bezafibrate (Bezalip), ciprofibrate (Modalim), fenofibrate (Lofibra, Tricor, Triglide), gemfibrozil (Apo-Gemfibrozil, Lopid, Novo-Gemfibrozil).

Interaction Type and Significance
≈≈≈ **Drug-Induced Nutrient Depletion, Supplementation Therapeutic, with Professional Management**
⊕✗ **Bimodal or Variable Interaction, with Professional Management**
◇◇ **Drug-Induced Effect on Nutrient Function, Supplementation Contraindicated, Professional Management Appropriate**
? **Interaction Possible but Uncertain Occurrence and Unclear Implications**

Probability: Evidence Base:
2. Probable   ▽ Mixed

Effect and Mechanism of Action

Even as it binds other nutrients, such as iron, and tends to produce malabsorption, clofibrate is hypothesized to improve copper nutriture. Leslie M. Klevay, a researcher who has studied copper metabolism extensively, described clofibrate as a "cholesterotropic and cuprotropic" substance. He has observed that clofibrate lowers plasma cholesterol and enhances copper metabolism. Thus, Klevay and others have proposed that clofibrate reduces hypercholesterolemia, at least in part, through its effect on copper deficiency.[15,16] This effect is mediated by an increase in hepatic copper. Possibly as a result of such actions, however, clofibrate has a poor safety profile with significant risk of liver damage, as well as other adverse effects, including increased risk of cancer and pancreatitis. In research involving rats, Fields et al.[17] and others have reported that administration of clofibrate reduces the activity of the lipogenic enzyme glucose-6-phosphate dehydrogenase (G6PD), even though total hepatic lipid was not reduced. Further, clofibrate did not affect hepatic lipid concentration, and the pathology associated with copper deficiency when fructose was fed was not prevented by the consumption of clofibrate. Also, the tendency for hypercholesterolemic people to be more likely to be malnourished in copper than normocholesterolemic people may influence differential responses among various populations and manifest as a change in copper metabolism in response to the drug.

Research

Clofibrate is consistently recognized as altering copper metabolism. However, various researchers have arrived at differing conclusions as to whether the net effect of clofibrate therapy is to enhance or deplete copper status, whether observed changes reflect the drug's action or the metabolic alterations associated with pathology, and the degree to which the interaction is clinically significant.[16,18] Clofibrate may bind copper and reduce absorption, but it also tends to elevate tissue levels, particularly in the liver. In particular, although research consistently indicates that clofibrate is active in animals malnourished in copper, it is still uncertain whether observed changes reflect changes in cholesterol metabolism induced by clofibrate because of a change in copper metabolism or other processes, and how such laboratory findings illuminate clinical practice involving humans.

Nutritional Therapeutics, Clinical Concerns, and Adaptations

Copper supplementation may be appropriate. Periodic monitoring is advised.

ESTROGENS, PROGESTINS, AND ESTROGEN-PROGESTIN COMBINATIONS

Oral Contraceptives: Monophasic, Biphasic, and Triphasic Estrogen Preparations (Synthetic Estrogen and Progesterone Analogs)

Ethinyl estradiol and desogestrel (Desogen, Ortho-TriCyclen).
Ethinyl estradiol and ethynodiol (Demulen 1/35, Demulen 1/50, Nelulen 1/25, Nelulen 1/50, Zovia).
Ethinyl estradiol and levonorgestrel (Alesse, Levlen, Levlite, Levora 0.15/30, Nordette, Tri-Levlen, Triphasil, Trivora).
Ethinyl estradiol and norethindrone/norethisterone (Brevicon, Estrostep, Genora 1/35, GenCepth 1/35, Jenest-28, Loestrin 1.5/30, Loestrin1/20, Modicon, Necon 1/25, Necon 10/11, Necon 0.5/30, Necon 1/50, Nelova 1/35, Nelova 10/11, Norinyl 1/35, Norlestin 1/50, Ortho Novum 1/35, Ortho

Novum 10/11, Ortho Novum 7/7/7, Ovcon-35, Ovcon-50, Tri-Norinyl, Trinovum).
Ethinyl estradiol and norgestrel (Lo/Ovral, Ovral).
Mestranol and norethindrone (Genora 1/50, Nelova 1/50, Norethin 1/50, Ortho-Novum 1/50).
Related, internal application: Etonogestrel/ethinyl estradiol vaginal ring (Nuvaring).

Hormone Replacement Therapy (HRT): Estrogen-Containing and Synthetic Estrogen and Progesterone Analog Medications

HRT, estrogens: Chlorotrianisene (Tace); conjugated equine estrogens (Premarin); conjugated synthetic estrogens (Cenestin); dienestrol (Ortho Dienestrol); esterified estrogens (Estratab, Menest, Neo-Estrone); estradiol, topical/transdermal/ring (Alora Transdermal, Climara Transdermal, Estrace, Estradot, Estring FemPatch, Vivelle-Dot, Vivelle Transdermal); estradiol cypionate (Dep-Gynogen, Depo-Estradiol, Depogen, Dura-Estrin, Estra-D, Estro-Cyp, Estroject-LA, Estronol-LA); estradiol hemihydrate (Estreva, Vagifem); estradiol valerate (Delestrogen, Estra-L 40, Gynogen L.A. 20, Progynova, Valergen 20); estrone (Aquest, Estragyn 5, Estro-A, Estrone '5', Kestrone-5); estropipate (Ogen, Ortho-Est); ethinyl estradiol (Estinyl, Gynodiol, Lynoral).

HRT, estrogen/progestin combinations: Conjugated equine estrogens and medroxyprogesterone (Premelle cycle 5, Prempro); conjugated equine estrogens and norgestrel (Prempak-C); estradiol and dydrogesterone (Femoston); estradiol and norethindrone, patch (CombiPatch); estradiol and norethindrone/norethisterone, oral (Activella, Climagest, Climesse, FemHRT, Trisequens); estradiol valerate and cyproterone acetate (Climens); estradiol valerate and norgestrel (Progyluton); estradiol and norgestimate (Ortho-Prefest).

HRT, estrogen/testosterone combinations: Esterified estrogens and methyltestosterone (Estratest, Estratest HS).

Interaction Type and Significance

◇◇   **Drug-Induced Effect on Nutrient Function, Supplementation Contraindicated, Professional Management Appropriate**

Probability: Evidence Base:
3. Possible   ○ **Preliminary**

Effect and Mechanism of Action

Oral contraceptives (OCs) and other exogenous female hormone medications have been shown to elevate intracellular copper and serum copper levels in humans and thereby potentially contribute to alterations in glucose metabolism, oxygen metabolism, and a woman's mental and emotional well-being. Although estrogens are known to affect copper absorption and metabolism, progestins in OCs are believed to be the primary determinant of elevated copper levels.

With regard to hormone replacement therapy (HRT), knowledge continues to evolve as to the respective roles of estrogen, in its various forms, and progestins. The issues and evidence concerning OCs inherently influences and sets the stage for an emerging understanding of interactions between combined HRTs and copper and their clinical implications.

Research

Studies have consistently found OC use positively associated with increased absorption of copper and increased serum copper and ceruloplasmin levels.[19-22] Even though higher serum copper concentration in women using OCs is well known, uncertainty still surrounds the influence of newer progestin compounds in OCs on serum copper concentration. In a study involving low-estrogen preparations, Liukko et al.[23] noted that copper levels rose significantly in women while using OCs over a 2-year period, but returned to initial levels after the OCs were discontinued. Johnson et al.[24] observed that OCs elevated plasma copper, enzymatic ceruloplasmin, and SOD activity, but not copper absorption and biological half-life, in women age 20 to 39. In a more recent epidemiological study (1998) of 610 nonpregnant and nonlactating women (18-44 years old), Berg et al.[25] reported that although elevated serum copper concentration was found in users of all OC types, elevation was more pronounced among women taking OCs with antiandrogen progestins (56% elevation) than with desogestrel (46%), norethisterone/lynestrenol (42%), or levonorgestrel (34%), after adjusting for multiple covariaters/variables (e.g., age, smoking, alcohol intake).

The effects of hormonal interventions on copper absorption and metabolism occur within a context influenced by gender and life stage. In their study of 44 healthy postmenopausal women, 50 to 60 years old, 18 of whom were treated by oral combined HRT for at least 2 years, and 26 of whom were untreated, Bureau et al.[26] examined plasma trace-mineral levels (Zn, Se, Cr, Mn, Cu), red blood cell antioxidant enzymes (Cu-Zn SOD, Se-GPX, Cu), and urinary excretion (Zn, Cr, Mg, Ca). Plasma copper concentrations were higher in women treated by HRT, whereas erythrocyte copper levels were not modified. Zinc, selenium, and manganese plasma levels; activities of Cu-Zn-SOD; and GSH-PX in erythrocytes were not statistically different between the two groups. The authors interpreted this as suggesting that HRT provides beneficial effects on trace-mineral status related to menopause. In their study of the effects of age and gender on copper absorption, biological half-life, and status, Johnson et al.[24] observed that among younger individuals, 20 to 59 years old, absorption was greater in women (71%) than in men (64%), but that the difference between men and women was negligible among those age 60 to 83. Likewise, biological half-life of ^{67}Cu ranged from 13 to 33 days and differed between men and women age 20 to 59, but not between men and women age 60 to 83. Such findings illuminate the changes in women's metabolism as they age and pass through their reproductive years and into menopause.

Although a causal relationship has not been demonstrated, recent epidemiological studies have shown an increased mortality from cardiovascular diseases in individuals with higher serum copper levels. In 1991, in an epidemiological study of Finnish men, Salonen et al.[27] concluded that high copper status, reflected by elevated serum copper concentration, is an independent risk factor for ischemic heart disease. This issue is of particular interest in the light of recent findings of an increased risk of venous thromboembolism in users of OCs containing newer progestins such as desogestrel, compared with users of other OCs. Further, Reunanen et al.,[28] in a nested case-control study (1996) within a prospective population study, found high serum copper and low serum zinc levels significantly associated with increased mortality from all cardiovascular diseases, particularly coronary heart disease.

Given the recent upheavals in medical consensus and practice guidelines, the emerging research picture, and the as-yet unclear clinical implications of HRT in relation to cardiovascular health and risk, the issues of copper status deserve further attention as part of the continued research.

Nutritional Therapeutics, Clinical Concerns, and Adaptations

At this time, evidence is inadequate to warrant routine monitoring of copper concentrations in female patients using estrogen and progestin medications in the absence of other specific cardiovascular risk factors. OCs can raise serum copper levels, but it is not clear whether or to what degree this occurs at the tissue level. Women using OCs may have increased needs for zinc based on potential depletion, as well as greater needs for folate and vitamins B_{12} and B_6. Individual evaluation of safe and effective hormone dosage levels is necessary. Pending such individualized assessment, patients requesting advice on copper intake might be well advised to refrain from additional supplementation in the absence of therapeutic imperatives involving depletion or deficiency status; zinc coadministration may be appropriate in some cases.

Ethambutol

Evidence: Ethambutol (Myambutol).
Extrapolated, based on similar properties: Isoniazid (isonicotinic acid hydrazide, INH; Laniazid, Nydrazid); combination drugs: isoniazid and rifampicin (Rifamate, Rimactane); isoniazid, pyrazinamide, and rifampicin (Rifater).

Interaction Type and Significance

☼   **Prevention or Reduction of Drug Adverse Effect**
◇≈≈ **Drug-Induced Adverse Effect on Nutrient Function, Coadministration Therapeutic, with Professional Management**
⊕⊕ **Beneficial or Supportive Interaction, with Professional Management**

Probability:	Evidence Base:
2. Probable	● Consensus

Effect and Mechanism of Action

The antimycobacterial agent ethambutol (EMB) forms chelate complexes with the bivalent metal ions (copper and zinc) participating in RNA biosynthesis or stabilization. Clinical research and case reports have consistently found that the optic neuropathy associated with ethambutol results from its effect on copper metabolism. Both ethambutol and its fellow antituberculosis agent isoniazid have been implicated as causes of reduced visual acuity, visual field defects, and disturbances of color vision.

Research

Findings from animal studies indicate that ethambutol alters trace-mineral metabolism through its chelating action. Binding of copper(II) and zinc(II) by 2,2'-(ethylenediimino)-dibutyric acid (EDBA), the metabolic oxidation product of dextro-2,2'-(ethylenediimino)-di-1-butanol (ethambutol), may account for many of the adverse effects of EMB treatment. In particular, ethambutol produced significant decreases in heart copper, kidney zinc, plasma zinc, and liver copper and zinc, not attributable to changes in dietary intake.[9,29]

The principal adverse effect of ethambutol is an optic neuropathy with clinical features closely paralleling a mitochondrial hereditary optic neuropathy (Leber's). As noted, EMB and isoniazid have been implicated in reduced visual acuity, visual field defects, and color vision disturbances. Research consistently indicates that chelation of copper causes EMB-induced optic neuropathy by precluding normal cytochrome-c oxidase activity and mitochondrial metabolism in the optic nerve. An in vitro study by Kozak et al.[30] (1998) suggests that if copper were given to patients to prevent EMB-induced optic neuropathy, such supportive supplementation would not compromise EMB's bacteriostatic properties against *Mycobacterium tuberculosis* and *Mycobacterium avium*. In concluding their study of 42 Congolese patients with tuberculosis receiving ethambutol treatment, Kaimbo et al.[31] emphasized the importance of color vision examinations in the detection of the complications of EMB treatment.

Nutritional Therapeutics, Clinical Concerns and Adaptations

Coadministration of copper with ethambutol may reduce adverse effects, particularly on the optic nerve and related functions, typically associated with EMB use. Monitoring of visual function is generally appropriate during ethambutol therapy. Supervision is advisable but may not be necessary because no known adverse effects are associated with concomitant copper intake. However, given the consistent evidence of EMB's copper-binding properties, individuals taking concomitant copper are advised to allow at least a 2-hour interval after taking ethambutol to avoid diminished therapeutic effect from the nutrient. The therapeutically appropriate level of copper would be 1 to 2 mg per day.

Famotidine and Related Histamine (H₂) Receptor Antagonists

Evidence: Famotidine (Pepcid, Pepcid AC, Pepcid RPD). Extrapolated, based on similar properties: Cimetidine (Tagamet, Tagamet HB), nizatidine (Axid, Axid AR), ranitidine (Zantac); combination drug: ranitidine, bismuth, and citrate (Tritec).
See also Antacids and Cimetidine.

Interaction Type and Significance

≈≈≈ **Drug-Induced Nutrient Depletion, Supplementation Therapeutic, Not Requiring Professional Management**

Probability: Evidence Base:
3. Possible   ○ **Preliminary**

Effect and Mechanism of Action

The normally acidic environment of the stomach facilitates optimal absorption of copper and other nutrients. Famotidine may induce a copper deficiency by inhibiting copper absorption and precipitating dietary copper.

Research

Famotidine may reduce absorption of copper by interfering with normal gastrointestinal (GI) physiology and function.[5,32]

Nutritional Therapeutics, Clinical Concerns, and Adaptations

Repeated use of famotidine, or other H₂ receptor antagonists (H₂RAs), over an extended period may tend to promote a deficiency of affected nutrients, such as copper. Nevertheless, evidence is lacking to support the conclusion that clinically significant adverse effects of copper deficiency due to famotidine are common. Nevertheless, individuals who regularly use famotidine, or another H₂RA medication, for an extended time may benefit from 1 to 2 mg of copper daily, possibly in the form of a multivitamin/mineral formula, taken at least 2 hours away from the drug.

Nonsteroidal Anti-Inflammatory Drugs (NSAIDs)

COX-1 inhibitors: Diclofenac (Cataflam, Voltaren); combination drug: diclofenac and misoprostol (Arthrotec); diflunisal (Dolobid), etodolac (Lodine), fenoprofen (Dalfon), furbiprofen (Ansaid), ibuprofen (Advil, Excedrin IB, Motrin, Motrin IB, Nuprin, Pedia Care Fever Drops, Provel, Rufen); combination drug: hydrocodone and ibuprofen (Reprexain, Vicoprofen); indomethacin (indometacin; Indocin, Indocin-SR), ketoprofen (Orudis, Oruvail), ketorolac (Acular ophthalmic, Toradol), meclofenamate (Meclomen), mefenamic acid (Ponstel), meloxicam (Mobic), nabumetone (Relafen), naproxen (Anaprox, Naprosyn), oxaprozin (Daypro), piroxicam (Feldene), salsalate (salicylic acid; Amigesic, Disalcid, Marthritic, Mono Gesic, Salflex, Salsitab), sulindac (Clinoril), tolmetin (Tolectin).
COX-2 inhibitor: Celecoxib (Celebrex).

Interaction Type and Significance

☼ **Prevention or Reduction of Drug Adverse Effect**
⊕ **Potential or Theoretical Beneficial or Supportive Interaction, with Professional Management**

Probability: Evidence Base:
3. Possible   ▽ **Mixed**

Effect and Mechanism of Action

Copper complexes of NSAIDs are more effective in their anti-inflammatory effect and less toxic than the parent NSAID substances. Based on these observations, Sorenson[33] proposed that copper complexes of NSAIDs are their active metabolites. However, continuing research by Berthon, Brumas, Miche, and associates indicates that the extra anti-inflammatory activity induced by copper on NSAIDs appears to be independent of any Cu(II)-NSAID association in vivo. On the contrary, the binding of inactive substances with copper(II) at inflammatory sites seems to be essential to their activation by copper. Parallel investigations suggest that the apparent copper potentiation of NSAIDS may be caused by copper interactions with endogenous histidine.[34-36]

Research

Kishore[37] reported that administration of copper aspirinate to arthritic rats for 20 days increased hepatic copper concentrations. Such animal models of inflammation have also shown that the copper chelate of aspirin is active at one-eighth the effective amount of aspirin. These copper complexes are less toxic than the parent compounds as well. Based on such findings, speculation has been raised that copper supplementation might enhance the anti-inflammatory effects of NSAIDs while reducing their ulcerogenic effects. However, the ability of NSAIDs to influence copper metabolism is still poorly understood, and apart from the proposed SOD-like activity of copper salts in vivo, knowledge is limited as to how copper-NSAID interactions participate in the regulation of the inflammatory process. Interactions between copper and anti-inflammatory medications deserve continued research, especially within the context of deepening our understanding of copper absorption and metabolism and the inflammatory responses of the immune system.

Clinical Implications and Adaptations

Copper complexes may be more active than parent NSAIDs, but concomitant copper will not necessarily result in or amplify such effects. Coadministration of 1 to 2 mg/day of copper might enhance the anti-inflammatory activity of NSAIDs while reducing potential adverse effects caused by such medications. However, such action is not based on a clear, consistent, and substantive pattern of evidence; some research questions such a conclusion. Nevertheless, the risk of adverse effects from low levels of copper intake would be negligible and probably less than the potential risk of adverse effects typically associated with use of NSAIDs.

Penicillamine and Related Chelating Agents

Deferasirox (Exjade), desferoxamine (desferrioxamine mesilate, desferoxamine mesylate; Desferal), EDTA (ethylenediaminetetraacetic acid), penicillamine (Cuprimine, Depen), tetrathiomolybdate (TM), trientine (trien, trienthylene tetramine; Syprine).

Interaction Type and Significance

◇◇   **Drug-Induced Effect on Nutrient Function, Supplementation Contraindicated, Professional Management Appropriate**

≈◇◇   **Drug-Induced Nutrient Depletion, Supplementation Contraindicated, Professional Management Appropriate**

Probability: Evidence Base:
1. Certain   ● Consensus

Effect and Mechanism of Action

Penicillamine, trientine (trienthylene tetramine), and tetrathiomolybdate are chelating agents that bind metals and carry them out of the body. Tetrathiomolybdate was initially developed as a less toxic copper chelator than penicillamine and is now considered the treatment of choice for Wilson's disease, with zinc acetate maintenance after the copper levels are sufficiently low. Oral administration of copper, as well as aluminum, iron, and magnesium salts, and possibly other minerals (e.g., calcium, zinc), may decrease the GI absorption and bioavailability of these chelating agents, and vice versa. The medication's chelation of polyvalent metal ions resulting in a nonabsorbable complex constitutes the operative mechanism.

Research

Penicillamine is used to treat people with Wilson's disease, cystinuria, and severe rheumatoid arthritis. Wilson's disease (WD) is an autosomal recessive disease that causes excessive copper deposition in the liver, basal ganglia, kidney, cornea, and other tissues, with resultant hepatic, neurological, and visual sequelae. Medical research continues to clarify the pathophysiology of WD, with major advances in recent years. The key strategy of current conventional medical treatment focuses on reducing the amount of copper in the liver and other tissues by administering both copper-chelating agents and a low-copper diet. Although major progress has been achieved in the treatment of WD, significant controversy remains as to the optimal treatment of individuals in the various stages of the disease. Specifically, the relative roles of penicillamine, trientene, and tetrathiomolybdate in the initial treatment of the symptomatic patient with WD continue to be researched, debated, and emergent.[9,38,39] Copper control using these agents has also emerged as an antiangiogenic anticancer therapy.[40,41]

Penicillamine prevents the formation or promotes the solubilization of copper-rich particles occurring in lysosomes of hepatocytes and Kupffer cells in the livers of individuals with WD. Once chelated with D-penicillamine, copper can then be excreted into urine. However, research indicates that the mobilization of copper by D-penicillamine is limited because of the binding of the metal to metallothionein in liver cytosol. This form of copper, even at relatively high concentrations, appears to be well tolerated.[42,43]

Penicillamine use is associated with numerous adverse effects, often severe, such as systemic lupus erythematosus (SLE) and nephrotic syndrome, which occur in 20% to 25% of all patients. In cases where D-penicillamine has to be withdrawn, trientine becomes the drug of choice and is generally considered to be as effective as penicillamine. Trientine is sometimes administered as a first-choice drug to individuals with neurological symptoms.[42,44]

Again, among the primary therapeutic uses of chelating agents such as penicillamine and trientine is the treatment of WD, in which toxic deposits of copper accumulate. Penicillamine is also used to treat individuals with cystinuria and severe rheumatoid arthritis.[33,38,45]

Copper also plays an essential role in promoting angiogenesis. Tumors that become angiogenic acquire the ability to enter a phase of rapid growth and exhibit increased metastatic potential, the major cause of morbidity and mortality in cancer patients. Human and animal research on breast, lung, and other cancers indicates that copper deficiency induced by chelating agents, such as tetrathiomolybdate, significantly impairs tumor growth and angiogenesis through suppression of nuclear factor kappa B (NF-κB), contributing to a global inhibition of NF-κB–mediated transcription of proangiogenic factors.[46,47] NF-κB expression is also associated with the development of both chemotherapy and radiation resistance in cancer cells.

Note: Given the high risk of teratogenicity, based on animal studies, and the known adverse effects associated with many chelating agents, Brewer et al.[48] and other researchers have investigated the treatment of WD using tetrathiomolybdate, followed by zinc monotherapy or complementary use of zinc salts, using zinc in particular during pregnancy and with children.

Clinical Implications and Adaptations

Given the therapeutic objective of reducing toxic levels of copper in the body by increasing urinary excretion of the mineral, individuals with WD should minimize dietary intake of copper and avoid consuming copper supplements of any kind, even in the small doses found in most multivitamin/mineral formulas. In individuals taking any of these chelating agents to reduce copper levels, the consumption of any supplemental copper would obviously have an adverse effect on the drug's performance.

If copper (or iron) supplementation is incidental to the consumption of other medications or supplements or therapeutically indicated in some extraordinary circumstance, substances containing such minerals should be taken 2 hours before or after penicillamine, trientine, or tetrathiomolybdate to minimize interference with the medication's effects.

Note: Clinicians should also be aware of chlorophyllin, a water-soluble copper complex of chlorophyll that is becoming increasingly popular as a nutritional supplement. Chlorophyllin has antimutagenic and anticarcinogenic properties, but it is also a source of copper and needs to be considered as part of the standard supplement inventory inquiry.

Valproic Acid and Related Anticonvulsant Medications (AEDs)

Evidence: Divalproex semisodium, divalproex sodium (Depakote), sodium valproate (Depacon), valproate semisodium, valproic acid (Depakene, Depakene Syrup).
Similar properties but evidence lacking for extrapolation: Carbamazepine (Carbatrol, Tegretol), clonazepam (Klonopin), clorazepate (Tranxene), ethosuximide (Zarontin), ethotoin

(Peganone), felbamate (Felbatol), fosphenytoin (Cerebyx, Mesantoin), levetiracetam (Keppra), mephenytoin, mephobarbital (Mebaral), methsuximide (Celontin), oxcarbazepine (GP 47680, oxycarbamazepine; Trileptal), phenobarbital (phenobarbitone; Luminal, Solfoton), phenytoin (diphenylhydantoin; Dilantin, Phenytek), piracetam (Nootropyl), primidone (Mysoline), topiramate (Topamax), trimethadione (Tridione), vigabatrin (Sabril), zonisamide (Zonegran).

Interaction Type and Significance

≈≈   **Drug-Induced Nutrient Depletion, Supplementation Therapeutic, with Professional Management**

◇≈≈ Drug-Induced Adverse Effect on Nutrient Function, Coadministration Therapeutic, with Professional Management

Probability:	Evidence Base:
4. Plausible	◉ Emerging

Effect and Mechanism of Action

Valproic acid (VPA) may induce increased excretion of copper into the bile, thereby disrupting the homeostatic balance of copper and causing abnormalities in serum copper concentration.

Research

In several studies of children with epilepsy being treated with VPA, serum copper levels remained unchanged relative to control groups.[49-53] Subsequently, however, Kaji et al.[54] investigated serum zinc and copper levels in epileptic children treated with VPA and/or other antiepileptic drugs (AEDs). They found that patients "treated with VPA monotherapy had significantly lower levels of serum Cu" than normal controls, as did those "treated with VPA in addition to some other AED," whereas those "treated with AEDs except for VPA" exhibited serum copper concentrations "not statistically different from those of control subjects." These researchers suggested that physicians should watch for potential symptoms of copper deficiency, even though none of their patients showed any symptoms of copper deficiency at the time of the study.[54] Suzuki et al.[55] reported that long-term anticonvulsant therapy could induce alterations in both the metabolism and the distribution of copper, zinc, and magnesium, and that gender was a significant factor in the resultant effects.

Clinical Implications and Adaptations

No definitive evidence has emerged as to the prevalence or clinical significance of copper depletion or deficiency resulting from valproic acid. Physicians prescribing VPA, especially in children, should consider coadministration of copper to restore proper trace-mineral balance and avoid possible deficiency. Inadequate consumption of copper through dietary sources is common. Copper (and zinc) status should be monitored, particularly in epileptic children taking valproate derivatives. Coadministration of copper at 1 to 3 mg daily may be beneficial, especially for individuals taking zinc supplements.

Zidovudine (AZT) and Related Reverse-Transcriptase Inhibitor (Nucleoside) Antiretroviral Agents

Evidence: Zidovudine (azidothymidine, AZT, ZDV, zidothymidine; Retrovir).

Extrapolated, based on similar properties: Abacavir (Ziagen), didanosine (ddI, dideoxyinosine; Videx), dideoxycytidine (ddC, zalcitabine; Hivid), lamivudine (3TC, Epivir), stavudine

(D4T, Zerit), tenofovir (Viread); zidovudine combination drugs: zidovudine and lamivudine (Combivir); abacavir, lamivudine, and zidovudine (Trizivir).

Protease inhibitors: Amprenavir (Agenerase), atazanavir (Reyataz), brecanavir, darunavir (Prezista), fosamprenavir (Lexiva), indinavir (Crixivan), nelfinavir (Viracept), ritonavir (Norvir), saquinavir (Fortovase, Invirase), tipranavir (Aptivus); combination drugs: lopinavir and ritonavir (Aluvia, Kaletra); saquinavir and ritonavir (SQV/RTV).

Interaction Type and Significance

≈≈   **Drug-Induced Nutrient Depletion, Supplementation Therapeutic, with Professional Management**

⊕   **Potential or Theoretical Beneficial or Supportive Interaction, with Professional Management**

☼   **Prevention or Reduction of Nutrient Adverse Effect**

◇   **Adverse Drug Effect on Nutritional Therapeutics, Strategic Concern**

Probability:	Evidence Base:
3. Possible	▽ Mixed

Effect and Mechanism of Action

Coadministration of zinc during AZT therapy will tend to deplete copper during extended therapy. The antagonistic relationship between copper and zinc might be a concern, given the importance of zinc for immune status.

Research

Preliminary human research by Baum et al.[56] published in 1991 suggested AZT therapy might cause decreased levels of zinc and copper along with a significant increase in red cell folate. The level of plasma zinc appeared to be particularly important in maintaining immune function in the zidovudine-treated group. Also in 1991, Graham et al.[57] reported that higher serum copper and lower serum zinc levels predicted progression to acquired immunodeficiency syndrome (AIDS) independently of baseline CD4+ lymphocyte level, age, and calorie-adjusted dietary intakes of both nutrients. Allavena et al.[58] observed alterations in parameters of several trace minerals during AZT treatment but reported that copper values were within normal limits. More recently, however, in a 2001 paper on survival in a cohort of HIV-1–infected homosexual men, Lai et al.[59] reported that although plasma zinc inadequacy or the plasma copper/zinc ratio may be useful predictors of survival in human immunodeficiency virus type 1 (HIV-1) infection, plasma levels of copper were not significantly associated with mortality. In a study involving 86 subjects with known HIV infection, Jimenez-Exposito et al.[60] found that AIDS patients with active opportunistic infection showed significantly lower serum concentrations of vitamin A and significantly higher serum concentrations of copper. They concluded that these findings were correlated with various inflammatory parameters more than with nutritional status.

Nutritional Therapeutics, Clinical Concerns, and Adaptations

The clinical significance of these findings remains unclear with regard to dietary intake of copper and potential therapeutic effects of an interaction between copper and zidovudine. Copper appears to play an important role in the immune system's inflammatory response, but no conclusive evidence has emerged indicating that copper coadministration would be therapeutically beneficial. However, any extended supplementation of zinc might induce a copper deficiency and would suggest a need for countervailing copper, 1 to 2 mg/day. Ultimately, the evidence at this point indicates the importance of monitoring nutritional status of individuals with HIV infection, whether or not they are undergoing retroviral therapy such as with zidovudine.

NUTRIENT-NUTRIENT INTERACTIONS

Iron

The metabolic pathways and functions of copper and iron are intertwined, and the minerals have many similarities and some significant interactions. Copper stimulates intestinal absorption and improves utilization of iron, whereas iron can inhibit copper absorption. Both are transition elements that can participate in redox reactions; both can also be sequestered by proteins and thus prevent undesirable redox reactions. Iron deficiency can contribute to increased concentrations of copper in tissues, and copper deposition can be a significant risk in some anticancer therapies aimed at altering iron status.

Molybdenum

Within integrative chemotherapy regimens, as well as the treatment of Wilson's disease, administration of tetrathiomolybdate, which contains molybdenum at the center of four chelating sulfhydryl groups, can serve as an effective copper-chelating agent with significantly fewer adverse effects than most conventional copper chelators.

Vitamin C

Vitamin C intake at pharmacological doses for extended periods can lead to a depletion of copper, in the absence of compensatory copper intake supplementation.

Zinc

Zinc significantly interferes with copper absorption.[61] Zinc induces intestinal cell metallothionein, which binds copper and prevents its transfer into blood. eventually the intestinal cells die and slough, taking the trapped copper with them in the stool, thus preventing intestinal absorption of copper. Prolonged intake of supplemental zinc, particularly longer than 1 month, warrants compensatory copper, except for individuals with Wilson's disease and those whose therapeutic strategy employs zinc as an anticopper agent. Copper supplements should be taken at least 2 hours after zinc supplements.

The 61 citations for this monograph, as well as additional reference literature, are located under Copper on the CD at the back of the book.

Nutrient-Drug Interactions and Drug-Induced Nutrient Depletions

Iron

Nutrient Name: Iron.

Synonyms: Iron salts; fer; ferric sulfate; ferrous carbonate anhydrous, ferrous citrate, ferrous fumarate, ferrous gluconate, ferrous glutamate, ferrous glycinate, ferrous glycine sulphate, ferrous lactate, ferrous picolinate, ferrous pyrophosphate, ferrous succinate, ferrous sulfate; carbonyl iron; iron-polysaccharide, iron dextran, iron-ovotransferrin, iron sorbitol, iron sucrose, sodium ferric gluconate.

Elemental Symbol: Fe.

Summary

Drug/Class Interaction Type	Mechanism and Significance	Management
Acetylsalicylic acid (ASA, aspirin) ☼/≈≈	Aspirin causes gastrointestinal (GI) irritation and bleeding, which may be slight but acts cumulatively with chronic use to increase risk of iron deficiency and anemia. Iron supplementation can reverse adverse hematological effects of ASA therapy.	Short-term iron may be appropriate if deficiency or depletion present; separate intake, monitor. Address dietary and lifestyle factors contributing to inflammation and pain.
Angiotensin-converting enzyme (ACE) inhibitors ◇◇/☼/⊕✗/✗✗	Coadministration of iron can abolish cough induced by ACE inhibitors, possibly by inhibiting NO synthase activity in bronchial epithelial cells. However, iron and ACE medications may bind and reduce absorption of both agents. IV iron may be appropriate in certain anemic hemodialysis patients treated with an ACE inhibitor but this treatment is controversial, complicated, and risky.	Coadminister, when indicated. Separate intake by 3 or more hours. IV iron requires active supervision by experienced provider(s), with broad antioxidant support.
Antacids and gastric acid—suppressive medications Histamine (H₂) receptor antagonists Proton pump inhibitors (PPIs) ☼/≈≈/◇◇	Inhibition of gastric acid environment can inhibit reduction of ferric iron and reduce absorption and bioavailability of dietary iron. History of GI bleeding and increased risk of iron depletion common in patient population. Some agents may bind with iron and impair absorption of either or both substances. Adverse effects on iron status may be slow to develop and difficult to assess.	Short-term iron may be appropriate if deficiency or depletion present; separate intake, monitor. Address dietary and lifestyle factors contributing to dyspepsia, GERD, and ulcers.
Bile acid sequestrants ◇◇/≈≈≈/◇	Simultaneous intake of iron and bile sequestrants may result in binding and reduced absorption due to formation of poorly absorbed chelate complexes. Drug action may be impaired with interaction. Evidence is limited and inconsistent regarding probability and significance of iron depletion.	Low risk of significant interaction if oral intake separated by at least 2 hours.
Bisphosphonates ◇◇/≈≈	Binding may occur with simultaneous intake and inhibit absorption and bioavailability of both agents. Decreased therapeutic activity probable with interaction; minimal effect with separation of intake. Limited evidence on long-term effects.	If iron is indicated, separate intake by 2 or more hours to avoid interference. Monitor iron status.
Carbidopa, levodopa Antiparkinsonian medications ◇◇/≈≈	Simultaneous intake of carbidopa or levodopa and iron (especially ferric) may result in binding and reduced absorption due to formation of poorly absorbed chelate complexes. Medication may also cause autoxidation to ferric form.	Iron may be contraindicated in this patient population. If indicated, separate intake by at least 2 hours and monitor iron status.
Cefdinir Cephalosporin antibiotics ◇◇	Chelation between cephalosporin antibiotics and iron likely to impair absorption and bioavailability of both agents if ingested concurrently. Decreased therapeutic activity with interaction; minimal effect with separation of intake. Iron depletion plausible with extended use, but not established or probable. Caution warranted regarding supplementation during infection.	Discontinue iron or separate intake during short-term therapy. Mineral supplementation may be appropriate with extended therapy but caution warranted; separate intake by several hours.
Chloramphenicol ☼/◇≈≈/◇	Chloramphenicol can inhibit erythropoiesis and red cell maturation, thus delaying or impeding iron therapy; it can also cause aplastic anemia. Dosage levels < 25-30 mg/kg are usually effective without adversely affecting bone marrow.	Discontinuation of chloramphenicol may be necessary if treating patients with anemia. Largely replaced by alternatives as a standard treatment in recent years.
Chlorhexidine ✗✗	Concurrent intake of chlorhexidine and iron may stain teeth.	If iron is indicated, separate intake by at least 2 hours to avoid interaction.
Clofibrate ◇◇/≈≈/◇	Chelation between clofibrate and iron likely to impair absorption and bioavailability of both agents if ingested concurrently.	If iron is indicated, separate intake by 3 hours to avoid interference. Monitor iron status.
Desferoxamine ☼/◇◇/✗✗	Desferoxamine is a chelating agent applied to treat overload and intoxification involving iron and other metals. It binds to iron and increases iron excretion. Intake of iron (supplemental or as iron-rich foods) is contraindicated, as contrary to the therapeutic intent.	Discontinue supplemental iron and decrease dietary intake immediately. Close supervision and monitoring necessary. Supplementation with other nutrients may be appropriate; separate intake by several hours.
Dimercaprol ✗✗✗	Dimercaprol is used as an antidote in arsenic, cadmium, lead, and mercury poisoning in inpatient settings. Iron intake during dimercaprol therapy may cause kidney damage but is often appropriate after such treatment.	Avoid supplemental iron during dimercaprol therapy. Close supervision and monitoring necessary. Supplementation with iron may be appropriate 24 hours or more following conclusion of dimercaprol.
EDTA ☼/◇◇/✗✗	EDTA is a chelating agent applied to treat overload and intoxification involving iron and other metals. It binds to iron and increases iron excretion. Intake of iron (supplemental or as	Avoid supplemental iron and decrease dietary intake. Close supervision and monitoring contrary necessary. Supplementation with

Summary

Drug/Class Interaction Type	Mechanism and Significance	Management
	iron-rich foods) is contraindicated, as opposed to the therapeutic intent. Some iron chelates containing EDTA are used for iron fortification.	iron and other nutrients may be appropriate with extended therapy; separate intake by several hours.
Erythropoiesis-stimulating agents ⊕⊕/⊕✗/✗✗/✗✗✗	Synergistic interaction often used in treatment of oncology patients with functional iron deficiency or anemia but remains controversial. Coadministration may enhance epo-induced erythropoiesis, but risk of adverse effects is significant if applied prematurely, with inadequate iron stores, during anemia of chronic inflammation, or in unstable oncology patients. Further research warranted. Iron administration in hemodialysis patients is often contraindicated, although oral heme iron may be effective.	Assess endogenous EPO level. Coadminister iron with iron deficiency if no response to initial EPO therapy, under close supervision and monitoring of iron status, especially stores. Oral forms may be safer than IV administration.
Fluoroquinolone/quinolone antibiotics ✗✗/◇◇/≈≈	Chelation between this class of antibiotics and iron likely to impair absorption and bioavailability of both agents; similarly with other minerals. Decreased therapeutic activity with interaction; minimal effect with separation of intake. Iron deficiency and effects of iron depletion plausible with extended use, but not established or probable. Iron-ovotransferrin combines directly with gut transferrin receptors and minimizes risk of binding to drug. Caution warranted regarding supplementation during infection.	Avoid iron or separate intake during short-term therapy. Iron-ovotransferrin may be most effective form. Mineral supplementation may be appropriate with extended therapy, but caution warranted regarding iron, even with established depletion; separate intake by several hours.
Hyoscyamine ≈≈/☼/◇	Hyoscyamine can impair iron absorption, but mechanism, occurrence, and clinical significance not fully elucidated. Potential for decreased therapeutic activity with simultaneous intake. Iron depletion and effects of iron depletion plausible with extended, use but not established or probable.	Iron supplementation with iron or other appropriate minerals may be appropriate with extended therapy; separate intake by several hours.
Indomethacin Nonsteroidal anti-inflammatory drugs (NSAIDs) ≈≈/◇◇/☼/⊕✗/✗	NSAIDs, especially indomethacin, can cause GI irritation and bleeding, which may be slight but acts cumulatively with chronic use to increase risk of iron deficiency and anemia. Iron supplementation can reverse adverse hematological effects of NSAID therapy.	Short-term iron may be appropriate if deficiency or depletion present; separate intake, monitor. Address dietary and lifestyle factors contributing to inflammation and pain.
Interferon alpha ✗✗✗	Iron excess can contribute to inflammatory processes, support infectious agents, and reduce response to interferon. Iron reduction can enhance positive outcomes in interferon therapy. Phlebotomy may enhance interferon therapy outcomes, as may low-iron diet.	Avoid supplemental iron and recommend low-iron, vegetarian diet. Close supervision and monitoring necessary. Phlebotomy may be appropriate.
Levothyroxine Thyroid hormones ✗✗/◇◇/≈≈/⊕⊕	Thyroid therapy may be enhanced with iron coadministration. However, simultaneously ingested thyroxine and iron likely to bind to form poorly soluble chelate complex and thereby impair absorption and bioavailability of both agents. Decreased therapeutic activity with interaction; minimal effect with separate intake. Consensus regarding probability of binding, but evidence lacking for iron depletion, plausible with extended use.	Comorbid conditions may require both agents. Separate intake by several hours to avoid binding and interference. Monitor TSH; may need to adjust dosage levels.
Methyldopa ✗✗/◇◇/≈≈	Simultaneously ingested methyldopa and iron likely to bind to form poorly soluble chelate complex and thereby impair absorption and bioavailability of both agents. Decreased antihypertensive activity probable with interaction. Decreased interference with separation of intake. However, medication may also cause autoxidation to the ferric form. Iron depletion and effects of iron depletion plausible with extended use, but not established or probable.	If iron is indicated, separate intake by at least 2 hours to avoid interference.
Neomycin ≈◇◇/⊕✗/⊕	Neomycin known to impair absorption of iron and many other nutrients; concurrent intake may alter drug activity. Clinical significance may vary depending on individual's iron status. Iron deficiency and effects of nutrient depletion probable with extended use; adverse effect improbable with short-term or topical use. Caution warranted regarding supplementation during infection.	Iron supplementation with iron or other appropriate nutrients may be appropriate with extended therapy, but caution warranted regarding iron, even with established depletion; separate intake by several hours.
Oral contraceptives (OCs) ⊕⊕/◇◇	OCs may support iron status and reduce need for supplementation by reducing menstrual blood loss. Serum ferritin, serum transferrin, serum iron, TIBC, MCH, and MCHC levels may be greater, but RBC and hematocrit levels often lower in OC users. Systemic implications of exogenous hormones, in diverse formulations and with chronic administration, on multiple levels of iron metabolism and storage not fully elucidated. Continued research into responses among variable individuals to these complex medications is warranted.	Women using OCs may have reduced need for iron supplementation, although possibly higher needs for folate and vitamins B_{12} and B_6. Individual evaluation of safe and effective hormone dosage levels necessary. Periodic assessment of serum ferritin, ferritin saturation, and/or serum transferrin receptor levels may be warranted.
Penicillamine ✗✗/◇◇/⊕✗/≈≈	Penicillamine is a chelating agent applied to treat overload and intoxification involving copper, iron, and other metals. It binds to iron and increases iron excretion. Intake of iron (supplemental or as iron-rich foods) can bind medication doses when ingested concurrently. However, abrupt discontinuation of ongoing iron intake may lead to rapid elevation in circulating penicillamine levels and resultant nephrotoxicity. Iron intake may also be contraindicated, as opposed to the therapeutic intent, i.e., copper chelation.	Avoid concurrent iron and dietary intake; tapered reduction needed in discontinuing supplemental iron. Close supervision and monitoring necessary. Supplementation with iron and other nutrients may be appropriate with extended therapy if depletion detected; separate intake by several hours.
Sulfasalazine ◇◇/≈≈/◇	When ingested concurrently, iron can bind to sulfasalazine, interfering with its breakdown into 5-aminosalicylic acid (5ASA) and sulfapyridine. This pharmacokinetic interaction can reduce absorption, bioavailability, and therapeutic activity of the prodrug, its constituents, and the nutrient, but can be minimized by separation of intake. Iron	Separate intake by several hours to avoid binding and interference. Iron supplementation may be warranted if bleeding, anemia, and/or iron depletion established,

Continued

Nutrient-Drug Interactions and Drug-Induced Nutrient Depletions

Summary

Drug/Class Interaction Type	Mechanism and Significance	Management
	depletion possible with extended use, particularly in patient population with ulceration and GI bleeding, but not established.	but caution is appropriate to avoid aggravating inflammation.
Tetracycline antibiotics ◇◇/≈≈/◇	Chelation between iron and tetracycline-class antibiotics and impaired absorption of both to clinically significant degree probable with concurrent intake. Iron intake, even small amounts, can significantly impair antimicrobial activity. General consensus despite minimal direct evidence. Iron depletion with extended tetracycline use but evidence lacking. Caution warranted regarding supplementation during infection.	Discontinue iron (including iron-rich foods) or separate intake during short-term therapy. Iron supplementation may be appropriate with extended therapy, but caution warranted, even with established depletion; separate intake by several hours.
Trientine ✗✗/◇◇/⊕✗/≈≈	Trientine is a chelating agent applied to treat copper overload and toxicity, particularly in Wilson's disease. Simultaneous ingestion with iron likely to bind to form poorly soluble chelate complex and thereby impair absorption and bioavailability of both agents. Anemia is common adverse effect of trientine due to increased iron excretion, as well as decreased iron absorption, with children, menstruating women, and pregnant women at greatest risk.	Separate intake by several hours to avoid binding and interference. Iron supplementation may be warranted if anemia and/or iron depletion established; separate intake by several hours.

NO, Nitric oxide; *IV*, intravenous; *GERD*, gastroesophageal reflux disease; *EPO*, erythropoietin; *TSH*, thyroid-stimulating hormone; *TIBC*, total iron-binding capacity; *MCH*, mean corpuscular hemoglobin; *MCHC*, MCH concentration; *RBC*, red blood cell.

NUTRIENT DESCRIPTION

Chemistry and Forms

Oxidation states: Ferric (Fe^{3+}) iron, ferrous (Fe^{2+}) iron. Heme and nonheme.

Physiology and Function

Iron is an essential mineral that plays a vital role in numerous essential biochemical pathways. The principal functions of iron involve DNA synthesis and cell formation, oxygen sensing and cellular uptake, oxygen transport and storage within blood and muscle, electron transfer and the conversion of glucose to adenosine triphosphate (ATP), both antioxidant and beneficial pro-oxidant functions, and regulation of intracellular iron. Within the human body, iron occurs primarily in functional forms, such as proteins, particularly hemoglobin and myoglobin, and in transport and storage forms, such as transferrin, ferritin, and hemosiderin. Iron is also a constituent of numerous enzymes, amino acids, hormones, and neurotransmitters. Iron is a key component of enzymes responsible for oxidative phosphorylation and ATP generation in the mitochondria and for synthesis of serotonin and dopamine. Iron is essential for the synthesis of carnitine, a critical compound in fatty acid metabolism, and for the operation of the cytochrome P450 system and other cytochromes. It also acts as a cofactor in the synthesis of collagen and elastin.

Iron absorption is highly dependent on maintenance of the normal biochemical environment and coordination of upper gastrointestinal (GI) function. Iron must be in ferrous form to be absorbed. When iron is found in meat, it is in the *heme* form. When the source of iron is from plants or from animal products such as milk, eggs, and cheese, it is referred to as *nonheme* iron. In the heme form, once it is cleaved from the food, iron may be converted to hemin (Fe^{3+}), which can be directly absorbed intact by the mucosal cell into the blood. Absorption of heme iron is about 10 times that of nonheme iron, depending on whether body stores are replete. In the nonheme form, iron must be cleaved from its food source, then reduced from the ferric to the ferrous form, facilitated by gastric hydrochloric acid, before it can be absorbed. Likewise, ascorbic acid, found in foods and supplements, increases absorption by keeping the ferrous form from oxidizing to ferric in the gastric environment. Iron absorption is a slow process, taking between 2 and 4 hours, and occurring principally in the duodenum and proximal jejunum. Iron is absorbed from the small intestine in different forms at 5% to 15% of intake. Absorption percentages, as opposed to excretion, are largely responsible for regulation of body iron content and respond to levels of body iron stores. Thus, low body iron levels lead to improved absorption.

Iron is oxidized back to ferric state for transport and then transported within the mucosal cell and in the blood bound to the protein transferrin. Transferrin is usually saturated to about one-third its total iron-binding capacity (TIBC). If no iron is needed, transferrin remains saturated and less is absorbed from the intestinal mucosal cells. The transferrin that remains in the cells eventually is sloughed away with the mucosal cells at the end of their 2- to 3-day life cycle. If iron is needed, the transferrin is less saturated when it reaches the intestinal mucosal cells, and more iron passes from the mucosal cell to the transferrin. Thus, the degree of saturation of transferrin is also used as a measurement of body stores of iron. Iron is stored in the liver, spleen, and bone marrow as ferritin and hemosiderin. The normal human body contains 3 to 4 grams of iron (40-50 mg/kg body weight), 75% of which (~ 36 mg/kg) is present in metabolically active compounds. A storage pool maintains the remaining 25% (~ 10 mg/kg in men and ~ 5 mg/kg in menstruating women) in a form that is readily available for use if metabolically active iron is depleted for any reason.

The body's capacity to eliminate iron is limited and, once absorbed, largely occurs through blood loss. Under normal conditions, the largest loss of iron is through bleeding in menstruating women; although considerably greater than other channels, these iron losses vary widely from individual to individual. Very small amounts of iron are also excreted through sweat and normal exfoliation of hair, skin, and nails. Most iron expelled in the feces is nonabsorbed iron from dietary intake.

Hemoglobin and myoglobin are proteins involved in the transport and storage of oxygen that contain heme, an iron-based compound. *Hemoglobin* is the primary protein responsible for oxygen transport in red blood cells (RBCs) and constitutes approximately two thirds of the iron in the human body. Hemoglobin functions to acquire oxygen efficiently and rapidly during its short contact in oxygenated lung tissue, transporting that oxygen from the lungs throughout the circulatory system and releasing it as needed into the target tissues. *Myoglobin* is the primary protein responsible for oxygen transport and regulation of short-term oxygen storage within myocytes and for the coordination of oxygen influx with the physiological demands of muscle function. Iron's ability to shift between its ferrous or reduced state (Fe^{2+}) and its oxidized ferric state (Fe^{3+}) enables it to hold or release oxygen and empowers its functional activity in electron transport and energy production.

Iron plays a critical role in the body's ability to sense oxygen and dynamically respond to variable conditions. Prolyl hydroxylase is an iron-dependent enzyme that participates in regulating the body's response to hypoxic conditions, such as high altitude or impaired function caused by lung disease. In particular, hypoxia inducible factors (HIFs) are transcription factors that respond to decreases in cellular oxygen tension characteristic of hypoxic conditions, by binding to genetic response elements that encode various proteins involved in compensatory responses to hypoxia, and increase their synthesis. Thus, in response to cellular oxygen tension, prolyl hydroxylase will either rapidly degrade HIF-alpha subunits or bind them to HIF-beta subunits to create an active transcription factor capable of entering the nucleus and binding to specific response elements on genes.

Iron, in both heme and nonheme forms, is part of several enzymes involved in electron transport, cellular energy production, and cellular detoxification. Cytochromes are heme-containing compounds critical to mitochondrial electron transport in the synthesis of ATP. In the liver the cytochrome P450 family of enzymes, in particular, metabolizes a wide range of biological molecules and exogenous toxins, including detoxification and metabolism of pharmaceuticals. NADH dehydrogenase and succinate dehydrogenase are among several enzymes containing nonheme iron involved in energy metabolism. Iron is also prominent in the synthesis of carnitine, an amino acid that plays an essential role in the metabolism of fatty acids. Thus, in a state of iron deficiency, an individual will fatigue more readily because of inadequate accessible oxygen and impaired synthesis of ATP.

Iron is well known for its tendency to cause oxidative damage, but it is also part of the antioxidant enzymes *catalase* and *peroxidase,* which serve to quench potentially damaging reactive oxygen species (ROS). These heme-containing enzymes catalyze the conversion of hydrogen peroxide to water and oxygen and thus prevent its buildup within cells. *Myeloperoxidase,* another heme-containing enzyme, catalyzes neutrophils to synthesize hypochlorous acid, an ROS, to be used within the immune system's response to pathogenic bacteria.

Iron is intimately involved in a number of other physiological and biochemical processes at cellular and systemic levels. DNA synthesis requires the activities of ribonucleotide reductase, an iron-dependent enzyme. Iron storage and metabolism are managed by key proteins within self-regulatory processes coded by short sequences of nucleotides found in the messenger RNA (mRNA), known as "iron response elements," in response to changing iron storage levels. In particular, *iron regulatory proteins* (IRPs) can bind to iron response elements and affect mRNA translation, thereby regulating the synthesis of specific proteins. Thus, iron binds to IRPs to a greater or lesser degree, depending on iron supply to influence relative levels of ferritin, the central iron storage protein; translation of mRNA that regulates enzymatic control of heme synthesis in immature RBCs; and synthesis of transferrin receptors. Iron is

also a constituent of the enzymes that initiate the synthesis of serotonin and dopamine. Lastly, iron is essential in the synthesis of collagen and elastin.

NUTRIENT IN CLINICAL PRACTICE
Known or Potential Therapeutic Uses

Treatment of iron deficiency anemia constitutes the dominant use of supplemental iron within conventional medicine. Standard practice recognizes the increased risks of iron depletion associated with menstrual blood loss but typically responds only reactively and in the narrowest sense of anemia. Modern schools of natural medicine more often recognize the potential value of iron-rich foods and botanical preparations as a tonic therapy within a comprehensive strategy.

Historical/Ethnomedicine Precedent

In the classical medical tradition of Western culture, iron was considered the metal of Mars, and associated with vitality, the qualities of heat and fire, the blood, and inflammatory processes. Historically, traditions of natural medicine have emphasized enhancement of iron intake as part of a broader approach toward enriching the blood through provision of multiple minerals within the context of single herbs, herbal formulae, and nutrient-rich foods. Herbal formulae that "build the blood" have played central roles within many classical and folk herbal traditions around the world, especially in conjunction with strategies to regulate the menstrual cycle and improve hormonal balance, treat or prevent fatigue, and improve stamina and fertility.

Possible Uses

Alzheimer's disease, anemia, athletic performance (with deficiency only), attention deficit–hyperactivity disorder (ADHD), canker sores, celiac disease (with deficiency only), childhood cognitive development (with deficiency), cough, depression (with deficiency), dermatitis herpetiformis, human immunodeficiency virus (HIV) support, infertility (female) (with deficiency only), iron deficiency anemia, lactation support, menorrhagia (heavy menstruation) (with deficiency only), presurgery and postsurgery support (with deficiency, or after major surgery), pregnancy and postpartum support, restless legs syndrome (with deficiency).

Deficiency Symptoms

Iron deficiency is the most common nutrient deficiency in the United States (U.S.) and the world. Mild degrees of iron deficiency are common in U.S. toddlers, teenage girls, and women of childbearing age, although full-fledged iron deficiency anemia remains rare.[1] Most cases of iron deficiency appear according to well-known patterns of susceptibility, malnutrition, depletion, and exacerbation. Nevertheless, because of the numerous risk factors associated with excess iron intake, use of supplemental iron to prevent or treat any of these patterns associated with iron deficiency must be assessed based on individual characteristics, needs, and susceptibilities.

Although iron deficiency is the primary nutritional disorder among humans and perhaps the most studied form of nutritional deficit within conventional medicine, a comprehensive and coherent understanding of its effects and influences, both frank and subtle, immediate and long-term, is just beginning to emerge into a coherent and comprehensive model. Iron deficiency anemia is the most overt and well-known symptom of iron deficiency. However, several gradations of iron depletion, including stages below the threshold and before the appearance of overt pathology, may contribute to physiological dysfunction and adversely affect quality of life. Thus, contrary to common assumptions, an individual does not have to be anemic to be iron deficient.[2] Furthermore, it is also critical to remember that iron deficiency anemia is not the only form of anemia, that other forms of anemia tend to appear in the same population(s), and that factors other than iron status contribute to iron deficiency anemia. In particular, folate and vitamin B_{12} status, as well as confounding factors such as drug-induced depletion patterns, must be considered to adequately diagnose suspected anemia.

Cellular responses to iron deprivation are poorly understood. Emerging evidence indicates that iron deficiency reprograms cellular genetic expression. Puig, Askeland, and Thiele[3] found that a deficiency of iron altered the expression of more than 80 genes in *Saccharomyces cerevisiae* (yeast) cells, which were chosen because of the similarity of their genome to that of humans. They observed that Cth2, a protein overproduced by iron-deficient cells, binds to the mRNA of over 80 genes and targets it for degradation or destruction by specifically down-regulating mRNAs encoding proteins that participate in many iron-dependent processes. Through this proposed mechanism, iron deficiency controls a posttranscriptional regulatory process that coordinately drives widespread metabolic reprogramming. The authors concluded: "We discovered that iron deprivation actually reprograms the metabolism of the entire cell. Literally hundreds of proteins require iron to carry out their proper function, so without this nutrient, there is a complete reorganization of how cellular processes occur."[3]

Iron deficiency may be modeled in the following three levels of increasing severity[4,5]:

1. Storage iron depletion. Tissue iron stores are depleted, but the functional iron supply is not limited.
2. Early functional iron deficiency. The supply of functional iron is low enough to impair RBC formation, but not sufficiently low to cause measurable anemia.
3. Iron deficiency anemia. Available iron is insufficient to support normal RBC formation, resulting in the microcytic and hypochromic anemia characteristic of iron deficiency. Both inadequate oxygen delivery due to anemia and suboptimal function of iron-dependent enzymes can produce symptoms at this more severe stage of iron deficiency.

Most of symptoms associated with iron deficiency result from the associated anemia; these include fatigue, weakness, pallor, tachycardia, palpitations, dyspnea on exertion, decreased endurance, and excess lactic acid production. Reduced hemoglobin and myoglobin levels associated with iron deficiency will impair physical exertion capacity and athletic performance by limiting oxygen delivery to tissues, reducing oxidative metabolism in mitochondria, diminishing mitochondrial content of cytochromes and other iron-dependent enzymes, and undercutting electron transport and ATP synthesis. Nonhematological effects resulting from iron deficiency include glossitis, taste bud atrophy, canker sores, nail spooning (koilonychia), brittle nails, hair loss, diminished immune function and increased susceptibility to infection, impaired intellectual performance, neurological dysfunction, and increased sensitivity to chill. Plummer-Vinson syndrome, characterized by the formation of webs of tissue in the throat

and esophagus and difficulty swallowing, can occur in some advanced cases, possibly corresponding to a genetic predisposition. Children may also manifest behavioral disturbances such as attention deficit–hyperactivity disorder (ADHD) and breath-holding spells. Restless legs syndrome, initial seizure, pica, and pagophagia (excessive ice consumption, characterized in particular by chewing of ice) have also been associated with iron deficiency. Fatigue, weakness, anorexia, and pica may be caused by tissue depletion of iron-containing enzymes and not by decreased levels of blood hemoglobin.

Conditions contributing to iron deficiency, particularly from blood loss or malabsorption, include diarrhea, ulcers, ulcerative colitis, Crohn's disease, celiac disease, parasitic infections, hemorrhoids, GI cancers, menorrhagia, accidents, injuries, and surgery. Other factors influencing iron absorption and deficiency include hydrochloric acid secretion and gastric pH, decreased dietary intake, blood loss (both internal and external, as in menorrhagia), calcium intake, caffeine intake, high–phytic acid fiber foods, vitamin A, genetic variability, and iron storage levels.

Populations particularly at risk for compromised iron status include infants and children, age 6 months to 4 years, especially those living in inner cities or other impoverished circumstances; rapidly growing adolescents, especially females after menarche; pregnant women; individuals with acute or chronic blood loss due to medication-induced ulcers or intestinal parasites; frequent blood donors; individuals, especially children, with *Helicobacter pylori* infection (even without GI bleeding); populations exposed to environmental contaminants, especially lead; and individuals who engage in regular, intense exercise, particularly daily endurance training. All these factors are exacerbated in the context of ongoing menstrual cycles; menstruating women require approximately twice as much iron intake as men to replace their monthly losses due to menses. Although iron deficiency is not usually caused by a lack of iron in the diet alone, vegan or vegetarian diet or dietary intake may increase the risk of deficiency because of less relative bioavailability of iron from plant versus animal sources, at least in some individuals. Nutriture status of all nutrients, including iron, is compromised with poverty or lifestyle choices characterized by high intake of processed and refined foods or other forms of malnutrition.

Dietary Sources

The hemoglobin and myoglobin consumed within meat, poultry, oysters, and fish are the primary sources of heme iron in the diet. Approximately 40% of the iron in animal foods is heme iron and 60% is nonheme iron. Heme iron provides up to one third of total absorbed dietary iron, even though it accounts for only 10% to 15% of the iron potentially available in the diet. Nonheme iron is an inorganic compound, less easily absorbed, and derived from plant foods, dairy products, dried fruit, molasses, leafy green vegetables, and wine. Overall, absorption of heme iron can be up to 10 times that of nonheme iron, depending on whether body stores are replete. In the U.S., most grain products are fortified with iron. Iron fortification of cereal, using microencapsulated ferrous fumarate flakes, appears to achieve high iron bioavailability and can serve as an effective means of enhancing hemoglobin nutriture for infants and children.[6]

Many foods, beverages, and supplements have been shown to affect the bioavailability and absorption of iron. Foods that contain heme iron usually also provide nonheme iron, and the presence of the heme iron will enhance absorption of nonheme iron within the same foods or from foods consumed concurrently. In contrast to heme iron, the absorption of which is influenced less by other dietary factors, the absorption of nonheme iron is strongly influenced by enhancers and inhibitors ingested at the same time. Iron absorption, especially nonheme iron, can be inhibited by concomitant intake of *phytate* (phytic acid, as found in unleavened wheat products, whole-wheat bran, wheat germ, oats, some rye crackers, nuts, beans, cacao powder, vanilla extract, and many other high-fiber foods), *tannins* (found in tea and coffee), *polyphenols* (as in green tea, rosemary, and red wine), calcium-rich foods, soy protein, and egg yolk. Conversely, the absorption of nonheme iron is also enhanced by concurrent ingestion of various organic acids, particularly ascorbic acid, but also citric, malic, tartaric, and lactic acids. Certain soy-containing foods (e.g., tofu, miso, tempeh), some soy sauces, vitamin A, and alcohol (other than red wine) can also increase iron absorption. In general, iron absorption from all forms may be influenced most by relative iron nutriture and storage status.

Ferrous salts are more efficiently absorbed than ferric salts. Acidic foods (e.g., tomato sauce) cooked in iron cookware may also provide a source of dietary iron, although not necessarily the optimal form. Alcohol, but not red wine, can increase the absorption of ferric, but not ferrous, iron.

Nutrient Preparations Available

Ferrous citrate, ferrous fumarate, ferrous gluconate, ferrous glutamate, ferrous glycinate, ferrous glycine sulfate, ferrous lactate, ferrous picolinate, ferrous succinate, ferrous sulfate; carbonyl iron; ferric sulfate.

A number of supplemental iron preparations are available, and different forms provide different proportions of elemental iron, with differing bioavailability characteristics. Ferrous fumarate is 33% elemental iron, ferrous sulfate (monohydrate) 33%, ferrous sulfate (heptahydrate) 23%, and ferrous gluconate 12% elemental iron. In general, absorption of elemental iron is very poor. Ferrous iron is much better absorbed than ferric iron. Heme iron is far better absorbed than nonheme. Absorption of organic chelates is probably the next highest, followed by organic salts (e.g., ferrous gluconate). Inorganic salts (e.g., ferrous sulfate) are the least well absorbed.

Diverse users absorb, tolerate, and respond to the various forms of iron to varying degrees and with differential responses. Iron supplements can be challenging to those who need to take them because when isolated, the nutrient is not easy to digest and can readily lead to nausea, constipation, or both. Nonheme iron is the predominant type of iron present in nutritional supplements. Ferrous forms (usually as the sulfate, gluconate, or fumarate salt) are readily absorbed without the need for acid. Although ferrous sulfate is the form of nonheme iron used most frequently, ferrous succinate is more often recommended. Ferrous fumarate and iron-EDTA may be more bioavailable than ferrous sulfate, particularly in individuals with low (or impaired) gastric acidity. Enteric coating is sometimes used with ferrous sulfate to delay tablet dissolution and moderate adverse effects, but bioavailability may be compromised. Combining iron with certain mineral-rich herbs, such as yellow dock (*Rumex crispus*), dandelion root (*Taraxacum officinale*), alfalfa leaf (*Medicago sativa*), and nettles tops (*Urtica dioica*), may enhance absorption, buffer irritant effects, and expand the nutritive effect beyond iron alone.

Dosage Forms Available

Capsule; capsule, time-release; liquid; tablet.

Intravenous (IV) iron forms: Iron dextran (DexFerrum, Imferon), iron sucrose (Venofer), sodium ferric gluconate (Ferrlecit).

Source Materials for Nutrient Preparations

Most are inorganic and organic salts, chelates, and synthetic polymeric matrices. Botanical extracts of iron-rich plants. Some heme iron concentrates have been used in clinical trials, but generally are not commercially available.

Dosage Range

The doses of iron discussed in this monograph represent elemental iron unless stated otherwise.

Adult

Dietary: In the U.S. the average adult daily diet of premenopausal and postmenopausal women provides 12 mg/day and of pregnant women about 15 mg/day. In the United Kingdom (U.K.) the average daily dietary intake for adult women is 12.9 mg/day. For men in the U.S. the average adult daily diet provides 16 to 18 mg elemental iron daily; in the U.K., 14.5 mg. Supplemental/Maintenance:

Men: 8 mg/day
Women, nonpregnant, nonlactating, age 19 to 50 years: 18 mg/day
Women, age 19 to 51 and older: 8 mg/day

During pregnancy, the metabolic needs of the developing fetus and placenta, as well as a significant expansion of blood volume, increase iron utilization. Conversely, iron requirements are potentially reduced during pregnancy by cessation of menstruation and increased efficiency of absorption. Consequently, iron intake may not need to be any greater than for other adult women, and routine iron supplementation is not necessarily required in pregnancy. Nevertheless, within context of care by a qualified health care professional, pregnant women may benefit from iron supplementation during the last 3 to 6 months of pregnancy. In particular, prenatal prophylactic iron supplementation before 20 weeks' gestation may help pregnant women increase the birth weight of their infants.[7] Iron status should be monitored in all pregnant women.

In general, routine supplementation of iron on a daily basis is not recommended. It is generally advised that use of iron supplements be avoided unless clinically indicated, such as low serum ferritin or microcytic, hypochromic anemia. Excess iron has been implicated in free-radical damage. These cautions do not extend consumption of iron-rich foods in moderation for most individuals. Notably, the dietary iron intake of the majority of premenopausal and pregnant women in the U.S. is lower than the recommended dietary allowance (RDA) and the dietary intake of many men is greater than the RDA. Many multivitamin-mineral preparations contain 18 mg of iron, which may result in excessive iron intake for certain individuals. Pharmacological/Therapeutic: 10 to 200 mg/day.

In treatment of iron deficiency, 100 mg/day is a common recommended amount for an adult; dosage is generally reduced after the frank deficiency is corrected. Administration of therapeutic levels is generally recommended for 3 to 4 months after correction of iron deficiency anemia, to replace iron stores. Toxic: 100 mg/day (in absence of iron deficiency).

The tolerable upper intake level (UL) for iron is 45 mg/day for non-iron-deficient adolescents and adults over age 14 years, including pregnant and breastfeeding women, according to standards set by the Food and Nutrition Board (FNB) of the U.S. Institute of Medicine. This UL is based on the prevention of GI distress and is generally understood not to apply to individuals being treated with iron under supervision of a qualified health care professional.

Pediatric (<18 Years)

Dietary (AI, adequate intake):

Infants, birth to 6 months: 0.27 mg/day (AI, adequate intake)
Infants, 7 to 12 months: 11 mg/day (AI)
Children, 1 to 3 years: 7 mg/day (AI)
Children, 4 to 8 years: 10 mg/day (AI)
Children, 9 to 13 years: 8 mg/day (AI)
Adolescents, 14 to 18 years: 15 mg/day (for females); 11 mg/day (for males)

Supplemental/Maintenance: Otherwise-healthy infants born without iron deficiency benefit from iron supplementation, according to the findings of an intervention trial.[8]
Pharmacological/Therapeutic: 10 to 50 mg/day, depending on body weight, condition, and other individual factors, under medical supervision.
Toxic: 2.0 to 2.5 g can be lethal in a 10-kg child. Deaths in children have occurred from ingesting as little as 200 mg to as much as 5.85 g of iron.[9]

Laboratory Values

Current diagnostic markers for iron deficiency are not highly sensitive, unless the deficiency is severe. Bone marrow iron is often considered the "gold standard" of iron stores but is rarely practical in most clinical situations. Serum ferritin concentration provides the most accurate diagnostic method to assess iron stores and confirm iron deficiency, but only if the values are low. Iron deficiency can accompany elevated serum ferritin levels when acute or chronic inflammatory states are present, because ferritin is one of the acute-phase reactants.

One can traditionally obtain a serum iron and serum iron-binding capacity and divide the former by the latter to determine the transferrin saturation. If iron/iron-binding capacity is less than 10%, there is a probability of iron deficiency. A more modern approach to this diagnosis is to measure the serum ferritin; iron deficiency can usually be excluded as a diagnosis if serum ferritin is more than 220 μg/L. However, if it is less than 220, it is judicious to obtain a serum transferrin receptor (sTfR) level. This measures the soluble receptors of transferrin in the circulation, receptors that bind to the available iron. If this value is 28 mg/L or higher, there is a significant probability of iron deficiency.[10] Ongoing developments in knowledge of how iron deficiency influences cellular genetic expression may soon provide diagnostic markers of increased sensitivity by pinpointing the genes affected by iron deprivation to provide a genetic fingerprint of how varying levels of iron deprivation are expressed in different patients.[3]

It is often necessary to assess ferritin, percentage transferrin saturation, and sTfR levels for an accurate assessment of iron status, because ferritin can be falsely elevated by a number of conditions, including pregnancy, inflammatory conditions (e.g., arthritis), malignancy, skin conditions, irritable bowel disease, and acute/chronic infections, both viral and bacterial.

Areas to exclude as causes of anemia include iron deficiency anemia, nutritional anemias due to B_{12} and folic acid deficiency, drug-induced anemia, alcohol-induced bone marrow toxicity, acute and chronic hemolysis, other illnesses affecting RBC production, and malignant infiltration of the bone marrow.

Serum Ferritin
Normal: 12 to 200 μg/L.

Serum ferritin is the measure of iron status that provides the most accurate indicator of tissue stores and can serve as an effective screening tool. However, it can be elevated with inflammation or infection independent of iron status. Serum ferritin greater than 225 μg/L can generally be interpreted as ruling out iron deficiency anemia. When serum ferritin is less than 220 μg/L, the soluble transferrin receptor (sTfR) level can be used to determine if the patient has upregulated transferrin receptors. Some practitioners of natural therapeutics recommend that males ideally should not have a ferritin level much more than 80 μg/L, unless they are actively engaged in strenuous athletic training or exercise regimens, to minimize iron-catalyzed oxidative stress.

Serum Iron
Normal: 9 to 29 mmol/L.

Serum iron provides an insensitive indicator of iron status, declining only after tissue stores are completely exhausted.

Transferrin Saturation
Transferrin saturation of less than 16% of available binding sites indicates iron deficiency.

Some practitioners of natural therapeutics recommend that transferrin saturation not be greater than 45%, especially with a history of heart disease, diabetes, or cancer. Transferrin saturations greater than 60% are highly suggestive of hereditary hemochromatosis, or another form of iron overload, and should be thoroughly investigated with genotyping and/or liver biopsy to assess hepatic iron stores.

Serum Transferrin Receptor
Also known as soluble transferrin receptor (sTfR). Levels greater than 8 mg/L indicate deficiency in standard diagnostic usage. However, some experienced practitioners of nutritional therapeutics use 28 mg/L as the level for demarcating iron deficiency. Values greater than 28 mg/L are also consistent with iron deficiency with corrections for altitude.

Measurement of serum transferrin receptor is a new marker of iron metabolism that reflects body iron stores and total erythropoiesis. Unlike serum ferritin, the sTfR is not an acute-phase reactant, so it is not elevated in response to acute or chronic inflammatory disease.[10] Thus, it serves as a reliable marker of iron status when iron deficiency is associated with chronic disorders, such as inflammation, infection, or malignancy. In situations of iron deficiency, the avidity and number of soluble transferrin receptors (i.e., sTfR) increases in proportion to tissue iron deficit. Thus, soluble TfR levels are decreased in situations characterized by diminished erythropoietic activity and are increased when erythropoiesis is stimulated by hemolysis or ineffective erythropoiesis. Measurements of sTfR are very helpful in investigating the pathophysiology of anemia, quantitatively evaluating the absolute rate of erythropoiesis and the adequacy of marrow proliferative capacity for any given degree of anemia, and to monitor the erythropoietic response to various forms of therapy, in particular allowing one to predict the response early, when changes in hemoglobin are not yet apparent. Iron status also influences sTfR levels, which are considerably elevated in iron deficiency anemia but remain normal in the anemia of inflammation, and thus may be particularly valuable in the differential diagnosis of microcytic anemia, especially when identifying concomitant iron deficiency in a patient with inflammation, because ferritin values are then generally normal. Elevated sTfR levels are also the characteristic feature of functional iron deficiency, a situation defined by tissue iron deficiency despite adequate iron stores. The sTfR/ferritin ratio can thus describe iron availability over a wide range of iron stores. With the exception of chronic lymphocytic leukemia (CLL), high-grade non-Hodgkin's lymphoma, and possibly hepatocellular carcinoma, sTfR levels are not increased independent of iron status in patients with malignancies.[11]

Erythrocyte Protoporphyrin

Recent research indicates that erythrocyte protoporphyrin (EP) can provide a useful screening tool for determining iron deficiency. Using the receiver operating characteristic (ROC) curve to characterize the sensitivity and specificity of hemoglobin and EP measurements in screening for iron deficiency, Mei et al.[12] found EP "consistently better than measurements of hemoglobin for detecting iron deficiency" in preschool children, age 1 to 5 years. However, in nonpregnant women, they found "no significant difference between EP and hemoglobin in ROC performance for detecting iron deficiency."

SAFETY PROFILE
Overview

Adverse effects resulting from ingestion of iron supplements occur frequently and often manifest with common dosage levels. However, iron toxicity is relatively rare and predominantly occurs acutely as a result of overdose. In the U.S., iron is the leading cause of accidental poisonings in children. In response, child-resistant safety packaging is legally required for all iron-containing products. Even so, the incidence of iron poisonings in young children increased dramatically in 1986. Many of these children obtained the iron from a child-resistant container opened by themselves or another child, or left open or improperly closed by an adult.[13]

Nutrient Adverse Effects
General Adverse Effects

In adults, early symptoms of supplemental iron toxicity include GI irritation, nausea, vomiting, and abdominal pain. Constipation is the most frequently reported adverse effect associated with some forms of iron, even when therapeutically indicated, and may lead to fecal impaction, particularly in the elderly. Conversely, an exacerbation of diarrhea can occur in individuals with inflammatory bowel disease and may be accompanied by bleeding. Liquid iron preparations may blacken the teeth. Signs and symptoms of overload include grayish skin, headache, shortness of breath, fatigue, dizziness, and weight loss. More advanced toxic effects associated with acute excessive iron intake include weakness, fatigue, pallor, arrhythmia, tachycardia, cardiovascular collapse, cyanosis, seizures, and coma.

Intravenous iron, administered in some cases of severe anemia in an inpatient setting, can lead to headache, fever, lymphadenopathy, joint pain and inflammation, hives, exacerbation of rheumatoid arthritis, hemolytic reactions (often associated with acute back pain and renal injury), and (rarely) anaphylaxis.

Adverse Effects Among Specific Populations

Individuals with insulin resistance syndrome, diabetes, or hepatitis C may be particularly susceptible to iron overload. Iron overload triples mortality in people with elevated transferrin saturation.[14]

Supplementing iron can be quite dangerous for individuals with hereditary hemochromatosis, hemosiderosis, polycythemia, iron-loading anemias, and other conditions involving excessive storage of iron. Excessive absorption of iron from dietary sources may occur in response to excessive formation of red blood cells. *Hereditary hemochromatosis* (HH) is a genetic disorder that affects up to 1 in 200 individuals of northern European descent and is characterized by increased intestinal absorption of iron leading to progressive deposition of iron-containing pigments in the liver and other tissues. If untreated, tissue iron accumulation may lead to bronzing of skin, cirrhosis, cardiomyopathies, diabetes, conduction irregularities, testicular atrophy, and arthritis. The HFE gene and the mutation resulting in HH were identified in 1996, but the precise role of the protein encoded by the HFE gene in intestinal iron absorption has yet to be fully elucidated.[15,16] Supplemental iron is generally contraindicated in individuals with HH, but they are usually not advised to avoid iron-rich foods, depending on their degree of iron overload at diagnosis and their response to iron unloading on repeated phlebotomies. Sub-Saharan African hemochromatosis is a variant that appears to require both high iron intake and an as-yet unidentified genetic factor.[17]

Hemosiderosis is characterized by excessive iron deposits in hemosiderin, the normal iron storage protein. Long-term use of iron at high dosage levels can cause hemosiderosis that clinically resembles hemochromatosis.

Patients with sideroblastic anemia, pyruvate kinase deficiency, thalassemia major, and similar conditions are particularly at risk of iron overload when treated for anemia with numerous transfusions. Iron overload is significantly less common in individuals with hereditary spherocytosis and thalassemia minor, unless they are administered excessive amounts of iron after being misdiagnosed as iron deficient. Emerging information suggests the existence of a Mediterranean form of hemochromatosis, not involving the HFE gene, and with a genetic association unknown at this time, distinct from HH and thalassemias. Treatment for iron overload is by phlebotomy, typically weekly removal of 500 mL of blood until mild iron deficiency is induced. Transfusion-dependent states, however, require iron chelation, generally with regular overnight subcutaneous infusions of deferoxamine mesylate (Desferal).

In a randomized, placebo-controlled trial involving children age 1 to 35 months living in Zanzibar, Sazawal et al.[18] found that "supplementation with iron and folic acid in preschool children in a population with high rates of malaria can result in an increased risk of severe illness and death." Routine prophylactic iron supplementation in such situations should be avoided pending further research. However, within the context of an active program "to detect and treat malaria and other infections, iron-deficient and anaemic children can benefit from supplementation."

Pregnancy and Nursing

Low-dose iron supplements are generally safe and effective in pregnancy.[19] Iron supplementation during pregnancy and lactation should be undertaken only under the supervision of a health care professional trained and experienced in nutritional therapeutics.

Infants and Children

Infants and children are especially vulnerable to iron toxicity. Doses as low as 60 mg/kg can be fatal.

Contraindications

Iron preparations are generally contraindicated for individuals diagnosed with a variety of conditions, including hemochromatosis, hemosiderosis, transfusion-dependent thalassemia or other transfusion-dependent states, other conditions associated with iron overload, peptic ulcer, inflammatory bowel disease or other GI disease, diverticulitis, and intestinal stricture. Patients receiving hemodialysis for end-stage renal disease (ESRD) are particularly susceptible to oxidative stress and carotid artery intima media thickening as a result of iron administration, especially without concomitant vitamin E.[20,21]

Prophylactic iron (and folic acid) may be contraindicated for children in malarial environments.[18]

Iron supplements are generally inappropriate for individuals with a history of any unusual or allergic reaction to iron, or medicines, foods, dyes, or preservatives containing iron.

Precautions and Warnings

Conservative principles of practice suggest that regular iron supplementation be avoided in any individual who has not demonstrated iron deficiency anemia or low iron stores. Such caution is warranted because of the frequency of undetected HH, the pervasive pathophysiology of inflammation and oxidative stress, and emerging concerns about the more subtle effects of chronic excess iron intake. Chronic iron administration increases vascular oxidative stress and accelerates arterial thrombosis.[22] Thus, for example, iron supplementation appears particularly to increase risks of vascular disease and thrombosis for smokers with hypercholesterolemia.[23]

Some patients have a serious allergic reaction to IV iron dextran (Imferon), and therefore patients must be monitored especially closely during the first two Imferon administrations using a test dose of 25 mg for each session. After the second test dose is given, the administered dose can be increased to 100 mg. Intravenous sodium ferric gluconate (Ferrlecit) does not contain dextran, and this significant concern regarding anaphylactic reactions is essentially negligible.

Numerous researchers and reviewers have proposed, and sometimes proved, links between excess iron and the development or exacerbation of numerous pathological conditions, including increased risk of infection and inflammatory processes (e.g., pulmonary tuberculosis, pelvic endometriosis), heart disease (e.g., carotid atherosclerosis, coronary disease, myocardial infarction), autoimmune processes (e.g., diabetes, rheumatoid arthritis, systemic lupus erythematosus), neurodegenerative diseases (e.g., Alzheimer's disease, Parkinson's disease, Huntington's disease), and cancer (especially hepatocellular carcinoma and colorectal cancer).[23-46] Most of these associations are not conclusively supported by a review of well-done human studies, and some have been disproved, but many are consistent with known patterns of physiology, epidemiology, and pathogenesis. This important area of conflicting data, experience, and opinions will undoubtedly continue to be the subject of clinical trials and meta-analyses.

INTERACTIONS REVIEW

Strategic Considerations

Iron deficiency is the most common micronutrient deficiency in the world, and iron is the nutrient most often prescribed by conventional physicians as an active therapeutic intervention. However, the principles underlying and clinical practices framing such administration have not yet matured into a comprehensive and coherent approach for safe and effective prescribing in daily clinical practice. As with the inflammation it can induce and the free radicals it often generates, the classical metaphor of iron as a "hot" mineral can be applied therapeutically, serving well in suitable circumstances at the appropriate amounts, but just as easily causing a ripple of multiple adverse effects when insufficient, excessive, or simply inappropriately situated. Given the risks of iron depletion and iron overload and the multiple interaction patterns involving iron, deeper analysis of the research data and clinical practices reveals that universal declarations of efficacy, risk, and response patterns do not adequately convey the complexity of individual variability, patient subgroups, and conflicting needs. Thus, iron exemplifies the need for personalized and evolving therapeutic strategies within an integrative model when multiple therapies and coordinated care among various health care providers are involved.

Iron might be seen as a warrior whose sword cuts both ways. It produces heat, agitation, and invigoration, which can convey vitality, sustain activity, and embody vigor, but also carries the risk of oxidative stress, irritation, inflammation, and infection. Although iron depletion is common and has been given more attention than any other nutrient deficiency in conventional medical practice, the methods of evaluation and the standards for augmentation (or reduction) remain controversial. Depleted tissue iron stores are often missed in susceptible individuals because the clinical focus almost exclusively centers on frank iron deficiency anemia rather than functional parameters. Conversely, iron excess or overload, or even inappropriately timed administration, will tend to increase susceptibility to, or aggravate inflammatory processes and promote an environment favorable to, pathogenic microorganisms. The physiological response to infection and neoplasm is to make iron as unavailable as possible to the invading cells, which results in the functional iron deficiency, often seen with acute or chronic infections, and malignancies. Although not rigorously investigated with careful clinical research, much clinical experience suggests that it is often unwise to override this physiological adaptation with oral, and particularly parenteral, iron administration.

Accurate laboratory evaluation of iron status is multifactorial, often making it difficult and elusive to assess functional iron levels, metabolic processes, and depletion and overload states. It is often necessary to assess ferritin, percentage transferrin saturation, and sTfR levels for an accurate assessment of iron status, because ferritin can be falsely elevated by a number of conditions, including pregnancy, inflammatory conditions (e.g., arthritis), malignancy, skin conditions, irritable bowel disease, and chronic infections, both viral and bacterial.

Many minerals and metals are known to bind with a wide range of medications to form insoluble complexes that impair absorption and bioavailability, but with no other common nutrient as much as with the iron salts. Although this phenomenon has been studied widely, the body of evidence indicates that adverse effects on therapeutic efficacy of either agent involved can usually be effectively avoided by separating oral intake by at least 2 hours. Nevertheless, direct inquiry and frank discussion with patients regarding supplement use is critical because simultaneous intake over an extended period could adversely impact therapeutic action and confuse monitoring. Further, unsupervised alterations in intake habits, especially sudden discontinuation of iron that had been taken simultaneously, could result in a rapid elevation in effective dose levels of other agents, thus creating unintended consequences. As always, physician-patient communication, interdisciplinary collaboration, and reinforcement of trust, honesty, and respect for patient choices will always enhance the therapeutic process and support positive clinical outcomes.

The volatility of iron within human physiology, its complex interactions with a wide range of medications and nutrients, and the adverse implications of not maintaining dynamic equilibrium all attest to the critical importance of attentiveness to the changing needs of the individual patient whenever dealing with iron, its intake, and reverberations throughout the economy of the organism.

NUTRIENT-DRUG INTERACTIONS

Acetylsalicylic Acid (Aspirin)

Acetylsalicylic Acid (acetosal, acetyl salicylic acid, ASA, salicylsalicylic acid; Arthritis Foundation Pain Reliever, Ascriptin, Aspergum, Asprimox, Bayer Aspirin, Bayer Buffered Aspirin, Bayer Low Adult Strength, Bufferin, Buffex, Cama Arthritis Pain Reliever, Easprin, Ecotrin, Ecotrin Low Adult Strength, Empirin, Extra Strength Adprin-B, Extra Strength Bayer Enteric 500 Aspirin, Extra Strength Bayer Plus, Halfprin 81, Heartline, Regular Strength Bayer Enteric 500 Aspirin, St. Joseph Adult Chewable Aspirin, ZORprin); combination drugs: ASA and caffeine (Anacin); ASA, caffeine, and propoxyphene (Darvon Compound); ASA and carisoprodol (Soma Compound); ASA, codeine, and carisoprodol (Soma Compound with Codeine); ASA and codeine (Empirin with Codeine); ASA, codeine, butalbital, and caffeine (Fiorinal); ASA and extended-release dipyridamole (Aggrenox, Asasantin).

See also Indomethacin and Related Nonsteroidal Anti-inflammatory Drugs (NSAIDs).

Interaction Type and Significance

☼ **Prevention or Reduction of Drug Adverse Effect**

≈≈ **Drug-Induced Nutrient Depletion, Supplementation Therapeutic, with Professional Management**

Probability:	Evidence Base:
2. Probable to 1. Certain	● Consensus

Effect and Mechanism of Action

Aspirin's activity in inhibiting the effects of cyclooxygenase (COX) extends beyond those functions involved in inflammatory responses. In the stomach the enzyme's products build bicarbonate and mucus buffers against stomach acidity, without which the risk of ulceration can increase 20-fold. Gastrointestinal (GI) bleeding caused by aspirin results in iron loss, which can create a state of iron deficiency if aspirin is taken regularly. Iron supplementation can reverse iron depletion induced by aspirin-related blood loss.

Research

In a 1973 study involving 13 healthy subjects, Leonards et al.[47] demonstrated that sodium salicylate tablets and aspirin tablets caused GI bleeding and that the blood loss in volunteers administered aspirin was appreciably greater (5.6 vs. 1.2 mL/day above control values).[47] Subsequently, Palme and Koeppe[48] compared the GI blood loss caused by the acetylsalicylic acid (ASA) and benorilate (4-acetamidophenyl-2-acetoxybenzoate, Benortan) in Wistar rats and human subjects by measuring the total body iron retention. Their findings indicate that the daily iron loss under ASA is significantly higher (almost doubled) than that under benorilate.

Nutritional Therapeutics, Clinical Concerns, and Adaptations

Chronic aspirin ingestion is a frequent cause of iron deficiency and anemia. Gastrointestinal bleeding is a universal and virtually unavoidable adverse effect associated with aspirin consumption. It can cause ulcerations, abdominal burning, pain, cramping, nausea, gastritis, and even serious GI bleeding and liver toxicity. Sometimes, stomach ulceration and bleeding can occur without abdominal pain. Black tarry stools, weakness, and dizziness on standing may be the only signs of internal bleeding. Often there are no externally observable symptoms or obvious blood in the stool.

Physicians prescribing aspirin, or working with patients who self-administer analgesics, are advised to be alert to signs of GI blood loss and iron depletion caused by aspirin intake. Likewise, it is essential to inform patients that aspirin, in any amount, causes gastric bleeding to some degree and to educate them regarding the associated risks. In general, iron supplementation should not be undertaken, and should be actively discouraged, unless iron deficiency has been clinically established. More broadly, patients may benefit from discussing the limitations of protracted palliative therapy for chronic pain and inflammation and engaging in the process of identifying and addressing the causes of pain within a more fundamental and proactive long-term therapeutic strategy.

Iron deficiency anemia (IDA) is readily identified by a low hemoglobin and serum ferritin concentration, although it is not excluded by a normal serum ferritin. Serum transferrin receptor measurements can provide a useful alternative for distinguishing IDA from the anemia of chronic disease because the serum receptor concentration is usually elevated in patients with IDA but normal in patients with anemia from inflammation or neoplasia. Screening for fecal occult blood is prudent with suspected GI blood loss, even when the suspicion of physiological IDA from other known risk factors is high. A gastric delivery system for oral iron that eliminates nausea and vomiting and improves iron absorption when given with food may be appropriate with patients who experience adverse effect from oral iron supplements.

Angiotensin-Converting Enzyme (ACE) Inhibitors

Evidence: Captopril (Capoten), enalapril (Vasotec).
Extrapolated, based on similar properties: Benazepril (Lotensin); combination drug: benazepril and amlodipine (Lotrel); captopril combination drug: captopril and hydrochlorothiazide (Acezide, Capto-Co, Captozide, Co-Zidocapt); cilazapril (Inhibace); enalapril combination drugs: enalapril and felodipine (Lexxel), enalapril and hydrochlorothiazide (Vaseretic); fosinopril (Monopril), lisinopril (Prinivil, Zestril); combination drug: lisinopril and hydrochlorothiazide (Prinzide, Zestoretic); moexipril (Univasc), perindopril (Aceon), quinapril (Accupril), ramipril (Altace), trandolapril (Mavik).
Evidence, iron forms: Ferric gluconate, ferrous sulfate.
Extrapolated, iron forms, based on similar properties: Iron dextran complex, iron sucrose.
Nutrient forms with similar properties but evidence lacking for extrapolation: Ferrous fumarate, ferrous gluconate, polysaccharide-iron complex.

Interaction Type and Significance

◇◇ **Impaired Drug Absorption and Bioavailability, Precautions Appropriate**

☼ **Prevention or Reduction of Drug Adverse Effect**

⊕✗ **Bimodal or Variable Interaction, with Professional Management**

✗✗   Minimal to Mild Adverse Interaction—Vigilance
        Necessary

Coadministration Benefit
Probability: Evidence Base:
2. Probable   ◉ Emerging

Coadministration Risk
Probability: Evidence Base:
4. Plausible or   ● Emerging
    2. Probable

Effect and Mechanism of Action

Supplemental iron salts may diminish absorption and bio-availability of ACE inhibitors, and vice versa. The mechanism of this interaction has yet to be fully elucidated but is likely caused, at least in part, by binding within the intestines to form a poorly absorbed stable chelation complex.[49] Dry cough, and resultant patient nonadherence, is the most common limiting factor of ACE inhibitors. The mechanism that induces ACE inhibitor–induced dry cough involves inhibition of the metabolism of inflammatory proteins known as *kinins* (e.g., bradykinin), but it has not yet been fully elucidated. Another contributing factor to ACE inhibitor–induced cough may be the increased generation of nitric oxide (NO), which acts as a proinflammatory substance on bronchial epithelial cells. Iron coadministration inhibits cough associated with ACE inhibitors, most likely by acting as an inhibitor of NO synthase activity in bronchial epithelial cells. The erythropoietin-lowering effects of enalapril treatment may also aggravate anemia in renal transplant recipients. Concomitant iron might reverse this adverse effect but can increase risks of oxidative stress if given without counterbalancing antioxidant support. However, ACE inhibitors may enhance the adverse effect and toxicity of iron salts, particularly administered parenterally. Outside the specific context of ACE inhibitor therapy, administration of intravenous (IV) iron to anemic patients on hemodialysis can lead to an "oversaturation" of transferrin, and as a result, non-transferrin-bound, redox-active iron can induce lipid peroxidation.[20]

Research and Reports

In a double-blind, placebo-controlled, crossover study involving seven healthy adult volunteers, Schaefer et al.[49a] observed that concomitant administration of captopril (25 mg) and ferrous sulphate (300 mg) resulted in a 37% decrease in area under the curve (AUC) plasma levels for unconjugated captopril compared with placebo. The authors suggested that the observed decrease could be caused by an interaction in the GI tract subsequent to simultaneous ingestion.

Dry cough has been reported to occur in 5% to 39% of patients undergoing ACE inhibitor therapy, and in most cases the drug needs to be discontinued because of this adverse effect. Lee et al.[50] conducted a randomized, double-blind, placebo-controlled trial involving 19 patients who had developed ACE inhibitor–induced cough to determine if iron could ameliorate the cough, hypothetically by inhibiting NO-induced inflammation of bronchial epithelial cells. After an initial 2-week observation period, the subjects were randomized to a daily morning dose of 256 mg ferrous sulfate as a tablet or placebo for 4 weeks. The researchers evaluated data from cough diaries, scoring the daily severity of the symptom, as well as blood cell count and serum iron and ferritin concentration between the two periods. Mean daily cough scores during the observation and treatment periods showed a significant reduction in cough scores with iron coadministration but not with placebo. Three subjects in the iron group demonstrated almost complete cough abolition. Interestingly, the authors reported no significant changes in laboratory data in either group.

A bimodal pattern of interaction appears to occur with the administration of IV iron in patients being treated with ACE inhibitors, particularly in the context of hemodialysis. In several studies of hypertensive patients with renal failure (or transplant) on dialysis, mild exacerbation of anemia has been observed during treatment with enalapril.[51-54] Gossmann et al.[55] have suggested that ACE inhibitor–related anemia in renal transplant recipients seems to result from the erythropoietin-lowering effect of this group of drugs. However, administration of iron salts presents numerous risks in this patient population. During a 13-month period, Rolla et al.[56] reported aggravated adverse effects, including erythema, abdominal cramps, nausea, vomiting, and hypotension, in three enalapril-treated patients after IV ferric gluconate administration. During that same period, 15 other patients, none of whom were undergoing ACE inhibitor therapy, demonstrated no similar adverse events while receiving IV ferric gluconate. The authors suggested that enalapril might exaggerate the known adverse effects of IV iron by inhibiting the degradation of bradykinin, substance P, or other presumed inflammatory mediators of such iron-related effects. Notably, coadministration of vitamin E may attenuate oxidative stress induced by IV iron in patients on hemodialysis. In a randomized crossover design involving 22 patients, Roob et al.[20] investigated the effects on lipid peroxidation of 100 mg iron(III) hydroxide–sucrose complex, either with or without a single oral dose of 1200 IU of all-racemic alpha-tocopheryl acetate administered 6 hours before hemodialysis. They observed that vitamin E supplementation led to a 68% increase in plasma alpha-tocopherol concentrations and significantly reduced the AUC (0-180 minutes) of plasma malondialdehyde (MDA) to cholesterol and peroxides to cholesterol ratios. These findings suggest that an integrative strategy using several nutrients, such as ascorbic acid, folic acid, beta-carotene, and vitamin E, acting as an antioxidant network might serve to buffer potential adverse effects of IV iron salts and potentially enhance overall treatment outcomes in patients undergoing hemodialysis, particularly with concomitant ACE inhibitors. Further research in the form of well-designed clinical trials may be warranted to test these possible synergies.

Nutritional Therapeutics, Clinical Concerns, and Adaptations

Physicians prescribing ACE inhibitors are advised to educate patients regarding the risk of adverse effects, including drug-induced cough and anemia, and to inform them that coadministration of an oral iron supplement may reduce such symptoms. However, to avoid absorption problems inhibiting bioavailability of both substances, patients should wait at least 2 hours after administration of the medication before taking iron.

Supplementation of any minerals by patients with renal failure or on dialysis can be dangerous and should only be done within the context of close medical supervision. Patients receiving ACE inhibitor therapy may experience an exaggeration of adverse effects often associated with IV administration of iron salts; monitor closely for adverse effects such as nausea, vomiting, and hypotension.

Antacids and Gastric Acid—Suppressive Medications

Antacids: Aluminum carbonate gel (Basajel), aluminum hydroxide (Alternagel, Amphojel); combination drugs: aluminum hydroxide, magnesium carbonate, alginic acid, and sodium bicarbonate (Gaviscon Extra Strength Tablets, Gaviscon Regular Strength Liquid, Gaviscon Extra Strength Liquid); aluminum hydroxide and magnesium hydroxide (Advanced Formula Di-Gel Tablets, co-magaldrox, Di-Gel, Gelusil, Maalox, Maalox Plus, Mylanta, Wingel); aluminum hydroxide, magnesium trisilicate, alginic acid, and sodium bicarbonate (Alenic Alka, Gaviscon Regular Strength Tablets); calcium carbonate (Titralac, Tums); magnesium hydroxide (Phillips' Milk of Magnesia MOM); combination drugs: magnesium hydroxide and calcium carbonate (Calcium Rich Rolaids); magnesium hydroxide, aluminum hydroxide, calcium carbonate, and simethicone (Tempo Tablets); magnesium trisilicate and aluminum hydroxide (Adcomag trisil, Foamicon); magnesium trisilicate, alginic acid, and sodium bicarbonate (Alenic Alka, Gaviscon Regular Strength Tablets); combination drug: sodium bicarbonate, aspirin, and citric acid (Alka-Seltzer).

Histamine (H₂) receptor antagonists:
Evidence: Cimetidine (Tagamet; Tagamet HB).
Extrapolated, based on similar properties: Famotidine (Pepcid RPD, Pepcid, Pepcid AC), nizatidine (Axid, Axid AR), ranitidine (Zantac); combination drug: ranitidine, bismuth, and citrate (Tritec).
Similar properties but evidence lacking for extrapolation:
Proton pump inhibitors: Esomeprazole (Nexium), lansoprazole (Prevacid, Zoton), omeprazole (Losec, Prilosec), pantoprazole (Protium, Protonix, Somac), rabeprazole (AcipHex, Pariet).

Interaction Type and Significance

☼ **Prevention or Reduction of Drug Adverse Effect**
≈≈ **Drug-Induced Nutrient Depletion, Supplementation Therapeutic, with Professional Management**
◇◇ **Impaired Drug Absorption and Bioavailability, Precautions Appropriate**

Probability:
2. Probable to
1. Certain

Evidence Base:
◉ Emerging but
▽ Mixed

Effect and Mechanism of Action

The mechanisms proposed vary with the agent in question and the form of iron involved. All iron-antacid interactions are affected by the physiological premise that hydrochloric acid in the stomach reduces ferric iron to ferrous iron, the required form for absorption. By inhibiting acid secretion or neutralizing the normally acidic gastric environment, acid-suppressive agents will tend to reduce the absorption of dietary iron. Conversely, the iron status of patients with iron depletion due to internal bleeding from ulcers could also benefit from the therapeutic action of such medications. Finally, iron and some medications can bind to each other and inhibit absorption of both agents.

Scientific knowledge of the full set of factors and mechanisms involved in the various interactions in question is limited, inconsistent, and often of questionable relevance to clinical practice. In vitro experiments investigating the interactions of oral hematinics and antacid suspensions indicate that aluminum hydroxide can precipitate iron as hydroxide and ferric

ions become intercalated into the aluminum hydroxide crystal lattice.[57] Carbonates can interact with iron to form poorly soluble iron complexes.[58] Ferrous sulfate can change into less easily absorbable salts, or its polymerization may increase, in the presence of magnesium trisilicate.[59] Histamine (H₂) receptor antagonists (H₂RAs) appear to be more problematic than other antacids, at least in light of currently available evidence. Cimetidine, and probably to a lesser extent ranitidine, can potentiate the action of oral anticoagulants of both coumarin and indanedione structure, through a dose-dependent, reversible inhibition of cytochrome P450, and if international normalized ratio (INR) is not closely monitored and adjusted appropriately, can cause hemorrhagic complications that further compromise iron status.[60] Furthermore, H₂RAs are considered efficient chelators of Fe^{2+}, and each agent will decrease absorption of the other by binding iron in the GI tract.[61] More recently, there has been concern that long-term use of proton pump inhibitors (PPIs) might impair the normal hematological process and result in iron deficiency by reducing stomach acid levels.

The adverse effect on absorption of food from iron, particularly ferric nonheme forms as found in plants and dairy products, is likely to be greater than from most iron contained in supplements, which is more often of the ferrous form and is readily absorbed without the need for acid. The degree and clinical significance of this interaction can be influenced by genetics, iron source, concomitant food constituents, timing of intake, duration of medication use, digestive health, aging, and other factors.

Research

A wide range of experimental and clinical studies in the scientific literature have reported that pharmacologically reducing the acidity of the gastric environment will inherently impair normal gastric function and inhibit absorption of iron and, to a lesser degree, zinc, calcium, and other minerals.[62-67] Although the basic theme of impaired acidity underlies all permutations involved, the evidence cannot easily be analyzed as a coherent data set because of a variety of confounding factors, including significant variety in forms of iron used, iron doses ranging from minimal to relative overdoses, variable mechanism of action and dose of medications, initial iron status and medical conditions (or health) of subjects, the history and severity of any pathology present, lack of dietary consistency, and durations of treatment ranging from experimental single administrations to extended periods representative of clinical practice. Timing of intake and duration of use appear to influence the clinical significance of the interaction to the greatest degree.

Aluminum Hydroxide, Calcium Carbonate, Magnesium Hydroxide, Magnesium Trisilicate, Sodium Bicarbonate, and Combinations. Most experiments have assessed short-term pharmacokinetic effects of simultaneous iron and antacid administration. In an experiment involving iron-replete healthy subjects, Benjamin et al.[58] (1967) and Rastogi et al.[68] (1976) observed poor absorption of iron in the presence of sodium bicarbonate or aluminum hydroxide, respectively. Ekenved et al.[69] found that an antacid containing aluminum and magnesium hydroxides along with magnesium carbonate reduced absorption of ferrous sulfate and ferrous fumarate (both containing 100 mg ferrous iron) by 37% and 31%, respectively. Hall and Davis[59] administered magnesium trisilicate (35 g) to nine subjects, who were given 5 mg of isotopically labeled ferrous sulfate (5 mg), and observed a reduction in iron from 30% to 12% on average but from 67% to 5% in one individual. In 1986, O'Neil-Cutting and Crosby[70] published findings from a small-dose iron tolerance test involving 22 mildly iron-deficient (menstruation or blood donation) but healthy subjects to compare absorption of iron with and without various antacids. They found that sodium bicarbonate (1 g) and calcium carbonate (500 mg) caused the plasma iron increase to decline by 50% and 37% compared with the controls, respectively, except when the calcium carbonate was present in a tableted multivitamin-mineral formulation. The authors suggested that the competitive binding of iron by ascorbic acid in the multivitamin-mineral tablet facilitated uninhibited absorption of the iron. In contrast, they observed that 1 teaspoonful of a magnesium hydroxide/aluminum hydroxide antacid did not significantly decrease absorption at 2 hours of simultaneously ingested iron (10 or 20 mg ferrous sulfate). In a prospective, unblinded, randomized trial involving 16 healthy, fasting male subjects, Snyder and Clark[71] investigated the effect of administering magnesium hydroxide, in a 5:1 MgOH/Fe ratio, on a supratherapeutic dose of ferrous sulfate, containing a 10-mg/kg dose of elemental iron, ingested 30 minutes later, by measuring serum iron levels at hourly intervals for 6 or 7 hours. The mean peak serum iron level was 300.8 µg/dL in the control group and 272.5 µg/dL in the experimental group, but mean serum iron levels at each time point and peak serum iron levels did not differ significantly between groups. This experiment was subsequently criticized in a letter by Wallace et al.[72] on the basis that iron absorption was not measured for an adequate period to rule out a reduction in iron absorption.

Histamine (H₂) Receptor Antagonists. The inhibition of gastric secretion by the H₂RAs alters the stomach environment for significantly longer periods than simple antacids and can cause malabsorption of dietary iron (and cobalamin), although not necessarily of iron in supplemental form, such as ferrous sulfate. Furthermore, patients with internal bleeding from ulcers demonstrate improved iron status as a result of the intended therapeutic action of the medications. Lastly, evidence from multiple sources indicates that H₂RAs can act as efficient chelators of Fe^{2+} such that coadministration might result in binding and reduced bioavailability of both substances. Macdougall et al.[73] conducted a controlled clinical trial investigating the prevention of bleeding from gastric erosions in patients with fulminant hepatic failure using antacids and H₂ blockers. They found that intragastric pH recordings taken at 2-hour intervals in the treated group could be consistently maintained above 5.0 with the H₂RAs metiamide and cimetidine, as opposed to patients receiving antacids. In the group receiving H₂ blockers only, 1 of 26 patients bled, compared with 13 (54%) of the controls, a highly significant difference. Blood transfusion requirements were significantly less in those treated with H₂RAs. Campbell et al.[61] performed experiments in vitro and in vivo using isolated perfused rat jejunal tissue to examine the binding of iron and cimetidine. They used a dose of cimetidine paralleling a human dose of 300 mg, with the ferrous sulfate doses equivalent to 150- and 300-mg doses. They observed complete inhibition of cimetidine absorption with the higher ferrous sulfate dose, whereas the lower dose of ferrous sulfate caused a 63% reduction in cimetidine absorption. Furthermore, in vitro iron in its ferrous form rapidly oxidized to the ferric form, which then binds to cimetidine. In a prospective, open, multicenter clinical trial, Bianchi et al.[74] studied the effects of concurrent use of famotidine, nizatidine, or ranitidine on response to administration of iron succinyl–protein complex (2400 mg, equivalent to 60 mg iron, twice daily) in a group of patients with iron deficiency or iron deficiency anemia.

These researchers observed no significant alteration in iron absorption at the end of 60 days. In this situation the healing of the ulcers, and attendant decreased blood loss, may have improved the iron status of treated individuals.

Partlow and two teams of researchers conducted two studies on the effects of H₂ blockers on absorption of ferrous sulfate. In an in vitro experiment, they found that cimetidine and famotidine bind with iron and that ranitidine did so to a much lesser degree.[75] In a second study, Partlow et al.[76] conducted a series of three experiments investigating the interaction between ferrous sulfate and H₂ blockers and the potential impairment of absorption (of both agents) caused by binding. They observed that the reductions in the AUC and the maximum serum levels (C_{max}) of cimetidine were small (<16%) when healthy subjects were administered ferrous sulfate, 300 mg, either as a tablet or in solution. Similarly, they observed very small (<10%) reductions in the AUC and C_{max} of famotidine when 40 mg was administered concurrently with 300 mg ferrous sulfate, as a tablet. Overall, these experiments of short duration have tended to show minimal adverse effects on iron absorption and status as well as on drug availability. Thus, Stockley's review[77] of the subject concludes that evidence is inadequate to confirm a clinically significant reduction of supplemental iron by H₂ blockers. However, extended or repetitive use of H₂RAs may contribute to the occurrence of iron (and/or cobalamin) deficiency anemia.[60]

Despite long-standing knowledge of the intimate and essential role that gastric pH plays in the conversion of ferric to ferrous iron and subsequent bioavailability and absorption, controversy has continued unabated as to whether the suppression of gastric acid is likely to induce a clinically significant effect on iron nutriture and risk of iron depletion and deficiency. In part, this results from the predominant study of ferrous sulfate as a form of medicinal iron rather than a study of food sources, and a methodological emphasis on studies that often last only 1 day, sometimes as long as 2 months, but rarely reflect the extended duration of medication use common in clinical practice. Likewise, the body of available evidence indicates that any reduction in the serum levels of cimetidine and famotidine due to iron are small and clinically irrelevant. Remarkably, given the widespread use of such agents over extended periods, the issue of iron supplementation in individuals receiving acid-suppressive therapies has been the subject of only limited human research.

Reports

An unconfirmed report published by Esposito[78] briefly described a reduction in clinical response to ferrous sulfate (600 mg/day) in three patients taking cimetidine (1 g) and attributed it to the "prolonged periods" of elevated intragastric pH after cimetidine, as previously reported by Macdougall et al.[73] After 2 months' treatment, anemia and altered iron metabolism persisted, even though the ulcers resolved. In a subsequent letter, Rosner[79] noted that the proposed mechanism involved was unconvincing because the iron in ferrous sulfate is Fe^{2+}, not ferric Fe^{3+}, and thus not needing an acidic environment for absorption.

Nutritional Therapeutics, Clinical Concerns, and Adaptations

The clinical implications of the interaction between gastric acid–suppressive therapies and iron intake and function operate at two levels. The most immediate and probable pharmacokinetic issue of chelation and decreased absorption and bioavailability affects both iron and pharmaceutical agents. The longer-term and more variable issues of decreased iron absorption and bioavailability, potentially leading to depletion and deficiency, are subject to more variability in terms of occurrence, severity, and consequences. The former is easily avoided through education regarding the timing of intake. The latter may be offset through iron supplementation or alteration in dietary sources of iron intake, but may only partially address the potential adverse effects of chronic suppression of gastric acid activity.

Stabilization of iron status is central among the many benefits of medical treatment of gastric bleeding, and subsequent enhancement of iron intake may be appropriate in select cases. Anemia due to blood loss is common among the users of antacids and gastric acid–suppressive medications because many have ulcers. Proper medical evaluation of blood and tissue iron status and presence of internal blood loss from GI bleeding are necessary preliminaries to consideration of iron supplementation. Professional supervision and regular monitoring are appropriate once it has been determined that iron administration is appropriate. It is important to inform patients of limitations and risks of acid suppression on an extended basis, including increased susceptibility to *Helicobacter pylori* and other infections, impaired protein digestion and other adverse effects of hypochlorhydria, and disruption of normal GI ecology.[80-86] In clinical practice, complementary approaches for supporting renewal of gastric mucosa typically include deglycyrrhizinated licorice (DGL), zinc carnosine, cabbage leaf *(Brassica oleracea),* craneshill root *(Geranium maculatum),* marshmallow root *(Althaea officinalis),* and slippery elm bark *(Ulmus rubra).* Ultimately, changes in causative and exacerbating factors underlying dyspepsia and reflux need to be addressed through education about the importance of thorough chewing and relaxing while eating; the inherent risks of excessive portion size and eating late in the evening; the value of paying attention to individual responses to particular foods, food combinations, and eating patterns; potential roles of *H. pylori;* and the influence of stress. Overall, the adverse effect on absorption of iron from food, particularly ferric forms as found in plants, is likely to be greater than on ferrous forms, as found in many iron supplements. Thus, the initial action of these medications in providing a gastric environment more suitable toward healing of ulcerations and resolution of internal bleeding may tend to result in minimal adverse effect on iron status. This situation could, however, change as the continued elevation of gastric pH results in decreased iron absorption from some food sources, particularly ferric iron.

In the event that iron administration is determined to be necessary, a typical adult dose is 100 mg of elemental iron daily. Iron preparations should be taken at least 2 hours before or after antacid medications, particularly cimetidine, sodium bicarbonate, or calcium, to avoid interference with iron absorption (and in some cases drug absorption). In general, gastric acidity is not required for absorption of supplements containing ferrous iron. However, because carbonyl iron requires adequate stomach acid for absorption, concomitant use of PPIs may suppress its absorption. Ferrous fumarate and iron-EDTA may be more bioavailable than ferrous sulfate, particularly in individuals with low (or impaired) gastric acidity. Simultaneous intake of vitamin A and C (> 200 mg/day) may enhance absorption. Increased intake of plant foods and herbs rich in iron and other minerals may be more appropriate than iron supplements for some individuals because of tolerance, compliance, and bioavailability factors. Furthermore, because iron levels in the body are regulated by absorption, rather than by excretion, individuals with low body iron levels, including

iron deficiency, can demonstrate increased absorption efficiency, often in the range of 10% to 20%.

Bile Acid Sequestrants

Evidence: Cholestyramine (Locholest, Prevalite, Questran), colestipol (Colestid).
Extrapolated, based on similar properties: Colesevelam (Welchol).

Interaction Type and Significance
◇◇ **Impaired Drug Absorption and Bioavailability, Precautions Appropriate**
≈≈≈ **Drug-Induced Nutrient Depletion, Supplementation Therapeutic, Not Requiring Professional Management**
◇ **Adverse Drug Effect on Nutritional Therapeutics, Strategic Concern**

Probability:
2. Probable

Evidence Base:
◉ **Emerging** but
▽ **Mixed**

Effect and Mechanism of Action
When ingested together, iron and cholestyramine or colestipol can bind to form a chelation complex that is poorly absorbable.[63,87] In the process of sequestering intestinal bile acids, these agents may contribute to iron depletion and potential deficiency with long-term use.[88,89] Impaired absorption and resultant decreased bioavailability of the drug could reduce its therapeutic activity.

Research
The body of research regarding the pattern of interactions between iron and bile acid sequestrants is limited, potentially contradictory, and sometimes not focused on key questions of clinical relevance. Using a rat model, Thomas et al.[90] observed that cholestyramine reduced intestinal absorption of a single 100-μg dose of ferrous sulfate by half. Subsequently, this same team extended their research by demonstrating diminished iron stores after prolonged cholestyramine administration.[91] Several years later, in vitro experiments by Leonard et al.[87] demonstrated that cholestyramine and colestipol can both bind iron citrate. The amount of iron citrate bound by colestipol ranged from 95% to 98%. Cholestyramine bound 24% to 97% of the iron citrate in a pH-dependent manner. In another animal study, Watkins et al.[88] found that cholestyramine-fed rats had a net negative balance for calcium and a lower net positive balance for iron, magnesium, and zinc than the controls. These researchers attributed the reported disturbance in iron balance to diminished iron absorption caused by resin binding. Schlierf et al.[92] investigated the availability of minerals and vitamins in young patients with familial hypercholesterolemia administered colestipol over a 5-year period. They reported a lack of significant alterations in plasma levels of iron (as well as of calcium, sodium, parathyroid hormone, and water-soluble and fat-soluble vitamins, except for changes in carotenoid and vitamin E levels paralleling lipoprotein concentrations). The researchers' observation that the treatment was effective in lowering cholesterol levels by 19% indicates that any mutual binding that might have occurred did not significantly impair drug activity.

Notably, no human trials have examined the effect of the observed pharmacokinetic interactions on long-term patterns of depletion in tissue iron stores (as opposed to plasma levels), the influence of intake timing, or the variable responses in patients with preexisting iron depletion or anemia. In a review of cholesterol-lowering agents, Torkos[89] suggested that an iron deficiency can result from long-term use of colestipol.

Nutritional Therapeutics, Clinical Concerns, and Adaptations
Physicians prescribing bile acid sequestrants are advised to inform patients of the probable pharmacokinetic interaction between iron and these agents and to recommend separating oral intake by at least 2 hours. Such measures usually allow concurrent use of both agents without interfering with the intended therapeutic activity of either. Despite the lack of solid evidence, many practitioners of nutritional therapeutics recommend regular use of a multivitamin-mineral formula to patients on long-term bile acid sequestrant therapy as a preventive measure in light of the diverse body of evidence indicating significant probability of associated, multiple nutrient deficiency patterns, particularly with fat-soluble vitamins. Such safe and low-cost measures appear judicious pending the emergence of more conclusive evidence based on well-designed, long-term clinical trials.

Bisphosphonates

Alendronate (Fosamax), clodronate (Bonefos, Ostac), etidronate (Didronel), ibandronate (Bondronat, Boniva), pamidronate (Aredia), risedronate (Actonel), tiludronate (Skelid), zoledronic acid (Zometa).

Interaction Type and Significance
◇◇Impaired Drug Absorption and Bioavailability,
     Precautions Appropriate
≈≈ Drug-Induced Nutrient Depletion,
     Supplementation Therapeutic, with Professional
     Management

Probability:	Evidence Base:
2. Probable	● Consensus

Effect and Mechanism of Action
Absorption of bisphosphonates occurs through passive diffusion in the stomach and upper small intestine and is very low and variable (1%-10%). Simultaneous ingestion of cations such as iron (or calcium/magnesium) can result in chelation that significantly reduces absorption and bioavailability of both substances.[93]

Research
Evidence from clinical trials specifically investigating the interaction between iron and bisphosphonates is lacking. Nevertheless, this interaction represents the consensus position within the standard pharmacological literature.[93,94]

No research or case reports were found focusing on potential iron depletion resulting from simultaneous intake of these substances over an extended period.

Clinical Implications and Adaptations
Oral iron preparations need to be taken at least 2 hours away from the bisphosphonate to avoid pharmacokinetic interference. It is generally recommended that oral bisphosphonates be taken with a full glass (6-8 ounces) of plain water on an empty stomach, avoiding the recumbent position for at least 30 minutes to prevent potential severe esophageal irritation associated with incomplete transfer of the tablet to the stomach.

Carbidopa, Levodopa, and Related Antiparkinsonian Medications

Carbidopa (Lodosyn), levodopa (L-dopa; Dopar, Larodopa); combination drugs: levodopa and benserazide (co-beneldopa; Madopar); levodopa and carbidopa (Atamet, Parcopa, Sinemet, Sinemet CR); levodopa, carbidopa, and entacapone (Stalevo).

Interaction Type and Significance
◇◇Impaired Drug Absorption and Bioavailability,
     Precautions Appropriate
≈≈ Drug-Induced Nutrient Depletion,
     Supplementation Therapeutic, with Professional
     Management

Probability:	Evidence Base:
2. Probable	● Consensus

Effect and Mechanism of Action
Iron, especially ferric iron, can bind strongly to carbidopa or levodopa, and the resulting insoluble chelation complexes can significantly reduce absorption and bioavailability of both substances.[49,95-97]

Ferrous iron, such as ferrous sulfate, is formed from ferric iron when it is reduced under the influence of the acidic pH of the GI environment. However, ferrous iron undergoes auto-oxidation to the ferric form in the presence of methyldopa and levodopa. The formation of these complexes is rapid at high pH (i.e., pH 9), and the rate slows considerably as the pH is lowered (e.g., pH 4). A variety of iron-methyldopa complexes can be formed between pH 4 and 9. Complexation is absent below pH 2. Together these processes can result in both catechol oxidation and production of the toxic hydroxyl radical.[96]

Research
The pioneering research done by Campbell, Hasinoff, and Greene has established the basis for consensus regarding these issues within the pharmacological literature. In a rat model, Campbell et al.[98] observed that ferrous sulfate significantly reduced L-dopa absorption by 22.6% in the duodenum and 23.9% in the jejunum, on average. Furthermore, the authors noted a tendency for ferrous sulfate to cause a greater reduction in L-dopa absorption as the buffer pH increased. They concluded that "the combined results are compatible with the chemical model of increased L-dopa–iron binding as pH increases." Chelation was investigated as a mechanism in iron-induced reduction in levodopa bioavailability in a study involving eight healthy subjects who were administered a single dose of levodopa (250 mg), with and without a single dose of ferrous sulfate (325 mg). When the serum levodopa levels were measured, these researchers observed a 55% decline in peak serum levodopa levels (from 3.6 to 1.6 nmol/L) and a reduction in the AUC by 51% (from 257 to 125 nmol.min/mL). Notably, subjects who had demonstrated the highest peak levels and greatest absorption demonstrated the largest reductions in the presence of ferrous sulfate.[95] Similarly, in a study involving nine patients with Parkinson's disease being treated with Sinemet (100/25 tablet), Campbell et al.[97] found that coadministration of a single dose of ferrous sulfate resulted in a decrease in the AUC of carbidopa by more than 75% and of levodopa by 30%. However, despite an apparently strong relationship observed between reductions in levodopa AUC and reductions in Sinemet efficacy, the average reduction in Sinemet efficacy associated with ferrous sulfate did not achieve

statistical significance. Thus, these authors reported that some patients manifested a worsening of their Parkinson's symptomatology and concluded that the effect on Sinemet availability, when taken concurrently with ferrous sulfate, appears to be clinically significant in some, but not all, patients.[97]

More broadly, an emerging pattern of evidence indicates that chronic iron intake may be contraindicated in patients who would typically be prescribed these medications. Diverse findings suggest that glutathione depletion, oxidative stress, and possibly other factors resulting from iron excess may play a significant role in the pathophysiology of Parkinson's and other neurodegenerative diseases.[42,45,99,100] As noted by Gotz et al.[45]: "Glial iron is mainly stored as ferric iron in ferritin, while neuronal iron is predominantly bound to neuromelanin. Iron overload may induce progressive degeneration of nigrostriatal neurons by facilitating the formation of reactive biological intermediates, including reactive oxygen species, and the formation of cytotoxic protein aggregates." Thus, apart from short-term response in cases involving confirmed comorbid depleted iron stores or iron deficiency anemia, a more appropriate therapeutic strategy might invoke iron chelators in the prevention or treatment of Parkinson's disease in individuals with iron overload, or even with physiological iron stores in the higher ranges of normal.[46,101,102]

Clinical Implications and Adaptations

Despite a relatively consistent body of evidence, the clinical significance of the interaction between iron preparations and levodopa or carbidopa is not fully known. Physicians prescribing levodopa or carbidopa are advised to caution these patients against taking iron supplements outside the context of medical supervision and monitoring. Simultaneous intake can decrease absorption and bioavailability of both substances, which may result in impaired control of Parkinson's symptomatology and interfere with medically appropriate iron support.

In cases where a comprehensive strategy calls for inclusion of both agents as medically necessary and appropriate, intake should be separated by at least 2 hours to avoid impairing their activity. Otherwise, conservative principles of practice suggest that coadministration be discouraged pending substantive research clearly defining mechanisms of action, parameters of effect, and respective risks and benefits.

Cefdinir and Related Cephalosporin Antibiotics

Evidence: Cefdinir (Omnicef).
Extrapolated, based on similar properties: Cefaclor (Ceclor), cefadroxil (Duricef), cefamandole (Mandol), cefazolin (Ancef, Kefzol), cefepime (Maxipime), cefixime (Suprax), cefoperazone (Cefobid), cefotaxime (Claforan), cefotetan (Cefotan), cefoxitin (Mefoxin), cefpodoxime (Vantin), cefprozil (Cefzil), ceftazidime (Ceptaz, Fortaz, Tazicef, Tazidime), ceftibuten (Cedax), ceftizoxime (Cefizox), ceftriaxone (Rocephin), cefuroxime (Ceftin, Kefurox, Zinacef), cephalexin (Keflex, Keftab), cephapirin (Cefadyl), cephradine (Anspor, Velocef); imipenem combination drug: imipenem and cilastatin (Primaxin I.M., Primaxin I.V.); loracarbef (Lorabid); meropenem (Merrem I.V.).

Interaction Type and Significance

◇◇Impaired Drug Absorption and Bioavailability,
    Precautions Appropriate

Probability:	Evidence Base:
2. Probable	◉ **Emerging,** treated as ● **Consensus**

Effect and Mechanism of Action

Supplemental iron salts may diminish absorption and bioavailability of cefdinir and related cephalosporin antibiotics, and vice versa. The mechanism of this interaction has yet to be fully elucidated but is likely caused, at least in part, by binding within the GI tract to form a poorly absorbed, stable chelation complex.[77,103,104]

Research

In a randomized three-way crossover study involving healthy male volunteers, Ueno et al.[103] compared the effects on concentration curve [AUC (0-12)] of cefdinir (200 mg) alone, ingested simultaneously with two tablets of iron ion, and followed 3 hours later by two tablets of iron ion preparation. They observed that the AUC (0-12) of cefdinir with concurrent iron and the AUC (3-12) with delayed iron were both significantly smaller than that with cefdinir alone. However, there were no differences in AUC (0-3) between cefdinir alone and with delayed iron. These researchers interpreted their findings to suggest that the impaired absorption of cefdinir was caused by formation of a chelation complex.

More recently, in an in vitro experiment comparing the effects of calcium polycarbophil granules and iron(III) citrate on cefdinir, Kato et al.[105] found that, in contrast to the calcium compound, "the release of cefdinir from the cellulose membrane in the presence of iron ions was slower than in the absence of iron ions."

Clinical Implications and Adaptations

Physicians prescribing cefdinir or related oral cephalosporin antibiotics are advised to caution these patients against taking iron supplements within 3 hours of the medication. A general caution regarding iron supplementation outside the context of medical supervision and monitoring may also be appropriate with some patients. Simultaneous intake can decrease absorption and bioavailability of the antibiotic, which may impair its antimicrobial activity.

Clinically significant iron depletion caused by simultaneous intake of these substances is improbable over the limited time such medications are typically administered.

Chloramphenicol

Chloramphenicol (Chloromycetin).

Interaction Type and Significance

☼   **Prevention or Reduction of Drug Adverse Effect**

◇≈≈ **Drug-Induced Adverse Effect on Nutrient Function, Coadministration Therapeutic, with Professional Management**

◇   **Adverse Drug Effect on Nutritional Therapeutics, Strategic Concern**

Probability:	Evidence Base:
2. Probable or **3. Possible**	● **Consensus**

Effect and Mechanism of Action

At serum levels of 25 µg/mL or more, chloramphenicol can inhibit protein synthesis and cause a reversible bone marrow depression. Although much milder than the irreversible form, in which chloramphenicol can cause aplastic anemia, this more common and possibly unrelated adverse effect can interfere with the activity of iron (or vitamin B_{12}) in the treatment of anemia.

Research and Reports

The adverse effects of chloramphenicol on erythropoiesis and red blood cell (RBC) maturation have been well documented for more than 50 years. In 1954, Rigdon et al.[106] first documented anemia produced by chloramphenicol in the duck. In their study of the effect of chloramphenicol on erythropoiesis, Saidi et al.[107] observed that 10 of 22 patients being treated with iron dextran for iron deficiency anemia failed to demonstrate the expected hematological response when coadministered chloramphenicol. Likewise, four patients being treated with vitamin B_{12} for pernicious anemia were refractory to therapy until chloramphenicol was discontinued. McCurdy[108] reported bone marrow toxicity in series of patients with liver disease after exposure to chloramphenicol. Jiji et al.[109] (1963) published a report of reversible erythropoietic toxicity in healthy volunteers associated with chloramphenicol and its sulfamoyl analog. Two years later, Scott et al.[110] conducted a controlled double-blind study of the hematological toxicity of chloramphenicol and, based on their findings, suggested that drug dosage levels of 25 to 30 mg/kg are usually sufficient for effectively treating infections while minimizing the risk of elevating serum levels to 25 µg/ml or greater, at which bone marrow suppression occurs.

Nutritional Therapeutics, Clinical Concerns, and Adaptations

Chloramphenicol may impair the therapeutic effects of iron administration. A decline in the reticulocyte count will indicate inadequate RBC maturation. As recommended by Scott et al.,[110] dosage levels below 25 to 30 mg/kg may be safe and effective, whereas higher doses increase risks of drug-induced adverse effects. Iron coadministration may be judicious in some cases when extended chloramphenicol is anticipated. Consideration of alternative antimicrobials may be warranted in the treatment of individuals diagnosed with depleted iron stores or iron deficiency anemia or otherwise at elevated risk for adverse effects on erythropoiesis and iron function.

Chloramphenicol, although used in some countries such as Mexico, is used extremely rarely in the U.S., and then only in the hands of infectious disease specialists when no alternatives exist. It is not generally available because of the risk of aplastic anemia associated with its use (a life-threatening complication quite different from simple bone marrow suppression).

Chlorhexidine

Chlorhexidine (Chlorohex, Corsodyl, Eludril, Oro-Clense, Peridex, Periochip, Periogard Oral Rinse).

Interaction Type and Significance

**✗ ✗   Minimal to Mild Adverse Interaction—Vigilance
        Necessary**

Probability:	Evidence Base:
2. Probable to 1. Certain	**● Consensus**

Effect and Mechanism of Action

Tooth staining is an adverse effect associated with both chlorhexidine and ingestion of iron in liquid preparations. Concurrent intake may increase the probability and severity of dental staining.

Research

The mechanism and significant probability of this interaction are accepted as consensus within the pharmacological literature, even though the body of direct evidence from controlled clinical

trials is relatively limited. In a controlled study using analytical electron microscopy, Warner et al.[111] demonstrated that individuals administered iron immediately after using chlorhexidine developed severe dental staining within 2 weeks. They noted that enhanced levels of sulfur and transition metals, particularly iron, were found in stained regions, whereas unstained regions contained low sulfur and metal levels similar to those treated with water or nonstaining agents.

Clinical Implications and Adaptations

Physicians prescribing chlorhexidine, in liquid dosage forms, are advised to inform patients to prevent this adverse effect by separating intake of iron (as well as sulfur or other transition metals) by at least 1 hour before or 2 hours after using the drug.

Clofibrate

Clofibrate (Atromid-S).

Interaction Type and Significance

**◇ ◇ Impaired Drug Absorption and Bioavailability,
       Precautions Appropriate**

**≈ ≈   Drug-Induced Nutrient Depletion,
        Supplementation Therapeutic, with Professional
        Management**

**◇   Adverse Drug Effect on Nutritional Therapeutics,
        Strategic Concern**

Probability:	Evidence Base:
2. Probable	**○ Preliminary**, treated as **○ Consensus**

Effect and Mechanism of Action

Clofibrate can bind to iron (and other nutrients) within the GI tract to form a chelation complex that is poorly absorbed and reduces bioavailability of both substances.[112]

Research

Clinical research directly investigating this iron-clofibrate interaction is limited. However, the pharmacological literature accepts this pharmacokinetic interaction as representing a consensus position based on the principles involved and general knowledge of the agents involved.

Nutritional Therapeutics, Clinical Concerns, and Adaptations

Physicians prescribing clofibrate are advised to inform patients of the probable pharmacokinetic interaction between iron and the medication and to recommend separating oral intake by at least 3 hours. Such measures should allow concurrent use of both agents without interfering with the intended therapeutic activity of either. In general, conservative principles of practice warrant advising patients against taking iron supplements without specific, well-founded therapeutic need and outside the context of medical supervision and monitoring.

Desferoxamine

Desferoxamine (desferrioxamine mesilate, desferoxamine mesylate; Desferal).
Similar properties but evidence lacking for extrapolation: Deferasirox (Exjade).

Interaction Type and Significance

☼   Prevention or Reduction of Nutrient Adverse Effect

**◇ ◇ Drug-Induced Effect on Nutrient Function,
       Supplementation Contraindicated, Professional
       Management Appropriate**

✗✗ Minimal to Mild Adverse Interaction—Vigilance Necessary

Probability: Evidence Base:
1. Certain   ● Consensus

Effect and Mechanism of Action

Desferoxamine mesylate (Desferal) is the chelator of choice for acute iron intoxication and of chronic iron overload caused by transfusion-dependent anemias. It is also used to decrease aluminum accumulation in patients with kidney failure. Desferoxamine can be administered intramuscularly, subcutaneously, or intravenously.

Because desferoxamine is administered to individuals with dangerously high levels of iron, it would be counterproductive to supplement or coadminister iron.

Research

It is self-evident that patients with acute or chronic iron excess being treated with desferoxamine to chelate and remove excess iron should avoid iron supplementation as well as iron-rich foods. Thus, no specific research studies have ever combined desferoxamine with iron coadministration because the interaction is obvious.

Clinical Implications and Adaptations

Chelation with desferoxamine or other agents requires appropriate training and proper monitoring. Assessment of nutrient status is appropriate, and clinical responses will vary accordingly. Iron supplementation would exacerbate the condition of patients prescribed desferoxamine. Thus, iron-containing products of any type are contraindicated in individuals receiving appropriate desferoxamine therapy and specifically need to be avoided during such treatment. Physicians who administer desferoxamine for chelation of heavy metals or other clinical applications routinely supplement their patients with minerals of nutritional importance. Patients undergoing iron removal therapy should be made aware that they should avoid over-the-counter (OTC) multivitamin-mineral preparations that contain iron.

Dimercaprol

Dimercaprol (British antilewisite [BAL], dicaptol, dithioglycerol, sulfactin).
Similar properties but evidence lacking for extrapolation: Other metal chelators, such as DMPS (2,3-dimercapto-1-propanesulfonic acid) or DMSA (2,3-dimercaptosuccinic acid).

Interaction Type and Significance

✗✗✗ Potentially Harmful or Serious Adverse Interaction—Avoid

Probability: Evidence Base:
2. Probable   ● Consensus

Effect and Mechanism of Action

Dimercaprol is an effective antidote in arsenic, cadmium, lead, and mercury poisoning and is most efficient if administered intramuscularly immediately after exposure to the metal. Dimercaprol's mechanism of action involves the formation of toxic complexes with iron, cadmium, selenium, and uranium. Nevertheless, dimercaprol cannot be used in poisoning from iron, cadmium, tellurium, selenium, vanadium, or uranium; it is also contraindicated in poisoning from elemental mercury vapor.

Research

Research into this interaction is implicitly contained within the clinical trials, case reports, and clinical experience of the therapeutic application of dimercaprol.

Clinical Implications and Adaptations

Physicians administering dimercaprol need to avoid iron administration out of sequence. Iron therapy is often administered 24 hours or more after the last dose of dimercaprol. However, the concomitant intake of iron and dimercaprol can result in serious renal injury. Warnings to patients to avoid iron supplements would seem reasonable but are usually unnecessary because this medication is typically administered in emergency or inpatient settings.

EDTA

EDTA (Ethylenediaminetetraacetic acid).

Interaction Type and Significance

☼ **Prevention or Reduction of Nutrient Adverse Effect**
◇◇ **Drug-Induced Effect on Nutrient Function, Supplementation Contraindicated, Professional Management Appropriate**
✗✗ Minimal to Mild Adverse Interaction—Vigilance Necessary

Probability: Evidence Base:
1. Certain   ● Consensus

Effect and Mechanism of Action

EDTA binds to iron (and other minerals) and thereby increases iron excretion. EDTA may be used to treat iron overload, although it is much less efficient than desferoxamine. Conversely, chelation therapy with EDTA could induce or exacerbate depleted iron stores if compensatory nutrient augmentation is appropriate but not provided.

Research

The chelation function of EDTA is central to its primary pharmacological action in therapeutic application.

Conversely, iron chelates, such as ferric EDTA, sodium iron EDTA [NaFe(III)EDTA], and ferrous bisglycinate, have been proposed as promising alternatives to iron salts for food fortification based on recent studies involving healthy and at-risk infants and children.[113,114] Continued research is warranted.

Clinical Implications and Adaptations

Chelation with EDTA or other agents requires appropriate training and proper monitoring. Assessment of iron status is appropriate, and clinical responses will vary accordingly. When properly administered, EDTA chelation is considered unlikely to result in adverse reactions caused by iron depletion. Physicians who administer EDTA for chelation of heavy metals or other clinical applications routinely coadminister minerals of nutritional importance as part of a strategic therapeutic protocol.

Erythropoiesis-Stimulating Agents

Epoetin alpha (EPO, epoetin alfa, recombinant erythropoietin; Epogen, Eprex, Procrit), epoetin beta (NeoRecormon), darbepoetin alpha (darbepoetin alfa; Aranesp).
See also Vitamin C monograph.

Interaction Type and Significance

⊕⊕   **Beneficial or Supportive Interaction, with Professional Management**

⊕✗   **Bimodal or Variable Interaction, with Professional Management**

✗✗   **Minimal to Mild Adverse Interaction—Vigilance Necessary**

✗✗✗   **Potentially Harmful or Serious Adverse Interaction—Avoid**

Probability: Evidence Base:
2. Probable   ◉ Emerging, ▽ Mixed

Effect and Mechanism of Action

Erythropoietin is an endogenous peptide, produced primarily by the kidneys, which drives erythropoiesis in the bone marrow. It became available as a recombinant peptide hormone for therapeutic use in the 1980s.

Approximately 50% of oncology patients develop anemia, with that incidence rising dramatically in patients with more advanced cancer or in those receiving chemotherapy and/or radiation therapy. Within conventional oncology, *recombinant human erythropoietin* (rHuEpo) represents the standard of care in managing cancer therapy-related anemia and fatigue, increasing hemoglobin levels, reducing transfusion need, and improving patient quality of life. Likewise, rHuEpo may correct anemia in chronic renal failure (CRF) patients, in iron-deficient erythropoiesis associated with the anemia of chronic disease (ACD), and in primary bone marrow dysfunction states, such as myelodysplastic syndrome. By stimulating erythropoiesis, erythropoietin may increase synthesis of RBCs, thereby increasing metabolic need for iron. Iron coadministration, intravenous/parenteral or oral, could improve the response to erythropoietin or rHuEpo in cases of iron-deficient erythropoiesis by delivering adequate iron to the bone marrow.

Research

Since the late 1980s, rHuEpo has provided a safe and effective option for treating cancer-related anemia and fatigue. Recent research confirmed that epoetin beta, 30,000 IU once weekly, is equally effective as the conventional 10,000 IU three times weekly in alleviating cancer-related anemia.[115] Nevertheless, erythropoietin therapy exhibits variable response rates, and 30% to 50% of patients did not respond adequately to treatment in some trials. True iron deficiency is the most common cause of an inadequate response to rHuEpo in CRF patients. However, in oncology patients, this failure may be caused by factors related to the underlying disease, adverse effects of chemotherapy or radiotherapy, functional iron deficiency, or some combination.[116,117] Thus, in cases of functional iron deficiency, patients may not respond to rHuEpo when iron availability is inadequate to the demands of erythropoietin-induced erythropoiesis, despite the presence of adequate bone marrow iron stores.

Since the emergence of rHuEpo as a standard treatment, concomitant iron has often been proposed as an important therapeutic option in optimizing the response of cancer-related anemia to rHuEpo.[118] Guidelines published by the American Society of Clinical Oncology and American Society of Hematology recommend iron repletion in patients receiving rHuEpo when functional iron deficiency is present, based on indirect evidence and biological inferences.[117] A growing body of literature regarding chronic renal failure patients has shown that iron coadministration can correct functional iron deficiency and may improve erythropoietin response, with IV iron doing so more effectively than oral iron.

Markowitz et al.[119] conducted a double-blind, placebo-controlled trial to evaluate the effectiveness of oral iron therapy in 49 hemodialysis patients receiving rHuEpo. They divided the subjects into two groups, based on adequate or deficient iron stores, and treated them for 3 months with 150 mg elemental iron (polysaccharide complex) or placebo, twice daily. Over 5 months they observed that iron-replete patients, in both oral iron and placebo subgroups, demonstrated decreasing iron stores; that is, oral iron failed to maintain their iron stores. Furthermore, compared to iron-replete patients, iron-deficient patients had a significantly greater dropout rate because of adverse effects, even though responses to the side effect questionnaire were equivalent, suggesting poor medication compliance. Beguin[116] found that oral iron is largely ineffective in the treatment of anemia in chronic diseases other than cancer, mainly because of the development of iron deficiency, which significantly limits the efficacy of rHuEpo therapy.

Oral iron products in patients with ESRD have been largely abandoned, and the safety of IV iron preparations has improved with the introduction of new-generation compounds that have significantly reduced incidence of allergenicity. Since its approval, sodium ferric gluconate complex (SFGC) has largely displaced iron dextran as the primary form of IV iron, which had been associated with significant adverse reactions, including anaphylaxis and death. Adverse reactions to SFGC are uncommon in hemodialysis patients, including both iron dextran–sensitive and dextran-tolerant patients.[120] These findings indicate that dextran, rather than iron, is the cause of most reactions to iron dextran administration.

Iron deficiency is the most common cause of suboptimal response to rHuEpo in chronic hemodialysis patients. Intravenous iron can improve hemoglobin response, help maintain adequate iron stores, and decrease erythropoietin dosage requirements in hemodialysis patients and patients with anemia of kidney disease. In 1997, Kooistra et al.[121] investigated the effects of iron availability, inflammation, and aluminum on iron absorption in 19 chronic hemodialysis patients on maintenance erythropoietin (rHuEpo) therapy. They concluded that iron absorption is decreased in hemodialysis patients with elevated C-reactive protein (CRP) values and higher levels of aluminum ingestion. Iron absorption correlated significantly with transferrin saturation and CRP in the iron-deficient group, and with serum ferritin in the iron-replete group. Auerbach et al.[122] conducted a randomized trial involving 43 hemodialysis patients receiving rHuEpo (epoetin alpha) to investigate three iron dextran infusion methods for anemia. They reported no significant differences in efficacy and safety (as measured by time to the maximum hemoglobin and adverse reactions) when they compared subjects who received IV iron dextran as a total-dose infusion, 500-mg infusion to total dose, or 100-mg bolus to total dose, in each case during the dialysis procedure.

In a trial involving 24 patients of an outpatient dialysis center, Vankova et al.[123] reported significant improvements obtained by tracking hematocrit, transferrin saturation, and ferritin levels and adjusting iron and rHuEpo dosage accordingly. In 23 patients (96%), transferrin saturation levels were within the recommended range after treatment. Hematocrit increased from 27.7% to 35.7%, with the recommended value of 33% being achieved in 18 patients. Overall, the weekly dose of rHuEPO fell from 3958 IU to 2042 IU, and the average dose of iron administered was 157 mg per week. Similarly, Chang et al.[124] conducted a 12-month IV iron substitution trial in 149 iron-replete chronic hemodialysis patients receiving subcutaneous rHuEpo therapy. They maintained the available iron pool with 100 mg iron every 2 weeks or 1 month, depending on serum ferritin and transferrin saturation levels, with the rHuEpo dosage titrated depending on hematocrit levels. After 12 months these researchers reported increases in the hematocrit, serum ferritin, and transferrin saturation along with a 25% reduction in rHuEpo requirement. The authors concluded that maintaining high levels of serum ferritin and transferrin saturation could further reduce the requirement of erythropoietin in chronic hemodialysis patients, but cautioned that "the long-term effect of iron overloading...must be further evaluated in contrast to the economic saving."[124]

However, oral heme iron may provide an effective option for iron therapy in hemodialysis patients because it is absorbed by patients with high ferritin levels, it has fewer adverse effects, and its absorption is stimulated by erythropoietin administration. In an open, 6-month, prospective evaluation of heme iron in 37 hemodialysis patients who had been on maintenance IV iron therapy, Nissenson et al.[125] discontinued the IV iron and replaced it with oral heme iron. Among the 28 subjects who completed the study, the authors observed an initial slight reduction in average transferrin saturation, which subsequently reversed, and a significant reduction in average serum ferritin level was seen at months 4 through 6. No significant changes were seen in average transferrin saturation or hematocrit. The authors concluded that heme iron polypeptide successfully replaced IV iron therapy in a majority of hemodialysis patients during the 6-month study period, maintained target hematocrits with no concomitant use of IV iron, and thus was associated with a significant increase in rHuEpo efficiency.

Ongoing research is examining the role of concomitant IV iron during epoetin therapy with the aim of further improving the effectiveness of epoietins in anemia treatment. A study published in 2004 was the first controlled trial confirming that iron should be coadministered intravenously rather then orally in cancer patients with chemotherapy-related anemia. In a prospective, multicenter, open-label, randomized trial involving 157 patients, Auerbach et al.[126] found that IV iron optimizes the response to rHuEpo in cancer patients with chemotherapy-related anemia. In addition to rHuEpo, 40,000 U subcutaneously once weekly, subjects received (1) no iron; (2) 325 mg iron orally twice daily; (3) iron dextran, repeated 100-mg IV bolus; or (4) iron dextran total-dose infusion (TDI). They reported that subjects in all four groups showed hemoglobin (Hb) increases from baseline with mean Hb increases for both IV iron groups were greater than for no-iron and oral iron groups. Patients in both groups receiving IV iron demonstrated higher hematopoietic responses (68%) than did those in the groups receiving no iron (25%) and oral iron (36%). Furthermore, subjects in the IV iron group showed increases in energy, activity, and overall quality of life from baseline, compared with a decrease in energy and activity for the no-iron group and no change in activity or overall quality of life for the oral iron group. The authors concluded that rHuEpo increases Hb levels and improves quality of life in patients with chemotherapy-related anemia, and that coadministration of IV iron significantly increased the magnitude of improvement for both outcomes. Patients were not followed long term to determine whether the therapy had any positive or negative impact on cancer specific survival. In a letter, Pedrazzoli et al.[127] responded with a cautionary approach: "Because of absence of iron stores, in this subset of patients, it is clinically cautious to postpone treatment with erythropoietic agents until iron stores are replenished or to treat iron deficiency aggressively along with rHuEpo therapy." In contrast, in a randomized, double-blind, placebo-controlled trial

involving 351 head and neck cancer patients with anemia undergoing radiotherapy, Henke et al.[128] found that epoetin beta corrected anemia but did not improve cancer control or survival, and in fact, locoregional progression-free survival was poorer with epoetin beta than with placebo. Moreover, whether concomitant iron can increase the proportion of patients without iron deficiency responding to erythropoietic agents remains the subject of ongoing controversy and an area in need of further elucidation within the field of rHuEpo therapy for anemia of cancer.

Anemia of chronic disease (ACD) is a frequent complication of chronic inflammation in rheumatoid arthritis and other conditions. The cytokine interleukin-6 (IL-6) mediates hypoferremia (anemia) of inflammation by inducing the synthesis of the iron-regulatory hormone hepcidin.[129,130] Arndt et al.[131] investigated the concomitant use of rHuEpo and parenteral iron to correct iron-deficient erythropoiesis (IDE) in patients diagnosed with anemia of chronic disease. They treated 30 rheumatoid arthritis patients with ACD using subcutaneous rHuEpo, 150 IU/kg twice weekly. Intravenous iron (200 mg iron sucrose once weekly) was coadministered in cases of IDE, as defined by the presence of two of three criteria: saturation of transferrin 15% or less, hypochromic erythrocytes 10% or more, and serum ferritin concentration 50 μg/L or less. The authors reported that all 28 subjects who completed the trial met the treatment goal of successful correction of anemia, with an increase of the median Hb concentration from 10.3 to 13.3 g/dL, and concluded that such coadministration of erythropoietin and iron was safe, effective, and well tolerated in all patients.

Nutritional Therapeutics, Clinical Concerns and Adaptations

Physicians administering erythropoietin are advised to exercise caution in the coadministration of iron, especially IV iron within the context of oncological care. Combination therapy using erythropoietin and iron is controversial and awaits greater evolution of clinical research, particularly specificity to individuals, conditions, and stages of treatment.[116] The erythropoietic response is a tactical element within the broader therapeutic strategy and, although evoking apparent short-term benefits using narrow parameters of hematological response, may be irrelevant or deleterious, even counterproductive, to achieving the desired clinical outcome, such as the strategic goal of eliminating cancer.[132] Thus, this intervention could be beneficial or adverse, depending on the particulars of the case.

Most anemia is cancer patients is the "anemia of chronic inflammation," which although sometimes similar in presentation to iron deficiency, is part of a protective response, similar to that in acute infection; the body "locks down" iron to keep it out of circulation to counter the proliferative process, because most malignant cells and pathogenic bacteria require iron for rapid proliferation. Erythropoietin (EPO) is most appropriate in anemic cancer patients, and then only after assessing the endogenous EPO level and determining that it is not already extremely elevated. Iron is coadministered most safely and effectively only when there has been no or only minor response to initial EPO therapy. It is essential to monitor iron status and to address either true or functional iron deficiency before and during rHuEpo therapy to optimize the effect of rHuEpo in cancer patients. It must also be kept in mind that oncology patients with limited iron stores may become iron deficient as a result of erythropoiesis stimulated by EPO therapy, which then limits further response unless iron is supplied. The IV route shows significantly greater efficacy than the oral route with inorganic iron preparations. Oral administration of heme iron should also be investigated in this population.

Coadministration of ascorbic acid may also be indicated in certain cases, especially involving resistance to EPO in hemodialysis patients with functional iron deficiency.

Fluoroquinolone (4-Quinolone) Antibiotics

Evidence: Ciprofloxacin (Ciloxan, Cipro), gatifloxacin (Tequin), levofloxacin (Levaquin), norfloxacin (Noroxin), ofloxacin (Floxin, Ocuflox), sparfloxacin (Zagam).

Minimally affected: Lomefloxacin (Maxaquin).

Extrapolated, based on similar properties: Cinoxacin (Cinobac, Pulvules), enoxacin (Penetrex), lomefloxacin (Maxaquin), moxifloxacin (Avelox), nalidixic acid (Neggram), trovafloxacin (alatrofloxacin; Trovan).

Related but evidence against extrapolation: Fleroxacin.

Nutrient form with similar properties but evidence indicating no or reduced interaction effects: Iron-ovotransferrin.

Interaction Type and Significance

✗✗ **Minimal to Mild Adverse Interaction—Vigilance Necessary**

◇◇ **Impaired Drug Absorption and Bioavailability, Precautions Appropriate**

≈≈ **Drug-Induced Nutrient Depletion, Supplementation Therapeutic, with Professional Management**

Probability: Evidence Base:
1. **Certain** or **2. Probable**   ● **Consensus**
   variable

Effect and Mechanism of Action

Iron and the 3-carbonyl and 4-oxo functional groups on quinolone antibiotics can bind within the GI tract to form a poorly absorbed, stable chelation complex, for example, a ferric ion–ciprofloxacin complex. A similar pharmacokinetic interaction can also occur with other divalent metal cations, such as aluminum, calcium, copper, magnesium, manganese, and zinc, as well as mineral-based antacids.[49,133-141] This binding process can interfere to varying degrees with the absorption, bioavailability, and activity of both the antimicrobials in this class and the orally administered iron.

In contrast to most forms of iron, iron-ovotransferrin can combine directly with the transferrin receptors of intestinal cells, and thus may release only minimal amounts of elemental iron into the gut to bind with the quinolones.[142,143]

However, an experiment using a rat model to examine the pharmacokinetics and pharmacodynamics aspects of the interaction between oral ferrous sulfate and IV ciprofloxacin suggested that the observed effects may only partially be attributable to direct physical interaction in the GI tract.[144]

Research

In vitro experiments first demonstrated the pattern of interaction between quinolones and metals in an aqueous medium and the resultant effects on antimicrobial activity. Subsequently, changes in oral bioavailability and alterations in therapeutic efficacy have been the focus of many previous interaction studies involving metal cations and quinolones. Thus, through multiple lines of research, the ability of multivalent cations to reduce the absorption and serum levels of oral quinolone antibiotics is well established.

Iron salts, particularly ferrous fumarate, gluconate, and sulfate, can reduce the absorption of ciprofloxacin, gatifloxacin, levofloxacin, norfloxacin, ofloxacin, and sparfloxacin from the GI tract to a degree that can interfere with therapeutic activity. In contrast, iron only minimally affects lomefloxacin, and separation of intake renders insignificant any interaction between gemifloxacin and ferrous sulfate. Iron does not appear to interact significantly with fleroxacin. Notably, iron-ovotransferrin appears to exert no adverse effect on quinolone absorption because of its direct binding to intestinal transferrin receptors. Thus, in his review of the various interactions between iron and members of this drug class, Stockley[77] summarizes the body of evidence as revealing a pattern of descending order in the degree to which the serum levels of the various quinolone antibiotics can become subtherapeutic and thus subject to clinically significant interaction, as follows:

Norfloxacin > levofloxacin > ciprofloxacin > gatifloxacin > ofloxacin > sparfloxacin > lomefloxacin.

Ciprofloxacin. Many studies have confirmed that compounds containing elemental iron can greatly decrease absorption of ciprofloxacin, with demonstrated reductions in the AUC and C_{max} of 30% to 90%. Several studies have documented this effect with ferrous sulfate.[135,138,145] For example, in a four-way crossover trial with 12 healthy volunteers, Polk et al.[133] (1989) observed a clinically significant reduction in the absorption of oral doses of ciprofloxacin (500 mg) when administered with ferrous sulfate (325 mg orally three times daily) or a multivitamin-mineral formulation containing zinc. Notably, peak concentrations of ciprofloxacin with ferrous sulfate regimen were below the minimum inhibitory concentration (MIC) for 90% of strains of many organisms normally considered susceptible to the antimicrobial activity of ciprofloxacin. Also in 1989, Lode et al.[146] demonstrated a pharmacokinetic interaction between oral ciprofloxacin/ofloxacin and iron glycine sulfate. A year later, Brouwers et al.[147] published research showing decreased ciprofloxacin absorption with concomitant administration of ferrous fumarate. Kara et al.[135] investigated clinical and chemical interactions between ciprofloxacin and iron preparations and found impairment of absorption with ferrous gluconate and a multimineral preparation containing iron, magnesium, zinc, calcium, copper, and manganese (Centrum Forte). They reported that when ferrous ion was mixed with ciprofloxacin, rapid spectral changes occurred in a manner consistent with oxidation of the ferrous form of iron to its ferric form, followed by rapid formation of a Fe^{3+}-ciprofloxacin complex. Ciprofloxacin seems to bind to ferric ion in a ratio of 3:1 by interacting with the 4-keto and 3-carboxyl groups on ciprofloxacin. These authors concluded that the formation of a ferric ion–ciprofloxacin complex was most likely responsible for the reduction in ciprofloxacin bioavailability in the presence of iron. In contrast, iron-ovotransferrin, a novel iron formulation in which iron ions are bound to ovotransferrin, has been found to have no significant effect on the absorption of ciprofloxacin from the GI tract and thus only minimally effects the drug's margin of efficacy.[142,143]

However, based on findings from an experiment using a rat model to examine the pharmacokinetics and pharmacodynamics of the interaction between oral ferrous sulfate and IV ciprofloxacin, Wong et al.[144] suggested that the observed effects may only partially be attributable to direct physical interaction in the GI tract. Further research is warranted to investigate the concern that oral iron might interfere even with parenteral fluoroquinolones.

Fleroxacin. In a study involving 12 volunteers, Sorgel et al.[148] observed that ferrous sulfate (equivalent to 100 mg elemental iron) exerted no significant effect on the pharmacokinetics of fleroxacin.

Gatifloxacin. Shiba et al.[149] conducted a study of gatifloxacin pharmacokinetics involving six healthy volunteers that showed coadministration of ferrous sulfate (160 mg) and gatifloxacin (200 mg) produced a 49% decrease in the C_{max} and 29% decrease in the AUC of gatifloxacin.

Gemifloxacin. Allen et al.[150] observed no significant alterations in pharmacokinetics and bioavailability when they administered gemifloxacin (320 mg) to 27 healthy volunteers either 2 hours after or 3 hours before ferrous sulfate (325 mg).

Levofloxacin. Shiba et al.[151] reported that ferrous sulfate, when taken concurrently, inhibited levofloxacin absorption and reduced bioavailability by 79%.

Lomefloxacin. Lehto and Kivisto[152] demonstrated that coadministration of ferrous sulfate (equivalent to 100 mg elemental iron) with lomefloxacin (400 mg) reduced the lomefloxacin C_{max} by approximately 28% and the AUC by approximately 14%.

Moxifloxacin. In their review of moxifloxacin, Balfour and Wiseman[140] concluded that bioavailability of the medication is substantially reduced by coadministration with an iron preparation or antacid.

Norfloxacin. In a single-dose study assessing the pharmacokinetic interactions of norfloxacin with iron and metallic agents, Okhamafe et al.[134] reported a 97% reduction in bioavailability with iron. Campbell et al.[153] found that ferrous sulfate reduced the urinary recovery of norfloxacin by 55%; similar effects occurred with zinc sulfate. Subsequently, in eight normal subjects, Lehto et al.[138] observed that ferrous sulfate reduced the AUC of a single 400-mg dose of norfloxacin by 73% and the C_{max} by 75%. Similarly, Kanemitsu et al.[154,155] noted a 51% reduction in the norfloxacin AUC with ferrous sulfate.

Ofloxacin. In a study involving 12 healthy subjects, Lode et al.[146] found that an iron-glycine-sulfate complex (containing 200 mg elemental iron) reduced the bioavailability of ofloxacin (400 mg) by 36%. However, in an experiment with nine healthy volunteers, Martinez Cabarga et al.[156] observed only an 11% decrease in GI absorption of ofloxacin (200 mg) with coadministration of ferrous sulfate (1050 mg). In a 1994 study with eight healthy subjects, Lehto et al.[138] observed that coadministration of ferrous sulfate (100 mg elemental iron) reduced the AUC and C_{max} after a single dose of ofloxacin (400 mg) by 25% and 36%, respectively.

Sparfloxacin. In a single-dose study assessing the effect of ferrous sulfate on the pharmacokinetics of sparfloxacin, Kanemitsu et al.[154,155] reported that 525 mg ferrous sulfate (170 mg elemental iron) reduced the AUC of sparfloxacin (200 mg) by 27% in six subjects.

Iron Depletion. Iron depletion resulting from chelation by this class of medications has not been studied per se. Although plausible, such an adverse effect on iron status is highly improbable, given the normal physiological controls on iron levels, variable absorption rates, and the limited duration of standard fluoroquinolone antibiotic use. Long-term quinolone therapy and simultaneous oral iron intake in the face of iron deficiency could theoretically contribute to lack of tissue repletion. It is not clear whether or not long-term oral fluoroquinolone antibiotic therapy might cause iron deficiency in certain persons, such as menstruating women, by preventing dietary iron absorption.

Nutritional Therapeutics, Clinical Concerns, and Adaptations

The reduction of fluoroquinolone activity by concomitant iron is the primary established interaction between these two groups of agents; the potential depletion of iron through the same mechanisms is plausible, but it is generally improbable in standard clinical usage. Both directions of interaction and decreased bioavailability can be adequately avoided through proper patient education and dose timing.

Physicians treating patients for serious infections with quinolone antibiotics should advise that they refrain from ingesting iron supplements or using multivitamin-mineral formulations containing iron or other divalent mineral cations during the course of therapy, to avoid interfering with the absorption and thus the antimicrobial action of the medication.

Iron intake can usually be temporarily halted in most patients but can be continued with separation of intake timing in those for whom iron repletion has been confirmed as necessary to their therapeutic strategy. If this is not possible, administration of the medication 2 hours before or 6 hours after ingestion of an oral iron preparation is suggested and can effectively minimize risk of an adverse interaction (i.e., antibiotic malabsorption). This recommendation also applies to intake of iron-rich or iron-fortified foods. Monitor for decreased therapeutic effects of oral quinolones if inadvertently administered simultaneously with oral iron supplements. A special iron formulation, in which iron ions are bound to ovotransferrin, is less likely than the usual iron salts to reduce drug absorption.

Hyoscyamine

Hyoscyamine (Anaspaz, A-Spas S/L, Cystospaz, Cystospaz-M, Donnamar, ED-SPAZ, Gastrosed, Levbid, Levsin, Levsinex, Levsin/SL).

Interaction Type and Significance

≈≈ **Drug-Induced Nutrient Depletion, Supplementation Therapeutic, with Professional Management**

☼ **Prevention or Reduction of Drug Adverse Effect**

◇ **Adverse Drug Effect on Nutritional Therapeutics, Strategic Concern**

Probability:	Evidence Base:
4. Plausible	○ **Preliminary**

Effect and Mechanism of Action

Hyoscyamine impairs absorption of ferrous citrate. The mechanism of this interaction has not been fully elucidated but may be caused by the drug's anticholinergic activity.

Research

Orrego-Matte et al.[157] found that absorption of ferrous sulfate, which is usually well absorbed, was impaired in individuals administered hyoscyamine.

Nutritional Therapeutics, Clinical Concerns, and Adaptations

Physicians prescribing hyoscyamine are advised to ask patients if they are taking supplements containing iron. Concomitant intake could limit the therapeutic activity and clinical efficacy of either agent. Long-term coadministration could potentially contribute to depletion of iron stores, particularly in individuals presenting with or susceptible to iron deficiency. If iron administration is clinically warranted, separation of intake is appropriate to avoid interference with absorption.

Indomethacin and Related Nonsteroidal Anti-Inflammatory Drugs (NSAIDS)

Evidence: Indomethacin (indometacin; Indocin, Indocin-SR).
Extrapolated, based on similar properties:
COX-1 inhibitors: Diclofenac (Cataflam, Voltaren); combination drug: diclofenac and misoprostol (Arthrotec); diflunisal (Dolobid), etodolac (Lodine), fenoprofen (Dalfon), furbiprofen (Ansaid), ibuprofen (Advil, Excedrin IB, Motrin, Motrin IB, Nuprin, Pedia Care Fever Drops, Provel, Rufen); combination drug: hydrocodone and ibuprofen (Reprexain, Vicoprofen); ketoprofen (Orudis, Oruvail), ketorolac (Acular ophthalmic, Toradol), meclofenamate (Meclomen), mefenamic acid (Ponstel), meloxicam (Mobic), nabumetone (Relafen), naproxen (Aleve, Anaprox, Naprosyn), oxaprozin (Daypro), piroxicam (Feldene), salsalate (salicylic acid; Amigesic, Disalcid, Marthritic, Mono Gesic, Salflex, Salsitab), sulindac (Clinoril), tolmetin (Tolectin).
COX-2 inhibitor: Celecoxib (Celebrex).

Interaction Type and Significance

≈≈ **Drug-Induced Nutrient Depletion, Supplementation Therapeutic, with Professional Management**
◇◇ **Drug-Induced Effect on Nutrient Function, Supplementation Contraindicated, Professional Management Appropriate**
☼ **Prevention or Reduction of Drug Adverse Effect**
⊕✗ **Bimodal or Variable Interaction, with Professional Management**
✗ **Potential or Theoretical Adverse Interaction of Uncertain Severity**

Nutrient Depletion

Probability: | Evidence Base:
2. Probable | ● Consensus

Coadministration Benefit

Probability: | Evidence Base:
4. Plausible | ○ Preliminary

Effect and Mechanism of Action

The activity of NSAIDs in inhibiting the effects of cyclooxygenase (COX) extends beyond those functions involved in inflammatory responses. In the stomach the enzyme's products build bicarbonate and mucus buffers against stomach acidity, without which the risk of ulceration can increase 20-fold. In general, NSAIDs can damage the epithelium of the stomach as well as the small and large intestines, causing ulceration, increased small intestine permeability, chronic bleeding, and eventually iron deficiency.[158-160] Oral indomethacin is one of the most damaging NSAIDs in this regard. Iron coadministration may provide a means of countering the nutrient depletion effect of such medications.

Indomethacin's primary action is prostaglandin inhibition through the COX pathway. Indomethacin causes anemia by two possible mechanisms: (1) peptic ulceration or GI bleeding and (2) interference with normal iron metabolism and erythropoiesis. Curiously, edible black ink derived from black iron oxide is often used as a nonmedicinal ingredient in indomethacin capsules.

Both NSAIDs and iron can cause GI irritation; thus, concomitant use represents a potential additive adverse effect. Excessive iron intake can also contribute to inflammatory processes.

Research

Iron loss resulting from GI bleeding is well established as an adverse effect associated with indomethacin or other NSAIDs. Additionally, according to a nested case-control analysis of multiple linked health care databases conducted by Canadian researchers, patients taking warfarin at the same time as selective COX-2 inhibitors or nonselective NSAIDs have an increased risk of hospitalization for upper GI hemorrhage.[161]

Animal research indicates that prostaglandins are necessary for normal iron metabolism and for erythropoiesis.[162,163] Notably, indomethacin has also been associated with aplastic anemia.[164-166]

Although widely discussed as if evidence based, the specific use of iron coadministration to reverse this depletion pattern has not been the subject of significant human research, as indicated by a search of the scientific literature.

Lactoferrin is a glycoprotein present in human breast milk and other body fluids and is available as a supplement derived from bovine whey protein, which has been shown to act as an antioxidant, anti-inflammatory, and bactericidal agent as well as having an immunomodulatory effect. In a study presented at the Digestive Disease Week meeting on May 20, 2001, Dr. Troost observed the concomitant administration of this form of iron with indomethacin to iron-deficient women resulted in an additional increase in intestinal permeability. Furthermore, he reported: "When iron is bound to lactoferrin, it is not able to catalyze free radical formation."[167] In related research, Troost et al.[168] conducted a randomized crossover dietary intervention involving 15 healthy volunteers to determine whether administration of recombinant human lactoferrin (rhLF) inhibits NSAID-induced gastroenteropathy in vivo as a model for disorders associated with increased permeability of the stomach and small intestine. They demonstrated that intestinal permeability after the administration of indomethacin and lactoferrin was significantly reduced compared with the permeability observed after ingestion of indomethacin and placebo, underscoring rhLF's potential as a GI-protective agent; in contrast, gastroduodenal permeability did not differ between the two interventions. These researchers concluded that "oral recombinant human lactoferrin supplementation during a short-term indomethacin challenge reduced the NSAID-mediated increase in small intestinal permeability and hence may provide a nutritional tool in the treatment of hyperpermeability-associated disorders." The authors noted that the protective mechanism of lactoferrin is still undetermined, but it may be related to its ability to bind strongly to iron, thus acting as an antioxidant.[168]

Nutritional Therapeutics, Clinical Concerns, and Adaptations

Physicians prescribing NSAIDs for extended use are advised to monitor for blood loss and iron depletion; frank questioning of patients regarding self-medication is also necessary. In cases where both iron and indomethacin (or another NSAID) are required, based on established iron deficiency or tissue depletion, the patient should be advised to take the substances with food to reduce stomach irritation and bleeding risk. In cases of existing GI irritation, the use of iron-rich foods and herbs may be more efficacious and better tolerated. Investigation to identify and therapeutic intervention to address the causes of inflammatory processes are fundamental in individuals with chronic inflammation.

Interferon Alpha

Interferon alpha (Alferon N, Intron A, Roferon-A); combination drug: interferon alfa-2b and ribavirin (Rebetron).

Interaction Type and Significance

✗✗✗ Potentially Harmful or Serious Adverse Interaction—Avoid

Probability:	Evidence Base:
2. Probable	◉ Emerging

Effect and Mechanism of Action

Pathogenic microorganisms such as the hepatitis C virus require iron to replicate. Reduction of iron levels, particularly in the liver, appears to inhibit viral replication and increase efficacy of interferon therapy, especially within the context of complementary measures, such as adding cytokines and antivirals. Iron supplementation would counter this therapeutic approach: moreover, reducing iron intake is consistent with the therapeutic strategy.

Research

Hepatic iron concentration has consistently been observed as being directly correlated with the response to interferon therapy in patients with chronic hepatitis C infection. In 1981, Blumberg et al.[169] first reported that patients with hepatitis B viral infection who had higher serum iron or ferritin levels were more likely to develop chronic infections than those with lower levels, who more often experienced spontaneous resolution of their infections. Patients with chronic hepatitis C have high frequencies of elevated levels of serum ferritin, iron, and transferrin saturation, and these higher levels are generally associated with decreased likelihood of response to interferon therapy. Notably, complete responders to interferon, on average, demonstrate lower hepatic iron concentrations than do noncomplete responders.[170,171] Hayashi et al.[172] reported that bloodletting through repeated venesection reduced iron levels to a degree sufficient to cause significant improvement in serum alanine transaminase (ALT) levels in subjects with chronic active hepatitis C and excess hepatic iron. In two studies, research teams led by Fong[173] (1998) and Fontana[174] (2000) observed that iron reduction through phlebotomy, combined with interferon alpha, reduces liver inflammation, but not fibrosis. Although not statistically significant, their findings indicate that this combination appears to reduce the viral load and may improve sustained response. Notably, ribavirin, which tends to cause anemia (via direct bone marrow suppression), was not part of either treatment protocol being investigated.

In a multicenter, prospective, randomized, controlled trial involving 96 patients with chronic hepatitis C who have previously not responded to interferon, Di Bisceglie et al.[175] compared iron reduction by phlebotomy with iron reduction followed by re-treatment with interferon. They concluded that, "although prior phlebotomy therapy does not improve the rate of sustained response to interferon retreatment, it does result in less liver injury manifested by a decrease in serum transaminase activity and a slight improvement in liver histopathology." In the first randomized, controlled study on the effect of phlebotomy before long-term and high-dose interferon therapy in naive patients with hepatitis C virus–related chronic liver disease, Fargion et al.[176] assessed the outcomes of 114 subjects who were randomized to receive interferon alone or interferon preceded by phlebotomy. In both groups, interferon was given at a dose of 6 mU three times a week for 4 months, followed by 3 mU three times a week for 8 months. The virological sustained response rate in the interferon-only group was 15.8% compared with 28.1% in the iron-depletion group. Patients who underwent phlebotomy tended to respond better to interferon therapy than patients without iron reduction. The difference in sustained response rates between the treatment groups was almost significant for subjects with hepatic iron concentrations no greater than 1100 µg/g dry weight. In contrast to earlier studies indicating that iron removal can improve the histological and virological response to short-term interferon therapy, this latest research demonstrates an improved sustained response when longer courses and higher doses of interferon therapy are administered.

Although the body of literature on use of iron reduction therapy together with interferon suggests the possibility of an effective cure rate of about 75% to 80%, which might be enhanced through the addition of cytokines and antivirals such as ribavirin, trials are evolving from being inconclusive toward consensus.

In India, phlebotomy is not socially acceptable as a means of reducing iron overload to improve the efficacy of interferon therapy. Tandon et al.[177] investigated the efficacy of an indigenous, low-iron, vegetarian diet in reducing serum Fe levels in 19 patients with hepatitis B–related and hepatitis C–related chronic liver disease. One group of 10 subjects had normal (< 25 µmol/l) baseline serum Fe levels, whereas another nine had high (> 25 µmol/l) serum Fe levels. All the subjects were advised to eat a low-Fe rice-based diet, which decreased the daily Fe intake by approximately 50%. All patients complied with the dietary regimen, and at 4 months, significant reductions from baseline were seen in serum Fe and transferrin saturation index (TSI) in both groups, although earlier in those subjects with the higher initial serum Fe levels. Serum ferritin levels, however, were reduced only in the group with lower initial serum Fe levels and not in those with higher initial serum Fe levels. The ALT levels were reduced significantly in both groups. These authors concluded that a low-iron diet results in significant reductions in serum Fe and TSI levels, regardless of baseline Fe levels, and recommended that such a diet should be evaluated to improve the efficacy of interferon therapy in patients with hepatitis B/C–related chronic liver disease.

In a potentially related area, in a pilot study involving 11 patients with chronic hepatitis C virus (HCV) infection, Tanaka et al.[178] found that bovine lactoferrin, 1.8 to 3.6 g daily for 8 weeks, suppressed ALT levels and viral load (as indicated by HCV RNA concentrations) in three of four patients with low pretreatment serum concentrations of HCV RNA. However, seven patients with high pretreatment concentrations showed no significant changes in these indices. The authors suggested that bovine lactoferrin, a subfraction of milk whey protein belonging to the iron transporter family, could be used with any combination of antiviral therapies, including interferon plus ribavirin, without adverse effects.

Clinical Implications and Adaptations

Iron supplementation is generally contraindicated during interferon therapy for viral hepatitis. Physicians treating individuals with hepatitis C virus are advised to consider a strategy of iron reduction, including dietary changes and modification of the nutritional support regimen to minimize iron intake, as well as more direct interventions, such as phlebotomy.

Levothyroxine and Related Thyroid Hormones

L-Triiodothyronine (T_3): Cytomel, liothyronine sodium, liothyronine sodium (synthetic T_3), Triostat (injection).
Levothyroxine (T_4): Eltroxin, Levo-T, Levothroid, levothyroxine (synthetic), levoxin, Levoxyl, Synthroid, thyroxine, Unithroid.

L-Thyroxine and L-triiodothyronine ($T_4 + T_3$): animal levothyroxine/liothyronine, Armour Thyroid, desiccated thyroid, Westhroid.

L-Thyroxine and L-triiodothyronine (synthetic $T_4 + T_3$): Euthroid, Euthyral, liotrix, Thyar, Thyrolar.

Dextrothyroxine (Choloxin).

Evidence: Ferrous sulfate; levothyroxine.

Interaction Type and Significance

✗✗   **Minimal to Mild Adverse Interaction—Vigilance Necessary**

◇◇**Impaired Drug Absorption and Bioavailability, Precautions Appropriate**

≈≈   **Drug-Induced Nutrient Depletion, Supplementation Therapeutic, with Professional Management**

⊕⊕   **Beneficial or Supportive Interaction, with Professional Management**

Coadministration Risk
Probability:
2. Probable

Evidence Base:
● **Consensus**

Coadministration Benefit
Probability:
3. Possible

Evidence Base:
○ **Preliminary**

Effect and Mechanism of Action

Limited but pharmacologically sound evidence indicates that thyroxine and iron (as ferrous sulfate) can bind to form a poorly soluble, stable complex when ingested simultaneously. Consequently, dietary and supplemental iron may reduce the GI absorption of oral levothyroxine, potentially adversely affecting therapeutic response in patients being treated for primary hypothyroidism.[49,179] Simultaneous intake could also contribute to iron depletion in susceptible individuals by impairing iron absorption.

Iron deficiency may contribute to decreased thyroid hormone synthesis and impaired thermoregulation.[180] Iron coadministration may enhance thyroid function, particularly in individuals with iron depletion or deficiency.

Research

Campbell et al.[179,181] observed that the addition of ferrous sulfate to levothyroxine in vitro will produce a poorly soluble, purple, iron-levothyroxine complex.

Clinical observations suggest that a similar pharmacokinetic interaction occurs with in the human gut and is likely to impair absorption and bioavailability of both agents when ingested within the allotted time frame. Thus, in an experiment involving 14 patients with established primary hypothyroidism on stable thyroxine replacement, Campbell et al.[179] observed a reduction in the efficacy of thyroid hormone, as indicated by an increase in thyroid-stimulating hormone (TSH) levels from 1.6 to 5.4 mU/L (although the free thyroxine index did not change significantly), when ferrous sulfate (300 mg) and the usual thyroxine dose were simultaneously ingested for a 12-week period. Thus, 9 of the 14 patients demonstrated an aggravation of their hypothyroid symptoms.

Iron deficiency anemia has been associated with lower plasma thyroid hormone. Beard et al.[180] conducted several intriguing clinical trials looking at the synergistic relationship between iron administration and thyroid function. In an experiment, they exposed 10 women with iron deficiency anemia, eight with depleted iron stores (nonanemic), and 12 control women, all of similar percentage body fat, to a 28° C water bath to test the hypothesis that iron deficiency anemia impairs thermoregulatory performance. They observed that iron administration given to iron-deficient women was associated with improved thyroid function, as indicated by partially normalized plasma thyroid hormone concentrations, and decreased need for thyroid medication. Later, they found that 27 mg/day of iron supplementation helped maintain normal thyroid hormone levels in obese patients put on a very-low-calorie diet.[182] However, using a rodent model, these researchers also found that plasma thyroid hormone kinetics in iron deficiency anemia are corrected by simply providing more thyroxine.[183]

Reports

Schlienger[184] reported the case of a woman with hypothyroidism, stable on levothyroxine, who demonstrated a significant elevation in TSH levels after administration of ferrous sulfate. Subsequently, the dosage of her levothyroxine was raised from 175 to 200 µg per day. In another case, Shakir et al.[184a] described a patient with primary hypothyroidism whose previously effective dose of levothyroxine sodium was impaired subsequent to her beginning treatment with ferrous sulfate. Initially, the patient was restabilized by increasing the dose of L-thyroxine. However, she later became hyperthyroid at that higher dosage level when she discontinued the iron supplementation.[184]

Clinical Implications and Adaptations

Physicians prescribing exogenous thyroid hormone preparations to individuals with primary hypothyroidism are advised to inform these patients to avoid unsupervised iron supplementation and, when concurrent iron administration is indicated by established iron deficiency or depleted iron stores, to separate intake by at least 2 hours to avoid pharmacokinetic interaction that could reduce absorption and bioavailability of both agents. Because hypothyroidism and iron deficiency anemia may coexist, more frequent thyroid function testing is recommended in patients treated concurrently with iron and L-thyroxine. Research suggests that individuals wanting to enhance thyroid function and increase thermogenic effects may benefit from concomitant iron, especially if they have been diagnosed with iron deficiency.

Methyldopa

Methyldopa (Aldomet); combination drugs: methyldopa and chlorothiazide (Aldoclor); methyldopa and hydrochlorothiazide (Aldoril).

Evidence: Ferrous gluconate, ferrous sulfate.

Interaction Type and Significance

✗✗   **Minimal to Mild Adverse Interaction—Vigilance Necessary**

◇◇**Impaired Drug Absorption and Bioavailability, Precautions Appropriate**

≈≈   **Drug-Induced Nutrient Depletion, Supplementation Therapeutic, with Professional Management**

Probability:
2. Probable

Evidence Base:
◉ **Emerging**

Effect and Mechanism of Action

Limited but consistent research has found that iron binds strongly to methyldopa, producing ferric iron–methyldopa complexes, and thereby reduces the absorption and bioavailability of both the methyldopa and the iron salt.[49,185]

Thus, the pharmacokinetic interaction could reduce the antihypertensive effects of methyldopa and might contribute to compromised iron status, particularly in individuals with iron deficiency or susceptible to depleted iron stores.

Ferrous iron, such as ferrous sulfate, is formed from ferric iron when it is reduced under the influence of the acidic pH of the GI environment. However, ferrous iron undergoes auto-oxidation to the ferric form in the presence of methyldopa and levodopa. The formation of these complexes is rapid at high pH (i.e., 9), whereas the rate slows considerably as the pH is lowered (e.g., 4). A variety of iron-methyldopa complexes can be formed between pH 4 and 9. Complexation is absent below pH 2. Together, these processes can result in both catechol oxidation and production of the toxic hydroxyl radical.[96]

Research

Campbell et al.[186] conducted a randomized crossover trial involving 12 normal subjects in which they administered a 500-mg tablet of methyldopa (2.37 mmol) with and without ferrous sulfate (325 mg) and measured absorption and excretion of methyldopa. When ferrous sulfate and methyldopa were coadministered, they observed a decrease in the proportion of methyldopa excreted as "free" methyldopa (49.5% vs. 21.1%), a significant increase in the proportion excreted as methyldopa sulfate (37.8% vs. 65.8%), and a decrease in the percentage of methyldopa absorbed (29.1% vs. 7.88%). Together these factors resulted in an 88% reduction in the quantity of "free" methyldopa excreted. Ferrous gluconate (600 mg) produced similar effects. These researchers also found that concurrent intake of ferrous sulfate and methyldopa for 2 weeks produced an increase in both systolic and diastolic blood pressure in four of five hypertensive subjects receiving chronic methyldopa therapy, with substantial increases in blood pressure seen in three of the patients. A decrease in blood pressure occurred in all patients after ferrous sulfate was discontinued.[186]

Subsequently, Campbell[185] and another team used a rat model to investigate the mechanism(s) by which ferrous sulfate (and sodium sulfate) reduces methyldopa absorption. They observed that ferrous sulfate reduced methyldopa absorption by 52.9% when they injected solutions of 14C methyldopa alone and with ferrous sulfate or sodium sulfate in vivo into closed duodenal segments. In the presence of methyldopa, iron in its ferrous form rapidly oxidizes to the ferric form, in vitro. "The ferric form of iron binds strongly to methyldopa, presumably resulting in the decreased methyldopa absorption." Methyldopa was stable in vivo and in vitro, in the presence of ferrous sulfate and sodium sulfate.

Clinical Implications and Adaptations

Physicians prescribing methyldopa are advised to inform patients to avoid unsupervised iron supplementation and, when concurrent iron administration is indicated by established iron deficiency or depleted iron stores, to separate intake by at least 2 hours to avoid pharmacokinetic interaction that could reduce absorption and bioavailability, and thus therapeutic activity, of methyldopa. Concomitant use, with simultaneous or proximate intake, could also potentially, over time, contribute to or aggravate iron deficiency or depletion of iron stores in susceptible individuals.

Neomycin

Neomycin (Mycifradin, Myciguent, Neo-Fradin, NeoTab, Nivemycin).

Interaction Type and Significance

≈◇◇ **Drug-Induced Nutrient Depletion, Supplementation Contraindicated, Professional Management Appropriate**

⊕✗ **Bimodal or Variable Interaction, with Professional Management**

⊕ **Potential or Theoretical Beneficial or Supportive Interaction, with Professional Management**

Probability:
2. Probable

Evidence Base:
○ Preliminary

Effect and Mechanism of Action

Neomycin may impair the absorption of iron and many other nutrients.[77,187]

Research

Jacobson et al.[188] coadministered neomycin and ferrous citrate to six nonanemic subjects in an experimental malabsorption syndrome study. They observed marked reduction in iron absorption in four subjects but increased iron absorption in the other two subjects, both of whom initially demonstrated low serum iron levels. These findings suggest that an individual's initial iron status may play a pivotal role in their response to iron absorption under the influence of neomycin.

Nutritional Therapeutics, Clinical Concerns, and Adaptations

Physicians prescribing neomycin for an extended period are advised to monitor iron status and consider the potential need for iron supplementation in individuals susceptible to iron depletion. Oral intake should be separated by at least 2 hours if iron supplementation is determined to be clinically appropriate for a given patient. However, it is generally inappropriate to administer iron during an infection because iron may enhance pathogenic activity and contribute to the inflammatory process. Short-term use, such as preparation for surgery using oral neomycin, is unlikely to result in clinically significant iron deficiencies.

Oral Contraceptives: Monophasic, Biphasic, and Triphasic Estrogen Preparations (Synthetic Estrogen and Progesterone Analogs)

Ethinyl estradiol and desogestrel (Desogen, Ortho-TriCyclen).
Ethinyl estradiol and ethynodiol (Demulen 1/35, Demulen 1/50, Nelulen 1/25, Nelulen 1/50, Zovia).
Ethinyl estradiol and levonorgestrel (Alesse, Levlen, Levlite, Levora 0.15/30, Nordette, Tri-Levlen, Triphasil, Trivora).
Ethinyl estradiol and norethindrone/norethisterone (Brevicon, Estrostep, Genora 1/35, GenCept 1/35, Jenest-28, Loestrin 1.5/30, Loestrin1/20, Modicon, Necon 1/25, Necon 10/11, Necon 0.5/30, Necon 1/50, Nelova 1/35, Nelova 10/11, Norinyl 1/35, Norlestin 1/50, Ortho Novum 1/35, Ortho Novum 10/11, Ortho Novum 7/7/7, Ovcon-35, Ovcon-50, Tri-Norinyl, Trinovum).
Ethinyl estradiol and norgestrel (Lo/Ovral, Ovral).
Mestranol and norethindrone (Genora 1/50, Nelova 1/50, Norethin 1/50, Ortho-Novum 1/50).
Related, internal application: Etonogestrel/ethinyl estradiol vaginal ring (Nuvaring).

Interaction Type and Significance

⊕⊕ **Beneficial or Supportive Interaction, with Professional Management**

◇◇ **Drug-Induced Effect on Nutrient Function, Supplementation Contraindicated, Professional Management Appropriate**

Probability: Evidence Base:
2. Probable   ◉ **Emerging**

Effect and Mechanism of Action

Oral contraceptive (OC) use is associated with decreased menstrual blood loss and potentially a reduced need for supplemental iron if increased iron stores result.

Research

The volume of blood loss associated with menstrual flow is usually decreased among certain women using OCs, but evidence of associated benefits in iron stores is less definite. Several early studies and reviews reported that OCs have beneficial effects on iron status, even though clinical research investigating the effects of OCs on iron metabolism was largely scarce.[189-191] For example, in 1984, Tyrer[192] presented the conventional position in summarizing that OCs have been "shown to decrease the physiologic levels of six nutrients—riboflavin, pyridoxine, folacin, vitamin B_{12}, ascorbic acid and zinc." However, they followed with the optimistic conclusion: "Women who take OCs and have adequate diets need little or no supplemental vitamins." After further noting that OCs are associated with increased levels of vitamin C, iron, copper, and vitamin A, the author suggested: "Vitamin and mineral increases caused by OCs do not require treatment." Thus, iron supplementation would be considered less important to women using OCs and experiencing decreased menstrual blood loss than to those not having their menstrual processes altered with exogenous hormones.

Frassinelli-Gunderson et al.[193] compared serum ferritin and other parameters of iron status in 46 women using OCs for 2 or more years continuously and 71 women who never took OCs. They found that the mean serum ferritin level for the OC users was significantly higher, 39.5 ng/mL, compared to a mean level of 25.4 ng/ml in the control group. Serum transferrin, serum iron, TIBC, mean corpuscular hemoglobin (MCH), and MCH concentration (MCHC) levels were also significantly greater among the OC users. However, significantly lower RBC and hematocrit levels were found for OC users, whereas other parameters, such as hemoglobin, mean corpuscular volume (MCV), and percent transferrin saturation, were not significantly different between the groups. OC users also reported decreased menstrual cycle blood losses and a higher heme iron content in their diet. Palomo et al.[194] found that use of OCs was not associated with hemoglobin decrease, but they did observe a significant rise in saturation of transferrin. Masse and Roberge[195] investigated the effect of low-dose OC use for at least 1 year on iron metabolism and body iron status in 64 active and healthy adult women. The serum iron concentration was significantly higher in OC users than an age-matched control group. However, they found that serum ferritin, a marker for body iron stores, was marginal in both OC users and control subjects, even though mean dietary iron intake was adequate in both groups. These researchers noted that this finding indicated an underlying "high prevalence of deficient-iron reserves among subjects" that was not correlated to dietary iron content. These researchers concluded that their findings "commanded a discussion on the pertinence of evaluating the total dietary iron intake and on the sensitivity of biochemical methods used to assess the iron status."[195]

Steegers-Theunissen et al.[196] conducted a study of the effects of long-term use of OCs containing less than 50 µg of estrogen (sub-50 OCs) on the kinetics of folic acid monoglutamate, vitamin B_{12} levels, and iron status in 29 OC users and in 13 non-OC-user controls. OC users showed significantly higher TIBC. The OC users also demonstrated significantly lower serum vitamin B_{12} concentrations and significantly lower median serum folate concentration at 210 minutes after oral folate loading compared with the control group, but the authors concluded that even with these "significant effects upon folate kinetics and vitamin B_{12} levels, the folate and vitamin B_{12} status does not seem to be at risk."[196]

Mooij et al.[197] compared the effects of multivitamin supplementation on serum ferritin and hematological parameters in 28 women using OCs (sub-50 OCs) and 31 non-OC users over three consecutive cycles. Comparison of the baseline values on days 3 and 23 of the first cycle of the two groups revealed that the parameters of serum iron status were all significantly increased for the OC users compared to the non-OC control group, even though there were no significant different hematological parameters from OC use. Multivitamin supplementation was started on day 1 of the second cycle and continued daily throughout three consecutive cycles until the end of the study. The multivitamin was associated with a significantly decreased MCHC in both groups, increased MCV, and significantly increased serum iron and TIBC, whereas serum ferritin decreased during multivitamin supplementation and hematocrit and MCH remained unaltered.

Recent reviews continue to state that enhancement of iron status is among the noncontraceptive benefits of OCs.[198,199] However, human research has yet to emerge investigating the clinical implications of apparent pharmacogenomic variability in responses to synthetic, exogenous hormones such as OCs and their influence on menstrual flow, blood loss, and iron metabolism.

Nutritional Therapeutics, Clinical Concerns, and Adaptations

Physicians prescribing OCs are advised to monitor the iron status of these female patients with periodic assessment of serum ferritin, ferritin saturation, and serum transferrin receptor levels. Increased iron levels in the blood are not necessarily a problem, but decreased monthly blood loss could potentially result in increased iron stores over time. Consequently, premenopausal women using OCs may have a decreased need for supplemental iron. Evaluation of iron status is essential before initiation of iron supplementation. Regular monitoring of folate and vitamins B_{12} and B_6 is also recommended in such women, and preventive supplementation is usually advisable.

Penicillamine

Penicillamine (D-Penicillamine; Cuprimine, Depen).

Interaction Type and Significance

✗✗   Minimal to Mild Adverse Interaction—Vigilance Necessary

◇◇Impaired Drug Absorption and Bioavailability, Precautions Appropriate

⊕✗   Bimodal or Variable Interaction, with Professional Management

≈≈   Drug-Induced Nutrient Depletion, Supplementation Therapeutic, with Professional Management

Probability: Evidence Base:
1. Certain   ● **Consensus**

Effect and Mechanism of Action

The chelation function of penicillamine is central to its primary pharmacological action in therapeutic application. Penicillamine and iron bind together, thereby increasing iron excretion and impairing bioavailability and reducing therapeutic activity of penicillamine.[200]

Penicillamine may be used to treat iron overload. Conversely, chelation therapy with penicillamine aimed at removal of other metals could induce or exacerbate depleted iron stores if compensatory nutrient augmentation is appropriate but not provided.

Research

After administering single 500-mg oral doses of penicillamine to six healthy men, Osman et al.[201] observed that penicillamine levels were reduced to 35% of those from a fasting dose. Stockley[77] reported that the absorption of penicillamine can be reduced as much as two-thirds by the concurrent use of oral iron preparations.

Reports

Harkness and Blake[202] described four cases of penicillamine-induced kidney damage that occurred when concomitant iron therapy was stopped, presumably as a result of increased penicillamine absorption and toxicity.

Clinical Implications and Adaptations

Physicians prescribing penicillamine therapy are advised to question patients regarding use of supplements containing iron and other minerals and to caution against initiation of such substances or their abrupt, unsupervised discontinuation. Chelation with penicillamine or other agents requires appropriate training and proper monitoring. Assessment of iron status is appropriate, and clinical responses will vary accordingly.

During the course of penicillamine therapy, iron deficiency can often develop, especially in children and menstruating women. In Wilson's disease, this may be a result of adding the effects of the low-copper diet, which is probably also low in iron, and the penicillamine to the effects of blood loss or growth. In cystinuria, a low-methionine diet may contribute to iron deficiency because it is inherently low in protein.

In certain circumstances, physicians who administer penicillamine for chelation of copper or other metals or for other clinical applications should coadminister minerals of nutritional importance in accordance with the therapeutic strategy and individual patient needs. When properly administered, penicillamine chelation is considered unlikely to result in adverse reactions from iron depletion. Great caution needs to be exercised when changing the level of iron intake in individuals taking penicillamine. Adverse reactions have been reported in which the prescribing physician was unaware that a patient was using concomitant supplemental iron and responded to the lack of therapeutic response to penicillamine by increasing the drug dose, after which the patient discontinued the self-prescribed iron supplementation.

Orally administered iron has been shown to reduce the effects of penicillamine. If necessary, iron may be given in short courses, but at least 2 hours, or preferably 8 hours, should elapse between administration of penicillamine and oral intake of iron supplements or other iron-containing products.

Note: Tetrathiomolybdate is much less toxic than penicillamine (or trientine) and is emerging as the copper chelator of choice for Wilson's disease. However, it has not yet obtained final approval as a new drug. Tetrathiomolybdate probably has the same interaction with iron as the other copper chelators, but substantive evidence is lacking.

Sulfasalazine

Sulfasalazine (Salazosulfapyridine, salicylazosulfapyridine, suphasalazine; Apo-Sulfasalazine, Azulfidine, Azulfidine EN-Tabs, PMS-Sulfasalazine, Salazopyrin, Salazopyrin EN-Tabs, SAS).

Interaction Type and Significance

◇◇Impaired Drug Absorption and Bioavailability, Precautions Appropriate

≈≈ Drug-Induced Nutrient Depletion, Supplementation Therapeutic, with Professional Management

◇ Adverse Drug Effect on Nutritional Therapeutics, Strategic Concern

Probability:	Evidence Base:
2. Probable or 1. Certain	● Consensus

Effect and Mechanism of Action

Despite long-standing clinical application, scientific understanding of sulfasalazine, its mechanisms, and actions is incomplete. Sulfasalazine is a prodrug that is broken down by gut bacteria into 5-aminosalicylic acid (5ASA) and sulfapyridine. Although the therapeutic activity of 5ASA has been established to some degree, controversy surrounds the role and significance of sulfapyridine. A systemic immunosuppressant effect appears to be involved, but much of the anti-inflammatory activity may result from local effects on the bowel. After oral administration, 33% of the sulfasalazine is absorbed, about 33% of the 5ASA is absorbed, and all the sulfapyridine is absorbed.

Iron and sulfasalazine tend to bind in the digestive tract to form a chelate that is poorly absorbed. Consequently, the concurrent ingestion of these substances can interfere with metabolism of the prodrug into its constituents and lead to their decreased absorption and bioavailability, as well as that of iron.[203]

Research

Clinical research directly investigating the interaction between sulfasalazine and iron is limited. However, the pharmacological literature accepts the existence of this pharmacokinetic interaction as representing a consensus position, based on the principles involved and general knowledge of the agents.

Iron depletion resulting from chelation by concomitant sulfasalazine has not been studied per se. Such an adverse effect on iron status is not improbable, even with the normal physiological controls on iron levels and variable absorption rates, in light of the typically extended duration of standard sulfasalazine use. Clinical concern for iron deficiency is reasonable given the high incidence of blood loss and tissue iron depletion in individuals being treated with sulfasalazine for conditions such as ulcerative colitis or Crohn's disease. Thus, long-term sulfasalazine therapy and simultaneous oral iron intake in the face of iron deficiency could theoretically contribute to lack of tissue repletion, if care is not taken to separate intake of the two agents. Furthermore, evidence is lacking to determine whether or not long-term oral sulfasalazine therapy might cause or aggravate iron deficiency in certain persons, such as menstruating women, by preventing dietary iron absorption.

Evidence is lacking as to interactions between iron and other members of the sulfonamide class of drugs.

Nutritional Therapeutics, Clinical Concerns, and Adaptations

Physicians prescribing sulfasalazine are advised to inform patients of the probable pharmacokinetic interaction between iron and the medication and to recommend separating oral intake by at least 3 hours. Such measures should allow concurrent us of both agents without interfering with the intended therapeutic activity of either. In general, conservative principles of practice warrant advising patients against taking iron supplements without specific, well-founded therapeutic need and outside the context of medical supervision and monitoring. Such cautions are particularly relevant in a patient population characterized by inflammation, even in the presence of blood loss and significant probability of anemia.

Tetracycline Antibiotics

Demeclocycline (Declomycin), doxycycline (Atridox, Doryx, Doxy, Monodox, Periostat, Vibramycin, Vibra-Tabs), minocycline (Dynacin, Minocin, Vectrin), oxytetracycline (Terramycin), tetracycline (Achromycin, Actisite, Apo-Tetra, Economycin, Novo-Tetra, Nu-Tetra, Sumycin, Tetrachel, Tetracyn); combination drugs: chlortetracycline, demeclocycline, and tetracycline (Deteclo); bismuth, metronidazole, and tetracycline (Helidac).

Interaction Type and Significance

◇◇Impaired Drug Absorption and Bioavailability, Precautions Appropriate

≈≈ Drug-Induced Nutrient Depletion, Supplementation Therapeutic, with Professional Management

◇ Adverse Drug Effect on Nutritional Therapeutics, Strategic Concern

Probability:
2. Probable or 1. Certain

Evidence Base:
● Consensus

Effect and Mechanism of Action

Tetracycline-class medications are primarily absorbed in the stomach and upper small intestine. When ingested concurrently, tetracyclines tend to form insoluble chelates with iron salts and other polyvalent metal cations, including calcium, magnesium, and zinc. This pharmacokinetic interaction can impair absorption and bioavailability of both agents, reduce the therapeutic activity of the antibiotic, and adversely affect iron balance.[204,205]

Research

Clinical research directly investigating this interaction is limited. However, the pharmacological literature accepts this pharmacokinetic interaction as representing a consensus position based on the principles involved and general knowledge of the agents involved.

Ingestion of iron supplements or iron-rich foods within a time frame allowing for binding in the gut can depress drug levels to such a degree that their therapeutic effectiveness is significantly reduced or neutralized. This adverse interaction can be avoided by maximally separating intake to minimize contact between the agents.[77]

Iron depletion resulting from chelation by antibiotics in the tetracycline class has not been the subject of substantial study. Although plausible, such an adverse effect on iron status is highly improbable with short-term tetracycline antibiotic use, given the normal physiological controls on iron levels and variable absorption rates. However, long-term tetracycline therapy and simultaneous oral iron intake in the face of iron deficiency could theoretically contribute to lack of tissue repletion. Evidence is lacking to determine whether or not long-term oral tetracycline antibiotic therapy might cause iron deficiency in certain persons, such as menstruating women, by preventing dietary iron absorption.

Nutritional Therapeutics, Clinical Concerns, and Adaptations

Iron in the form of preparations and iron-rich foods should generally be avoided while using drugs in the tetracycline class of antibiotics. Conservative principles of practice warrant advising patients against taking iron preparations without specific, well-founded therapeutic need and outside the context of medical supervision and monitoring. Such cautions regarding iron intake are particularly relevant during an infection because iron may enhance pathogenic activity and contribute to the inflammatory process.

In cases where iron administration is warranted, physicians prescribing tetracycline antibiotics are advised to inform patients of the probable pharmacokinetic interaction between iron and the medication and to recommend separating oral intake by at least 3 hours. Such measures should allow concurrent us of both agents without interfering with the intended therapeutic activity of either. Monitoring of iron status is warranted with extended administration.

Trientine

Trientine (Trien, trienthylene tetramine; Syprine).

Interaction Type and Significance

✗✗ Minimal to Mild Adverse Interaction—Vigilance Necessary

◇◇Impaired Drug Absorption and Bioavailability, Precautions Appropriate

⊕✗ Bimodal or Variable Interaction, with Professional Management

≈≈ Drug-Induced Nutrient Depletion, Supplementation Therapeutic, with Professional Management

Probability:
1. Certain

Evidence Base:
● Consensus

Effect and Mechanism of Action

Trientine is primarily used as a chelating agent in patients with Wilson's disease who are intolerant of penicillamine, to reduce the toxic load of excess copper on the liver, brain, and other organs. Iron from supplements or iron-rich foods can bind to trientine when ingested concurrently, thereby impairing trientine bioavailability and reducing its therapeutic activity (copper chelation) while increasing iron excretion.

Research

The chelation function of trientine is central to its primary pharmacological action in therapeutic application, and its interaction with iron is well established. Anemia is a common adverse effect associated with trientine and is more likely to occur in children, menstruating women, and pregnant women, who usually have greater needs for iron nutriture than other patients.

Nutritional Therapeutics, Clinical Concerns, and Adaptations

Although clinical experience with trientine is limited, it is generally agreed that use of iron and mineral nutrients concurrently with trientine may impair absorption and decrease therapeutic activity of the medication. Physicians prescribing trientine always need to ask patients about supplement use and track dietary intake patterns of copper and other minerals; close supervision and regular monitoring are essential throughout the period of drug administration. Copper levels are typically monitored in patients undergoing trientine therapy, with determination of free serum copper being the most reliable index for monitoring treatment. Adequately treated patients will usually have less than 10 µg free copper/dL serum.

Close monitoring of iron status is also warranted in patients, especially children and menstruating or pregnant women, with a known history of or a high susceptibility to iron deficiency anemia or tissue iron depletion. Except for potential interference with iron absorption caused by the chelating activity of the medication, patients following the low-copper diet appropriate to Wilson's disease are at increased risk of insufficient dietary intake of iron and other key nutrients. In patients with an established need for concomitant iron or other mineral supplementation, iron is usually prescribed in short courses, and patients are advised to separate oral intake by at least 2 hours to minimize any incidence of mutual interference.

Note: Tetrathiomolybdate is much less toxic than trientine (or penicillamine) and is emerging as the copper chelator of choice for Wilson's disease. However, it has not yet obtained final approval as a new drug. Tetrathiomolybdate probably has the same interaction with iron as the other copper chelators, but substantive evidence is lacking.

THEORETICAL, SPECULATIVE, AND PRELIMINARY INTERACTIONS RESEARCH, INCLUDING OVERSTATED INTERACTIONS CLAIMS

Allopurinol

Allopurinol (Oxypurinol; Aloprim, Apo-Allopurinol, Lopurin, Purinol, Zyloprim).

Allopurinol is a xanthine oxidase inhibitor used to prevent gout and to lower blood levels of uric acid in certain oncology patients undergoing chemotherapy. Allopurinol should always be used with caution during lactation and in patients with liver or renal disease.

Preliminary evidence from animal experiments indicates that concurrent intake of allopurinol and iron preparations could potentially result in an adverse interaction involving excess hepatic iron storage.[206-209] For example, in a study involving hyperthermic rat liver perfusion, Powers et al.[210] reported that allopurinol, as an inhibitor of the xanthine oxidase/reductase enzyme system, can both slow mobilization of iron from ferritin and reduce the oxidative stress associated with xanthine oxidase activity, which generates superoxide radicals. However, these effects have never been observed clinically in humans.

Based on a highly cautious approach to the limited data available, physicians might find it judicious to monitor ferritin levels in patients taking chronic allopurinol and iron supplements (in iron-deficient patients) because of a possible adverse interaction.

Amphetamines and Related Stimulant Medications

Amphetamine aspartate monohydrate, amphetamine sulfate, dextroamphetamine saccharate, dextroamphetamine sulfate; D-amphetamine, Dexedrine.
Methylphenidate (Metadate, Methylin, Ritalin, Ritalin-SR; Concerta).
Mixed amphetamines: Amphetamine and dextroamphetamine (Adderall; dexamphetamine).
Pemoline (Cylert).

Konofal et al.[211] found that iron deficiency is a clinically significant factor in many children diagnosed with attention deficit–hyperactivity disorder (ADHD), and that iron supplementation may improve therapeutic outcomes in certain cases. These findings suggest that further research is warranted into the role of iron nutriture and metabolism in the pathophysiology of ADHD and the potential for enhanced therapeutic efficacy from administration of supplemental iron along with

conventional medications in cases where iron deficiency is diagnosed as a comorbid condition.

Dipyridamole

Dipyridamole (Permole, Persantine).

Dipyridamole is an older antiplatelet drug, often combined with aspirin before the availability of ticlopidine (Ticlid) and clopidogrel (Plavix) to prevent strokes, with warfarin (Coumadin) to prevent clotting after heart valve replacement, or used alone. Dipyridamole might reduce the oxidative damage caused by iron, particularly iron-induced platelet aggregation.

In vitro research indicates that dipyridamole inhibits platelet aggregation induced by iron and oxygen-derived free radicals. De la Cruz et al.[212] observed that "ferrous salts (Fe2+) induced 34% platelet aggregation which was inhibited (79.6%) by a concentration of dipyridamole of 10 microM. Dipyridamole inhibited ferrous-induced lipid peroxidation with IC-50 values of 17.5 microM."

An emerging body of evidence indicates that excess iron intake by individuals who are not iron deficient might cause tissue damage that could then contribute to heart disease.[33]

Well-designed human trials might be appropriate to investigate this potential therapeutic application of dipyridamole in reducing the effects of iron-induced oxidative damage on by platelet aggregation. Administration of dipyridamole with the specific aim of countering the effects of iron is unsupported at this time and requires supportive evidence from substantive research.

Haloperidol

Haloperidol (Haldol).

Use of haloperidol is associated with decreased blood levels of iron.[213] Ben-Shachar and Youdim[214] observed that dopamine D_2 receptor subsensitivity, a feature of iron deficiency, is absent in iron-deficient rats administered haloperidol, and that biochemical and behavioral D_2 receptor supersensitivity is relatively greater than in control, haloperidol-treated animals. These researchers found that haloperidol (5 mg/kg daily for 21 days), as well as chlorpromazine (10 mg/kg daily for 21 days), caused a significant reduction (20%-25%) in liver nonheme iron stores compared with values in control rats. However, haloperidol had no effect in iron-deficient rats whose liver iron stores had been almost totally depleted. The authors interpreted these findings to suggest that lower iron levels may result in an increase in free haloperidol available to the dopamine D_2 receptor.

No definitive research has emerged to confirm the occurrence or clarify the clinical significance of this interaction between haloperidol and iron in humans. Pending more conclusive findings from well-designed clinical trials or consistent, substantive, and well-documented case reports, physicians prescribing haloperidol are advised to ask patients about their supplement use and recommend that they avoid supplements containing iron unless iron deficiency has been diagnosed. Monitoring of haloperidol levels may be warranted if iron status is altered or dietary intake significantly changes.

Methotrexate

Methotrexate (Folex, Maxtrex, Rheumatrex).

Concern has been raised that concomitant oral iron intake might alter absorption and therapeutic activity of methotrexate. In a randomized, double-blind, placebo-controlled crossover study, Hamilton et al.[215] compared the urinary excretion of unmetabolized methotrexate in 10 patients with rheumatoid arthritis who were administered methotrexate, 7.5 mg weekly, and either ferrous sulfate, 300 mg twice daily, or placebo for 1 week. No significant difference was observed in average 24-hour urine excretion of methotrexate between the two groups.

Pending further research, the probability of a clinically significant interaction between methotrexate and supplemental iron can be considered as improbable. Nevertheless, it might be judicious to advise patients for whom both agents are medically appropriate to separate intake by at least 3 hours to avoid any as-yet undocumented pharmacokinetic interference with absorption of either agent.

Pyrimethamine/Sulfadoxine

Pyrimethamine (Daraprim); combination drug: sulfadoxine and pyrimethamine (Fansidar).

Deficiencies in vitamin A, zinc, iron, folate, and other micronutrients are responsible for a substantial proportion of malaria morbidity and mortality. Iron deficiency and *Plasmodium falciparum* malaria are the two main causes of anemia in young children in regions endemic for this disease, even though malaria infection itself does not contribute to iron deficiency. However, Stockley[77] reports that iron may delay the therapeutic activity of pyrimethamine/sulfadoxine in eradicating *P. falciparum* or *Plasmodium vivax*, the malaria parasite. Thus, the determination of nutritional status and the appropriate timing of nutritional support can be of critical importance in promoting positive clinical outcomes.

In a trial of two-by-two factorial design, Verhoef et al.[216] randomly assigned 328 anemic but symptom-free Kenyan children into four groups of equal size to receive either iron or placebo and sulfadoxine-pyrimethamine (SP) or placebo. Hematological indicators of iron status and inflammation at the end of the follow-up and occurrence of malaria attacks served as primary outcomes. Analyses were by intention to treat. These researchers observed that after 12 weeks, the groups administered iron plus SP, iron alone, or SP alone had higher hemoglobin concentrations than the group given placebo. Coadministration of iron and SP also lowered the proportion with anemia from 100% at baseline to 36% at 12 weeks, and with iron deficiency from 66% at baseline to 8% at 12 weeks. Survival analysis revealed no evidence of substantially increased risk of malaria after iron administration.

Desai et al.[217] conducted a randomized, placebo-controlled trial involving 546 anemic children age 2 to 36 months in a malaria-endemic area of western Kenya. All children used bednets and received a single dose of SP on enrollment, followed by either intermittent preventive treatment (IPT) with SP at 4 and 8 weeks and daily iron for 12 weeks, daily iron and IPT with SP placebo, IPT and daily iron placebo, or daily iron placebo and IPT with SP placebo (double placebo). After assessing the mean hemoglobin concentration at 12 weeks, compared with that for the double-placebo group, these researchers determined that IPT reduced the incidence of malaria parasitemia and clinic visits, but iron provided no additional preventive benefit. Furthermore, although the combination of IPT and iron was most effective in treating mild anemia and IPT prevented malaria, with IPT "the hematological benefit...added to that of a single dose of SP and bednet use was modest."[217] However, in a subsequent cluster-randomized clinical trial investigating iron dosing in the treatment of anemia in preschool children, this research team found that, after initial antimalarial treatment with a single SP dose, 6 weeks of daily iron supplementation results in superior hematological responses, particularly hemoglobin concentrations, than does twice-weekly iron administration, regardless of whether adherence can be ensured.[218]

Iron supplementation can play an important role in the recovery of patients, especially malnourished children, after treatment for malaria. However, iron coadministration in cases of anemia associated with malaria is controversial. Introduction of weekly iron may be appropriate starting 2 weeks after the malaria is controlled. However, in children who have been severely malnourished or ill, especially edematous, it is advisable to withhold iron until the child is recovering (e.g., loss of edema, weight gain, no hepatomegaly), even if iron deficiency anemia has been diagnosed. Iron should not be administered until they regain their appetite, regardless of the hemoglobin level. These children generally have very low levels of transferrin, a high iron saturation, stainable iron in their marrow and liver, and high levels of iron excretion after desferrioxamine. Thus, iron should be initiated when the children start to grow rapidly, have resynthesized their transferrin, and have reversed the oxidized intracellular environment. Measuring GSH and NADPH longitudinally can guide the timing of iron introduction. Monitoring for iron overload is warranted, but the probability of this occurring in the affected patient populations is low. Life-threatening anemia (in the range of 3 g/dL) will usually require transfusion, but great caution and careful supervision are required so as not to precipitate cardiac failure.

Folic acid administration is warranted in many individuals because anemia is endemic in susceptible populations, particularly children, and the causes of anemia are multifactorial.

Stanozolol

Stanozolol (Winstrol).

In a letter, Taberner[219] reported that stanozolol therapy was associated with iron deficiency. Sixteen patients taking 10 mg stanozolol daily in a trial of fibrinolytic enhancement therapy in intermittent claudication experienced a significant fall in mean cell hemoglobin (MCH) after 3 months of treatment. The red blood cell (RBC) count did not change significantly, but hemoglobin (Hb) and mean cell volume (MCV) also declined, contrary to an expected rise in Hb and RBC count. After exclusion of one patient who was iron deficient at baseline, six patients remained on therapy for a year or more. Four of these had dietary histories indicating insufficient iron nutriture and demonstrated RBC indices suggestive of iron deficiency, later confirmed by biochemical measurement and ferritin assay. In one of these four patients, stanozolol was discontinued without iron supplementation; the RBC indices and iron status returned to normal. No GI bleeding or evidence of fecal blood loss was observed to account for the iron deficiency. The increase in muscle bulk induced by the anabolic steroids was hypothesized to cause utilization of iron at the expense of Hb, subsequently reflected in a change in RBC Hb. The author concluded by recommending that "patients taking stanozolol for long periods should have RBC indices and liver function monitored regularly".[219]

Warfarin

Warfarin (Coumadin, Marevan, Warfilone).

Iron (as well as magnesium and zinc) can bind with warfarin, potentially decreasing absorption and activity of both agents.[220] However, these potential effects have never been confirmed by conclusive findings from well-designed clinical trials or consistent, substantive, and well-documented case reports.

According to a nested case-control analysis of multiple linked health care databases conducted by Canadian researchers, patients taking warfarin at the same time as selective COX-2 inhibitors or nonselective NSAIDs have an increased risk of hospitalization for upper GI hemorrhage.[161] Patients in such situations would be at increased risk of iron deficiency anemia or tissue iron depletion because of chronic blood loss.

Although the pharmacological principles of an interaction involving binding of warfarin by concurrent ingestion of common mineral nutrients are well founded, the frequency of occurrence and clinical significance of this potential interaction are uncertain. Physicians prescribing warfarin should be aware of the possible risk of reduced effectiveness of treatment in patients taking nutrient formulations containing iron, magnesium, and zinc. Separating oral intake of warfarin and such minerals by at least 2 hours will usually provide adequate protection from unwanted interference.

NUTRIENT-NUTRIENT INTERACTIONS

Calcium

Calcium in foods or supplements may reduce absorption of iron, especially heme iron. When ingested concurrently, substantial doses of calcium (as carbonate, phosphate, or citrate) can significantly decrease iron absorption, by as much as 62%.[221-226] The available findings suggest that the effects of this pharmacokinetic interaction may be clinically insignificant at calcium intake levels of 1000 to 1500 mg/day, as indicated by serum ferritin levels, in individuals who are neither iron deficient nor demonstrating malabsorption.[227-229]

Available evidence indicates that the absorption of iron in multimineral formulations containing iron and calcium is probably not significantly altered. Nevertheless, separating oral intake of calcium and iron supplements by 2 hours or more may reduce the adverse effects of potential pharmacokinetic interference with absorption of either or both nutrients.

Copper

Iron and copper exhibit a multifaceted synergistic relationship within human physiology. Adequate copper nutriture appears necessary for normal iron absorption and metabolism, iron transport to the bone marrow, and RBC formation. Animals deficient in copper tend to accumulate hepatic iron. Anemia is a clinical sign of copper deficiency. However, simultaneous oral administration of copper and iron in large doses may impair the absorption of either or both nutrients.

Fiber

When consumed concurrently, fiber (particularly phytic acid-containing fiber, as from cereal brans) can reduce iron absorption. Other fibers, such as that from psyllium seed, have minimal if any effect on iron or other mineral absorption.

Folate

Iron and folate work together in many aspects of human physiology, particularly RBC formation and function. Coadministration of iron and folate is common in the prevention and treatment of anemia, but proper diagnostic assessment is essential to determine causal factors.

Thompson et al.[230] at the Cancer Foundation of Western Australia found a protective association between maternal iron or folate supplementation in pregnancy and the risk of common acute lymphoblastic leukemia (ALL) in a population-based case-control study of children from birth to age 14 years and living in Western Australia from 1984 to 1992. For iron alone, the odds ratio was 0.75; only one mother took folate without iron. Further analyses of folate use with or without iron showed that the protective effect varies little by

time of first use of supplements or for how long they were taken.

Manganese

When iron and manganese are ingested together, the absorption of manganese may be impaired. In a study involving 47 women, Davis et al.[231] observed that increased dietary intake of nonheme iron, typical of supplemental formulations, was associated with decreased manganese status. Notably, foods that contain significant amounts of manganese (green vegetables, breads, and cereals) often have significant amounts of nonheme iron and therefore greater probability of impaired manganese absorption. In contrast, heme iron intake was positively correlated with hematological status and had no consistent effect on nutritional status in regard to manganese. Similarly, Finley[232] reported that young women with high iron status, as indicated by serum ferritin concentration, had relatively poor absorption and retention of manganese.

In a review of manganese research, Freeland-Graves[233] recommended that oral intake of iron and manganese be separated by 4 hours, or taken at a different time of day, to avoid absorption problems. However, these findings might also suggest that multimineral formulations containing both iron and manganese could be more effective in preventing manganese deficiency than iron-only preparations.

Pancreatic Enzymes

Iron absorption may potentially be reduced by concomitant use of pancreatic extracts.

Phosphorus/Phosphate Supplements

Calcium phosphate (Tribasic); potassium phosphate; sodium phosphates.

After oral administration, divalent cations, such as iron salts, can bind to orally administered phosphate in the GI tract, potentially reducing the absorption and bioavailability of phosphate supplements. Administering oral phosphate preparations at least 1 hour before, or 2 hours after, oral iron salt intake can reduce the probability and significance of this interaction and maximize the therapeutic effect of the phosphate.

Taurine

In a double-blind, randomized trial involving 51 female university students with iron deficiency anemia (IDA), Sirdah et al.[234] reported a possible beneficial additive effect associated with coadministration of oral taurine (1000 mg/day) and slow-release iron sulfate (325 mg/day), as indicated by changes in hemoglobin concentrations and normalization of iron deficiency markers. No significant adverse effects were reported. They noted that, at baseline, mean serum taurine was significantly lower in the IDA subjects than in the controls.

Vitamin A

Vitamin A improves the absorption and utilization of iron, and vitamin A deficiency may exacerbate iron deficiency anemia. Vitamin A also prevents the inhibition of iron absorption by coffee and tea.[228] Two studies, one focusing on iron metabolism and protein status in children and the other involving pregnant women in West Java with nutritional anemia, found that coadministration of vitamin A enhanced treatment of iron deficiency anemia and improved iron status. The concomitant administration of vitamin A and iron ameliorated anemia more effectively than either iron or vitamin A alone.[235,236] Likewise, in a study of Mexican preschoolers at high risk for deficiency of vitamin A, iron, and zinc, Muñoz et al.[237] demonstrated that supplementation with iron, or iron and zinc, improved indicators of vitamin A status. More recently, Zadik et al.[237a] reported that combined vitamin A and iron supplementation is as efficient as hormonal therapy in constitutionally delayed children.

Vitamin C (Ascorbic Acid)

Vitamin C, in supplemental formulations or vitamin C–rich foods, can strongly enhance the absorption of nonheme iron in the GI tract by reducing dietary ferric iron (Fe^{3+}) to ferrous iron (Fe^{2+}), forming a highly absorbable iron–ascorbic acid complex, and increasing bioavailability of the iron twofold to threefold.[62,77,238-241] This effect, however, appears to be influenced by gastric pH, bile function, and other dietary constituents, very dose dependent, and relatively minor at ascorbic acid doses under 200 mg, even in individuals with low iron stores.[62,242,243] However, ascorbic acid can prevent the dose-dependent inhibitory effects of polyphenols and phytates on nonheme-iron absorption.[244] Furthermore, ascorbate stabilizes the iron cores of ferritin in cells and impairs ferritin degradation and autophagic uptake of ferritin clusters into lysosomes.[245]

Iron deficiency anemia affects one third to half of children in the developing world. Zlotkin et al.[6] found that adding "sprinkles," ferrous fumarate and ascorbic acid microencapsulated in a thin, soy-based coat, to weaning foods can be an effective tool in reducing rates of anemia in susceptible children.

Vitamin E

Evidence: Ferrous sulfate, iron dextran complex.
Extrapolation: Ferric gluconate, ferrous fumarate, ferrous gluconate, iron sucrose, polysaccharide-iron complex.

Concomitant administration of vitamin E may diminish the therapeutic effects and mitigate the adverse effects of iron salts.

In an early study, Melhorn and Gross[246] observed a decrease in the hematological response to iron administration (iron dextran, 5 mg/kg/day for 3 days, followed by oral ferrous sulfate beginning on the seventh day) in children with iron deficiency anemia when oral vitamin E (200 IU) was coadministered on iron days 1 through 3. They reported that the reticulocyte response in patients receiving vitamin E was 4.4%, versus 14.4% in those not receiving vitamin E.

Large doses of iron may increase requirements for vitamin E. Roob et al.[20] found that the antioxidant activity provided by concomitant vitamin E can attenuate oxidative stress induced by IV iron in patients on hemodialysis.

Zinc

When administered orally, at the same time, iron and zinc can mutually reduce absorption. In particular, the ingestion of iron in high doses on an empty stomach can inhibit the absorption of zinc from simultaneous oral intake. However, supplemental iron does not appear to significantly inhibit zinc absorption in the presence of food. Similarly, iron-fortified foods do not appear to significantly alter zinc absorption.[228,229]

Zago and Oteiza[247] reported that the antioxidant activity of zinc may ameliorate oxidative stress induced by iron. Furthermore, the inhibition of Fe^{2+}-induced lipid oxidation by either alpha-tocopherol or epicatechin was increased by the simultaneous addition of zinc.

HERB-NUTRIENT INTERACTIONS

Herbs Containing Tannins And Polyphenols

Black tea, green tea *(Camellia sinensis)*.
Coffee *(Caffea arabica, Caffea canephora, Caffea robusta)*.

Coffee, black or green tea, chamomile, and many other plants, some commonly consumed as beverages, contain significant levels of polyphenols and tannins that can significantly impair absorption of iron by binding with iron to form insoluble complexes. In particular, phenolic compounds from plants consumed as foods and beverages are released during digestion and can complex with nonheme iron in the intestinal lumen, rendering it unavailable for absorption.

Black tea polyphenols are more inhibitory than the polyphenols from herb teas, cocoa, or wine, possibly because of their higher content of galloyl esters. Hurrell et al.[248] studied the effects of different polyphenol-containing beverages on nonheme iron absorption from a bread meal, containing a mere 2.1 mg iron, in adult human subjects from the erythrocyte incorporation of radiolabeled Fe. They tested beverages that contained different polyphenol structures and were rich in either phenolic acids (e.g., chlorogenic acid in coffee), monomeric flavonoids (as found in chamomile [*Matricaria recutita* L.], vervain [*Verbena officinalis* L.], lime flower [*Tilia cordata* Mill.], peppermint [*Mentha piperita* L.], and other common herb teas, as well as pennyroyal [*Mentha pulegium* L.]; or complex polyphenol polymerization products (such as black tea and cocoa). All beverages were potent inhibitors of iron absorption and reduced absorption in a dose-dependent fashion depending on the content of total polyphenols. Compared with a water control meal, beverages containing 20 to 50 mg total polyphenols per serving reduced iron absorption from the bread meal by 50% to 70%. Herbal beverages containing 100 to 400 mg total polyphenols per serving reduced iron absorption by 60% to 90%. Black tea inhibited iron absorption by 79% to 94%, peppermint tea by 84%, pennyroyal by 73%, cocoa 71%, vervain 59%, lime flower 52%, and chamomile by 47%. Black tea was more inhibitory than cocoa, chamomile, vervain, lime flower, and pennyroyal at an identical concentration of total polyphenols. The addition of milk to coffee or tea did not significantly influence their inhibitory nature. Despite the relatively low dose of iron tested, the researchers concluded that these findings demonstrate that black tea, coffee, cocoa, and a variety of herbal teas can be potent inhibitors of iron absorption.[248]

The effect of coffee's inhibition of iron absorption from supplemental or dietary sources may contribute to iron deficiency anemia, particularly in pregnant women; such effects might potentially reduce the levels of iron in breast milk to a clinically significant degree. Morck et al.[249] demonstrated that coffee inhibits iron absorption in a concentration-dependent fashion with simultaneous ingestion and when coffee was taken 1 hour later in iron-replete human subjects. In a controlled study involving pregnant low-income women in Costa Rica who consumed more than 450 mL coffee daily, Muñoz et al.[250] observed an association between coffee consumption and reductions in maternal hemoglobin levels and hematocrits, as well as similar effects in their infants, despite daily supplementation with ferric sulfate 200 mg (i.e., 60 mg elemental iron) and folate (500 μg). Iron deficiency anemia (hemoglobin < 11 g/dL) was demonstrated in almost one quarter of the coffee-drinking mothers compared with none of the non-coffee-drinking mothers in the control group. Iron levels in breast milk were one-third lower in mothers who consumed coffee.

Merhav et al.[251] report a much higher incidence of microcytic anemia among infants in Israel who consumed 50 to 750 mL tea per day (median, 250 mL). On studying 122 healthy infants, they found that the percentage of tea-drinking infants with microcytic anemia was significantly higher than that of the non–tea-drinking infants (32.6% vs. 3.5%). The tea drinkers had significantly lower mean Hb and MCV levels than the non–tea drinkers. However, in a study involving 10 iron-deficient children who consumed 150 mL of tea per day, Koren et al.[252] reported no significant alterations in absorption of iron at daily doses of 2 to 15.8 mg/kg.

These preliminary findings suggest a pattern of impaired iron absorption and bioavailability of potentially meaningful dimensions, even in the presence of iron supplementation. Further research is warranted to determine the incidence and clinical import of these observations. In the meantime, healthcare providers are advised to recommend limited consumption of coffee, tea and other tannin-containing beverages by pregnant or lactating women as well as nursing infants or children drinking herbal beverages.

Samman et al.[253] reported that green tea or rosemary extract, added to foods, reduces nonheme iron absorption by as much as 26%. This apparently significant interaction may be clinically efficacious in the treatment of individuals with iron overload diseases, such as hemochromatosis.

The 256 citations for this monograph, as well as additional reference literature, are located under Iron on the CD at the back of the book.

Nutrient-Drug Interactions and Drug-Induced Nutrient Depletions

Magnesium

Nutrient Name: Magnesium.
Elemental Symbol: Mg.

Drug/Class Interaction Class	Mechanism and Significance	Management
Albuterol Beta-2-adrenoceptor agonist bronchodilators ⊕⊕	Supplementation enhances albuterol efficacy and counters hypomagnesemia. Variable significance, ranging from minimal, preventive to significant, urgent.	Coadminister. Monitor.
Aminoglycoside antibiotics ≈≈/☼	Drug-induced tubular damage, impaired magnesium absorption. Magnesium important with extended therapy.	Coadminister. Monitor.
Amphetamines and stimulant medications Dextroamphetamine Methylphenidate ⊕⊕	Magnesium salts may enhance drug retention and availability; drugs may elevate magnesium levels; mutual increased effect. Improved drug kinetics and enhanced Mg status and effect on Ca/Mg ratio may benefit clinical outcomes.	Coadminister. Monitor. Possible decrease of drug dose.
Amphotericin B ≈≈≈☼	Hypomagnesemia caused by renal magnesium wasting and impaired reabsorption. Hydration and nutrients nephroprotective.	Coadminister. Monitor. Consider liposomal amphotericin B.
Bisphosphonates ◇◇/◇	Minerals and bisphosphonate chelate; reduced absorption and bioavailability. Immediate onset, usually moderate severity, gradual effect.	Modify timing to prevent chelation.
Calcium channel blockers ⊕✗/✗✗✗/✗✗/≈≈	Reduced ionic calcium availability to muscle cells; more hypotensive. Possible synergy. Caution: increased risk in pregnancy.	Consider coadministration. Closely monitor.
Cisplatin ≈≈≈/◇	Cisplatin impairs renal tubules' ability to conserve magnesium, resulting in clinically significant hypomagnesemia.	Evaluate magnesium and potassium status, renal function. Coadminister. Monitor.
Colchicine ≈≈≈	Colchicine may impair absorption of magnesium and other nutrients, potentially causing depletion and adverse effects. Plausible mechanism, but minimal evidence.	Consider supplementing with multivitamin/mineral formulation containing magenesium, with extended colchicine therapy. Separate intake.
Corticosteroids, oral ≈≈≈/◇	Magnesium depletion and impaired absorption. Associated with steroid-induced bone loss.	Supplement minerals during extended steroids.
Cyclosporine ≈≈≈/☼/◇	Severe hypomagnesemia, renal magnesium wasting, nephrotoxicity.	Coadminister. Regularly monitor renal function and RBC Mg levels.
Digoxin ≈≈≈/☼/◇/◇◇	Digoxin decreases Mg and increases loss, increasing risk of digitalis toxicity. Magnesium and digoxin may chelate; reduced absorption and bioavailability of both. Immediate and potentially severe as well as cumulative depletion effects; potential mutual interference.	Coordinated use with separated administration. Closely monitor.
Diuretics, loop and thiazide ≈≈≈/☼/◇	Diuretics inhibit magnesium absorption and increase excretion, amplifying potassium depletion. Cumulative adverse effect of mineral depletion; rapid correction may require intravenous or intramuscular administration of magnesium.	Evaluate magnesium and potassium status, renal function. Coadminister long-term. Monitor.
Estrogens Estrogen replacement therapy (ERT) Oral contraceptives (OCs) ≈≈≈/◇	Exogenous estrogen may shift magnesium to soft tissue and bone, lowering serum levels and body stores. Magnesium depletion may amplify, and supplementation may moderate, possible adverse effects from PMS to bone and heart.	Conservative to supplement for short-term and long-term preventive and protective effects.
Fentanyl ⊕⊕/☼	Coadministration of intravenous magnesium sulfate may enable reducing analgesic dosage requirements, possibly by resetting nerve activation thresholds. Encouraging preliminary research indicates further study warranted, including trials using oral magnesium.	Coadministration of magnesium, usually IV, may be beneficial. Closely monitor.
Fluoroquinolone/quinolone antibiotics ◇◇/◇	Magnesium and fluoroquinolones may chelate; reduced absorption and bioavailability of both. Evidence of potential interference derived from magnesium antacids.	Adjust timing to avoid simultaneous or close oral administration.
Foscarnet ≈≈	Renal impairment caused by foscarnet may be responsible for adverse effect on magnesium, calcium, potassium, and phosphorus. Depletion sequelae are common and can be rapid and severe.	Frequently monitor magnesium and other electrolytes. Administer magnesium as indicated.
Insulin ⊕⊕	Diabetics tend toward magnesium deficiency; magnesium can improve insulin sensitivity and secretion. Both risks and benefits tend to increase gradually.	Coadminister. Monitor.
Lithium carbonate ◇◇	Lithium and magnesium may compete. Concomitant intake may elevate magnesium levels but adverse effects unlikely. No indication of interference with drug activity.	Monitor.
Macrolide antibiotics ≈≈≈/☼	Erythromycin and other macrolide antibiotics may interfere with absorption of magnesium and other nutrients, especially with extended treatment. Mechanism plausible but evidence preliminary or inconclusive.	Consider nutrient supplementation with extended macrolide therapy. Separate intake.

Summary

Drug/Class Interaction Class	Mechanism and Significance	Management
Misoprostol ✗✗/◇◇	Probable additive effect of magnesium, increasing diarrhea. Misoprostol's adverse effects on gastrointestinal tract may be aggravated.	Temporarily avoid magnesium, if possible.
Neuromuscular blocking agents ✗✗/⊕✗/⊕⊕	Magnesium salts can increase and prolong agent effects. Unintentional additive effects may be severe; coordinated use may allow lower drug doses.	Assess magnesium status. Consider coadministration. Monitor closely.
Pentamidine ≈≈/☼	Pentamidine can decrease magnesium levels and produce adverse effects, especially on cardiac function. Evidence minimal but mechanisms reasonable.	Assess and monitor magnesium (and potassium) status initally and during treatment. Coadminister as indicated, possibly preventively.
Penicillamine ◇◇/◇/⊕✗	These agents tend to complex; may reduce magnesium absorption. Simultaneous intake may interfere with and inhibit activity of both agents. High doses of penicillamine for extended period can inactivate and deplete magnesium.	Assess magnesium status. Adjust timing to separate oral administration if magnesium strategically necessary.
Quinidine Antiarrhythmic drugs ⊕⊕/☼/≈≈	Quinidine-induced arrhythmias aggravated by electrolyte abnormalities; MgSO4 reverses torsades de pointes by unknown mechanism. Hypomagnesemia may increase quinidine adverse effects, especially with hypokalemia.	Assess magnesium and potassium status. Consider coadministration. Monitor closely.
Sodium polystyrene sulfonate (SPSS) ≈≈/◇	SPSS may alter magnesium levels and contribute to depletion. Compensatory magnesium may prevent or reverse potential adverse effects. Evidence minimal but mechanism(s) plausible.	Consider magnesium coadministration, especially if magnesium strategically significant.
Sotalol Beta-1-adrenoceptor antagonists ☼/⊕/◇◇	Magnesium salt may reduce drug absorption and availability; drug effect on magnesium (and other minerals) may increase adverse effects; MgSO4 reverses torsades de pointes by unknown mechanism. Intentional coadministration can be acute therapy or long-term supportive; unintentional interference may be gradual.	Coordinated use may be beneficial but need separate administration; closely monitor.
Sulfonylurea Hypoglycemics ✗✗/✗✗✗/⊕✗/⊕/⊕⊕	Magnesium may increase drug activity on glucose. Diabetics tend toward magnesium deficiency; Mg can improve insulin sensitivity and secretion. Enhanced drug response may excessively lower glucose or may facilitate therapeutic strategy.	Coadminister. Monitor. Titrate drug dose.
Tetracycline antibiotics ◇◇/◇/⊕✗	Tendency to chelate may reduce (or enhance) absorption of both; mixed evidence. Coadministration carries risk of (increased) adverse effects but may be efficacious in some uses.	Adjust timing to separate oral administration if magnesium strategically necessary.
Theophylline/aminophylline ◇≈≈/◇/⊕⊕	Theophylline may deplete magnesium and aggravate magnesium status. Patient population tends to be magnesium deficient, and magnesium can support therapeutic outcome.	Assess magnesium status. Consider coadministration. Monitor closely.
Warfarin Oral vitamin K antagonist anticoagulants ◇◇/✗✗/◇	Binding and formation of chelate complexes may reduce absorption and activity of both agents. Evidence mixed but suggests negligible impact on drug activity, especially with separation of oral intake. Further research warranted.	Separate intake by at least 2 hours. Monitor closely.

RBC, Red blood cell; *PMS*, premenstrual syndrome.

NUTRIENT DESCRIPTION

Chemistry and Forms

Magnesium ascorbate, magnesium aspartate, magnesium chloride, magnesium citrate, magnesium fumarate, magnesium gluconate, magnesium glycerophosphate, magnesium glycinate, magnesium hydroxide, magnesium malate, magnesium oxide, magnesium pidolate, magnesium succinate, magnesium sulfate.

Physiology and Function

Magnesium functions as a structural cofactor or as an allosteric activator of enzyme activity in more than 300 enzyme reactions in the body, including those related to the transfer of phosphate groups, all reactions that require adenosine 5'-triphosphate (ATP; i.e., mitochondrial oxidative phosphorylation), glycolysis, fatty acid oxidation and amino acid metabolism, and the replication and transcription of DNA, synthesis of RNA, and translation of messenger RNA (mRNA). Magnesium is the second most abundant intracellular cation and the fourth most prevalent cation in the body. The normal body magnesium content is approximately 1000 mmol, or 22.66 g, of which 50% to 60% resides in bone. Magnesium affects many cellular functions, including transport of potassium (K^+) and calcium (Ca^{++}) ions, and modulates signal transduction, energy metabolism, and cell proliferation. The magnesium cation (Mg^{++}) is also required for cellular energy metabolism and plays an important role in cell proliferation and membrane stabilization, nerve signal transduction, ion transport, and calcium metabolism. Magnesium decreases coagulation and acts as a calcium channel blocker. Magnesium regulates the absorption of calcium and is involved in the structural integrity of bones and teeth. If it is deficient in the bones, the bones may be dense but brittle because of poor trabecular integrity. Magnesium regulates the contractility of cardiac muscle. It is concentrated 18 times greater in heart muscle than in the bloodstream, and decreased levels in heart tissue increase susceptibility to coronary spasms. Magnesium has a relaxing effect on smooth muscle and may be helpful in relaxing the smooth muscle of the bronchioles and the arterioles. Consequently, magnesium deficiency can produce a variety of metabolic abnormalities and clinical consequences.

Serum magnesium concentration is maintained within a narrow range by the small intestine and kidneys. Total body magnesium (TBMg) depends mainly on gastrointestinal absorption and renal excretion. Many factors regulate magnesium absorption. Intestinal absorption is inversely proportional to the amount ingested. As calcium intake decreases, Mg^{++} absorption increases. Magnesium absorption occurs primarily in the jejunum and ileum via active carrier-mediated transport (partly dependent on vitamin D and parathyroid hormone [PTH]) and passive diffusion. The rate of magnesium absorption varies from as low as 24% to as high as 85%. Plasma Mg^{++} concentration is the major regulator of magnesium reabsorption within the kidney, serving as the principal organ in magnesium regulation. About 100 mg is excreted daily into the urine. In contrast to other ions, 60% to 70% of Mg^{++} reabsorption occurs in the thick ascending loop of Henle. Even so, the distal tubule is the major site of magnesium regulation, although it normally reabsorbs only 10% of filtered Mg^{++}. Both hormonal and nonhormonal factors influence Mg^{++} reabsorption in the loop of Henle and distal tubule, including PTH, calcitonin, glucagon, and vasopressin levels; magnesium restriction; acid-base changes; and potassium depletion. In plasma magnesium self-regulatory processes, the Ca^{++}/Mg^{++}-sensing receptor induces inhibition of loop transport in response to hypermagnesemia, whereas hypomagnesemia stimulates transport. Hypercalcemia and the rate of sodium chloride reabsorption can also influence reabsorption. Under conditions of magnesium deprivation, both organs increase their fractional absorption of the nutrient. Magnesium distribution constantly but gradually shifts between stores in bone or muscle and the extracellular fluid (ECF). In situations of magnesium depletion, resulting in negative magnesium imbalance, ECF will give up the initial losses, and serum Mg^{++} concentrations will rapidly fall. A compensatory reduction will then occur in urinary Mg^{++} concentrations unless there is magnesium wasting for other reasons. Finally, over several weeks, equilibration utilizing the bone stores will take place.

NUTRIENT IN CLINICAL PRACTICE

Known or Potential Therapeutic Uses

Magnesium has primarily been used in, and investigated for, the treatment of cardiovascular disease, diabetes, migraine, muscular spasm and irregular contractility, osteoporosis, and premenstrual syndrome. Usage ranges from daily dietary and supplemental intake to intravenous infusion for critical care. The value of this mineral in promoting health and treating disease is gradually coming into greater appreciation, as are the implications of its involvement in interactions with pharmaceutical agents. For example, a recent large study confirmed that greater levels of dietary magnesium intake appear to be associated with a reduced risk of coronary heart disease.[1]

Possible Uses

Alcohol withdrawal, angina, anxiety, asthma, atherosclerosis, autism, cardiac arrhythmias, cardiomyopathy, cardiovascular disease, celiac disease, chronic fatigue syndrome (CFS), chronic obstructive pulmonary disease (COPD), congestive heart failure, constipation, Crohn's disease, depression, diabetes mellitus, dysmenorrhea, eclampsia, eosinophilia-myalgia syndrome, epilepsy, fatigue, fibromyalgia, gastrointestinal spasms or cramping (acute), glaucoma, hearing loss (especially noise-related), hyperactivity, hypercholesterolemia, hypertension, hypocalcemia, hypoglycemia, hypokalemia, insomnia, intermittent claudication, kidney stones, lead toxicity, low levels of high-density lipoprotein (HDL) cholesterol, menopause, migraine, mitral valve prolapse, muscle cramping (especially nocturnal), multiple sclerosis, myocardial infarction (acute), osteoporosis, premenstrual syndrome (PMS), Raynaud's disease, retinopathy, sickle cell disease, stress response, stroke, torticollis, toxemia of pregnancy, urinary urge incontinence.

Deficiency Symptoms

There is significant disagreement as to the prevalence of clinically significant, although possibly subclinical, magnesium deficiency among the healthy subpopulations in developed societies. Nevertheless, the incidence of inadequate magnesium nutriture among susceptible subpopulations is widely recognized. A survey conducted by the U.S. Department of Agriculture showed that the daily dietary magnesium intake of many Americans (up to 75%) falls below the recommended dietary allowance (RDA),[2] which would mean that magnesium is among the most commonly deficient nutrients in that population. Suboptimal magnesium intake adversely affects a wide range of tissues, particularly those of the heart, nerves, and kidneys; many experts would say that all tissues are compromised by such a status. A diet high in processed and packaged foods tends to be magnesium poor because magnesium is found predominantly in whole, unprocessed foods.

Hypomagnesemia is frequently encountered in hospitalized patients and is seen in up to two thirds of patients admitted to intensive care units.[3] One survey of predominantly female urban African Americans found a 20% overall prevalence of magnesium deficiency.[4] Chronic degenerative diseases, such as diabetes, hyperlipidemia, hypertension, renal disease, asthma, and heart failure, are often associated with, and even potential causes of, magnesium deficiency, usually resulting from loss of magnesium from the gastrointestinal (GI) tract or the kidney. Alcoholism, severe burns, and other debilitative or traumatized states are also strongly linked to compromised magnesium status. Other GI causes include protein-calorie malnutrition, intravenous administration of Mg-free fluids and total parenteral nutrition, acute or chronic watery diarrhea, short bowel syndrome, bowel fistula, acute pancreatitis, continuous nasogastric suctioning, malabsorption steatorrhea, and extensive bowel resection. A rare inborn error of metabolism (primary intestinal hypomagnesemia), characterized by a selective defect in magnesium adsorption, is another known cause. The renal causes include Bartter's and Gitelman's syndromes, postobstructive diuresis, post–acute tubular necrosis, renal transplantation, and interstitial nephropathy.[5-8] Hypomagnesemia may also accompany other disorders, including phosphate depletion, hungry-bone syndrome after parathyroidectomy, correction of chronic systemic acidosis, postobstructive nephropathy, renal transplantation, and the diuretic phase of acute tubular necrosis.[6] Many medications, particularly aminoglycosides, furosemide, and amphotericin-B, can also cause or contribute to magnesium depletion.

Hypomagnesemia is known to produce a wide variety of clinical presentations. Clinically, neuromuscular hyperexcitability may be the first symptom to manifest in individuals with hypomagnesemia. Magnesium deficiency is associated with hypocalcemia and hypokalemia, fatigue, lethargy and apathy, anxiety, insomnia, irritability, weakness, convulsions, delirium and coma, muscle spasm, tremor and tetany, high blood pressure, atherosclerosis, cardiomyopathy, cardiac spasm, cardiac arrhythmias, tachycardia, supraventricular ectopy, sudden cardiac death, insulin resistance, sugar cravings, nerve conduction problems, anorexia, nausea, vomiting, abdominal pains, paralytic ileus, dysmenorrhea, PMS, and poor nail growth.[5,9-12]

Dietary Sources

The magnesium content in foods varies widely, as does the soil content of magnesium. Nuts (almonds, cashews, Brazil), soybeans, brewer's yeast, buckwheat, and wheat bran are rich sources of magnesium, with 200 to 400 mg per 100 g of food.

Moderate sources include corn, peas, carrots, barley, oats, rye, wheat, rice bran, pecans, filberts, pistachios, black walnuts, green leafy vegetables (kale, endive, chard beet tops), celery, alfalfa, figs, apples, lemons, peaches, almonds, whole grains (millet, cornmeal, wheat germ, barley, buckwheat, oats), tahini, sunflower seeds, brown rice, sesame seeds, black-eyed peas, lima beans, tofu, lentils, potato, sweet potato, peas, brussels sprouts, broccoli, cauliflower, avocado, dates, banana, blueberries, grape juice, cantaloupe, orange juice, and milk.

Nutrient Preparations Available

Magnesium citrate, magnesium gluconate, and magnesium lactate are more soluble and bioavailable than magnesium oxide.

Magnesium chloride is more soluble than magnesium oxide, gluconate, citrate, hydroxide, and sulfate and does not require stomach acid for solubility, but its use is limited because of its hygroscopic properties.

Magnesium hydroxide (milk of magnesia).

Magnesium sulfate (Epsom salts).

Dosage Forms Available

Capsule, liquid, powder, spray, tablet, injectable (prescription only), intravenous (inpatient).

Dosage Range
Adult

Dietary: 300 to 400 mg/day (Dietary Reference Intake; DRI)

Pregnant or lactating females: 450 to 550 mg/day (DRI)

Supplemental/Maintenance: 250 to 500 mg/day.

Pharmacological/Therapeutic: 50 to 2500 mg/day; 5 to 6 g have been used under close medical supervision.

Toxic: Single doses of 800 mg may cause diarrhea. Significantly lower doses can be toxic in renally impaired individuals.

Pediatric (< 18 Years)

Dietary: Infants, 0-6 months: 50 mg/day (DRI)

Infants, 7-12 months: 70 mg/day (DRI)

Children, 1-10 years: 150 to 250 mg/day (DRI)

Adolescents, 11-18 years: 300 to 400 mg/day (DRI)

Supplemental/Maintenance: Not established.

Pharmacological/Therapeutic: Not established.

Toxic: Not established.

Laboratory Values

Consensus is lacking as to what constitutes an abnormally low plasma magnesium concentration [Mg^{++}] and how to best assess magnesium depletion in critical tissues. Some authorities contend that measuring serum magnesium concentration and urinary magnesium excretion is usually sufficient in most cases to diagnose magnesium deficiency.[5] However, serum magnesium is a very poor indicator of how much magnesium is actually in the tissues, particularly cardiac tissue, which normally has much higher concentrations of magnesium than typical of serum. Measuring white blood cell (WBC) magnesium may provide a more sensitive indicator of tissue levels. An anionic

magnesium measurement, pioneered by Drs. Burton and Bella Altura at Down-State University of New York in Brooklyn, appears to be a considerably more accurate indicator of tissue levels of magnesium than either WBC or red blood cell (RBC) measurements. Koivisto and other researchers at Helsinki University Hospital in Finland assert that spot serum ionized magnesium reveals depletion poorly, and that the most reliable method for evaluating magnesium status is the magnesium loading test. In cases of depletion, uptake of magnesium is increased by 20% to 50%, reaching 6% of normal magnesium status; normally, it represents less than 1% of the TBMg.[13] A recently developed in vitro blood load test using a magnesium-stable isotope appears to offer an accurate assessment of magnesium status, based on initial animal research.[14] Sublingual buccal cell scrapings analyzed with x-ray fluorescence spectroscopy, developed by Burton Silver, have been shown to correlate well with cardiac tissue levels; this is considered the best clinically available test by many magnesium experts.[15]

Urinary Magnesium

Urinary magnesium provides a sensitive measure of magnesium status.

Deficiency: Excretion of less than 1 mmol/day indicates magnesium deficiency.

Leukocyte magnesium levels may reflect tissue levels.

Normal range: 3.0 to 4.0 ±0.09 fmol/cell.

Serum Ionized Magnesium

Serum ionized magnesium is a superior index, compared to serum levels, because the ionized portion of blood magnesium is not affected by variables that alter serum proteins.

Normal range: 0.5 to 0.66 mmol/L.

Serum Magnesium

Serum magnesium is an insensitive index of body magnesium stores; levels fall only with advanced deficiency.

Normal range: 0.75 to 1.05 mmol/L.

Occasionally, parenteral magnesium load test can be used to assess magnesium status.

SAFETY PROFILE
Overview

Magnesium has a very high therapeutic index, and hypermagnesemia is rare and usually iatrogenic, most commonly after intravenous (IV) magnesium, resulting from magnesium-containing laxatives or antacids, or rarely with intramuscular (IM) injection. Magnesium excess and toxicity most often result in diarrhea, drowsiness, weakness, and lethargy but may lead to depression of the central nervous system (CNS) and possibly death. Those most at risk are the elderly and patients with GI disorders or renal insufficiency.[16] Treatment of hypermagnesemia primarily consists of discontinuation of magnesium intake and introduction of calcium administration, but hemodialysis may be necessary in some cases.

Nutrient Adverse Effects
General Adverse Effects

Toxicity from oral ingestion of magnesium supplements is highly improbable in individuals with normal renal function, other than the potential for osmotic diarrhea. Clinical manifestations of hypermagnesemia include hypotension, nausea, vomiting, urinary retention, bradycardia, respiratory depression, depressed mental status, and electrocardiographic (ECG) abnormalities. Diarrhea is the most common adverse effect from oral magnesium supplements but is not associated with parenteral administration. Excessive oral magnesium intake can actually lead to a magnesium deficiency if it causes chronic diarrhea. Magnesium also competes with calcium and may induce a calcium deficiency if calcium intake levels are already low. About 800 mg of elemental magnesium will generally cause loose stools, but some individuals may tolerate much higher doses. Different forms of magnesium, such as magnesium glycinate, may be tolerated better as well. Slow-release forms of magnesium (e.g., Slo-mag), may be helpful in elevating the intracellular levels of magnesium. Individuals with kidney failure must be cautious about magnesium supplementation because they may experience elevated serum levels with associated toxicity symptoms.

Intravenous magnesium, because of its effect on smooth muscles, may cause hypotension along with dizziness and fainting. It may also cause respiratory depression or depletion of potassium with high doses and rapid infusion.

Intramuscular injections can often be painful and may cause a persistent lump if injection does not go deep enough to reach the muscle tissue. After the magnesium is loaded into the syringe, a small amount of 2% lidocaine can be drawn into the tip of the syringe to ease the reaction.

Adverse Effects Among Specific Populations
Gitelman's syndromes.

Pregnancy and Nursing
No problems have been reported with normal intake during pregnancy and lactation.

Infants and Children
No problems have been reported with normal intake in infants and children.

Contraindications

Individuals with impaired kidney function can accumulate magnesium, which is potentially fatal. Some medications, such as aminoglycosides and amphotericin-B, cause both renal tubular damage and magnesium depletion patterns.

Individuals with high-grade atrioventricular blocks or bifascicular blocks must avoid magnesium supplementation because it could slow cardiac conduction.

Precautions and Warnings

Magnesium supplementation may theoretically alter glucose regulation to such a degree as to be problematic for individuals with hypoglycemia or diabetes. Gradual introduction and increase of dosage will generally prevent complications. Close supervision and regular monitoring may be appropriate.

INTERACTIONS REVIEW
Strategic Considerations

Although oral magnesium, as with many minerals, can bind and reduce bioavailability of many medications, the primary interactions of clinical significance derive from depletion and deficiency of this critical nutrient. Dietary magnesium deficiency is relatively common in the modern world, much more than usually expected, and its implications penetrate many aspects of human physiology, with the cardiovascular lesions being the most

common arena of adverse effects. Inadequate dietary intake may affect the young and the aged, the poor and the institutionalized, the alcoholic and the malnourished, but iatrogenic causes of magnesium depletion produce many of the most severe outcomes. Clinically significant alterations in serum concentrations of Mg^{++} (and K^+) not only are frequently observed in acute or severely ill patients, especially in emergency rooms or intensive care wards, but also are a common adverse effect of many medications. Accurate assessment of magnesium status can be elusive but is critical because many symptoms of magnesium deficiency are nonspecific, and their effective correction requires early detection and intervention. In particular, digitalis and diuretics can intensify an underlying magnesium deficiency, leading to cardiac arrhythmias that are refractory unless magnesium is integrated into the therapeutic regimen. Furthermore, magnesium functions in association with other key minerals in supporting cardiovascular homeostasis, and these nutrients must often be administered in concert. Diuretic-treated hypertensive patients are particularly susceptible to potassium depletion and a resulting increased incidence of ventricular ectopy and sudden death. In such cases, potassium administration alone is inadequate, and concomitant magnesium is essential to intracellular potassium repletion and cardiovascular stabilization. Individuals receiving diuretic therapy, especially those with congestive heart failure, are also prone to chloride loss leading to metabolic alkalosis; this state interferes with potassium repletion, and the combination of potassium, magnesium, and chloride is often appropriate.

Ultimately, the disruptions of magnesium availability and function have their greatest impact on those populations most at risk for their adverse consequences. Furthermore, because the primary adverse effects of magnesium intake occur in individuals with compromised renal function, it is important that kidney function be assessed initially and monitored regularly, along with magnesium status. Importantly, the pharmacokinetic interaction between magnesium and many medications, involving formation of chelated complexes, reduces absorption and bioavailability of both agents. Both the nutrient and the drug presumably play important roles in the therapeutic strategy, so the separation of their administration by 2 to 4 hours avoids the interference and enables both agents to express their full activity.

NUTRIENT-DRUG INTERACTIONS

Albuterol/Salbutamol and Related Beta-2-Adrenoceptor Agonists (Inhalant Bronchodilators)

Evidence: Albuterol (salbutamol; Albuterol Inhaled, Proventil, Ventolin); combination drug: albuterol and ipratropium bromide (Combivent); rimiterol (Pulmadil)
Extrapolated, based on similar properties: Fenoterol (Berotec), isoetharine (Arm-A-Med, Bronkosol, Bronkometer), isoproterenol (isoprenaline; Isuprel, Medihaler-Iso), levalbuterol (Xopenex), metaproterenol (Alupent), pirbuterol (Exirel), rimiterol (Pulmadil), salmeterol (Serevent, Combination drug: Advair), terbutaline (Brethaire, Brethine, Bricanyl), tulobuterol (Brelomax).
See also Theophylline/Aminophylline.

Interaction Type and Significance

⊕⊕ **Beneficial or Supportive Interaction, with Professional Management**

Probability:	Evidence Base:
2. Probable	◉ Emerging

Effect and Mechanism of Action

Magnesium can enhance the therapeutic efficacy of albuterol, and potentially other adrenergic bronchodilators, as a delivery vehicle, as a concomitant therapy, or simply as nutrient support in the treatment of individuals with asthma. Both agents exercise a bronchodilatory effect that can be amplified by coadministration. Albuterol therapy is associated with significant hypokalemia but apparently does not directly deplete magnesium levels.

Research

Magnesium deficiency is associated with the occurrence and severity of asthma, particularly airway hyperreactivity, wheeze, and impairment of lung function. Hypomagnesemia is common in chronic asthmatic individuals, and those with low serum magnesium tend to have more hospitalizations than chronic asthmatic persons with normal magnesium; hypomagnesemia is also associated with more severe asthma.[17]

Human studies indicate that coadministration of albuterol and magnesium can invoke synergistic effects in the treatment of asthma, but concerns have been raised that adrenergic bronchodilators may adversely affect magnesium (and potassium) levels. Magnesium sulfate is considered an effective bronchodilator in the treatment of acute, moderate to severe asthma when administered intravenously, and it can be safely administered to patients with stable asthma by inhalation.[18-20] However, Lipworth et al.[21] found that inhaled albuterol caused no significant change in magnesium level, but it did produce hypokalemic and hyperglycemic effects of probable clinical significance, especially during acute exacerbations of airflow obstruction.

The therapeutic effects of and supportive interactions between albuterol and magnesium have been researched in various permutations. In vitro experimental data show that magnesium increases beta-receptor affinity to agonists. Clinical research comparing inhaled magnesium sulfate and albuterol (salbutamol sulfate) in the treatment of patients with acute asthma has found that both agents produced significant bronchodilatory effects, but that the duration from the albuterol was longer than that of the magnesium (e.g., 6 hours vs. 1 hour).[22,23] In a randomized, double-blind, controlled trial involving 35 patients with acute asthma, Nannini et al.[24] found that isotonic magnesium sulfate, as a vehicle for nebulized albuterol, increased the peak flow response to treatment compared with salbutamol plus normal saline. In a small, double-blind, placebo-controlled trial involving six patients with asthma, Rolla et al.[25] observed that a mild sustained increase in serum magnesium level, using IV magnesium infusion, increases the bronchodilating effect of low doses of albuterol, possibly through an increased beta-receptor affinity. They found, however, no effect on the maximum bronchodilating effect of albuterol. Subsequently, in a double-blind placebo-controlled trial involving 52 emergency care patients, Hughes et al.[26] demonstrated an enhanced bronchodilator response using isotonic magnesium as an adjuvant to nebulized albuterol in the treatment of severe asthma. The clinical relevance of these findings remains contentious, particularly whether the use of isotonic magnesium confers any additional improvement to optimized nebulized bronchodilator therapy with albuterol and ipratropium, standard first-line therapies for the treatment of acute severe asthma. No clinical trials have yet been published exploring any potential differential clinical response to acute albuterol therapy in individuals regularly supplementing with pharmacologically efficacious doses of magnesium compared with those not taking magnesium

regularly for asthma (or other comorbid conditions); clinical trials into such integrative options are warranted.

In 2005 the *Cochrane Review* published a meta-analysis examining the evidence regarding the use of inhaled magnesium sulfate in conjunction with inhaled beta-2 agonists. They concluded that there was good evidence that nebulized magnesium sulfate was safe and effective and that it should be considered as a combined therapy with beta-2 agonists. The authors noted that magnesium sulfate was most useful in situations where the asthmatic exacerbations were severe.[27]

Nutritional Therapeutics, Clinical Concerns, and Adaptations

Magnesium can provide an efficacious adjuvant to conventional care for patients with asthma, including coadministration of magnesium sulfate with albuterol in emergency care settings. Concomitant use, especially in acute care and through IV infusion, will inherently be appropriate only under qualified medical care informed by an integrative approach to, and necessary training in, such synergistic therapeutic options. Close monitoring of potassium and magnesium levels, and possible coadministration of either or both, is appropriate when administering beta-2-adrenoceptor agonists, such as albuterol/salbutamol, levalbuterol, and rimiterol, as inhalant bronchodilators or especially as IV infusions. Within conventional practice, bronchodilators are almost never used alone (except for pure exercise-induced bronchospasm), and some treatment directed at airway inflammation, predominantly inhaled corticosteroids, is considered a necessary part of asthma management.

Amikacin (Amikin), gentamicin (G-mycin, Garamycin, Jenamicin), kanamycin (Kantrex), neomycin (Mycifradin, Myciguent, Neo-Fradin, NeoTab, Nivemycin), netilmicin (Netromycin), paromomycin (monomycin; Humatin), streptomycin, tobramycin (AKTob, Nebcin, TOBI, TOBI Solution, TobraDex, Tobrex).

Interaction Type and Significance

≈≈ **Drug-Induced Nutrient Depletion, Supplementation Therapeutic, with Professional Management**
☼ **Prevention or Reduction of Drug Adverse Effect**

Probability:	Evidence Base:
2. Probable	● **Consensus**

Effect and Mechanism of Action

Aminoglycoside antibiotics can induce magnesium depletion and deficiency-related symptoms by several mechanisms. Neomycin impairs absorption of oral magnesium.[28,29] Aminoglycosides can inhibit hormone-stimulated Mg^{++} uptake in distal convoluted tubule cells.[30] Gentamicin can cause increased urinary magnesium loss.[31,32] Renal tubular damage and nonoliguric renal insufficiency are well-known nephrotoxic adverse effects resulting from aminoglycosides, particularly gentamicin and tobramycin, and can lead to hypomagnesemia, usually combined with hypocalcemia, hypokalemia, and alkalosis.[31,33-35] Such tubular damage may occasionally be reversible in the absence of any change in the renal function.[36]

Research

Numerous animal studies have demonstrated hypomagnesemia, as well as hypocalcemia, hypokalemia, and alkalosis, as a result of aminoglycoside-induced renal tubular damage.[30,35,37,38]

Keating et al.[39] reported that 17 oncology patients developed a complex metabolic syndrome of 2 to 8 weeks' duration, characterized by hypocalcemia, hypomagnesemia, and hypokalemia, after administration of several aminoglycoside antibiotics, including tobramycin, gentamicin, amikacin, and sisomicin. The authors attributed these adverse outcomes to the nephrotoxic effects of the aminoglycoside and noted the possible potentiating action of chemotherapeutic agents, particularly doxorubicin. Twelve patients died before recovering from the metabolic stress, and five patients developed progressive renal impairment. Kes and Reiner[31] described renal wasting of magnesium and symptomatic hypomagnesemia, hypocalcemia, and hypokalemia in seven patients after gentamicin therapy. They noted a pattern of "excessive and inappropriate urinary excretion of magnesium and potassium in the presence of subnormal serum concentrations" and suggested that adverse effects were most likely in older patients given large doses of gentamicin over extended periods. Aminoglycosides and platinum together are particularly responsible for tubular damage.

Akbar et al.[40] have noted that hypomagnesemia may be especially common among children with cystic fibrosis who have a history of repeated use of aminoglycosides.

Reports

Kelnar et al.[41] reported the case of a 12-year-old boy who developed renal wasting of magnesium, calcium, and potassium, with secondary hypomagnesemia, hypocalcemia, and hypokalemia (without hyperaldosteronism) after treatment with high-dose gentamicin over 4 months. They recommended that prolonged courses of gentamicin not be administered if less toxic antibiotics are suitable, and that, when it is given, plasma magnesium, calcium, and potassium levels be monitored during and after treatment.

Slayton et al.[42] reported a case of tetany in a child with acquired immunodeficiency syndrome (AIDS) who developed magnesium, calcium, and potassium depletion, requiring prolonged replacement therapy, subsequent to a 3-week course of IV tobramycin. Adams et al.[43] reported hypomagnesemic tetany associated with repeated courses of IV tobramycin in a patient with cystic fibrosis.

Nutritional Therapeutics, Clinical Concerns, and Adaptations

Physicians prescribing aminoglycosides, particularly on a repeated or chronic basis, should regularly monitor kidney function along with magnesium and potassium status, especially in individuals in high-risk groups, such as children and the elderly. Nutritional support may restore normal levels of magnesium, as well as potassium or other related minerals; prophylactic administration may be appropriate in susceptible populations. Individuals taking neomycin are generally at less risk of adverse effects as a result of magnesium depletion. Clinically significant drug-induced magnesium depletion is an uncommon but important complication of gentamicin therapy. However, in patients receiving IV tobramycin, close monitoring of calcium, magnesium, and potassium levels and the consideration of mineral replacement are especially warranted. Serum creatinine, blood urea nitrogen (BUN), and creatinine clearance should be measured before initiating therapy and monitored throughout treatment. In this regard, many nutritionally oriented practitioners find that testing magnesium levels in RBCs is much more reliable than testing serum magnesium, even though low serum levels virtually always reflect serious intracellular compartment deficits. In individuals with a low threshold for osmotic diarrhea, parenteral magnesium replacement may be the only effective way to replenish the intracellular compartment. Careful assessment should precede administration of magnesium or potassium and then preferably within the context of integrative care involving health care professionals trained and experienced in both conventional pharmacology and nutritional therapeutics.

Magnesium supplementation is often medically appropriate to prevent or correct depletion patterns associated with the various aminoglycosides. Even though conclusive evidence demonstrating the unqualified need for therapeutic supplementation is lacking, 250 to 400 mg daily would generally provide a safe, protective dose of magnesium for individuals receiving neomycin for more than 2 to 3 days. Administration of magnesium in the dosage range of 300 to 500 mg daily is usually appropriate for individuals prescribed more potent aminoglycosides but requires evaluation of renal function testing and other individual characteristics. Magnesium augmentation can be risky in patients with compromised renal function and is usually contraindicated in such cases. It is also important to note that magnesium is needed to maintain intracellular potassium, as well as calcium homeostasis, becasue PTH production is magnesium dependent.

Amphetamines and Related Stimulant Medications

Amphetamine aspartate monohydrate, amphetamine sulfate, dextroamphetamine saccharate, dextroamphetamine sulfate; D-amphetamine, Dexedrine.
Methylphenidate (Metadate, Methylin, Ritalin, Ritalin-SR; Concerta).
Combination drug: Mixed amphetamines: amphetamine and dextroamphetamine (Adderall; dexamphetamine).

Interaction Type and Significance

⊕⊕ **Beneficial or Supportive Interaction, with Professional Management**

Probability:
3. Possible

Evidence Base:
◉ **Emerging**

Effect and Mechanism of Action

Magnesium may favorably alter the kinetics of mixed amphetamines and thereby enhance their retention and bioavailability. Medications in this class appear to elevate plasma magnesium levels and favorably shift the calcium/magnesium ratio. Further, the independent therapeutic effects of both agents on various forms of hyperactivity may result in an additive or synergistic effect, pharmacological and/or functional.

Research

Magnesium salts, specifically magnesium hydroxide in the context of antacids, alter the pharmacokinetics of amphetamines so as to enhance retention of such medications, thereby increasing their activity.[44] Conversely, in a double-blind placebo-controlled study of methylphenidate and dextroamphetamine in hyperactive boys, Schmidt et al.[45] found that plasma magnesium levels were significantly higher and calcium/magnesium ratio was significantly lower after 3 weeks of dextroamphetamine treatment, compared with the baseline or placebo condition. These authors cited other research suggesting that concomitant magnesium may enhance learning and the therapeutic response to stimulants. In particular, they proposed that the lowering of the calcium/magnesium ratio may play a significant role in the therapeutic action of stimulants such as dextroamphetamine.

The significant association observed between magnesium deficiency and hyperactivity has led to promising research into the role of magnesium as a component of an integrative approach to the treatment of this cluster of conditions.[46] Starobrat-Hermelin and Kozielec[47] assessed magnesium levels (in blood serum, RBCs, and hair) in 116 children with recognized attention deficit–hyperactivity disorder (ADHD) and determined that 95% demonstrated some form of magnesium deficiency, most frequently in hair (77.6%), RBCs (58.6%), and blood serum (33.6%). Subsequently, this same research team conducted a clinical trial in which they administered 200 mg/ day magnesium to 50 of these children, who had been diagnosed with both ADHD and magnesium deficiency, but not to 25 similarly diagnosed controls. They concluded that the children treated with magnesium, independently of other mental disorders coexisting with hyperactivity, demonstrated an increase in magnesium contents in hair and a significant decrease of hyperactivity, compared with their clinical state before magnesium administration and with the control group.[48] These findings suggest that coadministration of magnesium and mixed amphetamines might produce beneficial clinical outcomes, and that controlled clinical trials into such integrative options is warranted.

Nutritional Therapeutics, Clinical Concerns, and Adaptations
Physicians prescribing mixed amphetamines can reasonably suggest the option of concomitant magnesium. Given the potential effect on pharmacokinetics, close supervision and regular monitoring are advised, and reduction of the medication dosage may be appropriate if magnesium enhances bioavailability. Coordinated treatment involving health care professionals trained and experienced in both conventional pharmacology and nutritional therapeutics may serve to ensure safety and enhance clinical outcomes. A dosage of magnesium in the range of 200 to 400 mg per day, depending on age, weight, diet, and comorbid conditions, would typically be appropriate.

Amphotericin B

Amphotericin B (AMB; Fungizone).

Interaction Type and Significance
≈≈≈ **Drug-Induced Nutrient Depletion, Supplementation Therapeutic, Not Requiring Professional Management**
☼ **Prevention or Reduction of Drug Adverse Effect**

Probability:
2. Probable

Evidence Base:
● Consensus

Effect and Mechanism of Action
Renal toxicity is a common and serious adverse effect of conventional amphotericin B. Renal impairment manifests as a decrease in glomerular filtration and damage to tubular function.[49] Hypomagnesemia due to renal magnesium wasting can result from cumulative dosages of amphotericin B, most likely from a tubular defect in magnesium reabsorption.[50] Hydration and administration of depleted nutrients, particularly magnesium and potassium, may prevent or reduce such adverse effects.

Research
Barton et al.[50] documented the effect of amphotericin B on magnesium metabolism in 10 adults being treated for systemic fungal infections. After relatively small cumulative dosages of amphotericin B, renal magnesium wasting (as evidenced by

fractional magnesium excretion and serum magnesium level) and mild to moderate hypomagnesemia appeared to manifest by the second week of therapy, peak by the fourth week, and then plateau. Follow-up data in three subjects, from 1 year after discontinuation of amphotericin B therapy, showed that serum magnesium level and fractional magnesium excretion were restored to pretreatment levels and indicate that the magnesium wasting was reversible.

Mayer et al.[49] tested the hypothesis that administration of potassium and magnesium corresponding to the amounts lost by the kidneys, as well as sufficient hydration, are necessary to prevent renal function damage. In subsequent clinical trials, they found that the nephrotoxicity of amphotericin B therapy can be significantly reduced through minimal nephroprotective measures, including hydration and administration of magnesium and other ionic minerals susceptible to depletion.[51,52]

Because of the toxicity of amphotericin B, a modified lipid complex variant of the drug was introduced. The liposomal amphotericin B formulation appears to be well tolerated and effective in treating systemic fungal infections, without the high occurrence of severe adverse effects associated with conventional amphotericin B therapy.[53-55]

Reports
Clinicians have published case reports of tetany and other adverse effects of hypomagnesemia and hypokalemia caused by IV administration of amphotericin B.[56-58]

Nutritional Therapeutics, Clinical Concerns, and Adaptations
Physicians prescribing extended courses of amphotericin B may find it prudent to recommend magnesium administration (e.g., IV or 300 mg/day orally). Monitoring of magnesium levels and compensatory administration may be especially appropriate in patients with cardiovascular conditions or pathophysiological dysfunction in whom magnesium depletion might have clinically significant impact. Vigorous hydration and IV administration of magnesium, potassium, and sodium, as described by Mayer and Doubek, in the context of close monitoring of renal function and magnesium and other ionic levels, are appropriate for inpatient or oncological care settings where IV amphotericin B is being administered for systemic fungal infections. Use of the liposomal form of amphotericin B may reduce risk of adverse effects and complications.

Bisphosphonates

Evidence: Alendronate (Fosamax), risedronate (Actonel), tiludronate (Skelid).
Extrapolated, based on similar properties: Clodronate (Bonefos, Ostac), etidronate (Didronel).
Related but evidence against extrapolation: Pamidronate (Aredia), zoledronic acid (Zometa).

Interaction Type and Significance
◇◇ **Impaired Drug Absorption and Bioavailability, Precautions Appropriate**
◇ **Adverse Drug Effect on Nutritional Therapeutics, Strategic Concern**

Probability:
2. Probable

Evidence Base:
● Consensus

Effect and Mechanism of Action
Some oral magnesium compounds may interfere with the absorption and bioavailability of the various bisphosphonate

derivatives. Magnesium salts may interfere with absorption of tiludronate. This pharmacokinetic interaction typically is immediate in onset but of moderate severity. According to manufacturers, simultaneous ingestion of divalent cations will interfere with absorption of the various bisphosphonates by forming insoluble (nonabsorbable) chelates; specifically, the bioavailability of tiludronate is reduced 60% by supplements or antacids containing magnesium (or aluminum) and 80% by calcium.

The occurrence of insoluble chelates will also reduce the bioavailability of the magnesium and interfere with its therapeutic efficacy.

Research

The apparently unpublished research cited by the manufacturers of these agents and secondary references primarily focuses on magnesium in the context of antacids. However, the various extrapolations underlying the cautions are reasonable and consistent with generally accepted pharmacological research and principles regarding chelation properties of orally administered minerals.

Nutritional Therapeutics, Clinical Concerns, and Adaptations

In patients undergoing therapy with bisphosphonates, concurrent but segregated administration of magnesium (and calcium) enables an integrative approach to therapeutics. Oral magnesium, as well as other mineral supplements or related antacids, should be taken at least 2 hours before or 30 minutes after oral administration of bisphosphonate derivatives to minimize interference with the drug's absorption. Conversely, patients taking magnesium for therapeutic purposes will derive greater benefit from the nutrient by avoiding its binding with the bisphosphonate agent.

Calcium Channel Blockers

Evidence: Felodipine (Plendil), nifedipine (Adalat, Adalat CC, Nifedical XL, Procardia, Procardia XL).
Extrapolated, based on similar properties: Amlodipine (Norvasc); combination drug: amlodipine and benazepril (Lotrel); bepridil (Bapadin, Vascor), diltiazem (Cardizem, Cardizem CD, Cardizem SR, Cartia XT, Dilacor XR, Diltia XT, Tiamate, Tiazac); felodipine combination drugs: felodipine and enalapril (Lexxel), felodipine and ramipril (Triapin); gallopamil (D600), isradipine (DynaCirc, DynaCirc CR), lercanidipine (Zanidip), nicardipine (Cardene, Cardene I.V., Cardene SR); nifedipine combination drug: nifedipine and atenolol (Beta-Adalat, Tenif); nimodipine (Nimotop), nisoldipine (Sular), nitrendipine (Cardif, Nitrepin), verapamil (Calan, Calan SR, Covera-HS, Isoptin, Isoptin SR, Verelan, Verelan PM); combination drug: verapamil and trandolapril (Tarka).

Interaction Type and Significance

⊕✗   **Bimodal or Variable Interaction, with Professional Management**

✗✗✗   **Potentially Harmful or Serious Adverse Interaction—Avoid**

✗✗   **Minimal to Mild Adverse Interaction—Vigilance Necessary**

≈≈   **Drug-Induced Nutrient Depletion, Supplementation Therapeutic, with Professional Management**

Probability: Evidence Base:
3. Possible   ◉ Emerging

Effect and Mechanism of Action

Both calcium channel blockers and magnesium can reduce the amount of ionic calcium available to muscle cells. Their concomitant use can result in an additive effect, thereby enhancing their hypotensive effect and decreasing cardiac function. Felodipine therapy is also associated with increased magnesium excretion.

Research

Magnesium's central role in regulating calcium metabolism contributes to its ability to lower blood pressure[59] and may account for its reputed efficacy in the treatment of glaucoma.[60] Both calcium channel blockers and magnesium are used to treat a range of cardiovascular conditions, especially arrhythmias and angina, and individuals with such conditions (e.g., variant angina)[61] often demonstrate magnesium deficiency. In a rodent study, Mervaala et al.[62] found that the cardiovascular effects of low-dose felodipine and ramipril could be enhanced by regular administration of a magnesium-enriched salt, in place of sodium. However, Davis et al.[63] reported that the synergistic effect from combining magnesium sulfate and calcium channel blockers may decrease cardiac function and increase the risk of cardiac toxicity in pregnant women.

Reports

Two published case reports have described the development of muscular weakness and subsequent paralysis in pregnant women who were being treated for preeclampsia with concomitant oral nifedipine and IV magnesium sulfate.[64,65] In one case, cessation of the magnesium resulted in the resolution of the adverse symptoms within 25 minutes. In the other case, the paralytic state reversed after IV administration of calcium gluconate. Waisman et al.[66] reported a potentiation effect in two pregnant patients who were receiving methyldopa and IV magnesium and developed transient hypotension within 1 hour after administration of oral nifedipine.

Nutritional Therapeutics, Clinical Concerns, and Adaptations

The concomitant use of calcium channel blockers and magnesium can produce an additive effect that has the potential to be detrimental or beneficial, depending on patient characteristics, pathophysiological processes, and clinical management. Initial evaluation and regular monitoring of magnesium (and potassium) levels are necessary when the patient's history and cardiac risk factors indicate that magnesium might be clinically appropriate as part of the therapeutic strategy, as well as to counter drug-induced magnesium depletion. In particular, both magnesium and calcium channel blockers may have roles to play in the prevention and treatment of hypertension during pregnancy, especially preeclampsia, but their concomitant use should be discouraged except under close supervision and regular monitoring. The coordinated use of a calcium channel blocker and oral magnesium may provide greater efficacy while allowing reduced dosage of the drug and reducing the risk of adverse effects. However, collaboration by health care professionals trained and experienced in both conventional pharmacology and nutritional therapeutics is essential given the potential synergy of these combined agents and attendant risks. In most cases the typical therapeutic dosages of magnesium for adults are in the range of 250 to 350 mg per day.

Cisplatin

Cisplatin (*cis*-Diaminedichloroplatinum, CDDP; Platinol, Platinol-AQ).

Interaction Type and Significance

≈≈≈ Drug-Induced Nutrient Depletion,
      Supplementation Therapeutic, Not Requiring
      Professional Management

◇   Adverse Drug Effect on Nutritional Therapeutics,
      Strategic Concern

Probability: Evidence Base:
2. Probable   ● Consensus

Effect and Mechanism of Action

Cisplatin can induce clinically significant hypomagnesemia by increasing urinary excretion of magnesium, through its toxic effects on the kidneys, and possibly by a direct injury to mechanisms of magnesium reabsorption in the ascending limb of Henle's loop as well as the distal tubule.[67-70] This drug-induced impairment of the renal tubules' ability to conserve magnesium may persist for months, or possibly years, after discontinuing the drug.[71] Cisplatin may also cause excessive excretion of potassium that will amplify the adverse effects of magnesium depletion, and vice versa.[72,73]

Research

Numerous animal and human studies, as previously cited, have documented the occurrence, mechanisms, and sequelae of cisplatin's nephrotoxic effects on magnesium (and potassium) status. One British study found higher serum magnesium concentration levels in children given IV magnesium before and after administration of cisplatin than in those give magnesium only after the cisplatin.[74] These researchers concluded that magnesium supplements should be given to patients receiving cisplatin during the precisplatin hydration period to prevent hypomagnesemia. An unrecognized and untreated magnesium deficiency can lead to refractory potassium depletion. Rodriguez et al.[75] and Whang et al.[73] documented cases of refractory hypokalemia following cisplatin therapy that failed to respond to potassium administration until hypomagnesemia was recognized and corrected.

Reports

Van de Loosdrecht et al.[76] reported the case of seizures in a male patient with disseminated testicular cancer caused by cisplatin-induced hypomagnesemia.

Nutritional Therapeutics, Clinical Concerns, and Adaptations

Physicians prescribing or administering cisplatin are advised to evaluate magnesium and potassium status, as well as renal function, before initiating therapy and throughout its course; some clinicians would recommend continuing such monitoring through posttherapy follow-up examinations. The research cited suggests that coadministration of magnesium be initiated before beginning chemotherapy and that supplemental potassium be added if indicated. A collaborative approach based on principles of integrative care and involving health care professionals trained and experienced in both conventional pharmacology and nutritional therapeutics is recommended to enhance safety and efficacy.

Colchicine

Colchicine

Interaction Type and Significance

≈≈≈ Drug-Induced Nutrient Depletion,
      Supplementation Therapeutic, Not Requiring
      Professional Management

Probability: Evidence Base:
4. Plausible   ☐ Inadequate

Effect and Mechanism of Action

Colchicine has been linked to impaired absorption of magnesium.[77]

Research

Published research has documented colchicine-induced depletion of calcium, potassium, and other nutrients and reported that such absorption-related depletion patterns resolved subsequent to cessation of colchicine therapy. Clinical trials investigating and confirming specific effects by colchicine on magnesium are lacking.

Nutritional Therapeutics, Clinical Concerns, and Adaptations

Individuals prescribed colchicine would most likely benefit from daily supplementation with a high-potency multivitamin/mineral formulation to compensate for these interactions. Separate oral intake by at least 2 hours.

Corticosteroids, Oral

Betamethasone (Celestone), cortisone (Cortone), dexamethasone (Decadron), fludrocortisone (Florinef), hydrocortisone (Cortef), methylprednisolone (Medrol) prednisolone (Delta-Cortef, Orapred, Pediapred, Prelone), prednisone (Deltasone, Liquid Pred, Meticorten, Orasone), triamcinolone (Aristocort).
Similar properties but evidence indicating no or reduced interaction effects: Inhaled or topical corticosteroids.

Interaction Type and Significance

≈≈≈ Drug-Induced Nutrient Depletion,
      Supplementation Therapeutic, Not Requiring
      Professional Management

◇   Adverse Drug Effect on Nutritional Therapeutics,
      Strategic Concern

Probability: Evidence Base:
2. Probable   ◉ Emerging

Effect and Mechanism of Action

Long-term use of corticosteroids is associated with depletion of magnesium and decrease in serum and bone levels.[22,78,79] Magnesium deficiency adversely influences calcium and vitamin D metabolism and is primarily associated with hypocalcemia[80]; bone loss is a significant adverse effect of long-term steroid therapy.

Magnesium trisilicate has been reported to interfere with GI absorption of dexamethasone in healthy male volunteers, as indicated by the increased urinary excretion of 11-hydroxycorticosteroids.[81] However, magnesium trisilicate is a poorly absorbable form of magnesium never used as a nutrient source, although sometimes used in laxative preparations.

Research

Using adult male rats, Simeckova et al.[78] found that prednisolone caused a significant decrease in bone magnesium content. In a clinical trial involving 95 patients with chronic airway obstruction, Rolla et al.[22] found a significant negative correlation between serum magnesium and the length of oral steroid therapy; diuretics were also associated with a significantly lower serum magnesium level. Atkinson et al.[79] conducted a clinical trial involving 56 children with acute lymphoblastic leukemia (ALL) to investigate abnormalities in mineral homeostasis and bone mass. They found that more than 70% of children had abnormally low plasma 1,25-dihydroxyvitamin D, 73% had low osteocalcin (a reflection of vitamin K status), and 64% had hypercalciuria, at diagnosis, indicating an effect of the leukemic process on vitamin D metabolism and bone turnover. During remission induction, treatment with high-dose steroid (prednisone or dexamethasone) resulted in further reduction in plasma osteocalcin and elevated PTH levels. Despite normal dietary intake and absorption of magnesium, 84% of children developed hypomagnesemia (of whom 52% were hypermagnesuric) by 6 months; plasma 1,25-dihydroxyvitamin D remained abnormally low in 70%. The authors attributed the altered magnesium status to renal wasting of magnesium after cyclical prednisone therapy and treatment with aminoglycoside antibiotics. Magnesium coadministration for up to 16 to 20 weeks normalized plasma magnesium in only half the children treated for hypomagnesemia.

Nutritional Therapeutics, Clinical Concerns, and Adaptations

Magnesium can provide an important therapeutic component within integrative care for many pathological and dysfunctional conditions, such as asthma and irritable bowel syndrome, which are often treated with corticosteroids. Physicians prescribing oral corticosteroids for longer than 2 weeks should discuss with their patient the potential benefit of concomitant magnesium to counter the depleting effects of the drug(s). A typical dose in such situations would be 300 to 400 mg of magnesium daily. A multimineral formulation would add support against parallel depletions of other vulnerable minerals; however, clinically effective levels of potassium require a prescription. Any such mineral preparations should be taken at least 2 hours before or 30 minutes after oral corticosteroids to minimize risk of interference with absorption of the medication.

Cyclosporine

Cyclosporine (Ciclosporin, cyclosporin A, CsA; Neoral, Sandimmune, SangCya).

Interaction Type and Significance

≈≈≈ **Drug-Induced Nutrient Depletion, Supplementation Therapeutic, Not Requiring Professional Management**

☼   **Prevention or Reduction of Drug Adverse Effect**

◈   **Adverse Drug Effect on Nutritional Therapeutics, Strategic Concern**

Probability: Evidence Base:
1. Certain   ⊙ **Emerging**

Effect and Mechanism of Action

Cyclosporin A (cyclosporine) is a highly potent immunosuppressive agent for solid-organ transplantation, but its use carries significant risk of varied adverse effects. In addition to magnesium depletion and its sequelae, cyclosporine's adverse effects include nephrotoxicity, hepatotoxicity, hypertension, neurotoxicity, and gum hyperplasia.[82] Magnesium may reduce the severity of some of the drug's toxic effects, especially its nephrotoxicity.

Severe hypomagnesemia and renal magnesium wasting are associated with the use of cyclosporine and many of its toxic effects. In particular, systemic depletion of magnesium appears to play a significant role in the pathogenesis of cyclosporine-induced neurotoxicity and produces a high risk of seizures.[82-94]

Research

Pere et al.[95] reported beneficial effects of dietary magnesium and potassium on cardiac and renal morphological features in cyclosporin A–induced damage in spontaneously hypertensive rats. In a series of rodent studies, Asai et al.[96] showed that correction of cyclosporine-induced hypomagnesemia by magnesium coadministration ameliorates chronic cyclosporin A (CsA) nephropathy by inhibiting gene expression of fibrogenic molecules. Subsequently, they demonstrated that CsA induced a decline in glomerular filtration with characteristic striped fibrosis, but that magnesium abolished precedent interstitial inflammation, possibly through inhibition of chemoattractant expression and consequently, attenuated tubulointerstitial fibrosis.[97]

Thompson and June and colleagues documented association between cyclosporine neurotoxicity and hypomagnesemia[83] and the correlation of hypomagnesemia with the onset of cyclosporine-associated hypertension[85] in marrow transplant patients. These researchers concluded that their findings suggested that such adverse effects may be prevented with or treated by magnesium replacement.

Vannini et al.[90] investigated kidney function and magnesium status in 109 renal transplant patients receiving cyclosporine, with allografts functioning stably for more than 6 months and plasma creatinine levels of less than 200 μmol/L, as well as 15 renal transplant patients not receiving cyclosporine and 21 healthy volunteers. They found that the cyclosporine patients showed significantly lower total and ionized circulating magnesium values than the two control groups, and that these deficiencies appeared to be permanent. They also noted that plasma total and ionized magnesium levels were significantly lower among cyclosporine patients treated concurrently with insulin or oral hypoglycemic agents.

Low total serum magnesium concentration has been reported in transplant recipients on cyclosporine therapy, and this is a risk factor for hypertension and cardiac death, especially after renal transplant. In a study involving 31 post–renal transplant patients, Thakur et al.[94] found that mean total serum magnesium in posttransplant patients was significantly lower than in 16 chronic renal failure patients who had not yet received a transplant as controls, and that an inverse correlation existed between total serum magnesium and blood CsA concentration. Systolic and diastolic blood pressures were also higher in the cyclosporine-treated patients.

Reports

Numerous published case reports have described aspects of cyclosporine-associated neurotoxicity in recipients of solid-organ and bone marrow transplants, especially in relation to magnesium wasting. Ozkaya et al.[98] reported a case of a 16-year-old renal transplant patient who developed tremor, tinnitus, and peripheral facial paralysis during oral CsA treatment; her serum magnesium level was below the normal range. Al-Rasheed et al.[99] reported on a girl who had idiopathic renal magnesium wasting secondary to suspected Gitelman's syndrome and CsA neurotoxicity after a heart transplant. The child had acute progressive encephalopathy, intractable seizures, quadriparesis, and extensive bilateral cortical involvement on neuroimaging. Many of these symptoms improved dramatically 2 days after discontinuing CsA, and she was fully ambulatory after 6 weeks. This drug-induced neurotoxicity was exacerbated by hypomagnesemia. The authors emphasized that caution was especially important in administering cyclosporine to transplant patients with Gitelman's syndrome or other acquired magnesium homeostasis disorders because of the possible increased risk of neurotoxicity.

Nutritional Therapeutics, Clinical Concerns, and Adaptations

Magnesium coadministration prevents magnesium deficiency and subsequent neurotoxicity resulting from CsA; it may also reduce the severity of nephrotoxicity. In the event of cyclosporine-induced depletion, the prescribing physician should be consulted before any form of magnesium administration is initiated. Renal function testing is advised at baseline and at 6-month intervals, through creatinine clearance and albumin excretion, along with assessment of markers NAG and ALP (D-glucosaminidase and alkaline phosphatase, respectively) for tubular toxicity. Furthermore, initial evaluation and regular monitoring of magnesium levels are necessary in individuals undergoing cyclosporine therapy. Nutritionally oriented physicians generally find that monitoring RBC magnesium levels, rather than serum magnesium, is a more accurate method for diagnosing a deficiency.

Digoxin and Related Cardiac Glycosides

Evidence: Digoxin (Digitek, Lanoxin, Lanoxicaps, purgoxin). Extrapolated, based on similar properties: Deslanoside (cedilanin-D), digitoxin (Cystodigin), ouabain (g-strophanthin).

Interaction Type and Significance

≈≈≈ **Drug-Induced Nutrient Depletion, Supplementation Therapeutic, Not Requiring Professional Management**
☼ **Prevention or Reduction of Drug Adverse Effect**
◇ **Adverse Drug Effect on Nutritional Therapeutics, Strategic Concern**
◇◇ **Adverse Drug Effect on Nutritional Therapeutics, Strategic Concern**

Coadministration Risk

Probability: Evidence Base:
4. Plausible   ▽ **Mixed**

Nutrient Depletion

Probability: Evidence Base:
2. Probable   ● **Consensus**

Effect and Mechanism of Action

Digoxin decreases intracellular magnesium and causes increased urinary magnesium loss. Hypomagnesemia may predispose to digitalis toxicity.

Oral magnesium compounds may interfere with digoxin absorption and bioavailability. Conversely, the occurrence of insoluble chelates will also reduce the bioavailability for the magnesium and interfere with its therapeutic efficacy.

Research

Digoxin decreases intracellular magnesium and reabsorption of magnesium from the kidneys, causing increased urinary magnesium loss, and digitalis (and diuretics) can intensify an underlying magnesium deficiency.[5,100-103] Magnesium deficiencies induced by concomitant diuretic use are especially common in individuals prescribed digoxin.[104,105] Adequate magnesium concentration enhances digoxin's antiarrhythmic activity, particularly by diminishing ventricular response during atrial fibrillation. However, hypomagnesemia inhibits the therapeutic efficacy of digoxin in controlling atrial fibrillation and can increase the risk of cardiac glycoside toxicity, particularly refractory arrhythmias.[73,106-108]

Magnesium is also necessary to intracellular potassium repletion in diuretic-treated hypertensive patients.

Magnesium intake, particularly in the form of antacids such as magnesium trisilicate, may result in adsorption of digoxin, reduced absorption in the GI tract, and decreased bioavailability,[109] although most likely only to a negligible degree.[110-112] In single-dose studies with 10 healthy volunteers, Brown and Juhl[109] found that antacids containing magnesium hydroxide, and particularly magnesium trisilicate, substantially reduced digoxin absorption, apparently through physical adsorption of digoxin by the antacids in the GI tract. However, subsequent research by D'Arcy and McElnay[112] determined that magnesium trisilicate did not significantly interfere with digoxin absorption. Using an in vitro model, previously proven to correlate well with absorption across a physiological membrane in vivo,[110] research by McElnay et al.[111] suggests that magnesium carbonate only weakly impairs digoxin absorption. Overall, research findings are inconclusive.

Reports

Kinlay and Buckley[113] described a patient with digoxin toxicity, associated with ventricular tachycardia, who achieved a more stable junctional rhythm after IV magnesium sulfate (two doses of 10 mmol).

Nutritional Therapeutics, Clinical Concerns, and Adaptations

Digoxin and magnesium both play important therapeutic roles in the treatment of heart failure and related conditions. Normal magnesium levels need to be maintained during digoxin treatment. Given that individuals taking digoxin are especially likely to demonstrate hypomagnesia, supervised nutrient support can be even more important. Hypomagnesemia is known to produce a wide variety of clinical presentations, including neuromuscular irritability, cardiac arrhythmias, and increased sensitivity to digoxin.

Many physicians are aware of the need to monitor and prescribe for potassium depletion but do not consider the issue of magnesium deficiency unless serum levels fall below acceptable levels. Furthermore, many physicians experienced in nutritional assessment consider serum magnesium to be a very poor indicator of how much magnesium is actually in the intracellular compartment. Serum magnesium concentration is maintained within a narrow range by the kidney and small intestine; under conditions of magnesium deprivation, both organs increase their fractional absorption of magnesium. If magnesium depletion continues, the bone store contributes by exchanging part of its content with extracellular fluid. The serum [Mg^{++}] can be normal in the presence of intracellular Mg^{++} depletion, and the occurrence of a low level usually indicates significant magnesium deficiency. Hypomagnesemia is frequently encountered in hospitalized patients and most often in those admitted to intensive care units. The detection of magnesium deficiency can be increased by monitoring RBC magnesium levels, measuring [Mg^{++}] in the urine, or using the parenteral magnesium load test. Assessment of magnesium status may be appropriate but is often not essential since deficiency status is not required for patients to benefit from magnesium administration. However, renal function testing is advisable before initiating such treatment because increased magnesium intake can carry significant risks in patients with renal insufficiency and is usually contraindicated in such cases.

Physicians prescribing digoxin should discuss with their patient the potential benefit of concomitant magnesium as part of a program of integrative care and to counter the depleting effects of the medication. A typical dose in such situations would be 300 to 500 mg of magnesium daily, depending on the individual's diet, age, genetic predisposition, medications, and other factors. Refractory hypokalemia and hypocalcemia can be caused by concomitant hypomagnesemia and can potentially be corrected with magnesium therapy.[80,104] A multimineral formulation would add support against parallel depletions of other vulnerable minerals. To avoid potential interference with digoxin absorption, mineral preparations should be taken at least 2 hours before or after digoxin. Clinical care within an integrative setting might also emphasize a diet rich in minerals, vitamins, and antioxidants and incorporate fish oil, hawthorn (*Crataegus oxyacantha*), L-carnitine, coenzyme Q10, and other nutrients as part of an evolving and individualized approach to cardiovascular therapeutics.

Diuretics: Loop Diuretics and Thiazide Diuretics

Loop diuretics: Bumetanide (Bumex), ethacrynic acid (Edecrin), furosemide (Lasix), torsemide (Demadex).
Thiazide diuretics: Bendroflumethiazide (bendrofluazide; Naturetin); combination drug: bendrofluazide and propranolol (Inderex); benzthiazide (Exna), chlorothiazide (Diuril), chlorthalidone (Hygroton), cyclopenthiazide (Navidrex); combination drug: cyclopenthiazide and oxprenolol hydrochloride (Trasidrex); hydrochlorothiazide (Aquazide, Esidrix, Ezide, Hydrocot, HydroDiuril, Microzide, Oretic); combination drugs: hydrochlorothiazide and amiloride (Moduretic); hydrochlorothiazide and captopril (Acezide, Capto-Co, Captozide, Co-Zidocapt); hydrochlorothiazide and enalapril (Vaseretic); hydrochlorothiazide and lisinopril (Prinzide, Zestoretic); hydrochlorothiazide and losartan (Hyzaar); hydrochlorothiazide and metoprolol (Lopressor HCT); hydrochlorothiazide and spironolactone (Aldactazide); hydrochlorothiazide and triamterene (Dyazide, Maxzide); hydroflumethiazide (Diucardin), methyclothiazide (Enduron), metolazone (Zaroxolyn, Mykrox), polythiazide (Renese), quinethazone (Hydromox), trichlormethiazide (Naqua).
See also Quinidine and Related Antiarrhythmic Drugs.

Interaction Type and Significance

≈≈≈ **Drug-Induced Nutrient Depletion, Supplementation Therapeutic, Not Requiring Professional Management**
☼ **Prevention or Reduction of Drug Adverse Effect**
◇ **Adverse Drug Effect on Nutritional Therapeutics, Strategic Concern**

Probability: Evidence Base:
2. Probable   ● **Consensus**

Effect and Mechanism of Action

Loop and thiazide diuretics, to varying degrees, inhibit passive magnesium absorption and increase urinary excretion of magnesium, as well as sodium and potassium, and usually deplete blood levels of magnesium.[5,114-121] In turn, the drug-induced magnesium deficiency can contribute to further potassium depletion. Furthermore, hypokalemia reduces magnesium transport in the distal tubule, increasing urinary magnesium excretion.[122] Ultimately, the relationship between these two patterns of depletion can be difficult to determine, and practically, they need to be treated together in most patients.[73,101,104,105] Although loop and thiazide diuretics inhibit Mg^{++} reabsorption, the tendency to hypomagnesemia may be moderated because of increased proximal tubular reabsorption of Mg^{++} induced by the volume depletion.[6]

Research

Diuretics are generally prescribed to individuals with congestive heart failure (CHF) and other conditions typically associated with hypomagnesemia and other electrolyte imbalances that may increase myocardial electrical instability, as well as risk of malignant arrhythmias and sudden death.[123-126] In particular, hypomagnesemia and hypokalemia occur in a high percentage of patients receiving thiazide monotherapy.[127] Generally, potassium depletion in diuretic-treated hypertensive patients has been linked to an increased incidence of ventricular ectopy and sudden death. In such cases, potassium alone is generally inadequate, and concomitant magnesium administration is required to reestablish intracellular potassium repletion.[73,105] The associated tendency of patients receiving diuretic therapy, especially those with CHF, to chloride loss and subsequent metabolic alkalosis also interferes with potassium repletion. Consequently, the combination of magnesium and potassium (and possibly chloride) is often appropriate.[128]

The extent of magnesium depletion inherently depends on the interaction between the patient's individual physiology and the pharmacological characteristics of the particular diuretic, its drug class, dosage, duration of therapy, and other factors.[129] Furthermore, the time frame of symptom manifestation can vary significantly since extended drug-induced depletion may cause magnesium recruitment from bones to sustain blood levels; tissue levels may be profoundly depleted, even though serum levels are still normal such that low serum levels usually suggest a significant or severe deficiency status.[5,130] Magnesium depletion and hypomagnesemia are common among furosemide-treated patients with chronic CHF. Cohen et al.[131] analyzed clinical, biochemical, and ECG variables relating to serum magnesium aberrations and outcomes in 404 consecutive patients diagnosed with CHF and previously treated with furosemide for at least 3 months. Hypomagnesemia was found in 50 patients (12.3%) and ultimately, after adjustment for renal failure, old age, and severity of CHF, emerged as being significantly associated with shorter survival.

Individuals with Gitelman's syndrome, associated with hypocalciuria and a defect in the gene encoding for the thiazide-sensitive Na^+/Cl^- cotransporter, are particularly at risk for hypomagnesemia and hypokalemia caused by primary renal tubular Mg^{++} wasting.[6-8]

Dorup et al.[132] examined 76 consecutive patients receiving diuretic therapy for 1 to 17 years for arterial hypertension or CHF and found that muscle concentrations of magnesium, potassium, and sodium-potassium pumps were significantly reduced compared with matched controls. When 36 patients with depleted muscle magnesium and/or potassium levels were subsequently given oral magnesium hydroxide for 2 to 12 weeks or 26 weeks, magnesium muscle parameters initially increased, but muscle concentrations of magnesium, potassium, and sodium-potassium pumps did not normalize, in most cases, until after 26 weeks of magnesium administration. Thus, the authors concluded that at least 6 months of oral magnesium therapy appeared to be necessary to restore diuretic-induced disturbances in the concentrations of magnesium, potassium, and sodium-potassium pumps in skeletal muscle.[132]

Ruml and Pak[128] investigated the effect of potassium magnesium citrate, magnesium citrate, and potassium citrate on thiazide-induced hypokalemia and magnesium loss in 62 healthy subjects. They found that all three mineral compounds increased serum potassium concentration compared with that resulting from thiazide alone, and that potassium magnesium citrate and potassium citrate, but not magnesium citrate, significantly increased urinary pH and citrate values. They concluded that potassium magnesium citrate not only corrects thiazide-induced hypokalemia, but also may avert magnesium loss while providing an alkali load. In a related trial, Ruml et al.[133] tested the efficacy of three different dosages of a potassium and magnesium combination, including up to 800 mg/day of magnesium, and found that four tablets daily (24 mEq potassium, 12 mEq magnesium, 36 mEq citrate) was adequate to overcome hypokalemia and magnesium loss induced by thiazide (50 mg/day) and increased urinary pH and citrate. Likewise, after administering oral magnesium citrate (300 mg daily for 30 days) to 10 patients with severe CHF maintained on high-dose furosemide, Cohen et al.[134] observed a significant increase in peripheral blood mononuclear cell magnesium content and serum potassium levels, whereas the other related parameters remained unchanged.

Parallel attempts at addressing the depleting effects of diuretics have not been as straightforward or as effective as mineral supplementation. Triamterene, a potassium-sparing diuretic, has sometimes been combined with hydrochlorothiazide as a means of mitigating potassium and hydrogen loss. Although often effective at partly compensating for the kaliuretic effect of hydrochlorothiazide, many diabetic patients thus treated either remained or became hypokalemic.[135] However, sometimes the combination of hydrochlorothiazide and lisinopril, an angiotensin-converting enzyme (ACE) inhibitor, has been found to be effective in attenuating thiazide-induced potassium loss, thereby reducing magnesium wasting, because of lisinopril's ability to reduce production of aldosterone. Likewise, in some cases a magnesium-potassium-sparing diuretic such as amiloride (e.g., 5-10 mg) may negate the potassium-wasting effect of 40 mg furosemide.[5] However, Dorup[129] reported that such a furosemide-amiloride combination still produced hypomagnesemia in 12% of those thus treated. Importantly, the combined use of magnesium supplementation and potassium-sparing diuretic(s) could theoretically introduce a risk of hypermagnesemia, although the likelihood of this seems unlikely with normal renal function and oral supplementation.

Nutritional Therapeutics, Clinical Concerns, and Adaptations

In practice, it is generally advisable to coadminister both potassium and magnesium when prescribing any potassium-depleting diuretic, except in those with renal insufficiency. Severe magnesium deficiency may require IM or IV magnesium sulfate or chloride to achieve rapid correction. For long-term care, administration of magnesium at 300 to 600 mg daily is usually appropriate, depending on the individual's diet, age, genetic predisposition, and medications and other factors. Magnesium deficiency status can be evaluated by monitoring RBC magnesium levels, measuring $[Mg^{++}]$ in the urine, using x-ray spectroscopy of sublingual cell scrapings, or using the parenteral magnesium load test. Assessment of magnesium status may be appropriate but is often not essential because deficiency status is not required for patients to benefit from magnesium administration. However, since magnesium augmentation can be risky, and is usually contraindicated, in patients with renal insufficiency, kidney function tests are critical before initiating, and periodically during, concomitant repletion therapy.

As indicated by research findings, concomitant magnesium needs to be maintained for 6 months to compensate for any drug-induced tissue depletion pattern and during and possibly after relevant diuretic therapy. A typical dose for most individuals would be 300 to 500 mg of magnesium daily. A multimineral formulation would add support against parallel depletions of other vulnerable minerals. In the event that diarrhea appears during magnesium administration, switching to magnesium gluconate or glycinate may alleviate this adverse effect. Beyond magnesium and potassium, clinical care within an integrative setting might also emphasize a diet rich in minerals, vitamins, and antioxidants and incorporate dandelion (*Taraxacum officinale*, as a mineral-rich nutritive diuretic), essential fatty acids, coenzyme Q10, calcium, and other elements as part of an evolving and individualized approach to cardiovascular therapeutics involving health care professionals trained and experienced in multiple therapeutic disciplines.

ESTROGENS AND ESTROGEN-PROGESTIN COMBINATIONS

Oral Contraceptives: Monophasic, Biphasic, and Triphasic Estrogen Preparations (Synthetic Estrogen and Progesterone Analogs)

Ethinyl estradiol and desogestrel (Desogen, Ortho-TriCyclen). Ethinyl estradiol and ethynodiol (Demulen 1/35, Demulen 1/50, Nelulen 1/25, Nelulen 1/50, Zovia). Ethinyl estradiol and levonorgestrel (Alesse, Levlen, Levlite, Levora 0.15/30, Nordette, Tri-Levlen, Triphasil, Trivora). Ethinyl estradiol and norethindrone/norethisterone (Brevicon, Estrostep, Genora 1/35, GenCept 1/35, Jenest-28, Loestrin 1.5/30, Loestrin1/20, Modicon, Necon 1/25, Necon 10/11, Necon 0.5/30, Necon 1/50, Nelova 1/35, Nelova 10/11, Norinyl 1/35, Norlestin 1/50, Ortho Novum 1/35, Ortho Novum 10/11, Ortho Novum 7/7/7, Ovcon-35, Ovcon-50, Tri-Norinyl, Trinovum). Ethinyl estradiol and norgestrel (Lo/Ovral, Ovral). Mestranol and norethindrone (Genora 1/50, Nelova 1/50, Norethin 1/50, Ortho-Novum 1/50). Related, internal application: Etonogestrel/ethinyl estradiol vaginal ring (Nuvaring).

Hormone Replacement Therapy (HRT): Estrogen-Containing and Synthetic Estrogen and Progesterone Analog Medications

HRT, estrogens: Chlorotrianisene (Tace); conjugated equine estrogens (Premarin); conjugated synthetic estrogens (Cenestin); dienestrol (Ortho Dienestrol); esterified estrogens (Estratab, Menest, Neo-Estrone); estradiol, topical/transdermal/ring (Alora Transdermal, Climara Transdermal, Estrace, Estradot, Estring FemPatch, Vivelle-Dot, Vivelle Transdermal); estradiol cypionate (Dep-Gynogen, Depo-Estradiol, Depogen, Dura-Estrin, Estra-D, Estro-Cyp, Estroject-LA, Estronol-LA); estradiol hemihydrate (Estreva, Vagifem); estradiol valerate (Delestrogen, Estra-L 40, Gynogen L.A. 20, Progynova, Valergen 20); estrone (Aquest, Estragyn 5, Estro-A, Estrone '5', Kestrone-5); estropipate (Ogen, Ortho-Est); ethinyl estradiol (Estinyl, Gynodiol, Lynoral).
HRT, estrogen/progestin combinations: Conjugated equine estrogens and medroxyprogesterone (Premelle cycle 5, Prempro); conjugated equine estrogens and norgestrel (Prempak-C); estradiol and dydrogesterone (Femoston); estradiol and norethindrone, patch (CombiPatch); estradiol and norethindrone/norethisterone, oral (Activella, Climagest, Climesse, FemHRT, Trisequens); estradiol valerate and cyproterone acetate (Climens); estradiol valerate and norgestrel (Progyluton); estradiol and norgestimate (Ortho-Prefest).
HRT, estrogen/testosterone combinations: Esterified estrogens and methyltestosterone (Estratest, Estratest HS).
Similar properties but evidence indicating no or reduced interaction effects:
Progestin-only oral contraceptives, implants, and postcoital contraceptives: Etonogestrel, implant (Implanon),

levonorgestrel, implant (Jadelle, Norplant; Norplant-2); levonorgestrel, oral postcoital contraceptive (Duofem, Escapelle, Levonelle, Levonelle-2, Microlut, Microval, Norgeston, Nor-Levo, Plan B, Postinor-2, Vika, Vikela); medroxyprogesterone, injection (Depo-Provera, Depo-subQ Provera 104); medroxyprogesterone, oral (Cycrin, Provera); NES progestin, implant (ST-1435, Nestorone); norethindrone, oral (norethisterone; Aygestin, Camila, Errin, Jolivette, Micronor, Nor-QD, Ortho-Micronor); norethindrone, injectable (NET EN; Noristerat); norgestrel, oral (Ovrette).

Interaction Type and Significance

≈≈≈ **Drug-Induced Nutrient Depletion, Supplementation Therapeutic, Not Requiring Professional Management**

◇ **Adverse Drug Effect on Nutritional Therapeutics, Strategic Concern**

Probability:
3. Possible

Evidence Base:
◉ **Emerging**

Effect and Mechanism of Action

Exogenous estrogen, as oral contraceptive (OC) or estrogen replacement therapy (ERT), enhances magnesium uptake and utilization by soft tissues and bone, thereby moving magnesium from the blood, lowering serum levels, and depleting body stores of magnesium.[136-138]

Research

Decreased levels of serum magnesium have been associated with OCs, in pregnancy, and during ERT in postmenopausal women.[139,140] Seelig[138] has suggested that one mechanism by which estrogen provides cardiovascular support is through its effects on magnesium, particularly the resistance of young women to heart disease and osteoporosis. She also notes that "estrogen-induced shifts of Mg can be deleterious when estrogen levels are high and Mg intake is suboptimal. The resultant lowering of blood Mg can increase the Ca/Mg ratio, thus favoring coagulation. With Ca supplementation in the face of commonly low Mg intake, risk of thrombosis increases." In a controlled clinical study involving 25 healthy women at varying age and duration of menopause and 15 healthy, cycling women of childbearing age, Muneyyirci-Delale et al.[141] found that serum levels of magnesium were inversely related to the serum level of estrogen in both groups.

The use of OCs is associated with unfavorable alterations in magnesium status. In a controlled study, Olatunbosun et al.[142] found that women being administered exogenous estrogen in OC form had significantly lower serum magnesium levels as circulating magnesium shifted from serum to tissues. In a later clinical study of 32 women, mean age 24.2 years, administered an OC containing ethinyl estradiol (0.03 mg) and levonorgestrel (0.15 mg), Blum et al.[137] reported a 26% decrease in serum magnesium after 6 months compared to baseline levels; no clinical signs of magnesium deficiency were observed among these women. Subsequently, Hameed et al.[143] studied serum mineral levels in 50 women taking OCs (Lofeminal) and 50 taking injectable contraceptive (depot medroxyprogesterone acetate and Norigest) and found that there was significant decrease in serum levels of calcium, magnesium, and phosphorus in women taking OCs but significant increase in these minerals in women taking injectable contraceptives.

In a preliminary trial, Herzberg et al.[144] found that osteoporotic postmenopausal women demonstrated reduced urinary excretion of zinc, magnesium, and hydroxyproline after HRT (conjugated estrogens and medroxyprogesterone) for 1 year. Combined use of estrogen and calcium increases the need for magnesium, particularly in the treatment of osteoporosis.[136]

Nutritional Therapeutics, Clinical Concerns, and Adaptations

Although the clinical research thus far has not focused specifically on the clinical implications of the interaction between estrogen and magnesium, the basic trend suggested by relevant findings points in a clear and relatively consistent direction. Premenstrual syndrome (PMS) and other gynecological conditions are associated with, or more likely to result in, aggravated symptoms or adverse outcomes in the presence of compromised magnesium status, particularly when estrogen dominance or exogenous estrogens are present. The signs of symptomatic hypomagnesemia and those of PMS and related conditions share many features, including appetite loss, nausea and vomiting, sleepiness, weakness, muscle spasms, tremors, and personality changes. Thus, magnesium deficiency is associated with increased risk of PMS,[145,146] and magnesium supplementation can play an important role in preventing and treating PMS,[147,148] particularly in those with hypomagnesemia. Likewise, magnesium and estrogen (at least endogenous estrogen) both have important roles to play toward the therapeutic goals of preventing osteoporosis and supporting cardiovascular health.

The coadministration of magnesium and exogenous estrogen requires an individualized, flexible, and evolving approach to integrative care and clinical management to achieve the desired clinical outcomes effectively. Further research into the characteristic, mechanism, and clinical implications of the interaction between magnesium and estrogen is clearly warranted by its potential importance with both preventive and therapeutic agendas. Pending the outcome of such focused study, supplementation with magnesium, 250 to 350 mg per day, can provide a safe support against estrogen-induced stress on magnesium function and potential drug-induced depletion. Likewise, the coadministration of the two agents might prove advantageous, especially in reducing the risk of adverse effects of exogenous estrogen. Within the practice of integrative medicine, other approaches to supporting hormonal balance and liver conjugation of estrogen are often considered as appropriate to the characteristics and needs of the particular patient, such as exercise, vitamin B6, natural progesterone, chaste tree (Vitex agnus-castus), and Chinese herbal formulae such as Xiao Chai Hu Tang or Xiao Yao San.

Fentanyl

Fentanyl (Actiq Oral Transmucosal, Duragesic Transdermal, Fentanyl Oralet, Sublimaze Injection).

Interaction Type and Significance

⊕⊕ **Beneficial or Supportive Interaction, with Professional Management**

☼ **Prevention or Reduction of Drug Adverse Effect**

Probability:
2. Probable

Evidence Base:
○ **Preliminary**

Effect and Mechanism of Action

Not specified; speculatively, magnesium may reset nerve activation thresholds, thus lessening the level of anesthesia necessary to prevent pain.

Research

In a randomized double-blind study involving 46 patients, split into two groups, undergoing arthroscopic knee surgery under total IV anesthesia, Konig et al.[149] found that in a clinical setting with almost identical levels of surgical stimulation, IV magnesium sulfate administration significantly reduced intraoperative and postoperative analgesic requirements using fentanyl for induction and postoperative analgesia, compared with isotonic sodium chloride solution administration.

Nutritional Therapeutics, Clinical Concerns, and Adaptations

Fentanyl is an opioid analgesic administered intravenously or through a patch. Further research is warranted to explore the positive findings in this preliminary clinical trial of the synergistic interaction between fentanyl and magnesium sulfate during surgery. Related research into whether oral magnesium administration might interact similarly in patients using fentanyl patches remains to be done. Since all opioids significantly slow intestinal peristalsis, which frequently results in constipation when used for more than a few days, the laxative effects of oral magnesium can also be used as part of a program to normalize bowel function during opioid analgesic therapy.

Fluoroquinolone (4-Quinolone) Antibiotics, Particularly Ciprofloxacin

Evidence: Ciprofloxacin (Ciloxan, Cipro).
Extrapolated, based on similar properties: Cinoxacin (Cinobac, Pulvules), enoxacin (Penetrex), gatifloxacin (Tequin), levofloxacin (Levaquin), lomefloxacin (Maxaquin), moxifloxacin (Avelox), nalidixic acid (Neggram), norfloxacin (Noroxin), ofloxacin (Floxin, Ocuflox), sparfloxacin (Zagam), trovafloxacin (alatrofloxacin; Trovan).

Interaction Type and Significance

◇◇ **Impaired Drug Absorption and Bioavailability, Precautions Appropriate**
◇ **Adverse Drug Effect on Nutritional Therapeutics, Strategic Concern**

Probability: Evidence Base:
2. Probable   ○ Preliminary

Effect and Mechanism of Action

Magnesium salts may decrease the absorption of fluorinated quinolone antibiotics. Numerous studies have demonstrated that antacids containing magnesium, and by extension other magnesium compounds, readily chelate with and reduce absorption of fluoroquinolone antibiotics when administered concurrently.[150-155] Specifically, the antimicrobials appear to be rendered inactive when the 3-carbonyl and 4-oxo functional groups characteristic of medications in this class form chelates with multivalent metal cations, particularly aluminum, magnesium, calcium, iron, and zinc, but also copper, manganese, and possibly sodium.[153,155-166] For example, the absorption of ciprofloxacin is reduced by 50% to 90% in the presence of antacids containing magnesium and aluminum.

Research

Although there is general agreement as to the pattern of interaction between fluoroquinolones and multivalent cations, no published research has specifically involved magnesium supplements. Numerous minerals are known to form chelated complexes with fluoroquinolone antibiotics, or otherwise significantly reduce their absorption and bioavailability (AUC).

Research involving magnesium has largely focused on antacids containing magnesium (or conclusions have been extrapolated from research involving aluminum-based antacids).[152,156,157,164,167-174] Given the nature of the apparent mechanism of action and the consensus on the pharmacological principles involved, the probability of similar interactions occurring with magnesium supplements can be reasonably extrapolated from the observed phenomena. Nevertheless, despite similarities, the evidence available on the degree of reduction in fluoroquinolone C_{max} and AUC attributable to aluminum-based antacids cannot reasonably be extrapolated to magnesium supplements.

Clinical Implications and Adaptations

Physicians prescribing fluoroquinolone antibiotics should instruct patients to take magnesium and other mineral supplements (as well as related antacids) as far apart as possible from the medications (at least 6 hours before or 2 hours after antibiotics is usually adequate) to avoid the potential interaction. It is important to note that this interaction concern is only relevant to oral administration of both agents.

Foscarnet

Foscarnet (Trisodium phosphonoformate hexahydrate; Foscavir).

Interaction Type and Significance

≈≈ **Drug-Induced Nutrient Depletion, Supplementation Therapeutic, with Professional Management**

Probability: Evidence Base:
2. Probable   ◉ Emerging

Effect and Mechanism of Action

Magnesium depletion, acute ionized hypocalcemia and hypomagnesemia, hypokalemia, and hypo/hyperphosphatemia are common and often severe adverse effects associated with IV foscarnet. The mechanisms by which foscarnet induces these changes, especially in ionized cations, are not completely understood, although renal impairment is the major toxicity of Foscavir. Foscarnet causes increased elimination of magnesium and other electrolytes in the urine and induces changes in plasma concentrations of total and ionized calcium and magnesium. Foscarnet binds preferentially to the magnesium ion.[175] Foscarnet-induced ionized hypomagnesemia might contribute to ionized hypocalcemia by impairing excretion of preformed PTH or by producing target organ resistance.[176]

Research

In a clinical trial involving 13 male HIV-positive patients who had no active cytomegalovirus (CMV)–associated disease, Noormohamed et al.[175] observed significant foscarnet-induced changes in plasma concentrations of total and ionized calcium and magnesium. The maximal decreases in ionized calcium and magnesium were much more rapid and larger than changes in the plasma concentrations of total calcium and magnesium, and the relative changes in the plasma concentration of ionized magnesium were greater than those of ionized calcium.

In a small study of solid-organ transplant recipients with ganciclovir-resistant CMV infection, Mylonakis et al.[177] reported that magnesium depletion occurred in all six patients within 72 to 96 hours after initiating treatment with a combination of ganciclovir and daily IV foscarnet.

Huycke et al.[176] conducted a randomized, double-blind, placebo-controlled crossover trial involving 12 patients with AIDS and CMV disease to investigate the effect of IV magnesium sulfate on foscarnet-induced ionized hypocalcemia and hypomagnesemia. Parenteral MgSO$_4$, administered in increasing doses, reduced or eliminated foscarnet-induced, acute ionized hypomagnesemia. However, it had no discernible effect on foscarnet-induced, ionized hypocalcemia or associated symptoms, despite significant increases in serum PTH levels.

Reports

In 1993, Gearhart and Sorg[178] reported the first known case of severe hypomagnesemia and other electrolyte disorders (hypocalcemia, hypokalemia, hypophosphatemia) in a patient with AIDS being treated for an exacerbation of CMV retinitis with foscarnet. The symptoms of muscle twitches, tremulousness, and anxiety resolved, and laboratory indices returned to normal after administration of magnesium and other electrolytes and discontinuation of foscarnet.

Nutritional Therapeutics, Clinical Concerns, and Adaptations

Although the general consensus is that foscarnet causes magnesium depletion, the issue of an effective therapeutic response to foscarnet-induced hypomagnesemia and hypocalcemia remains unresolved. Physicians prescribing and administering foscarnet are advised to monitor magnesium and other electrolytes frequently during foscarnet therapy. Huycke et al.[176] concluded that routine IV administration for patients with normal serum magnesium levels is not recommended during treatment with foscarnet. However, divergent opinions remain as to the accuracy of various methods of assessing magnesium. The duration of treatment with foscarnet will generally affect both the clinical implications of the magnesium depletion pattern and the appropriate diagnostic approach. Furthermore, Gearhart and Sorg[178] noted that concomitant therapy with antianxiety medications may mask the symptoms of electrolyte disorders and should be undertaken with caution. Further research into the clinical significance of these issues and integrative therapeutic options is clearly warranted.

Insulin

Animal-source insulin (Iletin); human analog insulin (Humanlog); human insulin (Humulin, Novolin, NovoRapid, Oralin).

Interaction Type and Significance

⊕⊕ **Beneficial or Supportive Interaction, with Professional Management**

Probability:
2. Probable

Evidence Base:
◉ **Emerging**

Effect and Mechanism of Action

Glucosuria-related hypomagnesuria, nutritional factors and hyperinsulinemia-related hypermagnesuria all contribute to the well-established tendency for magnesium deficiency in patients with diabetes mellitus. Magnesium improves insulin sensitivity as well as insulin secretion in patients with type 2 diabetes.[179]

Research

Diabetes is associated with low magnesium status,[180] and general consensus has existed since the early 1990s on the recognition of "strong associations ... between magnesium deficiency and insulin resistance."[181]

Most researchers have found that magnesium improves insulin sensitivity as well as insulin secretion in patients with

type 2 diabetes.[182] In a small clinical trial involving eight older, non–insulin-dependent diabetes mellitus (NIDDM) subjects, Paolisso et al.[183] demonstrated that long-term magnesium administration (2 g/day) can elevate plasma magnesium levels and improve insulin response and action. In a subsequent double-blind trial, dosage appeared crucial, with 1000 mg/day magnesium producing a favorable effect that was not obtained with half that dosage.[184] Eibl et al.[185] showed that a 3-month course of replacement therapy with oral magnesium corrected hypomagnesemia in patients with type 2 diabetes. Johnsen et al.[186] similarly reported that well-regulated NIDDM patients with marked magnesium deficiency responded favorably to oral magnesium. Two studies of the effect of magnesium administration on glucose tolerance in nondiabetic elderly subjects produced mixed results.[187,188]

Nadler et al.[11] found that healthy subjects receiving a low-magnesium diet, adequate to demonstrate reductions in both serum magnesium and intracellular free magnesium in RBCs, produced a significant decrease in insulin sensitivity as well as increased thromboxane synthesis. In a clinical trial involving 16 subjects with insulin-dependent type 1 diabetes mellitus and 30 healthy controls, Sjogren et al.[189] found that oral administration of magnesium hydroxide (500 mg/day) reduced insulin requirements, without changing levels of glycosylated hemoglobin (HbA$_{1c}$) and glucose, and corrected muscular magnesium and potassium deficiency in the diabetic patients. However, a decade later, in a clinical trial with 50 moderately controlled, insulin-requiring type 2 diabetic patients, randomized to 15 mmol oral magnesium or placebo daily for 3 months, De Valk et al.[190] reported that plasma [Mg^{++}] was higher after magnesium than after placebo, but that significant differences were lacking with regard to erythrocyte [Mg^{++}], glycemic control, lipids, or blood pressure.

Diabetic patients with severe retinopathy have a lower plasma magnesium level than those without retinopathy,[191] and a prospective study demonstrated that plasma magnesium concentration are inversely related to occurrence or progression of retinopathy.[192]

Nutritional Therapeutics, Clinical Concerns, and Adaptations

Insulin and magnesium represent important elements of a comprehensive repertoire of therapeutic options appropriate for consideration within a personalized and evolving program of care for individuals with diabetes and cardiovascular sequelae, along with dietary changes, exercise, alpha-lipoic acid, chromium, and omega-3 fatty acids such as fish oil. Initial assessment of renal function and magnesium status as well as regular monitoring and adjustment of insulin levels are important before beginning administration of oral magnesium, which is typically prescribed in the range of 200 to 600 mg of elemental magnesium per day.

Lithium Carbonate

Lithium carbonate (Camcolit, Carbolith, Duralith, Eskalith, Li-Liquid, Liskonum, Litarex, Lithane, Lithobid, Lithonate, Lithotabs, PMS-Lithium, Priadel).

Interaction Type and Significance

◈◈ **Drug-Induced Effect on Nutrient Function, Supplementation Contraindicated, Professional Management Appropriate**

Probability:
4. Plausible

Evidence Base:
○ **Preliminary**

Effect and Mechanism of Action

Magnesium and lithium are chemically related and appear to interact and sometimes compete within various physiological functions.[193-195] The consumption of lithium carbonate may cause high blood levels of magnesium.[196-198]

Research

Ramasamy and de Freitas[194] have observed competition between Li$^+$ and Mg^{++} for ATP in human erythrocytes in vitro using a 31P NMR and optical spectroscopy study. Herzberg and Herzeberg[198] reported a significant gender difference in mean plasma magnesium levels in 44 depressed patients. The authors concluded that such findings suggested an unknown interaction between lithium and magnesium and that magnesium metabolism could play an important role in bipolar disorder and the mode of action of lithium. In a small clinical trial, researchers found that antacids containing magnesium hydroxide did not significantly alter bioavailability of lithium carbonate in six healthy subjects.[199]

Nutritional Therapeutics, Clinical Concerns, and Adaptations

Although based on reasonable pharmacological principles and representing a plausible likelihood of occurrence, the clinical significance of the proposed interaction between lithium and magnesium remains largely unstudied. Nevertheless, physicians prescribing lithium carbonate are advised to ask such patients if they are taking magnesium. Initial assessment of magnesium status (and renal function) and regular monitoring of both lithium levels and magnesium levels are important to avoid excessive magnesium levels, if it is determined that both agents are therapeutically appropriate and strategically necessary.

Macrolide Antibiotics

Azithromycin (Zithromax), clarithromycin (Biaxin), dirithromycin (Dynabac), erythromycin, oral (EES, EryPed, Ery-Tab, PCE Dispertab, Pediazole); troleandomycin (Tao).

Interaction Type and Significance

≈≈≈ **Drug-Induced Nutrient Depletion, Supplementation Therapeutic, Not Requiring Professional Management**

☼ **Prevention or Reduction of Drug Adverse Effect**

Probability:
4. Plausible

Evidence Base:
○ **Preliminary**

Effect and Mechanism of Action

Some macrolide antibiotics, including erythromycin, may interfere with the absorption and activity of magnesium and other nutrients, particularly with extended treatment.

Research

The evidence pertaining to the effects of most macrolide antibiotics on magnesium is strongly suggestive but remains preliminary or inconclusive.[200]

Nutritional Therapeutics, Clinical Concerns, and Adaptations

Physicians prescribing extended courses of erythromycin or other macrolide antibiotics may find it prudent to recommend magnesium supplementation (e.g., 300 mg/day orally) given the potential for interference with magnesium absorption and functions. Monitoring of magnesium levels and compensatory supplementation may be especially appropriate for patients

with cardiovascular conditions or pathophysiological dysfunction in whom magnesium depletion might be clinically significant.

Misoprostol

Misoprostol (Cytotec); combination drug: misoprostol and diclofenac (Arthrotec).

Interaction Type and Significance

✗✗ **Minimal to Mild Adverse Interaction—Vigilance Necessary**

◇◇ **Drug-Induced Effect on Nutrient Function, Supplementation Contraindicated, Professional Management Appropriate**

Probability:
2. Probable

Evidence Base:
○ **Preliminary,** but treated as ● **Consensus**

Effect and Mechanism of Action

The most common adverse effect associated with misoprostol, a prostaglandin E$_1$ analog, is mild, transient diarrhea, often accompanied by abdominal cramps. Excessive magnesium intake can also cause diarrhea. Concomitant use of the two agents might result in an additive effect and subsequent occurrence or aggravation of diarrhea or other adverse effects.[201]

Research

No specific evidence; possibility of occurrence is considered pharmacologically self-evident.

Nutritional Therapeutics, Clinical Concerns, and Adaptations

Physicians prescribing misoprostol are advised to inform patients of the risk of diarrhea associated with the medication and the potential aggravation of adverse effects by concomitant magnesium intake. Drug-induced diarrhea can usually be minimized by administration of misoprostol after meals and at bedtime. Magnesium administration might be temporarily held in abeyance in some cases where the nutrient is considered strategically important but secondary in importance to the misoprostol in terms of tactical therapeutics.

Neuromuscular Blocking Agents

Evidence: Rocuronium, suxamethonium (succinylcholine), tubocurarine, vecuronium.
Extrapolated, based on similar properties: Atracurium, cisatracurium, doxacurium, metocurine iodide, mivacurium, pancuronium, pipecuronium.

Interaction Type and Significance

✗✗ **Minimal to Mild Adverse Interaction—Vigilance Necessary**

⊕✗ **Bimodal or Variable Interaction, with Professional Management**

⊕⊕ **Beneficial or Supportive Interaction, with Professional Management**

Probability:
2. Probable

Evidence Base:
◉ **Emerging**

Effect and Mechanism of Action

Magnesium salts, particularly magnesium sulfate given parenterally, can increase and prolong (up to eightfold) the effects of neuromuscular blocking agents.[202-207] Many substances alter the pharmacokinetics of neuromuscular blockers, especially those that depend on renal excretion, such as magnesium. Furthermore, some degree of additive effect is also operative because magnesium itself exerts significant neuromuscular blocking activity. These effects are at least partly caused by magnesium's marked inhibitory effect on acetylcholine release.[208]

Research

In a study involving women with toxemia of pregnancy undergoing cesarean birth, Morris and Giesecke[202] reported that patients receiving IV magnesium required approximately 65% of the dosage of succinylcholine (compared with those not receiving magnesium) to achieve adequate neuromuscular blocking activity.

Nutritional Therapeutics, Clinical Concerns, and Adaptations

Concomitant use of IV magnesium may enable neuromuscular blocking activity to be achieved with lower doses of neuromuscular blockers. Beyond such intentional coadministration, this interaction pattern is primarily of clinical significance in patients with increased serum magnesium concentrations; in such patients, unintentional additive effects could be of major severity. Physicians administering neuromuscular blocking agents are advised to assess initial magnesium status and closely monitor parameters of both substances if present together.

Penicillamine

Penicillamine (D-Penicillamine; Cuprimine, Depen).

Interaction Type and Significance

◇◇ **Impaired Drug Absorption and Bioavailability, Precautions Appropriate**

◇ **Adverse Drug Effect on Nutritional Therapeutics, Strategic Concern**

⊕✗ **Bimodal or Variable Interaction, with Professional Management**

Probability:	Evidence Base:
2. Probable	◉ Emerging

Effect and Mechanism of Action

Penicillamine and magnesium salts tend to form complexes, resulting in reduced magnesium absorption and inhibited activity of both substances. However, magnesium administration may reduce adverse effects of penicillamine in individuals who are magnesium deficient or who have become magnesium depleted due to action of the drug.

Research

The primary action of penicillamine is chelation of minerals and inhibition of their absorption and bioavailability. Formation of such complexes with magnesium inherently reduces availability of penicillamine for its intended therapeutic action. In a randomized crossover trial involving six healthy men given a single 500-mg oral dose of penicillamine, Osman et al.[209] observed that coadministration of a magnesium-containing antacid reduced the peak plasma level of penicillamine to 66% of those with the fasting dose. However, the antacid used contained both magnesium hydroxide and aluminum hydroxide, and the researchers did not attempt to distinguish the respective effects of the two components.

Use of high doses of penicillamine over an extended time can result in significant inactivation of magnesium and subsequent depletion. Seelig[210] hypothesized that autoimmune complications of D-penicillamine could result from magnesium and zinc depletion and pyridoxine inactivation. In a clinical trial involving more than 50 patients on long-term high-dose penicillamine therapy for advanced stages of autoimmune diseases, she found that coadministration of magnesium, along with zinc, pyridoxine, and vitamins B_1, B_{12}, and E, resulted in fewer adverse reactions than usual for patients treated with penicillamine alone.

Nutritional Therapeutics, Clinical Concerns, and Adaptations

Physicians prescribing penicillamine are advised to assess magnesium (and zinc) status at the initiation of treatment, especially when anticipating long-term high-dose penicillamine therapy. When magnesium has been determined to represent an essential element of the therapeutic strategy for the given patient, penicillamine should be administered at least 2 hours away from magnesium preparations (or magnesium-containing antacids).

Pentamidine

Pentamidine (NebuPent, Pentacarinat, Pentam 300, Pneumopent).

Interaction Type and Significance

≈≈ **Drug-Induced Nutrient Depletion, Supplementation Therapeutic, with Professional Management**

☼ **Prevention or Reduction of Drug Adverse Effect**

Probability:	Evidence Base:
3. Possible	○ Preliminary

Effect and Mechanism of Action

Pentamidine, an antiprotozoal medication, is known to decrease magnesium levels.[5]

Research

In vitro research suggests that pentamidine binds to a magnesium-binding site of the ribozyme in the target microbe. Zhang et al.[211] demonstrated that pentamidine inhibits catalytic activity of group I intron Ca.LSU from the transcripts of the 26S rRNA gene of *Candida albicans* by altering RNA folding.

Reports

Cortes et al.[212] reported two cases of hypocalcemia and hypomagnesemia associated with pentamidine therapy in patients with human immunodeficiency virus (HIV) infection. Otsuka et al.[213] reported a case in which torsades de pointes developed subsequent to pentamidine therapy for *Pneumocystis carinii* pneumonia in a patient with acute myelogenous leukemia. Torsades de pointes resolved with administration of magnesium sulfate and discontinuation of the IV pentamidine; however, sinus bradycardia and prolonged QT interval persisted. The authors recommended "careful monitoring of the electrocardiogram" during IV pentamidine therapy.

Nutritional Therapeutics, Clinical Concerns, and Adaptations

Physicians prescribing pentamidine are advised initially to assess and then regularly monitor magnesium (and potassium) status and administer compensatory nutrients as appropriate. Complementary therapies to support healthy cardiovascular and immune systems are usually appropriate in an integrative approach to treatment of immunocompromised individuals.

Quinidine and Related Antiarrhythmic Drugs

Evidence: Quinidine (Quinaglute, Quinidex, Quinora). Extrapolated, based on similar properties: Amiodarone (Cordarone, Pacerone), disopyramide (Norpace), dofetilide (Tikosyn), flecainide (Tambocor), ibutilide (Corvert), procainamide (Procan-SR, Pronestyl), sotalol (Betapace, Betapace AF, Sorine).
See also Sotalol and Related Beta-1-Adrenoceptor Antagonists (Beta-1-Adrenergic Blocking Agents).

Interaction Type and Significance

⊕⊕   **Beneficial or Supportive Interaction, with Professional Management**
☼   **Prevention or Reduction of Drug Adverse Effect**
≈≈   **Drug-Induced Nutrient Depletion, Supplementation Therapeutic, with Professional Management**

Probability:	Evidence Base:
2. Probable	○ **Preliminary**

Effect and Mechanism of Action

Quinidine, and other antiarrhythmic drugs, may worsen cardiac rhythm disorders and increase the risk of death, especially in individuals with a history of a heart attack. In particular, quinidine causes torsades de pointes under certain conditions, particularly hypokalemia, hypomagnesemia, and other electrolyte abnormalities. Potent suppression of a potassium channel subunit current by quinidine is a likely contributor to torsades de pointes arrhythmias.[214] Magnesium may prevent or reverse such quinidine-induced aggravation of cardiac arrhythmias. However, research into antacid-drug interactions shows that intragastric release of free aluminum and magnesium ions can induce potent effects on drug pharmacokinetics and GI function, particularly with drug-induced changes in GI motility or alterations in gastric and urinary pH. Direct adsorption by magnesium, or other mineral salts, may also result in decreased drug bioavailability, although not necessarily to a clinically significant degree.[215]

Research

Hypomagnesemia, especially in the presence of hypokalemia or other electrolyte abnormalities, is associated a range of adverse effects, including quinidine-related torsades de pointes, and interference with the antiarrhythmic activity of quinidine. Mutations in a gene encoding a potassium channel subunit (HERG) can be related to the long-QT (LQT) syndrome characteristic of torsades de pointes, a polymorphic ventricular arrhythmia. Pharmacological suppression of repolarizing potassium currents is also a mechanism causing the acquired LQT syndrome. Intravenous magnesium sulfate is often effective in reversing torsades de pointes induced by quinidine or other drugs, but the molecular basis of the mechanism involved in this action is not fully understood. In an in vitro study, Po et al.[214] found that increasing extracellular Mg^{++} did not relieve the inhibition of HERG currents by quinidine, but did cause additional suppression. These authors concluded that modulation of this important K^+ current is not the mechanism by which IV magnesium terminates drug-induced LQT and torsades de pointes. Further research into electrolyte function in cardiac tissue, related drug interactions and depletion, and individual genomic and pharmacogenomic variability is warranted and can benefit from an integrative approach to multidisciplinary therapeutic interventions.

Nutritional Therapeutics, Clinical Concerns, and Adaptations

Within a comprehensive therapeutic repertoire, quinidine and magnesium represent important options appropriate for consideration in crafting a program of care for individuals with arrhythmias and other cardiovascular conditions. Treatment of arrhythmias, hypertension, or other cardiovascular conditions using medications that do not deplete vital nutrients or otherwise introduce electrolyte abnormalities is preferable, especially patients at risk of arrhythmias or receiving drugs such as quinidine. Regular monitoring and appropriate nutrient administration are important therapeutic tools when recourse to more deleterious agents is deemed necessary. Low potassium and magnesium concentrations not only contribute to or cause cardiac arrhythmias, but also interfere with the efficacy or enhance the toxicity of many drugs typically used to treat patients with heart disease. Physicians prescribing quinidine, especially in conjunction with potassium-depleting diuretics, are advised initially to assess and then periodically monitor potassium and magnesium status and consider recommending coadministration of both minerals. Clinical care within an integrative setting might also emphasize a diet rich in vitamins, minerals, and antioxidants and incorporate hawthorn (*Crataegus oxyacantha*), L-carnitine, coenzyme Q10, and other nutrients as part of an individualized and evolving approach to cardiovascular therapeutics.

Sodium Polystyrene Sulfonate

Sodium Polystyrene Sulfonate (SPSS)

Interaction Type and Significance

≈≈   **Drug-Induced Nutrient Depletion, Supplementation Therapeutic, with Professional Management**
◇   **Adverse Drug Effect on Nutritional Therapeutics, Strategic Concern**

Probability:	Evidence Base:
4. Plausible	○ **Preliminary**

Effect and Mechanism of Action

Sodium polystyrene sulfonate (SPSS), often administered for the acute and chronic treatment of hyperkalemia, may alter magnesium levels and interfere with the therapeutic effects of magnesium. SPSS appears to increase sodium levels because of exchange for calcium and magnesium, thereby increasing susceptibility to magnesium depletion.[216]

Research

In vitro research investigating methods for reducing potassium intake indicates that, when used in hyperkalemia as a pretreatment for making a low-potassium formula, SPSS appears to lower calcium and magnesium levels while elevating sodium levels.[216]

Nutritional Therapeutics, Clinical Concerns, and Adaptations

Concomitant administration of SPSS may reduce the efficacy of therapeutic or supplemental magnesium intake and could potentially induce a nutrient depletion pattern impacting magnesium. Such repercussions may simply need to be taken into account when adopting SPSS as an appropriate therapeutic tactical element and introduce no significant clinical complications. However, compensatory magnesium intake may be necessary if magnesium constitutes an essential component of the therapeutic strategy and long-term SPSS is contemplated.

Nutrient-Drug Interactions and Drug-Induced Nutrient Depletions

Sotalol and Related Beta-1-Adrenoceptor Antagonists (Beta-1-Adrenergic Blocking Agents)

Oral forms (Systemic)
Evidence: Sotalol (Betapace, Betapace AF, Sorine)
Extrapolated, based on similar properties: Acebutolol (Sectral), atenolol (Tenormin); combination drugs: atenolol and chlortalidone (Co-Tendione, Tenoretic), atenolol and nifedipine (Beta-Adalat, Tenif); betaxolol (Kerlone), bisoprolol (Zebeta), carteolol (Cartrol), esmolol (Brevibloc), labetalol (Normodyne, Trandate), metoprolol (Lopressor, Toprol XL); combination drug: metoprolol and hydrochlorothiazide (Lopressor HCT); nadolol (Corgard), nebivolol (Nebilet), oxprenolol (Trasicor), penbutolol (Levatol), pindolol (Visken), propranolol (Betachron, Inderal LA, Innopran XL, Inderal); combination drug: propranolol and bendrofluazide (Inderex); timolol (Blocadren).
See also Quinidine and Related Antiarrhythmic Drugs.

Interaction Type and Significance

☼ **Prevention or Reduction of Drug Adverse Effect**
⊕ **Potential or Theoretical Beneficial or Supportive Interaction, with Professional Management.**
◇◇ **Impaired Drug Absorption and Bioavailability, Precautions Appropriate**

Probability:	Evidence Base:
3. Possible	◉ **Emerging**

Effect and Mechanism of Action

Magnesium compounds may reduce absorption and bioavailability of some beta blockers. Unintentional coadministration of some beta blockers, such as sotalol, and a magnesium-containing antacid appear to reduce serum levels of the drug.[217] However, beta blockers can induce numerous metabolic disturbances, including dose-related decreases in plasma potassium, phosphate, and corticosteroids and significant hypocalcemia and hypomagnesemia, that may result in excessive cardiac depressant effects, such as bradycardia, asystole, and sinus arrest. In particular, sotalol can produce an arrhythmia known as torsades de pointes. Intravenous magnesium sulfate can be effective in reversing torsades de pointes and has been observed to abolish inadequate kinetics of frequency adaptation of the Q-aT interval,[218] but the molecular basis of this effect is not understood.[214] Further, magnesium can theoretically exert many effects similar to those of a calcium channel blocker, so standard cautions regarding the potential for an additive interaction with beta blockers may be relevant to magnesium administration.

Research

Magnesium appears to be an effective adjuvant to beta-blocker therapy, especially in cases involving arrhythmia or atrial fibrillation. As with other antiarrhythmic drugs, beta blockers can also induce ventricular arrhythmias. Stark et al.[218] investigated the effects of sotalol alone and in combination with $MgSO_4$ and the Q-aT interval during abrupt changes in heart rate. In an animal experiment, they found that sotalol led to inadequate kinetics of rate adaptation of the Q-aT interval (indicated by high amplitude of Q-aT interval change, especially within first beat after abrupt change in pacing rate) and that magnesium sulfate abolished this adverse effect. Frick et al.[219] investigated the effect of administering sotalol and magnesium on the incidence of atrial fibrillation after elective direct-current cardioversion of persistent atrial fibrillation. They found that

occurrence of atrial fibrillation was significantly reduced by the administration of sotalol or magnesium individually, but that combination therapy was even more effective. Subsequently, in a randomized clinical trial with 207 consecutive coronary artery bypass patients, Forlani et al.[220] determined that the concomitant administration of sotalol and magnesium can prevent atrial fibrillation, a common complication after coronary artery bypass grafting.

Reports

In at least two published reports, IV magnesium effectively treated torsades de pointes in individuals taking sotalol.[221,222]

Nutritional Therapeutics, Clinical Concerns, and Adaptations

Research on coadministration of magnesium with sotalol appears promising, but available evidence is inadequate to warrant a general recommendation that individuals prescribed sotalol also take an oral magnesium supplement to prevent known adverse effects. When the patient's history and cardiac risk factors indicate that magnesium coadministration might be clinically appropriate, initial and regular monitoring of magnesium (and potassium) levels is necessary. Nevertheless, prudence suggests that any magnesium preparation should be taken at least 2 hours away from sotalol or related medications, even though the cautionary research is based on magnesium-containing antacids. Such metabolic monitoring is inherently part of critical care situations where IV magnesium (sulfate) may be indicated.

Sulfonylurea Hypoglycemics

Acetohexamide (Dymelor), chlorpropamide (Diabinese), glimepiride (Amaryl), glyburide (glibenclamide; Diabeta, Glynase Prestab, Glynase, Micronase, Pres Tab), glipizide (Glucotrol; Glucotrol XL), tolazamide (Tolinase), tolbutamide (Orinase; Tol-Tab); combination drugs: glipizide and metformin (Metaglip), glyburide and metformin (Glucovance).

Interaction Type and Significance

✗✗ **Minimal to Mild Adverse Interaction—Vigilance Necessary**
✗✗✗ **Potentially Harmful or Serious Adverse Interaction—Avoid**
⊕✗ **Bimodal or Variable Interaction, with Professional Management**
⊕ **Potential or Theoretical Beneficial or Supportive Interaction, with Professional Management**
⊕⊕ **Beneficial or Supportive Interaction, with Professional Management**

Probability:	Evidence Base:
3. Possible	○ **Preliminary**

Effect and Mechanism of Action

Magnesium intake may improve insulin sensitivity and secretion.[179] Concomitant ingestion of magnesium hydroxide, observed primarily in the form of antacids, with glipizide and glyburide can significantly enhance the rate and extent of absorption and efficacy of both medications and thereby facilitate early insulin and glucose responses.[223-226] These pharmacokinetic and pharmacodynamic interactions, as well as the cumulative effect of two therapies that can effectively alter blood glucose response, result in a potentially significant combination that might excessively lower blood glucose levels or enable more effective therapy or modification of dosage regimen.

Research

Diabetes is associated with low magnesium status,[180] and general consensus has existed since the early 1990s on the recognition of "strong associations ... between magnesium deficiency and insulin resistance."[181]

Most researchers have found that oral magnesium improves insulin sensitivity as well as insulin secretion in patients with type 2 diabetes.[182] In a small clinical trial involving eight older, non-insulin-dependent diabetes mellitus (NIDDM) subjects, Paolisso et al.[183] demonstrated that long-term magnesium administration (2 g/day) can elevate plasma magnesium levels and improve insulin response and action. In a subsequent double-blind trial, dosage appeared crucial, with 1000 mg/day of magnesium producing a favorable effect that was not obtained with half that dosage.[184] Eibl et al.[185] showed that a 3-month course of replacement therapy with magnesium corrected hypomagnesemia in patients with type 2 diabetes. Johnsen et al.[186] similarly reported that well-regulated NIDDM patients with marked magnesium deficiency responded favorably to oral magnesium. Two studies of the effect of magnesium supplementation on glucose tolerance in nondiabetic elderly subjects produced mixed results.[187,188]

Looking at a group of poorly controlled type 2 diabetic patients with hypomagnesemia, hypermagnesuria, and hypercalciuria, McBain et al.[227] observed that treatment with glipizide was associated with a significant rise in serum magnesium levels. Numerous pharmacological studies have demonstrated that the rate and extent of absorption of glipizide and glyburide, as well as their efficacy, are significantly enhanced by the concomitant administration of magnesium hydroxide.[223-226] For example, in a randomized trial with eight healthy people, Kivisto and Neuvonen[224] found that 850 mg magnesium hydroxide accelerated absorption of glipizide and increased early insulin and glucose responses.

Nutritional Therapeutics, Clinical Concerns, and Adaptations

The clinical implications of potential interaction(s) between magnesium and sulfonylurea drugs, particularly glipizide, glimepiride, and glyburide, largely depend on physician-patient communication and clinical management based on a coherent strategy. Magnesium can play an important role within a comprehensive, individualized, and evolving approach to clinical management of insulin resistance, dysglycemia, diabetes, and cardiovascular sequelae in conjunction with very-low-fat (and/or high-protein) diet, aerobic exercise, and appropriate weight reduction, as well as a coordinated nutraceutical program including chromium, multiple networked antioxidants (including mixed tocopherols and alpha-lipoic acid), soluble fiber, and possibly taurine.[228] Within a clinical context of collaboration by health care professionals trained and experienced in both conventional pharmacology and nutritional therapeutics, using magnesium in conjunction with sulfonylurea drugs at least can address the probability of magnesium deficiency in the susceptible individuals and may enhance the blood glucose–lowering effects of the medication. However, such concomitant use outside of integrative therapeutics and regular monitoring may increase the risk of hypoglycemia from an excessive additive interaction.

Tetracycline Antibiotics

Demeclocycline (Declomycin), doxycycline (Atridox, Doryx, Doxy, Monodox, Periostat, Vibramycin, Vibra-Tabs), minocycline (Dynacin, Minocin, Vectrin), oxytetracycline (Terramycin), tetracycline (Achromycin, Actisite, Apo-Tetra, Economycin, Novo-Tetra, Nu-Tetra, Sumycin, Tetrachel, Tetracyn); combination drugs: chlortetracycline, demeclocycline, and tetracycline (Deteclo); bismuth, metronidazole, and tetracycline (Helidac).

Interaction Type and Significance

◇ ◇ **Impaired Drug Absorption and Bioavailability, Precautions Appropriate**

◇ **Adverse Drug Effect on Nutritional Therapeutics, Strategic Concern**

⊕✗ **Bimodal or Variable Interaction, with Professional Management**

Probability:	Evidence Base:
2. Probable	● **Consensus**

Effect and Mechanism of Action

Magnesium salts can chelate with tetracycline medications and thereby interfere with their absorption and possibly reduce their bioavailability and effectiveness; although one study suggests that the complexed tetracycline may be more bioavailable.[229-236] This interaction occurs not only with supplemental magnesium but also with many antacids (e.g., Pepto-Bismol) that contain aluminum-magnesium hydroxide. Conversely, the formation of such complexes inherently reduces magnesium absorption and bioavailability and could contribute to magnesium depletion over an extended period. Furthermore, in vitro studies indicate that chelates of magnesium and tetracycline may play a role in the toxicity of tetracycline.

Research

The findings of Neuvonen[229] (1976) are typical of most subsequent research in concluding that tetracyclines form chelates with divalent and trivalent cations, including iron, aluminum, magnesium, and calcium. The team of Lambs, Brion, and Berthon has written extensively in the area of metal ion–tetracycline interactions. One paper states that simultaneous ingestion of minocycline and magnesium (as well as calcium, iron, or zinc) can decrease the absorption of both the medication and the mineral.[232] In another paper, however, they reported that although magnesium-tetracycline complexes are likely to form, the resulting complex may actually be more bioavailable than uncomplexed tetracycline because of a higher degree of membrane diffusion.[231]

Nutritional Therapeutics, Clinical Concerns, and Adaptations

In general, physicians prescribing tetracycline-class antibiotics should advise their patients to avoid using magnesium-based antacids and supplemental magnesium unless a patient's clinical care demands otherwise. Neuvonen[229] noted that the "pharmacokinetic interactions in absorption of tetracyclines [are] likely to be clinically significant in cases where the infecting pathogens are moderately resistant to tetracyclines and relatively high serum concentrations are needed for proper bacteriostasis." Nevertheless, tetracycline and antacids are often used together in combination therapies for *Helicobacter pylori* infection.

It is generally recommended that tetracycline be taken on an empty stomach, with a full glass of water, 1 hour before or 2 hours after ingestion of any supplements, food, or other drugs. However, an interval of 3 hours between the ingestion of tetracyclines and minerals such as magnesium is usually more effective in preventing this potential interaction.

Theophylline/Aminophylline

Theophylline/aminophylline (Phyllocontin, Slo-Bid, Slo-Phyllin, Theo-24, Theo-Bid, Theocron, Theo-Dur, Theolair, Truphylline, Uni-Dur, Uniphyl); combination drug: ephedrine, guaifenesin, and theophylline (Primatene Dual Action). See also Epinephrine in Theoretical, Speculative, and Preliminary Interactions Research.

Interaction Type and Significance

◇≈≈**Drug-Induced Adverse Effect on Nutrient Function, Coadministration Therapeutic, with Professional Management**

◇ **Adverse Drug Effect on Nutritional Therapeutics, Strategic Concern**

⊕⊕ **Beneficial or Supportive Interaction, with Professional Management**

Probability:	Evidence Base:
2. Probable	◉ Emerging

Effect and Mechanism of Action

Theophylline therapy is associated with magnesium depletion in the chronic asthmatic patient population characterized by magnesium deficiency. Magnesium can be an effective bronchodilator and, in various forms, is used in the treatment of chronic and acute asthma.

Research

Preliminary evidence indicating that theophylline can promote hypomagnesemia and hypokalemia concurs with clinical observations of a tendency for individuals taking this medication to develop potassium and magnesium deficiency.[237,238] In a study involving 869 patients treated with theophylline, Flack et al.[239] found that patients with measurable theophylline (concentrations >5.5 μmol/L) had a higher risk of hypokalemia, hyponatremia, hyperglycemia, hypophosphatemia, and hypomagnesemia than individuals in a control group of 350 inpatient and outpatient adults and children with no history of reactive airways disease or theophylline exposure.[239] Likewise, in a study of 93 chronic stable asthmatic patients on regular follow-up in an asthma clinic, Alamoudi[17] found that magnesium deficiency is associated with the occurrence and severity of asthma, particularly airway hyperreactivity, wheeze, and impairment of lung function. This paper concluded that hypomagnesemia is common in chronic asthmatic patients, and those with low serum magnesium tend to be hospitalized more than those with normal magnesium. Hypomagnesemia is also associated with more severe asthma.

Reports

Numerous case reports have documented hypomagnesemia and its respiratory, neurological, and cardiac sequelae subsequent to chronic theophylline therapy or theophylline overdose.[240-243] Chevalier et al.[244] reported the case of a patient with ischemic heart disease complicated by left ventricular failure and chronic asthma who had ventricular tachycardia induced by theophylline overdose and responded to IV magnesium chloride.

Nutritional Therapeutics, Clinical Concerns, and Adaptations

Magnesium as a nutritional therapy in chronic care and as an infusion in emergency care can play an important role in an integrative approach to the prevention and treatment of asthma, particularly to prevent or reverse hypomagnesemia

resulting from, and or act therapeutically in concert with, theophylline therapy. Administration of oral magnesium (300-600 mg/day) is often appropriate for individuals with asthma (or other magnesium-responsive conditions), in whom theophylline use over an extended period might induce magnesium depletion and interfere with magnesium's therapeutic or preventive action. Physicians prescribing theophylline are advised initially to assess and then regularly monitor magnesium status and correspondingly test renal function in individuals at risk for compromised ability to tolerate sustained magnesium administration, if determined to be appropriate. Magnesium sulfate infusions may be efficacious in the emergency care of individuals with acute asthma exacerbations, either in conjunction with beta-2 agonists via nebulizer, IV aminophylline, corticosteroids, or other first-line conventional therapies or in nonresponders.[245]

Warfarin and Related Oral Vitamin K Antagonist Anticoagulants

Evidence: Warfarin (Coumadin, Marevan, Warfilone).
Extrapolated, based on similar properties: Anisindione (Miradon), dicumarol, ethyl biscoumacetate (Tromexan), nicoumalone (acenocoumarol; Acitrom, Sintrom), phenindione (Dindevan), phenprocoumon (Jarsin, Marcumar).

Interaction Type and Significance

◇◇ **Impaired Drug Absorption and Bioavailability, Precautions Appropriate**

✗✗ **Minimal to Mild Adverse Interaction—Vigilance Necessary**

◇ **Adverse Drug Effect on Nutritional Therapeutics, Strategic Concern**

Probability:	Evidence Base:
4. Plausible	▽ Mixed

Effect and Mechanism of Action

Magnesium, as well as other minerals such as iron and zinc, may bind with warfarin or dicumarol.[246] However, the evidence is mixed as to whether such chelation reduces or enhances absorption and activity of dicumarol anticoagulants.[226,247] Formation of such complexes might also reduce magnesium absorption and bioavailability and could interfere with the effectiveness of oral magnesium as a preventive or therapeutic agent. Magnesium also exerts some degree of effect on the warfarin-albumin interaction.

Research

Testing four antacid preparations using an in vitro experimental model, McElnay et al.[248] found that magnesium trisilicate, a poorly absorbable form of magnesium never used as a nutrient source, although sometimes used in laxative preparations, decreased intestinal absorption of warfarin sodium by 19%. However, Neuvonen and Kivisto[226] reviewed the relevant literature and noted that magnesium hydroxide, as an antacid, increased absorption of dicumarol most likely because of chelate formation. In contrast, antacids containing both aluminium hydroxide and magnesium hydroxide appeared to produce no net change in the absorption of dicumarol, with aluminium hydroxide counterbalancing the enhancing effect of magnesium hydroxide.[249] Following the work of van der Giesen and Wilting[250] on the magnesium effect on the warfarin-albumin interaction, Perez Gallardo[251] conducted an in vitro experiment investigating the binding of warfarin to human serum albumin in the presence of several concentrations of calcium and magnesium, as chloride compounds.

He found that the free fraction of warfarin remained constant until calcium or magnesium reached concentrations of 50 mmol/L, at which point the binding fell to 92%. He concluded that displacement of bound warfarin can be expected only if the plasma concentrations of calcium or magnesium and chloride are significantly elevated.

Clinical Implications and Adaptations

Although the chemistry of common mineral nutrients binding warfarin is well founded, the frequency of occurrence is uncertain, its nature remains unclear and effects potentially variable, and conclusive evidence of the clinical significance of this interaction is lacking. Nevertheless, physicians prescribing warfarin are advised to recommend to patients that they separate warfarin administration from intake of magnesium (or iron or zinc) supplements (or magnesium-containing antacids) by at least 2 hours. Physician-patient communication is especially important in the event that individuals undergoing anticoagulant therapy are taking magnesium or any other mineral supplements. Regular monitoring of international normalized ratio (INR) is critical so that warfarin levels can be adjusted accordingly.

THEORETICAL, SPECULATIVE, AND PRELIMINARY INTERACTIONS RESEARCH, INCLUDING OVERSTATED INTERACTIONS CLAIMS

Captopril

Captopril (Capoten); combination drug: captopril and hydrochlorothiazide (Acezide, Capto-Co, Captozide, Co-Zidocapt).

Both captopril (an ACE inhibitor) and magnesium can be used in the treatment of hypertension. Captopril increases lymphocyte magnesium levels, although possibly only in patients with preexisting low levels.[252,253] This report of an observed interaction may be considered as preliminary or clinically insignificant. However, the therapeutic role of magnesium can be especially important in the population who would most likely be prescribed captopril. In particular, individuals with CHF, such as those noted in the research, tend both to be deficient in magnesium and to benefit therapeutically from magnesium. Thus, the issue of initial and regular monitoring of magnesium levels, along with cardiac function and other prognostic parameters, is essential to effective management of integrative therapeutics.

Cholestyramine

Cholestyramine (Locholest, Prevalite, Questran).

In animal research, cholestyramine produced an increased urinary excretion of magnesium, as well as other metabolic alterations.[254] A pattern of magnesium depletion resulting from this potential interaction could be counterproductive to the overall therapeutic strategy and detrimental to achieving the desired clinical outcomes (i.e., reducing mortality from cardiovascular disease). Supplementation with oral magnesium, typically 300 to 400 mg per day, preferably as part of a balanced multimineral formulation, could prevent nutrient depletion and deficiency. Evaluation of initial magnesium status and regular monitoring may be appropriate in some patients, especially anyone at risk of compromised renal function. Supplementation with fat-soluble vitamins is generally also indicated in patients taking cholestyramine.

Cycloserine

Cycloserine (Seromycin).

Cycloserine may interfere with absorption of magnesium (and calcium).[255] On the other hand, pharmacokinetics of cycloserine are minimally affected by magnesium-containing antacids[256] and thus at least as unlikely to be affected by supplemental magnesium. The probability of occurrence and clinical significance of these potential interactions remain uncertain pending substantive evidence from controlled clinical trials. Concomitant magnesium may be appropriate to address the potential for magnesium depletion with cycloserine use over an extended period and might be particularly relevant in patients with cardiovascular disease, asthma, or other conditions that tend to be magnesium-sensitive.

Docusate

Docusate (Colace, Surfak).

A single case report suggests that chronic use of docusate as a stool softener during and after pregnancy resulted in hypomagnesemia in a woman and her newborn infant.[257] The clinical significance and probability of occurrence of this potential interaction remains uncertain pending substantive evidence from controlled clinical trials. Supplemental magnesium may be appropriate to address the potential for magnesium depletion with docusate use over an extended period, particularly in patient populations at increased risk of magnesium deficiency.

Epinephrine

Epinephrine (Adrenaline, epi; Adrenalin, Ana-Gard, AsthmaHaler, AsthmaNefrin, Bronchaid, Bronkaid Mist, Brontin Mist, Epifin, Epinal, EpiPen, Epitrate, Eppy/N, Medihaler-Epi, Primatene Mist, S-2, Sus-Phrine; epinephrine, injectable: Adrenalin Chloride Solution, EpiPen Auto-Injector).

Hormones associated with stress response, including epinephrine, are known to reduce intracellular concentrations of potassium and magnesium.[258] Thus, endogenous catecholamine release during stress or acute illness can contribute to the hypomagnesemia, such as that seen in acutely ill patients.[259] In particular, catecholamines can intensify cellular magnesium depletion. The detrimental and mutually enhancing effects of catecholamine excess and magnesium deficiency can be particularly deleterious to the myocardium. Animal research has shown that magnesium supplementation can reduce the ultrastructural features of myocardial damage induced by epinephrine without an effect on changes in intracellular distribution of calcium induced by epinephrine.[260] Also, magnesium is indicated for surgery of pheochromocytoma based on its calcium channel–blocking properties and its activity of lowering the release of epinephrine.[261] Even though controlled human trials investigating the effects of epinephrine administration on magnesium status are lacking, physicians prescribing epinephrine for extended periods can consider whether supplementing magnesium is appropriate, especially in individuals susceptible to magnesium depletion and its potential sequelae.

Histamine (H₂) Receptor Antagonists

Cimetidine (Tagamet; Tagamet HB), famotidine (Pepcid RPD, Pepcid, Pepcid AC), nizatidine (Axid, Axid AR), ranitidine (Zantac); ranitidine, bismuth, and citrate (Tritec).

Concerns regarding potential interaction between H₂ blockers, particularly ranitidine, and magnesium does not primarily originate with a drug-nutrient interaction per se. Instead, research on the interaction between magnesium hydroxide and ranitidine has found that some antacids reduce the bioavailability of the H₂ receptor antagonists. This is particularly true when ranitidine is used at the same time as high doses of the relevant antacids. Bachmann et al.[262] found that among healthy subjects (i.e., who would not normally use the drug) a magnesium-aluminum hydroxide antacid decreased ranitidine absorption by 20% to 25% when the two substances were taken at the same time.

In relation to antacid use, the potential for interaction can be reduced by taking the H_2 blocker at least 2 hours before or after any antacid containing aluminum or magnesium. There is concern that a multivitamin/mineral supplement containing magnesium could have the same effect, especially if the magnesium is in the form of magnesium hydroxide. In such cases, caution would advise taking the H_2 blocker at least 2 hours before or after the magnesium-containing supplement.

Hydroxychloroquine and Chloroquine

Hydroxychloroquine (Plaquenil), chloroquine (Aralen, Aralen HCl).

Research involving chloroquine[263] suggests that oral magnesium intake may reduce blood levels of hydroxychloroquine and thereby decrease its effectiveness. Pending clinical trials providing more conclusive evidence and clarification, physicians prescribing hydroxychloroquine for conditions such as arthritis are advised to instruct patients to take magnesium preparations separate from these medications.

Isoniazid and Related Antitubercular Agents

Isoniazid (isonicotinic acid hydrazide, INH; Laniazid, Nydrazid); combination drugs: isoniazid and rifampicin (Rifamate, Rimactane); isoniazid, pyrazinamide, and rifampicin (Rifater).

Isoniazid appears to interfere with the activity of many nutrients, including magnesium. Human trials indicate that coadministration of magnesium-based antacids does not significantly alter isoniazid parameters.[264] Supplementation with a multivitamin/mineral formulation is advised for individuals undergoing long-term isoniazid therapy.

Magnesium-Containing Antacids

Magnesium carbonate combination drug: magnesium carbonate, aluminum hydroxide, alginic acid, and sodium bicarbonate (Gaviscon Extra Strength Tablets, Gaviscon Regular Strength Liquid, Gaviscon Extra Strength Liquid); magnesium hydroxide (Phillips' Milk of Magnesia MOM); combination drugs: magnesium hydroxide and aluminum hydroxide (Advanced Formula Di-Gel Tablets, Co-Magaldrox, Di-Gel, Gelusil, Maalox, Maalox Plus, Mylanta, Wingel); magnesium hydroxide and calcium carbonate (Calcium Rich Rolaids); magnesium hydroxide, aluminum hydroxide, calcium carbonate, and simethicone (Tempo Tablets); magnesium trisilicate and aluminum hydroxide (Adcomag trisil, Foamicon); magnesium trisilicate, alginic acid, and sodium bicarbonate (Alenic Alka, Gaviscon Regular Strength Tablets).

Concomitant use of supplemental magnesium and these antacids for an extended period might theoretically induce a magnesium excess. However, apart from individuals with compromised renal function, this is doubtful in light of general knowledge of magnesium, its minimal toxicity, and the difficulty in accumulating excessive magnesium levels in tissue.

The potential for interactions involving antacids depends on the chemistry and physical properties of the antacid preparation. The intragastric release of free aluminum and magnesium ions has potent effects on GI function and on drug pharmacokinetics. Antacid-drug interactions may occur secondary to changes in GI motility or alterations in gastric and urinary pH. Direct adsorption also results in decreased drug bioavailability.[215]

Mycophenolate

Mycophenolate (CellCept).

Oral magnesium salts, particularly within antacids, can inhibit absorption of mycophenolate, an immunosuppressive agent. However, even though a magnesium-containing antacid can reduce absorption and lower AUC of mycophenolic acid 15% and C_{max} by 37% (compared with fasting), and plasma mycophenolic acid parameters similarly, such "changes are small in comparison with the interpatient variability and are not likely to have clinically major effects."[265]

Metformin and Related Biguanides

Evidence: Metformin (Dianben, Glucophage, Glucophage XR). Extrapolated, based on similar properties: Buformin (Andromaco Gliporal, Buformina); metformin combination drugs: glipizide and metformin (Metaglip); glyburide and metformin (Glucovance); phenformin (Debeone, Fenformin).

Looking at a group of poorly controlled type 2 diabetic patients with hypomagnesemia, hypermagnesuria, and hypercalciuria, McBain et al.[227] observed that patients treated with metformin therapy demonstrated reduced urinary magnesium excretion but remained hypomagnesemic and hypercalciuric. Given the known associations between magnesium levels and insulin sensitivity, controlled clinical research is warranted. Pending such trials, the clinical significance of this potential interaction remains unclear.

Nitrofurantoin

Nitrofurantoin (Furadantin, Macrobid, Macrodantin).

Mannisto[266] reported that coadministration of nitrofurantoin (100 mg) and a magnesium-aluminum antacid reduced the bioavailability of the nitrofurantoin by approximately 25%. In a study with six healthy male subjects, Naggar and Khalil[267] observed that magnesium trisilicate, a poorly absorbable form of magnesium never used as a nutrient, but sometimes used in combination with other mineral salts as a laxative, reduced the rate and extent of intestinal absorption and thus the bioavailability of nitrofurantoin. An in vitro experiment showed that magnesium oxide, a form of magnesium often used in supplements, exhibited intermediate adsorptive powers. After administering oral nitrofurantoin (200 mg) to 11 subjects in five different suspension materials, Soci and Parrott[268] found that the viscosity effect of colloidal magnesium aluminum silicate slowed absorption and urinary excretion of the medication, thus delaying the time of the maximum excretion rate without a decrease in bioavailability. The clinical significance of these findings remains unclear, particularly their relationship, if any, to magnesium supplements. Nevertheless, physicians prescribing nitrofurantoin may find it prudent to recommend to patients that magnesium in any form be taken at least 2 hours away from the medication.

Potassium-Sparing Diuretics

Amiloride (Midamor), spironolactone (Aldactone), triamterene (Dyrenium).
Combination drugs: amiloride and hydrochlorothiazide (Moduretic); spironolactone and hydrochlorothiazide (Aldactazide); triamterene and hydrochlorothiazide (Dyazide, Maxzide).
See Diuretics: Loop Diuretics and Thiazide Diuretics.

Magnesium deficiency tends to be common among individuals undergoing diuretic therapy, and magnesium supplementation often plays an important role in prevention and treatment of cardiovascular conditions for such patients. According to preliminary studies involving rats, amiloride has a magnesium-sparing effect in addition to its potassium-sparing effect.[269] Consequently, individuals who take a magnesium supplement while also taking amiloride possibly could theoretically build up excessively high levels of magnesium. Thus the concurrent use of hydrochlorothiazide and amiloride would make this accumulation unlikely given the magnesium-depleting action of hydrochlorothiazide; for example, 5 to 10 mg of amiloride may negate the potassium-wasting effect of 40 mg of furosemide.[5] Nevertheless, Dorup et al.[132] reported that a furosemide-amiloride combination still produced hypomagnesemia in 12% of those treated with such a regimen. Similarly, triamterene may inhibit the urinary excretion of magnesium, according to preliminary research in animals. Initial assessment and regular monitoring of renal function and magnesium status are important to appropriate clinical management of individuals being administered both a potassium-sparing diuretic and a magnesium supplement.

Sulfamethoxazole and Related Sulfonamide Antibiotics

Sulfamethoxazole (Gantanol).
Related: Sodium sulfacetamide (AK-Sulf, Bleph-10, Sodium Sulamyd), sulfanilamide (AVC), sulfasalazine (Salazosulfapyridine, salicylazosulfapyridine, suphasalazine; Apo-Sulfasalazine, Azulfidine, Azulfidine EN-Tabs, PMS-Sulfasalazine, Salazopyrin, Salazopyrin EN-Tabs, SAS), sulfisoxazole (Gantrisin); combination drug: sulfamethoxazole and trimethoprim (cotrimoxazole, co-trimoxazole, SXT, TMP-SMX, TMP-sulfa; Bactrim, Bactrim DS, Cotrim, Septra, Septra DS, Sulfatrim, Uroplus); triple sulfa (Sultrin Triple Sulfa).

Sulfonamides, including sulfamethoxazole, can decrease absorption of magnesium, as well as of calcium and vitamin B$_{12}$. Although this potential depletion patterns may not be clinically significant when prescribing sulfamethoxazole for less than 2 weeks, physicians prescribing the medication for longer than 2 weeks are advised to monitor magnesium status and supplement when indicated.

RELATED INTERACTION ISSUES

Antacids containing magnesium are involved in many well-known and clinically significant interactions. In such uses, magnesium functions as part of a pharmaceutical agent that, although often self-prescribed and available without a prescription, does not function as a nutrient. Thus, such substances will be treated as drugs rather than nutrients based on their drug class, mechanism of action, therapeutic intent, and commercial channels of distribution and will not be addressed as nutrient-drug interactions.

The more soluble (i.e., better absorbed) chelates of magnesium probably have less influence on absorption of drugs and other compounds. Some research suggests that drug-magnesium complexes may actually be better absorbed and increase bioavailability of both agents. As always, titration of any medication, as well as regular monitoring of electrolyte status, including magnesium and potassium, is essential to safe and effective implementation of integrative therapeutics.

NUTRIENT-NUTRIENT INTERACTIONS

Alcohol

High alcohol intake increases renal excretion of magnesium, and hypomagnesemia is very common in alcoholics (e.g., 30% of alcoholic patients admitted to hospital care).

Calcium

Magnesium intake from food and supplements is associated with bone mineral density.[270] However, high calcium intake may inhibit magnesium absorption. Such competition does not appear to exert a significant effect on overall magnesium status.[271-273] Calcium supplementation, as well as cessation of magnesium administration, is typically used in treating hypermagnesemia.

Iron

Numerous in vitro, animal, and human studies have raised the issue of interactions between magnesium and iron.[159,274] In a clinical trial involving 111 healthy women ages 18 to 40 years, of whom 45 were either iron deficient or iron deplete, Newhouse et al.[275] observed that although therapeutic iron dose (320 mg elemental iron daily as Slow-Fe tablets) for 12 weeks was successful in raising mean serum ferritin values and did not significantly effect serum zinc and magnesium levels during the supplementation period, there was a downward trend through the discontinuation phase; at 18 and 24 weeks, serum zinc and magnesium levels were significantly lower than baseline. These researchers also noted that oral contraceptive use was associated with elevated serum copper and ferritin values and lowered serum magnesium levels.

Rodent studies, single-dose experiments using healthy subjects, and a clinical trial involving two groups of pregnant women with moderately reduced hemoglobin levels showed that concomitant iron gluconate and magnesium-L-aspartate hydrochloride were well tolerated, stabilized hemoglobin levels, and moderated progesterone-induced constipation (during pregnancy), without interfering with iron absorption.[276]

Manganese

Individuals supplementing with manganese may need concomitant supplemental magnesium.

Phosphate

Individuals with high phosphorus intake may experience decreased magnesium absorption. After oral administration, magnesium and other divalent cations can bind to oral phosphate in the GI tract, reducing bioavailability and therapeutic effect of both substances.[6,277] This interaction can usually be avoided by separating oral intake of the two substances by 2 hours. Increased dosage of magnesium may also be medically appropriate for preventive or therapeutic purposes in some individuals.

Potassium

Potassium and magnesium deficiency often occur together and need to be treated concomitantly.[3,101,104,127,129] For example, magnesium (and sometimes sodium) supplementation often needs to accompany potassium supplementation to correct intracellular potassium depletion in hypertensive patients who develop ventricular ectopy and other potassium deficiency effects subsequent to diuretic therapy.[105] However, some research shows that such coadministration may not provide efficacy beyond that of potassium alone in the treatment of some conditions, such as ventricular extrasystoles.[278] Most individuals who benefit from magnesium supplementation also often benefit from potassium supplementation or increased dietary potassium intake. Initial assessment and regular monitoring of renal function and potassium status are important to safe and effective administration of both minerals. Clinically effective levels of potassium require a physician's prescription. A diet rich in fruits, vegetables, and whole grains provides several grams of potassium daily.

Nutrient-Drug Interactions and Drug-Induced Nutrient Depletions

Vitamin B₁ (Thiamine)

One case report described a patient in whom cardiac beriberi with polyneuritis developed after protracted use of large amounts of magnesium trisilicate,[279] a poorly absorbable form of magnesium never used as a nutrient, but sometimes used in combination with other mineral salts as a laxative, and widely used as a flowing agent in the tableting and food industries.

Vitamin B₆ (Pyridoxine)

Pyridoxine is necessary for cellular accumulation of magnesium (and zinc), and its presence increases the amount of magnesium that can enter cells. Concurrent administration of both nutrients may enhance therapeutic efficacy.

Vitamin D

Magnesium bioavailability appears to be enhanced by vitamin D.

Zinc

Supplementation with zinc may increase magnesium intake needs, possibly through an inhibitory effect on magnesium absorption and adverse effect on magnesium metabolic balance.[277]

The 279 citations for this monograph, as well as additional reference literature, are located under Magnesium on the CD at the back of the book.

Potassium

Nutrient Name: Potassium.
Synonym: Kali.
Elemental Symbol: K.
Forms: Potassium aspartate, potassium bicarbonate, potassium chloride, potassium citrate, potassium gluconate, potassium iodide, potassium-R-lipoate, potassium orotate, potassium para-aminobenzoate.

Summary

Drug/Class Interaction Type	Mechanism and Significance	Management
Albuterol, rimiterol Beta-2-adrenoceptor agonist bronchodilators ≈≈/☼	Oral or intravenous albuterol, rimiterol, and related beta-2-adrenoceptor agonists can deplete potassium and other nutrients, possibly to a clinically significant degree. Hypokalemia due to these drugs, particularly in combination with steroids or digoxin, may contribute to arrhythmias or aggravate asthma. Evidence is lacking to determine frequency of occurrence or confirm benefits of potassium coadministration.	Monitor regularly. Coadministration of potassium (and magnesium) may prevent or correct nutrient depletion.
Amiloride Antikaliuretic-diuretic agent ✗✗/✗✗✗/◇◇	As a potassium-sparing diuretic, amiloride carries implicit risk of hyperkalemia when combined with significant increase in potassium intake, especially with compromised renal function and concomitant ACE inhibitor therapy. Probability of adverse events with concurrent use of potassium supplements, salt substitutes, or food sources generally recognized; risk of acute and severe event with rapid increase in intake.	Limit potassium intake, and avoid rapid and significantly increased intake, outside professional supervision. Closely monitor high-risk patients.
Aminoglycoside antibiotics ≈≈/☼	Aminoglycosides can cause renal tubular damage and induce hypokalemia; renal failure is also potentiated by potassium depletion. Case reports and animal studies available; small but recognized risk for elderly and compromised persons. Evidence from clinical trials lacking to confirm benefits of concomitant potassium.	Concurrent potassium may prevent or correct adverse effects with long-term or repeated drug therapy. Monitor.
Amphotericin B ≈≈/☼	Amphotericin can cause potassium depletion, especially with steroids; hypokalemia is possible, particularly with drug-induced renal damage or rapid infusion. Not common but widely recognized.	Concurrent potassium may prevent or correct adverse effects with long-term or repeated drug therapy. Monitor.
Angiotensin-converting enzyme (ACE) inhibitors ✗✗/✗✗✗/◇◇	Significant risk of hyperkalemia when potassium intake increased during ACE inhibitor therapy, especially with compromised renal function or diabetes. Probability of acute and severe adverse events with concurrent use of potassium supplements, salt substitutes, or food sources generally recognized, particularly with rapid increase in intake.	Limit potassium intake, and avoid rapid and significantly increased intake, outside professional supervision. Closely monitor high-risk patients.
Beta-adrenoceptor antagonists ✗✗/✗✗✗	Beta blockers can elevate potassium levels and may cause hyperkalemia. A variety of mechanisms may be involved, but not fully elucidated. Frequency unknown, but potentially severe consequences.	Potassium generally contraindicated but may be indicated in certain circumstances. Monitor potassium closely with beta blockers.
Carbonic anhydrase inhibitors ≈≈	Carbonic anhydrase inhibitors generally decrease renal blood flow and glomerular filtration rate. However, other than furosemide and acetazolamide, limited evidence indicates they do not appear to affect potassium status adversely in most individuals. Potential for significant disequilibrium in carbon dioxide transport; low probability but high risk.	Concurrent potassium may prevent or correct adverse effects with long-term or repeated drug therapy. Monitor, especially for acidosis.
Cisplatin ≈≈/⊕✗/✗✗	Renotubular damage is common with cisplatin and may cause wasting of potassium and other minerals. Resulting hypokalemia may be refractory without concomitant administration of potassium and magnesium. Risk of clinically significant adverse effects widely recognized.	Concurrent potassium and magnesium may prevent or correct depletion. Protect renal function. Closely monitor electrolyte status.
Colchicine ◇≈≈	Colchicine can impair absorption and increase loss of potassium (and other nutrients). Coadministration of potassium may prevent or correct clinically significant adverse effects. Minimal research but widely accepted as possible or probable.	Coadministration of potassium and other nutrients may prevent or correct adverse effects with long-term or repeated drug therapy. Monitor.
Corticosteroids, oral ≈≈/☼	Oral corticosteroids can deplete potassium and other nutrients, possibly to clinically significant degree. Hypokalemia due to these drugs, particularly in combination with other agents affecting potassium status, may contribute to edema, arrhythmias, or aggravate asthma. Widely recognized, but minimal evidence and lack of consensus as to clinical significance. Benefits of potassium coadministration unproven.	Consider coadministration of potassium and other nutrients, may prevent or correct adverse effects with long-term therapy. Monitor, especially with renal impairment.
Cyclosporine ◇◇	Cyclosporine-induced nephrotoxicity and other mechanisms can cause hyperkalemia, most often in patients with compromised renal function. Onset of effects can be rapid or gradual. Varied attempts at reducing drug toxicity and its effects on renal function and potassium metabolism, but mixed results and no consensus as to effective corrective measures.	Close monitoring of allograft patients is always essential. Potassium generally contraindicated, but coadministration may be indicated; caution imperative.

Nutrient-Drug Interactions and Drug-Induced Nutrient Depletions

Continued

Nutrient-Drug Interactions and Drug-Induced Nutrient Depletions

Summary

Drug/Class Interaction Type	Mechanism and Significance	Management
Digoxin Cardiac glycosides ◇≈≈/⊕✗	Hypokalemia increases risk of digoxin toxicity, but digoxin impairs potassium function, and overdose can cause hyperkalemia. Increased risk in patients taking diuretics. Interplay with magnesium; increased risks with dual depletion.	Consider coadministration of potassium, magnesium, and other nutrients, especially through food sources; may prevent or correct adverse effects. Monitor, especially with diuretics and renal impairment.
Diuretics, potassium depleting Loop and thiazide diuretics ≈≈/☼	Potassium-wasting diuretics inherently increase risk of potassium depletion and hypokalemia. Generally accepted as inherent risk of clinically significant adverse effects. Concomitant ACE inhibitor therapy or other polypharmacy often used to mitigate depletion.	Coadministration of potassium and other nutrients, as food or supplements, can prevent or correct depletion and sequelae. Monitor.
Laxatives Stool softeners ≈≈≈/☼	Through various mechanisms, laxatives or stool softeners can deplete potassium and other nutrients, more often with repeated use. However, hypokalemia occasionally possible with short-term cathartic use, as in procedure preparation. Generally recognized as possible risk, but corrective measures inconsistently applied. Increased risk of adverse effects in cardiac patients, especially with concomitant diuretics or other potassium-depleting drugs.	Review diet and exercise; advise improvements as indicated. Coadministration of potassium and other nutrients may prevent or correct adverse effects with long-term or repeated drug therapy. Monitor.
Losartan Angiotensin II receptor antagonists ✗✗/✗✗✗/◇◇	All angiotensin II receptor antagonists inherently carry risk of hyperkalemia. Through effects on renin-angiotensin system and aldosterone, losartan may cause clinically significant elevations in potassium levels. Effect on potassium is universal and widely recognized. However, severity may vary, and clinically significant events are uncommon.	Avoid extra potassium, especially rapid and significantly increased intake, outside professional supervision. Monitor regularly.
Nonsteroidal anti-inflammatory drugs (NSAIDs) ✗✗/✗✗✗/◇◇	Various NSAIDs alter potassium metabolism through a range of mechanisms, many only partially understood, but many resulting from drug-induced nephrotoxicity. Severe potassium-related adverse effects with NSAIDs are uncommon but not rare; they may be acute and reversible, but chronic renal failure possible.	Limit potassium intake, and avoid rapid or significantly increased intake; professional supervision indicated. Closely monitor high-risk patients.
Quinidine Antiarrhythmic drugs ≈≈/☼	Hypokalemia of various origins can significantly increase risk of acute cardiac irregularities and adverse reactions to antiarrhythmic drugs, especially when accompanied by hypomagnesemia.	Closely monitor; restore electrolyte balance, particularly magnesium and potassium, whenever disturbed or depleted by diuretics, vomiting, diarrhea, or other causes.
Spironolactone, triamterene ◇◇/✗✗	Potassium-sparing diuretics (spironolactone, triamterene) carry implicit risk of hyperkalemia if potassium intake significantly increased, especially with compromised renal function or concomitant ACE inhibitor. Probability of acute and severe adverse events with concurrent use of potassium supplements, salt substitutes, or food sources generally recognized. Frequently coadministered with potassium-depleting diuretics based on known activity.	Limit potassium intake, and avoid rapid and significantly increased intake; professional supervision indicated. Closely monitor high-risk patients.
Trimethoprim-sulfamethoxazole ◇◇/✗✗/✗✗✗	Trimethoprim, alone or with sulfamethoxazole, can elevate potassium levels, sometimes causing hyperkalemia, through one or more mechanisms involving renal function. Severe adverse effects are uncommon but not rare; they may be acute and reversible, but chronic renal failure possible. Risk minimal to moderate for most patients but increased in AIDS patients or others with compromised physiological function or polypharmacy affecting renal function.	Limit potassium intake, and avoid rapid or significantly increased intake, outside professional supervision. Closely monitor high-risk patients.

NUTRIENT DESCRIPTION

Chemistry and Forms

Potassium aspartate, potassium bicarbonate, potassium chloride, potassium citrate, potassium gluconate, potassium orotate, potassium tartrate.

Physiology and Function

Cell membrane excitability, ion transport, and energy production are central functions of potassium in human physiology. Potassium, sodium, and chloride are the essential dietary minerals that serve as the major electrolytes in the human body within a triangular equilibrium. Directly and through these relationships, potassium participates in the regulation of water balance, osmotic equilibrium, acid-base balance, and blood pressure, and it plays a critical role in the contractility of smooth, cardiac, and skeletal (striated) muscle, particularly through its contribution to nerve function and carbohydrate and protein metabolism. It participates in glucose metabolism through its involvement with insulin in the movement of blood glucose into cells and conversion of blood glucose into glycogen for storage in the muscles and liver.

Potassium (K^+) is the principal cation in intracellular fluid, whereas sodium (Na^+) is the principal extracellular cation. Potassium concentrations are tightly regulated both inside and outside of cells, with a differential of 30 times, and this sodium-potassium concentration gradient creates the membrane potential on which all contractility and nerve function depend.

Water balance is maintained by using ion pumps in the cell membrane, especially the sodium-potassium-adenosinetriphosphatase (Na^+, K^+-ATPase) pumps, to move potassium into cells in exchange for sodium being pumped out of cells. The proper functioning of nerve impulse transmission, muscle contraction, and cardiac function all require tight control of cell membrane potential. The critical function of these ion pumps is demonstrated in their exchange activities, accounting for 20% to 40% of the resting energy expenditure (of ATP) in a typical adult. The activity of the adenosine triphosphate (ATP)–sensitive K^+ channel plays an important role in mitochondrial cell-signaling pathways for ischemic protection and gene transcription, "roles that appear to depend on the ability of mitochondrial K(ATP) opening to trigger increased mitochondrial production of reactive oxygen species."[1] Beyond Na$^+$, K$^+$-ATPase, potassium is required as a cofactor in the activity of only a few other enzyme systems, such as pyruvate kinase, central to carbohydrate metabolism. Potassium is also essential for proper kidney and adrenal function.

Potassium salts are inherently highly soluble, and dietary potassium intake is readily absorbed, 85% to 98%, principally in the small intestine. Average body content of potassium is 180 grams, and the intracellular fluid holds approximately 98% of the total body potassium. Dietary potassium is primarily excreted in the urine ($\sim$ 77%-90%), with minimal renal capacity for conservation and minimal elimination of unabsorbed and intestinally secreted potassium eliminated via feces. The correlation between dietary potassium intake and urinary potassium content is high ($r = 0.82$). Small amounts of potassium are excreted, along with other electrolytes, through perspiration and saliva.

NUTRIENT IN CLINICAL PRACTICE
Known or Potential Therapeutic Uses

Potassium is among the nutrients more frequently prescribed in conventional medical practice, particularly in the context of hypertension and drug-induced depletion, as well as diarrhea and other causes of acute electrolyte depletion or disequilibrium. Although the legal limitation of potassium in over-the-counter (OTC) preparations to 99 mg in the United States is unique, much higher dosage levels are often prescribed in conjunction with potassium-wasting diuretics, or simply are attainable through consumption of a few pieces of fruit daily (or many electrolyte-rich "sports" drinks). Professional supervision and regular monitoring of serum potassium concentrations are appropriate whenever potassium is coadministered with conventional medications. Notably, perioperative outcomes are better in cardiac surgery patients with adequate potassium levels than those in patients with low preoperative serum potassium levels, who are at increased risk of developing arrhythmias and more likely to require cardiopulmonary resuscitation.[2] Conversely, hyperkalemia can occur when excess potassium accumulates because of decreased urinary potassium excretion as a result of diminished renal elimination, or more rarely, acute excessive intake. Apart from unintended effects of potassium-sparing diuretics, acute or chronic renal failure and hypoaldosteronism constitute the most common causes of hyperkalemia. Hemolysis, traumatic tissue damage, severe burns, and tumor lysis syndrome may also produce hyperkalemia as a result of a rapid shift of intracellular potassium into general circulation.

Historical/Ethnomedicine Precedent

The simple admonition to eat plenty of fruits and vegetables, especially those grown in soil rich with minerals, represents a time-honored recommendation that would encompass a healthful dietary potassium intake.

Possible Uses

Allergies, asthma, atherosclerosis, cancer, cardiac arrhythmia, congestive heart failure, Crohn's disease, diabetes mellitus (mild), diarrhea (especially in infants), electrolyte depletion, glaucoma, hypertension, hypokalemia, inflammatory bowel disease, muscle cramping and spasms, muscle fatigue and weakness, nephrolithiasis, osteoporosis, premenstrual syndrome, stroke, ulcerative colitis.

Deficiency Symptoms

Potassium deficiency can lead to a broad range of adverse effects across multiple body systems. These effects primarily derive from alterations in membrane potential and cellular metabolism and include muscle weakness, fatigue, listlessness, irritability, apprehension, mental confusion, drowsiness, nerve conduction irregularities, respiratory failure, reduced or absent reflexes, paralysis, cardiac disturbances (particularly arrhythmia), hypotension, muscle cramping and spasms, anorexia, nausea, abdominal bloating, delayed gastric emptying, constipation, paralytic ileus, polydypsia, and polyuria. Severe hypokalemia can be fatal as a result of cardiac arrhythmias and muscular paralysis. Electrocardiographic (ECG) changes accompanying hypokalemia are ST depression, flat T waves, U waves, and dysrhythmias. The pulse will alternate between fast and slow. It is necessary to monitor for digitalis toxicity in digitalized patients.

Most incidents of hypokalemia (i.e., abnormally low plasma potassium concentration) result from excessive loss of potassium, but inadequate or unbalanced intake can make a significant contribution. Thus, gross deficiencies of potassium are most often associated with use of potassium-depleting diuretics or glucocorticoids but can also result from severe or prolonged vomiting, diarrhea or perspiration, gastrointestinal (GI) disturbances caused by parasites, ostomy, laxative abuse or food reactions, some forms of renal disease, or other metabolic disturbances (e.g., acidosis) associated with alcoholism, anorexia nervosa, bulimia, rapid weight loss, congestive heart failure, chronic obstructive pulmonary disease, diabetes mellitus, or magnesium depletion. To a lesser degree, because potassium losses increase with perspiration, exercise and heat exposure, particularly hot humid climate, can adversely affect potassium status. In another clinical scenario, fluid shifting from the extracellular to the intracellular fluid compartment as a result of elevated insulin levels in the treatment of diabetic ketoacidosis is the most common cause of a drop in serum potassium levels. Subsequently, potassium is pulled from the intracellular space to the serum and then excreted through the kidneys in the hyperglycemic phase. At that point, serum potassium levels appear elevated, even though the stores are being lost with polyuria. Consequently, in the absence of replacement, serum potassium can drop to dangerously low levels if insulin is administered to reduce the hyperglycemia and potassium returns to the intracellular space. In a less dramatic process, potassium can become depleted during periods of stress as the adrenal glands secrete increased levels of adrenaline, which pulls potassium from the cells to be lost by the kidneys' excretion. Similarly, overproduction of corticosteroids resulting from Cushing's syndrome, hyperaldosteronism, or other endocrine disorders (or exogenous administration) can provoke sodium retention and increase potassium excretion.

Absolute potassium deficiency is relatively rare, but relative potassium deficiency (i.e., in relation to sodium excess) is common, even in those with apparently healthy diets. In 2001 the Third National Health and Nutrition Examination Survey (NHANES-III) found that the modern American diet, especially when dominated by salt and processed foods, contains an average of 2300 mg of potassium daily for adult females and 3100 mg daily for adult males; slightly more than minimum daily requirements but approximately one-quarter to one-third the estimated daily potassium intake of hunter-gatherers or other "primitive" diets. Moreover, with daily potassium intake in modern diets being half as much as the typical daily sodium intake, most experts recommend significantly higher levels of dietary potassium, for example, a ratio of at least 5:1 or optimally 10:1 potassium/sodium intake or more, especially in the form of fresh fruits and vegetables. Dietary intake for reducing risk of hypertension, heart disease, and stroke is at least in the range of 4 to 5 g daily. Thus, even though low dietary intakes of potassium will generally not produce hypokalemia, insufficient dietary potassium probably increases significantly the risk of a wide range of chronic diseases, especially in the context of an imbalanced or poor-quality diet.

Several commonly consumed substances may induce lowered potassium levels. Caffeine and tobacco can reduce potassium absorption. Apart from the major adverse impact on potassium status associated with sodium intake, magnesium can also cause increased excretion of potassium in the stool with excess intake. Rare case reports describe hypokalemia subsequent to continued intake of large doses of licorice; the herb (but usually not the candy) contains glycyrrhizic acid, which can increase urinary excretion of potassium in a manner similar to aldosterone.

Dietary Sources

Fruits and vegetables are generally the richest dietary sources of potassium, and an individual who eats a diet high in these can have a high potassium intake (8-11 g/day). Notably, however, U.S. Department of Agriculture (USDA) data (2004) documented changes in food composition for 43 garden crops indicating that the nutrient content of many vegetables and fruits declined significantly from 1950 to 1999.[3]

Bananas, orange juice, prunes and prune juice, raisins, avocados, cantaloupes, peaches, tomato juice, potatoes (baked with skin), soy flour, white beans, lima beans (cooked), lentils (cooked), acorn squash (cooked), parsnips (cooked), turnips (cooked), artichokes (cooked), and spinach (cooked) contain more than 300 mg of potassium per serving. Other foods providing moderate amounts of potassium include oranges, tomatoes, other fruits and vegetables, mint leaves, molasses, whole grains, sunflower seeds, almonds, flounder, salmon, cod, milk, chicken, and red meat.

Common herbs also considered sources of potassium include red clover, sage, catnip, hops, horsetail, nettle, plantain, and skullcap.

The potassium/sodium ratio in foods varies considerably and is more influential than the potassium content per se. Beans, peas, potatoes, grains, nuts, and fruits are among the foods with the highest potassium/sodium ratio. Thus, bananas or navy beans contain more than 1000 times more potassium than sodium, and Brazil nuts or corn contain more than 700 times more potassium than sodium. In comparison, eggs, beef, and fish contain 6 to 10 times more potassium than sodium, and spinach, celery, and beets contain only about 2.5 to 4 times more potassium than sodium, as do whole milk, chicken, and lamb. Many health care professionals advise using potassium chloride, rather than sodium chloride, as a seasoning to shift the potassium/sodium balance.

Nutrient Preparations Available

Potassium preparations can be potassium salts (chloride and bicarbonate), potassium bound to various mineral chelates (e.g., aspartate, citrate), or food-based potassium sources. Forms of potassium used as supplemental nutrients or as pharmaceutical agents include potassium aspartate, potassium bicarbonate, potassium chloride (oral, effervescent, or injection), potassium citrate, potassium gluconate, potassium iodide (oral solution or syrup), potassium-R-lipoate, potassium orotate, and potassium para-aminobenzoate. Potassium gluconate and potassium citrate are the most common supplemental forms. Potassium is administered parenterally when oral replacement is not possible or if hypokalemia is life threatening. Intravenous (IV) administration without cardiac monitoring should not exceed 10 mEq/hr.

Available forms are composed of potassium bound to other nonmetallic substances that render it chemically stable. Pure potassium is never available as a supplement or prescription item because it is a highly reactive metal that spontaneously ignites when exposed to water. Potassium bicarbonate or citrate is the form most conducive to a reduced risk of kidney stones.[4,5] Among the chelated forms used orally, potassium citrate is generally better tolerated (and possibly more efficacious), whereas potassium chloride is less well tolerated, although it is used as a substitute for table salt and, in solution, for IV administration. A large amount given rapidly after sedation and neuromuscular paralysis is used as part of execution by lethal injection because it stops cardiac electrical activity and thus cardiac function.

Prescription preparations of potassium usually contain an inorganic form of potassium, usually potassium chloride, along with nonnutritive additives, and are dispensed as timed-release tablets, liquids, powders, and effervescent tablets, typically in the dosage range of 1.5 to 3 g (20-40 mEq) daily. Potassium iodide is also the preferred agent recommended by some governmental bodies as a protective measure against iodine-131 radiation-induced thyroid cancer in cases of nuclear radiation contamination.

Potassium is available generically from numerous manufacturers as an over-the-counter (OTC) product, but it is limited to 99 mg per serving as a nutritional supplement, which is small compared with the U.S. Institute of Medicine's recommendation for a dietary intake of 4700 mg daily. More significant quantities of supplemental potassium require a physician's prescription. Notably, so-called salt substitutes, such as Morton Salt Substitute, Lite Salt, No Salt, and Nu-Salt, are basically potassium chloride at the dosage level of 530 mg of potassium per ⅙ teaspoon.

Dosage Forms Available

Divided doses, taken with or near food, throughout the day are generally best for availability and tolerance.

Over-the-counter potassium supplements, singly or within multivitamin/mineral formulations, typically contain 99 mg of potassium per recommended daily dose, the legal nonprescription limit in the United States, as established by the Food and Drug Administration (FDA), for non-food-based forms. Notably, so-called salt substitutes, such as Morton Salt Substitute, Lite Salt, No Salt, and Nu-Salt, are basically potassium chloride at the dosage level of 530 mg potassium per ⅙ tsp.

Dosage Range

Adult

Dietary: A daily intake of 2000 mg (51 mEq) is generally considered an adequate (i.e., minimum) requirement of potassium for adult men and women, including for pregnant and nursing women. The need to ensure a (minimal) daily potassium intake of 2.5 to 3.5 g, a supply from fruits and vegetables (chiefly as citrate or malate, through daily intake of 0.6-0.8 mg/kg) represents the underlying rationale for the often-repeated "5 to 10 servings per day" recommendations from official bodies. Many practitioners experienced in nutritional medicine recommend 6 to 9 g from food sources as an optimal daily intake.

In 2004 the Food and Nutrition Board (FNB) of the U.S. Institute of Medicine established, for the first time, a recommended adequate intake (AI) level of 4700 mg (120 mEq) per day of potassium for adult, based on intake levels that have been found to lower blood pressure, reduce salt sensitivity (particularly in African-American men), and minimize the risk of kidney stones. However, the AI for potassium during lactation is set at 5100 mg (130 mEq)/day (4700 + 400 mg).[6] In the United Kingdom the average adult daily diet provides 2562 mg for women and 3279 mg for men.

Supplemental/Maintenance: No dosage level has been officially established for use as a dietary supplement. Potassium supplementation is not normally necessary in the presence of a balanced diet.

Pharmacological/Therapeutic: An oral dose of 1500 to 4000 mg daily, with plenty of fluid, is usually indicated in correction of mild deficiency or to lower blood pressure. More broadly, therapeutic doses can range from 100 to 6000 mg per day.

As a prescription medication, potassium is usually measured according to milliequivalents (mEq) or millimoles (mmol) rather than as milligrams (mg). To convert mg of elemental potassium to mEq, take mg and divide it by 39.0983 (atomic weight of potassium). For example, 90 mg is equivalent to 2.30 mEq, and 99 mg is equivalent to 2.53 mEq. Conversely, if you know the mEq, multiply by 39.0983 to find the elemental potassium weight in mg. For example, 2 mEq is equal to 78.0 mg. A typical therapeutic dosage of potassium is between 10 and 20 mEq, three to four times daily; professional supervision is recommended.

Toxic: Daily intakes exceeding 17 g, difficult to obtain from oral supplements, would be required to produce potassium toxicity. Hyperkalemia from oral administration is virtually unknown in individuals with normal renal function. Thus, the U.S. FNB noted that in "otherwise healthy individuals (i.e., individuals without impaired urinary potassium excretion from a medical condition or drug therapy), there is no evidence that a high level of potassium from foods has adverse effects," and concluded that "a Tolerable Upper Intake Level (UL) for potassium from foods is not set for healthy adults."[6]

Pediatric (<18 Years)

Dietary: As of 2004, official U.S. recommendations for AI were established for the first time[6]:

Children, 1 to 3 years: 3000 mg (77 mEq)/day
Children, 4 to 8 years: 3800 mg (97 mEq)/day
Children, 9 to 13 years: 4500 mg (115 mEq)/day
Children, 14 to 18 years: 4700 mg (120 mEq)/day

Supplemental/Maintenance: Usually not recommended for children under 12 years of age with healthy, balanced diet.
Pharmacological/Therapeutic: Not established.
Toxic: Not established.

Laboratory Values

The accuracy of laboratory assessment of potassium status is severely limited because most potassium in the human body is within cells. Consequently, measuring levels of free potassium in the serum will only detect deficiency in extreme depletion states. Measurement of potassium levels in red blood cells (RBCs), white blood cells (WBCs), or other intracellular tissues can provide a more accurate index of tissue potassium stores and thus reveal potassium insufficiency more readily.

Serum Potassium (K⁺)

Normal levels are 3.5 to 5.0 mmol/L. (To convert mg of elemental potassium to mEq, take mg and divide it by 39.0983 [atomic weight of potassium].) Low serum potassium levels may reflect a shift to intracellular space or to depletion from the total body stores. Hyperkalemia is indicated by an increase in the serum potassium concentration above 5.5 mEq/L (plasma potassium >5.0).

Urinary Potassium (24 Hour)

Normal levels are 26 to 123 mmol/day.

Ranges depend on dietary intake. Because potassium excretion in the urine varies with intake and concentrations are affected by fluid intake, 24-hour measurement of urinary potassium provides a more consistent value.

Erythrocyte Potassium

Normal levels are approximately 100 mmol/L RBCs. This test most accurately reflects tissue stores.

Note: *Pseudohyperkalemia* is defined as a difference between serum and plasma potassium greater than 0.4 mmol/L. Cases have been reported in which potassium is released from platelets, WBCs, or RBCs into the serum as blood clots, giving a falsely high value. This has occurred in polycythemia rubra vera, other myeloproliferative disorders with a high hematocrit or high platelet count, release of potassium from platelets during coagulation, RBC hemolysis during or after collection, and a protracted interval between blood sampling and separation of serum. Such misleading findings can be avoided, and a more accurate estimation obtained, by use of plasma instead of serum.[7]

SAFETY PROFILE
Overview

At moderate or high dosage levels, potassium salts taken orally can cause symptoms of nausea, vomiting, abdominal discomfort, diarrhea, and ulcers. A single dose of several hundred milligrams in tablet form can produce gastric irritation, especially when ingested on an empty stomach, with potassium chloride particularly well known for adverse effects, even in liquid forms. Microencapsulated forms are generally better tolerated. In contrast, modified-release preparations (e.g., potassium chloride with enteric coating) have been associated with GI ulceration. Adverse effects can usually be prevented or reduced by taking potassium with meals. Potassium in dietary forms, at any intake level, is generally not associated with adverse effects, except that occasionally, ingestion of potassium-rich fruit has been reported to produce hyperkalemia in the context of potassium-sparing diuretics and ACE inhibitor medications. Most adverse effects associated with potassium result from depletion and deficiency. Chronic renal insufficiency requires dietary restriction of potassium (and magnesium) with careful monitoring of blood levels.

Nutrient Adverse Effects

Gastrointestinal (GI) symptoms constitute the most common adverse effects associated with nondietary potassium intake, with nausea, vomiting, abdominal discomfort, and diarrhea quite common and ulceration less frequent. When indicated, high-potency potassium chloride tablets should only be administered in a slow-release form (e.g., Slow K), to minimize the risk of GI distress or bleeding ulcers often attributable to the high amounts of chloride in the tablets.

The most serious adverse reaction to potassium is hyperkalemia. Abnormally elevated serum potassium concentrations [K$^+$] occur when potassium intake exceeds the capacity of renal elimination. The accumulation of excess potassium can occur with decreased urinary potassium excretion due to acute or chronic renal failure, hypoaldosteronism, or the use of potassium-sparing diuretics, ACE inhibitors, or other drugs. More acutely, a shift of intracellular potassium into the circulation, most often resulting from hemolysis or sudden tissue damage, can also cause hyperkalemia. Thus, hyperkalemia is almost always caused by metabolic derangement due to pathophysiology (especially compromised kidney function) or medications that interfere with metabolic feedback systems; close monitoring is always appropriate when treating such patients.

A toxic reaction with severe hyperkalemia could potentially result from rapid ingestion of oral doses greater than 17 g (434 mEq) by individuals not acclimated to high intake, even with normal renal function.[6] Ingestion of a dose this size would be difficult and unlikely to occur unintentionally.

Potassium is generally considered to be neither a mutagen nor a carcinogen in standard forms at typical doses.

Adverse Effects Among Specific Populations

Individuals with compromised renal function, especially chronic renal failure, are at greatest risk for complications.

Pregnancy and Nursing

Specific data on potassium administration or supplementation in pregnancy and nursing are lacking. However, typical supplemental dosage levels are at or below recommended dietary intake levels or doses from typical intake of many common (and healthful) foods.

Infants and Children

Specific data on potassium administration or supplementation in infants and children are lacking. However, typical supplemental dosage levels would be at or below recommended dietary intake levels or doses from typical intake of many common (and healthful) foods.

Contraindications

Limited risk with food-level doses, but excessive doses should be avoided outside professional supervision and close monitoring: Addison's disease; compromised renal function, especially chronic renal failure; heart block; peptic ulcer; GI ulceration or obstruction; acute dehydration; severe burns.

Precautions and Warnings

Concurrent medications that alter potassium metabolism or interfere with potassium regulation, except with supervision and monitoring, including amiloride, spironolactone, triamterene, or other potassium-sparing diuretics, and ACE inhibitors such as captopril, enalapril, or lisinopril. Note that in such cases, consumption of foods providing potassium at recommended level (4.5-4.7 g/day) may develop excessive potassium levels. Caution also warranted in individuals undergoing trimethoprim-sulfamethoxazole therapy.

The 2004 recommendations from the U.S. FNB state: "Overall, because of the concern for hyperkalemia and resultant arrhythmias that might be life-threatening, the proposed AI [Adequate Intake: 4700 mg per day for adults] should not be applied to individuals with chronic kidney disease, heart failure, or type 1 diabetes, especially those who concomitantly use ACE inhibitor therapy. Among otherwise healthy individuals with hypertension on ACE inhibitor therapy, the AI should apply as long as renal function is unimpaired."[6]

INTERACTIONS REVIEW
Strategic Considerations

A cursory review of standard information on the therapeutic applications, effects and risks, interactions, and depletion patterns associated with potassium typically focuses on hypertension, diabetes, and renal disease, or frank hypokalemia/hyperkalemia, often to the exclusion of the diverse effects of numerous medications on the key physiological functions of potassium and its many clinical applications. A deeper and broader review of the scientific literature looking at therapeutic applications beyond mere "supplementation" reveals both subtle and profound, gradual and rapid, obvious and complex effects of potassium insufficiency, deficiency, or excess, even when not necessarily at the threshold of hypokalemia or hyperkalemia. Health care professionals applying the information available through such an integrative analysis can discover many opportunities for enriching their therapeutic repertoire and enhancing clinical outcomes while avoiding or carefully navigating some of the more problematic encounters between potassium and various drugs, particularly in the context of treating patients with chronic disease or metabolic maladaption.

Potassium is one of the primary mineral nutrients, which, along with magnesium, are the most susceptible to drug-induced depletion. Such depletion patterns, particularly in early stages, are typically difficult to detect at the intracellular level, where hypokalemia can be most significant, especially for normal cardiac muscle and electrical activity. Potassium-wasting diuretics, particularly the thiazide and loop diuretics, represent the most widely recognized examples of medications that inherently increase risks of potassium depletion and hypokalemia. However, long-term, repeated, and high-dose use of numerous pharmaceutical agents, such as beta-2-adrenoceptor agonists, colchicine, amphotericin B, and laxatives or stool softeners, can impair potassium absorption, deplete potassium, and interfere with its physiological activity. Hypokalemia resulting from these drugs, particularly in combination with steroids or digoxin, may contribute to edema, acute cardiac rhythm irregularities, aggravation of asthma, or other adverse responses. Compensatory increase in potassium intake can usually, but not always, prevent or correct drug-induced adverse effects, and sometimes the corrective remedy is simply regular intake of several pieces of potassium-rich fruit. However, in situations such as cyclosporine-induced nephrotoxicity and hyperkalemia, adverse effects can be either rapid or gradual in onset, and attempts at mitigating drug toxicity through nutrient support can be of limited effectiveness. Likewise, the risks accompanying diuretic therapy or renal impairment can become unpredictable and complex, especially when interacting with agents such as digoxin, which can intrinsically impair potassium function; digoxin toxicity increases with hypokalemia, and digoxin overdose can cause hyperkalemia. In this case, as in many others, the intimate relationship between potassium and magnesium (as well as other key nutrients) reveals itself in physiology, therapeutics, interactions, and parallel depletion patterns and demonstrates the need for a comprehensive risk assessment and nutrient support strategy. As with many drug-induced depletion patterns, evidence of benefit from nutrient coadministration is often present in clinical practice but lacking in the scientific literature. Close monitoring is imperative in patients with intertwined pathologies, multiple medications, and comorbidities such as renal impairment, cardiac conditions, organ allografts, or other complicating factors.

Serum/plasma concentrations indicate critical deficiency or excess and disequilibrium or dysregulation, but potassium depletion at the intracellular level is difficult to detect with conventional laboratory assessment of blood constituents. Increasing potassium intake with potassium-rich foods, salt substitutes, and supplements is generally indicated and effective, although increased vigilance is necessary in the setting of compromised renal function or other medications altering potassium status.

Mineral wasting caused by renal tubular damage occurs in patients being treated with cisplatin or aminoglycosides, particularly in elderly and compromised populations, and hypokalemia often results. potassium depletion can further potentiate renal insufficiency or failure in such cases. Concurrent potassium therapy may prevent or correct adverse effects with long-term or repeated drug therapy, but evidence is limited. With cisplatin, however, refractory hypokalemia may require concomitant administration of both potassium and magnesium, possibly because of the magnesium dependence of the Na^+,K^+-ATPase membrane "pump" enzyme. Some agents, such as carbonic anhydrase inhibitors, can decrease renal blood flow and glomerular filtration rate. However, other than furosemide and acetazolamide, these may not adversely impact potassium status in most individuals. Nevertheless, given the potential for significant disequilibrium in carbon dioxide and bicarbonate transport, risks may be significantly elevated in certain individuals.

Hypokalemia, whether from disease, drugs, or physiological degeneration, can increase risks associated with many pharmaceutical agents that require stable levels of potassium and other key nutrients. For example, hypokalemia of various origins can significantly increase risk of acute cardiac rhythm irregularities and adverse reactions to quinidine and other antiarrhythmic drugs, especially when accompanied by hypomagnesemia.

Certain medications lead to increased potassium levels and potential for hyperkalemia, with the attendant risk of severe adverse events, sometimes acute, often chronic. Notably, hyperkalemia was virtually unknown except in renal failure until introduction of several drug classes in recent years. This rapid escalation of occurrence of hyperkalemia represents a major challenge in the chronic care of patients with multiple intertwined and complex patterns of dysfunction and disease, debilitation, and comedication.

In the context of certain medical conditions and comedications, some drugs can create or aggravate a risk of hyperkalemia and the potential for sudden onset of severe symptoms. Amiloride or other potassium-sparing diuretics carry an implicit risk of hyperkalemia when combined with a significant increase in potassium intake, especially with compromised renal function and concomitant ACE inhibitor therapy. Likewise, beta-adrenergic blockers can also elevate potassium levels and cause hyperkalemia through uncertain and often unpredictable mechanisms. Similarly, losartan and other angiotensin II receptor antagonists inherently carry a risk of hyperkalemia.

In these cases, potassium intake needs to be limited and patients educated as to the various sources (and relative dosages) of potassium. Some medications, such as trimethoprim, alone or in combination with sulfamethoxazole, can elevate potassium levels and may occasionally cause hyperkalemia, usually through effects on renal function; although uncommon and often reversible, severe adverse effects can be acute, and

renal failure is possible. High-risk patients, such as those with compromised physiological function, with human immunodeficiency virus (HIV) infection, or receiving polypharmacy affecting renal function, should always be monitored closely. Perhaps more importantly than any absolute prohibition, patients need to avoid rapid or significantly increased potassium intake (e.g., new use of salt substitute) outside professional supervision.

As a mineral, potassium has variable risk for pharamacokinetic interference in which binding between the drug and potassium impairs bioavailability and decreases therapeutic effect of both agents. Risks of clinically significant adverse effects are generally minimized by separating oral intake by several hours.

In a few cases, administration of potassium is relatively contraindicated in patients with specific pathological conditions or being treated with specific medications. Nevertheless, such contraindication is often cautionary, and coadministration of these agents is safe, or even beneficial in certain patients, but requires regular monitoring and close supervision by health care professionals trained and experienced in the various modalities and their integrative application.

NUTRIENT-DRUG INTERACTIONS

Albuterol/Salbutamol, Rimiterol, and Related Beta-2-Adrenoceptor Agonists

Evidence: Intramuscular (IM), intravenous (IV), and subcutaneous (SC) forms: Albuterol (salbutamol), rimiterol (Pulmadil).

Extrapolated, based on similar properties: IM, IV, and SC forms: Fenoterol (Berotec), isetharine (Arm-A-Med, Bronkosol, Bronkometer), pirbuterol (Exirel), salmeterol, tulobuterol (Brelomax).

Similar properties but evidence indicating no or reduced interaction effects: Inhalation forms: Albuterol (Albuterol Inhaled, Proventil, Ventolin); combination drug: albuterol and ipratropium bromide (Combivent); isoproterenol (isoprenaline; Isuprel, Medihaler-Iso), levalbuterol (Xopenex), metaproterenol (Alupent), salmeterol (Serevent, combination drug: Advair), terbutaline (Brethaire, Brethine, Bricanyl).

See also Ephedrine and Theophylline sections.

Interaction Type and Significance

≈≈ **Drug-Induced Nutrient Depletion, Supplementation Therapeutic, with Professional Management**

☼ **Prevention or Reduction of Drug Adverse Effect**

Probability:	EvidenceBase:
3. Possible	◉ **Emerging**

Effect and Mechanism of Action

Albuterol, administered by IM, IV, and SC routes, is associated with decreased levels of serum/plasma potassium, as well as of calcium, magnesium, and phosphate.[8]

Research

In an experiment investigating nontherapeutic metabolic and cardiovascular effects of therapeutic doses of beta-2-adrenoceptor agonists, Phillips et al.[9] administered IV infusions of salbutamol (albuterol) and rimiterol to four healthy male subjects. In response to "equivalent molar amounts of salbutamol and rimiterol," they observed "dose-related decreases in plasma potassium, phosphate and corticosteroids" as well as "significant" hypocalcemia, hypomagnesemia, hyperlactatemia, and ketonemia and dose-related increases in plasma glucose, renin activity, serum insulin, and heart rate. They noted that with either drug, "special care is required for patients who may have abnormal glucose tolerance, potassium depletion, or be predisposed to lactic acidosis," and suggested that rimiterol "may be preferable for infusion because of its short plasma half-life."[9] Spector[8] reported that "beta adrenergic agonists can lower serum potassium levels predominantly when they are administered by the parenteral route." In particular he noted that dose-related hypokalemia has been demonstrated with albuterol given by the IM, IV, and SC routes, as well as with SC epinephrine. He further cautioned that comedication with agents such as corticosteroids, theophylline, diuretics, and digoxin could exacerbate potassium status and recommended further research into the "hypokalemic effect of all forms of beta agonists in view of their possible contribution toward arrhythmias and asthma deaths."[8] Subsequently, in a study of the effects of oral albuterol on serum and skeletal levels of digoxin in four healthy subjects, Edner and Jogestrand[10] observed a parallel reduction in the serum potassium concentration (0.58 mmol/L) and serum digoxin concentration, compared with control measurements.

Nutritional Therapeutics, Clinical Concerns, and Adaptations

The possibility of adverse effects on potassium status from albuterol, rimiterol, or related beta-2-adrenergic bronchodilators has been consistently demonstrated, but evidence is lacking as to the frequency of this effect or the efficacy of interventions to prevent or diminish it. The observed adverse effects on potassium levels are less likely to occur with use of albuterol via oral inhalation, the most common form of administration, particularly with occasional application in acute episodes. Clinical trials are warranted to determine the clinical significance of these effects of albuterol on potassium status and whether supportive coadministration of potassium and other minerals is safe and efficacious, as well as the comparative effects of food versus supplemental/prescribed sources. Pending substantive research findings, physicians prescribing albuterol, particularly those administering it parenterally, are advised to monitor potassium levels and consider potassium coadministration if indicated by direct findings or other factors associated with increased risk.

Amiloride

Amiloride (Midamor)
Combination drug: Amiloride and hydrochlorothiazide (Moduretic).
See also Spironolactone and Triamterene.

Interaction Type and Significance

✗✗   **Minimal to Mild Adverse Interaction—Vigilance Necessary**

✗✗✗   **Potentially Harmful or Serious Adverse Interaction—Avoid**

◇◇   **Drug-Induced Effect on Nutrient Function, Supplementation Contraindicated, Professional Management Appropriate**

Probability:	Evidence Base:
2. **Probable** or	● **Consensus**
1. **Certain**	

Effect and Mechanism of Action

Amiloride hydrochloride is an antikaliuretic-diuretic agent, which as a pyrazine-carbonyl-guanidine is unrelated chemically to other diuretics, including potassium-sparing agents. Because of its intended action of reducing urinary excretion of potassium, amiloride can produce a state of inappropriately elevated potassium levels, especially with concomitant angiotensin-converting enzyme (ACE) inhibitor therapy.[11,12] Further, exogenous sources of potassium, including potassium-rich foods such as fruit or food seasoning containing potassium chloride, can contribute to potassium accumulation in the presence of amiloride. Except for hyperkalemia (serum potassium levels >5.5 mEq/L), amiloride is generally thought to be well tolerated, and reports of significant adverse effects are infrequent.

Research and Reports

Published research is lacking, and case reports of hyperkalemia are generally uncirculated because this interaction is considered axiomatic, and coadministration is always accompanied by cautions of inherent risk.

Note: As a result of its potassium-sparing activity, amiloride is often prescribed in conjunction with medications, such as thiazides and amphotericin B, that cause electrolyte disturbances, especially potassium wasting, to mitigate these potentially dangerous adverse effects. These patterns of compensatory coadministration are discussed in the context of the respective medication(s) involved.

Clinical Implications and Adaptations

Amiloride is often prescribed because of demonstrated hypokalemia, but the risk of hyperkalemia warrants frequent monitoring when an ACE inhibitor and amiloride are administered concomitantly. Patient education is critical because potassium-rich foods are generally considered desirable for individuals wanting to enhance their cardiovascular health, and salt substitutes may be misconstrued as appropriate. Thus, despite good intentions, consuming even several pieces of fruit per day can be problematic for some individuals in the context of potassium-sparing agents such as amiloride. Regular monitoring and highly specific and practical dietary counseling are essential, with patients having even mildly compromised renal function at greatest risk.

Aminoglycoside Antibiotics, Including Gentamicin, Neomycin, and Tobramycin

Amikacin (Amikin), gentamicin (G-mycin, Garamycin, Jenamicin), kanamycin (Kantrex), neomycin (Mycifradin, Myciguent, Neo-Fradin, NeoTab, Nivemycin), netilmicin (Netromycin), paromomycin (monomycin; Humatin), streptomycin, tobramycin (AKTob, Nebcin, TOBI, TOBI Solution, TobraDex, Tobrex).

Interaction Type and Significance

≈≈   **Drug-Induced Nutrient Depletion, Supplementation Therapeutic, with Professional Management**

☼   **Prevention or Reduction of Drug Adverse Effect**

Probability:	Evidence Base:
2. **Probable**	● **Consensus**

Effect and Mechanism of Action

Hypokalemia, as well as hypocalcemia, hypomagnesemia, and alkalosis, is a predictable outcome of renal tubular damage from aminoglycosides. Moreover, gentamicin-induced renal failure is potentiated by potassium depletion. Potassium administration may reduce the sequelae of aminoglycoside-induced hypokalemia but introduces significant risks in at-risk patient populations.

Research and Reports

Renal tubular damage is a well-established toxic effect of aminoglycosides, such as gentamicin, which has been demonstrated in animal studies and described in case reports. Clinically significant depletion of potassium (and magnesium) or other metabolic disturbances are assumed to be uncommon complications but are more likely to occur in elderly patients administered large doses over extended periods.[13-17] Findings from clinical trials specifically investigating coadministration of potassium, alone or with synergistic nutrients, in the prevention or treatment of aminoglycoside toxicity are lacking in the published literature.

Nutritional Therapeutics, Clinical Concerns, and Adaptations

Physicians prescribing aminoglycosides on a chronic or repeated basis are advised to monitor closely for depletion of potassium and magnesium and other metabolic disturbances resulting from renal tubular damage and to consider prophylactic or compensatory nutritional support for such individuals. Serum creatinine, blood urea nitrogen (BUN), and creatinine clearance should be measured before initiating therapy and should be monitored throughout treatment, along with serum potassium and magnesium levels. Only after such assessment should increased intake of potassium (from dietary or supplemental sources) be undertaken, and then only under close supervision.

Enhancing potassium levels in response to potential compromise by aminoglycosides may be necessary and appropriate but needs to be approached with caution and care. Potassium levels can most easily be increased through consumption of several pieces of fruit each day. Slow-K, Micro-K, and K-dur are typical examples of the potassium preparations prescribed by physicians. However, increasing potassium intake by any means is usually contraindicated and often dangerous in patients with reduced kidney function, especially those on dialysis. Magnesium may also be appropriate for its general role in cardiovascular health; its tendency to be depleted by aminoglycosides, other drugs, and their adverse effects; and its role in maintaining intracellular potassium. Similar precautions regarding renal function apply to magnesium as well as potassium.

Amphotericin B (AMB; Fungizone)

Amphotericin B (AMB; Fungizone)
Similar properties but evidence indicating no or reduced interaction effects: Liposomal amphotericin, injection (AmBisome, Fungisome).

Interaction Type and Significance

≈ ≈   **Drug-Induced Nutrient Depletion, Supplementation Therapeutic, with Professional Management**

☼   **Prevention or Reduction of Drug Adverse Effect**

Probability: Evidence Base:
2. Probable   ◉ **Emerging**

Effect and Mechanism of Action

Amphotericin B is a macrocyclic antifungal agent, similar in structure to nystatin, administered both systemically and topically for fungal infections. Amphotericin B is well known for inducing electrolyte disturbances. In particular, hypokalemia and potassium depletion (as well as magnesium wasting) are frequent complications of amphotericin B therapy, especially when combined with oral corticosteroids.[18,19] Moreover, potassium depletion appears to potentiate amphotericin B–induced toxicity to renal tubules.[20]

Hyperkalemia from rapid infusion or high doses in renally compromised patients is also possible, with attendant risks and adverse effects.

Research

Early research demonstrated reversible concentration-dependent loss of intracellular potassium in vitro and hyperkalemic ventricular arrhythmias in dogs.[21-26] Craven and Gremillion[27] reported two episodes of ventricular fibrillation with progressive hyperkalemia (up to 8-8.4 mEq/L) in an anuric patient during rapid infusion of high-dose amphotericin B (1.4 mg/kg over 45 minutes). They subsequently conducted animal experiments investigating risk factors of ventricular fibrillation during rapid amphotericin B infusion. First, they noted that prolonged infusion (≥3 hours) and concurrent hemodialysis "each prevented the development of hyperkalemia and ventricular arrhythmia." Thus, in trials involving two anuric patients receiving 4-hour infusions of amphotericin B during dialysis (0.7 and 1.0 mg/kg), they observed that peak amphotericin B concentrations in serum were lower and that serum potassium levels were maintained in the normal range. Likewise, in eight patients with normal renal function who received lower doses (0.7 ± 0.2 mg/kg) over 45 minutes, peak concentrations of amphotericin B in serum were also lower, with only slight increases in the serum potassium level. The authors thus recommended that "rapid infusion of amphotericin B not be used in patients with impaired potassium excretion unless accompanied by hemodialysis and careful potassium monitoring."[27]

Findings from a rodent study conducted by Bernardo et al.[20] suggest that "potassium depletion does not influence the acute renovascular effects of amphotericin B but potentiates its [renal] tubular toxicity."

Although substantive evidence is minimal, in some cases amiloride is combined with amphotericin B to prevent or mitigate the adverse effects of amphotericin B–induced hypokalemia and hypomagnesemia, especially in patients at high risk for complications resulting from these electrolyte disorders.[28] Other potassium-sparing agents might provide similar activity, but research is lacking.

Limited clinical research indicates the importance of regulating potassium, preventively or in response to observed hypokalemia, using amiloride and potassium coadministration. In a randomized clinical trial involving 20 neutropenic patients with various hematological disorders, Smith et al.[29] compared the prophylactic use of oral amiloride, 5 mg twice daily, concomitantly with IV amphotericin B (vs. amphotericin B alone) and demonstrated a decrease in potassium wasting. "Patients receiving amiloride had a significantly higher plasma potassium (p <.01), a significantly lower urinary potassium loss (p <.01), and required significantly less potassium chloride supplementation to maintain their plasma potassium within the normal range."[29] Subsequently, Bearden and Muncey[30] investigated the effect of amiloride (5-10 mg twice daily for 14.7 ± 12.6 days) in 19 oncology patients exhibiting marked electrolyte wasting from amphotericin B at 0.67 ± 0.30 mg/kg for a mean of 21.9 days (range, 7-57 days). They found that mean serum potassium concentrations increased in the 5 days before and after administration and reported a trend toward decreased potassium supplementation. Notably, these researchers adopted a more conservative approach than that of Smith et al.,[29] in that "amiloride was added to amphotericin B treatment only when patients began to exhibit excessive potassium requirements." Nevertheless, they concluded: "Early utilization of amiloride may be considered in patients with underlying risk factors for hypokalaemia (i.e., leukaemia, cisplatin use, diuretics) in whom a prolonged course of amphotericin is anticipated.... This retrospective study suggests that amiloride may benefit patients by decreasing total potassium requirements and supplementation, as well as increasing serum potassium concentrations." They also cautioned that the "addition of another medication to a patient population receiving multidrug therapy is not recommended in all instances, and should be considered on a case-by-case basis."[30]

Pasic et al.[31] studied the safety and efficacy of liposomal amphotericin B (mean daily dose, 5 mg/kg; 2-6 mg/kg) in 15 pediatric patients receiving bone marrow transplants for primary immunodeficiency (PID). Of these, four developed mild hypokalemia, which resolved with increased potassium administration.

Reports

Hypokalemia is a frequently reported adverse effect of amphotericin B therapy, but hypokalemia-associated rhabdomyolysis tends to be a rare occurrence. Da Silva et al.[32] reported on a 10-year-old boy with hypokalemic rhabdomyolysis in the lower extremities after 1 week of amphotericin B therapy. Initial laboratory tests revealed a "serum potassium of 1.7 mEq/L and a serum creatinine phosphokinase of 3937 U/L plus myoglobulinuria." The patient "progressed to achieve full regression of muscular weakness after one week" after fluid expansion and IV potassium replacement.

Nutritional Therapeutics, Clinical Concerns, and Adaptations

Physicians administering amphotericin B, whether in standard or liposomal form, are advised to be watchful for electrolyte disturbances, particularly depletion of potassium and magnesium. Such events are common and can be predicted in many patients, especially with extended or repeated amphotericin therapy. Amphotericin is almost always administered in inpatient hospital settings. Careful and frequent monitoring of serum electrolytes is required in all patients. Coadministration of potassium and possibly magnesium as a preventive, or at least reactive, measure is fundamental to comprehensive and judicious care, particularly in patients at high risk for potassium depletion. Amiloride is sometimes coadministered during amphotericin B therapy to decrease potassium wasting and can be considered a therapeutic option. It is noteworthy that amphotericin-induced potassium depletion can cause serious complications through its secondary effects on other medication, such as a potential increase in digitalis toxicity.

Angiotensin-Converting Enzyme (ACE) Inhibitors

Benazepril (Lotensin); combination drug: benazepril and amlodipine (Lotrel); captopril (Capoten); combination drug: captopril and hydrochlorothiazide (Acezide, Capto-Co, Captozide, Co-Zidocapt); cilazapril (Inhibace), enalapril (Vasotec); enalapril combination drugs: enalapril and felodipine (Lexxel); enalapril and hydrochlorothiazide (Vaseretic); fosinopril (Monopril), lisinopril (Prinivil, Zestril); combination drug: lisinopril and hydrochlorothiazide (Prinzide, Zestoretic); moexipril (Univasc), perindopril (Aceon), quinapril (Accupril), ramipril (Altace), trandolapril (Mavik).

Interaction Type and Significance

✗ ✗   Minimal to Mild Adverse Interaction—Vigilance Necessary

✗ ✗ ✗   Potentially Harmful or Serious Adverse Interaction—Avoid

◇ ◇   Drug-Induced Effect on Nutrient Function, Supplementation Contraindicated, Professional Management Appropriate

Probability: Evidence Base:
2. Probable   ● Consensus

Effect and Mechanism of Action

The ACE inhibitors can increase serum levels of potassium in certain individuals, particularly those with diabetes or compromised renal function.[33-35] The increased levels of intracellular potassium and magnesium associated with ACE inhibitor therapy may be an important mechanism by which ACE inhibitors reduce arrhythmias.[36-38] Some ACE inhibitors, such as enalapril, can significantly inhibit plasma aldosterone concentration and urinary excretion of aldosterone.[39] In general, these effects appear to be similar for long-acting ACE inhibitors such as enalapril and short-acting ACE inhibitors such as captopril.

The concomitant use of potassium with an ACE inhibitor drug increases the risk of hyperkalemia, especially with rapid introduction.[12] Potassium levels may become further elevated with simultaneous use of potassium-sparing diuretics, potassium-based salt substitutes, very-low-calorie diets, and NSAIDs (which reduce renal excretion of ACE inhibitors).[40-42] All these risks are amplified in the context of renal insufficiency.

Research

The concomitant use of ACE inhibitor and potassium-sparing diuretic therapy is a contraindication rather than a potassium interaction; in such cases, both potassium and potassium-sparing medications should be avoided. For example, Burnakis and Mioduch[43] noted the significant risk of hyperkalemia in patients receiving combined therapy with captopril and potassium. Chiu et al.[12] conducted a retrospective chart review of five patients, all with diabetes and older than 50, who were seen for hyperkalemia in emergency care after having amiloride HCl/hydrochlorothiazide added to an ACE inhibitor drug regimen 8 to 18 days before presenting. They stated that these findings "highlight the dangers of a precipitous rise in serum potassium levels in patients at risk for renal insufficiency, already receiving an angiotensin-converting enzyme (ACE) inhibitor, who are given a potassium-sparing diuretic."

Ohya et al.[39] administered enalapril (5 mg once daily) and captopril (12.5 mg three times daily) to 11 patients with mild essential hypertension and normal renal function for 1 week each in a crossover design, to compare effects of long-acting (enalapril) and short-acting (captopril) ACE inhibitors on serum electrolytes and circadian rhythm of urinary electrolyte excretion in relation to aldosterone status. Both agents "significantly decreased urinary K excretion" while "not significantly alter[ing] serum K level." Notably, the amplitude of urinary K excretion was decreased by both drugs, although the circadian rhythm (acrophase) was not affected by either drug. Both enalapril and captopril "significantly reduced blood pressure" (to a similar degree) while enalapril, but not captopril, "significantly inhibited plasma aldosterone concentration and urinary aldosterone excretion." Thus, although the primary finding of this trial was that "enalapril caused more sustained inhibition of aldosterone secretion" than captopril, they also noted that "both drugs showed similar effects on the K homeostasis in patients with mild essential hypertension."[39]

Nevertheless, the effects of ACE inhibitor therapy on potassium and magnesium may play an important role in their therapeutic effect. O'Keeffe et al.[36] investigated the effect of captopril therapy on lymphocyte potassium and magnesium concentrations in patients with congestive heart failure (CHF). They compared lymphocyte potassium and magnesium in 18 patients taking furosemide and potassium for CHF before and 3 months after the introduction of captopril to 32 healthy controls. Nine of the treatment subjects exhibited decreased baseline lymphocyte magnesium and potassium concentrations, despite similar plasma electrolyte levels. Notably, there was a "significant increase in both lymphocyte potassium and magnesium levels" after 3 months' treatment with captopril and furosemide in these patients. Furthermore, nine patients "who had been taking a potassium-sparing combination diuretic also had an increase in lymphocyte magnesium" after the introduction of captopril. These authors concluded that "increased intracellular potassium and magnesium may be one mechanism whereby [ACE] inhibitors reduced arrhythmias and improve survival" in CHF patients.[36] In contrast, however, some of these same researchers subsequently examined the effect of 6 months' captopril (or nifedipine) therapy on lymphocyte magnesium and potassium levels in 28 patients treated for hypertension. They observed "no difference in serum or lymphocyte concentrations in the two groups compared to 45 healthy, normotensive controls."[37]

Overall, as summarized by Shionoiri[41] in a review of pharmacokinetic drug interactions involving ACE inhibitors (1993): "When ACE inhibitors are given, hyperkalaemia may occur in patients with renal insufficiency, those taking potassium supplements or potassium-sparing diuretics, and in diabetic patients with mild renal impairment."

Reports

Numerous case reports have been published describing hyperkalemia in patients undergoing ACE inhibitor therapy.[35,44-46] Stoltz and Andrews[40] described severe hyperkalemia during very-low-calorie diets and ACE inhibitor use. Ray et al.[42] reported two cases of severe hyperkalemia resulting from the concomitant use of salt substitutes (KCl) in hypertensive patients taking ACE inhibitors, in what they warned was "a potentially life threatening interaction." Serum potassium stabilized in the normal range after cessation of the salt substitute in each case. The authors concluded that "without vigilance the contribution of the salt substitute to hyperkalaemia would have been overlooked and an ACE inhibitor erroneously withdrawn."[42]

Clinical Implications and Adaptations

Health care professionals treating patients taking an ACE inhibitor are strongly encouraged to counsel these individuals to avoid unsupervised increases in potassium intake, in the form of supplements but also as high-potassium foods (e.g., fruit) or salt substitutes, on the basis of the increased risk for problematic reactions. A clinically significant increase in blood potassium levels represents an uncommon yet potentially serious adverse effect associated with ACE inhibitors. The importance of frank inquiry and detailed inventory of concomitant (or even occasional) medications, diet, nutrients and herbs cannot be overemphasized. Close supervision and regular monitoring are essential, particularly in individuals with compromised renal function. The prescription of potassium chloride or potassium-sparing medications is generally contraindicated during ACE inhibitor therapy.

Beta-Adrenoceptor Antagonists (Beta-Adrenergic Blocking Agents)

Evidence: **Nonselective agents (oral systemic forms):** Alprenolol, carteolol (Cartrol), levobunolol (AKBeta, Betagan),

mepindolol, metipranolol (OptiPranolol), nadolol (Corgard), oxprenolol (Trasicor), penbutolol (Levatol), pindolol (Visken), propranolol (Betachron, Inderal LA, Innopran XL, Inderal); combination drug: propranolol and bendrofluazide (Inderex); sotalol (Betapace, Betapace AF, Sorine); timolol (Blocadren).

Similar properties but evidence indicating no or reduced interaction effects:

Beta-1-selective agents: Acebutolol (Sectral), atenolol (Tenormin); combination drugs: atenolol and chlortalidone (Co-Tendione, Tenoretic); atenolol and nifedipine (Beta-Adalat, Tenif); betaxolol (Kerlone), bisoprolol (Zebeta); combination drug: bisoprolol and hydrochlorothiazide (Ziac); esmolol (Brevibloc), metoprolol (Lopressor), nebivolol (Nebilet).

Mixed alpha-1/beta-adrenergic antagonists: Carvedilol (Coreg), celiprolol, labetalol (Normodyne, Trandate).

Beta-2-selective agents: Butoxamine (weak alpha-adrenergic agonist activity).

Related but evidence against extrapolation: Beta-adrenergic blocking ophthalmic drops: Betaxolol (Betoptic), carteolol (Cartrol, Ocupress), levobunolol (AKBeta, Betagan), metipranolol (OptiPranolol), timolol (Timoptic).

Interaction Type and Significance

✗ ✗   **Minimal to Mild Adverse Interaction—Vigilance Necessary**

✗ ✗ ✗   **Potentially Harmful or Serious Adverse Interaction—Avoid**

Probability: Evidence Base:
2. Probable   ○ **Preliminary**

Effect and Mechanism of Action

Nonselective beta blockers inhibit both beta-1-adrenergic and beta-2-adrenergic receptors. Carvedilol, celiprolol, and labetalol exhibit mixed antagonism of both beta-adrenergic and alpha-1-adrenergic receptors.

In general, beta-adrenergic blockers can cause moderate increase in serum potassium concentrations and may lead to hyperkalemia. Beta-adrenergic blockade can enhance the rise and prolong the elevation in serum potassium without decreasing urinary potassium excretion.[47] "Beta-adrenergic mechanisms seem to be concerned in the extrarenal handling of the potassium-load," and beta blockade in humans can particularly impair extrarenal disposal of an acute potassium load.[47,48] This increase "cannot be explained by the retention of potassium in the organism, and is probably caused by the redistribution of potassium from intracellular to extracellular compartments." Further, the action inhibited by beta-blockade appears to function "presumably by inducing an increased uptake of potassium in muscular cells and liver cells" through beta-adrenergic mechanisms that are "probably of the beta 2-type."

Research

In contrast to beta-adrenergic agonists, which are often used to treat acute hyperkalemia, beta blockers can cause profound elevations of serum potassium. In an experiment involving nine healthy subjects, Rosa et al.[47] investigated the role of catecholamines in the regulation of potassium homeostasis by administering IV potassium chloride (0.5 mEq/kg) in the presence and absence of propranolol. The initial potassium infusion elevated serum potassium by 0.6 ± 0.09 mEq/L, and the addition of propranolol "augmented the rise (0.9 ± 0.05 mEq per liter) and prolonged the elevation in serum potassium without decreasing urinary potassium excretion." The authors concluded that "Beta-adrenergic blockade impairs ... extrarenal disposal of potassium load" and that such findings "suggest that in patients with impaired potassium disposal, the risk of hyperkalemia may be increased when sympathetic blockade is induced."[47]

In a review (1983) of the effect of adrenergic blockade on potassium concentrations in different conditions, Lundborg[48] cautioned that in theory "there are several conditions in which it is important to have a defence against hyperkalaemia from exogenous or endogenous sources, for example, during heavy physical exercise, after a potassium-rich meal, or after traumatic tissue damage." He concluded: "Available data indicate that non-selective beta-blockade increases serum potassium concentrations during and after heavy exercise and during coronary bypass."

Reports
Arthur and Greenberg[49] described the cases of three renal transplant recipients who "developed potentially life-threatening hyperkalemia" after IV administration of labetalol for post-operative hypertension.

Clinical Implications and Adaptations
Physicians prescribing beta-adrenergic blockers are advised to caution patients to avoid potassium in supplements, medications, and salt substitutes. Moreover, eating large servings of fruit rich in potassium, such as bananas, is generally contraindicated without prior discussion and ongoing monitoring. Nevertheless, enhanced potassium intake may be appropriate in certain patients comedicated with potassium-depleting diuretics or after an episode of vomiting or diarrhea. Close supervision and regular monitoring of potassium levels and other relevant clinical parameters are essential, especially with changes in medication regimens, diet, and intake of natural agents such as herbs or nutrients. Again, as noted by Lundborg,[48] the risk of hyperkalemia is increased after heavy physical exercise, a potassium-rich meal, or traumatic tissue damage, all of which may cause a rapid elevation in circulating potassium levels, which can be exacerbated in patients taking beta-blocker medications.

Carbenoxolone (CBX)

See Licorice in Herb-Nutrient Interactions.

Carbonic Anhydrase Inhibitors, Potassium Depleting

Evidence: Acetazolamide (Diamox), diclofenamide (dichlorphenamide; Daranide), dorzolamide (Trusopt); combination drug: dorzolamide and timolol (Cosopt); furosemide (BAN, frusemide, INN; Lasix), methazolamide (Glauctabs, Neptazane).
Similar properties but evidence lacking for extrapolation: Brinzolamide (Azopt), topiramate (Topamax), zonisamide (Zonegran).
See also Diuretics, Potassium Depleting.

Interaction Type and Significance

≈ ≈   **Drug-Induced Nutrient Depletion, Supplementation Therapeutic, with Professional Management**

Probability:
4. Plausible

Evidence Base:
▽ Mixed

Effect and Mechanism of Action
The enzyme carbonic anhydrase catalyzes the reversible reaction involving the hydration of carbon dioxide and the dehydration of carbonic acid with attendant potassium loss. Agents with diverse mechanisms act as carbonic anhydrase inhibitors in the treatment of a variety of conditions, most of which involve fluid regulation, including those involving intraocular pressure. For example, acetazolamide achieves alkalinization of the urine and promotion of diuresis through its action on this reversible hydration-dehydration reaction in the kidneys and resultant renal loss of bicarbonate (HCO_3^-), along with sodium, water, and potassium. In high doses, all carbonic anhydrase inhibitors cause some decrease in renal blood flow and glomerular filtration rate. In general, with the exception of specific agents such as furosemide (which is also a loop diuretic) and acetazolamide, methazolamide and most other drugs in this class tend to have a weak and transient diuretic effect and are not used as systemic diuretics.

Research
Clinical trials investigating the systemic effect of carbonic anhydrase inhibitors on potassium status are lacking. Although acetazolamide is used for its diuretic action in the treatment and prevention of high-altitude pulmonary edema, and furosemide is well known as a loop diuretic, most agents in this class are used in the treatment of ocular conditions such as glaucoma. Consequently, the limited available data indicate that in most cases the degree of potassium loss is unlikely to be of clinical significance, even with chronic administration, barring other dominant influences or confounding factors.

Nutritional Therapeutics, Clinical Concerns, and Adaptations
Physicians prescribing carbonic anhydrase inhibitors, with the significant exceptions of furosemide and acetazolamide for systemic cardiovascular conditions, can generally assume that adverse effects on potassium status are improbable in most patients not taking other potassium-depleting medications or otherwise compromised. As a cautionary suggestion, and for the benefit of overall nutritional status, health care professionals can reiterate support for the healthful practice of regularly consuming plentiful fresh fruits and vegetables and decreasing intake of salt (specifically sodium) and processed foods. Monitoring is important because excessive alkalinization of the urine and metabolic acidosis (resulting from decreases in plasma bicarbonate) may lead to a disequilibrium in carbon dioxide transport in the erythrocytes.

Cisplatin

Evidence: Cisplatin (*cis*-diaminedichloroplatinum, CDDP; Platinol, Platinol-AQ).
Similar properties but evidence indicating no or reduced interaction effects: Carboplatin (Paraplatin), oxaliplatin (Eloxatin).

Interaction Type and Significance

≈ ≈   **Drug-Induced Nutrient Depletion, Supplementation Therapeutic, with Professional Management**

⊕ ✗   **Bimodal or Variable Interaction, with Professional Management**

✗ ✗   **Minimal to Mild Adverse Interaction—Vigilance Necessary**

Probability:
1. Certain

Evidence Base:
 ◉ **Emerging** to
● **Consensus**

Effect and Mechanism of Action

Cisplatin can induce renal functional damage and cause chronic tubulopathy, characterized by magnesium and potassium wasting, reduced calcium excretion, metabolic alkalosis, and a strong tendency to hypomagnesemia and hypokalemia. In this common complication an unrecognized and untreated magnesium depletion can lead to a potassium depletion that is refractory to repletion with potassium alone.[50] The resulting hypokalemia can be corrected only with concomitant administration of magnesium with potassium.[51] Thus, this interaction demonstrates the critical role that magnesium plays in maintaining intracellular potassium.

Cisplatin and related chemotherapeutic agents cause renal toxicity to varying degrees. Coadministration of potassium, magnesium, or other nutrients adversely affected by these drugs is constrained by compromised urinary excretion and may be contraindicated in some patients with borderline renal function.

Research

Limited but consistent research findings parallel and confirm clinically based consensus regarding the effects of cisplatin in depleting potassium. Buckley et al.[52] documented hypomagnesemia in 66 patients receiving a five-drug combination chemotherapy regimen containing low-dose cisplatin. They observed that 38 (76%) of 50 patients receiving treatment every 4 weeks became hypomagnesemic during treatment, and that the incidence increased with the cumulative cisplatin dose, ranging from 41% after a single course to all patients receiving six cycles of therapy. Notably, patients receiving the combination at a longer interval (8 vs. 4 weeks) between cycles exhibited a lower incidence. The authors thus reported that the incidence and severity of hypomagnesemia was dose dependent. They also noted that the higher incidence of hypomagnesemia observed in this study might be related to an interaction of cisplatin with one or more of the drugs in the combined regimen.[52] Bianchetti et al.[53] studied renotubular handling of potassium, sodium, calcium, phosphate, hydrogen ions and glucose, and urinary concentrating ability in three children (age 8-11 years) with renal magnesium loss, persisting for longer than 2 years after discontinuation of cisplatin treatment for neuroblastoma, and compared these findings with group of healthy children serving as controls. Apart from renal magnesium wasting, there was a clear tendency toward reduced calciuria associated with normal or slightly elevated plasma calcium, and plasma potassium levels "tended to be low" (3.4-3.7 mmol/L). Plasma chloride was normal, and plasma "creatinine levels, glucosuria and phosphaturia, and urinary concentrating capacity were adequate." They noted that overall patterns in these children were similar to those observed in three children (age 4½-13 years) with primary renotubular hypomagnesemia-hypokalemia and hypocalciuria. Thus, the authors concluded that "cisplatin may induce renal functional damage identical to that found in primary renotubular hypomagnesaemia-hypokalaemia with hypocalciuria."[53]

Reports

Rodriguez et al.[50] described "two patients with hypomagnesemia-associated refractory hypokalemia following cisplatin therapy." They found that potassium administration failed to correct the potassium deficit and "profound hypokalemia persisted until hypomagnesemia was recognized and corrected" after the eleventh and ninth days, respectively. Based on these clinical experiences, the authors recommended that "both serum K ion and Mg levels should routinely be assessed in patients who require cisplatin therapy."

Nutritional Therapeutics, Clinical Concerns, and Adaptations

Physicians administering cisplatin will want to monitor electrolyte status closely and will usually need to coadminister a wide range of nutrients, including potassium, to mitigate adverse effects and optimize therapeutic outcome. In clinical practice, adverse effects on potassium status are considered a certainty with cisplatin. Carboplatin has considerably less renal toxicity (but more marrow suppression), and oxaliplatin also has less renal toxicity but more neurotoxicity. Given the high probability of renal damage with these agents, regular monitoring of renal function is obligatory, and nutrient administration can proceed only within the constraints of such systemic limitations, particularly resultant compromise of urinary excretion of potassium and magnesium. Thus, many oncologists treating with standard-dose cisplatin routinely include potassium and magnesium in the pre/post–IV hydration fluid.

In a review of the relationship between magnesium deficiency and potassium depletion refractory to repletion, Whang et al.[51] concluded by recommending that "(1) serum Mg be routinely assessed in any patients in whom serum electrolytes are necessary for clinical management and (2) until serum Mg is routinely performed, consideration should be given to treating hypokalemic patients with both Mg as well as K to avoid the problem of refractory K repletion due to coexisting Mg deficiency."

Further research may be warranted to determine factors influencing degree of risk and adverse effects among patients treated with cisplatin and to develop clinical guidelines for integrative therapeutics incorporating nutritional support.

Colchicine

Colchicine

Interaction Type and Significance

◇≈≈ **Drug-Induced Adverse Effect on Nutrient Function, Coadministration Therapeutic, with Professional Management**

Probability:
3. Possible or
2. Probable

Evidence Base:
● **Consensus**, though
○ **Preliminary**

Effect and Mechanism of Action

Colchicine can impair absorption of potassium (and other nutrients) and may increase potassium loss (as well as loss of other minerals, e.g., calcium and magnesium).[54,55] Depletion can be prevented or corrected with nutrient coadministration.

Research

For decades, colchicine has been widely viewed as likely to cause potassium loss.[54] However, clinical trials specifically investigating and confirming this adverse effect are lacking.

Nutritional Therapeutics, Clinical Concerns, and Adaptations

Physicians prescribing colchicine, especially for an extended period and in patients at greater risk for overall compromised nutritional status, are advised to monitor for imbalances and depletions in potassium and other nutrients. Colchicine is a potent anti-inflammatory often used as therapy in acute attacks of gout, which carries significant toxicity. It is sometimes used on a more chronic basis for rare disorders such as familial Mediterranean fever. Conservative practice also suggests consideration of preventive or corrective coadministration of potassium, as well as magnesium, calcium, and beta-carotene. Vitamin B_{12} may also be indicated if neuropathies develop. Dietary changes, especially restricting purine intake and reducing alcohol consumption, as well as adding cherry juice, can also be therapeutic in the treatment of individuals with gout.

Corticosteroids, Oral

Betamethasone (Celestone), cortisone (Cortone), dexamethasone (Decadron), fludrocortisone (Florinef), hydrocortisone (Cortef), methylprednisolone (Medrol) prednisolone (Delta-Cortef, Orapred, Pediapred, Prelone), prednisone (Deltasone, Liquid Pred, Meticorten, Orasone), triamcinolone (Aristocort).
Similar properties but evidence indicating no or reduced interaction effects: Inhaled or topical corticosteroids.

Interaction Type and Significance

≈≈   **Drug-Induced Nutrient Depletion,**
        Supplementation Therapeutic, with
        Professional Management
☼   **Prevention or Reduction of Drug Adverse Effect**

Probability:	Evidence Base:
3. Possible	◉ **Emerging**

Effect and Mechanism of Action

Oral corticosteroids increase urinary excretion of potassium and can cause hypolkalemia.[56-58] The mineralocorticoid action of cortisol causes a decrease in serum potassium concentration, together with stimulation of intestinal sodium absorption and an increase in serum sodium concentration, the combination of which can lead to water retention, weight gain, and increased risk of hypertension. Although used for its mineralocorticoid effects, fludrocortisone is classified as a glucocorticoid and an aldosterone agonist with physiological effects similar to but more potent than hydrocortisone. In general, these adverse effects vary with agent, dosage, duration, and comedications.

Potassium depletion may contribute to the mineralocorticoid-induced sodium retention. Conversely, potassium administration can augment urinary sodium excretion, attenuate mineralocorticoid-induced sodium retention, and reverse hyperaldosteronism.[59-63]

Research

The effects of oral corticosteroids on urinary excretion of potassium is well established, but consensus is lacking (and specific research absent) regarding the clinical significance of this influence.[57] Nevertheless, there is risk of hypokalemia during prolonged, high-dose corticosteroid therapy.[56,64]

The role of external potassium balance in modulating mineralocorticoid-induced sodium retention in humans remains uncertain. However, in a small trial involving eight healthy subjects treated with fludrocortisone, Krishna and Kapoor[61] demonstrated that potassium administration can ameliorate mineralocorticoid-induced sodium retention and enhance urinary sodium excretion. Conversely, fludrocortisone is used to treat interdialytic hyperkalemia in dialysis patients or may be useful, in combination with spironolactone, to correct sodium and potassium losses in secretory diarrhea.[65,66]

Nutritional Therapeutics, Clinical Concerns, and Adaptations

Physicians prescribing oral corticosteroids, especially for an extended period and in patients at greater risk for overall compromised nutritional status, are advised to monitor for imbalances and depletions in potassium and other nutrients. The minimal available evidence suggests that clinically significant potassium depletion is possible in some patients depending on the patient's general health, including diet, exercise, and other key physiological influences, and the potency of the particular agent(s) applied. In patients whose potassium status may be at risk, the consumption of fruit, vegetables, and other foods rich in potassium is usually the simplest and most effective means of preventing or correcting potential potassium depletion associated with long-term steroid therapy.

Cotrimoxazole (Sulfamethoxazole and Trimethoprim)

See Trimethoprim-Sulfamethoxazole.

Cyclosporine

Cyclosporine (Ciclosporin, cyclosporin A, CsA; Neoral, Sandimmune, SangCya).

Interaction Type and Significance

◇◇   **Drug-Induced Effect on Nutrient Function,**
        Supplementation Contraindicated, Professional
        Management Appropriate

Probability:	Evidence Base:
3. Possible	◉ **Emerging**

Effect and Mechanism of Action

Cyclosporine, an inhibitor of calcineurin, can induce hyperkalemia through different mechanisms, most notably immunosuppressant-induced nephrotoxicity, and chronic progressive tubulointerstitial fibrosis/arteriopathy in particular.[67] "Cyclosporin A (CsA)–induced hyperkalemia is caused by alterations in transepithelial K^+ secretion resulting from the inhibition of renal tubular Na^+,K^+-ATPase activity."[68] An obvious cause, found in many cases, derives from CsA-induced nephrotoxicity, a well-known adverse effect, that "causes a reduction in glomerular filtration rate through vasoconstriction of the afferent glomerular arterioles and may result in acute renal failure."[69] "Calcineurin inhibitor-induced acute renal failure may occur as early as a few weeks or months after initiation of cyclosporin therapy."[67] Nevertheless, other individuals exhibiting adequate kidney function have developed hyperkalemia, possibly because of tubular resistance to aldosterone.[69] Overall, dose-related renal tubule dysfunction, tubulointerstitial fibrosis/arteriopathy, and secondary hypoaldosteronism are considered the primary reasons for CsA-associated hyperkalemia, but no conclusive evidence has emerged to provide a comprehensive explanation for this phenomenon.

Reports and Research

Cyclosporin A and other immunosuppressive drugs are generally known to "induce either hypoaldosteronism or pseudo-hypoaldosteronism presenting with hyperkalemia and metabolic acidosis" after renal transplantation.[70]

Caliskan et al.[69] reported four cases of cyclosporine-associated hyperkalemia in allogeneic blood stem cell transplant patients "despite adequate kidney function." The authors proposed that hyperkalemia was caused by renal tubule dysfunction and secondary hypoaldosteronism. Takami et al.[71] reported the cases of two patients with advanced renal cell carcinoma who developed hyperkalemia during CsA therapy after allogeneic hematopoietic stem cell transplantation. They noted that this adverse effect occurred despite adequate renal function; both patients developed hyperkalemia, and cyclosporine, "the only pharmaceutical agent to which this electrolyte abnormality could be attributed," contributed to "tubular resistance to aldosterone." They also suggested that "the presence of a single functional kidney may be a risk factor for isolated hyperkalemia" resulting from cyclosporine.

In a 1995 study involving 24 renal transplant recipients 6 months after transplantation, Laine and Holmberg[72] investigated renal and adrenal mechanisms in cyclosporine-induced hyperkalemia observed in 11 of these patients. "The TTKGs [transtubular potassium concentration gradients] were low normal or reduced in both normo- and hyperkalaemic patients implying inhibition of K^+ secretion." The hyperkalemic patients received more CsA, and serum potassium concentration correlated with CsA dose. Notably, adrenal function exhibited "no clear effect," and the authors of this relatively early study concluded that hyperkalemia "was not fully explained by renal mechanisms."

In a 1999 prospective study of 49 kidney allograft recipients who received transplants before age 5 years, Qvist et al.[73] documented "excellent long-term graft survival and good graft function" 5 to 7 years after renal transplantation. Nevertheless, the authors noted that whereas "sodium handling remained intact, ... hyperuricemia was seen in 43-67%; 17-33% showed abnormal handling of potassium; and most patients had a subnormal concentrating capacity."

Higgins et al.[74] studied and compared the frequency and severity of nephrotoxicities, hyperkalemia, and hyponatremia in renal transplant recipients treated with cyclosporine versus tacrolimus. In this retrospective study they investigated sodium and potassium handling in 125 patients initially treated with cyclosporine ($n = 80$) or tacrolimus ($n = 45$) during the first 90 days after renal transplantation. They observed that serum potassium levels were higher in patients treated with tacrolimus than in those treated with cyclosporine, noting that hyponatremia was more likely in subjects with hyperkalemia.

Dangerous disturbances in potassium status and concentrations in patients being treated with cyclosporine have been reported repeatedly, and polypharmacy using several different agents has been used to reverse these adverse effects. Thyroxine is known to enhance renal cortical Na^+,K^+-ATPase activity. In a rodent experiment, You et al.[68] found that coadministration of thyroxine "prevented CsA-induced hyperkalemia and reduced creatinine clearance, Na^+,K^+-ATPase activity, and severity of the histologic changes in the renal tubular cells." Limited research indicates that ACE inhibitors or angiotensin II type I receptor antagonists such as losartan may be effective and well tolerated in the treatment of hypertension in renal transplant recipients at heightened risk of hyperkalemia and hyperuricemia from decreased renal blood flow and glomerular filtration rate associated with a single kidney and concomitant cyclosporine use.[75] One study noted that "in this high-risk population, the effects on serum potassium levels are less marked with losartan than with enalapril."[76] In a clinical trial involving 21 renal transplant patients under CsA therapy and 12 healthy controls, Heering et al.[70] investigated the relationship between renal allograft function under CsA therapy and plasma aldosterone concentration, potassium and water homeostasis, and mineralocorticoid receptor (MR) expression level in peripheral leukocytes. They concluded that "aldosterone resistance in kidney transplantation is in part induced by a down-regulation of mineralocorticoid receptor expression." They also noted that administration of fludrocortisone reversed hyperkalemia and metabolic acidosis without significant effect on MR expression. Similarly, Singer et al.[77] described the prompt reversal of hyperkalemia and other "severe life-threatening complications" through

administration of glibenclamide in three critically ill patients who developed "potassium-channel syndrome" after receiving cyclosporine or other drugs with K(ATP) channel-opening properties. Thus, although several strategies have been evaluated to attenuate cyclosporine-induced nephropathy, evidence of their efficacy remains preliminary.

Clinical Implications and Adaptations

Physicians treating allograft patients with cyclosporine will generally be monitoring for renal damage and associated hyperkalemia and other disturbances in electrolyte balance. Concomitant potassium in such patients is generally contraindicated, and frank inquiry as to lifestyle practices, including a thorough inventory of dietary and supplement intake, is essential to comprehensive management of such patients.

Digoxin and Related Cardiac Glycosides

Digoxin (Digitek, Lanoxin, Lanoxicaps, purgoxin). Extrapolated, based on similar properties: Deslanoside (cedilanin-D), digitoxin (Cystodigin), ouabain (g-strophanthin); foxglove plant (*Digitalis lanata*).

Interaction Type and Significance

◇≈ ≈   **Drug-Induced Adverse Effect on Nutrient Function, Coadministration Therapeutic, with Professional Management**

⊕✗   **Bimodal or Variable Interaction, with Professional Management**

Probability: Evidence Base:
2. Probable   ● Consensus

Effect and Mechanism of Action

The central role of potassium in maintaining proper function of cardiac (and other) muscles is a basic physiological precept in clinical medicine. The safe use of digoxin requires stable blood potassium levels because hypokalemia may predispose to digitalis toxicity and dangerous cardiac arrhythmias. However, digoxin impairs potassium transport from the blood into cells.[78] Furthermore, potassium depletion, induced by concomitant diuretic use and often secondary to hypomagnesemia, is quite common among individuals treated with digoxin. Conversely, an overdose of digoxin can cause a potentially fatal hyperkalemia.

Reports and Research

As early as 1960, in a paper on the relationship between digitalis and potassium in the context of surgery, Lown et al.[78] discuss impaired potassium transport from the blood into cells caused by digoxin. In reporting on correlations with serum digoxin level in five cases of suicidal and accidental digoxin ingestion, Smith and Willerson[79] noted that potentially fatal hyperkalemia can result from an overdose of digoxin.

In 1985, Whang et al.[80] published their findings on the frequency of hypomagnesemia in hospitalized patients receiving digitalis. In measuring serum sodium, magnesium, and potassium levels in 136 serum samples sent to the laboratory for digoxin assay, they found that hyponatremia occurred most frequently (21%), followed by hypomagnesemia in 19%, hypokalemia in 9%, and hypermagnesemia in 7%. They noted that the "twofold frequency of hypomagnesemia" compared to hypokalemia "indicates that clinicians are more attuned to avoiding hypokalemia than hypomagnesemia in patients receiving digitalis," and added that their "observation suggests that hypomagnesemia may be a more frequent contributor than hypokalemia to induction of toxic reactions to digitalis." Thus, they concluded that electrolyte monitoring, both of magnesium and potassium, is critical "in patients receiving digitalis, who often are also receiving potent diuretics."

Schmidt et al.[81] found that the impairment of extrarenal potassium homeostasis by heart failure and digoxin treatment may be counterbalanced by exercise. Based on the finding that "extrarenal potassium handling is altered as a result of digoxin treatment," the authors proposed that this is "likely to reflect a reduced capacity of skeletal muscle Na/K-ATPase for active potassium uptake because of inhibition by digoxin (similar to that seen with beta-blockers), adding to the reduction of skeletal muscle Na/K-ATPase concentration induced by heart failure *per se*." Consequently, however, "in heart failure patients, improved haemodynamics induced by digoxin may . . . increase the capacity for physical conditioning."

Nutritional Therapeutics, Clinical Concerns, and Adaptations

Physicians prescribing digoxin or related cardiac glycosides need to monitor for potassium (and magnesium) depletion. Unsupervised use of potassium supplements (or even high intake of potassium-rich foods) is generally contraindicated during digitalis therapy. However, when coadministration of potassium may be indicated, particularly in the context of potassium-depleting diuretics, oral preparations may not be as effective or as well tolerated as consistent dietary consumption of fruit and other foods rich in potassium. Education and support for a regular program of moderate exercise can be therapeutically valuable in most patients and consistent with broader knowledge of cardiovascular health and risk factors. Close supervision and regular monitoring are inherently appropriate in all digitalized patients.

Diuretics, Potassium Depleting, Including Loop and Thiazide Diuretics

Loop diuretics: Bumetanide (Bumex), ethacrynic acid (Edecrin), furosemide (Lasix), torsemide (Demadex).

Thiazide diuretics: Bendroflumethiazide (bendrofluazide; Naturetin); combination drug: bendrofluazide and propranolol (Inderex); benzthiazide (Exna), chlorothiazide (Diuril), chlorthalidone (Hygroton), cyclopenthiazide (Navidrex); combination drug: cyclopenthiazide and oxprenolol hydrochloride (Trasidrex); hydrochlorothiazide (Aquazide, Esidrix, Ezide, Hydrocot, HydroDiuril, Microzide, Oretic); combination drugs: hydrochlorothiazide and amiloride (Moduretic); hydrochlorothiazide and captopril (Acezide, Capto-Co, Captozide, Co-Zidocapt); hydrochlorothiazide and enalapril (Vaseretic); hydrochlorothiazide and lisinopril (Prinzide, Zestoretic); hydrochlorothiazide and losartan (Hyzaar); hydrochlorothiazide and metoprolol (Lopressor HCT); hydrochlorothiazide and spironolactone (Aldactazide); hydrochlorothiazide and triamterene (Dyazide, Maxzide), hydroflumethiazide (Diucardin), methyclothiazide (Enduron), metolazone (Zaroxolyn, Mykrox), polythiazide (Renese), quinethazone (Hydromox), trichlormethiazide (Naqua).

Thiazide-like diuretics: Indapamide (Lozol).

See also Carbonic Anhydrase Inhibitors, Potassium Depleting, and Quinidine and Related Antiarrhythmic Drugs.

Interaction Type and Significance

≈≈ **Drug-Induced Nutrient Depletion, Supplementation Therapeutic, with Professional Management**

☼ **Prevention or Reduction of Drug Adverse Effect**

Probability:	Evidence Base:
1. Certain	● Consensus

Effect and Mechanism of Action

Thiazide, loop, and similar diuretics are often referred to as "potassium depleting" because by definition they increase potassium excretion with diuresis; in practice, they concurrently deplete magnesium at the cellular level.[82] The diuretic-induced magnesium deficiency can lead to refractory potassium depletion but may not be detectable through routine serum magnesium determinations.[51,83]

Research

Potassium wasting with these medications is axiomatic, and hypokalemia is a common finding in those taking diuretic medications, especially the elderly. Avoiding hypokalemia is generally agreed to be beneficial in several cardiovascular disease states, including acute myocardial infarction, heart failure, and hypertension. Nevertheless, data from direct research into diuretic-induced hypokalemia are limited. Moreover, clinically significant differences in the severity of effects on potassium status between high-dose and low-dose diuretics, as well as oral versus intravenous administration, have been proposed. Furthermore, the available research does provide some important insights that depart from common assumptions.

Not all patients receiving treatment with "potassium-depleting" diuretics necessarily develop clinically significant (or at least readily detectable) decreases in potassium concentrations. In three yearly multicenter surveys involving 18,872 patients with initially normal baseline serum potassium, Zuccala et al.[84] investigated older age and in-hospital development of hypokalemia in the 4035 patients who started receiving loop diuretics during their hospital stay. After adjusting for a number of variables, age and use of parenteral (but not oral) loop diuretics were associated with hypokalemia. The authors concluded that "older age is independently associated with the in-hospital development of hypokalemia, particularly among patients taking loop diuretics" and recommended monitoring of serum potassium levels "when older patients are treated with these agents."

Franse et al.[85] analyzed data of 4126 participants in a 5-year, randomized, placebo-controlled clinical trial of chlorthalidone-based treatment of isolated systolic hypertension in older persons to determine whether hypokalemia that occurs with low-dose diuretics is associated with a reduced benefit on cardiovascular events. They found that after "adjustment for known risk factors and study drug dose, the participants who received active treatment and who experienced hypokalemia had a similar risk of cardiovascular events, coronary events, and stroke as those randomized to placebo." However, "within the active treatment group, the risk of these events was 51%, 55%, and 72% lower, respectively, among those who had normal serum potassium levels compared with those who experienced hypokalemia." Thus, they concluded that subjects who had hypokalemia after 1 year of treatment with a low-dose diuretic "did not experience the reduction in cardiovascular events achieved among those who did not have hypokalemia." Besides demonstrating that treatment with a thiazide diuretic led to a reduction in serum potassium levels in some participants, these findings indicate that patients exhibiting decreased potassium levels were also more likely to experience cardiovascular events, such as heart attacks, heart failure, sudden cardiac death, stroke, and aneurysm.

The interrelationship between potassium (K) and magnesium (Mg) depletion patterns is an important topic with significant implications for normal electrolyte balance and cardiac function. In a 1992 paper, Whang et al.[51] reviewed experimental and clinical observations supporting the view that uncorrected Mg deficiency impairs repletion of cellular K. "[C]onsistent with the observed close association between K and Mg depletion," they found that concomitant "Mg deficiency in K-depleted patients ranges from 38% to 42%." Although this refractory "K repletion due to unrecognized concurrent Mg deficiency can be clinically perplexing," they note that it "may be operative in … patients receiving potent loop diuretics" as well as other medications. Based on these findings, they recommend that "(1) serum Mg be routinely assessed in any patients in whom serum electrolytes are necessary for clinical management and (2) until serum Mg is routinely performed, consideration should be given to treating hypokalemic patients with both Mg as well as K to avoid the problem of refractory K repletion due to coexisting Mg deficiency."[51]

The complications arising from the effects of potassium depletion have broad implications for an at-risk cardiovascular patient population. For example, low preoperative serum potassium levels can adversely influence perioperative outcomes in cardiac surgery patients. Wahr et al.[2] conducted a prospective, observational, case-control study to determine the prevalence of abnormal preoperative serum potassium levels and whether such abnormal levels are associated with adverse perioperative events. Analyzing data gathered from 24 diverse U.S. medical centers in a 2-year period, they found that perioperative arrhythmias occurred in 1290 (53.7%) of 2402 patients and that "serum potassium level less than 3.5 mmol/L was a predictor" of serious perioperative arrhythmia, intraoperative arrhythmia, and postoperative atrial fibrillation/flutter, and "these relationships were unchanged after adjusting for confounders." These authors concluded: "Although interventional trials are required to determine whether preoperative intervention mitigates these adverse associations, preoperative repletion is low cost and low risk, and our data suggest that screening and repletion be considered in patients scheduled for cardiac surgery."[2]

Ruml et al.[86] conducted two clinical trials investigating the effect of varying doses of potassium-magnesium citrate on thiazide-induced hypokalemia and magnesium loss. In subjects first administered hydrochlorothiazide, 50 mg daily, these researchers found that three different "dosages of potassium-magnesium citrate significantly increased serum potassium concentration, with > 80% of subjects regaining normal values despite continued thiazide therapy." They concluded that potassium-magnesium citrate "not only corrects thiazide-induced hypokalemia, but also may avert magnesium loss while providing an alkali load." However, "higher dosages," such as 70 mEq potassium, 35 mEq magnesium, and 105 mEq citrate per day, are "probably required for the prevention of magnesium loss and adverse symptoms of thiazide therapy."[87]

Nutritional Therapeutics, Clinical Concerns, and Adaptations

In practice, it is generally advisable to coadminister both potassium and magnesium when prescribing any potassium-depleting diuretic, except in cases involving those with renal insufficiency. For long-term care, coadministration of potassium in the dosage range of several hundred milligrams to several grams per day is usually appropriate, depending on the individual's diet, age, genetic predisposition, medications,

and other factors. Potassium deficiency status can be evaluated by monitoring RBC potassium levels or, more conventionally, serum potassium concentration. Assessment of potassium status may be appropriate but is often not essential, because low serum potassium is not required for patients to benefit from potassium coadministration. However, since administration of potassium (and/or magnesium) can be risky, and is usually contraindicated, in patients with renal insufficiency, kidney function tests are critical before initiating, and periodically through the course of, concomitant repletion therapy.

Administration of potassium, magnesium, or other electrolyte needs to be maintained for 6 months to compensate for any drug-induced tissue depletion pattern and throughout the duration of, and possibly after conclusion of, relevant diuretic therapy. A typical complementary magnesium dose for most individuals would be in the range of 300 to 500 mg per day, preferably as magnesium citrate, malate, gluconate, or glycinate. A multimineral formulation would add support against parallel depletions of other vulnerable minerals. Beyond potassium and magnesium, clinical care within an integrative setting might also emphasize a diet rich in minerals, vitamins, antioxidants, and essential fatty acids as part of an evolving and individualized approach to cardiovascular therapeutics involving health care professionals trained and experienced in multiple therapeutic disciplines.

Ipecac

See Ipecac in Herb-Nutrient Interactions.

Laxatives and Stool Softeners

Fast-acting laxative agents: Glycerin-containing suppositories (Fleet), magnesium-containing products (Phillips' Milk of Magnesia Magnesium Citrate Solution); bisacodyl tablets (Dulcolax), monobasic sodium phosphate monohydrate and dibasic sodium phosphate heptahydrate (Fleet Phospho-soda Oral Saline Laxative), senna (*Cassia senna, Cassia argustifolia;* Black-Draught, Fletcher's Castoria, Gentlax, Senexon, Senna-Gen, Senekot, Senolax).

Enemas: Bisacodyl enemas (Dulcolax), monobasic sodium phosphate monohydrate and dibasic sodium phosphate heptahydrate (Fleet enema).

Slow-acting laxative agents: Bulk-forming laxatives: Methylcellulose (Citrucel), polycarbophil (FiberCon), psyllium (Metamucil, Konsyl-D).

Stool softeners: Docusate (Colace, Surfak), mineral oil (Agoral, Kondremul Plain, Milkinol, Neo-Cultol, Petrogalar Plain).

Prescription laxative agents: Lactulose (Chronulac), polyethylene glycol (Miralax), polyethylene glycol–electrolyte solution (CoLyte, GoLYTELY, NuLytely).

Interaction Type and Significance

≈≈≈ **Drug-Induced Nutrient Depletion, Supplementation Therapeutic, Not Requiring Professional Management**

☼ **Prevention or Reduction of Drug Adverse Effect**

Probability:
3. Possible or
  2. Probable

Evidence Base:
▽ **Mixed** and
○ **Preliminary**

Effect and Mechanism of Action

Excessive or repeated use of any laxative can deplete potassium (and a wide range of other nutrients) through a variety of mechanisms, including impaired absorption and altered transit time. Short-term use of cathartic laxatives, as in the context of colon cleansing for radiological examinations, can cause acute drops in serum potassium that may be particularly dangerous in patients on diuretic or digitalis therapy and those with cardiac conditions or otherwise susceptible to arrhythmias.[88] Among its several actions, docusate administration stimulates net secretion of potassium.[89] Mineral oil, as a lipid solvent, may interfere with normal absorption of potassium and other nutrients and absorb many substances. Inherently, these factors are aggravated in the context of compromised nutritional intake and limited physical activity. Potassium coadministration, through dietary or supplemental prescription intake, can usually prevent or reverse any disturbances in potassium status.

Stimulant-type laxatives such as bisacodyl may both reduce potassium absorption and cause excessive potassium loss, as well as sodium depletion and hyperreninemia, most probably through two mechanisms: (1) loss of potassium as a result of stimulation of mucus secretion in intestinal mucosa and (2) a "dual effect of potassium on aldosterone secretion, with renin as a mediator."[90-93] Thus, hypokalemia can result from abuse or chronic bisacodyl use.

Reports and Research

Fleming et al.[92] reported the case of a patient "with marked chronic hypokalemia (potassium, 1.7 to 2;3 meq/litre) and sodium depletion secondary to laxative abuse and dietary inadequacy."

Moriarty et al.[89] used an intestinal perfusion technique to investigate the mechanism of action of docusate in the human jejunum and observed that it "stimulated net secretion of water, sodium, chloride and potassium and inhibited net absorption of glucose and bicarbonate."

In a prospective study involving 320 patients, Ritsema and Eilers[88] investigated the impact of colon cleansing before procedures on serum potassium concentrations and the efficacy of potassium administration in preventing serious hypokalaemia. Of the four subject subgroups, two were being treated with diuretics, and one of those also received potassium. "Hypokalaemia was present prior to cleansing in six (11%), and after cleansing in 20 (36%) of the 55 patients in the group 1 patients on diuretics but without potassium supplements. There was, after cleansing, no significant fall in serum potassium in the group 2 patients on diuretics who received potassium supplements." Notably, no hyperkalemia resulted from potassium coadministration. Likewise, both subgroups not receiving diuretics, one of which received a 2-day preparation of 15 g magnesium sulfate and 10 mg bisacodyl twice daily and the other a 1-day preparation of 2.4 mg sennoside, exhibited a "significant fall of the mean level of serum potassium." Thus, the authors concluded that "both 1 day and 2 days of cleansing with cathartics may result in a significant fall in serum potassium, which can be prevented by oral potassium supplements." In particular, they noted that administration of 15 mL of potassium chloride with 0.9 mmol K/mL three times daily during the preparation "in patients on diuretics may be prudent to avoid the risk of cardiac arrhythmia."[88]

Nutritional Therapeutics, Clinical Concerns, and Adaptations

Individuals using laxatives or stool softeners on a regular basis, especially outside the context of professional supervision, should be encouraged to increase their consumption of fresh fruits and vegetables as a means of preventing or reversing nutrient depletion. Repeated use of laxatives, other than bulking

fibers such as psyllium seed husks, for longer than 7 days should be discouraged and root causal factors addressed. Healthful dietary practices will reduce the likelihood and severity of constipation and the need for laxatives or stool softeners in most individuals, especially when combined with increased intake of healthy oils and whole grains and regular exercise. Acute prophylactic potassium administration is judicious in some clinical situations, such as short-term use of laxatives before diagnostic procedures. Regular use of a high-quality multivitamin/mineral formulation will often be indicated and beneficial in preventing and correcting multiple nutritional insufficiencies in individuals using these medications, especially the elderly, institutionalized, or otherwise nutritionally compromised individuals. In general, nutritional supplements are most effectively assimilated when taken separate from fiber, mineral oils, or other substances that may potentially impair their absorption.

Losartan and Related Angiotensin II Receptor Antagonists

Evidence: Losartan (Cozaar), combination drug: losartan and hydrochlorothiazide (Hyzaar).
Extrapolated, based on similar properties: Candesartan (Atacand); combination drug: candesartan and hydrochlorothiazide (Atacand HCT); eprosartan (Teveten), irbesartan (Aprovel, Avapro, Karvea); combination drug: irbesartan and hydrochlorothiazide (Avalide); olmesartan (Benicar), telmisartan (Micardis), valsartan (Diovan); combination drug: valsartan and hydrochlorothiazide (Diovan HCT).
See also Angiotensin-Converting Enzyme (ACE) Inhibitors.

Interaction Type and Significance

✗✗ **Minimal to Mild Adverse Interaction—Vigilance Necessary**
✗✗✗ **Potentially Harmful or Serious Adverse Interaction—Avoid**
◇◇ **Drug-Induced Effect on Nutrient Function, Supplementation Contraindicated, Professional Management Appropriate**

Probability:	Evidence Base:
2. Probable or	● **Consensus**
1. Certain	

Effect and Mechanism of Action

Losartan and its active metabolite, E-3174, affect the renin-angiotensin system and reduce aldosterone activity by selectively blocking the binding of angiotensin II to angiotensin I receptors found in vascular smooth muscle and other tissues, causing vasodilation and inhibiting retention of sodium and water by the kidneys, thus decreasing blood volume. Neither losartan nor its active metabolite inhibits angiotensin converting enzyme, and, in fact, as these agents inhibit the pressor effect of angiotensin II the removal of the negative feedback of angiotensin II causes a significant rise in plasma renin activity, and a resultant rise in angiotensin II plasma concentration, in hypertensive patients. Consequently, losartan may cause increases in blood potassium levels that can be clinically significant.[94] Increasing potassium intake (food, supplements, prescription, salt substitute) concurrent with an angiotensin II receptor antagonist may lead to hyperkalemia and the resulting adverse effects.

Research

As the first angiotensin II receptor antagonist (ARB) to be marketed for the treatment of hypertension, losartan has been the subject of more research than others drugs in this class. Nevertheless, "ARB-related hyperkalemia is class- and not compound-specific." Thus, as summarized by Sica[95] in a 2006 review of the effects of antihypertensive therapy on potassium homeostasis, that ARBs, as with ACE inhibitors, "will increase the serum K⁺ value in virtually all treated subjects, but only to a degree (0.1-0.2 mEq/L) that is barely discernible clinically," and proposed that hyperkalemia in such cases "remains highly definitional in nature."

Hyperkalemia is a known adverse effect of losartan. In controlled hypertensive trials with losartan monotherapy and losartan-hydrochlorothiazide (Hyzaar), a serum potassium greater than 5.5 mEq/L occurred in 1.5% and 0.7% of patients, respectively.[96] Nevertheless, in such research no patient discontinued losartan or losartan-hydrochlorothiazide therapy because of hyperkalemia.[97] Moreover, in a study of the efficacy and tolerability of losartan in hypertensive patients with chronic renal insufficiency, Toto et al.[98] reported that hyperkalemia (>6 mEq/L) requiring discontinuation of losartan occurred in only one patient (of 112 subjects). However, in another study focusing on patients with type 2 diabetes and proteinuria, significantly more patients in the losartan group developed hyperkalemia (losartan 24.2% vs. placebo 12.3%; $p <$ 0.001).[99]

Reports

Numerous reports, published and unpublished, describe hyperkalemia in patients receiving losartan or other angiotensin II receptor antagonist drugs, particularly in the context of potassium-sparing diuretics and compromised renal status.[100-105] Miyahara et al.[106] reported a case of intraoperative hyperkalemia induced with administration of an angiotensin II receptor antagonist and intake of dried persimmons, a fruit high in potassium.

Clinical Implications and Adaptations

Health care professionals treating patients taking an angiotensin II receptor antagonist (ARB) are strongly encouraged to counsel these individuals to avoid unsupervised increases in potassium intake, in the form of supplements but also as high-potassium foods (e.g., fruit) or salt substitutes, on the basis of the increased risk for problematic interactions. A clinically significant increase in blood potassium levels represents an uncommon yet potentially serious adverse effect associated with ARB drugs. The importance of frank inquiry and detailed inventory of concomitant (or even occasional) medications, diet, nutrients, and herbs cannot be overemphasized. Close supervision and regular monitoring are essential, especially in individuals with compromised renal function. The prescription of potassium chloride or potassium-sparing medications is generally contraindicated during angiotensin II receptor antagonist therapy.

Magnesium-Containing Antacids

See Magnesium in Nutrient-Nutrient Interactions.

Nonsteroidal Anti-Inflammatory Drugs (NSAIDs)

COX-1 inhibitors: Diclofenac (Cataflam, Voltaren); combination drug: diclofenac and misoprostol (Arthrotec); diflunisal (Dolobid), etodolac (Lodine), fenoprofen (Dalfon), furbiprofen (Ansaid), ibuprofen (Advil, Excedrin IB, Motrin, Motrin IB, Nuprin, Pedia Care Fever Drops, Provel, Rufen); combination drug: hydrocodone and ibuprofen (Reprexain, Vicoprofen); indomethacin (indometacin; Indocin, Indocin-SR), ketoprofen

(Orudis, Oruvail), ketorolac (Acular ophthalmic, Toradol), meclofenamate (Meclomen), mefenamic acid (Ponstel), meloxicam (Mobic), nabumetone (Relafen), naproxen (Aleve, Anaprox, Naprosyn), oxaprozin (Daypro), piroxicam (Feldene), salsalate (salicylic acid; Amigesic, Disalcid, Marthritic, Mono Gesic, Salflex, Salsitab), sulindac (Clinoril), tolmetin (Tolectin).

COX-2 inhibitor: Celecoxib (Celebrex).

Interaction Type and Significance

✗✗   **Minimal to Mild Adverse Interaction—Vigilance Necessary**

✗✗✗   **Potentially Harmful or Serious Adverse Interaction—Avoid**

◇◇   **Drug-Induced Effect on Nutrient Function, Supplementation Contraindicated, Professional Management Appropriate**

Probability:	Evidence Base:
3. Possible,	⊙ Emerging
5. Improbable	

Effect and Mechanism of Action

Many anti-inflammatory agents affect potassium metabolism, but through a variety of mechanisms with the potential to produce a range of different effects, including severe reactions of rapid-onset hyperkalemia in acute renal failure. The effects of NSAIDs on prostaglandin production appear central to many adverse reactions. For example, indomethacin inhibits renal prostaglandin synthesis, which in turn reduces renin-aldosterone levels and potassium excretion and subsequently elevates serum potassium levels, potentially causing hyperkalemia. Similarly, ibuprofen can impair renal function and thus elevate blood potassium levels, particularly in elderly persons or those with preexisting renal compromise.[107] "Generally, the renal failure with NSAIDs is acute and reversible, though analgesic nephropathy with papillary necrosis and chronic renal failure are reported."[108]

Research

In a prospective, randomized, crossover trial, Whelton et al.[109] compared the renal effects of ibuprofen, piroxicam, and sulindac in patients with asymptomatic renal failure. "All three regimens suppressed renal prostaglandin production." In contrast to the other two NSAIDs, they observed excessive elevations of serum potassium by the eighth day (beyond those tolerated in the study design) that required withdrawal of treatment in 3 of 12 subjects who received ibuprofen, 800 mg three times daily. Further, when these three patients were rechallenged with ibuprofen, 400 mg three times daily, "two again developed evidence of acute renal deterioration." The authors concluded that "a brief course of ibuprofen, a compound widely used on a nonprescription basis, may result in acute renal failure in patients with asymptomatic, mild chronic renal failure."

Reports

Poirier[108] reported a "probable case of acute, reversible renal failure and hyperkalemia, after an increase in dose of ibuprofen." After reviewing other cases of renal dysfunction associated with NSAIDs, the author concludes: "Electrolytes, blood urea nitrogen, and serum creatinine levels need to be monitored in high-risk patients with predisposing factors and for chronic, long-term use of drugs that inhibit prostaglandin synthesis."

Clinical Implications and Adaptations

Potassium intake should be limited during NSAID therapy because potassium levels may rise in an unregulated manner, potentially reaching clinically significant hyperkalemia. Health care professionals treating patients using NSAIDs are strongly encouraged to counsel these individuals to avoid unsupervised increases in potassium intake, in the form of supplements but also as high-potassium foods (e.g., fruit) or salt substitutes, on the basis of the increased risk for problematic interactions. Although their use is widespread and largely unregulated, the high frequency of adverse reactions to NSAIDs is generally underestimated by patients and often forgotten by health care professionals. Apart from hepatotoxicity, which continues to be a major risk factor, the adverse effects of these agents on renal function need to be considered in all individuals with chronic use and even in some individuals with occasional use. A clinically significant increase in blood potassium levels represents an uncommon yet potentially serious adverse effect associated with NSAID therapy.

As previously noted, adverse reactions, although reversible, can be sudden and severe, particularly in those with compromised renal function. As summarized by Poirier[108]: "Possible predisposing factors to renal deterioration include the amount of drug consumed, presence of compromised renal blood flow, underlying renal insufficiency, nephrotoxic drug combinations, and high urinary prostaglandin excretion." Thus, regular monitoring is important in all patients using NSAIDs and close supervision may also be essential in those at high risk for adverse reactions. Principles of conservative practice recommend that health care professionals assess and correct the causes and aggravating factors involved in chronic inflammatory responses and educate patients to minimize use of anti-inflammatory medications.

Quinidine and Related Antiarrhythmic Drugs

Evidence: Quinidine (Quinaglute, Quinidex, Quinora).
Extrapolated, based on similar properties: Amiodarone (Cordarone), disopyramide (Norpace), dofetilide (Tikosyn), flecainide (Tambocor), ibutilide (Corvert), procainamide (Pronestyl, Procan-SR), sotalol (Betapace, Betapace AF, Sorine).
See also Digoxin and Related Cardiac Glycosides.

Interaction Type and Significance

≈≈ **Drug-Induced Nutrient Depletion, Supplementation Therapeutic, with Professional Management**
☼ **Prevention or Reduction of Drug Adverse Effect**

Probability: Evidence Base:
3. Possible   ○ Preliminary or
                          ◉ Emerging

Effect and Mechanism of Action

The antiarrhythmic drugs with class 1A cardiac activity slow cardiac conduction and lengthen the QT interval. As with other antiarrhythmic drugs, quinidine may worsen cardiac rhythm disorders and increase the risk of death, especially in individuals with a history of a heart attack. More broadly, intracellular potassium and magnesium levels are intrinsic to electrical stability, and high and low levels of these anions, both within the cells and in the serum, predispose to cardiac rhythm disturbances; therefore, antiarrhythmic drugs of all classes (1A, 1C, and 3) can interact with medicines that affect potassium (and magnesium) levels.

Individuals with low blood levels of potassium (and magnesium), caused by diuretics, vomiting, or other stressors, may develop serious cardiac adverse effects, such as arrhythmias, in response to quinidine. In particular, quinidine causes torsades de pointes under certain conditions, particularly hypokalemia, hypomagnesemia, and other electrolyte abnormalities. Potent suppression of a potassium channel subunit current by quinidine is a likely contributor to torsades de pointes arrhythmias.[110] Thus, arrhythmias "may develop in hypokalemia due to enhanced normal automaticity, abnormal automaticity, or slowed conduction; moreover, hypokalemia is associated with enhanced digitalis toxicity, quinidine-related torsades de pointes, and interference with the antiarrhythmic activity of quinidine."[111]

With simultaneous intake, direct adsorption by potassium or other mineral salts could theoretically result in decreased drug bioavailability, although not necessarily to a clinically significant degree.[112]

Research

Hypokalemia, especially in the presence of hypomagnesemia or other electrolyte abnormalities, is associated with a range of adverse effects, including quinidine-related torsades de pointes, and interference with the antiarrhythmic activity of quinidine. Here, once again, the critical importance of the interrelationship between potassium and magnesium is a recurrent theme.

Mutations in a gene encoding a potassium channel subunit (HERG) can be related to the long-QT (LQT) syndrome characteristic of torsades de pointes, a polymorphic ventricular arrhythmia. Pharmacological suppression of repolarizing potassium currents is also a mechanism causing the acquired LQT syndrome.[110]

Roden and Iansmith[111] concluded their paper on the effects of low potassium or magnesium concentrations on isolated cardiac tissue by proposing that, in individuals with hypertension, "treatment that controls hypertension without causing electrolyte abnormalities is preferable for patients who are at risk of arrhythmias, or who are receiving drugs such as digitalis or quinidine."

Further research into electrolyte function in cardiac tissue, related drug interactions and depletions, and individual genomic and pharmacogenomic variability is warranted and can benefit from an integrative approach to multidisciplinary therapeutic interventions.

Report

Teplick et al.,[113] as well as other authors,[114] have reported cases of esophagitis caused by oral potassium chloride ("slow KCl" liquid and tablets) and quinidine tablets, separately. The concomitant use of these agents could theoretically increase the probability of adverse reactions. The authors noted that in "all reported cases caused by KCl tablets, left atrial enlargement was present as the result of mitral stenosis."[113]

Nutritional Therapeutics, Clinical Concerns, and Adaptations

Physicians prescribing quinidine or related antiarrhythmic drugs, especially in conjunction with potassium-depleting diuretics, are advised initially to assess and then periodically monitor potassium and magnesium status, keeping in mind that serum concentrations do not accurately reflect intracellular levels. Coadministration of potassium and other nutrients may prevent or correct nutrient depletion that could create or amplify adverse drug effects. In contrast to magnesium, rapid repletion of potassium by the IV route is not used in the treatment of acute arrhythmias.

Within a comprehensive therapeutic repertoire, quinidine, potassium, and magnesium represent important options appropriate for consideration in crafting a long-term program of care for individuals with arrhythmias, hypertension, and other cardiovascular conditions. Treatment using medications that do not deplete vital nutrients or otherwise introduce electrolyte abnormalities is preferable, especially patients who at risk of arrhythmias or receiving drugs such as quinidine. Regular monitoring and appropriate nutritional support are important therapeutic tools when recourse to more deleterious agents is deemed necessary. Low potassium and magnesium concentrations not only contribute to or cause cardiac arrhythmias, but deficiencies of these minerals can also interfere with the efficacy or enhance the toxicity of many drugs used to treat patients with heart disease. Clinical care within an integrative setting might also emphasize a diet rich in vitamins, minerals, and antioxidants and incorporate hawthorn *(Crataegus oxyacantha),* L-carnitine, coenzyme Q10, and other nutrients as part of an individualized and evolving approach to cardiovascular therapeutics.

Spironolactone and Triamterene

Spironolactone (Aldactone); combination drug: spironolactone and hydrochlorothiazide (Aldactazide); triamterene (Dyrenium); combination drug: triamterene and hydrochlorothiazide (Dyazide, Maxzide).

Interaction Type and Significance

◇◇   **Drug-Induced Effect on Nutrient Function, Supplementation Contraindicated, Professional Management Appropriate**

✗✗   **Minimal to Mild Adverse Interaction—Vigilance Necessary**

Probability: Evidence Base:
2. Probable to   ● Consensus
   1. Certain

Effect and Mechanism of Action

In contrast to potassium-wasting diuretics, spironolactone and triamterene, along with amiloride, constitute a drug class of diuretic agents that, by design, conserve potassium. Spironolactone inhibits the action of aldosterone and other mineralocorticoids, causing the kidneys to excrete sodium and fluid while retaining potassium. Triamterene achieves its diuretic effect by inhibiting the reabsorption of sodium in exchange for potassium and hydrogen ions in the distal renal tubule and thus maintains or increases sodium excretion and reduces loss of potassium, hydrogen, and chloride ions. Because triamterene is not a competitive antagonist of aldosterone, its dosing is determined by the kaliuretic effect of concomitantly administered drugs and the response of the individual patient, rather than being proportionate to the level of mineralocorticoid activity. Thus, triamterene can prevent diuretic-induced potassium loss comparable to 3.1 to 4.7 g (80-120 mmol) of potassium daily. Consequently, these medications are often used in combination with hydrochlorothiazide or other kaliuretic drugs to mitigate potassium wasting.

Conversely, increased potassium intake (foods, supplements, prescription, salt substitutes) could lead to excessive elevation of potassium levels in patients being treated with these medications, especially with concomitant ACE inhibitors or other medications that alter potassium metabolism. Arrhythmias and other adverse effects of hyperkalemia can be severe and are sometimes rapid in onset.

In addition to hypertension, potassium-sparing medications are used in the treatment of cirrhotic patients with ascites as well as those with Conn's, Bartter's, and Liddle syndromes and hirsutism.

Research

Spironolactone and triamterene intentionally reduce urinary excretion of potassium while enhancing sodium excretion. As potassium-sparing diuretics, these agents can produce a state of hyperkalemia (i.e., inappropriately elevated potassium levels). When used in combination with a thiazide diuretic, hyperkalemia (>5.4 mEq/L) has been reported as ranging from 4% in patients less than 60 years of age to 12% in patients 60 years and older, with an overall incidence of less than 8%. Arrhythmias and other cardiac irregularities are among the adverse effects associated with hyperkalemia. Conversely, concern has been raised about potential risks of hypokalemia among some patients using triamterene, even though hypokalemia is a less common occurrence with the use of triamterene than with non-potassium-sparing diuretics.

In a random crossover study, Jackson et al.[115] investigated the influence of spironolactone (50 and 100 mg daily), triamterene (100 and 200 mg daily), potassium chloride (32 and 64 mmol daily), and placebo on plasma potassium and other variables in nine hypertensive patients taking bendrofluazide, a thiazide diuretic (10 mg daily). They observed that spironolactone and triamterene had "significant and parallel dose-response curves for plasma potassium, with a relative potency for triamterene:spironolactone of 0.25:1, significantly lower than the accepted 0.5:1 ratio," while also lowering serum sodium, bicarbonate, and body weight and increasing serum urea and creatinine levels. Potassium chloride "increased plasma potassium above placebo values, but the dose-response was not significant and was not parallel with those of the potassium-sparing drugs." Notably, seven of nine patients "remained hypokalaemic despite treatment with 64 mmol potassium chloride daily."

Sawyer and Gabriel[116] studied progressive hypokalemia in 80 elderly patients with heart failure taking three thiazide potassium-sparing diuretic combinations over 36 months. Compared with amiloride and spironolactone, the "triamterene-containing preparation was discontinued most frequently (6/44) because of hypokalaemia (plasma potassium less than 3.0 mmol/L)." The median fall in plasma potassium over 3 years in those patients not withdrawn because of hypokalemia was "similar in each case (P greater than 0.05) and possibly failed to reach significance because of the withdrawal rate (9%)," and the "trend was for a greater fall in those patients taking triamterene." The authors concluded that the "spironolactone-containing preparation may be the least unsatisfactory of the three."

In a randomized study, Schnaper et al.[117] evaluated the efficacy of three drug regimens (hydrochlorothiazide and 20 mmol potassium; hydrochlorothiazide and 40 mmol potassium; or hydrochlorothiazide and triamterene) in patients rendered hypokalemic by hydrochlorothiazide while maintaining blood pressure control. Among 447 hypertensive patients, most with a history of diuretic-induced hypokalemia, 252 developed diuretic-induced hypokalemia while receiving hydrochlorothiazide (50 mg/day). In all groups, mean serum levels of potassium increased within 1 week and "showed no further change thereafter." Although each "regimen provided continued control of mild to moderate hypertension," the hydrochlorothiazide/triamterene and hydrochlorothiazide plus 40 mmol of potassium combinations were "significantly more effective in restoring serum potassium levels" than was the combination of hydrochlorothiazide and 20 mmol of potassium. Furthermore, the authors reported that "significant increase in magnesium levels was observed only in the group treated with the hydrochlorothiazide/triamterene combination."

Reports

In at least one case, reported by Stepan et al.,[118] a patient has caused unintended hyperkalemia (and diarrhea) through surreptitious ingestion of potassium-sparing diuretics, with attendant decreased sodium absorption and elevated serum aldosterone levels.

Clinical Implications and Adaptations

Health care professionals treating patients with a potassium-sparing diuretic are strongly encouraged to counsel these individuals to avoid unsupervised increases in potassium intake, in the form of supplements but also as high-potassium foods (e.g., fruit) or salt substitutes, on the basis of the increased risk for problematic interactions. A clinically significant increase in blood potassium levels represents a potentially serious adverse effect associated with potassium-sparing diuretics. The importance of frank inquiry and detailed inventory of concomitant (or even occasional) medications, diet, nutrients, and herbs cannot be overemphasized. Close supervision and regular monitoring are essential, particularly when coadministered with an ACE inhibitor or in individuals with compromised renal function.

Trimethoprim-Sulfamethoxazole

Sulfamethoxazole and trimethoprim (cotrimoxazole, co-trimoxazole, SXT, TMP-SMX, TMP-sulfa; Bactrim, Bactrim DS, Cotrim, Septra, Septra DS, Sulfatrim, Uroplus). Related: Sulfamethoxazole (Gantanol), trimethoprim (Proloprim, Trimpex).

Interaction Type and Significance

◇◇ **Drug-Induced Effect on Nutrient Function, Supplementation Contraindicated, Professional Management Appropriate**

✗✗ **Minimal to Mild Adverse Interaction—Vigilance Necessary**

✗✗✗ **Potentially Harmful or Serious Adverse Interaction—Avoid**

Probability:
3. Possible or
2. Probable

Evidence Base:
◉ Emerging

Effect and Mechanism of Action

Trimethoprim or trimethoprim-sulfamethoxazole (TMP-SMX) may elevate potassium concentration, possibly to the point of hyperkalemia, which although reversible may be severe; these agents also can increase serum creatinine and BUN.[94,119-121] "Trimethoprim (an organic cation) acts like amiloride and blocks apical membrane sodium channels in the mammalian distal nephron."[120] Inhibition of sodium channels in A6 distal nephron cells by trimethoprim appears to play a role in the drug's potassium-sparing diuretic activity.[120] Consequently, the transepithelial voltage is reduced and potassium secretion inhibited, resulting in decreased renal potassium excretion and hyperkalemia.

Research

A small but consistent body of research findings indicates that trimethoprim or TMP-SMX can elevate potassium levels and tend to cause hyperkalemia, particularly in patients with compromised renal function or other major medical problems (e.g., AIDS).

Over several years, Velazquez, Alappan, Perazella, et al.[120-123] have conducted a series of trials and published several papers examining the issue of hyperkalemia during TMP-SMX therapy. In conjunction with a rodent experiment, they investigated the effects of trimethoprim-containing drugs on sodium channels in the distal nephron and renal potassium excretion in 30 patients with acquired immunodeficiency syndrome (AIDS). They found that trimethoprim "increased the serum potassium concentration by 0.6 mmol/L (95% Cl, 0.29 to 0.95 mmol/L) despite normal adrenocortical function and glomerular filtration rate," and that 15 of the 30 subjects exhibited serum potassium levels greater than 5 mmol/L during trimethoprim treatment.[120] In a prospective chart review of 105 hospitalized patients with various infections, 80 of whom were treated with standard-dose TMP-SMX, they observed that serum potassium concentration in the treatment group increased about 5 days after TMP-SMX therapy was initiated. In contrast, the serum potassium concentration in the control group decreased nonsignificantly over 5 days. Thus, they reported that standard-dose TMP-SMX therapy used to treat various infections "leads to an increase in serum potassium concentration," based on the findings that a "peak serum potassium concentration greater than 5.0 mmol/L developed in 62.5% of patients; severe hyperkalemia (peak serum potassium concentration > or = 5.5 mmol/L) occurred in 21.2% of patients." They concluded that patients treated with standard-dose TMP-SMX "should be monitored closely for the development of hyperkalemia, especially if they have concurrent renal insufficiency (serum creatinine level > or = 106 μmol/L)."[122] Subsequently, in a prospective, randomized clinical study involving 97 outpatients, they investigated the effect of standard-dose TMP-SMX combination treatment on serum potassium concentrations. They observed that after 5 days, subjects receiving TMP-SMX (TMP, 320 mg/day; SMX, 1600 mg/day) "developed a statistically significant rise in the serum potassium concentration as compared with the control group," who received other antibiotics. "However, severe hyperkalemia (K^+ ≥5.5 mmol/L) occurred in only 3 patients (6%) treated with trimethoprim-sulfamethoxazole," and "none of the subgroups of treated patients developed clinically important hyperkalemia." The authors interpreted these findings as suggesting that "outpatients, in contrast to [AIDS] patients and hospitalized patients with mild renal insufficiency, develop severe or life-threatening hyperkalemia less commonly when treated with this antimicrobial regimen." Nevertheless, they cautioned that "outpatients having risk factors which may predispose to the development of hyperkalemia should be carefully monitored" when treated with TMP-SMX.[123]

Reports

Hyperkalemia has been reported in patients receiving high-dose trimethoprim as well as standard-dose TMP-SMX therapy.[119,120,124] Velazquez et al.[120] and Greenberg et al.[119] described increases in serum potassium concentration of 0.6 mmol/L and 1.1 mmol/L., respectively, in AIDS patients administered high-dose trimethoprim (20 mg/kg/day). Three other cases of hyperkalemia in elderly patients receiving standard-dose TMP-SMX therapy were subsequently reported.[125-127] Koc et al.[128] published a case report of severe hyperkalemia in two renal transplant recipients treated with standard-dose TMP-SMX.

Clinical Implications and Adaptations

Physicians prescribing trimethoprim or TMP-SMX are strongly encouraged to counsel these individuals to avoid unsupervised increases in potassium intake, in the form of supplements but also as high-potassium foods (e.g., fruit) or salt substitutes, on the basis of the increased risk for problematic interactions. A clinically significant increase in blood potassium levels represents a potentially serious adverse effect associated with trimethoprim or TMP-SMX therapy. The importance of frank inquiry and detailed inventory of concomitant (or even occasional) medications, diet, nutrients, and herbs cannot be overemphasized. Close supervision and regular monitoring are essential, particularly with long-term use in individuals with compromised renal function or other significant physiological burdens and those taking other medications that might alter potassium metabolism.

THEORETICAL, SPECULATIVE, AND PRELIMINARY INTERACTIONS RESEARCH, INCLUDING OVERSTATED INTERACTIONS CLAIMS

Acetylsalicylic Acid (Aspirin)

Acetylsalicylic acid (acetosal, acetyl salicylic acid, ASA, salicylsalicylic acid; Arthritis Foundation Pain Reliever, Ascriptin, Aspergum, Asprimox, Bayer Aspirin, Bayer Buffered Aspirin, Bayer Low Adult Strength, Bufferin, Buffex, Cama Arthritis Pain Reliever, Easprin, Ecotrin, Ecotrin Low Adult Strength, Empirin, Extra Strength Adprin-B, Extra Strength Bayer Enteric 500 Aspirin, Extra Strength Bayer Plus, Halfprin 81, Heartline, Regular Strength Bayer Enteric 500 Aspirin, St. Joseph Adult Chewable Aspirin, ZORprin); combination drugs: ASA and caffeine (Anacin); ASA, caffeine, and propoxyphene (Darvon Compound); ASA and carisoprodol (Soma Compound); ASA, codeine, and carisoprodol (Soma Compound with Codeine); ASA and codeine (Empirin with Codeine); ASA, codeine, butalbital, and caffeine (Fiorinal); ASA and extended-release dipyridamole (Aggrenox, Asasantin).

Similar properties: Salsalate (salicylic acid; Amigesic, Disalcid, Marthritic, Mono Gesic, Salflex, Salsitab).

High-dose aspirin may cause hypokalemia.[129] The effects of chronic aspirin intake on potassium status have not been documented. Clinically significant adverse effects are improbable in otherwise-unmedicated individuals with a well-balanced diet rich in fruits and vegetables, but are possible in the context of other risk factors, such as declining function with physiological aging, diet poor in nutrients and high in processed foods, comedication with potassium-depleting medications, or individual pharmacogenomic variations affecting any of these influences.

Amphetamines and Related Stimulant Medications

Amphetamine aspartate monohydrate, amphetamine sulfate, dextroamphetamine saccharate, dextroamphetamine sulfate; D-amphetamine, Dexedrine; combination drug: mixed amphetamines: amphetamine and dextroamphetamine (Adderall; dexamphetamine).

Amphetamine may theoretically disrupt potassium channels and thereby contribute to some of the adverse cardiac effects associated with these drugs.[130,131] However, potassium channel function and dietary intake of potassium are not necessarily related. Focused research with well-designed clinical trials may be warranted to determine the existence, probability and circumstances, severity, and clinical significance of any such interaction.

Calcium Channel Blockers

Amlodipine (Norvasc); combination drug: amlodipine and benazepril (Lotrel); bepridil (Bapadin, Vascor), diltiazem (Cardizem, Cardizem CD, Cardizem SR, Cartia XT, Dilacor XR, Diltia XT, Tiamate, Tiazac), felodipine (Plendil); combination drugs: felodipine and enalapril (Lexxel); felodipine and ramipril (Triapin); gallopamil (D600), isradipine (DynaCirc, DynaCirc CR), lercanidipine (Zanidip), nicardipine (Cardene, Cardene I.V., Cardene SR), nifedipine (Adalat, Adalat CC, Nifedical XL, Procardia, Procardia XL); combination drug: nifedipine and atenolol (Beta-Adalat, Tenif); nimodipine (Nimotop), nisoldipine (Sular), nitrendipine (Cardif, Nitrepin), verapamil (Calan, Calan SR, Covera-HS, Isoptin, Isoptin SR, Verelan, Verelan PM); combination drug: verapamil and trandolapril (Tarka).

See also Angiotensin-Converting Enzyme (ACE) Inhibitors and Beta-Adrenoceptor Antagonists.

Calcium signaling appears to play a role in both renal and external handling mechanisms involved in potassium regulation. Both verapamil and nifedipine, at pharmacological doses, can impair aldosterone production, but chronic administration of verapamil (but not nifedipine) appears to attenuate aldosterone responsiveness to angiotensin II in vivo after potassium loading. Calcium channel blockers may improve extrarenal potassium disposal. In a review (1991) of the effects of calcium channel blockers on potassium homeostasis Freed et al.[132] noted: "Clinically, there are no reports of either hyperkalemia or hypokalemia with the routine therapeutic use of these agents given alone." The authors concluded that review of the "data indicates that current evidence implicating this class of drugs in the pathogenesis of disordered potassium regulation remains equivocal." The authors reported the "development of hyperkalemia in a patient with chronic renal failure following the initiation of therapy with the calcium channel blocker diltiazem: however, numerous other etiologies may also have contributed to the development of hyperkalemia in this case."

Lavin et al.[37] examined the effect of 6 months' nifedipine (or captopril) therapy on lymphocyte magnesium and potassium levels in 28 patients treated for hypertension. They observed "no difference in serum or lymphocyte concentrations in the two groups compared to 45 healthy, normotensive controls."

Epinephrine and Related Beta-Adrenergic Agonists

Ephedrine (Adrenaline, Epi; Adrenalin, Ana-Gard, Asthma-Haler, AsthmaNefrin, Bronchaid, Bronkaid Mist, Brontin Mist, Epifin, Epinal, EpiPen, Epitrate, Eppy/N, Medihaler-Epi, Primatene Mist, S-2, Sus-Phrine; epinephrine, injectable: Adrenalin Chloride Solution, EpiPen Auto-Injector.

Based on the function of epinephrine/adrenaline as a "stress hormone," some secondary literature has suggested that elevated levels may reduce intracellular concentrations of potassium and magnesium and thus could be associated with hypokalemia.[133] In some discussions, adrenaline and beta-adrenergic agonists are lumped together, even though adrenaline is both an alpha-adrenergic and a beta-adrenergic agonist. Moreover, patients almost never use adrenaline on an ongoing basis; it is almost exclusively used in allergic reactions and other acute care situations, with the possible exception of Primatene mist (inhaled adrenaline OTC drug), which has been linked to asthma deaths, presumably from arrhythmias. Evidence from clinical trials or qualified case reports is lacking, and proposed mechanisms have not been confirmed in relation to exogenous intake of epinephrine as a pharmaceutical agent.

Pending substantive research findings, it seems prudent that individuals using epinephrine on a repeated basis be counseled to maintain a diet high in potassium (as well as vitamin C and magnesium) or should consider regular use of a multinutrient formulation containing these nutrients. In general, close supervision and regular monitoring are warranted in patients prescribed adrenaline or related beta-adrenergic agonists, particularly with repeated use in individuals with compromised renal function, a history of cardiac irregularities or other significant physiological burdens, and taking other medications that might alter potassium metabolism.

Fluoroquinolone (4-Quinolone) Antibiotics

Cinoxacin (Cinobac, Pulvules), ciprofloxacin (Ciloxan, Cipro), enoxacin (Penetrex), gatifloxacin (Tequin), levofloxacin (Levaquin), lomefloxacin (Maxaquin), moxifloxacin (Avelox), nalidixic acid (Neggram), norfloxacin (Noroxin), ofloxacin (Floxin, Ocuflox), sparfloxacin (Zagam), trovafloxacin (alatrofloxacin; Trovan).

Several minerals can decrease the absorption of fluorinated quinolone antibiotics by chelating with these antibiotics when administered simultaneously. In such situations, the antimicrobials appear to be rendered inactive when the 3-carbonyl and 4-oxo functional groups characteristic of medications in this class form chelates with multivalent metal cations, particularly aluminum, magnesium, calcium, iron, and zinc, but also copper, manganese, and possibly sodium.

There is general agreement as to the pattern of interaction between fluoroquinolones and multivalent cations, as discussed in the monographs for several minerals. However, no published research (case reports or clinical trials) has specifically found that potassium acts in this way or adversely affects fluoroquinolone antibiotics by any other known mechanism.

Nevertheless, physicians prescribing fluoroquinolone antibiotics should instruct patients to take any mineral supplements (as well as related antacids) as far apart as possible from the medications, although a margin of at least 6 hours before or 2 hours after the antibiotics is usually adequate, to avoid the potential interaction. It is important to note that this interaction concern is only relevant to oral administration of both agents.

Haloperidol (Haldol)

Haloperidol (Haldol)

Haloperidol has variously been observed to induce both hyperkalemia and hypokalemia.[134,135] The clinical significance of changes in potassium concentrations due to haloperidol remains unclear, and specific evidence from relevant clinical trials is lacking.

Physicians prescribing haloperidol should consider disturbances in potassium metabolism and status among the potential adverse effects discussed with patients and monitored during therapy. Physicians should caution against rapid increases or decreases in potassium intake, from supplements, salt substitutes, or food sources (e.g., fruit), and any significant changes in potassium intake should be professionally supervised. The limitations of using serum potassium levels to detect intracellular potassium concentrations should be kept in mind when watching for adverse drug reactions.

Heparin

Heparin (Calciparine, Hepalean, Heparin Leo, Minihep Calcium, Minihep, Monoparin Calcium, Monoparin, Multiparin, Pump-Hep, Unihep, Uniparin Calcium, Uniparin Forte).

Related but evidence lacking for extrapolation:
Heparinoids: Danaparoid (Orgaran), fondaparinux (Arixtra). **Low-molecular-weight heparins:** Ardeparin (Normiflo), dalteparin (Fragmin), enoxaparin (Lovenox), tinzaparin (Innohep).

Heparin therapy may increase serum potassium levels and has been associated with hyperkalemia.[94,136] Physicians administering heparin are advised to consider potential elevations in potassium levels and caution against rapid increases or decreases in potassium intake, from supplements, salt substitutes, or food sources (e.g., fruit). Any significant changes in potassium intake should be professionally supervised. Focused research with well-designed clinical trials may be warranted to determine the existence, probability and circumstances, severity, and clinical significance of any such interaction.

Insulin

Animal-source insulin: Iletin; human analog insulin: Humanlog; human insulin: Humulin, Novolin, NovoRapid, Oralin.

Matsumura et al.[137] reported the case of 47-year-old man with type 2 diabetes mellitus who experienced severe electrolyte disorders (including hypokalemia, hypophosphatemia, and hypomagnesemia) after attempting suicide by subcutaneously injecting a massive dose (2100 U) of insulin. Although this unique and extreme incident appears to carry minimal relevance to typical diabetic patients, this report has been mentioned as an example of a potential interaction between insulin and potassium. Pending well-qualified case reports or other scientific data indicating clinically significant interactions, further research does not seem warranted.

Notably, one of the standard treatments for life-threatening hyperkalemia is administration of glucose and insulin, which moves large amounts of potassium from the serum to the intracellular compartment to assist in rapidly lowering serum potassium.

Pseudoephedrine, Phenylpropanolamine, and Related Decongestants

Phenylpropanolamine (Acutrim, Dex-A-Diet, Dexatrim, Phenldrine, Phenoxine, PPA, Propagest, Rhindecon, Unitrol); combination drugs: Ami-Tex LA, Appedrine, Contac 12 Hour, DayQuil Allergy Relief, Dex-A-Diet Plus Vitamin C, Diadex Grapefruit Diet Plan, Dimetapp, Entex LA, Robitussin CF, Tavist-D, Triaminic-12.
Pseudoephedrine (Afrinol, Cenafed, Chlor Trimeton, Decofed, Dimetapp Decongestant, Drixoral, Efidac, Genaphed, PediaCare Infant Drops, Ridafed, Sudafed, Sudrine, Suphedrin, Triaminic A.M.).

Unsupported statements scattered through secondary literature mention the possibility of hypokalemia being associated with use of pseudoephedrine, phenylpropanolamine, and related decongestants. Published evidence from clinical trials is lacking to substantiate the occurrence of any such interaction, as is documentation of any proposed or proven mechanism of action.

The sympathomimetic effects of these medications may be similar to effects of the beta-2 agonists.

Tetracycline Antibiotics

Demeclocycline (Declomycin), doxycycline (Atridox, Doryx, Doxy, Monodox, Periostat, Vibramycin, Vibra-Tabs), minocycline (Dynacin, Minocin, Vectrin), oxytetracycline (Terramycin), tetracycline (Achromycin, Actisite, Apo-Tetra,

Economycin, Novo-Tetra, Nu-Tetra, Sumycin, Tetrachel, Tetracyn); combination drugs: chlortetracycline, demeclocycline, and tetracycline (Deteclo); bismuth, metronidazole, and tetracycline (Helidac).

Potassium may interact with tetracycline antibiotics in several ways. As with many minerals, but not as strongly as others, potassium may form chelates with tetracyclines, thereby impairing absorption of both agents. Tetracycline may interfere with the activity of potassium. Finally, self-limiting esophagitis and renal damage, adverse effects associated with tetracyclines, may be aggravated by concomitant potassium or may produce hyperkalemia from nephrotoxic effects, respectively.[113,114,138]

In 1965, Mavromatis[139] published a case describing tetracycline-induced nephropathy confirmed by renal biopsy. This apparently unique report has germinated a concern that tetracycline might cause hypokalemia because of its nephrotoxic effects. Evidence to substantiate this as an adverse event of any frequency is lacking but reinforces the recurrent admonition to monitor renal function and watch for hyperkalemia in at-risk patients.

Teplick et al.,[113] as well as other authors, reported several cases of esophagitis caused by oral potassium chloride ("slow KCl" liquid and tablets), tetracycline capsules, and doxycycline capsules, separately.[114,138] The concomitant use of these agents could theoretically increase the probability of adverse reactions. The authors noted that in "all reported cases caused by KCl tablets, left atrial enlargement was present as the result of mitral stenosis."[113]

Only minimal evidence from clinical trials or qualified case reports is available documenting or substantiating these possible interactions. This lack of confirmation in the literature suggests that such interactions are rare and of minimal clinical significance.

Physicians prescribing tetracycline-class antibiotics for longer than 2 weeks are advised to monitor renal function closely in patients with compromised renal function. Clinically significant potassium depletion is improbable in most individuals with short-term use of these medications. It is generally recommended that tetracycline antibiotics be taken on an empty stomach, with a full glass of water, 1 hour before or 2 hours after ingestion of any supplements, food, or other drugs. However, separating intake of antibiotics from mineral intake may be particularly important given the propensity to chelation between minerals and many medications. Further, potassium chloride should generally be taken with plenty of water and an upright position maintained for at least 1 hour after ingestion to avoid esophageal irritation; other forms of potassium may be tolerated more readily.

Theophylline/Aminophylline and Related Beta-2 Sympathomimetics (Oral and Inhalant)

Dyphylline (Dilor, Lufyllin), fenoterol (Berotec), oxytriphylline (Choledyl), salbutamol (Airomir, Apo-Salvent), terbutaline (Brethaire, Brethine, Bricanyl), theophylline/aminophylline (Phyllocontin, Slo-Bid, Slo-Phyllin, Theo-24, Theo-Bid, Theocron, Theo-Dur, Theolair, Truphylline, Uni-Dur, Uniphyl); combination drug: ephedrine, guaifenesin, and theophylline (Primatene Dual Action).

Although still unresolved after contentious debate for over 20 years, it appears that beta-2 sympathomimetic drugs can affect potassium status to the point of inducing hypokalemia, but that clinically significant adverse effects are improbable in most individuals.[140] As summarized by Cayton[141] in a letter: "The beta2 receptor has an important role in potassium homoeostasis, and hypokalaemia is a physiologically and pharmacologically predictable consequence of treatment with beta2 sympathomimetic bronchodilator drugs, which has been well documented in normal and asthmatic subjects."

In a clinical trial involving four groups of four healthy young subjects each, Haalboom et al.[142] investigated the effects on plasma potassium after inhalation of fenoterolin, a beta-2 agonist. Plasma potassium levels decreased significantly in subjects from the three groups who received fenoterol, whereas levels were unchanged in the placebo group. Based on these preliminary findings, the authors cautioned: "Inhalation of beta 2-agonists may be dangerous, especially in patients under stress—e.g., during an acute asthmatic attack, when the plasma potassium concentration would already be subnormal as the result of raised circulating adrenaline levels."[142] However, in a series of published letters, Smith, Berkin, and others replied that although "it is not disputed that acute beta2 agonist administration lowers the plasma potassium, the clinical relevance of this is not established." Citing prior research, they added: "Perhaps more importantly, the effect of chronic beta2 agonist dosing on plasma K appears to be negligible."[143-145]

Physicians treating patients using beta-2 sympathomimetic bronchodilator drugs are advised to monitor potassium levels, keeping in mind that serum concentrations can reveal hypokalemia but do not accurately reflect intracellular levels, and to be watchful for indications of potassium deficiency. The risk of compromised potassium status is often already heightened in patients with asthma taking steroids or those being treated with digoxin/diuretics for congestive heart failure. Concomitant nutritional support with potassium and magnesium may be beneficial in many of these patients but requires professional supervision and regular monitoring, at least initially, and on a continued basis in any individuals with compromised renal function. Well-designed clinical trials investigating this potentially dangerous adverse effect may be warranted to determine the existence, probability and circumstances, severity, and clinical significance. Discovery, compilation, and analysis of qualified case reports are also warranted.

Thioridazine

Thiorodazine (Mellaril).

Ventricular arrhythmias associated with use of thioridazine in alcohol withdrawal may be caused by alterations in electrical activity within the heart.[146] Coadministration of potassium might reduce the incidence and severity of such adverse effects, but substantive evidence from clinical trials and qualified reports is lacking.

NUTRIENT-NUTRIENT INTERACTIONS

Magnesium and Magnesium-Containing Antacids

Magnesium carbonate combination drug: magnesium carbonate, aluminum hydroxide, alginic acid, and sodium bicarbonate (Gaviscon Extra Strength Tablets, Gaviscon Regular Strength Liquid, Gaviscon Extra Strength Liquid); magnesium hydroxide (Phillips' Milk of Magnesia MOM); combination drugs: magnesium hydroxide and aluminum hydroxide (Advanced Formula Di-Gel Tablets, Co-Magaldrox, Di-Gel, Gelusil, Maalox, Maalox Plus, Mylanta, Wingel); magnesium hydroxide and calcium carbonate (Calcium Rich Rolaids); magnesium hydroxide, aluminum hydroxide, calcium carbonate, and simethicone (Tempo Tablets); magnesium trisilicate and aluminum hydroxide (Adcomag trisil, Foamicon); magnesium trisilicate, alginic acid, and sodium bicarbonate (Alenic Alka, Gaviscon Regular Strength Tablets).

Magnesium plays a critical role in potassium metabolism. The dynamic and interdependent relationship between potassium and magnesium is demonstrated throughout the literature examining the physiology, pharmacology, therapeutics, and interactions of these key minerals, most critically with regard to cardiac electrical activity.[147] Magnesium depletion may be a cause of potassium deficiency, and magnesium coadministration is often necessary to correct refractory potassium repletion.[51,148] However, administration of potassium may increase the need for magnesium intake. Conversely, increased magnesium intake may cause a fall in serum potassium concentrations unless potassium intake is also increased.

The risk of cardiac arrhythmias or adverse effects due to the depletion of or interaction between these electrolytes is heightened in individuals taking potassium-depleting diuretics or digoxin or otherwise at risk of developing potassium deficiency becasue of chronic diarrhea, vomiting, or other factors.[80,104] Physicians treating individuals with such elevated risk, especially those with cardiac irregularities, are advised to encourage patients to maintain a regular and ample intake of foods rich in potassium, particularly fruits and vegetables, and to avoid changes in intake of either nutrient, especially rapid increases of supplemental forms, outside the context of medical supervision and regular monitoring.

HERB-NUTRIENT INTERACTIONS

Diuretic Herbs

Botanical agents with a diuretic action may or may not inherently deplete potassium or other nutrients, and some, such as dandelion leaf *(Taraxacum)*, may actually enhance mineral levels. The plant part(s) used, preparation, dosage, and clinical context all influence the mechanism by which any single herb or botanical combination achieves diuresis and the degree of depletion of potassium or other electrolytes. In general, a huge gap exists between the collective clinical experience of trained prescribers of botanical medicines and the relevant scientific literature of well-designed, adequately powered clinical trials as well as qualified case reports. Nevertheless, such effects and the limitations in the available data are discussed here to a limited degree and more thoroughly in the monographs on the major plant medicines in clinical use.

Ipecac

Ipecac *(Cephaelis ipecacuanha)*.

Repeated use of ipecac as an emetic can excessively lower serum potassium levels.[149] Health care professionals treating individuals with eating disorders or engaged in unsupervised rapid weight loss programs should caution them regarding the potential adverse effects of electrolyte imbalances and potentially dangerous practices associated with bulimia and other eating disorders. Increased consumption of fruit and potassium-containing mineral formulations may be appropriate pending suspension of such behavior.

Licorice Root

Licorice root *(Glycyrrhiza glabra, G. uralensis, G. echinata, G. pallidiflora)*; carbenoxolone (CBX); deglycyrrhizinated licorice, DGL.
See also Licorice monograph.

Licorice root from several species has been used in various forms in the traditional practices of European, American, and Chinese herbal medicine for centuries, if not millennia, and has generally been regarded as safe with professional evaluation and supervision. Nevertheless, high-dose chronic intake of herbal products containing licorice with the glycyrrhizin constituent present can cause pseudoaldosteronism, in certain susceptible individuals, characterized by elevated blood pressure, hypokalemia, and fluid retention, resulting from mineralocorticoid activity. Intake of more than 1 g of glycyrrhizin daily, the amount in approximately 10 g of licorice root, is considered adequate to produce clinically significant adverse effects.[150] Consequently, individuals with a history of or predisposition to hypertension are encouraged to use herbal medications containing non-deglycyrrhizinated (i.e., glycyrrhizin-containing) licorice (non-DGL) only under the supervision of health care professionals trained and experienced in herbal medicine and with active collaboration with the prescribing physician(s) whenever diuretics or cardiac medications are involved.

In contrast, licorice extracts that have been deglycyrrhizinated, and thus are typically labeled as "DGL," do not induce these effects, nor do most of the "licorice" confectionary products, because they generally do not contain actual licorice root.

Senna

Senna (*Cassia senna, Cassia angustifolia;* Black-Draught, Fletcher's Castoria, Gentlax, Senexon, Senna-Gen, Senokot, Senolax).
See Laxatives and Stool Softeners.

The 150 citations for this monograph, as well as additional reference literature, are located under Potassium on the CD at the back of the book.

Selenium

Nutrient Name: Selenium.
Elemental Symbol: Se.
Related Substances: Seleocysteine, selenomethionine; selenium aspartate; sodium selenite.

Summary

Drug/Class Interaction Type	Mechanism and Significance	Management
Chemotherapy ⊕⊕/☼	Selenium, as part of an antioxidant formulation, appears to reduce adverse effects of chemotherapy in treatment of ovarian cancer, most likely by reducing oxidative stress and enhancing activity of glutathione peroxidase system. Further clinical trials warranted.	Coadministration appears to provide benefit without impairment of therapeutic efficacy.
Cisplatin ☼/⊕⊕	Selenium can reduce nephrotoxicity and adverse effects on white blood cells associated with cisplatin, apparently without inhibiting antineoplastic activity of cisplatin. Bioactivation of selenite into selenols is a glutathione-dependent process that enables formation of protective cisplatin-selenol complex.	Coadminister, with supervision and monitoring. High selenium levels required may be toxic. Watch for interference with drug activity.
Clozapine ≈≈≈	Clozapine may decrease selenium levels; this may contribute to adverse effects associated with the drug, including agranulocytosis, decreased glutathione, and effects on the heart.	Coadminister selenium at modest levels. Monitor.
Corticosteroids, oral ≈≈≈	Inflammatory conditions may be associated with low selenium status. High-dose oral corticosteroids increase urinary selenium loss and may lower plasma selenium levels. Selenium enhancement can also support immune function and reduce risk of oxidative DNA damage.	Coadminister selenium with extended high-dose oral corticosteroid therapy.
Doxorubicin ☼/◇≈≈	Selenium may reduce doxorubicin-induced cardiotoxicity without interfering with the drug's antiproliferative effect, possibly by increasing cardiac mitochondrial glutathione peroxidase activity and reducing myocardial malondialdehyde content. Coadministration, at typical doses, is considered nontoxic and unlikely to interfere with therapeutic action of doxorubicin.	Selenium may be more effective when given before doxorubicin exposure. Assess cardiac performance during treatment.
Oral contraceptives (OCs) ◇≈≈/≈≈≈	OCs may decrease selenium levels. Selenium enhancement might reduce oxidative DNA damage and genomic instability, thereby reducing risk of hormone-associated cancer.	Coadminister, especially with selenium-deficient diet.
Valproic acid ◇≈≈/≈≈≈/☼	Valproic acid may decrease plasma selenium levels. Concomitant selenium may enhance antioxidant activity, particularly glutathione peroxidase, and decrease drug-induced toxic effects (e.g., hepatotoxicity) related to oxidative metabolites.	Coadminister, especially in children.

NUTRIENT DESCRIPTION

Physiology and Function

Selenium is an essential trace mineral in the human body, even though it was generally considered a toxic element until the 1950s. Dietary intake of selenium largely determines selenium levels in the body, and the mineral is found in variable amounts in some foods depending on its presence in the soil. The various forms of selenium are absorbed differently in the digestive tract and are retained for different durations. L-(+)selenomethionine is most readily absorbed and exhibits a significantly slower whole-body turnover rate, especially compared with inorganic selenite. These metabolic characteristics provide for efficient use of the selenium contained in methionine.

Selenium plays a key role in numerous metabolic pathways, most notably those exerting an antioxidant action. Selenium is metabolized to methylselenium and S-methylselenocysteine, its bioactive metabolites; it then acts at the level of nuclear transcription factors, signal transduction, cell cycle checkpoints, and cellular apoptosis. Selenium also appears to act as a substitute for sulfur in key signaling enzymes such as tyrosine kinase. In the form of selenocysteine, selenium is incorporated into selenoproteins, which play a central role in cellular antioxidant defenses and serve to neutralize free radicals and reduce risk of cancer and cardiovascular disease. In particular, *glutathione peroxidase* (GSH-Px, GPX), a selenium-dependent enzyme containing four atoms of selenium, recycles glutathione, reducing lipid peroxidation by

catalyzing the reduction of peroxides, neutralizing hydrogen peroxide, and providing anti-inflammatory properties. Within several metabolic pathways, selenium acts as a cofactor, sometimes in the form of selenocysteine. Selenium also potentiates the antioxidant effects of vitamin E. Plasma selenium concentrations influence thyroid hormone levels, particularly the conversion of thyroxine (T_4) to the more active triiodothyronine (T_3), through its effect on the key regulatory enzyme iodothyronine deiodinase; lowered selenium levels are associated with impaired peripheral conversion of T_4 to T_3. Selenium's role in thyroid hormone activation exerts a special role in peripheral tissues. Thioredoxin reductase, a selenium- and NADPH-dependent flavoenzyme, is involved in intracellular reduction of substrates and appears essential to the mineral's anticancer activity. Selenium also participates in immune and detoxification functions by increasing T lymphocytes, enhancing natural killer cell activity, regulating production of immunoglobulin G (IgG) and tumor necrosis factor, and detoxifying heavy metal toxins, including mercury and cadmium.

The effects of selenium deficiency have been brought into focus through epidemiological studies in areas where the soil is particularly lacking in selenium, most notably the Chinese province of Keshan and Finland. Thus, the multifocal myocarditis of Keshan disease provides a stark study of the pathogenesis and pathology of frank selenium deficiency. Elevated rates of cancer in Finland exemplify the strong association between low dietary intake of selenium and increased risk of malignant disease. Diets high in processed foods are similarly depleted of selenium. Numerous studies have documented an association between selenium intake and serum concentrations and the risk and severity of a wide range of cancers. Other symptoms of selenium deficiency include destructive changes to the heart and pancreas, pseudoalbinism, macrocytosis, increased red blood cell (RBC) fragility, immune system dysfunction, myositis, elevated creatine kinase derived from muscles, whitening of the fingernail beds, and a peculiar form of osteoarthropathy known as Kashin-Beck disease.

NUTRIENT IN CLINICAL PRACTICE

Known or Potential Therapeutic Uses

Apart from treatment of deficiency patterns, selenium is most widely known and universally respected as a cancer-preventive nutrient. Although not generally considered an antioxidant per se, selenium forms an integral part of the antioxidant system related to the superfamily of antioxidant enzymes that includes glutathione perioxidase (GSH-Px). Selenium's antioxidant role is critical in many ways, but its cytotoxic and antitumor activities cannot be wholly attributable to such properties. Maximal GSH-Px activity requires only minimal amounts of selenium. Significantly higher levels of selenium, approximately 10 times as much, are necessary to reach levels at which this trace element begins to exercise its cancer prevention effects.[1]

Historical/Ethnomedicine Precedent

Selenium has not been used historically as an isolated nutrient.

Possible Uses

Asthma, atherosclerosis, cardiac arrhythmia, cardiomyopathy, cataracts, childhood infectious diseases, colorectal cancer (risk reduction), depression, dermatitis herpetiformis, diabetic retinopathy, Down syndrome, food intolerance, gingivitis, human immunodeficiency virus and acquired immunodeficiency syndrome (HIV/AIDS) support, hepatitis, heavy metal toxicity, hospital-acquired infections in very-low-birth-weight infants (preventive), hypothyroidism, liver cirrhosis, lung cancer (risk reduction), macular degeneration, Osgood-Schlatter disease, pancreatic insufficiency, Pap smear (abnormal), parenteral nutrition (adjunctive), phenylketonuria (if deficient), prostate cancer (risk reduction), rheumatoid arthritis, retinopathy, surgery preparation/recovery support.

Dietary Sources

Brazil nuts are the single best food source of selenium. Herring, tuna, sardines, calf liver, soybeans, yeast, garlic, and eggs are good sources. Whole grains, especially wheat, can be excellent dietary sources of selenium but provide variable amounts depending on selenium levels in soil where cultivated.

Nutrient Preparations Available

Selenomethionine, selenocysteine, selenium-rich yeast, and selenium aspartate are organic forms of selenium and are preferable. Sodium selenite is the primary inorganic form of selenium and is generally considered less bioavailable.

Dosage Forms Available

Tablet, injection.

Source Materials for Nutrient Preparations

Yeast; organic selenium, selenite.

Dosage Range

Adult

Dietary: Average U.S. daily intake: 100 µg/day.
Supplemental/Maintenance: An adult intake of 100 to 300 µg/day is often recommended, depending on exposure to environmental toxins and individual risk assessment.
Pharmacological/Therapeutic: 50 to 200 µg/day, can be up to 1000 µg/day.
Toxic: Greater than 900 µg/day.

The U.S. National Academy of Sciences recommends that selenium intake not exceed 400 µg daily, unless the higher intake is monitored.[2] Daily intakes of up to 400 to 500 µg daily appear to be safe in healthy adults, although certain increased risks may be associated.

Note: Men apparently require higher levels of selenium intake than women, possibly because stores are lost with ejaculation.

Pediatric (<18 Years)

Pharmacological/Therapeutic: Usual dosage for children: 30 to 150 µg/day, or 1.5 µg per pound of body weight.

Laboratory Values

Blood Glutathione Peroxidase Activity

Blood glutathione peroxidase (GSH-Px) activity is a sensitive assay. The GSH-Px activity of RBCs can be expressed as international units per gram of hemoglobin.

Activity less than 30 IU/g hemoglobin indicates deficiency.

Serum Selenium

Serum selenium levels are transient.
Normal range is 0.9-1.9 µmol/L.

Many clinicians consider blood and urinary levels as inadequate indicators of selenium intake and tissue levels.

SAFETY PROFILE

Overview

Selenium has a narrow margin of safety. Although it is generally considered safe at typical supplement levels of 100 to 200 µg/day; 800 µg/day is probably the highest long-term daily dose that can be taken without the development of toxicity in most people. There are variations in the toxic dose, as with other nutrients, but selenium must be used with caution. Daily dosages exceeding 900 µg have been associated with adverse effects in some individuals.[3] Estimates from cattle and other animals show that the toxic long-term dose is probably closer to 2.4 to 3 mg/day. This would lead to symptoms such as liver, skeletal, and cardiac muscle damage.

General Adverse Effects

High blood levels of selenium can result in a condition called *selenosis*.

Dosages greater than 1000 µg of selenium daily for an extended period have been associated with toxic signs that include depression, nervousness, emotional instability, lethargy, weight loss, nausea, vomiting, garlic-like breath and sweat, metallic taste in mouth, digestive irritation, peripheral neuropathies, dermatitis, hair loss, loss of teeth, and fingernail damage or loss. Rare cases of thrombocytopenia and hepato-renal dysfunction have been reported.

Signs and symptoms of severe overdose include fever, increased respiratory rate, gastrointestinal (GI) distress, paralysis, myelitis, and, potentially in extreme cases, death.

There have been no reports of death attributed to selenium toxicity in humans; however, fatal overdoses have been reported in livestock. Reports of selenium overdose in humans indicate resolution of adverse effects on cessation of intake.

Limited secondary research suggests that supplemental intake of selenium, 200 μg/day, for 7.7 years (average) may be associated with an increased risk of developing type 2 diabetes mellitus.[3a]

Contraindications

Individuals with low thyroid function or iodine deficiency–induced goiter are reported to be at an increased risk of symptom exacerbation with selenium supplementation.[4] Selenium supplementation in individuals with a history of nonmelanoma skin cancer may raise the risk of squamous cell cancer.[5]

High hair selenium levels in children have been associated with learning disabilities and behavioral problems.

INTERACTIONS REVIEW
Strategic Considerations

The wide-ranging roles of selenium in healthy human physiology and the well-known adverse effects of selenium deficiency warrant our attention as a valuable agent in health optimization and disease prevention, as well as a potentially critical ally in disease management using conventional pharmacology. In particular, clinicians must consider the selenium depletion patterns associated with many pathologies and suspected to be aggravated by some pharmacological agents. Selenium's role in cancer prevention has always suggested to clinicians that it might prove to be of therapeutic benefit as a component of cancer therapy. Although the direct treatment of cancer using selenium within an integrative model is just emerging, the use of selenium coadministration within a chemotherapeutic regimen has been the subject of extensive, but still often inconclusive, research. It has been widely demonstrated that alterations in selenium levels directly affect the concentration and activity of glutathione peroxidases. Results from animal experiments indicate that selenium compounds, as well as other antioxidant nutrients such as vitamin E, are protective against lethality and other radiation effects, although to a lesser degree than some synthetic protectors.[6] Further, the strong association recognized between selenium deficiency and cardiomyopathy suggests use of this crucial trace mineral in limiting known cardiotoxic effects of medications such as doxorubicin.

Many of the issues discussed reveal a need for human clinical trials, first to ascertain efficacy and then, on confirmation, to flesh out the particulars of integrative care models using the knowledge, skills, and experience of clinicians experienced in both conventional pharmacology and nutritional therapeutics. Researchers may find value in looking to studies such as the Polish clinical trial investigating selenium deficiency and concomitant administration of selenium (200 μg/day) and antioxidant nutrients for 3 months in women with ovarian cancer undergoing multidrug chemotherapy. Selenium nutrient coadministration was associated with significantly increased serum and hair concentrations of selenium and significantly higher activity of GSH-Px.[7] Further, Last et al.[8] retrospectively analyzed total selenium content in 100 sera of patients with aggressive B-cell non-Hodgkin's lymphoma who had received

anthracycline-based chemotherapy, radiotherapy, or both. They determined that serum selenium concentration at presentation is a prognostic factor, predicting positively for dose delivery, treatment response, and long-term survival. The authors concluded that selenium supplementation might offer a novel therapeutic strategy in the treatment of aggressive non-Hodgkin's lymphoma.

NUTRIENT-DRUG INTERACTIONS

Chemotherapy (Cytotoxic Agents)

Evidence:Cisplatin (*cis*-diaminedichloroplatinum, CDDP; Platinol, Platinol-AQ), cyclophosphamide (Cytoxan, Endoxana, Neosar, Procytox).

Related but evidence lacking for extrapolation: Alkylating agents: Busulfan (Myleran), carboplatin (Paraplatin), chlorambucil (Leukeran), dacarbazine (DIC, DTIC, DTIC-Dome, imidazole carboxamide), ifosfamide (Ifex, Mitoxana), mechlorethamine (Mustargen, nitrogen mustard), melphalan (Alkeran), oxaliplatin (Eloxatin), phenylalanine mustard (Melphalan), pipobroman (Vercyte), streptozocin (Zanosar), temozolomide (Temodar), thiotepa (Thioplex), uracil mustard (uramustine).

See also Cisplatin and Doxorubicin

Interaction Type and Significance
⊕⊕ **Beneficial or Supportive Interaction, with Professional Management**
☼ **Prevention or Reduction of Drug Adverse Effect**

Probability:	Evidence Base:
2. Probable	○ **Preliminary**

Effect and Mechanism of Action
Selenium can reduce oxidative stress and enhance activity of the glutathione peroxidase (GSH-Px) system.

Research
Sieja and Talerczyk[9] found that selenium supplementation positively influences oxidative stress (as evidenced by lowered levels of the oxidative stress marker malondialdehyde), enhances the GSH-Px system, and decreases the morbidity of patients with ovarian cancer undergoing chemotherapy. Their study involved the proprietary formulation Protecton Zellactiv (Smith Kline Beecham, Fink Naturarznei GmbH). In a clinical trial involving 62 patients with ovarian cancer, after standard debulking surgery, all patients were treated with adjuvant cyclophosphamide and cisplatin chemotherapy. Half the patients were randomized to receive, concurrently with the chemotherapy, either the antioxidant formula containing beta-carotene (25,000 IU), vitamin C (200 mg), vitamin E (27 IU), riboflavin (4.5 mg), niacin (45 mg), and selenium (200 μg) or the same formula without selenium, for 3 months. Patients who received both the antioxidant vitamins and the selenium for 3 months were noted to have significant increases in serum selenium concentration, GSH-Px in erythrocytes (RBCs), and white blood cell (WBC) numbers and a decrease of hair loss, flatulence, abdominal pain, weakness, malaise, and loss of appetite.[9]

Nutritional Therapeutics, Clinical Concerns, and Adaptations
The encouraging findings from this small trial support the need for further large, well-designed clinical trials to investigate integrative therapeutic strategies using selenium with and without

other antioxidant nutrients (e.g., Protecton Zellactiv) in conjunction with chemotherapeutic agents. Safe and effective implementation of this therapeutic strategy requires close supervision and regular monitoring within the context of integrative care involving health care professionals trained and experienced in both conventional pharmacology and nutritional therapeutics.

Cisplatin

Cisplatin (*cis*-Diaminedichloroplatinum, CDDP; Platinol, Platinol-AQ).
Extrapolated, based on similar properties: Carboplatin (Paraplatin), oxaliplatin (Eloxatin).
See also Chemotherapy (Cytotoxic Agents).

Interaction Type and Significance

☼ **Prevention or Reduction of Drug Adverse Effect**
⊕⊕ **Beneficial or Supportive Interaction, with**
        Professional Management

Probability:	Evidence Base:
3. Possible	◉ Emerging

Effect and Mechanism of Action

Selenium appears capable of playing a protective role in the treatment of cancer patients by reducing the nephrotoxicity and WBC-lowering effects typically encountered as an adverse effect of chemotherapy regimens employing cisplatin. Cisplatin exerts its antitumor activity through an interaction with DNA, which results in the formation of bidentate adducts. An important adverse effect of cisplatin therapy is nephrotoxicity. Cisplatin also causes changes in selenium levels and GSH-Px activities. The protective effect observed with administration of selenium correlates with higher levels of selenium in the kidney (about eight times) and with higher levels of glutathione in the kidney, both compared to tumors. Selenite is metabolized into selenols, specifically into methylselenol and glutathionyl-selenol; this bioactivation of selenite into selenols is a glutathione-dependent process. Baldew et al.[10] proposed in 1991 that the formation of a cisplatin-selenol complex (from methylselenol) takes place in the kidney, thereby preventing cisplatin from exerting its nephrotoxic activity. Selenium may also bind with platinum and inactivate the antineoplastic platinum coordination complexes in a manner similar to sulfur, with which it shares many chemical properties.

Research

The research team led by Vermeulen and Baldew conducted a number of studies into the interaction between selenium and cisplatin. A paper published in 1988 reported cisplatin-induced changes of selenium levels and GSH-Px activities in blood of testis tumor patients.[11] The next year, in research using rodents, they determined that administration of sodium selenite (2000 μg/kg), 1 hour before cisplatin therapy, greatly reduced the nephrotoxic effects associated with the medication without altering antitumor activity.[12] In 1993 this team reported a reduction of cisplatin nephrotoxicity in rodents after administration of sodium selenite and noted a lack of interaction at the pharmacokinetic level of both compounds. Sodium selenite, in doses protecting against the nephrotoxicity of cisplatin, did not significantly affect areas under the plasma concentration-time curve (AUC) from 0 to 6 hours or the initial plasma half-lives of cisplatin and total platinum in plasma.[13] An animal study by Ohkawa et al.[14] similarly found that sodium selenite reduced toxicity from cisplatin in mice.

In a randomized controlled trial with 41 subjects, Chinese researchers investigated the effects of Seleno-Kappacarrageenan, a selenium-containing formulation, as an agent for reducing the nephrotoxicity and bone marrow suppression induced by cisplatin. Administration of the selenium compound, at 4000 μg/day, in conjunction with a cisplatin regimen, resulted in significantly reduced kidney damage, significantly elevated peripheral WBC counts, and significantly less required volumes of blood transfusion compared with controls. Even though researchers observed no toxicity attributable to the Seleno-Kappacarrageenan, the dosage of selenium administered in this study would generally be considered as potentially toxic, if given frequently, and only appropriate under expertly supervised conditions.[15]

A study conducted in Finland, a country known for selenium-poor soil, investigated the potential benefits of selenium and vitamin E in conjunction with cytotoxic chemotherapy in the treatment of 41 women with ovarian cancer. The chemotherapy regimen consisted of cisplatin in combination with either doxorubicin and cyclophosphamide or melphalan. The 29 patients administered nutrients were divided into three groups receiving 200 μg/day sodium selenate, 300 mg/day vitamin E, or both. Sodium selenate alone and combined with vitamin E significantly increased the serum selenium levels, but the activity of serum glutathione peroxidase (GSH-Px) increased significantly only in the selenium-treated and vitamin E–treated patients with low initial GSH-Px activity. Sodium selenate alone significantly decreased the capacity of the platelets to produce thromboxane A_2 (which should result in decreased platelet activation); it also increased high-density lipoprotein cholesterol levels and prevented the elevation of creatine kinase typically associated with cytotoxic chemotherapy. The therapeutic benefits of selenium coadministration appeared to be particularly evident in patients with low initial selenium levels.[16]

In a 1997 review article, Olas and Wachowicz[17] concluded that administration of sodium selenite reduces cisplatin toxicity without inhibiting the antineoplastic activity of cisplatin. Nevertheless, some of the potentially efficacious effects of selenium, such as reducing myelosuppression, suggest the potential for interference with the antitumor activity of cisplatin. Further, sodium thiosulfate is routinely used to deactivate cisplatin. Some head and neck cancer protocols infuse cisplatin intra-arterially through a major artery perfusing the tumor, then inject sodium thiosulfate intravenously, to complex with and deactivate the drug once in the venous circulation. Given the interchangeability of selenium and sulfur, this could also apply to selenium, but since selenium's doses are orders of magnitude less than for sulfur, the stoichiometry would argue against selenium having major interference. This proposition deserves to be rigorously tested in well-designed randomized clinical trials with well-matched patient populations that are large enough to detect even modest gains or losses of therapeutic efficacy.

Nutritional Therapeutics, Clinical Concerns, and Adaptations

Although selenium coadministration represents a valuable option for adjunctive use with cisplatin, the selenium dosages used in many of the cited studies represent a potentially toxic dosage level. Administration of selenium during chemotherapy using cisplatin and carboplatin warrants caution. Some of the potentially beneficial actions of selenium, such as reducing myelosuppression, suggest the as-yet unproven potential for interference with the action of platinum chemotherapy agents. Thus, safe and effective implementation of this therapeutic strategy requires close supervision and regular monitoring within the context of integrative care involving health care professionals trained and experienced in both conventional pharmacology and nutritional therapeutics. The collective research findings indicate that selenium appears to be most efficacious when administered 1 hour before cisplatin therapy. Selenium dosage, form, and mode of administration should be determined based on the unique and evolving needs of the individual being treated in coordination with the overall therapeutic strategy. Daily dosages in the range of 200 to 600 µg are considered as generally effective and safe over an extended time. Much higher intermittent doses, up to 4 mg, given 1 hour before platinum chemotherapy, appear to be well tolerated, and are unlikely to lead to toxic accumulation of selenium, unless relatively high doses are also chronically administered.

Clozapine

Clozapine (Clozaril).

Interaction Type and Significance
≈≈≈ **Drug-Induced Nutrient Depletion, Supplementation Therapeutic, Not Requiring Professional Management**

Probability:
2. Probable

Evidence Base:
○ Preliminary

Effect and Mechanism of Action
Clozapine use appears to decrease blood levels of selenium and may contribute to drug-related adverse effects, particularly agranulocytosis.

Research
In a cross-sectional pilot study, Linday et al.[18] investigated the possible role of abnormalities in the body's antioxidant defense system in the pathogenesis of clozapine-associated agranulocytosis, an uncommon adverse effect. They observed that plasma selenium levels were lowest in individuals undergoing clozapine therapy or experiencing postclozapine agranulocytosis; plasma GSH-Px levels were also lowest in the postclozapine agranulocytosis group. A subsequent study using a novel in vitro assay technique revealed that clozapine and its stable metabolites are not cytotoxic per se but are bioactivated to cytotoxic metabolites that may play a role in the pathogenesis of clozapine agranulocytosis. They noted that bioactivation of clozapine (and its metabolite demethylclozapine) was accompanied by depletion of intracellular glutathione.[19]

In a 2003 study, researchers gathered random venous blood samples to compare selenium levels in four groups: individuals diagnosed with mood disorder, schizophrenics treated with clozapine, schizophrenics not treated with clozapine, and a healthy control group. They found that selenium concentrations in plasma and RBCs were significantly lower in schizophrenic patients treated with clozapine compared with all other groups. The authors noted that low selenium concentrations in clozapine-treated patients may be important in the pathogenesis of life-threatening cardiac adverse effects associated with clozapine.[20]

Nutritional Therapeutics, Clinical Concerns, and Adaptations
The cumulative evidence indicates that clozapine may deplete selenium and glutathione, and that an association may exist between such status and susceptibility to clozapine-induced agranulocytosis. At this time, there is no conclusive evidence to confirm or negate the need for, or benefit from, selenium administration in individuals undergoing therapy with clozapine or other atypical neuroleptic medications. Given the protective antioxidant function of selenium in general and potentially in prevention of known adverse effects of clozapine, the conservative course of action would be to offer the patient the option of coadministering modest amounts of selenium (e.g., 100-200 µg/day) during clozapine therapy.

Corticosteroids, Oral

Betamethasone (Celestone), cortisone (Cortone), dexamethasone (Decadron), fludrocortisone (Florinef), hydrocortisone (Cortef), methylprednisolone (Medrol) prednisolone (Delta-Cortef, Orapred, Pediapred, Prelone), prednisone (Deltasone, Liquid Pred, Meticorten, Orasone), triamcinolone (Aristocort).

Interaction Type and Significance
≈≈≈ **Drug-Induced Nutrient Depletion, Supplementation Therapeutic, Not Requiring Professional Management**

Probability:
2. Probable

Evidence Base:
● Consensus

Effect and Mechanism of Action
High-dose oral corticosteroids increase urinary selenium loss and may lower plasma selenium levels. Some clinicians have also noted that individuals with chronic inflammatory conditions tend to have a preexisting compromised selenium status that would make them particularly susceptible to depletion by steroid medications.[21,22]

Research
Experimental and clinical studies suggest that selenium modulates inflammatory and immune responses. Low selenium levels are common among individuals with inflammatory rheumatic diseases, although such status does not correlate with disease severity. Peretz et al.[21,22] studied the plasma selenium levels, erythrocyte selenium levels, and activity of the selenoenzyme GSH-Px in erythrocytes of patients with rheumatoid arthritis (RA) and acute inflammatory arthritis. They determined that sustained oral corticosteroid therapy, particularly at high doses (20-60 mg prednisolone daily), was significantly related to the depressed plasma selenium levels of some patients with RA.[21,23]

Nutritional Therapeutics, Clinical Concerns, and Adaptations
Chronically low selenium levels are associated with diverse pathologies characterized by inflammation and immune dysfunction, including rheumatic disorders.[24] Deficiency of this trace mineral may lead to oxidative DNA damage.[25] The use of corticosteroid medications may further compromise selenium status in some treated individuals. Prevention of marginal selenium deficiency or reversal of steroid-induced depletion by moderate supplementation might enhance host defense mechanisms, facilitate symptom amelioration, and support systemic healing processes. Further research is needed to establish selection criteria and refine methods for ascertainment of appropriate dosage of selenium to obtain the desired stimulatory or inhibitory effect relevant to the disease state and therapeutic strategy. When prescribing glucocorticoid medications and seeking to invoke potential benefits of concomitant selenium, typical therapeutic dosages of selenium are in the range of 100 to 200 µg daily. At this time, no research appears to

indicate that concurrent selenium might interfere with the therapeutic action of steroid medications.

Doxorubicin and Related Anthracycline Chemotherapy

Evidence: Doxorubicin (Adriamycin, Rubex).
Extrapolated, based on similar properties: Daunorubicin (Cerubidine), epirubicin (Ellence, Pharmorubicin), idarubicin (Idamycin, Zavedos), mitoxantrone (Novantrone, Onkotrone). Similar properties but evidence lacking for extrapolation: Dounorubicin, liposomal (DaunoXome); doxorubicin, pegylated liposomal (Caelyx, Doxil, Myocet).

Interaction Type and Significance

☼ **Prevention or Reduction of Drug Adverse Effect**
◇≈≈ **Drug-Induced Adverse Effect on Nutrient Function, Coadministration Therapeutic, with Professional Management**

Probability: Evidence Base:
2. Probable   ◉ **Emerging**

Effect and Mechanism of Action

Doxorubicin is a highly effective antineoplastic agent, but cardiotoxicity, acute and chronic, is an adverse effect occurring in up to one third of the patients treated after a cumulative dose of 300 mg/m^2, and increasing sharply beyond a cumulative dose of 360 mg/m^2. The resultant irreversible and dose-dependent cardiomyopathy limits its clinical usefulness. Doxorubicin's toxicity results in significant part from free-radical generation and the resultant oxidative stress. Selenium significantly reduces toxicity of doxorubicin without reducing its antitumor activity. Although inorganic selenium lacks direct antioxidant properties, the glutathione peroxidases and other circulating selenoproteins play a central role in cellular antioxidant functions. Selenium coadministration with drug delivery, typically as part of an antioxidant combination, can inhibit doxorubicin-induced decreases in myocardial vitamin E and GSH-Px, reduce oxidative stress, and reduce or prevent doxorubicin-induced cardiotoxicity.[26-28]

Cardiotoxicity of anthracycline chemotherapy agents is multifactorial and also involves oxidative stress partly mediated by an iron-catalyzed Fenton reaction; iron-chelating agents have been shown to decrease doxorubicin cardiac toxicity. Two conditions of cardiotoxicity have been recognized. The first is a dose-independent idiosyncratic phenomenon appearing immediately after anthracycline administration and is based on a pericarditis-myocarditis syndrome in patients without previous cardiac disease. The second condition is dose related and characterized by progressive decline of left ventricular systolic function, as assessed by the ejection fraction on nuclear medicine and echocardiographic studies, which may lead to congestive heart failure (CHF). Diastolic dysfunction may also lead to CHF, with or without concomitant compromise of left ventricular ejection fraction. On pathological examination, progressive anthracycline-related cardiac damage may include restrictive endomyocardial disease, characterized by fibrous thickening of the endomyocardium, and dilated cardiomyopathy, as a result of myocardial fibrosis and hypertrophy of surviving myocytes. Symptoms can appear many years after completion of chemotherapy, although sequential assessment of left ventricular systolic and diastolic function will show compromise long before symptomatic CHF ensues. Risk of anthracycline-induced CHF is increased by radiotherapy fields that involve all or part of the heart.[29-31]

Cardiac toxicity is similar between equipotent doses of doxorubicin and daunorubicin, slightly lower for epirubicin, and only one-sixth that of doxorubicin for equipotent doses of mitoxantrone. Doxil and DaunoXome (liposomal doxorubicin and daunorubicin, respectively) have negligible cardiotoxicity, presumably because of minimal cardiac exposure to the active drug with the pharmacokinetics of the liposome-encapsulated preparation.

Research

Within conventional oncology, the anthracycline antibiotic doxorubicin (Adriamycin) is considered one of the most effective chemotherapeutic agents against a variety of cancers, but its utility is seriously curtailed by its cardiotoxic action and the attendant risk of developing cardiomyopathy and heart failure. Studies investigating the possible beneficial role of selenium in relation to doxorubicin toxicity have focused on two issues: selenium deficiency in laboratory animals and the effects of selenium administration in several experimental models.

Most authors,[32-35] but not all,[36,37] have reported that in rats, selenium deficiency contributes to an aggravation of doxorubicin cardiotoxicity. In these animal studies, researchers mainly reported that toxic effects in selenium-deficient rats resulted from the effect of lipid peroxidation or free-radical generation on several direct or indirect mechanisms, including DNA oxidative damage and mitochondrial alterations.

Studies on selenium supplementation have focused on its anticancer effects or its effects on the cardiotoxicity of doxorubicin. In the latter regard, conclusions have varied in several animal models. Van Vleet et al.[38] failed to find any significant evidence of cardioprotection after injecting dogs with selenium during a course of doxorubicin. In a study using mice, Hermansen and Wassermann[39] reported that selenium provided no significant protection against toxic effects from intraperitoneal injections of doxorubicin. Researchers in other animal studies reported that selenium administration provided cardioprotective effects against doxorubicin-induced toxicity. Van Vleet and Ferrans[40] injected rabbits with both doxorubicin and selenium once a week for 17 weeks and found that rabbits thus treated with selenium showed improved survival rates and reduced symptoms of cardiomyopathy. Van Vleet et al.[41] described positive outcomes, including delayed onset of leukopenia and prolonged survival, after selenium was administered to pigs receiving doxorubicin for 13 weeks. Dimitrov et al.[42] found that selenium abrogated doxorubicin-induced cardiotoxicity in rabbits without interfering with the drug's antiproliferative effect. Examination of animals that had received selenium showed increased selenium levels in the plasma and the heart muscle, as well as preservation of normal heart histology.[42] Finally, Boucher et al.[43] demonstrated several positive responses indicating reduction in doxorubicin cardiotoxicity after treating rats injected with intraperitoneal doxorubicin, twice weekly for 3 weeks, with 3 weeks of oral selenium, using standard food enriched with 2500 µg selenium/kg. The animals given selenium showed significantly increased levels of cardiac mitochondrial GSH-Px activity, reduced myocardial malondialdehyde content, and no increase in the degree of structural alterations to sarcomeres induced by doxorubicin.

These mixed results may reveal more about variable responses to doxorubicin and selenium among different species, as well as the influence of different dosages, treatment lengths, and delivery forms of selenium, than about the anticancer or cardioprotective effects of selenium. Generally, selenium was more effective when given before doxorubicin exposure.

In an in vitro study, Vadgama et al.[44] investigated the effects of administering doxorubicin and selenium together to several tumor cell lines. They reported that selenium increased the doxorubicin effect in most of the cell lines, including increased levels of apoptosis and decreased DNA synthesis.

Nutritional Therapeutics, Clinical Concerns, and Adaptations

In considering the paramount issue of doxorubicin-induced cardiotoxicity, the parameters of the individual patient's health status, risk factors, prognosis, and therapeutic preferences must be weighed within a process of informed decision making. Safe and effective implementation of this therapeutic strategy requires close supervision and regular monitoring within the context of integrative care involving health care professionals trained and experienced in both conventional pharmacology and nutritional therapeutics. Cardiac performance must be assessed before doxorubicin therapy begins, during treatment, and as part of regular follow-up after chemotherapy has concluded. The animal studies reviewed indicate that pretreatment selenium was more effective in limiting doxorubicin toxicity. Selenium dosage, form, and mode of administration need to be determined based on the unique and evolving needs of the individual being treated, in coordination with the overall therapeutic strategy. Daily dosages in the range of 200 to 600 µg are considered as generally effective and safe over an extended period. A conservative approach to clinical management suggests that selenium administration may provide protective influences and assist the therapeutic process, with little or no known risk that such nutrient coadministration might be toxic or interfere with the pharmacological action of the primary treatment.

Oral Contraceptives: Monophasic, Biphasic, and Triphasic Estrogen Preparations (Synthetic Estrogen and Progesterone Analogs)

Ethinyl estradiol and desogestrel (Desogen, Ortho-TriCyclen). Ethinyl estradiol and ethynodiol (Demulen 1/35, Demulen 1/50, Nelulen 1/25, Nelulen 1/50, Zovia). Ethinyl estradiol and levonorgestrel (Alesse, Levlen, Levlite, Levora 0.15/30, Nordette, Tri-Levlen, Triphasil, Trivora). Ethinyl estradiol and norethindrone/norethisterone (Brevicon, Estrostep, Genora 1/35, GenCept 1/35, Jenest-28, Loestrin 1.5/30, Loestrin1/20, Modicon, Necon 1/25, Necon 10/11, Necon 0.5/30, Necon 1/50, Nelova 1/35, Nelova 10/11, Norinyl 1/35, Norlestin 1/50, Ortho Novum 1/35, Ortho Novum 10/11, Ortho Novum 7/7/7, Ovcon-35, Ovcon-50, Tri-Norinyl, Trinovum). Ethinyl estradiol and norgestrel (Lo/Ovral, Ovral). Mestranol and norethindrone (Genora 1/50, Nelova 1/50, Norethin 1/50, Ortho-Novum 1/50). Related, internal application: Etonogestrel/ethinyl estradiol vaginal ring (Nuvaring).

Interaction Type and Significance

◇≈≈ **Drug-Induced Adverse Effect on Nutrient Function, Coadministration Therapeutic, with Professional Management**

≈≈≈ **Drug-induced Nutrient Depletion, Supplementation Therapeutic, Not Requiring Professional Management**

Probability:	Evidence Base:
3. Possible	◉ Emerging

Effect and Mechanism of Action

Human research indicates that oral contraceptives (OCs) are associated with decreased serum selenium concentrations,[45]

possibly attributable to interference with selenium absorption.

Research

Heese et al.[45] conducted a study in South Africa involving 200 female students, half of whom had been taking a low-dosage triphasic OC for a minimum of 3 months; the others were using no OCs. Women using OCs demonstrated differences in mean serum selenium concentrations that were statistically significant.

L'Abbe et al.[46] measured the activity of the enzyme glutathione peroxidase (SeGSHPx) as an indicator of selenium status in a large sample of healthy, free-living Canadians. They observed that estrogen use significantly elevated erythrocyte SeGSHPx, non-SeGSHPx, and total activities in both premenopausal and postmenopausal women.

Nutritional Therapeutics, Clinical Concerns, and Adaptations

Although the evidence shows that OCs may be associated with decreased levels of selenium and other micronutrients, the clinical significance of these actions regarding cancer susceptibility and other health risks remains unclear. However, deficiency of this trace mineral may contribute to increased oxidative DNA damage and genomic instability and is considered a significant factor in setting the stage for carcinogenesis.[25] Given the ever-growing literature on the beneficial role of selenium in the prevention of cancer, especially breast cancer, the adverse implications of contraceptive-induced decreases in selenium levels become increasingly significant.

Apart from supplementation of selenium, intake levels primarily depend on the levels of selenium in the soil where foods have been grown. Health care professionals providing care to women using OCs may want to discuss the potential benefits of compensatory selenium intake and present clinical options. Many practitioners experienced in nutritional therapeutics recommend 100 to 200 µg of selenium as the appropriate daily adult dose for cancer prevention; such a dosage level would also be generally considered adequate to address the additional depletion pattern possible from OCs. However, the character of an individual's diet, geographic locale, family history, personal medical history and health status, and other aspects of individual susceptibility, particularly pharmacogenomic variability of estrogen sensitivity and liver metabolic processes, need to be considered in determining individual risk severity and the relative need for such nutrient support.

Valproic Acid

Divalproex semisodium, divalproex sodium (Depakote), sodium valproate (Depacon), valproate semisodium, valproic acid (Depakene, Depakene Syrup).

Interaction Type and Significance

◇≈≈ **Drug-Induced Adverse Effect on Nutrient Function, Coadministration Therapeutic, with Professional Management**

≈≈≈ **Drug-Induced Nutrient Depletion, Supplementation Therapeutic, Not Requiring Professional Management**

☼ **Prevention or Reduction of Drug Adverse Effect**

Probability:	Evidence Base:
4. Plausible	◉ Emerging

Effect and Mechanism of Action

Valproic acid (VPA) may decrease plasma selenium levels and interfere with related normal physiological functions based on the medication's expected pharmacological actions. Researchers have produced mixed evidence as to the clinical significance of potential selenium (and glutathione) deficiency and its relative impact for different individuals and within different patient populations. Children undergoing anticonvulsant therapy using VPA may be particularly vulnerable to the hepatotoxicity and other adverse effects typically associated with the medication. Concomitant selenium intake may prevent or reduce adverse effects experienced by some individuals undergoing VPA therapy, at least in part by countering drug-induced depletion. Selenium-dependent antioxidant activity, particularly involving GSH-Px, appears to play a critical role in protecting against specific oxidative metabolites of VPA associated with the drug's toxicity.[47-49]

Research

Recent studies suggest that membrane lipid peroxidation may be causally involved in some forms of epilepsy, and that conventional anticonvulsant treatment may adversely affect selenium-dependent antioxidant systems. Although a significant body of evidence demonstrates that VPA adversely impacts selenium and glutathione levels, other researchers have reported minimal depletion of selenium and negligible clinical implications. Research indicates that VPA's cytotoxic activity is the result of generation of hydrogen peroxide and the production of highly reactive hydroxyl free radicals. Buchi et al.[50] found that the free-radical scavenging action of alpha-tocopherol (vitamin E) and N,N′-diphenyl-p-phenylenediamine (DPPD) protected against lipid peroxidation and hepatotoxicity caused by VPA in rats. Conclusive findings from clinical trials specifically investigating the severity or clinical significance of these effects or the appropriate dosage and specific therapeutic benefits of selenium supplementation have yet to be published.

In 1984, Hurd et al.[47] examined several aspects of altered trace-metal status resulting from anticonvulsant therapy using VPA. They found that administering VPA to rats produced a one-third reduction of hepatic selenium and significant reductions of plasma levels of both selenium and zinc. Also, decreased plasma selenium levels characterized patients treated chronically with VPA as their sole anticonvulsant medication. Further, in addressing the disproportionate incidence of hepatotoxicity and other adverse effects among children, these researchers suggested that this "could be due to decreased selenium concentrations when mechanisms for protection against peroxidative damage are not fully developed."

Several research teams have investigated plasma trace element, plasma GSH-Px, and superoxide dismutase (SOD) levels in epileptic children receiving antiepileptic drug therapy. Kurekci et al.[51] found plasma selenium concentrations (as well as those of copper, zinc, manganese, and magnesium) of patients undergoing valproate (or carbamazepine) monotherapy were not statistically different from those of control subjects, but that plasma GSH-Px activities in the VPA group were higher than in the control group, and the difference was statistically significant. Subsequently, Graf et al.[49] compared antioxidant enzyme activities in 15 children with a history of serious adverse experience (SAE) related to VPA therapy to those of 35 patients with good clinical tolerance of VPA, and 50 healthy, age-matched subjects. In patients who had SAEs, GSH-Px was significantly depressed, and glutathione reductase (GSSG-R) was significantly elevated relative to values for the other groups. Selenium and zinc concentrations were lower in SAE patients than in controls. The authors concluded that

individual susceptibility played a critical role in SAEs caused by VPA therapy and that selenium-dependent antioxidant activity appeared to be central to that protective function. In 2002, Verrotti et al.[52] published their findings from a clinical trial of sodium valproate and carbamazepine (CBZ) therapy for 1 year on serum selenium, copper, zinc, GSH-Px, and SOD levels in 36 epileptic children. They reported no initial differences in levels of all parameters studied between controls and epileptic subjects and that, after 1 year of medication, patients treated with VPA and CBZ continued to show normal values.

Conclusive judgments as to the interaction between VPA and selenium await further evidence from human clinical trials. Hepatotoxicity and other adverse effects attributable to VPA appear to be related to a number of known and unknown factors, including, in some measure, diminished antioxidant capacity resulting from depleted selenium and glutathione levels, age-related immaturity of necessary detoxification functions, and individual pharmacogenomic variability in tolerance of VPA and its metabolites.

Nutritional Therapeutics, Clinical Concerns, and Adaptations

Valproic acid, along with other forms of conventional anticonvulsant therapy, is associated with drug-induced nutrient depletion and deficiency patterns adversely affecting a wide range of micronutrients, including selenium. Use of VPA produces numerous adverse effects, especially on the liver, but no conclusive evidence has emerged to demonstrate the clinical role of selenium, or other micronutrients supporting antioxidant and detoxification processes, in countering these adverse effects or in the treatment of the underlying pathology of epilepsy.

Preliminary evidence indicates a potential risk of selenium deficiency associated with VPA in some individuals and groups, even though there may be no consensus as to its prevalence or clinical significance. Inadequate presence of selenium in dietary sources is common, especially in areas where soils are selenium deficient. Whether or not sufficient evidence exists to support use of concomitant selenium in relation to the direct adverse effects of VPA therapy, a general consensus exists that sustained selenium deficiency, and other nutrient depletion patterns, constitute an enhanced and avoidable risk for susceptibility to cancer and other chronic diseases. In particular, selenium deficiency may contribute to increased oxidative DNA damage, and genomic instability is considered a significant factor in setting the stage for carcinogenesis. Thus, administration of selenium at levels of 200 to 400 µg per day, depending on age, weight, and health status, may be beneficial in terms of reducing specific adverse effects caused by anticonvulsant treatment with VPA, as well as broader increased risk factors. Physicians prescribing VPA are advised to discuss the risks, especially adverse effects and potential depletion patterns, associated with VPA treatment and suggest options for supportive nutritional interventions, particularly antioxidants and selenium, or refer to a physician or other health care professional experienced in nutritional therapies.

THEORETICAL, SPECULATIVE, AND PRELIMINARY INTERACTIONS RESEARCH, INCLUDING OVERSTATED INTERACTIONS CLAIMS

Bleomycin

Bleomycin (Blenoxane).

Recent research indicates that selenium might interfere with the antineoplastic action of bleomycin, an antibiotic used in the treatment of various cancers. Bleomycin is known to damage DNA by free-radical mechanisms. In two rat studies published in 2001, Desai et al.[53,54] found that selenium may inhibit the therapeutic action of bleomycin, most likely by enhancing the catalytic function of glutathione peroxidase.

HMG-CoA Reductase Inhibitors (Statins)

Atorvastatin (Lipitor), fluvastatin (Lescol, Lescol XL), lovastatin (Altocor, Altoprev, Mevacor); combination drug: lovastatin and niacin (Advicor); pravastatin (Pravachol), rosuvastatin (Crestor), simvastatin (Zocor); combination drug: simvastatin and extended-release nicotinic acid (Niaspan).

Recent studies suggest that antioxidant nutrients may interfere with the therapeutic action of 3-hydroxyl-3-methylglutaryl coenzyme A (HMG-CoA) reductase inhibitors, popularly known as statins, particularly simvastatin (Zocor), in combination with niacin. The synergistic interaction between simvastatin and niacin has been shown to be effective in reducing low-density lipoprotein (LDL) cholesterol and increasing high-density lipoprotein (HDL) cholesterol levels in individuals with hyperlipidemia, particularly in the context of personal history of cardiac events, malignant family history of heart disease, elevated inflammatory index markers (IIMs), or other high-risk factors.[55] At this point, evidence from clinical trials, particularly two papers published in 2001 by Cheung, Brown, et al.[56,57] at the University of Washington, suggests that coadministration of antioxidants (including selenium) may diminish this combination medication's effectiveness in elevating HDL cholesterol. However, evidence thus far indicates that the interaction observed was between one or more of the antioxidants used and niacin, rather than involving the statin agent directly. Furthermore, no evidence has emerged to indicate that selenium in particular is responsible for this putative undesirable effect.

NUTRIENT-NUTRIENT INTERACTIONS

S-adenosylmethionine (SAMe)

The toxicity of selenium at high dosages, especially in its inorganic forms, is largely attributable to its depletion of SAMe reserves. SAMe is the body's principal methyl donor, and the metabolism of inorganic selenium requires both extra methyl donors and higher levels of antioxidants on its way to becoming methylselenol.

Total Parenteral Nutrition (TPN)

Numerous researchers and clinicians have reported deficiency and depletion patterns involving a wide range of micronutrients, particularly trace elements, in patients receiving TPN, especially over extended periods. Selenium can prevent adverse effects, particularly cardiomyopathy. A 1997 German review concluded: "The dietary parenteral selenium requirement can be calculated on the basis of the maximal gene expression of the selenoprotein plasma glutathione peroxidase (plGPx). In total parenteral nutrition a daily requirement of 0.01 μmol/Kg body weight for adults and 0.025 μmol/Kg body weight for children can be seen as adequate and safe."[58] Similarly, a 1996 Japanese review of the subject concluded: "Requirement of trace elements for human adults from TPN estimated as follows. Zinc: 3-4 mg/day, copper: 0.02-0.05 mg/day, iron: 1-2 mg/day, manganese: 0.15-0.80 mg/day, selenium: 0.02-0.05 mg/day, chromium: 0.01-0.015 mg/day, molybdenum: 0.075-0.250 mg/day and iodine: 0.070-0.140 mg/day."[59]

Vitamin E

Selenium potentiates the antioxidant activity of vitamin E. Selenium and vitamin E act synergistically and are more effective when taken together.

HERB-NUTRIENT INTERACTIONS

Milk Thistle (Silybum marianum) and Alpha-Lipoic Acid

Berkson[60] reported that symptomatic hepatitis C patients with elevated transaminases who were placed on a "conservative triple antioxidant" therapy comprising alpha lipoic acid, selenium, and Silybum marianum (milk thistle) were spared hepatic transplantation, showed improved laboratory indices, and returned to normal working life. Multi-antioxidant therapy combining alpha lipoic acid with other antioxidant agents, such as selenium and the herb milk thistle, is synergistic in hepatitis C therapy and may provide a cost-effective alternative approach, even in individuals with a poor prognosis.

The 61 citations for this monograph, as well as additional reference literature, are located under Selenium on the CD at the back of the book.

Zinc

Nutrient Name: Zinc.
Elemental Symbol: Zn.
Forms: Zinc acetate, zinc arginate, zinc ascorbate, zinc aspartate, zinc carbonate, zinc citrate, zinc gluconate, zinc glycerate, zinc glycinate, zinc histidinate, zinc lactate, zinc methionate, zinc monomethionine, zinc oxide, zinc picolinate, zinc selenate, zinc sulfate, zinc undecylenate.

Nutrient-Drug Interactions and Drug-Induced Nutrient Depletions

Summary

Drug/Class Interaction Type	Mechanism and Significance	Management
Amphetamines Related stimulant medications Methylphenidate ⊕⊕⊕	Zinc may directly benefit patients with ADHD, and coadministration with mixed-amphetamine salts may provide enhanced therapeutic effects. Benefit may be more probable in older and heavier individuals with low zinc and free fatty acid levels, but research indicates children may also benefit. Adverse effects unlikely. Further research warranted.	Coadminister, when indicated. Complement with low-dose copper with long-term use.
Androgens ⊕⊕	Zinc is key to normal male sexual function, including testosterone formation, spermatogenesis, and prostate function, as well as ovulation and fertilization in females. Deficiency can cause hypogonadism, and administration can elevate testosterone levels, raise sperm counts, and enhance action of androgen therapy, especially when pretreatment zinc levels are low. Adverse effects unlikely. Further research warranted.	Consider coadministration for synergistic effect. Complement with low-dose copper with long-term use.
Antibiotics, oral ⊕⊕/⊕✗/✗	Zinc plays central role in immunocompetence and may enhance acute immune response. Combination of oral antibiotics and zinc may benefit some patients, particularly those with compromised zinc status, but may be contraindicated in treatment of pneumonia during hot weather. Further research warranted.	Coadminister, when indicated, in infants and children, especially with poor zinc nurture. Routine pediatric prophylaxis may be contraindicated.
Antibiotics, topical ⊕⊕	In addition to zinc's general activity in supporting healthy skin and immune function, its bacteriostatic activity against *Propionibacterium acnes* and its role in polymorphonuclear leukocyte chemotaxis are beneficial in treating inflammatory acne. Coadministration of zinc, topical or oral, with topical antibiotics may enhance treatment of acne vulgaris. Adverse effects unlikely. Further research warranted.	Consider coadministration of oral zinc for synergistic effect. Complement with low-dose copper with long-term use.
Antidepressants, tricyclic Antidepressants, selective serotonin reuptake inhibitor (SSRI) ⊕⊕	The central nervous system and hippocampal and cortical neurons, in particular, rely on high concentrations of zinc to modulate the excitatory (glutamatergic) and inhibitory (GABAergic) amino acid neurotransmission pathways. Administration of zinc increases levels of synaptic pool zinc in hippocampus and promotes changes in brain similar to antidepressants. Zinc deficiency may contribute to depression, and coadministration may potentiate activity of antidepressant medications by one or more mechanisms. Further research warranted.	Consider coadministration of oral zinc for synergistic effect. Complement with low-dose copper with long-term use.
Captopril, enalapril Angiotensin-converting enzyme (ACE) inhibitors ≈≈/☼	ACE inhibitors possess a prominent zinc-binding moiety that binds to zinc ions. Zinc depletion at tissue levels and possibly deficiency can occur, with effects of captopril being more rapid than those of enalapril. Concomitant zinc can prevent or reverse depletion. Adverse effects unlikely. Further research warranted.	Watch for clinical signs of zinc depletion; lab tests often unreliable. Coadminister to prevent depletion. Complement with low-dose copper during long-term use.
Chlorhexidine ☼/⊕⊕	Coadministration of zinc can enhance binding affinity, reduce severity of chlorhexidine-induced staining, and enhance plaque-inhibiting effect.	Combining zinc with chlorhexidine indicated for reducing adverse effects and increasing efficacy.
Ciprofloxacin Fluoroquinolone/quinolone antibiotics ✗✗/◇◇/≈≈≈/☼	Binding may occur with simultaneous intake and inhibit absorption and bioavailability of both agents. Decreased therapeutic activity probable with interaction; minimal effect with separation of intake. Limited evidence on long-term effects.	Avoid zinc, or separate intake during short-term therapy. Separate intake by several hours.
Clobetasol Corticosteroids, topical ⊕⊕	Coadministration of zinc and clobetasol (and biotin) may enhance therapeutic effect in treatment of inflammatory dermatological conditions.	Consider coadministration, with biotin, for synergistic effect. Complement with low-dose copper with long-term use.
Corticosteroids, oral ≈≈/✗	Adenohypophyseal-adrenocortical network helps maintain circulating zinc and mobilize zinc from tissue stores. Internal or exogenous glucocorticoids can affect zinc metabolism. In particular, oral corticosteroids can elevate urinary zinc excretion and lower serum zinc levels. Coadministration of zinc may prevent or reverse depletion, but research is needed to rule out potential interference or adverse effects.	Coadminister to prevent depletion. Complement with low-dose copper with long-term use. Watch for clinical signs of zinc depletion with extended steroid therapy; lab tests often unreliable.
Estrogens, conjugated Oral contraceptives (OCs) Medroxyprogesterone Estrogen replacement therapy (ERT) ≈≈≈/⊕⊕	OCs may decrease serum levels of zinc. However, conjugated estrogens and medroxyprogesterone may reduce previously elevated urinary zinc excretion in osteoporotic postmenopausal women. Further research is warranted to determine varying effects of different estrogen compounds in their respective patient populations.	Women using OCs may have increased needs for zinc based on potential depletion, as well as possibly higher needs for folate and vitamins B_{12} and B_6. ERT may enhance zinc status. Individual evaluation of safe and effective hormone dosage levels necessary.

Summary

Drug/Class Interaction Type	Mechanism and Significance	Management
Histamine (H₂) receptor antagonists Antacids Gastric acid—suppressive medications ≈≈≈	Agents that interfere with normal acid environment of the stomach can impair zinc absorption and reduce availability; although among H₂ blockers, cimetidine appears to be an exception. Adverse effects on zinc status may be slow to develop and difficult to assess. Administration of zinc can prevent or reverse depletion and enhance healing of gastric tissue damaged by ulceration.	Coadministration of zinc can aid in gastric tissue repair and prevent possible depletion. Consider cimetidine. Separate intake by at least 2 hours to avoid compromised gastric pH. Complement with low-dose copper with long-term use.
Loop diuretics ≈≈	Loop diuretics can increase urinary zinc excretion, but probably to a lesser degree than thiazide diuretics. Adverse effects from zinc administration unlikely. Further research warranted.	Consider concomitant zinc to prevent depletion. Watch for clinical signs of zinc depletion with extended diuretic therapy; lab tests often unreliable. Complement with low-dose copper with long-term use.
Metronidazole (vaginal) ⊕⊕	Combination of metronidazole and zinc may exert greater therapeutic activity in trichomoniasis than either agent alone. Adverse effects unlikely. Further research warranted.	Consider coadministration for synergistic effect, especially with recurrent trichomoniasis or compromised immune status.
Nonsteroidal anti-inflammatory drugs (NSAIDs) ◇ ◇/≈≈/⊕ ✗/⊕	NSAIDs and other anti-inflammatory agents may increase urinary zinc excretion and contribute to zinc depletion. NSAIDs may complex with zinc (and other metals) and decrease absorption and bioavailability of these substances. Many individuals with inflammatory conditions tend to have low zinc levels. Concomitant administration may provide enhanced therapeutic effects, but intake should be separated. Further research into potential synergy as well as possible nutrient depletion with long-term NSAID use warranted.	Consider concomitant zinc to prevent depletion and possibly enhance effects. Watch for clinical signs of zinc depletion with extended NSAID therapy; lab tests often unreliable. Separate intake by 2 or more hours. Complement with low-dose copper with long-term use.
Penicillamine ⊕⊕/⊕ ✗/◇ ◇/≈≈/✗	Penicillamine is a chelating agent applied to treat overload and intoxification involving copper, iron, and other metals. Zinc reduces copper levels by inducing intestinal cell metallothionein, which then forms a mucosal block, preventing copper absorption and increasing copper excretion in the stool. Concurrent use of penicillamine and zinc may enhance copper limitation and therapeutic outcomes in treatment of Wilson's disease. However, oral zinc intake may bind medication doses when ingested concurrently, reducing absorption of both agents. Penicillamine may deplete zinc, even with timing precautions. Further research warranted.	Consider concomitant zinc to enhance effects for reducing copper levels, with separated intake. Close supervision and monitoring necessary. Supplementation with multiple nutrients may be appropriate with extended therapy if depletion detected; separate intake by several hours.
Potassium-sparing diuretics ⊕ ✗/◇ ◇/≈≈	Potassium-sparing diuretics affect zinc in diverse ways. Amiloride may cause zinc accumulation by reducing urinary excretion, whereas triamterene may increase urinary zinc excretion in short term and may cause depletion with extended use. Amiloride is sometimes combined with thiazide diuretic to reduce zinc loss. Further investigation warranted into potential depletion effects with long-term use.	Consider concomitant zinc to prevent depletion and possibly enhance effects. Monitor for clinical signs of zinc depletion with any long-term diuretic therapy; lab tests often unreliable. Separate intake by 2 or more hours. Complement with low-dose copper with long-term use.
Radiotherapy ☼	Preceding or concurrent zinc may prevent or reduce loss or alteration of taste sensation and hasten recovery with radiation therapy to head and neck. Adverse effects unlikely. Further research warranted.	Consider concomitant zinc to prevent, mitigate, or reverse adverse effects on taste sensation.
Tetracycline antibiotics ◇ ◇/⊕ ✗/◇ ≈≈	Chelation between zinc and tetracycline-class antibiotics (other than doxycycline) and impaired absorption of both agents, to clinically significant degree, possible with concurrent intake. Zinc intake, even small amounts, could impair antimicrobial activity. General consensus despite minimal direct evidence. Zinc depletion possible with extended tetracycline use, but evidence lacking.	Discontinue zinc (including zinc-rich foods), or separate intake during short-term therapy. Consider doxycycline. Zinc supplementation may be appropriate with extended therapy, but caution warranted, even with established zinc depletion; separate intake by several hours.
Thiazide diuretics ≈≈	Thiazide diuretics can increase urinary zinc excretion, possibly causing clinically significant deficiency. Coadministration of amiloride may mitigate this adverse effect, whereas concurrent use of ACE inhibitor may exacerbate zinc loss.	Concomitant zinc may be appropriate if depletion occurs or deficiency develops. Monitor for clinical signs of zinc depletion with any long-term diuretic therapy; lab tests often unreliable. Complement with low-dose copper with long-term use.
Valproic acid Anticonvulsant medications (AEDs) ≈≈	Zinc may play a role in activity of anticonvulsants. Risk of decreased zinc levels is greater with VPA, alone or in combination with other anticonvulsant agents. Further, VPA can alter homeostasis of both zinc and copper and may cause depletion of either or both. Research into protective benefits of zinc coadministration limited, and further investigation warranted.	Concomitant zinc may be appropriate if depletion occurs or deficiency develops. Monitor for clinical signs of zinc depletion with any long-term AED therapy, especially VPA; lab tests often unreliable. Complement with low-dose copper with long-term use.
Warfarin Oral vitamin K antagonist anticoagulants ◇ ◇/✗ ✗/◇	Binding may occur with simultaneous intake and inhibit absorption and bioavailability of both agents. Decreased therapeutic activity probable with interaction; minimal effect with separation of intake. General consensus despite minimal direct evidence. Evidence on long-term effects lacking.	Concomitant zinc may be appropriate if depletion occurs or deficiency develops. Monitor for clinical signs of zinc depletion with any long-term AED therapy, especially VPA; lab tests often unreliable.

Continued

Summary

Drug/Class Interaction Type	Mechanism and Significance	Management
		Complement with low-dose copper with long-term use.
Zidovudine (AZT) Nucleoside or nonnucleoside (analog) reverse-transcriptase inhibitors (NRTIs or NNRTIs) ≈≈/⊕⊕/⊕ X/X	Zinc is central to numerous immune functions, but AZT may deplete zinc levels. In addition, zinc deficiency may diminish drug effectiveness because zidovudine and other NRTIs require thymidine kinase, a zinc-dependent enzyme, for conversion to active triphosphate form. Moreover, HIV-infected populations tend to be zinc deficient. Conversely, elevated zinc status may not always be beneficial, and limited evidence suggests adverse effects in certain patients, especially at later stages of disease. Zinc coadministration appears to provide protective benefits, particularly in patients with diarrhea and opportunistic infections caused by *Pneumocystis* carinii and *Candida*. Further investigation warranted.	Concomitant zinc may be appropriate if depletion occurs or deficiency develops. Monitor for clinical signs of zinc depletion with any long-term HAART therapy, especially AZT; lab tests often unreliable. Complement with low-dose copper with long-term zinc use.

ADHD, Attention deficit–hyperactivity disorder; *GABA*, gamma-aminobutyric acid; *AED*, antiepileptic drug; *HIV*, human immunodeficiency virus; *HAART*, highly active antiretroviral therapy.

NUTRIENT DESCRIPTION

Chemistry and Forms

Zinc acetate, zinc arginate, zinc ascorbate, zinc aspartate, zinc carbonate, zinc citrate, zinc gluconate, zinc glycerate, zinc glycinate, zinc histidinate, zinc lactate, zinc methionate, zinc monomethionine, zinc oxide, zinc picolinate, zinc selenate, zinc sulfate, zinc undecylenate.

Physiology and Function

Zinc is required throughout the human body for protein synthesis, DNA synthesis, cell division, hormonal activity, neurotransmitter signaling, and other critical functions. Zinc's essential role in many biological processes is illustrated by its participation in the activity of up to 300 enzymes, in all known classes. Although its activity in immune function has often received the greatest attention, zinc is required for normal physiological functioning of most body systems, particularly growth and development, neurological function, and reproduction, as well as numerous catalytic, structural, and regulatory functions at the cellular level.

Absorption of zinc occurs both by carrier-mediated and energy-dependent saturable processes and by simple (nonsaturable) diffusion throughout the length of the small intestine, primarily in the jejunum. Absorption is regulated homeostatically, in a range of 2% to 70%, depending on concomitant intake and zinc status in healthy individuals, and is optimal at an intragastric pH of 3 or less because solubility of zinc salts is affected by pH.[1] Zinc is actively transported with albumin, amino acids, and an α_2-macroglobulin; transport is regulated, in part, by sulfur-containing amino acids. Bioavailability is mainly influenced by zinc status and form; however, red wine, soy protein, and glucose can enhance zinc absorption, and iron, copper, calcium, fiber, and phytates (a component of cereal grain fiber) can inhibit absorption. Elimination of zinc is primarily through the feces, with minor amounts excreted through the urine and perspiration.

The average adult human body contains a total of 1.4 to 2.5 grams of zinc, with 60% to 65% stored in skeletal muscle, 30% in bone, particularly marrow, and 4% to 6% in the skin. The brain (especially the hippocampus and cerebral cortex) is the organ with the highest zinc concentrations, with enzymatic zinc (85%-95%) and synaptic zinc constituting two separate pools of brain zinc. Zinc is also found in relatively high concentrations in the eye (particularly iris, macula of retina, and choroid), liver, spleen, pancreas, kidney, prostatic fluid, and spermatozoa. Both red blood cells (RBCs) and white blood cells (WBCs) contain relatively high concentrations of zinc.

Zinc is a cofactor in the synthesis of proteins, fats, and cholesterol, and as a metalloenzyme activator, zinc is associated with the activity of more enzymes than any other mineral. Carboxypeptidase is necessary for the digestion of dietary proteins. Several dehydrogenases require zinc, including alcohol, retinol, and sorbitol dehydrogenase. Carbonic anhydrase, a zinc enzyme, catalyzes the interconversion of carbon dioxide (CO_2) and bicarbonate (HCO_3^-) and thereby contributes to acid-base balance in RBCs. Cytochrome c is essential to electron transport and energy production. Superoxide dismutase (SOD), which contains both zinc and copper, inactivates free radicals in cytosol. Alkaline phosphatase (ALP) liberates inorganic phosphates for use in bone metabolism. The activity of these enzymes may be hampered by disruptions in zinc availability that are subclinical in degree (far short of frank deficiency) and conversely, are enhanced by increased zinc nutriture.

The immune, antioxidant, and detoxification systems require zinc, in ready availability and broad distribution, to maintain their functions at healthy levels. Immune function depends directly on zinc status in many ways through its central role in the production, regulation, activity, and equilibrium of both cellular and humoral immune responses, particularly as mediated by the thymus gland. Zinc participates in the regulation of a wide range of immune functions, including T lymphocytes, CD4 cells, natural killer (NK) T cells, interleukin-2 (IL-2), and SOD. As early manifestations of zinc deficiency, lymphopenia and thymic atrophy follow quickly on decreases in precursor T and B cells in the bone marrow, and IL-2 production by helper T (Th) lymphocytes will drop as lymphocyte proliferation decreases and cell-mediated immune function declines. Thus, decreases in available zinc may contribute to a premature transition from efficient Th1-dependent cellular immune activity to Th2-dependent humoral immune functions. The presence of adequate Zn^{2+} and nitrogen oxide tilt the thymic balance toward Th1 and IL-2 as nitrogen oxide releases Zn^{2+} from metallothionein, an intracellular storage molecule, and together they cooperate with glutathione (GSH) and GSSG, its oxidized form, to regulate immune responses to antigens. Conversely, a shift toward Th2 will be characterized by elevations in levels of IL-4, IL-6, IL-10, leukotriene-B$_4$ (LTB$_4$), and prostaglandin E$_2$ (PGE$_2$). Zinc is well known as a cofactor for SOD, a key antioxidant enzyme, but it also functions as a cofactor for alcohol metabolism and delta-6-desaturase (involved in PGE$_1$ synthesis). Among its activities in protecting against heavy metal toxicity, such as cadmium and lead, zinc's unique relationship with copper gives it a special capacity in countering toxic accumulation in Wilson's disease. Vitamin A levels are also regulated by a zinc-controlled release of hepatic stores.

Zinc plays diverse regulatory and support roles throughout the endocrine and reproductive systems as well as cell growth and differentiation processes. Proper functioning of genetic activities at many levels requires zinc, including the synthesis of DNA and RNA, protein synthesis, cellular division, and gene expression. Moreover, in its antioxidant capacity, zinc protects DNA from damage caused by oxidative stress. Zinc is necessary for the maturation of sperm, for ovulation, and for fertilization and normal fetal development. Zinc inhibits the activity of 5-alpha-reductase, the enzyme that irreversibly converts testosterone to dihydrotestosterone, a form that strongly binds to prostate tissue and thus contributes to hypertrophy. The hypogonadism observed in zinc deficiency may be related to impaired leptin secretion, which is also associated with zinc deficiency. Zinc promotes the conversion of thyroxine (T$_4$) to triiodothyronine (T$_3$) and enhances vitamin D activity. Thus, zinc plays a central role in normal growth and maturation, at cellular and systemic levels.

Synaptic zinc plays a modulatory role in synaptic neurotransmission. In the brain, zinc-containing neurons are found primarily in limbic and cerebrocortical systems. All neurons bearing synaptic zinc are glutamatergic. Synaptically released zinc plays a central role in brain excitability through modulation of ionic channels and amino acid receptors, including alpha-amino-3-hydroxy-5-methyl-4-isoxazole propionic acid (AMPA), N-methyl-D-aspartate (NMDA), and gamma-aminobutyric acid (GABA) receptors. In particular, zinc acts as a potent antagonist of the glutamate-NMDA receptor. Zinc also induces *brain-derived neurotrophic factor* (BDNF) gene expression in the hippocampal/cortical neurons.[2] Anorexia, dysphoria, impaired learning, diminished cognitive function, and other behavioral disturbances and mood disorders, as well as some neurological disorders (e.g., epilepsy, Alzheimer's disease), can be associated with zinc depletion and alterations of brain zinc homeostasis.[3,4]

Zinc participates in the somatic interface with the environment through both the superficial tissues and the sensory organs. In addition to its presence in the skin and release through perspiration, the presence of zinc in the nails and hair is also notable (with deficiency indicated by leukonychia). Zinc's crucial role in skin health and wound healing is inherently related to its physiological and therapeutic activity in epithelial tissue. As mentioned, zinc is particularly concentrated in various components of the eye, where it is essential to dark adaptation and night vision. It also participates in the regulation of sensory perception through taste and smell. Not only is zinc crucial for taste perception, especially of salt, but taste response (or lack thereof) to zinc itself is predictive of deficiency status.

NUTRIENT IN CLINICAL PRACTICE
Known or Potential Therapeutic Uses

Proposed therapeutic and preventive uses of zinc range from the more common, and often self-prescribed, administration for prevention and mitigation of the common cold, treatment of acne and other dermatological conditions, enhancement of wound healing and immune response, to more clinical applications for high-risk mothers and malnourished infants, HIV and other viral infections, diminished fertility and reproductive gland function, gastric and bowel conditions, macular degeneration and other ophthalmologic diseases, and inflammatory processes such as rheumatoid arthritis. Notably, zinc administration can enhance muscular strength and endurance in healthy individuals, even in the absence of zinc deficiency.[5] Pharmacological doses of zinc are administered for the treatment of acrodermatitis enteropathica (clinical zinc deficiency caused by congenital zinc malabsorption), to ascertain level of zinc absorption, and Wilson's disease, to prevent the copper accumulation in tissues. Effective treatment of mild or moderate zinc depletion typically requires months of zinc administration to reverse, and severe zinc depletion can require a year or more to resolve in some cases.

Historical/Ethnomedicine Precedent

Recorded use of zinc dates back to Egypt, circa 2000 BCE, in the Western medical tradition. Known primarily for its use in skin lotions in both classical and folk traditions, its presence as zinc ore in calamine lotion is perhaps its most familiar form in recent popular memory and usage. *Zincum metallicum* and other forms of zinc were introduced into homeopathic medicine by Franz (1827), provings were conducted by Hahnemann (1839), and a large and systematic catalog of toxicology was assembled in the materia medica texts of Allen and others throughout the 1800s; these agents have been included in the official *Homeopathic Pharmacopeia of the United States* for more than 100 years. In the 1870s, W.H. Burt,[6] a highly respected homeopathic physician, wrote: "Zinc corresponds to diseases of the nervous system, the same as Iron does to diseases of the blood."

Although often selected because of their morphological similarity to male sexual organs (or "signature"), the recommendation of mussels (especially oysters and geoducks), seeds, and nuts as male tonics in many traditional systems of nutritional therapy may derive, at least in good part, from relatively high concentrations of zinc (and essential fatty acids). In pharmacognosy, the standard term for seed is *semen*, with both meanings related to substances rich in zinc.

Possible Uses

Acne vulgaris, acrodermatitis enteropathica, ageusia or hypogeusia (loss or diminishment of taste sensation), amenorrhea, anorexia nervosa, anosmia (lack of ability to smell), aphthous stomatitis (topical), athletic performance, attention deficit–hyperactivity disorder (ADHD), benign prostatic hyperplasia, birth defects (risk reduction), cataracts, celiac disease, cervical dysplasia, childhood intelligence (deficiency), cirrhosis (deficiency), common cold, contact dermatitis, Crohn's disease, cystic fibrosis, dermatitis herpetiformis (deficiency), diaper rash, diabetes mellitus (types 1 and 2), diarrhea (including with HIV), diverticulitis, Down syndrome, eczema, gastric ulcer healing, gastritis, halitosis, hepatitis, herpes simplex infection, HIV support, hypoglycemia, hypothyroidism, immune support/enhancement, infection, insulin resistance syndrome, lead and cadmium toxicity, macular degeneration, male infertility, male sexual function, minor injuries, night blindness, Osgood-Schlatter disease (with selenium), osteoarthritis, otitis media (recurrent), peptic ulcer, periodontal disease, pharyngitis, psoriasis, radiation therapy support, rheumatoid arthritis, sickle cell anemia, skin ulcers, thalassemia (deficiency), ulcerative colitis, warts, Wilson's disease, wound healing (oral and topical).

Deficiency Symptoms

Primary (dietary) zinc deficiency in humans was first described in patients with alcoholic cirrhosis (in 1956) and then in rural Iranian children and Iranian and Egyptian farmers with inadequate nutritional intake in the early 1960s. Primary deficiency has largely been considered a significant risk in individuals and populations with malnourishment or compromised physiology. However, awareness continues to grow as to the full extent of at-risk populations from a broad range of age groups, socioeconomic conditions, and living situations. Foods grown in nutrient-depleted soil and processed foods are often low in zinc. In addition to protein/calorie-restricted diets, potential deficiencies from diets replete with zinc-poor foods but limited in foods rich in highly bioavailable zinc are often aggravated by foods that are rich in inhibitors of zinc absorption. Infants, impoverished and elderly persons with poor nutritional status, and those consuming excessive alcohol or with renal and hepatic disease are clearly susceptible, but seemingly healthy individuals with unbalanced nutritional intakes, elevated demands, or adverse genetic characteristics may be equally at risk. Survey data indicate that more than 60% of adults (≥ 20 years) in the United States do not consume dietary zinc at the level of the recommended dietary allowance (RDA). Even by following the U.S. Department of Agriculture (USDA) food pyramid recommendations of the past several decades, an individual will not obtain adequate zinc intake on a daily basis. Moreover, some young women who avoid red meat contribute, at least in part, to their being both zinc and iron deficient. Thus, the typical diet in developed countries usually provides insufficient zinc for healthy function, with infants, adolescents, women, and the elderly at greater risk.[7-10] The prevalence of primary zinc deficiency is estimated at 25% to 49% of the world's population.[11,12]

Mild zinc deficiency is fairly common and can have a significant and pervasive impact within a short time. The supply of zinc within the human body operates with a small margin of error relative to metabolic needs. The very small amount of zinc that functions as the "exchangeable zinc pool" in the human body is sufficient for only a few days without intake. Even with the relative inaccessibility of zinc deposits in bone or muscle tissue, excess zinc intake in the short-term is not usually retained (because of decreased absorption or rapid excretion). Consequently, consistent zinc intake is essential to maintain zinc metabolism within the narrow parameters between healthy function and systemic repercussions of insufficiency. Thus, a zinc-poor diet, poor assimilation, interfering agents, and an increase in physiologic demands can result in adverse effects within a short period. Nevertheless, scientific knowledge of the pathogenic mechanisms and complete characteristics of zinc deficiency remain incomplete.

A wide range of conditions can contribute to compromised zinc nutriture, insufficiency, and conditioned (secondary) deficiency. *Acrodermatitis enteropathica* is an inherited (autosomal recessive) disease characterized by zinc malabsorption and resulting in eczematoid skin lesions, alopecia, diarrhea, and concurrent bacterial and yeast infections. The life stages characterized by rapid growth, particularly pregnancy and lactation, childhood, and adolescence, are potentially as vulnerable as the hospitalized or institutionalized elderly person. Multiple

pregnancies or shifts in growth rate, as well as infection or malignancy, can further aggravate disequilibrium in zinc metabolism. Likewise, deficient zinc intake can occur with chronic dieting, as well as poorly planned vegan, vegetarian, and semivegetarian diets. Excessive iron, calcium, or grain intake, particularly with simultaneous ingestion, may also interfere with zinc absorption, particularly because of phytic acid content of cereal grains. Impaired zinc absorption also occurs in individuals with gastrointestinal (GI) disorders, including diarrhea, pancreatic insufficiency, celiac sprue or other malabsorption syndromes, inflammatory bowel disease, Crohn's disease, and ulcerative colitis. Likewise, injuries or inflammatory conditions, such as burns, wound healing, dermatitis, rheumatoid arthritis, and chronic inflammatory diseases, that increase interleukin-1 (IL-1) can rapidly deplete available zinc due to increased utilization, thus producing short-term adverse effects. Hemorrhage, hemolytic anemias (e.g., sickle cell disease, thalassemia), superficial losses, excessive diuresis, or GI tract wastage into stool can also produce rapid zinc loss sufficient to cause systemic problems. Renal insufficiency predisposes to excess zinc excretion. Macular degeneration, type 2 diabetes mellitus, malignant melanoma, congestive heart failure, and other degenerative conditions are also associated with zinc deficiency. The variety of conditions that can adversely affect zinc status, together with the delicate balance of zinc available within the human organism, render zinc nutriture critical and the consequences of deficiencies pervasive and potentially significant.

The classic clinical presentation of severe zinc deficiency is characterized by diarrhea, poor wound or ulcer healing, dermatitis, psychiatric disturbances, weight loss, intercurrent or recurrent infection, alopecia, and hypogonadism (in males). Immunodepression, muscle pain, and fatigue are also among the first and most important signs and symptoms of zinc deficiency, and immune function can be depressed in humans with even mild zinc deficiency. In general, any rapidly growing cells can be affected in initial stages. Thus, compromised health of epithelial tissues, manifesting as impaired wound healing, dermatitis, rough skin, inflammatory acne, poor nail health, increased incidence of infections, diminished immune response, and elevated intolerance to environmental toxins may also indicate impaired zinc status. Anosmia and reduced taste acuity can also suggest zinc deficiency and may manifest only through poor appetite. Photophobia, night blindness, nystagmus, or decline in visual acuity may signal diminished zinc availability affecting the eyes, resulting, at least in part, from decreased ability to mobilize retinol from the liver. Diminished fertility, particularly with impaired spermatogenesis or ovulation, menstrual irregularities, weight loss, impaired glucose tolerance, and increased lipid peroxidation are among the predictable but often-unrecognized consequences of deficiencies in physiological functions dependent on zinc nutriture. Also less obvious, but more insidious in outcomes, are longer-term changes that can result from poor zinc status, such as slow or stunted growth and delayed puberty or other sexual development, as well as irritability, anxiety, depression, difficulty with concentration and cognitive function, impaired learning, or other psychoneurological conditions. Zinc deficiency before and during pregnancy may contribute to intrauterine growth retardation and congenital fetal abnormalities. In rat studies, zinc deficiency during pregnancy results in lifelong immune abnormalities in the offspring despite adequate zinc intake from birth, which requires three generations of normal zinc nutriture to reverse.[13]

Dietary Sources

Seafood and red meat (especially liver and other organ meats) are the richest dietary sources of zinc, with a single oyster providing about 8 to 15 mg zinc. Poultry and eggs provide moderate amounts of dietary sources of zinc. Whole grains, nuts, and seeds provide smaller amounts of zinc, ranging from 0.2 to about 3 mg per serving, with notable sources being sunflower and squash seeds, wheat germ, hard-wheat berries, wheat bran, buckwheat, rice bran, millet, whole-wheat flour, oatmeal, brown rice, cornmeal, and sprouted grains. However, the zinc in plant foods, particularly whole-grain cereals and soy protein, can bind to phytic acid to form an insoluble zinc-phytate complex and thus is usually less bioavailable. Breads, breakfast cereals, and nutrition bars are often fortified with substantial amounts of zinc. Other food sources of zinc include hard cheese, peanuts, soy meal, black-eyed peas, green beans, chickpeas, lima beans, spinach, green onion, and green leafy vegetables. In general, food processing removes or destroys a high proportion of zinc, as well as other trace elements. The presence of certain amino acids, such as cysteine and histidine, may enhance absorption of zinc from foods.

Nutrient Preparations Available

Numerous forms of zinc are available, as previously listed. Zinc sulfate is an inexpensive form most often used in clinical trials. Many experienced practitioners of nutritional therapeutics, however, prefer to administer organically bound or chelated forms (e.g., zinc acetate, zinc citrate, gluconate, zinc glycerate, zinc monomethionine, zinc orotate, zinc picolinate, zinc-protein hydrolysate), based on a lower incidence of gastric irritation and (presumed) superior bioavailability and utilization. In general, zinc acetate provides the most bioavailable form of zinc, across a broad range of gastric pH.

Lozenges generally contain zinc gluconate, zinc gluconate-glycinate, or zinc acetate. The efficacy of various lozenges correlates with their relative *iZn* dosage, the sum of all positively charged *(ionized)* zinc species for zinc compounds at physiologic pH of 7.4.[14] Although all others forms are available over the counter (OTC) as nutritional supplements, zinc acetate is considered a prescription item because of its use in the treatment of Wilson's disease, although zinc acetate lozenges are available as an OTC drug for upper respiratory infection (URI) treatment.

The various forms of oral zinc are salts with differing zinc content. For example, zinc sulfate contains 23% elemental zinc and zinc gluconate 14.3% elemental zinc. Thus, the amount of zinc in some typical supplemental forms is as follows: zinc amino acid chelate, 100 mg/g; zinc gluconate, 130 mg/g; zinc orotate, 170 mg/g; and zinc sulfate, 227 mg/g. A typical zinc sulfate dose of 220 mg provides approximately 55 mg of elemental zinc. However, solubility and ionizability of the various salts of can have major impact on bioavailability.

Dosage Forms Available

Capsule, injectable, intranasal gel, intranasal spray, liquid, lozenge, tablet, topical. Parenterally, zinc is usually included as a component of total parenteral nutrition (TPN).

For optimal absorption, oral zinc should usually be ingested between meals. However, if adverse GI effects occur, consumption with meals may be adequate and effective. In general, oral zinc intake should be separated from ingestion of high-fiber foods to minimize impairment of absorption, as well as high-dose calcium or iron supplements. Likewise, the antiviral activity of zinc lozenges may be impaired by certain flavorings, sweeteners, or other additives.

Source Materials for Nutrient Preparations

Zinc acetate and zinc chloride are derived from mineral salts consisting of zinc and chloride or zinc nitrate and acetic anhydride, respectively. Zinc carbonate is derived from smithsonite or zincspar. Chelates such as zinc citrate, zinc gluconate, zinc lactate, zinc orotate, zinc picolinate, and zinc selenate are derived from smithsonite or other rock processed with citric acid, gluconic acid, lactic acid, orotic acid, picolinic acid, or selenic acid, respectively. Zinc oxide is derived from zincite and zinc phosphate from hopeite.

Dosage Range

The issue of zinc dosage is unclear and eludes scientific knowledge necessary to establish a basis for widely agreed conclusions. Dietary supplements typically contain 5 to 50 mg (elemental zinc) per daily dose. Moderate intake of 15 to 50 mg daily can be used safely to provide for physiological requirements and prevent deficiency. Short-term, repeated use of zinc lozenges containing higher doses (e.g., 13-25 mg each), with up to 10 lozenges daily, is generally well tolerated for several-day periods. Therapeutic application of zinc at 50 mg, one to three times daily, may be appropriate for certain conditions, such as copper overload in Wilson's disease, under the supervision of a health care professional. The presence of zinc in some fortified foods may alter the equation for any given individual based on consumption, but is often offset by impaired bioavailability resulting from certain dietary constituents and how they affect certain forms of zinc.

Adult

Dietary: The U.S. RDA for zinc is 15 mg per day for adult men and 12 mg per day for adult women, but average daily intake in developed societies is typically only 60% to 70% of that amount, with the average adult daily diet in the United Kingdom providing 11.7 mg for men and 8.7 mg for women. The official U.S. recommendations for daily intake in pregnant women is 11 mg (13 mg if ≤18 years old) and 12 mg for nursing women (14 mg if ≤18 years old).
Supplemental/Maintenance: 15 to 50 mg per day, preferably with copper.

In some respects, however, zinc intake beyond adequate dietary intake is sometimes considered inappropriate unless indicated, given "almost no gap for supplementation" above the RDA and the reference dose (RfD) for safe intake of zinc, although, as noted, usually a gap exists between average daily dietary intake and the recommended daily intake.[12] Few data are available on optimal zinc intakes (as assessed by function of zinc-dependent enzymes in free-living human subjects), and it is likely that optimal intakes vary considerably depending on age, lifestyle, and various states of health and disease.
Pharmacological/Therapeutic: 50 to 350 mg (elemental zinc) per day.

Oral doses as high as 220 mg zinc sulfate three times daily have been used in trials of zinc for the prevention of crisis in sickle cell anemia, and twice daily for 12 weeks to correct zinc deficiency in cirrhotic patients with symptoms of deficiency (e.g., blunted taste/smell).[15,16] In a trial involving patients with chronic fatigue syndrome, 135 mg/day was administered for 15 days (along with 2 mg copper daily) to correct zinc deficiency.[17]

Toxic: Toxicity can occur at levels as low as 60 mg/day (with prolonged intake) but is more frequently associated with doses higher than 300 mg/day. Prolonged intake at doses higher than 150 mg/day may be associated with adverse effects. The official U.S. tolerable upper limit (UL) for adults (≥19 years) is 40 mg, including pregnant or nursing women, although it is 34 mg/day if such women are 18 years old or younger.[18] This amount includes dietary intake and thus may vary considerably with high consumption of fortified foods or foods naturally rich in zinc.

Pediatric (<18 Years)

Dietary: Zinc concentrations in breast milk are relatively low, but such zinc is highly absorbable. Official U.S. recommendations for daily intake follow[18]:

> Infants, birth to 6 months: 2 mg/day
> Infants, 7 to 12 months: 3 mg/day
> Children, 1 to 3 years: 3 mg/day
> Children, 4 to 8 years: 5 mg/day
> Children, 9 to 13 years: 8 mg/day
> Adolescents, 14 to 18 years: 9 mg/day for females; 11 mg/day for males

Clinical experience with adolescents suggests that much larger amounts may be required during growth spurts (up to 40 mg/day).

Supplemental/Maintenance: Usually not recommended for children under 12 years of age with healthy, balanced diet, without excessive dietary phytates.

Pharmacological/Therapeutic: 5 to 40 mg per day, for specified periods.

Trials investigating zinc supplementation in infants born small for gestational age (SGA) typically use 5 mg zinc sulfate daily, often combined with other nutrients.[19] Zinc acetate (10 mg twice daily for 5 days) has been used successfully in infants and young children with severe acute lower respiratory infection.[20] Several prominent trials have found efficacy of low-dose oral zinc in acute and persistent diarrhea in children under 5 years of age in developing countries.

Toxic: 150 mg/day on a chronic basis, or acutely with doses greater than 200 mg daily. However, the toxic dose of zinc depends primarily on dose and duration, and also varies with status and absorption, weight, and concomitant intake. Single intravenous (IV) doses of 1 to 2 mg zinc/kg body weight have been given to adult leukemia patients without toxic manifestations. Consensus as to toxic dose in clinical applications has not been established, and plasma levels sufficient to produce symptoms of toxic manifestations are not known.

Tolerable upper intake levels (UL) for zinc follow[18]:

> Infants, 0 to 6 months: 4 mg/day
> Infants, 7 to 12 months: 5 mg/day
> Children, 1 to 3 years: 7 mg/day
> Children, 4 to 8 years: 12 mg/day
> Children, 9 to 13 years: 23 mg/day
> Adolescents, 14 to 18 years: 34 mg/day

Laboratory Values

Overview

Clinicians and researchers broadly agree that clinical presentation and response to zinc administration provide the most accurate means of assessing zinc status and confirming deficiency status.

Thereafter, retesting (e.g., plasma zinc) and reevaluation of symptoms after 4 to 6 months of treatment are usually effective for determining if dosages need adjustment. In a review, Hambridge[21] (2003) concluded that there is a "compelling demand for improved zinc biomarkers" based on numerous characteristics peculiar to the physiology of zinc in the human organism. "More specific markers of zinc status are needed, and their relationships to zinc-dependent cellular functions and the distribution and allocation of zinc to the different organ systems need to be clarified." Some physicians experienced in nutritional therapeutics consider measuring the leukocyte zinc level as the best laboratory method for determining zinc status.[22] Most clinicians and researchers do not consider hair a reliable form of analysis for measuring tissue levels of zinc.[23] Moreover, some clinicians observe that urine and hair tissue levels are often elevated in patients with zinc deficiency because of dysfunction in zinc metabolism and high rates of excretion.

Erythrocyte Zinc

Most of the zinc measured as erythrocyte zinc is incorporated in carbonic anhydrase. Although some studies report detection of depletion through low levels, erythrocyte zinc has been generally regarded as not readily depleted and therefore not accurately indicative of zinc status.[24]

Hair Zinc

Some clinicians have suggested that analysis of hair zinc concentrations might reveal associations between low hair zinc levels and zinc depletion status. However, numerous factors, such as age, growth rate, and dietary intake of phytates and meat, can confound analysis and decrease this test's ability to consistently determine impaired zinc status or inadequate intake.[23,25-29] Antidandruff shampoos often incorporate zinc as well, which can greatly elevate hair zinc levels.

Plasma Zinc

The range for normal plasma levels for zinc is 58 to 106 μg/dL. In blood plasma, zinc is bound to albumin (80%) and to α_2-macroglobulin (20%). Plasma zinc levels appear to follow a circadian rhythm, with the highest values occurring late morning, at approximately 10 AM. Plasma zinc can be normal even when plasma albumin is low, because albumin normally contains many unsaturated binding sites.

Plasma zinc and serum zinc are often used in clinical and research settings but are physiologically insensitive and of limited diagnostic value. Hambridge[21] observed: "Plasma zinc is currently the most widely used and accepted biomarker of zinc status despite poor sensitivity and imperfect specificity.... One reason that plasma zinc does not accurately reflect the volatile relationship between zinc intake and absorption is that homeostatic control of plasma zinc concentrations can occur while moderate changes are occurring in the zinc content of one or more of the pools of zinc that exchange rapidly with zinc in plasma." Furthermore, the decline that occurs as a recognized component of the acute-phase response in infections represents at least one important limitation affecting the specificity of plasma zinc as an index of zinc status.[30,31] Severe acute zinc deficiency states, such as untreated acrodermatitis enteropathica, may reveal profoundly depressed plasma zinc levels. However, mild zinc deficiencies that can adversely affect physiological function may appear as plasma zinc concentrations within the normal range, as with growth-limiting zinc deficiency states in young children.[26] Various studies have conflicting findings and mixed conclusions regarding an association between zinc intake and plasma zinc.

Nevertheless, concentrations less than 70 µg zinc/dL plasma can serve as a useful predictor of growth response to zinc supplementation, and beneficial effects of zinc administration in the prevention and management of diarrhea can be predicted using lower cutoff values. Plasma levels less than 70 µg/dL might constitute a better definition of deficiency state.

Red Cell Membrane Zinc

Metallothionein levels in erythrocytes respond to administration of zinc as well as restricted dietary intake.[32] Thus, RBC membrane zinc may be a sensitive indicator of zinc depletion, but its practical implementation on a widespread basis is considered unlikely given the complexity of sample preparation. A parallel situation appears with monocyte, neutrophil, or platelet zinc.[33-36]

Serum Zinc

Serum zinc concentration less than 33 µg/dL indicates zinc deficiency. Serum levels 33 to 50 µg/dL indicate marginal zinc status. The normal range for serum zinc is 67 to 124 µg/dL, although this varies between clinical laboratories.

Serum zinc is considered an insensitive marker of physiological zinc status, for the same reasons previously stated in relationship to plasma zinc.

White Blood Cell Zinc

The levels of zinc in leukocytes or lymphocytes appears to reflect zinc status accurately, particularly in relation to key zinc-related functions such as immune function, life stage, and growth processes. For example, leukocyte (WBC) zinc is reflective of fetal growth and associated with maternal muscle zinc concentration. Likewise, activity of lymphocyte ecto-5'-nucleotidase is a sensitive indicator of zinc status.[12,37-41]

Assessment of gene expression of zinc-dependent genes in lymphocytes (specifically cellular zinc transporter hZip1) offers promise as a biomarker of expression of the cellular zinc response to zinc intake and bioassay for zinc status.[42]

Zinc Tally

In this quick and simple screening method for evaluating zinc status, the absence of the typical metallic taste of zinc, after placing 2 teaspoons of a 0.1% solution of zinc sulfate heptahydrate in the patient's mouth and holding it there for 10 seconds, suggests deficiency. An immediate taste perception indicates that zinc status may be adequate; conversely, lack of zinc taste suggests deficiency.

Zinc Tolerance Test

In this test an oral load of 50 mg elemental zinc is administered, after a baseline plasma zinc measurement, and plasma zinc is remeasured 120 minutes later. A twofold to threefold increase in plasma zinc indicates zinc deficiency. Zinc supplements need to be avoided for 24 hours before sampling of plasma.

CD4+/CD8+ T-Lymphocyte Ratio and Thymulin Activity

The CD4+/CD8+ T-lymphocyte ratio and thymulin activity have been advanced as potential immunological tests for zinc deficiency, but evidence confirming their accuracy is lacking.

Other findings possibly consistent with zinc insufficiency, but also resulting from other causes, include the following[43]:

- Elevated anserine and carnosine peptides, with low levels of essential amino acids, in urine or plasma amino acid analysis.
- Elevated phosphoserine and phosphoethanolamine in urine amino acid analysis.

- Elevated lactic acid in plasma or urine (lactic acid dehydrogenase also is zinc dependent).
- Elevated or normal linolenic acid, but low gamma-linolenic acid, consistent with weak delta-6-desaturase activity (zinc dependent).

SAFETY PROFILE
Overview

Zinc dosage beyond the RDA is not established, and the perpetually marginal nature of zinc nutriture leaves a relatively small dosage range and tight time frame for safe and effective use of zinc between suboptimal and potentially toxic intake levels, particularly with extended use outside a balanced nutrient regimen. The affinity of zinc for certain tissues appears to result in a pattern of benefit and toxicity converging (e.g., immune system, possibly prostate). The dose typically used for short-term immune stimulation as a lozenge (13-25 mg each) would be excessive for continued use with oral intake and could impair immune function (at >150-300 mg/day). Likewise, 25 to 30 mg daily has been used to improve pregnancy outcomes in low-income pregnant women and pregnant teenagers, but a significantly higher dose could have potentially adverse effects during pregnancy, especially on embryogenesis.

Zinc is perhaps the least toxic mineral nutrient at usual doses but can be strikingly toxic at very high doses associated with industrial exposure. Notably, major authorities on zinc physiology, requirements, and safety acknowledge the limited scope of scientific knowledge as to its physiological functions, the multiple variables affecting bioavailability, dynamic relationships between zinc and other minerals, parameters governing insufficiency and toxicity, and methods of assessing functional zinc levels.

Nutrient Adverse Effects
General Adverse Effects

Zinc is generally considered relatively nontoxic at low to moderate levels typical of supplemental use: less than 50 mg elemental per day. Given the narrow gap between potentially insufficient and excessive levels, both deficiency and toxicity can vary significantly among individuals based on tissue and circulating levels, historic intake, zinc pool status, recent or active infection, blood loss or other depletion factors, dietary interactions, and other variables. Gastrointestinal upset and nausea are quite common when zinc supplements, especially zinc sulfate, are taken on an empty stomach. More importantly, zinc administration, especially lacking in compensatory copper support, can produce adverse effects rapidly (as with deficiency), which grow in intensity based on dose and duration and influenced by other variables. The primary toxic effects of zinc, typically associated with prolonged intake at levels greater than 150 mg daily, include copper deficiency anemia, depressed immune function, and reduced high-density lipoprotein (HDL) cholesterol levels.

Topical zinc preparations are generally considered safe and unlikely to produce any adverse effects. However, anosmia has been reported with zinc nasal spray and in rare cases has been reported to be severe or permanent.[44]

The primary effects of zinc toxicity can occur with doses higher than 150 mg/day on a chronic basis or acutely with doses greater than 200 mg daily. They include diarrhea, nausea, vomiting, metallic taste in the mouth, dizziness, drowsiness, incoordination, and lethargy. Gastric erosion and hematuria with chronic high-dose use have been reported but not confirmed. Ingestion of 10 to 30 g of zinc sulfate can be lethal in adults. However, acute zinc toxicity is extremely rare because ingestion of the amounts required for toxicity symptoms (2 g/kg) will usually provoke vomiting before toxic dose levels are attained. Impairment of copper absorption can begin at daily doses as low as 50 mg elemental zinc, with copper depletion accruing over time and manifesting as low serum copper and ceruloplasmin levels, microcytic anemia, and neutropenia; iron deficiency is also possible. Immune function can become impaired, HDL cholesterol levels decrease, and total cholesterol levels increase with daily doses over 300 mg/day for extended periods, but possibly as low as 150 mg/day, perhaps as a result of induced copper deficiency.[45-49] Subsequently, zinc-induced copper deficiency has been associated with cases of reversible acquired sideroblastic anemia, cardiac arrhythmias, and bone marrow depression. Such reports have involved chronic intake of 450 to 1600 mg daily, and many such cases are properly characterized as zinc abuse, with ingestion of coins being the source of zinc in one individual.[50-55] Inhalation of zinc oxide in certain industrial settings and the use of galvanized pipes for drinking water are also known causes of excess zinc exposure.

Short-term frequent use of zinc lozenges can occasionally produce digestive upset, local oral irritation, and unpleasant taste; typically reversible with cessation.[49,56]

Adverse Effects Among Specific Populations

One study from India suggests that the concomitant use of zinc and oral antibiotics in the acute management of pneumonia of infants or children may delay recovery during the hot season, particularly in the absence of zinc deficiency.[57]

Two preliminary papers by Bush et al.[58,59] discussed the possibility of zinc aggravating amyloid formation in individuals with Alzheimer's disease. However, subsequent research articles and reviews have concluded that zinc does not cause or exacerbate Alzheimer's disease symptoms, and may enhance mental function by improving platelet membrane microviscosity.[60,61]

Genotoxicity

"Zinc is apparently neither a mutagen nor a carcinogen."[12,62] However, in one study analyzing data from a larger trial, researchers reported a slight increase in the relative risk of prostate cancer among men who used zinc supplements for more than 10 years, particularly at doses greater than 100 mg elemental zinc daily.[63]

Pregnancy and Nursing

Maternal nutritional zinc deficit "can have permanent negative effects on the growth of offspring," and zinc administration at typical dose levels may be beneficial during pregnancy. However, excess zinc intake "during embryogenesis can be teratogenic or lethal," and premature birth and stillbirth have been reported when women consumed 100 mg three times daily during the third trimester.[12,62,64] The use of supplemental zinc by nursing mothers over an extended period, without compensatory copper support, could contribute to zinc-induced copper deficiency in breastfed infants. Nevertheless, no reports or studies in the scientific literature show any adverse effects on fetal development from supplemental zinc, at typical doses, in well-nourished mothers or in infants who are breastfed.

Contraindications

No contraindications have been established for zinc.

Precautions and Warnings

Extended use of zinc without copper carries a warning. The recommended ratio of zinc to copper is 15:1 to 20:1. This ratio is higher in elderly persons, who, in the United States, tend to have high copper levels and low zinc levels because of a history of chronic ingestion of water carried through copper pipes.

INTERACTIONS REVIEW
Strategic Considerations

Three simple and consistent themes are recurrent among the various interactions between zinc and pharmacological agents. First, as a mineral/metal, zinc tends to chelate with many substances when ingested simultaneously or in temporal proximity. This potential problem is easily avoided through patient education and clinical management; individuals should separate intake, preferably taking zinc at least 2 hours before or 4 hours after such medications. Second, in all situations except the treatment of individuals with Wilson's disease, the default prudent measure with any long-term application of zinc is to avoid zinc-induced copper deficiency by periodically monitoring serum copper levels and coadministering low-dose copper (1-3 mg/day). Third, within the human organism, zinc is volatile with an ever-shifting distribution between pools. Thus, establishing zinc deficiency or monitoring the impact of any agent on functional zinc status is difficult and unreliable. Consequently, at usual dosage levels and with attentiveness to clinical manifestations of zinc deficiency (or excess), coadministration of zinc within a therapeutic strategy carries minimal risk of adverse interactions, other than copper depletion and the predictable chelation phenomena common to most minerals when ingested with other substances.

Numerous pharmaceutical agents are associated with adverse effects, both subtle and overt, of zinc depletion. Consequently, numerous clinical situations occur in which coadministration of zinc may improve zinc nutriture, related physiological functions, and clinical manifestations, even when prior conventional laboratory assessment had revealed no measurable signs of depletion, insufficiency, or deficiency. These recurrent patterns indicate two probable phenomena: zinc can provide benefit in the absence of depletion, detected or not, and conventional laboratory methods currently applied for assessing zinc status are insensitive and inadequate to clinical demands. Our limited knowledge of the many functions of zinc is repeatedly revealed in the sparsity and limited depth of both the observations of zinc-related benefits and interactions and the mechanisms involved.

Many widely used pharmaceutical agents contribute to zinc depletion, usually through binding and increased urinary zinc excretion. Thus, coadministration of zinc may reduce depletion effects or prevent other adverse effects associated with a wide range of medications used to treat hypertension, inflammation, and other conditions. Particularly with chronic use, thiazide diuretics increase urinary zinc excretion, as do loop diuretics, although probably to a lesser degree. Although patients treated with angiotensin-converting enzyme (ACE) inhibitors (especially captopril) at clearly are risk for zinc depletion, the effects of potassium-sparing diuretics on zinc are diverse and complicated. Furthermore, amiloride is often combined with a thiazide diuretic to reduce mineral loss, but amiloride may cause zinc accumulation by reducing urinary excretion. In contrast, triamterene can increase urinary zinc excretion in the short-term and cause depletion with extended use. In patients treated with antacids and gastric acid–suppressive medications, long-term drug therapy can impair zinc absorption and reduce availability by interfering with the normal acid environment of the stomach; although cimetidine appears to be an exception among H_2 blockers. With these drugs, administration of zinc can prevent or reverse depletion and enhance healing of gastric tissue damaged by ulceration. When coadministered with nonsteroidal anti-inflammatory drugs (NSAIDs), zinc may reduce risk of adverse effects on zinc status while providing protective effects and contributing to enhanced therapeutic outcomes.

Oral corticosteroids and valproic acid, alone or in combination with other anticonvulsant agents, represent examples of medications that can deplete zinc, but for which evidence of benefit from concomitant zinc is limited or lacking.

Evidence of variable strength suggests a probable synergy or other benefit from concomitant zinc administration with a wide range of conventional interventions, including mixed amphetamines, androgens, clobetasol (and potentially other topical corticosteroids), metronidazole (in treating trichomoniasis), and chlorhexidine-zinc oral rinse. In the treatment of individuals with Wilson's disease, concomitant zinc may enhance the therapeutic activity of penicillamine in reducing copper levels, although intake needs to be separated. Zinc therapy can be applied to reduce adverse effects to taste sensation in patients receiving radiation therapy, particularly to the head and neck.

In several areas the coadministration of zinc with conventional therapies appears to produce mixed effects, depending on patient characteristics, with full implications as yet unclear. For example, in women of reproductive age, oral contraceptives may decrease serum levels of zinc; conversely, osteoporotic postmenopausal women taking conjugated estrogens and medroxyprogesterone may exhibit reductions in previously elevated urinary zinc excretion. Zidovudine (AZT) and related antiretroviral agents present another complicated situation where divergent responses are common. In a patient population often characterized by zinc insufficiency, zinc coadministration may reduce drug-related adverse effects, add protective benefits (particularly in patients with diarrhea and opportunistic infections), provide no significant benefit, or even potentially elevate the risk of complications.

Numerous clinical situations allow for possible synergy, particularly in individuals or populations at greater risk for compromised zinc or broader nutritional status. The areas of antibiotic therapy, oral or topical, and antidepressant medications, particularly tricyclic and selective serotonin reuptake inhibitor (SSRI) antidepressants, offer significant potential for continued research into integrative therapeutic applications.

In many situations, zinc (as well as most other minerals) tends to bind with other substances and thereby decrease bioavailability and therapeutic action or nutritive value of both agents. Separation of intake remediates this problem. Antibiotics from the tetracycline class (other than doxycycline) or fluoroquinolone class (particularly ciprofloxacin) and warfarin or related oral vitamin K antagonist anticoagulants stand as primary examples of situations commonly accepted as involving a significant risk of pharmacokinetic interference.

Zinc may play a central role in the intimate relationships between the immune system and the mental-emotional states traditionally ascribed to the central nervous system (CNS). The body of scientific knowledge emerging within the field of psychoneuroimmunology may render obsolete conventional parsing of academic disciplines, which often are inadequate in conveying the totality of complex physiological functioning

inherent in clinical medicine. A more comprehensive model can provide a forum for further research into the broader functions of zinc that transcend narrow categorization and defy reductionist analysis.

NUTRIENT-DRUG INTERACTIONS

Amphetamines and Related Stimulant Medications

Amphetamine (amphetamine aspartate monohydrate, amphetamine sulfate), dextroamphetamine (dextroamphetamine saccharate, dextroamphetamine sulfate; D-amphetamine; Dexedrine).
Mixed amphetamines: amphetamine and dextroamphetamine (Adderall; dexamphetamine).
Extrapolated, based on similar properties: Methylphenidate (Metadate, Methylin, Ritalin, Ritalin-SR; Concerta).

Interaction Type and Significance

⊕⊕⊕ **Beneficial or Supportive Interaction, Not Requiring Professional Management**

Probability:	Evidence Base:
2. Probable or	○ **Preliminary**, maybe
3. Possible	◉ **Emerging**

Effect and Mechanism of Action

Zinc nutriture and physiology are important in mood and brain function and may play an independent role in physiology related to attention deficit–hyperactivity disorder (ADHD), particularly in individuals of older age and higher weight with low zinc and free fatty acids levels. Mechanisms apart from correcting zinc deficiency have not been investigated or elucidated. However, data derived from research into depression and CNS function are relevant. In particular, zinc plays an important role in neurotransmission in the brain by modulating the activity of glutamate and gamma-aminobutyric acid (GABA) receptors.[65] Furthermore, hippocampal and cortical neurons, noted for high concentrations of zinc, "possess mechanisms for Zn^{2+} uptake and storage in synaptic terminals" and for stimulation of release of Zn^{2+} ions along with neurotransmitters. "Zn^{2+} modulates predominantly the excitatory (glutamatergic) and inhibitory (GABA-ergic) amino acid neurotransmission pathways in CNS."[66]

Research

Limited research suggests that zinc may provide independent benefit in patients with ADHD and may complement conventional therapy using mixed-amphetamine salts. Studies have suggested a correlation between zinc deficiency and pathophysiology of ADHD.[67-69] In a double-blind, placebo-controlled study involving 400 children (72 girls, 328 boys, mean age 9.61 years), Bilici et al.[70] found that zinc sulfate (150 mg daily for 12 weeks) was "significantly superior to placebo in reducing symptoms of hyperactivity, impulsivity and impaired socialization in patients with ADHD. However, full therapeutic response rates of the zinc and placebo groups remained 28.7% and 20%, respectively." The authors added that "the hyperactivity, impulsivity and socialization scores displayed significant decrease in patients of older age and high BMI score with low zinc and free fatty acids (FFA) levels."[70] In a paper published later that same year (2004), Akhondzadeh et al.[71] reported findings from a 6-week, double-blind, randomized trial involving 44 children (26 boys and 18 girls), age 5 to 11 years, comparing methylphenidate (1 mg/kg/day) plus zinc sulfate (15 mg elemental zinc daily) to methylphenidate plus placebo in the treatment of ADHD. Outcomes, as assessed using Parent and Teacher ADHD Rating Scale scores, "improved with zinc sulfate," and the difference between the two protocols was significant, "as indicated by the effect on the group, the between-subjects factor." The difference in frequency of adverse effects between the two groups was "not significant." The authors concluded that their findings demonstrated that zinc coadministration "might be beneficial in the treatment" of children with ADHD, and that further investigations using different doses of zinc are required to replicate these findings.[71]

Nutritional Therapeutics, Clinical Concerns, and Adaptations

Physicians treating individuals diagnosed with ADHD are advised to consider nutritional support independently or in concert with the pharmacological therapies, such as methylphenidate or mixed amphetamines. The evidence for benefit from zinc is positive but limited, and use would generally be considered as a component of a broader nutritional strategy rather than adequate as a monotherapy. Nevertheless, the use of concomitant zinc at a low dosage level, 10 to 40 mg elemental zinc daily depending on weight and age, may be beneficial and is generally safe and unlikely to produce clinically significant adverse effects.

Health care professionals experienced in nutritional therapies typically emphasize reduced sugar intake and other blood glucose stabilization measures, removal of artificial additives (especially dyes) from diet, observation of intolerance to potentially reactive foods, and coadministration of nutrients, on a personalized basis, such as essential fatty acids (eicosapentaenoic acid [EPA], docosahexaenoic acid [DHA], gamma-linolenic acid [GLA], linoleic acid), oligomeric proanthocyanidins (e.g., pine bark, grape seed extract), magnesium, chromium, L-carnitine, and B vitamins.

Androgens

Fluoxymesterone (Halotestin); testosterone cypionate; methyltestosterone (Android, Methitest, Testred, Virilon).
Related but evidence lacking for extrapolation: Methyltestosterone combination drug: methyltestosterone and esterified estrogens (Estratest, Estratest HS); testolactone (Testolacton; HSDB 3255, SQ 9538; Fludestrin, Teolit, Teslac, Teslak).

Interaction Type and Significance

⊕⊕ **Beneficial or Supportive Interaction, with Professional Management**

Probability:
3. Possible

Evidence Base:
○ **Preliminary**

Effect and Mechanism of Action

Various androgens are administered clinically for treatment of diverse conditions. Zinc plays a key role in normal male sexual development, prostate function, and the maturation of sperm, as well as ovulation and fertilization. Further, zinc deficiency can cause hypogonadism, with a possible contribution from impaired leptin secretion.[72] Zinc may raise serum testosterone and dihydrotestosterone levels and sperm counts in some men, particularly those with low sperm counts, possibly by stimulating testosterone production in Leydig cells.[73-75]

Coadministration of zinc during androgen treatment (e.g., infertile men with insufficient sperm motility) may enhance the efficacy of treatment, and in fact, zinc appears to be essential

for such functions. The mechanisms of action involved in this synergistic interaction have not been fully elucidated.

Research

Limited evidence from clinical trials indicates that coadministration of zinc with androgens may enhance therapeutic outcomes, particularly in males with low baseline zinc levels. Castro-Magana et al.[76] investigated the role of zinc in boys with constitutional growth delay, familial short status, and delayed appearance of secondary sexual characteristics. They measured hair and serum zinc levels in boys with growth delay and short status initially and then again after administering methyltestosterone. They determined that "zinc levels in boys beyond stage 3 of genital development are significantly higher than in stage 1 and 2," and they observed "a linear relationship between zinc levels and serum testosterone concentration (up to 250 ng/dL)." Moreover, they found that "methyltestosterone administration raised the zinc concentration in serum and hair, especially in boys with constitutional growth delay." Thus, a synergistic relationship between zinc and testosterone function was suggested, in that "increased endogenous production or exogenous supply of testosterone [is] associated with increased zinc levels." These authors concluded that "the relative testosterone deficiency and hypogonadotropism seen in constitutional growth delay may result in decreased zinc levels, which in turn could cause a further delay in the appearance of secondary sexual characteristics and greater growth retardation."

Subsequently, Takihara et al.[77] compared the effects of 3 months of zinc therapy (zinc sulfate, 220 mg twice daily), low-dose androgen therapy (fluoxymesterone, 5-10 mg daily), and combination therapy (zinc sulfate and low-dose fluoxymesterone) on sperm motility and seminal zinc concentration in infertile patients with decreased motility and different zinc concentrations. They found that low-dose androgen therapy "increased seminal zinc concentrations and sperm motility, only when pretreatment seminal zinc concentrations were low. Furthermore, patients with low seminal zinc concentrations and poor sperm motility showed greater improvement of sperm motility and seminal zinc levels in response to zinc sulfate along with fluoxymesterone than they did to fluoxymesterone alone or zinc sulfate alone, possible due to a synergistic effect of zinc and androgen."

These consistent but preliminary findings suggest that further research through well-designed and adequately powered clinical trials is warranted, with a focus on determining safety parameters and significators of pretreatment zinc status.

Nutritional Therapeutics, Clinical Concerns, and Adaptations

Physicians treating patients with androgen therapy are advised to assess zinc status and coadminister a highly bioavailable zinc salt preparation (e.g., 55 mg elemental zinc twice daily) when indicated. Judicious standards of practice suggest monitoring for adverse effects of excessive zinc and coadministration of copper (1-3 mg daily, depending on baseline plasma or serum zinc/copper ratio).

Antibiotics and Antimicrobial Agents (Systemic)

Aminoglycoside antibiotics: Amikacin (Amikin), gentamicin (G-mycin, Garamycin, Jenamicin), kanamycin (Kantrex), neomycin (Mycifradin, Myciguent, Neo-Fradin, NeoTab, Nivemycin), netilmicin (Netromycin), paromomycin (monomycin; Humatin), streptomycin, tobramycin (AKTob, Nebcin, TOBI, TOBI Solution, TobraDex, Tobrex).

Beta-lactam antibiotics: Methicillin (Staphcillin); aztreonam (Azactam injection); carbapenem antibiotics: meropenem (Merrem I.V.); combination drug: imipenem and cilastatin (Primaxin I.M., Primaxin I.V.); penicillin antibiotics: amoxicillin (Amoxicot, Amoxil, Moxilin, Trimox, Wymox); combination drug: amoxicillin and clavulanic acid (Augmentin, Augmentin XR, Clavulin); ampicillin (Amficot, Omnipen, Principen, Totacillin); combination drug: ampicillin and sulbactam (Unisyn); bacampicillin (Spectrobid), carbenicillin (Geocillin); cloxacillin (Cloxapen), dicloxacillin (Dynapen, Dycill), mezlocillin (Mezlin), nafcillin (Unipen), oxacillin (Bactocill), penicillin G (Bicillin C-R, Bicillin L-A, Pfizerpen, Truxcillin), penicillin V (Beepen-VK, Betapen-VK, Ledercillin VK, Pen-Vee K, Robicillin VK, Suspen, Truxcillin VK, V-Cillin K, Veetids), piperacillin (Pipracil); combination drug: piperacillin and tazobactam (Zosyn); ticarcillin (Ticar); combination drug: ticarcillin and clavulanate (Timentin).

Cephalosporin antibiotics: Cefaclor (Ceclor), cefadroxil (Duricef), cefamandole (Mandol), cefazolin (Ancef, Kefzol), cefdinir (Omnicef), cefepime (Maxipime), cefixime (Suprax), cefoperazone (Cefobid), cefotaxime (Claforan), cefotetan (Cefotan), cefoxitin (Mefoxin), cefpodoxime (Vantin), cefprozil (Cefzil), ceftazidime (Ceptaz, Fortaz, Tazicef, Tazidime), ceftibuten (Cedax), ceftizoxime (Cefizox), ceftriaxone (Rocephin), cefuroxime (Ceftin, Kefurox, Zinacef), cephalexin (Keflex, Keftab), cephapirin (Cefadyl), cephradine (Anspor, Velocef); imipenem combination drug: imipenem and cilastatin (Primaxin I.M., Primaxin I.V.); loracarbef (Lorabid), meropenem (Merrem I.V.).

Fluoroquinolone (4-quinolone) antibiotics: Cinoxacin (Cinobac, Pulvules), ciprofloxacin (Ciloxan, Cipro), enoxacin (Penetrex), gatifloxacin (Tequin), levofloxacin (Levaquin), lomefloxacin (Maxaquin), moxifloxacin (Avelox), nalidixic acid (Neggram), norfloxacin (Noroxin), ofloxacin (Floxin, Ocuflox), sparfloxacin (Zagam), trovafloxacin (alatrofloxacin; Trovan).

Macrolide antibiotics: Azithromycin (Zithromax), clarithromycin (Biaxin), dirithromycin (Dynabac), erythromycin oral (EES, EryPed, Ery-Tab, PCE Dispertab, Pediazole), troleandomycin (Tao).

Sulfonamide antibiotics: Sodium sulfacetamide (AK-Sulf, Bleph-10, Sodium Sulamyd), sulfamethoxazole (Gantanol), sulfanilamide (AVC), sulfasalazine (salazosulfapyridine, salicylazosulfapyridine, suphasalazine; Apo-Sulfasalazine, Azulfidine, Azulfidine EN-Tabs, PMS-Sulfasalazine, Salazopyrin, Salazopyrin EN-Tabs, SAS), sulfisoxazole (Gantrisin); combination drug: sulfamethoxazole and trimethoprim (cotrimoxazole, co-trimoxazole, SXT, TMP-SMX, TMP-sulfa; Bactrim, Bactrim DS, Cotrim, Septra, Septra DS, Sulfatrim, Uroplus); triple sulfa (Sultrin Triple Sulfa).

Miscellaneous antibiotics: Bacitracin (Caci-IM), chloramphenicol (Chloromycetin), chlorhexidine (Peridex), clindamycin, oral (Cleocin); colistimethate (Coly-Mycin M), dapsone (DDS, diaminodiphenylsulphone; Aczone Gel, Avlosulfon), furazolidone (Furoxone), lincomycin (Lincocin), linezolid (Zyvox), nitrofurantoin (Macrobid, Macrodantin), trimethoprim (Proloprim, Trimpex), vancomycin (Vancocin).

Interaction Type and Significance

⊕⊕ **Beneficial or Supportive Interaction, with Professional Management**

⊕✗ **Bimodal or Variable Interaction, with Professional Management**

✗ **Potential or Theoretical Adverse Interaction of Uncertain Severity**

Coadministration Benefit	
Probability:	Evidence Base:
2. Probable or **3. Possible**	▽ **Mixed**

Coadministration Risk	
Probability:	Evidence Base:
3. Possible	○ **Preliminary**

Effect and Mechanism of Action

Administration of zinc may prevent or, in conjunction with standard oral antibiotic therapy and vitamin A, may enhance the acute treatment and accelerate recovery of infants and children with pneumonia.[78,79] The role of zinc in immune function, generally by restoring immunocompetence and specifically as an acute-phase reactant, is presumed to provide the primary mechanism of action. However, such effect may occur only to the degree that nutrient coadministration corrects inadequate zinc intake or preexisting zinc deficiency.

During the "hot season," concomitant zinc may delay recovery of some children and infants being treated for pneumonia with standard oral antibiotics. The mechanism of such a potential adverse effect has not been elucidated.[57]

Research

The body of evidence on the effects of zinc in preventing and treating pneumonia, diarrhea, and other common diseases in malnourished infants and children is emerging and suggestive of a pattern of benefit but, as yet, mixed and incomplete. In a meta-analysis of randomized controlled trials, Bhutta et al.[78] found that zinc supplementation in children in developing countries is associated with substantial reductions in the rates of pneumonia and diarrhea. In a randomized controlled trial involving 2482 children age 6 months to 3 years in an urban slum, Bhandari et al.[80] found that zinc supplementation (with infants receiving 10 mg elemental zinc daily and older children 20 mg daily) "substantially reduced the incidence of pneumonia" in children who received single pharmacological dose of vitamin A (100,000 IU for infants and 200,000 IU for older children) at enrollment. In contrast, that same year (2002), in a double-blind, randomized controlled trial involving children age 9 months to 15 years in Calcutta, Mahalanabis et al.[81] found that children with severe measles accompanied by pneumonia did not demonstrate any additional benefit, beyond that provided by antibiotics and vitamin A palmitate (100,000 IU dose), from coadministration of zinc acetate (containing 20 mg elemental zinc) twice daily for 6 days.

Subsequently, in a double-blind, placebo-controlled clinical trial involving 270 children age 2 to 23 months in a Bangladesh hospital, Brooks et al.[79] compared the effects of concomitant elemental zinc (20 mg/day) versus placebo in combination with the hospital's standard antimicrobial management. Children in the zinc treatment group demonstrated reduced duration of severe pneumonia, including duration of chest indrawing, accelerated respiratory rate (>50 breaths/min), and hypoxia, and a shortened duration of overall hospitalization, with a mean reduction equivalent to one hospital day for both severe pneumonia and time in hospital. Less benefit was observed in children with wheezing. These researchers concluded that coadministration of "20 mg zinc per day accelerates recovery from severe pneumonia in children, and could help reduce antimicrobial resistance by decreasing multiple antibiotic exposures, and lessen complications and deaths where second line drugs are unavailable."[79] However, in a later, randomized, double-blind, placebo-controlled clinical trial involving 299 children, also age 2 to 23 months, being treated for severe pneumonia with standard antibiotic therapy in a hospital in southern India, Bose et al.[57] reported a lack of therapeutic benefit from 10 mg zinc sulfate, versus placebo, twice a day during hospitalization. Specifically, they observed "no clinical or statistically significant differences in the duration of tachypnea, hypoxia, chest indrawing, inability to feed, lethargy, severe illness, or hospitalization." Moreover, they reported "significantly longer duration of pneumonia in the hot season" in subjects treated with concomitant zinc.

The conflicting findings from this study compared with previous trials indicate that the value of zinc in preventing or correcting zinc deficiency may be the pivotal variable in the therapeutic response. Furthermore, the unexpected possibility of adverse effects, as seen in the "hot season" subgroup analysis, suggests the inadequacy of data underlying recommendations for routine administration of zinc in the treatment of pneumonia in young children in the developing world and the need for continued research with an emphasis on zinc-deficient populations.

Nutritional Therapeutics, Clinical Concerns, and Adaptations

Physicians treating infants and children with pneumonia, or other severe acute lower respiratory infection, are advised to consider coadministration of zinc, and possibly vitamin A, with standard antibiotic therapy in patients demonstrating or at high risk for compromised zinc status. A dose of 10 mg elemental zinc twice daily is typical but can vary depending on the child's age and weight. Current scientific knowledge suggests that such doses are unlikely to produce any adverse effects during a short course of treatment, but limited data suggest greater caution in hot climates. Methods for determining zinc deficiency are generally considered unreliable, so patient history and clinical presentation are usually the best predictors of zinc deficiency. Health care professionals are also advised to educate parents to shift dietary intake patterns away from foods with a high phytate-to-zinc ratio in order to increase the bioavailability of dietary zinc. In general, zinc acetate provides the most bioavailable form of zinc, across a broad range of gastric pH. The potential for a pharmacokinetic interaction involving binding between zinc and the antibiotic agent suggests that separating oral intake by 2 to 4 hours would be prudent.

Antibiotics, Topical

Erythromycin 3% and benzoyl peroxide 5% topical gel (Benzamycin).
Clindamycin, topical (Cleocin T, Clindaderm).

Interaction Type and Significance

⊕⊕ **Beneficial or Supportive Interaction, with Professional Management**

Probability:
2. Probable

Evidence Base:
○ **Preliminary**

Effect and Mechanism of Action

The important role of zinc in immune function and the health of the skin is well established.[82] Zinc is effective in the treatment of inflammatory acne, and zinc salts have demonstrated bacteriostatic activity against *Propionibacterium acnes*.[83] Zinc appears to exert a specific action on inflammatory cells, especially granulocytes, where the mechanism involved in zinc's "anti-inflammatory action is related to inhibition of

polymorphonuclear leukocyte chemotaxis induced by a decreased granulocyte zinc level."[84,85]

Concomitant administration of zinc, oral and/or topical solution, may enhance the efficacy of topical antibiotics in the treatment of acne vulgaris.

Research

A limited but consistent body of evidence indicates that erythromycin-zinc combination therapy is effective in the treatment of acne. In a double-blind, randomized, multicenter study involving 122 patients with acne vulgaris, Habbema et al.[86] evaluated the efficacy of a 4% erythromycin and zinc combination lotion (Zineryt) versus 2% erythromycin lotion (Eryderm). During visits at 0, 1, 2, 4, 8, and 12 weeks, they examined subjects and determined that treatment with erythromycin-zinc "combination lotion was more effective than with 2% erythromycin as regards the reduction in number of the acne lesions and the severity grade of the acne." Subsequently, Schachner et al.[87] conducted a 12-week double-blind trial to determine the safety and efficacy of a 4% erythromycin plus 1.2% zinc acetate formulation versus its vehicle. They continued the study for 40 weeks after the initial 12-week double-blind phase by switching vehicle-treated patients to active treatment and continuing to give patients treated with active drug the same treatment. Investigators reported "statistically significant differences" during the first 12 weeks "in the efficacy of the erythromycin-zinc compared with vehicle for acne severity grades (global assessment) and for papule, pustule, and comedo counts." Moreover, following crossover, the subjects who had been receiving vehicle-only (placebo) treatment and then had been switched to active therapy duplicated the improvement of the first group treated with erythromycin-zinc. The authors reported "no clinical problems with superinfection or secondary infection" during 1 year of treatment in the 39 female patients (of the initial 73).[87]

Dreno et al.[88] also conducted in vivo and in vitro studies investigating the combination of topical erythromycin and oral zinc gluconate in the treatment of patients with inflammatory acne. In a trial involving 30 patients with inflammatory acne, they found that treatment with zinc gluconate (30 mg daily for 2 months) resulted in "a reduction in the number of inflammatory lesions after a 2-month treatment whether or not *Propionibacterium acnes* carriage was present," as demonstrated in bacteriological samples taken at onset, day 30, and day 60. Further, they observed that in vitro "addition of zinc salts in the culture media of *Propionibacterium acnes* reduced resistance of *Propionibacterium acnes* strains to erythromycin." Thus, the authors concluded that the concomitant action of oral zinc salts acting systemically and topical erythromycin treatment "seems an interesting option in the light of an increasing number of patients carrying erythromycin resistant *Propionibacterium acnes* strains."

Nutritional Therapeutics, Clinical Concerns, and Adaptations

The scientific evidence, both broad and specific, indicates that health care professionals treating patients with acne, especially inflammatory acne, should consider integrating zinc into their therapeutic strategy. Whether by oral dose or combined in a topical preparation with an antibacterial agent, zinc can exert a beneficial effect directly and synergistically on the skin environment and broader immune function and on the pathological processes and pathogenic agents. A typical dose would be in the range of 20 to 40 mg elemental zinc per day orally and/or 1% to 2% topically. Continued zinc supplementation after cessation of antibiotics may be indicated in many patients as part of a comprehensive and individualized long-term strategy emphasizing dietary changes, hormonal modulation, and other interventions appropriate to the patient's characteristics and evolving needs. Patients who have a history of multiple courses of oral antibiotics will often also benefit from coadministration of probiotic bacterial flora over an extended period, at least in part through effects on digestive and immune function.

Antidepressants, Including Tricyclic Antidepressants and Selective Serotonin Reuptake Inhibitor (SSRI) Antidepressants

Evidence: Amitriptyline (Elavil), citalopram (Celexa), clomipramine (Anafranil), fluoxetine (Prozac, Sarafem).
Extrapolated, based on similar properties:
Tricyclic antidepressants: Amitriptyline combination drug: amitriptyline and perphenazine (Etrafon, Triavil, Triptazine); amoxapine (Asendin), desipramine (Norpramin, Pertofrane), doxepin (Adapin, Sinequan), imipramine (Janimine, Tofranil), nortriptyline (Aventyl, Pamelor), protriptyline (Vivactil), trimipramine (Surmontil).
Selective serotonin reuptake inhibitor (SSRI) antidepressants: Escitalopram (S-citalopram; Lexapro), fluvoxamine (Faurin, Luvox), paroxetine (Atropax, Deroxat, Paxil, Seroxat), sertraline (Zoloft).

Interaction Type and Significance
⊕⊕ **Beneficial or Supportive Interaction, with Professional Management**

Probability: Evidence Base:
2. Probable   ◉ **Emerging**

Effect and Mechanism of Action
Among its many functions, zinc is an important modulator of the CNS. In particular, hippocampal and cortical neurons, noted for high concentrations of zinc, "possess mechanisms for Zn^{2+} uptake and storage in synaptic terminals" and for stimulation of release of Zn^{2+} ions along with neurotransmitters. "Zn^{2+} modulates predominantly the excitatory (glutamatergic) and inhibitory (GABA-ergic) amino acid neurotransmission pathways in CNS."[66] Thus, zinc deficiency impairs neurological function and is associated with depression.[4,89-91]

Administration of zinc in patients diagnosed with depression may provide direct benefit and appears to enhance the effect of some conventional antidepressant medications, particularly those affecting monoamine transmitter reuptake or metabolism, at least in part by acting as a modulator of glutamatergic transmission.[4,92] Chronic zinc administration, as well as most "clinically effective antidepressants," induce expression of the gene coding for brain-derived neurotrophic factor (BDNF) and an increase in cortical (but not hippocampal) BDNF messenger RNA (mRNA) level; tranylcypromine, a classic antidepressant, increases BDNF mRNA level in both brain regions. Zinc administration also increases levels of synaptic pool zinc in the hippocampus.[2,4] Moreover, changes in the brain, particularly a phenomenon known as "mossy fiber sprouting," that occur with electroconvulsive shock (ECS), are associated with an increase in the synaptic zinc level in the hippocampus after such therapy and parallels effects of chronic but not acute zinc treatment.[3] "Chronic treatment with citalopram (but not with imipramine or ECS) significantly (approx 20%) increased the serum zinc level. Chronic treatment with both drugs slightly (by approx 10%) increased the zinc level in the hippocampus and slightly decreased it in the cortex, cerebellum and basal forebrain." Chronic imipramine treatment enhances the ability of zinc to inhibit the NMDA

receptor complex in the cerebral cortex, but not in the hippocampus, but such effects appear to be species specific.[93] Notably, chronic ECS may also induce a significant increase in zinc levels in the hippocampus (30%), as well as an 11% to 15% increase in zinc in other brain regions.[94] Another mechanism of action may derive from zinc's "antagonistic action on group I metabotropic glutamate receptors or potentiation of AMPA receptors which both may attenuate the NMDA receptor function."[4,95,96] Zinc may also exert an antidepressant action through its direct inhibition of glycogen synthase kinase-3β, which has been proposed as a target for treatment of affective (bipolar) disorder.[97] Thus, zinc acts as a natural modulator of amino-acidergic neurotransmission, particularly as an antagonist of the glutamate/N-methyl-D-aspartate (NMDA) receptor, and zinc administration may correct derangements of zinc homeostasis so that its presence may be necessary for, and its coadministration may potentiate, the therapeutic effects of many conventional antidepressants.

Research
McLoughlin and Hodge[89] initially published data reporting hypozincemia in patients with primary depressive disorders. Subsequently, one study by Maes et al.[90] showed significantly lower serum zinc levels in individuals diagnosed with major depression, compared with nondepressed controls, and intermediate zinc levels in those with minor depression. In another study, however, these researchers found no correlation between these parameters among treatment-resistant patients.[98] Further correlations have been observed between the serum level of zinc and the severity of illness in individuals with unipolar depression, as defined in the Hamilton Depression Rating Scale. The hypothesis that zinc status, as indicated by serum zinc concentrations, may be a sensitive and specific marker of depression is also supported by findings showing that lowered serum zinc concentrations may be normalized after successful antidepressant treatment.[4,89,98-100]

In a series of in vitro and animal studies and human trials spanning nearly a decade, Polish researchers have investigated the function of zinc in relation to depression and the interactions between zinc and conventional antidepressants. They showed a similar "antidepressant-like performance" in mice and rats subjected to the forced-swim test, but also found differences in the effects of imipramine on locomotor function and in the responses of these two rodent species to chronic imipramine treatment that suggest the existence of species-dependent adaptive mechanisms involving zinc sites at the NMDA receptor complex.[93,101,102] Further, a rodent model showed that the addition of low-dose zinc could potentiate the activity of antidepressants when administered at dosages too low to be effective and could synergistically achieve an antidepressant effect.[101,103] In one innovative study, Nowak et al.[104] demonstrated that the alteration in zinc interaction with NMDA receptors may be involved in psychopathology underlying suicidal attempts by showing a statistically significant (26%) reduction in the potency of zinc to inhibit NMDA receptor activity in the hippocampal, but not cortical, tissue of suicide subjects. Subsequently, these researchers conducted a placebo-controlled, double-blind pilot study investigating the efficacy of concomitant zinc (25 mg Zn^{2+}) and standard antidepressant pharmacotherapy using tricyclic antidepressants or SSRIs, specifically clomipramine, amitriptyline, citalopram, or fluoxetine, in the treatment of fourteen patients who fulfilled *Diagnostic and Statistical Manual of Mental Disorders* (4th edition, *DSM-IV*) criteria for major (unipolar) depression. Initially, after an initial washout period and throughout

12 weeks of treatment with antidepressant drugs and zinc or antidepressant drugs and placebo, they assessed therapeutic response to intervention using the Hamilton Depression Rating Scale and the Beck Depression Inventory. Subjects in both groups demonstrated an improvement in depressive symptoms at the second week, but the zinc-antidepressant group showed a statistically significant improvement in both measures, compared with the antidepressant-placebo group, at 6 and 12 weeks. The authors concluded that their findings, although preliminary, constituted "the first demonstration of the benefit of zinc supplementation in antidepressant therapy" and suggested that the effect "may be related to modulation of glutamatergic or immune systems by zinc ion."[92] Continued investigation of this interaction and its clinical implications is clearly warranted.

Greater refinement in methodology, to account for individual patient characteristics (e.g., clinical variation in condition, pharmacogenomics, personal history, lifestyle characteristics), will render future findings more robust and relevant to the dynamic and nuanced realities of treating the diverse presentations of depression. More broadly, further research, possibly framed within the more expansive model of psychoneuroimmunology, is warranted to investigate the potentially pivotal role of zinc in the interrelationships between the "immune system" and CNS function and thereby reveal the overarching unity of these supposedly discrete "systems" within human physiology and health, dysfunction and disease.

Nutritional Therapeutics, Clinical Concerns, and Adaptations

Health care professionals treating individuals diagnosed with depression, particularly physicians prescribing SSRI or tricyclic antidepressants, are advised to consider the potential value of zinc administration as part of a comprehensive, evolving, and individualized therapeutic strategy. The emerging body of scientific evidence strongly suggests that zinc may independently benefit many such patients, even outside compromised zinc status, and may enhance the efficacy of conventional antidepressant regimens, including pharmaceutical antidepressants and possibly electroconvulsive therapy. Pending further research, and the establishment of sensitive assays of zinc depletion, physiologic zinc administration, typically 25 to 40 mg elemental zinc daily, is generally considered safe and sufficient to achieve therapeutic effect. Coadministration of folic acid, DHEA, EPA (fish oil), inositol, or other synergistic nutritional support may also be efficacious with certain patients. Concomitant use of botanical medications, such as *Hypericum perforatum* (St. John's wort), *Ginkgo biloba, Rhodiola rosea, Withania somnifera* (Ashwaganda), is controversial and may be useful but requires assessment, prescribing, and management by a health care professional trained and experienced in botanical therapeutics, in coordination with the physician prescribing any pharmacotherapy.

Calcium-Based Antacids

See Calcium in Nutrient-Nutrient Interactions.

Captopril, Enalapril, and Related Angiotensin-Converting Enzyme (ACE) Inhibitors

Evidence: Captopril (Capoten), enalapril (Vasotec).
Extrapolated, based on similar properties: Benazepril (Lotensin); combination drug: benazepril and amlodipine (Lotrel); captopril combination drug: captopril and hydrochlorothiazide (Acezide, Capto-Co, Captozide, Co-Zidocapt); cilazapril (Inhibace); enalapril combination drugs: enalapril and felodipine (Lexxel); enalapril and hydrochlorothiazide (Vaseretic); fosinopril (Monopril), lisinopril (Prinivil, Zestril); lisinopril and hydrochlorothiazide (Prinzide, Zestoretic); moexipril (Univasc), perindopril (Aceon), quinapril (Accupril), ramipril (Altace), trandolapril (Mavik).

Interaction Type and Significance

≈≈ **Drug-Induced Nutrient Depletion, Supplementation Therapeutic, with Professional Management**

☼ **Prevention or Reduction of Drug Adverse Effect**

Probability:	Evidence Base:
2. Probable	● Consensus

Effect and Mechanism of Action

The ACE inhibitors possess a prominent zinc-binding moiety that binds to zinc ions in the active site of the ACE molecule. Drugs within the class of ACE inhibitors can be classified according to the ligand of the zinc ion of ACE and according to the excretion route of their active moiety. Thus, captopril has a sulfhydryl moiety as the zinc-binding ligand, whereas enalapril has a carboxyalkyl dipeptide moiety. Both captopril and enalapril are excreted primarily through the kidneys, but enalapril has a much longer duration of action than captopril. Gradual zinc depletion occurs as zinc is bound to the ACE inhibitor and can lead to zinc insufficiency. Some of the adverse effects associated with ACE inhibitors, such as hypogeusia, coincide with known characteristics of zinc depletion and may derive, at least in part, from the effect of these agents on zinc status.

Research

Several studies have demonstrated that captopril (and, at a slower pace, enalapril) is likely to cause significant urinary zinc loss, which over several months can lead to zinc depletion with attendant decreased red blood cell (RBC) zinc concentrations and reduced taste acuity (hypogeusia), even in the absence of adverse changes in serum zinc levels. In 1987, O'Connor et al.[105] reported that serum zinc was unaffected by captopril treatment of hypertension. However, the next year, Abu-Hamdan et al.[106] documented changes in taste acuity and zinc metabolism in a trial involving 31 hypertensive male patients treated with captopril. In comparing 11 long-term, high-dose captopril recipients (>6 months, 266 mg/day), six short-term captopril recipients (<6 months, 104 mg/day), and 14 noncaptopril controls, they found that, compared to controls, the long-term captopril group had significantly higher taste detection and recognition thresholds, lower plasma zinc, and higher urinary zinc excretion. The short-term captopril group did not differ significantly from the noncaptopril group, except for altered taste-recognition thresholds. Notably, two long-term captopril patients reported improved taste acuity and demonstrated "almost normalized zinc parameters" after discontinuing captopril.

Subsequently, Golik et al.[107] conducted two trials comparing the effects of captopril and enalapril on zinc metabolism in hypertensive patients. First, in a small retrospective study, they assessed several parameters of zinc metabolism in 13 patients with essential hypertension, of whom six were chronically taking captopril, seven were taking enalapril, and six were untreated, as well as nine healthy controls. Although serum zinc levels were comparable in all groups, the captopril-treated subjects exhibited significantly increased 24-hour urinary zinc excretion compared with the three other groups.

Further, subjects in both the captopril and the enalapril group exhibited a significant increase in the zinc/creatinine ratio in 24-hour urine, which was significantly greater in the captopril group. Notably, even though plasma zinc concentrations were comparable in all groups, subjects in the captopril group demonstrated significantly decreased RBC zinc values compared with those in the three other groups. The authors concluded that "(1) although both captopril and enalapril produce renal zinc loss, this loss is far greater in patients receiving captopril; and (2) captopril administration over 3 months or more generates RBC zinc depletion."[107] Several years later, in a prospective trial involving 44 subjects, these researchers investigated the effects of chronic captopril and enalapril treatment on zinc metabolism in hypertensive patients. They measured and compared zinc levels in serum, 24-hour urine samples, and peripheral blood monocytes at baseline and after 6 months in 10 patients newly diagnosed with essential hypertension who were randomly divided for ACE therapy, with 16 receiving captopril only and 18 receiving enalapril only, as well as 10 healthy subjects serving as controls. They found that patients in the captopril- and enalapril-treated groups demonstrated significantly decreased intramonocytic zinc levels over the same period, but that only subjects in the captopril-treated group showed a significant enhancement of 24-hour urinary zinc excretion after 6 months of treatment. Thus, the authors concluded: "Treatment of hypertensive patients with captopril or enalapril may result in zinc deficiency."[108]

Subsequently, Peczkowska[109] confirmed that ACE inhibitor therapy may adversely affect zinc metabolism. Although not statistically significant, serum zinc decreased more significantly in a group treated with captopril after 8 weeks of therapy than in a group receiving benazepril. Collectively, these findings indicate that captopril can cause clinically significant zinc depletion over several months, which may not be detectable through serum zinc assay. Other ACE inhibitors probably have a similar effect on zinc metabolism, although zinc depletion at the tissue level apparently occurs at a slower rate and possibly to a lesser degree.

In related research, Golik et al.[110] also determined that individuals with type 2 diabetes mellitus and congestive heart failure "excrete larger amounts of zinc, which may eventually lead to zinc deficiency." These findings bear directly on the data relating to hypertensive medications, given the widespread use of ACE inhibitors for heart failure and the high incidence of hypertension among these patient populations.

Nutritional Therapeutics, Clinical Concerns, and Adaptations
Physicians prescribing captopril or other ACE inhibitors are advised to discuss supportive coadministration of zinc (50 mg elemental zinc twice daily) to counter probable nutrient depletion. The risk attendant to such supplementation is minimal and its characteristics well known. Establishing zinc depletion through laboratory assessment is not considered sensitive enough to be clinically reliable because of the limitations of testing methods in the face of metabolic flux characteristic of zinc physiology. Clinical signs of zinc deficiency are more reliable but tend to manifest only with advanced deficiency, usually after subclinical depletion has adversely affected function. Patients who develop ACE inhibitor–associated cough, frequently cited as a cause of nonadherence, may also experience amelioration with iron supplementation.[111] Concomitant synergistic minerals (e.g., magnesium) as well coenzyme Q10 and hawthorn (Crataegus) could potentially further enhance therapeutic outcomes in the treatment of hypertension, heart failure, and related cardiovascular disease. Copper is

generally advisable to balance the potential depletion by zinc. However, to avoid absorption problems inhibiting bioavailability of both ACE inhibitors and zinc (as well as other nutrients), patients should wait at least 2 hours after administration of the medication before taking any supplements.

Supplementation of any minerals by patients with renal failure or on dialysis can be dangerous and should only be done within the context of close medical supervision. Patients receiving ACE inhibitor therapy may experience an exaggeration of adverse effects often associated with intravenous administration of iron salts; monitor closely for adverse effects such as nausea, vomiting, and hypotension. Notably, potassium is usually contraindicated with ACE inhibitors because they greatly decrease renal potassium excretion.

Chlorhexidine

Chlorhexidine (Chlorohex, Corsodyl, Eludril, Oro-Clense, Peridex, Periogard Oral Rinse).
Similar properties but evidence indicating no or reduced interaction effects: Periochip.

Interaction Type and Significance
☼ **Prevention or Reduction of Drug Adverse Effect**
⊕⊕ **Beneficial or Supportive Interaction, with Professional Management**

Probability: Evidence Base:
2. Probable   ○ **Preliminary**

Effect and Mechanism of Action
Chlorhexidine is known to cause staining of teeth when used as a rinse in dental care. The combination of zinc or other metal ions in solution with chlorhexidine can reduce the severity of such staining and enhance the plaque-inhibiting effect of the treatment. Zinc and other metal ions, such as tin (usually in the form of stannous fluoride), have the same receptor sites as chlorhexidine in the oral cavity, such that binding affinity for chlorhexidine is greater when the ions were applied together.

Research
The research into this interaction is preliminary in nature and limited in scope but consistent in its findings and their rationale. Waler and Rolla[112] investigated the plaque-inhibiting effect of chlorhexidine in combination with zinc (and tin) in a group of students. They observed that "chlorhexidine and zinc (0.2% and 0.3% respectively) gave a plaque inhibiting effect slightly better than chlorhexidine alone" and superior to pre-rinses with metal ions or chlorhexidine first and metal ions afterward. They concluded that "the metal ions and chlorhexidine have the same receptor sites in the oral cavity, chlorhexidine exhibiting the stronger affinity when the ions were applied together."

Subsequently, in a 6-month, randomized, stratified double-blind parallel study with 208 participants, Sanz et al.[113] investigated the effect of a dentifrice containing chlorhexidine and zinc on plaque, gingivitis, calculus, and tooth staining. Of the three test groups, the two receiving chlorhexidine as part of their treatment (with or without zinc) exhibited "significant reductions in plaque and gingivitis (gingival index and number of bleeding sites)... compared with the control group," but tooth staining was also higher. The group treated with the chlorhexidine-zinc rinse exhibited "significantly less staining compared with the positive control." These authors concluded that the chlorhexidine-zinc dentifrice "will contribute to a significant improvement in oral hygiene with less staining compared with using a 0.12% chlorhexidine rinse." Further clinical trials are warranted given the positive findings of these preliminary studies. The stability and acidic nature of these formulations in clinical practice are among the potential concerns deserving attention.

Nutritional Therapeutics, Clinical Concerns, and Adaptations

Dental professionals administering chlorhexidine are advised to consider adding zinc, usually as zinc sulfate heptahydrate, to their chlorhexidine preparation. No significant adverse effects, other than the probable bad taste, are to be expected. Direct evidence is lacking to confirm the efficacy of oral zinc administration alone in achieving similar preventive effects. Perhaps more importantly, clinicians should educate patients that brushing before applying the dentifrice is the most effective way to reduce chlorhexidine staining, because chlorhexidine adheres to plaque. Likewise, cultivating a healthy oral environment, by reducing acidity and supporting healthy oral flora, is also essential to preventing caries and erosion.

Ciprofloxacin and Related Fluoroquinolone (4-Quinolone) Antibiotics

Evidence: Ciprofloxacin (Ciloxan, Cipro), norfloxacin (Noroxin); 8-hydroxyquinoline.
Extrapolated, based on similar properties: Cinoxacin (Cinobac, Pulvules), enoxacin (Penetrex), gatifloxacin (Tequin), levofloxacin (Levaquin), lomefloxacin (Maxaquin), moxifloxacin (Avelox), nalidixic acid (Neggram), ofloxacin (Floxin, Ocuflox), sparfloxacin (Zagam), trovafloxacin (alatrofloxacin; Trovan).

Interaction Type and Significance

✗ ✗ **Minimal to Mild Adverse Interaction—Vigilance Necessary**

◇ ◇ **Impaired Drug Absorption and Bioavailability, Precautions Appropriate**

≈ ≈ ≈ **Drug-Induced Nutrient Depletion, Supplementation Therapeutic, Not Requiring Professional Management**

☼ **Prevention or Reduction of Drug Adverse Effect**

Coadministration Risk
Probability:
1. **Certain** or
   2. **Probable** (depending on agent and timing)

Evidence Base:
● **Consensus** but
○ **Preliminary**

Coadministration Benefit
Probability:
4. **Plausible**

Evidence Base:
○ **Preliminary**

Effect and Mechanism of Action

Zinc salts and the 3-carbonyl and 4-oxo functional groups on quinolone antibiotics can bind within the gastrointestinal (GI) tract to form a poorly absorbed, stable chelation complex. This binding process, which may not be limited to the gut, can interfere to varying degrees with the absorption, bioavailability, and activity of both the antimicrobials in this class and the orally administered preparations containing zinc.[114-120]

In one permutation of this interaction with a related quinolone, coadministration of zinc oxide may form chelates that inhibit the antibacterial activity or even counteract the antimycotic activity of 8-hydroxyquinoline, but may also mitigate allergic reactions to the 8-hydroxyquinoline.[121]

Research and Reports

In vitro experiments first demonstrated the pattern of interaction between quinolones and metals in an aqueous medium and the resultant effects on antimicrobial activity. Subsequently, changes in oral bioavailability and alterations in therapeutic efficacy have been the focus of many previous interaction studies involving metal cations and quinolones. Thus, through multiple lines of research, the ability of multivalent cations to reduce the absorption and serum levels of oral quinolone antibiotics is generally considered well established.

Evidence from clinical trials focusing on zinc-quinolone interactions is limited. Most of the evidence used to predict direct, one-to-one interactions between zinc and various quinolone agents is extrapolated from findings based on research involving iron and based on similar chemistry and presumed mechanisms of action. Similarly, calcium, magnesium, manganese, and copper, as well as milk and calcium-fortified juices, inhibit absorption of fluoroquinolones. Much of the remaining data derive from studies using multimineral preparations, usually with iron the primary interacting agent. The situation with case reports is similar. In a four-way crossover trial with 12 healthy volunteers, Polk et al.[114] (1989) observed a clinically significant reduction in the absorption of orally administered doses of ciprofloxacin (500 mg) when administered with a multivitamin-mineral formulation containing zinc, or ferrous sulfate (325 mg orally three times daily). Notably, peak concentrations of ciprofloxacin with ferrous sulfate regimen were below the minimum inhibitory concentration (MIC) for 90% of strains of many organisms normally considered susceptible to the antimicrobial activity of ciprofloxacin. Kara et al.[116] investigated clinical and chemical interactions between ciprofloxacin and iron preparations and found impairment of absorption with a multimineral preparation containing iron, magnesium, zinc, calcium, copper, and manganese (Centrum Forte). In an experiment involving eight healthy volunteers, each receiving a different metal ion, Campbell et al.[117] found that zinc sulfate reduced the urinary recovery of norfloxacin by 56%, just slightly more than ferrous sulfate. In reviewing the available data, Stockley[122] concluded: "There seems to be very little data about the zinc/quinolone interaction, but zinc appears to interact like iron so that the same precautions suggested for iron should be followed."

The particular interaction between zinc oxide and 8-hydroxyquinoline, a related quinoline, is more nuanced, although the data are rather limited. In a case report and subsequent trial involving 13 patients, Fischer[121] found that zinc oxide in a base reduced the eczematogenic effects associated with 8-hydroxyquinoline compared with an ointment using a paraffin base without zinc. However, this combination also inhibited the antibacterial and antimycotic activity of the medication and appeared to promote the growth of *Candida albicans*. Consequently, this interaction, particularly chelate formation, can interfere with the therapeutic effects of the 8-hydroxyquinoline to the degree that substantially "little or no antibacterial properties" remain.[122,123]

Zinc depletion resulting from chelation by this class of medications has not been studied per se. Although plausible, such an adverse effect on zinc status is highly improbable given the limited duration of standard fluoroquinolone antibiotic use. Long-term quinolone therapy and simultaneous oral zinc intake in the face of zinc deficiency could theoretically contribute to lack of tissue repletion. It is unclear whether long-term oral fluoroquinolone antibiotic therapy might cause clinically significant zinc depletion in certain vulnerable populations by preventing dietary zinc absorption.

Nutritional Therapeutics, Clinical Concerns, and Adaptations

The reduction of fluoroquinolone activity by simultaneously ingested zinc salts is a widely accepted, although not necessarily well-documented, interaction between these two groups of agents; the potential depletion of zinc through the same mechanisms is plausible but generally improbable in standard clinical use. Both directions of interaction and decreased bioavailability can be adequately avoided through proper patient education and dose timing. Notably, even with iron, the degree of interaction effect depends greatly on the particular quinolone agent involved, as well as timing of oral intake(s). Inherently, such separation of intake is irrelevant with combined topical formulations, and evidence indicates that the effectiveness of topical quinolone preparations may be compromised by the addition of zinc.

Patients with acute infections, diagnosed or presumed, frequently self-administer zinc because of its immune-supporting activity and often fail to inform their health care professionals. Physicians treating patients for serious infections with quinolone antibiotics should advise that they refrain from ingesting zinc supplements, or using multivitamin-mineral formulations containing zinc or other divalent mineral cations, during the course of therapy to avoid interfering with the absorption and thus the antimicrobial action of the medication.

Zinc intake can usually be temporarily halted in most patients but can be continued with separation of intake timing in those for whom concomitant zinc supplementation has been confirmed as necessary to other therapeutic needs. If this is not possible, administration of the medication 2 hours before or 6 hours after ingestion of an oral zinc or multimineral supplement is suggested and can effectively minimize risk of an adverse interaction (i.e., antibiotic malabsorption). This recommendation may also apply to intake of zinc-rich or zinc-fortified foods. Monitor for decreased therapeutic effects of oral quinolones if inadvertently administered simultaneously with oral zinc or multimineral supplements.

Clobetasol and Related Topical Corticosteroids

Evidence: Clobetasol (clobetasol topical; Cormax, Dermoval, Dermotyl, Dermovate, Dermoxin, Eumosone, Lobate, Olux, Temovate, Temovate E, Topifort).
Related, no evidence for extrapolation: Alclometasone (Aclovate, Modrasone), amcinonide (Cyclocort), beclomethasone, betamethasone dipropionate/valerate (betamethasone topical; Alphatrex, Beta-Val, Betaderm, Betanate, Betatrex, Diprolene AF, Diprolene, Diprosone, Luxiq, Maxivate, Teladar, Uticort, Valisone), clobetasone (Eumovate), clocortolone (clocortolone pivalate topical; Cloderm), desonide (DesOwen, Tridesilon), desoximetasone (Topicort, Topicort LP), desoxymethasone, dexamethasone (Aeroseb-Dex, Decaderm, Decadron, Decaspray), diflorasone (Apexicon, Florone, Maxiflor, Psorcon), diflucortolone (Nerisona, Nerisone), fluocinolone (Derma-Smoothe/FS, Fluonid, Synelar, Synemol), fluocinonide (Fluonex, Lidex, Lidex-E, Lonide, Vanos), fludroxycortide (flurandrenolone), fluocortolone (Ultralan), flurandrenolide (Cordran, Drenison), fluticasone (Cutivate), halcinonide (Halog), halobetasol (Ultravate); hydrocortisone 17-butyrate/acetate/probutate/ valerate (hydrocortisone topical; Acticort100, Aeroseb-HC, Ala-Cort, Ala-Scalp HP, Allercort, Alphaderm, Bactine, Beta-HC, Caldecort Anti-Itch, Cetacort, Cort-Dome, Cortaid, Cortef, Cortifair, Cortizone, Cortone, Cortril, Delacort,

Dermacort, Dermarest, DriCort, DermiCort, Dermtex HC, Epifoam, Gly-Cort, Hi-Cor, Hydro-Tex, Hytone, LactiCare-HC, Lanacort, Lemoderm, Locoid, MyCort, Nutracort, Pandel, Penecort, Pentacort, Proctocort, Rederm, S-T Cort, Synacort, Texacort, Westcort); mometasone (Elocon, mometasone topical), triamcinolone (Aristocort, Triderm, Kenalog, Flutex, Kenonel, triamcinolone topical); triamcinolone and nystatin (Mycolog II).

Interaction Type and Significance

⊕⊕ **Beneficial or Supportive Interaction, with Professional Management**

Probability:	Evidence Base:
3. Possible	○ **Preliminary**

Effect and Mechanism of Action

Clobetasol is a synthetic glucocorticoid derived from cortisol. Possessing significant corticosteroid activity and minor mineralocorticoid activity, it is used clinically for its activity as a topical anti-inflammatory and immunosuppressant, particularly for corticosteroid-responsive dermatoses, and systemically in replacement therapy for adrenal insufficiency. Zinc has demonstrated beneficial effects in supporting healthy skin and immune function generally, and facilitating tissue repair in particular, as does biotin, with which it can be combined. Coadministration of zinc and topical clobetasol, along with other synergistic nutrients such as biotin, may provide for enhanced therapeutic effect in the treatment of inflammatory dermatological conditions.

Research

Limited research suggests a potential synergistic effect may be obtained from combining zinc and clobetasol, especially as part of a more comprehensive therapeutic strategy. In a published letter, Camacho and Garcia-Hernandez[123a] reported that children with alopecia areata exhibited greater improvement when administered a treatment combining topical clobetasol with zinc aspartate (100 mg daily) and biotin (20 mg daily) than did children treated with oral corticosteroids. These findings are promising but primarily serve to indicate that further research is warranted.

Nutritional Therapeutics, Clinical Concerns, and Adaptations

Physicians treating inflammatory dermatological conditions such as alopecia areata with clobetasol or related topical corticosteroids may find that the addition of zinc, especially with other synergistic nutrients such as biotin, may enhance the therapeutic efficacy of the intervention. Patients should be advised of the preliminary nature of the scientific evidence, but also of the underlying rationale of the combination and the relatively low additional risk. In particular, such an approach may provide greater benefit and lesser adverse effects than oral corticosteroids.

Cisplatin

Cisplatin (cis-Diaminedichloroplatinum, CDDP; Platinol, Platinol-AQ).
See EDTA in Theoretical, Speculative, and Preliminary Interactions Research.

Corticosteroids, Oral, Including Prednisone

Betamethasone (Celestone), cortisone (Cortone), dexamethasone (Decadron), fludrocortisone (Florinef), hydrocortisone (Cortef), methylprednisolone (Medrol) prednisolone (Delta-Cortef, Orapred, Pediapred, Prelone), prednisone

Nutrient-Drug Interactions and Drug-Induced Nutrient Depletions

(Deltasone, Liquid Pred, Meticorten, Orasone), triamcinolone (Aristocort).

See also Clobetasol and Related Topical Corticosteroids.

Interaction Type and Significance

≈≈ **Drug-Induced Nutrient Depletion, Supplementation Therapeutic, with Professional Management**

✗ **Potential or Theoretical Adverse Interaction of Uncertain Severity**

Nutrient Depletion
Probability: Evidence Base:
3. Possible   ◉ Emerging or
                                    ● Consensus

Nutrient Interference
Probability: Evidence Base:
6. Unknown   ☐ Inadequate

Effect and Mechanism of Action

Zinc modulates acute immune response and promotes normal tissue repair. The adenohypophyseal-adrenocortical network plays a critical role in maintaining circulating zinc and in mobilizing zinc stores from tissue stores.[124] Under adrenocorticotropic hormone (ACTH) stress, the reaction of cortisol release is physiological, whereas the serum zinc level decreases significantly.[125] Thus, zinc metabolism can be significantly affected by both internal processes such as inflammation and exogenous influences such as glucocorticoid administration.

Oral corticosteroid medications, particularly at high doses, can cause increased urinary excretion of zinc and reduced serum zinc levels; significant effect is less probable with short-term, low-level corticosteroid administration.[124,126] Effects also vary through the course of steroid administration.

Zinc has been said to impair or interfere with the activity of corticosteroids or other immunosuppressant drug regimens because of its "immunostimulant" activity. No specific mechanism of action or other scientific data have been provided to support such assertions. This oversimplification likely derives from a misunderstanding of zinc's role in the immune system. Zinc deficiency is a documented cause of immune dysfunction, and zinc repletion restores normal immune function; however, zinc has not been demonstrated to act as an immune "stimulant."

Research

The scientific data on the interaction between corticosteroids and zinc have evolved over 30 years but still provide an incomplete understanding of the mechanisms involved and their clinical implications, especially with regard to the stages of immune response, tissue repair, and the role of the pituitary/adrenal axis in zinc metabolism. In 1971, Briggs et al.[126] reported that short-term, low-level prednisolone (5 or 10 mg/day) did not significantly effect serum zinc concentrations. That same year, Flynn et al.[124] published their findings on the effects on zinc during use of corticosteroids as vasodilators in the treatment of low-cardiac-output syndrome (LCOS) in patients with major burns (with or without LCOS) and surgical patients (with LCOS) compared with 30 elective or emergency surgery patients acting as controls. They noted that earlier researchers had found that elevated "serum and urine corticosteroids and, eventually, adrenocortical exhaustion have been reported in the early stages in severe burns," and that serum zinc "is also

raised during the first day after the burn and starts to decrease rapidly after the seventh day."[127,128] Intravenous (IV) corticosteroids were administered in pharmacological doses to the major burn patients with LCOS (hydrocortisone, 800 mg every 6 hours) and in a vascular-surgery patient with LCOS (dexamethasone phosphate, 200 mg, equivalent to 8.0 g cortisone). They observed that "massive doses of steroids rapidly lower serum-zinc levels" in seriously ill burn patients and differentiated that response from the response to low-dose steroids as reported by Briggs. "The extent of pituitary/adrenal shutdown is likely to play a vital role in the differences between high and low dose effects." Both controls who underwent surgery and "major burn and L.C.O.S. patients receiving nonsteroid therapy had similar zinc patterns (i.e., increased zinc with the stress during the first days after injury or onset of L.C.O.S.)." However, only patients who received large doses of steroids exhibited rapid zinc loss. "Falls of 30-75 mcg per 100 ml were recorded as little as 1 hour after a single bolus of corticosteroids." Based on these and other findings, the authors concluded that the "actions of large doses of corticosteroids in major burn and L.C.O.S. patients point to a role for the adenohypophyseal/adrenocortical system in maintaining circulating zinc levels.... Increases and decreases in serum-zinc are linked to stress-induced activation and steroid-produced deactivation of the pituitary/adrenal axis" and as such indicate a central role of the pituitary/adrenal axis in regulating serum zinc changes and mobilizing body zinc stores.[124] Subsequent research by Fodor et al.[125] confirmed "that the zinc metabolism probably depends on glucocorticoidal controls."

Likewise, Yunice et al.[129] conducted an experiment comparing the effects of varying doses of a short-acting (methylprednisolone) and a long-acting (dexamethasone) synthetic glucocorticoid on extent and duration of alterations in plasma zinc and copper concentrations in normal humans. They observed increases in plasma zinc (and copper) levels shortly after IV administration of either steroid. However, plasma zinc concentrations decreased below control levels by 12 hours, and no significant decrease was noted beyond 48 hours; "the extent and duration of the depression depended on the dosage of the steroid administered." The authors concluded that their findings suggested "serum zinc levels may depend on ACTH-adrenal interactions."

In related research, Fell et al.[130] tracked zinc mobilization in two patients after hip replacement surgery and correlated it with muscle catabolism. They measured large increases in the daily excretion of zinc-65 (^{65}Zn), total zinc, and nitrogen, with the maximum excretion occurring about 10 days after surgery and observed a "good correlation between the increased excretion of ^{65}Zn and total zinc, indicating the tissue origin of the latter as skeletal muscle." Because ^{65}Zn is a radioactive form used only in research, these findings offer data more toward developing physiological knowledge than directly applicable to clinical monitoring of normal ^{64}Zn.

More broadly, research investigating the connections between endogenous steroid regulation and zinc metabolism might reveal valuable insights into the possible role of zinc status in the adverse effects of elevated cortisol, steroid release, and other components of stress response physiology that adversely affect immune function.

No evidence from clinical trials or qualified case reports substantiates broad assertions that zinc should not be administered concomitantly with corticosteroids or other immunosuppressant drug regimens because of its "immunostimulant" activity. Further research would be warranted should preliminary findings strongly indicate the occurrence of such a phenomenon.

Nutritional Therapeutics, Clinical Concerns, and Adaptations

Physicians prescribing oral corticosteroids are advised to consider the potential benefit of coadministering zinc as a therapeutic synergist and, in patients taking long-term steroids, for prevention of depletion. The available evidence indicates that zinc plays an important role in physiological response to trauma and participates in immune and tissue repair functions, as in cases involving severe burns. Moreover, both acute and chronic use of steroids can contribute to zinc depletion patterns. In some cases, depletion is more probable with administration for longer than 2 weeks. In other situations, however, acute depletion, especially in the context of injuries or pathologies putting high demands on physiological zinc metabolism, acute high-dose steroids may cause zinc depletion with greater potential for clinically significant adverse effects.

A daily dose of 15 to 50 mg elemental zinc per day, within the context of appropriate supervision, will generally facilitate healing and prevent depletion without introducing substantial risk of significant adverse effects. Although serum zinc was used for assessment in some relevant research, expert consensus agrees that no sensitive laboratory method exists for detecting zinc depletion in tissue stores and zinc pools. The theoretical concern that zinc might counteract intentional immunosuppressant activity lacks substantive evidence-based support and, even if true, might be beneficial in some cases and only potentially detrimental in others, depending on the condition being treated, patient characteristics, therapeutic strategy, and phase of treatment intervention. Further research through well-designed and adequately powered trials is warranted to determine safety and efficacy, mechanisms, indications, and treatment guidelines.

ESTROGENS, PROGESTINS, AND ESTROGEN-PROGESTIN COMBINATIONS

Oral Contraceptives: Monophasic, Biphasic, and Triphasic Estrogen Preparations (Synthetic Estrogen and Progesterone Analogs)

Ethinyl estradiol and desogestrel (Desogen, Ortho-TriCyclen). Ethinyl estradiol and ethynodiol (Demulen 1/35, Demulen 1/50, Nelulen 1/25, Nelulen 1/50, Zovia). Ethinyl estradiol and levonorgestrel (Alesse, Levlen, Levlite, Levora 0.15/30, Nordette, Tri-Levlen, Triphasil, Trivora). Ethinyl estradiol and norethindrone/norethisterone (Brevicon, Estrostep, Genora 1/35, GenCept 1/35, Jenest-28, Loestrin 1.5/30, Loestrin1/20, Modicon, Necon 1/25, Necon 10/11, Necon 0.5/30, Necon 1/50, Nelova 1/35, Nelova 10/11, Norinyl 1/35, Norlestin 1/50, Ortho Novum 1/35, Ortho Novum 10/11, Ortho Novum 7/7/7, Ovcon-35, Ovcon-50, Tri-Norinyl, Trinovum). Ethinyl estradiol and norgestrel (Lo/Ovral, Ovral). Etonogestrel/ethinyl estradiol vaginal ring (Nuvaring). Mestranol and norethindrone (Genora 1/50, Nelova 1/50, Norethin 1/50, Ortho-Novum 1/50). Related, internal application: Etonogestrel/ethinyl estradiol vaginal ring (Nuvaring).

Hormone Replacement Therapy (HRT), Estrogens

Chlorotrianisene (Tace); conjugated equine estrogens (Premarin); conjugated synthetic estrogens (Cenestin); dienestrol (Ortho Dienestrol); esterified estrogens (Estratab, Menest, Neo-Estrone); estradiol, topical/transdermal/ring (Alora

Transdermal, Climara Transdermal, Estrace, Estradot, Estring FemPatch, Vivelle-Dot, Vivelle Transdermal); estradiol cypionate (Dep-Gynogen, Depo-Estradiol, Depogen, Dura-Estrin, Estra-D, Estro-Cyp, Estroject-LA, Estronol-LA); estradiol hemihydrate (Estreva, Vagifem); estradiol valerate (Delestrogen, Estra-L 40, Gynogen L.A. 20, Progynova, Valergen 20); estrone (Aquest, Estragyn 5, Estro-A, Estrone '5', Kestrone-5); estropipate (Ogen, Ortho-Est); ethinyl estradiol (Estinyl, Gynodiol, Lynoral).

Medroxyprogesterone-containing HRT and contraceptives: Medroxyprogesterone, oral (Cycrin, Provera); conjugated equine estrogens and medroxyprogesterone (Premelle cycle 5, Prempro).

Progestin/Progestogen-Only Oral Contraceptives, Implants, and Postcoital Contraceptives

Related, evidence lacking for extrapolation: Etonogestrel, implant (Implanon); levonorgestrel, implant (Jadelle, Norplant; Norplant-2); levonorgestrel, oral postcoital contraceptive (Duofem, Escapelle, Levonelle, Levonelle-2, Microlut, Microval, Norgeston, NorLevo, Plan B, Postinor-2, Vika, Vikela); medroxyprogesterone, injection (depot medroxyprogesterone acetate, DMPA; Depo-Provera, Depo-subQ Provera 104); NES progestin, implant (ST-1435, Nestorone); norgestrel, oral (Ovrette).

Hormone Replacement Therapy

Related, evidence lacking for extrapolation:
Estrogen/progestin combinations: Conjugated equine estrogens and norgestrel (Prempak-C); estradiol and dydrogesterone (Femoston); estradiol and norethindrone, patch (CombiPatch); estradiol and norethindrone/norethisterone, oral (Activella, Climagest, Climesse, FemHRT, Trisequens); estradiol valerate and cyproterone acetate (Climens); estradiol valerate and norgestrel (Progyluton); estradiol and norgestimate (Ortho-Prefest).
Estrogen/testosterone combinations: Esterified estrogens and methyltestosterone (Estratest, Estratest HS).
See also Androgens.

Interaction Type and Significance

≈≈≈ **Drug-Induced Nutrient Depletion, Supplementation Therapeutic, Not Requiring Professional Management**
⊕⊕ **Beneficial or Supportive Interaction, with Professional Management**

Probability:
2. **Probable** or
4. **Plausible**

Evidence Base:
○ **Preliminary**

Effect and Mechanism of Action

The use of oral contraceptives (OCs) may be associated with decreased serum levels of zinc.[131] Conversely, conjugated estrogens and medroxyprogesterone may reduce previously elevated urinary zinc excretion (as well as magnesium) in osteoporotic postmenopausal women.[132] No specific mechanisms have been established to explain the various observed interactions phenomena, singly or collectively.

Research

The effects of exogenous estrogens on zinc levels can vary depending on the form and dose of estrogen administered, concomitant agents in formulation, patient characteristics (including life stage), and therapeutic intent. A significant incidence of zinc deficiency has been documented in females of all ages in a broad range of socioeconomic conditions, with the greatest risk in premature infants; low-income urban infants, children, adolescents, and women of childbearing age; and populations with a high-cereal diet.[8]

Dorea et al.[131] assessed serum levels of zinc and copper in 44 women of the same age group, 24 of whom were taking OCs and 20 serving as controls. They observed that "serum zinc was significantly lower while serum copper was significantly higher for women taking the oral contraceptive agents," but that there was "no significant correlation between the serum zinc and copper levels" in either group. In general, adolescents in the United States tend to have inadequate intake of zinc and other micronutrients, with dietary intakes of zinc less than 75% of the U.S. RDA in more than one-third and less than 50% using nutritional supplements.[9]

In a trial involving 37 postmenopausal women, some of whom exhibited signs of osteoporosis, Herzberg et al.[132] compared serum and urinary zinc levels before and after 6 and 12 months of treatment with estrogen replacement therapy (ERT) consisting of conjugated estrogens (0.625 mg) and medroxyprogesterone acetate (5 mg). They observed a "consistent negative association ... between changes in bone mineral density and urinary zinc excretion in the osteoporosis group" and an association between ERT and "reduced excretion of zinc, magnesium, and hydroxyproline in the elevated zinc excretion group." In particular, urinary zinc excretion decreased 35% after 3 months and 26% after 1 year of ERT. In contrast, serum levels of zinc (as well as magnesium, calcium, and phosphate, but not alkaline phosphatase) "showed only negligible changes during ERT." Noting this significant decrease in urinary zinc excretion after 3 months of ERT, the authors concluded that this "change was more pronounced in women with osteoporosis and elevated zinc excretion" and was associated with changes in bone metabolism rather than variation in diet.

Nutritional Therapeutics, Clinical Concerns, and Adaptations

Physicians prescribing exogenous estrogen preparations may consider the potential value of coadministering zinc, with the effect and rationale varying for different populations using estrogen for different purposes. In women using OCs, coadministration of a multimineral/multivitamin formulation containing zinc, as well as vitamin B$_6$ and folic acid, may reduce adverse effects of the medication, including nutrient depletion. The probability that such nutritional support will be beneficial is generally greater in patients with compromised nutritional intake. Women treated with ERT may derive benefit against osteoporotic tendencies with concomitant zinc, particularly if they have compromised nutrient intake and signs if osteoporosis. The use of concomitant zinc at a physiologic dosage level, 15 to 40 mg elemental zinc daily, is generally safe and unlikely to produce any clinically significant adverse effects. Moreover, in women receiving concomitant androgen therapy, the addition of zinc may enhance therapeutic outcomes. Further research through well-designed and adequately powered clinical trials may be warranted to establish risk factors and parameters of benefit to shape clinical guidelines for integration of zinc and other nutrients into therapeutic strategies using exogenous estrogens.

Histamine (H$_2$) Receptor Antagonists and Related Antacids and Gastric Acid–Suppressive Medications

Evidence: Famotidine (Pepcid RPD, Pepcid, Pepcid AC), ranitidine (Zantac).
Similar properties but evidence lacking for extrapolation: Nizatidine (Axid, Axid AR); combination drug: ranitidine, bismuth, and citrate (Tritec).

Similar properties but evidence indicating no or reduced interaction effects: Cimetidine (Tagamet, Tagamet HB).
Extrapolated, based on similar properties:
Antacids: Aluminum carbonate gel (Basajel), aluminum hydroxide (Alternagel, Amphojel); combination drugs: aluminum hydroxide, magnesium carbonate, alginic acid, and sodium bicarbonate (Gaviscon Extra Strength Tablets, Gaviscon Regular Strength Liquid, Gaviscon Extra Strength Liquid); aluminum hydroxide and magnesium hydroxide (Advanced Formula Di-Gel Tablets, Co-Magaldrox, Di-Gel, Gelusil, Maalox, Maalox Plus, Mylanta, Wingel); aluminum hydroxide, magnesium trisilicate, alginic acid, and sodium bicarbonate (Alenic Alka, Gaviscon Regular Strength Tablets); calcium carbonate (Titralac, Tums); magnesium hydroxide (Phillips' Milk of Magnesia MOM); combination drugs: magnesium hydroxide and calcium carbonate (Calcium Rich Rolaids); magnesium hydroxide, aluminum hydroxide, calcium carbonate, and simethicone (Tempo Tablets); magnesium trisilicate and aluminum hydroxide (Adcomag trisil, Foamicon); magnesium trisilicate, alginic acid, and sodium bicarbonate (Alenic Alka, Gaviscon Regular Strength Tablets); combination drug: sodium bicarbonate, aspirin, and citric acid (Alka-Seltzer).
Proton pump inhibitors: Esomeprazole (Nexium), lansoprazole (Prevacid, Zoton), omeprazole (Losec, Prilosec), pantoprazole (Protium, Protonix, Somac), rabeprazole (AcipHex, Pariet).
See also Calcium and Calcium-Based Antacids in Nutrient-Nutrient Interactions.

Interaction Type and Significance

≈≈≈ **Drug-Induced Nutrient Depletion, Supplementation Therapeutic, Not Requiring Professional Management**

Probability:
2. Probable

Evidence Base:
○ **Preliminary** to
◉ **Emerging**

Effect and Mechanism of Action

The solubility of the diverse zinc salts is affected by pH, which may vary between pH 1 and 7 under various physiological conditions in the stomach. Zinc absorption is optimal at an intragastric pH of 3 or less.[1] Thus, by reducing gastric acid secretion, H$_2$ blockers (as well as proton pump inhibitors, and possibly antacids) can exert both direct and indirect effects on the absorption of zinc and result in depletion over time.

Through its important role in the healthy function of mucous membranes and recovery from injury, zinc supports the repair of damaged gastric tissue.

Research

The basic physiological premises of gastric pH environment effects on zinc absorption are generally agreed on, but research-based evidence into the clinical implications of this interaction, although consistent, is limited. Using a rodent model, Pinelli et al.[133] found that cimetidine and nizatidine may reduce zinc absorption by decreasing gastric acid secretion and can deplete zinc levels in the prostate gland. In a series of experiments involving 16 healthy subjects, Sturniolo et al.[134] compared the effects of inhibition of gastric acid secretion by ranitidine and cimetidine on zinc absorption. First, they performed a zinc tolerance test (ZTT, with ZnSO$_4$, 220 mg orally), then administered cimetidine (1 g daily for 3 days), and observed decreased zinc absorption. Next, they administered oral doses of ranitidine (300 mg) daily for 6 days, 3 days before testing and 3 days during the test; they also administered 500 mg cimetidine to these subjects. Overall, they observed that the "areas under the plasma concentration curves for zinc were significantly reduced after ranitidine…, but not after cimetidine administration. Gastric acid was also reduced after ranitidine, but not after cimetidine (500 mg) administration, suggesting that gastric acid secretion plays a role in the regulation of zinc absorption in man."[134] In a two-way, four-phase, crossover study involving 10 healthy subjects (five males and five females), Henderson et al.[1] investigated the effect of intragastric pH on zinc absorption. After a 9-hour fast, they administered a single oral dose of 50 mg elemental zinc as the acetate or the oxide salt and under either high or low intragastric pH conditions while continuously monitoring intragastric pH using a Heidelberg capsule pH detector-transmitter. "During the high pH phases, single oral doses of famotidine 40 mg oral suspension were administered before the zinc to raise the intragastric pH above 5. Intragastric pH < or = 3 was maintained in the low pH phases." They found that the "highest zinc plasma concentrations occurred with the acetate salt at a low intragastric pH, while the lowest plasma concentrations occurred with the oxide salt at a high intragastric pH." Subsequently, in vitro tests verified the importance of pH to the dissolution of these salts.[1]

Notably, numerous clinicians and researchers have reported benefits for gastric tissue damaged by ulceration. In a double-blind trial involving 18 patients with benign gastric ulcers and no evidence of zinc deficiency, Frommer[135] found that subjects administered zinc sulfate (220 mg orally three times daily) "had an ulcer healing rate three times that of patients treated with placebo," and that "complete healing of ulcers occurred more frequently in the patients taking zinc." These findings suggest that zinc may have independent therapeutic value in the treatment of individuals with gastric ulcer disease and related conditions, and that coadministration might provide synergistic effects.

Nutritional Therapeutics, Clinical Concerns, and Adaptations
Physicians prescribing H_2 blockers (as well as proton pump inhibitors or antacids) are advised to coadminister elemental zinc, 50 to 75 mg daily (preferably as the acetate), to prevent the probable adverse effect of zinc depletion with chronic suppression of gastric acid.

Loop Diuretics

Bumetanide (Bumex), ethacrynic acid (Edecrin), furosemide (Lasix), torsemide (Demadex).

Interaction Type and Significance
≈≈ **Drug-Induced Nutrient Depletion, Supplementation Therapeutic, with Professional Management**

Probability:
4. Plausible or
  3. Possible

Evidence Base:
○ **Preliminary**

Effect and Mechanism of Action
The use of loop diuretics may result in increased urinary excretion of zinc.

Research
In a small, randomized trial, Wester[136] compared urinary zinc excretion in nine patients during treatment with bendroflumethiazide, chlorthalidone, and hydrochlorothiazide with that in nine patients treated with bumetanide, furosemide, and triamterene. He observed that in patients receiving loop diuretics, "urine zinc concentration diminished and the total amount of zinc excretion increased much less than during therapy with the thiazides." Based on these preliminary findings, the author concluded that "the observed increased urinary losses of zinc deserve further attention."

Nutritional Therapeutics, Clinical Concerns, and Adaptations
Physicians prescribing a loop diuretic are advised to consider preliminary data suggesting that these medications may deplete zinc through increased urinary excretion. The risk of clinically significant zinc deficiency has not been established, but the probability of adverse effects is greater in individuals with compromised nutrient intake and concomitant medications that adversely affect zinc status. Dietary intake of zinc is often inadequate and zinc status impaired in many populations likely to be prescribed diuretics, such as patients with heart failure. Pending further research, medically supervised coadministration of zinc at a moderate dosage level, 40 to 80 mg elemental zinc once daily, is advisable as generally safe, unlikely to produce any clinically significant adverse effects, and potentially beneficial. Monitoring serum copper periodically and coadministering low-dose copper (e.g., 1-3 mg/day) are judicious means of guarding against zinc-induced copper deficiency with long-term zinc administration.

Metronidazole, Vaginal

Metronidazole, Vaginal (MetroGel-Vaginal)

Interaction Type and Significance
⊕⊕ **Beneficial or Supportive Interaction, with Professional Management**

Probability:
4. Plausible

Evidence Base:
○ **Preliminary**

Effect and Mechanism of Action
The reported antitrichomonal properties of zinc sulfate appear to combine with metronidazole to produce an additive or synergistic interaction exerting greater therapeutic effect. No specific mechanism of action has been established.

Research
In a retrospective case analysis, Houang et al.[137] reported the successful treatment of four patients with chronic recurrent trichomoniasis, without evidence of reinfection, using a combination of "zinc sulfate douching (1%) followed by a metronidazole 500 mg suppository per vaginale twice daily and 200 to 400 mg three times a day orally. The douching and suppository were used prophylactically for 3 nights after menstruation for some months." These clinicians found that the addition of zinc sulfate douche greatly increased therapeutic efficacy in four patients "who had a history of 4 months to 4 years of culture-positive symptomatic trichomoniasis and received a variety of therapies before referral" and for whom vaginal metronidazole treatment alone had been ineffective. All four subjects remained asymptomatic and exhibited normal results in clinical and laboratory examinations at 2 to 5 months after treatment.

Further research with well-designed and adequately powered clinical trials may be warranted to confirm the efficacy of a combination zinc sulfate douche and metronidazole regimen in the treatment of vaginal trichomoniasis, as well as vaginal infection involving other organisms.

Nutritional Therapeutics, Clinical Concerns, and Adaptations

Physicians treating women with vaginal trichomoniasis, especially recurrent or recalcitrant, are advised to consider concomitant prescription of zinc sulfate douche (1%) with metronidazole gel suppository. Adverse effects from zinc or from the combined intervention are unlikely to be greater than those associated with metronidazole alone, and the synergistic effect from coadministration may hasten or potentiate the treatment.

Nonsteroidal Anti-Inflammatory Drugs (NSAIDs)

COX-1 inhibitors: Diclofenac (Cataflam, Voltaren), combination drug: diclofenac and misoprostol (Arthrotec), diflunisal (Dolobid), etodolac (Lodine), fenoprofen (Dalfon), furbiprofen (Ansaid), ibuprofen (Advil, Excedrin IB, Motrin, Motrin IB, Nuprin, Pedia Care Fever Drops, Provel, Rufen); combination drug: hydrocodone and ibuprofen (Reprexain, Vicoprofen); indomethacin (indometacin; Indocin, Indocin-SR), ketoprofen (Orudis, Oruvail), ketorolac (Acular ophthalmic, Toradol), meclofenamate (Meclomen), mefenamic acid (Ponstel), meloxicam (Mobic), nabumetone (Relafen), naproxen (Aleve, Anaprox, Naprosyn), oxaprozin (Daypro), piroxicam (Feldene), salsalate (salicylic acid; Amigesic, Disalcid, Marthritic, Mono Gesic, Salflex, Salsitab), sulindac (Clinoril), tolmetin (Tolectin).

COX-2 inhibitor: Celecoxib (Celebrex).

Interaction Type and Significance

◇◇ **Impaired Drug Absorption and Bioavailability, Precautions Appropriate**

≈≈ **Drug-Induced Nutrient Depletion, Supplementation Therapeutic, with Professional Management**

⊕✗ **Bimodal or Variable Interaction, with Professional Management**

⊕ **Potential or Theoretical Beneficial or Supportive Interaction, with Professional Management**

Nutrient Interference
Probability:
4. Plausible

Evidence Base:
○ **Preliminary**

Nutrient Depletion
Probability:
4. Plausible or
3. Possible

Evidence Base:
○ **Preliminary**

Effect and Mechanism of Action

Low zinc levels may be associated with inflammatory conditions such as rheumatoid arthritis (RA).[138] Anti-inflammatory agents such as NSAIDs may increase zinc excretion and contribute to zinc depletion.[138,139]

Although not fully elucidated, zinc and other metals may complex with some NSAIDs to decrease absorption and bioavailability of both agents.[138,140] Other mechanisms are also probable but unknown.

Research

Data from human studies indicate that NSAIDs can increase urinary zinc excretion but differ as to whether serum zinc levels, a marginally accurate marker, may reflect these alterations. Elling et al.[139] conducted a study using healthy volunteers to assess the effect of naproxen, as a representative NSAID, on zinc metabolism. They observed a

"significant increase in the urinary zinc excretion rate" in subjects administered naproxen, "with a mean increase in the order of 35%," which fell toward normal at the end of treatment and returned to normal after withdrawal of naproxen. Notably, the "serum zinc concentration was virtually unchanged" during the treatment period. Although noting that the mechanism by which naproxen induces hyperzincuria was "not known" at the time, the authors suggested that increased zinc excretion could result from "protein binding interaction or a direct renal action of naproxen implying a decrease in the maximum tubular reabsorption capacity (Tmax)." They concluded that trials of longer duration, particularly involving patients with RA, "are needed, however, in order to evaluate the possibility of a zinc depletion."[139] That same year (1980), Balogh et al.[138] investigated total plasma zinc levels in patients with RA being treated with a variety of medications. They found "significantly lower zinc levels in patients with rheumatoid arthritis on nonsteroidal anti-inflammatory drugs than in patients on levamisole and penicillamine." Moreover, zinc levels "correlated positively with serum albumin, and there was an inverse correlation between zinc levels and both ESR and globulin concentration in all rheumatoid patients." The authors concluded that their findings "support the hypothesis that low plasma zinc level in rheumatoid arthritis is one of the nonspecific features of inflammation."[138]

Dendrinou-Samara et al.[140] conducted in vitro experiments that demonstrated the formation of complexes between anti-inflammatory medications and Zn(II), as well as other metal ions. In particular, they synthesized and characterized complexes of "Zn(II), Cd(II) and Pt(II) metal ions with the anti-inflammatory drugs, 1-methyl-5-(p-toluoyl)-1H-pyrrole-2-acetic acid (Tolmetin), alpha-methyl-4-(2-methylpropyl) benzeneacetic acid (Ibuprofen), 6-methoxy-alpha-methylnaphthalene-2-acetic acid (Naproxen) and 1-(4-chlorobenzoyl)-5-methoxy-2-methyl-1H-indole-3-acetic acid (indomethacin)." They noted that "antibacterial and growth inhibitory activity is higher than that of the parent ligands."

Nutritional Therapeutics, Clinical Concerns, and Adaptations

Health care professionals are advised to consider coadministration of zinc when providing care to individuals using NSAIDs or other anti-inflammatory agents on a chronic basis for the treatment of inflammatory conditions such as RA. Broad and specific data indicate that these patients are at increased risk of compromised zinc status because of their nutrient intake and pathophysiological changes, and that these agents may further deplete zinc. Such depletion patterns may not be easily detected through standard laboratory tests; for example, serum zinc may not predictably reveal zinc deficiency in tissue or cells. Specific evidence-based research is lacking to confirm efficacy, but the use of concomitant zinc at physiologic levels, 15 to 40 mg elemental zinc daily, is generally safe and unlikely to produce any clinically significant adverse effects. However, separation of intake by at least 2 hours is prudent given the limited but pharmacologically reasonable data suggesting the possibility of chelate formation with simultaneous intake.

Penicillamine

Penicillamine (D-penicillamine; Cuprimine, Depen).
Extrapolated, based on similar properties: Tetrathiomolybdate (investigational).

Interaction Type and Significance

⊕⊕   **Beneficial or Supportive Interaction, with Professional Management**

⊕✗   **Bimodal or Variable Interaction, with Professional Management**

◇◇   **Impaired Drug Absorption and Bioavailability, Precautions Appropriate**

≈≈   **Drug-Induced Nutrient Depletion, Supplementation Therapeutic, with Professional Management**

✗   **Potential or Theoretical Adverse Interaction of Uncertain Severity**

Coadministration Benefit

Probability:
2. Probable

Evidence Base:
◉ Emerging to
● Consensus

Coadministration Risk

Probability:
4. Plausible to
2. Probable

Evidence Base:
○ Preliminary

Effect and Mechanism of Action

Wilson's disease is a rare but potentially fatal autosomal recessive inherited disease of copper accumulation in the liver in which a defect in a copper-transport adenosine triphosphatase results in a failure of biliary excretion of excess copper.

Zinc and penicillamine can both be used in the treatment of individuals with Wilson's disease because of their effects of lowering copper levels, although by different mechanisms.[141-143] Zinc produces its unique anticopper action by inducing intestinal cell metallothionein, which then forms a mucosal block, preventing copper absorption and increasing copper excretion in the stool. "Because this mechanism blocks not only the absorption of food copper but the reabsorption of large amounts of endogenously secreted copper, zinc serves to remove copper from the body as well as prevent its reaccumulation."[142] On the other hand, penicillamine can effectively increase urinary excretion of copper and reverse positive copper balance through its action as a chelating drug, but is also known for adverse effects.

However, the simultaneous intake of zinc and penicillamine may result in impaired efficacy and nutrient depletion. When ingested close together, penicillamine and zinc, as a supplement or through zinc-rich or zinc-enriched foods, may bind, resulting in reduced bioavailability of both agents. Moreover, penicillamine, through its chelating effect, may cause an unintentional increase in urinary excretion of zinc, along with the intended copper excretion. Effects will vary with mode of administration; the maximal plasma penicillamine concentrations achieved with oral penicillamine are only one-fifth that achieved by injection.[144]

Research

Different forms of zinc have been used in the treatment of Wilson's disease, with zinc acetate used directly and zinc sulfate combined with penicillamine. Anderson et al.[141] reviewed trials and case reports concerning zinc acetate as maintenance therapy in patients initially treated with a chelating agent. They concluded: "Although studies evaluating large populations are lacking, zinc therapy has demonstrated exceptional safety and efficacy over a period of 40 years.... Zinc acetate is an effective maintenance therapy for patients with Wilson's disease."

They further noted that with its "negligible toxicity, compared with that of previously approved treatments, zinc acetate is considerably safer than other treatments and can be used during pregnancy and for the treatment of presymptomatic patients." They cautioned, however, that "data do not support its use as monotherapy in patients with acute neurologic or hepatic disease."

Li et al.[143] conducted a clinical trial, with long-term follow-up (4-11 years) of 31 children, investigating combined therapy with "large-dose zinc sulfate and low-dose penicillamine" in children with Wilson's disease (hepatolenticular degeneration, HLD). During the active phase of treatment, they treated symptomatic pediatric patients with "large-dose zinc sulfate (100-150 mg, <6 yr; 150-200 mg, 6-8 yr; 200-300 mg, 9-10 yr; 300 mg, >10 yr; 3 times a day) in addition to low-dose penicillamine (8-10 mg/kg/d)." Presymptomatic patients received zinc sulfate alone, as did patients receiving maintenance therapy when clinical improvement was achieved. They reported that "blood concentrations of copper were persistently lower than normal" and that "urine copper excretion of 24 hours was significantly lower than that before the combined therapy in all patients," and it became normal in five cases (16%) after 6 months of treatment, and in 26 cases (84%) after 1 to 2 years of treatment. They also observed "higher blood concentrations of zinc" in 20 subjects (65%), with "higher urine zinc excretion ... in 25 cases (81%) once or more times during the therapy." They concluded that combined treatment with "large-dose zinc sulfate and low-dose penicillamine is an effective, safe and cheap treatment for children with HLD."

Thus, the limited data from clinical trials indicate that zinc and penicillamine can be safely and effectively used together as part of a long-term strategy in the treatment of copper accumulation diseases, particularly Wilson's disease, but that timing and dosage need to be adjusted at different phases of the treatment based on patient response.

Nutritional Therapeutics, Clinical Concerns, and Adaptations

Physicians treating individuals with Wilson's disease may enhance clinical outcomes and reduce adverse effects through implementation of an integrative therapeutic strategy combining zinc and chelating agents such as penicillamine or tetrathiomolybdate (investigational). Oral zinc sulfate and zinc acetate have both been used successfully in clinical trials. However, many clinicians consider zinc sulfate an inferior form with limited bioavailability. Zinc acetate, on the other hand, has superior bioavailability but may require a prescription, mainly because of its use in treating Wilson's disease. In all cases, the timing of zinc administration will depend on patient condition and response, with some researchers and clinicians relying primarily on chelating agents during the more severe stages of treatment and using zinc primarily for maintenance once a patient has stabilized or in presymptomatic patients. Zinc and copper chelators are best used sequentially rather than simultaneously because copper chelators also chelate zinc, although they are sometimes used concurrently. In all cases, separation of intake by at least 2 hours is recommended to minimize the risk of the two agents complexing and becoming less bioavailable. Close clinical management by trained and experienced health care professionals, with supervision and regular monitoring, is essential. Further study is warranted and probable given the body of evidence and practice supporting coadministration and sequential administration.

Potassium-Sparing Diuretics

Evidence: Amiloride (Midamor), triamterene (Dyrenium). Similar properties but evidence indicating no or reduced interaction effects: Amiloride combination drug: amiloride and hydrochlorothiazide (Moduretic).

Similar properties but evidence lacking for extrapolation: Spironolactone (Aldactone), spironolactone and hydrochlorothiazide (Aldactazide), triamterene and hydrochlorothiazide (Dyazide, Maxzide).

Interaction Type and Significance

⊕✗   **Bimodal or Variable Interaction, with Professional Management**

◇◇   **Drug-Induced Effect on Nutrient Function, Supplementation Contraindicated, Professional Management Appropriate**

≈≈   **Drug-Induced Nutrient Depletion, Supplementation Therapeutic, with Professional Management**

Nutrient Depletion

Probability:
3. Possible or
2. Probable

Evidence Base:
○ Preliminary to
◉ Emerging

Coadministration Risk

Probability:
4. Plausible or
3. Possible

Evidence Base:
▽ Mixed,
○ Preliminary

Effect and Mechanism of Action

Potassium-sparing diuretics demonstrate varied effects on zinc metabolism. Amiloride may induce zinc accumulation (and potential toxicity) by significantly reducing zinc excretion; however, this effect appears to be dose related and may not compensate for zinc loss caused by concomitant diuretics such as hydrochlorothiazide. Conversely, triamterene appears to increase urinary zinc excretion in the short term and may cause depletion over time. Overall, the mechanisms by which thiazide diuretics affect zinc metabolism are incompletely known, although their blocking of reabsorption in the distal tubule is a plausible extrapolation from the known mechanism involving magnesium.

Research

Wester[145] conducted several studies of experiments investigating the effects of various diuretics on urinary zinc excretion and tissue levels of zinc. In one paper he reported that 2 weeks of treatment with triamterene increased urinary zinc excretion by 18% compared with baseline.[136]

The situation with amiloride is both more complicated and less clear in its implications. In a review, Reyes et al.[146] suggest that a 10-mg dose of amiloride can significantly reduce urinary zinc excretion, but not 5 mg. Such an effect introduces the potential for excess zinc accumulation, although the effect is dose related, and the patient population is characterized by a relatively high incidence of inadequate zinc nutriture. Moreover, decreased zinc excretion does not inherently result in elevated zinc levels, given the homeostatic regulation of zinc absorption and the dynamic metabolic processes of zinc pools.

Two trials have investigated the effects of an amiloride-thiazide combination on zinc metabolism and nutriture, with mixed conclusions. Golik et al.[146a] compared serum zinc levels and urinary zinc excretion in 15 patients with essential hypertension taking a combination of hydrochlorothiazide and amiloride as chronic monotherapy, eight patients maintained with hydrochlorothiazide alone, and eight control subjects. Although "serum zinc values were statistically comparable in all three groups," they found that "urinary zinc excretion was abnormally elevated in the two patient groups." These authors concluded that, at least "in the dosage used, amiloride did not have a zinc-sparing effect." That same year (1987), Verho et al.[146b] published a paper reporting their findings in a double-blind, parallel-group study comparing the effects of hydrochlorothiazide (50 mg) plus amiloride (5 mg) once daily versus piretanide (6 mg) once or twice daily on serum levels of zinc and other trace elements over 3 months in subjects with mild to moderate hypertension. They concluded that 3 months' therapy with "a thiazide-potassium sparer diuretic combination is safe without producing any disturbances in the serum levels of trace elements," based on the findings that urinary zinc excretion stayed within normal levels. The use of serum zinc to evaluate effects on zinc status in both studies limits the utility of conclusions based on their findings, but suggests that the depleting effects of the thiazide agent and the zinc-conserving effects of the potassium-sparing diuretic may neutralize each other in some cases. Nevertheless, the effects of these agents on tissue zinc stores and zinc pools deserve further research to determine the long-term effects of these drugs in a patient population with a relatively high incidence of subclinical zinc deficiency.

Nutritional Therapeutics, Clinical Concerns, and Adaptations

Physicians prescribing potassium-sparing diuretics are advised to monitor zinc status closely in all patients. However, early symptoms of zinc deficiency, such as hypogeusia (decreased taste sensation), hyposmia (decreased olfactory sensation), diminished male sexual function, increased incidence of infections, slower wound healing, and white spots in fingernails, may be more useful than relying on monitoring of zinc levels in serum or elsewhere, because consensus is lacking as to an adequate laboratory standard for accurate assessment. Patients should be instructed to report any such occurrences. Triamterene can readily cause zinc depletion in the short term and with chronic use and, despite some suggestions to the contrary, the risk of zinc depletion with amiloride cannot be excluded, particularly in individuals with potential risk of marginal zinc status and increased susceptibility to zinc toxicity. Thus, coadministration of zinc at physiologic levels, 15 to 40 mg elemental zinc daily, may be indicated in patients receiving long-term triamterene and possibly other potassium-sparing diuretics.

The risk of zinc accumulation with amiloride use remains controversial, but close supervision and regular monitoring are always judicious in patients at greater risk for zinc toxicity, such as occurs with pregnancy, alcoholism, or renal insufficiency. Inherently, the probability of such risk being clinically significant would be greater in patients taking amiloride at a higher dose. Combining a thiazide diuretic with amiloride to mitigate its possible adverse effects may not provide a safe and simple remedy because these drugs deplete not only zinc but also other nutrients. Moreover, the mechanisms through which thiazide diuretics affect the metabolism of zinc and other minerals have not been fully elucidated, and the physiological effects of this proposed "pharmacological balancing act" have not been confirmed by substantive evidence from high-quality clinical trials.

Radiotherapy

Radiotherapy, external radiation therapy.

Interaction Type and Significance

☼ **Prevention or Reduction of Drug Adverse Effect**

Probability:
2. Probable

Evidence Base:
○ **Preliminary**

Effect and Mechanism of Action

Loss or alteration of taste sensation is a common adverse effect of radiation therapy in oncology patients, particularly in those receiving external radiotherapy (ERT) to the head and neck region. Zinc is known to play a central role in taste sensation, as well as the synergistic function of olfaction. Coadministration of zinc during and after radiotherapy may mitigate adverse effects on taste sensation and support recovery from such damage.

Research

Limited research indicates that administration of zinc during or after radiotherapy may reduce adverse effects of radiation on taste perception, but that benefit is less likely in patients experiencing loss of taste perception resulting from hemodialysis. Ripamonti et al.[147] investigated the administration of oral zinc sulfate in preventing and correcting taste abnormalities for four taste qualities in cancer patients before, during, and after receiving radiotherapy to the head and neck region. They randomized 18 patients to receive either zinc sulfate tablets (45 mg per dose) or placebo three times daily "at the onset of subjective perception of taste alterations during the course of ERT and up to 1 month after ERT termination." After noting that "taste acuity for one or more taste qualities was already impaired before ERT," they reported that "taste alterations were experienced at least once for a minimum of 3 of the 8 measured thresholds by 100% of the patients" during ERT treatment, and that "33.3% of the patients became aware of some alteration within the first week of treatment." When treatment (or placebo) was initiated after appearance of such adverse effects, they found that "patients treated with placebo experienced a greater worsening of taste acuity during ERT treatment compared with those treated with zinc sulfate," and that "one month after ERT was terminated, the patients receiving zinc sulfate had a quicker recovery of taste acuity than those receiving placebo." In particular, "statistically significant differences between the two groups emerged for urea detection and sodium chloride recognition thresholds during ERT treatment and for sodium chloride, saccharose, and hydrogen chloride recognition thresholds after the termination of ERT treatment." These researchers concluded that "pharmacologic therapy [with zinc] is effective and well tolerated; it could become a routine in clinical practice to improve the supportive care of patients with taste alterations resulting from head and neck cancer."[147]

In relevant but unrelated research, Matson et al.[148] conducted a double-blind, randomized, placebo-controlled study involving 15 stable hemodialysis patients. They found that zinc sulfate, 220 mg daily for 6 weeks, "does not improve the disturbance of taste perception," particularly for the sour modality, in hemodialysis patients.

These two preliminary studies indicate that further research is warranted through well-designed clinical trials investigating the mechanisms of action in preventing and recovering taste sensation, how that differs in relation to iatrogenic cause, and whether prophylactic zinc coadministration might produce better outcomes than reactive prescribing.

Nutritional Therapeutics, Clinical Concerns, and Adaptations

Physicians administering radiotherapy, particularly to patients with head and neck cancers, may prevent or reverse alteration or loss of taste sense, which often occurs as a result of such therapy, through concomitantly prescribing 40 to 60 mg elemental zinc daily. Use of zinc at this dosage level is unlikely to produce any adverse effects, if complemented with low-dose copper, or interfere with conventional oncological therapies.

Tetracycline Antibiotics

Evidence: Demeclocycline (Declomycin), minocycline (Dynacin, Minocin, Vectrin), tetracycline (Achromycin, Actisite, Apo-Tetra, Economycin, Novo-Tetra, Nu-Tetra, Sumycin, Tetrachel, Tetracyn); combination drugs: chlortetracycline, demeclocycline and tetracycline (Deteclo); bismuth, metronidazole and tetracycline (Helidac).
Extrapolated, based on similar properties: Oxytetracycline (Terramycin).
Similar properties but evidence indicating no or reduced interaction effects: Doxycycline (Atridox, Doryx, Doxy, Monodox, Periostat, Vibramycin, Vibra-Tabs).
See also Antibiotics and Antimicrobial Agents (Systemic).

Interaction Type and Significance

◇◇ **Impaired Drug Absorption and Bioavailability, Precautions Appropriate**
⊕✗ **Bimodal or Variable Interaction, with Professional Management**
◇≈≈ **Drug-Induced Adverse Effect on Nutrient Function, Coadministration Therapeutic, with Professional Management**

Probability:
3. Possible or
2. Probable

Evidence Base:
● **Consensus**

Effect and Mechanism of Action

Tetracycline and some related antibiotics tend to form relatively insoluble chelates with zinc salts (and other divalent and trivalent metal ions) and thereby impair absorption and therapeutic activity of both agents.[149,150] In contrast to other members of the tetracycline class, doxycycline and zinc do not appear to interact to a clinically significantly degree.[151]

Research

The scientific literature on the effects of zinc on bioavailability of tetracycline antibiotics is generally considered as constituting a well-documented consensus, although specific research from human trials is limited. Penttila et al.[151] conducted a crossover study involving seven volunteers to compare the effect of zinc sulfate on the absorption of tetracycline and doxycycline. They reported that when a single dose of zinc sulfate (45 mg elemental zinc) was given simultaneously with tetracycline hydrochloride (500 mg) or doxycycline chloride (200 mg), the "serum concentration of tetracycline, the area under the serum tetracycline concentration-time curve and the excretion of tetracycline in urine were reduced by about 30%... from the respective control values," but the "absorption of doxycycline was not influenced significantly." Overall, they concluded that the "clinical significance of the zinc-tetracycline interaction seems to be of limited importance." Andersson et al.[152,153] published similar findings regarding intestinal absorption of zinc in their study of eight healthy volunteers administered 50 mg elemental zinc orally. That same year (1976), Mapp and McCarthy[154] found that "absorption of 250 mg phosphate-potentiated tetracycline hydrochloride was reduced by 75% when administered concurrently with 220 mg zinc sulphate."

Minimal research has focused on the effects of tetracycline on zinc absorption and clinical implications of long-term use. In rodent studies, administration of tetracycline was reported to result in increased elimination rate of zinc, which could originate in zinc-tetracycline interactions in blood plasma. However, after "using clinical data relative to fasting subjects as taken from the literature" to perform computer simulations of zinc-tetracycline interactions in the GI fluid, Brion et al.[155] concluded that "no significant effect can be expected from tetracyclines on the distribution of zinc in plasma at the usual therapeutic levels." Nevertheless, the authors added that "zinc-tetracycline interactions have been found to be determining factors for the bioavailabilities of the metal as well as of the antibiotic in the gastrointestinal fluid." No studies have been conducted to determine the effects of chronic or repeated tetracycline antibiotics on zinc status and function in humans.

Weimar et al.[156] and Michaelsson et al.[157] demonstrated that patients with dermatitis herpetiformis, acne, psoriasis, and Darier's disease have low epidermal zinc concentrations. Notably, "mean serum zinc concentration was, however, significantly decreased only in men with dermatitis herpetiformis."[156]

Clinical Implications and Adaptations

Physicians prescribing tetracycline antibiotics are advised to ask patients about their supplement use and to tell them to separate intake of zinc supplements, multimineral formulation, and zinc-rich food (as well as other mineral intake) by at least 2 hours before or 4 hours after the medication. Such precautions would also prevent the potential depletion of zinc by the tetracyclines by avoiding chelate formation. In patients being treated for acne, especially inflammatory acne, coadministration of 30 to 45 mg elemental zinc daily, as zinc acetate, citrate, gluconate, or other highly bioavailable forms, may be indicated and can be efficacious, assuming compliance with intake separation. Zinc sulfate has been less effective and associated with greater incidence of adverse effects.[84,156-159] When both agents are indicated, consider prescribing doxycycline, a noninteracting tetracycline.

Thiazide Diuretics

Bendroflumethiazide (bendrofluazide; Naturetin); combination drug: bendrofluazide and propranolol (Inderex); benzthiazide (Exna), chlorothiazide (Diuril), chlorthalidone (Hygroton), cyclopenthiazide (Navidrex); combination drug: cyclopenthiazide and oxprenolol hydrochloride (Trasidrex); hydrochlorothiazide (Aquazide, Esidrix, Ezide, Hydrocot, HydroDiuril, Microzide, Oretic), hydroflumethiazide (Diucardin), methyclothiazide (Enduron), metolazone (Zaroxolyn, Mykrox), polythiazide (Renese), quinethazone (Hydromox), trichlormethiazide (Naqua).

Similar properties but evidence lacking for extrapolation: Spironolactone (Aldactone); combination drugs: hydrochlorothiazide and amiloride (Moduretic); hydrochlorothiazide and captopril (Acezide, Capto-Co, Captozide, Co-Zidocapt); hydrochlorothiazide and enalapril (Vaseretic); hydrochlorothiazide and lisinopril (Prinzide, Zestoretic); hydrochlorothiazide and losartan (Hyzaar); hydrochlorothiazide and metoprolol (Lopressor HCT); spironolactone and hydrochlorothiazide (Aldactazide); triamterene and hydrochlorothiazide (Dyazide, Maxzide).

See also Amiloride in Potassium-Sparing Diuretics.

Interaction Type and Significance

≈≈ **Drug-Induced Nutrient Depletion, Supplementation Therapeutic, with Professional Management**

Probability:	Evidence Base:
3. Possible	○ **Preliminary**

Effect and Mechanism of Action

Thiazide diuretics can increase urinary zinc excretion and result in zinc loss with either single-dose or long-term use.[146,160] Long-term thiazide therapy may cause significant zinc depletion, particularly in individuals with preexisting impaired zinc status, compromised nutrient intake, or medical conditions susceptible to zinc deficiency.[136,161] The mechanism of thiazide diuretics' effect on zinc is poorly understood, but these agents act primarily on the initial portion of the distal convoluted tubule in the nephron; hormone-mediated processes may also be involved.

Research

In a small, randomized trial, Wester[136] compared urinary zinc excretion in nine patients during treatment with bendroflumethiazide, chlorthalidone, and hydrochlorothiazide with that in nine patients treated with bumetanide, furosemide, and triamterene. He observed that in patients receiving thiazide diuretics, "the zinc concentration rose by 30% and the total amount of zinc excretion increased by 60%." Based on these preliminary findings, the author concluded that "the observed increased urinary losses of zinc deserve further attention."

In a review, Reyes[160] cautioned that the probability of a clinically significant zinc deficiency with thiazide diuretics is greater in pregnant women and individuals with hepatic cirrhosis, diabetes mellitus, GI disorders, renal insufficiency, and alcoholism, that is, conditions associated with diminished total body zinc levels. Likewise, in related research, Golik et al.[110] determined that individuals with type 2 diabetes mellitus and congestive heart failure "excrete larger amounts of zinc, which may eventually lead to zinc deficiency." These findings bear directly on the data relating to hypertensive medications, given the use of diuretics for heart failure and the high incidence of comorbid hypertension among these patient populations.

The combination of amiloride with a thiazide combination, as a means of mitigating the adverse effects of both agents on zinc metabolism and nutriture, is discussed in the Potassium-Sparing Diuretics section. Similarly, the concomitant use of hydrochlorothiazide and ACE inhibitors may further exacerbate zinc loss; this interaction is reviewed in Captopril, Enalapril, and related Angiotensin-Converting Enzyme (ACE) Inhibitors.

Nutritional Therapeutics, Clinical Concerns, and Adaptations

Physicians prescribing thiazide diuretics are advised to coadminister zinc (50-100 mg elemental zinc daily) to compensate for possible drug-induced zinc loss and prevent zinc depletion. Monitoring for zinc deficiency is appropriate but is compromised by the limited sensitivity of laboratory assessment in accurately detecting depletion of zinc at the tissue level. Advise patients to watch for signs of zinc depletion, especially those at greater risk for compromised nutrient intake or other factors likely to impair zinc status.

Coadministration of folic acid, magnesium, potassium, and calcium may also be appropriate to prevent adverse effects from thiazide diuretic on the physiological levels and functions of these nutrients and to advance the broader therapeutic goals of enhancing cardiovascular health.

Valproic Acid and Related Anticonvulsant Medications (AEDs)

Evidence: Divalproex semisodium, divalproex sodium (Depakote), sodium valproate (Depacon), valproate semisodium, valproic acid (Depakene, Depakene Syrup).
Similar properties but evidence lacking for extrapolation: Carbamazepine (Carbatrol, Tegretol), clonazepam (Klonopin), clorazepate (Tranxene), ethosuximide (Zarontin), ethotoin (Peganone), felbamate (Felbatol), fosphenytoin (Cerebyx, Mesantoin), levetiracetam (Keppra), mephenytoin, mephobarbital (Mebaral), methsuximide (Celontin), oxcarbazepine (GP 47680, oxycarbamazepine; Trileptal), phenobarbital (phenobarbitone; Luminal, Solfoton), phenytoin (diphenylhydantoin; Dilantin, Phenytek), piracetam (Nootropyl), primidone (Mysoline), topiramate (Topamax), trimethadione (Tridione), vigabatrin (Sabril), zonisamide (Zonegran).

Interaction Type and Significance
≈≈ Drug-Induced Nutrient Depletion, Supplementation Therapeutic, with Professional Management

Probability: Evidence Base:
4. Plausible   ▽ Mixed

Effect and Mechanism of Action
Valproic acid (VPA) can alter zinc and copper homeostasis and may cause depletion of either or both minerals, not necessarily reflected in serum levels. The anticonvulsive activity of VPA on the brain may be "mediated through its effect on the metabolism of Zn in the brain and the concomitant changes in the activity of the zinc-dependent enzymes glutamic acid decarboxylase and carbonic anhydrase."[162]

Research
Animal and human studies of VPA's effect on zinc status have produced mixed findings. Using a rodent model, Hurd et al.[163] found that VPA administration for 1 week produced significant depletion of plasma levels of zinc, as well as selenium. In a study of 15 children with primary epilepsy receiving long-term VPA treatment, Lerman-Sagie et al.[162] found that serum and urine levels of zinc and copper levels were within normal limits, but erythrocyte zinc content was significantly lower than controls matched for age and gender. The authors interpreted their findings as suggesting that the antiseizure effect of valproate may be related to and/or mediated by its effect on zinc-dependent CNS enzymes. Subsequently, Kaji et al.[164] investigated measured serum zinc and copper levels in epileptic children treated with VPA and/or other antiepileptic drugs (AEDs). They found that in "contrast to the reported results of animal experiments, serum Zn levels were not altered in patients with VPA treatment." Notably, patients "treated with VPA monotherapy had significantly lower levels of serum Cu" than normal controls, as did those "treated with VPA in addition to some other AED." Those "treated with AEDs except for VPA" exhibited serum copper concentrations "not statistically different from those of control subjects." However, in a later trial involving 51 children with epilepsy, Sozuer et al.[165] observed that

patients treated with VPA, as monotherapy or in combination with carbamazepine, exhibited significantly lower levels of serum zinc than in the two control groups, consisting of seven untreated epileptic and 12 normal children. Because serum zinc and copper "concentrations of the untreated epileptics were not significantly different from those of normal controls," the authors concluded that "serum trace metal homeostasis may be affected by AED therapy, but not by the convulsive disorder itself."

Reports
In a letter, Simpson and Bryce-Smith[166] reported cutaneous manifestations of zinc deficiency during treatment with anticonvulsants.

Nutritional Therapeutics, Clinical Concerns, and Adaptations
Physicians prescribing VPA, as monotherapy or in combination with other AEDs, will want to be watchful for deficiencies of zinc and numerous other key nutrients, especially in children and women of childbearing age. Given the lack of reliable measures of zinc deficiency, it is particularly important to instruct patients to be alert to signs of zinc deficiency, such as alterations in taste or smell sensation and increased frequency of infections. Although specific evidence-based research is lacking to confirm drug-induced depletion or efficacy of coadministration, the use of concomitant zinc at a low dosage level, 30 to 50 mg elemental zinc daily, would be prudent and is generally safe and unlikely to produce any clinically significant adverse effects. In children a dose of 10 mg elemental zinc twice daily is typical but can vary depending on the child's age and weight. Complementary daily copper, $\frac{1}{15}$ to $\frac{1}{20}$ the dose of zinc, would prevent copper deficiency resulting from the medication or the zinc intake.

Warfarin and Related Oral Vitamin K Antagonist Anticoagulants

Anisindione (Miradon), dicumarol, ethyl biscoumacetate (Tromexan), nicoumalone (acenocoumarol; Acitrom, Sintrom), phenindione (Dindevan), phenprocoumon (Jarsin, Marcumar), warfarin (Coumadin, Marevan, Warfilone).

Interaction Type and Significance
◇◇ Impaired Drug Absorption and Bioavailability, Precautions Appropriate
✗✗ Minimal to Mild Adverse Interaction—Vigilance Necessary
◇ Adverse Drug Effect on Nutritional Therapeutics, Strategic Concern

Probability: Evidence Base:
4. Plausible   ▽ Mixed or
                        ○ Preliminary

Effect and Mechanism of Action
Zinc, as well as other minerals such as iron and zinc, may bind with warfarin or dicumarol and reduce bioavailability of the medication.[167,168] Formation of such complexes might also reduce zinc absorption and bioavailability and could potentially interfere with the effectiveness of oral zinc as a preventive or therapeutic agent.

Research and Reports
Despite recurrent descriptions of this interaction as "well documented," a search of the scientific literature provides no clinical trials or substantive case reports directly investigating or confirming evidence from in vitro experiments or extrapolations from interactions involving iron, calcium, or other minerals. Although reasonably predictable from a

pharmacokinetics perspective, research into this area would be valuable given the large number of patients using nutritional supplements that contain zinc or other metals.

Clinical Implications and Adaptations

The chemistry of common mineral nutrients binding warfarin is well founded, but the frequency of occurrence is uncertain, its nature remains unclear, and conclusive evidence of the clinical significance of this interaction is lacking. Nevertheless, physicians prescribing warfarin are advised to recommend to patients that they separate warfarin administration from intake of zinc (or iron or magnesium) supplements by at least 2 hours. Regardless, physician-patient communication is especially important in the event that individuals undergoing anticoagulant therapy are taking zinc or any other mineral supplements. Nutritional support, including zinc, may be indicated in many patients likely to be on warfarin therapy given the high incidence of inadequate zinc nutriture among elderly and institutionalized individuals. Regular monitoring of international normalized ratio (INR) is critical so that warfarin levels can be adjusted accordingly when concomitant intake is deemed appropriate.

Zidovudine (AZT) and Related Nucleoside or Nonnucleoside (Analog) Reverse-Transcriptase Inhibitors (NRTIS or NNRTIS) Antiretroviral Agents

Evidence: Zidovudine (azidothymidine, AZT, ZDV, zidothymidine; Retrovir).

Extrapolated, based on similar properties: Azidothymidine combination drugs: abacavir, lamivudine, and zidovudine (Trizivir); zidovudine and lamivudine (Combivir); didanosine (ddI, dideoxyinosine; Videx), dideoxycytidine (ddC, zalcitabine; Hivid), lamivudine (3TC, Epivir), stavudine (D4T, Zerit), tenofovir (Viread).

Interaction Type and Significance

≈≈ **Drug-Induced Nutrient Depletion, Supplementation Therapeutic, with Professional Management**

⊕⊕ **Beneficial or Supportive Interaction, with Professional Management**

⊕✗ **Bimodal or Variable Interaction, with Professional Management**

✗ **Potential or Theoretical Adverse Interaction of Uncertain Severity**

Probability: Evidence Base:
3. Possible   ◉ Emerging

Effect and Mechanism of Action

Zinc plays a central role in many immune functions, including T-cell division, maturation, differentiation, and function; lymphocyte response to mitogens; programmed cell death of lymphoid and myeloid origins; gene transcription; and biomembrane function. Thymulin, a zinc-bound hormone, and Cu/Zn superoxide dismutase, as well as congenital or acquired zinc deficiencies, are associated with immune abnormalities and increased susceptibility to infectious diseases.[169] AZT may deplete zinc (and other nutrients). Populations likely to have a high incidence of HIV infection may also be more likely to exhibit compromised zinc status, possibly due to malnutrition, progression of the pathology, or excessive ejaculation.[170-173] "AIDS subjects suffer from reduced zinc bioavailability, more severe in stage IV than in stage III."[174]

Zidovudine may deplete plasma zinc levels; conversely, adequate zinc levels may enhance therapeutic response to AZT treatment.[175] Zinc deficiency may diminish drug effectiveness because zidovudine requires thymidine kinase, a zinc-dependent enzyme, for conversion to its active triphosphate form.[170,175] Notably, individuals with HIV infection, particularly later stages of AIDS, tend to exhibit elevated cooper levels.[176]

Research

In a 1991 longitudinal study involving 37 HIV-positive participants, 15 treated with ZDV (AZT, 500-1200 mg/day) and 22 serving as untreated, CD4 level–matched controls, Baum et al.[175] found significantly decreased mean plasma levels of zinc (and copper) in a "large proportion" of AZT-treated subjects after 12 months of antiviral therapy. Hematological and plasma nutrient levels were similar in both groups before treatment, but after therapy, "drug-treated subjects demonstrated alterations in hematological and nutritional parameters." The authors noted that the "level of plasma zinc appeared to be particularly important in maintaining immune function in the ZDV-treated group. Whereas ZDV-treated subjects with adequate zinc levels displayed a significant increase in the response of peripheral blood lymphocytes to mitogens, this enhancement was not demonstrated in zinc-deficient, ZDV-treated participants or in untreated individuals whose lymphocyte response significantly declined over time, despite adequate zinc status." The authors concluded that their findings "reveal a zidovudine-induced effect on nutritional parameters, indicating the importance of monitoring nutritional status with drug therapeutic regimens."[175] Subsequent papers by Baum et al.[169] and Bogden et al.[176] have emphasized the key physiological roles of zinc and the importance of zinc status in HIV infection, providing evidence that compromised nutritional and antioxidant status begins early in HIV-1 infection and may contribute to disease progression.

Although some survey data indicate that higher zinc intake may be associated with worse outcomes in HIV-positive individuals (regardless of AZT therapy), other trials suggest a potential synergistic benefit from coadministration in patients treated with AZT. In a survey of 281 HIV-positive homosexual/bisexual men, Tang et al.[177] reported that increased intake (from food and supplements) of "zinc was monotonically and significantly associated with an increased risk of progression to AIDS." In a follow-up paper the authors reported that "any intake of zinc supplements, however, was associated with poorer survival" and suggested that further "studies are needed to determine the optimal level of zinc intake in HIV-1-infected individuals."[178] Conversely, in a study investigating the relationship between zinc deficiency and survival in HIV-positive homosexual men, Campa et al.[179] found that higher zinc levels were associated with better immune function and higher CD4+ cell counts, while zinc deficiency was associated with greater incidence of HIV-related mortality. Subsequently, Mocchegiani et al.[174] conducted a clinical trial involving 17 AZT-treated stage III subjects with generalized lymphadenopathy and 12 stage IV/subgroup C1 AIDS patients, with 18 stage III subjects with generalized lymphadenopathy and 10 stage IV/subgroup C1 subjects treated only with AZT serving as controls. Stage III and stage IV/C1 patients administered zinc sulfate (200 mg daily for 30 days) exhibited an "increase or a stabilization in the body weight and an increase of the number of CD4+ cells and the plasma level of active zinc-bound thymulin," and the "frequency of opportunistic infectious episodes in the 24 months following entry into the study was reduced after zinc supplementation in stage IV C1 subjects (11 infections versus 25 in controls) and delayed in stage III zinc-treated subjects (1 infection/24 months versus 13 infections/24 months in controls)." Notably, the beneficial effect of zinc on opportunistic infections was "restricted to infections due to *Pneumocystis carinii* and *Candida,* whereas no variations have been observed in the frequencies of *cytomegalovirus* and *toxoplasma* infections." The authors concluded that these data "may support the benefit of zinc as an adjunct to AZT therapy in AIDS pathology."[174]

In a randomized, double-blind, placebo-controlled trial involving 96 children with HIV-1 infection in South Africa, Bobat et al.[180] found that administering 10 mg daily of elemental zinc, as sulfate, reduced watery diarrhea significantly and lowered the incidence of pneumonia (compared to placebo), without adversely affecting (i.e., increasing) plasma HIV-1 viral load. In a randomized controlled trial involving 159 HIV-infected adults in Peru, with at least a 7-day history of diarrhea, Carcamo et al.[181] found that 2 weeks of treatment with 50 mg zinc twice daily does not reduce or eliminate persistent diarrhea in adults infected with HIV. The authors added: "Longer treatment or follow-up beyond 2 weeks might have revealed treatment benefit.... Among children, however, benefits of zinc supplementation on diarrhea have been evident after the fourth day of supplementation."

Nutritional Therapeutics, Clinical Concerns, and Adaptations

Physicians treating HIV-infected individuals with AZT or related antiretroviral regimens should always assess nutritional status, particularly dietary intake and use of antioxidant and other supplements, and consider coadministration of zinc, selenium, glutathione/N-acetylcysteine, and other nutrients that may be beneficial. Multiple factors, including the underlying pathology, concomitant health and lifestyle factors, comorbid conditions, and the multiple medications often used, strongly suggest high susceptibility to compromised nutritional status, which may be further exacerbated by drug-induced nutrient depletion patterns.

Moderate-dose to high-dose zinc, 50 to 100 mg elemental zinc daily, may counter preexisting deficiency, reduce effects of drug-induced depletion, and facilitate the activity of AZT. Coadministration of 1 to 2 mg of copper may be appropriate (but may be contraindicated if serum/plasma levels are already high) to neutralize the potential risk of adverse effects on the immune system from the long-term zinc. Laboratory assessment of zinc status may be less than ideal, but regular monitoring of the nutritional and metabolic status of such patients is essential, including instructing the patient to be attentive to signs of possible zinc deficiency. Clinical management of HIV-positive patients using multiple treatment modalities in an individualized and evolving integrative strategy requires close collaboration and regular coordination among health care professionals trained and experienced in conventional pharmacology and nutritional therapeutics.

THEORETICAL, SPECULATIVE, AND PRELIMINARY INTERACTIONS RESEARCH, INCLUDING OVERSTATED INTERACTIONS CLAIMS

Acetylsalicylic Acid (Aspirin) and Related Anti-Inflammatory Analgesic Medications

Acetylsalicylic acid (acetosal, acetyl salicylic acid, ASA, salicylsalicylic acid; Arthritis Foundation Pain Reliever, Ascriptin, Aspergum, Asprimox, Bayer Aspirin, Bayer Buffered Aspirin, Bayer Low Adult Strength, Bufferin, Buffex, Cama Arthritis Pain Reliever, Easprin, Ecotrin, Ecotrin Low Adult Strength, Empirin, Extra Strength Adprin-B, Extra Strength Bayer Enteric 500 Aspirin, Extra Strength Bayer Plus, Halfprin 81, Heartline, Regular Strength Bayer Enteric 500 Aspirin, St. Joseph Adult Chewable Aspirin, ZORprin); combination drugs: ASA and caffeine (Anacin); ASA, caffeine, and propoxyphene (Darvon Compound); ASA and carisoprodol (Soma Compound); ASA, codeine, and carisoprodol (Soma Compound with Codeine); ASA and codeine (Empirin with Codeine); ASA, codeine, butalbital, and caffeine (Fiorinal); ASA and extended-release dipyridamole (Aggrenox, Asasantin).
Salsalate (Salicylic acid; Amigesic, Disalcid, Marthritic, Mono Gesic, Salflex, Salsitab).
Indomethacin (Indometacin; Indocin, Indocin-SR).
See also Nonsteroidal Anti-inflammatory Drugs (NSAIDs); similar mechanisms involved.

In a 1982 letter, Ambanelli et al.[182] reported that intake of 3 g aspirin daily can induce changes in serum and urinary zinc, observable beginning 3 days after initiation of aspirin; indomethacin was also implicated. Such an effect would generally be considered reasonably predictable based on scientific knowledge of the respective properties and activities of these agents. Further research would be warranted to determine the risks, clinical implications, and responsible countermeasures in individuals using aspirin chronically.

Conversely, in vitro experiments conducted by Kim et al.[183] demonstrated attenuation of Zn^{2+} neurotoxicity by aspirin attributed to the prevention of synaptically released Zn^{2+} entry into neurons, primarily through voltage-gated Ca^{2+} channels (VGCC), which can mediate pathological neuronal death. The authors noted that "aspirin derivatives lacking the carboxyl acid group did not reduce Zn^{2+} neurotoxicity" and interpreted these findings as suggesting "that aspirin prevents Zn^{2+}-mediated neuronal death by interfering with VGCC, and its action specifically requires the carboxyl acid group." Further research may be warranted to determine potential clinical implications of these observations.

Bile Acid Sequestrants

Evidence: Cholestyramine (Locholest, Prevalite, Questran).
Extrapolation: Colesevelam (WelChol), colestipol (Colestid).

Cholestyramine and other bile acid sequestrants are known to bind a multitude of nutrients, including zinc and other key minerals, in the gut, impairing bioavailability to the degree that depletion and deficiency may occur. However, research is limited and primarily derived from animal studies. Using a rodent model to investigate alterations in calcium, magnesium, iron, and zinc metabolism by cholestyramine, Watkins et al.[184] found that, compared to controls, cholestyramine-fed rats exhibited "a lower net positive balance for magnesium, iron, and zinc" and "a decreased urinary zinc." The authors hypothesized: "Alterations in calcium, magnesium, and zinc metabolism might be explained by inadequate vitamin D absorption from the intestine followed by an increased secretion of parathyroid hormone." Regardless of the limited human research, concern for adverse effects on nutrient status in patients being treated with bile acid sequestrants is widespread among clinicians and researchers, and concomitant support with broad-spectrum multivitamin-mineral supplements is considered judicious, with the caveat that intake needs to be at least 2 hours before or 4 hours after the medication.

Bisphosphonates

Alendronate (Fosamax), clodronate (Bonefos, Ostac), etidronate (Didronel), ibandronate (Bondronat, Boniva), pamidronate (Aredia), risedronate (Actonel), tiludronate (Skelid), zoledronic acid (Zometa).

With simultaneous intake, numerous minerals, including zinc, may bind with bisphosphonates and impair the absorption of all agents involved.

Although reasonable and consistent with present pharmacokinetic knowledge concerning other minerals, evidence from clinical trials directly substantiating the chelation interaction between zinc and bisphosphonates is lacking.

Preliminary data indicate other probable interactions between bisphosphonates and zinc. Adami et al.[185] found that IV bisphosphonate administration "induced an acute-phase response (APR) irrespective of the underlying disease, manifested by a fall in circulating lymphocyte number and serum zinc concentration and in a rise in C-reactive protein." Notably, in postmenopausal women with osteoporosis, alendronate significantly reduces the concentrations of urinary zinc. Thus, comparison of zinc excretion and biochemical markers of bone remodeling have been proposed in the assessment of the effects of alendronate and calcitonin on bone in postmenopausal women with osteoporosis.[186]

Health care professionals treating individuals on bisphosphonate therapy for osteoporosis should inform patients of this probable chelation interaction and instruct them to separate oral intake, ingesting the zinc (and other minerals) 1 hour before or 2 hours after the bisphosphonate.

Zinc chelation may play a role in novel cancer therapies involving use of bisphosphonates to chelate zinc and thereby inhibit matrix metalloproteinases (MMPs), a family of zinc-dependent proteinases involved in the degradation of the extracellular matrix, a process on which cancer metastasis is believed to depend.[187-189] In an in vitro experiment, Boissier et al.[190] reported that bisphosphonates inhibited MMP proteolytic activity by breast and prostate carcinoma cells, and that this inhibitory effect of bisphosphonates on MMP activity was completely reversed in the presence of excess zinc. These areas of zinc-bisphosphonate interaction are currently being investigated.

Clofibrate and Related Fibrates

Evidence: Clofibrate (Atromid-S).
Related: Bezafibrate (Bezalip), ciprofibrate (Modalim), fenofibrate (Tricor, Triglide, Lofibra), gemfibrozil (Apo-Gemfibrozil, Lopid, Novo-Gemfibrozil).

In addition to its antihyperlipidemic activity, clofibrate is known to alter serum protein patterns, including proteins associated with key minerals.[191] Using a rodent model, Powanda et al.[192] detected a "significant decrease in plasma zinc ... after the rats were fed the 1.25% clofibrate diet for 1 week," as well as "a significant decrease in hepatic zinc." However, clofibrate did not affect the plasma concentration of α_2-macroglobulin, although it did "selectively decrease the plasma concentration of two trace metal carrier proteins, transferrin and ceruloplasmin." The authors noted that the observed reduction in the hepatic concentration of zinc "may merely be the result of a redistribution to achieve a new systemic equilibrium." However, they also speculated that "the depression in plasma zinc reflects the marked decrease in transferrin, which is known to bind zinc, or is caused by the displacement of zinc from albumin by clofibrate." Thus, despite offering several possible explanations for these findings, they declared that the "decrease in plasma zinc remains to be explained."[192]

Further research into the interaction between clofibrate and zinc is not readily discoverable through a standard search of the scientific literature. Follow-up research may be warranted given the increased knowledge of the manifold roles of zinc that has emerged since publication of this single paper.

Cyclosporine

Cyclosporine (Ciclosporin, cyclosporin A, CSA; Neoral, Sandimmune, SangCya).

Several secondary reference texts have declared, without citing specific and substantive evidence, that zinc should not be administered concomitantly with cyclosporine or other immunosuppressant drug regimens because of its "immunostimulant" activity. Emerging knowledge of the complex and nuanced function of zinc as a modulator of immune function in its interplay within the dynamic network and signaling model, such as suggested in the work of Candace Pert, Michael Ruff, and other pioneers of psychoneuroimmunology, as well as the continually shifting nature of its distribution, suggest that a simple characterization of zinc as "stimulating" the immune system is unlikely to offer a comprehensive explanation for the diverse effects observed in clinical practice and research settings. Consequently, a blanket contraindication of zinc coadministration appears speculative without substantive human research findings or qualified case reports documenting adverse effects, preferably with a clear elucidation of the mechanism(s) of action. Further research is warranted, with clinical supervision and monitoring being critical in the meantime, as always with patients undergoing any immunosuppressive therapy.

Dopamine Receptor Antagonists

Metoclopramide (Reglan), olanzapine (Symbyax, Zyprexa).

In vitro studies with zinc suggest that it appears to modulate antagonist drug interactions with the D_1 dopamine receptor and the dopamine transporter.[193,194] However, direct evidence, from clinical trials or substantive case reports, of a clinically significant adverse effect on the therapeutic activity of drugs that rely on dopamine receptor antagonists is lacking at this time. In an experimental setting, Schetz et al.[194] demonstrated "the effect of zinc on the binding of D_1- and D_2-selective antagonists to cloned dopamine receptors and show that the inhibition by zinc is through a dose-dependent, reversible, allosteric, two-state modulation of dopamine receptors." They found that zinc "exerts a low-affinity, dose-dependent, EDTA-reversible inhibition of the binding of subtype-specific antagonists primarily by decreasing the ligands' affinity for their receptors," and suggested that "the mechanism of zinc inhibition appears to be allosteric modulation of the dopamine receptor proteins." Based on data from multiple investigators indicating that zinc "retards the functional effects of antagonist at the D_2L receptor in intact cells," research findings have been interpreted to "suggest that synaptic zinc may be a factor influencing the effectiveness of therapies that rely on dopamine receptor antagonists."[193,194] These in vitro studies suggest that zinc may interact with drugs that rely on dopamine receptor antagonists and indicate that further clinical research is warranted to determine the character and clinical significance of such an interaction.

Gillin et al.[195] (1982) studied patients with acute and chronic schizophrenia, on or off treatment with various major tranquilizers, looking for significant deviations from normal in concentrations of zinc or copper in serum, urine, or gastric fluid, in serum ceruloplasmin or in hair zinc. Although depletion of body zinc and increases in brain copper have been associated with severe changes in mentation and personality, they found no differences. Research has already been reviewed to indicate that measurement of zinc deficiencies is unreliable and tentative, with multiple pools existing in the body and their concentrations not necessarily relating to levels found in plasma, urine, gastric fluid, or hair. Insufficient data exist even to guide zinc clinic trials because schizophrenia may be a heterogenous condition. Ten years later, Andrews[196] (1992) suggested that male transmission of risk, the parental age effect, racial differences in birth seasonality, the disturbed gender ratios in the offspring of schizophrenic mothers, and the association between diabetes and schizophrenia are explained by changes to zinc homeostasis. The primary site of action of zinc deficiency was proposed to be the putative ZFY sex-determining system. Zinc deficiency was also linked to other mental disorders. During the 1970s, Pfeiffer and Bacchi[197] reported successful outcomes in 95% of more than 400 patients diagnosed with pyrroluria-type schizophrenia using vitamin B_6 and zinc.

EDTA

EDTA (Ethylenediaminetetraacetic acid).

In vitro experiments suggest that concomitant use with zinc might increase the cytotoxicity of cisplatin in the presence of EDTA, compared with cisplatin alone.[198]

Ethambutol

Ethambutol (Myambutol).

Ethambutol is an antibiotic used therapeutically in the treatment of tuberculosis that can affect trace-metal metabolism through its action as a chelating agent. Using a rodent model, Solecki et al.[199] investigated the effects of ethambutol on tissue concentrations and balance of zinc, copper, iron, and manganese. They observed that ethambutol "produced significant decreases in heart copper, kidney zinc, plasma zinc, and liver copper and zinc not due to the associated reduced food intake." No human trials or qualified case reports have appeared in the scientific literature to confirm this possible interaction in humans or determine its clinical significance.

Folic Acid

Folic acid, folinic acid.

In addition to its availability as orally administered nutritional supplements, folic acid at doses greater than 1 mg is available in tablet and injectable forms with a prescription. Despite preliminary reports and unsubstantiated statements in the secondary literature indicating that folic acid administration can reduce blood levels of zinc, two reviews of folic acid safety concluded that such an adverse effect is improbable.[200,201] Pending confirmation by more substantive evidence, physicians prescribing folic acid at supplemental levels or in prescription doses do not need to recommend compensatory coadministration of zinc. Nevertheless, monitoring serum/plasma levels and watching for clinical signs of zinc insufficiency (e.g., decreased smell/taste) would be prudent when folic acid is administered at higher therapeutic levels for an extended time; in cases where long-term zinc supplementation is added, low-dose copper may also be indicated.

Hydralazine

Hydralazine (Apresoline).

The scientific literature provides very limited data on the potential interaction between zinc and hydralazine, and available research is convoluted by numerous confounding variables. Fjellner[202] described a 58-year-old woman with long-standing hypertension and leg ulcers and mild joint involvement of 3 years, being treated for 6 years with hydralazine (30-200 mg/day) and propranolol (120-640 mg/day) as well as thyroxine and several other medications, who developed multisystemic manifestations of a lupus erythematosus–like syndrome within 1 week after introduction of oral zinc sulfate (200 mg three times daily). Clinical improvement, including healing of the oral ulcers and remission of the fever and abdominal distress, occurred on cessation of zinc intake. Notably, however, the patient's condition persisted until all the medications except thyroxine were discontinued. Clearly, attributing a multifactorial aggravation in a single case to an interaction between zinc and hydralazine would be speculative, at best, and extrapolating that to a generalized pharmacological phenomenon would be an ill-founded misrepresentation of the very limited data available, particularly since hydralazine is known to be capable of producing drug-induced lupus on its own. It is also notable that the dose of zinc in this case report was extremely high. Vigilance for similar case reports may be warranted so that a pattern of incidence and common risk factors might be elucidated.

Interferon Alfa (Interferon Alpha)

Interferon alfa (Interferon alpha; Alferon N, Intron A, Roferon-A); combination drug: interferon alfa-2b and ribavirin (Rebetron).

Necrolytic acral erythema is a rare skin disorder categorized as a form of necrolytic erythema, along with acrodermatitis enterohepatica (congenital disorder of zinc metabolism), and apparently linked to infection with hepatitis C virus. Khanna et al.[203] described the case of a "43-year-old black woman who presented with a 4-year history of tender, flaccid blisters localized to the dorsal aspect of her feet," which was subsequently diagnosed as necrolytic acral erythema and chronic hepatitis C. Although her serum zinc level was normal, she was "successfully treated with interferon alfa-2b and zinc." In a review of the literature on necrolytic acral erythema, these authors found four cases (of seven) "treated with variable success using oral zinc sulfate and amino acids, whereas 2 were successfully treated with interferon alfa," even though "serum zinc levels were normal in all patients in whom they were measured." The dose of oral zinc sulfate administered ranged from 60 to 440 mg per day and "was effective to varying degrees" in five (of eight) patients, including the authors' original patient. In focusing on the interferon-zinc synergy they noted that in one case, "interferon alfa alone resulted in almost complete clearance of lesions," whereas in the two other cases, "the addition of interferon alfa to oral zinc resulted in total clearance." The authors interpreted the collective evidence from their case report and literature review to suggest that "interferon alfa alone may be sufficient to treat necrolytic acral erythema or may enhance the effect of oral zinc."[203] Further research appears to be warranted to investigate the mechanism(s) involved in this possible interaction, elucidate any relationship to zinc deficiency or faulty zinc metabolism as well as other forms of necrolytic erythema, and establish clinical guidelines, if confirmed to be effective.

Nystatin

Nystatin (Mycostatin, Nilstat, Nystex).

In a single in vitro study, Grider and Vazquez[204] found that nystatin, a sterol-binding drug known to inhibit potocytosis, inhibited zinc uptake in both normal and acrodermatitis enteropathica (AE) fibroblasts. They noted that "reduced cellular uptake of zinc was associated with its internalization, not its external binding." The authors concluded that "nystatin exerts its effect on zinc uptake by reducing the velocity at which zinc traverses the cell membrane, possibly through potocytosis," and that "the AE mutation also affects zinc status by reducing zinc transport." These preliminary findings, if confirmed by further research, suggest that individuals on nystatin therapy, especially for an extended period, may be at risk for zinc depletion and that zinc coadministration may be indicated; the potentially beneficial effects of zinc on immune function may provide added benefit, particularly in the presence of compromised zinc status.

NUTRIENT-NUTRIENT INTERACTIONS

Antioxidant Nutrients

An emerging body of evidence largely indicates that zinc in conjunction with an antioxidant network strategy, particularly one emphasizing lutein and anthocyanoside-rich plants such as bilberry *(Vaccinium myrtillus)*, may prevent or slow the advance of macular degeneration.[205-216] Research continues in this important area.

Calcium and Calcium-Based Antacids

Numerous reports suggest that calcium at high doses (e.g., >1500 mg/day) may significantly impair zinc absorption. Animal research suggests interference with zinc uptake by intestinal mucosa due to counter–ion binding to mucus glycoproteins as a possible mechanism.[217] However, this possible effect appears to be of limited clinical significance, especially if calcium is taken with food, which may improve the gastric environment. Further, the effect of calcium on gut pH, whether as supplement or as calcium-based antacids, can interfere with zinc absorption by altering gastric pH away from optimal (i.e., low) pH range, as noted in the discussion of Histamine (H_2) Receptor Antagonists.

In an early experiment, Pecoud et al.[218] investigated the effect of foodstuffs on the absorption of zinc sulfate by administering single doses of zinc sulfate to healthy young volunteers, either in the fasting state or with various types of meals. They observed that "dairy products (milk and cheese) and brown bread decreased zinc absorption, as indicated by a significant drop in peak serum zinc levels." Subsequently, however, other researchers have found that increases of calcium, within dietary sources or as calcium carbonate or hydroxyapatite, did not significantly alter zinc balance and retention in the presence of meals.[219,220]

In a study involving nine patients on hemodialysis and 11 controls, Hwang et al.[221] studied the effects of calcium carbonate and calcium acetate, both known phosphate binders, on intestinal zinc absorption by measuring 1-hour and 2-hour serum zinc levels after oral administration of 50 mg of elemental zinc as zinc gluconate, with or without concomitant administration of 2 g calcium carbonate (800 mg elemental calcium) or 3 g calcium acetate (750 mg elemental calcium). They observed that intestinal zinc absorption after an oral zinc challenge decreased in patients on hemodialysis with concomitant administration of calcium acetate, but calcium carbonate did not decrease intestinal zinc absorption in either group.

In contrast to these earlier studies, later research has used physiological doses of zinc and calcium more typical of the amounts found in meals. For example, in an experiment involving nine healthy female college-age students, Argiratos and Samman[222] observed that the plasma zinc AUC after simultaneous ingestion of zinc with calcium carbonate and calcium citrate (600 mg elemental calcium) was significantly lower than that after ingestion of zinc alone, reflecting a 72% and 80% reduction, respectively, in zinc absorption. The authors concluded that the "decrease in zinc absorption following the ingestion of zinc with different forms of calcium suggests that an antagonistic competition occurred between the minerals and that elemental calcium is the inhibiting factor."

In a trial involving 44 hemodialysis patients, Hwang et al.[223] found that short-term and long-term uses of calcium acetate (containing 25.35 mmol elemental calcium daily) did not change hair and serum zinc concentrations over an 8-month period. The authors noted that even though daily calcium did "not significantly interfere with zinc absorption and storage" in hemodialysis (HD) patients, the "comparable hair zinc content in the presence of decreased serum zinc concentrations indicates that the metabolic processing of zinc in HD patients is different from that of normal individuals."

Overall, the available data indicate that an antagonistic relationship between calcium and zinc may adversely affect zinc bioavailability with simultaneous intake in a fasting state, but that the presence of substantial food or separation of intake can minimize any such pharmacokinetic interaction. The resulting recommendation that patients ingest their zinc with a meal, but preferably not one high in phytates (e.g., grains, soy), or at least 2 hours away from calcium preparations is consistent with other known pharmacological principles and optimal clinical practices.

Copper

The complex interaction between these two pivotal minerals is well documented and generally agreed on but often oversimplified. Zinc significantly interferes with copper absorption and thus can cause copper deficiency or be therapeutic in the treatment of individuals with Wilson's disease.[47,48,52,224-227] Zinc induces intestinal cell metallothionein, which binds copper and prevents its transfer into blood; eventually the intestinal cells die and slough, taking the trapped copper with them in the stool, thus preventing intestinal absorption of copper. However, the combined presence of these two minerals in Cu/Zn superoxide dismutase indicates that they do not relate only competitively. Such key complementary activity, along with the whole arena of metalloenzymes, is only beginning to become the subject of research with practical clinical significance.

Prolonged intake of supplemental zinc, particularly longer than 1 month, warrants compensatory copper supplementation, typically 1 to 3 mg daily, except for individuals with Wilson's disease or when the therapeutic strategy employs zinc as an anticopper agent. The typical recommended ratio of zinc to copper is 10:1 to 20:1, with relatively higher zinc allowable in some elderly patients, who, at least in the United States, tend to have a history of ingesting water carried through copper pipes, and who tend to have a diet higher in copper and lower in zinc. Baseline serum copper and zinc levels, although not necessarily reflective of various metabolic pools, can nevertheless be useful in guiding the relative dosing of these two minerals where appropriate. Copper preparations should be taken at least 2 hours apart from zinc preparations.

L-Cysteine

The luminal phase of zinc intestinal absorption may be mediated by low-molecular-weight substances, with amino acids being primary candidates for this role through the formation of complexes with zinc. A significant proportion of plasma zinc exists complexed with amino acids. Zinc absorption may be enhanced by concomitant intake of the amino acid L-cysteine through the formation of a complex.[228] However, one study found that L-cysteine stimulates zinc uptake in rat but not in human erythrocytes.[229] Notably, L-cysteine may also help mobilize and excrete copper. Some clinicians suggest that L-cysteine is a CNS excitotoxin with potentially damaging effects, but that coadministration with zinc may block such effects. Pending further research, this potential interaction is most accurately characterized as speculative.

Folic Acid

See section in Theoretical, Speculative, and Preliminary Interactions Research.

Glutamine and Probiotic Bacterial Flora

Many clinicians experienced in natural medicine and integrative therapeutics place major importance on the phenomenon of excessive intestinal permeability, also known as *dysbiosis* or "leaky gut syndrome," diagnosed by alterations in the differential absorption of lactulose and mannitol. This syndrome can occur in patients with Crohn's disease or other GI pathology and potentially in large segments of the population whose gut ecology has been disrupted by the adverse effects of antibiotics and other stressors on healthy intestinal flora. Probiotics and glutamine are among the core treatment elements typically used in therapeutic regimens to restore gut wall integrity and normal intestinal flora colonization.

Sturniolo et al.[230] administered oral zinc sulfate (110 mg three times a day) for 8 weeks to 12 patients "with quiescent Crohn's disease who had been in remission for at least 3 months and had increased intestinal permeability on two separate occasions within the last 2 months." They found that "the lactulose/mannitol ratio was significantly higher before supplementation than after," and that during follow-up 12 months later, 10 patients "had normal intestinal permeability and did not relapse; of the remaining two who had increased intestinal permeability, one relapsed." The authors concluded that their "findings show that zinc supplementation can resolve permeability alterations in patients with Crohn's disease in remission" and that "improving intestinal barrier function may contribute to reduce the risk of relapse in Crohn's disease."

L-Histidine

Histidine is involved with the regulation of zinc levels. Both zinc and L-histidine are known competitors of intestinal copper uptake, and concomitant L-histidine intake may enhance the absorption of zinc.[231] Moreover, L-histidine can stimulate zinc uptake by erythrocytes.[229] In a study investigating zinc-dependent cognitive function, Keller et al.[232] found that coadministration of L-histidine during dietary zinc repletion improved short-term memory in zinc-restricted young adult male rats.

Iron

Interactions between iron and zinc appear to occur both during intestinal absorption and throughout the body after absorption. Iron and zinc may compete for absorption because of similarities in physicochemical properties and potentially shared absorptive pathways, such that bioavailability and therapeutic activity of both agents could potentially be reduced with simultaneous intake. Intestinal divalent metal transporter-1 (DMT1) has been proposed as a possible site, but others have noted that zinc is not transported by the DMT1.[233] This possible pharmacokinetic interaction can be difficult to manage clinically because iron and zinc deficiencies occur together in various populations and may have to be addressed concurrently, especially among women and children

in developing countries. In a review of literature investigating the interplay between iron and zinc at the level of enterocyte and neural tissues, Kordas and Stoltzfus[233] reported complex and paradoxical findings but clear patterns of probability. Their in vitro research indicates that iron may inhibit zinc absorption in some cells at very high ratios of iron to zinc, but not vice versa. Consequently, they proposed "a shift in thinking about iron-zinc interactions from the level of enterocyte to other sites/systems in the body [such as the nervous system] that may be equally relevant for the outcome and interpretation of supplementation trials."

Various studies have reported diverse interactions between zinc and iron, depending on forms, preparation, and doses administered; concomitant intake; protocol design; subject life phase (e.g., pregnancy); and trace-element status of subjects. Solomons[234] observed that inorganic iron competed for absorption with zinc when given to adults in solution in ratios greater than two to one. However, iron did not significantly affect zinc absorption when they administered Atlantic oysters, providing 54 mg "organic" zinc (vs. inorganic zinc sulfate). Thus, "the evidence for competitive interaction of zinc and iron was strongest with nonheme iron and inorganic zinc."[235] In human experiments, Rossander-Hulten et al.[236] compared the effect of zinc on iron absorption both in solution and in a hamburger meal and observed no inhibitory effect, "suggesting different pathways for the absorption of zinc and iron." They did, however, find that an "intraluminal interaction may occur, because a fivefold excess of zinc to iron (15 mg Zn/3 mg Fe) reduced iron absorption by 56% when given in a water solution but not when given with a hamburger meal." Nevertheless, they noted that "fractional iron absorption is strongly dose dependent." Similarly, using a rodent model, Peres et al.[237] demonstrated that inhibition of zinc absorption by iron depended on their ratio and the deficiency/repletion status of each mineral in the animals. "Between 2:1 and 5:1 a dose dependent inhibition of zinc absorption occurred and reached a plateau beyond this ratio. In iron deficient animals no changes in zinc uptake, mucosal retention and absorption compared to normal animals occurred at ratio 2:1." Meadows et al.[238] studied the oral bioavailability of zinc in nonpregnant adults before and 24 hours after 2 weeks of oral administration of iron and folic acid. They found that "bioavailability was greatly reduced, and the shape of the plasma curves suggested that this was due to impairment of the intestinal absorption of zinc." The authors interpreted their findings as suggesting that "the reduced bioavailability of zinc occurs because of interelement competition in the bowel wall" and cautioned that this phenomenon "might induce zinc depletion." O'Brien et al.[239] reported that zinc absorption was significantly reduced in fasting pregnant Peruvian women administered inorganic iron or inorganic iron plus zinc, compared with nonsupplemented women. However, they also noted that plasma zinc concentrations were also lower in women administered only iron, compared with controls.

In contrast, other researchers observed smaller improvements in hemoglobin and serum ferritin concentrations in Indonesian children administered both iron and zinc than in children given iron alone.[240,241] Similarly, Donangelo et al.[242] found that concomitant zinc (22 mg daily as zinc gluconate and 100 mg iron daily as ferrous sulfate) can lower measures of iron status in nonanemic young women with low iron reserves. In reviewing the literature on interactive effects of iron and zinc on biochemical and functional outcomes in supplementation trials, Fischer Walker et al.[243] concluded that "zinc supplementation alone does not appear to have a clinically important negative effect on iron status. However, when zinc is given with iron, iron indicators do not improve as greatly as when iron is given alone.... Although some trials have shown that joint iron and zinc supplementation has less of an effect on biochemical or functional outcomes than does supplementation with either mineral alone, there is no strong evidence to discourage joint supplementation."

Zinc is often combined with other nutrients, including iron, in the prevention and treatment of nutritional deficits and resulting health problems among impoverished infants and children, especially in nonindustrial societies. In a longitudinal, double-blind, placebo-controlled trial, Muñoz et al.[244] found that coadministration of zinc (20 mg/day), iron (20 mg/day), or the combination for 6 months improved indicators of vitamin A status, particularly higher plasma retinol and transthyretin, compared with placebo, in Mexican preschoolers.

Fortunately, analysis of these complex findings produces some clear and consistent clinical guidelines. The body of evidence indicates that clinically significant adverse pharmacokinetic interactions can be avoided by separating intake of iron and zinc by at least 2 hours, outside the context of meals, or minimized by ingesting the nutrients with a meal, particularly one containing meat, which tends to be rich in both iron and zinc. These guidelines are most important in individuals at risk for compromised nutrient status, of either mineral or generally, with particular concern in pregnant women being supplemented with iron and thus potentially increasing risk of adverse effects, including intrauterine growth retardation and congenital abnormalities related to exacerbated zinc deficiency.

Magnesium

Zinc may exert inhibitory effects on magnesium balance and magnesium absorption in humans.[245] Separating oral intact by at least 2 hours will generally mitigate any impairment of bioavailability of either mineral.

See also Histamine (H$_2$) Receptor Antagonists and related Antacids and Gastric Acid–Suppressive Medications.

Manganese

In experiments on competitive inhibition of iron absorption by manganese and zinc in humans, Rossander-Hulten et al.[236] found significant differences in the effect of the two minerals on manganese absorption, both in solution and in a hamburger meal. They observed that manganese "inhibited iron absorption both in solutions and in a hamburger meal" and that "fractional iron absorption is strongly dose dependent." Conversely, in "the same experiment with zinc, no inhibitory effect was observed, suggesting different pathways for the absorption of zinc and iron." However, an "intraluminal interaction may occur, because a fivefold excess of zinc to iron (15 mg Zn/3 mg Fe) reduced iron absorption by 56%

when given in a water solution but not when given with a hamburger meal."[236] Thus, although the impact of manganese on zinc absorption appears to be significantly less than on iron availability, separating oral intact by at least 2 hours will generally mitigate any impairment of bioavailability of either mineral.

N-Acetylcysteine (NAC)

N-acetylcysteine (NAC), particularly with high doses administered intravenously, as used clinically for acetaminophen poisoning, can complex with zinc, possibly increasing zinc absorption but also increasing urinary zinc excretion.[246] Coadministration of zinc (and copper) may be prudent in individuals using NAC on a long-term basis.

Vitamin B$_2$ (Riboflavin)

Zinc absorption may be impaired in riboflavin deficiency. Supportive data are lacking to confirm this possible interaction.

HERB-NUTRIENT INTERACTIONS

Ashwagandha

Ashwagandha *(Withania somnifera)*, boswellia *(Boswellia serrata)*, turmeric *(Curcuma longa)*.

In a randomized, double-blind, placebo-controlled, crossover study in 42 patients with osteoarthritis, Kulkarni et al.[247] reported clinical efficacy, including a "significant drop in severity of pain ... and disability score," after treatment with a herbomineral formulation containing roots of *Withania somnifera,* the stem of *Boswellia serrata,* rhizomes of *Curcuma longa,* and a zinc complex (Articulin-F). Although the contribution of zinc to the clinical efficacy observed cannot be determined with this research design, further research through well-designed and adequately powered clinical trials may be warranted.

Bloodroot

Bloodroot *(Sanguinaria canadensis)*.

Several studies have investigated and supported a synergistic interaction between zinc and sanguinaria in the treatment of plaque, halitosis, and gingivitis.[248-253]

Evening Primrose Oil

Evening Primrose Oil *(Oenothera biennis)*.

Weak evidence from preliminary research indicates that concomitant administration of zinc and evening primrose oil may be beneficial in the treatment if individuals diagnosed with attention deficit–hyperactivity disorder.[254]

The 257 citations for this monograph, as well as additional reference literature, are located under Zinc on the CD at the back of the book.

Arginine

Nutrient Name: Arginine.
Synonym: L-Arginine.

Summary

Drug/Class Interaction Type	Mechanism and Significance	Management
Antihypertensive medications Angiotensin-converting enzyme (ACE) inhibitors Potassium-sparing diuretics ⊕✗/✗/⊕⊕	Possible additive effect on potassium levels, phosphorus levels, vascular dilation, and blood pressure from concomitant administration. Resultant tendency toward elevated potassium levels and lowered blood pressure could theoretically produce cardiovascular instability or therapeutic benefit, depending on patient variability, communication and compliance, and therapeutic strategy.	Well-managed coadministration possibly appropriate, with close supervision and regular monitoring.
Cyclosporine ☼	L-Arginine, as substrate for nitric oxide (NO) synthesis, may alter vasodilator mechanism(s), particularly NO blockade, possibly responsible for cyclosporine-induced vascular dysfunction, and by enhancing NO levels, decrease cyclosporine nephrotoxicity.	Coadminister, if appropriate. Close supervision and regular monitoring warranted.
Sildenafil Phosphodiesterase-5 inhibitors ⊕⊕	Vasodilation involved in erection requires NO and arginine is the precursor of NO synthesis. NO enables therapeutic action of sildenafil, which may be enhanced by arginine intake, especially in men with low levels or abnormal metabolism of NO.	Coadminister; consider evaluating NO status. Communication, observation, and occasional management appropriate.
Theophylline, aminophylline ⊕	Increased arginase activity and NO deficiency can contribute to airway reactivity. Arginine is substrate for NO synthesis. Preliminary evidence indicates that theophylline or aminophylline could theoretically create a beneficial additive or synergistic effect by reducing arginase activity and increasing arginine's availability to be converted to NO.	Coadminister, if appropriate. Close supervision and regular monitoring warranted.

NUTRIENT DESCRIPTION

Chemistry and Forms

Arginine is a complex amino acid often found at the active (or catalytic) site in proteins and enzymes because of its amine-containing side chain. With four nitrogen atoms per molecule, it is the most abundant nitrogen carrier in humans and animals.

Physiology and Function

Arginine's primary function is generally considered to be the transport, storage, detoxification, and excretion of nitrogen, in particular, and metabolism of protein, in general, through the urea cycle. Arginine is also the substrate for nitric oxide synthase and arginase, two important metabolic pathways. Nitric oxide (NO), a key vasodilator, neurotransmitter, and cell-signaling molecule, is formed by the three different nitric oxide synthases from the N-guanido terminal of the amino acid L-arginine and from molecular oxygen. Nitric oxide synthase (NOS) also converts arginine to citrulline. Arginase converts arginine to ornithine and urea. Arginase I and arginase II control the transformation of arginine into ornithine, which subsequently forms proline and polyamines, which exert multiple effects on connective tissue, smooth muscle, and mucus synthesis. The NOS and arginase pathways interfere with each other through substrate competition.

As the precursor to NO, arginine plays a key role in the circulatory and respiratory systems, particularly endothelial function, vasodilation, and airway physiology. Arginine also functions as a key immunomodulator, particularly increasing the number of T cells, enhancing T cell function, and supporting tissue regeneration. Recent studies have reported increases in arginase in conditions including reperfusion injury, asthma, psoriasis, arthritis, and human breast cancer. Helper T cell type 2 (Th2) cytokines induce arginase expression. During allergic inflammation, increased interleukin-4 (IL-4) and/or IL-13 expression results in increased expression of arginase and amplification of the arginase-dependent pathway, with concomitant suppression of NO generation. Furthermore, in relation to neuroendocrine function, arginine strongly influences adrenal and pituitary functions, especially through stimulation of catecholamines, norepinephrine, insulin and glucagon, prolactin, and growth hormone (GH). Lastly, arginine is involved in synthesis of spermine and spermidine, polyamines required for cell division and growth, and numerous aspects of reproductive function. Hepatic metabolism of arginine produces hydrogen ions (H^+).

Arginine is generally considered a conditionally essential amino acid because adult humans can generally synthesize it de novo from ornithine, glutamine, glutamate, and proline. However, arginine must be obtained through the diet during the juvenile period in humans and in those not synthesizing adequate amounts to meet metabolic demands, especially after acute trauma, burns, or surgery and during infections, chronic illness, or wound healing. In all situations, dietary intake remains the primary determinant of plasma arginine levels, since the rate of arginine biosynthesis does not increase to compensate for depletion or inadequate supply.

NUTRIENT IN CLINICAL PRACTICE

Known or Potential Therapeutic Uses

Arginine's central role in promoting NO formation forms the basis of its therapeutic effect in the treatment of cardiovascular disease, asthma, interstitial cystitis, female sexual dysfunction, and male erectile dysfunction. In particular, a growing body of research has focused on arginine's ability to induce vasodilation and improve endothelial function through its role as a substrate for NO synthesis. Arginine hydrochloride has been used clinically in correcting severe metabolic alkalosis because of its high chloride content. Findings from preliminary double-blind trials indicate the efficacy of arginine in the treatment of acquired immunodeficiency syndrome (AIDS) cachexia, angina, congestive heart failure (CHF), endothelial function in type 1 diabetes, erectile dysfunction, hypertension, and other conditions. Arginine has also been used therapeutically to enhance several aspects of healthy function, including supporting wound healing and resistance to infection; elevating production of GH and related hormones; increasing exercise tolerance, lean muscle mass, and total strength; improving sperm motility and sexual vitality; and reducing low-density lipoprotein (LDL) cholesterol.

Historical/Ethnomedicine Precedent

Arginine has not been used historically as an isolated nutrient.

Possible Uses

Angina, athletic performance, burns, chronic renal failure, congestive heart failure, cystic fibrosis, enhancing formation of muscle mass, erectile dysfunction, female infertility (in vitro fertilization), gastritis, hepatic insufficiency, human immuno-deficiency virus (HIV) support, hypercholesterolemia, hypertension, inflammatory bowel disease, immunity enhancement, intermittent claudication (intravenous only), interstitial cystitis, male infertility (oligospermia), metabolic alkalosis, peripheral vascular disease, surgery preparation and recovery, trauma, wound healing enhancement.

Deficiency Symptoms

Arginine deficiency is uncommon and is usually related to overall protein malnutrition (especially protein deficiency), compromised health status or elevated physiological stress (e.g., burns, injury, infection), excessive ammonia production, or enzyme deficiency. Primary symptoms include rash, hair loss, poor wound healing, constipation, fatty liver, and cirrhosis.

Dietary Sources

The best dietary sources of arginine are meat (especially lamb), peanuts, soybeans, hazelnuts, shrimp, eggs, and milk products. Other foods containing significant mounts of arginine include: almonds, cashews, Brazil nuts, filberts, pecans, sesame and sunflower seeds, walnuts, raisins, coconut, gelatin, chicken, chocolate, brown rice, barley, buckwheat, corn, and oats.

Lysine competes with arginine for absorption, so a diet low in lysine may enhance the effects of arginine intake.

Dosage Forms Available

Capsules, powder, or tablets, containing a salt of L-arginine, such as L-arginine hydrochloride, or arginine glutamate; the free base amino acid is also sometimes used, although it is more problematic to use in a capsule or tablet because it is very hygroscopic.

   Well absorbed orally, with time to peak serum concentration approximately 2 hours.
   Best taken away from meals, in divided doses, throughout day.
   Intravenously administered for pituitary function test.

Dosage Range

Adult

Dietary: Optimal levels of intake have not been established.
Supplemental/Maintenance: 1.5 to 6.0 grams per day, usually 2 to 3 g/day; best in divided doses because absorption of doses greater than 3 g is usually poor. Arginine can be synthesized endogenously, and supplementation is usually not necessary for most individuals.
Pharmacological/Therapeutic: Researchers and practitioners of nutritional therapeutics have used a wide range of dosages, from 2 to 30 g daily, with 6 g daily being representative for most conditions. For example, 6 to 15 g daily has been used in CHF treatment. Long-term use is usually not advisable.

Pediatric (<18 Years)

Dietary: Optimal levels of intake have not been established.
Supplemental/Maintenance: Usually not administered as a nutritional supplement to children.
Pharmacological/Therapeutic: Usually not administered therapeutically to children, except possibly in relation to burns, injuries, or surgery; in such cases, dosage levels would be proportional to typical adult doses by weight.

Laboratory Values

Research laboratory methods for measuring NOS activity are available, but they are not used clinically to any significant degree. Serum and urine amino acid profiles are available, but not likely to be clinically relevant to the status of arginine-derived NO production capability, because more factors are involved than simply the amount of arginine present in tissues and body fluids. Therefore, effects of arginine supplementation are best judged clinically. Various measures of circulatory and endothelial function are most likely to show changes if supplemental arginine enhances NOS activity, as well as blood pressure, erectile function, and exercise tolerance.

SAFETY PROFILE
Overview

Dosage levels of 1 to 6 g per day generally are well tolerated by healthy adults. Adverse effects are estimated to occur in 1% to 10% of patients administered arginine, with more severe reactions associated with intravenous (IV) administration.

Nutrient Adverse Effects
General Adverse Effects

Minor gastrointestinal (GI) distress is occasionally associated with supplemental intake; headache also may occur. Excessive doses of arginine (>40 g/day) may cause diarrhea, most likely as a result of poor absorption at higher dosage levels. Rapid IV infusion may produce flushing.

Despite numerous studies demonstrating the immune-enhancing activity of arginine, including research with breast cancer, some researchers have suggested that high doses of arginine can increase the growth of cancer cells in humans.[1-4] Clinicians with experience in integrative oncology have observed that amino acids, particularly arginine, can have opposite effects at different stages in the disease process, for tissues at different sites, and for different individuals. Further research into such aspects of nutritional therapeutics within cancer prevention and treatment are warranted to delineate such patterns and determine their implications in developing therapeutic strategies. However, pending such studies, the influence of arginine on growth of cancers can generally be qualified as unpredictable.

Adverse Effects Among Specific Populations

Individuals with a history of gastritis, reflux esophagitis, or peptic ulcer disease may experience exacerbations with arginine administration, possibly from stimulation of gastrin. However, the evidence for such concern is mixed.

Hyperphosphatemia can be induced by arginine in patients with severe hepatic disease and kidney problems. The maximum safe dosage levels for arginine administration in individuals with compromised hepatic function have not been established.

Pregnancy and Nursing

Data on long-term safety for arginine administration in pregnant or lactating women are lacking, and maximum safe dosage levels have not been established.

Infants and Children

Data on long-term safety for arginine administration in infants and children are lacking, and maximum safe dosage levels have not been established.

Contraindications

Administration of L-arginine after acute myocardial infarction (MI) may lead to worsened clinical outcomes or death, particularly in older patients with diffuse atherosclerosis, and should be avoided except under the direct supervision of a physician trained and experienced in such interventions.[5] As a possible explanation for these results, it has been hypothesized that L-arginine may only help to alleviate vascular stiffness in patients with preexisting L-arginine deficiency. Continued research is warranted to clarify the role of L-arginine in cardiovascular health.

Avoidance of arginine supplementation by individuals with active or past herpes simplex virus (HSV) infections has often been asserted based on the theory that elevated arginine levels might stimulate viral replication or provoke an outbreak, especially in the context of low lysine levels. Although supported by broad anecdotal reports and older in vitro data,[6] evidence from clinical trials is lacking to confirm elevated susceptibility and validate this contraindication. Nevertheless, caution is warranted. If herpetic reactivations consistently occur shortly after initiating arginine administration or otherwise increasing intake, clinical anecdotes have suggested that a therapeutic trial of coadministration with equal amounts of L-lysine may be useful. Currently, no clinical evidence indicates whether or not L-lysine coadministration may interfere with L-arginine's bioavailability, based on the known competition between the two amino acids for intestinal absorption.

Arginine administration is generally contraindicated in individuals with hepatic or renal failure, except when clinically appropriate and then only under direct medical supervision.[7]

Individuals with a known history of hypersensitivity to arginine generally need to avoid supplemental intake.

Precautions and Warnings

Arginine administration, at usual dosage levels, is generally considered safe in individuals with stable type 2 diabetes mellitus.

However, regular monitoring of blood glucose levels is appropriate in diabetic individuals supplementing with arginine because of possible effects on insulin and glucagon.[6]

INTERACTIONS REVIEW
Strategic Considerations

Despite positive findings from a range of disparate studies, scientific research on the therapeutic use of arginine has not matured; evidence of interactions involving arginine, based on well-designed clinical trials and documented case reports, is uneven and often absent. In many cases, well-known pharmacological principles enable us to predict many probable patterns of interaction, but the body of evidence articulating mechanisms, actions, and efficacy has not yet produced a consistent set of clinically applicable knowledge and related practices. Medical conditions and pharmaceutical agents that deplete or impair arginine status inherently influence relationships between NO and arginase and their interdependent levels and functions and consequently affect cardiac, muscular, and respiratory tissues and processes of growth, inflammation, and expansion/contraction. Interactions involving arginine are primarily characterized by their beneficial effect in supporting the therapeutic strategy and reducing drug adverse effects; such action inherently invokes the occasional bimodal interaction that carries potential for adverse or supportive character largely dependent on communication, observation, and responsive clinical management. Thus, for example, drugs that reduce arginase activity would theoretically increase arginine's availability to be converted to NO. Further research into this apparent bimodal activity of NO, and arginine, is warranted because some aspects of current knowledge suggest that excess NO levels might be involved in chronic inflammatory disorders. Any resulting evidence of peroxynitrate/nitrite formation from NO in situations of increased oxidative stress in the context of inadequate antioxidant reserves would suggest that clinicians give further attention to antioxidant reserves when administering arginine.

In some respects, arginine has already established a role for itself within the inpatient clinical setting, more so than in conventional outpatient care. Within critical care guidelines, arginine hydrochloride is considered a fourth-line treatment for uncompensated metabolic alkalosis after sodium chloride, potassium chloride, and ammonium chloride supplementation has been optimized. The immunomodulatory actions of arginine in nourishing hospitalized patients represent an area of continued research and significant potential benefit. Research on *immunonutrition* using arginine as part of parenteral formulas in combination with other nutrients has focused on mucosal barrier function, cellular defense, and local or systemic inflammation; results have been promising but mixed.

Within nutritional pharmacology and integrative therapeutic strategies, arginine is primarily used as a component of multifactorial interventions to promote detoxification (especially excretion of ammonia), stimulate immune function and modulate inflammation, aid wound healing, enhance healthy function of cardiac and vascular tissue, and promote secretion of several hormones, including glucagon, insulin, and GH. Thus, the emerging concept of immunonutrition as a proactive component of an integrative therapeutic strategy represents a convergence of conventional practice and nutritive therapies, with further research inevitable.

NUTRIENT-DRUG INTERACTIONS

ANTIHYPERTENSIVE MEDICATIONS

Angiotensin-Converting Enzyme (ACE) Inhibitors

Benazepril (Lotensin), combination drug: benazepril and amlodipine (Lotrel); captopril (Capoten); captopril and hydrochlorothiazide (Acezide, Capto-Co, Captozide, Co-Zidocapt); cilazapril (Inhibace), enalapril (Vasotec); combination drugs: enalapril and felodipine (Lexxel); enalapril and hydrochlorothiazide (Vaseretic); fosinopril (Monopril), lisinopril (Prinivil, Zestril), lisinopril and hydrochlorothiazide (Prinzide, Zestoretic); moexipril (Univasc), perindopril (Aceon), quinapril (Accupril), ramipril (Altace) trandolapril (Mavik).

Potassium-Sparing Diuretics

Amiloride (Midamor), spironolactone (Aldactone), triamterene (Dyrenium).
Combination drugs: amiloride and hydrochlorothiazide (Moduretic), spironolactone and hydrochlorothiazide (Ald-acta-zide), triamterene and hydrochlorothiazide (Dyazide, Maxzide).

Interaction Type and Significance

⊕✗   **Bimodal or Variable Interaction, with**
        Professional Management
✗   **Potential or Theoretical Adverse Interaction of**
        Uncertain Severity
⊕⊕   **Beneficial or Supportive Interaction, with**
        Professional Management

Probability: Evidence Base:
4. Plausible   ○ Preliminary

Effect and Mechanism of Action

Hyperkalemia and hypotension are uncommon but potentially serious adverse effects associated with angiotensin-converting-enzyme (ACE) inhibitors, as a class (especially when combined with a potassium sparing diuretic or aldosterone antagonist), as well as with other antihypertensive agents.[8-10] Arginine administration can elevate potassium levels and produce arterial dilation. Intravenous arginine infusions can be used to treat metabolic alkalosis (in patients unresponsive to sodium chloride or potassium chloride supplementation) and are particularly known to induce hyperkalemia; they are also employed in laboratory testing for GH deficiency. Insulin and GH are also both responsive to arginine intake. Concomitant administration of arginine and antihypertensive medications (e.g., ACE inhibitor, potassium-sparing diuretic) could result in an additive effect on potassium levels, phosphorus levels, vascular dilation, and blood pressure lowering.

Research

Key factors that contribute to the potential interaction between arginine and ACE inhibitors have been the subject of human research, but comprehensive research is still in preliminary stages. Coadministration of arginine with ACE inhibitors alone or with other antihypertensive agents could potentially enhance the therapeutic effect on hypertension. However, unsupervised concomitant use of ACE inhibitors and arginine could result in excessive arginine levels, which would primarily manifest as excessive arterial dilation and inadvertent hypotension, through an additive effect.

In a small clinical trial involving 19 normal subjects, Massara et al.[11] noted that plasma phosphorus fell significantly; in 11 of 12 subjects, plasma potassium levels rose significantly after a 0.5 g/kg

arginine infusion. In another small, controlled trial, Pezza et al.[12] found that hypertensive patients refractory to enalapril and hydrochlorothiazide responded favorably when arginine (2 g three times daily orally) was coadministered. In a double-blind trial involving 35 patients with essential hypertension, Abbott and Bakris[13] observed improved arterial dilation in subjects who received 6 g L-arginine in a one-time dose versus placebo (although it not did not change blood pressure immediately). No clinical trial or formal interactions research has been performed specifically investigating the effects of concomitant arginine and ACE inhibitor administration.

Nutritional Therapeutics, Clinical Concerns, and Adaptations

Physicians prescribing antihypertensive medications such as ACE inhibitors or potassium-sparing diuretics are advised to ask patients about possible arginine supplementation and, if deemed clinically appropriate, closely supervise and regularly monitor such individuals for possible interactions between these agents. The nature of the possible interaction is variable, potentially beneficial or adverse, and still largely uncertain; effects in any given individual are likely to be influenced by such factors as dosage, timing, general health status, comorbid conditions, and pharmacogenomic variability. Physicians providing IV arginine should exercise special caution in administering such diagnostic procedures or therapeutic interventions to individuals who are also taking ACE inhibitors.

Caution and careful management are warranted in any patient supplementing with arginine while taking antihypertensive medications. Well-designed clinical trials comparing the effects of concomitant administration of antihypertensive medications and arginine are warranted to further determine arginine's ability to complement conventional antihypertensive therapy, determine parameters of appropriate usage and contraindications, and elucidate therapeutic protocols for effective integrative therapeutics.

Cyclosporine

Cyclosporine (Ciclosporin; cyclosporin A, CsA; Neoral, Sandimmune, SangCya).

Interaction Type and Significance

☼ **Prevention or Reduction of Drug Adverse Effect**

Probability: Evidence Base:
4. Plausible   ▽ Mixed

Effect and Mechanism of Action

L-Arginine is the substrate for nitric oxide (NO) synthesis. A diminished role of the NO/cyclic guanosine monophosphate (cGMP)–mediated vasodilator mechanism, particularly NO blockade, may be responsible for cyclosporine-induced vascular dysfunction. Nitric oxide can decrease cyclosporine nephrotoxicity; it can also have both effector (cytotoxic) and regulatory roles in immune function. L-Arginine is also the substrate for both nitric oxide synthase (NOS), which produces NO, and a component in the experimental NOS inhibitor, N-nitro-L-arginine-methyl ester (L-NAME); both substances have been shown to modify acute cyclosporin A (CsA)–induced intrarenal vasoconstriction.

Research

Arginine has many beneficial effects on the kidneys and may be beneficial in many forms of renal disease, including hypertension and ureteral obstructive nephropathy. A series of studies using a rat model indicate that oral administration of L-arginine can prevent chronic cyclosporine nephrotoxicity through effects on NO metabolites and cGMP.[14-16] Initially, Andoh et al.[14] found that "chronic CsA nephrotoxicity can be aggravated by NO blockade and ameliorated by NO enhancement." Later, Lee et al.[16] conducted in vitro experiments using tissue isolated from the thoracic aorta of normal rats and those acutely treated with CsA to investigate vascular relaxation response to acetylcholine and tissue levels of NO metabolites and cGMP. They found that acute treatment with CsA in vitro greatly attenuated the vasorelaxation response to acetylcholine and that such response was completely restored by L-arginine. The vascular accumulation of NO metabolites in response to acetylcholine was decreased significantly by CsA, but coadministration of L-arginine prevented this effect. While CsA decreased cGMP accumulation in response to acetylcholine (and sodium nitroprusside), acetylcholine-stimulated cGMP generation was restored, although not completely, by L-arginine, but it did not affect sodium nitroprusside–stimulated cGMP generation. After chronic CsA treatment in the whole animal, the vasorelaxation response to acetylcholine was decreased significantly, along with tissue levels of NO metabolites; administration of L-arginine preserved this effect. The authors concluded: "CsA causes an L-arginine-sensitive vascular dysfunction which is associated with impaired generation of NO and cGMP."[16] Other research with animals indicates that arginine may inhibit tumor growth by activating macrophage cytotoxic effects.[17]

Zhang et al.[18] conducted a randomized, double-blind clinical trial involving 11 young renal allograft recipients, age 11 to 22 years, with chronic renal transplant dysfunction treated with CsA. The subjects were randomly assigned to a 6-week treatment period with placebo, followed by two subsequent 6-week periods with L-arginine supplementation (0.1 g/kg/day) or 6-week treatment with L-arginine, followed by two subsequent 6-week periods with placebo. At the end of each treatment period, 24-hour blood pressure readings were taken, and glomerular filtration rate (GFR), renal perfusion function (RPF; PAH clearance), and urinary excretion of protein, albumin, nitrate, cGMP, and urea were evaluated. These researchers found that subjects receiving arginine did not demonstrate significant changes in GFR, RPF, proteinuria/albuminuria, mean systolic/diastolic blood pressure, compared with placebo. These researchers concluded that arginine administration "did not improve renal function and did not decrease proteinuria in CsA-treated renal allograft recipients with chronic transplant dysfunction possibly because of inhibition of NO-cGMP forming mechanism."[18] Given the negative results of this small clinical trial, with the suggestive preclinical data, clinicians might consider the question of how a trial might be designed with a stronger opportunity for a positive outcome. Higher doses, longer term, starting arginine vs. placebo concurrent with CsA, or other design variants might enable investigators to determine if CsA nephropathy can be prevented, if correction is not obtainable. Arginine may also increase oxidative stress by forming peroxynitrite radicals (NO reacting with superoxide radicals), so some measure of oxidative stress and correction with either dietary or supplemental antioxidants may be needed to demonstrate benefit.

Nutritional Therapeutics, Clinical Concerns, and Adaptations
The body of research on arginine can reasonably be interpreted as supporting the general hypothesis that arginine may provide a salutary effect to renal function, particularly in individuals whose kidneys are in a compromised state. However, the mixed character and preliminary state of the available research data suggest that sufficient evidence is lacking to support coadministration of L-arginine as likely to offer significant definite benefit to patients undergoing cyclosporine therapy. Well-designed clinical trials comparing different dosage levels of arginine and pretreatment versus coadministration are warranted to further determine arginine's ability to mitigate adverse effects of CsA therapy and elucidate therapeutic protocols for effective integrative therapeutics.

Sildenafil and Related Phosphodiesterase-5 Inhibitors

Evidence: Sildenafil (Viagra).
Extrapolated, based on similar properties: Tadalafil (Cialis), vardenafil (Levitra).

Interaction Type and Significance
⊕⊕   **Beneficial or Supportive Interaction, with Professional Management**

Probability:	Evidence Base:
3. Possible	◉ Emerging

Effect and Mechanism of Action
The vasodilation necessary to an erection depends on NO.[19] The vasodilatory effect of arginine, as an enhancer of NO production, is broadly accepted. Sildenafil is generally considered to require the presence of NO for its effectiveness.[20,21] Other phosphodiesterase-5 (PDE-5) inhibitors, such as tadalafil and vardenafil, have exactly the same mechanism of action, varying only in pharmacokinetic parameters.

Research
Research into the therapeutic value of arginine in the treatment of men with erectile dysfunction (ED) is in preliminary stages, but the findings thus far support the hypothesis that enhancement of NO status can be efficacious, especially in men with NO deficiency or metabolic dysfunction.

In a small preliminary trial, Zorgniotti and Lizza[22] found that 6 of 15 men with ED demonstrated improvement after taking arginine, 2800 mg/day, for 2 weeks, versus no reported improvement with placebo. Subsequently, in a prospective randomized, double-blind, placebo-controlled trial, Chen et al.[23] administered arginine, 5 g/day, or placebo to 50 men with ED for 6 weeks. Plasma and urine nitrite and nitrate (designated NOx), both stable metabolites of NO, were determined at the end of the placebo run-in period and after 3 and 6 weeks. Nine of 29 (31%) patients taking L-arginine, as well as 2 of 17 controls, reported a significant subjective improvement in sexual function. However, plasma and urine NOx levels, which served as objective variables, remained unchanged. All nine patients who had subjectively improved sexual performance after being treated with L-arginine had initially demonstrated low urinary NOx, levels of which had doubled at the end of the study. Thus, these researchers concluded that arginine was particularly effective at providing significant subjective improvement in sexual function in men with organic ED who had abnormal NO metabolism, particularly decreased NOx excretion or production.

In a randomized trial involving 116 men who had undergone non-nerve-sparing radical pelvic surgery (64 prostatectomies and 52 cystectomies), Mantovani et al.[19] compared erectile function in those treated with sildenafil alone versus those administered both sildenafil and L-arginine. An initial 50-mg dose was inefficient in both groups (using Buckling test for evaluation), but 100-mg doses gave significant results

(Buckling test >500) in both groups, especially those receiving the combined treatment.

Nutritional Therapeutics, Clinical Concerns, and Adaptations

Physicians prescribing sildenafil for the treatment of ED are advised to discuss with patients the potential benefits of concomitant arginine therapy. Based on preliminary evidence, a beneficial interaction between sildenafil and supplemental arginine appears to be possible as a result of the additive effects of the actions of these substances on NO function, especially in individuals with abnormal NO metabolism. Such simultaneous administration could alter the effects and the dosage levels and timing appropriate to safe and effective therapeutic application of sildenafil. Of note, the effects of arginine on NO production are best produced by chronic administration, whereas the effects of sildenafil and the other PDE-5 inhibitors, occur with acute (i.e., on-demand) administration. Suggested arginine dosage levels have not been definitively established, although clinical experience suggests that 6 g daily is a reasonable target. Thus, close supervision and regular monitoring are appropriate, even though evidence is lacking to suggest a significant risk of adverse reactions. Well-designed clinical trials investigating the effects of arginine alone and together with PDE-5 inhibitors are warranted to further determine arginine's ability to complement conventional therapy, determine parameters of appropriate usage and possible contraindications, determine effective dosage levels, and elucidate therapeutic protocols for effective integrative therapeutics.

Theophylline/Aminophylline

Theophylline/aminophylline (Phyllocontin, Slo-Bid, Slo-Phyllin, Theo-24, Theo-Bid, Theocron, Theo-Dur, Theolair, Truphylline, Uni-Dur, Uniphyl); combination drug: ephedrine, guaifenesin, and theophylline (Primatene Dual Action).

Interaction Type and Significance

⊕   **Potential or Theoretical Beneficial or Supportive Interaction, with Professional Management**

Probability: Evidence Base:
4. Plausible   ○ **Preliminary**

Effect and Mechanism of Action

Nitric oxide deficiency appears to play a major role in inducing airway hyperreactivity and other aspects of asthma pathogenesis. In particular, a relative deficiency of NO caused by increased arginase activity and altered L-arginine homeostasis is a major factor in the pathology of asthma.[24] Based on research of arginine metabolism and caffeine action, the therapeutic action of theophylline (aminophylline) may be attributable, at least in part, to their effect in increasing cellular levels of cyclic adenosine monophosphate (cAMP) and thereby depressing arginase activity.[25] Drugs that reduce arginase activity would theoretically increase arginine's availability to be converted to NO. Administration of arginine in the context of methylxanthine therapy could create a beneficial additive or synergistic effect against pathophysiological components of asthma by enhancing NO levels.

Research

These bronchodilator drugs are primarily used in the treatment of asthma, for which arginine's central role is becoming increasingly clear within the scientific literature and medical research. Nitric oxide is a critical regulator of airway physiology, including airway and vascular smooth muscle tone.[26] The NOS and arginase pathways interfere with each other through substrate competition. A review of recent research indicates that a deficiency of beneficial, bronchodilating, constitutive NOS (cNOS)–derived NO is important in allergen-induced airway hyperresponsiveness, and that increased arginase activity and decreased cellular uptake of L-arginine appear to play a key role.[24] Interpreting the findings of Zimmermann et al.,[27] based on a mouse model, Vercelli[28] showed that "NO inhibition resulted from substrate competition," because expression of arginase, but not NOS, was altered in the lungs of the allergen-challenged mice. Meurs et al.[29] found that increased arginase activity underlies allergen-induced deficiency of cNOS-derived NO and airway hyperresponsiveness. Arginase expression appears to be controlled by Th2 cytokines, central mediators of allergic asthma.[30] During allergic inflammation, increased IL-4 and/or IL-13 expression results in increased expression of arginase and amplification of the arginase-dependent pathway, with concomitant suppression of NO generation.[28] In particular, "while these enzymes are constitutively expressed, NOS-2 is an inducible enzyme independent of calcium and highly induced in inflammatory diseases such as allergic asthma, where NO may act beneficial or deleterious depending on the site … and amount of generation."[26] The emerging connections between the NO pathway, inflammatory response, and collagen generation "make arginine metabolism a rising star in the asthma firmament."[28]

Wechsler et al.[31] demonstrated an increased NO concentration in exhaled air in patients with asthma and observed an association with the asthmatic phenotype, in particular, NOS-1 genotype. Morris et al.[32] measured amino acid levels, arginase activity, and NO metabolites in the blood of asthmatic patients, as well as NO in exhaled breath. They found that "although levels of virtually all amino acids were reduced, asthmatic patients exhibited a striking reduction in plasma arginine levels compared to non-asthmatic normal controls." These researchers concluded: "High arginase activity in asthmatic patients may contribute to low circulating arginine levels, thereby limiting arginine bioavailability and creating a nitric oxide deficiency that induces hyperreactive airways."

The compiled findings could be interpreted to support the hypothesis that arginine could serve as a therapeutically efficacious component of a comprehensive strategy for the treatment of individuals with asthma, or at least some subpopulation, whether refractory to conventional care or defined by one or more genomic factors. Further, given the known and emerging knowledge of the mechanisms of action exerted by methylxanthines, a beneficial interaction appears pharmacologically plausible from concomitant administration of arginine with these agents.

Nutritional Therapeutics, Clinical Concerns, and Adaptations

Physicians prescribing theophylline (or other methylxanthines) might consider discussing with patients the possible benefits of arginine administration, if deemed clinically appropriate. The nature of the possible interaction is variable, with possibly beneficial but also potential (although as yet unknown) adverse effects, in any given individual and likely to be influenced by such factors as dosage, timing, general health status, comorbid conditions, and pharmacogenomic variability. Close supervision and regular monitoring of such individuals for therapeutic response and potential adverse interactions are warranted.

Asthma is a disease of inherent complexity and variability that remains a major medical and scientific challenge despite intense research efforts and a growing number of affected individuals.

Although inhaled corticosteroids and beta-2-agonist broncho-dilators have become the mainstay of asthma therapy, a complete understanding of the pathogenetic mechanisms of the disease, as well as diverse and difficult to define factors of individual variability in susceptibility, presentation, and exacerbation, continues to elude researchers. Caution and careful management are warranted when modifying the therapeutic intervention in any patient with asthma, especially those taking bronchodilators, whether inhaled or systemic. Well-designed clinical trials investigating the effects of arginine alone and together with theophylline (or other methylxanthines) are warranted to further determine arginine's ability to complement conventional bronchodilator therapy, determine parameters of appropriate usage and contraindications, and elucidate therapeutic protocols for effective integrative therapeutics.

THEORETICAL, SPECULATIVE, AND PRELIMINARY INTERACTIONS RESEARCH, INCLUDING OVERSTATED INTERACTIONS CLAIMS

Estrogen-Progestin Combinations

Oral Contraceptives: Monophasic, Biphasic, and Triphasic Estrogen Preparations (Synthetic Estrogen and Progesterone Analogs)

Hormone Replacement Therapy, Estrogen-Containing and Synthetic Estrogen and Progesterone Analog Medications

The concomitant use of an estrogen-progestin combination and an arginine preparation might theoretically result in increased toxicity effects because of resultant effects on GH response and glucagon and insulin effects. Although this interaction appears plausible, there is a lack of evidence from clinical trials and well-documented case reports characterizing such an interaction, defining its frequency and context of occurrence, or establishing its clinical implications.

Nitrates

Amyl nitrate, isosorbide dinitrate (ISDN, Isordil, Sorbitrate); combination drug: hydralazine and isosorbide dinitrate (BiDil); isosorbide mononitrate (Imdur, ISMN, ISMO, Isotrate, Monoket).

Members of the nitrate family of drugs are used to prevent angina. Human research has shown that arginine, as an NO precursor, also is potentially beneficial for individuals with angina or other cardiovascular conditions. An interaction between nitrate medications and arginine could potentially result from the additive effects of the similar actions of these substances if taken concomitantly. Such simultaneous administration could alter the effects and the dosage levels and timing appropriate to safe and effective therapeutic application of these agents.[33] Evidence from clinical trials or documented case reports is lacking at this time to confirm this theoretically possible interaction or characterize its frequency, context, or severity.

Pentoxifylline

Pentoxifylline (Pentoxil, Trenta).

Based on research of arginine metabolism and caffeine action, the therapeutic action of pentoxifylline may be attributable, at least in part, to the shared effect of methylxanthines in increasing cellular levels of cAMP and thus depressing arginase activity and increasing arginine's availability for conversion to NO.[25] Evidence from clinical trials or documented case reports is lacking at this time to confirm this theoretically possible interaction or characterize its frequency, context, or severity. Pentoxifylline's documented, though modest, enhancement of compromised circulation would theoretically synergize with arginine's ability to enhance endothelial function and vasodilation by optimizing NO production. Well-designed clinical trials to explore such possible synergy would seem indicated.

NUTRIENT-NUTRIENT INTERACTIONS

Lysine

Within the world of nutritional anecdotes, the antagonistic relationship between L-lysine and L-arginine has taken on almost self-evident status, particularly within the context of preventing herpes simplex by administering lysine and reducing arginine intake. However, although the evidence supporting such conclusions is emerging, it remains inconclusive.

Arginine and lysine compete for absorption into cells, so increased intake of either amino acid can decrease levels of the other. Consequently, a diet low in lysine can enhance effects of arginine supplementation because lysine competes with arginine for absorption. Furthermore, increased arginine intake is reputed to enhance arginine status, together with the benefits and risks attendant to such an environment. This competitive relationship appears to be founded on reasonable pharmacological principles.

Anecdotal reports based on consumption of foods with a high arginine/lysine ratios (e.g., nuts, peanuts, chocolate) and in vitro research dating back to 1964 indicate that HSV has a high requirement for arginine and lysine inhibits viral replication.[6] Findings from several clinical trials of varying size and design have generally supported the hypothesis that lysine intake reduces the recurrence rate of HSV infections.[34-38]

Although the available evidence is strongly suggestive rather than conclusive, conservative practice warrants approaching arginine and lysine as metabolic competitors and therefore requiring that diet and supplemental intake be adjusted in accordance with clinical objectives. The immune-enhancing functions of arginine are well known, but it appears judicious to advise decreasing arginine intake and increasing lysine intake with susceptible individuals, to prevent or resolve herpes simplex outbreaks. Further research with large, well-designed clinical trials is warranted to advance and clarify the metabolic relationship between these two amino acids, define factors of individual variability in response patterns and disease susceptibilities, and develop balanced and comprehensive guidelines for evidence-based clinical application of these key nutrients.

Omega-3 Fatty Acids (Fish Oils)

In a 6-month, prospective, randomized, double-blind controlled study involving 64 HIV-infected outpatients (with CD4 lymphocyte count $\geq 100 \times 10^6/L$), Pichard et al.[39] found that the addition of arginine and omega-3 fatty acids did not improve immunological parameters, compared with a group receiving only the base multinutrient oral supplement; body weight increased in both groups. The synergy between omega-3 fatty acids and arginine in supporting wound healing and tissue regeneration warrants further research and development of evidence-based clinical guidelines.

See also Parenteral and Enteral Nutritional Formulations.

Ornithine

Interest in the potentially beneficial synergy between arginine and ornithine largely derives from knowledge of arginine's function as a precursor of ornithine and their respective roles in GH secretion. Approximately 50% of arginine intake is rapidly converted to ornithine, primarily through the action of arginase. Ornithine can subsequently be metabolized to glutamate and proline, or into the polyamine pathway, under the action of ornithine decarboxylase.[40]

Coadministration of arginine and ornithine, often with other nutrients, has been suggested as a means of enhancing GH levels and thereby increasing development of muscle tissue and lean body mass, increasing gains in strength, and decreasing proportional body fat, primarily within the context of athletic training and body building.

Elam[41] reported that coadministration of arginine and ornithine (500 mg each twice daily, five times weekly) in a controlled clinical trial involving adult males, in conjunction with resistance exercise, produced a significant decrease in body fat. Subsequently, in a double-blinded clinical trial framed around a 5-week progressive strength-training program, Elam observed that a arginine-ornithine combination (1 g each, orally, five times weekly) scored significantly higher gains in total strength and enhancement of lean body mass compared to controls administered vitamin C and calcium as placebo. Elam et al.[42] also noted that arginine and ornithine enhanced recovery from chronic physiological stress by quelling tissue breakdown, as evidenced by lower urinary hydroxyproline levels.

However, Marcell et al.[43] found that acute arginine administration (5 g orally 30 minutes before exercise) did not stimulate basal or augment exercise-induced GH secretion in either young or old adults and may actually have impaired GH secretion in young adults.

Further research comparing timing, duration, and dosage levels of combined supplementation with arginine and ornithine through clinical trials of adequate size and appropriate design is warranted to elucidate the relationship of these nutrients in building lean body mass, particularly muscle tissue, and facilitating breakdown of adipose tissue.

Parenteral and Enteral Nutrition Formulations Containing Antioxidants, Fatty Acids, and Other Nutrients

Arginine is often used with nutrients as part of multi-ingredient immunonutrition-parenteral formulas administered to patients who are recovering from injury, burns, or surgery or otherwise critically ill. Three meta-analyses found that immunonutrition results in notable reductions in infection rate and length of hospital stay, with greater benefit observed in surgical than critically ill patients. However, there was an overall lack of significant impact on outcomes, particularly mortality, and at least one study indicated significant risk of increased mortality in critically ill patients receiving immunonutrition, especially when sepsis was involved.[44-49] "A biphasic response with an early hyperinflammatory response followed by an excessive compensatory response associated with immunosuppression" is seen in many critically ill patients.[49] Several clinical trials have reported positive outcomes (as indicated by measures of immune function) in oncology and trauma recovery patients administered formulations containing arginine, glutamine, omega-3 fatty acids, RNA or nucleotides, and other nutrients, typically in the form of enriched enteral diets.[50-54]

In a prospective, multicenter, single-blind, randomized trial, Caparros et al.[55] investigated the effect on nosocomial infections and outcome of early enteral nutrition in 220 critically ill intensive care unit (ICU) patients with a high-protein diet enriched with arginine, fiber, and antioxidants, compared with a standard high-protein diet. These researchers found that critically ill patients fed a high-protein diet enriched with arginine, fiber, and antioxidants had a significantly lower catheter-related sepsis rate than patients fed a standard high-protein diet. Further, although there were no differences in mortality or ICU and hospital length of stay between the two groups, the patients fed the study diet for more than 2 days showed a trend toward decreased mortality.

The preliminary nature and sometimes contradictory findings of studies thus far conducted suggest that different nutrient formulations may be appropriate for varying patient populations, Continued research into these integrative approaches to nutritional support within inpatient care settings, in general, and critical care, in particular, through large, well-designed clinical trials, is clearly warranted.

See also Omega-3 Fatty Acids (Fish Oils).

HERB-NUTRIENT INTERACTIONS

Yohimbe

Yohimbe *(Pausinystalia yohimbe; Corynanthe yohimbe (Corynanthejohimbe).*

The major identified alkaloid in yohimbe is *yohimbine*, an alkaloid that blocks alpha-adrenergic outflow, thereby increasing parasympathetic tone. This can promote erectile function, as well as have blood pressure–lowering effects. Purified yohimbine is a prescription drug in the United States, but it is also found in herbal preparations at lower doses.

In a double-blind, placebo-controlled, three-way crossover, randomized clinical trial involving 45 men with ED, Lebret et al.[56] compared the efficacy and safety of the combination of L-arginine glutamate (6 g) and yohimbine hydrochloride (6 mg) with that of yohimbine hydrochloride (6 mg) alone and that of placebo, administered orally, 1 to 2 hours before intended sexual intercourse. Based on the findings from this pilot study, these researchers concluded that "the on-demand oral administration of the L-arginine glutamate (6 g) and yohimbine (6 mg) combination is effective in improving erectile function in patients with mild to moderate erectile dysfunction," as measured by Erectile Function Domain scores and patients' assessment of efficacy.

Well-designed clinical trials investigating the combined effects of arginine and yohimbe derivatives are warranted to further determine safety and efficacy, determine parameters of appropriate usage and possible contraindications, determine effective dosage levels, and elucidate therapeutic protocols for effective integrative therapeutics.

The 56 citations for this monograph, as well as additional reference literature, are located under Arginine on the CD at the back of the book.

Carnitine

Nutrient Name: Carnitine.
Synonyms: L-Carnitine, levocarnitine; vitamin BT.
Forms: Acetyl-L-carnitine (ALC), L-acetylcarnitine (LAC); propionyl-L-caritine (PLC), L-propionylcarnitine (LPC).
Related Substance: D-Carnitine (synthetic isomer).

Summary

Drug/Class Interaction Type	Mechanism and Significance	Management
Allopurinol ⊕⊕	Carnitine deficiency is characteristic of Duchenne muscular dystrophy, particularly affecting mitochondrial metabolism and muscle tissue. Allopurinol restores carnitine levels in such individuals. Coadministration of carnitine could theoretically enhance this intervention.	Treat with allopurinol; consider carnitine coadministration.
Doxorubicin Anthracycline chemotherapy ≈≈/☼	Cardiotoxicity is a common and irreversible adverse effect of doxorubicin therapy, sometimes acute, often chronic or delayed. Coadministration of carnitine before, during, and after chemotherapy can prevent and reduce cardiomyopathy and other toxic effects, partly because of its role in supporting fatty acid oxidation and cardiac function. Nutrient support is nontoxic and unlikely to interfere with doxorubicin's therapeutic activity.	Coadminister; closely monitor cardiac and renal function. Consider liposomal forms.
Isotretinoin Retinoids ☼	Carnitine can prevent or reduce adverse effects of isotretinoin, particularly myalgia and hypertriglyceridemia, partly because of its role in supporting fatty acid oxidation, mitochondrial metabolism, and hepatic detoxification. Nutrient support is nontoxic and unlikely to interfere with therapeutic activity of retinoids.	Coordinated use with separated administration; closely monitor.
Levothyroxine Thyroid hormones ✗✗/⊕✗/☼	Carnitine inhibits thyroid hormone nuclear uptake and may partially block activity of thyroid hormone. Carnitine contraindicated in hypothyroidism (frank or subclinical) but valuable with hyperthyroidism, endogenous or iatrogenic.	Caution against carnitine supplementation in hypothyroid states. Administer with monitoring when thyroid hormone antagonist appropriate.
Nitroglycerin ⊕⊕/⊕✗/✗	Carnitine can support cardiac function and reduce ischemia and angina through its action on mitochondrial metabolism, fatty acid oxidation, and myocardial function. Coadministration of carnitine may reduce incidence and severity of angina and enable reduced nitroglycerin dosage. Theoretical risk of additive response.	Coadminister carnitine; monitor.
Pivampicillin, pivmecillinam Pivalate prodrugs ≈≈	Pivalate prodrugs cause carnitine depletion through urinary excretion of pivaloylcarnitine. Depletion inherent but of minimal clinical significance in most individuals with short-term drug intake. Adverse effects can be acute and potentially significant in susceptible individuals (e.g., infants and children, carnitine deficient, AEDs), but adverse effects primarily associated with chronic or recurrent use. Carnitine support can prevent or reverse depletion and adverse sequelae.	Carnitine coadministration may be prudent but usually unnecessary.
Simvastatin HMG-CoA reductase inhibitors (statins) ⊕⊕/☼	Statin therapy is generally ineffective (and sometimes counterproductive) in reducing lipoprotein(a) and its atherogenic and prothrombotic effects. L-carnitine appears efficacious in lowering lipoprotein(a) levels, particularly in patients with type 2 diabetes. Several trials show therapeutic benefits from L-carnitine, particularly in combination with simvastatin, in treating this form of dyslipidemia. No adverse effects have been reported.	Coadminister L-carnitine within comprehensive program, including statin.
Valproic acid (VPA) Anticonvulsant medications ≈≈/☼/⊕	Anticonvulsant medications (AEDs), particularly VPA, deplete carnitine and can cause clinically significant deficiency with long-term use, especially in children and with polytherapy. Other factors in patient population, besides drug effect, may contribute to compromised carnitine status. Coadministration of carnitine can prevent or reverse adverse medication effects but may be unnecessary in many patients.	Coadminister carnitine; monitor.
Zidovudine (AZT) Reverse-transcriptase inhibitor (nucleoside) antiretroviral agents ◇≈≈/≈≈/☼/⊕	Carnitine deficiency is characteristic of HIV infection, notably affecting mitochondrial metabolism, fatty acid oxidation, and immune function. Carnitine can prevent or reduce adverse effects of AZT and related antiviral medications, particularly accumulation of lipid droplets within muscle fibers from poor utilization of long-chain fatty acids.	Coadminister carnitine; monitor.

AEDs, Antiepileptic drugs; *HIV,* human immunodeficiency virus.

NUTRIENT DESCRIPTION

Chemistry and Forms

Carnitine (3-hydroxy-4N-trimethylammoniumbutanoate) is a naturally occurring quaternary amine. Forms include acetyl-L-carnitine (ALC; L-acetylcarnitine, LAC) and propionyl-L-carnitine (PLC; L-propionylcarnitine, LPC).

Physiology and Function

Carnitine (levocarnitine, L-carnitine) is considered to be a nonessential amino acid, although in certain situations it is considered conditionally essential (e.g., dialysis patients, premature and very-low-birth-weight infants, coronary artery disease). The highest concentrations of carnitine are found in the heart, muscles, liver, and kidney. The major biochemical function of carnitine is to act as a transmembrane carrier of long-chain fatty acids to the interior of mitochondria. It plays a major role in the utilization of fats in energy production at the mitochondrial level through the beta-oxidation of branched-chain amino acids and ketoacids. Carnitine also participates in transportation of acyl-coenzyme A (CoA) compounds. The activated long-chain fatty acyl-CoA esters in the cytosol are able to be transported to the mitochondrial matrix only by combining with carnitine. Beta-oxidation, the primary metabolic process by which fatty acids, branched-chain amino acids, and ketoacids (as acyl-coA esters) are used as fuel for cellular energy, occurs in the mitochondria. Thus, carnitine functions as an important physiological mediator of fatty acid and protein metabolism. Carnitine also enables hepatic detoxification and excretion of chemicals, including drugs, and improves glucose disposal and may reduce insulin resistance. Carnitine is instrumental in the production and release of acetylcholine.

Carnitine from dietary sources is rapidly absorbed from the intestinal tract by both passive and active transport. Although it exhibits vitamin-like properties, carnitine is a small amino acid derivative that can be synthesized de novo in the liver, brain, and kidneys using lysine and methionine in a process requiring vitamins C, B_6, and niacin. Exogenous intake may be necessary during periods of increased demand or increased loss. Acetyl-L-carnitine (ALC), the acetylated derivative of L-carnitine, is particularly localized in muscles, brain, and testicles.

NUTRIENT IN CLINICAL PRACTICE

Known or Potential Therapeutic Uses

Carnitine's central role in muscle function and fat metabolism has drawn the attention of clinicians and researchers to clinical applications related to these roles. Carnitine is proposed for increasing endurance and improving cardiac performance based on its known action of enhancing the efficiency of energy production in muscle tissue in general and the myocardium in particular. Human research has focused on therapeutic application of carnitine, especially as propionyl-L-carnitine (PLC), in the treatment of angina, myocardial insufficiency, peripheral claudication, and other conditions related to arterial insufficiency. Cardiac L-carnitine content, essential for mitochondrial fatty acid transport and adenosine triphosphate (ATP)–diphosphate (ADP) exchange, decreases during ischemia. Furthermore, acetyl-L-carnitine (ALC) has been administered for slowing, and even partially reversing, nerve and brain deterioration associated with the aging process. Thus, the primary potential clinical uses for carnitine include claudication, Alzheimer's disease, myocardial insufficiency, and renal dialysis. Hyperlipidemia, male infertility, athletic performance, and weight loss have also been the subjects of therapeutic claims and evolving investigations, although results have been more mixed.

During pregnancy, infancy, and breastfeeding (i.e., situations of high energy demands), the physiological need for L-carnitine can exceed the capacity for endogenous synthesis. Consequently, L-carnitine is often used as a supplement with breast milk or infant formula for low-birth-weight (LBW) infants (either preterm or full term).

Possible Uses

Attention deficit–hyperactivity disorder (ADHD), alcohol dependence, Alzheimer's disease, angina pectoris, anorexia nervosa, arrhythmias, atherosclerosis, athletic performance (enhancement), cardiac ischemia, cardiac surgery (recovery), cataracts, chronic fatigue syndrome, chronic obstructive pulmonary disease (COPD), congestive heart failure (CHF; propionyl-L-carnitine), dementia, depression in elderly (acetyl-L-carnitine), diabetes mellitus, diabetic cardiac autonomic neuropathy, erectile dysfunction, human immunodeficiency virus (HIV) infection, hyperactivity in fragile X syndrome, hypercholesterolemia, hyperthyroidism, hypertriglyceridemia, infertility (male), intermittent claudication, myocardial infarction, myocardial insufficiency (e.g., CHF or cardiomyopathy), Peyronie's disease, Raynaud's disease, renal dialysis, seizure disorders, weight loss.

Deficiency Symptoms

Carnitine deficiency is characterized by inadequate tissue levels, resulting in impaired tissue fatty acid oxidation. Other symptoms of a relative deficiency may include elevated blood lipids, abnormal liver function, chronic muscle weakness, reduced energy, impaired glucose control, cardiomyopathy, encephalopathy, and recurrent episodes of coma.[1]

Absolute carnitine deficiency is unlikely because of endogenous synthesis. Primary systemic carnitine deficiency is caused by a defect in the specific high-affinity carnitine transporter, which is expressed in most tissues and is responsible for bringing carnitine into the cytosol. This carnitine uptake defect is rare and is characterized by progressive infantile-onset carnitine-responsive cardiomyopathy, weakness, recurrent hypoglycemic hypoketotic encephalopathy, and failure to thrive.[2] Several inherited metabolic disorders, especially organic acidurias and disorders of beta-oxidation, can cause secondary carnitine deficiency.[3,4]

Carnitine deficiency can result from numerous factors, independently or in combination, and will contribute to further sequelae and increased risk factors. Deficiency can result from high fat diets and insufficient supply of precursors for synthesis (methionine, lysine, niacin, vitamins C and B_6). Individuals who have a limited intake of meat and dairy products tend to have lower L-carnitine intakes. However, even long-term vegans usually do not display signs of carnitine deficiency. Seizure disorders, diabetes mellitus, cirrhosis, illness, and infection (e.g., HIV), strenuous exercise, trauma, pregnancy and lactation, and other conditions characterized by increased physiological stress are associated with decreased carnitine levels. A carnitine deficiency can also result from oxygen deprivation, which can occur in some cardiac conditions.[5] Carnitine deficiency may play a role in the development of retinopathy, hyperlipidemia, neuropathy, or complications of diabetes.[6] Many prescription medications may also have an adverse effect on carnitine levels and functions.

Dietary Sources

As implied by its name, carnitine is primarily found in foods of animal origin, and to a lesser extent, in foods of plant origin. Meat, milk, eggs, and dairy products are the richest sources of dietary carnitine intake, with beef being the most abundant. Generally, the redder the meat, the higher is the carnitine content. Cereals, fruit, and vegetables are relatively poor dietary sources.

Nutrient Preparations Available

Carnitine is administered as one of three salts of L-carnitine: L-carnitine (for heart and other conditions), propionyl-L-carnitine (for heart conditions), and acetyl-L-carnitine (for Alzheimer's disease). The dosage is the same for all three forms, typically 500 mg to 1 g three times daily.

Note: Only pure L-carnitine should be used as a supplement or therapeutic agent.

Dextrocarnitine (D-carnitine), or the DL-mixture, may interfere with the normal function of the levo (L-) isomer and produce signs of deficiency.

Dosage Forms Available

Capsule, powder, tablet.

Source Materials for Nutrient Preparations

Synthesized.

Dosage Range

Adult

Dietary: No dietary reference intake (DRI) or recommended dietary allowance (RDA) has been established for carnitine. The average omnivorous diet provides approximately 100 to 300 mg of carnitine per day.
Supplemental/Maintenance: 1500 to 4000 mg per day in divided doses, when supplementation is indicated. Optimal levels of intake have not been established.
Pharmacological/Therapeutic: 150 mg to 1 g three times daily.
Toxic: No toxicities have been reported or suspected as being associated with carnitine.

Pediatric (<18 Years)

Dietary: No DRI or RDA has been established for carnitine.
Supplemental/Maintenance: Usually not necessary, although often administered to LBW infants (preterm or full term) with breast milk or infant formula and in children receiving long-term total parenteral nutrition (TPN). Optimal levels of intake have not been established.
Pharmacological/Therapeutic: 50 mg to 1 g three times daily. One clinical trial involving children diagnosed with ADHD used 50 mg/kg twice daily, up to a maximum of 4 g daily.[7]
Toxic: No reported adverse effects have been specifically related to children.

SAFETY PROFILE

Overview

L-Carnitine is quite safe, with no significant adverse effects reported, even at high doses.

Nutrient Adverse Effects

General Adverse Effects

Rarely, gastrointestinal (GI) complaints such as nausea and vomiting have been reported with the use of L-carnitine.[8] Sleeplessness may occur if taken before bed.

Pregnancy and Nursing

Adverse effects are not predicted, and reports are lacking. However, the lack of controlled studies involving pregnant or lactating women prevents any claims of safety and suggests that supplementation should be avoided during such life stages.

Infants and Children

Adverse effects are not predicted, and reports are lacking. Supplementation is not recommended unless otherwise indicated as essential.

Contraindications

Individuals with low or borderline-low thyroid levels should avoid carnitine supplementation because it may impair the action of thyroid hormone.[9,10] This proposed effect is primarily extrapolated from research involving patients being treated for goiter with exogenous hormone.

Precautions and Warnings

DL-Carnitine may produce muscle weakness; the D isomer should be avoided because it may interfere with the activity of L-carnitine and thus is potentially toxic.

INTERACTIONS REVIEW

Strategic Considerations

The activity of carnitine suggests significant potential in preventing and treating many conditions, particularly in supporting healthy cardiovascular function. Combination therapy with a statin drug can be particularly effective in reducing lipoprotein(a) levels, especially in patients with type 2 diabetes. However, several common medications and drug classes can increase carnitine excretion or interfere with its activity. Continued development of carnitine therapy in treatment of ischemic disease is probable given its potential to limit anoxic damage while simultaneously reducing peripheral arterial resistance.[11] Furthermore, it may inhibit platelet-activating factor (PAF), thus potentially contributing an antithrombotic effect. Arterial insufficiency can decrease carnitine content of heart muscle cells. Carnitine is used conventionally in critical care and cancer surgery and has been found to benefit elderly and other high-risk patients undergoing elective cardiac surgery.[12]

In regard to neurological conditions and carnitine, emerging evidence supports further research into its value in treating individuals with Alzheimer's disease.[13] Anticonvulsant medications tend to increase carnitine excretion, thus suggesting a potential role for coadministration in seizure disorders. Its immune-enhancing activity and potential efficacy during infections is countered by the adverse effects exerted on it by some chemotherapeutic agents and antiviral drugs, especially antiretroviral nucleoside analogs. Carnitine inhibits entry of thyroid hormone into certain cells and can be used to prevent adverse effects of thyroid therapy for goiter.[9,10]

NUTRIENT-DRUG INTERACTIONS

Allopurinol

Allopurinol (Oxypurinol; Aloprim, Apo-Allopurinol, Lopurin, Purinol, Zyloprim).

Interaction Type and Significance

⊕⊕   **Beneficial or Supportive Interaction, with Professional Management**

Drug Benefit Probability:	Evidence Base:
2. Probable to	● Consensus
1. Certain	

Nutrient-Drug Interactions and Drug-Induced Nutrient Depletions

Nutrient Coadministration

Probability:	Evidence Base:
4. Plausible	☐ Inadequate

Effect and Mechanism of Action

Carnitine is essential for intramitochondrial metabolism of long-chain fatty acids. Researchers have proposed that Duchenne muscular dystrophy (DMD) involves alterations leading to blockage of the inosine monophosphate (IMP) to adenylsuccinate purine pathway. Allopurinol inhibits xanthine oxidase (thus favoring restoration of IMP synthesis) and slows degradation of purines through its effects on adenosine deaminase and purine nucleotide phosphorylase, two key enzymes.[14] These effects favor restoration of energy charge and thus of membrane integrity, thereby reducing transmembrane losses of essential metabolites. Coadministration of L-carnitine could theoretically benefit individuals with DMD and enhance therapeutic effects of allopurinol.

Research

Individuals with DMD exhibit severely depressed muscle carnitine levels, i.e., approximately 16.5 times lower than in normal subjects.[15] Such patients also exhibit severely depressed levels of all adenine and guanine nucleotides and some of their metabolites, and ATP levels are approximately 40 times lower than in normal subjects.[16] Carnitine deficiency in the muscle of DMD patients may be related to this observed ATP deficiency because muscle cells take up carnitine from the serum by a process of active transport.[17,18]

In the first of several studies, Castro-Gago et al.[14] found that the activity levels of adenosine deaminase and purine nucleotide phosphorylase were more than double in the serum of untreated DMD patients than in normal patients, thus leading to increased rates of purine catabolism. They reported that allopurinol treatment reduces activities to normal or below-normal levels.

Camina et al.[16] determined levels of purines, purine metabolites, related enzymes, and carnitine in muscle of eight untreated DMD patients, 12 allopurinol-treated DMD patients, and 12 age-matched controls. Together with several other beneficial changes to IMP and related metabolites, allopurinol restored acylcarnitine to normal levels, resulting in improved muscle strength, and significantly increased free carnitine levels.

Evidence based on clinical trials is lacking thus far to determine whether L-carnitine coadministration might enhance this beneficial effect of allopurinol and at what dosage level, if any, an adverse additive effect might occur.

Nutritional Therapeutics, Clinical Concerns, and Adaptations

Health care professionals treating individuals with DMD are advised to discuss the effects of the disease process on carnitine status and its implications for their health. Administration of allopurinol may constitute a valuable component of a comprehensive therapeutic strategy in the treatment of such individuals. Clinical evidence is lacking to confirm whether concomitant use of carnitine might improve efficacy of such an approach. However, available research indicates that carnitine is unlikely to produce any adverse effects and suggests that muscle function and strength in such patients would generally benefit from increased carnitine levels, which are known to result from carnitine administration.

Doxorubicin and Related Anthracycline Chemotherapy

Evidence: Doxorubicin (Adriamycin, Rubex).
Extrapolated, based on similar properties: Daunorubicin (Cerubidine), epirubicin (Ellence, Pharmorubicin), idarubicin (Idamycin, Zavedos), mitoxantrone (Novantrone, Onkotrone). Similar properties but evidence lacking for extrapolation: Daunorubicin, liposomal (DaunoXome); doxorubicin, pegylated liposomal (Caelyx, Doxil, Myocet).

Interaction Type and Significance

≈≈   **Drug-Induced Nutrient Depletion, Supplementation Therapeutic, with Professional Management**
☼   **Prevention or Reduction of Drug Adverse Effect**

Nutrient Depletion

Probability:	Evidence Base:
2. Probable to **1. Certain**	● Consensus

Coadministration Benefit

Probability:	Evidence Base:
4. Plausible to **2. Probable**	◉ Emerging to ● Consensus

Effect and Mechanism of Action

Doxorubicin is a highly effective antineoplastic agent, but cardiotoxicity (acute and chronic) is an adverse effect occurring in up to one third of patients treated after a cumulative dose of 300 mg/m^2 and increasing sharply beyond a cumulative dose of 360 mg/m^2. The resultant irreversible and dose-dependent cardiomyopathy limits its clinical usefulness. Research indicates that doxorubicin inhibits fatty acid oxidation in part secondary to inhibition of carnitine palmitoyl transferase 1 (CPT-1) and depletion of L-carnitine, its substrate, in cardiac tissue after acute (in vitro) or chronic (in vivo) administration. L-Carnitine also plays a role in fatty acid oxidation independent of CPT-1 or fatty acid chain length. Acute exposure to doxorubicin can cause a concentration- and time-dependent inhibition of CPT-1-dependent long-chain fatty acid oxidation (i.e., of palmitate). Chronic doxorubicin exposure can inhibit palmitate oxidation as much as 40%. Doxorubicin can also acutely inhibit medium- and short-chain fatty acid oxidation, which is independent of CPT-1.[19]

Cardiotoxicity of anthracycline chemotherapy agents is multifactorial and also involves oxidative stress, in part mediated by an iron-catalyzed Fenton reaction; iron-chelating agents have been shown to decrease doxorubicin cardiac toxicity. Two conditions of cardiotoxicity have been recognized. The first is a dose-independent idiosyncratic phenomenon appearing immediately after anthracycline administration and is based on a pericarditis-myocarditis syndrome in patients without previous cardiac disease. The second condition is dose related and characterized by progressive decline of left ventricular systolic function, as assessed by the ejection fraction on nuclear medicine and echocardiographic studies, which may lead to congestive heart failure (CHF). Diastolic dysfunction may also lead to CHF, with or without concomitant compromise of left ventricular ejection fraction. On pathological examination, progressive anthracycline-related cardiac damage may include restrictive endomyocardial disease, characterized by fibrous thickening of the endomyocardium, and dilated cardiomyopathy, as a result of myocardial fibrosis and hypertrophy of surviving myocytes. Symptoms can appear many years after completion of chemotherapy, although sequential assessment of left ventricular systolic and diastolic function will show compromise long before symptomatic CHF ensues. Risk of anthracycline-induced CHF is increased by radiotherapy fields that involve all or part of the heart.[20-22]

Carnitine is well known for its central roles in fatty acid oxidation, mitochondrial integrity and metabolism, cardiovascular function, and muscle tissue (especially myocardium) metabolism. Its depletion impairs these normal activities, and its presence provides protective effects on these tissues and activities. In particular, acute or chronic administration of L-carnitine may abolish the doxorubicin-induced inhibition of palmitate oxidation and reverse acute inhibition of medium- and short-chain fatty acid oxidation by doxorubicin.[19]

Cardiac toxicity is similar between equipotent doses of doxorubicin and daunorubicin, slightly lower for epirubicin, and only one-sixth that of doxorubicin for equipotent doses of mitoxantrone. Doxil and DaunoXome (liposomal doxorubicin and daunorubicin, respectively) have negligible cardiotoxicity, presumably because of negligible cardiac exposure to the active drug with the pharmacokinetics of the liposome-encapsulated preparation.

Research

A wide range of both in vitro and animal research has demonstrated that L-carnitine can prevent or reduce doxorubicin-related cardiac damage.[23-25] Alberts et al.[26] reported that carnitine significantly decreased doxorubicin-induced cardiotoxicity at both acute high dose and chronic intermittent low dose without decreasing antitumor activity or increasing bone marrow toxicity, based on a mouse model. The findings of an in vitro experiment conducted by Maccari and Ramacci[27] using rat heart tissue indicate that the L-diastereoisomer of carnitine is specific in its reparatory effect against doxorubicin cardiotoxicity, as indicated by heart rate, coronary flow, and contractile force; they noted that the dextrorotatory form (D-carnitine) was totally inactive. These authors ascribed this benefit to the "natural role played by this substance in metabolic processes."

Abdel-aleem et al.[19] investigated the acute and chronic effects of doxorubicin on fatty acid oxidation in isolated cardiac myocytes. Acute exposure to doxorubicin produced a concentration- and time-dependent inhibition of CPT-1-dependent long-chain fatty acid oxidation of palmitate. Chronic doxorubicin exposure (18 mg/kg) inhibited palmitate oxidation 40% and to a similar extent seen in vitro with 0.5 mM doxorubicin. Conversely, acute or chronic administration of L-carnitine completely abolished the doxorubicin-induced inhibition of palmitate oxidation. Furthermore, medium- and short-chain fatty acid oxidation was also inhibited acutely by doxorubicin and could be reversed by L-carnitine, even though they are independent of CPT-1. Doxorubicin also significantly decreased oxidation of the CPT-1-dependent substrate palmitoyl-CoA by 50% in isolated rat heart mitochondria, but only at concentrations greater than 1 mM, which is higher than clinically relevant doxorubicin concentrations.

Similarly, Sayed-Ahmed et al.[28] reported that propionyl-L-carnitine (PLC) reversed cardiotoxic effects in isolated cardiac myocytes and rat mitochondria perfused with doxorubicin (5 mM) without affecting therapeutic effects. For example, daily administration of PLC to doxorubicin-treated rats resulted in complete reversal of drug-induced increase in cardiac enzymes, except lactate dehydrogenase (LDH), which was only reversed by 66%. In cardiac tissue homogenate, doxorubicin caused a significant 53% increase in malonedialdehyde (MDA), a marker of oxidative stress, and a significant 50% decrease in reduced glutathione (GSH), a fundamental intracellular peptide

antioxidant; levels. In contrast, PLC induced a significant 33% decrease in MDA and a significant 41% increase in GSH levels. Daily administration of PLC to doxorubicin-treated rats completely reversed the increase in MDA and the decrease in GSH induced by doxorubicin to normal levels. Overall, PLC therapy completely protected against doxorubicin-induced inhibition of mitochondrial beta-oxidation of long-chain fatty acids. PLC also exerted or induced a significant antioxidant defense mechanism against doxorubicin-induced lipid peroxidation of cardiac membranes. PLC did not interfere with the antitumor activity of doxorubicin while providing these beneficial effects.[28]

Mijares and Lopez[29] determined that acute exposure to doxorubicin impaired intracellular Ca^{++} handling and induced a concentration-dependent elevation of diastolic calcium concentration ($[Ca^{++}]$) in isolated cardiomyocytes loaded with fura-2/AM (acetoxymethyl ester). These adverse effects were not prevented by pretreatment with L-carnitine. However, L-carnitine at 10 μM concentration in the culture medium of the cardiomyocytes fully inhibited the increase in $[Ca^{++}]$ induced by this anthracycline derivative. These results indicate that acute exposure to doxorubicin impairs intracellular Ca^{++} handling and that L-carnitine exerts a cardioprotective effect, in part by preventing the doxorubicin-induced elevation in diastolic Ca^{++} concentration.

The cardiotoxicity of doxorubicin can be of rapid onset and endure for decades, often without cardiac complaints. In a longitudinal assessment of cardiac function in 22 patients treated with anthracycline chemotherapy for osteogenic sarcoma or malignant fibrous histiocytoma, Brouwer et al.[30] found systolic dysfunction in more than a quarter of the patients and diastolic dysfunction in almost half after two decades (median, 22 years). Moreover, cardiac dysfunction was progressive, as measured at 9, 14, and 22 years.[30]

Although limited by their small size and preliminary character, clinical trials have similarly found beneficial effects from coadministration of carnitine with doxorubicin therapy. De Leonardis et al.[31] studied nine patients receiving a cumulative dose (200-490 mg/m²) of doxorubicin using creatine kinase levels to evaluate acute cardiotoxicity and electrocardiography and echocardiography to evaluate myocardial contractility for chronic cardiotoxicity. Based on their findings, they proposed "systematic use of L-carnitine as adjuvant therapy ... during doxorubicin administration" to be cardioprotective. Subsequently, Chavez et al.[32] reported that the cardiotoxic effects of doxorubicin were not observed in children treated with a combination of doxorubicin (cumulative dose, 30-60 mg/kg) and carnitine (1-2 g/day).

Nutritional Therapeutics, Clinical Concerns, and Adaptations

Physicians administering doxorubicin therapy are advised to consider pretreatment and concomitant use of L-carnitine as a safe measure with significant probability of preventing or reducing the cardiotoxic effect of this powerful antineoplastic agent. A typical therapeutic dosage of L-carnitine would be in the range of 1 to 3 g daily, given orally in two divided doses commencing before doxorubicin therapy, continued throughout therapy, and for several years after treatment, especially if the cumulative dose of doxorubicin is greater than 360 mg/m², if the patient has also received thoracic radiation with exposure of all or part of the cardiac volume, or if sequential assessment of left ventricular ejection fraction and/or diastolic function reveal significant decline from pretreatment values. L-Carnitine is not a potent antioxidant, as is coenzyme Q10 (ubiquinone), another nutrient that helps abrogate doxorubicin cardiotoxicity, but which is controversial because at least some of the antineoplastic effect of doxorubicin may be mediated by free-radical production, which can be inhibited by antioxidants. (See Coenzyme Q10 monograph.) The body of evidence indicates that L-carnitine is essentially nontoxic and unlikely to interfere with the efficacy of chemotherapeutic treatment.

Acute cardiotoxicity can be evaluated by creatine kinase, particularly the cardiac-specific MB isoenzyme. Chronic cardiotoxicity can be monitored using electrocardiography and the left ventricular performance by computed M-mode echocardiography measuring the ejection fraction and by MUGA scan (nuclear medicine technique for measuring cardiac ejection fraction), both of which are reliable and highly sensitive, noninvasive parameters for evaluating myocardial contractility.

Anecdotal clinical experience has indicated that therapeutic benefit in existing doxorubicin-induced cardiomyopathy with clinical CHF can be obtained by therapeutic use of L-carnitine, coenzyme Q10, taurine, magnesium, fish oil, and hawthorn (Crataegus) leaf/flower and berry extracts, at least in some cases. Conventional pharmacological management includes angiotensin-converting enzyme (ACE) inhibitors, diuretics, and sometimes digoxin. Integrative management with these nutrients, botanicals, and pharmaceuticals may be of greatest clinical benefit when applied by individuals experienced both in nutritional and conventional medicine. Randomized controlled clinical trials in this area would be of great interest.

Isotretinoin and Related Retinoids

Evidence: Isotretinoin (13-cis retinoic acid; Accutane).
Extrapolated, based on similar properties: Acitretin (Soriatane), bexarotene (Targretin), etretinate (Tegison), tretinoin (All-Trans-Retinoic Acid, ATRA, Atragen, Avita, Renova, Retin-A, Vesanoid, Vitinoin).

Interaction Type and Significance

☼   **Prevention or Reduction of Drug Adverse Effect**

Probability:	Evidence Base:
4. Plausible to	○ Preliminary to
2. Probable	◉ **Emerging**

Effect and Mechanism of Action

The specific mechanism of action underlying the protective effect of carnitine in relation to retinoids is unknown. The hepatotoxic action of isotretinoin can cause abnormalities in liver function, as well as elevations in serum cholesterol and muscle pain and weakness.[33,34] The resultant symptoms are similar to the main characteristics of carnitine deficiency (e.g., myalgia, weakness, hypotension). The growing body of scientific knowledge about the role of carnitine in hepatic detoxification functions should lead to a better understanding of the interaction between carnitine and retinoids.

Carnitine is well known for its central role in fatty acid oxidation in mitochondria and L-carnitine, in particular, serving as the substrate of CPT-1. Two major isoforms of acetyl-CoA carboxylase (ACC) are present in mammals. The 275-kDa beta form (ACC-β) is predominantly in heart and skeletal muscle, whereas the 265-kDa alpha form (ACC-α) is the major isoform in lipogenic tissues such as liver and adipose tissue. ACC-β plays a major role in controlling fatty acid oxidation by means of the ability of malonyl-CoA to inhibit CPT-1, a rate-limiting enzyme of fatty acid oxidation in mitochondria.[35]

Research

Georgala et al.[36] investigated the use of L-carnitine to reduce the adverse effects of isotretinoin, specifically myalgia; 230 patients with cystic acne were treated with isotretinoin (0.5 mg/kg/24 hours). They divided the patients who reported muscular symptoms into two groups; 20 subjects received L-carnitine (100 mg/kg/24 hours orally), and another 20 received placebo. Among these patients, they noted that carnitine blood levels (both total and free, acylcarnitine) were "remarkably decreased at the onset of their muscular symptoms," along with "the well known increases of their liver enzymes and lipids." Furthermore, among those patients receiving isotretinoin but not reporting myalgia, they found that laboratory tests showed elevated liver enzymes and lipids along with a decrease in blood carnitine levels and a "remarkable increase" of urinary carnitine excretion. Subjects receiving concomitant L-carnitine, without isotretinoin discontinuation or reduction, reported the disappearance of their muscular symptoms within 5 to 6 days and exhibited normalization in liver enzymes and carnitine levels at the 45th day of their combined therapy. In contrast, the patients who received placebo along with the isotretinoin continued to report myalgias.

Nutritional Therapeutics, Clinical Concerns, and Adaptations

Physicians prescribing retinoids are advised to monitor liver enzymes, blood lipids, and carnitine levels and to request that patients report any adverse symptoms characteristic of retinoid toxicity. Prophylactic coadministration of L-carnitine provides a safe protective measure with a reasonable probability of efficacy. A typical therapeutic dosage of L-carnitine would be 1 to 2 g daily, given orally in two divided doses.

Levothyroxine and Related Thyroid Hormones

L-Triiodothyronine (T_3): Cytomel, liothyronine sodium, liothyronine sodium (synthetic T_3), Triostat (injection).
Levothyroxine (T_4): Eltroxin, Levo-T, Levothroid, levothyroxine (synthetic), levoxin, Levoxyl, Synthroid, thyroxine, Unithroid.
L-Thyroxine and L-triiodothyronine ($T_4 + T_3$): animal levothyroxine/liothyronine, Armour Thyroid, desiccated thyroid, Westhroid.
L-Thyroxine and L-triiodothyronine (synthetic $T_4 + T_3$): Euthroid, Euthyral, liotrix, Thyar, Thyrolar.
Dextrothyroxine (Choloxin).

Interaction Type and Significance

✗✗   **Minimal to Mild Adverse Interaction—Vigilance Necessary**
⊕✗   **Bimodal or Variable Interaction, with Professional Management**
☼   **Prevention or Reduction of Drug Adverse Effect**

Probability:	Evidence Base:
4. Plausible to	◉ **Emerging** to
2. Probable	● **Consensus**

Effect and Mechanism of Action

Carnitine may partially block activity of thyroid hormone, at least in part by inhibiting thyroid hormone entry into the nucleus of hepatocytes, neurons, and fibroblasts.[9] Cellular levels of L-carnitine decrease in several diseases, including hyperthyroidism.[37]

Thyroid hormone controls carnitine status through modifications of gamma-butyrobetaine hydroxylase activity and gene expression. In particular, thyroid hormones interact with lipid metabolism by increasing long-chain fatty acid oxidation through activation of carnitine-dependent fatty acid import into mitochondria. Thyroid hormones also increase carnitine bioavailability.[38]

Research

Based on animal experiments and unblinded studies in a few hyperthyroid patients from about 45 years ago, carnitine has been considered a peripheral antagonist of thyroid hormone action, at least in some tissues. More recent research has clarified and expanded scientific knowledge of the physiological properties underlying this interaction. Salvatore Benvenga, MD, and fellow researchers at the University of Messina, School of Medicine, Italy, have conducted extensive research into various aspects of the interaction between carnitine and thyroid hormone.

Data from in vitro experiments by Benvenga et al.[9] using three thyroid hormone–responsive cell lines demonstrate that carnitine acts as a peripheral antagonist of thyroid hormone (TH) action, with a site of inhibition at or before the nuclear envelope. These researchers noted: "We are aware of no inhibitor of TH uptake that has such a markedly different effect on the nuclear versus whole-cell uptake."

In an early uncontrolled study, DeFelice and Gilgore[39] observed clinical amelioration of thyrotoxicosis based on the antagonistic effect of carnitine in hyperthyroidism. In a randomized, double blind, placebo-controlled clinical trial involving 50 women being treated for benign goiter under a fixed, thyroid-stimulating hormone (TSH)–suppressive dose of L-T_4 for 6 months, Benvenga et al.[10] demonstrated that 2 or 4 g/day oral L-carnitine both reversed and prevented symptoms of hyperthyroidism and exerted a beneficial effect on bone mineralization. They also proposed its use in the treatment of thyroid storm. Thus, they concluded that "hyperthyroidism depletes the body deposits of carnitine and since carnitine has no toxicity, teratogenicity, contraindications and interactions with drugs, carnitine can be of clinical use."

Report

Benvenga et al.[40] published a report describing the case of a hyperthyroid patient taking low doses of a conventional antithyroid drug, methimazole (10-15 mg/day), and L-carnitine (2 g/day in two doses) who survived three successive storms, which were associated with potentially life-threatening precipitating factors (post–influenza myocarditis and thrombophlebitis). They remarked that "although L-carnitine does not prevent relapses of thyrotoxicosis, its use should be considered in thyrotoxic patients when intervening factors may precipitate a thyroid storm."

Nutritional Therapeutics, Clinical Concerns, and Adaptations

Physicians treating patients with hyperthyroidism, endogenous or iatrogenic, are advised to consider administering oral L-carnitine with dosage in the range of 1 to 2 g twice daily. Such administration can reverse carnitine depletion associated with hyperthyroid states and support cardiovascular health, which is often compromised in such cases. Confirmatory clinical trials are lacking, but prudence suggests caution in administration of carnitine to individuals with low or borderline thyroid status. Physicians prescribing thyroid hormone are advised to query patients as to supplement use and counsel avoidance of concomitant carnitine. Regular monitoring is appropriate when both agents are clinically indicated.

Nitroglycerin and Related Nitrates

Nitroglycerin (glyceryl trinitrate, GTN; Deponit, Minitran, Nitrek, Nitro-Bid, Nitro-Dur, Nitro-Time, Nitrodisc, Nitrogard, Nitroglyn, Nitrolingual, Nitrol, Nitrostat, Transderm-Nitro, Tridil).

Extrapolated, based on similar properties: Isosorbide dinitrate (ISDN, Isordil, Sorbitrate); combination drug: hydralazine and isosorbide dinitrate (BiDil); isosorbide mononitrate (Imdur, ISMN, ISMO, Isotrate, Monoket).

Interaction Type and Significance

⊕⊕　**Beneficial or Supportive Interaction, with Professional Management**

⊕✗　**Bimodal or Variable Interaction, with Professional Management**

✗　　**Potential or Theoretical Adverse Interaction of Uncertain Severity**

Probability:	Evidence Base:
4. Plausible or	○ **Preliminary** to
2. Probable	◉ **Emerging**

Effect and Mechanism of Action

An additive pharmacological effect, as well as a broader supportive synergy, appears to be involved in the combined use of L-carnitine and glyceryl trinitrate (nitroglycerin), although specific research is lacking as to the mechanism(s) of action. DeFelice and Kohl[41] have proposed that is one of several possible mechanisms for L-carnitine's benefit in cardiac ischemia and infarction. Nitroglycerin vasodilates, reduces cardiac afterload (i.e., work), and thus increases oxygen availability to ischemic myocardium. Increasing carnitine availability may prevent a limited availability of fatty acids and ketoacids for beta-oxidation and ATP production within cardiac myocytes, which depend exclusively on this fuel source. If nitroglycerin restores oxygen, and carnitine restores fuel, the metabolic processes will function more effectively.

Research

Several clinical trials have demonstrated that carnitine administration contributes to reduced angina symptoms and related cardiac events and decreased usage of antianginal medications, particularly glyceryl trinitrate. Garzya and Amico[42] reported that oral L-carnitine, 2 g/day, was associated with reduced anginal attacks and decreased glyceryl trinitrate consumption. In experiments with models of myocardial infarction, Tishkin et al.[43] "established that carnitine chloride reduced the size of an ischemic zone, prevented oxidative metabolism, lowered ATP and creatine phosphate levels, inhibited lactate and free fatty acid accumulation in the ischemic myocardium." They also found that concomitant administration of carnitine chloride "with nitrong and isoptin increased the anti-ischemic potency of the former."

In a 1983 review of natural physiological agents in the management of acute myocardial infarction, McCarty[44] proposed that carnitine infusion could improve the bioenergetics of ischemic myocardium by relieving inhibition of mitochondrial adenine nucleotide.

Cacciatore et al.[45] conducted a randomized controlled trial involving 200 patients, 40 to 65 years of age, with exercise-induced stable angina that investigated the therapeutic effect of L-carnitine (2 g/day) in conjunction with their already-instituted therapy over a 6-month period. Compared with the control group, the patients receiving carnitine demonstrated a significant reduction in the number of premature ventricular contractions at rest, as well as an increased tolerance during ergometric cycle exercise, as demonstrated by an increased maximal cardiac frequency, increased maximal systolic arterial blood pressure, and therefore also increased double cardiac product and reduced ST-segment depression during maximal effort. These changes were accompanied by a reduction in the consumption of cardioactive drugs and improvement in cardiac function and resultant performance, as shown by an increase in the number of patients belonging to class I of the New York Heart Association (NYHA) classification. Furthermore, plasma lipid levels showed improvement laboratory analysis. These researchers concluded that "L-carnitine undoubtedly represents an interesting therapeutic drug for patients with exercise-induced stable angina."

In isometric contraction experiments using rabbit thoracic aorta and cultured bovine aortic endothelial cells (BAEC), Inoue et al.[46] investigated the effect of palmitoyl-L-carnitine (PLC) on endothelium dependent relaxation. They observed that PLC (1-20 μM) inhibited endothelium-dependent relaxation induced by acetylcholine and substance P in a dose-dependent manner, while having no effect on resting tension and glyceryl trinitrate–induced relaxations. Furthermore, although bradykinin, another endothelium-dependent relaxant, induced a biphasic Ca^{++} transient in BAEC, pretreatment of these cells with PLC (5-10 μM) inhibited bradykinin-induced Ca^{++} transients. The authors concluded that the inhibitory effect of PLC on endothelium-dependent relaxation results from the suppression of the intracellular calcium signal transduction in endothelial cells and speculated that PLC "may be an important mediator of the impaired vascular endothelial function in myocardial ischaemia."

Nutritional Therapeutics, Clinical Concerns, and Adaptations

Physicians treating patients with angina are advised to consider administering oral L-carnitine, 1 to 2 g twice daily, in concert with nitroglycerin or related intervention. Although further research through well-designed clinical trials is warranted, the available evidence indicates that the established benefits of carnitine administration on cardiac health, particularly myocardial mitochondrial function, may combine effectively with conventional therapies such as nitroglycerin. Physicians treating patients with angina or related cardiovascular conditions are advised to discuss the potential benefits of carnitine administration and the possible advantages of combining it with their conventional therapies. Nevertheless, even though carnitine is generally considered as essentially nontoxic, regular monitoring is appropriate given the slight (and unproven) risk of an excessive additive response contributing to destabilization.

Coordination of care between health care professionals trained and experienced in both conventional pharmacology and nutritional therapies may provide for the most safe and effective approach to integrative therapeutics. Concomitant use of coenzyme Q10, taurine, magnesium, fish oil, and hawthorn (Crataegus) leaf/flower and berry extracts may also be appropriate in some cases.

Pivalate Prodrugs

Cefcapene pivoxil, cefditoren pivoxil (Spectracef), cefetamet pivoxil, pivampicillin (Pondocillin), pivmecillinam (Selexid). Extrapolated, based on similar properties:

Adefovir dipivoxil (experimental anti-viral drug, with activity against hepatitis B and other viruses).
Pivanex (pivalate prodrug of butyrate, experimental cancer drug).

Interaction Type and Significance

≈≈ **Drug-Induced Nutrient Depletion, Supplementation Therapeutic, with Professional Management**

Nutrient Depletion
Probability:
4. Plausible or
    2. Probable

Evidence Base:
▽ **Mixed** to
◉ **Emerging**

Coadministration Benefit
Probability:
4. Plausible to
    2. Probable

Evidence Base:
▽ **Mixed** to
◉ **Emerging**

Effect and Mechanism of Action

Pivalate (trimethylacetic acid) is used to generate prodrugs to increase oral bioavailability. After oral administration, all pivalate prodrugs are broken down in the GI tract during absorption and hydrolyzed to pivalic acid and the active agent by nonspecific esterases present in most body tissues. The resultant pivaloyl moiety causes carnitine depletion through the increased urinary excretion of carnitine as pivaloylcarnitine.

After hydrolysis of the prodrug, pivalate (as with other carboxylic acids) can be activated inside cells for further metabolism by acyl-CoA synthases to form pivaloyl-CoA. However, unlike other coenzyme A thioesters, pivaloyl-CoA cannot be oxidized to carbon dioxide in human cells. Consequently, pivaloyl-CoA accumulates in cells and acts as a substrate for a variety of acyl-CoA transferases. The kidneys are primarily responsible for excreting the pivaloyl conjugates that are generated by reactions. Subsequently, the dominant route of pivalate elimination is through formation and urinary excretion of pivaloylcarnitine. This increased carnitine excretion introduces potentially significant risk of perturbing normal cellular function because of the important roles of carnitine in cellular homeostasis.[47]

Research

The increased carnitine excretion caused by pivalate prodrugs is generally accepted as axiomatic. Carnitine deficiency or inborn errors of metabolism resulting in significant carnitine deficiency are among the standard contraindications for pivalate prodrugs. It is generally agreed that long-term treatment or frequently repeated treatment courses using pivalate prodrugs should be used with caution because of increased excretion of carnitine in urine and a reduction of serum carnitine. Nevertheless, the clinical significance of this interaction, the characteristics of patients at increased risk for depletion and adverse sequelae, and the conditions and factors influencing such effects remain unresolved and occasionally controversial.

The limited duration of therapy using most drugs made with pivalic acid and the availability of carnitine from endogenous synthesis and dietary sources reduce the probability of clinically significant carnitine depletion in most cases. Tissue total carnitine content will only be impacted as the urinary losses are sustained over time, and several months of continued pivalate exposure will usually be necessary to impact the liver carnitine pool significantly and lead to depletion of the large muscle carnitine stores. However, Holme et al.[48] note that patients with carnitine deficiency can have serious, even fatal, clinical manifestations and caution that the "risk of adverse effects from prodrugs that give rise to pivalic acid should be seriously considered, particularly in patients under metabolic stress."

For example, treatment with pivalic acid–liberating antibiotics (e.g., pivampicillin) for 22 and 30 months in children resulted in total muscle carnitine depletion to 10% of reference values. However, no adverse clinical effects were observed or reported, which could be associated with primary or secondary carnitine deficiency. Serum carnitine was significantly reduced after pivampicillin treatment at the highest recommended doses for 7 to 10 days, but levels returned to the normal range within 2 weeks after discontinuing the medication. Despite these reductions in serum carnitine, total body stores of carnitine were reduced by approximately 10%. Thus, the increased excretion of carnitine associated with the use of pivampicillin and other pivalate prodrugs is considered to be without clinical significance in short-term treatment. The frequency with which adverse effects that could be related to carnitine deficiency occur is similar to that of other antibiotics not liberating pivalic acid.[47]

A study conducted by Diep et al.[49] found that replenishment of carnitine levels using normal dietary sources was slow after long-term treatment with pivalate antibiotics. Long-term treatment with pivampicillin and pivmecillinam for 6 to 24 months in five adults and one child reduced the total serum carnitine concentrations to 3.7 to 14.0 μmol/L (reference value: 25-66 μmol/L). In two cases, muscle carnitine was reduced to 0.3 to 0.7 μmol/g wet weight (reference value: 3-5 μmol/g). All patients reported asthenia and muscle symptoms with weakness and pain. One patient developed signs of carnitine depletion in the liver. Serum carnitine levels recovered slowly after cessation of therapy and reached normal concentrations after 6 to 12 months on a normal diet without carnitine supplement. All symptoms caused by carnitine depletion disappeared after the serum carnitine reached 20 μmol/L.

The effects of pivalic acid on carnitine can adversely impact mitochondrial function and metabolic processes in muscles, lungs, and other tissues. In a preliminary study, researchers observed that carnitine administration was associated with preferential elimination of pivalate through formation of pivaloylcarnitine.[50] Subsequently, in a study involving 10 children, Melegh et al.[51] coadministered carnitine (1 g/day) during the latter 4 days of an 8-day course of pivampicillin. Pivampicillin treatment was associated with formation and urinary excretion of pivaloylcarnitine, and administration of carnitine aided the elimination of pivalate as its carnitine ester. These researchers observed that pivampicillin treatment resulted in inhibited oxidation of fats as metabolic fuel and increased utilization of carbohydrates, but that carnitine partially reversed this drug effect by promoting the elimination of the pivaloyl moiety from the body.

Abrahamsson et al.[52] administered pivaloyl-conjugated antibiotics to healthy subjects for 54 days to study the effect of carnitine depletion on physical working capacity. The mean carnitine concentration in serum decreased from 35.0 to 3.5 μmol/L, and in muscle from 10 to 4.3 μmol/g noncollagen protein (NCP). The concentration of 3-hydroxybutyrate in serum slightly increased at submaximal exercise in tests performed before and after 54 days' administration of the drug, an effect attributed to decreased fatty acid oxidation in the liver. Consumption of muscle glycogen

also decreased, suggesting decreased glycolysis in the skeletal muscle. However, the concentration of ATP and creatine phosphate did not significantly decrease during exercise, indicating that adequate energy was available for muscle function. Carnitine depletion appeared to affect cardiac function given observed reductions in the work at maximal oxygen uptake and maximal heart rate. Cardiac muscle is an obligate user of fatty acid beta-oxidation as its fuel source (which requires carnitine for transport), as opposed to skeletal muscle, which stores glycogen for anaerobic glycolysis as its initial fuel source.

Nutritional Therapeutics, Clinical Concerns, and Adaptations

In most cases, physicians prescribing pivalate prodrugs for short-term use can safely assume that these medications will not cause clinically significant carnitine depletion. Conventional practice does not recommend either measurement of serum carnitine or concomitant administration of prophylactic carnitine as a general measure for patients prescribed pivalic acid–liberating prodrugs for short-term (acute) use. Almost 1 billion treatment days experience with pivalate prodrugs was accumulated worldwide between 1996 and 2001. Despite such widespread usage, published reports of clinical toxicity have been limited to patients with long-duration treatment.

Coadministration of L-carnitine may be appropriate during treatment with these medications in patients demonstrating or at risk for carnitine deficiency or diagnosed with cardiovascular disease, seizure disorder, or HIV infection. Such protective use is generally considered safe and unlikely to interfere with drug efficacy. If used, administration of at least fourfold molar excess of carnitine (vs. pivalate) is advisable,[53] which in most cases would be adequately provided by 1.5 to 2 g twice daily. Notably, pivalate prodrugs intended for chronic use, such as the antiretroviral adefovir dipivoxil, incorporate carnitine as part of the dosing regimen.[54]

Several important cautions and contraindications arise from the possible adverse effects of these medications on carnitine status. Pivalate prodrugs should be avoided in patients with known or suspected carnitine deficiency. Prudence suggests that use of pivalate prodrugs be avoided in children less than 3 months of age because endogenous carnitine production may not yet be fully developed during the first months of life. Concurrent treatment with valproic acid is also contraindicated, especially in children. In Sweden, pivampicillin is also contraindicated in patients with very small muscle mass. Selection of alter-native pharmacological agents may also be judicious in some cases.

Simvastatin and Related HMG-COA Reductase Inhibitors (Statins)

Evidence: Simvastatin (Zocor).
Atorvastatin (Lipitor), fluvastatin (Lescol, Lescol XL), lovastatin (Altocor, Altoprev, Mevacor); combination drug: lovastatin and niacin (Advicor); pravastatin (Pravachol), rosuvastatin (Crestor); simvastatin combination drug: simvastatin and extended-release nicotinic acid (Niaspan).

Interaction Type and Significance

⊕⊕   **Beneficial or Supportive Interaction, with Professional Management**
☼   **Prevention or Reduction of Drug Adverse Effect**

Probability:
3. Possible or
  2. Probable

Evidence Base:
◉ **Emerging**

Effect and Mechanism of Action

Interventions to reduce lipoprotein(a) [Lp(a)] concentration are important given its atherogenic/prothrombotic properties and associations with both coronary artery and cerebrovascular disease. Statin therapy, as well as fibrates and resins, are generally considered incapable of reducing Lp(a) levels and may in many cases contribute to an increase in Lp(a) levels, even while lowering total cholesterol and low-density lipoprotein (LDL) cholesterol levels. Among conventional pharmaceutical interventions, only nicotinic acid (2-4 g/day) is known to reduce Lp(a). However, L-carnitine can lower plasma Lp(a) levels.

Research

A series of clinical trials conducted by Italian researchers have demonstrated the efficacy of L-carnitine in lowering Lp(a) and a synergistic interaction between L-carnitine and statin therapy in lipid-lowering strategies, especially in individuals with type 2 diabetes. In a double-blind, placebo controlled study, Sirtori et al.[55] found that L-carnitine (2 g/day) significantly reduced Lp(a) levels in subjects with hyper-Lp(a) (i.e., serum Lp(a) levels of 40-80 mg/dL). Two years later, in a study involving patients with type 2 diabetes and hyperlipidemia, Brescia et al.[56] reported that combined therapy with simvastatin (20 mg/day) and L-carnitine (2 g/day) demonstrated greater lipid-lowering efficacy than simvastatin alone, particularly in lowering triglyceride levels. Subsequently, in a trial involving 94 subjects newly diagnosed with type 2 diabetes mellitus being managed through dietary restriction alone, Derosa et al.[57] observed significantly lower plasma Lp(a) levels, compared with placebo, after 3 and 6 months of L-carnitine (2 g/day). Based on these findings, Solfrizzi et al.[58] conducted an open, randomized, parallel-group study involving 52 patients with type 2 diabetes mellitus, triglyceride serum levels less than 400 mg/dL (<4.5 mmol/L), and Lp(a) serum levels greater than 20 mg/dL (>0.71 mmol/L). Subjects were randomized into two groups of equal size and administered either simvastatin alone (20 mg/day) or simvastatin plus L-carnitine (2 g/day) orally for 60 days. The investigators reported that "Lp(a) serum levels increase[d] from baseline to 60 days in the simvastatin group alone versus a significant decrease in the combination group." No differences between the two groups were observed regarding LDL cholesterol, non-HDL cholesterol, and apoB serum levels. The consistent pattern of evidence from these trials indicates that the combination of L-carnitine with statin therapy can enhance therapeutic management of hyperlipidemia, particularly in individuals with type 2 diabetes.

Nutritional Therapeutics, Clinical Concerns, and Adaptations

Physicians treating individuals with hyperlipidemia characterized by elevated Lp(a), particularly the context of type 2 diabetes, are advised to consider a comprehensive approach founded on regular exercise and a healthy diet and combining L-carnitine, as well as fish oil, chromium, and niacin (as inositol hexaniacinate), with conventional lipid management interventions such as statin therapy. As previously noted, L-carnitine is unlikely to produce any adverse effects on the therapeutic action of a statin drug and may in fact mitigate potential adverse effects on Lp(a) status. Enthusiastic support for improved diet, invigorating exercise, and other healthy lifestyle changes are fundamental to an effective integrative strategy for optimizing healthy function, reversing patterns of dyslipidemia and dysglycemia, and reducing risk of cardiovascular disease.

Valproic Acid and Related Anticonvulsant Medications

Evidence: Divalproex semisodium, divalproex sodium (Depakote), sodium valproate (Depacon), valproate semisodium, valproic acid (Depakene, Depakene Syrup).
Extrapolated, based on similar properties: Carbamazepine (Carbatrol, Tegretol), clonazepam (Klonopin), clorazepate (Tranxene), diazepam (Valium), ethosuximide (Zarontin), ethotoin (Peganone), felbamate (Felbatol), fosphenytoin (Cerebyx, Mesantoin), gabapentin (Neurontin), levetiracetam (Keppra), mephenytoin, mephobarbital (Mebaral), methsuximide (Celontin), oxcarbazepine (GP 47680, oxycarbazepine; Trileptal), phenobarbital (phenobarbitone; Luminal, Solfoton), phensuximide (Milontin), phenytoin (diphenylhydantoin; Dilantin, Phenytek), piracetam (Nootropyl), primidone (Mysoline), tiagabine (Gabitril), topiramate (Topamax), trimethadione (Tridione), vigabatrin (Sabril), zonisamide (Zonegran).

Interaction Type and Significance

≈≈   **Drug-Induced Nutrient Depletion, Supplementation Therapeutic, with Professional Management**

☼   **Prevention or Reduction of Drug Adverse Effect**

⊕   **Potential or Theoretical Beneficial or Supportive Interaction, with Professional Management**

Nutrient Depletion
Probability: Evidence Base:
2. Probable to   ▽ **Mixed** to
   1. Certain   ● **Consensus**

Coadministration Benefit
Probability: Evidence Base:
4. Plausible to   ▽ **Mixed** to
   2. Probable   ◉ **Emerging**

Effect and Mechanism of Action

Significant but incomplete evidence indicates that valproic acid (VPA) depresses renal absorption of both free carnitine and acylcarnitine. Other anticonvulsants appear to depress renal absorption of acylcarnitine only. Carnitine depletion may play a central role in the hepatotoxicity of VPA as well as the interference with fatty acid oxidation widely recognized as an adverse effect of VPA. Antiepileptic drugs (AEDs) may also affect carnitine and its functions by other mechanisms.

Research into the pharmacokinetics of VPA's adverse impact on free-carnitine levels suggest accelerated hepatic degradation of VPA as a result of enzyme induction with VPA metabolism.[59] VPA is extensively metabolized by the liver through glucuronic conjugation and oxidative pathways (P450) to produce biologically active metabolites. Half-life can range from 5 to 24 hours because of first-order kinetics. The three major metabolites of VPA are 2-EN-VPA, 4-EN-VPA, and propionic acid derivatives. The 4-EN-VPA may mediate reversible hepatotoxicity, which causes elevation of aminotransferases. Propionic acid derivatives may precipitate hyperammonemia by three different mechanisms, one of which is by interacting with carnitine, acting as a mitochondrial cofactor in the transport and metabolism of long-chain fatty acids.[60]

In treatment of acute VPA toxicity, including coma, L-carnitine's mechanism of action is hypothesized to derive from its ability to decrease elevated ammonia levels. Carnitine coadministration may counterbalance adverse drug effects of extended AED therapy, but such benefit may vary depending on the agent(s) being used, dosing and duration of therapy, patient age and health status, initial carnitine balance, and other factors.

Research

The body of evidence investigating interactions between anticonvulsant medications and carnitine is strong and largely consistent in its findings, but conclusive assessment of clinical implications is difficult because of significant limitations in the research. Carnitine depletion characterizes most of the medications in this drug class, or at least many of the patients. However, many studies failed to assess carnitine status before initiation of anticonvulsant therapy. Broader evidence suggests that individuals prescribed these medications may already be at higher risk for preexisting compromised carnitine status.[1,61]

Valproic acid causes carnitine deficiency, notably in infants and children with epilepsy. Prolonged treatment with VPA, more than other anticonvulsants, enhances renal losses of carnitine esters, lowers serum carnitine levels, and results in secondary carnitine deficiency. In most cases these decreased carnitine levels have no obvious pathological significance, and most children manifest no symptoms of carnitine deficiency. However, anticonvulsant-induced depletion may occasionally cause symptoms of carnitine deficiency such as severe cardiac dysfunction. Typical adverse effects reported in patients treated with VPA include anemia, fatigue, hyperammonemia, hypotonia, lethargy, unexplained stupor, and carnitine-responsive cardiomyopathy. Recurrent episodes of a Reye's-like syndrome with low concentrations of carnitine in liver and muscle, reduced plasma glucose levels, and ketone bodies are among the most serious consequences of carnitine depletion.[62] Coulter[63] hypothesized in a 1984 letter that carnitine depletion plays a central role in VPA's hepatotoxicity. Dreifuss and Langer[62] proposed that the risk of AED-related liver damage increases in children under 24 months of age. Melegh and Trombitas[64] described lipid globule accumulation with ultrastructural abnormalities of mitochondria in the skeletal muscle of seven children treated with VPA. They attributed these lipid deposits to inhibited mitochondrial fatty acid oxidation, a carnitine-dependent process.

Several preliminary studies and controlled trials have demonstrated dramatic reductions in serum carnitine levels and related adverse effects associated with anticonvulsant medications, especially among pediatric patients receiving multidrug therapy. Morita et al.[65] measured decreases in the serum concentrations of total and free carnitine in patients who had received multiple doses of AEDs, especially those receiving sodium valproate, but also those receiving other medications. Nevertheless, no abnormal losses of carnitine in urine were observed. Several factors that may be relevant to the hypocarnitinemia were surveyed statistically. Further analysis revealed that in all the patients, levels of total carnitine and free carnitine were inversely correlated with the dosages of sodium valproate, and that dosage of sodium valproate was the most critical negative contributor to carnitine status. Furthermore, these researchers found that poor muscle volume and coadministration of phenytoin with sodium valproate enhanced hypocarnitinemia. Rodriguez-Segade et al.[66] conducted a study with 183 adult outpatients and 49 controls in which 77% of subjects taking VPA demonstrated a deficiency of free carnitine (i.e., >2 SD below the mean). In contrast, such deficiency was observed in 27% of subjects receiving combined phenytoin-phenobarbital therapy, 23% taking carbamazepine, and 16% receiving phenytoin monotherapy.

In a clinical trial involving 37 children, Zelnick et al.[67] assessed blood carnitine levels before and after therapy using several different anticonvulsant medications. They found that carnitine levels decreased significantly from baseline values only in children receiving VPA; total blood carnitine dropped from 45.3 µM before treatment to 34.9 µM after treatment among those subjects. In contrast, total blood carnitine dropped from 45.7 µM pretreatment to 43.4 µM posttreatment among subjects administered carbamazepine and from 44.9 µM pretreatment to 42.1 µM posttreatment among subjects in the phenobarbital group.[68] Castro-Gago et al.[68] measured serum carnitine levels in 32 epileptic children before and during treatment with VPA, carbamazepine, and phenobarbital. They found that both free-carnitine and total-carnitine levels declined significantly with respect to pretreatment levels in all three treated groups. Levels dropped most markedly and consistently in the VPA-treated group, 35% of whom exhibited carnitine deficiency (i.e., total carnitine <30 µmol/L) by the twelfth month of treatment. In none of the three groups were serum carnitine levels significantly correlated with the serum concentration of the anticonvulsant drug. Based on these findings, the authors recommended that physicians prescribing any of these drugs to children monitor their serum carnitine levels.

In contrast, Hug et al.[69] studied 471 children of various ages on eight variations of AED monotherapy and polytherapy (with 32 healthy controls, age 1 to 16 years). They found that phenobarbital monotherapy more significantly reduced carnitine levels than VPA monotherapy. "Only for phenobarbital was there an inverse correlation between the serum concentration of the drug and that of carnitine concentration." Total carnitine and free carnitine were deficient in the following percentages of patients receiving AED monotherapy: phenobarbital (36% total; 21% free), VPA (23% total; 9% free), phenytoin (12% total; 8% free), and carbamazepine (8% total; 1% free). For patients receiving AED polytherapy, the percentages were VPA-carbamazepine (44% total; 22% free), phenobarbital-phenytoin (37% total; 16% free), phenobarbital-carbamazepine (18% total; 6% free). Although both Zelnick et al.[67] and Castro-Gago et al.[68] reported decreased serum carnitine levels among individuals using VPA, Zelnick found no such association for phenobarbital, but Castro-Gago found such an effect. Subsequently, Verotti et al.[70] questioned whether the depletion of carnitine and the increase in blood ammonia levels (both caused by VPA) are actually related to each other. Their investigation found that the depletion of carnitine was significantly more severe when epileptic individuals were taking VPA together with other antiseizure medications.

The risk of carnitine depletion and drug-induced deficiency may reflect the disease severity, broader health condition, and nutritional status of patients being treated with anticonvulsants more than the adverse effects of the medications themselves. De Vivo et al.[71] reviewed many clinical trials demonstrating an association between anticonvulsant therapy and decreased carnitine levels, especially in children and particularly involving VPA. They concluded that younger children (1-10 years) treated with VPA tend to demonstrate a more significant decrease in carnitine concentrations than older children (10-18 years) and advised L-carnitine coadministration in certain cases, particularly infants and young children (especially those <2 years) diagnosed with neurological disorders and receiving VPA and multiple anticonvulsants. Earlier, Van Wouwe[1] had noted that before VPA therapy, plasma free-carnitine values were age dependent and increased during childhood. Hirose et al.[72] conducted a randomized, case-control study involving 45 children with epilepsy, age 6 to 21 years, who were treated with VPA monotherapy and were free of abnormal neurological findings or nutritional problems; an age-matched group of

45 children without epilepsy served as the control group. Although serum VPA concentration exhibited a weak negative correlation with both total and free serum carnitine, there was no significant difference in total and free serum carnitine levels between the VPA-treated and control groups; plasma ammonia levels were the same in the two groups. These researchers concluded that children on a regular diet receive sufficient carnitine intake to adequately meet their daily carnitine requirement, that valproate therapy does not deplete carnitine levels in otherwise healthy children, and that VPA-induced carnitine deficiency is not likely to occur in this population.

Hiraoka et al.[73] studied the pharmacokinetics of decreases in the blood free-carnitine level as an adverse effect of VPA administered to epileptic patients in connection with changes in the VPA disposition. They observed that serum free-carnitine level in patients taking at least one of phenobarbital, phenytoin, and carbamazepine in addition to VPA was significantly lower than that in the group given only these other agents without VPA. Subjects medicated only with VPA also tended to have a lower serum free-carnitine level than controls, although not to a significant degree. Among all the patients taking VPA with or without other AED(s), a significantly positive correlation was observed between the serum free-carnitine level and the value of dose and level ratio (L/D) of VPA. Such findings indicate that both the serum free-carnitine concentration and the L/D value of VPA were remarkably reduced in patients receiving both VPA and another AED. The researchers interpreted these results to suggest that enzyme induction by and accelerated hepatic degradation of VPA plays a role in the reduction of free carnitine levels, which is then reflected in free-carnitine deficiency.

Plasma carnitine levels are often low in people taking VPA for extended periods. Coadministration of carnitine may normalize low carnitine levels associated with anticonvulsant therapy, especially children taking VPA. Even so, concomitant carnitine therapy for patients undergoing long-term AED therapy remains contentious, and research findings have yet to evolve to an established level of consistency, refinement, and clarity to form a consensus or enable formulation of well-founded clinical algorithms. Ohtani et al.[74] compared plasma carnitine and blood ammonia concentrations in 25 severely handicapped patients, age 3 to 21 years, with those of 27 age-matched control subjects. Of the handicapped patients, 14 were treated with anticonvulsant drugs, including VPA; the remaining 11 patients were treated with drugs other than VPA. They found that plasma carnitine concentrations were lower and blood ammonia values were higher in VPA-treated patients than in the untreated patients and control subjects, and that plasma carnitine concentrations exhibited a significant inverse relationship with both VPA dosage and blood ammonia values. Both carnitine deficiency and hyperammonemia were corrected after oral administration of DL-carnitine (50 mg/kg/day) for 4 weeks.

Ater[60] reported that carnitine appeared to be protective against the drug-induced liver damage for which children treated with anticonvulsants are at high risk. Subsequently, Freeman et al.[75] conducted a placebo-controlled, double-blind, crossover study involving 47 children with seizures being treated with either VPA or carbamazepine that attempted to assess changes in "well-being," as perceived by parents, after oral carnitine coadministration (100 mg/kg). They found that well-being scores improved weekly for all children (i.e., when either placebo or carnitine was administered), and that none of the analyses of improved well-being achieved statistical significance. These researchers concluded that available evidence indicated that prophylactic coadministration of carnitine to children taking anticonvulsant medications for alleviating common, nonspecific symptoms was not warranted. Furthermore, they noted that, as of 1994, there were no reliable clinical or laboratory tests for determining symptomatic carnitine deficiency caused by anticonvulsant administration, and that further research was needed to develop methods for identifying children in need of carnitine coadministration.

Melegh, Pap, et al.[76] compared 10 randomly selected subjects with age- and gender-matched controls in a randomized trial measuring energy metabolism in children receiving long-term VPA therapy. Eight of the treated subjects showed an altered fuel consumption pattern, including a significant reduction in the amount of fats oxidized and a shift to increased utilization of carbohydrates. Carnitine coadministration for a month (50 mg/kg/day as oral solution, divided equally into two or three doses) reversed this pattern as the respiratory quotient decreased, oxidation of fats increased, and consumption of carbohydrates decreased. Van Wouwe[1] demonstrated that "prolonged" VPA treatment results in secondary carnitine deficiency in children. He compared samples of plasma drawn at the onset of and after 9 months of continuous VPA treatment in 13 children and found that mean plasma free carnitine decreased by 40%, plasma total carnitine decreased by 20%, and the esterified/free-carnitine ratio increased by 40%. Biochemical evidence of carnitine deficiency appeared in 6 of the 13 subjects, although clinical symptoms, primarily fatigue and excessive sleepiness, were observed in only two. The author concluded that a "dose of 15 mg/kg body weight is effective to reverse the clinical symptoms of carnitine deficiency within a week" and advised carnitine coadministration in children complaining of fatigue during prolonged VPA therapy. He also noted that the "dose to prevent deficiency is not yet established." Gidal et al.[77] found that carnitine (50 mg/kg) protected children from valproate-induced, transient hyperammonemia.

Carnitine therapy may do more than only protect against AED-induced depletion and resulting adverse effects. Research by Sakemi and Takada[78] indicates that concomitant administration of L-carnitine during VPA therapy may potentiate the activity of VPA. They reported that L-carnitine coadministration increased carnitine concentrations significantly in serum and liver but not in the brain, and that the resultant increase of serum free-VPA concentrations by concomitant carnitine apparently caused free-VPA concentrations in the brain to increase. Overall, the research literature reveals an understanding that carnitine has an effect on the performance and toxicity of VPA, but no clear agreement as to a potential therapeutic role for carnitine has emerged.

Currently available clinical trials exhibit mixed and conflicting results and cast doubt on the efficacy of carnitine administration as a generic prescription for individuals taking AEDs. However, no clinical trial has yet addressed the issues of carnitine depletion and carnitine administration over an extended time. These medications are often prescribed for years or decades, and the risk of cumulative depletion patterns and their clinical implications have yet to be adequately addressed. Long-term, well-designed clinical trials are warranted to investigate the adverse effects on carnitine level and function and compensatory concomitant carnitine administration, particularly with reference to specific age groups, contextual pathological and nutritional status, and various anticonvulsant agents. Adequate tools for assessing carnitine status are critical to accurate and clinically applicable findings.

Apart from issues of chronic depletion and corrective replacement therapy, intravenous (IV) carnitine is among the interventions used in acute VPA-induced hepatotoxicity and overdose; high-flux hemodialysis and charcoal hemoperfusion are also used in such situations.[79]

Reports

Several case reports have described VPA-related carnitine deficiency causing abdominal pain in children. For example, Shuper et al.[79] reported on a pediatric patient with intractable epilepsy who had a complete remission of severe VPA-induced abdominal pain immediately after administration of L-carnitine, 300 mg/day.

Houghton and Bowers[80] reported a case of VPA overdose in a woman with polysubstance overdose and a history of alcoholism and hepatitis B and C. Several interventions were necessary to address the multiple toxicities involved and the sequence of risk and immediacy. L-Carnitine at 100 mg/kg/day was administered to correct hyperammonemia and encephalopathy and continued until serum ammonia and VPA levels had normalized.

Nutritional Therapeutics, Clinical Concerns, and Adaptations

In consideration of research available at this time, physicians prescribing valproic acid, phenobarbital, or related anticonvulsant medications may find it prudent to coadminister oral L-carnitine prophylactically or monitor carnitine blood levels and coadminister L-carnitine as indicated. Susceptibility to adverse effects appears to be greater in three groups: infants and young children receiving VPA, patients receiving anticonvulsant polytherapy (especially those <2 years), and individuals with severe neurological conditions, compromised nutritional status, or other medical conditions characterized by compromised liver function or systemic overload. Concurrent treatment with pivalate prodrugs is contraindicated because of increased urinary carnitine excretion. Although higher-dose carnitine (3-7 g/day) likely would prevent deficiency, there is little clinical experience in this area and no available clinical research to serve as a guideline. Serum carnitine levels should be monitored during long-term anticonvulsant therapy. Concomitant administration of L-carnitine may be advisable for some patients. Nevertheless, clinically significant deficiencies of carnitine appear to be uncommon, and no conclusive evidence has confirmed that most individuals benefit from carnitine supplements.

In 1998, a panel of pediatric neurologists and experts on L-carnitine coadministration strongly recommended oral L-carnitine for all infants and children taking VPA, as well as for adults with carnitine deficiency syndromes, people with VPA-induced hepatic and renal toxicity, people on kidney dialysis, and premature infants on TPN. Oral carnitine in three to four divided doses totaling 100 mg/kg, up to a maximum of 2 g/day, represents a consensus dosage level. However, physicians prescribing anticonvulsant medications should advise patients to refrain from starting any supplemental use of carnitine outside the context of regular supervision and close monitoring by health care professionals trained and experienced in both conventional pharmacology and nutritional therapeutics.

In acute VPA toxicity, use of IV L-carnitine remains investigational but can be considered in patients with coma, central nervous system (CNS) depression, evidence of hepatic dysfunction, and hyperammonemia. In such patients, L-carnitine may be initiated at 50 to 100 mg/kg/day (up to maximum dose of 2 g/day) to correct hyperammonemia and encephalopathy.

Such therapy would be continued until serum ammonia and VPA levels had normalized.

Zidovudine (AZT) and Related Antiretroviral Agents, Reverse-Transcriptase Inhibitor (Nucleoside)

Evidence: Didanosine (ddI, dideoxyinosine; Videx); dideoxycytidine (ddC, zalcitabine; Hivid), stavudine (d4T, Zerit), tenofovir (Viread); zidovudine (azidothymidine, AZT, ZDV, zidothymidine; Retrovir); combination drugs: zidovudine and lamivudine (Combivir); abacavir, lamivudine, and zidovudine (Trizivir).
Extrapolated, based on similar properties Abacavir (Ziagen), lamivudine (3TC, Epivir).

Interaction Type and Significance

◇≈≈ **Drug-Induced Adverse Effect on Nutrient Function, Coadministration Therapeutic, with Professional Management**

≈≈ **Drug-Induced Nutrient Depletion, Supplementation Therapeutic, with Professional Management**

☼ **Prevention or Reduction of Drug Adverse Effect**

⊕ **Potential or Theoretical Beneficial or Supportive Interaction, with Professional Management**

Nutrient Depletion
Probability:
2. Probable to
1. Certain

Evidence Base:
◉ **Emerging** to
● **Consensus**

Coadministration Benefit
Probability:
4. Plausible to **2. Probable**

Evidence Base:
▽ **Mixed** to ◉ **Emerging**

Effect and Mechanism of Action

Antiretroviral drugs are well known to cause mitochondrial toxicity, peripheral neuropathy, and other significant adverse effects. L-Carnitine normally plays a major role in the transport of long-chain fatty acids across the inner mitochondrial membrane and facilitates the beta-oxidation of fatty acids.

Reduced levels of carnitine in serum and muscle are found in most patients treated with antiretroviral therapy using AZT and related agents. These agents are well known for causing muscle damage, notably mitochondrial myopathy characterized by depletion of mitochondrial DNA, enzymatic defects in the respiratory chain system, poor utilization of long-chain fatty acids, and accumulation of lipid droplets within the muscle fibers.[81-84] Thus, reduced muscle carnitine levels, resulting from decreased carnitine uptake by the muscle, are associated with depletion of energy stores within the muscle fibers.

Destructive changes have been observed in other critical sites. Didanosine (ddI), stavudine (d4T), and zalcitabine (ddC) are relatively strong inhibitors of g-polymerase and thus cause a time- and dose-dependent decrease in the intracellular levels of mitochondrial DNA.[85] Acetyl-carnitine deficiency and impairment of mitochondrial DNA synthesis are also crucial to the pathogenesis of axonal peripheral neuropathy, a severe dose-limiting toxicity often associated with didanosine, zalcitabine, and stavudine.[86,87] With regard to zalcitabine (ddC), ddCDP-choline appears to be the zalcitabine metabolite primarily responsible for mitochondrial toxicity.[87] Carnitine depletion has also been observed in peripheral blood mononuclear cells (PBMCs) of HIV-infected individuals.[88] Disrupted mitochondrial membrane potential (along with increased oxidant stress) also appears in the CD4 and CD8 cells of asymptomatic HIV-infected subjects with advanced immunodeficiency treated with AZT and ddI.[84]

Coadministration of L-carnitine may restore carnitine levels, correct disrupted mitochondrial transmembrane potential, and decrease apoptotic CD4 and CD8 lymphocytes to support immune function and limit or reverse some of the adverse effects of these medications.

Research

The adverse effects of AZT and related antiretroviral nucleoside analogs, particularly on carnitine levels, have been well established in over a decade of research and clinical observations. Their implications for patient health and therapeutic outcomes have also become increasingly clear.

Several studies published in 1994 focused on carnitine depletion in HIV patients and linked it to the action of antiretroviral nucleoside analogs. In an in vitro study using human muscle tissue, Semino-Mora et al.[84] observed depopulation of Leu-19–positive myotubes and destructive changes in mitochondria, including accumulation of lipid droplets, when exposed to AZT at concentrations of 250 μM and higher. Dalakas et al.[81] examined the degree of neutral fat accumulation and muscle carnitine levels in the muscle biopsy specimens from 21 patients with AZT-induced myopathic symptoms of varying severity. They described a pattern of "DNA-depleting mitochondrial myopathy" associated with zidovudine (AZT) use, which is "histologically characterized by the presence of muscle fibers with 'ragged-red'-like features, red-rimmed or empty cracks, granular degeneration, and rods (AZT fibers)." This muscle cell damage caused by AZT results in accumulation of lipid droplets within the muscle fibers from poor utilization of long-chain fatty acids. Reduced muscle carnitine levels, from decreased carnitine uptake by the muscle, are associated with depletion of energy stores within the muscle fibers. De Simone et al.[86] reported carnitine depletion in PBMCs of 20 male patients with advanced AIDS and normal serum levels of carnitines. Campos and Arenas[83] also published a letter reporting muscle carnitine deficiency associated with AZT-induced mitochondrial myopathy.

Preliminary but growing evidence indicates that the L-carnitine may mitigate mitochondrial toxicity associated with zidovudine (AZT) and other nucleoside analogs, provide independent therapeutic benefits on HIV infection parameters, and complement conventional chemotherapeutic regimens in HIV-infected patients.

In a randomized, placebo-controlled clinical trial involving 20 male patients with advanced AIDS (stage IV-CI), De Simone et al.[86] randomly assigned subjects to receive either oral L-carnitine (6 g/day) or placebo for 2 weeks. AIDS patients exhibited cellular carnitine depletion (with concentrations of total carnitine in PBMCs lower than in healthy controls), even though serum carnitine levels were within normal range. These researchers found that treatment with high-dose L-carnitine was associated with a significant trend toward the restoration of appropriate intracellular carnitine levels and strongly improved proliferative responsiveness by lymphocytes in the S and G_2-M stages to mitogens. They also observed a strong reduction in serum triglycerides in the L-carnitine group at the end of the trial compared with baseline levels, which would be expected from improved efficiency of fatty acid transport and utilization.

In an in vitro experiment using human muscle tissue, Semino-Mora et al.[84] found that the addition of L-carnitine (5 mM) to muscle cultures pretreated with AZT (0.0027 to

135 μg/mL) preserves the integrity and volume of mitochondria, prevents AZT-associated destruction of human myotubes, preserves structural integrity and volume of mitochondria, and prevents the accumulation of lipids.[89] Such findings suggest that L-carnitine provides independent therapeutic benefit through its effects on immune system function rather than on the pathogen itself.[90]

Uncontrolled apoptosis plays a critical role in the loss of T lymphocytes in HIV-infected individuals. The Fas/Fas ligand system and ceramide, an endogenous mediator of Fas-triggered apoptosis, appear to be particularly important in the progression of HIV infection. The signal transduced by the Fas receptor involves the activation of an acidic sphingomyelinase, sphingomyelin breakdown, and ceramide production. Disruption of mitochondrial transmembrane potential is an early, irreversible step in the effector phase of apoptosis that allows identification of an additional pool of lymphocytes irreversibly committed to undergo apoptosis, despite still lacking the morphological features typical of apoptosis. Both in vitro and in vivo research show that L-carnitine inhibits Fas-induced apoptosis and ceramide production.[86,91]

Moretti, Alesse, et al.[91] conducted a series of studies investigating the relationship of carnitine to lymphocyte apoptosis, oxidant stress, and immune function in subjects infected with HIV. In a pilot study, they administered daily infusions of L-carnitine (6 g) for 4 months to 11 asymptomatic HIV-1-infected subjects, who had refused antiretroviral treatment despite experiencing a progressive decline in CD4 counts, and monitored immunological and virological measures (as well as safety) at the start of the treatment and then on days 15, 30, 90, and 150. L-Carnitine administration resulted in an increase in absolute CD4 counts, which was statistically significant on days 90 and 150 ($p = 0.010$ and $p = 0.019$, respectively). They also observed a positive but not significant trend in the change in absolute counts of CD8 lymphocytes and a gradual but strongly significant ($p = 0.001$) decrease in the frequency of apoptotic CD4 and CD8 lymphocytes at the end of the study compared to baseline. Cell-associated levels of ceramide also exhibited a strong decline ($p = 0.001$) at the end of the study. L-Carnitine also corrected previously disrupted mitochondrial transmembrane potential. No evidence of L-carnitine toxicity was observed, and no dose reductions were necessary. There was no clinically relevant change in HIV-1 viremia.

In a subsequent trial involving 20 asymptomatic HIV-infected subjects with advanced immunodeficiency, Moretti et al.[88] compared the effects of either zidovudine (AZT) and didanosine (ddI) or the same regimen plus L-carnitine over 7 months. As previously, they measured immunological and virological parameters at baseline and after 15, 60, 120, and 210 days of treatment. They found significant reductions in apoptotic CD4 and CD8 cells, lymphocytes with disrupted mitochondrial membrane potential, and lymphocytes undergoing oxidant stress in subjects treated with AZT and ddI plus L-carnitine compared with subjects receiving only the antiviral agents. Fas and caspase-1 were downexpressed and p35 overexpressed in lymphocytes from patients of the L-carnitine group. CD4 and CD8 counts and viremia showed no significant difference between the groups. No evidence of toxicity from L-carnitine was recognized. They concluded that coadministration of L-carnitine "is safe and allows apoptosis and oxidant stress to be greatly reduced in lymphocytes from subjects treated with AZT and DDI."

In an in vitro experiment, Rossi et al.[87] investigated mitochondrial toxicity and peripheral neuropathy caused by

2′,3′-dideoxycytidine (ddCyd; zalcitabine). 2′,3′-Dideoxycytidine 5′-diphosphocholine (ddCDP-choline) is among the metabolites of zalcitabine found in a concentration-dependent manner after incubating human cells with the antiretroviral drug. Uptake of ddCDP-choline into mitochondria is more efficient than dideoxyCTP uptake (the triphosphocholine metabolite), suggesting that ddCDP-choline is the metabolite of zalcitabine responsible for mitochondrial toxicity. Furthermore, these researchers reported that, in the cell-free system investigated, 3.0 mM L-carnitine inhibited the uptake of both ddCTP and ddCDP-choline by mitochondria, and when added to U937 cells grown in the presence of 0.25 μM zalcitabine, 3.0 mM L-carnitine partially abrogated the mitochondrial toxicity of zalcitabine.

Nevertheless, in a 2003 review of antiretroviral nucleoside analog reverse-transcriptase inhibitors (NRTIs), Walker[85] concluded that "in established mitochondrial toxicity, cessation of the offending NRTI remains the most effective therapeutic intervention because vitamin cocktails and L-carnitine have, at best, only a marginal effect." He also notes: "Mitochondrial toxicity cannot yet be adequately monitored and predicted."

Nutritional Therapeutics, Clinical Concerns, and Adaptations

Physicians treating HIV-infected individuals may provide therapeutic benefit by administering L-carnitine regardless of whether they are prescribing AZT or other nucleoside analogs concurrently. Findings from clinical trials and related research support the significant probability that concomitant carnitine therapy may enhance immune function, mitigate the pathological process, prevent the development of myotoxicity, and reduce adverse effects of conventional antiviral therapies. A typical therapeutic dosage of L-carnitine would be in the range of 1 to 3 g daily. However, a large proportion of patients may require an initial dosage of up to 6 g daily to restore carnitine levels, especially if they have become depleted by antiviral medications. The body of evidence indicates that L-carnitine is essentially nontoxic and unlikely to interfere with the efficacy of conventional treatment.

THEORETICAL, SPECULATIVE, AND PRELIMINARY INTERACTIONS RESEARCH, INCLUDING OVERSTATED INTERACTIONS CLAIMS

Calcium Channel Blockers

Amlodipine (Norvasc); combination drug: amlodipine and benazepril (Lotrel); bepridil (Bapadin, Vascor), diltiazem (Cardizem, Cardizem CD, Cardizem SR, Cartia XT, Dilacor XR, Diltia XT, Tiamate, Tiazac), felodipine (Plendil); combination drugs: felodipine and enalapril (Lexxel); felodipine and ramipril (Triapin); gallopamil (D600), isradipine (DynaCirc, DynaCirc CR), lercanidipine (Zanidip), nicardipine (Cardene, Cardene I.V., Cardene SR), nifedipine (Adalat, Adalat CC, Nifedical XL, Procardia, Procardia XL); combination drug: nifedipine and atenolol (Beta-Adalat, Tenif); nimodipine (Nimotop), nisoldipine (Sular), nitrendipine (Cardif, Nitrepin), verapamil (Calan, Calan SR, Covera-HS, Isoptin, Isoptin SR, Verelan, Verelan PM); combination drug: verapamil and trandolapril (Tarka).

Many studies have demonstrated the value of L-carnitine in the prevention and treatment of cardiovascular disorders. Some clinicians experienced in nutritional therapeutics have suggested that coadministration of carnitine during calcium channel blocker therapy might introduce an additive or synergistic beneficial effect. Evidence from clinical trials is lacking to support

this speculation. However, the pharmacological principles underlying this proposal are reasonable and in accordance with known activities and effects of both agents. Research through well-designed clinical trials may be warranted to explore this potential supportive interaction.

Physicians treating individuals with significant risk for or known presence of cardiovascular disease are advised to discuss with their patients the potential benefits of carnitine. L-Carnitine and L-propionyl-carnitine are the forms most often used for prevention and treatment of cardiovascular conditions, with typical therapeutic dosages in the range of 1 to 3 g daily.

Cisplatin, Ifosfamide, and Related Chemotherapy

Cisplatin (*cis*-diaminedichloroplatinum, CDDP; Platinol, Platinol-AQ).
Ifosfamide (Ifex, Mitoxana).

In a preliminary study involving nonanemic cancer patients, Graziano et al.[92] found that concomitant administration of L-carnitine (2 g twice daily) for 7 days relieved chemotherapy-induced fatigue in 90% of subjects who had been treated with cisplatin or ifosfamide. These findings are limited by the lack of a placebo group in the study, which would have enabled accounting for spontaneous resolution of fatigue. Further research through well-designed clinical trials is warranted.

Gentamicin

Gentamicin (G-mycin, Garamycin, Jenamicin).

Based on reports that hearing is improved when L-carnitine is administered to infants with neurological disorders, Kalinec et al.[93] investigated the effectiveness of L-carnitine for preventing the ototoxic effects typically associated with gentamicin therapy. They administered L-carnitine, 100 mg/kg/day, to pregnant guinea pigs beginning either 2 weeks before or simultaneously with gentamicin, 100 mg/kg/day for 7 days. Not only did the administration of L-carnitine prevent neonatal mortality, but it also prevented hearing loss associated with the antibiotic. Thus, using auditory brainstem responses, the authors found that the auditory threshold of untreated offspring was 21 dB, compared with 30 db in those treated with gentamicin but that those treated with L-carnitine starting before or at the same time as gentamicin, demonstrated hearing thresholds restored to 23 db and 21 dB, respectively. Furthermore, confocal microscopy and scanning electron microscopy revealed that L-carnitine ameliorated the significant damage of outer hair cells induced by gentamicin. Further study, using cell culture of an auditory cell line highly sensitive to ototoxic drugs and other biochemical testing, indicated that apoptosis was the mechanism by which gentamicin produced its damaging effects, specifically through upregulation of the Harakiri (Hrk) gene, a proapoptotic member of the Bcl-2 family of proteins, mediated by activation of ERK1/2 and inhibition of the JNK pathways. Their findings suggested that L-carnitine exerted its protective action by preventing inhibition of JNK and the consequent upregulation of Hrk, thus blocking cell death. Based on these findings, these investigators have planned a clinical trial to investigate the ability of L-carnitine to prevent gentamicin-induced ototoxicity.

Propranolol and Related Beta-1-Adrenoceptor Antagonists (Beta-1-Adrenergic Blocking Agents)

Propranolol and Related Beta-1-Adrenoceptor Antagonists (Beta-1 Adrenergic Blocking Agents).
Propranolol (Betachron, Inderal LA, Innopran XL, Inderal) Related: Acebutolol (Sectral), atenolol (Tenormin), atenolol

combination drugs: atenolol and chlortalidone (Co- Tendione, Tenoretic), atenolol and nifedipine (Beta-Adalat, Tenif), sotalol (Betapace, Betapace AF, Sorine); betaxolol (Kerlone), bisoprolol (Zebeta), carteolol (cartrol), esmolol (Brevibloc), labetalol (Normodyne, Trandate), metoprolol (Lopressor, Toprol XL); combination drug: metoprolol and hydrochlorothiazide (Lopressor HCT), nadolol (Corgard), nebivolol (Nebilet), oxprenolol (Trasicor), penbutolol (Levatol), pindolol (Visken), propranolol combination drug: propranolol and bendrofluazide (Inderex), timolol (Blocadren)

Many studies have demonstrated the value of L-carnitine in the prevention and treatment of cardiovascular disorders. Ferro et al.[94] reported on the case of a 52-year-old man with dilated cardiomyopathy in whom concomitant treatment with L-carnitine and propranolol restored cardiac function, with a 50% reduction in mitral EPSS (E point septal separation), from 20 to 10 mm, and a decrease from 60 to 57 mm in diastolic diameter. These clinicians concluded that their "experience suggests promising benefits in adopting beta blockers combined with L-carnitine therapy in myocardial failure secondary to dilated cardiomyopathy."

After reviewing the literature on the treatment of hypertrophic cardiomyopathy, Ferro et al.[94] also proposed that the protective action of beta-blocking agents against chronic catecholamine stimulation may be enhanced by the combination with L-carnitine. Notably, L-carnitine plays a synergistic role by acting as an important source of energy because of fatty acid oxidation and by avoiding the accumulation of lipids in the blood plasma and myocardium.

Physicians prescribing beta-blocker therapy are advised to discuss with their patients the potential benefits of concomitant carnitine. L-Carnitine and L-propionyl-carnitine are the forms most frequently used for prevention and treatment of cardiovascular conditions, with typical therapeutic dosages in the range of 1 to 3 g per day.

NUTRIENT-NUTRIENT INTERACTIONS

Alpha-Lipoic Acid

Hagen et al.[95] demonstrated improved memory and metabolic function and decreased oxidative stress in old rats fed the combination of acetyl-L-carnitine and lipoic acid.

Coenzyme Q10, Fish Oil, Magnesium, and Taurine

Carnitine, coenzyme Q10, fish oil, magnesium, and taurine are critical nutrients in maintaining healthy cardiovascular function, muscle, and brain tissue and can play a valuable therapeutic role in the treatment of cardiovascular disease and other conditions and the support of CNS function. Health care professionals trained and experienced in nutritional therapies often use multiple nutrients together. These agents are all considered essentially nontoxic. Clinical trials investigating their synergistic effects are clearly warranted.

HERB-NUTRIENT INTERACTIONS

Hawthorn

Hawthorn, *Crataegus laevigata* (Poir) DC., *Crataegus monogyna* Jacq. (Lindm.), *Crataegus oxyacantha L.* (for *C. laevigata*).

Concomitant administration of carnitine and *Crataegus* is common practice among health care professionals trained and experienced in the synergistic use of nutrients and herbs in supporting healthy cardiovascular function and treating cardiovascular conditions. Clinical trials investigating the clinical efficacy of combined therapy using these two agents are lacking, as is research into mechanisms underlying interactions between them. Hawthorn is generally considered essentially nontoxic. Clinical trials investigating their synergistic effects are clearly warranted.

The 95 citations for this monograph, as well as additional reference literature, are located under Carnitine on the CD at the back of the book.

Methionine

Summary

Drug/Class Interaction Type	Mechanism and Significance	Management
Acetaminophen ☼/⊕⊕⊕	Methionine appears to reduce toxic effects of acetaminophen, especially on liver. Long-term, well-designed clinical trials are warranted.	Coadminister, possibly within same dose.
Levodopa (L-dopa) ✗✗/✗✗✗/⊕✗/⊕⊕	Methionine administration (500-1000 mg/day) may benefit individuals with Parkinson's disease, but high doses (> 4 g/day) may interfere with action of levodopa. Multinutrient support is important to protect against elevated homocysteine (Hcy) associated with Parkinson's disease and possibly aggravated by levodopa therapy. Long-term, well-designed clinical trials are warranted.	Consider administration of methionine at low to midrange doses along with folate, B₆, and B₁₂; monitor serum total Hcy. Monitor for interference with levodopa via symptoms.

NUTRIENT DESCRIPTION

Chemistry and Forms

DL-Methionine, L-methionine.

Physiology and Function

Methionine is an essential sulfur-containing amino acid that facilitates and helps initiate the translation of messenger RNA (mRNA) by being the first amino acid incorporated into the N-terminal position of all proteins. The terminal methyl group of the methionine side chain often participates in biochemical methyl transfer reactions, making methionine a member of the "methyl donor" class of biochemicals.

S-adenosylmethionine (SAMe) is intimately involved in the synthesis of brain chemicals and also in detoxification reactions. Methionine is converted into SAMe, which is considered to be the activated form of methionine. This occurs in the first step of the metabolism of methionine, which requires energy in the form of adenosine triphosphate (ATP). In this activation of methionine, an adenosyl moiety is transferred from the ATP molecule. SAMe is one of the most potent methyl donors and is involved in many methylation reactions. Its methyl group, which is attached in a sulfonium linkage with high-energy characteristics, may be donated to any of a large number of methyl-group acceptors in the presence of the appropriate enzyme. DNA methylation influences the expression of many genes and depends on the availability of methyl groups from SAMe. SAMe is intimately involved in the synthesis of neurotransmitters and also in detoxification reactions.

Along with inositol, choline (tetramethylglycine), and betaine (trimethylglycine), methionine is considered a member of the group of compounds called lipotropics that are closely involved in lipid metabolism. Transmethylation metabolic pathways closely interconnect choline, methionine, methyltetrahydrofolate (methyl-THF), and vitamins B₆ and B₁₂. Methionine can be formed from homocysteine using methyl groups from methyl-THF, or using methyl groups from betaine that are derived from choline. Through interrelated pathways, methyl-THF can be formed from one-carbon units derived from serine or from the methyl groups of choline via dimethylglycine, and choline can be synthesized de novo using methyl groups derived from methionine (via SAMe).

Methionine regulates several sulfur-containing compounds in the body that play an important role in liver detoxification processes and the synthesis of structural proteins and enzymes. It acts as a sulfur donor and, as such, is the source of sulfur for biosynthesis of cysteine. Methionine is also the precursor for the synthesis of cystine and taurine and is one of three amino acids required for the synthesis of creatine. Methionine may serve as a precursor for the synthesis of glutathione, which is the substrate for glutathione peroxidase, a crucial antioxidant enzyme. Methionine assists in the metabolism of homocysteine and helps reduce histamine levels.

NUTRIENT IN CLINICAL PRACTICE

Known or Potential Therapeutic Uses

Methionine is an essential amino acid which is primarily administered to enhance liver functions such as detoxification and lipid metabolism and to support the function of the central nervous system (CNS) and neurotransmitters. In nutritional therapeutics, methionine can be used to increase levels of SAMe, reduced glutathione (GSH), taurine, and N-acetylcysteine (NAC) and to promote detoxification of xenobiotics via the sulfation pathway.

Historical/Ethnomedicine Precedent

Not used historically as an isolated nutrient.

Possible Uses

Acrodermatitis enteropathica, AIDS-related dementia, AIDS-related nervous system degeneration, fat maldigestion, human immunodeficiency virus (HIV) support, liver detoxification, migraine headaches, pain control, pancreatitis, Parkinson's disease, radiation effects, schizophrenia, urinary tract infections, weight loss, Wilson's disease.

Deficiency Symptoms

Typical symptoms associated with methionine deficiency include hair loss, hepatic dysfunction, poor skin tone, and toxic elevation of metabolic waste products.

Methionine deficiency is usually related to overall protein malnutrition. Individuals with acquired immunodeficiency syndrome (AIDS) demonstrate low levels of methionine. Experimentally, a methionine deficiency causes premature atherosclerosis in monkeys, especially if they are also deficient in vitamin B_6. Methionine deficiency can also cause a folate deficiency since a deficiency causes 5-methyl-THF to accumulate in the liver. Lower methionine intake during pregnancy has been associated with neural tube defects in newborns.

Dietary Sources

Dairy products, fish, and meat (beef, chicken, pork, liver) are considered the richest dietary sources of methionine. Sunflower seeds, pumpkin seeds, sesame seeds, and lentils are also good sources of methionine. Egg yolks are particularly high in sulfur. Methionine and cysteine make up 91% of the sulfur in the yolk. Endogenous gut flora may be able to synthesize significant amounts. Homocysteine in the diet can eliminate the requirement for methionine.

Soybeans are a poor source, and soy-based infant formulas are generally low in methionine.

Dosage Forms Available

Capsule, powder, tablet; oral and intravenous (IV) administration.

Source Materials for Nutrient Preparations

Most L-methionine in supplements is produced by bacterial fermentation processes in a growth medium, from which the amino acid is then purified. Methionine used in supplements is frequently of the DL form, which implies chemical synthesis, thus resulting in a racemic mixture.

Dosage Range
Adult
Dietary: No reference (recommended) daily intake (RDI) has been established. Average intake in the United States is 2.7 to 5 g per day.
Supplemental/Maintenance: Dietary sources of methionine are usually adequate so supplemental methionine is usually not considered necessary. Optimal levels of intake have not been established but probably are 800 to 1000 mg daily, depending on weight, diet, and related factors.
Pharmacological/Therapeutic: 500 to 3000 mg per day.
Toxic: No toxic dose level has been reported.

Pediatric (< 18 Years)
Dietary: No minimal dietary requirement established.
Supplemental/Maintenance: Not currently recommended for children.
Pharmacological/Therapeutic: Specific treatment recommendations have not established.
Toxic: No toxic dosage level established specifically for infants and children.

Laboratory Values

Serum or Plasma Methionine
Range of normal levels for plasma methionine:
Children: 13 to 30 μmol/L
Adults: 16 to 30 μmol/L

SAFETY PROFILE
Overview

Methionine is usually tolerated well by most adults and generally considered to be free of adverse effects for most individuals at common dosage levels (e.g., 1-3 g/day). Toxicity is rare but possible with excessive dosage. Diets high in methionine may be associated with an increased occurrence of atherosclerosis, especially with concurrent deficiencies of vitamin B_6, vitamin B_{12}, and folic acid, resulting from elevations of blood homocysteine levels.

Nutrient Adverse Effects
General Adverse Effects
Nausea and gastrointestinal (GI) irritation are the primary signs of methionine toxicity, although occurrence is rare. Some sensitive individuals may experience gas, bloating, and digestive discomfort at levels as low as 500 mg per day. Other symptoms reportedly associated with methionine toxicity may include anorexia, ataxia, hyperactivity, reduced growth, hemosiderosis, and suppressed hematocrit. Extremely high doses may increase urinary calcium excretion and could potentially induce hallucinations. However, administration of up to 2 g daily for extended periods has not been associated with any serious adverse effects.

Rats fed methionine as 50% of dietary protein (equivalent human dose of 25 g/day) exhibited hyperactivity, anorexia, reduced growth, and iron accumulation in the spleen.

Pregnancy and Nursing
Evidence is lacking within the scientific literature to suggest or confirm any adverse effects related to fetal development during pregnancy or to infants who are breast-fed associated with methionine administration. Caution still advised.

Infants and Children
No adverse effects have been reported. However, sufficient research-based evidence is lacking to guarantee the safety of methionine in infants and children.

Contraindications

Avoid S-adenosylmethionine (SAMe) in Parkinson's disease; administration may aggravate symptoms caused by serotonergic effect.

Precautions and Warnings

Large intakes of methionine require higher intakes of methyl donor–related nutrients, such as B_{12}, folic acid, pyridoxine, choline (tetramethylglycine), betaine (trimethylglycine), and dimethylglycine. Large loads of dietary methionine without concomitant intake of these interdependent nutrients at adequate levels can increase the conversion of methionine to homocysteine (Hcy) and will result in higher levels of Hcy, a vasculotoxic product of intermediary metabolism. Need for methyl donor nutrients in relation to methionine intake varies according to pharmacogenomic determinants, such as methyl-THF reductase enzyme activity. In cases of strong family history of coronary heart disease, it would be judicious to check Hcy levels before and during methionine treatment, because of the potential homocysteinergic and atherogenic effects of methionine.

Animal research conducted by Toborek and Hennig[1] suggests that high dietary intake of methionine, in the presence of

B-vitamin deficiencies, may increase the risk for atherosclerosis by increasing blood levels of cholesterol and Hcy. Troen et al.[2] observed that apolipoprotein E–deficient mice fed methionine-rich diets developed significant atheromatous pathology in the aortic arch, even with normal plasma Hcy levels. These findings suggest that moderate increases in methionine intake are atherogenic in susceptible mice.

Administration may be inappropriate in individuals with osteoporosis because high dosage levels increase urinary excretion of calcium.

INTERACTIONS REVIEW
Strategic Considerations

The issue of methionine function and exogenous administration in individuals with Parkinson's disease and related degenerative neurotransmitter conditions remains unclear, inconclusive, and contentious. Preliminary research by Smythies and Halsey suggests that methionine (5 g/day) may help ameliorate some symptoms of Parkinson's disease. However, some authors have suggested that exogenous methionine, as with other amino acids, may interfere with the absorption or action of the levodopa, particularly in the treatment of individuals with Parkinson's disease. Several studies have reported elevated plasma levels of total Hcy, along with decreased methionine and SAMe, in patients treated long term with levodopa and dopa decarboxylase inhibitors (DDIs) as a result of alterations in levels of substrates of the O-methylation cycle.[3]

Several studies have investigated the use of methionine coadministration as a means of reducing toxicity caused by acetaminophen and suggested the probable benefits of such an integrative approach to prescribing.

Viewing methionine administration or supplementation within the larger context of wellness and therapeutics, it is important to note that increasing intake of methionine without providing for adequate intake of folic acid, vitamin B_6, and vitamin B_{12} can augment the conversion of methionine to Hcy and thereby increase cardiovascular risk.

NUTRIENT-DRUG INTERACTIONS

Acetaminophen

Acetaminophen (APAP, paracetamol; Tylenol); combination drugs: acetaminophen and codeine (Capital and Codeine; Phenaphen with Codeine; Tylenol with Codeine); acetaminophen and hydrocodone (Anexsia, Anodynos-DHC, Co-Gesic, Dolacet, DuoCet, Hydrocet, Hydrogesic, Hy-Phen, Lorcet 10/650, Lorcet-HD, Lorcet Plus, Lortab, Margesic H, Medipain 5, Norco, Stagesic, T-Gesic, Vicodin, Vicodin ES, Vicodin HP, Zydone); acetaminophen and oxycodone (Endocet, Percocet 2.5/325, Percocet 5/325, Percocet 7.5/500, Percocet 10/650, Roxicet 5/500, Roxilox, Tylox); acetaminophen and pentazocine (Talacen); acetaminophen and propoxyphene (Darvocet-N, Darvocet-N 100, Pronap-100, Propacet 100, Propoxacet-N, Wygesic); acetaminophen, butalbital, and caffeine (Fioricet).

Interaction Type and Significance

☼   **Prevention or Reduction of Drug Adverse Effect**
⊕⊕⊕   **Beneficial or Supportive Interaction, Not Requiring Professional Management**

Probability: Evidence Base:
2. Probable to 1. Certain   ◉ Emerging

Effect and Mechanism of Action

Methionine appears to reduce the toxic effects of acetaminophen (paracetamol), particularly on the liver, without adversely affecting (and possibly enhancing) the drug's pharmacokinetics and efficacy. Glutathione is most likely central to such activity, but the mechanisms involved have yet to be fully elucidated. The observed phenomenon might relate to empirical reports of methionine use in liver detoxification; however, the available evidence is not sufficient to support such an extrapolation. Further research is warranted to investigate the mechanisms of action responsible for the observed effects.

Research

Acetaminophen (paracetamol) poisoning is a major source of morbidity and mortality and represents one of the most common examples of adverse drug reactions in conventional medical practice. Numerous studies have demonstrated that coadministration of methionine may be effective in the treatment of acetaminophen toxicity. For more than a decade, various researchers and clinicians have proposed that methionine be incorporated into acetaminophen tablets routinely as a protective mechanism against acetaminophen-induced toxicity.

Skoglund and Skjelbred[4] conducted a randomized, single-blind, between-patient study comparing the onset of analgesia, duration, and efficacy of paracetamol versus a combination medication containing free paracetamol and its N-acetyl-methionate ester (SUR 2647) in outpatients after oral surgery. Using several subjective and objective assessments, the authors reported that median onset of analgesia for both groups was approximately equivalent (i.e., $\leq\frac{1}{2}$ hour) and that the duration of analgesia after the combination was greater than that for paracetamol (i.e., ≥ 5.5 hours vs. ≥ 2.5 hours). Furthermore, the combination regimen reduced pain significantly more than the paracetamol from $\frac{1}{2}$ to 3 hours after initiation of medication, but the mean pain scores did not show a significant difference during the remaining observation period. Subjects in both treatment groups reported mild to moderate drowsiness, but it was more common in subjects given the paracetamol/methionine combination.

Research by Neuvonen et al.[5] indicates that methionine might protect against the hepatotoxic effects of acetaminophen. Using a rat model, they compared the analgesic effect, toxicity, and kinetics of oral paracetamol with those of paracetamol + L-methionine (5:1). They reported that the presence of methionine did not significantly change the analgesic effect of paracetamol, but that methionine reduced the acute toxicity (LD_{50}) of paracetamol by 50% in nonfasted, fasted, and phenobarbital-pretreated mice. Subsequently, in a small, randomized crossover study involving 10 human subjects, they observed that coadministration of methionine (300 mg) did not alter the pharmacokinetics of paracetamol (1500 mg). Furthermore, they found that the "absorption of methionine from the combination tablets was rapid, peak concentrations occurred in plasma at 30 min and were 3-4 times higher than after paracetamol tablets not containing methionine."[5] In a later paper, some of these same researchers reviewed their findings and related data and rhetorically asked, "Why not add methionine to paracetamol tablets?"[6]

Based on these concerns and the emerging pattern of evidence supporting coadministration of methionine with acetaminophen, McAuley et al.[7] investigated whether methionine administration might adversely affect cardiovascular risk factors through its effect on endothelial function, plasma homocysteine (Hcy), and lipid peroxidation in 16 healthy volunteers. Their findings showed no significant difference in endothelial-dependent vascular responses after acute (250 mg orally), 1 month of low-dose (250 mg daily), or 1 week of high-dose (100 mg/kg daily) methionine. Plasma Hcy concentrations demonstrated no significant differences after acute or 1 month of low-dose methionine. However, Hcy concentrations significantly increased after 1 week of high-dose methionine (100 mg/kg) daily. Thus, methionine administration at dosage levels similar to those used in combination preparations with acetaminophen do not adversely affect plasma Hcy concentrations. The observation that high-dose methionine administration can cause elevated plasma Hcy concentrations in only 1 week is consistent with other research findings on methionine administration outside the context of synergistic nutrients.

Nutritional Therapeutics, Clinical Concerns, and Adaptations

Pending release of a commercial product combining acetaminophen and methionine, health care professionals are advised that it is reasonable to coadminister the two agents, particularly for patients who take acetaminophen on a long-term basis, such as for osteoarthritis. Although definitive conclusions from large, well-designed, controlled, double-blind clinical trials is lacking at this time, the evidence thus far available strongly indicates a pattern of clinical efficacy and lack of adverse effects associated with such coordinated use. Monitoring of Hcy would be judicious with long-term use in at-risk patients.

Levodopa

Levodopa (L-dopa; Dopar, Larodopa); combination drugs: levodopa and benserazide (co-beneldopa; Madopar); levodopa and carbidopa (Atamet, Parcopa, Sinemet, Sinemet CR); levodopa, carbidopa, and entacapone (Stalevo).

Interaction Type and Significance

✗✗   **Minimal to Mild Adverse Interaction—Vigilance Necessary**

✗✗✗   **Potentially Harmful or Serious Adverse Interaction—Avoid**

⊕✗   **Bimodal or Variable Interaction, with Professional Management**

⊕⊕   **Beneficial or Supportive Interaction, with Professional Management**

Probability: Evidence Base:
4. Plausible to **2. Probable**   ◉ **Emerging**

Effect and Mechanism of Action

Depletion of dopamine in the striatum of the brain plays a central role in the symptoms of Parkinson's disease. As a dopamine precursor, levodopa is able to cross the blood-brain barrier (BBB) to enter the CNS. After being decarboxylated to dopamine in the basal ganglia, L-dopa is able to replenish depleted dopamine stores and provide symptomatic relief. Methionine may diminish the therapeutic effect of levodopa through a mechanism that has not yet been elucidated but likely to involve S-adenosylmethionine, a methyl-activated metabolite of methionine.

Amino acids (in high-protein foods or as supplements) may compete with levodopa for transport across the BBB and thereby interfere with the drug's therapeutic activity.[8]

S-adenosylmethionine (SAMe) is a key metabolic contributor to the recycling of Hcy. Methylation of multiple intracellular molecules, including nucleic acids and proteins, uses SAMe as the donor, which is converted to S-adenosylhomocysteine

(SAH), which in turn is in equilibrium with Hcy. The regeneration of methionine, the precursor of SAMe, occurs in neurons exclusively through methionine synthase, which requires methyl-THF aznd vitamin B$_{12}$. Additionally, vitamin B$_6$ deficiency results in total-Hcy elevation by preventing the conversion by cystathionine synthase of Hcy to cystathionine.

Research

The use of methionine in patients with Parkinson's disease potentially presents both problems and opportunities as a component of an integrative therapeutic strategy and when used concomitantly with levodopa. Administration of L-methionine may benefit individuals with Parkinson's disease.[9,10] However, the available evidence is preliminary, contradictory, and unclear. In a preliminary clinical trial involving 15 patients who had obtained maximal improvement from L-dopa, carbidopa-levodopa, and/or anticholinergic compounds, Smythies and Halsey[10] found that 10 exhibited improvement on all measures except tremor and drooling when administered methionine (500 mg with 25 mg pyridoxine), starting at 1 g daily and gradually increasing to 5 g daily over 3 weeks. The authors cautioned that such nutrient therapy "should be avoided by patients on L-dopa or Sinemet." In a randomized, double-blind clinical trial lasting 8 days, Pearce and Waterbury[11] administered 4.5 g methionine daily or placebo to 14 Parkinson's patients who were clinically stable after at least 3 months of levodopa therapy (1.5-5.5 g/day); all subjects were restricted to 0.5 g/day dietary methionine. Concomitant methionine decreased the therapeutic effects of levodopa and exacerbated related symptoms, such as gait disturbances, increased tremor, and rigidity. The adverse effects disappeared when methionine was discontinued, although one patient declined to a state worse than at the study onset and required 7 to 10 days to recover fully. These preliminary findings suggest that high dosage levels of methionine ($\geq$ 4.5 g/day) may interfere with the therapeutic effects of levodopa, whereas lower doses may be compatible. The short duration of these studies limits the ability to extrapolate these findings over a longer period because of inability to assess whether symptoms would continue to worsen or might be modified by physiological adaptation over time.

In a clinical trial involving six children with dopamine deficiency, Surtees and Hyland[12] demonstrated that elevating levodopa concentrations in the CNS caused a fall in cerebrospinal fluid (CSF) SAMe concentration and a rise in CSF 3-methoxytyrosine concentration. No change was observed in CSF methionine concentration, and all patients had normal CSF 5-methyl-THF concentration. These findings suggest that levodopa depletes SAMe in the CNS and may also disrupt the homeostatic regulation of Hcy.

Parkinson's patients treated with levodopa often develop elevated plasma Hcy.[13-16] Levodopa metabolism via catechol-O-methyltransferase increases levels of the neurotoxin Hcy, which induces an axonal-accentuated degeneration in sensory peripheral nerves in vitro.[16] This pattern of drug-related elevation in plasma Hcy suggests at least one major factor in developing an understanding of the increased mortality caused by vascular disease in individuals diagnosed with Parkinson's disease.

Nutritional Therapeutics, Clinical Concerns, and Adaptations

The available evidence can be reasonably interpreted to suggest that physicians treating individuals with Parkinson's disease consider prescribing methionine at doses of 500 to 1000 mg daily, i.e., within the common range, for its possible benefits without introducing significant risk of interfering with the therapeutic activity of levodopa (or levodopa/carbidopa). In cases where methionine administration may be indicated, it is essential to monitor for reduced therapeutic effect of levodopa given the potential that methionine may inhibit levodopa's antiparkinsonian effects, especially at doses of 4.5 g/day or higher. In the event of an adverse interaction, the severity is generally moderate; the rate of onset is unknown. Given the well-established risk of elevated Hcy in such cases, health care professionals treating individuals with Parkinson's disease receiving levodopa therapy are advised to coadminister folate and vitamin B_{12}, both of which help recycle Hcy, as well as monitor fasting plasma Hcy levels.

Furthermore, concomitant tyrosine, phenylalanine, and tryptophan should be considered because levodopa can interfere with absorption of these three amino acids, thereby inducing deficiency. Notably, L-tyrosine is a direct precursor to levodopa. However, although concomitant therapy with L-tyrosine, L-phenylalanine, and L-tryptophan may be beneficial, intake needs to be separated from L-dopa by at least 2 hours because these amino acids can compete with L-dopa for absorption.

THEORETICAL, SPECULATIVE, AND PRELIMINARY INTERACTIONS RESEARCH, INCLUDING OVERSTATED INTERACTIONS CLAIMS

Vidarabine

Evidence: Vidarabine (Ara-A, arabinoside; Vira-A).
Similar properties but evidence lacking for extrapolation: Related nucleoside antivirals.

The most common use of vidarabine is as an ophthalmic preparation for the treatment of herpes simplex virus type 1 (HSV-1) and type 2 (HSV-2) in acute keratoconjunctivitis and recurrent superficial keratitis. The therapeutic action of vidarabine is achieved by interfering with viral DNA synthesis, specifically inhibition of S-adenosylhomocysteine hydrolase (SAH), methionine synthesis, and SAMe-dependent DNA methylation.[17-19] Vidarabine cannot be given orally because it is metabolized in the gut, so it is usually administered intravenously or topically.

The action of vidarabine indicates a potential risk for interfering with methionine function in humans and potentially inducing a depletion of methionine with extended use. Any such depleting effect on methionine status is likely to be gradual and cumulative, but evidence from human trials is lacking. Concomitant administration of methionine (or SAMe) could theoretically interfere with the therapeutic activity of vidarabine or related antiviral medications.

It has long been established that vidarabine is known to interfere with methionine synthesis, although recent and substantial research is lacking.[17,18] Human studies are lacking to determine whether vidarabine might induce clinically significant methionine depletion or whether methionine administration might interfere with the medication's antiviral activity. Further research is warranted.

Physicians prescribing vidarabine for an extended period are advised to discuss options for countering the potential adverse effects of this medication. Some nutritionally oriented

physicians have found value in monitoring serum methionine in their patients taking vidarabine. Close monitoring is warranted in cases where methionine administration is indicated so as to prevent potential reduction of drug efficacy.

NUTRIENT-NUTRIENT INTERACTIONS

Antioxidants

As with other antioxidants, methionine may work synergistically to produce an antioxidant network effect. In a small but well-controlled trial, Uden et al.[20] found that 2 g/day methionine in combination with several antioxidants reduced pain and recurrent attacks of pancreatitis in patients with chronic recurring pancreatitis. In a 20-week, double-blind, double-dummy crossover trial, these researchers provided treatment as two types of tablets containing daily doses of 600 µg organic selenium, 9000 IU beta-carotene, 0.54 g vitamin C, 270 IU vitamin E, and 2 g methionine. Of the 20 patients who adhered to the full protocol, six experienced an attack while on the placebo phase of the crossover trial, compared with none while on the active-treatment phase. Despite the small number of patients in the trial, these results were statistically significant in favor of the antioxidant phase, indicating that this is a large effect. Larger trials would be warranted for this difficult-to-manage clinical problem.

Folate, Vitamin B_6, and Vitamin B_{12}

Methionine works synergistically with folate, vitamin B_6, and vitamin B_{12} in the management of homocysteine (Hcy) and in regulating the relationships and facilitating the functions of these interconnected nutrients.

Animal studies suggest that, in the presence of B-vitamin deficiencies, high dietary intake of methionine may produce hypercholesterolemia and hyperhomocysteinemia, thereby elevating risk for atherosclerosis.[1] These observations have not been directly confirmed by human trials. However, McAuley et al.[7] found that 7 g methionine daily (i.e., megadoses) can elevate blood levels of Hcy in the absence of a deficiency of folic acid, B_6, or B_{12}.

Carmel et al.[21] studied Hcy metabolism in 22 patients with pernicious anemia (vitamin B_{12} deficiency). They found that only levels of total Hcy and cysteine were increased and only glutathione (glutamyl-cysteinyl-glycine) was decreased in cobalamin deficiency as a whole, compared with 17 control subjects. SAMe levels correlated only with methionine levels and cysteine levels only with cysteinylglycine in healthy subjects, but in cobalamin-deficient patients, SAMe correlated instead with cysteine, cysteinylglycine, and folate levels only. Significant differences appeared in clinically subgrouped cobalamin-deficient patients. The 11 B_{12}-deficient patients with neurological damage had higher mean levels of folate, SAMe, cysteine, and cysteinylglycine than did the 11 neurologically unaffected, B_{12}-deficient patients. In all patients, cobalamin therapy restored metabolic changes to normal.

The 21 citations for this monograph, as well as additional reference literature, are located under Methionine on the CD at the back of the book.

Phenylalanine

Nutrient Name: Phenylalanine.
Synonyms: DL-Phenylalanine (DLPA), D-phenylalanine (DPA), L-phenylalanine (LPA).
Related Substances: Tyrosine, aspartame.

Summary

Drug/Class Interaction Type	Mechanism and Significance	Management
Baclofen ◇◇	Baclofen intestinal transport is mediated, at least in part, by beta-, gamma-, and alpha-amino acid carriers and may be reduced by phenylalanine. Clinical significance uncertain.	Avoid simultaneous intake of baclofen with phenylalanine or even with high-protein meal.
Levodopa (L-dopa) ✗✗/◇◇/⊕✗/⊕	Levodopa and phenylalanine (alone or in high-protein foods) may compete for CNS transport when taken concomitantly and thereby reduce drug activity. Conversely, phenylalanine is precursor of L-tyrosine and thus L-dopa. Relative influence of countervailing factors may depend on baseline values, timing of administration, and other factors. Clinical significance uncertain. Long-term, well-designed clinical trials are warranted.	Coadministration, possibly with intake separated by several hours, may be beneficial with proper monitoring and management.
Methadone, morphine Oral narcotic analgesics, opiates ✗/⊕✗/⊕⊕	D-Phenylalanine (DPA) may increase circulating enkephalin levels by inhibiting breakdown of enkephalinase. Coadministration may enhance analgesic effect by this mechanism and by direct analgesic action of DPA. Adverse effects improbable. Well-designed clinical trials are warranted to investigate coadministration in treatment of chronic pain.	Coadministration may be beneficial with close monitoring and active management.
Naloxone ◇/✗✗/⊕✗	Naloxone may inhibit D-phenylalanine's analgesic effect.	Avoid concomitant use. Consider alternate options to phenylalanine for analgesia if naloxone is necessary.
Phenothiazine Butyrophenone neuroleptics Typical antipsychotics ✗✗✗	Exogenous phenylalanine could theoretically elevate levels of dopamine and other tyrosine-derived neurotransmitters. Concomitant administration with neuroleptics might increase risk of drug-induced tardive dyskinesia.	Avoid concomitant intake. Monitor closely if both agents determined to be appropriate and necessary.
Selegiline Monoamine oxidase (MAO-B) inhibitors ✗/⊕✗/⊕⊕	D-Phenylalanine (or LPA) can be converted to phenylethylamine and contribute to enhanced response when used concomitantly with selegiline. L-Phenylalanine (or DPA) could theoretically be converted to L-tyrosine and induce excessive levels of tyrosine and dopamine in presence of MAO-B inhibitor. Adverse effects improbable. Well-designed clinical trials are warranted to investigate safety and efficacy of coadministration.	Coadministration of DPA or DLPA may be beneficial with close monitoring and active management. MAO-B inhibitor dosage may need to be reduced.

CNS, Central nervous system.

NUTRIENT DESCRIPTION
Chemistry and Forms

L-Phenylalanine and DL-phenylalanine (DLPA) are the commercially available forms of phenylalanine. However, phenylalanine appears in the following three chemical forms:

L-Phenylalanine, the form of phenylalanine that occurs naturally in proteins within the human body.
D-Phenylalanine, a synthetic mirror image of L-phenylalanine.
DL-Phenylalanine, a synthesized racemic mixture of L-phenylalanine and D-phenylalanine.

Physiology and Function

L-Phenylalanine is an essential amino acid that serves as a precursor in the biosynthesis of other amino acids including L-tyrosine. It plays a critical role in related biochemical processes involving the synthesis of several important neurotransmitters, principally L-dopa, dopamine, epinephrine, and norepinephrine, as well as thyroxine and melanin. Through a different metabolic pathway, L-phenylalanine can also be converted to phenylethylamine (PEA). Phenylethylamine is a naturally occurring substance in the brain that appears to exert stimulant effects and elevate mood. It also influences the synthesis of many important brain neuropeptides, including vasopressin, adrenocorticotropic hormone (ACTH), somatostatin, enkephalin, and angiotensin II. Together with tryptophan, phenylalanine governs the release of the intestinal hormone cholecystokinin (CCK).

Hepatic conversion of phenylalanine to tyrosine can be impaired during infection, trauma, chronic illness, liver disease, or other forms of severe stress; thus making tyrosine a conditionally essential amino acid.

Because D-phenylalanine does not occur naturally, it cannot be converted to L-tyrosine, L-dopa, or norepinephrine and, when ingested, is primarily converted to phenylethylamine. D-Phenylalanine can increase levels of enkephalins by blocking enkephalinase, thereby inhibiting the breakdown of these opiate-like substances in the brain. This analgesic effect of D-phenylalanine is inhibited by naloxone.

DL-Phenylalanine does not occur naturally in the human body.

NUTRIENT IN CLINICAL PRACTICE
Known or Potential Therapeutic Uses

Therapeutically, phenylalanine is primarily known for its proposed antidepressant and analgesic effects. Thus far clinical trials of various design, power and clinical relevance have resulted in mixed results. DLPA should be taken only under medical supervision because of its strong effects on neurotransmitters, mood, and central nervous system (CNS) function. It is generally recommended that phenylalanine be taken 15 to 30 minutes before meals to avoid competition from protein-derived amino acids.

Historical/Ethnomedicine Precedent

Phenylalanine has not been used historically as an isolated nutrient.

Possible Uses

Clinical application varies according to form.

L-Phenylalanine: Appetite suppression, depression, vitiligo.
D-Phenylalanine: Depression, osteoarthritis, Parkinson's disease, rheumatoid arthritis, and pain from a variety of causes, such as chronic back pain, dental pain, menstrual cramps, and migraines.
DLPA: Alcohol withdrawal, depression, osteoarthritis, rheumatoid arthritis, and pain from a variety of causes (from action of D-phenylalanine).

Deficiency Symptoms

Frank phenylalanine deficiency is considered a very uncommon occurrence, and the potential for deficiency is primarily associated with very low protein intake. Typical symptoms of phenylalanine deficiency include fatigue, confusion, behavioral changes, decreased alertness, impaired memory, poor vascular health, eye disorders (e.g., bloodshot eyes, cataracts), changes in appetite, and weight gain.

Dietary Sources

Cheese and meats are the richest dietary sources of phenylalanine, with most protein-containing foods providing some L-phenylalanine, for example, beef, poultry, pork, fish, milk, yogurt, cheese, eggs, soy products (including tofu, soy flour, and soy protein isolate), and certain nuts and seeds.

D-Phenylalanine does not naturally occur in foods.

Aspartame (L-aspartyl-L-phenylalanine methyl ester) is a synthesized dipeptide, composed of aspartic acid and phenylalanine as the methyl ester. It is marketed as an ingredient in food products as NutraSweet and as an artificial sweetener (Equal).

Nutrient Preparations Available

Phenylalanine should generally be administered in the L-phenylalanine form, the naturally occurring isomer, as the preferred form in the treatment of all conditions other than pain and depression. In the treatment of these conditions, particularly chronic pain, D-phenylalanine exhibits unique activity in the CNS/brain and thus makes a critical contribution as part of DLPA. Thus, many health care professionals trained and experienced in nutritional therapeutics might suggest that DLPA is perhaps the only amino acid where the racemic mix is often clinically effective, or even preferable, in contrast to most amino acids, where the naturally occurring L-isomer is strongly if not exclusively recommended.

Dosage Forms Available

Capsule, powder, tablet; topical cream.

Source Materials for Nutrient Preparations

L-Phenylalanine is commercially produced by a bacterial fermentation process. DLPA and D-phenylalanine are synthesized.

Dosage Range

Adult

Dietary: Recommended dietary allowance (RDA): 14 mg per kg body weight per day, or about 1 g for a 70-kg adult.
Supplemental/Maintenance: Usually not necessary. Optimal levels of intake have not been established.
Pharmacological/Therapeutic: L-Phenylalanine is usually provided in doses of 500 mg, typically taken one to three times daily, preferably between meals. Doses of 100 to 200 mg daily are often used in the treatment of depression. The dosage range in most cases is 750 to 3000 mg daily for adults. Doses as high as 50 to 100 mg/kg have been used in studies of those with *vitiligo,* an autoimmune process in which melanocytes are destroyed, resulting in patches of depigmented skin.

DL-Phenylalanine (DLPA) is the most common form of phenylalanine used as a nutraceutical, typically in dosages ranging from 75 mg to 1500 mg daily. DLPA is 50% D-phenylalanine and 50% L-phenylalanine and generally comes in capsules containing 375 to 750 mg. One to two capsules are usually taken in the morning on waking, preferably on an empty stomach. Doses used in research on pain relief were 4 g before an acute painful episode, such as surgery, or 500 mg three times daily for chronic pain.
Toxic: The maximum safe dosage level of phenylalanine, in any form, has not been established. Doses in excess of 1500 mg/day may produce adverse effects.
Experienced practitioners of nutritional medicine generally caution that dosages of various forms of phenylalanine should never exceed 2400 mg/day. Concern has also been raised that prolonged use of any D-isomer amino acid may eventually exert a toxic effect.

Pediatric (< 18 Years)

Dietary: RDA (recommended dietary allowances):

Birth to 4 months: 125 mg/kg/day
5 months to 2 years: 69 mg/kg/day
3 to 12 years: 22 mg/kg/day
Adolescents, 14 to 18 years: 14 mg/kg/day

Supplemental/Maintenance: Not currently recommended for children.
Pharmacological/Therapeutic: Specific treatment recommendations have not established.
Toxic: No toxic dosage level established specifically for infants and children.

Laboratory Values

Serum or Plasma Phenylalanine
Range of normal levels for plasma phenylalanine:

Children: 26 to 86 μmol/L
Adults: 41 to 68 μmol/L

SAFETY PROFILE
Overview

L-Phenylalanine and DLPA are generally considered safe in most individuals at usual dosage levels. Some sources caution that DLPA should be taken only under medical supervision because of its potentially strong effects on neurotransmitters, mood, and CNS function. Although no serious adverse effects have been reported in humans taking phenylalanine, dosage levels greater than 1500 mg/day should be supervised by a health care professional trained and experienced in nutritional therapeutics.

Nutrient Adverse Effects
General Adverse Effects (Adults)

L-Phenylalanine. Animal studies have reported toxicity symptoms at dosage levels of 100 mg/kg or more. Burkhart and Burkhart,[1] two leading phenylalanine researchers, have expressed concerns about potential toxicity with high-dosage administration in humans.

DL-Phenylalanine. The maximum safe dosage level of DLPA is unknown. Within clinical trials 1500 mg/day or less of DLPA has not induced consistent toxicity in healthy subjects. Some researchers and clinicians have reported occasional anxiety, nausea, dyspepsia, and transient headaches. Cautions regarding LPA are most likely equally applicable to DLPA.

Adverse Effects Among Specific Populations

Phenylketonuria. Phenylketonuria (PKU) is an inherited error of metabolism caused by a deficiency in the enzyme phenylalanine hydroxylase (PAH; phenylalanine 4-monoxygenase). PAH utilizes tetrahydrobiopterin to convert phenylalanine into tyrosine, a critical step in dopamine biosynthesis. Loss of this enzyme results in mental retardation, organ damage, and unusual posture and in cases of maternal PKU, can severely compromise pregnancy as a result of the accumulation of phenylalanine and its neurotoxic metabolites. Classic PKU is an autosomal recessive disorder, caused by mutations in both alleles of the gene for PAH, found on chromosome 12. Mild hyperphenylalaninemia (phenylketonuria II) is a phenotypically mild form of PKU that will predominate when the individual is heterozygous for the two mutations of PAH.

In the United States, standards of practice mandate that newborns be tested for PKU during the initial 48 to 72 hours after delivery. If not diagnosed and treated before 3 weeks of age, PKU can cause severe, irreversible mental retardation.

Prudence suggests that high blood levels of phenylalanine (and tyrosine) be avoided in individuals with severe liver disease; such elevation may contribute to encephalopathy, mental impairment, and coma.

Pregnancy and Nursing

Phenylalanine is generally contraindicated because of potential adverse effects on the fetus.

Evidence is lacking in the scientific literature to suggest or confirm any adverse effects related to fetal development during pregnancy or to infants who are breast-fed associated with phenylalanine administration.

Infants and Children

Testing for PKU is critical before any administration. Otherwise, no adverse effects have been reported. However, sufficient research-based evidence is lacking to guarantee the safety of phenylalanine in infants and children.

Contraindications

Phenylalanine should not be taken by phenylketonuric individuals because they lack the enzyme necessary to metabolize phenylalanine.

Exogenous phenylalanine is generally considered contraindicated during pregnancy or while nursing.

Phenylalanine should be used with caution by people with hypertension; it may raise blood pressure in some individuals.

Phenylalanine (and tyrosine) should be avoided by individuals with cancer, especially pigmented melanoma.

Use of phenylalanine may be contraindicated for individuals with hyperthyroidism or schizophrenia, particularly when high dopamine levels are present in the brain. Exogenous phenylalanine (or tyrosine) administration could theoretically result in elevated brain dopamine levels and symptom aggravation.

Precautions and Warnings

L-Phenylalanine should not be taken with foods high in protein because it competes with other amino acids for a position on the same amino acid carrier.

Avoid concomitant administration of phenylalanine and tyrosine because of potential additive effects.

Some derivative sources suggest that phenylalanine should be avoided by individuals taking monoamine oxidase (MAO) inhibitors, presumably because of L-phenylalanine's role in synthesis of dopamine, norepinephrine, and epinephrine. However, this potential for an adverse interaction has not been substantiated by clinical studies; in fact, some research points to synergistic value of such a combination at appropriate dosage levels.

The use of phenylalanine-containing aspartame by individuals with Parkinson's disease is the subject of ongoing controversy. Ingestion of aspartame, the artificial sweetener, may induce a rapid increase in brain levels of phenylalanine. Aspartame is generally contraindicated in individuals with phenylketonuria (PKU). Statements implying that aspartame is "safe" in Parkinson's disease patients derive solely from a single-day, poorly designed study by Karstaedt and Pincus[2] involving 16 levodopa-treated patients with Parkinson's disease. Some clinicians and researchers have suggested that aspartame may be contraindicated in such individuals because of potential for rapid elevation of phenylalanine and effect on levodopa levels. Long-term, independent clinical trials are lacking.

INTERACTIONS REVIEW
Strategic Considerations

Management of *chronic pain* may constitute the most common use of phenylalanine in conventional medicine and the professional practice of natural therapeutics. Several trials of varying design quality, size, and power have been conducted with mixed findings.[3,4] Two preliminary studies suggest possible analgesic action of D-phenylalanine.[5,6] In contrast, Walsh and other researchers at the University of Texas published two critical articles. They noted potentially flawed design in a letter challenging the hypothesis of D-phenylalanine analgesic action via mediation of opiate receptors.[7] In a double-blind trial, they reported that using D-phenylalanine (250 mg four times daily) for 4 weeks was no more effective than placebo for 30 people with various types of chronic pain, including 13 individuals with low back pain.[8] That use of phenylalanine as pharmacological monotherapy is not representative of its application by health care professionals trained and experienced in nutritional therapeutics.

In a small, two-part, placebo-controlled clinical trial more relevant to typical integrative approaches, Kitade et al.[9] hypothesized that D-phenylalanine (DPA) might prolong analgesia induced by acupuncture through its known activity of blocking carboxypeptidase, an enzyme that degrades enkephalins (endogenous neuropeptides that bind to opiate receptors in the CNS). This team of Japanese researchers administered DPA (4 g/day) to individuals with chronic low back pain half an hour before they received acupuncture. The results were good or excellent for 18 of the 30, but not statistically significant because of small sample size. These researchers arrived at a similar conclusion when tooth extraction was performed on 56 patients under acupuncture anesthesia, with 18 subjects receiving 4.0 g DPA orally 30 minutes before treatment and 38 given placebo. These researchers also found that the combined DPA-acupuncture effect was slightly better when DPA was given on the previous day in three 0.5-g doses than a single 4-g dose administered 30 minutes before treatment.

The coadministration of DPA and conventional analgesics represents an integrative approach to care that warrants further research. DL-Phenylalanine (DLPA) is the most common form of phenylalanine administered for pain relief by health care professionals, at a typical dose of 1500 to 2500 mg per day. Further research employing placebo-controlled double-blind pain studies, as well as outcomes-based research for assessing multidisciplinary interventions, is warranted to evaluate the efficacy of phenylalanine in the treatment of pain syndromes and to determine dosage levels, synergies, and other aspects of therapeutic protocols for its effective integration into clinical care models.

Although not conclusively established by large, well-designed human trials, a solid theoretical foundation, broad anecdotal reports, and numerous preliminary studies suggest therapeutic benefit in using phenylalanine as part of a comprehensive therapy for depression. Administration of L- or DL-phenylalanine alone, with other nutrients, or with conventional medications and psychotherapy, can support healthy neurotransmitter levels by enhancing production of dopamine and norepinephrine. Health care professionals treating individuals diagnosed with depression are advised to query patients about self-medication; present evidence-based options for integrative therapies employing exercise, dietary changes, nutrient coadministration, botanical medicine, acupuncture, stress resilience training, and other appropriate therapies; and offer support in the form of supervision, monitoring, and collaboration with other health care providers.

Tardive dyskinesia (TD), a condition characterized by unusual, uncontrollable body movements, was first brought to the attention of the medical community in 1973 by Crane.[10] Since then, clinicians and researchers have studied this largely irreversible and untreatable neurological disorder in patients receiving long-term neuroleptic agents. In 1992 the American Psychiatric Association estimated that TD occurs in at least 5% of patients taking certain antipsychotic medications annually. Within 3 years, 15% of these patients develop TD, and its prevalence often exceeds 50% of all patients in long-term antipsychotic medication studies. The disease affects children and adults of all ages, with higher rates among older populations. In a controlled study, Yassa et al.[11] found that 41% of patients age 65 and older developed TD within 24 months. It is estimated that TD could affect as many as 1 million Americans. Concomitant use of conventional

antipsychotic medications and phenylalanine, a dopamine precursor, could theoretically increase the risk of developing neuroleptic-induced TD by elevating levels of dopamine, norepinephrine, and epinephrine. Phenylalanine supplementation, particularly when self-prescribed and unmonitored, should generally be avoided by individuals under treatment with antipsychotic agents, including phenothiazine and butyrophenone types and newer, atypical antipsychotic agents. In clinical trials, vitamin E has reduced the severity of TD, especially involuntary movements.[12,13] In a double-blind, placebo-controlled, crossover study, Lerner et al.[14] observed that coadministration of vitamin B$_6$ can control TD. Concomitant choline and lecithin may also reduce TD symptoms. Nutritional support can be therapeutically efficacious when appropriate to the individual being treated, strategically planned, and applied with monitoring within an integrative therapeutic framework.

The role of amino acid intake and therapeutics within integrative approaches to oncology is not well researched. Increased expression of various tyrosine kinase enzymes is key to growth and cell signaling in a wide variety of tumor types. A low-phenylalanine and low-tyrosine diet has shown some potential in limiting tumor growth in animal models. However, Harvie et al.[15] found that patients with advanced cancer do not appear to tolerate or accept such a diet. In a small pilot study involving 22 patients with advanced metastatic melanoma and 15 patients with metastatic breast cancer, the diet was restricted to 10 mg/kg/day each of phenylalanine and tyrosine in foods or supplements. Only three patients with metastatic melanoma and three with metastatic breast cancer agreed to start the diet. After 1 month, these researchers attempted to establish the effect of the diet on nutritional status; immune cell function; plasma levels of phenylalanine, tyrosine, and tryptophan; and quality of life, as measured by Hospital Anxiety and Depression scores. All the patients who followed the restricted diet reported adverse effects, particularly increases in anxiety and depression. Although slight increases in white cell counts and neutrophils were observed, patients on the diet also experienced declines in weight, with loss of fat and fat-free mass.

NUTRIENT-DRUG INTERACTIONS

Baclofen

Baclofen (Kemstro, Lioresal).

Interaction Type and Significance
◈◈   **Impaired Drug Absorption and Bioavailability, Precautions Appropriate**

Probability:
4. Plausible

Evidence Base:
○ **Preliminary**

Effect and Mechanism of Action
Baclofen is a skeletal muscle relaxant medicine that works by binding to gamma-aminobutyric acid type B (GABA-B) receptors in the CNS. Phenylalanine may reduce absorption of baclofen.

Research
In a series of experiments examining inhibition of baclofen absorption by beta-alanine, GABA, and leucine, a group of Spanish researchers found that baclofen intestinal transport was mediated, at least in part, by the beta-, gamma-, and

alpha-amino acid carriers.[16-21] Cejudo-Ferragud et al.[22] found that phenylalanine (up to 100 mM) decreased the absorption of isotonic perfusion solutions of baclofen (0.5 mM) by 67% in situ in rat small intestines.

Nutritional Therapeutics, Clinical Concerns, and Adaptations

Physicians prescribing baclofen should advise patients to avoid intake of phenylalanine or even a meal high in protein content 2 hours before or 4 hours after medication to prevent impaired drug absorption.

Levodopa

Levodopa (L-dopa; Dopar, Larodopa); combination drugs: levodopa and benserazide (co-beneldopa; Madopar); levodopa and carbidopa (Atamet, Parcopa, Sinemet, Sinemet CR); levodopa, carbidopa, and entacapone (Stalevo).

Interaction Type and Significance

✗✗　　Minimal to Mild Adverse Interaction—Vigilance Necessary

◇◇　　Impaired Drug Absorption and Bioavailability, Precautions Appropriate

⊕✗　　Bimodal or Variable Interaction, with Professional Management

⊕　　　Potential or Theoretical Beneficial or Supportive Interaction, With Professional Management

Probability:　　　　　　Evidence Base:
4. Plausible　　　　　　○ Preliminary

Effect and Mechanism of Action

Concomitant intake of amino acids as supplements or high-protein food may result in competition within CNS transport systems between levodopa and these nutrients, including phenylalanine.[23] Because phenylalanine is a precursor of L-tyrosine, a semi-essential amino acid that converts to L-dopa, an additive effect may occur with coadministration. The relative effect of these two influences has not been established and could be significantly altered by other variables, such as patient characteristics, baseline levels, and substance intake.

Research

High intake and elevated blood levels of amino acids, especially hyperphenylalaninemia, could induce blockade of the therapeutic effects of levodopa. In animal experiments, Wade and Katzman[24] observed that the large, neutral amino acid phenylalanine and L-dopa share a transport system into the brain. Consequently, researchers and clinicians assume that L-dopa levels in the brain would be inversely related to plasma neutral amino acid levels. In subsequent research, Nutt, Woodward, et al.[25] attributed the oscillating clinical response (the "on-off" phenomenon) seen in Parkinson's patients receiving L-dopa therapy to interference with absorption of levodopa by dietary amino acids and competition between large, neutral amino acids and levodopa for transport from plasma into the brain. They report that "bypassing absorption by constant infusion of the drug produced a stable clinical state lasting for twelve hours in all of six patients and for up to 36 hours in some. High-protein meals or oral phenylalanine, leucine, or isoleucine (100 mg per kilogram of body weight) reversed the therapeutic effect of infused levodopa without reducing plasma levodopa concentrations. Glycine and lysine at identical doses had no effect." In a subsequent clinical trial, these researchers[26] monitored the motor response and plasma and ventricular

cerebrospinal fluid (CSF) concentrations of L-dopa during intravenous (IV) infusions of L-dopa in two patients with advanced Parkinson's disease. They first observed that concentrations of L-dopa in ventricular CSF mirrored, but lagged behind, those in plasma. Then, during IV infusions of L-dopa following oral administration of phenylalanine, they noted that the duration of the motor response was greatly attenuated despite undiminished ventricular CSF levels of L-dopa. These researchers interpreted these findings to suggest that either L-dopa entry into ventricular CSF and the brain are "differentially affected by phenylalanine or that phenylalanine affects other steps in the motor response."

Nutritional Therapeutics, Clinical Concerns, and Adaptations

Physicians prescribing levodopa are advised to be aware of the possible responses to phenylalanine intake and their potential clinical implications. On the one hand, increased intake of phenylalanine (or L-tyrosine) might augment L-dopa levels. This potential additive response could be beneficial or detrimental depending on resultant levels, patient response, and clinical management. On the other hand, the simultaneous ingestion of phenylalanine and related amino acids, especially leucine and isoleucine, could interfere with levodopa pharmacokinetics and diminish its therapeutic effects.

The use of phenylalanine (or tyrosine) along with levodopa may represent a valuable integrative approach to the treatment of individuals with Parkinson's disease. Close monitoring of L-dopa levels is essential in cases where a therapeutic trial of such coadministration appears appropriate. Furthermore, administration of the two amino acids should be separated by at least 2 hours before or 4 hours after the medication to minimize risk of interference with absorption and transport and enhance endogenous L-dopa synthesis. Further research with well-designed, long-term clinical trials is warranted.

Methadone, Morphine, and Related Oral Narcotic Analgesics (Opiates)

Butorphanol (Stadol, Stadol NS), codeine sulfate, fentanyl (Actiq Oral Transmucosal, Duragesic Transdermal, Fentanyl Oralet, Sublimaze Injection), hydrocodone, hydromorphone (Dilaudid), levorphanol (Levo-Dromoran), meperidine (Demerol), methadone (Dolophine, Methadose), methadone hydrochloride (Dolophine, Methadose), morphine sulfate (Astramorph PF, Avinza, Duramorph, Infumorph, Kadian, MS Contin, MSIR, Oramorph SR, RMS, Roxanol, Roxanol Rescudose, Roxanol T), opium tincture, oxycodone (Endocodone, OxyContin, OxyIR, Percolone, Roxicodone), oxymorphone (Numorphan), paregoric, pentazocine (Talwin, Talwin NX), propoxyphene (Darvon; Darvon-N).
Combination drugs: Buprenorphine and naloxone (Suboxone); codeine and acetaminophen (Capital and Codeine; Phenaphen with Codeine; Tylenol with Codeine); codeine and acetylsalicylic acid (Empirin with codeine); codeine, acetylsalicylic acid, caffeine, and butalbital (Fiorinal); codeine, acetaminophen, caffeine, and butalbital (Fioricet); hydrocodone and acetaminophen (Anexsia, Anodynos-DHC, Co-Gesic, Dolacet, DuoCet, Hydrocet, Hydrogesic, Hy-Phen, Lorcet 10/650, Lorcet-HD, Lorcet Plus, Lortab, Margesic H, Medipain 5, Norco, Stagesic, T-Gesic, Vicodin, Vicodin ES, Vicodin HP, Zydone); hydrocodone and acetylsalicylic acid(Lortab ASA); hydrocodone and ibuprofen (Reprexain, Vicoprofen); opium and belladonna (B&O Supprettes); oxycodone and acetaminophen (Endocet, Percocet 2.5/325, Percocet 5/325, Percocet

7.5/500, Percocet 10/650, Roxicet 5/500, Roxilox, Tylox); oxycodone and acetylsalicylic acid (Endodan, Percodan, Percodan-Demi); pentazocine and acetaminophen (Talacen); pentazocine and acetylsalicylic acid (Talwin Compound); propoxyphene and acetaminophen (Darvocet-N, Darvocet-N 100, Pronap-100, Propacet 100, Propoxacet-N, Wygesic); propoxyphene and acetylsalicylic acid (Bexophene, Darvon Compound-65 Pulvules, PC-Cap); propoxyphene, acetylsalicylic acid, and caffeine (Darvon Compound).

Interaction Type and Significance

✗   **Potential or Theoretical Adverse Interaction of Uncertain Severity**
⊕✗   **Bimodal or Variable Interaction, with Professional Management**
⊕⊕   **Beneficial or Supportive Interaction, with Professional Management**

Probability:	Evidence Base:
2. Probable	○ **Preliminary**

Effect and Mechanism of Action

D-Phenylalanine (DPA) can limit the activity of enkephalinase, thereby inhibiting the breakdown of and increasing circulating levels of enkephalins, the endogenous neuropeptides with opiate-like activity in the brain.[4,27] Concomitant administration of opiate agent(s) and DPA could potentially produce an additive or synergistic effect as a result of DPA's effects on endogenous neurotransmitters and exogenous opiates. An adverse interaction is improbable because endorphins (i.e., enkephalins) do not suppress respiration; they would only potentiate the analgesic activity of opiates. Although premised on reasonable pharmacological principles, such interpretations are of necessity speculative, given the paucity of documented clinical data.

Research

Dove et al.[28] have conducted a series of animal experiments investigating the analgesic activity of DPA. In a mouse model, they determined that DPA produces dose-dependent analgesic effects, similar to well-established nonnarcotic analgesics, but with action significantly longer in duration. In rats they observed neither a tolerance to DPA after administration for 10 days, nor a development of drug dependence after treatment for 6 weeks. These researchers also reported that the analgesic action of DPA "has been demonstrated in hot-plate tests on mice that combining D-Phe with narcotic analgesics already with doses inactive on separate application." They observed that dosage of morphine could be reduced by half when combined with DPA, without reducing analgesic activity in rats. After 6 weeks of treatment, this combination "markedly lowered" typical adverse drug effects such as "dependence, behavioural disorders and growth retardation."[29]

In a review article, Russell and McCarty[30] discussed the activity of DL-phenylalanine (DLPA) greatly potentiating opiate analgesia as an example of "nutrient/pharmaceutical up-regulation of the endogenous analgesia system." Most available research indicates that the dosage of phenylalanine (DPA or DLPA) necessary for analgesic effect gradually declines over time with continued use.[3]

Nutritional Therapeutics, Clinical Concerns, and Adaptations

The administration of D-phenylalanine in conjunction with narcotic medications can be considered a reasonable option for integrative approaches to analgesia, especially in the treatment of chronic pain. Closely monitored therapeutic trials may show a safe, effective intervention in the treatment of severe and recalcitrant pain, pending well-designed, larger clinical trials. Available evidence suggests that such concomitant therapy may enable reduced opiate dosage, reduced adverse effects, and lessened susceptibility to the development of drug tolerance.

Naloxone

Naloxone (Narcan).

Interaction Type and Significance

◈   **Adverse Drug Effect on Nutritional Therapeutics, Strategic Concern**
✗✗   **Minimal to Mild Adverse Interaction—Vigilance Necessary**
⊕✗   **Bimodal or Variable Interaction, with Professional Management**

Probability:	Evidence Base:
1. Certain	● **Consensus**

Effect and Mechanism of Action

Naloxone hydrochloride acts as an opioid antagonist. D-Phenylalanine can limit the activity of enkephalinase, thereby inhibiting the breakdown and increasing circulating levels of enkephalins.[4,27]

Research

The inhibition of D-phenylalanine's analgesic effect by naloxone has been well established within pharmacology and physiology.[27,30,31] Naloxone has been clearly shown to block placebo pain responses, which are mediated by endorphins/enkephalins. DLPA can exert a placebo effect as well as a physiological response.

Nutritional Therapeutics, Clinical Concerns, and Adaptations

Physicians: prescribing naloxone are advised to query patients as to whether they may also be using D- or DL-phenylalanine for pain relief. During use of naloxone, such patients experience reduced therapeutic efficacy of the nutrient.

Phenothiazine and Butyrophenone Typical Antipsychotic (Neuroleptic) Medications

Phenothiazines: Acetophenazine (Tindal), chlorpromazine (Largactil, Thorazine), fluphenazine (Modecate, Permitil, Prolixin, Prolixin Decanoate, Prolixin Enanthate), mesoridazine (Serentil), methotrimeprazine (levomepromazine; Nozinan), pericyazine (Neuleptil), perphenazine (Trilafon); combination drug: perphenazine and amitriptyline (Etrafon, Triavil, Triptazine); prochlorperazine (Compazine, Stemetil), promazine (Sparine), promethazine (Phenergan, Promacot, Promethegan), propiomazine (Largon), thiethylperazine (Torecan), thioproperazine (Majeptil), thioridazine (Mellaril), trifluoperazine (Stelazine), triflupromazine (Vesprin).
Butyrophenone neuroleptics: Benperidol (Anquil, Benperidol-neuraxpharm, Frenactil, Glianimon), droperidol (Dridol, Inapsine), haloperidol (Haldol), melperon (Buronil), triperidol (Trifluperidol).

Interaction Type and Significance

✗✗✗   **Potentially Harmful or Serious Adverse Interaction—Avoid**

Probability:
2. Probable

Evidence Base:
⊙ **Emerging**

Effect and Mechanism of Action

Concomitant use of phenylalanine, a dopamine precursor, could theoretically increase the risk of developing neuroleptic-induced tardive dyskinesia (TD) by elevating levels of dopamine, norepinephrine, and epinephrine.

Research

Gardos et al.[32] observed a statistically significant correlation between Abnormal Involuntary Movements Scale (AIMS) total scores and plasma phenylalanine levels subsequent to a loading dose of 100 mg/kg phenylalanine. These researchers concluded that abnormalities in phenylalanine metabolism may contribute to the development and severity of TD in some unipolar depressed patients treated with neuroleptic medications. In a double-blind, placebo-controlled clinical trial involving 18 male schizophrenic patients with TD, Mosnik et al.[33] found that challenge with 100 mg/kg phenylalanine significantly exacerbated involuntary movements compared with placebo. In a subsequent experiment involving 25 patients, Schultz et al.[34] studied the magnitude of induced abnormal movements to assess factors influencing exacerbation of TD before and after oral administration of a phenylalanine challenge drink. They observed that lower fasting levels of phenylalanine and the severity of abnormal movements at baseline predicted greater movements in response to phenylalanine influx. This suggests that measuring fasting amino acid levels might enable clinicians to predict differences in vulnerability to drug-induced effects.

Nutritional Therapeutics, Clinical Concerns, and Adaptations

Physicians prescribing haloperidol and related typical antipsychotic medications should advise patients to avoid consumption of supplemental phenylalanine and other isolated nutrients that may act as neurotransmitter precursors. Assessment of fasting amino acid levels might provide insight into risk of susceptibility to such exacerbation.

Selegiline, Phenylethylamine, and Monoamine Oxidase (MAO-B) Inhibitors

MAO-B inhibitors: Selegiline (deprenyl, L-deprenil, L-deprenyl; Atapryl, Carbex, Eldepryl, Jumex, Movergan, Selpak); pargyline (Eutonyl), rasagiline (Azilect).
Phenylethylamine (PEA)
See MAO-A inhibitors in Theoretical, Speculative, and Preliminary Interactions Research.

Interaction Type and Significance

✗　　　**Potential or Theoretical Adverse Interaction of Uncertain Severity**

⊕✗　　**Bimodal or Variable Interaction, with Professional Management**

⊕⊕　　**Beneficial or Supportive Interaction, with Professional Management**

Probability:
2. Probable

Evidence Base:
⊙ **Emerging** or
● **Consensus**

Effect and Mechanism of Action

Phenylalanine, particularly the D isomer (DPA), can be converted to phenylethylamine (PEA), an endogenous neuroamine that appears to elevate mood. Such coadministration might also produce a synergistic effect on neurotransmitter status in the treatment of individuals with depression and possibly Parkinson's disease.

Phenylalanine, particularly the L isomer, is also the precursor of tyrosine, and elevations in phenylalanine levels can increase levels of tyrosine. Increased tyrosine levels could raise monoamine neurotransmitters if monoamine oxidase (MAO), the enzyme that breaks down dopamine, norepinephrine, and other monoamines, is inhibited. As a result, the concomitant intake of MAO inhibitors and exogenous D- and/or L-phenylalanine could theoretically produce adverse effects associated with excessive tyrosine-derived neurotransmitters or DPA-derived PEA. This could result in a hypertensive crisis and the attendant risk of a heart attack or stroke.

Research

The coadministration of selegiline with D-phenylalanine, or PEA, may alleviate depression and improve mood. Such effects are sustained and have been noted in some patients who are unresponsive to conventional antidepressant treatment.[35] Phenylethylamine is an endogenous neuroamine that has been linked to the regulation of physical energy and attention, and high doses are known to produce significant mood-elevating effects, often compared to those of cocaine or methamphetamine. Investigators have found that PEA increases attention and activity in animals and has been shown to relieve depression in 60% of depressed patients, as demonstrated by urinary excretion of phenylacetic acid.[36] Several researchers have proposed that PEA deficit may be the cause of a common form of depressive illness.[37]

Phenylethylamine can be synthesized from both D-phenylalanine and L-phenylalanine. With L-phenylalanine being preferentially converted to L-tyrosine, the direct conversion to PEA makes D-phenylalanine the preferred substrate for increasing the synthesis of PEA. Normally, MAO-B selectively metabolizes phenylethylamine to phenylacetic acid. 2-Phenylethylamine is a metabolite of the MAO inhibitor antidepressant phenelzine, and concentrations of PEA are greatly increased in brain after administration of MAO inhibitor antidepressants. Further, PEA may be a neuromodulator of catecholamine activity.[38]

In a clinical trial involving 155 patients diagnosed with unipolar depression, Birkmayer et al.[39] demonstrated that enhanced antidepressive efficacy and beneficial effects in 90% of outpatients and 80.5% of inpatients treated with 5 to 10 mg L-deprenyl (selegiline) and 250 mg L-phenylalanine, administered daily, both orally and intravenously. These researchers conclude that "this combined treatment has a potent antidepressive action based on the accumulation of L-phenylethylamine in the brain."

In 1986, Sabelli et al.[36] published clinical studies on the phenylethylamine hypothesis of affective disorder in which they reported that decreased urinary levels of PEA (suggesting a deficiency) have been found in a significant portion of patients with depression. In two subsequent trials, Sabelli et al.[40,41] reported that the combination of selegiline and phenylalanine provided for "rapid treatment of depression," and that phenylethylamine relieves depression after selective MAO-B inhibition. In a small trial, published in 1991, ten patients with severe, intractable depression were treated with a daily cocktail of low-dose selegiline/L-deprenyl (5 mg), vitamin B6 (100 mg), and L-phenylalanine (2-6 g). "Nine of 10 patients experienced mood elevation within hours of phenylalanine administration and 6 viewed their episodes of depression as terminated within 2 to 3 days."[40] Several years later, this research team coadministered PEA (10-60 mg/day orally) and selegiline (10 mg/day to prevent rapid PEA destruction) to 14 patients with major depressive episodes. They found that 12 patients maintained an initial antidepressant response after 20 to 50 weeks, and that the necessary therapeutic dosage of PEA was stable over time, did not produce tolerance, and was not associated with any significant pattern of adverse effects.[37]

In a related study involving 20 healthy, regularly exercising young men, Szabo et al.[42] found that 24-hour mean urinary concentration of phenylacetic acid increased by 77% after a 30-minute bout of moderate to high intensity aerobic exercise. These findings were interpreted to demonstrate, or at least suggest, that PEA, as reflected in phenylacetic acid levels, may be a key factor in the therapeutic effects of physical exercise on depression.

In an experiment using squirrel monkeys, Bergman et al.[43] observed that inhibition of MAO-B, with R-$(-)$-deprenyl or MDL 72974, enhances discriminative-stimulus and reinforcing-stimulus effects of beta-PEA (0.3-1.0 mg/kg), presumably by delaying its inactivation. These researchers concluded that "MAO-B inhibition leading to increased levels of beta-PEA may be useful, alone or in combination with other therapeutic agents, in the pharmacological management of selected aspects of drug dependence."

Nutritional Therapeutics, Clinical Concerns, and Adaptations

Selegiline is an irreversible and (relatively) selective MAO-B inhibitor used in the treatment of Parkinson's disease and reported to induce an excess of mortality. The preliminary research available indicates that coadministration of selegiline and phenylalanine (in the D form or as the combined DL mixture) may, under proper medical supervision, reduce the necessary therapeutic dosage of the MAO inhibitor, thereby decreasing risk of drug-induced adverse effects.

Further research with well-designed clinical trials is warranted in the complex area of efficacy and safety of combining phenylalanine (in either form or as the combined DL mixture) with either type of MAO inhibitor.

THEORETICAL, SPECULATIVE, AND PRELIMINARY INTERACTIONS RESEARCH, INCLUDING OVERSTATED INTERACTIONS CLAIMS

Monoamine Oxidase (MAO-A) Inhibitors

Isocarboxazid (Marplan), moclobemide (Aurorix, Manerix), phenelzine (Nardil), procarbazine (Matulane), tranylcypromine (Parnate).

Phenylalanine, particularly the L isomer, is the precursor of L-tyrosine, and elevations in phenylalanine levels can lead to increased levels of tyrosine. Levels of tyrosine-derived neurotransmitters could rise to excessive levels if MAO, the enzyme that breaks down dopamine and other monoamines, is inhibited. Thus, the concomitant intake of MAO inhibitors and exogenous D-phenylalanine could theoretically produce adverse effects associated with excessive tyrosine-derived neurotransmitters, most notably a hypertensive crisis and the attendant risk of heart attack or stroke.

Prudence warrants the avoidance of concomitant administration of phenylalanine and MAO-A inhibitors. Nevertheless, evidence from qualified reports or human trials is lacking to characterize the theoretical interaction between MAO-A inhibitors and phenylalanine or establish the frequency or conditions of its occurrence. The suggested mechanism of action indicates that the outcome of such an interaction would primarily be determined by dosage, patient pharmacogenomics, and clinical management. Further research with well-designed clinical trials is warranted in the complex area of efficacy and safety of combining phenylalanine (in either form or as the combined DL mixture) with either type of MAO inhibitor.

NUTRIENT-NUTRIENT INTERACTIONS

Branched-Chain Amino Acids: Isoleucine, Leucine, Valine

Branched-chain amino acids (BCAAs: isoleucine, leucine, and valine) compete with phenylalanine and other aromatic amino acids for absorption and transport across the blood-brain barrier into the brain. Separating intake of phenylalanine (by at least 2 hours) from amino acids and meals high in protein will reduce interference with bioavailability and therapeutic action.

Vitamin B_6 (Pyridoxine)

Vitamin B_6 plays a key role in processing all amino acids. L-Phenylalanine activity is enhanced by simultaneous administration of vitamin B_6 (20-50 mg twice daily), especially in the treatment of depression.[40,44]

Preliminary research involving children with PKU indicates the possibility of reduced turnover of vitamin B_6 in PKU.[45]

Tyrosine

Phenylalanine is a precursor of tyrosine, and elevations in either (and especially both) can lead to excessive elevations in dopamine and norepinephrine. Because of the possible additive effect, avoid unmonitored concomitant administration of phenylalanine and tyrosine in depression. Potential additive effect with phenylalanine could theoretically increase the possibility of adverse effects within the context of MAO inhibitor therapy, as previously discussed.

When observed, high phenylalanine levels may be the result of high protein intake or a block in the conversion of phenylalanine to tyrosine (as occurs in PKU). Iron, vitamin C, and niacin are necessary for this enzymatic step. Check tyrosine level and, if low, administer tyrosine and iron.

The 45 citations for this monograph, as well as additional reference literature, are located under Phenylalanine on the CD at the back of the book.

Tryptophan

Nutrient Name: Tryptophan.
Synonyms: 1-Alpha-amino-3-indolepropionic acid, indole-alpha-aminopropionic acid, L-tryptophan, tryptophane, Trp.

Summary

Drug/Class Interaction Type	Mechanism and Significance	Management
Allopurinol ⊕⊕	Allopurinol inhibits hepatic tryptophan pyrrolase activity, thereby (apparently) decreasing tryptophan breakdown and increasing levels of serotonin and melatonin. Coadministration of L-tryptophan and allopurinol may be effective in treating depression, especially refractory cases. Clinical significance probable, but evidence lacking consistency and rigor.	Caution. Concomitant use could be therapeutic with appropriate clinical management.
Clorazepate ✗	Potential competition between clorazepate and tryptophan may interfere with drug activity. Mechanism plausible but evidence minimal.	Monitor if concomitant use required. Separate intake.
Fluoxetine Selective serotonin reuptake inhibitor and selective norepinephrine reuptake inhibitor (SSRI and SNRI) antidepressants ✗✗/⊕✗/⊕⊕	Combination of tryptophan's effect as serotonin precursor and activity of SSRI in inhibiting serotonin reuptake creates inherent risk of excessively elevated serotonin levels. This additive effect can result in rapid onset of severe symptoms but might also be applied purposefully within a tightly managed therapeutic protocol.	Generally avoid concomitant use. Transitional or continued concomitant use possible with close supervision and regular monitoring.
Lithium ⊕⊕/☼	Lithium increases serotonin release and decreases metabolism. Genetic variation in tryptophan hydroxylase may play role in variable efficacy of lithium. Tryptophan administration may enhance the therapeutic efficacy of lithium and allow for reduced adverse drug effects by enabling lower lithium dosage. Evidence mixed.	Concomitant use could be therapeutic with appropriate clinical management.
Phenelzine Monoamine oxidase (MAO-A) inhibitors ✗✗✗	Serotonin is metabolized by MAO to 5-hydroxyindoleacetic acid, so combination of MAO inhibition and increased tryptophan intake carries high probability of resulting in clinically significant serotonin excess and major risk of serious adverse effects.	Avoid concurrent use.
Sibutramine Serotonin agonists ✗✗✗	Serotonin agonists can increase serotonergic effect of tryptophan as a serotonin precursor, resulting in clinically significant serotonin excess and major risk of serious adverse effects.	Avoid concurrent use of tryptophan, as well as other serotonin agonists or precursors.
Tricyclic antidepressants (TCAs) ✗✗/⊕✗/⊕⊕	Tryptophan can potentiate action of TCAs through its serotonergic effects, which could result in excessively elevated serotonin levels. This additive effect can result in rapid onset of severe symptoms but might also be applied purposefully within a tightly managed therapeutic protocol.	Caution. Concomitant use could be therapeutic with appropriate clinical management.

NUTRIENT DESCRIPTION

Chemistry and Form

Levotryptophan, L-tryptophan.

Physiology and Function

Tryptophan is one of eight essential amino acids that must be obtained from the diet. Its primary functions include its role in niacin synthesis and as a precursor to both serotonin and melatonin. Approximately 98% of dietary L-tryptophan is metabolized into nicotinic acid (niacin), and only a very small amount is metabolized into serotonin via the intermediary stage of 5-hydroxytryptophan (5-HTP). The unusual indole side chain of tryptophan serves as the nucleus of serotonin. Serotonin is synthesized through a two-step process involving a tetrahydrobiopterin-dependent hydroxylation reaction (catalyzed by tryptophan-5-monooxygenase) and then a decarboxylation catalyzed by aromatic L-amino acid decarboxylase. Tryptophan hydroxylase (TPH) is the rate-limiting biosynthetic enzyme in the serotonin pathway, regulates levels of serotonin, and is normally only about half-saturated. Serotonin is present at highest concentrations in platelets and in the gastrointestinal (GI) tract. Lesser amounts are found in the brain and the retina. Serotonin in the central nervous system (CNS) is metabolized by monoamine oxidase to 5-hydroxyindoleacetic acid (5-HIAA).

Melatonin (N-acetyl-5-methoxytryptamine) is derived from serotonin within the pineal gland and the retina, where the necessary N-acetyltransferase enzyme is found.

NUTRIENT IN CLINICAL PRACTICE

Known or Potential Therapeutic Uses

Anodyne, antidepressant, antihyperglycemic, antihypertensive, galactagogue, melatonin precursor, niacin precursor, sedative, serotonin precursor.

Possible Uses

Agalactia, anorexia, bulimia, appetite suppression, bipolar disorder, carcinoid syndrome, dementia, depression, fibromyalgia, Hartnup's disease, hypertension, insomnia, mania, menopausal symptoms, migraine headaches, obesity, pain syndromes, parkinsonism, phenylketonuria, psychosis, premenstrual syndrome, schizophrenia, serotonin deficiency syndrome.

Deficiency Symptoms

A deficiency of tryptophan may lead to depression, edema, hair depigmentation, insomnia, lethargy, liver damage, muscle loss, pellagra, slowed growth in children, and suicidal thoughts. Metabolic disturbances associated with tryptophan deficiencies are carcinoid syndrome and Hartnup's disease. Symptoms of serotonin deficiency syndrome (SDS) include nervousness, anxiety, sleep disorders, mood disorders, and excessive appetite.

Dietary Sources

Tryptophan is the least abundant amino acid in foods. It tends to be deficient in most dietary proteins and has an uneven distribution. The richest dietary sources include fish, meat, dairy, eggs, nuts, and wheat germ. The seeds of evening primrose are a particularly rich plant source of tryptophan. There is lingering controversy as to the degree to which dietary levels of tryptophan intake affect serotonin and melatonin levels.

Dosage Forms Available

Capsule.

Source Materials for Nutrient Preparations

Synthetic L-tryptophan is manufactured by a fermentation process using pure glucose as a substrate. The products of fermentation are then separated and purified by filtration and purification procedures.

Dosage Range

Adult

Dietary: Minimum daily requirements are estimated as 0.25 g for males and 0.15 g for females.

Average U.S. daily intake: 1.0 to 1.5 g.
Recommended dietary allowance (RDA): 200 mg per day.

Supplemental/Maintenance: Supplementation usually not necessary.
Pharmacologic/Therapeutic: 0.5 to 4.0 g per day, short-term use. Occasionally, doses of 8 to 12 g daily, given in three or four equally divided doses, are used in the treatment of depression.

When L-tryptophan is prescribed within the context of integrative clinical management, the dosage will typically start low and increase gradually as needed. Clinical response will often require 60 days to demonstrate full benefits. Daily dosage usually does not exceed 1 gram per 100 pounds of body weight (1 g/100 lb).
Toxic: 7 g per 150 lb body weight.

SAFETY PROFILE

Overview

L-Tryptophan is an essential amino acid generally considered to have a low risk of toxicity, when used at typical dietary or supplemental intake levels, barring contraindications.

Nutrient Adverse Effects

General Adverse Effects

Anorexia, dizziness, drowsiness, dry mouth, headache, nausea, sexual disinhibition.

Long-term supplementation or treatment with tryptophan may increase plasma levels of other amino acids, potentially resulting in various adverse effects.

Adults

Studies in humans have shown that 100 mg/kg/day of tryptophan, corresponding to 7 g/150 lb, can cause gastric irritation, vomiting, and head twitching. A dosage of 800 mg/kg given to rhesus monkeys did not produce detectable clinical adverse effects.

Although tryptophan is a naturally occurring substance in the body, controversies surround serious adverse reactions to reported contaminants in both L-tryptophan and 5-HTP.

Special Issues

During 1989, 35 deaths and many cases of severe allergic reaction, in the form of the eosinophilia-myalgia syndrome characterized by high eosinophil counts, scleroderma-like muscle pain, and thickening of the skin, were associated with consumption of tryptophan supplements. The Food and Drug Administration (FDA) removed L-tryptophan from the U.S. market by pursuant to these events. Subsequent investigation determined that a single manufacturer in Japan had employed a new bacterial strain to synthesize L-tryptophan, and that this bacterium had introduced toxic byproducts that contaminated particular batches of the product.

As a serotonin precursor, L-tryptophan intake could theoretically contribute to "serotonin syndrome," an excess accumulation of serotonin in the synapses, characterized by altered mental states, autonomic dysfunction, and neuromuscular abnormalities (see later discussion).

Mutagenicity

Animal tests involving oral or subcutaneous administration of L-tryptophan or its metabolites have not yielded evidence of statistically significant increases in incidence of neoplasms. However, evidence indicates that foods containing tryptophan may carry an increased risk of carcinogenicity, especially to breast and bladder tissues, when they have been charbroiled or heated to high temperatures.

Life Stage

Inadequate research-based evidence exists to demonstrate any particular age-related effects on pediatric or geriatric populations as a result of increased tryptophan intake.

Pregnancy and Nursing

Well-designed controlled clinical trials with human subjects have not been undertaken, nor have case reports been qualified and systematically analyzed, regarding effects of L-tryptophan during pregnancy or breastfeeding. In some animals the equivalent of 8 g per day was found to be teratogenic. However, L-tryptophan intake by pregnant women and lactating mothers has not been shown to cause birth defects or other pregnancy or lactation problems. It is not known whether L-tryptophan passes into breast milk. However, L-tryptophan has not been reported to cause problems in nursing babies. Nevertheless, caution should be used with supplementation or administration during pregnancy or breastfeeding, and any such usage during pregnancy should be supervised and closely monitored.

Laboratory Values

Tryptophan levels in the blood vary greatly when measured by different laboratories. Tryptophan can be measured by fluorometric and high-performance liquid chromatography (HPLC) techniques. Some experts believe chromatography may be the most accurate. Other, indirect methods can also be employed, such as the tryptophan load test. This test involves measuring a metabolite of tryptophan, xanthurenic acid, in the urine after a standard 2-g dose is given. The more xanthurenic acid found in the urine, the greater is the need for either vitamin B_6 or tryptophan.

Contraindications

Achlorhydria, bladder cancer, cataracts, diabetes mellitus, female infertility, pregnancy, psoriasis; sensitivity to L-tryptophan. May exacerbate rheumatoid arthritis.

Precautions and Warnings

L-Tryptophan is best taken with a low-protein, carbohydrate-rich meal or snack to minimize risk of digestive distress. Also, an insulin response to carbohydrate facilitates transfer of serum tryptophan into the CNS (thought to be the reason serotonin-deficient people crave carbohydrates). Minimizing concomitant protein intake decreases competition between tryptophan and other dietary protein–derived amino acids for transport through the blood-brain barrier.

INTERACTIONS REVIEW
Strategic Considerations

The therapeutic effects of L-tryptophan, especially as an antidepressant, are related to its ability to increase serotonin synthesis in the CNS. Emerging research indicates that baseline availability of L-tryptophan, prolactin, and large, neutral amino acids (LNAAs) are key factors that predict response to antidepressant treatment in major depression. The major concern with tryptophan supplementation or administration with regard to drug interactions is the risk of inducing serotonin syndrome. This potentially dangerous situation results from an excess serotonin availability in the CNS at the 5-HT1A receptor; some interaction with dopamine and 5-HT2 receptors is also likely to be involved. Clinical trials have demonstrated that L-tryptophan causes a significant increase in the level of the serotonin metabolite, 5-HIAA, in the lumbar cerebrospinal fluid, corresponding to an increased turnover of serotonin in the CNS.

Serotonin syndrome carries potentially serious clinical consequences and is characterized by the triad of altered mental status, autonomic dysfunction, and neuromuscular abnormalities. The serotonin syndrome is similar to the neuroleptic malignant syndrome and is usually differentiated by the setting of recent addition of a serotonergic agent. Specific symptoms can include agitation, anxiety, ataxia, confusion, delirium, diaphoresis, diarrhea, fever, hyperreflexia, myoclonus, incoordination, shivering, nausea, vomiting, or tremor. This phenomenon most often occurs in the presence of selective serotonin reuptake inhibitors (SSRIs), monoamine oxidase (MAO) inhibitors, opioids, and other serotonergic agents, when the serotonin system has been modulated by another serotonergic agent or compromised by illness. SSRIs, particularly fluoxetine, are most frequently involved in reported instances of drug interactions inducing serotonin syndrome; as a consequence of their long elimination half-life (1 week for fluoxetine), the risk of interactions persists for several days or even weeks after SSRI withdrawal.

Many clinicians and some researchers have investigated potential synergistic benefits from coadministration of tryptophan and various psychoactive pharmaceutical agents. Although the consequences of adverse effects can be clinically significant, the available evidence suggests that such risk is less probable, and adverse effects less severe, with tryptophan than with 5-HTP. Caution is requisite to use of tryptophan, in any dose, during antidepressant or other medication therapy, and this warrants close supervision and regular monitoring within an integrative context. 5-HTP should never be combined with SSRIs or MAO inhibitors in any dose, except possibly in a carefully monitored inpatient clinical research setting.

NUTRIENT-DRUG INTERACTIONS

Allopurinol

Allopurinol (Oxypurinol; Aloprim, Apo-Allopurinol, Lopurin, Purinol, Zyloprim).

Interaction Type and Significance

$\oplus\oplus$ **Beneficial or Supportive Interaction, with Professional Management**

Probability:	Evidence Base:
2. Probable	◉ Emerging

Effect and Mechanism of Action

Human and animal studies consistently indicate that allopurinol causes elevated brain levels of tryptophan.[1,2] Allopurinol is a xanthine oxidase inhibitor and is typically used to lower blood levels of uric acid to prevent gout and adjunctively with certain forms of chemotherapy. However, allopurinol also inhibits hepatic tryptophan pyrrolase activity and prevents the reduction in the indole levels induced by heme precursor 5-aminolevulinate (5-ALA). Daytime administration of 5-ALA can reduce brain tryptophan and serotonin levels because of saturation of liver tryptophan pyrrolase. Saturation of this enzyme with heme results in enhanced activity, leading to increased catabolism of tryptophan and thus making less tryptophan available to the brain. Thus, Daya et al.[3] demonstrated that 5-ALA alters brain tryptophan and serotonin levels without changing pineal serotonin and melatonin concentrations. It is hypothesized that increased levels of serotonin and melatonin, as a result of decreased tryptophan breakdown, can result in an antidepressant and analgesic effect.

Research

Over the decades, research on the effects of inhibition of tryptophan pyrrolase by allopurinol has elicited several distinct patterns but evolved to no certain conclusion. Many (but not all) studies have observed measurable effects of allopurinol on tryptophan metabolism.[4,5] Green et al.[6] investigated the effect of oral administration of allopurinol (300 mg daily) or nicotinamide (500 mg twice daily) on the metabolism of an oral L-tryptophan load (50 mg/kg). Their findings were interpreted to suggest that allopurinol and nicotinamide were unlikely to be of value as tryptophan pyrrolase inhibitors in vivo and therefore would not increase the therapeutic effect of L-tryptophan when given to treat depressive illness. However, Stern and Mendels[7] reviewed a preliminary study involving eight individuals diagnosed with refractory depression using a combination of L-tryptophan and allopurinol. The investigators reported that five of the trial participants demonstrated full remission. Throughout the course of study on this topic, the various authors have continued to stress the need for further, double-blind, controlled studies to evaluate the safety and efficacy of this combination therapy.

Nutritional Therapeutics, Clinical Concerns, and Adaptations

Controlled clinical trials will be necessary to determine whether the adjunctive use of allopurinol during tryptophan therapy can provide clinical efficacy in the treatment of depression or other conditions responsive to tryptophan supplementation. In the meantime, health care practitioners experienced in therapeutic nutrition and qualified in conventional pharmacology who might be interested in experimenting with this potential synergistic therapy at low dosage levels, and possible gradual escalation, are advised to supervise and regularly monitor any such patients. No investigators have expressed concern with adverse effects from this interaction, but such clinical practice is recommended as judicious.

Clorazepate

Clorazepate (Gen-Xene, Tranxene).

Interaction Type and Significance

✗   **Potential or Theoretical Adverse Interaction of Uncertain Severity**

Probability: Evidence Base:
4. Plausible   ☐ Inadequate

Effect and Mechanism of Action

L-Tryptophan and dipotassium clorazepate potentially compete, such that high intake of tryptophan might interfere with the intended therapeutic action of the medication.

Research

In vitro research by Coassolo et al.[8] demonstrated the competitive binding of L-tryptophan and dipotassium clorazepate, a benzodiazepine, for human serum albumin.

Clinical Implications and Adaptations

Further research, preferably human clinical trials, is needed to determine the probability, risk settings, and clinical significance of this plausibly significant interaction. Separate intake if concomitant use necessary.

Fluoxetine and Related Selective Serotonin Reuptake Inhibitor and Serotonin-Norepinephrine Reuptake Inhibitor (SSRI and SNRI) Antidepressants

Evidence: Fluoxetine (Prozac, Sarafem).
Extrapolated, based on similar properties: Citalopram (Celexa), duloxetine (Cymbalta), escitalopram (S-citalopram; Lexapro), fluvoxamine (Faurin, Luvox), paroxetine (Aropax, Deroxat, Paxil, Seroxat), sertraline (Zoloft), venlafaxine (Effexor).

Interaction Type and Significance

✗✗   **Minimal to Mild Adverse Interaction—Vigilance Necessary**

⊕✗   **Bimodal or Variable Interaction, with Professional Management**

⊕⊕   **Beneficial or Supportive Interaction, with Professional Management**

Probability: Evidence Base:
1. Certain   ◉ Emerging

Effect and Mechanism of Action

L-Tryptophan acts as a serotonin precursor, and the selective serotonin reuptake inhibitors (SSRIs) are designed to increase the functional level of serotonin in the brain by inhibiting its reuptake into the presynaptic neurons. Fluoxetine is a potent and selective inhibitor of presynaptic serotonin reuptake, therefore increasing the amount of serotonin in the synaptic cleft. Increased intake of L-tryptophan can potentially elevate levels of serotonin in the CNS. Such concomitant elevation of serotonin and inhibition of its reuptake presents both the opportunity for possible therapeutic synergy and the risk of potentially dangerous serotonin excess.

Research

In an early trial involving zimelidine for the treatment of depression, Walinder et al.[9] found that the administration of the relatively high dose of 45 mg per pound body weight of DL-tryptophan, a synthetic variation of L-tryptophan, did not result in adverse effects. Zimelidine is an SSRI medication, similar in action to paroxetine, that was withdrawn worldwide in September 1983 because of the risk of Guillain-Barré syndrome associated with its use.

Research into the relationship between tryptophan depletion and the therapeutic mechanisms and efficacy of SSRI medications provides useful data in understanding the tryptophan-SSRI interaction pattern. Short-term reduction in plasma tryptophan (tryptophan depletion) produces a relapse of depressive symptoms in 60% of previously depressed patients recently recovered with SSRI treatment. Barr et al.[10] investigated the hypothesis that SSRI treatment itself may confer vulnerability to the development of depressive symptoms during tryptophan depletion. They conducted a double-blind placebo-controlled involving six healthy individuals who underwent tryptophan depletion before and after 6 weeks of treatment with fluoxetine, 20 mg/day. Their findings showed no increased vulnerability to the mood-lowering effects of tryptophan depletion as a result of fluoxetine treatment. From these data the researchers determined that treatment with SSRIs alone does not produce the depressive effects of tryptophan depletion observed in SSRI-treated depressed and obsessive-compulsive disorder patients.

In a subsequent trial looking at the differential pathways of antidepressant action in desipramine and fluoxetine, Delgado et al.[11] studied 55 individuals diagnosed with, but not currently medicated for, depression who were randomly assigned to antidepressant treatment with either desipramine or fluoxetine, then administered amino acid drinks capable of inducing tryptophan depletion. Whereas eight (of 15) fluoxetine responders reported relapse of significant depressive symptoms, only one (of 15) of the desipramine responders and none of the control subjects relapsed. The researchers concluded that rapid depletion of plasma tryptophan transiently reverses the antidepressant response in many patients taking fluoxetine, but not desipramine, and that antidepressant response to fluoxetine appears to be significantly dependent on serotonin (5-HT) availability. An important finding of this study is that various SSRI antidepressants mediate their therapeutic effects through different mechanisms. Recent investigation by Porter et al.[12] into the connection between tryptophan availability and variable response to different antidepressant medications further demonstrates that patients with a tryptophan level below the mean improved significantly more than those with a higher level but with comparable serum steady-state drug levels.

Meltzer et al.[13] have found that fluoxetine potentiates the 5-HTP-mediated increase in plasma cortisol and prolactin secretion in subjects with major depression or with obsessive-compulsive disorder.

More directly, Levitan et al.[14] conducted a randomized, double-blind, placebo-controlled trial that examined the antidepressant and hypnotic effects of combining tryptophan and fluoxetine. In this small, preliminary clinical study, 30 individuals diagnosed with major depressive disorder were treated with fluoxetine and either tryptophan or placebo for 8 weeks. The investigators concluded that "combining 20 mg of fluoxetine with 2 g of tryptophan daily at the outset of treatment for major depressive disorder appears to be a safe protocol that may have both a rapid antidepressant effect and a protective effect on slow-wave sleep." The cumulative message of the assembled research strongly suggests that large-scale, well-designed clinical trials are warranted to confirm and clarify the emerging pattern indicated by the various findings.

No available report or trial evidence suggests an adverse interaction response when fluoxetine has been combined with a protein-rich diet containing significant levels of L-tryptophan.

Reports

Unsupervised coadministration of an SSRI agent with tryptophan carries a moderate risk for higher incidence of serotonin-associated unintended effects and adverse events. Specifically, reports have suggested that when taken in the form of a nutraceutical, L-tryptophan can interact adversely with fluoxetine, resulting in the following adverse effects, which are not associated with either drug alone: agitation, restlessness, poor concentration, nausea, diarrhea, and worsening of obsessive-compulsive disorder. These apparently interaction-induced symptoms disappeared as soon as the tryptophan was discontinued.[15-17] In a review of five case reports, Steiner and Fontaine[18] noted that signs and symptoms of CNS toxicity, both central and peripheral, developed within a few days of adding tryptophan (1-4 g/day) to ongoing fluoxetine therapy. Typical symptoms included nausea and vomiting, agitation, anxiety and restlessness, headache, dizziness, and increased perspiration.

Clinical Implications and Adaptations

A review of the evidence suggests an emerging, but not yet coherent and articulate, consensus supporting the proposition that L-tryptophan, in graduated dosages in the range of 2 to 4 g daily, can be used adjunctively with SSRI medications to enhance the clinical effectiveness of treatment for depression and other appropriate conditions. The ability of tryptophan to enhance, but not necessarily forcefully elevate, serotonin levels appears to exert a beneficial synergistic effect in conjunction with fluoxetine and some other SSRIs. However, the variable mechanisms of action among different SSRIs, along with individual pharmacogenomic variability, life stage and gender factors, and other metabolic influences, may account for differing therapeutic responses and occurrences of adverse effects.

Such an integrative therapeutic strategy warrants close supervision and regular monitoring within the context of coordinated care by health providers trained and experienced in both clinical nutrition and conventional pharmacology. However, the concomitant use of supplemental L-tryptophan and an SSRI such as fluoxetine outside such a context of active clinical management is contraindicated and potentially dangerous. A rapid onset of symptoms indicating an adverse response, particularly CNS toxicity, is highly probable in the event that a serotonin syndrome reaction or other adverse event does develop.

All available evidence strongly indicates that tryptophan-related data cannot be extrapolated to a clinical opportunity for safely combining 5-HTP and SSRI medications, and that all warnings and contraindications are amplified.

Lithium Carbonate

Lithium carbonate (Camcolit, Carbolith, Duralith, Eskalith, Li-Liquid, Liskonum, Litarex, Lithane, Lithobid, Lithonate, Lithotabs, PMS-Lithium, Priadel).

Interaction Type and Significance

⊕⊕ **Beneficial or Supportive Interaction, with Professional Management**

☼ **Prevention or Reduction of Drug Adverse Effect**

Probability:	Evidence Base:
2. Probable	◉ **Emerging**

Effect and Mechanism of Action

Lithium intake raises cortisol levels, and both lithium and supplemental tryptophan can elevate serotonin and cortisol levels as part of their therapeutic action. Concomitant use of these agents may induce excessively elevated serotonin levels and disrupt regulation of cortisol and other neuroendocrine substances.

Research

Lithium increases serotonin release and decreases metabolism. Despite lithium's proven efficacy as a long-term treatment for recurrent mood disorders (bipolar syndromes), individuals show a variable response, ranging from complete efficacy to no influence at all.[19,20] Serotonergic pathways appear to be of importance in the mechanisms of the action of lithium. Much recent research has focused on identifying possible predictors of response through molecular genetic studies. Recent research has observed an association between genetic variation in tryptophan hydroxylase (TPH) and aggressive and anger-related traits.[21] It is becoming apparent that clinical predictors account for about half the variance in lithium response, and genetic factors probably play a substantial role in both risk factors and response factors in affective disorders.[22-25]

In 1999, Serretti et al.[26] published one of several papers examining the possible association between the TPH gene variants and prophylactic efficacy of lithium in mood disorders. In a review from 2002, Serretti[27] reported that the functional polymorphism in the upstream regulatory region of the serotonin transporter gene (5-HTTLPR) has been associated with long-term efficacy of lithium in two independent studies; marginal associations have been reported for TPH and inositol polyphosphate 1-phosphatase (INPP1). Even though no unequivocal susceptibility gene for lithium efficacy has been identified, individual pharmacogenomic variability significantly influences response patterns. Within that context, manipulation of tryptophan metabolism and serotonin synthesis appears to play an important role.

In 1983, Brewerton and Reus[28] published the results of a small, double-blind clinical trial in which lithium therapy for bipolar disorder or schizoaffective disorders generated significantly enhanced outcomes with adjunctive administration of L-tryptophan, 2 to 4 g three times daily.

Reports

Clinical observations suggest that L-tryptophan can serve as a clinically effective adjunct to lithium therapy, particularly in the treatment of some individuals diagnosed as bipolar with mania or depression for whom lithium, alone or in combination with neuroleptics or tricyclics, has demonstrated limited or no effect.

Nutritional Therapeutics, Clinical Concerns, and Adaptations

L-Tryptophan offers a valuable adjunct to lithium therapy in the management of some individuals with bipolar affective disorders. In addition to enhanced therapeutic efficacy, such coordinated administration of lithium and L-tryptophan provides an opportunity to reduce lithium doses and decrease attendant adverse effects, particularly in controlling acute mania and other severe conditions for which higher, more toxic doses of lithium are often required. Concomitant therapy may also achieve therapeutic efficacy with some individuals previously unresponsive to lithium alone or in combination with other psychoactive agents.

Some bipolar patients have demonstrated an increased sensitivity to L-tryptophan administration, with adverse reactions occurring at levels as low as 1 to 2 g daily. Low initial dose levels, slow and graduated increases in dosage, and regular monitoring are important to safe and effective concomitant medication.

L-Tryptophan, when administered to individuals undergoing lithium therapy, might increase some adverse effects associated with lithium therapy by potentiating the lithium effect; these include nausea, vomiting, dermatological eruptions, psoriasis, and alopecia. Gradual reduction of lithium in chronic cases, such as treatment of bipolar disorder, not only may be valuable for reduction of typical adverse effects associated with lithium, but also may be necessary because of an increase in lithium concentrations resulting from potentiation by L-tryptophan. Monitoring lithium concentrations for at least 2 weeks after introduction of L-tryptophan or making changes in lithium dosage is appropriate with such individuals. Individuals being treated for acute mania may be particularly sensitive to exacerbations because of alterations in effective concentrations of lithium. In such cases it may be appropriate to decrease the lithium dosage, especially with doses above 900 to 1200 mg per day. Implementation of such integrative strategies warrants active supervision and close monitoring by health care professionals trained and experienced in clinical nutrition and conventional pharmacology. Pharmacogenomic variability, particularly involving TPH polymorphisms, appears to influence both individual susceptibility to bipolar disorder and related conditions and therapeutic response to lithium and L-tryptophan.

Phenelzine and Related Monoamine Oxidase (MAO) Inhibitors

Evidence: Phenelzine (Nardil).
Extrapolated, based on similar properties: MAO-A inhibitors: Isocarboxazid (Marplan), moclobemide (Aurorix, Manerix), procarbazine (Matulane), tranylcypromine (Parnate).
Related but evidence lacking for extrapolation: MAO-B inhibitors: Pargyline (Eutonyl), rasagiline (Azilect), selegiline (deprenyl, L-deprenil, L-deprenyl; Atapryl, Carbex, Eldepryl, Jumex, Movergan, Selpak).

Interaction Type and Significance

✗✗✗ **Potentially Harmful or Serious Adverse Interaction—Avoid**

Probability:
1. Certain

Evidence Base:
● Consensus

Effect and Mechanism of Action

The MAO-A inhibitor medications elevate serotonin concentrations because CNS serotonin is metabolized by monoamine oxidase (MAO) to 5-hydroxyindoleacetic acid (5-HIAA). Concomitant intake of L-tryptophan can then result in amplified serotonergic effects.

Research

Combined use of tryptophan and MAO inhibitors increases the risk of adverse drug effects. MAO inhibitors can induce potentiation of sympathomimetic substances and related compounds and result in a hypertensive crisis.

Reports

The most common adverse effects caused by the combination of L-tryptophan and MAO inhibitors are nausea, dizziness, and headache, usually immediately or shortly after coadministration. L-Tryptophan, 20 to 50 mg/kg, and MAO inhibitors, at standard therapeutic dosages, when taken together, have been reported to cause drowsiness, ethanol-like intoxication, hyperreflexia, and clonus. Levy et al.[29] documented three cases of multiple adverse effects from phenelzine-tryptophan combination treatment, including myoclonus, hyperreflexia, and diaphoresis.[29] Single case reports of adverse reactions to the drug combination include confusional states, hypomanic behavior, ocular oscillation, ataxia, and myoclonus.[30-33] On occasion, reactions have approached the severity of classic serotonin syndrome with tremor, hypertonus, myoclonus, and hyperreactivity. Reports concur that such symptoms resolve shortly after cessation of L-tryptophan intake; no detrimental long-term effects have been documented.

Clinical Implications and Adaptations

The concomitant use of tryptophan and MAO inhibitors represents a particularly high probability of clinically significant adverse effects and is strongly contraindicated. Individuals taking phenelzine or other MAO inhibitors should avoid unsupervised supplemental intake of L-tryptophan. Similar adverse reactions are known to occur with concomitant use of MAO inhibitors and sympathomimetic drugs (including amphetamines, cocaine, methylphenidate, dopamine, epinephrine, and norepinephrine) or related compounds (e.g., methyldopa, L-dopa, L-tyrosine, ephedra, ephedrine, pseudoephedrine, phenylalanine), as well as food sources of tyramine, such as red wine and aged cheese.

Sibutramine and Other Serotonin Agonists

Evidence: Sibutramine (Meridia, Reductil).
Extrapolated, based on similar properties: Almotriptan (Axert), buspirone (Buspar), dihydroergotamine (DHE-45), ergotamine, eletriptan (Relpax), frovatriptan (Frova), naratriptan (Amerge), rizatriptan (Maxalt), sumatriptan (Imitrex), zolmitriptan (Zomig).

Interaction Type and Significance:

✗✗✗ **Potentially Harmful or Serious Adverse Interaction—Avoid**

Probability:
1. Certain

Evidence Base:
● Consensus

Effect and Mechanism of Action

Serotonin agonists can enhance the serotonergic effect of other serotonin agonists, as well as serotonin precursors, thereby increasing the risk of augmenting serotonin activity to toxic levels.[34] In particular, the additive effect on serotonin activity resulting from concomitant use of L-tryptophan and pharmaceutical serotonin agonists presents a significant risk of inducing serotonin syndrome.

Reports

The product information provided by the manufacturer of sibutramine states that "because [sibutramine] inhibits serotonin reuptake, it should not be administered with other serotonin agonists."[35]

Clinical Implications and Adaptations

The concomitant use of L-tryptophan and agents that enhance serotonin activity is contraindicated and should be undertaken only in the context of close clinical supervision and regular monitoring. Adverse effects of a dangerous additive interaction are likely to be characterized by rapid onset of toxicity symptoms.

Tricyclic Antidepressants (TCAs)

Evidence: Clomipramine (Anafranil), imipramine (Janimine, Tofranil).
Extrapolated, based on similar properties: Amitriptyline (Elavil); combination drug: amitriptyline and perphenazine (Etrafon, Triavil, Triptazine); amoxapine (Asendin), desipramine (Norpramin, Pertofrane), doxepin (Adapin, Sinequan), nortriptyline (Aventyl, Pamelor), protriptyline (Vivactil), trimipramine (Surmontil).
Related, no longer on market: Zimelidine.

Interaction Type and Significance

✗✗   **Minimal to Mild Adverse Interaction—Vigilance Necessary**
⊕✗   **Bimodal or Variable Interaction, with Professional Management**
⊕⊕   **Beneficial or Supportive Interaction, with Professional Management**

Probability: Evidence Base:
2. Probable   ∇ Mixed

Effect and Mechanism of Action

L-Tryptophan can potentiate the action of tricyclic antidepressants (TCAs) through its serotonergic effects.

Research

A review of the research literature and clinical practice observations suggest clinically significant variability in the character and significance of interactions between L-tryptophan and various TCAs. Human clinical trials indicate that the dosage levels of L-tryptophan administration and the mechanism of action of the particular TCA affected the character and strength of potential interactions with TCAs. In a human trial, Chouinard et al.[36] enhanced imipramine therapy for bipolar disorder by expanding the therapeutic strategy to incorporate L-tryptophan (6 g/day) and niacinamide (1500 mg/day), compared with imipramine alone. Lower adjunctive doses of L-tryptophan (4 g/day) and niacinamide (1000 mg/day) suggested a significant but less efficacious effect in potentiating imipramine compared with the higher levels of administration.

However, when the higher levels of L-tryptophan and niacinamide were administered to individuals diagnosed with depression, evidence of synergistic benefit was lacking.

Related research on antidepressant therapy using other TCAs demonstrated that larger dosages of L-tryptophan did not contribute to increased therapeutic benefit, with 6 g daily failing to provide therapeutic effect, whereas 4 g daily demonstrated therapeutic efficacy.[37] In a placebo-controlled trial with 24 individuals, Walinder et al.[38] found "significantly more rapid improvement" in those administered L-tryptophan with clomipramine than in those given clomipramine with placebo for endogenous depression, "especially with regard to the depression-anxiety cluster of symptoms." In contrast, further research by Walinder et al.[9] found that tryptophan in combination with zimelidine was not superior to zimelidine with placebo with respect to antidepressant activity. Recent investigation by Porter et al.[12] and others into the connection between tryptophan availability and variable response to different antidepressant medications shows that patients with tryptophan level below the mean improved significantly more than those with a higher level but with comparable serum steady-state drug levels.

Thus, human clinical trials indicate that the dosage levels of L-tryptophan and preexisting endogenous blood levels of the amino acid, as well as the mechanism of action of the particular TCA, affected the character and strength of potential synergistic interactions between tryptophan supplementation and TCAs.

Nutritional Therapeutics, Clinical Concerns, and Adaptations

The coordinated administration of TCAs and L-tryptophan can achieve clinically significant synergistic effect within the context of an integrative therapeutic strategy. Pretreatment tryptophan depletion status and carefully calibrated dosages of L-tryptophan, typically 4 g daily, appear to be primary factors in determining probability of optimal effect. Once stabilization occurs, reduction of antidepressant levels can be considered if consistent with the expressed patient treatment goals, particularly with a history of adverse effects attributable to the TCA. Evolving personalized treatment protocols with close supervision and regular monitoring by health care professionals trained and experienced both in nutritional therapeutics and conventional psychopharmacology offer opportunities for deriving clinical benefits greater than what might be achieved by conventional antidepressant medications alone.

THEORETICAL, SPECULATIVE, AND PRELIMINARY INTERACTIONS RESEARCH, INCLUDING OVERSTATED INTERACTIONS CLAIMS

Numerous discussions have arisen as to whether data and conclusions from potential or documented interactions involving 5-HTP can be reasonably extended to L-tryptophan, or vice versa. However, a critical difference between tryptophan and 5HTP is that the 5-hydroxy form only requires decarboxylation to become 5-hydroxytryptamine (5-HT, serotonin). Tryptophan has much greater metabolic physiological flexibility; it can be made into niacin or serotonin, or melatonin via serotonin, whereas 5-HTP is committed to the serotonin pathway. As previously noted, approximately 98% of dietary L-tryptophan is metabolized into nicotinic acid (niacin). Further, some research indicates that eating a diet high in tryptophan does not significantly increase 5-HTP levels. Thus, in contrast to 5-HTP, tryptophan may be able to enhance, but not necessarily forcefully elevate, serotonin levels in such a way as to allow for systemic equilibration through negative-feedback loops within neurohormonal self-regulatory systems. Clinically, this means that 5-HTP has a much greater risk of resulting in a significant serotonin syndrome when combined with a pharmaceutical agent, particularly an SSRI or MAO inhibitor. In cases other than where evidence directly demonstrates such interactions involving tryptophan itself, such extrapolation (from interactions involving 5-HTP) warrants attention as "possible," but cannot be defined as an evidence-based interaction in the absence of direct data from human clinical trials, or at least case reports specifically involving L-tryptophan. Also, adverse reactions and interactions involving L-tryptophan are much less common than might have been the case before 1989, since L-tryptophan now requires a prescription, generally filled by a compounding pharmacy. 5-HTP is widely available in health food stores as a dietary supplement. This state of affairs is somewhat ironic because 5-HTP has a much narrower therapeutic dose range and is much more prone to cause adverse reactions (particularly nausea) than L-tryptophan. Time-release preparations of 5-HTP, which can be obtained from compounding pharmacists, largely avert problems with nausea.

Consult the 5-HTP monograph for interaction issues specifically involving that substance. Clinically, the behavior and interactions of tryptophan and 5-hydroxytryptophan are quite different. Experience with one should never be extrapolated to the other, despite their chemical similarity and metabolic relationship.

NUTRIENT-NUTRIENT INTERACTIONS

Large, Neutral Amino Acids: Tyrosine, Phenylalanine, Valine, Leucine, Isoleucine

Tryptophan competes with the other large, neutral amino acids (LNAAs)—tyrosine, phenylalanine, valine, leucine, and isoleucine—for transport across the blood-brain barrier. When tryptophan is therapeutically administered, it is usually given with vitamin B_6, apart from meals, with a small amount of carbohydrate to facilitate uptake by the brain. Tryptophan's action can also be supported by coadministration of vitamins B_3 and C, the other cofactors necessary for its metabolism.

The 38 citations for this monograph, as well as additional reference literature, are located under Tryptophan on the CD at the back of the book.

Nutrient-Drug Interactions and Drug-Induced Nutrient Depletions

Tyrosine

Nutrient Name: Tyrosine.
Synonym: L-Tyrosine
Related Substance: L-Phenylalanine.

Summary

Drug/Class Interaction Type	Mechanism and Significance	Management
Amphetamines Dextroamphetamine Methylphenidate ⊕⊕/≈≈/☼	Tyrosine administration may enhance dopamine synthesis through its role as a precursor of L-dopa. Coadministration of L-tyrosine may reverse or prevent tyrosine depletion caused by amphetamines and support activity of amphetamine therapy by enhancing precursor availability. Adverse effects improbable. Research with well-designed trials warranted.	Coadministration may enhance therapeutic outcomes within integrative strategy, particularly with tyrosine depletion. Supervise, monitor, and titrate.
Imipramine Tricyclic antidepressants (TCAs) ⊕⊕	Tyrosine is a precursor to many neurotransmitters, including dopamine. Coadministration of tyrosine and L-tryptophan with imipramine may facilitate withdrawal in cocaine addiction. Evidence mixed and limited. Further research warranted.	Consider coadministration with close supervision. Monitor and titrate.
Levodopa Antiparkinsonian medications ◇◇/⊕✗/◇≈≈/☼/⊕⊕	Tyrosine administration may enhance dopamine synthesis through its role as a precursor of L-dopa. L-Tyrosine may benefit Parkinson's patients. However, limited knowledge regarding potential issues of competition in absorption, transport system, and brain uptake suggests need for continued research.	Consider coadministration with close supervision and regular monitoring.
Levothyroxine Thyroid hormones ⊕⊕	L-Tyrosine is a precursor in endogenous synthesis of L-thyroxine. Additive interaction is probable from concomitant administration of exogenous thyroid hormone(s) and tyrosine, but possibly with minimal effect in individuals whose thyroid gland has atrophied from chronic use of synthetic thyroid medication. Adverse effects improbable. Research with well-designed trials examining various permutations warranted.	Coadministration may be beneficial. Monitor and titrate.
Monoamine oxidase (MAO) inhibitors ✗✗✗	MAO inhibitors can potentiate sympathomimetic substances and related compounds to induce a hypertensive crisis with potential risk of heart attack or stroke. Tyramine from food sources is usually implicated in such interactions, but tyramine can also be produced by intestinal bacteria from tyrosine through decarboxylation. This plausible but potentially dangerous interaction has not been confirmed by evidence from case reports or clinical trials.	Avoid concomitant use, also L-tryptophan, 5-HTP, and phenylalanine.
Oral contraceptives (OCs) ◇≈≈/≈≈/☼	Through effects on amino acid balance, exogenous estrogen and progestins can decrease plasma tyrosine levels, alter neurotransmitter levels, and potentially contribute to or exacerbate OC adverse effects, such as depression. Human research is limited and inadequate to determine occurrence of clinically relevant interactions or susceptibility factors. Adverse effects from coadministration improbable. Research with well-designed trials warranted.	Coadministration, with B-complex vitamins, may be beneficial unless otherwise contraindicated. Consider support for liver conjugation functions. Supervise and monitor.

5-HTP, 5-Hydroxytryptophan.

NUTRIENT DESCRIPTION
Physiology and Function

Tyrosine is a conditionally essential amino acid normally synthesized from phenylalanine, which is an essential amino acid. Hepatic conversion of L-phenylalanine to L-tyrosine can be impaired during infection, trauma, chronic illness, liver disease, or other forms of severe stress, thus making tyrosine a conditionally essential amino acid.

L-Tyrosine plays a critical role in the synthesis of neurotransmitters within the central nervous system (CNS). In particular, it serves as a precursor to L-dopa, dopamine, norepinephrine, and epinephrine, the brain concentrations of which depend on intake of tyrosine. The conversion of L-tyrosine into these neurotransmitters requires vitamin B_6, folic acid, and copper. Tyrosine also requires biopterin (a folate derivative), NADPH and NADH (metabolites of niacin), copper, and vitamin C. Tyrosine acts as an adaptogen through its role as a precursor of norepinephrine and epinephrine.

Several other key activities are among the known functions of tyrosine. Tyrosine is a precursor to thyroid hormones and catecholestrogens, compounds that have estrogen-like and catecholamine-like effects, as well as a constituent of amino sugars and amino lipids. It is also involved in the synthesis of enkephalins, important endogenous analgesic peptides in the endorphin family, and melanin, a pigment responsible for hair and skin color. Lastly, tyrosine binds free radicals and is considered a mild antioxidant.

NUTRIENT IN CLINICAL PRACTICE
Known or Potential Therapeutic Uses

Common uses include depression, thyroid nutriture, and alcohol withdrawal support. Individuals with phenylketonuria (PKU) are often treated with tyrosine to compensate for inborn errors of phenylalanine metabolism and resultant tendency to tyrosine deficiency.

Historical/Ethnomedicine Precedent

Tyrosine has not been used historically as an isolated nutrient.

Possible Uses

Addictions, alcohol withdrawal support, Alzheimer's disease, attention deficit disorder, cardiovascular disease, chronic fatigue, cocaine abuse and withdrawal, cognitive enhancement, dementia, depression, excessive appetite, fatigue, hypotensive crisis, hypothyroidism, impotence, jet lag, low libido, narcolepsy, Parkinson's disease, premenstrual syndrome, schizophrenia, stress disorders, weight loss.

Deficiency Symptoms

Because tyrosine is a precursor to thyroid hormones and catecholamines, a deficiency may lead to impaired thyroid function as well as low adrenal function. Some research indicates that tyrosine levels may be low in some individuals with depression. A lack of melanin caused by a tyrosine deficiency could predispose a person to skin cancer. Anyone experiencing a pattern of protein loss, especially over an extended period (e.g., with nephrotic syndrome), may develop a deficiency in tyrosine and other amino acids.

Dietary Sources

Dietary sources richest in tyrosine are fish, meat, dairy, eggs, nuts, wheat germ, and oats. Normally, tyrosine can be synthesized endogenously from L-phenylalanine.

Source of Supplemental Form

Most L-tyrosine in nutraceuticals is produced by bacterial fermentation processes in a growth medium, from which the amino acid is then purified.

Supplemental Form

Capsule, powder, tablet; solution, oral.

Tyrosine is best absorbed when ingested at least 30 minutes before meals, divided into three daily doses. Some manufacturers have claimed that acetyl-L-tyrosine (ALT) affects the brain more rapidly than any other form.

It is often recommended that tyrosine be taken together with a multivitamin-mineral complex because vitamins B_6, folate, and copper participate in the conversion of L-tyrosine into neurotransmitters.

Dosage Range

Adult
Dietary:

Recommended dietary intake (RDA): 7.3 mg/pound
body weight/day, approximately 1 g/day
Average daily intake in United States: 3.5 to 5 g

Supplemental/Maintenance: Supplementation is usually not necessary for most individuals. Optimal levels of intake have not been established.
Pharmacological/Therapeutic: 1 to 8 g/day.

Clinical trials have used 100 mg/kg body weight/day, which constitutes a large dose. When indicated, many health care providers experienced in nutritional therapeutics initiate treatment with 2 g per day and gradually increase the dose as appropriate. Use at therapeutic doses would typically be short term. The most common recommended dose is 500 to 1000 mg three times daily (before each of the three meals). Toxic: Usually not to exceed 12 g per day, the highest known safe level.

Pediatric (< 18 Years)
Dietary: No specific dietary recommendation has been established for tyrosine in children.
Supplemental/Maintenance: Not currently recommended for children.
Pharmacological/Therapeutic: Indicated when amino acid imbalance demonstrated by laboratory assessment. In particular, tyrosine is administered in patients with PKU once plasma tyrosine levels have been controlled. Other-wise, specific treatment recommendations have not been established.
Toxic: No toxic dosage level established specifically for infants and children.

Laboratory Values

Range of normal plasma tyrosine levels:

Children: 26 to 110 µmol/L
Adults: 45 to 74 µmol/L

SAFETY PROFILE
Overview

L-Tyrosine is usually tolerated well by most adults and generally considered to be free of adverse effects for most individuals at usual dosage levels of 2 to 3 g daily. L-Tyrosine has very low toxicity.

Nutrient Adverse Effects

General Adverse Effects
Nausea, diarrhea, vomiting, and nervousness are the primary effects associated with intake of high dosage levels of tyrosine in some reports. Migraine headache, elevated blood pressure, and mild gastric upset may also result from excessive levels of tyrosine (or tyrosine-derived neurotransmitters such as dopamine).

Adverse Effects Among Specific Populations
Use of tyrosine may be contraindicated for individuals with hyperthyroidism, Tourette's syndrome, or schizophrenia, particularly when high brain dopamine levels are present. Exogenous tyrosine (or phenylalanine) administration could theoretically result in elevated brain dopamine levels and symptom aggravation.

Exogenous tyrosine could theoretically promote cancer cell division in susceptible individuals. Many tumor cells overexpress tyrosine kinase enzymes; phosphorylated tyrosine functions as a cell-signaling molecule that drives DNA synthesis, cell growth, and division in these tumors.

Pregnancy and Nursing
Evidence is lacking within the scientific literature to suggest or confirm any adverse effects related to fetal development during pregnancy or to infants who are breast-fed associated with tyrosine administration. Caution still advised regarding supplementation with free-form L-tyrosine.

Infants and Children

No adverse effects have been reported. However, sufficient research-based evidence is lacking to guarantee the safety of tyrosine in infants and children.

Contraindications

Migraine.

L-Tyrosine is contraindicated in those with the inborn errors of metabolism, alkaptonuria and tyrosinemia types I and II.

Tyrosine (and phenylalanine) should be avoided by individuals with cancer, especially pigmented melanoma.

Tyrosine should be avoided by individuals taking monoamine oxidase (MAO) inhibitors because of its role in synthesis of dopamine, norepinephrine, and epinephrine.

L-Tyrosine is contraindicated in those hypersensitive to any component of an L-tyrosine-containing supplement.

Precautions and Warnings

Concomitant administration of phenylalanine and tyrosine at high dosage levels should be avoided outside of professional supervision due to potential additive effects. Food sources may contain both nutrients but typically would be considered safe at usual levels of intake.

INTERACTIONS REVIEW

Strategic Considerations

Tyrosine from direct dietary sources as well as that synthesized endogenously from phenylalanine provides adequate quantities for normal physiological functions in most healthy individuals with reasonable nutriture. Administration of tyrosine is uncommon in conventional medicine apart from prevention and treatment of tyrosine deficiency in individuals with PKU and occasionally as an adjunctive agent for individuals with Parkinson's disease. Oral dosage levels of 19.2 mg/kg daily, divided equally in meals, and 100 mg/kg daily in three divided doses are typical for PKU and Parkinson's patients, respectively. Prudent clinical management requires establishing controlled plasma tyrosine levels approximating the norm of 45 µmol/L before considering tyrosine administration. Furthermore, concomitant use of tyrosine and levodopa should be discouraged outside the context of medical supervision because levodopa may interfere with the absorption of tyrosine.

Although supportive evidence is largely inconclusive, many practitioners experienced in nutritional therapeutics routinely prescribe L-tyrosine, with other nutrients and botanicals, as part of a comprehensive strategy to support thyroxine, dopamine, and other neurotransmitters in the treatment of fatigue, depression, suboptimal thyroid function, and other conditions. Methods for establishing clinical indications and determining therapeutic response are largely anecdotal and unsystematic, with clinical research data limited and preliminary.

A review of the collective body of available evidence reveals several medications that may interact with tyrosine to produce clinically significant effects in certain patients. The potentially severe interaction with MAO inhibitors, including the risk of a hypertensive crisis and catastrophic sequelae, warrants a general contraindication of concomitant use. Physicians prescribing any of these medications should ask patients about supplemental use of tyrosine and advise that they be avoided or discontinued, except possibly under close supervision. However, most interactions involving tyrosine and conventional medications can be beneficial in appropriate circumstances, but usually warrant supervision, monitoring, and periodic adjustments. Thus, coadministration of tyrosine can often enhance clinical outcomes when used in conjunction with levodopa, levothyroxine, and oral contraceptives within an integrative strategy. Concomitant use with imipramine, mixed amphetamines, appetite suppressants, or opioid analgesics may be appropriate in some cases but requires close supervision and regular monitoring by health care providers trained and experienced in both conventional pharmacology and nutritional therapeutics. In many cases, tyrosine administration can work more effectively when complemented by folic acid, B vitamins, and other nutrients typically at suboptimal levels in the target patient populations, compromised with the primary pathology or comorbid conditions, depleted by typical medications, or otherwise supportive of the therapeutic intervention.

NUTRIENT-DRUG INTERACTIONS

Amphetamines and Related Stimulant Medications

Amphetamine (amphetamine aspartate monohydrate, amphetamine sulfate), dextroamphetamine (dextroamphetamine saccharate, dextroamphetamine sulfate, D-amphetamine, Dexedrine).

Methylphenidate (Metadate, Methylin, Ritalin, Ritalin-SR; Concerta).

Combination drug: Mixed amphetamines: amphetamine and dextroamphetamine (Adderall; dexamphetamine).

Extrapolated, based on similar properties: Modafinil (Provigil).

Related but no longer on market: Pemoline (Cylert).

See also Appetite-Suppressant Medications in Theoretical, Speculative, and Preliminary Interactions Research.

Interaction Type and Significance

⊕⊕　**Beneficial or Supportive Interaction, with Professional Management**

≈≈　**Drug-Induced Nutrient Depletion, Supplementation Therapeutic, with Professional Management**

☼　**Prevention or Reduction of Drug Adverse Effect**

Probability:	Evidence Base:
4. Plausible	○ **Preliminary**

Effect and Mechanism of Action

Both adrenergic stimulants and tyrosine have been used in the treatment of narcolepsy and attention deficit disorder (ADD) with hyperactivity. An increase in the availability of tyrosine, under certain conditions, may influence the synthesis and release of dopamine.

Research

Animal research indicates that tyrosine depletion attenuates the release of dopamine produced by amphetamine but not the release of noradrenaline. In a rodent model, Geis et al.[1] observed that rats exposed to amphetamines for 4 to 6 months, but not 35 days or less, reduced amphetamine self-administration after receiving tyrosine. These investigators hypothesized that tyrosine may be useful in certain individuals depending on their history of substance abuse. In an experiment using male rats, Woods and Meyer[2] reported that exogenous tyrosine potentiates the methylphenidate-induced increase in extracellular dopamine in the nucleus accumbens.

A dietary deficiency of tyrosine may impair the therapeutic activity of amphetamines by depleting the available reserves of neurotransmitters. In an experiment involving 15 healthy volunteers, McTavish et al.[3] administered D-amphetamine (20 mg orally) 2 hours after they had ingested either a nutritionally balanced amino acid mixture or one lacking tyrosine and phenylalanine, the catecholamine precursors. These researchers observed that plasma tyrosine levels were significantly lower in subjects who received the nutrient-depleted mixture, but that mean plasma amphetamine levels were higher. Nevertheless, subjects reported that the nutrient-depleted mixture decreased the subjective psychostimulant effects of amphetamine, as indicated by visual analog scales. However, the nutrient-depleted mixture failed to reduce the subjective anorectic effect of amphetamine. This attenuation of some subjective effects of amphetamine after tyrosine depletion suggests that adequate tyrosine intake from dietary protein or nutraceuticals is essential to achieve full therapeutic effect in individuals administered amphetamines. Further research through large, well-designed clinical trials may be warranted.

Nutritional Therapeutics, Clinical Concerns, and Adaptations

Physicians prescribing mixed amphetamines or related stimulants may consider coadministering L-tyrosine as part of an integrative therapeutic strategy. The potential therapeutic efficacy of either therapy may be enhanced by concomitant use, especially in individuals susceptible to or exhibiting a tyrosine deficiency. Prudent clinical management warrants supervision and regular monitoring within the context of collaborative care by health care professionals trained and experienced in both conventional pharmacology and nutritional therapeutics.

Imipramine and Related Tricyclic Antidepressants (TCAs)

Evidence: Imipramine (Janimine, Tofranil).
Extrapolated, based on similar properties: Amitriptyline (Elavil); combination drug: amitriptyline and perphenazine (Etrafon, Triavil, Triptazine); amoxapine (Asendin), clomipramine (Anafranil), desipramine (Norpramin, Pertofrane), doxepin (Adapin, Sinequan), nortriptyline (Aventyl, Pamelor), protriptyline (Vivactil), trimipramine (Surmontil).

Interaction Type and Significance

⊕⊕ **Beneficial or Supportive Interaction, with Professional Management**

Probability:
4. Plausible

Evidence Base:
○ **Preliminary**

Effect and Mechanism of Action:

L-Tyrosine functions as a precursor to L-dopa, dopamine, norepinephrine, and epinephrine, the brain concentrations of which depend on intake of tyrosine. Augmenting tyrosine intake may produce an additive effect.

Research

Chronic cocaine use is believed to cause catecholamine depletion, and similarities exist between cocaine withdrawal and major depression. Tyrosine is the dietary precursor to catecholamines, and administration has produced positive outcomes in small trials of its antidepressant efficacy. The synaptic loss of dopamine with cocaine abuse increases demands for dopamine synthesis, as evidenced by the increase in tyrosine hydroxylase

activity after cocaine administration. Consequently, a dopamine deficiency develops when precursor reserves are exhausted. Administration of the precursors of the depleted monoamine neurotransmitters L-tyrosine and L-tryptophan is postulated to promote their biosynthesis and thus restore neurotransmitter function. Precursors use a naturally regulated pathway in which the precursor is converted to the neurotransmitter only when needed, and then the body distributes the product on the basis of need. As dopamine is synthesized from precursors such as L-tyrosine, dopamine reserves are rebuilt, thus overcoming the dopamine depletion problem. Thus, a benefit in treating drug dependence has been hypothesized based on these premises as well as the possibility of reducing the severe depression that typically accompanies withdrawal. Acute and chronic amphetamine abuse presents a situation analogous to that associated with cocaine abuse.

Human studies investigating the use of tyrosine, alone or with tryptophan, in the treatment of cocaine addiction and withdrawal have arrived at mixed conclusions.[4-7] However, in one small study the combination of imipramine, tyrosine, and tryptophan was associated with a success rate greater than 74% in the treatment of chronic cocaine abuse.[8] Verebey and Gold[9] proposed a regimen involving concomitant administration of L-tyrosine, L-tryptophan, thiamine, riboflavin, niacin, pantothenic acid, pyridoxamine, ascorbic acid, folic acid, and cyanocobalamin for the treatment of cocaine addiction. Further research through large, well-designed clinical trials may be warranted.

Nutritional Therapeutics, Clinical Concerns, and Adaptations

Health care professionals treating individuals for cocaine abuse may consider supporting the withdrawal process through administration of key neurotransmitter precursors such as tyrosine and tryptophan, possibly in concert with imipramine. Although not yet validated by mature research or conclusive evidence, such concomitant administration of these agents may be therapeutically appropriate within the context of collaborative care by health care professionals trained and experienced in both conventional pharmacology and nutritional therapeutics and with close supervision and regular monitoring. Titration of medication dosage may be appropriate with significant therapeutic response to tyrosine; a tyrosine-induced excess is improbable.

Levodopa and Related Antiparkinsonian Medications

Evidence: Levodopa (L-dopa; Dopar, Larodopa).
Extrapolated, based on similar properties: Carbidopa (Lodosyn); levodopa combination drugs: levodopa and benserazide (co-beneldopa; Madopar); levodopa and carbidopa (Atamet, Parcopa, Sinemet, Sinemet CR); levodopa, carbidopa, and entacapone (Stalevo).

Interaction Type and Significance

◇◇ **Impaired Drug Absorption and Bioavailability, Precautions Appropriate**

⊕✗ **Bimodal or Variable Interaction, with Professional Management**

◇≈≈ **Drug-Induced Adverse Effect on Nutrient Function, Coadministration Therapeutic, with Professional Management**

☼ **Prevention or Reduction of Drug Adverse Effect**

⊕⊕ **Beneficial or Supportive Interaction, with Professional Management**

Adverse Interaction
Probability:
4. Plausible

Evidence Base:
☐ **Inadequate**

Adverse Effect on Nutrient
Probability:
2. Probable

Evidence Base:
● **Consensus**

Coadministration Benefit
Probability:
2. Probable

Evidence Base:
◉ **Emerging**

Effect and Mechanism of Action

L-Tyrosine is a semi-essential amino acid that converts to L-dopa (levodopa), and administration of tyrosine can increase dopamine levels. However, levodopa may interfere with the absorption of tyrosine by competitively inhibiting the transport system.[10] Furthermore, levodopa and aromatic amino acids such as tyrosine and tryptophan can compete for brain uptake, and simultaneous administration may decrease levels of both nutrients and the medication.[11]

Research

Tyrosine has been considered a potential tool in the treatment of Parkinson's disease, depression, and other related conditions based on its role as a neurotransmitter precursor. Rodent and human studies have demonstrated that L-tyrosine administration can enhance dopamine synthesis. Growdon et al.[12] measured levels of tyrosine and homovanillic acid, the major dopamine metabolite, in lumbar cerebrospinal fluid (CSF) of 23 patients with Parkinson's disease before and during ingestion of 100 mg/kg/day of tyrosine; nine subjects were coadministered 100 mg/kg/day of probenecid (to prolong half-life of tyrosine by slowing renal elimination) in six divided doses for 24 hours before each spinal tap, whereas the other 14 did not receive probenecid. These researchers observed that CSF tyrosine levels significantly increased in both groups after oral L-tyrosine administration, and that homovanillic acid levels significantly increased in the group of patients pretreated with probenecid. These findings indicate that "L-tyrosine administration can increase dopamine turnover in patients with disorders in which physicians wish to enhance dopaminergic neurotransmission."[12]

In a small preliminary trial, Lemoine et al.[13] prescribed L-tyrosine (45 mg/lb body weight) to five naive patients diagnosed after sleep polygraphy criteria and five patients receiving L-dopa and/or dopamine agonist as long-term treatment of Parkinson's disease. After 3 years of L-tyrosine treatment, several patients demonstrated better clinical results and significantly fewer adverse effects than subjects treated with L-dopa or dopamine agonists. These authors cautioned that further research would be required to determine the "theoretical long-term sparing neurons potentiality" of this approach.

Riederer[11] spectrofluorometrically assayed tyrosine and tryptophan in postmortem human brain areas of patients with Parkinson's disease treated orally with or without L-dopa plus the peripherally acting decarboxylase inhibitor benserazide. He observed that both tyrosine and tryptophan were significantly decreased after treatment with L-dopa and interpreted these findings as demonstrating a competitive action of L-dopa to other aromatic amino acids on human brain uptake. No research has been conducted to determine whether such depletion is clinically significant. Furthermore, evidence is lacking as to whether concomitant L-tryosine could prevent or reverse adverse effects, if any, and whether such coadministration would be safe and effective. Well-designed clinical trials are warranted.

Nutritional Therapeutics, Clinical Concerns, and Adaptations

Administration of L-tyrosine, or its precursor phenylalanine, may serve as a valuable adjunctive therapy in the treatment of Parkinson's disease or similar conditions. Coadministration of tyrosine may prevent or reverse nutrient depletion resulting from levodopa therapy. However, concomitant use of levodopa and L-tyrosine could introduce several complications and should be avoided except under close supervision, regular monitoring, and coordinated care by health care professionals trained and experienced in both conventional pharmacology and nutritional therapeutics. Although concomitant administration might enhance effectiveness and reduce adverse effects of levodopa therapy, it carries an attendant risk of inducing adverse effects by excessively elevating dopamine levels. In cases where tyrosine is indicated, ingestion of the two agents should be separated (e.g., at least 4 hours apart) to reduce interference with absorption and CNS uptake.

Levothyroxine and Related Thyroid Hormones

L-Triiodothyronine (T_3): Cytomel, liothyronine sodium, liothronine sodium (synthetic T_3), Triostat (injection).
Levothyroxine (T_4): Eltroxin, Levo-T, Levothroid, levothyroxine (synthetic), levoxin, Levoxyl, Synthroid, thyroxine, Unithroid.
L-Thyroxine and L-triiodothyronine ($T_4 + T_3$): animal levothyroxine/liothyronine, Armour Thyroid, desiccated thyroid, Westhroid.
L-Thyroxine and L-triiodothyronine (synthetic $T_4 + T_3$): Euthroid, Euthyral, liotrix, Thyar, Thyrolar.
Dextrothyroxine (Choloxin).

Interaction Type and Significance

⊕⊕ **Beneficial or Supportive Interaction, with Professional Management**

Probability:
2. Probable or
1. Certain

Evidence Base:
☐ **Inadequate,** but considered
● **Consensus**

Effect and Mechanism of Action

L-Tyrosine is a direct precursor to thyroxine. Coadministration of tyrosine and exogenous thyroid hormone(s) may produce an additive interaction.

Research

Evidence from clinical trials directly investigating coadministration of tyrosine and thyroid hormone is lacking. Nevertheless, the effect of tyrosine levels on thyroid function is considered axiomatic within conventional pharmacology. Physicians experienced in nutritional therapeutics report beneficial effects after administering tyrosine to support thyroid function and coadministering tyrosine with various forms of exogenous thyroid hormone in treating individuals with hypothyroidism.

Nutritional Therapeutics, Clinical Concerns, and Adaptations

With proper clinical management, coadministration of tyrosine with natural or synthetic thyroid medications represents a potentially valuable synergy in the treatment of individuals with subclinical or frank hypothyroid conditions. The administration of tyrosine, alone or in combination with synergistic agents such as iodine, is common within the professional practice of nutritional therapeutics. Concomitant administration of tyrosine may be therapeutically appropriate but requires supervision and regular monitoring within the context of collaborative care by health care professionals trained and experienced in both conventional pharmacology and nutritional therapeutics. Titration of medication dosage may be appropriate with significant therapeutic response to tyrosine; a tyrosine-induced hyperthyroid state is improbable. Conversely, any additive effect of augmented tyrosine intake may be minimal in individuals whose thyroid gland has atrophied because of chronic use of synthetic thyroid medication and subsequent decline in endogenous hormone synthesis.

Monoamine Oxidase (MAO) Inhibitors

MAO-A inhibitors: Isocarboxazid (Marplan), moclobemide (Aurorix, Manerix), phenelzine (Nardil), procarbazine (Matulane), tranylcypromine (Parnate).
MAO-B inhibitors: Rasagiline (Azilect), selegiline (deprenyl, L-deprenil, L-deprenyl; Atapryl, Carbex, Eldepryl, Jumex, Movergan, Selpak).

Interaction Type and Significance

✗✗✗   **Potentially Harmful or Serious Adverse Interaction—Avoid**

Probability:
2. Probable

Evidence Base:
○ **Preliminary**

Effect and Mechanism of Action

The MAO inhibitors act by inhibiting the activity of the enzyme monoamine oxidase, which normally breaks down central monoamine neurotransmitters to render them inactive. The potentiation of sympathomimetic substances and related compounds by MAO inhibitors may result in hypertensive crisis and potential risk of heart attack or stroke. Tyramine in foods (e.g., red wine, aged cheeses) is the pressor amine most often implicated in these reactions. Tyrosine is converted into tyramine through decarboxylation by bacteria in the bowel. Therefore, elevated levels of tyrosine could induce an increase in tyramine capable of causing a clinically significant interaction.

Research

Concomitant intake of an MAO inhibitor (including selegiline) and foods containing certain pressor amines, particularly tyramine, or pharmacological agents containing sympathomimetic agents, has been associated with potentially serious hyperadrenergic states.[14] Besides tyramine, other amines and amine precursors, such as tyrosine, dopamine, levodopa, and histamine, may also precipitate such interactions.[15] This interaction is severe but infrequent and is characterized by severe occipital and temporal headache, elevation of both systolic and diastolic blood pressures, neuromuscular excitation, neck stiffness, diaphoresis, and mydriasis, generally occurring within 2 hours of ingestion of the substances. Cardiac dysrhythmias, heart failure, or intracerebral hemorrhage can occur, but rarely do. Meperidine (Demerol) and dextromethorphan (in many OTC cough medicines) have both been associated with fatal interactions with the type A MAO inhibitors.

Reports

No case reports have been published documenting adverse interactions involving tyrosine and MAO inhibitors. However, several reports have described delirium, hypomania, myoclonus, hyperreflexia, and diaphoresis attributed to the combination of L-tryptophan and a MAO inhibitor.[16-18]

Clinical Implications and Adaptations

Physicians prescribing phenelzine and related MAO inhibitors need to advise patients to avoid concomitant intake of L-tyrosine, sympathomimetic drugs (including amphetamines, cocaine, methylphenidate, dopamine, epinephrine, and norepinephrine), or related compounds (including methyldopa, L-dopa, L-tryptophan, 5-HTP, and phenylalanine), as well as foods high in tyramine. Concomitant administration of tyrosine may be appropriate in the treatment of some individuals but requires close supervision and regular monitoring within the context of collaborative care by health care professionals trained and experienced in both conventional pharmacology and nutritional therapeutics.

Oral Contraceptives: Monophasic, Biphasic, and Triphasic Estrogen Preparations (Synthetic Estrogen and Progesterone Analogs)

Ethinyl estradiol and desogestrel (Desogen, Ortho-TriCyclen).
Ethinyl estradiol and ethynodiol (Demulen 1/35, Demulen 1/50, Nelulen 1/25, Nelulen 1/50, Zovia).
Ethinyl estradiol and levonorgestrel (Alesse, Levlen, Levlite, Levora 0.15/30, Nordette, Tri-Levlen, Triphasil, Trivora).
Ethinyl estradiol and norethindrone/norethisterone (Brevicon, Estrostep, Genora 1/35, GenCept 1/35, Jenest-28, Loestrin 1.5/30, Loestrin 1/20, Modicon, Necon 1/25, Necon 10/11, Necon 0.5/30, Necon 1/50, Nelova 1/35, Nelova 10/11, Norinyl 1/35, Norlestin 1/50, Ortho Novum 1/35, Ortho Novum 10/11, Ortho Novum 7/7/7, Ovcon-35, Ovcon-50, Tri-Norinyl, Trinovum).
Ethinyl estradiol and norgestrel (Lo/Ovral, Ovral).
Mestranol and norethindrone (Genora 1/50, Nelova 1/50, Norethin 1/50, Ortho-Novum 1/50).
Related, Internal Application: Etonogestrel/ethinyl estradiol vaginal ring (Nuvaring).

Interaction Type and Significance

◇≈≈   **Drug-Induced Adverse Effect on Nutrient Function, Coadministration Therapeutic, with Professional Management**
≈≈   **Drug-Induced Nutrient Depletion, Supplementation Therapeutic, with Professional Management**
☼   **Prevention or Reduction of Drug Adverse Effect**

Probability:
2. Probable

Evidence Base:
◉ **Emerging**

Effect and Mechanism of Action

The formation of brain noradrenaline depends on brain tyrosine levels, associated with the ratio in plasma of tyrosine to other large, neutral amino acids (LNAAs). The combination of estrogen and progestins in oral contraceptives (OCs) can decrease plasma levels of tyrosine so as to contribute to adverse effects of the medications (e.g., depression).

Research

Moller and colleagues have been investigating the effects of OC use on amino acid metabolism for more than 25 years. In 1981, they studied the relationship of this effect on tryptophan and tyrosine, in particular on the association between OC use and depression. They found that, compared to controls, the "estrogen-progestogen users showed elevated plasma levels of total tryptophan and decreased levels of tyrosine," and that there "was a clear trend that the incidence of adverse reactions was related to the decrease in tyrosine levels." Furthermore, "the plasma ratio of tryptophan to competing amino acids was increased in the estrogen-progestogen users, whereas the ratio of tyrosine to competitors was severely decreased suggesting a decreased brain tyrosine concentration." They noted that ethinyl estradiol was more potent than mestranol in its effect on plasma tyrosine.[19] In a subsequent series of published human studies, they demonstrated significantly increased plasma tyrosine transaminase activity, and significantly decreased plasma tyrosine and tyrosine/LNAA levels at midcycle and luteal phase, relative to the follicular phase, in women administered new-generation combined OCs compared with comparable controls. They observed that, after an oral protein load, the area under the curve in plasma of tyrosine and tyrosine/ LNAA in OC users at the luteal phase were 43% and 29%, respectively, of control levels. These results "suggest that the decreased tyrosine availability to the brain in OC users may result in a substrate-limited reduction of brain noradrenaline formation, which, secondarily, may contribute to disturbances of mood, coping mechanisms, and appetite in susceptible subjects."[20] These researchers interpreted the findings of their third study to "suggest that the metabolic effects of the new-generation combined OCs on neutral amino acids and cholesterol are only modest to slight, except for the effect on tyrosine, the brain noradrenaline precursor, which may cause disturbances of various noradrenaline-mediated central functions in susceptible individuals."[21]

Clinical Implications and Adaptations

Physicians prescribing OCs may find it prudent to suggest that patients supplement with L-tyrosine and B-complex vitamins, particularly if they are susceptible to or have experienced depression or other emotional adverse effects in relation to medication use. Botanical and nutrient support of liver conjugation may also be beneficial within the context of collaborative care by health care professionals trained and experienced in both conventional pharmacology and nutritional/botanical therapeutics. Such coadministration is generally considered safe and does not require regular monitoring.

THEORETICAL, SPECULATIVE, AND PRELIMINARY INTERACTIONS RESEARCH, INCLUDING OVERSTATED INTERACTIONS CLAIMS

Appetite-Suppressant Medications, Including Amphetamine, Ephedrine, and Phenylpropanolamine

See also Amphetamines and Related Stimulant Medications.

As a precursor of many neurotransmitters, tyrosine may increase the activity of exogenous sympathomimetic agents. In an animal model using hyperphagic rats, Hull and Maher[22] observed that L-tyrosine (200 and 400 mg/kg) potentiated the anorectic activity of amphetamine/AMPH (0.75, 1.25, or 1.75 mg/kg), ephedrine/EPH (5, 10, or 20 mg/kg), and phenylpropanolamine/PPA (5, 10, or 20 mg/kg) in a dose-dependent manner. This response pattern suggested increased catecholamine synthesis in stimulated neurons. Notably, the potentiation by L-tyrosine was attenuated when L-valine was coadministered. However, in a subsequent experiment, they found that L-tyrosine fails to potentiate several peripheral actions of the sympathomimetics, particularly peripherally mediated PPA-, EPH-, and AMPH-induced increases in

gastrointestinal transit time and retention and intrascapular brown adipose tissue thermogenesis. Lastly, these researchers demonstrated that although each of the mixed-acting sympathomimetics significantly increased mean arterial, systolic, and diastolic blood pressures when administered alone, the coadministration of L-tyrosine failed to potentiate the pressor responses of PPA, EPH, or AMPH in urethane-anesthetized rats. Thus, Hull and Maher[23] concluded that the potentiation of the mixed-acting sympathomimetics by L-tyrosine is "largely restricted to centrally mediated responses."

Research through well-designed clinical trials would be necessary to determine whether coadministration of L-tyrosine and sympathomimetic appetite-suppressant agents would produce similar results in humans. Even though pharmacologically plausible, the combined use of these agents cannot be supported by the available evidence.

Codeine, Methadone, Morphine, and Related Oral Narcotic Analgesics (Opiates)

Butorphanol (Stadol, Stadol NS), codeine sulfate, fentanyl (Actiq Oral Transmucosal, Duragesic Transdermal, Fentanyl Oralet, Sublimaze Injection), hydrocodone, hydromorphone (Dilaudid), levorphanol (Levo-Dromoran), meperidine (Demerol), methadone (Dolophine; Methadose), metha-done hydrochloride (Dolophine, Methadose), morphine sulfate (Astramorph PF, Avinza, Duramorph, Infumorph, Kadian, MS Contin, MSIR, Oramorph SR, RMS; Roxanol, Roxanol Rescudose, Roxanol T), opium tincture, oxycodone (Endocodone, OxyContin, OxyIR, Percolone, Roxicodone), oxymorphone (Numorphan), paregoric, pentazocine (Talwin, Talwin NX), propoxyphene (Darvon; Darvon-N).

Combination drugs: Buprenorphine and naloxone (Suboxone); codeine and acetaminophen (Capital and Codeine; Phenaphen with Codeine; Tylenol with Codeine); codeine and acetylsalicylic acid (Empirin with codeine); codeine, acetaminophen, caffeine, and butalbital (Fioricet); codeine, acetylsalicylic acid, caffeine, and butalbital (Fiorinal); hydrocodone and acetaminophen (Anexsia, Anodynos-DHC, Co-Gesic, Dolacet, DuoCet, Hydrocet, Hydrogesic, Hy-Phen, Lorcet 10/650, Lorcet-HD, Lorcet Plus, Lortab, Margesic H, Medipain 5, Norco, Stagesic, T-Gesic, Vicodin, Vicodin ES, Vicodin HP, Zydone); hydrocodone and acetylsalicylic acid (Lortab ASA); hydrocodone and ibuprofen (Reprexain, Vicoprofen); opium and belladonna (B&O Supprettes); oxycodone and acetaminophen (Endocet, Percocet 2.5/325, Percocet 5/325, Percocet 7.5/500, Percocet 10/650, Roxicet 5/500, Roxilox, Tylox); oxycodone and acetylsalicylic acid (Endodan, Percodan, Percodan-Demi); pentazocine and acetaminophen (Talacen); pentazocine and acetylsalicylic acid (Talwin Compound); propoxyphene and acetaminophen (Darvocet-N, Darvocet-N 100, Pronap-100, Propacet 100, Propoxacet-N, Wygesic); propoxyphene and acetylsalicylic acid (Bexophene, Darvon Compound-65 Pulvules, PC-Cap); propoxyphene, acetylsalicylic acid, and caffeine (Darvon Compound).

Research using a rodent model indicates that L-tyrosine may potentiate the analgesic effect of opiate medications. In an experiment exposing rodents to a hot plate, Hull et al.[24] found that the observed potentiation of morphine sulfate (10 mg/kg) and codeine sulfate (30 mg/kg) was positively correlated with increases in brain tyrosine concentrations. The L-tyrosine-induced potentiation was dependent on increased catecholamine synthesis, as determined by alpha-methyl-p-tyrosine pretreatment. Furthermore, blockade of L-tyrosine uptake into the brain by the coadministration of L-valine attenuated this potentiation. No other L-amino acid, except

L-tryptophan, was capable of mimicking the potentiating action of L-tyrosine. The authors concluded that these findings demonstrate that L-tyrosine "dose dependently potentiates the analgesic activity of opioids and are consistent with the requirement of the central conversion of L-TYR to catecholamines via TYR hydroxylase for this response."[24] In a subsequent study, Ali[25] observed that L-tyrosine (25, 50, 100, and 200 mg/kg), administered subcutaneously, dose-dependently potentiated the antinociceptive action of subcutaneous morphine (5 mg/kg).

Well-designed clinical trials would be necessary to determine whether L-tyrosine would potentiate the analgesic activity of opiates in humans.

NUTRIENT-NUTRIENT INTERACTIONS

5-Hydroxytryptophan (5-HTP)

Tyrosine levels are occasionally low in depressed patients. Several studies in the 1970s published encouraging findings showing potential benefit from the treatment of depression using tyrosine, especially when combined with 5-HTP.[26-29] However, subsequent research failed to demonstrate significant antidepressant activity on the part of L-tyrosine.[30] Further human trials are warranted to investigate the relative influences of variations in presentations of depression, associated neurotransmitter patterns, and pharmacogenomic variability, as well as practice management principles for shaping individualized and evolving therapeutic interventions.

Branched-Chain Amino Acids: Isoleucine, Leucine, Valine

Branched-chain amino acids (BCAAs: isoleucine, leucine, valine) compete with tyrosine and other aromatic amino acids for absorption and transport across the blood-brain barrier into the brain. Separating intake of tyrosine (by at least 2 hours) from other amino acids and meals high in protein will reduce interference with bioavailability and therapeutic action. Dietary carbohydrates increase the amount of tryptophan, tyrosine, and phenylalanine that reach the brain.

Iodine

L-Tyrosine is a direct precursor to thyroxine. The combined use of tyrosine and iodine, from dietary or supplemental sources, has been practiced within naturopathic medicine and other traditions of nutritional therapeutics for decades, based on the hypothesis that coordinated intake can support the endogenous synthesis of thyroid hormones. Nevertheless, evidence from clinical trials directly investigating coadministration of tyrosine and iodine is lacking. Long-term, well-designed clinical trials are warranted to determine the safety and efficacy of this therapeutic strategy.

Phenylalanine

L-Tyrosine is synthesized from L-phenylalanine. Coadministration could theoretically enhance the activity of both nutrients. However, concomitant administration of phenylalanine and tyrosine at high dosage levels should be avoided outside of professional supervision because of potential additive effects. Food sources may contain both nutrients but typically would be considered safe at usual levels of intake.

The 30 citations for this monograph, as well as additional reference literature, are located under Tyrosine on the CD at the back of the book.

Nutrient-Drug Interactions and Drug-Induced Nutrient Depletions

5-Hydroxytryptophan

Nutrient Name: 5-Hydroxytryptophan.
Synonyms: 5-HTP, L-5-hydroxytryptophan, L-5-HTP.
Related Substances: L-tryptophan; 5-hydroxytryptamine, 5-HT, serotonin.

Summary

Drug/Class Interaction Type	Mechanism and Significance	Management
D-Amphetamine Stimulant medications ⊕/☼	5-Hydroxytryptophan (5-HTP) may mitigate adverse effects associated with amphetamine therapy in schizophrenic patients through an unknown mechanism.	Concomitant use could be therapeutic with appropriate clinical management.
Carbidopa Antiparkinsonian medications ⊕⊕/⊕✗/✗✗	Coadministration of 5-HTP with carbidopa therapy may reduce intention myoclonus and related neuromuscular disorders by enhancing serotonin levels. Some individuals react with symptoms that include scleroderma-like lesions, based on enzyme variability.	Concomitant use could be therapeutic with appropriate clinical management and attention to individual pharmacogenomic response.
Chlorimipramine Tricyclic antidepressants ⊕/⊕✗/✗✗	Coadministration of chlorimipramine and 5-HTP can elevate serotonin and cortisol levels, possibly producing more favorable therapeutic response in treatment of depression than either agent alone; additive effects of concomitant use could be detrimental or beneficial, depending on clinical circumstances.	Concomitant use could be therapeutic or detrimental. Individualized assessment, flexible clinical management, close supervision, and regular monitoring required.
Lithium ⊕⊕/☼	Lithium may enhance 5-HTP-induced increase in serum cortisol concentration in bipolar or depressed patients. Concomitant administration of 5-HTP may improve clinical outcomes, especially in patients resistant to lithium therapy alone.	Concomitant use could be therapeutic, if indicated. Individualized assessment, close supervision, and regular monitoring required.
Sertraline Selective serotonin reuptake inhibitor (SSRI) antidepressants ✗✗✗/⊕✗/⊕	As a 5-HT precursor, 5-HTP administration can elevate serotonin levels. SSRIs inhibit serotonin uptake. Probable additive effect from combined use of these agents appears to be near-certain with adverse interactions of rapid onset and severe character, particularly serotonin syndrome. However, direct evidence from clinical trials or case reports is minimal, if not absent. Closely supervised coadministration suggested in select circumstances, but supportive evidence lacking and currently outweighed by suspected risks.	Avoid concomitant use because of probable risks.
Selegiline Monoamine oxidase (MAO-B) inhibitors ⊕⊕/⊕✗/✗	Small clinical trials indicate that coadministration of 5-HTP with selegiline in treatment of unipolar and bipolar depression may enhance MAO inhibition and clinical response through additive effect on serotonin.	Concomitant use could be therapeutic, if indicated. Individualized assessment, close supervision, and regular monitoring required.
Sibutramine Serotonin agonists ✗✗✗	As a 5-HT precursor, 5-HTP administration can elevate serotonin levels. As a serotonin agonist, sibutramine inhibits serotonin uptake. Probable additive effect from combined use of these agents induces significant risk of adverse interactions of rapid onset and severe character, particularly serotonin syndrome. However, direct evidence from clinical trials or case reports is minimal, if not absent.	Avoid concomitant use because of probable risks.
Sumatriptan, zolmitriptan Triptans ✗✗✗	As a 5-HT precursor, 5-HTP administration can elevate serotonin levels. As serotonin receptor agonists (5-HT1B/1D), triptans bind to and activate serotonin receptors. Probable additive effect from combined use of these agents induces significant risk of adverse interactions of rapid onset and severe character, particularly serotonin syndrome. However, direct evidence from clinical trials or case reports is minimal, if not absent.	Avoid concomitant use because of probable risks.

NUTRIENT DESCRIPTION

Chemistry and Form

5-hydroxytryptophan (5-HTP) is similar in structure to tryptophan except that an OH group has been added to the fifth group of the carbon ring. Subsequently, the amino acid decarboxylase enzyme converts 5-HTP to 5-hydroxytryptamine (5-HT, serotonin).

Physiology and Function

Within the human body, the amino acid L-tryptophan is converted into 5-HTP. Tryptophan is one of eight essential amino acids that must be obtained from the diet. Its primary functions include its role in niacin (vitamin B_3) synthesis and as a precursor to both serotonin and melatonin. Approximately 98% of dietary L-tryptophan is metabolized into nicotinic acid (niacin), and only a very small amount is metabolized into serotonin via the intermediary stage of 5-HTP. 5-Hydroxytryptamine (5-HT, serotonin) is a key neurotransmitter associated with sleep, mood, aggression, anxiety, locomotion, body temperature, feeding, and pain sensation. The central serotoninergic neuronal system is quite complex. Seven discrete major serotonin receptors, numbered 1 through 7, have been characterized; several of these have been further divided into A, B, and C subtypes. Each of these receptors binds serotonin, various drugs, and other ligands with varying avidity, and several of these serotonin receptor subtypes have functionally opposing roles, notably the effects of 5-HT1A and 5-HT2C receptor agonism on anxiety. The potent nausea-blocking agents used with many cancer chemotherapies specifically block the 5-HT3 receptor. The neuroendocrine effects of 5-HTP appear to be mediated through 5HT2A/5HT2C receptors.

5-Hydroxytryptophan crosses the blood-brain barrier (BBB, through a calcium-dependent mechanism) and affects hypothalamic-pituitary-adrenal activity by stimulating the central nervous system (CNS) synthesis and release of serotonin. Serotonin is synthesized in the CNS and gut using the unique indole moiety of tryptophan as its nucleus. Serotonergic neurons express the enzyme *tryptophan hydroxylase* (TPH), which catalyzes the conversion of tryptophan to 5-hydroxytryptophan. TPH is the rate-limiting biosynthetic enzyme in the serotonin pathway; it regulates levels of serotonin and is normally only about half-saturated. Serotonin is formed from tryptophan in a two-step process: after formation of 5-HTP by TPH, the final decarboxylation is catalyzed by aromatic L-amino acid decarboxylase (AADC), resulting in the conversion of 5-HTP to 5-HT (serotonin). The pineal gland is the major site for synthesis of *melatonin,* a methoxy derivative of tryptophan that modulates the sleep cycle, among other activities. The pineal gland also synthesizes serotonin, production of which is upregulated at night and controlled by beta-adrenergic signaling. Serotonin is present at highest concentrations in platelets and in the gastrointestinal (GI) tract. Lesser amounts are found in the brain and the retina. Serotonin in the CNS is metabolized by the monoamine oxidase (MAO) enzyme to 5-hydroxyindole-acetic acid (5-HIAA). Levels of 5-HIAA in cerebrospinal fluid (CSF) are believed to reflect serotonergic activity in the CNS. Urinary levels are probably a less precise reflection but may be clinically useful.

NUTRIENT IN CLINICAL PRACTICE
Known or Potential Therapeutic Uses

5-Hydroxytryptophan is primarily used in the treatment of anxiety, depression, insomnia, and other conditions typically associated with serotonin deficiency or dysregulatory states. Poldinger et al.[1] argue that, although 5-HTP appears to be treating depression, it may actually be treating a much broader condition, "serotonin deficiency syndrome." This syndrome may manifest in any of a variety of forms, including depression, anxiety, sleeplessness, aggressiveness, agitation, obsessive-compulsive traits, migraines, and other common behavioral disorders.

5-Hydroxytryptophan is well absorbed, with approximately 70% of an oral dose reaching the bloodstream. Subsequently, some exogenous 5-HTP is rapidly decarboxylated in the peripheral vasculature to form serotonin, and the remainder crosses the BBB and increases synthesis of serotonin within serotonergic neurons. Therapeutic use of 5-HTP bypasses the conversion of L-tryptophan into 5-HTP by TPH, the rate-limiting step in the synthesis of serotonin.

Research using infusions of radiolabeled 5-HTP and positron-emission tomography (PET) scanning found that significantly less 5-HTP crossed the BBB into the brains of depressed subjects than into the brains of normal controls. Such findings have been interpreted to suggest that the transport of 5-HTP across the BBB may be compromised in major depression.

5-Hydroxytryptophan was introduced into the U.S. market in 1994. L-Tryptophan had been tarnished in the late 1980s and early 1990s by toxic effects of contaminated material produced by one Japanese supplier. In contrast, the related compound 5-HTP could be used for a therapeutically similar effect, but without the attendant susceptibility to contamination; 5-HTP is not produced by microbial biosynthesis requiring subsequent purification steps.

Historical/Ethnomedicine Precedent

5-Hydroxytryptophan has not been used historically as an isolated nutrient.

Possible Uses

Aggressive behavior, alcohol addiction, anxiety, attention deficit–hyperactivity disorder, bipolar disorder, bulimia, childhood headaches, depression, Down syndrome, fibromyalgia, hepatitis, insomnia, migraine, narcolepsy, obesity, obsessive-compulsive disorder, pain syndromes, Parkinson's disease, premenstrual syndrome, rheumatoid arthritis, schizophrenia, seasonal affective disorder, sleep apnea, sleep disorder–related headaches (children), sleep paralysis, systemic lupus erythematosus, tension headaches, Tourette's syndrome, weight management.

Deficiency Symptoms

Standard definitions of deficiency states have not been established, given endogenous synthesis, and because the relationship between 5-HTP status and serotonin-shortage syndrome is controversial. However, many clinicians and researchers have considered anxiety, depression, insomnia, and other conditions as deriving from diminished serotonin status and therefore implicitly some measure of 5-HTP deficiency.

Dietary Sources

Diets low in tryptophan may result in reduced synthesis of serotonin and melatonin, but L-tryptophan from dietary sources does not directly influence or contribute to 5-HTP levels.

Dosage Forms Available

Capsule, tablet; typically containing 25, 50, or 100 mg.

Source Materials for Nutrient Preparations

An alcoholic extraction process is used to extract 5-HTP from the seeds of the *Griffonia simplicifolia,* an African plant. The resulting oily solid is then purified into a dry solid at 99% or higher purity levels.

Dosage Range
Adult

Dietary: Not applicable per se.
Supplemental/Maintenance: 5-HTP is usually not taken except for therapeutic purposes.
Pharmacological/Therapeutic: Oral: 50 to 100 mg one to three times daily; occasionally, doses up to 200 mg three times daily may be appropriate. Doses of 100 to 200 mg daily may be effective for many individuals, and dosages used in clinical trials have ranged from 150 to 900 mg daily over 2 weeks to 6 months. Dosages are usually divided throughout the day, with possible increased dosage before bedtime; 5-HTP is often taken only before bedtime to enhance sleep. Orally administered 5-HTP is considered to provide the most rapid absorption when taken on an empty stomach.

Toxic: Excessive oral intake of 5-HTP could theoretically induce a state of serotonin excess, but levels necessary to exceed such a threshold have not been established and would most likely vary significantly among individuals based on health status, comorbid conditions, and pharmacogenomics.

Pediatric (< 18 Years)

Dietary: Not applicable per se.

Supplemental/Maintenance: 5-HTP is usually not taken except for therapeutic purposes.

Pharmacological/Therapeutic: Data are lacking on dosage for 5-HTP administration in children. Such usage is not recommended in sources reviewed.

Toxic: Data are lacking on toxicity of 5-HTP in children.

Laboratory Values

Serotonin may be relevant and could be assessed via urinary levels of 5-hydroxyindoleacetic acid (5-HIAA), the chief breakdown metabolite of serotonin.

SAFETY PROFILE

Overview

Individuals taking higher doses of 5-HTP have reported anxiety, digestive upset, headache, lethargy, and muscle pain, with GI symptoms being the most common. Theoretically, serotonin syndrome could result from use of excessive levels of 5-HTP, especially in combination with medications, herbs, or other supplements that alter serotonin levels or impair regulation. Some individuals with compromised liver function might not be able to regulate 5-HTP properly and require close medical supervision. Further, contaminants reported in some commercially available sources of 5-HTP may be associated with symptoms similar to eosinophilia-myalgia syndrome (EMS), which was linked to contaminated tryptophan in the late 1980s and early 1990s; however, recent reports of such incidents are lacking.

Nutrient Adverse Effects

Nausea and mild GI distress are the most common adverse effects generally associated with 5-HTP intake. Such GI symptoms affect only a minority of users, and then only occasionally. They usually lessen or disappear in the first few days or weeks of use. Headache, drowsiness, anxiety, and generalized muscle pain have also been reported. Research indicates that the incidence of such adverse reactions is minimal and usually only associated with higher dosage levels than typically used. Careful dose titration for each individual will usually prevent or minimize the occurrence of nausea and other adverse effects. Anecdotal clinical experience has suggested that, in patients very sensitive to GI effects of 5-HTP, a time-release preparation of 5-HTP from a compounding pharmacy will overcome this problem.

Adverse Effects Among Specific Populations

Individuals diagnosed with liver disease or compromised liver function may have limited capacity to metabolize 5-HTP and should avoid concomitant use with substances known to impair hepatic function or cause liver damage. Likewise, individuals with scleroderma or other autoimmune diseases may be more susceptible to an adverse reaction to 5-HTP intake; such cases also require consultation with a health care professional trained and experienced in prescribing physiologic agents such as 5-HTP.

Genotoxicity and Teratogenicity

Pregnancy and Nursing

The safety of exogenous 5-HTP intake during pregnancy and breastfeeding has not been established at this time.

Infants and Children

Data are lacking regarding toxicity and safety parameters for 5-HTP administration in infants and children. A high level of caution is suggested, especially given concerns of adverse effects among children receiving selective serotonin reuptake inhibitor (SSRI) therapy. Such pharmacological manipulation of serotonin levels and regulatory processes is generally not recommended, and significant caution is warranted, especially given the continued reports of adverse effects (and limited efficacy) in children being treated with conventional antidepressants, particularly SSRIs.[2]

Sparse anecdotal clinical evidence suggests that 5-HTP is well tolerated and can be effective as an alternative in children for whom experienced clinicians have recommended SSRI therapy for anxiety and depression, or in pervasive developmental disorders. In the absence of clinical trials, such therapy should be undertaken only by clinicians experienced in child psychiatry/psychology, in concert with clinicians experienced with 5-HTP and other nutraceutical therapies. SSRIs and 5-HTP may be hazardous to combine in both children and adults.

Contraindications

Because of the generally accepted risk of excessive serotonin levels and resultant effects, it is usually recommended that 5-HTP not be taken concomitantly with antidepressant medications (SSRIs, tricyclics, MAO-A inhibitors) or other serotonin-modifying agents. Given the rapid action of orally administered 5-HTP and the potentially high risk of complications, such concomitant administration should be avoided, except possibly under close supervision of and regular monitoring by health care professionals trained and experienced in both conventional pharmacology and nutritional precursor therapeutics, preferably within the context of an inpatient research setting. Direct evidence of such adverse interactions is minimal, but caution is advisable.

Precautions and Warnings

It has occasionally been recommended that individuals with asthma avoid oral 5-HTP intake, based on the theory that the condition could be aggravated by elevating levels of any serotonin precursor, and that higher dosage levels in particular might increase the risk of exercise-induced asthma and fatigue. There is no substantial clinical evidence of this, but it should be kept in mind as a possibility, if a patient with underlying asthma were to experience exacerbation while taking 5-HTP. Given the pharmacokinetics involved, discontinuation of the 5-HTP should result in rapid resolution of the exacerbation, were this to occur.

Note: During the early 1990s a substance designated as "Peak X" was reportedly found in low concentrations in some 5-HTP preparations. Speculation arose that it might be linked to the EMS previously associated with contaminated batches of L-tryptophan, which contained larger amounts of "Peak X," although the exact structure of this component and a causative role in EMS were never definitively established. No substantive evidence ever confirmed a connection between this substance and alleged incidents of 5-HTP toxicity, nor was it ever conclusively proven to have caused or contributed to any adverse events or toxicity reactions.

INTERACTIONS REVIEW
Strategic Considerations

An evolving body of evidence indicates that 5-HTP may be as effective as many conventional medications in the treatment of depression, anxiety, insomnia and other neuroendocrine conditions, generally with fewer adverse effects. "In functional dimensional parlance, treating a serotonin deficiency is tantamount to treating all symptoms figuring as behavioral expressions of the serotonin-dependent psychological dysfunctions," write Poldinger, Calanchini, and Schwarz.[1]

For many years, a broad assumption in the medical literature is that drug-nutriceutical interactions involving 5-HTP represent significant risks of frequent occurrence, severe character, and seemingly self-evident pharmacological characteristics. Such interactions between 5-HTP and pharmacological agents could theoretically be relatively common because 5-HTP and many medications with which it may interact are used to treat the same conditions and patient populations. Oral ingestion of 5-HTP in animals and humans seems to be able to cause symptoms (primarily diarrhea) associated with elevated serotonin. In an experimental model, 5-HTP plus a MAO inhibitor has been shown to produce a syndrome similar to serotonin syndrome.[3] However, there is a surprising dearth of scientific evidence from controlled clinical trials or documented case reports supporting or detailing this interaction of presumably high probability. A significant number of the "interactions" attributed to 5-HTP are actually extrapolations derived from case reports and trials involving drugs, particularly those that interfere with serotonin metabolism or regulation, and as such function through a fundamentally different mechanism of action than the nutritive supply enhancement model of therapeutics employing 5-HTP. The lack of documented interactions involving 5-HTP, in contrast to SSRIs or other pharmacological agents directly manipulating serotonin levels by impairing the regulatory processes of serotonin breakdown, might be interpreted to suggest that enhancement of 5-HTP levels through oral intake, in contrast to SSRIs or other pharmacological agents directly manipulating serotonin levels, may enable serotonin production when needed, without forcing up serotonin levels when feedback systems signal saturation. No evidence has emerged to indicate that serotonin syndrome or other adverse interaction phenomena can result from combining an SSRI agent with a protein-rich diet containing significant levels of L-tryptophan. Although a naturally occurring intermediate, 5-HTP is normally self-regulated in the body, with elevated levels rarely reported. Most likely, if 5-HTP production is upregulated for some reason (e.g., SNPs, diet, lifestyle), causing increased serotonin production, the body compensates by upregulating serotonin reuptake, keeping everything in balance.

Nevertheless, the combined use of 5-HTP and antidepressant drugs (including tricyclics, MAO inhibitors, and SSRIs, as well as other serotonin agonists) all present a significant probability of increased risk of adverse effects. In particular, widespread warnings have cautioned against the risk of *serotonin syndrome,* a dangerous but relatively rare condition caused by excess serotonin levels that could theoretically result from simultaneous 5-HTP intake in individuals whose serotonin regulation has been impeded by such medications. This potentially dangerous situation results from excess serotonin availability in the CNS at the 5-HT1A receptor; some interaction with dopamine and 5-HT2 receptors is also likely to be involved. Serotonin syndrome carries potentially serious clinical consequences and is characterized by the triad of altered mental status, autonomic dysfunction, and neuromuscular abnormalities. The serotonin syndrome is similar to the neuroleptic malignant syndrome and is usually differentiated by the setting of recent addition of a serotonergic agent. Specific symptoms can include agitation, anxiety, ataxia, confusion, delirium, diaphoresis, diarrhea, fever, hyperreflexia, myoclonus, incoordination, shivering, nausea, vomiting, and tremor. This phenomenon most often occurs with SSRIs, MAO inhibitors, opioids, and other serotonergic agents, when the serotonin system has been modulated by another serotonergic agent or compromised by illness. SSRIs, particularly fluoxetine, are most often involved in reported drug interactions inducing serotonin syndrome; because of their long elimination half-life (1 week for fluoxetine), the risk of interactions persists for several days or even weeks after SSRI withdrawal. Simultaneously elevating serotonin levels through introduction of precursors while inhibiting serotonin uptake and breakdown risks interaction scenarios. 5-HTP should never be combined with SSRIs or MAO inhibitors at any dose, except possibly in a carefully monitored inpatient clinical research setting.

Conversely, the concomitant use of 5-HTP and serotonin antagonists is likely to reduce the effectiveness of these agents. Nevertheless, the likelihood and frequency of such adverse events, as well as the respective levels of drug and nutrient intake at which this toxic effect might occur, remain unknown.

More broadly, clinicians treating individuals with depression, insomnia, and related conditions face the more profound and demanding task of helping these patients restore their lives to a healthy level of functionality, stability, and resilience. Comprehensive positive clinical outcomes cannot be achieved simply by medicating patients in adverse or stressful life circumstances. The fundamental therapeutic interventions in such circumstances require that health care providers work together to reempower these individuals by encouraging and supporting lifestyle changes involving exercise and healthy diet, changes in dysfunctional work or relationship behaviors and patterns, psychological counseling, and the challenges of personal growth. Despite repeated promises of pharmacologically induced emotional well-being based on "correction" of "brain chemistry," clinicians face the daily challenge of viewing antidepressants or other psychopharmacological interventions as "bridge therapies" within a broader therapeutic strategy, as "crutches" that give way to free walking and renewed vigor and equilibrium.

Nutraceuticals and herbal therapeutics that enhance neurotransmitter status can play important primary or adjunctive roles in such a broader strategic approach. Such a multimodality approach can often provide safe and effective intervention during certain phases of the therapeutic process to "round out" pharmacology or as alternatives to medications that primarily preempt or interfere with self-regulatory feedback systems.

NUTRIENT-DRUG INTERACTIONS

Dextroamphetamine and Related Stimulant Medications

Evidence: Amphetamine (amphetamine aspartate monohydrate, amphetamine sulfate); dextroamphetamine, dextroamphetamine saccharate, dextroamphetamine sulfate; D-amphetamine; Dexedrine; combination drug: mixed amphetamines: amphetamine and dextroamphetamine (Adderall; dexamphetamine).
Similar properties but evidence lacking for extrapolation: Methylphenidate (Metadate, Methylin, Ritalin, Ritalin-SR; Concerta).

Interaction Type and Significance
⊕   **Potential or Theoretical Beneficial or
    Supportive Interaction, with Professional
    Management**
☼   **Prevention or Reduction of Drug Adverse Effect**

Probability: Evidence Base:
3. Possible   ○ **Preliminary**

Effect and Mechanism of Action
Serotonin may be involved in the modulation of psychotic symptoms in some forms of schizophrenia. Although frequently associated with aggressive behavior and other adverse effects, amphetamine use is generally not associated with symptoms of acute psychosis, except in individuals with schizophrenia. Administration of exogenous 5-HTP may mitigate adverse effects associated with therapeutic amphetamine use in schizophrenic patients through an unknown mechanism involving its role as a serotonin precursor.

Research
Amphetamines are well known to trigger acute schizophrenic breaks in susceptible individuals, which may require hospitalization. In an uncontrolled clinical trial, Irwin et al.[4] found that "preadministration with 5HTP significantly antagonized amphetamine-elicited elevations in thought disturbance, activation, and hallucinations" in schizophrenic patients.

No research appears to be available investigating potential synergy between 5-HTP and amphetamine agents in the treatment of broader patient populations or other conditions for which this drug class is employed (e.g., hyperactivity/ADHD).

Nutritional Therapeutics, Clinical Concerns, and Adaptations
Physicians prescribing D-amphetamine to patients diagnosed with schizophrenia or related psychiatric conditions are advised to consider the potential benefits of 5-HTP coadministration under close supervision. Such a situation is unusual and not likely to be encountered in most clinical settings.

Carbidopa and Related Antiparkinsonian Medications

Evidence: Carbidopa (Lodosyn).
Extrapolated, based on similar properties: Levodopa (L-dopa; Dopar, Larodopa); combination drugs: levodopa and benserazide (co-beneldopa; Madopar); levodopa and carbidopa (Atamet, Parcopa, Sinemet, Sinemet CR); levodopa, carbidopa, and entacapone (Stalevo).

Interaction Type and Significance
⊕⊕   **Beneficial or Supportive Interaction, with
      Professional Management**
⊕✗   **Bimodal or Variable Interaction, with Professional
      Management**
✗✗   **Minimal to Mild Adverse Interaction—Vigilance
      Necessary**

Supportive Interaction
Probability: Evidence Base:
2. Probable   ◉ **Emerging**

Adverse Effect
Probability: Evidence Base:
3. Possible   ○ **Preliminary**

Effect and Mechanism of Action
Abnormalities in tryptophan metabolism, particularly elevated kynurenine, have been associated with adverse dermatological reactions in some individuals administered both 5-HTP and carbidopa, which combines L-dopa with a peripheral decarboxylase inhibitor. It has been suggested that individuals with an abnormality in kynurenine hydrolase or another of the enzymes responsible for catabolizing kynurenine, an intermediate compound in tryptophan metabolism, might be susceptible to this reaction in the presence of carbidopa, when serotonin levels rise subsequent to 5-HTP intake.

Research
Some types of intention myoclonus are caused by a deficiency of brain 5HT (serotonin) and respond to serotonin precursor therapy (e.g., L-5-HTP). Clinical trials have found that the coadministration of carbidopa and 5-HTP may have a beneficial effect in the treatment of many individuals with intention myoclonus and related neuromuscular disorders. Growdon et al.[5] investigated the concomitant use of 5-HTP and carbidopa in eight individuals with posthypoxic intention myoclonus. They found a variable response depending on the individual and the form of myoclonus. These researchers concluded: "A patient's response to L-5-hydroxytryptophan therapy may be important in a diagnostic classification of myoclonic syndromes based on differences in indoleamine neurotransmitter function." Van Woert et al.[6] administered 5-HTP to 18 patients being treated for intention myoclonus caused by anoxia or other brain damage. Eleven derived more than 50% overall improvement during treatment with L-5-HTP and carbidopa. Cerebrospinal fluid 5-HIAA was 35% lower in patients with intention myoclonus than in controls. Combined therapy with L-5-HTP and carbidopa increased the concentration of serotonin metabolites in urine and CSF. These researchers postulated that "a deficiency of brain serotonin is causally related to intention myoclonus and that the therapeutic effect of L-5HTP and carbidopa may be due to the repletion of serotonin in regions of the brain where serotoninergic neurons have degenerated."[6] In subsequent research, Van Woert et al.[7] found that although fluoxetine alone provided no antimyoclonic effect when administered alone to four patients with intention myoclonus, a combination therapy using carbidopa, 5-HTP, and fluoxetine had a beneficial effect on serotonin in relation to intention myoclonus. Thus, "in two patients with intention myoclonus responsive to L-5HTP and carbidopa, fluoxetine reduced the required dose of L-5HTP to approximately one-third, with greater antimyoclonic activity, decreased side effects, and reduction in platelet 5HT and plasma 5-hydroxyindoleacetic acid and L-5HTP concentrations."[7]

A range of adverse effects have been noted in individuals being treated with such a regimen, including "persistent euphoria," early mania, rapid speech, restlessness, insomnia, aggressiveness, and diarrhea.

In a potentially relevant animal study, Bender and Smith[8] found that carbidopa inhibits kynurenine hydrolase, an enzyme involved in the biosynthesis of niacin.

In 1981, Magnussen et al.[9] measured the influence of L-aromatic amino acid decarboxylase inhibitors on single oral doses of L-5-HTP, as reflected in plasma concentrations of 5-HTP, 5-HT (serotonin), and 5-HIAA and the concentrations of serotonin in blood platelets. They observed that "carbidopa enhanced the rise in plasma concentrations of 5-HTP 5-15 fold and counteracted the increase in plasma 5-HIAA levels induced by 5-HTP alone. A single dose of the decarboxylase inhibitor was equipotent to 14 days' pretreatment."[9] In a follow-up study the next year, this research team determined that neurological patients receiving steady-state treatment with 5-HTP demonstrated accumulation of 5-HT in blood platelets and 5-HIAA in plasma in all patients, despite concomitant administration of the L-aromatic amino acid decarboxylase inhibitors, carbidopa and benserazide. There was no correlation between the 5-HTP dose and the circulating concentrations of the amino acid or its metabolites. Preliminary comparison of the carbidopa versus benserazide suggest the 5-HTP/carbidopa combination appeared superior to 5-HTP/benserazide in terms of biochemical and therapeutic effects.[10]

Reports

Magnussen et al.[11] published a case report that offers some potentially valuable clues in understanding this interaction. They described a patient successfully treated for posthypoxic intention myoclonus by long-term coadministration of 900 mg 5-HTP daily and 150 mg carbidopa. By administering methysergide (12 mg/day), they were able to block the therapeutic effect, thus indicating a specific serotoninergic function of precursor loading with 5-HTP. Further, coadministration of tryptophan (8 g/day) exerted no beneficial effect on the myoclonus, thereby suggesting a reduced tryptophan hydroxylase activity.

Sternberg et al.[12] reported a scleroderma-like illness that developed in a patient treated with L-5-HTP and carbidopa for intention myoclonus. The patient had high plasma kynurenine levels that remained high when the L-5-HTP/carbidopa combination was discontinued and rose further when the drug was reintroduced, suggesting that the drug revealed an abnormality in an enzyme that catabolizes kynurenine. Cessation of 5-HTP, along with introduction of 100 mg vitamin B$_6$ daily (which enhances decarboxylase activity), was associated with gradual resolution of the scleroderma-like condition. Subsequently, these researchers found that plasma kynurenine was also elevated in 7 of 15 patients with idiopathic scleroderma, but not in eight patients with intention myoclonus treated with L-5-HTP and a decarboxylase inhibitor and in whom scleroderma did not develop, or in 10 patients with Parkinson's disease treated with L-dopa and carbidopa. They concluded that high plasma serotonin and a metabolic abnormality associated with elevated kynurenine were important in the pathogenesis of some scleroderma-like disorders.

Joly et al.[12a] also published a case report of hardening of the skin similar to scleroderma and pseudobullous morphea during therapy with 5-HTP and carbidopa. Subsequently, Auffranc et al.[13] reported a case of sclerodermiform and poikilodermal syndrome in a male patient receiving carbidopa and 5-HTP.

This adverse reaction is not widely associated with concomitant use of carbidopa and 5-HTP and appears to be related to particular pharmacogenomic factors shared by the affected individuals, but of unknown frequency in the general patient population. Reports of such scleroderma-like conditions in association with 5-HTP intake appear to be confined to the context of carbidopa therapy, presumably related to the decarboxylase inhibitor component of carbidopa slowing transformation of 5-HTP into serotonin in the peripheral circulation, with consequent elevation of kynurenine in susceptible individuals.

Nutritional Therapeutics, Clinical Concerns, and Adaptations

The combined use of carbidopa and 5-HTP appears to be a potentially beneficial therapeutic tool in the treatment of at least some individuals with intention myoclonus. However,

physicians prescribing carbidopa should advise patients to avoid concomitant use of 5-HTP, except under coordinated care involving close supervision by a health care professional trained and experienced in nutritional therapeutics. Ideally, the emergence of pharmacogenomic testing will assist physicians by providing adequate information about the individual's ability to tolerate and benefit from the treatment combination.

Chlorimipramine and Related Tricyclic Antidepressants

Evidence: Chlorimipramine (clomipramine; Anafranil). Extrapolated, based on similar properties: Amitriptyline (Elavil); combination drug: amitriptyline and perphenazine (Etrafon, Triavil, Triptazine); amoxapine (Asendin), desipramine (Norpramin, Pertofrane), doxepin (Adapin, Sinequan), imipramine (Janimine, Tofranil), nortriptyline (Aventyl, Pamelor), protriptyline (Vivactil), trimipramine (Surmontil).

Interaction Type and Significance

⊕   **Potential or Theoretical Beneficial or Supportive Interaction, with Professional Management**

⊕✗ **Bimodal or Variable Interaction, with Professional Management**

✗✗ **Minimal to Mild Adverse Interaction—Vigilance Necessary**

Probability: Evidence Base:
2. Probable   ◉ **Emerging**

Effect and Mechanism of Action

Chlorimipramine is a halogenated derivative of imipramine that is more potent as a serotonin (5-HT) reuptake inhibitor than the parent compound. Both chlorimipramine and exogenous 5-HTP can elevate serotonin and cortisol levels, and their concomitant use could potentially result in excessive levels as a result of an additive effect.

Research

In a pioneering clinical trial, van Praag et al.[14] found that the combination of 5-HTP and clomipramine proved more effective than clomipramine alone in the treatment of patients with "therapy-resistant" depression. Subsequently, in a 28-day double-blind clinical trial involving 26 hospitalized, depressed patients who were randomized into two groups, Nardini et al.[15] found that those subjects who received chlorimipramine (50 mg/day), combined with L-5-HTP (300 mg/day), demonstrated significantly better response, quantitatively and qualitatively, than did those who received chlorimipramine plus placebo, according to several standard depression scoring systems.

Meltzer et al.[16] noted that serum cortisol concentration was significantly greater in unmedicated depressed and manic patients than in normal controls after administration of 5-HTP, 200 mg orally. Further, increases in serum cortisol levels greater than 5 µg/dL were significantly more frequent in both unmedicated depressed and manic patients than in the normal controls. Subsequently, this same research team, determined that in subjects with major depression or with obsessive-compulsive disorder, most tricyclic antidepressants (TCAs) do not increase 5-HTP-mediated cortisol release, in contrast to fluoxetine, which does potentiate such a 5-HTP-mediated increase in plasma cortisol and prolactin secretion.[17] However, in a small clinical trial involving seven patients with major depression, Sargent et al.[18] observed that cortisol response to 5-HTP was significantly increased after 8 weeks' treatment with clomipramine, "suggesting that clomipramine, like selective serotonin re-uptake inhibitors (SSRIs), enhances this 5-HT2 receptor mediated response."

Nutritional Therapeutics, Clinical Concerns, and Adaptations

The available literature indicates that the concomitant administration of clomipramine and 5-HTP may interact to elevate cortisol and serotonin levels. This effect could be therapeutically appropriate and efficacious or potentially risky, depending on the dosage levels, diagnosis, patient characteristics, and other factors. Any treatment program utilizing this combined action requires close supervision and regular monitoring and would be most safely and effectively undertaken within the context of the coordinated efforts of health care professionals trained and experienced in both conventional pharmacology and nutritional precursor therapeutics. Although the preliminary findings have been encouraging, further research with large, well-designed clinical trials is necessary to evaluate further the safety and efficacy of this integrative therapeutic option and to assist development of clinical guidelines.

Lithium Carbonate

Lithium carbonate (Camcolit, Carbolith, Duralith, Eskalith, Li-Liquid, Liskonum, Litarex, Lithane, Lithobid, Lithonate, Lithotabs, PMS-Lithium, Priadel).

Interaction Type and Significance

⊕⊕ **Beneficial or Supportive Interaction, with Professional Management**

☼ **Prevention or Reduction of Drug Adverse Effect**

Probability: Evidence Base:
3. Possible   ○ **Preliminary**

Effect and Mechanism of Action

Both lithium and exogenous 5-HTP can elevate serotonin and cortisol levels as part of their therapeutic action. Concomitant use of these agents may induce excessively elevated serotonin levels and disrupt regulation of cortisol and other neuroendocrine substances.

Research

Lithium increases serotonin release and decreases metabolism. Despite lithium's proven efficacy as a long-term treatment for recurrent mood disorders (bipolar syndromes), individuals show a variable response, ranging from complete efficacy to no influence at all.[19,20] Serotonergic pathways appear to be important to the mechanisms of action of lithium. Much recent research has focused on identifying possible predictors of response through molecular genetic studies. Recent research has observed an association between genetic variation in tryptophan hydroxylase (TPH) and aggression and anger-related traits.[21] Clinical predictors apparently account for about half the variance in lithium response, and genetic factors probably play a substantial role in both risk factors and response factors in affective disorders.[22-24]

In 1999, Serretti et al.[25] published one of several papers examining the possible association between the TPH gene variants and prophylactic efficacy of lithium in mood disorders. In a review from 2002, Serretti[26] reported that the functional polymorphism in the upstream regulatory region of the serotonin transporter gene (5-HTTLPR) has been associated with long-term efficacy of lithium in two independent studies; marginal associations have been reported for TPH and inositol polyphosphate 1-phosphatase (INPP1). Even though no unequivocal susceptibility gene for lithium efficacy has been identified, individual pharmacogenomic variability significantly influences response patterns. Within that context, manipulation of tryptophan metabolism and serotonin synthesis appears to play an important role.

Meltzer et al.[27] investigated the hypothesis that lithium carbonate may enhance serotonin receptor sensitivity, whereas TCAs and second-generation antidepressants diminish 5-HT receptor sensitivity. They found that serum cortisol levels were significantly increased after administration of 5-HTP, 200 mg orally, to subjects with affective disorders. Further, 3 to 5 weeks of treatment with lithium carbonate or a MAO inhibitor augmented the mean 5-HTP-induced increase in serum cortisol concentration in manic or depressed patients, respectively.

Reports

Documented case reports confirming interactions between lithium and 5-HTP are lacking. Clinical observations suggest that 5-HTP (or tryptophan) can serve as a clinically effective adjunct to lithium therapy, particularly in the treatment of some individuals diagnosed as bipolar with mania or depression, for whom lithium, alone or in combination with neuroleptics or tricyclics, has demonstrated limited or no effect.

Nutritional Therapeutics, Clinical Concerns, and Adaptations

5-Hydroxytryptophan administration potentially offers a valuable adjunct to lithium therapy in the management of some individuals with bipolar affective disorders. Besides enhanced therapeutic efficacy, such coordinated administration of lithium and 5-HTP provides an opportunity to reduce lithium doses and decrease attendant adverse effects, particularly in controlling acute mania and other severe conditions for which higher, more toxic doses of lithium are often required. Concomitant therapy may also achieve therapeutic efficacy with some individuals previously unresponsive to lithium alone or in combination with other psychoactive agents.

Controlled clinical trials involving coadministration of 5-HTP and lithium are lacking, so specific 5-HTP dosage recommendations cannot be made. However, in related research, some bipolar patients have demonstrated an increased sensitivity to L-tryptophan administration, with adverse reactions occurring at levels as low as 1 to 2 g daily. Based on functional parallels, low initial 5-HTP levels, slow and graduated increases in dosage, and regular monitoring are important to safe and effective concomitant medication.

5-Hydroxytryptophan, when administered to individuals undergoing lithium therapy, might increase some adverse effects associated with lithium therapy by potentiating the lithium effect; these include nausea, vomiting, dermatological eruptions, psoriasis, and alopecia. Gradual reduction of lithium in chronic cases, such as treatment of bipolar disorder, not only may be valuable for reduction of typical adverse effects associated with lithium, but also may be necessary because of an increase in lithium concentrations as a result of potentiation by 5-HTP. Monitoring of lithium concentrations for at least 2 weeks after introduction of 5-HTP or changes in lithium dosage is appropriate with such individuals. Individuals being treated for acute mania may be particularly sensitive to exacerbations because of alterations in effective concentrations of lithium. In such cases it may be appropriate to decrease the lithium dosage, especially with doses above 900 to 1200 mg per day. Implementation of such integrative strategies warrants active supervision and close monitoring by health care professionals trained and experienced in clinical nutrition and conventional pharmacology. Pharmacogenomic variability, particularly involving TPH polymorphisms, appears to influence both individual susceptibility to bipolar disorder and related conditions and therapeutic response to lithium and 5-HTP.

Selective Serotonin Reuptake Inhibitor and Serotonin-Norepinephrine Reuptake Inhibitor (SSRI and SNRI) Antidepressants

Evidence: Fluoxetine (Prozac, Sarafem), fluvoxamine (Faurin, Luvox), paroxetine (Aropax, Deroxat, Paxil, Seroxat).
Extrapolated, based on similar properties: Citalopram (Celexa), duloxetine (Cymbalta), escitalopram (S-citalopram; Lexapro), sertraline (Zoloft), venlafaxine (Effexor).
See Venlafaxine in Theoretical, Speculative, and Preliminary Interactions Research.

Interaction Type and Significance

✗✗✗ **Potentially Harmful or Serious Adverse Interaction—Avoid**

⊕✗ **Bimodal or Variable Interaction, with Professional Management**

⊕ **Potential or Theoretical Beneficial or Supportive Interaction, with Professional Management**

Probability:	Evidence Base:
2. Probable	○ Preliminary

Effect and Mechanism of Action

Selective serotonin reuptake inhibitor (SSRI) agents are designed to increase the functional level of serotonin in the brain by inhibiting its reuptake into the presynaptic neurons. SSRIs work acutely on synaptosomes in rat models but take several weeks to develop full antidepressant clinical effects in patients, which suggests the possibility of at least two different mechanisms. L-5-hydroxytryptophan (and L-tryptophan) are serotonin precursors that elevate serotonin stores.[28,29] Apparently eating a diet high in tryptophan does not significantly increase 5-HTP levels. However, the introduction of L-tryptophan, and especially 5-HTP, into the body through supplementation could increase available levels of serotonin and amplify the effects of any SSRI drugs.[30,31] This combination could potentially result in excessive levels of serotonin and produce an adverse reaction known as the "serotonin syndrome"; it could also alter the levels of other related hormones, such as cortisol, melatonin, and prolactin.[16,32] The serotonin syndrome is a potentially severe adverse drug interaction characterized by the triad of altered mental status, autonomic dysfunction, and neuromuscular abnormalities.

Research

Human research directly investigating 5-HTP intake is inconclusive in the context of conventional antidepressant therapy, despite widespread use of SSRIs and a presumption of consensus as to the high probability and serious risk of the interaction between SSRIs and 5-HTP. Several studies have favorably shown clinical efficacy and safety of 5-HTP compared with SSRIs and other conventional medications. In a 6-week, multicenter trial, for example, Poldinger et al.[1] reported 5-HTP to be as effective as fluvoxamine in treating severe depression. However, despite numerous data on adverse reactions, including serotonin syndrome, from patients taking SSRIs, limited direct evidence from controlled human clinical trials is available demonstrating the frequency, character, and severity of the presumed interaction between 5-HTP and SSRIs. Nevertheless, there have been reports of experienced clinicians

safely and effectively using graduated doses of 5-HTP with reduced SSRI doses as a transitional device in weaning patients off SSRIs.

Meltzer et al.[17] found that fluoxetine potentiates the 5-HTP-mediated increase in plasma cortisol and prolactin secretion in subjects with major depression or with obsessive-compulsive disorder.

Using a rat model, Dreshfield-Ahmad et al.[33] reported elevation of extracellular serotonin levels by 5-HTP loading after administration of WAY 100635 (a selective 5-HT1A antagonist) and fluoxetine. These researchers concluded that their findings "suggest that combining blockade of 5-HT1A autoreceptors with 5-HT uptake inhibition results in a synergistic increase in synthesis and release of 5-HT when precursor is administered."

The complex issue of potential adverse effects on neurotransmitter and hormonal self-regulatory processes, including endogenous 5-HTP synthesis, resulting from long-term administration of SSRIs, has yet to be fully addressed. Using a rat model. Yamane et al.[33a] observed a reduction in serotonin synthesis after acute and chronic treatments with paroxetine. Conversely, Kim et al.[34] found that long-term treatment of rats with sertraline upregulated mRNA and protein levels of the serotonin-synthesizing enzyme TPH. They concluded that, in addition to the known short-term action as a serotonin uptake inhibitor, sertraline also exerts a long-term effect on the serotonin neurotransmission by enhancing serotonin synthesis. A parallel effect was observed with fluoxetine, but not with the non-SSRI chlorpromazine.

Research conducted by Serretti et al.[35,36] indicates that the antidepressant therapeutic response to SSRIs, specifically paroxetine and fluvoxamine, may be mediated by variations in the TPH and serotonin transporter genes. Further investigation into such pharmacogenomic factors may not only shed light on SSRI safety and efficacy, but also enhance understanding of individual susceptibility to depression and variable response to 5-HTP, as well as the probability of adverse interactions with exogenous 5-HTP intake.

Reports

A search of the available literature reveals a single case report involving combined use of L-tryptophan and paroxetine that resulted in headache, sweating, dizziness, agitation, restlessness, nausea, vomiting, and other symptoms, which could be representative of serotonin syndrome. However, although appearing pharmacologically probable, documented case reports are lacking to confirm interactions between SSRIs and 5-HTP. Even with a shortage of formal scientific data and published case reports, however, many health care professionals, particularly those practicing nutritional therapeutics using precursor substances, have treated patients who have self-administered 5-HTP while taking SSRIs and experienced adverse reactions of varying degrees of severity.

Clinical Implications and Adaptations

Physicians prescribing SSRI drugs are advised to warn patients to avoid concomitant 5-HTP (or L-tryptophan) unless they are under the direct care and coordinated supervision of the prescribing physician and a health care professional trained and experienced in nutritional psychopharmacology. Even though a potentially valuable synergy could develop from the careful combining of 5-HTP (or L-tryptophan) with SSRIs, such experimentation would be premature and should be considered potentially dangerous until well-designed, controlled clinical trials have been conducted. Because only a small amount of ingested tryptophan is metabolized into serotonin, and because 5-HTP bypasses the rate-limiting step of serotonin synthesis (5-hydroxylation of tryptophan), the probability of untoward interactions between 5-HTP and SSRIs is higher than for tryptophan. At this time, tryptophan is available in the United States only by prescription through compounding pharmacies, despite tryptophan's therapeutic index being considerably higher than that of 5-HTP, which is widely available as an over-the-counter product.

Selegiline and Related Monoamine Oxidase (MAO) Inhibitors

Evidence: MAO-B inhibitors: Rasagiline (Azilect), selegiline (deprenyl, L-deprenil, L-deprenyl; Atapryl, Carbex, Eldepryl, Jumex, Movergan, Selpak).

Benserazide combination drug: Levodopa and benserazide (co-beneldopa; Madopar).

Similar properties but evidence lacking for extrapolation: MAO-A inhibitors: Isocarboxazid (Marplan), moclobemide (Aurorix, Manerix), phenelzine (Nardil), procarbazine (Matulane), tranylcypromine (Parnate).

See MAO-A Inhibitors in Theoretical, Speculative, and Preliminary Interactions Research.

Interaction Type and Significance
⊕⊕ **Beneficial or Supportive Interaction, with Professional Management**
⊕✗ **Bimodal or Variable Interaction, with Professional Management**
✗ **Potential or Theoretical Adverse Interaction of Uncertain Severity**

Probability: Evidence Base:
2. Probable   ◉ **Emerging**

Effect and Mechanism of Action
The combined use of 5-HTP and a MAO-B inhibitor may result in a possible additive interaction that could be beneficial or could increase risk.

Research
Selegiline is an irreversible selective MAO-B inhibitor without "cheese effect," the severe hypertensive/adrenergic activation interaction that occurs between MAO-A inhibitors and foods containing tyramine (e.g., aged cheeses, some red wines). Selegiline is the primary type B MAO inhibitor in clinical use; it is most widely used with levodopa and carbidopa to treat symptoms of Parkinson's disease. No research has been conducted on the multivariable interaction of 5-HTP in the context of such polypharmacy. However, in a series of studies, Mendlewicz and Youdim[37,38] investigated coadministration of selegiline and 5-HTP in the treatment of individuals with affective illness. In an open-trial study, selegiline was given to patients with unipolar and bipolar depression receiving L-5-HTP and benserazide, a peripheral decarboxylase inhibitor that inhibits conversion of 5-HTP to serotonin outside the CNS. Of 14 patients, 10 showed a positive response to this combination, and a correlation was found between the degree of platelet MAO inhibition and clinical response. In a double-blind controlled study, 18 affectively ill patients were randomized to a group who received selegiline, L-5-HTP, and benserazide; 21 patients received L-5-HTP and benserazide only; and 19 were given placebo. The subjects treated with selegiline and L-5-HTP demonstrated a significantly greater clinical improvement than placebo patients; such beneficial effect was not observed in patients treated with 5-HTP/benserazide

alone. These results are weakened by not having a selegiline-alone group, since an MAO inhibitor could certainly have antidepressant activity on its own.

Nutritional Therapeutics, Clinical Concerns, and Adaptations
Physicians prescribing selegiline may want to discuss with patients the potentially valuable synergy from administering 5-HTP with their psychopharmacological intervention. Generally, such integrative therapeutics are best undertaken within the context of collaborative care involving health care professionals trained and experienced in both conventional pharmacology and nutritional psychopharmacology; close supervision and regular monitoring are warranted. Although the preliminary findings have been encouraging, further research with large, well-designed clinical trials is necessary to evaluate further the safety and efficacy of this integrative therapeutic option and to assist development of clinical guidelines.

Sibutramine and Related Serotonin Agonists

Evidence: Sibutramine (Meridia, Reductil).
Extrapolated, based on similar properties: Almotriptan (Axert), buspirone (Buspar), dihydroergotamine (DHE-45), ergotamine, eletriptan (Relpax), frovatriptan (Frova), naratriptan (Amerge), rizatriptan (Maxalt), sumatriptan (Imitrex), zolmitriptan (Zomig).
See also Sumatriptan, Zolmitriptan, and Related 5-Hydroxytryptamine Receptor Agonists (Triptans)

Interaction Type and Significance
✗ ✗ ✗ **Potentially Harmful or Serious Adverse Interaction—Avoid**

Probability: Evidence Base:
2. Probable   ○ **Preliminary**

Effect and Mechanism of Action
Serotonin agonists can enhance the serotonergic effect of other serotonin agonists, as well as serotonin precursors, thereby increasing the risk of augmenting serotonin activity to potentially toxic levels. In particular, the additive effect on serotonin activity resulting from concomitant use of 5-HTP and pharmaceutical serotonin agonists presents a significant risk of inducing serotonin syndrome.

The product information provided by the manufacturer of sibutramine states that because sibutramine "inhibits serotonin reuptake, it should not be administered with other serotonin agonists."[39]

Research
Using a rat model, Heal et al.[40] found that the combination of sibutramine and fluoxetine, at doses less than 10 mg/kg, had no effect on 5-HTP accumulation in either frontal cortex or hypothalamus, whereas sibutramine (10 mg/kg intraperitoneally) and fluoxetine (10 mg/kg intraperitoneally) produced slow, prolonged increases of extracellular 5-HT (serotonin) in the anterior hypothalamus. Overall, in investigating the action of several agents, these researchers interpreted their findings to show that "sibutramine powerfully enhances central 5-HT function via its secondary and primary amine metabolites; this effect, like that of fluoxetine, is almost certainly mediated through 5-HT uptake inhibition."

Nevertheless, there remains a lack of scientific evidence from human studies directly supporting or detailing this pharmacologically probable interaction. No clinical trials have investigated the potential interaction between sibutramine and 5-HTP.

Reports

A search of the literature reveals no documented case reports confirming interactions between sibutramine and 5-HTP. Thus, scientific evidence is currently lacking as to the frequency, character, or severity of this potential interaction.

Clinical Implications and Adaptations

The concomitant use of 5-HTP and agents that enhance serotonin activity is contraindicated and, if determined to be necessary in a particular case, should only be undertaken from within the context of close clinical supervision and regular monitoring. Adverse effects of a dangerous additive or synergistic interaction are likely to be characterized by rapid onset of toxicity symptoms characteristic of serotonin syndrome.

Sumatriptan, Zolmitriptan, and Related 5-Hydroxytryptamine Receptor Agonists (Triptans)

Almotriptan (Axert), eletriptan (Relpax), frovatriptan (Frova), naratriptan (Amerge), rizatriptan (Maxalt), sumatriptan (Imitrex), zolmitriptan (Zomig).
See also Sibutramine and Related Serotonin Agonists.

Interaction Type and Significance

✗ ✗ ✗ Potentially Harmful or Serious Adverse Interaction—Avoid

Probability:	Evidence Base:
2. Probable	○ Preliminary

Effect and Mechanism of Action

Triptans are 5-hydroxytryptamine (5-HT1B/1D) agonists; they also activate the 5-HT1B receptors on coronary arteries, which is the basis for the potentially dangerous adverse effect of coronary spasm with use of triptans. Their antimigraine activity is attributed to stimulation of serotonin receptors in the brain. Serotonin agonists can enhance the serotonergic effect of other serotonin agonists, as well as serotonin precursors, thereby increasing the risk of augmenting serotonin activity to toxic levels. The introduction of exogenous 5-HTP into the context of pharmaceutical serotonin agonists carries a significant risk of an additive effect, resulting in excessive elevation of functional serotonin levels and potentially inducing serotonin syndrome.

Research

As a class, triptans are well known for a high degree of variability in their therapeutic action, numerous adverse effects, and frequent interactions with other agents. In a paper reviewing the safety and clinical use of triptans, Tepper[40a] wrote: "Some triptans have the potential for significant drug-drug interactions (sumatriptan, rizatriptan, and zomitriptan and monoamine oxidase inhibitors; rizatriptan and propranolol; zolmitriptan and cimetidine; and eletriptan and CYP3A4 metabolized medications and p-glycoprotein pump inhibitors)." In an important review paper, Saper[40b] simply declared: "What matters is not the differences between triptans, but the differences between patients."

Nevertheless, despite the apparently formulaic potential for clinically significant interactions, there remains a lack of scientific evidence from human studies directly supporting or detailing this pharmacologically probable interaction. No clinical trials have investigated the potential interaction between triptan agents and 5-HTP.

Reports

A search of the literature reveals no documented case reports confirming interactions between triptan selective serotonin receptor agonists and 5-HTP. Thus, scientific evidence is lacking as to the frequency, character, or severity of this potential interaction.

Clinical Implications and Adaptations

Triptans are a primary therapy for migraines within conventional practice, and several studies have demonstrated efficacy of 5-HTP in the treatment of migraines.[41-43] Consequently, there is a need for explicit communication and coordination to prevent the combined use of these agents, particularly with unsupervised patient self-care. Even though a potentially valuable synergy could develop from the careful combining of 5-HTP (or L-tryptophan) with triptans, such experimentation would be premature and should be considered potentially dangerous until well-designed, controlled clinical trials have been conducted.

The concomitant use of 5-HTP and agents such as triptan selective serotonin receptor agonists that enhance serotonin activity is contraindicated and, if determined to be therapeutically necessary in a particular case, should only be undertaken within the context of close clinical supervision and regular monitoring. Adverse effects of a dangerous additive interaction are likely to be characterized by rapid onset of toxicity symptoms.

THEORETICAL, SPECULATIVE, AND PRELIMINARY INTERACTIONS RESEARCH, INCLUDING OVERSTATED INTERACTIONS CLAIMS

"Atypical Antipsychotics"

Aripiprazole (Abilify, Abilitat), clozapine (Clozaril), olanzapine (Symbyax, Zyprexa), quetiapine (Seroquel), risperidone (Risperdal), ziprasidone (Geodon).

Atypical antipsychotics are often used "off label" for many conditions other than schizophrenia. They are well known to interact with serotonin as well as many other receptors. It is generally advisable to avoid concomitant use of these agents and 5-HTP.

Monoamine Oxidase (MAO-A) Inhibitors

Isocarboxazid (Marplan), moclobemide (Aurorix, Manerix), phenelzine (Nardil), procarbazine (Matulane), tranylcypromine (Parnate).

Despite a lack of data from clinical trials or well-documented case reports, the general consensus is that the combined use of 5-HTP and MAO-A inhibitors carries significant potential adverse reactions similar to serotonin syndrome. Adverse effects of a dangerous additive or synergistic interaction of this nature are likely to be characterized by rapid onset of toxicity symptoms.

Tramadol

Tramadol (Tramake, Ultram, Zamadol, Zydol).

Tramadol is a synthetic opiate receptor agonist/antagonist analgesic that also blocks serotonin reuptake in the brain. L-5-Hydroxytryptophan (and L-tryptophan) are serotonin precursors that elevate serotonin stores. Simultaneous use could amplify the effects of tramadol, excessively elevate functional levels of serotonin, and thereby possibly increase the risk of tramadol-induced adverse effects, including serotonin syndrome.

No clinical trials have investigated the potential interaction between tramadol and 5-HTP. Consequently, although pharmacologically plausible, research-based data are lacking as to the frequency, character, or severity of this potential interaction.

The literature contains numerous case reports of adverse interactions, including serotonin syndrome, in individuals taking tramadol and other antipsychotic and antidepressant medications, particularly fluoxetine and paroxetine.[44-51] However, documented case reports are currently lacking to confirm interactions between tramadol and 5-HTP.

Physicians prescribing tramadol should warn patients to avoid the use of concomitant 5-HTP unless they are under the direct care and coordinated supervision of the prescribing physician and a health care professional trained and experienced in nutritional psychopharmacology. Even though a potentially valuable synergy could develop from the careful combining of 5-HTP (or L-tryptophan) with tramadol, such experimentation would be premature and should be considered as carrying significant risk of adverse effects until well-designed, controlled clinical trials have been conducted.

Trazodone

Trazadone (Desyrel).

Trazodone is a weak serotonin reuptake inhibitor drug. Adverse reactions characterized as similar to serotonin syndrome have been reported in patients taking trazodone in conjunction with medications that increase CNS serotonin levels, notably SSRI drugs.[52-55] At this time, however, there is a lack of documented case reports confirming direct interactions between trazodone and 5-HTP.

The use of 5-HTP to wean patients off trazodone has been effectively employed within the context of collaborative and supervised integrative care. Nevertheless, concomitant use of trazodone and serotonin precursors such as 5-HTP is generally contraindicated, except perhaps under the direct care and coordinated supervision of health care professionals trained and experienced in both conventional pharmacology and nutritional psychopharmacology. This potentially valuable synergy warrants further investigation through well-designed, controlled clinical trials.

Venlafaxine

Venlafaxine (Effexor).
Similar Properties: Duloxetine (Cymbalta).

Venlafaxine is a phenethylamine bicyclic derivative, chemically unrelated to tricyclic, tetracyclic, or other available antidepressant agents. It is known to be a potent serotonin reuptake inhibitor (as well as a potent dopaminergic agonist) and has been associated with several cases of serotonin syndrome. As such, there is high probability of this medication interacting with exogenous 5-HTP and resulting in adverse effects because of excessively elevated functional levels of serotonin.

Nevertheless, scientific evidence is lacking to support or detail this pharmacologically probable interaction. No clinical trials have investigated the potential interaction between venlafaxine and 5-HTP. Likewise, a search of the literature reveals no documented case reports confirming direct interactions between venlafaxine and 5-HTP. Thus, scientific evidence is currently lacking as to the frequency, character, or severity of this potential interaction.

Physicians prescribing venlafaxine should warn patients to avoid the use of concomitant 5-HTP unless they are under the direct care and coordinated supervision of the prescribing physician and a health care professional trained and experienced in nutritional psychopharmacology. Even though a potentially

valuable synergy could develop from the careful dose titration of 5-HTP with venlafaxine, such experimentation would be premature and should be considered potentially dangerous until well-designed, controlled clinical trials have been conducted.

Zolpidem

Zolpidem (Ambien, Stilnoct).
Similar Properties: Eszopiclone (Lunesta).

Zolpidem is a hypnotic drug used for short-term treatment of insomnia. Reports describing nine cases of suspected adverse interaction between zolpidem and serotonin reuptake inhibitor antidepressants, including hallucinations of several hours' duration, have been published.[56] No clinical trials have investigated the potential interaction between zolpidem and 5-HTP. Likewise, a search of the literature reveals no documented case reports confirming direct interactions between zolpidem and 5-HTP.

Physicians prescribing zolpidem should warn patients to avoid the use of concomitant 5-HTP unless they are under the direct care and coordinated supervision of the prescribing physician and a health care professional trained and experienced in nutritional psychopharmacology. Even though a potentially valuable synergy could develop from the careful combining of 5-HTP with zolpidem, such experimentation would be premature and should be considered potentially dangerous until well-designed, controlled clinical trials have been conducted.

NUTRIENT-NUTRIENT INTERACTIONS

Melatonin

The concomitant use of 5-HTP and melatonin may result in additive effects. The two agents are often used together clinically based on such observed activity. This potentially valuable synergy warrants further investigation through well-designed, controlled clinical trials.

S-Adenosylmethionine (SAMe)

The concomitant use of 5-HTP and SAMe may result in additive effects because SAMe-mediated methylation appears to enhance CNS neurotransmitter synthesis. The two agents are often used together clinically based on such observed activity. This potentially valuable synergy warrants further investigation through well-designed, controlled clinical trials. Supervision and monitoring are warranted with coadministration pending conclusive research findings.

Tryptophan

The concomitant use of 5-HTP and L-tryptophan will probably result in some additive effects. Dietary sources of tryptophan have not been found to raise levels of 5-HTP. This potentially valuable synergy warrants further investigation through well-designed, controlled clinical trials.

Vitamin B6 (Pyridoxine)

Vitamin B_6 activates the decarboxylase enzyme that converts 5-HTP to serotonin in the bloodstream. The two agents are often used together clinically based on such observed activity. However, peripheral decarboxylation (potentially enhanced by B_6) may increase peripheral (outside the CNS) conversion of 5-HTP to serotonin, which then binds to gastrointestinal receptors, causing unpleasant side effects, such as nausea and diarrhea. In the analogous case of L-dopa (dihydroxyphenylalanine), a peripheral decarboxylase inhibitor is coadministered to prevent peripheral conversion of L-dopa to dopamine, so that more L-dopa is converted to dopamine within the CNS to drive the remaining dopaminergic neurons in parkinsonian brains. This explains the trade name "Sinemet" for carbidopa/L-dopa, literally, "without metabolizing," meaning in the extra-CNS compartment. For this reason, vitamin B_6 is contraindicated with carbipoda or benserazide and L-dopa combinations. Thus, an argument could be made that vitamin B_6 given with 5-HTP might be counterproductive. This potentially important interaction warrants further investigation through well-designed, controlled clinical trials. Supervision and monitoring are warranted with coadministration pending conclusive research findings.

HERB-NUTRIENT INTERACTION

St. John's Wort

St. John's Wort *(Hypericum perforatum)*.

The concomitant use of 5-HTP and *Hypericum perforatum* may result in additive effects, particularly in the treatment of mild to moderate depression. One of the multiple St. John's wort mechanisms of action appears to resemble SSRI-like activity. The two agents are often used together clinically based on such observed activity. A typical combination would provide 50 to 100 mg of 5-HTP and 150 to 300 mg of St. John's wort extract (standardized for 0.3% hypericin), three times daily. This potentially valuable synergy warrants further investigation through well-designed, controlled clinical trials.

The 60 citations for this monograph, as well as additional reference literature, are located under 5-Hydroxytryptophan on the CD at the back of the book.

Nutrient-Drug Interactions and Drug-Induced Nutrient Depletions

Alpha-Lipoic Acid

Nutrient Name: Alpha-lipoic acid.
Synonyms: Alpha lipoic acid, ALA, acetate replacing factor, biletan, lipoic acid, lipoicin, thiactacid, thioctan, thioctic acid.
Related Substance: Alpha-dihydrolipoic acid (DHLA); dihydrolipate.

Summary

Drug/Class Interaction Type	Mechanism and Significance	Management
Cisplatin, oxaliplatin Platinum chemotherapy ☼/⊕⊕	Alpha-lipoic acid (ALA) may protect neural and otic tissue from oxidative damage induced by platinum-based chemotherapy. Strong trend of evidence indicating clinically significant supportive interaction. Clinical protocols emerging.	Coadminister; timing and sequence may vary with agent. Supervise and monitor.
Gentamicin, amikacin Aminoglycoside antibiotics ☼/⊕⊕	ALA may protect kidney, liver, and inner ear tissues by providing antioxidant protection against aminoglycoside-induced free-radical generation and lipid peroxidation. Preliminary direct and consistent related evidence suggests that supportive interaction reasonably predictable as clinically significant.	Consider coadministration, especially with extended aminoglycoside use.
Haloperidol ☼/⊕⊕	ALA may provide antioxidant protection against hydrogen peroxide generation and oxidative stress due to excess dopamine turnover associated with haloperidol. Preliminary direct and consistent related evidence suggests that supportive interaction reasonably predictable as clinically significant.	Consider coadministration, especially with extended haloperidol use.
Irbesartan Angiotensin II receptor antagonists ⊕⊕	Concurrent use of ALA and irbesartan can produce an additive or synergistic response, producing improvements in endothelial function and reductions in markers of inflammation in patients with metabolic syndrome. Strategic interaction consistent with known activity of these agents on angiotensin II activity, proinflammatory processes, and oxidative stress.	Coadministration could support clinical outcomes in patients with metabolic syndrome, hypertension, or dysglycemic patterns. Monitor blood pressure, insulin response, and inflammatory markers.
Oral hypoglycemic agents Insulin ✗/⊕ ✗/⊕⊕	Concurrent use of ALA and oral hypoglycemic agents could theoretically produce an additive or synergistic response resulting in hypoglycemia due to ALA's supportive effect on glucose and insulin metabolism. Strategic interaction consistent with known activity of both agents, but consistent direct evidence of pharmacological interaction lacking.	Coadministration could support clinical outcomes in dysglycemic patients. Monitor blood glucose levels.

NUTRIENT DESCRIPTION

Chemistry and Forms

1,2-Dithiolane-3-pentanoic acid; 1,2-dithiolane-3-valeric acid; 6,8-thioctic acid; alpha-lipoic acid; 5-(1,2-dithiolan-3-yl) valeric acid.

Physiology and Function

Known by many names, alpha-lipoic acid (ALA) is a naturally occurring, fat-soluble and water-soluble, vitamin-like antioxidant and enzyme cofactor. It is involved in antioxidant protection and cell damage prevention, energy production and blood sugar regulation, growth stimulation and regulation of gene transcription, detoxification, and toxic metal chelation. Although the enzyme pathway for its de novo synthesis has not been fully elucidated, cysteine appears to be the source of sulfur, and octanoate serves as the intermediate precursor for the 8-carbon fatty acid. ALA is readily converted into dihydrolipoic acid (DHLA), its reduced form, in many tissues of the body. ALA is not required in the diet and therefore is not considered a true vitamin, because it can be synthesized by humans, as well as plants and other animals.

Lipoic acid was first isolated in 1951 by Reed and coworkers, in the course of research on "potato growth factor" in lactic acid bacteria, as a catalytic agent associated with pyruvate dehydrogenase; it serves as a coenzyme in the Krebs cycle and functions in the same manner as many B-complex vitamins. *Lipoamide*, the protein-bound form of the naturally

occurring isomer *R*-alpha-lipoic acid, where it is covalently attached through the carboxylic acid to lysine residues, is a required cofactor for several multienzyme complexes that catalyze energy metabolism reactions within mitochondria. The pyruvate dehydrogenase complex and the alpha-ketoglutarate dehydrogenase complex both catalyze reactions within the citric acid cycle. The alpha-ketoacid dehydrogenase complex catalyzes the metabolism of leucine, isoleucine, and valine, the three branched-chain amino acids. ALA also increases glucose transport and improves heart rate variability. Biliary excretion, electrochemically inactive degradation products, and complete utilization of ALA appear to be the primary substrate in the endogenous metabolism. Urinary excretion of ALA and its main metabolites does not play a significant role in ALA elimination.

Alpha-lipoic acid is a carboxy acid with two sulfur atoms that can be oxidized or reduced and thus, along with glutathione, is one of the thiol antioxidants. Lester Packer, PhD, of the University of California–Berkeley, and others demonstrated the potent antioxidant activity of ALA and described it as the "universal," "ideal," and "metabolic" antioxidant because of its unique ability to neutralize free radicals in both lipophilic and hydrophilic environments and operate effectively throughout all tissues, including the brain. The low molecular weight and lipophilicity of ALA also enables it to cross the blood-brain barrier and may contribute to its protective effects on brain and neural tissue. ALA directly supports the liver in its detoxifying functions and plays an important role enhancing the activity of the body's systemic "antioxidant network." ALA and dihydrolipoic acid (DHLA), also known as dihydrolipoate, both act as powerful antioxidants, protecting against oxidative damage by interacting with potentially damaging reactive oxygen and nitrogen species. In particular, the two forms work together to quench peroxynitrite radicals, an especially destructive class of free radicals consisting of both oxygen and nitrogen, which are known to play a role in the pathophysiology of chronic inflammation, atherosclerosis, lung disease, and neurological disorders. DHLA also enhances the uptake of cysteine by cells to enable increased glutathione synthesis and support intracellular glutathione levels. Furthermore, ALA and DHLA facilitate the synergistic relationship among antioxidants by regenerating ascorbic acid from dehydroascorbic acid, indirectly regenerating vitamin E, and reducing the oxidized forms of vitamin C, glutathione, and coenzyme Q10 to extend their metabolic life spans. Both ALA and DHLA may also chelate free metal ions, such as iron, copper, and arsenic, and prevent them from generating highly reactive free radicals that induce oxidative damage. Lastly, ALA (and DHLA) may play a role in repair of oxidative damage.

Alpha-lipoic acid also regulates signal transduction of nuclear factor kappa B (NF-κB), a transcription factor protein that binds to DNA and affects the rate of transcription of certain genes, with NF-κB-binding sites. By inhibiting the activation of NF-κB, ALA may influence a wide range of pathological processes, including inflammation, atherosclerosis, diabetes, hypertension, glaucoma, cancer, and acquired immunodeficiency syndrome (AIDS).

NUTRIENT IN CLINICAL PRACTICE
Known or Potential Therapeutic Uses

Alpha-lipoic acid has been used clinically to protect against oxidative stress, to enhance mitochondrial function, to support healthy liver and neurological function, and to reduce the cellular effects of aging. In a clinical trial investigating in vivo antioxidant activity of ALA in healthy humans, Marangon et al.[1] found that a 4-month course of 600 mg/day significantly decreased several biomarkers of oxidative stress compared to baseline. Pharmacokinetic studies of oral ALA suggest that it might be most effectively administered in divided doses throughout the day, rather than in a single daily dose, because it is rapidly absorbed, rapidly metabolized, and rapidly cleared from plasma and tissues.

Historical/Ethnomedicine Precedent

Alpha-lipoic acid has not been used historically as an isolated nutrient.

Possible Uses

Age-related macular degeneration, Alzheimer's disease (dementia), *Amanita* poisoning, antioxidant support, cancer, cataracts, cellular oxidative damage, diabetic polyneuropathy, glaucoma, hepatitis C, human immunodeficiency virus and acquired immunodeficiency syndrome (HIV/AIDS) support, insulin resistance, ischemia-reperfusion injury, metal chelation, neuralgias, surgical recovery, type 2 diabetes mellitus.

Deficiency Symptoms

De novo synthesis generally prevents ALA deficiency, which has not been described per se. Nevertheless, the destruction

of its cofactor form may play an important role in numerous pathophysiological processes. For example, individuals with primary biliary cirrhosis may have circulating antibodies to lipoamide-containing enzyme subunits.[2] Likewise, arsenic can render ALA inactive in arsenic toxicity by forming a complex with ALA in dehydrogenase enzymes.[3]

Dietary Sources

Limited quantitative information is available regarding ALA content in various food sources, and research into the relationship of dietary sources to circulating free ALA is in preliminary stages. Most dietary ALA is derived from lipoamide-containing enzymes and delivered as lipoyllysine (i.e., bound to lysine), which digestive enzymes may not effectively cleave.[3]

Foods that contain mitochondria, especially red meat, are believed to provide the highest levels of alpha-lipoic acid. Other animal sources include heart, liver, kidney, and skeletal muscle (i.e., red meat). Broccoli, spinach, tomatoes, and potatoes are rich plant sources of lipoyllysine, with yeast, peas, brussels sprouts, and rice bran having lower amounts.[4]

Nutrient Preparations Available

The *R*-isomer of alpha-lipoic acid is the form synthesized naturally and is the only form that functions as a cofactor for mitochondrial enzymes; it is currently commercially available. Previously, ALA was exclusively available as a 50/50 racemic mixture of the two optical isomers, *R*-alpha-lipoic acid and *S*-alpha-lipoic acid, as rendered by conventional chemical synthesis. *R*-ALA has greater bioavailability than *S*-ALA when administered orally and is reduced within the mitochondria to DHLA 28 times more rapidly, hypothetically providing significantly greater antioxidant activity.[5]

Dosage Forms Available

Capsule.

Dosage Range
Adult

Dietary: Alpha-lipoic acid is created in the human body and thus is not an essential nutrient. Consequently, humans are usually not deficient in ALA.
Supplemental/Maintenance: 20 to 50 mg/day.
Pharmacological/Therapeutic: 50 to 400 mg/day.

The amount of ALA used in research has ranged from 150 to 600 mg per day, with 600 mg/day being used to treat diabetic neuropathies and 150 mg/day for glaucoma.
Toxic: No upper limit (UL) dose has been established.

SAFETY PROFILE
Overview

Alpha-lipoic acid has been well tolerated and is considered to be extremely safe in the dosages typically used in clinical settings (e.g., 600 mg/day). When administered under medical supervision to patients with diabetic neuropathy, oral doses as high as 1200 mg/day (600 mg twice daily) for 2 years and 1800 mg/day (600 mg three times daily) for 3 weeks produced no adverse effects. No cases of toxicity from ALA overdose in humans have been published or otherwise reported. Nevertheless, no long-term studies have yet systematically evaluated the safety of ALA in healthy adults.

Nutrient Adverse Effects

General Adverse Effects

Skin rash (occasional).

Pregnancy and Nursing

There are no reports of adverse reactions. However, because no studies have confirmed the safety or documented any dangers of using ALA during pregnancy, nutraceutical intake should be avoided by pregnant or lactating women until safety has been demonstrated.

Contraindications

Use of ALA and other antioxidants is controversial during radiation therapy and some forms of chemotherapy.

Precautions and Warnings

Theoretically, as discussed later, orally administered ALA might enhance the effects of insulin and oral hypoglycemic agents and induce hypoglycemia.

INTERACTIONS REVIEW

Strategic Considerations

Although research into the biological activity of alpha-lipoic acid has been underway for more than 40 years, scientific knowledge of its potential role in clinical medicine has only recently begun emerging in a comprehensive and cohesive picture. The significant antioxidant activity of ALA and alpha-dihydrolipoic acid (DHLA), as well as other modes of biological activity, presents numerous apparent, and many as-yet undiscovered, opportunities for concomitant use with conventional medications, in both the prevention and the reduction of drug adverse effects, as well as through collaborative implementation of integrative strategies and by invoking beneficial or supportive interactions within the context of professional management. Even though *R*-ALA is the naturally occurring form and has superior pharmacokinetic characteristics, almost all human clinical trials of ALA administration have been performed using racemic ALA.[6] Furthermore, continued research into ALA's relative role in antioxidant networks will undoubtedly reveal deeper implications for its physiological functions and clinical applications. Thus, more refined research design is warranted to enable advancement of clinical knowledge concerning the therapeutic use and efficacy of alpha-lipoic acid.

NUTRIENT-DRUG INTERACTIONS

Cisplatin and Related Platinum Chemotherapy Compounds

Evidence: Cisplatin (*cis*-diaminedichloroplatinum, CDDP; Platinol, Platinol-AQ).
Extrapolated, based on similar properties: Carboplatin (Paraplatin), oxaliplatin (Eloxatin).

Interaction Type and Significance

☼   **Prevention or Reduction of Drug Adverse Effect**
⊕⊕   **Beneficial or Supportive Interaction, with Professional Management**

Probability: Evidence Base:
2. Probable   ◉ **Emerging**

Effect and Mechanism of Action

The antioxidant activity of alpha-lipoic acid appears to protect neural and otic tissue from oxidative damage associated with cisplatin, oxaliplatin and related agents, particularly with regard to renal systems and lipid peroxidation.

Research

Ototoxicity is a widely recognized and often severe adverse effect associated with cisplatin therapy. In an experimental model using rats, Rybak, Somani, et al.[7] investigated the effects of ALA (at variable doses of 25-100 mg/kg) on cisplatin-induced ototoxicity, compared with controls receiving no cisplatin. In their first published study, they concluded that ALA conferred significant, dose-dependent protection against cisplatin ototoxicity at all dose levels, and that such beneficial effect was further demonstrated by improved metabolic markers for glutathione and oxidative stress. The next year (2000) they came to similar conclusions. In particular, they observed that after cisplatin administration, renal superoxide dismutase, catalase, glutathione peroxidase (GSH peroxidase), and glutathione reductase activities decreased significantly, and malondialdehyde content doubled, and that these changes were reversed by increasing doses of ALA. They also found that renal platinum concentration increased after cisplatin administration, which they attributed as possibly decreased by chelation with lipoic acid. These findings suggest that the "graded doses of alpha-lipoic acid effectively prevented a decrease in renal antioxidant defense system and prevented an increase in lipid peroxidation, platinum content and plasma creatinine concentrations in a dose-dependent manner."[8] In a preliminary clinical trial, Gedlicka et al.[9] reported that ALA coadministration, including infusions, produced a significant pattern of amelioration of docetaxel/cisplatin-induced polyneuropathy.

Peripheral sensory neuropathy, with both acute and cumulative symptoms, is one of the most common and clinically significant adverse effects associated with oxaliplatin and other platinum-based chemotherapeutic regimens. Approximately 85% to 95% of patients receiving oxaliplatin experience acute transient neuropathy, particularly distal and peroral dysesthesia. Cumulative neuropathies, manifesting the dose-limiting toxicity of oxaliplatin, develop progressively in 10% to 18% of patients who have been administered a cumulative dose of 800 mg/m².[10] In a small, human clinical trial, Gedlicka et al.[11] found that ALA, 600 mg intravenously once weekly for 3 to 5 weeks, followed by 600 mg orally three times daily, effectively counteracted cumulative oxaliplatin-related peripheral sensory neuropathy (PNP). Eight of 15 (53%) patients reported that ALA effectively reduced the severity of this dose-limiting oxaliplatin-related adverse effect. These authors recommended further larger-scale, placebo-controlled research.

Nutritional Therapeutics, Clinical Concerns, and Adaptations

The emerging body of research strongly suggests that coadministration of ALA with platinum-based chemotherapeutic agents such as cisplatin and oxaliplatin may serve as a safe and effective adjuvant therapy capable of decreasing the neurological and ototoxic effects resulting from drug-induced oxidative damage. Because ALA can chelate heavy metals, careful randomized trials with both arms carefully stratified to have equivalent prognostic factors will be necessary to be certain that concomitant ALA therapy with platinum-based therapies (as well as other neurotoxic chemotherapies, e.g., taxanes, vinca alkaloids) does not compromise efficacy of the chemotherapy.

Patients offered such therapy should be informed of the preliminary work done, and that although ALA likely can provide neuroprotection from neurotoxic chemotherapy, we cannot be certain at this time that it would definitely not compromise chemotherapy efficacy. This is much less of an issue when palliative chemotherapy is involved, but when chemotherapy is given with curative intent, such as for germ cell tumors, careful monitoring of clinical response and full disclosure to the patient and family regarding current evidence are essential. Such integrative approaches to oncology care require a high level of collaboration among health care professionals trained and experienced in both conventional pharmacology and nutritional therapeutics, usually obtained only in multidisciplinary oncology clinics.

Gentamicin, Amikacin, and Related Aminoglycoside Antibiotics

Evidence: Amikacin (Amikin), gentamicin (G-mycin, Garamycin, Jenamicin).

Extrapolated, based on similar properties: Kanamycin (Kantrex), neomycin (Mycifradin, Myciguent, Neo-Fradin, NeoTab, Nivemycin), netilmicin (Netromycin), paromomycin (monomycin; Humatin), streptomycin, tobramycin (AKTob, Nebcin, TOBI, TOBI Solution, TobraDex, Tobrex).

Interaction Type and Significance

☼ **Prevention or Reduction of Drug Adverse Effect**
⊕⊕ **Beneficial or Supportive Interaction, with Professional Management**

Probability:	Evidence Base:
3. Possible	O **Preliminary**

Effect and Mechanism of Action

Free-radical generation and lipid peroxidation associated with gentamicin and other aminoglycosides play an important role in drug-induced damage to the liver, kidneys, and inner ear.[12] Alpha-lipoic acid can act as a powerful antioxidant and free-radical scavenger, especially against nephrotoxicity and ototoxicity.

Research

Sandhya and Varalakshmi[13] found that the intraperitoneal administration of gentamicin to rats is associated with an increased production of malondialdehyde (MDA), an end product of lipid peroxidation in the kidney, as well as decreased renal levels of glutathione (GSH) and decreased activity of superoxide dismutase (SOD), catalase (CAT), and glutathione peroxidase (GPx), three antioxidant systems in the kidney. In contrast, they observed that the coadministration of gentamicin and DL-alpha-lipoic acid decreased lipid peroxidation as well as increased GSH level and activity of SOD, CAT, and GPx. These authors concluded that "administration of DL-alpha-lipoic acid prevents lipid peroxidation, which may, at least partly, play an important role in the injury cascade of gentamicin-induced nephrotoxicity." Subsequently, Conlon et al.[14] conducted studies using guinea pigs to investigate the ability of ALA (100 mg/kg/day) to attenuate the cochlear damage induced by amikacin, 450 mg/kg/day intramuscularly. Their results showed that animals receiving ALA in combination with amikacin demonstrated a significant decrease in the severity of changes in cochlear function compared with animals receiving amikacin alone.

Nutritional Therapeutics, Clinical Concerns, and Adaptations

Aminoglycoside antibiotics are indicated in the treatment of serious systemic infections for which less toxic antibacterials are ineffective or contraindicated, but they are strongly associated with numerous toxicities, particularly involving the kidneys and nerves of the inner ear. Because the preliminary research on this topic has involved animals and not human patients, no conclusive recommendations can be offered. However, a diverse set of clinical studies has demonstrated ALA's role as a potent antioxidant and its ability to enhance protective systems in the kidneys, liver, and inner ear in a variety of situations. Therefore, although coadministration of ALA might be advisable for individuals being treated with aminoglycosides, the available research literature provides no specific indications as to the appropriate dosage for such concomitant use. Physicians prescribing gentamicin and related aminoglycosides are advised to work in close collaboration with health care professionals trained and experienced in nutritional therapeutics and closely monitor patients choosing to use ALA during and after aminoglycoside therapy.

Haloperidol

Haloperidol (Haldol).

Interaction Type and Significance

☼ **Prevention or Reduction of Drug Adverse Effect**
⊕⊕ **Beneficial or Supportive Interaction, with Professional Management**

Probability:	Evidence Base:
3. Possible	O **Preliminary**

Effect and Mechanism of Action

Haloperidol, a widely used neuroleptic, acts through blockade of dopamine receptors, leading to increased turnover of dopamine. Excessive production of hydrogen peroxide and thus generation of oxidative stress are predictable outcomes from such increased turnover of dopamine. The antioxidant activity of alpha-lipoic acid, as well as that of glutathione, may protect against and reverse free-radical damage.

Research

Using a rat model, Shivakumar and Ravindranath[15] demonstrated that chronic administration of haloperidol induced significant oxidative stress and thiol modification in brain tissue, particularly after the first month. However, after 6 months of haloperidol administration, the glutathione-protein thiol homeostasis was largely restored, and the concentration of lipid peroxidation products decreased. Subsequently, Balijepalli et al.[16] examined the effects of a variety of classic and atypical neuroleptic drugs and found that haloperidol was the most potent inhibitor of mitochondrial NADH ubiquinone oxidoreductase (complex I) activity. They found that in vitro treatment of mouse brain slices with haloperidol resulted in a loss of glutathione, and that pretreatment of slices with glutathione and ALA abolished haloperidol-induced loss of complex I activity.

Nutritional Therapeutics, Clinical Concerns, and Adaptations

Preliminary evidence indicates that coadministration of ALA (and/or glutathione) could potentially reduce depletion of naturally occurring glutathione and other adverse side effects caused by use of haloperidol. No definitive advice or dosage recommendations can be offered given the lack of clinical trials. Physicians prescribing haloperidol, and possibly related antiemetics and antipsychotics, are advised to work in close collaboration with health care professionals trained and experienced in nutritional therapeutics and closely monitor patients choosing to use ALA (and/or glutathione) during and after haloperidol therapy. ALA, typically at dosages of 20 to 50 mg per day, is frequently prescribed for general antioxidant protection, whereas 800 mg/day ALA and 150 mg/day glutathione are often administered in the treatment of other neurological conditions involving free-radical damage. ALA has no known toxic effects at such dosages and has never been shown to inhibit the therapeutic efficacy of haloperidol.

Irbesartan and Related Angiotensin II Receptor Antagonists

Evidence: Irbesartan (Aprovel, Avapro, Karvea).

Extrapolated, based on similar properties: Candesartan (Atacand), eprosartan (Teveten), losartan (Cozaar), olmesartan (Benicar), telmisartan (Micardis), valsartan (Diovan); combination drugs: candesartan and hydrochlorothiazide (Atacand HCT); irbesartan and hydrochlorothiazide (Avalide); losartan and hydrochlorothiazide (Hyzaar); valsartan and hydrochlorothiazide (Diovan HCT).

Interaction Type and Significance

⊕⊕   **Beneficial or Supportive Interaction, with Professional Management**

Probability: Evidence Base:
2. Probable   ○ **Preliminary**

Effect and Mechanism of Action

Increased angiotensin II activity, induction of a proinflammatory and oxidative state, and endothelial dysfunction are pathophysiological characteristics associated with metabolic syndrome; insulin resistance, obesity, hypertension, hypertriglyceridemia, and low HDL cholesterol are its clinical hallmarks. Concurrent use of ALA and irbesartan can produce an additive or synergistic response in reducing inflammation and oxidative damage in endothelial tissue. ALA's antioxidant activity may reduce endothelial tissue damage, support endothelial function, and protect insulin action through its action on oxidative stress. Irbesartan is an angiotensin II receptor (AT1 subtype) antagonist, effectively blocking the renin-angiotensin system, specifically the vasoconstrictor and aldosterone-secreting effects of angiotensin II by selectively binding to the AT1 angiotensin receptor. The mechanisms of this interaction appear to derive from the known activities of the individual agents but have yet to be fully elucidated.

Research

In a randomized, double-blind, placebo-controlled trial involving 58 patients with the metabolic syndrome, Sola et al.[17] investigated the effects of combining irbesartan and ALA on vasodilation and inflammation biomarkers. The subjects were administered irbesartan (150 mg/day), lipoic acid (300 mg/day), both irbesartan and ALA, or placebo. After 4 weeks' intervention, endothelium-dependent flow-mediated vasodilation of the brachial artery was increased by 67%, 44%, and 75% in the irbesartan, ALA, and irbesartan plus ALA groups, respectively, compared with the placebo group. Irbesartan and/or ALA administration was associated with statistically significant reductions in plasma levels of interleukin-6 and plasminogen activator-1. Similarly, levels of 8-isoprostane (a marker of oxidative stress) decreased in patients receiving irbesartan alone or in combination with ALA. No significant changes in blood pressure were observed in any of the study groups.

Nutritional Therapeutics, Clinical Concerns, and Adaptations

Physicians prescribing irbesartan for patients with hypertension are advised to consider coadministration of ALA and to discuss this therapeutic option with the patient. Further research through well-designed clinical trials is warranted to test and refine guidelines for clinical management of such concomitant therapy. Pending conclusive research, available evidence indicates that integration of this nutrient into an existing or new therapeutic strategy for blood pressure management, glucose stabilization, atherosclerosis prevention, and cardiovascular risk reduction introduces little, if any, probability of adverse effects and is relatively inexpensive to administer.

Oral Hypoglycemic Agents and Insulin

Evidence: Glyburide (Glibenclamide; Diabeta, Glynase, Glynase Prestab, Micronase, Pres Tab).

Extrapolated, based on similar properties: Chlorpropamide (Diabinese), glimepiride (Amaryl), glipizide (Glucotrol, Glucotrol XL), insulin (animal-source insulin: Iletin; human analog insulin: Humanlog; human insulin: Humulin, Novolin, NovoRapid, Oralin), metformin (Glucophage), tolazamide (Tolinase), tolbutamide (Orinase, Tol-Tab); combination drugs: glipizide and metformin (Metaglip); glyburide and metformin (Glucovance).

Interaction Type and Significance

✗   **Potential or Theoretical Adverse Interaction of Uncertain Severity**

⊕✗   **Bimodal or Variable Interaction, with Professional Management**

⊕⊕   **Beneficial or Supportive Interaction, with Professional Management**

Probability: Evidence Base:
4. Plausible   ▽ **Mixed**

Effect and Mechanism of Action

Numerous studies of ALA have investigated many aspects of its effect on glucose, insulin resistance, and diabetes. Theoretically, concomitant use of oral hypoglycemic agents or insulin and ALA could result in an additive or synergistic response on glucose and insulin levels.

Research

Alpha-lipoic acid and other antioxidants (e.g., vitamin C, vitamin E, N-acetylcysteine/NAC) may protect insulin action under oxidative stress. Animal studies have demonstrated that oral administration of ALA can prevent early glomerular injury in non–insulin-treated, streptozotocin diabetic rats. Furthermore, ALA can attenuate hyperglycemia and prevent hypertension, insulin resistance, and oxidative stress, while also preventing glomerular mesangial matrix expansion, in animal models of diabetes.[18,19] In a randomized, open, three-period crossover trial with 14 male and 10 female healthy volunteers, Gleiter et al.[20] reported finding a lack of interaction between ALA, glyburide, and acarbose. ALA did not alter glyburide pharmacokinetics to a clinically significant extent. Plasma insulin and glucose concentrations did not indicate a significant interaction between ALA and glyburide or ALA and acarbose.

Nutritional Therapeutics, Clinical Concerns, and Adaptations

The available evidence indicates that in some circumstances, concomitant use of ALA with oral hypoglycemic agents or insulin might result in an additive or synergistic response of uncertain clinical significance. The exact clinical effect has yet to be demonstrated, but the protective effects on tissues of diabetic animals strongly suggest the use of this significant substance as an adjunctive to oral hypoglycemics and insulin in a preventive mode.

In the event that such an interaction is active, it could be therapeutically advantageous, if applied in a coordinated manner involving collaboration, close supervision, and regular monitoring involving health care professionals trained and experienced in both conventional pharmacology and nutritional therapeutics, or it might result in adverse effects of unknown severity, if physician-patient dialogue is inadequate or multidisciplinary coordination insufficient. Further research in large, well-designed human trials is warranted to confirm the efficacy of ALA as part of a comprehensive approach to the care of patients with dysglycemia, insulin resistance, and diabetes and to develop clinical guidelines for integrative therapeutics.

THEORETICAL, SPECULATIVE, AND PRELIMINARY INTERACTIONS RESEARCH, INCLUDING OVERSTATED INTERACTIONS CLAIMS

Anesthesia, General

Anesthesia, general
Related but evidence lacking for extrapolation: Halogenated inhalational anesthetic agents: Desflurane (Suprane), enflurane (Ethrane), halothane (Fluothane), isoflurane (Forane), sevoflurane (Sevorane, Ultane).

Administration of alpha-lipoic acid (ALA) may be beneficial after surgery as a means of facilitating metabolic breakdown of anesthesia, analgesics, and other drugs and ameliorate any residual toxic effects. Postoperative care might include 100 mg ALA orally three times daily for 2 weeks. In some cases a similar dosage for 1 week preoperatively might provide a means of reducing adverse effects in particularly sensitive individuals. However, such preemptive usage would only be appropriate with agents that would not be interfered with or prematurely broken down by ALA.

Cyclophosphamide and Vincristine

Cyclophosphamide (Cytoxan, Endoxana, Neosar, Procytox), vincristine (Leurocristine, Oncovin, Vincasar PFS).

In a rat model, Berger et al.[21] reported that pretreatment with ALA showed no negative influence on the chemotherapeutic efficacy of cyclophosphamide against transplanted sarcoma or vincristine sulfate against transplanted carcinosarcoma. ALA significantly increased median survival time and lowered the toxic effects of vincristine compared to animals treated with vincristine alone. Evidence was lacking of any significant diminution of cyclophosphamide-induced toxic effects from adjuvant treatment with ALA. Subsequently, in a mouse model, Faust et al.[22] found that ALA significantly reduced the incidence of cytotoxic effects from cyclophosphamide, particularly drug-induced diabetes. These authors hypothesized that the anti-inflammatory action and protective effect of ALA on diabetes development might be attributed to enhanced scavenging of reactive oxygen species (ROS) reducing islet infiltration and inflammation. Further research into this potential supportive interaction is warranted in light of ALA's strong safety profile and the common occurrence and relative severity of cyclophosphamide-induced adverse effects, particularly iatrogenic diabetes.

Doxorubicin and Related Anthracycline Chemotherapy

Evidence: Doxorubicin (Adriamycin, Rubex).
Extrapolated, based on similar properties: Daunorubicin (Cerubidine), epirubicin (Ellence, Pharmorubicin), idarubicin (Idamycin, Zavedos), Mitoxantrone (Novantrone, Onkotrone).

Similar properties but evidence lacking for extrapolation: Daunorubicin, liposomal (DaunoXome); doxorubicin, pegylated liposomal (Caelyx, Doxil, Myocet).

The cardiotoxicity of doxorubicin can be of rapid onset and can endure for decades, often absent cardiac complaints. In a longitudinal assessment of cardiac function in 22 patients treated with anthracycline for osteogenic sarcoma or malignant fibrous histiocytoma, Brouwer et al.[23] found systolic dysfunction in more than a quarter of the patients and diastolic dysfunction in nearly half after two decades (median, 22 years). Moreover, cardiac dysfunction was progressive, as measured at 9, 14, and 22 years. Numerous animal studies have demonstrated ALA's ability to ameliorate myocardial toxicity, nephrotoxicity, and other effects of lipid peroxidation induced by doxorubicin.[24-29] If, as suggested, ALA provides a significant protective effect against toxicity induced by doxorubicin, it may therefore improve the therapeutic index of doxorubicin. Further research in well-designed human trials is warranted to confirm the efficacy of ALA as an adjuvant therapy within a comprehensive approach to chemotherapeutics and to develop clinical guidelines for such integrative therapeutics within oncological care.

Levothyroxine, Thyroid

L-Triiodothyronine (T$_3$): Cytomel, liothyronine sodium, liothyronine sodium (synthetic T$_3$), Triostat (injection).
Levothyroxine (T$_4$): Eltroxin, Levo-T, Levothroid, levothyroxine (synthetic), levoxin, Levoxyl, Synthroid, thyroxine, Unithroid.
L-Thyroxine and L-triiodothyronine (T$_4$ + T$_3$): animal levothyroxine/liothyronine, Armour Thyroid, desiccated thyroid, Westhroid.
L-Thyroxine and L-triiodothyronine (synthetic T$_4$ + T$_3$): Euthroid, Euthyral, liotrix, Thyar, Thyrolar.
Dextrothyroxine (Choloxin).

In rats, ALA (7.5 mg/100 g/day) inhibited enzymatic conversion of thyroxine (T$_4$) to triiodothyronine (T$_3$).[30] ALA coadministration with T$_4$ also had an apparent synergistic effect on serum cholesterol, producing significantly greater depression than T$_4$ alone. Blood hormone levels and thyroid function tests should be monitored for this potential interaction.

NUTRIENT-NUTRIENT AND HERB-NUTRIENT INTERACTIONS

Acetyl-L-Carnitine

The combined administration of ALA and acetyl-L-carnitine improved measures of memory in rats, particularly in the older animals.[31,32] Such findings are consistent with the known pharmacological activity of both agents on neural tissue, especially mitochondrial function, and further research involving well-designed human trials appears warranted.

Biotin

Biotin synthase and lipoate synthase share a very high sequence similarity, suggesting that both enzymes are strongly mechanistically related.[33,34] Some initial animal research indicated that chronic administration of ALA may interfere with the activities of biotin-dependent liver carboxylases in rats. However, subsequent research indicates that ALA may inhibit biotin uptake in some but not all conditions involving biotin transport systems.[35] Further research is required to determine if this phenomenon occurs in humans and if so whether it is clinically significant.[36] The role biotin deficiency might play in influencing such efficacy also deserves consideration.

Coenzyme Q10

As physiological allies within antioxidant networks, ALA, DHLA, and coenzyme Q10 facilitate, magnify, and reinforce each other's activity against ROS and oxidative damage, possibly achieving a superadditive effect of ubiquinone in combination with DHLA in preventing peroxidation of biomembranes.[37]

Copper

By chelating Cu^{2+} and other mechanisms, ALA and other antioxidants may provide significant protective activity against the free-radical damage associated with copper toxicity.[3,38-40] Pyruvate dehydrogenase is especially vulnerable to inhibition by oxygen free radicals and can play a central role in copper toxicity–induced neuronal death in Wilson's disease and possibly the pathogenesis of Alzheimer's and prion diseases.

Omega-3 Fatty Acids (Fish Oil)

Free radicals may be involved in causing toxicity in hyperoxaluric conditions. In an animal study, Lenin et al.[41] found that cellular antioxidant defenses can be increased by the coadministration of lipoate and a novel derivative, eicosapentaenoate-lipoate. Further clinical research is warranted to determine the efficacy of prophylactic treatment with ALA, eicosapentaenoic acid, and eicosapentaenoate-lipoate in preventing stone formation in the bladders of susceptible individuals.

Iron

By chelating Fe^{2+} and other mechanisms, ALA and other antioxidants may provide significant protective activity against the free-radical damage associated with iron toxicity.[3,38-40,42-49] For example, a clinical trial using the ethylenediamine salt of ALA on the indices of iron metabolism in patients with occupational pathologies found that the positive effects of ALA preparation in the patients with hyperferremia could be associated, at least partially, with normalization of iron exchange and reduction in the labile iron pool.[50]

Selenium and Milk Thistle (Silybum marianum)

Multiple-antioxidant therapy combining ALA with other agents, such as selenium and the herb milk thistle, is synergistic in hepatitis C therapy and may provide a cost-effective alternative approach, even in patients with a poor prognosis.[51]

Vitamin B₁ (Thiamine)

Individuals susceptible to thiamine deficiency, such as alcoholics, may derive increased benefit from concomitant vitamin B_1 and ALA. However, Gal[52] reported reversal of selective toxicity of ALA by thiamine in thiamine-deficient rats. Although no toxicity in humans has been suggested, further research into the relationships between these two important nutrients is warranted.

Vitamin E

Alpha-lipoic acid regenerates and thus extends the metabolic activity of vitamin E, particularly in the context of vitamin C administration.[3,6,53-58] Researchers have found that ALA may prevent symptoms of vitamin E deficiency, although not in the context of a vitamin E–deficient diet.[59]

Vitamin K

Vitamin K 2,3-epoxide reductase is the enzyme that recycles vitamin K back to its active form. This enzyme's activity in hepatic microsomes requires only a thiol cofactor, such as synthetic dithiothreitol (DTT). Both reduced lipoamide and reduced ALA stimulate microsomal vitamin K epoxide reduction, with kinetics comparable to those of synthetic DTT, suggesting that ALA is entirely capable of recycling oxidized vitamin K without relying on other cofactors. Thijssen et al.[60] found that hepatic microsomes contain NADH-dependent lipoamide reductase activity, which can provide reduced lipoamide for this purpose as well. These findings suggest that the vitamin K cycle obtains reducing equivalents from NADH through microsomal lipoamide reductase, and that ALA, vitamin K, and other nutritional cofactors may also provide synergistic beneficial actions in the treatment of mitochondrial disorders.[61]

The 61 citations for this monograph, as well as additional reference literature, are located under Alpha-Lipoic Acid on the CD at the back of the book.

Chondroitin Sulfate

Nutrient Name: Chondroitin sulfate.

Synonyms: Chondroitin, chondroitin sulphate, CS, CSA, CSC; ACS4-ACS6, CDS, chondroitin sulfate A, chondroitin sulfate C, chondroitin sulphate A sodium, chondroitin-4-sulfate, chondroitin-6-sulfate, chonsurid, condroitin, Condrosulf.

Related Substances: Chondroprotective agents, chondroitin sulfuric acid, GAG, galacotosaminoglucuronoglycan sulfate (Matrix), glycosaminoglycan, mesoglycan (heparan sulfate-52%, dermatan sulfate-35%, heparin-8%, chondroitin sulfate-5%).

Summary

Drug/Class Interaction Type	Mechanism and Significance	Management
Cisplatin Platinum chemotherapy ☼/⊕⊕	Complexing with chondroitin sulfate appears to alter pharmacokinetic properties of cisplatin and reduce nephrotoxicity without diminishing therapeutic efficacy. Consistent findings in animal and in vitro studies suggest that human trials are warranted.	Administration of cisplatin complexed with chondroitin may be beneficial. Close monitoring appropriate.
Nonsteroidal anti-inflammatory drugs (NSAIDs) ⊕⊕⊕/☼	Coadministration of chondroitin sulfate and NSAIDs may enable anti-inflammatory effect at lower drug doses. Concurrent use of chondroitin sulfate with NSAIDs appears to result in an additive or synergistic effect. More strategically, NSAIDs may promote cartilage destruction and impair cartilage repair.	Coadministration may enable decreased dose and shortened period of NSAID use.

NUTRIENT DESCRIPTION

Chemistry and Forms

Chondroitin sulfate (CS) is composed of a protein core covalently linked to complex of large-molecular-weight glycosaminoglycans (GAGs) and disaccharide polymers, large linear heteropolysaccharide chains composed of equimolar amounts of D-glucuronic acid, D-acetylgalactosamine, and sulfates in 10 to 30 repeating disaccharide units. These repeating chains of GAGs are found embedded with type II collagen fibers in cartilaginous tissue. Chondroitin sulfate structures appear in two primary forms: chondroitin sulfate A (CSA) or chondroitin-4-sulfate has a sulfate group in the 4 position of galactosamine, and chondroitin sulfate C (CSC) or chondroitin-6-sulfate has a sulfate group in the 6 position.

Physiology and Function

Chondroitin sulfate is normally synthesized endogenously and secreted by chondrocytes, but such endogenous production tends to decrease with age, thereby playing a role in the declining ability to maintain normal structure and function of joint cartilage typically associated with the aging process.

Chondroitin sulfates are widely distributed in tissues and fluids, particularly throughout connective tissue, joint cartilage, internal walls of blood vessels and skin, urinary bladder, and embryonic tissue tissues, as well as amniotic fluid, cornea, heart valves, placenta, synovial fluid, teeth, and umbilical cord. They are the most abundant GAGs in the body.

Among its several functions, CS is most well known for its central role in articular cartilage. The high concentration of CS in the collagen network provides structure and a load-bearing surface that is both tough and compliant. By absorbing water and holding nutrients, chondroitin enhances the thickness and elasticity of cartilage and increases its ability to absorb and distribute compressive forces. Chondroitin regulates formation of new cartilage matrix by stimulating chondrocyte metabolism and synthesis of collagen and proteoglycan and facilitating transport through the low-blood-flow environment.

In particular, chondroitins enhance levels of hyaluronic acid, a protective fluid that lubricates the joints. Furthermore, chondroitin sulfate inhibits the degradative action of elastase and hyaluronidase, synovial enzymes that participate in inflammation and contribute to cartilage destruction and loss of joint function by breaking down cartilage matrix and synovial fluid.

NUTRIENT IN CLINICAL PRACTICE

Known or Potential Therapeutic Uses

Evidence from clinical trials is gradually emerging to confirm the widespread anecdotal reports of chondroitin efficacy in the treatment of musculoskeletal injuries and degenerative joint disease, such as osteoarthritis. Administration of exogenous CS supplements the naturally occurring CS in maintenance of strong, flexible cartilage and support of healthy joint function. Some clinicians and researchers studying and treating osteoarthritis (OA) refer to CS as a "symptomatic slow-acting drug for osteoarthritis (SYSADOA)." Chondroitin sulfate addresses OA symptoms by reducing pain and increasing overall mobility while also slowing the pathological process by stabilizing and possibly improving bone and joint metabolism. Reports consistently indicate that response to treatment with chondroitin may have a delayed effect (typically reaching maximal effects after 2-6 months of regular use) compared with conventional analgesics, but that the therapeutic response exhibits longer duration (typically 3 months) after cessation of treatment. Evidence from human trials has thus far not matured sufficiently to determine whether chondroitin primarily slows or halts the process of cartilage destruction and joint damage or is capable of promoting repair and regeneration of damaged cartilage and reversal of arthritic changes, and if so, under what circumstances and treatment protocols.

As a compound rich in sulfur, and thus related to glucosamine sulfate, chondroitin may help cartilage by acting in a nutritive capacity to provide raw materials for tissue repair and regeneration.

Chondroitin may also lower blood cholesterol levels, prevent atherosclerosis, and reduce the risk of heart attacks in individuals who already have atherosclerosis.

The GAGs affect how the body processes oxalate and chondroitin intake is associated with reduced risk of stone formation by reducing urinary oxalate excretion.

Historical/Ethnomedicine Precedent

Many traditional cultures have encouraged the dietary consumption of connective tissue and use of bones in soups.

Possible Uses

Alzheimer's disease, angina, anti-inflammatory, atherosclerosis, chronic venous ulcers, connective tissue injury recovery, coronary artery disease (secondary prevention), gonarthrosis, heart disease, hypercholesterolemia, hyperlipidemia, interstitial cystitis, iron deficiency anemia, joint injury rehabilitation, leukemia, malaria, myocardial infarction, nephrolithiasis (oxalate stones), osteoarthritis (OA), osteoporosis, preterm labor prevention, snoring, sprain/strain injury.

Deficiency Symptoms

Chondroitin is not considered an essential nutrient because of endogenous synthesis. Consequently, consensus is lacking for characteristics of a chondroitin deficiency.

Dietary Sources

Animal cartilage is the only dietary source of chondroitin. The precise amount and bioavailability of chondroitin in foods is unknown.

Nutrient Preparations Available

Oral chondroitin sulfate is absorbed particularly rapidly in humans when it is dissolved in water before ingestion. It is rapidly degraded during its absorption and by extensive first-pass metabolism.[1,2] The active moiety remains unknown. In a double-blind clinical study published in 1992, L'Hirondel[3] demonstrated that up to 15% of oral chondroitin is absorbed intact through the digestive tract. Subsequent research determined that approximately 12% of oral CS becomes available to the joint tissues from the blood.[4] These studies have disproved previous speculation that oral chondroitin was not efficacious because of the large size of its molecules.

Different chondroitin products can very significantly in their chemical structure, thus affecting absorption and effectiveness. Chondroitin products with physically smaller molecules (<16,900 daltons) are more likely to provide superior bioavailability.[5] Thus, low-molecular-weight (LMW) CS is preferred. Findings from clinical trials using proprietary or otherwise specific forms of CS may not be reliably extrapolated to other products.

A review of two U.S. products conducted in 2000 reported that both had lower chondroitin levels than declared on the labels; similarly, 6 of 13 glucosamine and chondroitin combination products assayed contained low chondroitin levels.[6,7]

Dosage Forms Available

Capsule (often containing CS gel), tablet; often with glucosamine sulfate and or MSM; eyedrop solutions; intravesicular bladder administration; intramuscular (IM) injection; nasal spray; topical cream.

Source Materials for Nutrient Preparations

Chondroitin sulfate was first extracted and purified in the 1960s. Commercially available forms are usually manufactured from shark, pig, or bovine cartilage or bovine trachea, or by synthesis.

Dosage Range

Adult

Dietary: No minimal dietary requirement established.
Supplemental/Maintenance: 300 mg one to three times daily.
Pharmacological/Therapeutic: 300 to 1500 mg daily, usually in divided doses, as indicated by manufacturer recommendations and use in clinical trials. A typical dosage level for osteoarthritis is 400 mg three times daily. Researchers investigating atherosclerosis have sometimes initiated therapy administering 5 g twice daily, with meals, lowering the amount to 500 mg three times daily after a few months.
Toxic: No toxic dosage level established.

Pediatric (< 18 Years)

Dietary: No minimal dietary requirement established.
Supplemental/Maintenance: Not currently recommended for children.
Pharmacological/Therapeutic: Potential use in treating musculoskeletal injuries, but specific treatment recommendations have not been established.
Toxic: No toxic dosage level established specifically for infants and children.

Laboratory Values

Serum and synovial fluid levels have been used in clinical trials. Uesaka et al.[8] concluded that "synovial fluid levels of C4S and C6S may provide useful data in assessing the pathology of OA." However, du Souich and Verges[9] found that measuring plasma concentrations of CS "allows prediction of the maximal effect (Emax) elicited by the drug and the concentration eliciting 50% of Emax (EC50)."

SAFETY PROFILE

Overview

Chondroitin sulfate is generally well tolerated at usual dosage levels, and reports of serious adverse effects are absent. Nausea may occur at intakes greater than 10 g daily. However, no clinical trials have been of sufficient duration to assess conclusively the long-term safety of chondroitin administration.

Nutrient Adverse Effects

General Adverse Effects

Rare reports of gastrointestinal (GI) effects (diarrhea, constipation, abdominal pain) and headache constitute the primary known adverse effects. Rare reports attribute edema of legs and eyelids, arrhythmia, and alopecia.

In canine experiments, McNamara et al.[10] reported significantly decreased hematocrit, hemoglobin, white blood cell (WBC) count, and platelet count after 30 days' administration of chondroitin and suggested a potential risk of internal bleeding. However, no case reports or clinical trials have reported occurrences of bleeding in humans as a result of exogenous chondroitin intake.

Adverse Effects Among Specific Populations

A single case report describes an exacerbation of asthma attributed to use of a glucosamine-chondroitin supplement.[11]

Pregnancy and Nursing

No adverse effects have been reported. However, sufficient research-based evidence is lacking to guarantee the safety of chondroitin in pregnancy and breastfeeding. Pending conclusive findings, prudence suggests that chondroitin be avoided during pregnancy. Some commentators have suggested that the structural similarity between heparin and chondroitin is sufficient to warrant contraindication during pregnancy because heparin is contraindicated during pregnancy, except in women with protein C or S deficiency who are normally maintained on warfarin (Coumadin), which is indeed contraindicated in pregnancy, where heparin is substituted for the duration of the pregnancy.

Infants and Children

No adverse effects have been reported. However, sufficient research-based evidence is lacking to guarantee the safety of chondroitin in infants and children.

Contraindications

No qualified contraindications have been published. Out of caution, and despite a lack of substantive evidence, some commentators have suggested that individuals with bleeding problems, such as hemophilia, or temporarily at risk for bleeding during surgery or labor and delivery should avoid chondroitin. Pending conclusive findings, such speculation may deserve consideration, and chondroitin avoidance may be appropriate for short periods before and after surgery.

An emerging body of evidence suggests that exogenous CS be avoided by individuals with a history or high susceptibility of prostate cancer, breast cancer, or melanoma. Myers[12,13] reported the case of aggravated prostate cancer in an individual whose prostate cancer had been in remission until he initiated use of CS. In a review of relevant literature, Myers reported several studies that together could reasonably be interpreted to support his hypothesis that the chondroitin had exerted a tumor-promoting effect. Myers proposes that the action of CS involves formation of a complex with the protein *versican*, which along with *decorin*, is one of two proteins that CS is attached to in joint cartilage. Notably, prostate cancer cells, breast cancer cells, and melanoma cells also express versican on their surface. Thus, the introduction of exogenous chondroitin could increase levels of versican-chondroitin complex adhering to the surface of the cancer cells, facilitating their growth and metastasis.

De Klerk et al.[14,15] studied the concentration of GAGs in fetal, normal adult, and benign hyperplastic prostate tissue. They found that dermatan sulfate is the predominant GAG in the adult normal prostate, with the central zone exhibiting a slightly higher CS content than the peripheral zone and an increased CS content in benign prostatic hyperplasia (BPH).[14] Subsequently, they investigated GAGs in human prostatic cancer and observed that the concentration of CS was higher in cancerous prostate tissue than in normal prostate tissue.[15] In 1997, Ricciardelli et al.[16] noted that elevated stromal CS GAG predicts progression in early-stage prostate cancer. The following year these researchers investigated versican and decorin,

two proteins CS is attached to within the prostate, and found that versican may increase the spread of cancer, whereas decorin may suppress the spread of prostate cancer.[17] Then, in 1999, they observed that elevated levels of peritumoral CS predict a higher rate of recurrence after radical prostatectomy for early-stage prostate cancer and poor prognosis. Men demonstrating a high concentration of peritumoral CS had a 47% probability of recurrence within 5 years, in contrast to 14% in the men with low CS levels.[18] These issues were further explored in an in vitro study by Sakko, Ricciardelli, et al.[19] that examined whether versican, a recognized anti–cell adhesion molecule for various mesenchymal and nerve cell types, influences prostate cancer cell adhesion to extracellular matrix components. Further research involving versican purified from human prostate fibroblast conditioned medium confirmed its antiadhesive activity for prostate cancer cells. These researchers concluded that versican is an important modulator of tumor cell attachment to the interstitial stromal matrix of the prostate, the latter being an essential step in cancer cell motility and local invasion of the prostatic stroma.

At this point, no clinical trials or epidemiological studies have specifically determined whether administration of CS is carcinogenic or likely to aggravate existing prostate carcinoma. In particular, evidence is lacking to confirm a pattern of occurrence or mechanism of action linking chondroitin preparations and the development of CS-containing versican within tumors.

Pending substantive demonstration of safety, health care professionals treating men with prostate cancer or hyperplasia are advised to recommend glucosamine sulfate as a safe and effective substitute for chondroitin or for use as a monotherapy instead of in combination with CS. Similar considerations may be warranted for patients with a history of breast cancer or melanoma. No evidence suggests, nor have cautions been raised, that glucosamine contributes to the progression of prostate or other cancers.

Precautions and Warnings

Chondroitin could have a potential, although unproven and improbable, interaction with anticoagulant medications.

INTERACTIONS REVIEW
Strategic Considerations

Chondroitin sulfate has effectively graduated from the ranks of "alternative" therapies to the realm of standard care within recent years. Starting with its role in treating musculoskeletal disorders its potential scope for therapeutic application offers a promising future, especially within the context of multidisciplinary care using an integrative model.

Degenerative joint disease, more often referred to as osteoarthritis, is characterized by the progressive loss of functional articular cartilage and represents the most common type of arthritis worldwide. For example, osteoarthritis affects more than 20 million Americans, most of whom are over 45 years of age. Although conventional pharmacological therapies may provide palliative relief for many individuals, the shortage of effective clinical approaches for addressing the underlying disease process and pathophysiological changes has frustrated both health care providers and patients grappling with this painful degenerative process. During the past decade, a body of evidence from clinical trials and experimental studies has emerged supporting the use of CS and glucosamine sulfate, often in concert. Use of these agents, usually self-prescribed by patients, has grown steadily in the United States and Europe.

These cartilage extracts are considered as drugs in European continental countries and dietary supplements in the United States and England. Although many physicians initially relegated these agents to a questionable role based on their status as "nutritional supplements," maturation of the production system to the standards of Good Manufacturing Practices is evolving to match their proven efficacy and strong safety profile. Most importantly, chondroitin has demonstrated efficacy in halting the degenerative changes within joints to produce symptomatic efficacy (e.g., in knee OA), which is complemented by the structural and symptomatic efficacy of glucosamine sulfate. Furthermore, many literature-derived data show that CS could have an anti-inflammatory activity and a chondroprotective action by modifying the structure of cartilage and increasing both the concentration of hyaluronic acid and the viscosity of synovial fluid.

Several systematic reviews and meta-analyses have described the growing body of evidence documenting the therapeutic efficacy of CS in the treatment of OA. In a systematic quality assessment and meta-analysis of 15 clinical trials in the *Journal of the American Medical Association,* researchers concluded that glucosamine and CS "demonstrate moderate to large effects, but quality issues and likely publication bias suggest that these effects are exaggerated."[20] However, in a meta-analysis of seven trials investigating efficacy of chondroitin in the treatment of knee and hip OA also published in 2000, Leeb et al.[21] reported that in patients followed to 120 or more days, "CS was shown to be significantly superior to placebo" with respect to standard indices of pain and function. They concluded that "pooled data confirmed these results and showed at least fifty per cent improvement in the study variables in the CS group compared to placebo."[21] In a subsequent paper, Richy, Reginster, and a team of investigators from Belgium and France conducted seven individual, outcome-oriented meta-analyses using 15 randomized clinical trials selected from approximately 500 studies on the basis of high methodological quality. Although noting that quality scores in the chondroitin trials exhibited a mean of only 68.4%, they concluded: "Our work provides a clear, evidence-based advance regarding the interest in the wide use of glucosamine and chondroitin as disease-modifying compounds in the treatment of knee osteoarthritis through an accurate, conservative analysis of the most reliable experiments performed until now."[22]

In a series of interviews with several leading researchers and respected clinicians in the OA field, Hungerford[23] documented the emerging consensus supporting use of chondroitin (and glucosamine sulfate) among experienced clinicians. Noting that "chondrocytes are constantly replacing and repairing their environment," particularly "reversible lesions that occur during daily activities," Schenck and Verbruggen suggested that "90% of all patients with osteoarthritis can be treated nonoperatively." However, this repair capacity decreases with age and demanding activity because both the incorporation of sulfate into proteoglycans and the capacity to synthesize new molecules and large molecule aggregates decline with age. In response to these degenerative changes, support of normal function can be achieved using a nutritive approach. Thus, Hungerford[23] stated that in treating patients with OA, he generally uses LMW "chondroitin sulfate with glucosamine for symptomatic relief" and sees a response rate of "approximately 50%." These experts and others experienced in the care of individuals with degenerative joint changes (and injury-related joint repair) consistently emphasize that this synergistic approach should be expanded whenever possible to include individualized exercise programs and nutritional support.

Acupuncture, gentle joint mobilization, exercise programs, and botanical medicine represent other time-tested options of potential value in creating an evolving and personalized multidisciplinary therapeutic strategy for prevention and treatment.

NUTRIENT-DRUG INTERACTIONS

Cisplatin and Related Platinum Chemotherapy Compounds

Evidence: Cisplatin (*cis*-diaminedichloroplatinum, CDDP; Platinol, Platinol-AQ).
Extrapolated, based on similar properties: Carboplatin (Paraplatin), oxaliplatin (Eloxatin).

Interaction Type and Significance
☼   **Prevention or Reduction of Drug Adverse Effect**
⊕⊕ **Beneficial or Supportive Interaction, with Professional Management**

Probability: Evidence Base:
2. Probable   ◉ Emerging

Effect and Mechanism of Action
Cisplatin has a reputation as an effective antineoplastic agent, particularly against solid tumors such as testicular cancer, ovarian cancer, both small cell and non–small cell lung cancer, and head and neck cancer. However, renal, GI, and neurological toxicity limit its clinical application, with nephrotoxicity being the most common dose-limiting adverse effect. When administered as a complex, cisplatin and CS act to alter the pharmacokinetic properties of cisplatin and reduce the nephrotoxic effects usually associated with platinum-based chemotherapy.

Research
Hausheer et al.[24] investigated a variety of substances to address the fact that almost all platinum-protecting drugs have their own intrinsic toxicities, which can be additive to the toxicity of platinum-type drugs. They observed that the sulfate groups were highly favored to react with platinum species. Albertini et al.[25] demonstrated that chondroitin sulfate A (CSA, 4-sulfate) and chondroitin sulfate C (CSC, 6-sulfate) exhibited completely different physiological roles against copper-dependent oxidation of lipoprotein, probably because of the different Cu^{2+} binding ability of each form.

Subsequently, Zhang, Otagiri, et al.[26,27] conducted a series of studies exploring the application of CSA and CSC employed as to form complexes with cisplatin (CDDP) in reducing toxic effects of cisplatin monotherapy. They stated that the "purpose of the study is to apply both carboxylate and sulfate groups to form a complex via displacement of two labile chlorides of CDDP."[26] In their initial research, they "found that CSA with a mean molecular weight of 23 kDa was capable of increasing the plasma retention of CDDP while reducing its nephrotoxicity."[27] Later, using a rat model, Zhang et al.[26] compared the effects of two different doses of a cisplatin-CS complex with cisplatin monotherapy in reducing the nephrotoxic effects associated with cisplatin therapy, specifically comparing in vivo pharmacokinetics and in vitro cytotoxicity. They found that complexing cisplatin with either of two doses of chondroitin (2 and 5 mg/kg) altered the pharmacokinetic properties of cisplatin. This modified activity provided a protective effect by slowing the distribution and perfusion of cisplatin to tissues, particularly the kidneys, and reducing renal clearance while maintaining the same level of therapeutic activity. Their conclusion stated that this study provided "evidence that the sulfated position of chondroitin sulfates really affects the stability and the disposition of the CDDP complexes. The complex prepared with chondroitin sulfate A, with a molecular weight of over 20 kDa, is superior to that prepared by chondroitin sulfate C, because of improved pharmacokinetic properties and similar pharmacological activity to native drug."[26] Such consistent findings from these preliminary animal studies indicate that further clinical studies are warranted.

Nutritional Therapeutics, Clinical Concerns, and Adaptations

The emerging body of research strongly suggests that coadministration of CS with platinum-based chemotherapeutic agents such as cisplatin has the potential to serve as a safe and effective adjuvant therapy capable of decreasing the nephrotoxic effects resulting from drug-induced oxidative damage. Well-designed randomized trials with both arms carefully stratified to have equivalent prognostic factors will be necessary to be certain that concomitant chondroitin therapy with platinum-based therapies (as well as other neurotoxic chemotherapies, e.g., taxanes, vinca alkaloids) does not compromise efficacy of the chemotherapy. When offered such therapy, patients should be informed of the preliminary work done, and that although chondroitin likely can provide protection from nephrotoxic chemotherapy, we cannot be certain at this time that it would definitely not compromise chemotherapy efficacy. This is much less of an issue when palliative chemotherapy is concerned, but when chemotherapy is given with curative intent, such as for germ cell tumors, careful monitoring of clinical response and full disclosure to the patient and their family regarding current evidence are essential. Such integrative approaches to oncology care require a high level of collaboration among health care professionals trained and experienced in both conventional pharmacology and nutritional therapeutics, usually only obtained in multidisciplinary oncology clinics.

Nonsteroidal Anti-Inflammatory Drugs (NSAIDs)

COX-1 inhibitors: Diclofenac (Cataflam, Voltaren); combination drug: diclofenac and misoprostol (Arthrotec); diflunisal (Dolobid), etodolac (Lodine), fenoprofen (Dalfon), furbiprofen (Ansaid), ibuprofen (Advil, Excedrin IB, Motrin, Motrin IB, Nuprin, Pedia Care Fever Drops, Provel, Rufen); combination drug: hydrocodone and ibuprofen (Reprexain, Vicoprofen); indomethacin (indometacin; Indocin, Indocin-SR), ketoprofen (Orudis, Oruvail), ketorolac (Acular ophthalmic, Toradol), meclofenamate (Meclomen), mefenamic acid (Ponstel), meloxicam (Mobic), nabumetone (Relafen), naproxen (Aleve, Anaprox, Naprosyn), oxaprozin (Daypro), piroxicam (Feldene), salsalate (salicylic acid; Amigesic, Disalcid, Marthritic, Mono Gesic, Salflex, Salsitab), sulindac (Clinoril), tolmetin (Tolectin).
COX-2 inhibitor: Celecoxib (Celebrex).

Interaction Type and Significance

⊕⊕⊕ **Beneficial or Supportive Interaction, Not Requiring Professional Management**
☼ **Prevention or Reduction of Drug Adverse Effect**

Probability:	Evidence Base:
2. Probable	⦿ **Emerging**

Effect and Mechanism of Action

In addition to supporting formation, repair, and functionality of cartilage, tendons, bone, and joints, the nutritive activity of CS can counter the tendency of NSAID therapy to impair formation and repair of connective tissue and bone and joint rehabilitation.

Research

Numerous in vivo, animal, and human studies suggest that many NSAIDs exert deleterious effects on synthesis of vasodilator prostaglandins, joint perfusion, chondrocyte and proteoglycan metabolism, bone formation, cartilage synthesis, tendon-to-bone healing, and organization in articular cartilage, especially influencing the course of osteoarthritis.[28-34]

In a 1997 discussion of the issue of coadministration of NSAIDs and CS, Towheed and Hochberg[34a] noted that these agents provided a complementary (rather than directly pharmacologically additive) effect within a comprehensive strategy for treating OA and other musculoskeletal conditions. Leeb et al.[21] conducted a meta-analysis of seven randomized, placebo-controlled and double-blind or double-dummy trials involving a total of 703 patients (372 treated with CS and 331 controls) with OA of the knee and/or hip.[3,35-40] CS treatment duration varied from 3 to 12 months and prescribed daily CS doses ranged from 800 to 2000 mg. Because of substantial differences in reporting among the studies reviewed, the underlying therapy with NSAIDs and analgesics could not be evaluated on a clear-cut, quantitative basis. These authors noted that "CS was given along with analgesics or nonsteroidal anti-inflammatory drugs, making required dosage of comedication an important factor." Thus, "all seven publications reported statistically significant reductions in consumption of NSAIDs and/or analgesics compared to baseline in the CS groups and much less marked ones for placebo." They concluded that "CS in combination with analgesics or low-dose NSAIDs is superior to analgesics or NSAIDs alone over longer periods in the treatment of OA. Moreover, a reduction of the required daily dose of analgesics or NSAIDs could be achieved." Therefore, coadministration might enable reducing dose of these medications, especially in managing pain associated with osteoarthritis, and reduce risk of adverse effects associated with prolonged NSAID use.

In a short-term in vitro culture using cartilage specimens, El Hajjaji et al.[41] found that celecoxib, a cyclooxygenase (COX-2) selective inhibitor, increased the synthesis of hyaluronan (HA) and proteoglycans (PGs) in human cartilage explants with midrange severity of OA in a relatively dose-dependent manner. celecoxib also reduced the net loss of labeled HA and PG molecules from cartilage explants.

Jordan et al.[42] conducted a survey of 828 patients over 55 years of age with clinically diagnosed knee OA in two general-practice populations in Wessex, England, comparing conventional and complementary therapy use by a deprived urban population with that of an affluent rural population. They found a high prevalence of NSAID use, and in "the affluent population there were statistically more NSAIDs, [and] glucosamine and chondroitin sulphate were also used."

Nutritional Therapeutics, Clinical Concerns, and Adaptations

The body of available evidence clearly supports concomitant use of CS and NSAIDs as a therapeutic option of probable value in the treatment of OA and related conditions. Such an approach is well supported by consistent findings from the research literature and emerging standards of conscientious and innovative clinical practice, and it appears to offer enhanced combined efficacy at minimal risk and cost and, because of the ability to reduce NSAID dosage levels, a likelihood of reduced risk of adverse effects.

Nutrient-Drug Interactions and Drug-Induced Nutrient Depletions

Notably, discrimination in selecting the most efficacious anti-inflammatory agent appears to be critical, since both animal and human research indicate that aspirin and acetaminophen may interfere with the activity and efficacy of concomitant glucosamine sulfate (GS). Evidence to this point, as reviewed in the Glucosamine Sulfate monograph, suggests that coadministration of ibuprofen with GS may provide a synergistic therapeutic effect and that acetaminophen should be avoided. Thus, for example, a reasonable option where the activity of an NSAID seems indicated might be combining the standard dosage of CS (400 mg) and GS (500 mg) with ibuprofen (200 mg), three times daily, with phasing out of the ibuprofen to an as needed basis when clinically improved. This long-term clinical strategy thus shifts from symptom management to maintenance, with emphasis on tissue strengthening and maximal restoration of healthy function.

THEORETICAL, SPECULATIVE, AND PRELIMINARY INTERACTIONS RESEARCH, INCLUDING OVERSTATED INTERACTIONS CLAIMS

Heparin and Related Anticoagulant and Antiplatelet Medications

Anticoagulants, heparin, unfractionated (UFH): Heparin (Calciparine, Hepalean, Heparin Leo, Minihep Calcium, Minihep, Monoparin Calcium, Monoparin, Multiparin, Pump-Hep, Unihep, Uniparin Calcium, Uniparin Forte).
Anticoagulants, heparinoids: Danaparoid (Orgaran), fondaparinux (Arixtra).
Related:

Anticoagulants, low-molecular-weight (LMW) heparin: Ardeparin (Normiflo), certoparin (Mono-Embolex), dalteparin (Fragmin), enoxaparin (Clexane, Lovenox), nadroparin (Fraxiparine), tinzaparin (Innohep).

Anticoagulants, oral vitamin K antagonist anticoagulants: Anisindione (Miradon), dicumarol, ethyl biscoumacetate (Tromexan), nicoumalone (acenocoumarol; Acitrom, Sintrom), phenindione (Dindevan), phenprocoumon (Jarsin, Marcumar), warfarin (Coumadin, Marevan, Warfilone).

Observations of structural similarities in the chemical composition of CS and heparin have been extrapolated into speculative claims of a potential risk of adverse interactions in the presence of anticoagulant medications such as heparin (or warfarin), as well as antiplatelet agents, and warnings that chondroitin might be contraindicated in individuals with bleeding disorders. Chondroitin sulfate is a subcomponent of the antithrombotic danaparoid, which is classified as a "heparinoid" medication. Danaparoid sodium is a mixture of glycosaminoglycuronans, heparan sulfate, dermatan sulfate, and CS, isolated from porcine or other animal intestinal mucosa. Danaparoid is devoid of a heparin fraction; its antithrombotic effect is derived primarily from antithrombin III–mediated inhibition of factor Xa and to a significantly lesser extent by inactivation of factor IIa (thrombin). Dermatan sulfate (sometimes called chondroitin B sulfate) potentiates heparin cofactor II and may prolong bleeding time but is not used in treating joint pain or degeneration. Overall, the available data suggest that CS may potentially exert a mild anticoagulant effect.[43]

Several case reports have been published describing a possible augmentation effect, as indicated by an elevated international normalized ratio (INR), in patients taking formulations containing both GS and CS while undergoing anticoagulant therapy with oral vitamin K antagonist medication.[44,45]

The limited and nonqualified nature of the available data in these published reports supports caution and indicates that further investigation through well-designed clinical trials

is warranted. However, stark, generalized contraindications are not supported by the data available at this time. Health care providers treating individuals taking anticoagulant (or antiplatelet) medications are advised to caution patients against self-medication with CS and to monitor such patients in the event that CS administration is deemed clinically appropriate.

NUTRIENT-NUTRIENT INTERACTIONS

Glucosamine Sulfate

The number of studies supporting increased efficacy from concomitant administration of GS and CS in the treatment of joint pain and degenerative conditions has grown steadily in number and power. Most have found the combination more effective than either agent alone, particularly in OA treatment.[22,46-55] Although often limited by size and design, the findings from clinical trials remain consistent with known physiological function and reasonably predictable therapeutic activity.

Nevertheless, in the 4-year Glucosamine/chondroitin Arthritis Intervention Trial (GAIT) involving almost 1600 participants with documented knee OA, Clegg et al.[55,56] found that glucosamine hydrochloride (500 mg three times daily), CS (400 mg three times daily), or the combination for 24 weeks did not provide statistically significant relief (defined as a decrease in pain of at least 20%) from OA-associated pain among all subjects, compared to placebo and celecoxib (200 mg daily) as positive control. However, an analysis of the subgroup with initial moderate to severe pain (excluding those with mild pain) revealed relief with the combined nutrients at statistically significant levels compared to placebo (79.2% vs. 54.3%) or celecoxib (69.4%). Also, 60% of all subjects administered placebo reported 20% or greater pain reduction; this high response rate in the placebo group may have obscured a therapeutic response in subjects administered the glucosamine and/or CS, especially among subjects with initial mild pain. As with many similar trials, participants were allowed to use up to 4000 mg of acetaminophen daily for pain, except for the 24 hours before assessment, further confounding the data and possibly adversely affecting therapeutic response. Notably, however, resort to such "rescue" acetaminophen was relatively low, overall averaging fewer than two 500-mg tablets daily.[56,57] The pivotal clinical issue of disease progression (vs. pain relief), including joint function and regeneration, was not addressed in this study. Such elements of pathophysiology are central to the therapeutic strategy of nutritional interventions, such as those involving the sulfate compounds, and are illuminated by research demonstrating that meniscal pathology increases the risk of cartilage loss in patients with symptomatic knee OA.[58] Continued research is warranted, but changes in trial design might provide more meaningful clinical findings.

Manganese

Leffler et al.[47] conducted a 16-week, randomized, double-blind, placebo-controlled crossover trial involving 34 male subjects investigating the combined effects of glucosamine HCl (1500 mg/day), CS (1200 mg/day), and manganese ascorbate (228 mg/day) in the treatment of degenerative joint disease (DJD) of the knee or low back. They found, by several objective and subjective measures, that such short-term combination therapy "relieves symptoms of knee osteoarthritis" and "appears safe." In a 6-month, double-blind, placebo-controlled clinical trail involving 93 people with knee arthritis, Das and Hasmmand[49] found that a combination of glucosamine and chondroitin (along with manganese) was more effective than placebo. It is not possible to determine from such studies whether or not manganese contributes additively, synergistically, or not at all to the established clinical activity of glucosamine and chondroitin.

Some sources suggest that total daily intake of manganese from foods and supplements should not exceed 11 mg, the upper limit of safety for manganese established by the Food and Nutrition Board of the U.S. Institute of Medicine.

Vitamin D; Vitamins C and E

Epidemiological studies suggest that a low serum level of vitamin D and low dietary intake of both vitamins C and E in healthy individuals 50 years of age is a predisposing factor for occurrence of knee OA at age 70.[59]

HERB-NUTRIENT INTERACTIONS

Devil's Claw

Devil's Claw *(Harpagophytum procumbens)*.

Ginger

Ginger *(Zingiber officinale)*.

Traditional patterns of use in indigenous and classic medical practice suggest efficacy of these botanicals in the treatment of OA and related joint pain and degenerative conditions. Enhanced therapeutic benefits resulting from additive or synergistic effects of combined use with CS (as well as GS) are reasonably probable based on clinical anecdotal reports and known pharmacological activity. Further clinical trials of good design, adequate size, and extended duration are warranted to investigate efficacy and establish guidelines for therapeutic application. Adverse effects caused by toxicity, at usual dosage levels in appropriate conditions, are improbable based on currently available scientific data.

The 60 citations for this monograph, as well as additional reference literature, are located under Chondroitin Sulfate on the CD at the back of the book.

Coenzyme Q10

Nutrient Name: Coenzyme Q10.

Synonyms: Coenzyme Q, coQ10, ubidecarenone; co-enzyme Q10, coQ10-alpha-cyclodextrin, coenzyme Q (50), coQ, coQ(50), co-Q10, coQ-10, 2,3 dimethoxy-5 methyl-6-decaprenyl benzoquinone, mitoquinone, Q10, ubiquinone, ubiquinone-10, ubiquinone-Q10, vitamin q10, vitamin Q10.

Related Substance: Ubiquinol (QH).

Synthetic Analog: Idebenone (water soluble).

Trade Names: Andelir, Cavamax W8/CoQ10, Heartcin, Neuquinone, Taidecanone, UBTH, Udekinon.

Summary

Drug/Class Interaction Type	Mechanism and Significance	Management
Beta-1-Adrenoceptor Antagonists Antihypertensive medications ☼/⊕	Beta blockers and related agents inhibit, to varying degrees, coQ10-related mitochondrial enzymes in cardiac tissue. Resulting drug-induced depletion pattern can adversely affect cardiac patients who are, in general, characterized by compromised coQ10 status. CoQ10 does not appear to interfere with therapeutic action of these medications.	Coadminister oral coQ10. Monitor closely.
Chlorpromazine Thioridazine Phenothiazines ◇≈≈/☼	Phenothiazines appear to inhibit NADH-oxidase and succinoxidase, coQ10-related enzymes, and thereby contribute to pattern of adverse myocardial depressant effects associated with these agents. CoQ10 appears to mitigate adverse effects without diminishing therapeutic action of these medications.	Coadminister oral coQ10. Monitor closely.
Doxorubicin Anthracycline chemotherapy ◇≈≈/☼	Oxidative stress caused by anthracyclines often results in cardiotoxicity and other adverse effects from competitive inhibition of coQ10. CoQ10 supplementation can reduce free-radical damage and prevent anthracycline-induced cardiotoxicity. Clinical evidence is lacking to suggest coQ10 might interfere with therapeutic effect of anthracycline chemotherapy agents.	Coadminister oral coQ10. Monitor closely within context of integrative oncology care.
HMG-CoA reductase inhibitors (statins) ◇≈≈/≈≈/☼/⊕⊕	HMG-CoA reductase inhibitors lower coQ10 levels, to varying degrees, by directly interfering with coQ10 synthesis. Resulting depletion of coQ10 over time can potentially induce adverse effects on cardiac function, especially in individuals with susceptibility to or presence of chronic heart failure, but may be prevented with coQ10 coadministration, without diminishing therapeutic action of the statin. Research findings on clinical significance of statin-induced coQ10 depletion and potential benefits of coQ10 coadministration are mixed.	Consider coadministration of oral coQ10. Monitor closely within context of integrative cardiovascular care.
Sulfonylureas Oral hypoglycemic agents ☼/◇≈≈/≈≈	Hypoglycemic drugs may inhibit, to varying degrees, the coQ10 enzyme NADH-oxidase and thereby cause adverse effects on bioenergetics, ATP generation, and insulin biosynthesis. Diabetic individuals are more likely to be predisposed to compromised coQ10 status and elevated oxidative stress. CoQ10 support can mitigate drug-induced adverse effects and may enhance insulin function and cardiovascular health.	Coadminister oral coQ10. Closely monitor glucose levels.
Tricyclic antidepressants (TCAs) ◇≈≈/≈≈≈	TCAs can interfere with NADH-oxidase and succinoxidase, coenzyme Q10 enzymes, and may induce coQ10 deficiency. These actions may contribute to well-known association with cardiac adverse effects. Concomitant coQ10 administration appears to mitigate adverse effects without diminishing antidepressant activity.	Coadminister oral coQ10. Monitor closely.
Warfarin Oral vitamin K antagonist anticoagulants ?/X/X X	Available clinical trial evidence does not support concerns that coQ10 might interfere with warfarin function based on structural similarities to vitamin K and several anecdotal reports. Administration of coQ10 may be therapeutically appropriate for many individuals receiving coumarin therapy. Nevertheless, gradual changes in dosage levels of any medication or nutrient is critical to maintain INR within therapeutic range.	Coadminister oral coQ10 if indicated. Monitor INR closely within context of integrative cardiovascular care.

HMG-CoA, 3-Hydroxy-3-methylglutaryl coenzyme A; *NADH*, reduced form of nicotinamide adenine dinucleotide; *ATP*, adenosine triphosphate; *INR*, international normalized ratio.

NUTRIENT DESCRIPTION

Chemistry and Form

Coenzyme Q10 (coQ10) belongs to a family of compounds known as *ubiquinones*, all of which are characterized by a functional group known as a *benzoquinone*. Ubiquinones are fat-soluble molecules with between 1 and 12 isoprene (5-carbon) units. Among the 10 naturally occurring coenzyme Q compounds, the ubiquinone found in humans is known as coenzyme Q10 because of the distinctive "tail" of 10 isoprene units (containing 50 carbons in toto) attached to its benzoquinone "head."

Physiology and Function

In humans, coQ10 is synthesized in most tissues throughout the body. Three major steps are involved in the endogenous synthesis of coQ10: (1) synthesis of the benzoquinone structure from tyrosine or phenylalanine, (2) synthesis of the isoprene side chain from acetyl coenzyme A (CoA) via the mevalonate pathway, and (3) the condensation or merging of these two structures. 3-Hydroxy-3-methylglutaryl-CoA (HMG-CoA) reductase is the critical enzyme regulating coQ10 synthesis as well as cholesterol synthesis.

Coenzyme Q is highly soluble in lipids and is found in virtually all cell membranes, as well as lipoproteins. The primary biochemical action of coQ10 is as a coenzyme for numerous enzymes in the electron transport chain, a series of oxidation-reduction (redox) reactions involved in cellular respiration, where the presence of coQ in the inner mitochondrial membrane is required for the conversion of energy from carbohydrates and fats in the synthesis of adenosine triphosphate (ATP). Within the mitochondrial electron transport chain, coQ accepts electrons from reducing equivalents generated during fatty acid and glucose metabolism and transfers them to electron acceptors. Simultaneously, a proton gradient across that membrane results when coQ transfers protons outside the inner mitochondrial membrane. When the protons subsequently flow back into the mitochondrial interior, energy is released to form ATP.

Coenzyme Q10 has dual potential to enhance energy production by bypassing defective elements of the respiratory energy production chain and through its function as an antioxidant. Coenzyme Q can exist in three oxidation states: (1) the fully reduced ubiquinol form ($CoQH_2$), (2) the radical semiquinone intermediate (CoQH), and (3) the fully oxidized ubiquinone form (CoQ). Thus, in its central role as a pro-oxidant within mitochondria, coQ10 enables aerobic energy gain, promotes unilateral proton accumulation, and generates reactive oxygen species (ROS) involved in physiological signaling. Ubiquinone can execute reversible addition of single electrons and protons. Lysosomal membranes critical to cellular detoxification and recycling contain particularly high concentrations of coQ. Recent research indicates that lysosomal ubiquinone maintains the optimal pH for cellular recycling through its double function as proton translocator and radical source, particularly under certain metabolic conditions such as an acid pH. Alternately, a range of research demonstrates a pervasive and potent role of coenzyme Q10 in protecting membranes and DNA from oxidative damage from free radicals directly and through suppression of the formation of oxidized lipids and the consumption of alpha-tocopherol. As a lipophilic molecule, the reduced form of coQ, $coQH_2$, along with enzymes that are capable of reducing oxidized coQ back to $coQH_2$, is particularly concentrated in mitochondrial cell membranes, where it acts as a key cellular antioxidant and provides protection against free-radical damage. However, the type of biomembrane where ubiquinone exerts its free-radical, chain reaction—breaking activity can significantly affect this action's efficiency. Furthermore, $coQH_2$ regenerates alpha-tocopherol radicals back to the chain-breaking (i.e., antioxidant) form of vitamin E and thereby further contributes to the control of lipid peroxidation. This ability to counteract oxidative stress is particularly evident in its support of healthy cardiac tissue and its protection of endothelial function. Thus, coQ10's unique chemistry enables it to function both as a pro-oxidant and as an antioxidant.

NUTRIENT IN CLINICAL PRACTICE

Known or Potential Therapeutic Uses

Coenzyme Q10 can be synthesized in vivo by all living organisms, including humans, and thus is not defined as a vitamin. However, in some situations, the need for coQ10 may surpass the body's ability to synthesize it, so it may be regarded as "conditionally essential." CoQ10 is well absorbed by oral administration, as evidenced by significant increases in serum, plasma, and lipoprotein concentrations of coQ10 after oral intake.[1,2] However, evidence from animal and human research is mixed as to the degree to which oral intake elevates levels in various target tissues, and how that effect might vary depending on state of health, influence of aging, and presence of dysfunction, depletion, or pathology in particular tissues and systems.[3-7]

In 1958, Professor Karl Folkers elucidated the chemical structure of coQ10 and noted its potential in the treatment of cardiovascular disease. However, his employer, Merck, chose to sell the formula and patent to a Japanese firm in favor of promoting Diuril, a new product at the time aimed at the cardiovascular drug market. Thus, although coQ10 developed a strong presence in medical and supplement markets in Japan, its entry into clinical use in the United States has been delayed but is steady growing.

Possible Uses

Alzheimer's disease, angina, arrhythmia, breast cancer, cardiac bypass surgery, cardiomyopathy, cardiovascular disease, cerebellar ataxia (familial), chemotherapy support, chronic fatigue, chronic obstructive pulmonary disease (COPD), congestive heart failure (CHF), diabetes mellitus, diastolic dysfunction, fibromyalgia, gingivitis, human immunodeficiency virus (HIV) support, Huntington's disease, hypertension, immune deficiencies, insulin resistance syndrome, ischemia, lung cancer, male infertility, mitochondrial diseases, mitral valve prolapse, muscular dystrophies, myocardial infarction, neurodegenerative diseases, Parkinson's disease, periodontal disease, prostate cancer, renal failure, rhabdomyolysis.

Oral administration may also enhance aerobic capacity and muscle performance, especially in sedentary and elderly individuals. Conclusive evidence from large clinical trials has yet to be carried out to investigate this proposed action.

Deficiency Symptoms

The deficiency pattern associated with coQ10 has not been clearly defined, and it is widely assumed that endogenous production and a varied diet provide adequate coQ10 for most individuals. A deficiency may result from impaired synthesis caused by nutritional deficiencies, acquired defect in synthesis or utilization, or increased tissue needs resulting from illness. Most coQ10 in humans is internally synthesized. Genetic defects in coQ10 synthesis and metabolism are considered rare at this time. Deficiency can be caused or aggravated by depletion or deficiency of any of the many nutrients required within this 17-stage synthetic pathway, including riboflavin (vitamin B_2), niacinamide (vitamin B_3), pantothenic acid (vitamin B_5), pyridoxine (vitamin B_6), cobalamin (vitamin B_{12}), folic acid, vitamin C, and several trace elements. As might be expected, given the central role of the HMG-CoA reductase enzyme in the coQ10 synthetic pathway, HMG-CoA reductase inhibitors ("statins"), which are widely prescribed for management of dyslipidemias and cardiovascular disease, have been implicated as an iatrogenic cause of coQ10 deficiencies.

CoQ10 concentrations in various tissues decline with advancing age, and elderly individuals are known generally to have lower levels of coQ10.[8,9] Likewise, researchers have observed that the patient populations exhibiting many of the conditions coQ10 is used to treat more often demonstrate low levels of coQ10; these include cardiomyopathy, gingivitis and periodontal disease, heart failure, and HIV/AIDS. Many researchers and clinicians consider at least a CHF subset to represent a coQ10 deficiency disease, to a significant degree. Decreased plasma levels of coQ10 have also been observed in individuals with diabetes and cancer. Lastly, individuals with the genetic polymorphisms called the LPL and NQO1 genotypes exhibit decreased coQ10 redox ratios, reflective of impaired ability to convert ubiquinone to ubiquinol.[10]

Dietary Sources

Coenzyme Q10 is widely distributed in foods but in such small amounts that extraordinary serving sizes would be required to obtain intake levels typically provided by commercial preparations (e.g., 100 mg daily).

Organ meats (e.g., heart, liver), meat, poultry, and fish are the richest dietary sources of coenzyme Q10. Nuts provide relatively high levels, as do soybean and canola oils. Vegetables, fruits, eggs, and dairy products contain moderate levels of coQ10, with broccoli and spinach being relatively richer.

Studies in Denmark conducted during the 1990s found that average dietary intake of coQ10 was 3 to 5 mg per day.[11,12] Overall, dietary sources appear to provide most individuals with less than 10 mg/day. Foods are estimated to provide an average of 25% of plasma coQ10 in most individuals. Boiling appears to have little adverse effect, but frying destroys 14% to 32% of coQ10 in foods thus prepared. The precise dietary contribution to plasma coQ10 concentration is unknown in any given individual but is estimated to be approximately 25%.

Nutrient Preparations Available

Microcrystalline cellulose-coQ10 complex.

Complexing coenzyme Q10 with alpha-cyclodextrin may enhance bioavailability of coQ10 by approximately 35% compared to a microcrystalline cellulose-coQ10 complex.[13]

Ubiquinol (QH) is the converted active form of coQ10. The conversion rate of coQ10 (ubiquinone) to ubiquinol tends to decline with age, rendering lowered serum levels of ubiquinol. Furthermore, LPL and NQO1 genotypes are associated with impaired ability to conduct this conversion.[10] However, outside the body, ubiquinol is extremely unstable without certain stabilizing procedures because it will convert to coQ10 on exposure to oxygen.[14] Since ubiquinone must be reduced to become active, oral ubiquinol may provide bioavailability up to eight times as great as that of oral ubiquinone.

Dosage Forms Available

Powder-filled hard-shell capsule, soft-gel capsule, liposomal spray, tablet, chewable wafer.

Oral coenzyme Q10 should be taken with a meal with some fat content since it is fat-soluble. Absorption decreases in the absence of lipid. Some experts suggest taking coQ10 with a small amount of olive oil to increase absorption. There is some evidence that coQ10 in oil suspension provides better bioavailability than granular form.[15-17] Chewable forms may also provide greater bioavailability than capsules or tablets.

Source Materials for Nutrient Preparations

Yeast fermentation, or semisynthetic process.

Kaneka Corporation of Japan, which is the only company to use yeast fermentation in the production of coQ10, produces the natural all-*trans* Q, which is identical to the coQ10 occurring in nature and has succeeded in obtaining "generally recognized as safe" (GRAS) status from the U.S. Food and Drug Administration (FDA).[18]

Dosage Range
Adult

Dietary: No level has been established for optimal dietary intake of coenzyme Q10.

Supplemental/Maintenance: 25 to 60 mg twice daily.

Pharmacological/Therapeutic: Ranging from 30 to 60 mg twice daily to 50 to 100 mg two to three times daily, depending on condition and in concert with a health care professional trained in nutritional therapies. Daily dosage levels of 300 to 600 mg have been used in clinical and research settings in the treatment of conditions such as severe cardiovascular disease and advanced breast cancer. Administration of 60 to 100 mg per day will usually double plasma levels of coQ10 in adults. Evidence indicates that oral intake does not impair endogenous coQ10 synthesis.

Toxic: None established.

Pediatric (< 18 Years)

Coenzyme Q10 is usually not prescribed for infants or children.

Laboratory Values

Plasma and lymphocyte coenzyme Q10 and coenzyme Q10H$_2$ levels.

SAFETY PROFILE
Overview

All available evidence indicates that coenzyme Q10 is generally safe. No significant adverse effects or toxicities have been reported as being associated with oral intake of coQ10. CoQ10 in doses up to 900 mg daily is safe and well tolerated in healthy adults for 4 weeks.[19] Even continued doses of 600 mg/day for 30 months and 1200 mg/day for up to 16 months have not been associated with significant adverse effects.[20,21]

Nutrient Adverse Effects
General Adverse Effects

Occasional reports of mild nausea, gastrointestinal (GI) discomfort, anorexia, or skin eruptions have been reported with oral intake of coQ10. Other reported adverse effects include fatigue, insomnia, headache, dizziness, irritability, photosensitivity, dyspepsia, vomiting, diarrhea, dermatitis, or flulike symptoms. Reported adverse effects typically receded when oral coQ10 was stopped or dosage levels or format were modified. Dividing daily intake into two or three dosages may eliminate adverse effects, especially if more than 100 mg/day is being used.

Pregnancy and Nursing

Adverse effects are not predicted, and reports are lacking. However, the lack of controlled studies involving pregnant or lactating women precludes claims of safety and suggests that oral intake should be avoided during such life cycles.

Infants and Children

Adverse effects are not predicted, and reports are lacking. CoQ10 administration is not recommended unless otherwise indicated as essential.

Contraindications

No contraindications have been established for coQ10.

Precautions and Warnings

No precautions or warnings are known at this time for healthy individuals. Individuals with CHF or other serious cardiovascular conditions should only discontinue coQ10 under the supervision of the prescribing health care professional; withdrawal of coQ10 intake could potentially contribute to relapse.

Cautions have been voiced regarding coQ10 use by individuals with diabetes, hypoglycemia, hypertension, or liver disease. Evidence to substantiate clinically significant adverse events is limited. Supervision and appropriate monitoring are usually adequate in most cases.

INTERACTIONS REVIEW

Strategic Considerations

The primary clinical uses of coenzyme Q10 supported by human trials are in the treatment of CHF, angina pectoris, mitochondrial encephalopathies, mitochondrial cytopathies, chronic myalgic conditions, dystrophies, fibromyalgia, and Parkinson's disease. In such conditions characterized by mitochondrial dysfunction, the functions of coQ10 in mitochondrial bioenergetics and protection against oxidative stress appear to be paramount. CoQ10's strong antioxidant activity also enables it to function as an effective therapeutic ally when administered in conjunction with medications, such as doxorubicin, that cause adverse effects as a result of inducing oxidative damage. Virtually all antioxidants are capable of functioning as pro-oxidants, either when present in overwhelming quantity (e.g., high-dose intravenous ascorbate) or when present with inadequate antioxidant network partners in an environment of high oxidative stress (e.g., smokers with poor dietary antioxidant intake who are supplemented with synthetic beta-carotene). Perhaps the unique aspect of coQ10 is that it functions physiologically both as a pro-oxidant and antioxidant and can be regenerated back to its reduced or antioxidant form through normal cellular enzymatic processes.

Many pharmacological agents inhibit coQ10 synthesis, interfere with its function, and induce coQ10 deficiency states. In such circumstances, coadministration of coQ10 can prevent or reverse adverse drug effects, often in a manner that enhances therapeutic efficacy and improves clinical outcomes. In these situations, coQ10 carries no significant risks, and controversy as to its use is minimal.

Coenzyme Q10 is most widely used in the prevention and treatment of heart disease, more recently incorporated into acute cardiac care. For example, in an innovative placebo-controlled randomized trial involving 49 patients, Damian et al.[22] found that combining liquid coQ10 (250 mg followed by 150 mg three times daily for 5 days) with mild hypothermia immediately after out-of-hospital cardiac arrest and cardiopulmonary resuscitation (CPR) appears to improve survival and may prevent reperfusion injury and neurological damage in survivors. The astroglial protein S100 is an established biochemical marker of central nervous system (CNS) injury. Mean serum S100 protein 24 hours after CPR was significantly lower in the coQ10 group (0.47 vs. 3.5 ng/mL). Three-month survival in the coQ10 group was 68% versus 29% in the placebo group, and nine coQ10 patients survived with a Glasgow outcome scale of 4 or 5 (vs. five placebo patients). As for chronic cardiovascular conditions and attendant mortality risk, evidence is not unanimously in support of its efficacy, but as part of a lifestyle that includes regular exercise and a healthy diet (particularly omega-3 oils), coQ10 may help significantly decrease cardiovascular risk.[23] In particular, chronic CHF has reached epidemic proportions and is the single most common cause for hospitalization among individuals over age 65 in the United States; in more than half these patients, impaired left ventricular (LV) diastolic function plays a major role. CoQ10 appears to provide particular benefit in reversing diastolic impairment, including adverse effects on LV diastolic function associated with atorvastatin therapy.[24] This therapeutic action, as well as the broader role of coQ10 in the treatment of chronic cardiovascular conditions, leads directly into what may become a major controversy within medicine.

The issue of the interaction between statin drugs and coenzyme Q10 presents some of the most complex and timely clinical issues affecting coQ10 and its role in human health. HMG-CoA reductase inhibitors have demonstrated important and substantial cardiovascular clinical benefits, including reducing mortality; however, the impact of coQ10 depletion with long-term statin therapy ($\geq$20 years) is only beginning to be considered in a substantive manner, particularly concerning patients with heart failure. Nevertheless, in the first clinical research addressing some of these concerns, Go et al.[25] conducted a propensity-adjusted cohort study of all-cause death and hospitalization for heart failure during a median of 2.4 years of follow-up after initiation of statin therapy. They reported that among "adults diagnosed with heart failure who had no prior statin use, incident statin use was independently associated with lower risks of death and hospitalization among patients with or without coronary heart disease." Although encouraging, the short duration of follow-up in this study precludes any substantive conclusions regarding long-term safety of statin therapy.

The medical literature currently portrays statin therapy as a virtual "panacea" for prevention and treatment of cardiovascular conditions (and a multitude of other pathologies), but the parameters of the statin discussion have yet to expand beyond cholesterol and inflammation and incorporate comprehensive functional assessment of all risk factors. In a paper with potentially disturbing implications, Getz et al.[26] discussed the issue of estimating the high-risk group for cardiovascular disease in a well-defined Norwegian population according to European guidelines and the systematic coronary risk evaluation system. They raised concerns regarding the efficacy of applying the current cholesterol reduction goals (of total cholesterol below 180 mg/dL) being established as public policy in Europe and the United States. They noted that, in Norway, one of the world's healthiest countries, 85% of the men and more than 20% of the women over age 40 would need to be treated for high cholesterol under the American recommendations. Thus, in this population with relatively low rates of heart disease, "implementation of the 2003 European guidelines on

Nutrient-Drug Interactions and Drug-Induced Nutrient Depletions

prevention of cardiovascular disease in clinical practice would classify most adult Norwegians at high risk for fatal cardiovascular disease."[26] These observations prompted provocative responses in the scientific literature questioning the necessity, safety, and prudence of broad-based implementation of aggressive lipid-lowering standards. In particular, Ravnskov et al.[27] pointed out that application of these recommendations would result in the majority of the world's adult population being treated with statin drugs; to which they added, "As the risk to benefit ratio for a more drastic lowering of low density lipoprotein cholesterol is unknown, we question the wisdom of this advice." Notably, May et al.[28] found that a total cholesterol level approaching 200 mg/dL is associated with higher survival in patients with heart failure than levels below 140 mg/dL.

Paradoxical evidence showing both reduced cardiovascular risk, including heart attack and stroke, and stress on cardiac tissue induced by the inherent action of HMG-CoA reductase inhibitors has yet to withstand the test of time over decades. Although 20 years may be required for ongoing inhibition of endogenous ubiquinone synthesis resulting in mitochondrial interference and diastolic dysfunction to manifest as impaired hepatic, neurological, and cardiac dysfunction or frank cardiomyopathy resulting in chronic CHF, long-term statin use could represent a significant iatrogenic risk factor for some patients, particularly those with baseline coQ10 levels that are suboptimal or compromised by aging, malnutrition, drug depletions, genotypic susceptibility, and other adverse influences. Thus, for example, Tsivgoulis et al.[29] found that patients with asymptomatic neuromuscular disorders may have their condition precipitated by statin use.

Although statin therapy may reduce inflammation, as reflected by reduced C-reactive protein (CRP) concentrations, other critical cardiovascular risk factors such as lipoprotein(a), homocysteine, and fibrinogen are not modified to any significant degree by inhibition of HMG-CoA reductase. Moreover, preliminary research indicates that hypotheses of reduced atherosclerosis and calcific aortic stenosis through aggressive lipid-lowering therapies using statins may have been premature and overly optimistic in the face of mixed findings; in fact, statins appear to block the beneficial effects of exercise on intimal thickening.[30,31] Likewise, in the IDEAL study comparing high-dose atorvastatin with usual-dose simvastatin for secondary prevention after myocardial infarction (MI), Pedersen et al.[32] found that although aggressive lipid lowering significantly reduced the risk of other composite secondary endpoints and nonfatal acute MI, intensive lowering of low-density lipoprotein (LDL) cholesterol did not reduce coronary death or cardiac arrest with resuscitation, and that there were no differences in cardiovascular or all-cause mortality.

Thus far, the potential for integrative clinical strategies based on synergistic activities has been neglected and may be most deserving of thorough investigation. A thorough review of the literature of statin therapy that incorporates a frank appraisal of risk factors suggests that the growing enthusiasm for statin drugs over the past decade may eventually succumb to a harsh realization that they are appropriate for a relatively select patient population, specifically those with severe and recalcitrant hypercholesterolemia for whom other therapies have proved ineffectual. Notably, the issue of individual pharmacogenomic variability influencing efficacious or adverse responses to statin therapy is only beginning to be considered.[33] Furthermore, until continued concerns about neuropathies, skeletal myopathies, and cardiomyopathies known or suspected to be associated with long-term statin therapy, as

well as their potential for enhancing growth of subclinical malignancies through angiogenic and possibly immunomodulating mechanisms, are more fully investigated, the use of these widely prescribed, arguably overprescribed, medications should be more carefully considered, given the paucity of long-term studies of these agents, which, once instituted, will often be consumed for the lifetime of most patients. For example, in a retrospective case-control study, Wilke et al.[34] found that CYP3A genotype was associated with increased severity of atorvastatin-induced muscle damage, but not an increased risk for development of such adverse effects, as indicated by elevated serum creatine kinase (CK) levels. Thus, individuals who were homozygous for CYP3A5*3 demonstrated greater serum CK levels than patients who were heterozygous for CYP3A5*3, when concomitant lipid-lowering agents (gemfibrozil with or without niacin) were sequentially removed from the analysis. Similarly, in comparing nine haplotypes in the gene that carries the code for HMG-CoA reductase within both Caucasian and African Americans, Krauss et al.[35] found that treatment with simvastatin (40 mg) demonstrated significant genetic differences in statin response in lowering LDL cholesterol levels. Consequently, individuals who have a genetic problem with metabolizing statins could have a larger depletion of coQ10 (because of a higher level of the statin drug) and thus could have more problems. conversely, individuals who tolerate statins better may be metabolizing them faster, and thus their Q10 may not become as depleted. Moreover, half of all individuals who have heart attacks do not have hypercholesterolemia.

Meanwhile, other methods of cardiovascular disease risk reduction, such as a healthy and balanced diet, regular exercise, and omega-3 fatty acid supplementation, should be pursued vigorously as a coordinated broad response to multiple risk factors. In such an integrative approach, for example, the therapeutic benefits of statin therapy can be complemented or enhanced through coadministration of fish oil or L-carnitine.[36-43] Nevertheless, when Studer et al.[23] conducted a review of data on the efficacy and safety of different antilipidemic agents and diets on mortality, they found that fish oil and statins were the most effective interventions for lowering cardiac mortality risk, fish oil being superior to statin therapy in terms of lowering all-cause mortality, despite very modest effects on lipids.

However, other evidence has emerged that could complicate the picture. In a 6-year, randomized, controlled trial involving 140 middle-aged men, Rauramaa et al.[30] found that men undergoing statin treatment are significantly less likely to exhibit benefit from exercise in slowing atherosclerosis than those exercising but not taking statins. Intermittent exercise enhances coQ10 biosynthesis, resulting in higher coQ10 levels, and this could be a factor in the well-known health benefits of exercise. The findings from this study suggest that statins may neutralize the beneficial effect of exercise, at least in part, through their blocking of coQ10 biosynthesis. Levy and Kohlhaas[44] conducted a review of studies examining the effects of statin drugs, prescribed for reduction of cholesterol levels, on plasma concentrations of coQ10 and considerations regarding coadministration of coQ10 and concluded that "statin drug therapy does indeed reduce blood concentrations of coenzyme Q10." However, the authors determined that "due to the small number and dissimilar nature of studies available, the ability of the reviewers to draw any strong conclusions was limited." Nevertheless, "results from isolated studies suggest that statin drugs may induce mitochondrial dysfunction." Furthermore, "limited data suggest that supplementation with coenzyme Q10 may be beneficial in patients taking statin drugs who 1) have a family history of elevated cholesterol levels, or 2) have a family history of heart failure, or 3) are over 65 years of age. Further studies investigating the effects of statin drugs on the development of myotoxicity are warranted, particularly among high-risk populations."[44] Continued research is needed to investigate the long-expressed hypothesis that many of the other adverse effects associated with statins derive from its interference with coQ10 synthesis and function.

Administration of coQ10 alone or in conjunction with other agents, as part of an integrative therapeutic strategy, offers significant potential for enhancing clinical outcomes in individuals with a range of cardiovascular conditions. In particular, numerous researchers and clinicians have reported many cases of extraordinary clinical improvement in individuals with conditions such as CHF in which the expected progression is characterized by steady worsening and morbidity within 2 years under conventional therapy. At the least, incorporation of coQ10 into the therapeutic repertoire presents an opportunity to correct myocardial deficiency of coQ10 and enhance synthesis of coQ10-requiring enzymes, thereby extending the duration and enhancing the quality of life of such patients.

NUTRIENT-DRUG INTERACTIONS

Beta-1-Adrenoceptor Antagonists (Beta-1-Adrenergic Blocking Agents) and Related Antihypertensive Medications

Evidence: Metoprolol (Lopressor, Toprol XL), propranolol (Betachron, Inderal LA, Innopran XL, Inderal).
Extrapolated, based on similar properties: Acebutolol (Sectral), atenolol (Tenormin); combination drugs: atenolol and chlorthalidone (Co-Tendione, Tenoretic); atenolol and nifedipine (Beta-Adalat, Tenif); betaxolol (Kerlone), bisoprolol (Zebeta), carteolol (Cartrol), esmolol (Brevibloc), labetalol (Normodyne, Trandate); metoprolol combination drug: metoprolol and hydrochlorothiazide (Lopressor HCT); nadolol (Corgard), nebivolol (Nebilet), oxprenolol (Trasicor), penbutolol (Levatol), pindolol (Visken); propranolol combination drug: propranolol and bendrofluazide (Inderex); sotalol (Betapace, Betapace AF, Sorine), timolol (Blocadren).
Similar properties but evidence lacking for extrapolation: Other antihypertensive drugs.

Interaction Type and Significance

☼   **Prevention or Reduction of Drug Adverse Effect**
⊕   **Potential or Theoretical Beneficial or Supportive Interaction, with Professional Management**

Probability: Evidence Base:
3. Possible   ◉ Emerging

Effect and Mechanism of Action

Coenzyme Q10 plays a central role in energy production within the mitochondria of all cells but most critically in muscle cells, especially those of the heart. Propranolol and some other beta blockers inhibit, to varying degrees, enzymes in cardiac muscle, particularly NADH-oxidase and succinoxidase, that are dependent on coQ10 and indispensable for the bioenergetics of the myocardium.[45,46] Kishi et al.[47] reported that adrenergic blockers for beta receptors inhibited mitochondrial coQ10 enzymes to varying degrees.

Research

Kishi, Kishi, Folkers, et al.[46-49] have demonstrated with both in vitro and human studies and through reviews of the scientific literature that individuals with myocardial failure (dilated and restrictive cardiomyopathy and alcoholic heart disease) exhibit significantly decreased coQ10 levels compared to those with healthy myocardial tissue. Further, a strong association has been observed between the severity of the pathology and the degree of coQ10 deficiency.[46] Conversely, enhancement of coQ10 levels in the myocardium appears to counteract energy deficiency and reduce the tendency to and severity of myocardial dysfunction.

A range of antihypertensive medications have exhibited inhibitory effects on enzymes containing coQ10 in assays using mitochondrial preparations from beef myocardium.[47] Among beta blockers, propranolol demonstrates the most active inhibition of NADH-oxidase. Researchers have reported that adverse reactions related to depressed myocardial function associated with propranolol occurred in approximately 10% of 268 hospitalized patients receiving propranolol; adverse effects were reported at dosage levels as low as 30 mg daily or less.[47] In vitro research indicates that metoprolol is approximately 25% as inhibitory as propranolol; clonidine and hydralazine (both alpha-adrenergic blockers) exerted similar levels of effect. Timolol showed negligible inhibition of NADH-oxidase and exerted pharmacologically low cardiac-depressant effects. Five alprenolols showed inhibition that approached that of propranolol. The 1-isomer of alprenolol showed weak inhibition of another coQ10 enzyme, succinoxidase, but the other beta blockers were essentially noninhibitory to this enzyme.[48]

The common pattern of fatigue associated with beta-blocker drugs, particularly in the elderly and individuals with preexisting coQ10 deficiency, may derive from diminished myocardial contractility, decreased cardiac output, and other coQ10-related depression of myocardial function.[47] In an open study of 40 patients in severe heart failure (classes III and IV), almost two-thirds showed objective and subjective improvement when treated with 100 mg of coQ10 daily. Individuals with hypertension demonstrate coQ10 deficiencies regardless of whether or not they are taking antihypertensive agents.[47] In a small open study, three of five subjects taking propranolol complained of general malaise, whereas none of seven subjects receiving both propranolol and coQ10 reported similar adverse effects.[49] Hamada et al.[50] found that adverse effects on myocardial contractility (and coQ10 levels) associated with propranolol therapy in hypertensive patients were reduced when 60 mg of coQ10 daily was integrated into the treatment plan. In parallel research, Takahashi et al.[51] conducted a trial with 16 glaucoma patients in which they coadministered coQ10 (90 mg/day) during treatment with timolol eye preparation for 6 weeks. They reported that this complementary therapeutic approach reduced timolol-induced cardiovascular adverse effects while preserving intended effects on intraocular pressure.

Nutritional Therapeutics, Clinical Concerns, and Adaptations

Physicians prescribing beta blockers or related antihypertensive medications are advised to discuss adverse effects associated with these medications and the potential compensatory benefits of concomitant coQ10. Nutritionally oriented physicians and other health care providers often prescribe coQ10 for patients with cardiovascular conditions, or to prevent the occurrence of such in those concerned with or predisposed to such diseases. Therapeutic dosages of coQ10 for cardiovascular conditions range from 50 mg daily to 100 mg or more three times daily; such dosage levels would be appropriate within the context of conventional treatment of hypertension with beta blockers and most other antihypertensive medications.

Chlorpromazine, Thioridazine, and Related Phenothiazines

Evidence: Chlorpromazine (Largactil, Thorazine), thioridazine (Mellaril).

Extrapolated, based on similar properties: Acetophenazine (Tindal), fluphenazine (Modecate, Permitil, Prolixin, Prolixin Decanoate, Prolixin Enanthate), mesoridazine (Serentil), methotrimeprazine (levomepromazine; Nozinan), pericyazine (Neuleptil), perphenazine (Trilafon); combination drug: perphenazine and amitriptyline (Etrafon, Triavil, Triptazine); prochlorperazine (Compazine, Stemetil), promazine (Sparine), promethazine (Phenergan, Promacot, Promethegan), propiomazine (Largon), thiethylperazine (Torecan), thioproperazine (Majeptil), trifluoperazine (Stelazine), triflupromazine (Vesprin).

Interaction Type and Significance

◇≈≈ **Drug-Induced Adverse Effect on Nutrient Function, Coadministration Therapeutic, with Professional Management**
☼ **Prevention or Reduction of Drug Adverse Effect**

Adverse Effect
Probability:　　　　　　　Evidence Base:
3. Possible　　　　　　　⊙ Emerging

Nutrient Benefit
3. Possible　　　　　　　○ Preliminary

Effect and Mechanism of Action

Phenothiazines are associated with adverse effects on cardiac function in some individuals. In vitro, phenothiazines inhibit NADH-oxidase and succinoxidase. Furthermore, chlorpromazine has strong alpha-adrenergic blocking activity and can induce orthostatic hypotension.

Research

Folkers, Kishi, and other researchers demonstrated that thioridazine and related phenothiazine agents can induce adverse changes in cardiac activity in some individuals. Inhibition of myocardial respiration, particularly NADH-oxidase and succinoxidase, by phenothiazines and other psychotherapeutic drugs contributes significantly to these adverse myocardial depressant effects. Research indicates that coadministration of coQ10 can prevent or reverse these changes, but conclusive evidence from large, well-designed clinical trials is lacking.[49,52]

Nutritional Therapeutics, Clinical Concerns, and Adaptations

Current use of phenothiazines has largely moved beyond the more obvious adverse effects and nutrient depletion patterns associated with prescribing patterns of prior decades. However, pending further research, physicians prescribing thioridazine and related phenothiazine agents are advised to inform patients of potential adverse effects and the possible benefit of reducing adverse effects through coadministration of coenzyme Q10. A typical oral dose of 30 to 50 mg twice daily would generally be appropriate but should be tailored to the particular characteristics and evolving needs of the individual patient. No evidence is available and no suggestion has been made that such nutrient

support introduces any significant risk directly or through interference with the medication.

Doxorubicin and Related Anthracycline Chemotherapy

Evidence: Doxorubicin (Adriamycin, Rubex).

Extrapolated, based on similar properties: Daunorubicin (Cerubidine), epirubicin (Ellence, Pharmorubicin), idarubicin (Idamycin, Zavedos), mitoxantrone (Novantrone, Onkotrone). Similar properties but evidence lacking for extrapolation: Daunorubicin, liposomal (DaunoXome); doxorubicin, pegylated liposomal (Caelyx, Doxil, Myocet).

Interaction Type and Significance

◇≈≈ **Drug-Induced Adverse Effect on Nutrient Function, Coadministration Therapeutic, with Professional Management**
☼ **Prevention or Reduction of Drug Adverse Effect**

Probability:　　　　　　　Evidence Base:
1. Certain　　　　　　　● Consensus

Effect and Mechanism of Action

Anthracyclines generate free radicals that cause oxidative damage, particularly microsomal lipid peroxidation, through an iron-dependent process, which results in cardiotoxicity and adverse effects on other tissues. Doxorubicin also causes several other adverse effects, including (1) reduction of the coQ10 content within mitochondrial membranes, (2) inhibition of mitochondrial biosynthesis of coQ10, and (3) inhibition of mitochondrial synthesis coQ10-dependent enzymes, particularly succinoxidase and NADH-oxidase. Evidence indicates that such interference with coQ10 metabolic processes and depletion of coQ10 constitutes a major factor in the acute and chronic adverse effects associated anthracyclines, particularly doxorubicin-induced cardiotoxicity.[52-54]

The acute and chronic forms of cardiomyopathy induced by doxorubicin appear to derive from its specific effects on coQ10 synthesis and function, both immediate interference and metabolic sequelae. A single dose of doxorubicin causes inhibition of respiratory enzymes and rapidly induces a characteristic, acute cardiotoxicity.[55] Furthermore, not only can the cardiotoxicity of doxorubicin be of rapid onset, but it also can endure for decades, often absent cardiac complaints. Thus, in a longitudinal assessment of cardiac function in 22 patients treated with anthracyclines for osteogenic sarcoma or malignant fibrous histiocytoma, Brouwer et al.[56] found systolic dysfunction in more than a quarter of the patients and diastolic dysfunction in almost half after two decades (median, 22 years). Moreover, cardiac dysfunction was progressive, as measured at 9, 14, and 22 years.[56] This effect, sometimes reversible, appears to result, at least in part, from competition between the drug and coQ10, both of which contain a quinone group, for the enzymatic sites of the coenzyme. Doxorubicin may also cause enzyme inhibition through oxidation of coQ10, directly and through doxorubicin-induced ROS. Subsequent depletion of coQ10, with attendant loss of its physiological functions in electron transport and mitochondrial respiratory energetics, plays a major role in the loss of mitochondrial integrity and necrosis of cardiac myocytes characteristic of chronic doxorubicin-induced cardiotoxicity. Thus, coQ10 exhibits a unique ability to reduce free-radical formation induced by doxorubicin and to prevent resultant toxicity, particularly the chronic form; other antioxidants, such as vitamin C and alpha-tocopherol, do not provide a similar protective effect.[57]

Cardiac toxicity is similar between equipotent doses of doxorubicin and daunorubicin, slightly lower for epirubicin, and only one-sixth that of doxorubicin for equipotent doses of mitoxantrone. Doxil and DaunoXome (liposome-encapsulated doxorubicin and daunorubicin, respectively) exhibit negligible cardiotoxicity, presumably because of minimal cardiac exposure to the active drug with the pharmacokinetics of the liposome-encapsulated preparation.

Research

A broad consensus exists regarding the cardiotoxic effects of doxorubicin and its adverse effects on coQ10. Confirmatory evidence as to the extent to which introduction of exogenous coQ10 might mitigate such damage has developed more gradually.

Animal studies using rabbits found that mitochondrial degeneration is the most immediate and characteristic ultrastructural damage associated with the nonreversible cardiomyopathy induced by repeated exposure to doxorubicin.[58] All anthracyclines share cardiotoxicity to differing degrees, probably by the same mechanism. Using a rodent model, Shinozawa et al.[59] observed that among anthracyclines, aclarubicin had the smallest effect on rat liver microsomal lipid peroxidation, and the degree of this effect increased in the order of pirarubicin, doxorubicin, daunorubicin, and epirubicin.

Coenzyme Q10 demonstrated a protective effect against doxorubicin-induced damage to cardiac tissue in numerous animal experiments using mice, rats, and rabbits.[59-67] However, after confirming protective activity of coQ10 in conjunction with intraperitoneal administration of doxorubicin in mice, Schaeffer et al.[65] found that coQ10 failed to exhibit such a protective effect with intravenous anthracycline, as typical in clinical application with humans.

In reporting the findings of an experiment using a mouse model, Shinozawa et al.[68] observed that pretreatment with alpha-tocopherol significantly increased the tissue concentration of aglycone I (the major metabolite of doxorubicin) compared with saline placebo. They concluded that caution was required in the concomitant application of coQ10 and alpha-tocopherol with antitumor drugs, especially doxorubicin.[68] Some derivative literature has interpreted this statement as a contraindication of concomitant doxorubicin and coQ10 use. However, in two subsequent papers, these researchers noted that coadministration of coQ10 was associated with improved myocardial mitochondrial functions and "showed a significant decrease in mouse liver and heart microsomal lipid peroxidation" compared with doxorubicin-administered controls.[59,67]

In two studies (one in vitro and the other using rats) the addition of carnitine enhanced the protective effect of coQ10 in preventing anthracycline-induced cardiac damage.[69,70]

Iarussi et al.[71] demonstrated the protective effect of coQ on anthracycline-induced cardiotoxicity in a small study involving children being treated for acute lymphoblastic leukemia and non-Hodgkin's lymphoma.

Nutritional Therapeutics, Clinical Concerns, and Adaptations

Although further research with large, well-designed clinical trials is essential, coQ10 is already playing a role in many cancer treatment protocols employing multiple therapeutic modalities within an integrative clinical strategy. Administration of coQ10 before, during, and after chemotherapy with anthracyclines, particularly doxorubicin, is supported by scientific evidence and experienced clinicians; evidence of any interference by the nutrient on the therapeutic effect of the drug(s) is lacking and generally considered as unlikely. The usual dosage of coQ10 ranges from 50 to 100 mg orally twice

daily and inherently requires close supervision and regular monitoring. Physicians and other health care professionals may consider reviewing the potential for such synergistic therapies with appropriate patients and provide referral information to centers specializing in such integrative approaches.

HMG-CoA Reductase Inhibitors (Statins)

Evidence: Atorvastatin (Lipitor), lovastatin (Altocor, Altoprev, Mevacor), combination drug: lovastatin and niacin (Advicor), pravastatin (Pravachol), simvastatin (Zocor); combination drug: simvastatin and extended-release nicotinic acid (Niaspan). Extrapolated, based on similar properties: Fluvastatin (Lescol, Lescol XL), rosuvastatin (Crestor).

Interaction Type and Significance

◇≈≈ Drug-Induced Adverse Effect on Nutrient Function, Coadministration Therapeutic, with Professional Management
≈≈ Drug-Induced Nutrient Depletion, Supplementation Therapeutic, with Professional Management
☼ Prevention or Reduction of Drug Adverse Effect
⊕⊕ Beneficial or Supportive Interaction, with Professional Management

Probability: Evidence Base:
2. Probable   ● Consensus

Effect and Mechanism of Action

3-Hydroxy-3-methylglutaryl coenzyme A (HMG-CoA) is normally converted to mevalonate, the substrate for biosynthesis of both cholesterol and coQ10. Coenzyme Q10 is a component of the LDL and VLDL fractions of cholesterol. Statin drugs exert their action in lowering cholesterol synthesis by competitively inhibiting hepatic synthesis of HMG-CoA reductase, the rate-limiting step of mevalonate synthesis, and thereby limiting conversion of HMG-CoA to mevalonate. Thus, HMG-CoA reductase inhibitors lower coQ10 (ubiquinone) levels, in a dose-dependent relationship, as they lower cholesterol.[72-79] Statins are the only class of lipid-lowering agents that are known to block the synthesis of mevalonate.

Research

Researchers have developed a consistent body of evidence over time demonstrating the adverse effects of HMG-CoA reductase inhibitors on the synthesis and function of coQ10 and determining the variables influencing this depletion pattern and its clinical significance. The emerging research demonstrating the central importance of coQ10 in myocardial and endothelial function underlies the growing concern for adverse effects on cardiovascular function, particularly among individuals who have developed or are susceptible to coronary artery disease and heart failure, especially within the context of aging and associated tendencies to coQ10 deficiency.[79-82] Significantly, Langsjoen and Langsjoen[69] have noted that all large clinical trials of statin therapy have excluded patients with "class III and IV heart failure such that long term safety of statins in patients with heart failure has not been established."

Beginning with Willis et al.[82a] in 1990, animal studies have evaluated the effects of statins on coQ blood and tissue levels. In addition to documenting the adverse effects of statin-induced depletion of coQ9 and coQ10 (species dependent) on ATP and creatinine phosphate in myocardium, these researchers also investigated prevention or reversal of resultant deficiency states through coadministration of exogenous ubiquinone. Researchers further established that statins are the only class of lipid-lowering agents that directly impede the synthesis of mevalonate and therefore most directly interfere with coQ10 synthesis. Lipid-soluble statins (atorvastatin, cerivastatin, simvastatin, fluvastatin) showed more toxicity in this regard than water-soluble/hydrophilic statins (pravastatin).[83,84] In all animal studies where coQ10 was administered to the animals before initiation of statin therapy, the coQ10 blood and tissue depletion was completely prevented.

In 1990, Folkers et al.[72] first reported the interaction between statins and coQ10 in a small human trial that documented depletion of coQ10 by lovastatin and concluded that oral administration of coQ10 increased blood levels of coQ10 and was generally accompanied by an improvement in cardiac function. These researchers further suggested that coQ10 depletion might play a significant role in or be responsible for abnormal liver function and other adverse effects associated with statin use. Studies published in 1993 by Watts et al.[73] and Ghirlanda et al.[74] and later by De Pinieux et al.[75] (1996) confirmed the effects of HMG-CoA reductase inhibitors on blood levels of ubiquinone.

Nevertheless, some researchers have interpreted as clinically insignificant the degree of coQ10 depletion in some patient populations and questioned the need for compensatory coQ10 administration. In 1994, Laaksonen et al.[85] conducted inquiries into the effects of lovastatin and simvastatin on serum ubiquinone concentrations and found that after short-term lovastatin treatment, and after long-term simvastatin treatment, average serum ubiquinone levels were similar to those observed in a group of apparently healthy middle-aged men. However, in 1997, Mortensen et al.[76] conducted a randomized, double-blind clinical trial where serum levels of coQ10 were measured over a period of eighteen weeks in forty-five hypercholesterolemic individuals who had been prescribed the statin drugs lovastatin and pravastatin. A dose-related significant decline of the total serum level of coQ10 was found in both groups, with those taking lovastatin (20-80 mg/day) demonstrating the more pronounced decline. Likewise, Paloma'ki et al.[86] conducted a double-blind, placebo-controlled, crossover trial with 27 hypercholesterolemic men with coronary heart disease. During the 6-week treatment period using lovastatin (60 mg/day), ubiquinol content diminished by 13%, as measured by LDL phosphorus. However, in a later randomized, double-blind, placebo-controlled, crossover trial, Paloma'ki et al.[87] found that 180 mg coQ10 daily did not convincingly correct impaired defense against initiation of oxidation of LDL due to lovastatin treatment at 60 mg/day. They concluded that concomitant coQ10 only partially restored the drug-induced depletion of LDL ubiquinol and questioned the clinical benefits of coQ10 coadministration in individuals taking HMG-CoA reductase inhibitors, specifically lovastatin.

Bleske et al.[88] reported a lack of significant decline in measurable coQ10 in a randomized crossover study involving 12 healthy young normolipidemic volunteers treated with either pravastatin or atorvastatin for 4 weeks despite a significant decrease in LDL levels. Despite the short period involved and the dissimilarity between the test subjects and the typical patient population, these authors concluded: "Routine supplementation of CoQ10 may not be necessary when HMG-CoA reductase inhibitor therapy is administered." In contrast, Rundek et al.[89] conducted a prospective blinded study involving 34 subjects eligible for statin treatment according to standard criteria. After assessing baseline coQ10 status, investigators found that a decline in blood concentration of CoQ10 was already detectable after 14 days and had dropped

by approximately 50% (mean, 1.26 µg/mL vs. 0.62 µg/mL) after 30 days. "Even brief exposure to atorvastatin causes a marked decrease in blood CoQ10 concentration," the authors observed, and further noted: "Widespread inhibition of CoQ10 synthesis could explain the most commonly reported adverse effects of statins, especially exercise intolerance, myalgia, and myoglobinuria." These researchers proposed that future research might benefit from measurement of tissue levels of cQ10 and concluded by suggesting that coadministration with coQ10 may be appropriate.[89]

Thus, coQ10 depletion appears to be well tolerated in younger and healthier patients, particularly in the short term, but the collected data demonstrate detrimental cardiac effects, especially with preexisting cardiac dysfunction, when subjected to this drug-induced depletion pattern. Some evidence indicates that pravastatin may reduce coQ10 levels to a lesser degree than other HMG-CoA reductase inhibitors.[74,76] Of particular concern to many clinicians and coQ10 investigators are the statin-induced changes in diastolic LV performance because myocardial diastolic function is highly ATP dependent and therefore particularly susceptible to coQ10 depletion. In November 2002, at the third conference of the International Coenzyme Q10 Association, Silver et al.[77] presented the results of a small pilot study involving six hyperlipidemic patients undergoing statin therapy. They reported that after 6 months of statin therapy, 67% demonstrated abnormalities of diastolic function.

The effect of statins on coQ10 is not paralleled by similar adverse impact on other antioxidant substances. Yoshida et al.[90] reported that LDL cholesterol (LDL-C) levels declined with low-dose simvastatin, with no attendant drop in the antioxidant levels of LDL or elevation of oxidative susceptibility of LDL. Subsequently, in a 3-month trial involving 42 hypercholesterolemic male patients treated with different doses of atorvastatin, simvastatin, and pravastatin, Passi et al.[78] observed not only the desired drop in total cholesterol and LDL-C, but also a significant dose-dependent plasma (and lymphocyte) depletion of $coQ10H_2$ and coQ10, although no accompanying change in the $coQ10H_2/coQ10$ ratio. Other antioxidants, both lipophilic (alpha- and gamma-tocopherol, lycopene, beta-carotene) and hydrophilic (vitamin C, uric acid) as well as glutathione, polyunsaturated fatty acid (PUFA), copper, and zinc–superoxide dismutase, were spared drug-induced depletion. Concomitant vitamin E may partially offset the loss of coQ10 caused by lovastatin.[91]

Following up on the early work of Folkers et al.,[72] human studies by Bargossi et al.[92] and Miyake et al.[93] found that coadministration of 90 to 100 mg daily of coQ10 protects against declining blood levels of coQ10 caused by statins without interfering with lipid-lowering activity. Pettit et al.[94] demonstrated reversal of statin toxicity to human lymphocytes in tissue culture. Significantly, in terms of clinical strategy, both coQ10 and statins appear to have a protective effect on endothelial function.[84,95-97] Wong et al.[98] found that concurrent coQ10 did not diminish the anti-inflammatory effect attributed to statins.

Brady et al.[99] and Goldman et al.[100] conducted surveys investigating the use of statins among general practitioners in the United Kingdom. They found that 80% believed that 80% of their patients had achieved target cholesterol levels (≤5 mmol/L). However, such outcomes were achieved in only 65% of patients initially, with that rate increasing to 78% after uptitrations and switching medication. Moreover, only 46% of patients demonstrated cholesterol reduction of 25% to the target levels, increasing to 56% after uptitrations or switching medication. Notably, in response to such failure to achieve intended clinical outcomes, these practitioners stated that they would continue the unsuccessful therapy in 23.2% of such cases. These findings indicate that clinical guidelines are not being followed by many primary care physicians and that a significant gap exists between expectation and actual clinical results in statin prescribing. The issues of patient skepticism and compliance further complicate the realities of clinical application of statin therapy and reveal a significant departure from the scenarios envisioned in clinical trials and academic reviews.

Nutritional Therapeutics, Clinical Concerns, and Adaptations

Concomitant administration of coQ10 during statin therapy offers the opportunity to derive benefits from HMG-CoA reductase inhibitors while countering some of their more direct potential adverse effects and supporting broader clinical outcomes. Therapeutic dosages of coQ10 for cardiovascular conditions range from 50 mg daily to 100 mg or more three times daily. CoQ10 support is more important in elderly persons and those with a high susceptibility to or known history of cardiovascular disease, particularly heart failure. Genomic testing may be appropriate to elicit patterns of increased susceptibility to adverse effects of a particular statin drug or to impaired conversion of ubiquinone to ubiquinol. The need for coQ10 coadministration is dose dependent and should be initiated with statin therapy, if not earlier. Individuals prescribed statins that have a greater impact on coQ10, such as atorvastatin, may benefit from higher coQ10 dosage levels. A collaborative approach involving health care professionals trained and experienced in cardiology, nutrition, and other relevant modalities can provide optimal care for each individual through a customized and evolving program of integrative care. Thus, more broadly, strong emphasis needs to be placed on a comprehensive approach using proactive interventions that are safe and effective, such as regular exercise, stress reduction, healthy diet, omega-3 oils, L-carnitine, magnesium, L-taurine, and nutrient support emphasizing a network of antioxidant substances; consideration might also be given to potentially beneficial plant medicines, including *Crataegus* (hawthorn), garlic, and *Ginkgo biloba*.

It is noteworthy that, in apparent recognition of the significant adverse effects associated with statin-induced coQ10 depletion, two patents were awarded to Merck and Co. (now Merck, Sharp and Dohme) in 1990 for the combination of Mevacor in particular and statins in general with 1000 mg of coQ10. U.S. Patent No. 4,933,165 was issued for the following therapy: "A method of counteracting HMG-CoA reductase inhibitor-associated skeletal muscle myopathy in a subject in need of such treatment which comprises the adjunct administration of a therapeutically effective amount of HMG-CoA reductase inhibitor and an effective amount of Coenzyme Q10 to counteract said myopathy."[101] Merck is also the assignee for U.S. Patent No. 4,929,437, which applies to a pharmaceutical composition and method of counteracting elevated transaminase levels associated with HMG-CoA reductase inhibitor. The method described comprises the adjunct administration of an effective amount of a statin inhibitor and an effective amount of coQ10.[102] These actions indicate that Merck was convinced of the clinical value and market potential of administering coQ10 in conjunction with statins, at least enough to apply for and receive patents for that combination of therapies. Merck's patents would preclude other companies from combining coQ10 with other statins in a single-dose form. It is not clear why Merck thus far has chosen not to market such a combination with Mevacor (lovastatin).

Sulfonylureas and Related Oral Hypoglycemic Agents

Evidence: Acetohexamide (Dymelor), glyburide (glibenclamide; Diabeta, Glynase Prestab, Glynase, Micronase, Pres Tab), phenformin (Debeone, Fenformin), tolazamide (Tolinase)

Related but evidence lacking for extrapolation: Glimepiride (Amaryl), metformin (Dianben, Glucophage, Glucophage XR); combination drugs: glipizide and metformin (Metaglip); glyburide and metformin (Glucovance).

Similar properties but evidence indicating no or reduced interaction effects: Chlorpropamide (Diabinese), glipizide (Glucotrol, Glucotrol XL), tolbutamide (Orinase, Tol-Tab).

Interaction Type and Significance

☼   **Prevention or Reduction of Drug Adverse Effect**
◇≈≈ **Drug-Induced Adverse Effect on Nutrient Function, Coadministration Therapeutic, with Professional Management**
≈≈   **Drug-Induced Nutrient Depletion, Supplementation Therapeutic, with Professional Management**

Probability: Evidence Base:
2. Probable   ◉ **Emerging**

Effect and Mechanism of Action

Certain hypoglycemic drugs inhibit the coQ10 enzyme NADH-oxidase.

Research

Numerous studies have reported that coQ10 levels tend to be lower in individuals with type 2 diabetes mellitus than in the general population. For example, comparing the activity of succinate dehydrogenase–coQ10 reductase in leukocytes from blood samples, Kishi et al.[103] found that the mean percent deficiency of coQ10 was significantly greater (20% ± 0.7%) in 120 patients with diabetes than in healthy controls (16% ± 1.0%). Likewise, a mean percentage deficiency of approximately 20% was observed in 37 individuals whose condition was being treated by diet alone.

Kishi et al.[103] reported that acetohexamide, glyburide, phenformin, and tolazamide inhibit NADH-oxidase in vitro; however, tolbutamide, glipizide, and chlorpropamide had no inhibitory effect on NADH-oxidase or succinoxidase. In assessing patients under treatment, they further found that coQ10 deficiency was greater in individuals taking phenformin and tolazamide than in controls. Based on these observations, an even greater depletion pattern would theoretically occur in individuals administered acetohexamide and glyburide because they exert more potent inhibitory activity on coQ10 enzymes. Overall, the evidence thus far available suggests that the added effect of oral hypoglycemic agents on compromised coQ10 levels often characteristic of individuals with diabetes mellitus might exert a further adverse effect on bioenergetics, ATP generation, and insulin biosynthesis.

Concern has been raised that coadministration of coQ10 might destabilize patients under treatment for diabetes. In a randomized, double-blind trial involving hypertensive patients with coronary artery disease, Singh et al.[104] found that coadministration of 60 mg coQ10 twice daily in 30 of 59 total patients was associated with a significant decline in fasting and 2-hour plasma insulin and glucose levels, compared with controls receiving a B-vitamin complex. These researchers interpreted their findings as suggesting that "treatment with coenzyme Q10 decreases blood pressure possibly by decreasing oxidative stress and insulin response in patients with known hypertension receiving conventional antihypertensive drugs." Subsequently, in a randomized, double-blind, placebo-controlled, 2×2 factorial intervention involving 74 subjects with uncomplicated type 2 diabetes and dyslipidemia, Hodgson et al.[105] found that subjects who received 100 mg coQ orally twice daily (200 mg/day), with 200 mg fenofibrate each morning, for 12 weeks demonstrated a threefold increase in plasma coQ concentration and improved blood pressure and long-term glycemic control. Although not associated with reduced oxidative stress (assessed by plasma F2-isoprostane levels), as hypothesized, the primary effects attributable to coQ10 were significant decreases in systolic and diastolic blood pressure and hemoglobin A_{1c}.

Nutritional Therapeutics, Clinical Concerns, and Adaptations

Health care professionals treating individuals with diabetes and especially those being prescribed oral hypoglycemic agents, particularly acetohexamide and glyburide, are advised to consider coadministration of coenzyme Q10 (30-100 mg twice daily) as adjunctive therapy for the primary condition (and typical comorbid conditions) and to mitigate adverse effects of the medications. Close supervision and regular monitoring of glucose levels and blood pressure are warranted, especially while introducing coQ10 or changing dietary programs or dosage levels of any relevant medication. After a period of stabilization, gradual, staged reduction in dosage of oral hypoglycemic agents may be possible and appropriate with continued coadministration of coQ10. Attending health care providers are also encouraged to advise patients to be watchful for changes indicative of unstable blood glucose levels, especially acute fatigue, malaise, difficulty focusing, agitation, irritability, lethargy, cravings for sweets, and other characteristics of hypoglycemia.

Tricyclic Antidepressants (TCAs)

Evidence: Amitriptyline (Elavil).
Extrapolated, based on similar properties: Amitriptyline combination drug: amitriptyline and perphenazine (Etrafon, Triavil, Triptazine); amoxapine (Asendin), clomipramine (Anafranil), desipramine (Norpramin, Pertofrane), doxepin (Adapin, Sinequan), imipramine (Janimine, Tofranil), nortriptyline (Aventyl, Pamelor), protriptyline (Vivactil), trimipramine (Surmontil).

Interaction Type and Significance

◇≈≈ **Drug-Induced Adverse Effect on Nutrient Function, Coadministration Therapeutic, with Professional Management**

≈≈≈ **Drug-Induced Nutrient Depletion, Supplementation Therapeutic, Not Requiring Professional Management**

☼ **Prevention or Reduction of Drug Adverse Effect**

Probability: Evidence Base:
3. Possible   ◉ Emerging

Effect and Mechanism of Action

Tricyclic antidepressants (TCAs) are antagonistic to coenzyme Q10 enzymes NADH-oxidase and succinoxidase.[49] Furthermore, these agents are class I antiarrhythmics.[106] Drug-induced coQ10 deficiency may be a contributing factor to the cardiac adverse effects associated with TCAs.

Research

Tricyclic antidepressant drugs, including amitriptyline, particularly when given in high doses, have been reported to produce arrhythmias, sinus tachycardia, and prolonged conduction time.[49] TCAs inhibit NADH-oxidase and succinoxidase in vitro.[52] Myocardial infarction and stroke have also been reported with TCAs.[107,108] At this time, direct evidence of the frequency, circumstances, and severity of this interaction from large-scale, randomized human trials is lacking. However, the pharmacological principles of this interference/depletion pattern is widely accepted, particularly inhibition of myocardial respiration by psychotherapeutic drugs and its prevention by coQ10, as is restoration of healthy coQ10 levels through oral administration.[52]

Nutritional Therapeutics, Clinical Concerns, and Adaptations

Coadministration of coQ10 may prevent myocardial depression and other adverse effects on cardiac function associated with use of TCAs. Physicians prescribing TCAs are advised to discuss these risks and the potential benefits of concomitant coQ10 with their patients. CoQ10, 20 to 100 mg three times daily, can offset depletion resulting from TCA use and may reduce adverse effects and attendant cardiac risks.

Warfarin and Related Oral Vitamin K Antagonist Anticoagulants

Warfarin (Coumadin, Marevan, Warfilone).
Similar properties but evidence lacking for extrapolation: Anisindione (Miradon), dicumarol, ethyl biscoumacetate (Tromexan), nicoumalone (acenocoumarol; Acitrom, Sintrom), phenindione (Dindevan), phenprocoumon (Jarsin, Marcumar).

Interaction Type and Significance

? **Interaction Possible but Uncertain Occurrence and Unclear Implications**

✗ **Potential or Theoretical Adverse Interaction of Uncertain Severity**

✗✗ **Minimal to Mild Adverse Interaction—Vigilance Necessary**

Probability: Evidence Base:
5. Improbable   ▽ Mixed or
                                □ Inadequate

Effect and Mechanism of Action

Warfarin exerts its therapeutic effect by interfering with vitamin K metabolism. As quinones, coenzyme Q10 and various forms of vitamin K share a chemical structure. As a result of this vague structural similarity, coQ10 could theoretically interfere with the action of warfarin.[109,110]

Research and Reports

Although often presented as well documented and almost self-evident in derivative literature, the evidence supporting this proposed interaction is at best suggestive and fragmentary. The available data are lacking in substantive information necessary to predict the character and severity of any such adverse event. Furthermore, the frequency of alleged incidence is far below what would be predicted based on known usage patterns.

The medical literature contains at least four case reports describing decreased international normalized ratios (INRs) subsequent to the introduction of coQ10 in patients previously stabilized on warfarin therapy. When the individuals stopped taking the coQ10, their previous responsiveness to warfarin resumed.[111,112] Heck et al.[113] (2000) published a cautionary review of this potential interaction based on these available case reports.

Engelsen et al.[113a] conducted a small, randomized, double-blind, placebo-controlled, crossover trial in which patients stabilized on long-term warfarin therapy were administered coQ10. Concomitant use of warfarin and coQ10 did not significantly alter the warfarin dosage needed to maintain an INR in the acceptable range of 2.0 to 4.0 in these patients.

Emerging knowledge of the significant pharmacogenomic variability that influences warfarin activity, sensitivity, and resistance suggests that such possible interactions may occur only in patients with certain genotypes and that inconsistencies in the literature may reflect such variability.[114]

Nutritional Therapeutics, Clinical Concerns, and Adaptations

The clinical significance and frequency of occurrence of this interaction are uncertain, even though the theoretical foundation for this interaction is plausible and several case reports have appeared. Grounds for concern are amplified because of the high probability of overlap among the patient populations interested in coQ10 for cerebrovascular benefits and those being treated for the disorders for which warfarin is often prescribed. Physicians prescribing of warfarin should be aware of the possible risk of treatment effect alteration when coQ10 is coadministered and closely monitor any such patients for reduced effects. INR levels and prothrombin time (PT) should be checked with greater frequency during the first 2 weeks after either starting or stopping coQ10 to verify that the risk of bleeding or clotting (as reflected by INR value) is not being affected by the coQ10 doses. In general, it is important always to monitor PT twice weekly when medications, supplements, and diet are changed in any significant way; this is the safest and most reliable method of compensating for unexpected or idiosyncratic interactions in patients undergoing treatment with coumarin derivatives.

THEORETICAL, SPECULATIVE, AND PRELIMINARY INTERACTIONS RESEARCH, INCLUDING OVERSTATED INTERACTIONS CLAIMS

Fenofibrate, Gemfibrozil, and Related Fibrates

Bezafibrate (Bezalip), ciprofibrate (Modalim), clofibrate (Atromid-S), fenofibrate (Tricor, Triglide, Lofibra), gemfibrozil (Apo-Gemfibrozil, Lopid, Novo-Gemfibrozil).

No mechanism of action has been articulated for the phenomena reported in the available research, nor has available evidence indicated a consistent effect. It is generally accepted that the mechanism of action of fibrates in lowering cholesterol does not involve direct inhibition of mevalonate, the substrate for biosynthesis of both coenzyme Q10 and cholesterol.[73]

The evidence for this interaction is in preliminary stages, and understanding of its clinical implications is. In a randomized, placebo-controlled, crossover study involving 21 men with combined hyperlipidemia, Aberg et al.[115] found that 10 to 12 weeks of gemfibrozil treatment reduced serum coQ10 levels by more than 40%; alpha- and gamma-tocopherol as well as serum antioxidant levels also dropped. Also, normolipemic control subjects had significantly lower levels of ubiquinone and other antioxidants than placebo-treated patients, as part of an association between antioxidants and lipoprotein lipids. The authors concluded that the mechanisms and clinical significance of this finding were "unclear." In contrast, in a randomized, double-blind, placebo-controlled, 2 × 2 factorial

intervention involving 74 subjects with uncomplicated type 2 diabetes and dyslipidemias, Hodgson et al.[105] found that subjects who received 100 mg coQ10 orally twice daily (200 mg/day), with 200 mg fenofibrate each morning, for 12 weeks demonstrated a threefold increase in plasma coQ concentration and improved blood pressure and long-term glycemic control. Although not associated with reduced oxidative stress, as hypothesized, the primary effects attributable to coQ10 were significant decreases in systolic and diastolic blood pressure and hemoglobin A_{1c}. The specific influence of fenofibrate on coQ10 levels and outcome measures was not determined.

Another factor involving the impact of fibrate derivatives on coQ10 derives from their use in combination with statin drugs (HMG-CoA reductase inhibitors). Gemfibrozil, in particular, inhibits the glucuronidation of most statins (especially cerivastatin), thereby increasing their levels and the attendant risks, including interference with coQ10 synthesis and function. Fluvastatin appears to be the only statin with which gemfibrozil does not increase drug levels.

The evidence for a direct interaction between fibrates and coQ10 remains unclear and lacking direct investigation. Nevertheless, such preliminary status does not contradict the therapeutic value of coQ10 (e.g., 30-100 mg twice daily) in individuals with or at significant risk for cardiovascular conditions, particularly heart disease. Concomitant administration of fibrates and coQ10 may be medically appropriate as a preventive measure or a treatment intervention for many such individuals. Health care providers are advised to discuss such integrative approaches with patients as part of a comprehensive review of options toward a personalized and evolving therapeutic strategy.

Hydrochlorothiazide and Related Thiazide Diuretics

Hydrochlorothiazide (Aquazide, Esidrix, Ezide, Hydrocot, HydroDiuril, Microzide, Oretic).
Related: Bendroflumethiazide (bendrofluazide; Naturetin); combination drug: bendrofluazide and propranolol (Inderex); benzthiazide (Exna), chlorothiazide (Diuril), chlorthalidone (Hygroton), cyclopenthiazide (Navidrex); combination drug: cyclopenthiazide and oxprenolol hydrochloride (Trasidrex); hydrochlorothiazide combination drugs: hydrochlorothiazide and amiloride (Moduretic); hydrochlorothiazide and captopril (Acezide, Capto-Co, Captozide, Co-Zidocapt); hydrochlorothiazide and enalapril (Vaseretic); hydrochlorothiazide and lisinopril (Prinzide, Zestoretic); hydrochlorothiazide and losartan (Hyzaar); hydrochlorothiazide and metoprolol (Lopressor HCT); hydrochlorothiazide and spironolactone (Aldactazide); hydrochlorothiazide and triamterene (Dyazide, Maxzide); hydroflumethiazide (Diucardin), methyclothiazide (Enduron), metolazone (Zaroxolyn, Mykrox), polythiazide (Renese), quinethazone (Hydromox), trichlormethiazide (Naqua).

Hydrochlorothiazide exerts a mild to moderate inhibitory effect on NADH-oxidase.[47] Although preliminary indications suggest that a probable adverse effect of thiazide diuretics on coQ10 status, this interaction has not been investigated adequately to provide evidence sufficient to enable a well-founded assessment of its frequency, circumstances, severity, or clinical significance. Nevertheless, patients with chronic heart failure are consistently deficient in coQ10, typically proportionate to the severity of the cardiac dysfunction, and will generally benefit from coQ10 as part of a comprehensive therapeutic strategy.[46] No evidence is available to suggest that such nutritional support would interfere with the clinical effectiveness of diuretic therapy.

Levothyroxine and Related Thyroid Hormones

L-Triiodothyronine (T$_3$): Cytomel, liothyronine sodium, liothyronine sodium (synthetic T$_3$), Triostat (injection).

Levothyroxine (T$_4$): Eltroxin, Levo-T, Levothroid, levothyroxine (synthetic), levoxin, Levoxyl, Synthroid, thyroxine, Unithroid.

L-Thyroxine and L-triiodothyronine (T$_4$ + T$_3$): animal levothyroxine/liothyronine, Armour Thyroid, desiccated thyroid, Westhroid.

L-Thyroxine and L-triiodothyronine (synthetic T$_4$ + T$_3$): Euthroid, Euthyral, liotrix, Thyar, Thyrolar.

Dextrothyroxine (Choloxin).

The physiological interrelationship between coenzyme Q10 and thyroid function is multifaceted and has been investigated in many contexts. In the literature, plasma coQ10 determination has been discussed as a potentially useful diagnostic tool in differential diagnosis of thyroid diseases. Kotake et al.[116] observed protective effect of exogenously administered coQ10 on thyrotoxic heart in rabbits. Mancini et al.[117] demonstrated that coQ10 levels have a significant inverse correlation with thyroid hormone concentration in patients with spontaneous hyperthyroidism or hypothyroidism. Furthermore, exogenous administration of coQ10 may be beneficial in hyperthyroid patients with risk factors for heart failure.

Given these and other known patterns of mutual influence between coQ10 and thyroid hormone, oral coQ10 theoretically may affect thyroid hormone levels and alter the effects of levothyroxine or other thyroid medications. Evidence of any such direct interaction of clinically significance is lacking. Nevertheless, physicians or other health care professionals recommending coQ10 to individuals taking thyroid medication are advised to monitor such patients regularly. Clinical investigation of potential interactions, their character, and clinical implications is warranted.

Orlistat

Orlistat (alli, Xenical).

Depletion of coenzyme Q10 in individuals using orlistat has been suggested, but findings from clinical trials or other direct substantive evidence is lacking. Nevertheless, physicians prescribing orlistat as part of a comprehensive program for reducing obesity, hypercholesterolemia, or other cardiovascular risk factors are advised to consider and discuss with patients the potential benefits of 30 to 50 mg twice daily (or more) of coQ10. Further research is warranted to determine if the action of orlistat in interfering with fat digestion and assimilation might produce a substantial adverse effect on coQ10 synthesis and metabolism.

Pentoxifylline

Pentoxifylline (Pentoxil, Trental).

Portakal and Inal-Erden[118] reported that combined pentoxifylline and coQ10 pretreatment reduced ischemia-reperfusion damage in the rat liver, as indicated by hepatic glutathione and malondialdehyde levels. Treatment with pentoxifylline alone did not produce beneficial results.

Radiotherapy

Radiotherapy

Lund et al.[119] reported a reduced effect of radiation therapy on small cell lung cancer (SCLC) with concomitant coQ10 using a human SCLC xenograft into an immunodeficient nude mouse model. They observed interference with radiation

therapeutic effect at 40 mg/kg coQ, but not at 10 mg/kg. The 10-mg/kg dosage would be 600 to 800 mg coQ10 in average-sized patients, which is a frequently used dose range in integrative care of cancer patients. The 40-mg/kg dosage is equivalent to 2.8 g for a 70-kg person, a dose infrequently, if ever, used in nutritional oncology.

Zidovudine (AZT) and Antiretroviral Agents, Reverse-Transcriptase Inhibitor (Nucleoside)

Evidence: Zidovudine (azidothymidine, AZT, ZDV, zidothymidine; Retrovir); combination drugs: zidovudine and lamivudine (Combivir); abacavir, lamivudine and zidovudine (Trizivir).

Extrapolated, based on similar properties: Abacavir (Ziagen), didanosine (ddI, dideoxyinosine; Videx), dideoxycytidine (ddC, zalcitabine; Hivid), lamivudine (3TC, Epivir), stavudine (D4T, Zerit), tenofovir (Viread).

Zidovudine (AZT/ZDV) has been associated with "ragged-red" fiber myopathy because of its effects on myocyte mitochondria; this condition typically is reversible with cessation of the drug. Rosenfeldt et al.[120] reported the case of a 52-year-old male who first developed ragged-red fiber myopathy in 1985 while on effective ZDV-based combination antiretroviral therapy (ART), 14 years after diagnosis of HIV infection. The patient demonstrated "an excellent recovery" after administration of coQ10, known for its antioxidant activity in mitochondria, and was able to continue ART without disruption. The authors concluded that this response to coQ10 therapy "suggests a novel therapy for further investigation targeted at ZDV induced myopathy, potentially allowing continuation of antiviral treatments including ZDV."

NUTRIENT-NUTRIENT INTERACTIONS

L-Carnitine

Concomitant administration of coenzyme Q10 and L-carnitine may result in an additive effect.[69,70] Such a potential interaction likely would be beneficial, but direct evidence from human trials is lacking. Close supervision and regular monitoring are warranted at the initiation of and through the course of any such coadministration, particularly in individuals with serious heart disease or other cardiovascular conditions. Clinical investigation of potential interactions, their character, and clinical implications is warranted.

Vitamin B$_6$, Pyridoxine, Pyridoxal 5'-Phosphate

Pyridoxal 5'-phosphate is required in the conversion of tyrosine to 4-hydroxyphenylpyruvic acid; the formation of the quinone nucleus being the first step in coQ10 biosynthesis. Many researchers have noted the parallel decline in coQ10 and B$_6$ levels associated with aging. In a pilot study involving 29 patients and healthy volunteers, Willis et al.[121] observed strong positive correlations between blood levels of coQ10 and the specific activity of erythrocyte glutamine-oxaloacetic acid transaminase (EGOT) and between coQ10 and the percent saturation of EGOT with pyridoxal phosphate (PLP).[121] Further research is warranted to better understand this physiological relationship and the potential for synergistic therapeutics using nutritional interventions.

Vitamin E, Alpha-Tocopherol

Vitamin E and coQ10 function in complementary roles within physiological antioxidant networks as the principal fat-soluble antioxidants in membranes and lipoproteins. In particular, coQH$_2$, the reduced form of coQ, is capable of regenerating alpha-tocopherol. Alpha-tocopherol becomes oxidized whenever it neutralizes a free radical, such as a lipid hydroperoxyl radical, and consequently an alpha-tocopheroxyl radical appears. Subsequently, when coQH$_2$ reacts with the alpha-tocopheroxyl radical, alpha-tocopherol is regenerated and CoQH, the semiquinone radical, is produced. Thus, the formation of oxidized lipids and the consumption of alpha-tocopherol are suppressed while CoQH$_2$ is present.[122,123]

Some researchers have reported that vitamin E may reduce blood levels of coQ10. Coadministration of vitamin E and coQ10 would reasonably be predicted to have a mutually supportive effect, which would also enhance the broader activity of the physiological antioxidant network against oxidative stress. Further investigation into the physiological functions and therapeutic roles of vitamin E, coQ10, and other antioxidants is underway within both research and clinical settings and promises to deepen our understanding of their roles in physiology, health enhancement, and treatment of disease.

HERB-NUTRIENT INTERACTIONS

Ginkgo

Ginkgo *(Ginkgo biloba)*.

In an open, pilot study, Lister[124] reported significant improvements in the quality-of-life self-rating scores of 64% of individuals with clinically diagnosed fibromyalgia syndrome after administration of 200 mg coQ10 and 200 mg *Ginkgo biloba* extract daily for 84 days. Controlled clinical trials involving larger number of subjects with a placebo group are warranted to further investigate this potential therapeutic synergy and assess its clinical implications, particularly in treating individuals with mitochondrial dysfunction.

The 126 citations for this monograph, as well as additional reference literature, are located under Coenzyme Q10 on the CD at the back of the book.

Nutrient-Drug Interactions and Drug-Induced Nutrient Depletions

DHEA

Nutrient Name: DHEA (dehydroepiandrosterone).
Synonym: Prasterone.
Related Compound: Dehydroepiandrosterone sulfate (DHEA-S); 3-acetyl-7-oxo DHEA
(7-keto DHEA).

Nutrient-Drug Interactions and Drug-Induced Nutrient Depletions

Summary

Drug/Class Interaction Type	Mechanism and Significance	Management
Alprazolam, triazolam Benzodiazepines ✗✗/◇◇	Alprazolam has been observed to elevate circulating DHEA (while decreasing ACTH and cortisol). DHEA may reduce hepatic metabolism of these benzodiazepines by inhibiting CYP4A and CYP3A23, potentially raising levels. Clinical significance of this potential interaction is unclear, and supporting evidence is preliminary.	Coadministration does not appear to be contraindicated if otherwise appropriate. Drug levels and AUC may be increased. Supervise and monitor.
Amlodipine ⊕	Amlodipine increases serum DHEA-S and androstenedione levels (and decreases cortisol) in some individuals. This action may contribute to beneficial effect on glucose tolerance, insulin sensitivity, and cardiovascular risk.	Coadministration may be beneficial. Supervise and monitor.
Anticoagulant medications ✗/⊕✗	Evidence concerning this possible interaction is mixed and insufficient to determine any consistent pattern or assess clinical significance. Speculation of potential for increased clotting from DHEA is not substantiated by available evidence.	Coadministration does not appear to be contraindicated if otherwise appropriate. Supervise and monitor.
Anticonvulsant medications Carbamazepine, phenytoin ✗✗✗	Some antiepileptic drugs may decrease levels of DHEA and DHEA-S by inducing P450 enzymes, particularly CYP3A4. Exogenous DHEA may interfere with action of anticonvulsants and could theoretically increase risk of aggressive behavior by elevating androgen levels. mechanisms of possible interactions are as yet unclear, and substantive evidence is lacking regarding their clinical significance. Limited case reports of marginal quality suggest need for caution or avoidance.	Caution indicated and concurrent use contraindicated unless otherwise appropriate. Supervise and monitor.
Clonidine, fluoxetine ⊕⊕	DHEA may enhance activity of clonidine and fluoxetine by restoring response of beta-endorphin. Preliminary evidence suggests reasonable probability of clinically significant supportive interaction.	Coadministration may be beneficial unless otherwise contraindicated. Supervise and monitor.
Corticosteroids, oral ≈≈/⊕⊕	Corticosteroids can lower serum levels of DHEA and DHEA-S, as well as ACTH and other key hormones within interdependent regulatory systems. DHEA may enhance activity of prednisolone and counteract some adverse effects associated with long-term steroid therapy.	Coadministration may be protective and/or therapeutic with long-term steroid use, especially if otherwise indicated. Supervise and monitor.
Estrogens/progestins Hormone replacement therapy (HRT) Oral contraceptives (OCs) ✗✗/⊕✗/⊕	DHEA and estrogen play mutually supportive roles, which may be enhanced with exogenous administration of either or both substances and their precursors. Although reasonably grounded and supported by clinical experience and anecdotal reports, evidence supporting interaction is primarily suggestive, and understanding of its clinical significance preliminary and evolving.	Coadministration may be beneficial unless otherwise contraindicated. Supervise and monitor.
Methyltestosterone Androgens ⊕⊕/⊕✗/✗✗	DHEA can be converted into testosterone, and administration of exogenous DHEA, alone or with methyltestosterone (or testosterone), can increase testosterone levels. Coadministration may enhance therapeutic efforts to increase androgen levels. Mechanism clear and axiomatic, but clinical significance as yet uncertain and therapeutic guidelines evolving.	Coadministration may be beneficial unless otherwise contraindicated. Supervise and monitor.
Zidovudine (AZT) Reverse-transcriptase inhibitor (nucleoside) anti-retroviral agents ⊕⊕	DHEA levels tend to be low in HIV-infected individuals, and depression is common with this patient population. DHEA can enhance levels of testosterone, estradiol, insulin-like growth factor, and growth hormone, all of which can be associated with depression and debilitation. DHEA may also modulate inflammatory cytokines such as tumor necrosis factor. Coadministration of DHEA to HIV patients with nonmajor depression on antiretroviral regimens can significantly improve their psychological state.	Coadministration may be beneficial unless otherwise contraindicated. Supervise and monitor.

ACTH, adrenocorticotropic hormone; *CYP*, cytochrome P450; *AUC*, area under the curve; *HIV*, human immunodeficiency virus.

NUTRIENT DESCRIPTION

Chemistry and Forms

Dehydroepiandrosterone; dehydroepiandrosterone sulfate.

Physiology and Function

Dehydroepiandrosterone (DHEA) and its sulfate ester metabolite (DHEA-S) are among the most abundant steroids in the human body, yet their physiological roles remain largely unknown. DHEA is a naturally occurring steroid synthesized in the adrenal cortex, gonads, central nervous system (CNS), skin, and gastrointestinal (GI) tract and is a precursor for the synthesis of more than 50 hormones, including androgenic and estrogenic steroids.

Adrenal production and serum concentrations of DHEA are known to peak between ages 25 and 30 years and thereafter decrease with age, severe illness, and chronic stress. The main characteristic of DHEA is that its concentration in plasma varies throughout life, being low during early childhood and after age 60. Aging in humans is accompanied by a progressive decline in the secretion of DHEA and DHEA sulfate (DHEA-S), paralleling that of the growth hormone–insulin-like growth factor-I (GH-IGF-I) axis. Although the functional relationship of the decline of the GH-IGF-I system and catabolism is recognized, the biological role of DHEA in human aging remains undefined. DHEA has different effects in men, premenopausal women, and postmenopausal women, with associations often reversed for older men and women. DHEA and DHEA-S are metabolized by the hepatic cytochrome P450 (CYP450) enzyme system or via a cutaneous pathway, where it is metabolized by the skin and other tissues sensitive to sex steroids.

NUTRIENT IN CLINICAL PRACTICE

Known or Potential Therapeutic Uses

Low endogenous levels of DHEA and DHEA-S have consistently been associated with the aging process and diseases such as systemic lupus erythematosus (SLE), diabetes, and cancer. Consequently, DHEA administration has primarily been suggested to prevent or reverse such conditions. For example, by modulating endocrine parameters and synthesis of neuroactive steroids, low-dose DHEA (25 mg/day) administration increases adrenal hormone plasma levels in early and late menopause.[1] Likewise, DHEA monotherapy can be effective for midlife-onset major and minor depression.[2] However, Nair et al.[3] found that administration of DHEA in elderly subjects does not demonstrate "physiologically relevant beneficial effects" on markers for antiaging, such as body composition, physical performance, insulin sensitivity, or quality of life, although they did observe an increase in plasma levels of sulfated DHEA. The role of DHEA within hormone replacement therapy (HRT) and as an antiaging substance remains controversial and research preliminary.

Historical/Ethnomedicine Precedent

Antiaging and longevity tonic medications have been sought-after, proposed, and used throughout history worldwide in almost all civilizations. Such medications have often been associated with human reproductive function, hormones, and fluids. Needham discussed the use of crystallized medications derived from the collected urine of adolescents in ancient China. Early in the twentieth century, the adrenal glands came into focus with the research work of experimental physiologist Walter Cannon at the University of Chicago and his pioneering study of homeostasis and the autonomic nervous system. Clinical application of these concepts began with the work of Henry Harrower, Royal Lee, and others with the use of glandular preparations in therapeutic nutrition.

Possible Uses

Addison's disease, adrenal insufficiency, allergic disorders, Alzheimer's disease, andropause, anorexia nervosa, atherosclerosis, athletic performance enhancement, autoimmune diseases, cancer prevention, chronic fatigue syndrome, dementia, depression, diabetes mellitus (type 2), endothelial function, erectile dysfunction, fatigue, human immunodeficiency virus and acquired immunodeficiency syndrome (HIV/AIDS) support, hypercholesterolemia, hypogonadism, immune modulation, insulin sensitivity, longevity, menopause, multi-infarct dementia, multiple sclerosis, obesity, osteoporosis, Parkinson's disease, rheumatoid arthritis, Sjögren's syndrome, systemic lupus erythematosus (SLE), testosterone deficiency.

Dietary Sources

Animal proteins are the richest dietary sources of DHEA.

Nutrient Preparations Available

A semisynthetic form of DHEA is available as a nutraceutical. Some product surveys have found variable potency and quality in commercially available DHEA preparations.

Dosage Forms Available

Capsule, liquid, tablet, and sublingual form.

Source Materials for Nutrient Preparations

Soy or wild yams are used for extraction of a steroid precursor molecule, which is then chemically synthesized into DHEA (and a wide variety of other sex hormones).

Dosage Range

Adult

Dietary:
   Average American daily intake: DHEA per se is not a normal dietary component.
   Recommended dietary allowance (RDA): No RDA has been established.

Supplemental/Maintenance: Usually not necessary. Optimal levels of intake have not been established. Individuals who have not been diagnosed as having a hormonal deficiency pattern, preferably through laboratory tests, should usually not take DHEA.

Pharmacological/Therapeutic: There is no consensus among practitioners who prescribe DHEA as to an optimal dose. Some practitioners are routinely prescribing 10 to 30 mg per day for healthy men and 5 to 15 mg per day for healthy women, whereas others often prescribe 50 to 100 mg per day. Dosage is usually split into morning and late-afternoon doses. Much larger doses have been administered under close observation to patients with cancer, acquired immunodeficiency syndrome (AIDS), SLE, and other serious conditions. The metabolic fate of exogenous DHEA is variable and unpredictable because it can become one of many other hormones. Orally administered DHEA can also be metabolized by enzymes in the small intestine, causing biotransformation even before it has been absorbed. Even when using laboratory testing to evaluate appropriateness of and response to DHEA, no data yet exist on what constitutes a physiologic dose or an optimum serum level. Consequently, the judicious practice would be to err on the side of caution by using initial low doses of DHEA, following a conservative schedule for any dosage increase, and observing discrimination and vigilance in the use of supraphysiologic doses.

Beyond those who prescribe DHEA, its use is a controversial, but generally unexplored, issue. Opinions vary widely as to the benefits and risks of using hormones such as DHEA as nutraceutical therapies. Any such application should be monitored by a health care professional trained and experienced in nutritional therapeutics and is best undertaken after initially testing DHEA levels.

Toxic: No toxic dose has been established.

Pediatric (< 18 years)

DHEA is generally not considered therapeutically appropriate in children or adolescents, in the absence of conditions such as Addison's disease, and has not been well studied in such populations.

SAFETY PROFILE
Overview

The long-term safety of DHEA administration has not been established through well-done clinical studies involving human subjects from a variety of populations. The inherent tendency of DHEA to increase or otherwise alter healthy physiologic levels of a wide range of hormones suggests that unintended effects are highly probable and potentially adverse for some individuals in the absence of experienced clinical management.

Nutrient Adverse Effects
General Adverse Effects

Adults. Masculinization in women; altered secondary sexual characteristics in either gender.

Mutagenicity. Preliminary evidence and extrapolated hypotheses have been presented on both increased and decreased risk of angiogenesis and cancer in relation to endogenous and exogenous DHEA.

Adverse Effects Among Specific Populations

DHEA is often prescribed for biological aging, functional symptoms of aging, and prevention of functional degeneration hypothesized to derive from age-related depletion in hormonal levels. Given that the use of prescription medications increases with age, issues of potential interactions, adverse or beneficial, deserve special attention among the elderly population.

Pregnancy and Nursing

The safety of DHEA use during pregnancy and lactation has not been established, and such application is contraindicated because of potential impact on hormonal levels, regulatory systems, and fetal development.

Infants and Children

DHEA administration is generally contraindicated in children and adolescents because theoretically it may interfere with normal hormonal regulatory systems and developmental processes.

Contraindications

Given DHEA's potential effect on testosterone and estrogen levels, its use by individuals with personal or family history of prostate or breast cancer, or other hormonally mediated cancer, is contraindicated. Such recommendation is based more on caution and plausibility than on a consistent or well-developed body of evidence. The 7-keto variant of DHEA was developed to circumvent the metabolic pathways associated with such hormonally mediated adverse effects.

Testing

Serum or saliva. Monitoring free and sulfate levels is considered the most accurate method of tracking DHEA levels, but exogenous DHEA can become many other hormones. Orally administered DHEA can also be metabolized by enzymes in the small intestine, causing biotransformation even before it has been absorbed.

INTERACTIONS REVIEW
Strategic Considerations

DHEA is often prescribed for biological aging, functional symptoms of aging, and prevention of functional degeneration hypothesized to derive from age-related depletion in hormonal levels. Because use of prescription drugs increases with age, issues of potential interactions, adverse or beneficial, deserve special attention in elderly individuals.

The status of endogenous DHEA and DHEA-S constitutes a significant aspect of many health conditions, especially those associated with aging. A wide range of medications may significantly increase or decrease circulating concentrations of DHEA and DHEA-S by various mechanisms. Some drugs may affect the hypothalamic-pituitary axis by inhibiting adrenocorticotropic hormone (ACTH) and therefore lower DHEA and DHEA-S levels. Other medications induce CYP450 enzymes, hasten metabolism of DHEA and DHEA-S, and decrease circulating concentrations of the hormones. The ratio of DHEA and DHEA-S can also be altered by agents that affect sulfatase activity. Whether a disease state is associated with lower levels of endogenous DHEA and DHEA-S or a medication alters such concentrations, minimal clinical evidence exists to indicate whether oral administration is safe or effective, or problematic and contraindicated, in specific patient populations.

Whenever DHEA is being prescribed for primary therapeutic effect or to counter a potential endogenous deficiency or drug-induced depletion, close supervision and regular monitoring are important, as is coordination of pharmacological interventions within an integrative perspective.

NUTRIENT-DRUG INTERACTIONS

Alprazolam, Triazolam, and Related Benzodiazepines

Evidence: Alprazolam (Xanax), triazolam (Halcion).
Extrapolated, based on similar properties: Bromazepam (Lexotan), chlordiazepoxide (Librium), clonazepam (Klonopin, Rivotril), clorazepate (Gen-Xene, Tranxene), diazepam (Valium), estazolam (ProSom), flurazepam (Dalmane), lorazepam (Ativan), medazepam (Nobrium), midazolam (Hypnovel, Versed), oxazepam (Serax), prazepam (Centrax), quazepam (Doral), temazepam (Restoril).

Interaction Type and Significance

✗✗   **Minimal to Mild Adverse Interaction—Vigilance Necessary**
◇◇   **Drug-Induced Effect on Nutrient Function, Supplementation Contraindicated, Professional Management Appropriate**

Probability: Evidence Base:
4. Plausible   ☐ **Inadequate**, possibly
                                 ○ **Preliminary**

Effect and Mechanism of Action

Alprazolam is a gamma-aminobutyric acid (GABA) agonist known to decrease ACTH and cortisol concentrations. DHEA is secreted synchronously with cortisol by the adrenal glands and demonstrates diurnal variation. Meanwhile, concentrated in limbic regions, in levels much higher than other steroids, DHEA has been postulated to function as an excitatory neuroregulator, antagonizing GABA transmission, based largely on in vitro research. Further, in animal studies, DHEA has been reported to inhibit CYP4A and CYP3A23, which might reduce capacity for metabolism of alprazolam, triazolam, and related medications. Conversely, alprazolam appears to increase circulating DHEA concentrations. The effects of elevated DHEA levels on liver microsomal drug metabolism could lead to unintentionally elevated circulating levels of these benzodiazepine medications and thereby increase risks associated with adverse effects.

Research

In a study involving 28 healthy men, Kroboth et al.[4] observed that a single intravenous (IV) dose of alprazolam produced (1) significant increases in DHEA concentrations at 7 hours in both young and elderly men; (2) significant decreases in cortisol concentrations; and (3) no change in DHEA-S concentrations. In the authors' interpretation, such findings suggest that alprazolam modulates peripheral concentrations of DHEA and that DHEA and DHEA-S may have an in vivo role in modulating GABA receptor–mediated responses.

Preliminary studies on human liver microsomes in vitro and after administration of 200 mg DHEA daily for 2 weeks to 13 elderly men and women (>65 years old) suggest that DHEA can inhibit CYP3A-mediated metabolism of triazolam. In particular, the findings of Frye et al.[5] suggest that use of exogenous DHEA may thereby increase the risk for adverse effects of triazolam.

Clinical Implications and Adaptations

The interaction between elevated DHEA levels, endogenous or from oral administration, and benzodiazepines such as alprazolam or triazolam appears to be multifaceted and potentially of clinical significance, but currently available research findings are fragmentary and inconclusive. The alprazolam research indicates the value of further investigation into the relationships among DHEA, GABA, ACTH, and cortisol, especially in relation to pharmaceutical agents, but remains inadequate to provide a basis for clinically reliable and therapeutically applicable conclusions. Similar limitations in the research on triazolam call for further investigation into the character and significance of the plausible interaction with DHEA. Given the limited character of the various subject populations, their small number, and the preliminary nature of the experiments, it would be premature to declare the available studies as offering any conclusive evidence regarding potential interaction patterns. The evolution of research in this area points to the need for further investigation into the character of the plausible interactions and their significance.

Pending further research, it would be prudent to avoid concomitant DHEA in individuals on benzodiazepine therapy, particularly with alprazolam or triazolam, because of the theoretical risks of adverse effects from potentially inhibited drug metabolism, heightened DHEA levels, and further derangement of regulatory mechanisms. However, any potential interaction is likely to be slow in onset and manageable with appropriate supervision.

Amlodipine

Amlodipine (Norvasc); combination drug: amlodipine and benazepril (Lotrel).

Interaction Type and Significance

⊕   **Potential or Theoretical Beneficial or Supportive Interaction, with Professional Management**

Probability: Evidence Base:
3. Possible   **O Preliminary**

Effect and Mechanism of Action

This interaction has two elements: (1) the effect of androgenic hormones on cardiovascular risk factors in general, and the atherogenic process in particular, and (2) the relationship between amlodipine and these hormones.

Research

Beer et al.[6] found that amlodipine increases serum DHEA-S and androstenedione levels and decreases circulating cortisol in insulin-resistant, obese men with hypertension.

A literature review by Porsova-Dutoit et al.[7] concluded that men with low plasma DHEA and DHEA-S levels were susceptible to increased risk of developing a fatal cardiovascular event; in contrast, evidence was lacking for a protective role of DHEA and DHEA-S in women. The androgenic hormones, especially DHEA-S, can modify the lipid spectrum through their influence on enzymes such as glucose-6-phosphate dehydrogenase (G6PD). These hormones can inhibit human platelet aggregation, enhance fibrinolysis, slow down cell proliferation, improve endothelial function and insulin sensitivity, and reduce plasma levels of plasminogen activator inhibitor type 1 and tissue plasminogen activator antigen.[8,9]

Nutritional Therapeutics, Clinical Concerns, and Adaptations

The action by which amlodipine increases serum DHEA-S and androstenedione levels and decreases circulating cortisol may represent significant components of the mechanism by which the medication improves glucose tolerance and reduces serum insulin levels.

The effect of amlodipine on DHEA levels could potentially be beneficial in reducing cardiovascular risk factors, particularly insulin resistance and hypertension. However, no specific substantive evidence indicates that the potential enhancement of DHEA specifically provides benefit to patients prescribed amlodipine, or that further augmentation would be appropriate unless indicated by other clinical factors for given individuals.

Anticoagulant Medications

Oral Vitamin K Antagonist Anticoagulants: Anisindione (Miradon), dicumarol, ethyl biscoumacetate (Tromexan), nicoumalone (acenocoumarol; Acitrom, Sintrom), phenindione (Dindevan), phenprocoumon (Jarsin, Marcumar), warfarin (Coumadin, Marevan, Warfilone).
Direct Thrombin Inhibitors: Argatroban, bivalirudin (Angiomax), dabigatran etexilate (Rendix; investigational), desirudin (Iprivask, Revasc), hirudin, lepirudin (Refludan).
Heparin, Unfractionated (UFH): Heparin (Calciparine, Hepalean, Heparin Leo, Minihep Calcium, Minihep, Monoparin Calcium, Monoparin, Multiparin, Pump-Hep, Unihep, Uniparin Calcium, Uniparin Forte).
Heparinoids: Danaparoid (Orgaran), fondaparinux (Arixtra).
Low-Molecular-Weight (LMW) Heparin: Ardeparin (Normiflo), certoparin (Mono-Embolex), dalteparin (Fragmin), enoxaparin (Clexane, Lovenox), nadroparin (Fraxiparine), tinzaparin (Innohep).

Interaction Type and Significance

✗   **Potential or Theoretical Adverse Interaction of Uncertain Severity**
⊕✗   **Bimodal or Variable Interaction, with Professional Management**

Probability: Evidence Base:
4. Plausible   **∇ Mixed**

Effect and Mechanism of Action

The research literature investigating the relationship of endogenous DHEA-S levels, fibrinolysis, and coagulation offers mixed conclusions and provides inadequate evidence for determining a consistent mechanism of any potential interaction between supplemental DHEA and anticoagulant medications.

Research

This frequently mentioned adverse interaction is based on DHEA's supposed action as a blood thinner and as a potential cause of increased clotting. However, searches for primary research yield little direct substantive evidence of a consistent and clinically relevant pattern of interaction.

A study by Nilsson et al.[10] (1985) of 33 men undergoing major abdominal surgery investigated the role of steroid hormones in regulation of extrinsic fibrinolysis and found that DHEA-S levels were the single correlation that distinguished patients with postoperative deep vein thrombosis from those without this complication. However, they could offer no explanation in terms of hemostatic mechanisms for this finding.

Clinical Implications and Adaptations

This potential interaction is derived from studies that have reported DHEA affecting clotting. Such action raises concern that exogenous DHEA intake might alter the effects of anticoagulant medications and possibly the therapeutic dose.

If a strong relationship exists between increased cardiovascular risk and decreased DHEA/DHEA-S levels, particularly in men, it does not necessarily follow that administration will reduce such risk. However, if as proposed, DHEA provides a significant antiatherogenic effect and fibrinolytic action, the same mechanism might also confuse the predicted outcomes of anticoagulant dosing. Nevertheless, any such "excessive" DHEA intake would presumably be less likely in individuals with lower endogenous DHEA/DHEA-S levels and, as indicated by the research, could exert a differential effect in men versus women. Furthermore, regular INR testing and avoidance of any sudden or dramatic levels of DHEA intake would be critical elements of any therapeutic agenda incorporating DHEA concurrent with warfarin therapy, or a PTT/anti-Xa activity for any of the heparin-related compounds. Such gradual increase and decrease of DHEA dosing levels is typical of prescribing patterns when DHEA has been used clinically by health care professionals experienced in nutritional therapeutics; in cases involving anticoagulants, caution, close monitoring, and gradual prescription alterations would be even more necessary.

Anticonvulsant Medications, Including Phenobarbital, Phenytoin, and Valproic Acid

Carbamazepine (Carbatrol, Tegretol), clonazepam (Klonopin), clorazepate (Tranxene), divalproex semisodium, divalproex sodium (Depakote), ethosuximide (Zarontin), ethotoin (Peganone), felbamate (Felbatol), fosphenytoin (Cerebyx, Mesantoin), levetiracetam (Keppra), mephenytoin, mephobarbital (Mebaral), methsuximide (Celontin), phenobarbital (phenobarbitone; Luminal, Solfoton), phenytoin (diphenylhydantoin; Dilantin, Phenytek), piracetam (Nootropyl), primidone (Mysoline), sodium valproate (Depacon), topiramate (Topamax), trimethadione (Tridione), valproate semisodium, valproic acid (Depakene, Depakene Syrup), vigabatrin (Sabril), zonisamide (Zonegran).
Similar properties but evidence indicating no or reduced interaction effects: Oxcarbazepine (GP 47680, oxycarbamazepine; Trileptal).
Similar properties but evidence lacking for extrapolation: Acetazolamide (Diamox, Diamox Sequels).

Interaction Type and Significance

✗✗✗   Potentially Harmful or Serious Adverse Interaction—Avoid

Probability:	Evidence Base:
4. Plausible	☐ Inadequate

Effect and Mechanism of Action

Carbamazepine, phenytoin, and other CNS agents induce the P450 enzymes, particularly CYP3A4, that metabolize DHEA and DHEA-S and therefore decrease circulating concentrations of these hormones.[11-14] Although related to carbamazepine, opinion is mixed as to whether oxycarbamazepine induces hepatic phase I microsomal enymes.[15] Further, concomitant DHEA has been reported to interfere with the action of anticonvulsant medications. Additionally, some have suggested that DHEA should be deemed as sharing the same risk profile as anabolic steroids in their ability to aggravate or induce significant psychiatric difficulties, including mania, impaired cognition, and overt psychosis; evidence for any specific mechanisms has usually been lacking.

Research and Reports

Some preliminary human studies and scattered case reports indicate a possible role of elevated DHEA levels in cases of mania and aggravation of bipolar disorder diathesis.[16] Although some of this research focuses on endogenous levels, at least one frequently cited case report of an "interaction" involved oral DHEA and an anticonvulsant medication, even though the valproic acid (VPA) was prescribed in relation to symptoms presumed to be caused by the DHEA and was initiated after the DHEA intake was discontinued. In that case, Markowitz et al.[17] reported mania in an older man acutely admitted to a psychiatric facility with no previous personal or family history of bipolar disorder, apparently related to 6 months' prior use of 200 to 300 mg DHEA daily. The patient responded favorably to 7-day inpatient hospitalization and 500 mg VPA twice daily.[17] In another case report, Dean[18] reported on a 31-year-old man with a history of alcohol abuse, violent anger, and an unsubstantiated diagnosis of bipolar disorder, who became threatening after taking an estimated 100 mg (unprescribed) sertraline and 300 to 500 mg DHEA daily for several weeks. This patient improved with valproate therapy.[18]

Although not necessarily demonstrating an authentic adverse interaction involving exogenous DHEA, these events suggest that one action by which some anticonvulsant medications may suppress an episode of mania could be by lowering circulating DHEA-S concentrations. Such events do reinforce continued cautions against the use of multiple potentially psychoactive substances by individuals with a history of violence or unstable emotional states without close monitoring by a qualified health care professional.

Clinical Implications and Adaptations

Dehydroepiandrosterone is deeply involved in the hypothalamic-pituitary axis, limbic function, and cortisol cycles, so it is reasonable to look for associations between DHEA-S levels and mental-emotional disturbances. Elevated DHEA levels may inhibit the therapeutic action of anticonvulsant medications; concomitant use of DHEA, particularly in doses greater than 100 mg/day and among men under 40 years of age, is generally contraindicated. Such medications may lower circulating DHEA concentrations, but use of exogenous DHEA could theoretically lead to adverse effects. However, if an individual has been stable while taking both agents simultaneously, it would be prudent to maintain current levels unless otherwise indicated, and if cessation of DHEA intake is deemed appropriate, such changes should be gradual and closely monitored.

Clonidine and Fluoxetine

Clonidine (Apo-Clonidine, Catapres Oral, Catapres-TTS Transdermal Dixarit, Duraclon, Novo-Clonidine, Nu-Clonidine); combination drug: clonidine and chlorthalidone (Combipres); fluoxetine (Prozac, Sarafem).

Interaction Type and Significance
⊕⊕ **Beneficial or Supportive Interaction, with Professional Management**

Probability:	Evidence Base:
2. Probable	○ Preliminary

Effect and Mechanism of Action
DHEA may restore the response of beta-endorphin, a key neuropeptide, to clonidine and fluoxetine.

Research
As part of their investigation of endocrine, neuroendocrine, and behavioral effects of oral DHEA-S administration in postmenopausal women, Stomati et al.[19] evaluated plasma beta-endorphin levels in response to neuroendocrine tests using clonidine, fluoxetine, and naloxone. After 3 months of 50 mg/day DHEA-S, the women in this small study demonstrated a restored response of the beta-endorphin to clonidine and fluoxetine. The authors concluded that their research "suggests that DHEAS and/or its active metabolites modulates the neuroendocrine control of pituitary beta-endorphin secretion."

Nutritional Therapeutics, Clinical Concerns, and Adaptations
The previous research indirectly suggests a potential therapeutic benefit from coordinated use of DHEA adjunctively with clonidine or fluoxetine. However, although based on solid evidence, the cited research did not specifically address the issue of interactions between DHEA and these pharmaceutical agents. the rationale for this potential supportive interaction is consistent with known data, but further research is required to determine whether such concomitant use provides therapeutic efficacy and how best to coordinate such integrative therapeutic strategies, if clinical evidence supporting implementation of such a strategy should emerge.

Corticosteroids, Oral

Betamethasone (Celestone), cortisone (Cortone), dexamethasone (Decadron), fludrocortisone (Florinef), hydrocortisone (Cortef), methylprednisolone (Medrol) prednisolone (Delta-Cortef, Orapred, Pediapred, Prelone), prednisone (Deltasone, Liquid Pred, Meticorten, Orasone), triamcinolone (Aristocort). Similar properties but evidence lacking for extrapolation: Inhalant and topical corticosteroids.

Interaction Type and Significance
≈≈ **Drug-Induced Nutrient Depletion, Supplementation Therapeutic, with Professional Management**
⊕⊕ **Beneficial or Supportive Interaction, with Professional Management**

Probability:	Evidence Base:
1. Certain	◉ Emerging

Effect and Mechanism of Action
Oral corticosteroid therapy has been demonstrated to lower serum levels of DHEA and DHEA-S significantly.

Some corticosteroid agents, such as dexamethasone, affect the hypothalamic-pituitary-adrenal (HPA) axis by inhibiting ACTH and therefore decrease DHEA and DHEA-S concentrations. Beclomethasone and budesonide may also induce such an effect.

The presence of exogenous corticosteroids from use of prednisone or related drugs can confuse the internal hormonal regulatory processes. If the pituitary senses that corticosteroid levels are higher than normal, the regulatory feedback loops send a signal to decrease the production of ACTH and thus reduce the levels of several key hormones. As a consequence of these changes in hormonal balance, the internal stimulation to produce DHEA can often fall, androgen levels can rise, and the cascade of adverse effects, such as muscle wasting, ensue.

Several researchers have suggested that DHEA depletion might constitute an aspect of corticosteroid-induced osteoporosis. DHEA may also increase the effects of prednisolone.

Research
Relatively early research by Judd et al.[20] (1977) correlated dexamethasone administration with severely lowered serum concentrations of DHEA and DHEA-S. A later study by Smith et al.[21] (1994) found that beclomethasone administration for asthma suppressed DHEA-S in postmenopausal women. This particular pattern raises the concern as to the respective roles of corticosteroids and DHEA on bone density and iatrogenic osteoporosis, especially among postmenopausal women, and suggests the value of continued research to clarify this clinically important drug-induced adverse effect and potential adjunctive therapeutics using concomitant DHEA. Studies led by Riedel et al.[22] and Rosen et al.[23] found impaired well-being in patients with adrenal insufficiency despite adequate replacement of glucocorticoids and mineralocorticoids. Further, a landmark study of middle-aged subjects by Morales et al.[24] suggested that DHEA administration might positively influence well-being. Thus, effects of DHEA on well-being and mood became a plausible target for studies in adrenal insufficiency. A literature review conducted by Robinzon and Cutolo[25] focused on the issue of the clinical efficacy of DHEA replacement therapy adjunctively with glucocorticoid therapy and concluded that the evidence suggests that DHEA concomitant may counteract adverse effects caused by long-term administration of steroidal agents. As with much of the evolving research on therapeutic corticosteroids, the risk of interaction and nutrient depletion is significantly greater with oral medications than with inhalant and topical steroids. Nevertheless, studies by Nadeau et al.[26] and Toogood et al.[27] observed adverse effects on several key metabolic factors, including DHEA levels, subsequent to treatment with high-dose inhaled corticosteroids, particularly budenoside.

DHEA and DHEA-S levels tend to be low in individuals prescribed corticosteroids, before therapy,[25,28,29] and administration of DHEA adjunctively during (and possibly after) corticosteroid therapy does not appear to interfere with therapeutic action of the drug, and may enable reduction of medication levels, and thus adverse drug effects, without compromising therapeutic efficacy. Straub et al.[30] investigated and confirmed that individuals with chronic inflammatory diseases, for which corticosteroids are typically prescribed, demonstrated significantly lower serum concentrations of the sulfated form of DHEA (DHEA-S). Meno-Tetang et al.[30a] found that multiple dosing of 200 mg oral DHEA produced serum concentrations of DHEA and DHEA-S significantly greater than endogenous levels, while also increasing serum androstenedione and testosterone levels. Such effect did not alter either single-dose oral prednisolone pharmacokinetics or inhibition of cortisol secretion by prednisolone. In a more recent study (2002) involving 191 women undergoing corticosteroid therapy for systemic lupus erythematosus (SLE), Petri et al.[31] reported that concomitant administration of 200 mg DHEA daily allowed for reduced dosage of prednisone "for a sustained period of time while maintaining stabilization or a reduction of disease activity was possible in a significantly greater proportion of patients ..., compared with patients treated with placebo." Nordmark[32] and colleagues conducted a double-blind, randomized, placebo-controlled study involving 41 women with SLE who were taking at least 5 mg prednisolone daily. The investigators followed the women for 6 months, during which they took placebo, 30 mg of DHEA daily if age 45 or younger, or 20 mg of DHEA daily if age 46 or older. After the double-blind period, the investigators followed the women for an additional 6-month open phase and offered the treatment to all the patients. In findings presented at the European Congress of Rheumatology (EULAR) in June 2004, the researchers reported that serum levels of sulfated DHEA increased in women treated with DHEA; the mean level at baseline was subnormal, but levels were in the normal range after treatment. Both subjects and their partners reported improvement in several quality-of-life parameters in association with DHEA coadministration. No adverse effects were associated with DHEA use; however, high-density lipoprotein (HDL) cholesterol decreased and insulin-like growth factor (IGF-I) and hematocrit increased. Nordmark et al.[33] later published their final findings and concluded that "low dose DHEA treatment improves HRQOL [health-related quality of life] with regard to mental well-being and sexuality and can be offered to women with SLE where mental distress and/or impaired sexuality constitutes a problem."

The evidence for this pattern of drug-induced depletion appears consistent, but research has focused on only a few medications within this drug class. Therefore, caution must be exercised in extrapolating these research findings to all corticosteroid agents generally, particularly in light of the wide range of individual variability and key factors, such as gender, life stage, medical condition, and polypharmaceutical prescribing.

Nutritional Therapeutics, Clinical Concerns, and Adaptations

Although the evidence of corticosteroid therapy's adverse effect on DHEA/DHEA-S generally approaches consensus, there is only an emerging sense of therapeutic appropriateness concerning the efficacy and clinical protocols for compensatory DHEA administration.[34] As mentioned, the review by Robinzon and Cutolo[25] suggested the clinical benefit of concomitant DHEA, but such therapeutic approaches, particularly as part of a conscious and coherent integrative strategy, have not even broached consideration in standard clinical practice guidelines.

Individuals using corticosteroids for extended periods should consult with their prescribing physician and/or a nutritionally trained health care professional about the potential benefits of concomitant DHEA to prevent muscle wasting without losing the anti-inflammatory effect of prednisone. Laboratory tests can determine the degree to which endogenous DHEA has been adversely affected and suggest an appropriate dosage level, if needed.

Continued investigation is warranted to determine if and when concomitant DHEA may be beneficial to individuals using corticosteroids, both oral and inhaled, and at what levels, when deemed therapeutically appropriate.

ESTROGENS, PROGESTINS, AND ESTROGEN-PROGESTIN COMBINATIONS

Oral Contraceptives: Monophasic, Biphasic, and Triphasic Estrogen Preparations (Synthetic Estrogen and Progesterone Analogs)

Ethinyl estradiol and desogestrel (Desogen, Ortho-TriCyclen). Ethinyl estradiol and ethynodiol (Demulen 1/35, Demulen 1/50, Nelulen 1/25, Nelulen 1/50, Zovia). Ethinyl estradiol and levonorgestrel (Alesse, Levlen, Levlite, Levora 0.15/30, Nordette, Tri-Levlen, Triphasil, Trivora). Ethinyl estradiol and norethindrone/norethisterone (Brevicon, Estrostep, Genora 1/35, GenCep. 1/35, Jenest-28, Loestrin 1.5/30, Loestrin1/20, Modicon, Necon 1/25, Necon 10/11, Necon 0.5/30, Necon 1/50, Nelova 1/35, Nelova 10/11, Norinyl 1/35, Norlestin 1/50, Ortho Novum 1/35, Ortho Novum 10/11, Ortho Novum 7/7/7, Ovcon-35, Ovcon-50, Tri-Norinyl, Trinovum). Ethinyl estradiol and norgestrel (Lo/Ovral, Ovral). Mestranol and norethindrone (Genora 1/50, Nelova 1/50, Norethin 1/50, Ortho-Novum 1/50). Related, Internal Application: Etonogestrel/ethinyl estradiol vaginal ring (Nuvaring).

Hormone Replacement Therapy (HRT): Estrogen-Containing and Synthetic Estrogen and Progesterone Analog Medications

HRT, estrogens: Chlorotrianisene (Tace); conjugated equine estrogens (Premarin); conjugated synthetic estrogens (Cenestin); dienestrol (Ortho Dienestrol); esterified estrogens (Estratab, Menest, Neo-Estrone); estradiol, topical/transdermal/ring (Alora Transdermal, Climara Transdermal, Estrace, Estradot, Estring FemPatch, Vivelle-Dot, Vivelle Transdermal); estradiol cypionate (Dep-Gynogen, Depo-Estradiol, Depogen, Dura-Estrin, Estra-D, Estro-Cyp, Estroject-LA, Estronol-LA); estradiol hemihydrate (Estreva, Vagifem); estradiol valerate (Delestrogen, Estra-L 40, Gynogen L.A. 20, Progynova, Valergen 20); estrone (Aquest, Estragyn 5, Estro-A, Estrone '5', Kestrone-5); estropipate (Ogen, Ortho-Est); ethinyl estradiol (Estinyl, Gynodiol, Lynoral).

HRT, estrogen/progestin combinations: Conjugated equine estrogens and medroxyprogesterone (Premelle cycle 5, Prempro); conjugated equine estrogens and norgestrel (Prempak-C); estradiol and dydrogesterone (Femoston); estradiol and norethindrone, patch (CombiPatch); estradiol and norethindrone/norethisterone, oral (Activella, Climagest, Climesse, FemHRT, Trisequens); estradiol valerate and cyproterone acetate (Climens); estradiol valerate and norgestrel (Progyluton); estradiol and norgestimate (Ortho-Prefest).

HRT, estrogen/testosterone combinations: Esterified estrogens and methyltestosterone (Estratest, Estratest HS).

Interaction Type and Significance

✗✗   **Minimal to Mild Adverse Interaction—Vigilance Necessary**

⊕✗   **Bimodal or Variable Interaction, with Professional Management**

⊕   **Potential or Theoretical Beneficial or Supportive Interaction, with Professional Management**

Probability:	Evidence Base:
3. Possible	☐ Inadequate

Effect and Mechanism of Action

As a precursor steroid, DHEA can be converted into estrogen (or progesterone), and exogenous DHEA intake has been shown to increase levels of female reproductive hormones. Serum DHEA/DHEA-S concentrations are likely to be lower among women in the life stages during which HRT is typically prescribed. Exogenous estrogen compounds might also induce lowered levels of endogenous DHEA through their impact on endocrine regulatory mechanisms. Either pattern of disruption in normal homeostatic processes could cause symptoms of hormonal dysfunction and imbalance.

Research

Mortola and Yen[35] investigated the effect of 12-month DHEA replacement therapy in 14 women age 60 to 70 who received daily applications of a 10% DHEA cream. They observed a beneficial effect on vaginal epithelium maturation in most of the women attributable to the estrogenic effect of DHEA and significantly increased hip bone mineral density (BMD), accompanied by an increase in serum osteocalcin. In contrast, they noted a lack of estrogenic effect from the DHEA on the endometrial tissue, which remained atrophic in all women.[35] Nevertheless, no substantive evidence is available concerning the likelihood, significance, and outcome(s) of this plausible interaction for a range of medications and involving populations with varied characteristics.

Clinical Implications and Adaptations

Given the inherent nature of estrogen and DHEA, their combined use within a coordinated integrative strategy suggests a reasonable likelihood of value in enhancing therapeutic efficacy and possibly reducing potential adverse effects associated with HRT. However, by the same additive effect, concomitant administration of estrogen hormone therapies and DHEA, in theory, may induce increased adverse effects resulting from excessively elevated levels of either hormone. The combination of DHEA with compounded "tri-est" formulations (mixtures of estrone, estradiol, and estriol, often in a 1:1:8 ratio) has been used in clinical practice for many years by physicians implementing integrative therapeutics strategies. Even though preliminary clinical research suggests potential for emergent integrative therapeutics, particularly in the treatment of menopausal women, the direct effects of the potential interaction between exogenous estrogen medications and DHEA has not yet been studied in a thorough and systematic manner translatable into clear and consistent clinical practice guidelines. The concomitant use of these two therapeutic approaches could be either beneficial or adverse, depending on the individual, health status, relative dosage levels, and resultant blood and tissue levels. Close clinical management and regular monitoring by a health care professionals experienced in both conventional pharmacology and nutritional therapeutics are warranted during concomitant use of these substances.

Methyltestosterone and Related Androgens

Methyltestosterone (Android, Methitest, Testred, Virilon). Extrapolated, based on similar properties: Methyltestosterone combination drug: methyltestosterone and esterified estrogens (Estratest, Estratest HS).

Androgens: Fluoxymesterone (Halotestin), testolactone (Testolacton; HSDB 3255, SQ 9538; Fludestrin, Teolit, Teslac, Teslak), testosterone cypionate.

Interaction Type and Significance

⊕⊕　**Beneficial or Supportive Interaction, with Professional Management**
⊕✗　**Bimodal or Variable Interaction, with Professional Management**
✗✗　**Minimal to Mild Adverse Interaction—Vigilance Necessary**

Probability:　　　　Evidence Base:
2. Probable　　　◉ **Emerging**

Effect and Mechanism of Action

As a precursor steroid, DHEA can be converted into testosterone, and exogenous DHEA intake has been shown to increase levels of circulating androgens. Thus, administration of both methyltestosterone (or testosterone) and exogenous DHEA could each independently increase testosterone levels. Intentional additive interaction could be therapeutically efficacious, whereas uncoordinated concurrent use could theoretically induce excessive testosterone levels and attendant adverse effects and elevated risk factors.

Research

Many studies have demonstrated the effects of DHEA administration on androgen levels and noted differentials effects based on gender and age, preintervention deficiency states, health status, and other factors.[36-38] For example, in a randomized, placebo-controlled crossover trial, Morales et al.[39] administered a 50-mg nightly oral dose of DHEA to 13 men and 17 women, age 40 to 70, over 6 months. They reported a restoration of DHEA and DHEA-S serum levels to those found in young adults within 2 weeks of DHEA replacement, and a twofold increase in serum levels of androgens (androstenedione, testosterone, and dihydrotestosterone) in women, with only a small rise in androstenedione in men. Later, Wolfe et al.[40] administered 50 mg daily DHEA to 40 healthy elderly men and women, all of whom had low DHEA-S baseline levels. DHEA augmentation leads to a fivefold increase in DHEA-S levels in women and men. DHEA, androstenedione, and testosterone levels also increased significantly in both genders.

Despite the plethora of research relating to interrelationships between endogenous DHEA and steroid hormones, including testosterone, no substantive human clinical research has yet directly investigated the effects, methods, and implications of concomitant use of DHEA and testosterone (or methyltestosterone), either deliberately or unintentionally. The need for and potential value of such research are clearly indicated by patient needs, the extant literature, and emerging clinical practice, particularly in the turbulent and reconfiguring realm of hormone therapy related to menopause and other aspects of aging.

Nutritional Therapeutics, Clinical Concerns, and Adaptations

Simultaneous use of DHEA and testosterone presents a clinically significant, though as-yet inadequately investigated, example of the potential for a drug-nutraceutical interaction to induce beneficial or adverse effects and thereby require qualified clinical management. DHEA and testosterone are often prescribed together for menopausal women with diminished libido in conjunction with tri-est formulations within individualized compounded pharmaceutical preparations.[41] A similar but simpler approach is embodied in the combination drug Estratest/Estratest HS. Such formulations are typically individually formulated and prepared in conjunction with a compounding pharmacist, and the doses and constituent proportions evolve over time in response to therapeutic effect and clinical strategy. Recent research indicates that the apolipoprotein E (ApoE) gene determines serum testosterone and DHEA levels in postmenopausal women.[42] Thus, pharmacogenomic factors need to be considered in determining hormonal deficiency patterns, response to medications, and risk of adverse effects, including genetic susceptibility to and family history of breast cancer. In cases where methyltestosterone has been prescribed for men diagnosed with testosterone deficiency, DHEA therapy could also be considered as indicated. Endogenous levels, relative doses, mode of administration, health status, gender and life stage, concomitant polypharmacy, and other factors, as well as the as-yet inadequately predictable response of the individual's endocrine regulatory processes, will all influence the probability, clinical significance, and character of any resultant interaction.

While offering an opportunity for synergistic prescribing and innovative therapeutic strategies to individualized and evolving integrative care, concomitant use of testosterone (or methyltestosterone) and DHEA demands close supervision and regular monitoring. Even though methyltestosterone can be used in the treatment of breast cancer, such combined use would be therapeutically inappropriate and contraindicated for women (or men) with a personal or family history of or genetic susceptibility to breast cancer, because DHEA may also be converted to either estrogen or progesterone. Likewise, administration of either or both substances is contraindicated for men with a personal or family history of or genetic susceptibility to prostate cancer. DHEA is currently being studied as a potential primary and secondary chemopreventive agent in women at high risk for breast cancer, but results of these studies are not yet available.

Zidovudine (AZT) and Related Reverse-Transcriptase Inhibitor (Nucleoside) Antiretroviral Agents

Evidence: Zidovudine (azidothymidine, AZT, ZDV, zidothymidine; Retrovir); combination drugs: zidovudine and lamivudine (Combivir); abacavir, lamivudine, and zidovudine (Trizivir).
Extrapolated, based on similar properties: Abacavir (Ziagen), didanosine (ddI, dideoxyinosine; Videx); dideoxycytidine (ddC, zalcitabine; Hivid), lamivudine (3TC, Epivir), stavudine (D4T, Zerit), tenofovir (Viread).

Interaction Type and Significance

⊕⊕   **Beneficial or Supportive Interaction, with Professional Management**

Probability: Evidence Base:
2. Probable   ○ Preliminary

Effect and Mechanism of Action

Deficiencies in testosterone, estradiol, and growth hormone (GH) can be associated with depression or dysthymia. DHEA acts as a precursor to testosterone and estradiol, both of which are known to exert a beneficial effect on mood when administered exogenously. DHEA also increases available levels of insulin-like growth factor, which in turn can elevate GH levels. Furthermore, DHEA may modulate tumor necrosis factor and other inflammatory cytokines, an excess of which are associated with cachexia in HIV disease and cancer. These factors can be especially significant in individuals with HIV infection, in whom declines in DHEA levels can be associated with the progression to AIDS. Potential supportive effects of coadministration on therapeutic response to antiretroviral agents have been proposed, but mechanisms of action have not been elucidated or confirmed.

Research

Preliminary research in vitro and with mice has indicated a potential synergistic interaction from coordinated, concomitant use of AZT and DHEA, as indicated by enhanced effectiveness of AZT against HIV-infected cells and as part of cisplatin-based chemotherapy against colorectal adenocarcinoma.[43,44] Although encouraging, such laboratory studies suggest the value of further research, particularly randomized clinical trials, more than they offer a solid basis for clinical experimentation or evidence-based practice.

Subsyndromal major depressive disorder is common among HIV-positive adults, particularly physically ill patients undergoing current multidrug antiretroviral regimens (HAART). In a randomized, placebo-controlled trial, Rabkin et al.[45] administered either DHEA, using flexible dosing of 100 to 400 mg daily, or placebo to 145 patients with subsyndromal depression or dysthymia, 80% of whom were receiving concurrent antiretroviral treatment. Using both a Clinical Global Impression improvement rating and a final Hamilton Depression Rating Scale score, the response rate was 62% (43 of 64) for the DHEA group, compared to 33% (21 of 64) for the placebo patients. Few adverse events and no significant changes in CD4 cell count or HIV RNA viral load were reported in either treatment group. DHEA may be particularly important for HIV-positive pre-AIDS patients, because declining levels of DHEA have been associated with progression to AIDS in both cross-sectional comparisons of HIV-positive men and women at different stages of HIV illness and in longitudinal studies. Further, the authors noted: "The low attrition rate in this group of physically ill patients, together with requests for extended open-label treatment, reflect high acceptance of this readily available intervention."[45]

Nutritional Therapeutics, Clinical Concerns, and Adaptations

Physicians providing treatment to HIV-positive individuals exhibiting nonmajor depression are advised to consider coadministration of DHEA (100-200 mg twice daily), particularly in patients who are unwilling to use conventional antidepressants. The available research findings are limited but significant, and the probability of adverse effects is minimal. Further research through well-designed, adequately powered clinical trials, with more diverse subject population and long-term follow-up on maintenance of response or possible long-term endocrine or other effects of DHEA, appears warranted.

THEORETICAL, SPECULATIVE, AND PRELIMINARY INTERACTIONS RESEARCH, INCLUDING OVERSTATED INTERACTIONS CLAIMS

In their valuable review of the influence of hormones and pharmaceutical agents on DHEA-S concentrations, Salek et al.[46] noted that although exogenous DHEA intake increases circulating DHEA and DHEA-S concentrations, "the kinetics does not appear to be the same as with endogenous secretion."

Evidence indicates that a wide range of medications may lower DHEA and DHEA-S levels, but no adequate investigation has yet determined whether clinically significant depletion patterns result. Further, given the complex interdependencies among hormones and their multiple feedback systems, it is premature to speculate, in most circumstances, whether administration of DHEA might be therapeutically appropriate, even in instances of probable drug-induced depletion. Likewise, the adverse consequences of excess androgen concentrations and the likely attendant disruptions in related hormone levels and interrelationships emphasize the need for caution in considering dosage levels that might result in excessive concentrations of DHEA and DHEA-S. Such considerations are further complicated by the variable nature of DHEA concentration and functions in diverse human populations, especially based on gender and life stage, and by individual biochemical and pharmacogenomic variability, particularly in the context of disease, aging, and physiological dysfunction.

The action of endogenous DHEA and DHEA-S and exogenous oral DHEA on blood glucose and insulin levels, hepatic enzyme systems, atherogenesis, endothelial function, coagulation and fibrinolytic processes, sex steroid and other hormone levels, as well as myriad other metabolic functions creates many potential interactions with several classes of pharmaceutical agents. The scientific discourse and clinical research cannot yet substantively answer most of the potential questions as to whether these interactions are frequent or rare, significant or negligible, and adverse, neutral, or beneficial. Within this context of complexity and variability where animal and in vitro research are fundamentally inadequate to understand conclusively the therapeutics of DHEA, any discussion of interactions is inherently even more theoretical, extrapolated, and speculative.

Antidepressant and Stimulant Medications

Antidepressant and Stimulant Medications

Some broad concerns have been expressed declaring risks of adverse interactions from concomitant use of DHEA with antidepressants and CNS stimulants. Although such theoretical interactions are plausible, especially with extremely high doses of DHEA in unstable individuals outside the context of close clinical management, they are as yet not supported by a significant or substantial body of scientific evidence, especially drawn from clinical human studies. Some secondary sources have cited papers on "mania" supposedly associated with DHEA supplementation by Dean, Markowitz, and others, with unclear case reports and presumptions of linkage to intake of steroidal hormones other than DHEA. In their discussion of one case, Markowitz et al.[17] note that the association of mania with both tricyclic antidepressants and selective serotonin reuptake inhibitors was "well-known" but then explicitly declared as "speculative" the hypothesis that DHEA might induce mania based on such a possible mechanism and that of elevated androgenic steroid levels. Critical examination of the literature renders such concerns as potentially worthy of further investigation, but claims of definitive causation are premature and unsubstantiated. If, as suggested by some authors, DHEA exercises a serotonergic action on the CNS, such effect might function therapeutically but would form the basis of a potentially adverse additive interaction, in the absence of proper clinical management. Other writers have cited the numerous studies examining DHEA as potentially elevating mood and enhancing feelings of well-being in research on depression, Addison's disease, aging, menopause, and other conditions, as grounds for supposed risk of adverse interactions from a presumed additive effect. Any such assertions appear to be premature, speculative, and potentially misleading. Although the unsupervised use of DHEA in supraphysiologic doses by individuals under pharmacological therapy, especially those with a psychiatric diagnosis, is imprudent and deserving caution, substantial evidence of significant clinical risk is lacking.

Oral Hypoglycemic Agents and Insulin

Buformin (Andromaco Gliporal, Buformina), chlorpropamide (Diabinese), glimepiride (Amaryl), glipizide (Glucotrol; Glucotrol XL), glyburide (glibenclamide; Diabeta, Glynase, Glynase Prestab, Micronase, Pres Tab), insulin (animal-source insulin: Iletin, human analog insulin: Humanlog; human insulin: Humulin, Novolin, NovoRapid, Oralin), metformin (Dianben, Glucophage, Glucophage XR); combination drugs: glipizide and metformin (Metaglip); gyburide and

metformin (Glucovance); tolazamide (Tolinase), phenformin (Debeone, Fenformin), tolbutamide (Orinase, Tol-Tab).

Insulin acts as a physiological regulator of DHEA sulfate metabolism and lowers circulating DHEA-S concentrations, especially in men. Insulin administration has been found to decrease the concentration of circulating DHEA and DHEA-S. Meanwhile, DHEA can stimulate the production of insulin-like growth factor-1 (IGF-1), a hormone that stimulates anabolic metabolism, improves insulin sensitivity, and otherwise affects insulin- and glucose-related metabolic processes. Such relationships suggest that exogenous DHEA administration might alter blood glucose regulation and interact with several medications. Related research indicates that DHEA intake might reduce risk or enhance treatment of glucose dysregulation and could counter an insulin-induced DHEA depletion pattern. In the absence of informed supervision, such influences could disturb the intended effects of insulin, metformin, or oral hypoglycemics such as sulfonylureas and require modification in the therapeutic dose.

The findings of a small study by Lavallee et al.[47] involving infusion of DHEA and insulin suggest that insulin increases the metabolic clearance rate of DHEA by stimulating its conversion to DHEA fatty acid esters (DHEA-FA) and by enhancing uptake of DHEA-FA by peripheral tissues. Nestler et al.[48] investigated the effect of oral administration of metformin three times daily over 21 days on 28 nondiabetic men. Metformin administration resulted in significant reductions in serum insulin levels and concurrent increases in serum DHEA-S levels. Higher levels of DHEA-S may be part of the beneficial effects of metformin in relation to insulin and glucose regulation. DHEA use enhances endothelial function and insulin sensitivity in men. In a study of 24 older men with hypercholesterolemia, randomized to receive DHEA (25 mg/day) or placebo for 12 weeks, Kawano et al.[9] found that DHEA treatment, but not placebo, was associated with a significant improvement in endothelial function, an effect apparent within 4 weeks of beginning treatment. The DHEA augmentation also produced a significant drop in steady-state glucose levels, without altering insulin levels. The duration of DHEA use was inversely tied to levels of plasminogen activator inhibitor type 1, another protective effect within the cardiovascular system.

Even with this emerging insight into several mechanisms that may help explain DHEA's antiatherosclerotic effect, substantive evidence is still needed, based on human clinical studies using oral DHEA with insulin-dependent diabetic individuals, that directly confirms a consistent pattern of interaction, either adverse or beneficial. Pending further research, individuals undergoing insulin or metformin therapy are advised to avoid DHEA intake outside the context of integrative therapeutic care with close supervision and regular monitoring by health care professionals experienced in both conventional pharmacology and nutritional therapeutics.

Thyroid Hormones

L-Triiodothyronine (T$_3$): Cytomel, liothyronine sodium, liothyronine sodium (synthetic T$_3$), Triostat (injection).
Levothyroxine (T$_4$): Eltroxin, Levo-T, Levothroid, levothyroxine (synthetic), levoxin, Levoxyl, Synthroid, thyroxine, Unithroid.
L-Thyroxine and L-triiodothyronine (T$_4$ + T$_3$): animal levothyroxine/liothyronine, Armour Thyroid, desiccated thyroid, Westhroid.
L-Thyroxine and L-triiodothyronine (synthetic T$_4$ + T$_3$): Euthroid, Euthyral, liotrix, Thyar, Thyrolar.
Dextrothyroxine (Choloxin).

DHEA may potentiate thyroid medications. Animal studies, clinical reports, and reasonable interpretations of known endocrine interrelationships indicate a plausible interaction between thyroid medications (e.g., Synthroid) and orally administered DHEA. Such effect, whether additive or synergistic, might introduce an increased risk of iatrogenic thyrotoxicosis if unintentionally induced, or it might be used to reduce the dose of thyroid medication through concomitant, coordinated administration of DHEA. Because this interaction is plausible given present data and clinical experience, further research is recommended, and concomitant use should be only be undertaken within the context of a coordinated strategy of integrative therapeutics providing for close supervision and regular monitoring by health care professionals trained and experienced in both conventional pharmacology and nutritional therapy.

The 49 citations for this monograph, as well as additional reference literature, are located under DHEA on the CD at the back of the book.

Glucosamine Sulfate

Nutrient Name: Glucosamine sulfate.
Synonyms: Glucosamine sulphate; D-glucosamine sulfate potassium salt; GS.
Related Substances: Glucosamine hydrochloride, N-acetyl-D-glucosamine (NAG, N-A-G).

Summary

Drug/Class Interaction Type	Mechanism and Significance	Management
Acetaminophen Ibuprofen Nonsteroidal anti-inflammatory drugs (NSAIDs) ◇≈≈/◇/⊕✗/⊕⊕	Coadministration of glucosamine and NSAIDs may enable anti-inflammatory effect at lower drug doses. Concurrent use of glucosamine sulfate (GS) with ibuprofen or ketoprofen appears to result in synergistic effect; other NSAIDs may provide additive effect. Acetaminophen metabolism involves sulfation and thus consumes sulfate provided by GS for glycosaminoglycan synthesis; aspirin may similarly interact to induce subadditive effect. More strategically, NSAIDs may promote cartilage destruction and impair cartilage repair.	Consider ibuprofen rather than acetaminophen when using GS. Coadministration may enable decreased dose and shortened period of NSAID use.
Insulin Oral hypoglycemic agents ✗	Glucosamine might theoretically accelerate hexosamine pathway and inhibit liver glucokinase because of similarity between glucosamine-6-phosphate and glucose-6-phosphate glucosamine. Such effect might induce changes in glucose metabolism and contribute to insulin resistance. Glucosamine (sulfate or hydrochloride) administration may slightly elevate glucose levels in some individuals, but evidence indicates that it does not alter glucose metabolism, including that of diabetics, to a clinically significant degree, and that clinically significant interactions with insulin or oral hypoglycemic agents are improbable.	Administer glucosamine (sulfate) as indicated. Monitor glucose levels in diabetic individuals as customary.

NUTRIENT DESCRIPTION

Chemistry

D-Glucosamine (2-amino-2-deoxy-D-glucose) is a chemically defined, small molecule (molecular weight, 179.17 daltons) with a pK_a of 6.91. It is an amino-monosaccharide molecule, formed of glucose and an amine moiety, and one of the basic constituents of the disaccharidic units of articular cartilage glycosaminoglycans (GAGs). The amine is positively charged at physiologic pH and will hold a counter anion, either two chlorides or one sulfate.

See also Nutrient Preparations section.

Physiology and Function

Glucosamine plays a central role in determining the strength and resiliency of connective tissue. An amino sugar biosynthesized from glucose, glucosamine is one of the principal substrates used in the biosynthesis of macromolecules that comprise articular cartilage and thus a key compound within the ground substance that makes up connective tissue. Glucosamine is the preferred substrate for biosynthesis of mucopolysaccharides and bipolymers of the articulations and bones and has been reported to facilitate the hexosamine pathway of proteoglycan synthesis by the chondrocytes. It modulates interleukin-1 (IL-1)–induced activation of chondrocytes for cartilage rebuilding and stimulates production of proteoglycans (including therefore the proteic moiety) with a normal polymeric structure while simultaneously inhibiting proteoglycan degradation. Glucosamine also stimulates synthesis of GAGs and collagen, as well as synovial production of hyaluronic acid, which is critical to the lubricating and shock-absorbing properties of synovial fluid. Glucosamine sulfate (GS), in particular, can increase serum sulfate concentrations and thereby elevate synovial fluid sulfate concentrations and enable proteoglycan sulfation.[1] In addition to these nutritive and stimulating functions, GS also inhibits some cartilage-destroying enzymes, such as serine proteases collagenase and phospholipase A_2 (PLA_2), and the generation of cell-damaging superoxide radicals. Thus, GS exerts a mild anti-inflammatory effect by a mechanism of action other than the inhibition of the biosynthesis of prostaglandins, most likely inhibition of proinflammatory effects of the nuclear factor kappa B (NF-κB) pathway.

NUTRIENT IN CLINICAL PRACTICE

Known or Potential Therapeutic Uses

Glucosamine (sulfate) is primarily used to relieve symptoms, stop disease progression, and stimulate joint cartilage growth in the treatment of osteoarthritis (OA). In this role, GS acts as chondroprotective agent by stopping the pathogenic mechanism of OA, relieving its symptoms, and reducing its progression. Surveys show that it is one of the most widely used nutraceuticals in self-medication practices, especially among the elderly population.[2] Most,[3-12] but not all,[13] published studies, have shown positive effects on both joint pain and joint structure (e.g., joint space narrowing) in patients with OA, particularly of the knee, compared with nonsteroidal anti-inflammatory drugs (NSAIDs) or placebo. In addition to its beneficial activities on cartilage and chondrocytes, glucosamine has generally demonstrated mild anti-inflammatory properties and a favorable pharmacokinetic profile. Until recently, long-term studies on the effectiveness of GS have been lacking.

Historical/Ethnomedicine Precedent

No historical precedents have been reported.

Possible Uses

Cartilage injuries, gonarthritis, kidney stones, low back pain, minor injuries, osteoarthritis (OA), sprains and strains, temporomandibular joint (TMJ) dysfunction pain and joint noises, wound healing.

Deficiency Symptoms

There are no reports of a glucosamine deficiency, per se, in humans. The issue of sulfate deficiencies may deserve further attention.

Dietary Sources

Tempeh, a fermented soy product, is a food source of glucosamine.[14] However, significant amounts of glucosamine are not a normal constituent of most diets.

Nutrient Preparations Available

Commercially available glucosamine products are available in three forms. Glucosamine sulfate (GS) is the primary form used in clinical settings. However, many products labeled as "glucosamine" contain glucosamine hydrochloride. N-acetyl-D-glucosamine (NAG) is a related substance found in joints and connective tissue.

Glucosamine sulfate is the preferred form because of its very high absorption, ease of utilization, immediacy of incorporation into connective tissue matrix, and history of clinical studies. Sulfur is an essential nutrient for joint tissue, where it functions in the stabilization of the connective tissue matrix of cartilage, tendons, and ligaments. In particular, sulfation is an active metabolic process in cartilage, and the sulfate moiety seems to be essential to *sulfation,* an active metabolic process in cartilage. The sulfate moiety also seems to be essential to synovial fluid delivery to articular cartilage as well as improving efficacy of the synovial fluid by strengthening cartilage and aiding GAG synthesis.[3,15] Further, even though it is often used in clinical trials, evidence supporting efficacy of the hydrochloride (HCl) salt of glucosamine is weak and unclear, and its use is rarely recommended by experienced clinicians.[16]

Chitin is a polymer of D-glucosamine with randomly assigned D-glucosamine monomers having a chemically bonded "acetyl" group, giving rise to NAG units. After extraction from the exoskeletons of shrimp and other shellfish, chitin can be chemically modified with hydrochloric acid digestion and deacetylation to yield quite pure D-glucosamine HCl monomers. Combining glucosamine HCl with sulfuric acid yields glucosamine sulfate. Glucosamine sulfate is produced through a co-crystallization step with sodium chloride (NaCl), resulting in a GS-NaCl complex. Alternatively, potassium chloride (KCl) can be used as the co-crystallization agent. Although most clinical trials have focused on the NaCl-stabilized form, the form using KCl as a stabilizer may be preferable for most individuals, given general dietary tendencies toward excess sodium and inadequate potassium intake. However, this issue has not yet been studied in controlled trials. In either form, these mineral salts stabilize GS by decreasing oxidation and moisture absorption.

In contrast, glucosamine HCl is typically granulated to reduce moisture absorption from the air. Salts are usually not necessary for its crystallization, but polyvinylpyrrolidone and corn syrup are often used as binders for granule formation.[17]

Regarding the N-acetyl form of glucosamine, researchers have concluded that "glucosamine is a more efficient precursor of macromolecular hexosamine (glycosaminoglycans) than N-acetylglucosamine. It is possible that N-acetylglucosamine

does not penetrate the cell membranes and, as a result, is not available for incorporation into glycoproteins and mucopolysaccharides."[18] Further, clinical trials using NAG in the treatment of osteoarthritis are lacking.

Dosage Forms Available

Capsule, tablet, liquid, powder.

Source Materials for Nutrient Preparations

Supplemental glucosamine is usually derived from the processed exoskeletons of shellfish, such as shrimp, lobster, and crab. Glucosamine may also be synthesized. A novel source of the HCl form is fermented corn-derived glucose, although this may not be a preferred form.

Dosage Range

Adult

Dietary: Not appreciable.
Supplemental/Maintenance: Generally not considered as recommended on a preventive basis, but glucosamine is widely used by individuals with a history of or susceptibility to joint pain or injury.
Pharmacological/Therapeutic: 500 to 2000 mg daily, most often 500 mg three times daily (of GS) orally. Obese individuals may need to increase dosages by 20 mg/kg body weight daily.[19] Anecdotally, many clinicians experienced in treating pain and injuries with nutritional therapies report that doses at two to three times typical levels (i.e., 3000-4500 mg/day) for 3 to 5 days decreases pain and accelerates tissue repair immediately after injury.
Toxic: Glucosamine sulfate is generally considered nontoxic.

Pediatric (<18 Years)

Dietary: Not appreciable.
Supplemental/Maintenance: Not applicable.
Pharmacological/Therapeutic: Ehler-Danlos syndrome, Marfan syndrome.
Toxic: Glucosamine sulfate is generally considered nontoxic.

SAFETY PROFILE

Overview

In the majority of studies, oral GS at standard dosage levels appears to be safe, nontoxic, and well tolerated, with only minor, transient, and reversible adverse effects. Several studies have reported an incidence of adverse effects no greater than among subject receiving placebo.[4,10,20,21] A meta-analysis by the Cochrane Collaboration reported only 16 adverse events requiring withdrawal from investigation, of 1000 patients treated for OA with glucosamine in 16 clinical trials.[22] Injectable and parenteral forms have also generally demonstrated an excellent safety profile. Allergic reactions appear to be rare and when suspected may derive from the shellfish used as source material for most preparations.[23]

Nutrient Adverse Effects

General Adverse Effects

Rarely mild and transient gastrointestinal (GI) effects, including flatulence, abdominal bloating, indigestion, heartburn, nausea, and diarrhea. These symptoms are often reduced by taking GS with a meal.

Adverse Effects among Specific Populations

One study noted that the onset of possible adverse effects was significantly related to preexisting GI disorders and related treatments and to concomitant diuretic treatment.[20]

One unqualified case report of impaired kidney function in a 79-year-old woman with myasthenia gravis, also undergoing corticosteroid and immunosuppressive therapy, resolved with discontinuation of glucosamine.[24]

Pregnancy and Nursing

Although evidence or reports of adverse events associated with glucosamine administration during pregnancy or breastfeeding are lacking, no clinical studies have demonstrated safety in such populations.

Infants and Children

Evidence or reports of adverse events associated with glucosamine intake are lacking, but glucosamine administration is generally inappropriate for most children and should be avoided in those under 2 years of age.

Contraindications

None documented, with the exception of possible (and probably rare) allergic reactivity to shellfish.

Precautions and Warnings

Some individuals with preexisting peptic ulcers or other GI conditions may have increased susceptibility to adverse effects.

INTERACTIONS REVIEW

Strategic Considerations

In general, comprehensive formal drug interaction studies involving glucosamine compounds are lacking. At this time, potential or suspected interactions involving diuretics or oral hypoglycemic agents appear to be discredited, clinically insignificant, or exceptional. A review of the scientific literature indicates that NSAIDs are the drug class most likely to manifest a clinically significant pattern of interaction with GS, and different agents within that class may theoretically produce different outcomes. Although evidence indicates that acetaminophen may obstruct the therapeutic activity of glucosamine, research is warranted to investigate opportunities for possible synergy or additive therapeutic benefit from coadministration with certain NSAIDs, such as ibuprofen.

Over the years, evidence supporting the clinical effectiveness of GS in the treatment of OA has increased in number, depth, and quality. Nevertheless, published clinical guidelines for integrative therapeutics involving glucosamine in the treatment of OA remain nascent and out of step with the clinical practices that have matured based on anecdotes, outcomes, and collective experience. At this point, the position of glucosamine as a potential first-line agent for repair of damaged or degenerating joint cartilage is reaching consensus level, at minimum for patients with knee OA who have mild to moderate pain. Ongoing and future studies of structure-modifying anti-OA drugs such as GS and chondroitin sulfate (CS) present the opportunity for further confirming the efficacy of these agents and clarifying appropriate therapeutic protocols customized to meet the needs of individuals and their variable life stages, personal history, genetic predispositions, diagnoses, and prognoses.

More fundamentally, the challenge of integrative medical care for OA will be to investigate, analyze, and synthesize the therapeutic strengths and opportunities presented by the range of treatment modalities. The therapeutic approach to integrative care of OA cannot rely solely on natural substances such as glucosamine alone or, for that matter, on any exclusively pharmacological approach. Other nutritional and botanical approaches, such as S-adenosylmethionine (SAMe), vitamin E, vitamin B_3 (niacinamide), bromelain, green-lipped mussel *(Perna canaliculus)*, methylsulfonylmethane (MSM), cetyl myristoleate (CMO), topical capsaicin, turmeric *(Curcuma longa)*, ginger *(Zingiber officinale)*, devil's claw *(Harpagophytum procumbens)*, boswellia *(Boswellia serrata)*, and cat's claw *(Uncaria tomentosa)*, are beginning to be studied in well-designed clinical trials, as are interventions such as aerobic exercise, quadriceps exercises, and footwear modification. Although the role of NSAIDs continues to undergo reformation in light of its limitations and adverse effects, new cyclooxygenase-2 (COX-2) inhibitors may have a role in situational symptom management in patients for whom simple analgesia is inadequate. Intra-articular hyaluronate injections may also have a limited role. Furthermore, the patient population appears receptive to medical and lifestyle interventions, such as weight reduction, yoga, tai qi, massage, acupuncture, and manipulative therapies, which are often beyond the realm of the average physician's training and experience, but which may be able to play an important role in restoring mobility and enhancing vitality within the context of an integrative therapeutic strategy.

Gottlieb[25] calls for a fundamental reevaluation of the medical view of OA and presents a perspective that remains challenging in its comprehensive approach in his 1997 review article, "Conservative management of spinal osteoarthritis with glucosamine sulfate and chiropractic treatment":

> The rationales for using NSAIDs in the treatment of osteoarthritis is controversial and openly contested. Given the detrimental effects of NSAIDs on joints and other organs, their use should be discouraged and their classification as a first choice conservative treatment should be abolished. A truly effective and conservative approach to the treatment of osteoarthritis should include chiropractic manipulation [or other forms of joint mobilization and manipulation], essential nutrient supplementation, exogenous administration of glucosamine sulfate and rehabilitative stretches and exercises to maintain joint function. Because there is no correlation between pain levels and the extent of degeneration detected by radiographic or physical examination, conservative treatment should be initiated and sustained based on functional, objective findings and not strictly on how the patient feels. The use of NSAIDs should be limited to the treatment of gross inflammation and analgesics should only be used in the short-term when absolutely necessary for pain palliation. The present conservative approach could lead not only to a better quality of life but also to the saving of health care dollars by reducing the iatrogenic morbidity and mortality associated with NSAID use.

Thus, emerging approaches to treatment of OA may be prime ground for exploring the broad value, in terms of quality of life and meaningful outcomes standards, for multidisciplinary collaboration and integrative therapeutics.

NUTRIENT-DRUG INTERACTIONS

Acetaminophen, Ibuprofen, and Nonsteroidal Anti-Inflammatory Drugs (NSAIDs)

Acetaminophen (APAP, paracetamol; Tylenol); combination drugs: acetaminophen and codeine (Capital and Codeine; Phenaphen with Codeine; Tylenol with Codeine); acetaminophen and hydrocodone (Anexsia, Anodynos-DHC, Co-Gesic,

Dolacet, DuoCet, Hydrocet, Hydrogesic, Hy-Phen, Lorcet 10/650, Lorcet-HD, Lorcet Plus, Lortab, Margesic H, Medipain 5, Norco, Stagesic, T-Gesic, Vicodin, Vicodin ES, Vicodin HP, Zydone); acetaminophen and oxycodone (Endocet, Percocet 2.5/325, Percocet 5/325, Percocet 7.5/ 500, Percocet 10/650, Roxicet 5/500, Roxilox, Tylox); acetaminophen and pentazocine (Talacen); acetaminophen and propoxyphene (Darvocet-N, Darvocet-N 100, Pronap-100, Propacet 100, Propoxacet-N, Wygesic); acetaminophen, butalbital, and caffeine (Fiorcet).

COX-1 inhibitors (NSAIDs): Diclofenac (Cataflam, Voltaren), combination drug: diclofenac and misoprostol (Arthrotec), diflunisal (Dolobid), etodolac (Lodine), fenoprofen (Dalfon), furbiprofen (Ansaid), ibuprofen (Advil, Excedrin IB, Motrin, Motrin IB, Nuprin, Pedia Care Fever Drops, Provel, Rufen; combination drug: hydrocodone and ibuprofen (Reprexain, Vicoprofen), indomethacin (indometacin; Indocin, Indocin-SR), ketoprofen (Orudis, Oruvail), ketorolac (Acular ophthalmic, Toradol), meclofenamate (Meclomen), mefenamic acid (Ponstel), meloxicam (Mobic), nabumetone (Relafen), naproxen (Aleve, Anaprox, Naprosyn), oxaprozin (Daypro), piroxicam (Feldene), salsalate (salicylic acid; Amigesic, Disalcid, Marthritic, Mono Gesic, Salflex, Salsitab), sulindac (Clinoril), tolmetin (Tolectin).

COX-2 inhibitor (NSAID): Celecoxib (Celebrex).

Interaction Type and Significance

◇≈≈ **Drug-Induced Adverse Effect on Nutrient Function, Coadministration Therapeutic, with Professional Management**

◇ **Adverse Drug Effect on Nutritional Therapeutics, Strategic Concern**

⊕✗ **Bimodal or Variable Interaction, with Professional Management**

⊕⊕ **Beneficial or Supportive Interaction, with Professional Management**

Probability: Evidence Base:
3. Possible   ○ Preliminary

Effect and Mechanism of Action

Even when they temporarily relieve pain and reduce inflammation, NSAIDs may accelerate the progression of OA and similar connective tissue trauma, joint degeneration, or related disorders by promoting cartilage destruction and interfering with cartilage repair. However, this effect may vary among the different agents in this drug class. Glucosamine sulfate intake can significantly increase serum sulfate concentrations, required for GAG synthesis, and thereby elevate synovial fluid sulfate concentrations and enable proteoglycan sulfation. Acetaminophen metabolism involves sulfation and thus consumes the sulfate provided by GS and interferes with the therapeutic action of the nutrient.[1] Other NSAIDs appear to interact with GS to produce variable metabolic effects on the synovial environment and cartilage repair.

Research

Numerous in vivo, animal, and human studies suggest that many NSAIDs exert deleterious effects on synthesis of vasodilator prostaglandins, joint perfusion, chondrocyte and proteoglycan metabolism, cartilage synthesis, and organization in articular cartilage, especially influencing the course of OA.[26-32] Zupanets et al.[33] first investigated combining glucosamine and NSAIDs to determine if any resultant additive or synergistic effect might enable reduction of dosage levels

necessary to obtain anti-inflammatory activity and thereby reduce adverse effects associated with these agents. They found that lower doses of voltaren, indomethacin, and piroxicam could be used in conjunction with glucosamine to reduce experimentally induced inflammation in mice and attributed these phenomena to a "diverse influence of aminosugar on the anti-inflammatory effect of nonsteroidal anti-inflammatory drugs." In unrelated but potentially significant research, Shikhman et al.[34] found that adding either glucosamine or NAG to human cartilage in vitro reduced inflammatory changes and gene expression induced by two different cytokines (interleukin 1β and tumor necrosis factor). This focus on the glucosamine led to, or at least paralleled, a focus on the respective roles and relative efficacy of the sulfate and hydrochloride forms and the mechanisms of NSAIDs' apparent interference with healthy cartilage nutriture and repair.

In a study of the effect of glucosamine hydrochloride's effect on pain associated with OA of the knee, Houpt et al.[16] reported minimal efficacy in individuals concurrently taking up to 4000 mg acetaminophen daily. Interestingly, this and the GAIT studies are the primary published clinical trials involving glucosamine that are cited as lacking a beneficial outcome. Seeking to determine the relative importance of the sulfur component of GS, Hoffer et al.[1] and observed a significant increase in serum sulfate in subjects who received GS, versus sodium sulfate, after administering both compounds to healthy subjects, despite the elemental sulfate dose being doubled. The authors interpreted this increase in availability of sulfur compounds as critical to the delivery of critical nutrients to the synovium, which serves as the primary nutrient reservoir for cartilage that lacks significant direct blood supply. In particular, synovial fluid free sulfate appears to be essential to proteoglycan sulfation. These observations supported the researchers' hypothesis that sulfate, rather than glucosamine, was the critical component of GS in its action on cartilage formation. In the second phase of this experiment, serum sulfate levels fell in those administered both acetaminophen and GS. Given that acetaminophen metabolism involves sulfation, these authors suggested that the drug consumed the sulfate provided by GS and would presumably blunt its nutritive effect on synovial fluid and therapeutic efficacy. Finally, they measured the serum and knee synovial fluid sulfate concentrations in OA patients and found virtually identical concentrations in both compartments, thus confirming the interrelationship of nutrient levels, particularly sulfate, between blood and synovial fluid.[1] Thus, in retrospect, questions arise as to whether the acetaminophen in the Houpt study may have interfered with the subjects' obtaining the full measure of glucosamine's potential benefit and whether acetaminophen might interfere with the activity of glucosamine compounds by some mechanism other than affecting sulfation. Nevertheless, even in this study, as the authors noted: "After the end of the 8 week open label trial, 77% of the subjects were still taking glucosamine, although now obliged to pay for commercially available products."[16]

Subsequently, using a mouse model, Tallarida et al.[35] reported that commercial GS "administered as the sole agent (up to 500 mg/Kg, p.o.) was inactive in the mouse abdominal irritant test, but that certain combinations of glucosamine with nonopioid analgesics at the oral doses and ratios tested resulted in a synergistic (ibuprofen and ketoprofen), additive (diclofenac, indomethacin, naproxen, and piroxicam), or subadditive (aspirin and acetaminophen) antinociceptive interaction." Examining specific fixed ratios of glucosamine and certain NSAIDs, they found that combinations containing racemic ibuprofen and glucosamine in greater than 1:1 ratio (glucosamine/ibuprofen) were synergistic in the test and that combinations of 2:1 and 9:1 yielded plasma levels of ibuprofen that were no different from administration of ibuprofen alone. These authors suggested that their findings supported further research into synergistic coadministration of GS and certain NSAIDs to enhance pain relief while reducing adverse effects usually associated with higher doses of NSAIDs.[35] Despite the continued use of glucosamine hydrochloride in major clinical trials, their concluding declaration that these findings were "being pursued in clinical trials" provides encouragement that important initial steps are being taken toward clarifying these significant findings and critically exploring such integrative therapeutic innovations.

Clinical research into the efficacy of glucosamine in the treatment of joint pain, inflammation, and degeneration has evolved to the point where opportunities for integrative therapeutic combinations are now ripe for systematic investigation. Although glucosamine and NSAIDs might appear superficially to contribute to the same therapeutic goals—relief of joint pain and degeneration—the evidence indicates that their respective mechanisms of action, character of effect, and role in strategic clinical management may result in either cooperative or antagonist influences and divergent outcomes, depending at least in part on the particular NSAID employed. One important factor in whether glucosamine (particularly GS) and individual NSAIDs potentiate or interfere with one another depends on the role of sulfation in each particular drug's metabolism. Research is still preliminary and large, well-designed clinical trials are clearly warranted. However, the findings thus far further suggest that those engaged in research design for studies of glucosamine's effect on OA or other forms of joint pain, as well as clinicians, should not allow subjects to use acetaminophen as a "rescue" drug, as has sometimes occurred in the past. Thus, heavier users of acetaminophen might derive less benefit from GS by diverting sulfate for drug metabolism, because acetaminophen is metabolized by multiple pathways, including sulfation.

Nutritional Therapeutics, Clinical Concerns, and Adaptations

In light of the accumulated and evolving evidence, concomitant use of glucosamine and particular NSAIDs appears to be a potentially valuable therapeutic option in the treatment of conditions for which both agents are typically used. However, based on both animal and human research, discrimination in selecting the most efficacious NSAID appears to be critical. Evidence suggests that coadministration of ibuprofen with GS may provide a synergistic therapeutic effect and that acetaminophen should be avoided. Such approaches, while novel and exploratory, appear to offer enhanced combined efficacy at minimal risk and cost and, because of the ability to reduce NSAID dosage levels, a likelihood of reduced risk of adverse effects. A reasonable option where the activity of an NSAID seems indicated might be combining the standard dosage of GS (500 mg) with ibuprofen (200 mg), three times daily, with phasing out of the ibuprofen to an as-needed basis when clinically improved. This long-term clinical strategy thus shifts from symptom management to maintenance, with emphasis on tissue strengthening and maximal restoration of healthy function.

Oral Hypoglycemic Agents and Insulin

Buformin (Andromaco Gliporal, Buformina), chlorpropamide (Diabinese), glimepiride (Amaryl), glipizide (Glucotrol; Glucotrol XL), glyburide (glibenclamide; Diabeta, Glynase, Glynase Prestab, Micronase, Pres Tab), insulin (animal-source insulin: Iletin, human analog insulin: Humanlog; human insulin: Humulin, Novolin, NovoRapid, Oralin), metformin (Dianben,

Glucophage, Glucophage XR); combination drugs: glipizide and metformin (Metaglip), glyburide and metformin (Glucovance); tolazamide (Tolinase), phenformin (Debeone, Fenformin), tolbutamide (Orinase, Tol-Tab).

Interaction Type and Significance

✗ **Potential or Theoretical Adverse Interaction of Uncertain Severity**

Probability:
5. Improbable

Evidence Base:
◉ Emerging

Effect and Mechanism of Action

It has been hypothesized that because of the chemical similarity between glucosamine-6-phosphate and glucose-6-phosphate, glucosamine could activate the hexosamine pathway and induce inhibition of liver glucokinase and thereby cause clinically significant changes in glucose metabolism and potentially contribute to the development of insulin resistance.[36-45] If proven in humans, such effects might theoretically mean that glucosamine administration could decrease the effectiveness of insulin or other oral hypoglycemic agents used in the management of diabetes mellitus.

Research

Several preliminary animal studies suggested that glucosamine, often administered in relatively high dosage levels by continuous intravenous (IV) infusion, could accelerate the hexosamine pathway and lead to peripheral insulin resistance and decreased insulin secretion. Giaccari et al.[38] found that high-dose glucosamine infusions significantly (40%-50%) impaired glucose-induced insulin secretion (both first and second phases), greatly reduced muscle glucose 6-phosphate concentration and reduced insulin stimulation of both glycolysis and glycogen synthesis in rats. Rossetti et al.[37] found that in vivo glucosamine infusion induces insulin resistance in normoglycemic but not in hyperglycemic rats. Barzilai et al.[39] observed that glucosamine induced inhibition of liver glucokinase, which in turn impaired the ability of hyperglycemia to suppress endogenous glucose production. Virkamaki et al.[40] reported that activation of the hexosamine pathway by glucosamine in vivo induced insulin resistance and increased risk of glucose toxicity in skeletal muscle and other insulin-sensitive tissues. Collectively, these and other findings from animal studies suggested that exogenous glucosamine might alter glucose metabolism to such an extent as to aggravate insulin resistance and potentially adversely interact with insulin and other medications prescribed for glucose control. However, the speculative nature of these findings was generally acknowledged, especially in light of dosage levels, based on weight, that were beyond the range of normal therapeutic dosages and usually significantly higher than might ever be obtained in humans through oral administration.[46,47]

Human trials that have examined the effects of glucosamine intake, in various forms, on glucose metabolism have generally found evidence lacking of adverse effects on glycemic control. Noack et al.[5] found that glucose metabolism is not impaired by short-term GS intake, 500 mg three times daily, in a general population of 252 patients being treated for knee OA. In this multicenter, randomized, placebo-controlled, double-blind, parallel-group study, fasting plasma glucose levels were not modified over a 4-week treatment with GS or placebo,[5] nor were they modified in the small subset of subjects the authors thought could be defined as diabetic, "in whom mean plasma glucose concentrations fell both in the nine patients on glucosamine and the 14 given placebo."[46] In a large, 3-year, placebo-controlled OA study, researchers observed only a tendency for fasting blood glucose to decrease with glucosamine, compared with subjects receiving placebo for whom it remained stable. Although there were few diabetic patients in this long-term study, those with high baseline glucose concentrations, when analyzed separately, showed a tendency for similar results, with a fall in plasma glucose among those taking glucosamine.[48] In related research, Pouwels et al.[49] determined that short-term glucosamine infusion does not affect insulin sensitivity in healthy human subjects (*n*=18); thus, their findings did not support involvement of the hexosamine pathway in the regulation of insulin sensitivity in humans. In a focused and definitive study, the first placebo-controlled, double-blind trial of its kind, Scroggie et al.[47] evaluated the effects of glucosamine hydrochloride (1500 mg/day), together with chondroitin sulfate (1200 mg/day), versus placebo, for 90 days on glycemic control in a group of 34 mostly elderly patients with type 2 diabetes. They reported that mean hemoglobin A_{1c} levels, a marker for long-term blood-glucose control, remained relatively stable in the glucosamine group and decreased in the placebo group. In a double-blind clinical trial involving 19 healthy adults, Tannis et al.[50] administered 1500 mg GS or placebo daily for 12 weeks to test for glucosamine-induced glucose intolerance. Three-hour oral glucose tolerance tests were performed before the start of administration, at 6 weeks, and at the completion of administration. These researchers found no significant differences between fasted levels of serum insulin or blood glucose. They observed that GS treatment did not alter serum insulin or plasma glucose during the glucose tolerance tests, and that glycosylated hemoglobin (HbA_{1c}) measurements at the three time points showed no significant change over time, within or between treatments, ages, or gender. Collectively, these human trials provide significant evidence that oral glucosamine, at recommended dosage levels, does not result in clinically significant alterations in glucose metabolism in patients with type 2 diabetes mellitus and is unlikely to interact adversely with insulin or other oral hypoglycemic agents.

Nutritional Therapeutics, Clinical Concerns, and Adaptations

Given its favorable risk/benefit ratio, especially compared with NSAIDs, GS therapy offers an attractive option to both patients and physicians in the treatment of appropriate conditions. Thus, Scroggie et al.[47] concluded: "Since patients with diabetes are at risk for toxic effects from some of the current treatments for osteoarthritis (NSAIDs in particular), glucosamine may provide a safe alternative treatment for these patients." Nevertheless, introduction of new medications or significant alterations in existing prescriptions can disrupt glycemic control in patients being treated for type 2 diabetes. Thus far, the weight and direction of evidence indicates that GS, or related forms, does not pose a significant risk of disrupting clinical management of such patients. Even so, it would be judicious to monitor short-term and long-term markers of blood glucose control closely in such patients whenever there are significant changes in treatment of glucose-related or other conditions.

THEORETICAL, SPECULATIVE, AND PRELIMINARY INTERACTIONS RESEARCH, INCLUDING OVERSTATED INTERACTIONS CLAIMS

Diuretics

Potassium-Sparing Diuretics: Amiloride (Midamor), spironolactone (Aldactone), triamterene (Dyrenium); combination drugs: amiloride and hydrochlorothiazide (Moduretic); spironolactone and hydrochlorothiazide (Aldactazide); triamterene and hydrochlorothiazide (Dyazide, Maxzide).

Loop Diuretics: Bumetanide (Bumex), ethacrynic acid (Edecrin), furosemide (Lasix), torsemide (Demadex).

Thiazide Diuretics: Bendroflumethiazide (bendrofluazide; Naturetin); combination drug: bendrofluazide and propranolol (Inderex); benzthiazide (Exna), chlorothiazide (Diuril), chlorthalidone (Hygroton), cyclopenthiazide (Navidrex); combination drug: cyclopenthiazide and oxprenolol hydrochloride (Trasidrex); hydrochlorothiazide (Aquazide, Esidrix, Ezide, Hydrocot, HydroDiuril, Microzide, Oretic); combination drugs: hydrochlorothiazide and amiloride (Moduretic); hydrochlorothiazide and captopril (Acezide, Capto-Co, Captozide, Co-Zidocapt); hydrochlorothiazide and enalapril (Vaseretic); hydrochlorothiazide and lisinopril (Prinzide, Zestoretic); hydrochlorothiazide and losartan (Hyzaar); hydrochlorothiazide and metoprolol (Lopressor HCT); hydrochlorothiazide and spironolactone (Aldactazide); hydrochlorothiazide and triamterene (Dyazide, Maxzide); hydroflumethiazide (Diucardin), methyclothiazide (Enduron), metolazone (Zaroxolyn, Mykrox), polythiazide (Renese), quinethazone (Hydromox), trichlormethiazide (Naqua).

Thiazide-like Diuretics: Indapamide (Lozol).

Glucosamine sulfate (GS) is stabilized with a mineral salt and consequently contains relatively high amounts of potassium chloride (KCl) or sodium chloride (NaCl). The action of diuretics on potassium may result in increased potassium levels or decreased effective levels of GS. Furthermore, individuals taking diuretics for hypertension, or otherwise on a sodium-restricted diet, may be adversely affected by the elevated sodium intake resulting from a glucosamine preparation stabilized with sodium. Likewise, individuals on a potassium-restricted diet may experience adverse effects from concomitant use of a diuretic and glucosamine stabilized with potassium. For example, in a product containing 300 mg GS per one tablet serving, a 12% potassium level (12%-13.5%) for source GS (potassium salt) would contain 36 mg potassium (36-41 mg). The proportion and amount of the sodium content in a sodium-based glucosamine salt would be comparable.[51] In other words, approximately 200 mg sodium or potassium, respectively, are included in a daily dose of 1500 mg GS.

Although the pharmacological rationale for this potential interaction between diuretics and glucosamine sulfate appears to be reasonable and well founded, evidence as to its clinical significance and any pattern of occurrence remains inadequate. In concluding their study of oral GS in the management of arthrosis, Tapadinhas et al.[20] noted that glucosamine administration was generally well tolerated, but adverse effects were significantly related to concomitant diuretic treatment, as well as to preexisting GI disorders and related treatments.

Physicians prescribing diuretics are advised to ask patients about their use of glucosamine (and other supplements) and to monitor blood pressure regularly and measure potassium levels as appropriate. Some individuals taking diuretics may need to take higher doses of glucosamine to obtain the full therapeutic effect, usually 20 mg/kg daily.[19] Daily fruit or other concomitant potassium may also be appropriate for individual on long-term therapy with potassium-depleting diuretics.

NUTRIENT-NUTRIENT INTERACTIONS

Bromelain

Glucosamine sulfate and bromelain are often used together in clinical practice for the treatment of joint pain and inflammation of traumatic or degenerative origin. The mechanism and efficacy of any additive or synergistic interaction remain to be investigated in well-designed clinical trials. However, the rationale of supportive activity appears reasonable, especially in light of bromelain's more immediate anti-inflammatory effects complementing glucosamine's relatively gradual, long-term, and primarily nutritive action.

Chondroitin Sulfate

See also previous section on NSAIDs.

Numerous animal and human trials have used chondroitin sulfate (CS) together with glucosamine compounds, particularly GS, and most have found the combination more effective than either agent alone, particularly in the treatment of osteoarthritis (OA).[12,22,47,52-59] Nevertheless, in the 4-year Glucosamine/chondroitin Arthritis Intervention Trial (GAIT) involving almost 1600 participants with documented knee OA, Clegg et al.[59] found that glucosamine hydrochloride (500 mg three times daily), CS (400 mg three times daily), or the combination for 24 weeks did not provide statistically significant relief (defined as a decrease in pain of at least 20%) from OA-associated pain among all subjects, compared with placebo and celecoxib (200 mg daily) as positive control. However, an analysis of the subgroup with initial moderate to severe pain (i.e., excluding those with mild pain) revealed relief with the combined nutrients at statistically significant levels compared with placebo (79.2% vs. 54.3%) or celecoxib (69.4%). Also, 60% of all subjects administered placebo reported 20% or greater pain reduction; this high response rate in the placebo group may have obscured a therapeutic response in subjects administered the glucosamine and/or CS, especially among subjects with initial mild pain. As with many similar trials, participants were allowed to use up to 4000 mg acetaminophen daily for pain, except for the 24 hours before assessment, further confounding the data and possibly adversely affecting therapeutic response. Notably, however, resort to such "rescue" acetaminophen was relatively low, overall averaging fewer than two 500-mg tablets daily.[60,61] Interestingly, in most news accounts (both professional and lay), and even in the published abstract, the terms "glucosamine" and "glucosamine and chondroitin sulfate" are used, and only in the "Methods" section of the full text does the use of "glucosamine hydrochloride" (vs. glucosamine sulfate) become evident. The pivotal clinical issue of disease progression (vs. pain relief), including joint function and regeneration, was not addressed in this study. Such elements of pathophysiology are central to the therapeutic strategy of nutritional interventions such as the sulfate compounds and is illuminated by research demonstrating that meniscal pathology increases the risk of cartilage loss in patients with symptomatic knee OA.[62]

Chondroitin sulfate tends to be more chondroprotective than regenerative and, as a much larger molecule (compared to GS), may be difficult to absorb. Concern has also been raised that CS may also interfere with GS absorption. Further research to explore systematically the nature of the interaction and its clinical implications is warranted.

Manganese

Manganese is an essential cofactor in bone and cartilage formation and may enhance glucosamine utilization within chondrocytes. Concomitant administration of glucosamine and manganese may produce increased therapeutic effects.[53]

Methylsulfonylmethane

Methylsulfonylmethane (MSM), the isoxidized form of dimethyl sulfoxide (DSMO), is often used as a natural analgesic and anti-inflammatory agent. MSM and glucosamine are frequently coadministered in the treatment of musculoskeletal injuries, OA, and similar conditions. In a 12-week, randomized, double-blind, parallel, placebo-controlled trial involving 118 subjects, Usha and Naidu[63] demonstrated that oral "glucosamine" (500 mg three times daily, sulfate form inferred) and MSM (500 mg three times daily), individually and in combination, significantly improved signs and symptoms of OA compared with placebo. These researchers noted that the "onset of analgesic and anti-inflammatory activity was found to be more rapid with the combination" and concluded that together these agents provide "better and more rapid improvement in patients with osteoarthritis." Further research is warranted. In the meantime, MSM, alone and with glucosamine, is generally well tolerated and considered safe at usual dosage levels; it also lacks the characteristic odor associated with DMSO.

Oligomeric Proanthocyanidins

Oligomeric proanthocyanidins (OPCs), most widely provided by grape seed and pine bark extracts, bind to collagen and elastin and have been shown to protect these tissues from collagenases and elastinases (which are locally generated by the inflammatory cascade). Thus, OPCs may also synergize with the chondroprotective and nutritive effects of glucosamine sulfate.[64] Researchers have demonstrated that the Pycnogenol brand of pine bark extract can prevent cramps and muscular pain "in normal subjects, venous patients, athletes, claudicants and in diabetic microangiopathy."[65]

Omega-3 Fatty Acids, Especially Fish Oils, Eicosapentaenoic Acid, and Docosahexanoic Acid

The combination of glucosamine and fish oil, containing eicosapentaenoic acid (EPA) and docosahexanoic acid (DHA), may have an additive effect in the treatment of psoriasis,[66] and possibly other inflammatory conditions.

Vitamin C

Vitamin C is an essential component of collagen and the extracellular matrix of cartilage. Concomitant administration of glucosamine and vitamin C may produce increased therapeutic effects.

The 66 citations for this monograph, as well as additional reference literature, are located under Glucosamine Sulfate on the CD at the back of the book.

Inositol

Nutrient Name: Inositol.

Synonyms: *cis*-1,2,3,5-*trans*-4,6-cyclohexanehexol, cyclohexanehexol, hexahydroxycyclohexane, inositol monophosphate, mouse antialopecia factor, myo-inositol, vitamin B_8.

Related Substances: Inositol hexaphosphate, IP6, phytic acid; D-chiro-inositol; inositol hexaniacinate, inositol niacinate, inositol nicotinate (see Vitamin B_3 monograph).

Summary

Drug/Class Interaction Type	Mechanism and Significance	Management
Lithium ☼/⊕	Lithium inhibits inositol monophosphatase and depletes brain stores of inositol. Coadministration may reduce adverse effects associated with chronic lithium therapy, especially psoriasis and polydipsia-polyuria, without reducing treatment efficacy. Long-term, well-designed clinical trials are warranted.	Coadminister. Monitor.

NUTRIENT DESCRIPTION
Chemistry and Forms

First recognized as an essential nutrient in 1940, inositol is a sugar-like, water-soluble substance member of the B-vitamin complex. The nine isomers of inositol are ubiquitous, cyclic carbohydrates with a basic 6-carbon ring structure. Three forms of inositol occur in nature: phytic acid, free *myo*-inositol, and inositol-containing phospholipids. Phytic acid, the hexaphosphate ester of inositol, is present in the leaves and seeds of most plants. In mammal tissues, inositol appears as phosphorylated derivatives, various phosphoinositides, and in its free form. The highest concentrations of inositol are in the heart and brain, with free *myo*-inositol predominantly found in the brain and kidney, and phospholipid inositol (phosphatidylinositol) concentrated in liver, pancreas, skeletal muscle, and cardiac muscle.

Physiology and Function

Although the distribution of inositol within the human body has long been known, its functions and mechanisms of action have yet to be fully elucidated.

Inositol production occurs through three known pathways. Dietary sources primarily enter the system as phytate or phytic acid (inositol hexaphosphate, or IP6) in plant foods, which is converted in the intestinal tract through the action of endogenous bacterial flora. However, oral intake of inositol is considered a minor pathway. The majority of inositol is produced, as inositol monophosphate, via a receptor-mediated salvage system and from glucose-6-phosphate; these two pathways are regulated by polyphosphate-1-phosphomonoesterase, a lithium-sensitive enzyme.

Inositol plays key roles in lipid transport, hepatic fat metabolism and cell membrane function, nerve transmission, and neurotransmitter activity. Along with choline (tetramethylglycine), methionine and betaine (trimethylglycine), inositol is considered a member of the group of compounds called *lipotropics*, which are closely involved in lipid metabolism. As an essential component of phospholipids, phosphatidylinositol participates in regulating the function of cell membranes, where it is particularly important in mediating cellular responses to external stimuli and/or nerve transmission. Inositol with various numbers of bound phosphate groups are also widely involved in cell-signaling processes.

Phosphatidylinositol (PI) mediates the activity of numerous membrane enzymes through interactions with specific proteins. The PI cycle is a second-messenger system integral to the function of several noradrenergic, serotonergic, and cholinergic receptors. Thus, PI participates in the action of serotonin; low cerebrospinal fluid (CSF) levels of inositol have been observed in individuals diagnosed with depression. Phosphatidylinositol also facilitates the synthesis of arachidonic acid.

NUTRIENT IN CLINICAL PRACTICE
Known or Potential Therapeutic Uses

Inositol has been used in clinical trials with several central nervous system (CNS) disorders, such as Alzheimer's disease, binge eating, bulimia, depression, obsessive-compulsive disorder (OCD), and panic disorder, as well as concurrently with lithium treatment of bipolar disorder.

Historical/Ethnomedicine Precedent

Inositol has not been used historically as an isolated nutrient.

Possible Uses

Alzheimer's disease, bulimia, depression, diabetes mellitus, diabetic neuropathy, lithium-related psoriasis, OCD, panic disorder, pediatric respiratory depression syndrome, premenstrual dysphoric disorder, trichotillomania.

Deficiency Symptoms

Consensus is lacking on specific signs and symptoms of inositol deficiency. Deficiency is considered unlikely in most individuals because of its widespread occurrence in foods. However, loss of intestinal flora necessary for conversion of such plant sources to inositol could reduce inositol levels.

Individuals with diabetes have increased inositol excretion, whereas those with depression exhibit significantly lower-than-normal CSF levels of inositol.

Dietary Sources

Nuts, beans, seeds, whole grains (especially wheat and wheat bran), cantaloupe, and citrus fruits (especially oranges) are excellent plant sources of inositol in the form of phytate or phytic acid (inositol hexaphosphate, IP6). Organ meats are the richest animal sources.

Dosage Forms Available

Capsule, powder, tablet.

Source Materials for Nutrient Preparations

The dominant commercial process for producing *myo*-inositol is purification of phytic acid (IP6) from grain such as corn, and then dephosphorylating it with proprietary enzymes.

Dosage Range
Adult

Dietary: No dietary or nutritional requirement for inositol has been established. Average adult intake in the United States has been estimated at 1000 mg daily as phytate or phytic acid.

Supplemental/Maintenance: 100 to 1000 mg per day. Inositol usually is not recommended for general nutritional supplementation. Doses found in multivitamins, if at all present, are generally insufficient to exert any clinically significant effect.

Pharmacological/Therapeutic: 100 to 1000 mg per day, usually 250 to 500 mg twice daily; 12 to 18 g per day have been used in clinical trials investigating treatment of anxiety, depression, and obsessive-compulsive disorder. Palatnik et al.[1] (2001) found that 18 g daily was well tolerated with minimal adverse effects.

Toxic: No toxic dose level for inositol has been reported. Large amounts (>3 g), if quickly ingested, can have a laxative effect, similar to that of sugar alcohols (e.g., maltitol, xylitol).

Pediatric (<18 Years)

Dietary: No minimal dietary requirement for children has been established.

Supplemental/Maintenance: Inositol is not currently recommended for children.

Pharmacological/Therapeutic: Specific treatment recommendations have not established.

Toxic: No toxic dosage level for inositol has been established specifically for infants and children.

Laboratory Values

Blood and CSF inositol levels can be done in research laboratories, but are not in clinical use.

SAFETY PROFILE
Overview

No toxic effects reported or observed, even though some clinical trials have used a therapeutic dosage that equals about 18 times the average dietary intake. Gastrointestinal effects such as nausea and diarrhea are occasionally reported with larger doses. Because of the hypothetical possibility that inositol may exacerbate hypomanic or manic symptoms in those with bipolar disorder, these individuals should use larger amounts (>1 g) of inositol with caution and under medical supervision. There have been no long-term safety studies to confirm the lack of adverse effects with chronic administration.

Nutrient Adverse Effects
General Adverse Effects

No general adverse effects from inositol have been confirmed in the scientific literature.

Pregnancy and Nursing

The use of inositol in pregnant women remains controversial because of possible effects on oxytocin and uterine contractions.

Infants and Children

Evidence is lacking in the scientific literature to suggest or confirm any adverse effects related to fetal development during pregnancy or to breast-fed infants and associated with inositol administration. Caution still is advised.

Contraindications

Attention deficit–hyperactivity disorder (ADHD), chronic renal failure, schizophrenia; pregnancy.

Following up on research by Levine et al.[2] that found a lack of efficacy with the use of inositol in the treatment of schizophrenia, research by Jope et al.[3] and others indicates that schizophrenia involves elevated activity of the phosphoinositol signaling system; thereby suggesting that inositol administration may be contraindicated.

In a double-blind, crossover study involving 11 children with ADHD, Levine et al.[4] found that inositol administration was associated with a trend toward the aggravation of the disorder.

Preliminary, but pharmacologically plausible, evidence suggests inositol may trigger manic episodes in individuals diagnosed with bipolar disorder.[5] These individuals should use *myo*-inositol with caution and only under medical supervision because of the theoretical possibility of exacerbating hypomanic or manic symptoms.

The issue of inositol administration during pregnancy raises complex and as-yet unresolved issues. Animal experiments indicate that inositol may significantly reduce the incidence of embryonic neural tube defects, including those resistant to folate alone.[6,7] However, as reported by Phaneuf et al.,[8] oxytocin's clinical effectiveness is caused by the activation of phospholipase C to produce inositol-1,4,5-triphosphate, which in turn releases calcium from intracellular stores and stimulates uterine contractions. Consequently, inositol may stimulate uterine contractions. Using a rodent model, Chien et al.[9] also observed dose-related myometrial contractions related to activation of the phosphatidylinositol signaling system by calcium agonists. Further research is warranted; inositol administration during pregnancy should be avoided out of prudence until safety factors are clarified and confirmed.

Precautions and Warnings

It has been suggested that exogenous inositol may stimulate uterine contractions, but evidence from human research is lacking to demonstrate such an adverse effect.[10] Thus, the usefulness of inositol in preventing neural tube defects (as supported by animal experiments) is limited.

INTERACTIONS REVIEW
Strategic Considerations

Although much is known about the physiological roles of *myo*-inositol, therapeutic strategies using inositol remain largely within the realm of clinical trials, clinical experience, anecdote, and conjecture. *Myo*-inositol may have antidepressant and anti-anxiety activity, but the mechanism of action has yet to be fully elucidated. Furthermore, no clinically available means exist to assess inositol status, or even normal ranges of nutrient concentration in blood. Data are available on inositol levels in CSF, but routine lumbar punctures for determining inositol concentration are impractical. Dietary intake typically supplies about a gram per day but relies on bowel flora to dephosphorylate it, which is not necessarily a valid assumption given the disproportionate ratio of antibiotic/probiotic use among most patients. Endogenous synthesis from glucose is the major source, but this depends on assumptions as to how intact that pathway is in any given individual. Inositol synthesis and regulation also involve salvage-recirculating pathways known to be inhibited by lithium and perhaps other substances. Inositol and its phosphates are ubiquitous in cell-signaling pathways, and its phosphatides in membrane signaling.

Experienced clinicians report that a major proportion of individuals diagnosed with depression, anxiety/panic disorder, and OCD appear to improve when given prescribed inositol in multigram quantities per day. Unfortunately, the CSF level does not appear to predict who will and will not respond, even though it is known that inositol levels in CSF are lower in depressed patients than in euthymic individuals. This differential response may be influenced or determined by cofactors that are adequate in some individuals and low in others. One relevant action of inositol may derive from its apparent ability to reverse desensitization of serotonin receptors. As with other antidepressant agents, the logical course, treating patients with mild symptoms of depression, anxiety, and/or obsessive-compulsive thoughts/behavior, is to start with a low dose (1 g/day) and gradually increase to maximum dose (animals models have used 1.2 g/kg with no adverse effects).

NUTRIENT-DRUG INTERACTIONS

Lithium Carbonate

Lithium carbonate (Camcolit, Carbolith, Duralith, Eskalith, Li-Liquid, Liskonum, Litarex, Lithane, Lithobid, Lithonate, Lithotabs, PMS-Lithium, Priadel).

Interaction Type and Significance

☼ **Prevention or Reduction of Drug Adverse Effect**
⊕ **Potential or Theoretical Beneficial or Supportive Interaction, with Professional Management**

Probability:
2. Probable

Evidence Base:
◉ **Emerging**

Effect and Mechanism of Action

Lithium's activity in bipolar disease may involve depletion of brain stores of inositol through inhibition of inositol monophosphatase, the enzyme that returns inositol monophosphate back to *myo*-inositol.[11] Inositol can reverse or mitigate adverse effects of lithium therapy, such as psoriasis and polyuria-polydipsia syndrome and lithium-pilocarpine–induced seizures.[12] However, concern has been raised that such concomitant administration might interfere with the therapeutic effects of lithium by increasing the concentration of inositol, thereby causing a return of manic or depressive symptoms.

Research

In a 6-week randomized clinical trial involving 24 adult men and women with *DSM-IV* bipolar depression, Chengappa et al.[13]

compared inositol (12 g/day) with placebo and demonstrated that among the 22 subjects who completed the trial, six (50%) of the inositol-treated subjects showed improved depression, as indicated by a 50% or greater decrease in the baseline Hamilton Depression Rating Scale (HAM-D) score and a Clinical Global Improvement (CGI) scale score change of "much" or "very much" improved, compared to three (30%) subjects assigned to placebo. However, this study was underpowered to detect a statistically significant difference.

In a double-blind placebo-controlled study involving healthy volunteers and using magnetic resonance spectroscopy to measure the concentration of both *myo*-inositol and phosphomonoesters, Silverstone et al.[14] demonstrated that lithium therapy depletes brain stores of inositol by blocking the conversion of inositol monophosphates to *myo*-inositol, and that this effect is especially apparent after phosphoinositol cycle stimulation. Subsequently, using high-resolution nuclear magnetic resonance (NMR) spectroscopy, O'Donnell, Silverstone, et al.[15] observed a significant increase in the concentration of inositol monophosphates and a significant decrease in *myo*-inositol concentration in the brains of rats chronically treated with lithium (and/or sodium valproate) compared to saline-treated controls.

Polyuria-polydipsia syndrome is a common adverse effect associated with lithium therapy and can affect up to 60% of patients taking the medication for at least 1 year.[16,17] Preliminary research indicated that low-dose inositol could reverse polyuria-polydipsia in rats treated with lithium and that oral inositol (3 g/day) ameliorates lithium-induced polyuria-polydipsia as rated subjectively by patients.[11] Levine et al.[18] injected daily inositol or "artificial CSF i.c.v." to rats exhibiting lithium-induced polydipsia and observed that inositol i.c.v. reversed lithium-induced polydipsia, but that kidney inositol levels in lithium-treated rats were not different from controls. These findings suggest that inositol may alleviate symptoms of lithium-induced polydipsia via a central effect, but has no direct effect on lithium-induced polyuria. These researchers also conducted a double-blind crossover study involving seven patients that compared 6 g oral inositol daily versus placebo, each given for 2 weeks. Inositol did not reverse lithium-induced polyuria, as measured by 24-hour urine volume and urine specific gravity. However, subjective report of symptomatology was significantly improved in subjects taking inositol versus placebo, possibly resulting from alleviation of polydipsia.

Psoriasis is an adverse effect associated with long-term use of lithium in many patients. In a randomized, double-blind, placebo-controlled, crossover clinical trial, Allan et al.[19] compared the effects of inositol administration in 15 patients with psoriasis while undergoing lithium therapy with the effects in 11 patients with psoriasis not taking lithium. The inositol had a significantly beneficial effect on the psoriasis of patients taking lithium, in contrast to a lack of effect on psoriasis of patients not receiving lithium.

Some animal studies suggested that administration of pharmacological doses of inositol reverses behavioral effects of lithium.[20] Inositol derived from inositol phosphate breakdown appears to be recycled for use in membranous phosphatidylinositol. Belmaker et al.[21,22] proposed that inositol depletion was central to the action of lithium action and relevant to treatment of adverse effects associated with lithium therapy. Within this hypothesis, lithium's depletion of the recyclable inositol pool would affect hyperactivated systems while leaving isosystems unaffected. Berridge[23] similarly found that lithium only inhibits phosphoinositide-derived second messengers of activated systems. These findings and those of clinical trials consistently indicate that concomitant administration of inositol during lithium therapy does not interfere with the efficacy of the treatment of individuals with bipolar disorder.

Nutritional Therapeutics, Clinical Concerns, and Adaptations

Physicians prescribing lithium for patients with bipolar affective disorders are advised to consider concomitant inositol administration, especially when intractable psoriasis occurs and continued lithium therapy is deemed necessary. Inositol (e.g., 500 mg three times daily) could ameliorate adverse effects of lithium therapy without reducing the drug's therapeutic effectiveness; such nutrient administration may also provide therapeutic value independent of conventional pharmacological treatment.

Although the beneficial effects of inositol coadministration from clinical trials are encouraging, further research through well-designed clinical trials is warranted to investigate further the safety and efficacy of this combination and to develop clinical guidelines for therapeutic application. Pending findings from such investigations, it would be premature generally to recommend concomitant use of lithium and inositol for treatment or prevention of adverse effects.

THEORETICAL, SPECULATIVE, AND PRELIMINARY INTERACTIONS RESEARCH, INCLUDING OVERSTATED INTERACTIONS CLAIMS

5-Hydroxytryptamine Receptor Agonists (Triptans)

Almotriptan (Axert), eletriptan (Relpax), frovatriptan (Frova), naratriptan (Amerge), rizatriptan (Maxalt), sumatriptan (Imitrex), zolmitriptan (Zomig).

Triptans (5-hydroxytryptamine receptor agonists) are a primary pharmacological therapy for migraines within conventional practice. Theoretically, concomitant administration of high-dose *myo*-inositol and medications in this class may produce additive effects. Evidence from qualified case reports or human trials is lacking to determine the occurrence, conditions, and clinical significance of this potential interaction.

Careful monitoring is advised for concurrent or consecutive use of high-dose *myo*-inositol with triptans. Either or both agents should be discontinued if symptoms suggestive of serotonin syndrome develop. This has not been reported, but there is little clinical experience in this area. Human trials are warranted.

Antibiotics/Antimicrobials

Antibiotics and Antimicrobials

Intestinal microflora play a critical role in biosynthesis of many B vitamins, particularly converting phytate/phytic acid from dietary sources into inositol. The adverse impact of repeated courses or high doses of broad-spectrum antibiotics on these commensal microbiota, and thus conversion of phytic acid to inositol, is probable. However, evidence is lacking to determine the frequency, character, and implications of such effects. Current knowledge suggests that the probability of a clinically significant adverse effect is low for most individuals because this inositol production pathway accounts for a minor part of inositol formation. Nevertheless, specific evidence is lacking to disprove or confirm the occurrence and clinical implications of this potential interaction. Further research is warranted. Physicians prescribing broad-spectrum antibiotics are generally advised to restore healthy intestinal ecology by

administering diverse and vigorous cultures, providing 10 billion viable organisms daily of probiotic flora for a minimum of 3 weeks, although in many cases it may take 6 months of daily probiotic intake to reestablish optimal bowel flora.

Selective Serotonin Reuptake Inhibitor (SSRI) Antidepressants

Citalopram (Celexa), escitalopram (S-citalopram; Lexapro), fluoxetine (Prozac, Sarafem), fluvoxamine (Faurin, Luvox), paroxetine (Aropax, Deroxat, Paxil, Seroxat), sertraline (Zoloft).

In a randomized, controlled, double-blind augmentation trial, Nemets et al.[24] found that inositol coadministration did not improve depression in SSRI treatment failures. Comparing single-photon emission computed tomography (SPECT) on 14 subjects diagnosed with OCD before and after 12 weeks of treatment with inositol, Carey et al.[25] concluded that "inositol effects a clinical response through alternate neuronal circuitry to the SSRIs." Some research has suggested that inositol helps reverse desensitization of serotonin receptors.[26] Theoretically, high-dose *myo*-inositol might have additive effects with SSRIs and, in fact, has been recommended as an adjunctive therapy for people diagnosed with OCD who do not respond to SRIs (clomipramine and SSRIs).[27] Doses of 18 g/day have been well tolerated in conjunction with SSRIs for the treatment of OCD, although the addition of inositol did not provide any added benefit over SSRI alone.[28]

Careful monitoring is advised for concurrent or consecutive use of high-dose *myo*-inositol with SSRIs. Either or both agents should be discontinued if symptoms suggestive of serotonin syndrome develop. This has not been reported, but there is little clinical experience in this area.

Valproic Acid and Related Anticonvulsant Medications

Evidence: Divalproex semisodium, divalproex sodium (Depakote), sodium valproate (Depacon), valproate semisodium, valproic acid (Depakene, Depakene Syrup).
Extrapolated, based on similar properties: Carbamazepine (Carbatrol, Tegretol), clonazepam (Klonopin), clorazepate (Tranxene), ethosuximide (Zarontin), ethotoin (Peganone), felbamate (Felbatol), fosphenytoin (Cerebyx, Mesantoin), levetiracetam (Keppra), mephenytoin, mephobarbital (Mebaral), methsuximide (Celontin), oxcarbazepine (GP 47680, oxycarbamazepine; Trileptal), phenobarbital (phenobarbitone; Luminal, Solfoton), phenytoin (diphenylhydantoin; Dilantin, Phenytek), piracetam (Nootropyl), primidone (Mysoline), topiramate (Topamax), trimethadione (Tridione), vigabatrin (Sabril), zonisamide (Zonegran).

O'Donnell et al.[15] found that the brains of rats treated with sodium valproate exhibited a significant increase in the concentration of inositol monophosphates and a significant decrease in *myo*-inositol concentration compared with saline-treated controls. These unexpected results suggest that both lithium and sodium valproate may share a common mechanism of action in the treatment of bipolar disorder through actions on the phosphoinositol cycle.

Chengappa et al.[13] reported doses of 12 g/day inositol being well tolerated in combination with either valproic acid or carbamazepine.[13]

Clinical trials of concomitant use of valproate and *myo*-inositol in bipolar disorder would be of interest because inositol might be useful in preventing or treating the depressive cycles.

NUTRIENT-NUTRIENT INTERACTIONS

Calcium, Iron, and Zinc

Phytic acid or phytate, the form of inositol in plant food sources, has the strong ability to chelate multivalent metal ions, especially calcium, iron, and zinc. The resultant binding can produce very insoluble salts that are poorly absorbed from the gastrointestinal tract. Thus, high dietary intake of phytate can result in poor bioavailability of these minerals.

However, available evidence indicates that standard oral preparations of inositol do not exert a similar effect on absorption of these nutrients.[29]

The 29 citations for this monograph, as well as additional reference literature, are located under Inositol on the CD at the back of the book.

Summary

Drug/Class Interaction Type	Mechanism and Significance	Management
Benzodiazepines ≈≈/☼/⊕⊕	Benzodiazepines may suppress and/or deplete melatonin by one or more mechanisms, including suppression of the dark-induced increase of pineal N-acetyltransferase activity. Clinical significance unclear but disruption of sleep cycle dynamics could be significant. Coadministration of melatonin could be used for synergistic effect and/or to ameliorate withdrawal symptoms from benzodiazepine insomnia treatment by re-establishing a regular sleep cycle. Further research warranted based on encouraging preliminary findings.	Coadminister, especially if melatonin deficiency present. Coadminister for synergistic effect or transition, with supervision.
Beta1-Adrenoceptor Antagonists ≈≈≈/☼	With chronic use, beta blockers may suppress melatonin synthesis by blocking pineal adrenergic beta-1 receptors. Evidence of clinically significant adverse effect on sleep cycle, but may vary according to agent, patient, etc.	Coadminister to prevent or correct sleep disturbances.
Chemotherapy (and radiotherapy) ☼/⊕⊕	Coadministration of chemotherapeutic agents and high-dose melatonin can ameliorate adverse drug effects and enhance chemotherapy cytotoxicity. Diverse and preliminary consistent supportive evidence; probable clinical significance. Therapeutic methodology evolving.	Coadminister. Supervise and monitor.
Corticosteroids, oral ◇,≈≈/?	Exogenous corticosteroids may suppress melatonin synthesis and reduce amplitude of the rhythmic melatonin production. Melatonin may reduce adverse effects but could theoretically suppress corticosteroid activity. Evidence of interaction is suggestive but inconclusive.	Insufficient evidence to support generalized recommendation. Monitor for interference with drug activity if used concurrently.
Fluoxetine ≈≈/✗	Fluoxetine can decrease melatonin levels. Exogenous melatonin may neutralize intended inhibitory action on tryptophan-2,3-dioxygenase by fluoxetine. Preliminary evidence suggests reasonable probability of clinically significant adverse interaction. Consider alternative antidepressant if sleep disturbed.	Avoid concomitant use.
Fluvoxamine ⊕⊕	Fluvoxamine can significantly elevate serum melatonin concentrations, most likely by inhibiting melatonin breakdown by CYP450 enzymes. Fluvoxamine levels may also rise with concomitant use. Consistent and increasingly specific evidence of clinically significant additive interaction, contributing to probable beneficial response.	Consider coadministration; may enhance effect of either or both agents. Supervise and monitor.
Haloperidol Antipsychotics ☼	Melatonin may reduce symptoms of tardive dyskinesia (TD), including such adverse effects associated with long-term use of antipsychotic medications. Preliminary supportive evidence, but likely weak clinical significance.	Consider coadministration to ameliorate adverse effects (i.e., TD). Supervise and monitor.
Interleukin-2 (IL-2) ⊕⊕/☼	Potential mutually supportive antineoplastic activity and synergistic interaction between melatonin and IL-2 in oncological care. Possible reduction of adverse drug effects. Emerging pattern of supportive evidence; probable clinical significance. Therapeutic methodology evolving.	Consider coadministration; may enhance effect of either or both agents. Supervise and monitor.
Mirtazapine ◇◇/✗/⊕	Mirtazapine can significantly increase nocturnal melatonin secretion, which may be part of its therapeutic mechanism of action. Concomitant use could be beneficial, depending on case particulars, including facilitation of reduced drug dose or use in drug withdrawal. Adverse effects possible but considered unlikely. Evidence minimal but effects plausible.	Consider coadministration; supervise closely and monitor regularly.
Nonsteroidal anti-inflammatory drugs (NSAIDs) Acetylsalicyclic acid (aspirin, ASA) ☼/≈≈≈/◇≈≈	NSAIDs inhibit prostaglandin synthesis and thereby interfere with melatonin synthesis, suppress nocturnal melatonin levels, and may alter sleep patterns. Adverse effects unlikely with concomitant use. Evidence minimal but effects plausible.	Consider melatonin coadministration if sleep disruption occurs during anti-inflammatory therapy.
Tamoxifen ⊕⊕	Coadministration of tamoxifen and high-dose melatonin can ameliorate adverse drug effects and enhance chemotherapy cytotoxicity. Emerging body of supportive evidence; probable clinical significance. Therapeutic methodology evolving.	Coadminister. Supervise and monitor.

Continued

Summary

Drug/Class Interaction Type	Mechanism and Significance	Management
Triptorelin ⊕⊕	Melatonin may enhance efficacy of triptorelin, and may re-establish response after patients have become refractory. Mechanism(s) of action uncertain, but may include a direct cytostatic effect, or reduction of endogenous prolactin, IGF-1 (insulin-like growth factor-1), or other tumor-dependent growth factors. Preliminary evidence supportive and beneficial effects probable where indicated.	Consider coadministration; supervise closely and monitor regularly.
Verapamil ≈≈≈	Verapamil induces increased urinary melatonin excretion through its effect on liver and kidneys.	Consider coadministration to prevent or correct sleep disturbances.

NUTRIENT DESCRIPTION

Chemistry and Form

Melatonin is an amino acid–based (indole) hormone, produced in the brain by the pineal gland. It is synthesized from the amino acid tryptophan, which is converted to the neurotransmitter serotonin, which is then converted to melatonin.

Physiology and Function

Melatonin is the central hormone involved in the regulation of numerous environmental and body cycles. As the biological timekeeper of hormone secretion, melatonin functions as a hormonal interface between the body and the environment. The greatest regulatory influence involves the daily cycle of light and darkness; melatonin production by the pineal gland begins to rise slowly with nightfall, reaching its maximum between midnight and 3 AM. After its synthesis is triggered by various external environmental cues, melatonin integrates the environmental feedback of daily and seasonal cycles, sets the biological clock, and activates bodily functions associated with these cues. The most notable example is the circadian (24-hour) cycle of sleep and waking, in which darkness triggers melatonin production, which helps to engender a feeling of sleepiness, and light suppresses secretion. Thus, melatonin possesses both phase-shifting and sleep-promoting properties. Many other cycles influence melatonin production as well, such as the annual cycle of longer and shorter days and the monthly female reproductive cycle, and many events tied to these cycles are linked to melatonin. Melatonin is metabolized by the liver after a half-life of 30 to 50 minutes.

Melatonin acts on multiple systems, appears to be high on the hierarchy of regulatory hormones (i.e., it regulates hormones that regulate hormones), and demonstrates antioxidant, antiestrogenic, and oncostatic activity. For example, melatonin appears to be such a powerful regulator of the secretion of growth hormone (GH) and gonadotropic hormones (the hormones that regulate production of sex hormones such as estrogen and progesterone) that it is a crucial element in the timing of the female reproductive cycle; rising melatonin levels may bring on menstruation, and their decline may induce a surge of luteinizing hormone (LH) and ovulation. Thus, melatonin influences menarche; the frequency, timing, and duration of menstrual cycles; and menopause. It also introduces subtle changes according to external rhythms; for example, varying melatonin levels over the course of the year result in higher estrogen in the spring and summer and higher progesterone in the fall and winter.

Human lymphocytes synthesize and release large amounts of melatonin. This melatonin appears to play a central role in the regulation of the human immune system, possibly by acting as an intracrine, autocrine, and paracrine substance. Receptors have been reported on T and B lymphocytes, and melatonin has demonstrated immune-enhancing properties in many animal studies. Physiologically, melatonin opposes the degeneration caused by elevated levels of endogenous corticosteroids (e.g., protein catabolism, suppressed immune function, and altered blood glucose metabolism). The immunosuppressive activity of exogenous corticosteroids may also be moderated by melatonin.

Various studies have shown a correlation among melatonin, aging, and life span. One proposed rationale is that the ratio of serotonin to melatonin increases as a person ages, increasing the production of various chemicals that are linked with aging. Onset of melatonin's rhythmic patterns starts at approximately 3 months of age, and young children have the highest levels of nighttime melatonin. Levels rise and then gradually start to decline during adolescence. Adults generally exhibit a 37% decline, approximately, in daily melatonin output between 20 and 70 years of age. However, controversy surrounds whether such declines are as prominent in healthy adults. These secretion patterns may contribute to sleep disruption and the tendency to shift to earlier sleep in the evening and earlier rising in the morning in the elderly population.

Numerous researchers and clinicians have suggested that the increased use of artificial light and resulting extension of the daily photoperiod of light exposure over the past century has depressed melatonin secretion and elevated the incidence of cancer in industrialized societies.[1,2]

Melatonin also functions as a powerful antioxidant, particularly in neutralizing hydroxyl, the most damaging of all oxygen-based free radicals. Administration for this purpose may be inappropriate, however, because the antioxidant effects may be offset by hormonal disruption caused by taking large doses.

Studies have also shown that melatonin decreases the internal carotid pulsability index of premenopausal women[3] and, applied topically, can reduce skin damage inflicted by ultraviolet (UV) radiation.[4] Research does not support administration as a remedy for the effects of aging; it is probably more beneficial to protect oneself from influences that inhibit melatonin.

NUTRIENT IN CLINICAL PRACTICE

Known or Potential Therapeutic Uses

As a self-prescribed nutraceutical, melatonin is primarily used to induce sleep or adjust sleep cycles, especially with travel and schedule changes. Practitioners of nutritional therapeutics, particularly within the context of integrative medicine, often prescribe melatonin in the treatment of some forms of depression and hyperactivity, at low dosages, and as part of multimodality cancer treatment protocols, using high dosages.

Historical/Ethnomedicine Precedent

None known.

Possible Uses

Age-related cognitive decline, Angelman's syndrome (sleep disturbances only), attention deficit–hyperactivity disorder (ADHD), breast cancer, cluster headaches, colon cancer, coronary heart disease, depression, epilepsy, essential hypertension, glaucoma, insomnia, jet lag, lung cancer, migraine headaches, multiple sclerosis, myoclonus, nocturnal hypertension, oxidative stress in dialysis patients (preventive), postmenopausal osteoporosis, prostate cancer, sarcoidosis, seasonal affective disorder (SAD), sudden infant death syndrome (SIDS), sleep cycle disruption, tardive dyskinesia, tinnitus.

Deficiency Symptoms

Insomnia[5] and other sleep disturbances.

Dietary Sources

Melatonin appears in foods only in trace amounts.

Nutrient Preparations Available

Time-release forms may best approximate normal physiological secretion of melatonin,[6] which typically occurs over several hours during the night. Further, a limitation of non-time-release forms is that the half-life of oral melatonin is approximately 30 to 50 minutes.

Dosage Forms Available

Capsule, tablet, sublingual tablet, time-release tablet and capsule.

Source Materials for Nutrient Preparations

Melatonin used in preparations for oral administration is derived from animals or produced synthetically.

Dosage Range

Adult

Supplemental/Maintenance: Melatonin is usually not taken on a long-term basis as a general nutritional supplement, that is, outside situational appropriateness or therapeutic strategy.
Pharmacological/Therapeutic: 0.5 to 6.0 mg nightly; up to 40 mg per day in cancer therapy.
Toxic: Melatonin is generally considered nontoxic when used in accordance with proper dosing guidelines for appropriate conditions.

Pediatric (<18 Years)

Supplemental/Maintenance: Melatonin is generally not appropriate for children, other than short-term situational use (e.g., travel, jet lag).
Pharmacological/Therapeutic: Generally not appropriate, except with managed therapeutic protocols.

Toxic: Melatonin is generally considered nontoxic for children when used in accordance with proper dosing guidelines for appropriate conditions.

Laboratoary Values

Salivary melatonin concentration, urinary 6-hydroxymelatonin sulphate excretion rate, serum melatonin concentration.[7]

Note: Melatonin in a physiological setting is problematic to study, because a blood sample needs to be obtained between 3 and 4 AM without exposing the patient to light, in order to obtain a relevant measurement. Accurate interpretation of the assay requires a collection of normal levels arranged by age.

SAFETY PROFILE

Overview

Melatonin use is generally considered safe when used for appropriate conditions in accordance with standard dosage levels. Although certain predictable effects may occur, no substantive and consistent patterns of adverse effects or toxicity, based on clinical trials or qualified case reports, have been confirmed in the scientific literature. Long-term human studies on toxicity or subtle adverse effects have not been conducted. Evidence is lacking at this time of a feedback loop in which augmentation or replacement causes suppression. Nevertheless, as with administration of any exogenous hormone, regular use of melatonin over an extended period may interfere with self-regulatory mechanisms in hormonal systems.

Nutrient Adverse Effects

General Adverse Effects

Drowsiness is an expected outcome of taking melatonin, and being drowsy at inopportune times represents the most common adverse effect. Overuse or incorrect use of melatonin may disrupt circadian rhythms and sleep cycles. Morning sedation or drowsiness may indicate that the dosage used is excessive; if so, a lower dosage should reduce adverse symptoms. Somnambulism, disorientation, and vivid dreams have also been reported. Sleep disruption was observed in one small study.[8] Anxiety and irritability may occur in some individuals. Nocturnal asthma may be aggravated.[9,10]

Scattered and unqualified case reports have suggested exogenous melatonin intake as a factor in a variety of adverse phenomena, including transient psychosis, headache, abdominal cramps, decreased libido, infertility, and painful gynecomastia.[11-14] Subsequent investigation has yet to document and confirm significant patterns of adverse effects consistent with these reported individual reactions.[15-17]

Pregnancy and Nursing

Melatonin readily crosses the placenta, and its fetal effects are unknown; therefore, melatonin is not recommended during pregnancy. Given the intimate relationships between melatonin and reproductive hormones, use of melatonin by women who are pregnant is further contraindicated, pending substantive evidence of safety. The lack of research on the effects and safety of melatonin in infants warrants avoidance by mothers who are breastfeeding.

Infants and Children

An increased incidence of seizures in children with neurological disorders after melatonin administration has been reported but not confirmed.[18] Monitoring by a qualified health care professional is warranted when use in such populations is otherwise appropriate.

Contraindications

Driving and operation of machinery should be avoided while under the influence of melatonin. Daytime use may result in fatigue and decreased alertness; other contraindications include pregnancy and nursing; fibromyalgia (if elevated melatonin),[19] insulin sensitivity or diabetes,[3] and SAD.

Some highly experimental animal trials suggest that melatonin may be contraindicated for patients with autoimmune disorders such as rheumatoid arthritis, lupus, or multiple sclerosis.

Precautions and Warnings

General

Caution is advised given the limited knowledge of hormones and their interactions and the multiple influences melatonin exerts on other regulatory hormones.

Regular use for extended periods is not advised without supervision by a health care professional experienced in nutritional therapies.

Specific Populations

Elevated melatonin levels may inhibit ovulation; prudence suggests that melatonin should generally be avoided by women attempting to conceive.

Individuals diagnosed with depression, diabetes, fibromyalgia, or schizophrenia, especially when not deficient; adolescents; individuals undergoing corticosteroid therapy for anti-inflammatory or immune suppressive effects; individuals with nocturnal asthma may experience increased inflammation with elevated melatonin levels.

Many clinicians have observed a paradoxical effect, causing alertness and insomnia, from melatonin administration in approximately 5% of patients. With those individuals, melatonin can often be successfully dosed in the morning with no adverse effects (i.e., no drowsiness).

INTERACTIONS REVIEW
Strategic Considerations

In most clinical settings, and in the vast majority of self-prescribed use by the general public, melatonin is used to treat sleep disorders (3 mg time-release form) or regulate sleep cycles (e.g., travel across multiple time zones, changing work shift). Assays for deficiency status (or excess) are available, but most experienced practitioners use sleep quality (after correcting sleep hygiene as much as possible, and ruling out sleep apnea/nocturnal myoclonic leg jerks as problems) and response to melatonin (3 mg time-release form) as the primary criteria in clinical evaluation for melatonin sufficiency.

Although consideration of its physiological role raises suspicions that many medications may interfere with melatonin secretion, human research into such effects and their clinical implications is sparse and early in its evolution. Depletion of melatonin by some pharmaceutical agents can be easily corrected with coadministration, usually at low doses, if deficiency results. In a more proactive sense, melatonin may play an important role as a component of integrative care strategies in the treatment of hormone-related cancers and sleep disturbances.

NUTRIENT-DRUG INTERACTIONS

Benzodiazepines

Alprazolam (Xanax), bromazepam (Lexotan), chlordiazepoxide (Librium), clonazepam (Klonopin, Rivotril), clorazepate (Gen-Xene, Tranxene), diazepam (Valium), estazolam (ProSom), flurazepam (Dalmane), lorazepam (Ativan), medazepam (Nobrium), midazolam (Hypnovel, Versed), oxazepam (Serax), prazepam (Centrax), quazepam (Doral), temazepam (Restoril), triazolam (Halcion).

Interaction Type and Significance

≈≈   **Drug-Induced Nutrient Depletion, Supplementation Therapeutic, with Professional Management**
☼   **Prevention or Reduction of Drug Adverse Effect**
⊕⊕   **Beneficial or Supportive Interaction, with Professional Management**

Probability:	Evidence Base:
2. Probable	◉ **Emerging**

Effect and Mechanism of Action

Benzodiazepines may deplete melatonin by suppressing the dark-induced increase of pineal N-acetyltransferase activity, which catalyzes the rate-limiting step in melatonin synthesis.[20] Other researchers have proposed that melatonin suppression is attributable to benzodiazepine binding sites and gamma-aminobutyric acid (GABA)–ergic transmission in the human pineal gland, suprachiasmatic nuclei, and retina.[21]

The hypnotic effect of both triazolam and melatonin can be enhanced through an additive, or possibly synergistic, effect with concomitant use. Oral melatonin may enable reversal of tolerance to benzodiazepine hypnotics that is common with long-term benzodiazepine therapy.

Research

In a double-blind clinical trial, Monteleone et al.[22] reported that serum melatonin levels in six healthy men, observed at hourly intervals during the night, after diazepam administration, were significantly lower than the corresponding values after placebo. Subsequently, in an in vivo study, Wakabayashi et al.[20] found that subcutaneous (SC) injection of diazepam 1 hour before the start of darkness significantly suppressed nocturnal elevations of pineal N-acetylserotonin (NAS) and melatonin contents in rats and caused a 2-hour delay in reaching the maximum melatonin level in the dark phase. McIntyre et al.[21] observed a similar suppression of plasma melatonin (and cortisol) concentrations after evening alprazolam administration in six healthy human subjects.

Ferini-Strambi et al.[23] conducted a preliminary study on the effect of coadministration of melatonin (100 mg/day) and threshold doses of triazolam (0.125 mg) on the quality of sleep in healthy volunteers. They reported significant modulation of important parameters of sleep microstructure along with improved subjective sleep quality. The authors suggested that melatonin and low benzodiazepine doses could be used together to enhance the desired effects and avoid the residual, dose-related benzodiazepine effects (e.g., morning grogginess).

Cardinali et al.[24] conducted a double-blind placebo-controlled study involving 45 subjects to investigate the efficacy of melatonin in reducing anxiolytic benzodiazepine use in elderly adults (>80 years old) with minor sleep disturbance.

They found that the combination of anxiolytic benzodiazepines in low doses and melatonin (3 mg orally, non-time-release form) produced mixed results. Melatonin advanced sleep onset by approximately 28 minutes and decreased significantly the variability of sleep onset. However, they also noted a "general lack of changes in quality of wakefulness or sleep in patients taking melatonin or placebo" and even a decrease in sleep quality during the first 2 weeks with melatonin, as compared to placebo. These researchers concluded that their findings do "not support melatonin efficacy to reduce the use of benzodiazepines in low doses [which] contrasted with the demonstrable effectiveness of melatonin to reduce benzodiazepine consumption in insomniac patients when used in hypnotic amounts."[24]

Reports

Dagan et al.[25] reported the case of a 43-year-old woman on long-term benzodiazepine therapy for chronic insomnia who demonstrated improved sleep quality, reversal of benzodiazepine tolerance, and ability to cease use of benzodiazepine medications (without a recurrence of previous withdrawal symptoms) after only 2 days of melatonin (1 mg controlled-release form at bedtime). They suggested that adjunctive melatonin could be used to ameliorate withdrawal symptoms from benzodiazepine insomnia treatment by reestablishing a regular sleep cycle.

Nutritional Therapeutics, Clinical Concerns, and Adaptations

The therapeutic action of melatonin may interact synergistically to enhance the hypnotic effect of benzodiazepines. Physicians prescribing benzodiazepines can monitor patients for melatonin deficiency and prescribe oral melatonin as appropriate. Even without confirmed melatonin deficiency, melatonin augmentation can be presented to patients as a potential tool in facilitating withdrawal from benzodiazepine therapy by moderating adverse effects and assisting them to reestablish normal sleep cycles. Thus, successful use of melatonin and triazolam together enables exploration of decreasing the dosage level of the benzodiazepine and potentially weaning the patient off the medication if sleep has improved and stabilized.

These preliminary findings are encouraging, but further research is necessary to determine whether individuals taking triazolam or another benzodiazepine might also benefit from concomitant use of melatonin (3 mg time-release preparation before bedtime) to enhance efficacy of sleep promotion and minimize adverse effects such as morning grogginess. Such research could also focus on questions of patient variability, choice and dosage of benzodiazepine agent used, pace and method of transition, and guidelines for determining appropriateness of concomitant use or benzodiazepine withdrawal. Coadministration of such agents warrants close supervision and regular monitoring by health care professionals trained and experienced in both conventional pharmacology and nutritional therapeutics, preferably within an integrative care context, to avoid excessive sedation due to additive hypnotic effects from the combined agents.

Beta-1-Adrenoceptor Antagonists (Beta-1-Adrenergic Blocking Agents)

Oral forms (systemic).
Evidence: Atenolol (Tenormin), propranolol (Betachron, Inderal LA, Innopran XL, Inderal).
Extrapolated, based on similar properties: Acebutolol (Sectral); atenolol combination drugs: atenolol and chlorthalidone

(Co-Tendione, Tenoretic), atenolol and nifedipine (Beta-Adalat, Tenif), betaxolol (Kerlone), bisoprolol (Zebeta), carteolol (Cartrol), esmolol (Brevibloc), labetalol (Normodyne, Trandate), metoprolol (Lopressor, Toprol XL); combination drug: metoprolol and hydrochlorothiazide (Lopressor HCT); nadolol (Corgard), nebivolol (Nebilet), oxprenolol (Trasicor), penbutolol (Levatol), pindolol (Visken); propranolol combination drug: propranolol and bendrofluazide (Inderex); sotalol (Betapace, Betapace AF, Sorine), timolol (Blocadren).
Similar properties but evidence indicating no or reduced interaction effects: Carvedilol (Creg).
Related but evidence against extrapolation: Beta-adrenergic blocking eyedrops (Ophthalmic forms).

Interaction Type and Significance

≈≈≈ **Drug-Induced Nutrient Depletion, Supplementation Therapeutic, Not Requiring Professional Management**
☼ **Prevention or Reduction of Drug Adverse Effect**

Probability:	Evidence Base:
3. Possible	◉ Emerging

Effect and Mechanism of Action

Beta-adrenergic receptor antagonist agents appear to suppress melatonin synthesis with chronic use by blocking beta-1-adrenergic receptors in the pineal gland, specifically enzyme inhibition of serotonin N-acetyltransferase activity, along with the target beta-1 receptors in the heart.

Research

In an early animal study (1984), Steinlechner et al.[26] investigated the effect of propranolol in suppressing the normal nighttime rise in pineal melatonin levels in both Syrian hamsters and rats. Ten years later, Rommel et al.[27] examined the effect of 10 weeks' treatment with propranolol and ridazolol on melatonin synthesis and on sleep quality in 42 patients being treated for essential hypertension. Even though a 50% reduction of melatonin was observed, as measured by urinary sulfatoxymelatonin excretion rates before and after 6 and 10 weeks of beta-blocker administration, no significant adverse effects were reported in a standardized self-rating sleep inventory. These researchers suggested that pineal mechanisms were able to compensate for the drug-induced blockage of the β_1-adrenergic receptor transduction system and maintain the melatonin signal sufficiently to continue relatively normal sleep patterns. More recently, Stoschitzky et al.[28] conducted a randomized, double-blind, placebo-controlled, crossover study involving 15 healthy subjects, in which a 6-sulfatoxymelatonin (aMT6s) radioimmunoassay was performed subsequent to single oral doses of several beta blockers [(R)-propranolol, (S)-propranolol, (R)-atenolol, (S)-atenolol, (R,S)-carvedilol, (R,S)-verapamil] or placebo. They found that only the specifically beta-blocking (S)-enantiomers of propranolol and atenolol decreased the nocturnal production of melatonin and concluded that beta blockers decrease melatonin release through specific inhibition of β_1-adrenergic receptors and could thereby induce sleep disturbances.

Nutritional Therapeutics, Clinical Concerns, and Adaptations

Sleep disturbances are a well-known adverse effect of beta-adrenoreceptor blocker therapy. Physicians prescribing beta blockers are advised to query patients about changes in sleep patterns subsequent to medication. Assessment of melatonin levels for deficiency state can be confirmatory but may not be

Nutrient-Drug Interactions and Drug-Induced Nutrient Depletions

necessary. A clinical trial of melatonin (2-3 mg/day, preferably sustained-release preparation, before bedtime) may compensate for drug-induced depletion pattern and facilitate restoration of healthy sleep patterns. No evidence exists at this time to indicate that such melatonin intake would interfere with the therapeutic action of the beta blockers.

Chemotherapy and Radiotherapy

Including: Cisplatin (*cis*-diaminedichloroplatinum, CDDP; Platinol, Platinol-AQ), cyclophosphamide (Cytoxan, Neosar), docetaxel (Taxotere), doxorubicin (Adriamycin, Rubex), etoposide (Eposin, Etophos, VePesid, VP-16), fluorouracil (5-FU; Adrucil, Efudex, Efudix, Fluoroplex), gemcitabine (Gemzar), irinotecan (camptothecin-11, CPT-11; Campto, Camptosar), methotrexate (Folex, Maxtrex, Rheumatrex), paclitaxel (Paxene, Taxol), tumor necrosis factor alpha (TNF-α).
See also Interleukin 2 (IL-2), Tamoxifen, and Triptorelin.

Interaction Type and Significance

☼ **Prevention or Reduction of Drug Adverse Effect**
⊕⊕ **Beneficial or Supportive Interaction, with Professional Management**

Probability:	Evidence Base:
2. Probable	◉ **Emerging**

Effect and Mechanism of Action

Melatonin, at high dosages (typically 10-20 mg/day, often as high as 50 mg/day), has been used in combination with a variety of chemotherapeutic agents to ameliorate adverse drug effects and enhance chemotherapy cytotoxicity. At this point, published research indicates that melatonin's activity is attributable to its ability to reduce oxidative stress and inflammation, directly influence the neuroendocrine-immune system regulatory axis, promote apoptosis of cancer cells, and cause release of immunomodulating cytokines by activated T cells and monocytes.[29-34]

Research

Neri et al.[35] (1994) conducted a 12-month clinical trial in which 22 patients with metastatic renal cell carcinoma were treated with the combination of human lymphoblastoid interferon (IFN), 3 mega units (MU) intramuscularly three times per week, and melatonin, 10 mg/day orally, and then evaluated for response and toxicity. Three complete and four partial remissions (33%) were reported among the 21 evaluable patients, and nine achieved stable disease; five progressed. General toxicity was mild, with adverse effects generally of moderate severity and reversible. Several years later, these Italian researchers conducted immunoradiometric assays for tumor necrosis factor alpha (TNF-α); interleukins 1, 2, and 6 (IL-1, IL-2, IL-6); and interferon gamma (IFN-γ) after administering melatonin, 10 mg/day orally, for 3 months to 31 patients with advanced solid tumors (7 gastric, 9 enteric, 8 renal, 5 bladder, 2 prostate) who were unresponsive to chemotherapy and radiotherapy. After 3 months of therapy, marked by an absence of adverse reactions, 12 patients (39%) reported an improvement in their general well-being, demonstrated significant decrease of IL-6 circulating levels, and showed disease stabilization with no further growth of either the primary tumor or metastases.[31]

In a randomized preliminary study, Brackowski et al.[36] investigated the effects of TNF-α versus combined TNF-α and melatonin in the treatment of 14 advanced-cancer patients with metastatic solid tumors for whom no effective

conventional therapy was available. Those patients receiving melatonin were administered 40 mg/day orally, starting 7 days before the TNF-α. Five consecutive days of intravenous (IV) recombinant human TNF-α was then administered at 0.75 mg/day. Although many adverse effects of TNF-α therapy were common to both groups, lymphocyte mean number observed at the end of TNF-α infusion was significantly higher and asthenia and hypotension significantly less frequent in subjects receiving both agents. The authors concluded that this small trial suggested that melatonin coadministration offered a strong possibility of modulating TNF-α toxicity and biological activity. Nevertheless, while this study utilizing TNF-α is theoretically interesting, TNF-α as a therapy is strictly in the experimental phase and not being used clinically.

Over more than a decade, Lissoni et al.[37-42] have conducted a series of clinical trials investigating potential roles for melatonin within emerging integrative approaches to cancer care, with a focus on patients in a poor clinical state. Initially, they looked at using melatonin in conjunction with radiotherapy in treating patients with brain glioblastomas, reporting that this "radioneuroendocrine strategy...may prolong the survival time and improve the quality of life of patients" affected by this condition known for very poor prognosis.[37] In a small, randomized, controlled study involving 50 patients with unresectable brain metastases caused by solid neoplasms were treated with steroids and anticonvulsants as supportive care alone or in combination with 20 mg melatonin each evening. Among subjects receiving only steroids and anticonvulsants, 88% (21 of 26) died within 1 year, compared with 63% (15 of 24) in the group who also received melatonin. The survival at 1 year, free-from-brain-progression period, and mean survival time were significantly higher in patients who had received the melatonin, whereas steroid-induced metabolic and infective complications were significantly more frequent in those treated only with steroids and anticonvulsants.[38] In 1997, Lissoni et al.[39] published the results of a randomized study comparing combination cisplatin and etoposide chemotherapy versus cisplatin, etoposide and melatonin, "chemoendocrine therapy" as they have termed it, as a first-line treatment of advanced non–small cell lung cancer (NSCLC) patients. Although higher in patients receiving melatonin, improvement in the tumor response rate was not statistically significant. However, compared to subjects who received chemotherapy alone, patients treated with concomitant chemotherapy and melatonin demonstrated a significantly higher percentage of 1-year survival and greater tolerance of chemotherapy, particularly a significantly lower incidence of myelosuppression, neuropathy, and cachexia. Also in 1997, Lissoni et al.[40] conducted a clinical trial of 80 individuals with a range of advanced metastatic solid tumors and found that combining 20 mg melatonin each evening with various chemotherapeutic regimens measurably reduced several common chemotherapy-induced adverse effects. Subsequently, this same team of Italian researchers reported decreased toxicity and increased efficacy of cancer chemotherapy using melatonin in a randomized trial involving 250 patients with metastatic solid tumors. Chemotherapy consisted of cisplatin plus etoposide or gemcitabine alone for lung cancer; doxorubicin alone, mitoxantrone alone, or paclitaxel alone for breast cancer; 5-FU plus folinic acid for gastrointestinal tumors; and 5-FU plus cisplatin for head and neck cancers. Compared to patients treated with antineoplastic agents alone, those treated with melatonin (20 mg/day orally) and chemotherapy concomitantly demonstrated significantly higher 1-year survival rate and objective tumor regression rate, as well as reduced frequency of thrombocytopenia, neurotoxicity, cardiotoxicity, stomatitis, and asthenia.[41] Subsequent studies using melatonin in conjunction with conventional chemotherapy (e.g., irinotecan, etoposide, cisplatin) have carried these research findings into further development.[42,43]

More recent animal research has noted that melatonin may provide a protective effect against doxorubicin (Adriamycin) toxicity, cisplatin-induced acute renal injury, and doxorubicin-induced cardiotoxicity.[44-46]

Birdsall et al.[47] and Cancer Treatment Centers of America conducted an exploratory trial to investigate effects of concomitant naturopathic therapies on clinical tumor response to external beam radiation therapy for early-stage prostate cancer (tumor stages 1b through 2, N0,M0). External beam radiation therapy of up to 72 Gy was given to 22 patients on a conventional 8-week treatment regimen while the 13 patients in the naturopathic group received at least one antioxidant preparation, with the most frequent antioxidant naturopathic treatments including green tea extract, melatonin, and a high-potency multivitamin, vitamin C, or vitamin E. "All patients were monitored for at least 12 months (range 12-42) and no patient received concomitant hormonal therapy." The investigators reported that in the patients "who did not receive naturopathic [antioxidant] treatments, the median pretreatment PSA level was 5.4 ng/mL, the median PSA nadir was 0.66 ng/mL, and the median time to PSA nadir was 16.0 months," while in the "patients who did receive naturopathic treatments, the corresponding values were 5.8 ng/mL; 0.59 ng/mL; and 16.0 months." One tumor treatment failure occurred in the nonnaturopathic group "based on PSA elevation >2 ng from nadir which occurred at 14 months"; there were no treatment failures in the patients who received concomitant naturopathic regimens (*PSA*, prostate-specific antigen; *CAM*, complementary and alternative medicine). The authors noted as "also significant that 9/9 patients in the non-CAM group were considered to be low risk (based on pretreatment PSA levels of 4-10 ng) whereas 3 patients in the CAM group were classified as intermediate risk (PSA >10-20 ng) and 1 patient as high risk (PSA >20 ng)." Thus, the authors concluded that "concomitant naturopathic treatment does not appear to inhibit the capacity of external beam radiation therapy to control localized prostate cancer, and does not interfere with either the magnitude of the response, the velocity of the response, or its durability for at least 1 year." They added that these "results provide definitive evidence that antioxidant-based CAM modalities, designed to improve patient tolerance, quality of life, and possibly improve survival, do not inhibit tumor responses that depend on oxidative [tumor] killing mechanisms elicited by external beam radiation therapy."[47] Although encouraging, this small, retrospective study did not have sufficient power to draw any statistically significant conclusions. Similar studies involving much larger groups of patients receiving radiotherapy are warranted.

Nutritional Therapeutics, Clinical Concerns, and Adaptations
Further research with large, well-designed clinical trials is essential, but melatonin is already playing a role in many cancer treatment protocols employing multiple therapeutic modalities within an integrative clinical strategy. Many clinicians working with difficult cases have been offering this option to patients facing poor prognoses. Emerging clinical practices have begun to produce operative interventions based on collaboration of oncologists and other health care professionals experienced in both conventional pharmacology and nutritional therapeutics.

In many clinics providing integrative oncology care, melatonin has become part of therapeutic protocols used in the treatment of almost every cancer type and chemotherapy regimen, to mitigate adverse effects and enhance efficacy. Many such care facilities consider the human clinical trial data compelling enough to extrapolate using melatonin in most patients. The only patient population for whom many experienced practitioners do not routinely use melatonin is with hematological malignancies, because immune stimulation is potentially contraindicated.

The usual dosage of melatonin ranges from moderate (10 mg daily) to extremely high (>40 mg daily) and inherently requires close supervision and regular monitoring. Physicians and other health care professionals may consider reviewing the potential for such synergistic therapies with appropriate patients and provide referral information to centers specializing in such integrative approaches.

Corticosteroids, Oral

Betamethasone (Celestone), cortisone (Cortone), dexamethasone (Decadron), fludrocortisone (Florinef), hydrocortisone (Cortef), methylprednisolone (Medrol), prednisolone (Delta-Cortef, Orapred, Pediapred, Prelone), prednisone (Deltasone, Liquid Pred, Meticorten, Orasone), triamcinolone (Aristocort).

Interaction Type and Significance

◇≈≈ **Drug-Induced Adverse Effect on Nutrient Function, Coadministration Therapeutic, with Professional Management**

? **Interaction Likely but Uncertain Occurrence and Unclear Implications**

Probability:	Evidence Base:
4. Plausible	☐ Inadequate

Effect and Mechanism of Action
Physiologically, endogenous melatonin suppresses corticosteroid activity and opposes the degeneration caused by elevated levels of endogenous corticosteroids. However, in looking at exogenous intake, administration of corticosteroids, as dexamethasone, can suppress melatonin synthesis, at least in healthy subjects.

Research
Researchers found that melatonin protects rats from injurious effects of dexamethasone in a rat model.[48] In a small, controlled trial, researchers found that administration of a single dose of dexamethasone produced measurable depression of melatonin synthesis in 9 of 11 healthy subjects.[49] Animal studies have found that prolonged treatment with dexamethasone reduces the amplitude of the rhythmic melatonin production.[50]

In potentially related research, Pawlikowski et al.[51] conducted a study on the effects of 6 months' melatonin treatment on sleep quality and serum concentrations of cortisol, as well as estradiol, dehydroepiandrosterone sulfate (DHEA-S), and somatomedin C, in elderly women. They found that melatonin treatment (2 mg each evening) did not significantly change cortisol levels.

Nutritional Therapeutics, Clinical Concerns, and Adaptations
At this point, evidence as to the clinical significance of an apparent interaction between corticosteroids and melatonin is suggestive but inconclusive. Although short-term administration of a corticosteroid agent in an experimental setting may transiently reduce melatonin levels in healthy volunteers, little is known or can be extrapolated from such findings as to

Nutrient-Drug Interactions and Drug-Induced Nutrient Depletions

the potential effect of long-term corticosteroid therapy on melatonin levels and function in individuals experiencing various dysfunctional or pathological states. Sleep disturbances are a common adverse effect of steroid medications. Coadministration of exogenous melatonin may counter adverse effects of corticosteroids, including melatonin depletion. Exogenous melatonin could theoretically interfere with the action of corticosteroid medications; however, since corticosteroids are often prescribed for symptom control, such interference would be clinically obvious in those situations. Large, well-designed clinical trials are necessary to determine the character and implications of the interaction(s) between exogenous sources of these two key hormones.

Fluoxetine

Fluoxetine (Prozac, Sarafem).
Similar properties but evidence lacking for extrapolation: Citalopram (Celexa), duloxetine (Cymbalta), escitalopram (S-citalopram; Lexapro), fluvoxamine (Faurin, Luvox), paroxetine (Aropax, Deroxat, Paxil, Seroxat), sertraline (Zoloft), venlafaxine (Effexor).

Interaction Type and Significance

≈≈   **Drug-Induced Nutrient Depletion, Supplementation Therapeutic, with Professional Management**

✗   **Potential or Theoretical Adverse Interaction of Uncertain Severity**

Probability: Evidence Base:
2. Probable   ○ Preliminary

Effect and Mechanism of Action

Fluoxetine can decrease melatonin levels in humans by a mechanism that is as yet not fully understood. Selective serotonin reuptake inhibitors (SSRIs) inhibit, with varying degrees of inhibition potency, production of serotonin (5-HT) from 5-methoxytryptamine (5-MT), a metabolite and precursor of melatonin, normally catalyzed by polymorphic cytochrome P450 2D6 (CYP2D6). Based on findings of a study on the effect of administering 5-MT O-demethylase from liver microsomes extracted from CYP2D6-transgenic mice on serum 5-HT levels, Yu et al.[52] concluded that the "regeneration of 5-HT from 5-MT provides the missing link in the serotonin-melatonin cycle." They noted that up to 10% of the population lacks 5-MT O-demethylase and proposed that "this common inborn error in 5-MT O-demethylation to serotonin influences a range of neurophysiologic and pathophysiologic events."

In potentially related research, an animal model indicates that exogenous melatonin may interfere with tryptophan-2,3-dioxygenase activity, through chemical antagonism at the surface of the enzyme, and neutralize the intended inhibitory action on the enzyme by desipramine and fluoxetine. The therapeutic mechanism of desipramine and other tricyclics is unclear. However, the fundamental therapeutic mechanism of SSRIs is by definition blocking reuptake of 5-HT into the presynaptic nerve terminals after it has been secreted, thus prolonging and increasing the serotonergic tone. Tryptophan-2,3-dioxygenase is an enzyme expressed in both liver and brain tissue that is primarily responsible for catabolizing tryptophan. Its activity is not directly involved in the blocking of 5-HT reuptake in the brain. Thus, the implications of this finding for fluoxetine activity and melatonin levels remain unclear and inconclusive.

Research

In a 6-week case-control study with 20 age- and gender-matched subjects, half of whom had been diagnosed with seasonal affective disorder (SAD) and the other half healthy controls, Childs et al.[53] measured significant reductions in melatonin concentrations for both groups on administration of fluoxetine (20 mg/day). The authors noted the contrast with tricyclics and fluvoxamine, both of which increase melatonin. In an experimental rat study, Walsh and Daya[54] found that administration of exogenous melatonin counteracted the inhibitory effects of both desipramine and fluoxetine on hepatic tryptophan-2,3-dioxygenase activity and restored normal levels of enzyme activity in rats when administered in combination with either drug. The implications of this finding for the observed effect of fluoxetine decreasing melatonin levels are not clear or conclusive.

In related research, investigators found that changes in urinary excretion of 6-sulfatoxymelatonin, the principal metabolite of melatonin, distinguished antidepressant responders from nonresponders, with a significant increase observed in the former group and a significant decrease in the latter. The important role of enhanced noradrenergic function in determining clinical response to antidepressant pharmacotherapy was suggested by the high degree of correlation between clinical response and the change in 6-sulfatoxymelatonin excretion.[55]

Nutritional Therapeutics, Clinical Concerns, and Adaptations

At this time, no definitive evidence exists to confirm whether melatonin coadministration may be appropriate or contraindicated in individuals taking fluoxetine. A generalizable answer may be elusive in light of individual variations in melatonin status and pharmacogenomic variability in response to the antidepressant.

Well-designed human trials are warranted to determine if exogenous melatonin counteracts the effects of fluoxetine in humans and whether long-term fluoxetine use induces a clinically significant melatonin depletion pattern, particularly as manifested in new or aggravated sleep disturbances. If the former condition is confirmed, melatonin would be contraindicated in patients undergoing fluoxetine therapy. If the latter, physicians observing adverse effects on sleep might consider prescribing a different antidepressant, such as one that enhances melatonin levels or allows for adjuvant use when indicated. In the absence of high-quality clinical trials, at this time it would seem reasonable to undertake careful therapeutic trials of melatonin coadministration in patients on SSRI therapy who exhibit sleep disturbances. With good patient-practitioner communication, it should be clear if the previously obtained therapeutic effects of SSRI therapy are attenuated by concomitant melatonin, in which case it should be discontinued.

Fluvoxamine

Fluvoxamine (Faurin, Luvox).
Similar properties but evidence lacking for extrapolation: Citalopram (Celexa), duloxetine (Cymbalta), escitalopram (S-citalopram; Lexapro), fluoxetine (Prozac, Sarafem), fluvoxamine (Faurin, Luvox), paroxetine (Aropax, Deroxat, Paxil, Seroxat), sertraline (Zoloft), venlafaxine (Effexor).

Interaction Type and Significance

⊕⊕   **Beneficial or Supportive Interaction, with Professional Management**

Probability: Evidence Base:
2. Probable   ◉ Emerging

Effect and Mechanism of Action

Fluvoxamine can significantly elevate serum melatonin concentrations. More than other SSRI agents, fluvoxamine is a potent inhibitor of several cytochrome P450 (CYP) enzymes, particularly CYP1A2, a high-affinity enzyme that is almost exclusively responsible for the metabolism of melatonin to 6-hydroxymelatonin and N-acetylserotonin.[56-58] Thus, fluvoxamine appears to be a specific inhibitor of melatonin degradation, that is, 6-hydroxymelatonin formation via 6-hydroxylation, thereby enhancing bioavailability of oral melatonin. This effect on the pharmacokinetics of melatonin is further subject to significant individual variability in the activity of 5-MT O-demethylase, the key enzyme in the conversion of 5-methoxytryptamine (5-MT), a metabolite and precursor of melatonin, to serotonin (5-hydroxytryptamine, 5-HT), and the relative inhibition potency of fluoxetine on CYP2D6; 5-MT is a specific and high-turnover endogenous substrate of CYP2D6.[52]

Research

Numerous researchers and clinicians have reported that fluvoxamine increased melatonin levels, but the mechanism, degree, and significance of this effect are only gradually becoming apparent. In a clinical trial involving healthy subjects, von Bahr et al.[56] confirmed that fluvoxamine increases serum melatonin and determined that CYP1A2 and CYP2C19 hydroxylate melatonin. Grozinger, Hartter, et al.[59] (2000) assessed serum concentrations of melatonin and fluvoxamine in five healthy male volunteers (one whom was a CYP2D6-poor metabolizer) after administration of 5 mg melatonin either with or without coadministration of 50 mg fluvoxamine, 0 to 28 hours later. The combination of the two agents produced a 17-fold higher average area under concentration-time curve (AUC) and a 12-fold higher average serum peak concentration (C_{max}) of melatonin. Further, in the CYP2D6-poor metabolizer, the AUC and C_{max} of fluvoxamine were approximately three times higher and the half-life about two times higher, with a generally more pronounced and longer-lasting effect of fluvoxamine on the pharmacokinetics of melatonin. The authors concluded that this enhanced bioavailability of oral melatonin by coadministration of fluvoxamine was caused by inhibition of melatonin elimination, rather than increased melatonin production.[59] Subsequently, using human liver microsomes and recombinant human CYP isoenzymes in vitro, this research team found that melatonin is almost exclusively metabolized by CYP1A2 to 6-hydroxymelatonin and N-acetylserotonin, with a minimal contribution of CYP2C19, and that fluvoxamine potently inhibited both reactions.[57]

In related research, investigators found that changes in urinary excretion of 6-sulfatoxymelatonin, the principal metabolite of melatonin, distinguished antidepressant responders from nonresponders, with a significant increase observed in the former group and a significant decrease in the latter. The important role of enhanced noradrenergic function in determining clinical response to antidepressant pharmacotherapy was suggested by the high degree of correlation between clinical response and the change in 6-sulfatoxymelatonin excretion.[55]

Further more, SSRIs inhibit, with varying degrees of inhibition potency, production of serotonin (5-HT) from 5-MT, a metabolite and precursor of melatonin, normally catalyzed by polymorphic cytochrome P450 2D6 (CYP2D6). Based on findings of a study looking at the effect of administering 5-MT O-demethylase from liver microsomes extracted from CYP2D6-transgenic mice on serum 5-HT levels, Yu et al.[52] concluded that the "regeneration of 5-HT from 5-MT provides the missing link in the serotonin-melatonin cycle." They noted that up to 10% of the population lacks 5-MT O-demethylase and proposed that "this common inborn error in 5-MT O-demethylation to serotonin influences a range of neurophysiologic and pathophysiologic events."

Reports

The German team previously mentioned reported on a case where an individual with a low-amplitude melatonin profile demonstrated strongly inhibited melatonin metabolism in response to fluvoxamine therapy.[59]

Clinical Implications and Adaptations

The cumulative evidence consistently indicates that coadministration of fluvoxamine and melatonin results in significantly elevated levels of melatonin, and potentially of fluvoxamine, and provides a reasonable mechanism of action for such effects. Nevertheless, further clinical trials will be necessary to determine more fully the clinical significance of this interaction and the opportunities it might provide for an integrative therapeutic strategy, particularly in the treatment of pharmacogenomically appropriate individuals. Fluvoxamine might be used as an enhancer of melatonin, thereby offering new therapeutic possibilities of fluvoxamine. Likewise, in some situations, coadministration might enhance clinical response to fluvoxamine in otherwise–less responsive individuals. Such experimental combination therapy would warrant close supervision and regular monitoring by health care professionals trained and experienced in both conventional pharmacology and nutritional therapeutics.

Haloperidol and Related Antipsychotic Medications

Evidence: Haloperidol (Haldol).
Extrapolated, based on similar properties: Aripiprazole (Abilify, Abilitat), chlorpromazine (Largactil, Thorazine), clozapine (Clozaril), fluphenazine (Permitil, Prolixin, Prolixin Decanoate, Prolixin Enanthate), olanzapine (Symbyax, Zyprexa), prochlorperazine (Compazine, Stemetil), quetiapine (Seroquel), risperidone (Risperdal), ziprasidone (Geodon).

Interaction Type and Significance

☼ **Prevention or Reduction of Drug Adverse Effect**

Probability:
3. Possible

Evidence Base:
○ **Preliminary**

Effect and Mechanism of Action

Tardive dyskinesia (TD) is an adverse effect of long-term antipsychotic medications that occurs in up to 50% of patients hospitalized with chronic schizophrenia. The pathophysiology of TD is incompletely understood, but both dopamine receptor supersensitivity and oxidative stress–induced neurotoxicity in the nigrostriatal system have been implicated. The rationale for investigating melatonin is based on its activity as a potent antioxidant and its ability to attenuate dopaminergic activity in the striatum and dopamine release from the hypothalamus.

Research

In a double-blind, placebo-controlled, crossover study involving 22 patients with schizophrenia, Shamir et al.[60] found that subjects receiving melatonin (10 mg daily for 6 weeks) demonstrated less severe TD symptoms after they were treated with melatonin than after they received the inactive therapy. In an editorial accompanying the Shamir paper, Glazer et al.

speculated that melatonin might be suppressing TD symptoms instead of treating them, based on its proposed mechanism of action. Furthermore, they deemed the 30% or more reduction in symptom severity as "relatively weak" and thus not attaining a 50% standard of efficacy. These editorialists concluded: "From our perspective, the treatment value of melatonin for TD is questionable."

Nutritional Therapeutics, Clinical Concerns, and Adaptations
Coadministration of antipsychotic medications and melatonin may provide a valuable tool in increasing medication compliance among individuals diagnosed with schizophrenia, as many as 40% of whom stop taking their medications because of adverse effects. This first study to demonstrate clinically meaningful improvement of TD symptoms with melatonin offers encouragement for countering at least one of the more serious adverse effects of antipsychotic medications. However, although significant, the outcome may not represent a clinically adequate intervention for the treatment and prevention of TD. Larger clinical trials are warranted. Nevertheless, because evidence is lacking for any effective alternatives, physicians prescribing haloperidol and other antipsychotic medications have the option of discussing adjunctive use of melatonin with their patients undergoing pharmacological treatment for schizophrenia.

Interleukin-2 (IL-2)

Interleukin-2 (Aldesleukin, IL-2, interleukin-2, recombinant interleukin 2, rIL-2; Proleukin).

Interaction Type and Significance
⊕⊕ **Beneficial or Supportive Interaction, with Professional Management**
☼ **Prevention or Reduction of Drug Adverse Effect**

Probability:
2. Probable

Evidence Base:
◉ **Emerging**

Effect and Mechanism of Action
Melatonin directly influences the neuroendocrine-immune system regulatory axis, promotes release of cytokines by activated T cells and monocytes, and demonstrates significant antioxidant activity. Whereas some research indicates that melatonin may exert significant independent antineoplastic activity, its primary use in cancer therapy protocols has been in conjunction with conventional chemotherapy, particularly interleukin 2 (IL-2). Melatonin appears to potentiate and increase the efficacy of IL-2.

Research
The Italian research team of Lissoni, Barni, et al.[61-69] conducted a series of clinical trials over the past decade investigating the efficacy of melatonin in conjunction with or after low-dose IL-2 chemotherapy. In an early preliminary study involving 14 patients with advanced solid neoplasms, they found that the combination of IL-2 and oral melatonin rendered previously resistant tumors more responsive to IL-2 therapy by enhancing IL-2 antitumor immune effect and by increasing the susceptibility of cancer cells to the cytolysis mediated by IL-2-induced cytotoxic lymphocytes.[61] That same year (1994) they published an important paper in the *British Journal of Cancer* reporting the results of a larger, randomized clinical trial involving 80 patients with a range of locally advanced or metastatic solid tumors, other than renal cell cancer and melanoma. These patients, all of whom had

refused conventional chemotherapy or who had not responded to previous chemotherapy, received either low-dose IL-2 alone (3 million IU/day subcutaneously, 6 days a week for 4 weeks) or in combination with melatonin (40 mg/day orally at 8:00 PM, starting 1 week before IL-2). Whereas 3 of 41 patients treated with low-dose IL-2 plus melatonin demonstrated a complete response, none responded among those receiving IL-2 alone. Eight of 41 patients treated with both low-dose IL-2 and melatonin achieved a partial response, versus only one in the IL-2-only group. Tumor objective regression rate and mean increase in lymphocyte and eosinophil number were all significantly higher in the low-dose IL-2 plus melatonin group than in patients treated with only IL-2. Survival rate after 1 year was 19 of 41 in the group receiving both agents, versus only 6 of 30 in the IL-2 group.[61]

In subsequent years, this research team has further expanded its investigation into synergistic therapies with low-dose IL-2 and melatonin. Several studies have focused on decreased adverse effects, particularly immunosuppressive events, in addition to enhanced efficacy, from combined low-dose IL-2 and melatonin therapy, compared with various forms of interleukin therapy.[62-66] In 2000, Lissoni et al.[67] reported preliminary results suggesting that concomitant administration of SC low-dose IL-2 along with oral melatonin appeared to prolong the survival time in individuals with advanced hematological malignancies that had not responded to previous standard therapies, with results comparable to those previously reported using a more toxic immunotherapy, consisting of high-dose IL-2 alone. In exploring their long-term emphasis on psychoneuroimmunomodulation, these researchers conducted a study on the use of melatonin to abrogate the negative influence of opioids, particularly morphine-induced immunosuppression, on IL-2 immunotherapy in the treatment of renal cell cancer. Thirty patients with metastatic renal cell cancer undergoing subcutaneous IL-2 therapy were randomized to receive morphine alone or morphine plus melatonin (20 mg orally each evening). No diminished analgesic efficacy of morphine occurred among patients receiving the adjuvant melatonin, but percentage of partial responses achieved and 3-year survival percentage in patients in this group were significantly higher than among those receiving morphine alone.[68] In a related preliminary study, Lissoni et al.[69] observed that adding naltrexone (100 mg orally each morning), an opioid antagonist, significantly amplified the lymphocytosis obtained by the IL-2 and melatonin combination. Because the lymphocytosis represents the most important favorable prognostic variable predicting the anticancer efficacy of IL-2 immunotherapy, these authors proposed that further research into this novel synergistic approach to cancer neuroimmunotherapy, using IL-2 with both melatonin and naltrexone to activate T-helper type 1 (Th1) lymphocytes and suppress Th2 lymphocytes, respectively.

Nutritional Therapeutics, Clinical Concerns, and Adaptations
Further research with large, well-designed clinical trials is essential, but melatonin is already playing a role in many cancer treatment protocols employing interleukin along with other therapeutic modalities within an integrative clinical strategy. Many clinicians working with difficult cases have been offering this option to patients facing poor prognoses. Emerging clinical practices have begun to produce operative interventions based on collaboration of oncologists and other health care professionals experienced in both conventional pharmacology and nutritional therapeutics. The usual dosage of melatonin ranges from moderate (10 mg daily) to extremely high (>40 mg daily),

with 20 mg daily most common, and inherently requires close supervision and regular monitoring. It is also essential to note that the studies cited were primarily using low-dose IL-2, such as 3 million IU/day, in contrast to the standard dosing of IL-2, 30 to 60 million IU, which can be an extremely toxic regimen. Furthermore, many patients being treated with IL-2, at any dosage levels, will have to be managed in the intensive care unit (ICU) while receiving IL-2 and often can experience difficulty completing the optimal number of cycles. Consequently, the use of IL-2 in integrative oncology settings is quite limited. Physicians and other health care professionals may consider reviewing the potential for such synergistic therapies with appropriate patients and provide referral information to centers specializing in such integrative approaches.

Mirtazapine

Mirtazapine (Remeron).

Interaction Type and Significance

◇◇   **Drug-Induced Effect on Nutrient Function, Supplementation Contraindicated, Professional Management Appropriate**

✗   **Potential or Theoretical Adverse Interaction of Uncertain Severity**

⊕   **Potential or Theoretical Beneficial or Supportive Interaction, with Professional Management**

Probability: Evidence Base:
4. Plausible   ○ Preliminary

Effect and Mechanism of Action

Mirtazapine, an alpha-2-adrenoceptor antagonist form of non-selective serotonin reuptake inhibitor (NSRI), can significantly increase nocturnal melatonin secretion. This apparent existence of an α_2-adrenergic influence on melatonin secretion may play a significant role in the therapeutic action of mirtazapine.

Research

In a single, small study with 10 healthy volunteers, administration of mirtazapine significantly increased nocturnal melatonin secretion.[70]

Clinical Implications and Adaptations

Controlled research with a large, well-designed clinical trial is necessary to determine whether combining melatonin and mirtazapine might produce beneficial or adverse effects, particularly on the therapeutic action of mirtazapine in the treatment of individual with depression. Combined use could potentially enable mirtazapine to provide therapeutic effect at lower doses, if that activity is in part caused by elevated melatonin levels. Melatonin might also play a role in easing withdrawal symptoms and reestablishing a regular sleep cycle in individuals developing sleep disturbances during cessation of mirtazapine use. Evidence is lacking to suggest that combined use of melatonin and mirtazapine posing any significant risk. However, pending well-designed clinical trials, such coadministration warrants close supervision and regular monitoring by health care professionals trained and experienced in both conventional pharmacology and nutritional therapeutics, preferably within an integrative care context.

Nonsteroidal Anti-Inflammatory Drugs (NSAIDs) and Acetylsalicylic Acid (Aspirin)

COX-1 inhibitors (NSAIDs): Diclofenac (Cataflam, Voltaren); combination drug: diclofenac and misoprostol (Arthrotec); diflunisal (Dolobid), etodolac (Lodine), fenoprofen (Dalfon), furbiprofen (Ansaid), ibuprofen (Advil, Excedrin IB, Motrin, Motrin IB, Nuprin, Pedia Care Fever Drops, Provel, Rufen); combination drug: hydrocodone and ibuprofen (Reprexain, Vicoprofen); indomethacin (indometacin; Indocin, Indocin-SR), ketoprofen (Orudis, Oruvail), ketorolac (Acular ophthalmic, Toradol), meclofenamate (Meclomen), mefenamic acid (Ponstel), meloxicam (Mobic), nabumetone (Relafen), naproxen (Aleve, Anaprox, Naprosyn), oxaprozin (Daypro), piroxicam (Feldene), salsalate (salicylic acid; Amigesic, Disalcid, Marthritic, Mono Gesic, Salflex, Salsitab), sulindac (Clinoril), tolmetin (Tolectin).

COX-2 inhibitor (NSAID): Celecoxib (Celebrex).

Acetylsalicylic acid (acetosal, acetyl salicylic acid, ASA, salicylsalicylic acid; Arthritis Foundation Pain Reliever, Ascriptin, Aspergum, Asprimox, Bayer Aspirin, Bayer Buffered Aspirin, Bayer Low Adult Strength, Bufferin, Buffex, Cama Arthritis Pain Reliever, Easprin, Ecotrin, Ecotrin Low Adult Strength, Empirin, Extra Strength Adprin-B, Extra Strength Bayer Enteric 500 Aspirin, Extra Strength Bayer Plus, Halfprin 81, Heartline, Regular Strength Bayer Enteric 500 Aspirin, St. Joseph Adult Chewable Aspirin, ZORprin); combination drugs: ASA and caffeine (Anacin); ASA, caffeine, and propoxyphene (Darvon Compound); ASA and carisoprodol (Soma Compound); ASA, codeine, and carisoprodol (Soma Compound with Codeine); ASA and codeine (Empirin with Codeine); ASA, codeine, butalbital, and caffeine (Fiorinal); ASA and extended-release dipyridamole (Aggrenox, Asasantin).
See also Indomethacin.

Interaction Type and Significance

☼   **Prevention or Reduction of Drug Adverse Effect**

≈≈≈   **Drug-Induced Nutrient Depletion, Supplementation Therapeutic, Not Requiring Professional Management**

◇≈≈   **Drug-Induced Adverse Effect on Nutrient Function, Coadministration Therapeutic, with Professional Management**

Probability: Evidence Base:
4. Plausible   ○ Preliminary

Effect and Mechanism of Action

Inhibition of prostaglandin synthesis is an intended effect of nonsteroidal anti-inflammatory drugs (NSAIDs). Prostaglandins are involved in melatonin synthesis and sleep, as well as thermoregulation, in such a way that NSAID administration may inhibit melatonin synthesis. This activity provides a mechanism by which NSAIDs may alter sleep patterns.

Research

Murphy et al.[71] conducted a series of experiments in which they assessed the melatonin synthesis and body temperature (BT) in 75 subjects after administration of NSAIDs (aspirin and ibuprofen) or placebo at night in a within-subjects design. They found that normal nocturnal melatonin was suppressed, and BT decrease was attenuated, after NSAID administration versus after placebo. Lower melatonin levels were associated with a relative flattening of BT. The authors interpreted these findings as indicating that NSAID-induced prostaglandin synthesis inhibition and suppression of melatonin synthesis might explain some of the behavioral changes associated with NSAIDs, including changes in sleep.

Nutritional Therapeutics, Clinical Concerns, and Adaptations

Physicians prescribing NSAIDs are advised to ask patients to be watchful for adverse effects on sleep and to consider melatonin (3 mg 45 minutes before bedtime) in such situations. Individuals taking melatonin for sleep disturbances may need to increase their nightly dosage to compensate for suppression by NSAIDs or consider other options for treatment of inflammation-related symptoms.

Tamoxifen

Tamoxifen (Nolvadex).

Interaction Type and Significance

⊕⊕ **Beneficial or Supportive Interaction, with Professional Management**

Probability:	Evidence Base:
2. Probable	○ **Emerging**

Effect and Mechanism of Action

Melatonin coadministration may enhance clinical efficacy and reduce adverse effects of tamoxifen antiestrogen therapy. Melatonin may directly modulate estrogen receptor (ER) expression and inhibit breast cancer cell growth. At this point, published research indicates that melatonin's activity is attributable to its ability to reduce oxidative stress and inflammation, directly influence the neuroendocrine-immune system regulatory axis, promote apoptosis of cancer cells, and cause release of immunomodulating cytokines by activated T cells and monocytes.[29-34]

Research

Animal research has shown that melatonin can inhibit human breast cancer cell growth in vitro. Using the ER-positive human breast tumor cell line MCF-7 and other cell lines, Blask et al.[72] found that glutathione is required for melatonin's oncostatic action, and that coadministration offers the potential of enhancing synergistic therapeutic effects.

Several small human trials have found that the addition of melatonin to conventional tamoxifen therapy enhanced clinical outcomes and reduced adverse effects in the treatment of breast cancer. In a pilot phase II study, Lissoni et al.[73] investigated the effects of concomitant melatonin therapy in 14 women with metastatic breast cancer who had not responded to therapy with tamoxifen alone or progressed after initial stable disease. Melatonin was given orally at 20 mg each evening, every day starting 7 days before tamoxifen, which was given orally at 20 mg daily at noon. A partial response was achieved in four patients (28.5%), after a median duration of 8 months. The treatment was well tolerated in all cases, with no melatonin-induced enhancement of tamoxifen toxicity. Combined treatment was generally associated with decreased mean serum levels of insulin-like growth factor 1 (IGF-1). In a related study, Lissoni et al.[74] tested a similar tamoxifen-melatonin protocol in 25 patients with metastatic solid tumors, other than breast cancer and prostate cancer, for whom no other effective standard therapy was available. Three patients had a partial response, and a stable disease was achieved in 13 other patients, whereas the remaining nine patients progressed. Further, survival longer than 1 year was observed in seven patients (28%). Subsequent in vitro and animal research into the use of melatonin to enhance the clinical efficacy of tamoxifen, although potentially moderating adverse effects, has produced encouraging results.[75-78]

Nutritional Therapeutics, Clinical Concerns, and Adaptations

Concomitant administration of melatonin may induce objective tumor regressions in metastatic breast cancer patients refractory to tamoxifen alone. Further research with large, well-designed clinical trials is essential, but melatonin is already playing a role in many cancer treatment protocols employing tamoxifen along with other therapeutic modalities within an integrative clinical strategy. Many clinicians working with difficult cases have been offering this option to patients facing poor prognoses. Emerging clinical practices have begun to produce operative interventions based on collaboration of oncologists and other health care professionals experienced in both conventional pharmacology and nutritional therapeutics. The usual dosage of melatonin ranges from moderate (10 mg daily) to extremely high (>40 mg daily) and inherently requires close supervision and regular monitoring, preferably within the context of multidisciplinary care. Physicians and other health care professionals may consider reviewing the potential for such synergistic therapies with appropriate patients and provide referral information to centers specializing in such integrative approaches.

Triptorelin

Triptorelin (De-capeptyl Trelstar, Trelstar LA).

Interaction Type and Significance

⊕⊕ **Beneficial or Supportive Interaction, with Professional Management**

Probability:	Evidence Base:
2. Probable	○ **Preliminary**

Effect and Mechanism of Action

Triptorelin is a luteinizing hormone–releasing hormone (LHRH) analog that causes the testes/ovaries to shut down (after an initial increase in function) and is useful for treatment of hormone-sensitive cancers in men and premenopausal women. Concomitant use of melatonin appears to enhance clinical efficacy of triptorelin, although the mechanism of action is unknown. Melatonin may stimulate hormone receptor expression on both normal and cancer cells. Melatonin has apparently inhibited the growth of some cancer cell lines, including prostate cancer, either by exerting a direct cytostatic action or by decreasing the endogenous production of some tumor growth factors, such as prolactin and IGF-1.

Research

Fourteen consecutive metastatic prostate cancer patients with poor clinical conditions, refractory or resistant to a previous therapy with triptorelin alone, were given melatonin (20 mg orally each evening) with triptorelin intramuscular injections starting after 7 days and then repeated every 28 days. Eight of the patients (57%) demonstrated a decrease in PSA serum levels greater than 50%, and PSA mean concentrations significantly decreased in those receiving the combined triptorelin and melatonin therapy; mean serum levels of both prolactin and IGF-1, important tumor growth factors, also decreased significantly. Three of five patients with persistent thrombocytopenia before the study experienced a normalization of platelet number. Importantly, 9 of 14 patients (64%), who had been evaluated as being in poor clinical condition, achieved survival longer than 1 year.[79]

Nutritional Therapeutics, Clinical Concerns, and Adaptations

The findings from preliminary research suggests that the concomitant administration of melatonin may facilitate reversal of clinical resistance to triptorelin, and possibly other LHRH analogs, and improve drug response, outcomes, and quality of life in patients with metastatic prostatic cancer. Larger, well-designed clinical trials appear warranted.

Verapamil

Verapamil (Calan, Calan SR, Covera-HS, Isoptin, Isoptin SR, Verelan, Verelan PM).
Extrapolated, based on similar properties: Verapamil combination drug: trandolapril and verapamil (Tarka).

Interaction Type and Significance

≈≈≈ **Drug-Induced Nutrient Depletion,**
            Supplementation Therapeutic, Not Requiring
            Professional Management

Probability: Evidence Base:
2. Probable   ○ Preliminary

Effect and Mechanism of Action

Verapamil influences the renal and hepatic handling of melatonin, resulting in increased urinary melatonin excretion.

Research

After noting that individuals with primary hyperparathyroidism have higher serum melatonin concentrations during active disease than after surgical cure, Wikner et al.[80] conducted a three-part experiment to determine whether exogenous hypercalcemia, as induced by calcium channel blockers such as verapamil, would similarly inhibit nocturnal melatonin secretion. After eight healthy volunteers were treated, on separate occasions, with oral verapamil and placebo, verapamil increased urinary melatonin excretion significantly (by 67%), but did not alter excretion of 6-sulphatoxymelatonin, the primary melatonin metabolite excreted by the kidneys. Verapamil did not affect nocturnal melatonin secretion.

Nutritional Therapeutics, Clinical Concerns, and Adaptations

Although the mechanism of this proposed depletion pattern appears consistent with known research and pharmacological principles, its clinical significance remains undetermined at this time. Larger, well-designed clinical trials are warranted, preferably involving subjects with medical conditions for which verapamil would normally be prescribed. Pending such evidence, physicians prescribing verapamil or other calcium channel blockers may want to query relevant patients regarding sleep disruption as a potential adverse effect and discuss the option of corrective melatonin intake, usually 2 to 3 mg daily, before bedtime. Although evidence is lacking to indicate a significant risk from melatonin administration, close supervision and regular monitoring may be warranted in the event that the option to supplement is chosen, preferably within an integrative care context.

THEORETICAL, SPECULATIVE, AND PRELIMINARY INTERACTIONS RESEARCH, INCLUDING OVERSTATED INTERACTIONS CLAIMS

Anticoagulants

Anticoagulants
Melatonin may theoretically increase the risk of bleeding from anticoagulant medications such as warfarin. However, well-founded case reports and substantive evidence from well-designed clinical trials is lacking.

Bupropion, Desipramine, Tranylcypromine

Bupropion (Wellbutrin), desipramine (Norpramin, Pertofrane), tranylcypromine (Parnate).
The research by Walsh and Daya[54] previously discussed regarding fluoxetine and melatonin's interference with trypto-phan-2,3-dioxygenase activity could theoretically be extrapolated to related antidepressant medications. However, well-founded case reports and substantive evidence from well-designed clinical trials are lacking. Pending clarification, concurrent melatonin should be avoided outside the context of close supervision and regular monitoring by health care professionals trained and experienced in both conventional pharmacology and nutritional therapeutics, preferably within an integrative care context.

Clonidine; Methoxamine

Clonidine (Apo-Clonidine, Catapres Oral, Catapres-TTS Transdermal Dixarit, Duraclon, Novo-Clonidine, Nu-Clonidine); combination drug: clonidine and chlorthalidone (Combipres).
Methoxamine (Vasoxyl).
In an ex vivo experiment using thoracic aorta excised from male rats, melatonin reduced the efficacy, but not potency, of the contractile responses to methoxamine and clonidine by relaxing vascular smooth muscle. Low doses of melatonin appear to impair alpha-1- and alpha-2-adrenergic responses without changes in the beta-adrenergic response of vascular smooth muscle. The experimental data suggest that the inositol phosphate pathway may be involved in this relaxation, but the mechanism remains undetermined.[81]
Well-founded case reports and substantive evidence from well-designed clinical trials are lacking to suggest whether exogenous melatonin might substantively interfere with the effects of methoxamine and clonidine in humans. Pending clarification, concurrent melatonin should be avoided outside the context of close supervision and regular monitoring by health care professionals trained and experienced in both conventional pharmacology and nutritional therapeutics, preferably within an integrative care context.

Cyclosporine

Cyclosporine (Ciclosporin, cyclosporin A, CsA; Neoral, Sandimmune, SangCya).
Animal research using rats indicates that concomitant administration of melatonin during cyclosporin A therapy may reduce nephrotoxic effects of the drug, possibly by reducing oxidative stress.[82] Further research, moving toward clinical trials, appears warranted by the findings from this preliminary study.

Cytochrome 1A2 Isoenzyme Substrates

Caffeine, clozapine (Clozaril), haloperidol (Haldol), tacrine (tetrahydroaminoacridine, THA; Cognex), theophylline/aminophylline (Phyllocontin, Slo-Bid, Slo-Phyllin, Theo-24, Theo-Bid, Theocron, Theo-Dur, Theolair, Truphylline, Uni-Dur, Uniphyl); combination drug: ephedrine, guai-fenesin, and theophylline (Primatene Dual Action); other medications.
Research involving SSRIs (see previous section) suggests a high probability that melatonin, both at physiological levels and after oral administration, might result in interaction with drugs metabolized by CYP1A2.[20,56,58]

Cytochrome 2C9 Isoenzyme Substrates

NSAIDs, phenytoin (diphenylhydantoin; Dilantin, Phenytek), warfarin (Coumadin, Marevan, Warfilone), zafirlukast (Accolate, Accoleit, Vanticon), other medications.

In vitro data suggest melatonin may affect the disposition of drugs metabolized by the CYP2C9 isoenzyme system.[58]

Estrogens, Progestins, and Estrogen-Progestin Combinations

Hormone replacement therapy (HRT): Estrogen-containing and synthetic estrogen and progesterone analog medications. Oral contraceptives (OCs): Monophasic, biphasic, and triphasic estrogen preparations (synthetic estrogen and progesterone analogs).

Melatonin demonstrates antiestrogenic activity. More fundamentally, given current knowledge of the interplay between melatonin and female hormones, an interaction will likely be revealed with concerted investigation and well-designed clinical trials. The incidence of adverse and unintended effects from administration of exogenous hormones suggest the potential for some of those effects to be attributable, at least in part, to their influence on melatonin and the manner in which the physiological self-regulatory mechanisms of the endocrine system express themselves in daily, monthly, and annual cycles.

Indomethacin

Indomethacin (Indomethacin; Indocin, Indocin-SR).

In a rat model, Singh et al.[83] found that by scavenging of oxygen-derived free radicals, a combination of melatonin (20 mg/kg) and beta-carotene decreased the ulcer index and lipid peroxidation, and reduced the decrease in antioxidant enzyme levels, in exerting a protective effect against indomethacin-induced gastric injury.

Vitamin B₆—Depleting Drugs

Estrogen, hydralazine, 1-hydrazinophthalazine monohydrochloride; Apresoline; combination drugs: hydralazine and hydrochlorothiazide (Apresazide); hydralazine and isosorbide dinitrate (BiDil); loop diuretics, OCs, penicillamine (D-penicillamine; Cuprimine, Depen), theophylline; other drugs.

Drugs that deplete vitamin B₆ may induce a deficiency of pyridoxine that affects the tryptophan-serotonin-melatonin pathway and inhibits the synthesis of melatonin.[84-88] Pending large, well-designed clinical trials, physicians prescribing such medications may want to query relevant patients regarding sleep disruption as a potential adverse effect and discuss the option of corrective melatonin administration, usually 2 to 3 mg daily, before bedtime. The possibility that compensatory melatonin intake might interfere has yet to be investigated in a systematic manner. Close supervision and regular monitoring may be warranted if the option to coadminister melatonin is chosen.

Sedative Medications

Theoretically, concomitant use of sedative agents and oral melatonin may result in an additive effect and excessive central nervous system (CNS) sedation. Prudence suggests that such combinations be avoided outside the close supervision and regular monitoring by health care professionals trained and experienced in both conventional pharmacology and nutritional therapeutics.

NUTRIENT-NUTRIENT INTERACTIONS

Alcohol/Ethanol

Consumption of ethanol during the evening, in quantities comparable to typical social consumption, has been found to inhibit nocturnal melatonin secretion in a randomized, double-blind, crossover study involving healthy volunteers.[89] This observed depletion pattern might play a role in the sleep disturbances common to alcohol consumption, particularly on a chronic basis. Evidence is lacking to suggest that compensatory melatonin use might be beneficial or problematic.

Tryptophan

Tryptophan and melatonin synthesis and metabolism are intimately related, and tryptophan administration may help correct low-melatonin responses.

Vitamin B₆, Pyridoxine

A pyridoxine deficiency state may affect the tryptophan-serotonin-melatonin pathway and inhibit the synthesis of melatonin. Concomitant use of substances may be appropriate.

Vitamin B₁₂

Vitamin B₁₂ can influence melatonin secretion, although evidence is mixed as to the character and degree of that effect, particularly in different populations and settings. Vitamin B₁₂ may phase-advance the human circadian rhythm by increasing the light sensitivity of the circadian clock.[90]

The low vitamin B₁₂ status of many elderly patients may be related to their levels of melatonin. The beneficial effects of melatonin on sleep-wake cycles may be enhanced by 1.5 mg of vitamin B₁₂ (methylcobalamin) daily, presumably because of improved melatonin secretion.

HERB-NUTRIENT INTERACTIONS

Hypnotic Herbs

Some herbs used traditionally to induce or deepen sleep may have additive or synergistic interactions with melatonin. Physicians treating individuals choosing to combine melatonin with lemon balm (*Melissa officinalis*), hops (*Humulus lupulus*), valerian (*Valeriana officinalis*), passiflora (*Passiflora incarnata*), or similar herbs for the treatment of chronic or recalcitrant insomnia are advised to consult with or refer to health care professionals trained and experienced in botanical medicine and nutritional therapeutics. Proper diagnosis is always an essential prerequisite to any safe and effective treatment of a chronic condition.

The 90 citations for this monograph, as well as additional reference literature, are located under Melatonin on the CD at the back of the book.

Omega-3 Fatty Acids

Nutrient Name: Omega-3 fatty acids (ALA, DHA, EPA).

Synonyms: Alpha-linolenic acid (ALA), docosahexaenoic acid (DHA), eicosapentaenoic acid (EPA).

Synonyms, Collective: Essential fatty acids (EFAs); polyunsaturated fatty acids (PUFAs); omega-3s, n-3 fatty acids.

Fish Oils: Docosahexaenoic acid (DHA), eicosapentaenoic acid (EPA); cod liver oil; ethyl-omega-3 fatty acids.

Flaxseed and Flaxseed Oil *(Linum usitatissimum)*: Alpha linolenic acid, alpha-linolenic acid, ALA, type I flaxseed/flaxseed (51%-55% ALA), type II flaxseed/CDC-flaxseed (2%-3% ALA); alashi, brazen, common flax, flachssamen, flax, Graine de Lin, leinsamen, hu-ma-esze, Linaceae, linen flax, lini semen, lino, lino usuale, linseed, linseed oil, lint bells, linum, *Linum catharticum, Linum humile* seeds, keten, sufulsi, tesi-mosina, winterlien.

Alpha-linolenic acid (ALA): Canola/rapeseed, eichium oil, hemp seed oil, perilla, purslane; fiber.

Summary

Drug/Class Interaction Type	Mechanism and Significance	Management
Angiotensin-converting enzyme (ACE) inhibitors ⊕⊕	Fish oil may decrease immunological renal injury in patients with IgA nephropathy and thereby slow the decline in renal function. Research has been limited and findings mixed. Significant adverse effects or interference with drug efficacy appear improbable.	Consider coadministration of fish oils with ACE inhibitors in IgA nephropathy to reduce renal damage and slow disease progression. Closely monitor high-risk patients.
Anticonvulsant medications (AEDs) ⊕⊕	Concomitant use of fish oil with anticonvulsant drugs may enhance therapeutic action through mediation of inflammatory processes, shifting fatty acid balance away from arachidonic acid, and other, more general effects. Preliminary findings indicate reduced frequency of seizures with low omega-3 oil dosages. Limited duration of benefits suggests need to investigate dose, form, and other issues of administration. Significant adverse effects or interference with drug efficacy appear improbable.	Consider coadministration of fish oil with AEDs. Dose varies according to patient characteristics. Food sources also advisable.
Chemotherapy Cytotoxic agents ⊕⊕/☼	Fish oil may benefit oncology patients in many ways, particularly by reversing decreased appetite and weight loss associated with both cancer and chemotherapy. Mechanisms are uncertain, but EPA and DHA can alter proinflammatory cytokine production and acute-phase protein synthesis, as well as mitigate oxidative damage and drug toxicity and protect healthy cardiac function, without reducing drug efficacy. Findings suggest type of cancer and disease stage can influence degree of benefit.	Consider incorporating fish oil into cancer treatment protocols for patients with or at risk for cachexia, to restore appetite and prevent or recover weight loss, particularly in patients with low fish intake. Food sources also advisable. Close monitoring appropriate.
Cyclosporine ⊕⊕/☼	Coadministration of fish oil during cyclosporine therapy may support kidney function and reduce hypertension without adversely affecting drug activity, rates of rejection, or graft survival. Diverse mechanisms are likely, with preservation of microvascular endothelial function being central. Evidence is mixed regarding degree of benefit to renal function but largely favorable.	Consider coadministration. Dose varies according to patient characteristics. Food sources also advisable. Closely monitor renal function.
Etretinate ⊕⊕	Addition of fish oil may enhance therapeutic efficacy of oral etretinate for patients with recalcitrant psoriasis. Adverse effects from fish oil are improbable, but drug has limited use since being banned in the U.S. and Canada. Studies and reports on possible interactions with similar drugs are not available, but synergy with acitretin (which replaced etretinate in the U.S. and Canada) seems likely, given the similarity between these oral retinoids.	Consider coadministration. Other pharmacological agents with a superior safety profile may be preferable.
HMG-CoA reductase inhibitors (statins) ⊕⊕	Fish oil and statin therapy can provide a synergistic effect in mixed dyslipidemias, particularly with integrative strategy combining healthy diet, regular exercise, and customized nutrient support program. While improving numerous vascular characteristics and predictably reducing triglycerides, fish oil administration may increase LDL levels and decrease glycemic control. These potential adverse effects	Fish oil is important to integrative treatment of dyslipidemias and prevention of cardiovascular disease. Known benefits on triglycerides can complement other agents; these may be required to counter potential LDL-elevating effects of fish oil.

Summary		
Drug/Class Interaction Type	Mechanism and Significance	Management
	may be transient or related to patient-specific factors, but can be prevented with aerobic exercise and pectin fiber. Combination therapies to enhance risk reduction, increase therapeutic effect, and mitigate adverse effects may offer evolving and personalized options for cardiovascular care.	Support for exercise and healthy diet are central to any comprehensive program.
Selective serotonin reuptake inhibitor (SSRI) antidepressants ⊕⊕	Coadministration of fish oil, preferably with an increased proportion of DHA, may enhance therapeutic activity of antidepressant medications. Mechanisms not fully established but include critical role of EFAs in normal serotonin synthesis. Research limited and findings more often positive than not, but continued clinical trials anticipated. Adverse effects are improbable.	Combine with regular exercise, stress management, and healthy dietary changes for comprehensive approach. Ethyl ester or other preparation may be preferable. Food sources also advisable, particularly with prior low fish intake.
Sulfasalazine Corticosteroids, oral ⊕⊕/☼	Omega-3 fatty acids may reduce many symptoms of inflammatory bowel disease, especially through modulating inflammation, reducing oxidative stress, and altering phospholipid-membrane fatty acid composition. Concomitant therapy with sulfasalazine may exert multiple additive effects, particularly on balance between pro-oxidant and antioxidant mechanisms. Findings show effect on inflammation often limited, but consistent ability to reduce corticosteroid dose. Further research warranted.	Patients with inflammatory bowel conditions may benefit from omega-3 fatty acid monotherapy (ALA or fish oil) or as complement to sulfasalazine or other anti-inflammatory agents.

IgA, Immunoglobulin A; *AEDs*, antiepileptic drugs; *LDL*, low-density lipoprotein, *HMG-CoA*, 3-hydroxy-3-methylglutaryl coenzyme A.

NUTRIENT DESCRIPTION

Chemistry and Forms

Fish Oils: Docosahexaenoic acid (DHA), eicosapentaenoic acid (EPA); cod liver oil; ethyl-omega-3 fatty acids.

Flaxseed and Flaxseed Oil (*Linum usitatissimum*): Alpha linolenic acid, alpha-linolenic acid, ALA, type I flaxseed/flaxseed (51%-55% ALA), type II flaxseed/CDC-flaxseed (2%-3% ALA); alashi, brazen, common flax, flachssamen, flax, Graine de Lin, leinsamen, hu-ma-esze, Linaceae, linen flax, lini semen, lino, lino usuale, linseed, linseed oil, lint bells, linum, *Linum catharticum, Linum humile* seeds, keten, sufulsi, tesi-mosina, winterlien.

Alpha-linolenic acid (ALA): Canola/rapeseed, eichium oil, hemp seed oil, perilla, purslane; fiber.

Related Substances: DHA-45, ethyl-omega-3 fatty acids, Omacor; gamma-linolenic acid (GLA, as in borage, evening primrose, and black currant seeds), hemp seed oil, linoleic acid (LA), n-6 fatty acids, omega-6 fatty acids, omega-6s, omega-9s (from olive and macadamia nuts), vegetable oils.

Note: Omega-6 fatty acids are physiologically and clinically distinct and should not be confused with fatty acids of the omega-3 series.

Physiology and Function

The designation "omega" indicates at which position the first unsaturated (double) bond occurs at the noncarboxyl end of the molecule. Therefore, the first double bond in the omega-3 series is between the third and fourth carbon atoms, for the omega-6 series it is between the sixth and seventh carbon atoms, and for the omega-9 series, between the ninth and tenth carbon atom, from the noncarboxyl end of the molecule. There is no evidence that fatty acids from the omega-3, -6, and -9 series can be interconverted between series in the body.

Omega-3 fatty acids are essential to human physiology, particularly the immune system, circulatory system and central nervous system (CNS), and are obtained through foods and produced endogenously. Fish is the major dietary source of long-chain omega-3 polyunsaturated fatty acids (PUFAs), specifically the 20-carbon *eicosapentaenoic acid* (EPA) and the 22-carbon *docosahexaenoic acid* (DHA). Linoleic acid and linolenic acid are also essential fatty acids (EFAs). *Alpha-linolenic acid* (ALA) is an 18-carbon omega-3 polyunsaturated EFA that can serve as an essential precursor to both EPA and DHA. Humans are capable of synthesizing small amounts of EPA and DHA from ALA, but an as-yet undetermined dietary requirement of DHA and EPA is probable. Conversion of ALA by humans to the more active, longer-chain EPA and DHA is inefficient: less than 5% to 10% for EPA and less than 1% for DHA in men, whereas women can convert up to 9% of ALA to DHA, possibly because of the importance of DHA in fetal and infant nutriture.[1] Thus, total, ALA requirements may be higher for vegetarians than for nonvegetarians, because vegetarians must rely on conversion of ALA to EPA and DHA.[2] Algae-derived DHA supplements may also be an important nutrient source for vegetarians, particularly for men and weaned vegetarian children. EPA may be produced in vivo by beta-oxidation of DHA, although increased availability of algae-derived EPA supplements in the next few years is anticipated. Algae-derived omega-3 fatty acids will undoubtedly become increasingly important for nonvegetarians given the limited capacity of ocean fish stocks to sustain their populations in the face of increasing human demands and habitat destruction.

Linoleic acid, an EFA of the omega-6 series, which occurs naturally in many warm-weather vegetable oils, is the precursor of arachidonic acid (AA), which serves as substrate for inflammatory prostaglandins, thromboxane, and leukotrienes. Extensive research indicates that omega-3 fatty acids modulate inflammation and support healthy function of neural, cardiovascular, joint, and connective tissue. EPA modulates clotting and has a significant anti-inflammatory effect through its impact on prostaglandin metabolism.

The activity of omega-3 fatty acids in modulating immune function involves several important mechanisms. These oils play pivotal roles in the resolution of inflammatory processes through modulation of proinflammatory and prothombotic eicosanoid production (prostaglandins, thromboxane, and leukotrienes derived from AA) and reduction in interleukin-1 (IL-1) and other inflammatory cytokines. They are also directly involved in anti-inflammatory eicosanoid production. The partial replacement of AA with EPA in cell membrane lipids appears to play a key role in the activity and effects of omega-3 fatty acids. EPA acts as a substrate for the synthesis of the PG3 series of prostaglandins and increases production of these prostaglandins and thromboxane A_3 (TXA$_3$), which produce less inflammation than the PG2 series and TXA$_2$ (derived from AA), which they displace. Similarly, EPA acts as the source of series 5 leukotrienes, which have weaker inflammatory effects, while AA acts as the source of the more inflammatory series 4 leukotrienes. TXA$_3$, derived from EPA, is less potent in stimulating platelet aggregation than TXA$_2$, with attendant decrease in thrombotic risk. Furthermore, DHA inhibits the formation of the more inflammatory prostaglandins of the PG2 series, while EPA acts as a substrate for the synthesis of the less inflammatory prostaglandins of the PG3 series.

Fish oils benefit lipid metabolism and cardiovascular function through a variety of mechanisms not fully elucidated. Fish oils, by replacing other membrane fatty acids with omega-3 fats, improve blood flow characteristics, and also decrease platelet aggregation, all of which benefits individuals with atherosclerosis and at risk of clotting off a cerebral or coronary vessel. On the other hand, with individuals at risk for bleeding for other reasons, fish oils may slightly increase that tendency. The activity of EPA and DHA on peroxisome proliferator-activated receptor alpha (PPAR-α) appears to play a role in reducing triglycerides, modulating inflammatory reaction, and optimizing body composition.

These EFAs, particularly DHA, are highly concentrated in the brain's gray matter and retina and play a central role in neurological, cognitive, and behavioral development and function.[3,4] Brain cell membrane fluidity is essential for communication between neurons, and DHA helps maintain cell membrane fluidity as well as replenish brain tissue. Further, DHA supply in pregnancy affects placental expression of fatty acid transport proteins.[5] Consequently, infants who fail to receive adequate omega-3 fatty acids from their mothers during pregnancy are at increased risk for developing vision and CNS deficits.[6-8] Furthermore, deficiencies in DHA and EPA during early developmental stages, especially in infants deprived of DHA-rich breast milk, "may lower serotonin levels at critical periods of neurodevelopment and may result in a cascade of suboptimal development of neurotransmitter systems limiting regulation of the limbic system by the frontal cortex." Subsequently, the resulting deficits may produce residual developmental effects that "may be manifest as dysregulation of sympathetic responses to stress including decreased heart rate variability and hypertension, which in turn have been linked to behavioral dysregulation."[9] The full implications of these developmental perturbations and their significance in healthy function, dysfunction, and disease throughout childhood and adulthood have only begun to be understood.[8,10-12]

NUTRIENT IN CLINICAL PRACTICE
Known or Potential Therapeutic Uses
Omega-3 Fatty Acids
Angina, amyotrophic lateral sclerosis (risk reduction), arthritis, artherosclerosis, asthma, bipolar disorders, breastfeeding support, cancer, cardiovascular disease, cholesterol, chronic obstructive pulmonary disease (COPD), colon cancer, Crohn's disease, cystic fibrosis, depression, diabetes mellitus, dysmenorrhea, eczema, endometriosis, glaucoma, human immunodeficiency virus and acquired immunodeficiency syndrome (HIV/AIDS) support, hyperlipidemia, hypertension, hypertriglyceridemia, immune support, inflammatory bowel disease, mental disorders, migraine, multiple sclerosis, myocardial infarction, neonatal development, nephropathy, neurodegenerative disease, osteoarthritis, osteoporosis, phenylketonuria, photosensitivity, preeclampsia, pregnancy and postpartum support, presurgical and postsurgical support, psoriasis, Raynaud's syndrome, rheumatoid arthritis, sickle cell anemia, sudden cardiac death (risk reduction), systemic lupus erythematosus (SLE), ulcerative colitis.

EPA and DHA (Long Chain Omega-3s)
Acute myocardial infarction, acute respiratory distress syndrome (ARDS), age-related macular degeneration, aggressive behavior, agoraphobia, Alzheimer's disease, angina, anorexia nervosa, anthracycline-induced cardiac toxicity, anticoagulation, antiphospholipid syndrome, anxiety, arthritis, arthrosclerosis, asthma, attention deficit–hyperactivity disorder (ADHD), autoimmune nephritis, Behçet's syndrome, bipolar disorder, borderline personality disorder, breast cancer risk, breastfeeding support, burns, cachexia during chemotherapy, cancer treatment support, cardiovascular disease prevention, chronic fatigue syndrome, chronic obstructive pulmonary disease (COPD), cirrhosis, colorectal cancer risk, Crohn's disease, cystic fibrosis, dementia, depression, dermatomyositis, diabetes mellitus type 1, diabetes mellitus type 2, diabetic nephropathy, diabetic neuropathy, dyslexia, dyslipidemia, dysmenorrhea, dyspraxia, eczema, emphysema, endometriosis, exercise performance enhancement, fibrocystic breasts, gallstones, gingivitis, glaucoma, glomerulonephritis, glycogen storage diseases, gout, hepatorenal syndrome, human immunodeficiency virus and acquired immunodeficiency syndrome (HIV/AIDS) support, hypercholesterolemia, hyperlipidemia, hypertension, hypertriglyceridemia, hypoxia, ichthyosis, immune function, immunosuppression, inflammatory bowel disease, leprosy, leukemia, Lyme disease, malaria, male infertility, mastalgia, memory enhancement, menopausal symptoms, menstrual cramps, mental disorders, migraine, multiple sclerosis, myopathy, neck and low back pain, neonatal development, nephrolithiasis, nephropathy, neurodegenerative disease, neuropathy, night vision enhancement, obesity, omega-3 fatty acid deficiency, osteoarthritis, osteoporosis, panic disorder, peripheral vascular disease, phenylketonuria, photodermatitis, photosensitivity, postviral fatigue syndrome, preeclampsia, pregnancy and postpartum support, premature birth prevention, premenstrual syndrome, presurgical and postsurgical support, prostate cancer prevention, psoriasis, Raynaud's phenomenon, Refsum's syndrome, retinitis pigmentosa, Reye's syndrome, rheumatoid arthritis, schizophrenia, seizure disorder, sickle cell anemia, stroke prevention, sudden cardiac death (risk reduction), suicidal tendencies, systemic lupus erythematosus (SLE), tardive dyskinesia, tennis elbow, urolithiasis, ulcerative colitis, vision enhancement.

Alpha-Linolenic Acid (ALA)
Breast cancer, cardiovascular disease, diabetes mellitus, eczema, hypercholesterolemia, hyperlipidemia, hypertension, hypertriglyceridemia, laxative, lupus nephritis, menopause, menstrual breast pain, prostate cancer, psoriasis.

Deficiency Symptoms

Dry scaly skin, hair loss, immune system insufficiency, inflammation, poor wound healing; impaired vision, reduced childhood growth and impaired brain and eye development.

Dietary Sources

Alpha-Linolenic Acid (ALA)

Canola (rapeseed) oil, eggs (from hens fed flaxseed), hemp seed oil, eichium seed oil, flaxseed (linseed), perilla seed, pumpkin seed, purslane, walnuts, wheat germ.

Note: Safflower, sesame, and sunflower, and to a lesser degree soybean, contain ALA but also contain countervailing omega-6 fatty acids in significantly higher amounts.

DHA and EPA

Fish, fish oil; eggs (from hens fed DHA-rich algae); infant formula; margarine and milk fortified with EPA/DHA.

Fish oils and plant oils are the primary dietary sources of omega-3 fatty acids. The omega-3 fatty acids DHA and EPA are the key constituents in the oil found in cold-water fish. The high concentrations of omega-3 fatty acids in these fish may result from its "antifreeze" property. The richest sources of naturally occurring omega-3 oils include salmon, mackerel, halibut, sardines, and herring. The preparation of fish also influences its physiological and therapeutic actions, with "intake of tuna or other broiled or baked fish being associated with improved cardiac hemodynamics, but fried fish intake being associated with structural abnormalities indicative of systolic dysfunction and potential coronary atherosclerosis."[13] The liver of the cod, halibut, or shark is the primary source of fish liver oil, whereas herring, sardine, salmon, or anchovy flesh usually serves as the source of fish body oil. Other food from the oceans can also provide omega-3 oils. Some marine phytoplankton (microalgae) are good sources of DHA and can be obtained as nutritional products. New Zealand green-lipped mussels (*Perna canaliculus*) also contain omega-3 fatty acids and have been consumed by the Maori people of the South Pacific for centuries.[14] EPA/DHA has been added to "fortify" some foods, such as eggs, bread, margarines, and milk. Oil extracted from ocean krill (zooplankton) is also a rich source of EPA and DHA, available as a nutritional supplement, and in which EPA and DHA are uniquely bound in phospholipids, rather than triglycerides as in fish body/liver oils.

Fish liver oil, but not fish body oil, is also rich in vitamins A and D. For example, cod liver oil liquids normally provide concentrations of 750 to 1200 µg (2500-4000 units) vitamin A per 10 mL and 2.5 to 10 µg (100-400 units) vitamin D per 10 mL, although there is significant variability between brands, depending on multiple factors, including region, time of year, and processing. These vitamins are even more concentrated in halibut and shark liver oils. Shark liver oil is also rich in compounds called alkoxyglycerols, which are reputed to have protective effects from radiation therapy.[15,16] Oil from both body and liver of fish also contains some vitamin E.

Although they are readily available in many common foods, the ability to convert omega-3 fatty acids from vegetable sources to EPA within the human body is quite limited. ALA is found in a variety of plant foods, especially canola (rapeseed) oil, flaxseeds, flaxseed oil, pumpkin seeds, pumpkin seed oil, purslane, perilla seed oil, soybeans, soybean oil, walnuts, and walnut oil.

Nutrient Preparations Available

Fish oil products usually contain vitamin E and other antioxidant nutrients to reduce oxidative degradation and rancidity; this inherent problem may also be mitigated by extracting the oxygen from the capsule. Long-term intake of fish oil could theoretically cause a deficiency of vitamin E by increasing oxidative stress on fat-soluble antioxidants. Consequently, many commercial fish oil products contain additional vitamin E, which also acts as an antioxidant to prevent rancidity before ingestion.[17]

Variations on usual fish oil products have been developed for special populations. Fish oil preparations emphasizing DHA and containing no or lesser proportions of EPA are sometimes used with infants (or others) who generally do not need EPA. Enteric-coated, free–fatty acid preparations of purified EPA/DHA derived from fish oil are sometimes preferable for patients with Crohn's disease or other gastrointestinal (GI) conditions because of their reduced tendency to cause digestive distress. Omega-3 fatty acid ethyl esters are a slightly modified form of fish oil approved by the U.S. Food and Drug Administration (FDA) as a prescription treatment for hypertriglyceridemia either as monotherapy or in combination with statins or fibrates.[18]

Both EPA and DHA can be obtained from various algae. DHA-45 is an innovative proprietary source of DHA produced through a multistep fermentation and refining process using a nonpathogenic marine protist. The final product consists of approximately 45% DHA and is intended for use in food, but safety has not been fully established.[19] Martek produces DHA from cultured microalgae for use in infant formula and DHA products. Several European companies are planning to produce both EPA and DHA from algae, although at the time of this writing, these are not yet commercially available.

Flaxseed, flaxseed oil, and fish oil require refrigeration to maintain their integrity, even though many encapsulated fish oil products are stable at room temperature. Whole flaxseeds need to be consumed within 24 hours of being ground, or their unsaturated fatty acid constituents degrade through oxidation.

Dosage Forms Available

Fish oil: Capsule, gel cap, oil (liquid, often flavored with citrus or other fruit oils).
Flaxseed: Oil (liquid), powder, whole seeds.

For fish oil preparations, dosing should be based on the amount of EPA and DHA (omega-3 fatty acids) in a product, not on the total amount of fish oil. Commercial products vary in the amounts and ratios of EPA and DHA. A common amount of omega-3 fatty acids in fish oil capsules is 0.18 g (180 mg) of EPA and 0.12 g (120 mg) of DHA per gram of oil. Five grams of fish oil contains approximately 0.17 to 0.56 g (170-560 mg) of EPA and 0.072 to 0.31 g (72-310 mg) of DHA. Different types of fish contain variable amounts of omega-3 fatty acids; likewise, different types of nuts or oil contain variable amounts of ALA.

Flaxseed can be administered in several forms, as an oil in liquid medium or capsule, ground into powder, or mixed with liquid. See dosage section for further details.

Source Materials for Nutrient Preparations

Fish oil can be derived from a wide variety of fish species, each with different amounts and relative proportions of EPA and

DHA.[20] DHA and EPA are also commercially derived from both wild and cultivated algae.

Alpha-linolenic acid (ALA) can be obtained from a variety of nuts and vegetable oils, including canola oil, flaxseed/linseed oil, flaxseeds, olive oil, soybean oil, walnut oil, walnuts (English).[20]

Dosage Range

Optimal dosage has not been established. Over-the-counter (OTC) products typically provide 200 to 1500 mg combined EPA/DHA per dose. Clinical trials investigating fish oil therapeutics have often used 3 to 4 g daily (EPA/DHA), but doses of 1 to 2 g may be adequate, depending on the clinical application.

Dietary

Adult. No daily requirement for fish oil or EPA and DHA has been established. The adequate intake (AI) for ALA has been established as 1.6 g per day for men and 1.1 g per day for women. AIs represent the least amount needed to deter deficiency but do not take into account disease prevention. A healthy diet should provide at least 5 g total essential fatty acids daily. The dietary intake of omega-3/omega-6 fatty acids of most individuals is typically both low and imbalanced. The average American diet contains approximately 1.6 g omega-3 fatty acids per day, of which only 0.1 to 0.2 g comes from EPA and DHA and approximately 1.4 g (~90%) from ALA. Moreover, in Western diets, except for specific populations with unusually high fish intake, consumption of omega-6 fatty acids is about 10 to 40 times greater than that of omega-3 fatty acids. This high proportion of omega-6 fatty acid intake results largely from the widespread use of vegetable oils containing linoleic acid, a relatively recent dietary development, historically speaking. Increasing omega-3 fatty acid intake or decreasing intake of omega-6 fatty acids can improve the ratio, as well as health benefits, because omega-6 and omega-3 fatty acids compete for conversion into active metabolites.

The American Heart Association recommends that healthy adults with no history of heart disease eat fish at least twice weekly, preferably broiled or baked, not fried.[21] Fatty fish, in particular, are superior sources; these include anchovies, bluefish, carp, catfish, halibut, herring, lake trout, mackerel, pompano, salmon, striped sea bass, tuna (albacore), and whitefish. However, some fish need to be consumed in limited amounts because they contain high levels of mercury and other toxins. Swordfish, king mackerel, shark, and tilefish should be limited to 7 ounces per week (and avoided by pregnant women); tuna and red snapper should be limited to 14 ounces per week; salmon, catfish, mahi mahi, and canned tuna have no established restrictions. Consumption of plant-derived sources of ALA, such as tofu/soybeans, walnuts, flaxseed oil, and canola oil, is also recommended, although some experts have reservations about the euricic acid content of canola oil, which is a potentially problematic, very-long-chain fatty acid. Various national regulatory agencies, as well as the World Health Organization (WHO), recommend a daily dietary intake of 0.3 to 0.5 g EPA plus DHA and 0.8 to 1.1 g ALA (although this latter value is somewhat below the AI established for ALA).

Pregnancy and Nursing. Pregnant and lactating women are often advised to consume sufficient fish oils to provide at least 300 mg DHA daily to promote healthy neural and optical development in the child. Adequate DHA intake during pregnancy has also been associated with a decreased risk for postpartum depression.

Infants and Children. Although widely recognized for its critical role in development, no therapeutic protocols or standards of treatment have been established for the use of fish oils such as DHA by infants or children. An ample supply of DHA and AA enable healthy neurological and retinal development in infancy. Breast milk and brain tissue exhibit the highest naturally occurring concentrations of EPA and DHA in the human body, and breast-fed infants exhibit higher concentrations of erythrocyte DHA and AA than bottle-fed infants, with corresponding increases in visual acuity and developmental tests (vs. bottle-fed counterparts).[8,22] Infant formula is required by law in most developed countries, except the United States, to contain DHA. Formula should contain 0.35% DHA and less than 0.1% EPA.

ALA content in breast milk depends on maternal diet and may be adequate with proper nutrition, but it can vary considerably. Maternal intake of flax oil or fresh-ground seed can be used to increase ALA content in breast milk. Infant formula should contain 1.5% ALA.

A child's fatty acid intake may be enhanced and balanced through addition of freshly ground flaxseeds and flaxseed oil.

Supplemental/Maintenance

The recommendation for fish oil preparations is 3000 to 4000 mg fish oil per day, which is equivalent to approximately two to three servings of fatty fish per week. A single 1000-mg fish oil capsule typically contains 180 mg EPA and 120 mg DHA.

Supplementation is not necessary in children who are breast-fed because breast milk contains adequate amounts, assuming adequate maternal dietary intake. Infants not being breast-fed and other children can benefit from omega-3 fatty acids, but dosage levels have not been established. Exogenous DHA administration can increase levels of DHA in breast milk, and higher breast milk DHA levels increase the DHA in infants' cell membranes.[23-25] The metabolism of infants appears to have minimal need for EPA.

A typical dose for flaxseed can range from 1 tablespoon two to three times daily to 2 to 4 tablespoons once daily; usually ground and consumed with water; 100 g raw flaxseed provides 22,800 mg ALA.

Flaxseed oil can be dispensed in a liquid form, with a 15-ml tablespoon containing approximately 7 g ALA. A dose of 1 or 2 tablespoons of flaxseed oil daily is appropriate as a general recommendation. Refrigeration is essential to stable storage; integrity is significantly compromised with heating because of rapid oxidation of unsaturated bonds.

Flaxseed oil can also be distributed in a capsule form, with a typical 1000-mg capsule providing 500 mg ALA. Oral consumption of raw flaxseeds in doses up to 50 g daily for up to 4 weeks has been reported. Oral doses of 10 to 60 g daily have been used in several studies for periods of less than 2 weeks. A dose of 50 g flaxseeds is roughly equivalent to 250 g flaxseed flour.

Doses of soluble flaxseed mucilage/fiber as high as 60 to 80 g/kg body weight have been administered in research settings.

Pharmacological/Therapeutic

The appropriate range for an effective dose of omega-3 oils, regardless of the form or source, is under debate. Dosage suggestions in the literature range from 1 to 10 g per day. However, the appropriate dosage varies depending on the pathophysiology in question and the level of health in a given individual.

A maximum tolerated dose of 0.3 g/kg/day of fish oil capsules has been proposed; this tolerance is equivalent to 21 1-g capsules daily for a 70-kg (154-lb) patient.[26] Typical dosages of fish oil in therapeutic settings range from 3 to 9 g daily, but this is not the upper limit, and dosages in oncological settings are often 12 to 15 g/day, or more. Subjects in one clinical trial ingested 60 g daily. In essence, matching the dosage used in several major studies would require fish oil adequate to supply about 2 to 3 g EPA (2000-3500 mg) and about 1.0 to 2.5 g DHA (1000-2500 mg) daily. However, much higher doses have been used in some studies. The U.S. FDA classifies intake of up to 3 g/day omega-3 fatty acids from fish as "generally regarded as safe" (GRAS).

Children (2-12 years). Daily administration, typically about 1 teaspoon daily of ground flaxseeds or 1 teaspoon of fresh flaxseed oil, is often used in treating children with constipation.

Toxic. In their natural-occurring food contexts, omega-3 fatty acids possess an excellent safety profile and are considered generally nontoxic, particularly with single-dose or short-term application. Omega-3 fatty acids in OTC forms (i.e., free from contaminants) do not exhibit toxic levels in most individuals when used at standard doses. One study involving oncology patients being treated with concomitant fish oils for cachexia proposed a maximum tolerated dose of 21 g/day.[27] No maximum tolerated dose has been established for the general population or patients diagnosed with other conditions. However, the qualified health claim (for prevention of coronary heart disease) allowed for EPA/DHA by the FDA sets a maximum recommended intake of 2 g total EPA and/or DHA and suggests a maximum of 1 g, or about 3 g of usual-strength fish oil.

Contaminants do change the situation for many consumers of fish because methylmercury and other pollutants can represent significant health risks, especially in pregnancy, during breastfeeding, and throughout childhood development. Such contaminants are much less significant in fish oil products than with dietary consumption of fish meat.

Excessive intake of cod liver oil carries a risk of inducing vitamin A excess and thus is generally not considered a preferred source of EPA/DHA for long-term use. However, intakes of more than 1 ounce daily are necessary to provide excessive levels of vitamin A for most products. It would require extremely high intakes of fish liver oils to provide excessive intakes of vitamin D (>10,000 IU/day).

Laboratory Values

No clinical standards for laboratory evaluation of omega-3 fatty acid status have been established.

Fatty Acids, Nonesterified

Circulating nonesterified–fatty acid concentration is an independent factor for cardiac risk, especially sudden death in middle-aged men.[28] Omega-3 fatty acids are "preferentially stored in the Sn-2 position, from which they can be specifically and rapidly released by activated phospholipase A-2." However, free–fatty acid levels in plasma do not reliably reflect the immediate dietary consumption of fat because they primarily derive from the regulated turnover of lipid stores in adipose tissue by lipolysis and from phospholipids by phospholipases.[29]

Fatty Acid Composition of Serum Cholesterol Esters, Free Fatty Acids, Phospholipids, and Triglycerides

Blood levels of long-chain n-3 fatty acids have been used in clinical trials investigating the effects of omega-3 fatty acid

intake.[30,31] Such assays are not usually applied in routine clinical settings, although they are incorporated in various risk profile panels used by health care professionals specializing in nutritional therapeutics.

Red Blood Cell Membrane Fatty Acid Composition

Measurement of long-chain omega-3 fatty acids in red blood cell (RBC) membranes is a sensitive indicator of deficiency but remains investigational. This measurement has been used as an indicator of cardiac risk and other related susceptibility.[31] Low levels indicate deficiency, but specific reference ranges vary among laboratories.

Serum (or Plasma) Phospholipid

Fatty acid analysis of phospholipid concentration in serum (or plasma) may provide a useful biomarker for assessing nutritional status and EPA/DHA intakes in relation to potential risk.[32,33] Resulting data can then be presented as an "omega-3 fatty acid profile" with both an omega-3 score and a DHA score.

SAFETY PROFILE

Overview: Fish Oil

Fish oil intake is generally considered to be well tolerated with an excellent safety profile.[19,34] Few clinically significant adverse effects have been reported. Studies investigating the maximum tolerated dose and dose-limiting toxicities of fish oil found GI complaints, mainly nausea, loose stools, or diarrhea, as the predominant adverse effects. In clinical practice, fish-flavored aftertaste and eructations represent the adverse effects most often mentioned by patients using fish oils. Various clinical trials have suggested possible adverse effects from fish oil intake in specific patient populations.

The preeminent issue of toxicity affecting fish oils results not from the nutrients themselves but from damage to the fish and the environment in which they develop. Fish oils are free of intrinsic risks in their native state. However, growing concerns are widely expressed over the effects of pollution, especially the presence of mercury, toxic organochlorines, and polychlorinated biphenyls (PCBs) in seafood and large fish in particular, both directly (for humans, sealife, and the planet) and in effects on fish oil products.

In particular, fish meat may contain methylmercury, pesticides, and heavy metals, and caution is especially warranted in pregnant and lactating women and young children.[34] Methylmercury is known to cause neurological and developmental disorders.[35,36] Fish oils derived from wild fish are generally considered less likely to contain significant amounts of mercury and other heavy metals, although this is ultimately a relative safety factor because these toxic materials have permeated the environment to some degree. Moreover, methylmercury tends to accumulate more readily in fish meat than in fish oil. Consequently, fish oil products have generally been found to be largely free of mercury; a process known as *molecular distillation* is required for reliable removal of PCBs and other toxic pollutants. Unrefined fish oil preparations may still contain pesticides or other pollutants. Thus, products that are assayed for peroxides and environmental contamination are recommended. Overall, the significant risks associated with fish oil consumption, through dietary and nutraceutical sources, derive from contamination rather than from the nutrients themselves and, in fact, are generally more problematic in fish than in fish oil products.

The loss of biodiversity and destruction of ocean ecosystems constitute the other side of the fish contamination issue. Overfishing, destructive fishing practices, and destruction of habitats all represent huge problems reaching critical proportions.[37,38] Without significant and concerted global efforts to reverse these trends and establish sustainable practices, the availability of fish or omega-3 oils derived from fish may become obsolete and irrelevant. Advocating regular consumption of fish in the diet or products containing omega-3 fatty acids derived from fish on a global basis is unrealistic and inadvisable over the long term. Other technologies, such as those involving use of microalgae cultures, warrant aggressive research and rapid deployment.

Nutrient Adverse Effects

Eructations, nausea, dyspepsia, reflux, abdominal bloating and discomfort, flatulence, loose stools, diarrhea, and other minor GI complaints represent the most common adverse effects reported in individuals consuming fish oil products at typical levels, appearing in 1.5% to 5% of study subjects; severe diarrhea has been reported on rare occasions with the ingestion of high doses of fish oil supplements.[39-46] GI effects can be minimized if fish oils are taken with meals and if doses are started low and gradually increased; time-release preparations may also mitigate these complications. Such effects are generally considered improbable or inconsequential with dietary consumption of fish.

Caution should be used in regard to the dose of cod liver oil because of high vitamin A and D content. Large doses of vitamin A, particularly with rapid introduction, can be hepatotoxic (>20,000 IU/day combined with other hepatotoxic stress, e.g., chronic acetaminophen or alcohol use). Generally, the potential risk from vitamin D is considered greater in summer than in winter or cloudy climates, but this advisory may change given the emerging knowledge of pervasive vitamin D deficiency and insufficiency, versus previously dominant fears of vitamin D excess and toxicity.

The potential hematological effects of omega-3 fatty acids pose some of the more clinically significant effects in terms of unintended effects and interactions. Omega-3 fatty acids have multiple antithrombotic effects that may exert a bimodal effect (beneficial or adverse) depending on the individual, his or her physiology and medical conditions, and interactive medication effects. In particular, fish oils may decrease platelet aggregation, increase fibrinolysis, prolong bleeding time, and diminish von Willebrand factor, all of which concomitantly decrease thrombotic risk and increase bleeding risk. Daily doses of more than 3 g omega-3 fatty acids (9 g usual-strength fish oil) may increase the risk of bleeding, but there is a paucity of evidence to substantiate concerns of clinically significant bleeding risk at lower doses in most individuals.[47-49] Very high doses of omega-3 fatty acids in the form of fish oil, and at the intake level typical of indigenous Eskimo diet, could theoretically increase the risk of hemorrhagic stroke.[50] High-dose intake has also been associated with epistaxis and hematuria, usually in association with other anticlotting agents such as antiplatelet agents, as well as anticoagulants such as warfarin, or heparin.[51] Notably, in at least one study, hemostatic effects (opposite of increased bleeding risk) observed with dietary fish were not seen with fish oil products.[41] High levels of long-chain omega-3 fatty acids from marine sources reportedly may increase levels of plasminogen activator inhibitor type 1 (PAI-1), thus inhibiting endogenous fibrinolysis, with the attendant theoretical effect of increasing thrombotic risk. However, after careful assessment of this issue, Hansen et al.[52] concluded that, although dietary fat of any type somewhat raises PAI-1 levels, there is no difference between the

long-chain omega-3 oils and any other type of fat in this regard.

Fish oil can play an important role in a strategic approach to treatment of individuals with dyslipidemias, hypercholesterolemia, and dermatitis. Dose-dependent elevations in low-density lipoprotein (LDL) levels of 5% to 10% have been observed with increased intake of 1 g or more daily of omega-3 fatty acids, with more substantial elevations in individuals with familial combined hyperlipidemia.[53] However, these LDL-raising effects were not observed in all trials and appear to be transient, and a paradoxical LDL-lowering effect may be seen at high doses (e.g., 32 g fish oil daily).[41,43,54-57] Furthermore, coadministration of pectin or garlic may counteract this possible adverse effect.[58,59] Isolated reports indicate that mild elevations in alanine transaminase (ALT) levels may occur.[60] Although fish oils are often used in the treatment of inflammatory skin conditions, skin rashes have been reported on rare occasions.[54,61]

In one rodent study, omega-3 fatty acids were associated with metastatic progression of colon cancer.[62] Consequently, concerns have been raised about use of omega-3 fatty acids, through dietary sources or nutraceutical products, in patients with advanced stages of colorectal cancer. The majority of animal studies, however, have indicated an overall anticancer effect of dietary long-chain omega-3 fatty acids.

Adverse Effects Among Specific Populations

Individuals with allergy or hypersensitivity to fish, seafood, or nuts may react to omega-3 fatty acid or ALA products derived from these substances. Checking labeling and avoiding potentially problematic substances are advised.

Hypomania has been reported in patients with bipolar disorder or major depression after use of omega-3 oils.[63] Clinical studies, however, have shown a beneficial effect in both bipolar disorder and depression.[64-70] Rare reports of restlessness and formication (sensation of ants crawling on the skin) suggest the need for vigilance when introducing therapeutic agents in any case involving a psychiatric diagnosis.

Elevations in blood glucose levels have been reported with daily doses of fish oil greater than 3 g for extended periods. The frequency and severity of the potential risk of increased or unstable blood glucose levels appear to be of concern primarily in individuals with diabetes or hypertriglyceridemia, but research has not elucidated a clear and consistent understanding of this observed phenomenon. Addition of vitamin E or regular aerobic exercise (½ hour three times per week) may mitigate this possible potential impairment of glucose tolerance.[51,71,72]

Contraindications

An increased death rate in the fish oil–administered group was observed in a single study involving patients with implanted cardiac defibrillators.[73] In contrast, observations and trials conducted in the United States and Europe indicate that the predominant effect of high omega-3 consumption (e.g., 1000 mg daily from fish oil) is a reduction in risk of sudden cardiac death.[74,75]

Potential effects on female hormones have occasionally led to statements that the use of flaxseed or flaxseed oil during pregnancy and breastfeeding is contraindicated.[76] Evidence from clinical trials or qualified case reports is lacking, but animal studies have suggested possible adverse effects.

Precautions and Warnings

Patients being treated for cardiac arrhythmias, particularly with a history of sustained ventricular fibrillation or ventricular tachycardia, require close supervision when introducing fish oil preparations into their therapeutic regimen or significantly altering the dose or form. Complex and often bimodal responses are possible and vary depending on source (fish vs. fish oils), dose, and patient characteristics. For example, although some research indicates that individuals who ate fish had a reduced risk for developing atrial fibrillation, preliminary data suggest that a high level of fish consumption (five or more servings per week) is associated with an increased risk of atrial fibrillation in middle-age men.[77] However, fish consumption also protects against ventricular fibrillation and sudden cardiac death and helps to protect the coronary vessels.

Likewise, similar cautions are relevant in patients with hypertension, diabetes, or other cardiovascular disease. Although omega-3 fatty acids may be beneficial for many individuals with these conditions, regular monitoring and close supervision are appropriate when introducing any nutraceutical or pharmacological agent, altering dose or form, or interjecting new medications that might interact with the nutrient or comedications.

Individuals with familial combined hyperlipidemia may exhibit an increased incidence of spontaneous bleeding.[48,78]

Coincident ingestion of fat-soluble vitamins, specifically vitamins A, D, and E, can unintentionally elevate these levels through use of fish oil products. Attention to labels and cumulative dose is important to avoid adverse effects, although frank toxicity caused by supplemental intake at typical doses is unlikely, except in cases of regular use of fish liver oils. These oils are particularly rich in vitamins A and D, the concentrations of which can vary widely between products, depending on source of fish liver and processing of the product.

INTERACTIONS REVIEW

Strategic Considerations

The physiological, preventive, and therapeutic effects of omega-3 fatty acids are overwhelmingly positive, and most interactions between this nutrient class and conventional pharmaceutical agents are beneficial. Although not quite the panacea predicted by many early enthusiasts, the breadth of research into and possible clinical applications of fish oils (DHA, EPA) and ALA has grown at an astounding pace in the past few decades. These "discoveries" not only point to the fundamental and multifactorial roles that omega-3 fatty acids play in many aspects of human physiology, but also highlight the deficits and imbalances in the human diet in developed societies. Moreover, the manifold mechanisms by which omega-3 fatty acids support and modulate many physiological functions, while introducing few significant adverse effects, make them a particularly appropriate agent for integration with a broad range of pharmaceutical agents, particularly those that treat or increase oxidative damage or inflammation, neuroendocrine or immune dysregulation, or cardiovascular dysfunction. Recommendation of two or more servings of fish rich in omega-3 oils per week has become standard within conventional medicine and governmental policy, but clinical application of the benefits of fish oil and ALA in nutraceutical forms has yet to be integrated into conventional practice guidelines.

Research into the physiology and therapeutics of long-chain omega-3 fatty acids has grown steadily ever since Bang and Dyerberg reported the association between a diet rich in long-chain marine omega-3 fatty acids and reduced incidence of atherosclerotic heart disease in Greenland Eskimos.[79-81] However, the epidemiological associations of dietary fish intake and therapeutic effects (or risks) of omega-3 fatty acids and fish oil in the subsequent decades of literature are often intertwined and mixed without clarity or consistency in analyses and conclusions.[57,82] Most importantly, many key variables need to be taken into account in study design, in presentation of findings, and in dissemination of news. Variables such as proportions of preintervention dietary constituents, differentiation of dietary fish rich in omega-3s versus less oily fish, proportions of EPA and DHA in different preparations, and methods of extraction and purification can significantly alter findings and their clinical implications. However, these factors frequently are inadequately factored into meta-analyses, reviews, and news reports in both professional publications and the lay press.

The role of fish oil in development of the CNS and subsequent neurological and cognitive function is generally accepted.[83-88] In particular, DHA is pivotal through its activity as a major component of the phospholipid layer of neuronal membranes. Its roles in chloride and other ion channel opening at the synapse of neurons, increasing stability of neuronal functioning, influencing multiple gene expressions, modulating GABA responses, promoting dopamine and serotonin neurotransmission, increasing acetylcholine release, inhibiting multiple spikes in epileptiform activity, protecting against oxidative stress, and serving as an overall neuroprotectant, place DHA, and to a lesser extent its shorter-chain sibling EPA, at the center of ongoing and evolving neurocognitive science.[89-96] Surprisingly, however, the medical literature still contains lingering hesitations regarding the universal efficacy of increasing DHA during pregnancy and infant nutrient intake. In these areas the incomplete and sometimes contradictory evidence regarding the preventive properties of fish oil remains a source of controversy and investigation. Further research into the important supportive role of fish oil throughout the life cycle, from embryonic and infant development to preventing dementia in the elderly, continues to emerge, and the only remaining question is the degree to which conventional medicine can integrate this important nutritive strategy.

A broad consensus supports the proposition that fish and marine omega-3 fatty acid intake is associated with improved cardiovascular health. The central role of fish oil in risk reduction, prevention, and treatment of cardiovascular disease derives from broadly accepted functions and activities, including effects on inflammation and oxidation, membrane physiology and lipoprotein metabolism, blood vessel pliability and atherosclerotic plaque formation, platelet reactivity, and blood flow characteristics. Nevertheless, the efficacy and safety of fish oil administration for heart disease in general and patients with particular conditions remain controversial and uncertain, with data and interpretations suggesting a range of responses, from beneficial to potentially dangerous; some commentators interpret these contradictory findings to suggest that fish oil's benefit to individuals with heart disease is slight or nonexistent.[97-99] Consequently, according to various sources, fish and fish oil may reduce the risk, incidence, and severity of atherosclerosis, thrombosis, arrhythmias, atrial fibrillation, coronary heart disease, sudden cardiac death, heart failure, and stroke or may, on the other hand, potentially increase risk of sudden death from myocardial infarction in individuals with stable heart disease.[97,99-101] Nevertheless, in a review of data on the efficacy and safety of different antilipidemic agents and diets on mortality, Studer et al.[102] found that fish oil is superior to statin therapy for lowering overall cardiac mortality risk. They also found, regarding the fibrate class of antilipidemics (which historically preceded the statins), "any potential reduction in cardiac mortality from fibrates is offset by an increased risk of death from noncardiovascular causes."[102]

In addition to nutritive, antioxidant, and inflammatory modulation effects, the known antithrombotic effects of omega-3 fatty acids on platelet aggregation and blood viscosity suggest that administration may be beneficial in conjunction with surgical procedures such as prevention of restenosis after coronary angioplasty (PTCA) or prevention of graft failure after heart bypass surgery. Analyzing electrocardiographic (ECG) data from two prospective trials that included 52 heart transplant recipients, Harris et al.[103] found that administration of 1 to 3.4 g omega-3 fatty acid daily for 4 to 6 months reduced heart rates and prolonged QRS duration, even though these patients were presumably devoid of vagal innervation, suggesting that n-3 fatty acids may modify electrophysiological properties of the myocardium itself. Research into such integrative approaches, however, is still emerging and inconclusive, with findings that have been mixed and often less positive than expected.[46,104-109]

The potential small increase in bleeding risk, possibility of elevated LDL cholesterol level, and impact on glycemic control constitute the primary adverse effects consistently appearing in the literature, besides nausea, loose stools, and fishy eructations. These effects, however, are often transient, dose dependent, and preparation related and can usually be corrected by regular exercise and increasing dietary fibers such as pectin, especially within the context of a comprehensive strategy integrating lifestyle changes, improved diet, stress management, conventional medications, and specific nutrient/herb combinations.[59,72] Such synergistic approaches can be personalized and can evolve in response to the initiative and abilities, risks and needs, and susceptibilities and tolerances of the individual patient. As with other intersections of body systems and pathophysiology, individual pharmacogenomic variability, patient participation and compliance, and the therapeutic relationship play highly influential roles in determining risk severity, medication reactions, and therapeutic response. Although issues regarding potential for increased bleeding risk at high doses and possible elevation of LDL cholesterol level or reduced glycemic control will remain cause for concern and monitoring, these adverse effects are not axiomatic, universal, severe, or irremediable.

A review of the scientific and medical literature reveals broad support, with a strong and consistent underlying body of scientific evidence, for regular dietary intake of omega-3 fatty acids in amounts greater than currently in common use, with an accompanying reduction in omega-6 fatty acid intake (predominantly from warm-weather vegetable oils and grains) and a preferred emphasis on dietary fish consumption. The issue of shifting the balance between omega-3 and omega-6 fatty acids remains a central concern in epidemiological, dietary, and therapeutic contexts. The gross preponderance of omega-6 fatty acids in the typical American diet, especially through corn oil, is universally considered problematic in terms of physiological stress, particularly inflammatory thresholds, and as an impediment against the beneficial activities of fish oil and other omega-3 fatty acids.[93] Reducing the excess intake of omega-6 oils and shifting the balance of intake toward omega-3 oils can be beneficial in preventing or treating numerous pathological processes. For example, increasing omega-3 sources and reducing omega-6 intake may benefit several cardiovascular risk parameters.[110] Likewise, animal research indicates that increasing omega-3 fatty acid levels and decreasing omega-6 levels could

reduce the risk of prostate cancer through beneficial effects on prostate cell membrane composition, cyclooxygenase-2 (COX-2) activity, and lowering of prostaglandin E_2 (PGE_2) production.[111] The Mediterranean diet in particular has become the center of population studies on a broad level and more focused research in terms of particular constituents. In addition to its general emphasis on healthy dietary fats and a significantly higher proportion of omega-3 (vs. omega-6) fatty acids, this dietary approach is rooted in the regional ecosystem and provides a generous supply of whole grains, fresh fruits and vegetables, olive oil (rich in omega-9 fats, which are neutral in the omega-6/omega-3 equation), garlic, and other herbs, with high amounts of protein from fish and seafood and moderate amounts from meat.[112]

Overall, the body of evidence from scientific literature and clinical practice demonstrates the recurring need for a personalized, evolving, comprehensive therapeutic intervention, multidisciplinary in content and integrative in approach, toward the many areas of human physiology and health, as well as pathophysiology and disease that are affected by omega-3 fatty acids. Whether neurological health and cognitive function; inflammatory modulation, free-radical quenching, and immune function; or cardiovascular health and heart disease or stroke, this nutrient class exhibits a diverse range of direct effects and possibilities for therapeutic synergy.

The issue of toxic pollution attributable to humans, particularly methylmercury, dioxins, and PCBs, appears to be the most significant risk and limiting factor associated with dietary intake of omega-3 fatty acids from fish or fish-derived nutraceutical forms. Given the compromised state of oceanic ecologies and systemic damage to sealife, especially fisheries, a global policy of high dietary fish consumption seems unwise and unsustainable, and ultimately may prove irresponsible. Thus, the need arises for increased production and easier access to omega-3 fatty acids from nonfish sources. Shifting to nutraceutical forms of omega-3 intake leads to questions that rarely appear in looking at dietary sources, except among those small populations who consume fish or other sealife sources at high levels, sometimes referred to as "Eskimo" levels. A large and diverse set of well-designed, adequately powered, and long-duration clinical trials will be necessary to answer many of the lingering questions that have arisen from epidemiological and population studies, clinical interventions, and emergent integrative strategies.

This review has considered flaxseed and related plant sources of omega-3 fatty acids, particularly ALA, only in relation to those effects and interactions associated with the fatty acid constituents. Potential preventive, therapeutic, and interactions issues related to the fiber or lignan components, such as proposed laxative or anticancer properties, have not been considered.

In relation to possible interactions involving flaxseed, reasonable application of known pharmacological principles suggests that oral consumption of flaxseed (but not flaxseed oil) may impair absorption of drugs or other nutrients ingested at the same time. Such possible pharmacokinetic effects on bioavailability may be minimized by separating intake by 1 to 2 hours before or 2 to 4 hours after flaxseed ingestion, depending on dose and other variables.

NUTRIENT-DRUG INTERACTIONS

Angiotensin-Converting Enzyme (ACE) Inhibitors

Benazepril (Lotensin), captopril (Capoten), enalapril (Vasotec), enalapril combination drug: enalapril and felodipine

(Lexxel); fosinopril (Monopril), lisinopril (Prinivil, Zestril), moexipril (Univasc), perindopril (Aceon), quinapril (Accupril), ramipril (Altace), trandolapril (Mavik).

Interaction Type and Significance

⊕⊕ **Beneficial or Supportive Interaction, with Professional Management**

Note: Specifically in management of IgA nephropathic renal failure.

Probability:
2. Probable

Evidence Base:
◉ **Emerging**

Effect and Mechanism of Action

Although immunoglobulin A (IgA) nephropathy is the most common primary glomerulonephritis worldwide, the pathophysiology involved is incompletely understood. Eicosapentaenoic acid (EPA) and docosahexaenoic acid (DHA) appear to alter renal hemodynamics and inflammation by acting as substrates for cyclooxygenase (COX) and lipoxygenase (LOX) pathways and shifting the balance toward less potent inflammatory mediators than those produced through arachidonic acid (AA), the primary omega-6 substrate. Omega-3 fatty acids also can modulate inflammatory and immunological responses through eicosanoid-independent mechanisms, including interference with a number of effector pathways triggered by mesangial immune-complex deposition.[113-115] Overall, many of the effects of fish oils in renal disease appear to parallel those observed in preventing the development and progression of cardiovascular disease. Consequently, fish oil may decrease immunological renal injury in patients with IgA nephropathy and thereby slow the decline in renal function.

Coadministration of ACE inhibitor drugs to manage hypertension through angiotensin-converting enzyme (ACE) inhibition may further reduce the rate of renal progression caused by IgA nephropathy, at least in part, by reducing deleterious effects of hypertension.

Research

Fish oil may be beneficial in the treatment of individuals with IgA nephropathy, but findings have been mixed. Donadio, Bergstralh, Spencer, and colleagues in the Mayo Nephrology Collaborative Group have conducted a series of studies into the therapeutic effects of fish oil in treatment of 106 patients with IgA nephropathy. In a 2-year, multicenter, placebo-controlled, randomized trial, Donadio et al.[116] compared the efficacy of fish oil (12 g/day) with that of olive oil (as placebo) in patients with IgA nephropathy who had persistent proteinuria. They observed that 6% of subjects in the fish oil group and 33% in the placebo group exhibited increases of 50% or more in their serum creatinine concentrations during treatment, and that the annual median changes in these concentrations were 0.03 mg/dL (2.7 mmol/L) in the fish oil group and 0.14 mg/dL (12.4 mmol/L) in the placebo group. The authors noted that none of the subjects receiving fish oil discontinued treatment as a result of adverse effects. Ultimately, the cumulative percentage of patients who died or had end-stage renal disease was forty percent in the placebo group after four years and ten percent in the fish-oil group. The authors concluded that in "patients with IgA nephropathy, treatment with fish oil for two years retards the rate at which renal function is lost."[116] Subsequently, Donadio et al.[117] examined the long-term influence of fish oil treatment on renal progression, as indicated by serial serum creatinine and 24-hour urine protein measurements, in this same cohort of 106 patients

extending beyond the initial 2-year trial period. Using an increase of 50% or more in the serum creatinine as the primary endpoint and end-stage renal disease (ESRD) as the secondary endpoint, they reported that after a mean follow-up of 6.4 years, 17 patients in the fish oil group versus 29 in the placebo group reached the primary endpoint, and a total of 27 patients (8 in fish oil group vs. 19 in placebo group) developed ESRD. Notably, from an interactions perspective, blood pressure was controlled in all trial subjects through concomitant treatment with ACE inhibitors. Thus, with this long-term study, the authors concluded that "early and prolonged treatment with fish oil slows renal progression for high-risk patients with IgA nephropathy."[117]

Nutritional Therapeutics, Clinical Concerns, and Adaptations

Physicians treating patients with renal disease, specifically IgA nephropathy, are advised to consider administration of fish oil, in conjunction with ACE inhibitors, as a means of reducing renal damage and slowing disease progression. The 12-g/day doses used in some of the relevant research are much higher than typically used in other nononcological therapeutic contexts. However, patients with IgA nephropathy will inherently be closely supervised and regularly monitored. Further research with well-designed and adequately powered clinical trials appears warranted to confirm these consistent but preliminary findings.

Anticonvulsant Medications

Carbamazepine (Carbatrol, Tegretol), clonazepam (Klonopin), clorazepate (Tranxene), divalproex semisodium, divalproex sodium (Depakote), ethosuximide (Zarontin), ethotoin (Peganone), felbamate (Felbatol), fosphenytoin (Cerebyx, Mesantoin), levetiracetam (Keppra), mephenytoin, mephobarbital (Mebaral), methsuximide (Celontin), oxcarbazepine (GP 47680, oxycarbazepine; Trileptal), phenobarbital (phenobarbitone; Luminal, Solfoton), phenytoin (diphenylhydantoin; Dilantin, Phenytek), piracetam (Nootropyl), primidone (Mysoline), sodium valproate (Depacon), topiramate (Topamax), trimethadione (Tridione), valproate semisodium, valproic acid (Depakene, Depakene Syrup), vigabatrin (Sabril), zonisamide (Zonegran).

Interaction Type and Significance

⊕⊕ **Beneficial or Supportive Interaction, with Professional Management**

Probability:
4. Plausible or
2. Probable

Evidence Base:
○ **Preliminary**

Effect and Mechanism of Action

Long-chain omega-3 fatty acids "increase seizure thresholds, and lower inflammatory mediators, which are increased in patients with epilepsy" and thus "may be useful in the nonpharmacological treatment of patients with epilepsy."[118] Inflammatory mediators appear to play a major role in the pathophysiology of epilepsy, and omega-3 fatty acids can lower plasma inflammatory markers.[119-122] Omega-6 fatty acids, particularly AA, can inhibit sodium currents and synaptic transmission.[123] In contrast, omega-3 fatty acids not only shift the balance away from AA but exert anticonvulsant effects through their activity as anti-inflammatory mediators. Further, EPA reduces proinflammatory mediators by inhibiting phospholipase A_2 (PLA_2)] and COX-2 enzymes and is itself metabolized to form anti-inflammatory prostaglandins.[118,124,125]

Anticonvulsant medications, such as valproic acid and carbamazepine, may work in part by selectively inhibiting incorporation and turnover of AA, but not DHA, in brain cells.[126,127]

Research

In a very small, open clinical observation, Schlanger et al.[128] reported that a diet enriched with omega-3 fatty acids alleviates convulsion symptoms in patients with chronic epilepsy. In a 12-week, randomized, placebo-controlled, parallel group trial, Yuen et al.[118] investigated the effects of omega-3 fatty acid administration, using 1000 mg of encapsulated fish oil (with 171 mg EPA and 112 mg DHA, and <100 IU vitamin A and <40 IU vitamin D) three times daily, in 57 patients with refractory epilepsy and ongoing treatment with conventional antiepileptic drugs (AEDs). The authors observed a significant reduction in seizure frequency over the first 6 weeks of treatment in the omega-3 group, "but this effect was not sustained." The treatment group also exhibited "a significant increase in EPA and DHA concentrations and a reciprocal fall in arachidonic and linoleic acid concentrations." Notably, "no change in serum AED concentrations was detected." The authors suggested that "further studies are required to examine different omega-3 FA preparations, different doses, longer treatment duration, and larger sample sizes."[118]

Nutritional Therapeutics, Clinical Concerns, and Adaptations

Fish oil, as a rich source of EPA and DHA, is known to exert numerous beneficial effects on healthy nervous system and immune function, both nourishing these tissues and reducing inflammatory processes. Physicians treating patient with seizure disorders using anticonvulsant medications are advised to consider coadministration of omega-3 fatty acids. Although evidence reporting reduced frequency of seizures with low dosages is only preliminary, it does indicate that such nutrient support does not adversely affect drug levels. Further clinical trials are warranted to determine safety and efficacy of such synergistic interventions and establish efficacious parameters of dose, patient characteristics, and other influential factors.

Chemotherapy (Cytotoxic Agents)

Including: Bleomycin (Blenoxane), carboplatin (Paraplatin), cisplatin (cis-diaminedichloroplatinum, CDDP; Platinol, Platinol-AQ), cyclophosphamide (Cytoxan, Neosar), daunorubicin (Cerubidine), docetaxel (Taxotere), doxorubicin (Adriamycin, Rubex), etoposide (Eposin, Etophos, VePesid, VP-16), fluorouracil (5-FU; Adrucil, Efudex, Efudix, Fluoroplex), gemcitabine (Gemzar), irinotecan (camptothecin-11, CPT-11; Campto, Camptosar), methotrexate (Folex, Maxtrex, Rheumatrex), paclitaxel (Paxene, Taxol), pliamycin (Mithracin), tumor necrosis factor alpha (TNF-α), vinblastine (Alkaban-AQ, Velban, Velsar), vincristine (Leurocristine, Oncorvin, Vincasar PFS).

Interaction Type and Significance

⊕⊕ **Beneficial or Supportive Interaction, with Professional Management**

☼ **Prevention or Reduction of Drug Adverse Effect**

Probability:
3. Possible or
   2. Probable

Evidence Base:
▽ **Mixed**

Effect and Mechanism of Action

Cancer cachexia is "characterized by a lack of a normal anabolic response to the provision of apparently adequate nutrition" and "appears to result from a persistent response to illness stimulated by the cancer resulting in a proinflammatory cytokine and catabolic hormonal environment."[129] These phenomena, along with loss of appetite, adversely affect quality of life and survival in many patients.

Fish oil provides both a nutrient and an anti-inflammatory agent that may enhance benefits of concomitant nutritional intake and may reverse weight loss, with apparent gains in lean tissue and performance status, as well as facilitate normalization of the metabolic environment in patients with some forms of cancer.[130] Coadministration of fish oil during conventional oncology care may reduce loss of appetite and slow the rate of weight loss associated with many forms of chemotherapy, as well as cancer progression, and stabilize adipose tissue, muscle mass, and skeletal integrity.[129,131-135]

Essential fatty acids (EFAs) such as EPA and DHA can alter proinflammatory cytokine production and acute-phase protein synthesis. Fatty acids, especially those derived from fish oil, can alter the activity of cell membrane–bound enzymes (e.g., Na^+,K^+-ATPase, 5′-nucleotidase), levels of various antioxidants, p53 expression, and the concentrations of protein kinase C, and thereby may reduce inflammation and oxidative damage, mitigate tumor cell drug resistance, limit metastasis, and exert direct cytotoxic activity against a variety of tumor cells.[136-138] The effects of fish oil on cardiac function, including supporting normal heart rate variability, suggest that coadministration may also be protective in oncology care, particularly when specific agents or general poor health portend potential damage.[110,139-141]

Research

Fish oil consumption may reduce risk of oncogenesis in some cancer types, particularly breast, colon, renal cell, or prostate cancer.[142-156] However, greater intake of fish does not necessarily enhance survival rates (e.g., from breast cancer).[157]

Administration of fish oil to oncology patients may act in several beneficial ways. With nutrient support the patients may experience reduced severity of wasting common to the pathological processes. Furthermore, the use of these EFAs may reduce adverse effects associated with conventional cancer therapy or provide direct and indirect therapeutic activity against neoplastic diseases. Other agents with anti-inflammatory activity, such as nonsteroidal anti-inflammatory drugs (NSAIDs), or antioxidant activity might also be combined to achieve synergistic effects.

Progressive weight loss and reduced appetite are common features of many types of cancer and contribute not only to a poor quality of life and reduced response to chemotherapy, but also to a shorter survival time than patients with comparable tumors without anorexia and cachexia. Numerous surveys have found that oncology patients are among the patients with the highest rates of self-prescribing nutrients and herbs, with omega-3 fatty acids among the substances most often used.[150] Prevention or treatment of chemotherapy-induced cachexia may be the main reason why fish oil is used within integrative oncology regimens.

Das et al.[138] reported that EPA and gamma-linolenic acid (GLA) "can potentiate the cytotoxicity of vincristine, cisplatinum and doxorubicin on human cervical carcinoma (HeLa) cells in vitro. Alpha-linolenic acid (ALA), GLA, EPA, and docosahexaenoic acid (DHA) enhanced the uptake of vincristine by HeLa cells. In addition, DHA, EPA, GLA, and

DGLA [dihomogamma-linolenic acid, the direct precursor to prostaglandin E_1] were found to be cytotoxic to both vincristine-sensitive (KB-3-1) and -resistant (KB-ChR-8-5) human cervical carcinoma cells *in vitro*." Furthermore, "pre-incubation of vincristine-resistant cells with sub-optimal doses of fatty acids enhanced the cytotoxic action of vincristine." Overall, these fatty acids "enhanced the uptake and inhibited the efflux of vincristine and thus, augmented the intracellular concentration" of the antineoplastic agents.

In a series of investigations, Barber et al.[132] studied the efficacy of a fish oil–enriched nutritional preparation in attenuating the progression of the acute-phase protein (APP) response in weight-losing patients with advanced pancreatic cancer, a process believed to shorten survival in such patients. Using a sequential series design, they administered 2 g EPA and 1 g DHA daily to 18 patients with pancreatic cancer for 3 weeks to determine the effects of a fish oil–enriched nutritional formulation on the concentrations of a range of individual APPs; 18 other subjects received full supportive care alone, and six healthy subjects served as additional controls. "At baseline, albumin, transferrin and pre-albumin were significantly reduced and fibrinogen, haptoglobin, alpha-1-acid glycoprotein, alpha-1-antitrypsin, ceruloplasmin and C-reactive protein (CRP) were significantly elevated in the cancer patients compared with healthy controls, reflecting their roles as negative and positive acute phase proteins, respectively." Over the 4-week study period the only significant change in APP concentrations in the treated cancer group was an increase in transferrin. In contrast, there were further significant reductions in albumin, transferrin, and prealbumin and a significant increase in CRP concentration in the control cancer group. The authors stated that these findings "suggest that many positive and negative APP are altered in advanced pancreatic cancer" and that the APP response "tends to progress in untreated patients but may be stabilized by the administration" of a fish oil–enriched nutritional formulation in such a way as to reduce wasting.[132] In a related study, these researchers found that an "EPA-enriched supplement may reverse cachexia in advanced pancreatic cancer."[158]

Integration of fish oils into a comprehensive approach to oncology care may also help prevent or reduce the severity of other degenerative processes, such as decreased bone mineral density and drug-induced cardiac damage, common in this patient population. Scientific knowledge of the potential benefits of fish oils on cardiovascular health in general suggest that they may be beneficial in patients being treated with chemotherapeutic agents known for causing damage to cardiac tissue. In this situation the anti-inflammatory and antioxidant effects of fish oils are among the probable mechanisms of action and the typical response of increased heart rate variability among the desired results. Similarly, the ratio of omega-3 to omega-6 fatty acids appears to play a role in bone health, with higher omega-3 levels contributing to maintaining skeletal integrity during aging or other degenerative processes.[135] Direct evidence of these protective effects in patients with cancer is lacking, but reasonable inferences from broader or related research suggests that further study of these potential synergies is warranted.

In a phase II study involving the combination of "antioxidants, both in the diet and supplemented, pharmaconutritional support, progestagen, and anti-cyclooxygenase-2," Mantovani et al.[159] demonstrated "efficacy and safety" in 44 patients with "cancer-related anorexia/cachexia and oxidative stress." They evaluated data on four variables (clinical, nutritional, laboratory, quality of life) in 39 patients who completed 4 months of an integrative treatment regimen consisting of "diet with high polyphenols content (400 mg), antioxidant treatment (300 mg/d alpha-lipoic acid + 2.7 g/d carbocysteine lysine salt + 400 mg/d vitamin E + 30,000 IU/d vitamin A + 500 mg/d vitamin C), and pharmaconutritional support enriched with 2 cans per day (n-3)-PUFA (eicosapentaenoic acid and docosahexaenoic acid), 500 mg/d medroxyprogesterone acetate, and 200 mg/d selective cyclooxygenase-2 inhibitor celecoxib." They reported significant increases from baseline of body weight, lean body mass (LBM), and appetite; "important decrease of proinflammatory cytokines interleukin-6 (IL-6) and tumor necrosis factor-alpha, and a negative relationship worthy of note was only found between LBM and IL-6 changes," and "a marked improvement" in quality of life as assessed using several standard scoring systems. Of the 39 patients, 22 were determined to be "responders" or "high responders" at the end of the study. Based on these findings, the authors concluded that "the treatment was effective and more importantly was shown to be safe" and that "therefore, a randomized phase III study is warranted."[159]

Nutritional Therapeutics, Clinical Concerns, and Adaptations

Physicians treating patients with cancer who are exhibiting wasting or may be at increased risk of such complications are advised to develop a comprehensive nutritional support program within which fish oil may play a central role. Although the available evidence is largely preliminary or emerging in character, and not wholly characterized by favorable responses, there is little substantial data suggesting any adverse effects from coadministration of fish oils.

Cyclosporine

Cyclosporine (Ciclosporin, cyclosporin A, CsA; Neoral, Sandimmune, SangCya).

Interaction Type and Significance

⊕⊕ **Beneficial or Supportive Interaction, with Professional Management**
☼ **Prevention or Reduction of Drug Adverse Effect**

Probability:	Evidence Base:
2. Probable	⦿ **Emerging**

Effect and Mechanism of Action

Cyclosporine is an immunosuppressant agent often administered on a chronic basis after organ transplant and associated with a wide range of often-severe complications, particularly drug-induced nephrotoxicity, which manifests as dose-dependent acute azotemia and chronic (and typically irreversible) progressive renal disease. Thus, cyclosporine induces vasoconstriction and hypertension, as well as other adverse effects. Furthermore, atherosclerosis associated with hyperlipidemia and hypertension is a major cause of morbidity and mortality after renal transplant, and cardiovascular complications are responsible for about 40% of deaths in renal transplant recipients.

Coadministration of omega-3 oils appears to work by several mechanisms, including altering the prostaglandin profile, competitively reducing thromboxane A_2 (TXA_2) synthesis, shifting serum lipid concentrations, exerting vasodilatory effects on afferent arterioles in the glomeruli, decreasing systemic vascular resistance (SVR), and protecting against oxidative damage.[160-162] The combination of omega-3 fatty acids with cyclosporine may show promise against nephrotoxicity and hypertension in transplant patients, especially as prophylaxis.

Research

Findings from numerous clinical trials investigating coadministration of fish oil with cyclosporine after cardiac, liver, and renal transplant demonstrate improved renal function (i.e., glomerular filtration rate [GFR] and serum creatinine) and reduced incidence of hypertension compared with patients not treated with concomitant fish oil.[163-165] Nevertheless, other studies report more limited benefit regarding kidney function. Overall, circulating drug levels, rates of rejection, and graft survival have not been adversely affected.

Omega-3 polyunsaturated fatty acids (PUFAs) are generally recognized as beneficial for individuals with chronic renal insufficiency, but studies have shown some important differences between initial and longer-term responses and between responses in rejectors versus nonrejectors. In an early study with 14 subjects, Sweny et al.[160] reported that coadministration of fish oil preserves residual renal function in renal transplant recipients with chronic vascular rejection. Also in 1989, Stoof et al.[166] published the findings from a small preliminary study that found adding 6 g/day of fish oil "can reduce CyA-associated renal dysfunction in psoriasis patients."

Subsequently, Homan van der Heide, Bilo, and a team of Dutch researchers conducted a lengthy series of studies focusing on use of fish oil in allograft patients. In a double-blind, placebo-controlled, prospective, randomized clinical trial, these investigators followed the course of early postoperative rejection episodes in 21 stable cyclosporine-treated renal transplant recipients. They found that renal transplant recipients benefited from omega-3 fatty acids (6 g daily providing 30% EPA and 23% DHA) during cyclosporine therapy, versus placebo using corn oil (50% omega-6). After 3 months, blood pressure decreased in the omega-3 group, and GFR and renal blood flow increased by 20.3% and 16.4%, respectively. The authors concluded that their results showed that fish oil coadminstration "has considerable effects on renal function and blood pressure in stable CsA-treated renal transplant recipients."[167] In a later randomized prospective trial, they compared the effects of 1-month coconut oil (6 g daily) with 6 g daily fish oil (providing 30% EPA and 20% DHA as their methyl esters) on the incidence and course of early postoperative rejection in 88 first cadaveric, cyclosporine-treated renal transplant recipients. They reported that, while prerejection renal function and the decline of renal function during the rejection episode were similar before treatment, "the rejecting and fish oil-treated patients showed a significant better recovery of renal function after a histologically confirmed rejection episode," with creatinine clearance being 43 mL/min/1.73 m² in the fish oil + rejection group versus 27 mL/min/1.73 m² in the coconut oil + rejection group, and serum creatinine being 183 and 283 mmol/L, respectively. Notably, "nonrejecting fish oil-treated patients showed no better renal function than the nonrejecting coconut oil-treated patients," although "cyclosporine trough levels were significantly higher in the fish oil-treated group." However, even though fish oil favorably influenced renal function in the initial recovery phase after a rejection episode in cyclosporine-treated renal transplant recipients, the authors concluded that 1 month after grafting there is no difference in the incidence of rejection episodes, renal function in the absence of rejection, and decline in renal function during a rejection episode between the fish oil- and coconut oil-treated patients.[168]

Fish oil can prevent or reduce cyclosporine-induced nephrotoxicity and limit decline in glomerular filtration rate in allograft patients.[169] In 1991, Brouwer et al.[170] observed that fish oil (3 g daily for initial 6 weeks, then 6 g/day) ameliorates established cyclosporin A nephrotoxicity after heart transplantation. Badalamenti et al.[171] conducted a placebo-controlled, prospective, double-blind, randomized study to evaluate the renal effects of 12 g daily omega-3 fatty acids (vs. corn oil) on cyclosporine-induced nephrotoxicity in 26 liver transplant recipients. After 2 months, subjects in the fish oil group demonstrated a 22% increase in effective renal plasma flow, 33% increase in GFR, 17% increase in renal blood flow, and 20% decreased in calculated total renal vascular resistance; these parameters in the corn oil group were unchanged.

Following studies showing benefits of initiating fish oil at the time of engraftment, Bennett et al.[172] conducted a double-blind, placebo-controlled trial investigating the implications of the initial versus 16-week delay in the introduction of fish oil after allograft surgery. They reported that all observed occurrences of "acute CsA [cyclosporin A] nephrotoxicity occurred in placebo-treated patients without differences in whole blood CsA among toxic patients, other placebo patients, and EPA-treated recipients." Notably, diastolic blood pressure fell by 9 mm Hg during the second treatment period in subjects receiving 18 g EPA and by 10 mm Hg in those receiving 9 g EPA, but rose by 2 mm Hg in placebo patients receiving corn oil. Nevertheless, with delayed introduction, "there were no differences in glomerular filtration rate, renal blood flow, or creatinine clearance among groups" at the end of the study. Thus, these authors concluded that based "on our experience and that in the literature, administration of omega-3 fatty acids for purposes of kidney protection would seem to be most useful when started early after surgery," and that delayed administration was "associated with minor clinical benefits."[172]

The coadministration of fish oil may prevent or reduce hypertension in transplant patients treated with cyclosporine. Since the late 1980s, the effects of omega-3 fatty acids on hypertension after transplantation have been widely recorded, with positive positive in a majority of human studies. Most, but not all, clinical trials have shown that in allograft patients treated with cyclosporine immunosuppressant therapy, addition of 4 to 6 g daily of omega-3 fatty acids from fish oil can reduce hypertension, compared with placebo.[161,166,173,174]

Ventura et al.[161] conducted a randomized double-blind trial with 20 orthotopic cardiac transplant recipients showing that administration of fish oil may reverse changes in the prostaglandin profile and thereby counteract cyclosporine-induced hypertension related to vasoconstriction of the afferent arterioles in the glomeruli. Compared with omega-6 fatty acids (placebo group), subjects treated with omega-3 fatty acids (3 g/day) "demonstrated a significant reduction in mean arterial pressure (120 +/- 7 versus 102 +/- 7 mm Hg; P = .0001) associated with a decrease in systemic vascular resistance." Thus, the authors reported that omega-3 fatty acids appear to induce a "beneficial change in the prostaglandin profile" that provides a "vasodilatory effect" and thereby reduces "blood pressure by decreasing systemic vascular resistance." They concluded that "therefore, [fish oil] can be used as an adjuvant for the treatment of hypertension in cyclosporine-treated cardiac transplant recipients."[161]

In a subsequent randomized trial, Andreassen et al.[175] found that postoperative daily administration of 4 g/day omega-3 fatty acids in heart transplant recipients is "effective as hypertension prophylaxis, depending on increases in serum eicosapentaenoic and docosahexaenoic acids," compared with an equal dose of corn oil as placebo. These patients were being treated with an immunosuppressive regimen consisting of cyclosporine (6 mg/kg body weight), azathioprine (2 mg/kg/day), and prednisolone (0.2 mg/kg/day), as well as alpha-tocopherol (3.7 mg), beginning 4 days postoperatively and continuing for 6 months. Systolic blood pressure decreased in the omega-3 group and increased in the control group after 6 months. Although diastolic blood pressure increased in both groups, this increase was statistically significant in the control group. The authors noted that the "decrease in systolic blood pressure was inversely proportional to increases in concentrations of serum eicosapentaenoic and docosahexaenoic acid." Also, although after 6 months "the endothelial-dependent phase of the reactive hyperemic response remained unchanged in the treatment group, it decreased significantly in the placebo group." The authors suggested that "preservation of microvascular endothelial function...may contribute to the hypotensive role of omega-3 fatty acids."[175]

Holm et al.[176] found that omega-3 fatty acids improve blood pressure control and preserve renal function in hypertensive heart transplant recipients years after transplantation. In a double-blind trial, they studied 45 clinically stable hypertensive heart transplant recipients 1 to 12 years after transplantation who were randomized to receive either 3.4 g omega-3 fatty acids daily or placebo for 1 year. Although subjects in the placebo group demonstrated a nonsignificant increase in diastolic blood pressure of 3 ± 2 mm Hg and a 14% increase in SVR, those in the fish oil group exhibited "no change in blood pressure or systemic vascular resistance."[176] Interestingly, in a related study, these researchers also found that omega-3 fatty acids enhance tumor necrosis factor-alpha (TNF-α) levels in heart transplant recipients.[177]

Although most studies report clear benefits that include improved kidney function, not all studies have found long-term improvements with fish oil; evidence of renal benefits is lacking in findings from several trials beyond that previously discussed.[168,172] Hansen et al.[178] found no effect of dietary fish oil on renal hemodynamics, tubular function, or renal functional reserve in long-term renal transplant recipients in a 10-week study involving nine healthy volunteers and two groups (nine subjects each) of stable, long-term kidney-transplanted patients treated with maintenance low-dose CsA or without CsA. The authors concluded that "long-term renal transplant recipients treated with a low maintenance dose of CsA had a well-preserved renal functional reserve," and that concomitant "fish oil in these patients did not improve renal function." Similarly, in a randomized, placebo-controlled, double-blind trial, Kooijmans-Coutínho et al.[179] reported "no beneficial effect after renal transplantation" after comparing data from two groups of 25 recipients of primary cadaveric renal allografts who had been treated with CsA and 6 g/day fish oil or coconut oil for 3 months. One year after transplantation, they found no significant differences between the fish oil–treated group and the control patients regarding renal function, blood pressure and antihypertensive drug use, number of rejection episodes, and renal histopathological and immunohistochemical studies. Such conclusions, however, were qualified with reference to the dose of fish oil used and the limited time of treatment.

In a randomized clinical trial involving 30 patients who had received a first cadaveric renal transplant with delayed graft function, Santos et al.[162] administered 6 g fish oil daily, containing 30% EPA and 20% DHA, with 1 U vitamin E and 5 U vitamin A per gram, or placebo, beginning 2 days

postoperatively, for 12 months. Notably, beta-blocking agents, in combination with a diuretic or a centrally acting vasodilatory agent, were administered for hypertension, with calcium channel blockers and ACE inhibitors used only as a second-line treatment. The authors noted that "patients in the fish oil group required significantly less antihypertensive therapy to maintain similar blood pressure values." However, fish oil coadministration "did not have any beneficial effect on renal function, incidence of acute rejection episodes, or 1-year graft survival." Noting the contrast in these findings with those of other trials (except the one just discussed[179]), the authors qualified their conclusions by adding that renal "function as measured by GFR and creatinine clearance was consistently slightly better in the fish oil group, and it is possible that the power of the study was insufficient to detect a beneficial effect."[162]

Nutritional Therapeutics, Clinical Concerns, and Adaptations
Physicians treating organ allograft transplant patients with cyclosporine or other nephrotoxic immunosuppressant drugs are advised to consider coadministration of fish oil, particularly in patients exhibiting hypertension or renal damage. Prophylaxis against cyclosporin A nephrotoxicity may also be indicated. The amount of omega-3 oils used to elicit a beneficial response in hypertension has varied. Researchers have started with initial doses of 3 g daily for 6 weeks, followed by 6 g daily for up to 1 year; doses as high as 12 g daily have been used in research contexts. Inherently, initial treatment of allograft patients after transplant surgery requires direct supervision and close monitoring, and long-term care involves chronic immunosuppressant therapy with regular monitoring of blood pressure, kidney function, and drug levels. The available data suggest compatibility of such concomitant fish oil use with standard hypertensive medications, such as beta blockers or ACE inhibitors, but any polypharmaceutical intervention warrants individualized adjustments crafted to the needs and vulnerabilities of the given patient.

Etretinate

Evidence: Etretinate (Tegison).
Similar properties but evidence lacking for extrapolation: Acitretin (Soriatane).

Interaction Type and Significance
⊕⊕ **Beneficial or Supportive Interaction, with Professional Management**

Probability:	Evidence Base:
2. Probable	○ **Preliminary**

Effect and Mechanism of Action
Etretinate is an oral retinoid used in the treatment of recalcitrant psoriasis vulgaris. Omega-3 fatty acids are known for their anti-inflammatory activity, as well as their role in the integrity of cell membranes, and may have independent therapeutic value in the treatment of patients with inflammatory dermatological conditions. The combination of these agents may provide an additive or synergistic effect.

Research
In two small clinical trials, Danno et al.[180,181] first found that combining low-dose etretinate and EPA proved effective treatment for psoriasis. They concluded that "better and more rapid improvement was obtained with the combination therapy for 12 weeks than with low-dose etretinate monotherapy" and

noted that EPA "was safe, and adverse reactions due to low-dose etretinate were mild or tolerable." Notably, however, in the earlier study,[180] they found that, along with the etretinate combination therapies, CsA monotherapy also demonstrated "greater inhibitory effects on the endothelial expression of the adhesion molecules than the other monotherapies" tested.

Nutritional Therapeutics, Clinical Concerns, and Adaptations

Physicians prescribing oral etretinate for patients with recalcitrant psoriasis are advised to consider coadministration of fish oil for its probable value in enhancing the therapeutic efficacy of the intervention. However, etretinate is no longer commercially available in the United States and Canada. Etretinate has not been marketed in the U.S. for years because it remains in the body (stored in fatty tissue) for a very long time, with attendant teratogenic risk in females of childbearing age. In the U.S. it has been replaced by acitretin, which remains in the system for months rather than years; discontinuation of acitretin for 3 years before pregnancy is recommended, but no period of discontinuation before pregnancy may be safe for etretinate. Drinking alcohol, however, can convert acitretin into etretinate, which then persists in body fat for many years, perhaps decades. Further research with well-designed, adequately powered clinical trials is warranted to study the possible synergistic activity between fish oil omega-3 fatty acids and acitretin (soriatane), which is closely related to etretinate chemically, and likely functions via a similar mechanism of action.

It is also critical to warn all female patients of childbearing age of the potential teratogenic effects inherent to etretinate, acitretin, or other oral retinoids. Principles of conservative practice are moving toward a general contraindication of retinoids in female patients who could become pregnant. Fish oil, in contrast, may provide multiple benefits to pregnant or potentially pregnant women in terms of fetal development.

HMG-CoA Reductase Inhibitors (Statins)

Atorvastatin (Lipitor), fluvastatin (Lescol, Lescol XL), lovastatin (Altocor, Altoprev, Mevacor); combination drug: lovastatin and niacin (Advicor); pravastatin (Pravachol), rosuvastatin (Crestor), simvastatin (Zocor); combination drug: simvastatin and extended-release nicotinic acid (Niaspan).

Interaction Type and Significance

⊕⊕ **Beneficial or Supportive Interaction, with Professional Management**

Probability:
2. Probable

Evidence Base:
◉ **Emerging,** possibly
● **Consensus**

Effect and Mechanism of Action

Epidemiological and clinical evidence demonstrates that fish oil can lower plasma lipid levels, especially triglycerides. However, omega-3 fatty acids may cause small elevations in low-density lipoprotein (LDL) concentrations, with more substantial elevations in individuals with familial combined hyperlipidemia, but with a paradoxical lowering of LDLs at high doses (e.g., 32 g/day).[53,55] The mechanisms underlying the protective action of omega-3 PUFAs against coronary artery disease (CAD) remain to be established. However, their multiple cardiovascular effects appear to derive from numerous potential mechanisms, including lower levels of serum lipids, antithrombotic properties and relaxation in coronary arteries, enhanced arterial wall pliability, anti-inflammatory properties, reduced oxidative damage, antiplatelet-derived growth factor properties, natural

ligands for peroxisome proliferator-activated receptors (PPARs), and antiarrhythmic properties.[182-197]

Statin drugs reduce serum total cholesterol concentrations and the risk of CAD in individuals with hypercholesterolemia by interfering with the activity of the hepatic enzyme hydroxy-methylglutaryl–coenzyme A (HMG-CoA) reductase. These drugs alone, however, are usually not effective in reducing serum triglyceride concentrations, and they are known for dose-related adverse effects.

The concomitant administration of omega-3 fatty acids, through dietary or nutraceutical sources, during statin therapy could theoretically impair the LDL-lowering activity of agents in this drug class. However, coadministration may also have a cumulative therapeutic benefit for individuals with combined hyperlipidemia through complementary effects within a comprehensive lipid management strategy.

Research

Over the past 20 years or more, a broad range of clinical trials have usually, but not always, found that fish oil can reduce triglyceride levels by 25% to 44%.[56,57,198-203] Research indicates that dietary fish, fish oil, or EPA or DHA alone may further elevate high-density lipoprotein (HDL) cholesterol, reduce risk factors associated with atherothrombotic diseases (particularly CAD), and improve other aspects of lipid profile and cardiovascular health.[41,57,97,203-206] Conversely, numerous trials have reported elevations in LDL concentrations, although such increases may not persist.[57] Overall, when Studer et al.[102] conducted a review of data on the efficacy and safety of different antilipidemic agents and diets on mortality, they found that fish oil and statins were the most effective interventions for lowering cardiac mortality risk, fish oil being superior to statin therapy. The benefits of omega-3 fatty acids for risk reduction have been attributed to several factors, including moderating effects on heart arrhythmias, support of normal heart rate variability, and antithrombotic and anti-inflammatory properties.[102,110,140,141]

Most research shows that the concomitant administration of fish oil and a statin drug can produce a broader and more effective therapeutic effect in the treatment of dyslipidemic individuals, by lowering both cholesterol and triglyceride concentration, than either agent alone. In a preliminary trial, Nakamura et al.[207] confirmed the combined effects of HMG-CoA reductase inhibitors and "eicosapentaenoic acids" on serum lipid profile and plasma fatty acid concentrations in patients with hyperlipidemia. The authors administered 900 or 1800 mg per day of the ethyl ester of EPA to patients with hyperlipidemia who had been treated with HMG-CoA reductase inhibitors for 30 months (±6 months). They reported three significant findings after 3 months of combination therapy. Serum total cholesterol and triglyceride concentrations were significantly decreased (from 5.63 ± 0.23 mmol/L to 5.02 ± 0.20 mmol/L); serum HDL cholesterol concentrations were significantly increased (from 1.23 ± 0.12 mmol/L to 1.34 ± 0.13 mmol/L); and plasma EPA concentrations and the ratio to AA in plasma were also significantly increased (from 101.9 ± 8.1 mg/L to 181.8 ± 23.9 mg/L, and from 0.640 ± 0.075 to 1.211 ± 0.170, respectively). Thus, they concluded that these "results suggested that the combination therapy of HMG-CoA reductase inhibitors and eicosapentaenoic acid was effective for patients with hyperlipidemia."[207]

Clinical trials by Nordoy et al.,[208,209] as well as Contacos et al.[43] and Liu et al.,[206] have demonstrated additive therapeutic effects on hemostatic risk factors, postprandial hyperlipemia, serum lipid profile, plasma fatty acid concentrations, LDL subfractions, and plasma lipoproteins from coadministration of omega-3 fatty acids with simvastatin, pravastatin, and atorvastatin in patients with combined hyperlipemia. In the Japan EPA Lipid Intervention Study (JELIS), a large, prospective, randomized, open-label, blinded endpoint trial, Yokoyama and Origasa[97] studied the long-term use of highly purified EPA ethyl ester (600 mg three times daily), in conjunction with an HMG-CoA reductase inhibitor (either pravastatin or simvastatin), in preventing cardiovascular events in Japanese patients with hypercholesterolemia over a period lasting up to 5 years. Among their intermediate findings, they found that the combination of EPA and statins is an effective preventive measure against heart disease. They observed that each therapy alone successfully reduced the LDL to the same degree, approximately 26%. Moreover, they reported a 19% reduction risk among patients who experience sudden cardiac death, heart attack, or angina and who undergo coronary artery bypass surgery while treated with this combination therapy, versus statin therapy alone.

Several short-term and small studies, particularly those involving individuals with familial hypercholesterolemia, have produced less consistent findings on various lipid factors and suggested an increased risk of adverse effects, such as elevated LDL concentrations and spontaneous epistaxis, after treatment with variable doses of fish oil.[53,78] Ullmann et al.[210] reported additive effects with the combination of lovastatin and fish oil in patients with familial hypercholesterolemia. Balestrieri, Salvi, et al.[211] conducted a double-blind, placebo-controlled, randomized crossover trial involving 14 subjects affected by familial heterozygous hypercholesterolemia on chronic treatment with simvastatin. They observed that coadministration of fish oil ethyl ester (5.1 g/day) on lipid and lipoprotein serum concentrations did not produce "any significant variation" on total cholesterol, LDL cholesterol, HDL cholesterol, triglycerides, apoprotein B, apoprotein AI, or lipoprotein(a) during a 4-week treatment period. The authors interpreted their findings to "suggest that the possible favourable influence of fish oil on the progression of atherosclerosis in these high-risk patients might involve mechanisms which are different from lipid metabolism." This same group of Italian researchers conducted another small trial in which they administered six capsules of fish oil daily for 4 weeks to 10 patients (mean age, 49 ±14 years) "with heterozygous familial hypercholesterolemia who had high levels of lipoprotein (Lp)(a) (>30 mg/dl) and were receiving chronic treatment with simvastatin." Each 1-g "fish oil capsule contained almost 850 mg of omega-3 fatty acids with a ratio of eicosapentaenoic acid:docosahexaenoic acid of 1:1; the total daily dosage of omega-3 fatty acid was 5.1 gm/day." They reported that "mean serum Lp(a) levels did not change significantly" after 2 and 4 weeks of concomitant fish oil, and triglyceride levels decreased by 23% after 2 weeks (from 1.355 ± 0.38 mmol/L to 1.05 ± 0.35 mmol/L) and by 33% after 4 weeks (to 0.91 ± 0.18 mmol/L). Notably, total cholesterol and LDL cholesterol "showed a less pronounced but still statistically significant reduction of 8% (from 7.33 ± 2.55 mmol/L to 6.76 ± 1.31 mmol/L) and 9% (from 5.52 ± 1.98 mmol/L to 5.00 ± 1.67 mmol/L), respectively," after 2 weeks, followed by a "14% decrease in total cholesterol (to 6.30 ± 1.36 mmol/L) and LDL cholesterol (to 4.75 ± 1.49 mmol/L)" after 4 weeks. They observed a lack of significant change in HDL cholesterol concentrations. They cautioned that their findings of a positive "effect of fish oil on Lp(a) levels must be confirmed by double-blind, placebo-controlled studies before any definite conclusion can be drawn."[212]

In a 1991 review, Simopoulos[55] noted that in "patients with hyperlipidemia, omega 3 fatty acids decrease low-density lipoprotein (LDL) cholesterol if the saturated fatty acid content [of the diet] is decreased, otherwise there is a slight increase, but at high doses (32 g) they lower LDL cholesterol; furthermore, they consistently lower serum triglycerides in normal subjects and in patients with hypertriglyceridemia, whereas the effect on high-density lipoprotein (HDL) varies from no effect to slight increases." Thus, although fish oil therapy may alter LDL levels to varying degree, with the greatest risk being among individuals with familial hypercholesterolemia, such adverse effects are neither universal nor unaccompanied by beneficial effects, and may be strongly influenced by dose and diet.

The beneficial effects of integrative therapy combining omega-3 fatty acids and a statin drug (especially with concomitant aerobic exercise) appears to exert a particular influence among individuals with type 2 diabetes, particularly in controlling lipid levels, without significant risk of impairing glycemic control.[213] Kromhout et al.[213a] demonstrated an inverse relation between fish consumption and 20-year mortality from coronary heart disease (CHD) that may have particular relevance to triglyceride levels in the context of diabetes. Durrington et al.[202] investigated the triglyceride-lowering effectiveness, safety, and tolerability of 2 g daily of a proprietary concentrate of omega-3, long-chain PUFAs (Omacor), derived from fish oil but containing 84% of the total as opposed to an average of 35% in fish oil, over 1 year in 59 patients with established CHD and persisting hypertriglyceridemia (>2.3 mmol/L), despite simvastatin therapy (10-40 mg daily). The authors reported "a sustained significant decrease in serum triglycerides" (20%-30%) and in very-low-density lipoprotein (VLDL) cholesterol (30%-40%) in patients receiving omega-3 concentrate at 3, 6, and 12 months, compared with either baseline or placebo. The authors observed no deleterious effect on LDL or HDL cholesterol or on biochemical and hematological safety tests. Notably, the fish oil was well tolerated in general, and patients with diabetes in particular demonstrated no adverse effect on glycemic control. Overall, the subjects with diabetes exhibited a "decrease in serum triglyceride, which was at least as great as in non-diabetic patients." Thus, the authors concluded that "Omacor was found to be a safe and effective means of lowering serum triglycerides over one year in patients with CHD and combined hyperlipidaemia, whose triglycerides remained elevated despite simvastatin treatment."[202]

In response to preliminary data suggesting that fish oil may impair glycemic control in individuals with non-insulin-dependent diabetes mellitus (NIDDM), Dunstan et al.[72] conducted a controlled, 8-week trial to examine the effects of moderate aerobic exercise and a low-fat diet, including fish, on serum lipids and glycemic control in dyslipidemic NIDDM patients. The investigators randomly assigned 55 "sedentary NIDDM subjects (with serum triglycerides > 1.8 mmol/L and/or HDL cholesterol < 1.0 mmol/L) to a low-fat diet (30% daily energy intake) with or without one fish meal daily (3.6 g omega-3/day) and further randomized to a moderate (55-65% VO$_2$max) or light (heart rate < 100 bpm) exercise program." They reported that among the 49 subjects who completed the study, "moderate exercise improved aerobic fitness (VO$_2$max) by 12%," and fish consumption reduced triglycerides (0.80 mmol/L) and HDL$_3$ cholesterol (0.05 mmol/L) and increased HDL$_2$ cholesterol. Based on these findings, the authors concluded that a "reduced fat diet incorporating one daily fish meal reduces serum triglycerides and increases HDL$_2$ cholesterol in dyslipidemic NIDDM patients" and noted that potential omega-3-induced deterioration in glycemic control "can be prevented by a concomitant program of moderate exercise."[72]

The increased risk of cardiovascular disease in insulin-resistant, obese individuals is considered to result, at least in part, from hepatic accumulation of lipid substrates that perturb apolipoprotein B-100 (apoB) metabolism. In a placebo-controlled trial involving 48 subjects, Chan et al.[214] found that the combination of fish oil (4 g/day) and atorvastatin (40 mg/day) was effective in treating dyslipidemia in obese, insulin-resistant men. The authors demonstrated that atorvastatin significantly decreased plasma apoB-containing lipoproteins by increasing the fractional catabolic rate of VLDL-apoB, intermediate-density lipoprotein (IDL)–apoB, and LDL-apoB. Concurrently, they observed that fish oil significantly decreased plasma triglycerides and VLDL-apoB levels and decreased VLDL-apoB secretion rate; conversion of VLDL to LDL increased. Overall, the combination of atorvastatin and fish oil decreased VLDL-apoB secretion and increased the fractional catabolic rate of apoB in each lipoprotein fraction, compared with placebo, as well as the percent conversion of VLDL to LDL. Notably, none of the interventions altered insulin resistance. The investigators concluded that "atorvastatin increased hepatic clearance of all apoB-containing lipoproteins, whereas fish oils decreased hepatic secretion of [VLDL]-apoB. The differential effects of atorvastatin and fish oils on apoB kinetics support their combined use in correcting defective apoB metabolism in obese, insulin-resistant subjects."[214]

Although known for its anti-inflammatory activity, fish oil alone is not as effective as treatment with atorvastatin alone or a combination of atorvastatin and fish oil in reducing C-reactive protein (CRP) levels in dyslipidemic, obese individuals with visceral obesity and increased plasma high-sensitivity CRP.[215]

Shifting the dietary omega-6 to omega-3 ratio by increasing omega-3 sources and reducing omega-6 sources may also benefit several cardiovascular risk parameters.[110]

In related research, Wander et al.[216] conducted a double-blind crossover trial involving 48 women, equally divided between women using and not using hormone replacement therapy (HRT), to evaluate the effects of RRR-alpha-tocopheryl acetate (alpha-tocopheryl acetate) and HRT on the oxidative susceptibility of LDL in postmenopausal women consuming a 15-g fish oil product daily, versus placebo. They assessed LDL resistance to oxidative modification by calculating lag time, propagation rate, and maximum production of conjugated dienes. They observed that consumption of fish oil and alpha-tocopheryl acetate "increased plasma and LDL alpha-tocopherol contents significantly and lengthened lag time (at even the lowest concentration) but had no significant effect on propagation rate or maximum production compared with values measured after consumption of fish oil alone." Also, fish oil with placebo shortened lag time and slowed propagation rate in women both using and not using HRT. In their central finding, the authors observed that women "not using HRT had faster propagation rates and higher maximum production than women using HRT; after supplementation with fish oil and alpha-tocopheryl acetate these differences prevailed." Consequently, the authors concluded that the combination of fish oil and doses of alpha-tocopheryl acetate "as low as" 100 mg daily "increase the resistance of LDL to oxidation" and that "HRT and fish oil supplements may independently affect LDL oxidative susceptibility."[216]

Nutritional Therapeutics, Clinical Concerns, and Adaptations

Physicians treating individuals with combined dyslipidemia, particularly hypercholesterolemia and hypertriglyceridemia,

using statin therapy are advised to consider a comprehensive strategy combining pharmacological, nutritional, dietary, and lifestyle components customized to optimize lipid balance and metabolism, maximize patient participation and compliance, and secure a safe, sustainable, and effective intervention aimed at long-term health, prevention, and treatment. Eating a meal based around omega-3-rich fish two to three times a week is generally advisable, tempered only by risks of mercury or other toxic pollutants. In individuals with elevated risk for or diagnosed with cardiovascular disease, 1 to 3 g fish oil, at standard EPA/DHA proportions, in capsules or other nutraceutical forms represents a minimal daily dose, generally not needing professional supervision, whereas 4 to 6 g daily, or use of an equivalent concentrated product, is often indicated, but under the supervision of a health care professional. Continued research is warranted to clarify common and divergent effects of dietary fish, fish oils of standard composition, purified fish oils, and esterified EPA/DHA in both research and clinical settings.

The role of fish oil within such an integrative approach has been well established and can be optimized through coadministration of garlic, niacin (or inositol hexaniacinate), naturally occurring forms of vitamins A, E, and C, magnesium, potassium, and coenzyme Q10. For example, concomitant administration of garlic may provide a synergistic effect in lowering triglycerides while preventing the expected moderate fish oil–induced rise in LDL cholesterol.[58] The importance of regular exercise and a balanced diet rich in these nutrients cannot be overemphasized, and persistent and supportive cultivation of healthful behavioral changes cannot be underestimated.

By inhibiting the mevalonate pathway, the mechanism of action of statin drugs inherently impairs the endogenous synthesis of coenzyme Q10 (coQ10), an essential mitochondrial antioxidant produced through HMG-CoA reductase. Thus, as a protective measure, many health care professionals experienced in nutritional therapies prescribe coQ10 to prevent adverse effects from this action. Evidence is lacking, however, to prove a high incidence of broad-spectrum, clinically significant adverse effects (e.g., heart failure) or to confirm the advantages of concomitant prophylactic coQ10.[217]

Relatively small amounts of fish oil can have beneficial effects on plasma triglyceride levels in many hypertriglyceridemic patients. Importantly, however, doses used in clinical trials were typically 3 to 6 g per day, and the preparations used sometimes had modified proportions of DHA and EPA or were proprietary concentrated products. Further, although the medical literature, especially secondary and derivative material, carries an abundance of warnings that fish oil intake exceeding 3 g/day may increase the risk of bleeding, reports of such adverse effects are rare among the available primary clinical findings and qualified published case reports. If such events were common at a clinically significant level of severity, a sizable body of literature would be expected, not only amid the 30 years of clinical trials, but more broadly, given the widespread use of fish oil among the general public, especially within the population of patients with cardiovascular disease. Clearly, further research into the probability and circumstances of such potential adverse events is warranted given usage patterns and the reasonable pharmacological and physiological underpinning of the cause for concern. Overall, platelet antiaggregation and changes in cell membrane constituents may increase certain risks in some individuals or with certain pathologies; nevertheless, improved viscosity, arterial pliability, antiarrhythmic activity, and other properties are never mentioned as possible source of adverse reactions.

The potential for elevated LDL cholesterol and apoB levels and increased LDL/HDL cholesterol ratio suggests the need for careful monitoring of plasma lipoprotein changes during fish oil administration, as well as careful evaluation of their long-term benefits.

Selective Serotonin Reuptake Inhibitor (SSRI) Antidepressants

Citalopram (Celexa), escitalopram (S-citalopram; Lexapro), fluoxetine (Prozac, Sarafem), fluvoxamine (Faurin, Luvox), paroxetine (Aropax, Deroxat, Paxil, Seroxat), sertraline (Zoloft).
Similar properties but evidence lacking for extrapolation: Selective serotonin reuptake inhibitor/serotonin-norepinephrine reuptake inhibitor (SSRI/SNRI) antidepressants: Duloxetine (Cymbalta), venlafaxine (Effexor).

Interaction Type and Significance
⊕⊕ **Beneficial or Supportive Interaction, with Professional Management**

Probability: Evidence Base:
4. Plausible   ○ Preliminary

Effect and Mechanism of Action
Omega-3 fatty acids, particularly DHA, are a major component of neuronal tissue, particularly in the gray matter of the brain, and deficient states are associated with a wide range of neurological and psychological conditions. An epidemiological association has occasionally been proposed between populations with high rates of fish and fish oil consumption and low rates of depressive disorder.[218,219] Normal serotonin synthesis requires the availability of an ample supply of EFAs and as such provides for the intended activity of SSRIs in maintaining elevated levels of circulating serotonin as a primary mechanism of action in treating depression. The administration of omega-3 fatty acids, particularly fish oils, may enhance neurological activity and psychological states and complement or directly interact with SSRI medications in the treatment of individuals with depression, emotional lability, aggression, or other problematic behaviors.

Research
Although research into the effects of omega-3 fatty acids in the treatment of individuals with depression and a range of other mood disorders is rapidly emerging, the direct investigation of the concomitant administration of conventional antidepressants, particularly SSRIs, with therapeutic doses of omega-3 and other EFAs remains limited.

Using a rodent model, Kodas et al.[95] showed an association between chronic alpha-linolenic acid (ALA) deficiencies and decreased levels in overall serotoninergic neurotransmission. The authors reported that "chronic n-3 polyunsaturated fatty acid dietary deficiency induced changes in the synaptic levels of 5-HT both in basal conditions and after pharmacological stimulation with fenfluramine," and that higher "levels of basal 5-HT release and lower levels of 5-HT-stimulated release were found in deficient than in control rats." These neurochemical modifications were reversed once a balanced diet providing adequate EFAs was administered.

In a randomized, double-blind, placebo-controlled trial involving 36 subjects diagnosed with major depression, Marangell et al.[220] failed to show a significant effect of DHA monotherapy (2 g/day), versus placebo, after 6 weeks.

The limited human research directly investigating coadministration of omega-3 fatty acids, DHA, EPA, or fish oil in patients being treated with SSRI antidepressants suggest a probable benefit, but evidence is insufficient to support a broad, well-founded conclusion. In a double-blind, placebo-controlled trial involving 70 subjects with persistent/recalcitrant depression despite conventional therapy, Peet and Horrobin[221] found that coadministration of ethyl-EPA (a modified form of EPA) improved symptoms. Findings from several small, double-blind clinical trials indicate enhanced therapeutic benefits using ethyl-EPA or mixed EFAs.[222-224] In contrast, Silvers et al.[225] failed to observe therapeutic benefit with fish oil as an adjunctive intervention.

Nemets et al.[218] conducted a 4-week, parallel-group, double-blind study involving 20 patients diagnosed with major depressive disorder to study the effects of adding 1 g twice daily of ethyl ester of eicosapentaenoic acid (E-EPA) to maintenance medication treatment for recurrent unipolar depressive disorder of at least 3 months' duration. The authors reported "highly significant benefits" in subjects treated with omega-3 fatty acid compared with placebo by the third week of treatment; for example, 6 of 10 patients "receiving E-EPA but only one of 10 patients receiving placebo achieved a 50% reduction in Hamilton depression score." They further added that it was "not possible to distinguish whether E-EPA augments antidepressant action in the manner of lithium or has independent antidepressant properties of its own."[218]

Nutritional Therapeutics, Clinical Concerns, and Adaptations
Physicians prescribing SSRI medications are advised to consider coadministration of fish oil as a source of omega-3 fatty acids, especially in depressed patients who rarely or never eat fish or take OTC products containing fish oil. The weight of evidence from the scientific literature suggests that such nutritional support may have independent and additive beneficial effects. Findings indicating that fish oil might impair the therapeutic activity of SSRI antidepressant are unavailable, as are qualified case reports of adverse events. Nevertheless, even with the strong safety profile of fish oil therapy, professional supervision and regular monitoring are warranted.

Sulfasalazine (and Oral Corticosteroids)

Sulfasalazine (salazosulfapyridine, salicylazosulfapyridine, suphasalazine; Apo-Sulfasalazine, Azulfidine, Azulfidine EN-Tabs, PMS-Sulfasalazine, Salazopyrin, Salazopyrin EN-Tabs, SAS).

Interaction Type and Significance
⊕⊕ **Beneficial or Supportive Interaction, with Professional Management**
☼ **Prevention or Reduction of Drug Adverse Effect**

Probability: Evidence Base:
2. Probable or   ○ Preliminary
3. Possible

Effect and Mechanism of Action
Sulfasalazine is among the medications used in standard practice for treating inflammatory bowel disease (IBD). Omega-3 fatty acids, particularly ALA, may reduce symptoms of Crohn's disease, ulcerative colitis, and other forms of IBD through multiple mechanisms of action, including modulating inflammation, reducing oxidative stress, and altering phospholipid-membrane fatty acid composition. Nevertheless, the precise mechanisms of action of ALA and fish oil in many of these

observed effects are still controversial. Concomitant therapy with both sulfasalazine and omega-3 oils may provide increased therapeutic effect through complementary actions, especially if imbalances between pro-oxidant and antioxidant mechanisms and "excess production of reactive oxygen species (ROS) by inappropriate activation of phagocytic cells" play a significant role in the pathophysiology of IBD.[226]

Research

Available data on the efficacy of omega-3 fatty acids in the treatment of IBD are conflicting, and analysis suggests that discrepancies in the findings and conclusions may result to a large degree from the different study designs, e.g., choice of placebo, insufficient washout period, differing formulations and dosages of omega-3 PUFAs.[227] Most clinical studies of omega-3 fatty acids fail to control the dietary ratio of omega-6 to omega-3, which can have profound effects on inflammatory mediators, regardless of the level of omega-3 supplementation.

Two early clinical trials involving patients with active ulcerative colitis both found that coadministration of fish oils with standard medications allowed reductions in oral corticosteroid doses. However, they arrived at partly divergent conclusions as to whether the omega-3 fatty acids reduced disease markers and enhanced therapeutic outcomes and which patient populations displayed stronger responses. In a randomized, blinded, controlled study involving 87 patients, Hawthorne et al.[228] administered "20 ml HiEPA fish oil as [the] triglyceride (4.5 g of [total] eicosapentaenoic acid) or olive oil placebo daily" for 1 year, "in addition to standard drug therapy." The investigators determined that fish oil administration "significantly increased the eicosapentaenoic acid content of rectal mucosa to 3.2% of total fatty acids at six months, compared with 0.63% for patients on olive oil," as well as "increased synthesis of leukotriene B5, and 53% suppression of leukotriene B4 synthesis by ionophore-stimulated neutrophils." Overall, they reported "measurable, but only limited clinical benefit," with "a significant reduction in corticosteroid requirement after one and two months treatment" in "patients entering the trial in relapse (n = 53)," and "a trend towards achieving remission (off corticosteroids) faster in the patients on fish oil, although differences were not [statistically] significant." However, in "patients in remission at trial entry or during the trial (n = 69), there was no significant difference in the rate of relapse by log rank analysis." Thus, the authors concluded that fish oil coadministration "produces a modest corticosteroid sparing effect in active disease, but there is no benefit in maintenance therapy," with patient response noticeably varying depending on disease activity at the onset of combination treatment.[228] In contrast, Stenson et al.[229] conducted a multicenter, randomized, double-blind, placebo-controlled, crossover trial with 4-month treatment periods (fish oil and placebo) separated by a 1-month washout involving 24 patients with active ulcerative colitis, 18 of whom completed the study. Although all subjects continued ongoing treatment with prednisone and sulfasalazine, those in the treatment group received 18 fish oil capsules, containing a total of 3.24 g EPA and 2.16 g DHA. In contrast to subjects in the placebo group, who exhibited no significant change in any variable, those administered fish oil demonstrated a "significant decrease in rectal dialysate levels of leukotriene B4 from 71.0 to 27.7 pg/mL" and "significant improvements" in acute histology index and total histology index, "as well as significant weight gain," a desired outcome in this patient population. Moreover, among the seven patients who received concurrent treatment

with prednisone, "the mean prednisone dose decreased from 12.9 mg/d to 6.1 mg/d" during the fish oil supplementation period but "rose from 10.4 mg/d to 12.9 mg/d during the placebo diet period."[229]

Dichi et al.[230] compared the effects of omega-3 fatty acids and sulfasalazine in treatment of ulcerative colitis (UC) in a randomized crossover design trial involving 10 patients (five male, five female) with mild to moderate active UC. Subjects received either sulfasalazine (2 g/day) or omega-3 fatty acids (5.4 g/day) for 2 months. The authors reported that treatment with "omega-3 fatty acids resulted in greater disease activity as detected by a significant increase in platelet count, erythrocyte sedimentation rate, C-reactive protein, and total fecal nitrogen excretion." They concluded that "treatment with sulfasalazine is superior to treatment with omega-3 fatty acids in patients with mild to moderate active ulcerative colitis."[230] Subsequently, Barbosa[226] and members of the previous research team conducted a clinical trial using a randomized crossover design and involving nine patients (seven female and two male) with mild or moderately active UC. They investigated the effect of adding 4.5 g/day fish oil omega-3 fatty acids (or placebo) to their usual medication of sulfasalazine (2 g/day) for 2-month treatment periods separated by 2 months, when they received only sulfasalazine. Using nine healthy individuals as control subjects to compare oxidative stress status, the investigators demonstrated oxidative stress in patients "by significant decreases in TRAP and LPI levels, increased chemiluminescence induced by t-BuOOH, and higher SOD activity." Notably, treatment with "fish oil omega-3 fatty acids reverted the chemiluminescence induced by t-BuOOH and LPI to baseline levels but that did not occur when patients received only sulfasalazine." The authors interpreted their findings to indicate "plasma oxidative stress occurs in patients with UC, and there was a significant decrease when the patients used sulfasalazine plus fish oil omega-3 fatty acids." However, despite observed reductions in oxidative stress, "there was no improvement in most laboratory indicators, sigmoidoscopy, and histology scores." They concluded that "omega-3 fatty acids may act as free radical scavengers protecting the patients against the overall effect of oxidative stress."[226] The clinical implications of this effect, however, remain unclear.

Nutritional Therapeutics, Clinical Concerns, and Adaptations

Health care professionals treating individuals with inflammatory bowel conditions are advised to consider omega-3 PUFA therapy as either an independent intervention or as a complement to sulfasalazine, oral corticosteroids, or other anti-inflammatory agents. Although the available evidence is still preliminary and findings are mixed in some areas, the evidence from clinical trials generally indicates that fish oil, especially purified forms and time-release preparations, can enhance conventional therapies through symptom reduction and reduced medication requirements. Further research through well-designed, adequately powered clinical trials appears warranted. In studies of all pathophysiology that involves inflammation, an attempt should be made to control and standardize the omega-6 fat content of the diets within the clinical trial, because this may be a major confounder of clinical outcomes.

Dosing will depend on the type of omega-3 PUFA administered, the formulation and preparation, concomitant medications and doses, and individual patient characteristics. Standard fish oil formulations may contribute to abdominal bloating, flatulence, diarrhea, or other adverse GI effects similar to those of IBD. Time-release preparations of omega-3 fatty acids may be better tolerated in individuals with IBD.

THEORETICAL, SPECULATIVE, AND PRELIMINARY INTERACTIONS RESEARCH, INCLUDING OVERSTATED INTERACTIONS CLAIMS

Amphetamines and Related Stimulant Medications

Amphetamine (amphetamine aspartate monohydrate, amphetamine sulfate; dextroamphetamine); dextroamphetamine saccharate, dextroamphetamine sulfate; D-amphetamine, Dexedrine).

Methylphenidate (Metadate, Methylin, Ritalin, Ritalin-SR; Concerta).

Combination drug: Amphetamine and dextroamphetamine (Adderall; dexamphetamine).

Dopamine is a neurotransmitter involved in learning, attention, problem solving, and fine motor skills. DHA is a major component of neuronal membranes and is involved in the development of the mesocortical and mesolimbic dopamine systems. A deficiency of DHA may result in altered dopaminergic functioning.[10] The interrelatedness is currently being explored.

Anecdotal reports from some clinicians suggest that coadministering omega-3 fatty acids with conventional mixed-amphetamine therapy may enhance therapeutic effects in the treatment of individuals with attention deficit–hyperactivity disorder (ADHD). Evidence from clinical trials investigating the effects of omega-3 fatty acids with amphetamines is limited and does not support conclusions at this point. Voigt et al.[231] conducted a randomized, double-blind, placebo-controlled trial involving 63 children age 6 to 12 years with ADHD already being treated with "effective maintenance therapy with stimulant medication," who received concomitant DHA (345 mg/day) or placebo for 4 months. The observed that plasma "phospholipid DHA content of the DHA-supplemented group was 2.6-fold higher at the end of the study than that of the placebo group." However, using a variety of assessments, "there was no statistically significant improvement in any objective or subjective measure of ADHD symptoms," and it was concluded that such additional nutrient support "does not decrease symptoms of ADHD."

Antihypertensive Medications

Antihypertensive Medications

Evidence as to the hypotensive activity of fish oil is mixed, and use in clinical practice for treatment of hypertension is controversial.[42,232-237] Nevertheless, findings from several clinical trials indicates that a modest reduction in blood pressure from intake of omega-3 fatty acids seems likely.[238-244] Dose-dependent reductions in blood pressure of 2 to 5 mm Hg have been observed, with DHA exerting greater effects than EPA.[240,245] In a 6-week, double-blind, placebo-controlled involving 59 overweight men, Mori et al.[243] found that DHA, but not EPA, lowers ambulatory blood pressure and heart rate in humans. The ALA in flaxseed may theoretically also lower blood pressure.

The lack of a direct body of research focusing on coadministration and interactions has lead to speculative extrapolations and sometimes unreasonably foreboding warning that concomitant use of omega-3 PUFAs and standard antihypertensive medications could produce excessive reductions in blood pressure. The implied notion that such beneficial changes would be unnoticed and inherently dangerous verges on irresponsibly alarmist. Responsible implementation of integrative therapeutic strategies in the treatment of hypertension necessarily involves patient education, self-monitoring of blood pressure, and professional supervision. Nevertheless, caution is warranted in patients with hypotension or in those taking blood pressure–lowering medications without informing their prescribing physician of other interventions, pharmacological or otherwise.

Atypical Antipsychotics

Aripiprazole (Abilify, Abilitat), clozapine (Clozaril), olanzapine (Symbyax, Zyprexa), quetiapine (Seroquel), risperidone (Risperdal), ziprasidone (Geodon).

Numerous studies and a range of clinical experience during the past 30 years suggest the potential of omega-3 fatty acid therapy in the treatment of individuals diagnosed with schizophrenia.[84,223,246-257] Most patients are already being treated with atypical antipsychotic and/or neuroleptic medications. By reversing deficiency of EFAs and prostaglandins, positively influencing concentrations of AA, reducing oxidative damage, and other effects, the intake of fish oils or other nutrient sources can support healthy membrane and nerve function. Horrobin[253] noted that in "patients with schizophrenia, treatment with eicosapentaenoic acid (EPA) produced clinical improvement, but that improvement was greater at a dose of 2 g/day than at 4 g/day. The improvement was not significantly correlated with changes in either EPA or docosahexaenoic acid (DHA) but was highly significantly positively correlated with rises in red cell membrane AA." Further research through well-designed clinical trials specifically focusing on synergistic strategies appears warranted.

Bile Acid Sequestrants

Cholestyramine (Locholest, Prevalite, Questran), colesevelam (WelChol), colestipol (Colestid).

Bile acid resins and omega-3 fatty acids both reduce triglyceride levels, so an additive or synergistic effect might be reasonably predicted with their concomitant administration. However, a more comprehensive strategy will be necessary in treating many individuals given the tendency of fish oil to elevate LDL concentrations, although these changes typically range from negligible to slight, but occasionally can be substantial.

The primary mechanism of action employed by bile acid sequestrants involves inhibiting the absorption of fats and fat-soluble nutrients, both beneficial and problematic. This activity inherently impairs the bioavailability of omega-3 fatty acids and suggests that coadministration of fish oil preparations and a bile acid sequestrant would require separating intake of omega-3s (as well as fat-soluble vitamins) from the drug by at least 2 hours.

Available evidence suggests synergistic combinations of multiple nutrient and pharmaceutical combinations for the personalized treatment of dyslipidemias and the need for further investigation into efficacy and safety, dosage, and sequencing strategies.

Fibrates

Bezafibrate (Bezalip), ciprofibrate (Modalim), clofibrate (Atromid-S), fenofibrate (Lofibra, Tricor, Triglide), gemfibrozil (Apo-Gemfibrozil, Lopid, Novo-Gemfibrozil).

Omega-3 fatty acids may cause small elevations in LDL concentrations while lowering triglyceride (TG) levels. Fish oils also reduce inflammation and oxidative damage while enhancing arterial wall pliability. Consequently, the concomitant administration of omega-3 fatty acids may enhance the TG-lowering effects of fibrates, as well as nicotinic acid or resins.

The effects of this presumed interaction are generally accepted as self-evident in the secondary medical literature, although evidence from clinical trials directly investigating coadministration of fibrates and omega-3 fatty acids in relevant patient populations is lacking. In a single trial comparing treatment options for hypertriglyceridemia, van Dam et al.[258] found that both omega-3 "fatty acids and gemfibrozil markedly decreased TG levels in patients with severe hypertriglyceridaemia," but that gemfibrozil "decreased TG levels and increased HDL-C significantly more than n-3 fatty acids." However, in a review of data on the efficacy and safety of different antilipidemic agents and diets on mortality, Studer et al.[102] cautioned that "any potential reduction in cardiac mortality from fibrates is offset by an increased risk of death from noncardiovascular causes."

Physicians treating patient with hypertriglyceridemia can consider omega-3 fatty acids of probable therapeutic benefit, both independently and in conjunction with standard antihyperlipidemic medications such as fibrates. This is consistent with the broad body of literature showing that higher consumption of omega-3 fatty acids correlated with a lower risk of coronary heart disease and nonfatal myocardial infarction. Shifting the dietary omega-6 to omega-3 ratio by increasing omega-3 sources and reducing omega-6 sources may also benefit several cardiovascular risk parameters. Omega-3 fatty acids have an excellent safety profile at usual doses and can be used by most patients with minimal supervision and regular lipid monitoring. However, a comprehensive strategic approach under professional supervision will be required in patient with elevated LDL levels because fish oil may cause small elevations in LDL that contravene, to a limited but largely undetermined degree, the effects of statin therapy.

Heparin and Other Injectable Anticoagulants

Heparin and Other Injectable Anticoagluants

Warnings of a potential adverse interaction between heparin and omega-3 fatty acids, particularly from fish oil, are often encountered in the derivative literature. However, direct evidence of adverse effects from clinical trials or well-qualified case reports is lacking. Further, substantive evidence as to an operative mechanism of action is insufficient and often replaced with reliance on assertions of the "blood-thinning" action of fish oil. Heparins act by augmenting the effects of antithrombin, and the newer injectable anticoagulants are direct thrombin inhibitors. There is no evidence, in vitro, preclinical, or clinical, that omega-3 fatty acids interact either with thrombin or antithrombin. Given the mild antiplatelet effects of omega-3 fatty acids, concern for increased risk of bleeding is reasonable in the relevant patient population; ungrounded speculation, however, is not an adequate substitute for clinical evidence, given the potential severity of presumed risks and the probability of coadministration among the target patient population. Further research through well-designed clinical trials is warranted, as is vigilance and systematic compilation of adverse events data. Caution, close supervision, and regular monitoring are appropriate pending clarification of these critical issues, as would be expected in such cases.

Nicotinic Acid, Niacin, Vitamin B$_3$

Nicotinic Acid, Niacin, Vitamin B$_3$

The combination of omega-3 fatty acids and niacin/nicotinic acid may produce additive or synergistic effects in lowering triglyceride levels.[259,260] A personalized and evolving pharmacological intervention with the indicated drugs and nutrients can enhance the healthy diet and regular exercise habits that form the foundation of any comprehensive program of cardiovascular risk reduction and therapeutic intervention.

Nonsteroidal Anti-Inflammatory Drugs (NSAIDs)

COX-1 inhibitors: Diclofenac (Cataflam, Voltaren), diclofenac and misoprostol (Arthrotec), diflunisal (Dolobid), etodolac (Lodine), fenoprofen (Dalfon), furbiprofen (Ansaid), ibuprofen (Advil, Excedrin IB, Motrin, Motrin IB, Nuprin, Pedia Care Fever Drops, Provel, Rufen; combination drug: hydrocodone and ibuprofen (Reprexain, Vicoprofen)), indomethacin (Indocin, Indocin-SR), ketoprofen (Orudis, Oruvail), ketorolac (Acular ophthalmic, Toradol), meclofenamate (Meclomen), mefenamic acid (Ponstel), meloxicam (Mobic), nabumetone (Relafen), naproxen (Anaprox, Naprosyn), oxaprozin (Daypro), piroxicam (Feldene), salsalate (salicylic acid; Amigesic, Disalcid, Marthritic, Mono Gesic, Salflex, Salsitab), sulindac (Clinoril), tolmetin (Tolectin).
COX-2 inhibitor: Celecoxib (Celebrex)

Omega-3 fatty acids possess many properties that might be protective against the adverse effects of NSAIDs on gastric and gut mucosa and thus reduce the risk of drug-induced ulcers. Using a rodent model, al-Harbi et al.[261] found that acute administration of fish oil (5 and 10 mL/kg body weight) significantly protected the gastric mucosa against ulcers induced by NSAIDs, reserpine, and necrotizing agents. Such activity is reasonable and consistent with known pharmacological activity of omega-3 fatty acids, and adverse effects are improbable based on current knowledge. However, well-designed clinical trials are necessary before substantive conclusions can be made as to possible protective benefits against NSAID-induced ulcerative damage in humans.

Oral Hypoglycemic Agents and Insulin

Chlorpropamide (Diabinese), glimepiride (Amaryl), glipizide (Glucotrol; Glucotrol XL), glyburide (glibenclamide; Diabeta, Glynase, Glynase Prestab, Micronase, Pres Tab), insulin (animal-source insulin: Iletin; human analog insulin: Humanlog; human insulin: Humulin, Novolin, NovoRapid, Oralin), metformin (Glucophage), tolazamide (Tolinase), tolbutamide (Orinase, Tol-Tab); combination drugs: glipizide and metformin (Metaglip); glyburide and metformin (Glucovance).

Hypertriglyceridemia is associated with cardiovascular disease in diabetes, and the relevance of fish oil therapy in such populations initially appears as highly indicated. For example, as early as 1988, Schectman et al.[262] compared the effects of 4.0 and 7.5 g of omega-3 fatty acids in fish oil with a placebo of 12 g safflower oil over 1 month in a single-blind crossover design and concluded that "in NIDDM patients, dietary supplementation with omega-3 fatty acids induces a reduction in total plasma and VLDL triglyceride levels."

Research investigating the effects of omega-3 fatty acids on blood glucose levels in type 2 diabetic persons report mixed but generally favorable findings. Overall, despite some reports of slight elevations in fasting blood glucose levels, the use of fish oil does not appear inherently to cause persistent elevations in blood glucose levels in type 2 diabetic individuals.

In response to preliminary data suggesting that fish oil may impair glycemic control in individuals with NIDDM, Dunstan et al.[72] conducted a controlled, 8-week trial to examine the effects of moderate aerobic exercise and a low-fat diet, including fish, on serum lipids and glycemic control in dyslipidemic NIDDM patients. The investigators randomly assigned 55 "sedentary NIDDM subjects (with serum triglycerides > 1.8 mmol/L and/or HDL cholesterol < 1.0 mmol/L) to a low-fat diet (30% daily energy intake) with or without one fish meal daily (3.6 g omega-3/day) and further randomized to a moderate (55%-65% VO$_2$max) or light (heart rate < 100 bpm) exercise program." They reported that among the 49 subjects who completed the study, "moderate exercise improved aerobic fitness (VO$_2$max) by 12%," and fish consumption reduced triglycerides (0.80 mmol/L) and HDL$_3$ cholesterol (0.05 mmol/L) and increased HDL$_2$ cholesterol. Based on these findings, the authors concluded that a "reduced fat diet incorporating one daily fish meal reduces serum triglycerides and increases HDL$_2$ cholesterol in dyslipidemic NIDDM patients" and noted that potential omega-3-induced "deterioration in glycemic control can be prevented by a concomitant program of moderate exercise."[72]

Similarly, Sheehan et al.[59] conducted a trial in which subjects received 20 g fish oil daily, and usual daily fiber intake was increased with a 15-g pectin supplement at midpoint. They not only observed the expected beneficial effects on triacylglycerol and VLDL cholesterol levels, but also found that "diabetic control was maintained" during the 12-week study, and that total and LDL cholesterol concentrations "decreased significantly" with concomitant fish oil treatment and high fiber intake.

Administration of fish oil for dyslipidemia in patients with type 2 diabetes does not appear to result in significant long-term adverse effects. In two papers published in the late 1980s, Stacpoole et al.[51,263] reported dose-response effects of dietary fish oil on carbohydrate and lipid metabolism in hypertriglyceridemia and concluded that the increased insulin needs observed in some diabetic patients on long-term fish oil therapy were most likely derived from other dietary changes or weight gain. In an early review article, Harris[56] declared that the "safety of fish oils was also supported in these studies because problems with excessive bleeding and worsening glycemic control did not materialize." Subsequently, in a 1998 meta-analysis, Friedberg et al.[264] concluded that the "use of fish oil has no adverse affects on HbA$_{1c}$ in diabetic subjects and lowers triglyceride levels effectively by almost 30%," even though "this may be accompanied by a slight increase in LDL cholesterol concentration." Two years later, in a quantitative systematic review of the effects of fish oil administration on lipid levels and glycemic control in patients with type 2 diabetes, Montori et al.[213] concluded that fish oil administration in individuals with type 2 diabetes "lowers triglycerides, raises LDL cholesterol, and has no statistically significant effect on glycemic control." They suggested, however, that trials "with hard clinical end points are needed."

In a randomized, controlled trial investigating the effects of omega-3 PUFAs on glucose homeostasis and blood pressure in patients with essential hypertension, Toft et al.[265] concluded that fish oil, "in doses that reduce blood pressure and lipid levels in hypertensive persons, does not adversely affect glucose metabolism."

The occurrence of a clinically significant adverse interaction between fish oil and medications for glucose control appears improbable for most individuals at usual dosage levels. Overall, the literature suggests that adverse effects on glucose control caused by fish oil administration in type 2 diabetic individuals is possible but uncommon and possibly self-limiting. Further, the ability of aerobic exercise and increased fiber intake to neutralize adverse effects associated with fish oil intake suggests that other lifestyle interventions typical within a comprehensive integrative approach to management of type 2 diabetes will also serve to enhance the benefits and moderate the possible adverse effects of fish oil therapy. Notably, no clinical trials or qualified case reports have been presented as supporting the hypothesis

that fish oil coadministration might impair the therapeutic activity of oral hypoglycemic medications (or insulin). Nevertheless, health care professionals treating patients with type 2 diabetes will want to advise and support healthy lifestyle and dietary changes and monitor any significant changes in diet or intake of nutrients such as fish oil or flaxseed at therapeutic doses.

Oral Vitamin K Antagonist Anticoagulants

Anisindione (Miradon), dicumarol, ethyl biscoumacetate (Tromexan), nicoumalone (acenocoumarol; Acitrom, Sintrom), phenindione (Dindevan), phenprocoumon (Jarsin, Marcumar), warfarin (Coumadin, Marevan, Warfilone).

Omega-3 fatty acids may increase the anticoagulant properties of warfarin and related anticoagulant drugs, although the frequency and character of a clinically significant interaction appears to be less certain and severe than suggested in most of the secondary literature. Intake of 3 g or greater of omega-3 fatty acids daily may increase the risk of spontaneous bleeding, although there is little evidence of significant bleeding risk at lower doses.[48,78] When combined with dipyridamole, omega-3 fatty acid intake may have positive synergistic effects for the protection against heart diseases and stroke because this combination acts to reduce thrombosis, most likely through antiaggregatory effects on platelets.[266]

In a 1994 paper, Weksler[47] proposed that omega-3 fatty acids, at very high intake levels, appeared to have multiple antithrombotic effects. However, a subsequent study of hemostatic factors by Archer et al.[49] considered race, gender, age, and weight and systematically examined the effects of dietary ALA, EPA, and DHA in the Coronary Artery Risk Development in Young Adults (CARDIA) Study. They reported that "no significant associations were observed between those who consumed no fish versus those who consumed the highest level of dietary fish with respect to fibrinogen, factor VIII, or von Willebrand factor for any race-sex group. Comparisons of tertile 1 versus tertile 3 for dietary linolenic acid, eicosapentaenoic acid, and docosahexaenoic acid were also not significantly associated with fibrinogen, factor VII, factor VIII, or von Willebrand factor for any race-sex group." The authors concluded that their "data suggest that customary intakes of fish and n-3 fatty acids in populations that generally do not consume large amounts of these food items are not associated with [changes in] these hemostatic factors."[49] The amounts reported in this investigation were not the high doses used in much contemporary research, suggesting that anticoagulant effects reported in many studies may be dose dependent.

In a 2004 paper, Vanschoonbeek et al.[267] presented their findings from a study of the variable hypocoagulant effect of fish oil intake in humans, particularly focusing on modulation of fibrinogen level and thrombin generation. For 4 weeks they administered 3.0 g omega-3 PUFAs daily to 25 healthy, borderline-overweight males. They observed that fish oil intake "reduced plasma triglycerides and lowered platelet integrin activation, as well as plasma levels of fibrinogen and factor V, but had no effect on vitamin K–dependent coagulation factors." Notably, fish oil intake "reduced thrombin generation in the presence and absence of platelets" in a manner "correlated with the fish oil effect on fibrinogen and factor V levels" and "clustered around subjects with high fibrinogen carrying a structural fibrinogen alpha-chain polymorphism." The authors concluded that dietary "omega-3 PUFAs provoke a hypocoagulant, vitamin K–independent effect in humans, the degree of which may depend on [preexisting] fibrinogen level."[267]

More research is needed in this area to provide conclusive evidence of the omega-3 fatty acid interrelationship to antithrombotic effects and potential interaction with anticoagulant medications.

Health care professionals treating individuals with a history of or increased risk of stroke or clotting disorders or being treated with anticoagulant medications for other reasons are advised to conduct a frank discussion regarding nutrient, herb, and medication intake and thoroughly inventory all agents. Close supervision is usually unnecessary for most patients using omega-3 oils at typical doses, but regular international normalized ratio (INR) monitoring and dose titration are always critical in patients receiving oral vitamin K antagonist anticoagulants, especially with introduction, withdrawal, or change in dose of any pharmaceutical, nutraceutical, or herbal agent.

Salicylates and Related Antiplatelet Medications, Including Acetylsalicylic Acid and Monoclonal Antibody Antiplatelet Agents

Antiplatelet thromboprophylactics: Acetylsalicylic acid (acetosal, acetyl salicylic acid, ASA, salicylsalicylic acid; Arthritis Foundation Pain Reliever, Ascriptin, Aspergum, Asprimox, Bayer Aspirin, Bayer Buffered Aspirin, Bayer Low Adult Strength, Bufferin, Buffex, Cama Arthritis Pain Reliever, Easprin, Ecotrin, Ecotrin Low Adult Strength, Empirin, Extra Strength Adprin-B, Extra Strength Bayer Enteric 500 Aspirin, Extra Strength Bayer Plus, Halfprin 81, Heartline, Regular Strength Bayer Enteric 500 Aspirin, St. Joseph Adult Chewable Aspirin, ZORprin); combination drugs: ASA and caffeine (Anacin); ASA, caffeine, and propoxyphene (Darvon Compound); ASA and carisoprodol (Soma Compound); ASA, codeine, and carisoprodol (Soma Compound with Codeine); ASA and codeine (Empirin with Codeine); ASA, codeine, butalbital, and caffeine (Fiorinal); ASA and extended-release dipyridamole (Aggrenox, Asasantin); aminosalicylic acid: 5-amino-2-hydroxybenzoic acid, 5-ASA, mesalamine, asacol, salofalk, pentasa, mesalazine, m-aminosalicylic acid, para-aminosalicylic acid.

Similar properties but evidence lacking for extrapolation: Monoclonal antibody antiplatelet agents: Abciximab (ReoPro), eptifibatide (Integrelin), tirofiban (Aggrastat).

Fish oil improves blood flow characteristics by replacing other RBC and endothelial cell membrane fatty acids with omega-3 fats. This shift, along with other factors, reduces platelet-derived growth factor (PDGF), decreases platelet aggregation, inhibits the expression of vascular adhesion molecules, and stimulates relaxation of endothelial cells in the vasculature.[268] The multiple antithrombotic and eicosanoid-modifying effects of omega-3 PUFAs may increase the risk of bleeding under certain conditions, especially at higher dosage levels, but are probably also an important factor in the beneficial effect of dietary fish oil observed on cardiovascular disease.[47-49,108,267,269,270]

Omega-3 fatty acids could theoretically increase the antiplatelet aggregation effects of aspirin and other antiplatelet agents in a bimodal fashion, that is, beneficial with atherosclerosis and risk of clotting in a cerebral or coronary vessel, but problematic with bleeding disorders or in patients taking oral or injectable anticoagulants. Although the effects of omega-3 fatty acids on hemostatic variables have been widely discussed in the scientific literature for many years, the evidence supporting a pattern of clinically significant adverse interactions is lacking. The combination of aspirin and omega-3 fatty acids may be beneficial under certain circumstances (e.g., heart disease) but problematic in other conditions (e.g., warfarin therapy, von Willebrand's disease). A consensus has largely been achieved as

to the modulation of fibrinogen level and thrombin generation and resultant variable hypocoagulant effect of fish oil intake in humans. However, the clinical implications of these findings remain controversial, and broad generalizations remain elusive, particularly with regard to the little-researched area of interactions between omega-3 oils and antiplatelet agents.

Minimal evidence suggests that fish oil, flaxseed, and flaxseed oil may cause increased risk of bleeding complications. The secondary literature has made numerous declarations, usually without primary supporting citations, that intake of 3 g or greater of omega-3 fatty acids daily may increase the risk of bleeding; there is general agreement that significant bleeding is improbable at lower doses in most patients.[47-49]

In a double-blind, randomized, crossover study involving six healthy volunteers, Iacoviello et al.[271] observed that the combination of low-dose aspirin (40 mg/day) and omega-3 fatty acids (5.3 g/day) modulated the fibrinolytic response to venous occlusion and could be therapeutic in the treatment of some forms of coronary artery disease.

Fish oil appears to modulate inflammation in the GI tract in ways that might mitigate damage to the mucosal tissues inherent to use of salicylates, especially with chronic administration, and suggest a possible beneficial interaction. Although research concerning the benefits of omega-3 rich oils alone with Crohn's disease is controversial, some studies report a pattern of improvement in patients treated with fish oil.[272-274] A double-blind, randomized, placebo-controlled trial involving pediatric patients suggests that administration of omega-3 fatty acids, in combination with mesalazine (amino-salicyclic acid), acts as an effective measure for maintaining remission of Crohn's disease. The synergistic combination serves to strengthen the respective inhibitory roles within the anti-inflammatory cascade.[275] However, although the full range of effects exerted by fish oil on inflammation remains unclear, available evidence indicates that fish oil does not appear to affect C-reactive protein levels.[214]

Given the large number of individuals who use aspirin on a regular or occasional basis and the broad use of fish oil and flax, a number of qualified case reports of interactions events would be expected. The absence of such documented events supports the proposition that, pending substantive corroboration, any such interaction should be considered preliminary and theoretical and its clinical significance improbable. On the other hand, however, the occurrence of an interaction may be widespread but its effects negligible or beneficial, and thus unlikely to appear in published case reports.

Health care professionals treating individuals at risk for bleeding disorders or related complications are advised to conduct a frank discussion regarding nutrient and medication intake and thoroughly inventory all agents. Close supervision is usually unnecessary for most patients using omega-3 oils at typical doses, but regular monitoring would be judicious in any patients at risk for excessive bleeding.

NUTRIENT-NUTRIENT INTERACTIONS

Arginine

In a 6-month, prospective, randomized, double-blind controlled study involving 64 HIV-infected outpatients (with CD4 lymphocyte count $\geq 100 \times 10^6$/L), Pichard et al.[276] found that the addition of arginine and omega-3 fatty acids did not improve immunological parameters compared with a group receiving only the base multinutrient oral formulation; body weight increased in both groups.[276] The synergy between omega-3 fatty acids and arginine in supporting wound healing and tissue regeneration warrants further research and development of evidence-based clinical guidelines.

Iron and Vitamin B₆

The delta-6-desaturase enzyme complex is central to PUFA metabolism. The delta-6-desaturase enzyme complex requires iron for its activity. The transmethylation reaction of proteins is impacted by vitamin B_6 deficiency. Consequently, deficiencies of iron or vitamin B_6 can exert an adverse effect on PUFA metabolism.

In a trial involving 59 subjects, Krajcovicova-Kudlackova et al.[277] determined plasma PUFA content in "apparently healthy subjects of the general population with no consumption of fish" and low vitamin B_6 serum levels (<3 µg/L) or with low iron serum levels (men: <12 µmol/L; women: <10 µmol/L) and compared to a control group with normal vitamin B_6 and iron serum levels (i.e., within reference range). They observed that subjects in groups "with low vitamin B_6 and low iron levels," conversion of ALA to EPA and DHA was "significantly reduced." The authors noted that the "inhibition effect on fatty acid synthesis was more pronounced in subjects with low iron levels than in those with low vitamin B_6 levels" and that "conversion indices correlated significantly positively with vitamin B_6 or iron levels."

This reported interaction between omega-3 fats and other nutrients is only relevant to individuals on vegan diets who do not consume EPA and/or DHA directly through either fish oil or algae-derived DHA. The observed patterns may relate to cognitive, cardiovascular, and other benefits and risks associated with fish oil intake. Further investigation appears warranted.

Vitamin E

The apparent interactions between omega-3 fatty acids and vitamin E are complex, paradoxical, and insufficiently understood to support any firm conclusions. High dietary intake of PUFAs can induce decreased vitamin E levels.[278] Vitamin E is usually added to fish oil products to protect against degeneration caused by oxidative damage and in response to concerns that long-term use of fish oil at high dose levels may deplete vitamin E. Subsequently, the resulting product sometimes is considered a potential source of excessive vitamin E because of potential accumulation of this fat-soluble nutrient. Similarly, the "blood-thinning" effects of these two important nutrients may be of concern in patients at risk for or diagnosed with bleeding tendencies, but solid evidence of adverse additive effects is apparently lacking. The clinical significance of these proposed risks is belied by the apparent lack of large numbers of adverse events reports relative to the sizable number of individuals consuming these nutrients regularly. Nevertheless, the issues raised may deserve further research and could lead to deeper knowledge of these nutrients, their actions and effects, and any possible interactions (beneficial or adverse) or complications.

Vitamin E has also been shown to counteract the elevations in blood glucose sometimes seen with initiation of fish oil intake in individuals with type 2 diabetes.[71]

HERB-NUTRIENT INTERACTIONS

Ginkgo

Ginkgo (*Ginkgo biloba*)

Ginkgo biloba, as well as other botanicals such as ginger and feverfew, demonstrates antiplatelet effects and thus may increase the bleeding tendency associated with fish oil. However, no supporting clinical studies or qualified case reports have documented such an interaction as clinically significant. Nevertheless, further research may be warranted given the high probability of concomitant use, especially self-prescribed by patients outside professional supervision.

Ginseng, Chinese/Korean

Chinese/Korean Ginseng (*Panax ginseng*)

Based on presumptive and usually unarticulated mechanisms of action, claims that ginseng may increase the bleeding tendency associated with fish oil are occasionally found in secondary and derivative literature. However, substantive evidence from qualified case reports or clinical trials is lacking.

The 279 citations for this monograph, as well as additional reference literature, are located under Omega-3 Fatty Acids on the CD at the back of the book.

PABA

Nutrient Name: PABA (para-aminobenzoic acid).
Synonyms: Para-amino benzoic acid, p-aminobenzoic acid, pABA; Potaba.
Related Substance: Para-aminobenzoate.

Physiology and Function

Para-aminobenzoic acid (PABA) is a member of the vitamin-B complex but is not generally recognized as an official vitamin.

NUTRIENT IN CLINICAL PRACTICE
Possible Uses

Arthritis, dermatitis herpetiformis, dermatomyositis, hair graying, infertility (female), insomnia, pemphigus, Peyronie's disease, scleroderma, sunscreen (topical UV obstruction), vitiligo.

Deficiency Symptoms

None established.

Dietary Sources

Whole grains and foods of animal origin, particularly brewer's yeast, wheat germ, bran, and liver.

Nutrient Preparations Available

As a single-ingredient over-the-counter nutraceutical, PABA is usually 100 to 500 mg per dose. More often, small amounts of PABA may be contained within multivitamin or B-complex formulations. Potaba, the potassium salt of PABA, is available by prescription.

Dosage Forms Available

Capsule, tablet.

Dosage Range

Dietary: None established.
Supplemental/Maintenance: Dietary requirement not established.
Pharmacological/Therapeutic: Dosage in clinical trial has ranged from 300 mg to 12 g per day.
Toxic: Toxicity possible with greater than 400 mg PABA; extended use of several grams daily is more likely the range necessary to induce adverse symptoms.

SAFETY PROFILE
Overview

PABA is generally considered to be safe and free of adverse effects at doses up to 400 mg, but minor adverse effects have been reported at doses as low as 30 mg/day. Some symptoms may be attributable to its mildly acidic nature when taken orally; these generally do not occur with the potassium salt of PABA (Potaba). Most reports of significant adverse effects, such as vitiligo or elevated liver enzymes, have been associated with daily doses of 8 to 12 g daily.[1,2] Deaths have been reported at 20 g/day in children and as high as 48 g/day (for 6 days, followed by 7 months at 8 g/day).[3,4]

Nutrient Adverse Effects

Dermatitis, fever, hypoglycemia, itching, liver toxicity, loss of appetite, nausea, vomiting.

Contraindications

Individuals taking sulfonamides and sulfones.

INTERACTIONS REVIEW
Strategic Considerations

Increased PABA levels, resulting from increased endogenous production or increased exogenous (nutraceutical) sources, can cause increased resistance to sulfa drugs (sulfonamides and sulfones) through its effect on folic acid pathways. Patients receiving long-term sulfa drugs (e.g., HIV/AIDS patients on sulfa prophylaxis for *Pneumocystis*) are at risk for folic acid deficiencies; for example, megaloblastic anemia is a possible complication. Homocysteine levels often rise with ordinary courses of sulfa antibiotics.

NUTRIENT-DRUG INTERACTIONS

Sulfonamides, Sulfones, and Related Sulfa Antibiotics

Evidence: Dapsone (DDS, diaminodiphenylsulphone; Aczone Gel, Avlosulfon), sulfasalazine (salazosulfapyridine, salicylazo-sulfapyridine, suphasalazine; Apo-Sulfasalazine, Azulfidine, Azulfidine EN-Tabs, PMS-Sulfasalazine, Salazopyrin, Salazopyrin EN-Tabs, SAS); combination drug: sulfamethoxazole and trimethoprim (cotrimoxazole, co-trimoxazole, SXT, TMP-SMX, TMP-sulfa; Bactrim, Bactrim DS, Cotrim, Septra, Septra DS, Sulfatrim, Uroplus); sulfamethoxazole (Gantanol). Extrapolated, based on similar properties: Sodium sulfacetamide (AK-Sulf, Bleph-10, Sodium Sulamyd), sulfanilamide (AVC), sulfisoxazole (Gantrisin), triple sulfa (Sultrin Triple Sulfa).

Interaction Type and Significance

✗✗   Minimal to Mild Adverse Interaction—Vigilance Necessary
✗✗✗   Potentially Harmful or Serious Adverse Interaction—Avoid
≈◇◇   Drug-Induced Nutrient Depletion, Supplementation Contraindicated, Professional Management Appropriate

Probability:	Evidence Base:
2. Probable	● Consensus

Effect and Mechanism of Action
Sulfones and sulfonamides exert their antimicrobial action by competitively displacing para-aminobenzoic acid (PABA) from its binding site on 7,8-dihydropteroate synthase (DHPS), an enzyme critical for de novo synthesis of folic acid by many pathogenic microorganisms. Specifically, DHPS catalyzes the condensation of PABA with 6-hydroxymethyl-7,

8-dihydropterin-pyrophosphate to form 7,8-dihydropteroate and pyrophosphate. Consequently, sulfonamide and sulfone drugs cause cell death by depleting the folate pool necessary to microbial growth. Furthermore, extended use of sulfa drugs can result in depletion of PABA as well as depletion of folate and subsequent elevation of homocysteine. Conscientious physicians are advised to coadminister folic acid when they prescribe sulfa drugs.

Research

The phenomenon of sulfonamide-resistant infections was first discussed in the late 1960s, but the mechanism of action underlying the effectiveness of sulfa drugs only gradually became known, with increasing knowledge of the interaction between PABA and this important class of antibiotics.

In a 1966 clinical trial involving 39 volunteers subjected to mosquito-borne malaria infections, Degowin et al.[5] observed that PABA intake impaired the antimalarial activity of dapsone (DDS) against chloroquine-resistant *Plasmodium falciparum*. The five subjects receiving both PABA (1 g four times daily) and dapsone (25 mg daily) demonstrated acute malaria, in contrast to subjects given dapsone only, before and for 1 month after exposure, in whom malaria was suppressed. Irshaid et al.[6] (1993) found that PABA substantially inhibited the acetylation of dapsone (DDS) by whole blood taken from both slow and rapid acetylators. In 1994, McConkey et al.[7] showed that auxotrophs of *P. falciparum* were dependent on *p*-aminobenzoic acid for growth. That same year, Voeller et al.[8] described the interaction of *Pneumocystis carinii* DHPS with sulfonamides and diaminodiphenyl sulfone (dapsone) and clarified that DHPS is the target enzyme for the sulfonamide compounds. In a subsequent study of the pharmacokinetic parameters of elimination of sulfamoyl benzoic acids, sulfonamides, and penicillins via tubular secretion, Ehlert et al.[9] observed inhibition of the conjugation of PABA with glycine in vitro.

In a 1999 paper, Vinnicombe and Derrick[10] investigated the enzymatic mechanism and sulfonamide inhibition of DHPS from the pathogen *Streptococcus pneumoniae*. Using equilibrium binding assays, they showed that binding of the substrate PABA to DHPS was absolutely dependent on the presence of pyrophosphate, which acts as an analog of the second substrate 6-hydroxymethyl-7,8-dihydropterin pyrophosphate (DHPPP), and that the product of the reaction, dihydropteroate, was also able to bind to DHPS. Sulfonamides were capable of displacing PABA in a competitive manner. Thus, the authors determined that the specific target for sulfonamide inhibition of *S. pneumoniae* DHPS is the enzyme-DHPPP binary complex. Shortly thereafter, in an experiment using *Saccharomyces cerevisiae*, Castelli et al.[11] found that 15 sulfa drugs inhibited yeast growth in a manner indicating competition with PABA. Such competition resulted from direct addition of PABA or through increased expression of the PABA synthase gene.

Despite the axiomatic mechanism involved and the consistent evidence available in the interaction, its incidence and severity remain largely unclear.

Clinical Implications and Adaptations

Physicians prescribing sulfa drugs should advise patients to refrain from concomitant use of PABA, to avoid interference with the therapeutic activity of the medication. Although there is no known and agreed therapeutic ceiling for PABA dosing that would not interfere with sulfa therapy, daily doses greater than 100 mg twice daily are more likely to have a clinically significant effect. Whether it is also necessary to avoid B-complex or multivitamin formulas containing lower levels of PABA remains uncertain.

Further clinical research is warranted to determine the clinical significance of various dosage levels of pABA intake in relation to particular sulfa agents and respective pathogens, as well as the importance and implications of folate coadministration for patients undergoing long-term treatment with sulfones and sulfonamide antibiotics.

THEORETICAL, SPECULATIVE, AND PRELIMINARY INTERACTIONS RESEARCH, INCLUDING OVERSTATED INTERACTIONS CLAIMS

Chemotherapy and Radiation, Particularly Paclitaxel

Evidence: Paclitaxel (Paxene, Taxol).

Following reports that PABA might be capable of inhibiting the development of melanoma in vitro, Dr. Peter Brooks[12] and colleagues at New York University School of Medicine conducted research on highly melanotic B16F10 melanoma cells, as well as lung and breast carcinoma cells, using PABA alone and in conjunction with conventional cancer therapies. PABA alone had little effect on proliferation, but these researchers observed substantial inhibition of proliferation if the cells were treated with PABA and then treated with ionizing radiation and/or chemotherapy. Subsequent experiments with melanoma-bearing mice yielded similar results. In particular, a significant decrease in tumor progression was noted in tumors treated with PABA plus paclitaxel (Taxol) and/or ionizing radiation, compared with tumors left untreated or treated with paclitaxel alone. Although the mechanism of PABA action remains unknown, results of differential complementary DNA (cDNA) array analysis suggest that PABA upregulates cell cycle control genes and downregulates DNA repair enzymes. Such preliminary findings suggest a possible role for PABA in optimizing existing cancer therapies. These researchers have begun a clinical trial investigating concomitant administration of paclitaxel and PABA in the treatment of patients with melanoma.

Methotrexate

Methotrexate (Folex, Maxtrex, Rheumatrex).

As a dihydrofolate reductase (DHFR) inhibitor, methotrexate interferes with folic acid activation while PABA increases folate availability through its effect on DHPS. Consequently, PABA coadministration, or folic acid intake, has been found to interfere with the therapeutic activity of methotrexate in individuals being treated for cancer.[13] However, the action of methotrexate in the treatment of rheumatoid arthritis or psoriasis does not depend on folate suppression, so administration of PABA (as well as folic acid or folinic acid) is not contraindicated, even though it might lower methotrexate levels, and can be beneficial in reducing adverse effects associated with the drug.[14-21] Close supervision and regular monitoring are appropriate during any such coadministration. Further research into such concomitant therapeutic protocols is warranted.

The 21 citations for this monograph, as well as additional reference literature, are located under PABA on the CD at the back of the book.

Nutrient-Drug Interactions and Drug-Induced Nutrient Depletions

Policicsanol

Nutrient Name: Policosanol.

Summary

Drug/Class Interaction Type	Mechanism and Significance	Management
Acetylsalicylic acid (ASA, aspirin) Antiplatelet medications ✗✗/⊕✗/⊕⊕	Policosanol can inhibit platelet aggregation, but probability and intensity of clinically significant additive effect with antiplatelet medications are uncertain. Concomitant use could be therapeutically efficacious and enable lower drug dosage with proper management. Potential risk of excess additive effect.	Coadministration can be beneficial. May need to modify drug dosage. Monitor and titrate.
Anticoagulant medications ✗✗/⊕✗/⊕	Policosanol appears to inhibit platelet function, but not to alter coagulation parameters and is unlikely to interact with anticoagulant medications to produce an additive effect of clinical significance. Hemorrhage or inappropriate thinning are theoretically possible but have not been documented. Concomitant use could theoretically be therapeutically efficacious and enable lower drug dosage with proper management.	Coadministration may be beneficial (or potentially risky). May need to modify drug dosage. Monitor and titrate.
Beta-1-Adrenoceptor antagonists Antihypertensive medications ✗✗/⊕✗/⊕⊕	Policosanol can exert hypotensive effect, but probability and intensity of clinically significant additive effect with beta blockers are uncertain. Potential risk of additive effect and excess hypotensive action. Coadministration could be therapeutically efficacious and enable lower drug dosage with proper management.	Coadministration can be beneficial (or risky). May need to modify drug dosage. Monitor and titrate.
HMG-CoA reductase inhibitors (statins) ✗/⊕✗/⊕⊕	Both HMG-CoA reductase inhibitors and policosanol can inhibit cholesterol synthesis to varying degrees. Clinically significant additive or synergistic effect is possible, but research findings are preliminary and mixed. Concomitant use could potentially be therapeutically efficacious and enable lower statin dosage (and reduced adverse effects) with proper management, particularly within a personalized strategy. Minimal risk of detrimental additive effect.	Coadministration may be beneficial, typically within a strategy including coQ10, niacin, fish oil, and other agents. Monitor closely within context of integrative cardiovascular care. May need to modify drug dosage.

NUTRIENT DESCRIPTION

Chemistry and Form

Policosanol contains a natural mixture of eight long-chain aliphatic primary alcohols extracted from the wax of sugarcane (*Saccharum officinarum* L.). A similar complex of long-chain aliphatic alcohols can also be derived from rice bran and beeswax, although most of the existing clinical studies have been done with sugarcane-derived material. Octacosanol (18-carbon) is the predominant moiety, constituting approximately 60% of the mixture. Other important constituents include triacontanol (13%) and hexacosanol (6%). Minor components include tetracosanol, heptacocosanol, nonacosanol, dotriacontanol, and tetratriacontanol.

Physiology and Function

Policosanol decreases levels of cholesterol in serum as well as cholesterol content in various tissues, such as liver, heart, and fatty tissue. In numerous clinical trials, policosanol has demonstrated lipid-lowering efficacy comparable to statin drugs and offers the potential to suppress isoprenylation reactions much as statins do, without the attendant hepatotoxicity and other adverse effects typically associated with direct hydroxymethylglutaryl–coenzyme A (HMG-CoA) reductase inhibition. Other trials have produced less positive findings. Policosanol appears to reduce low-density lipoprotein cholesterol (LDL-C) and total cholesterol by inhibiting hepatic cholesterol synthesis before the formation of mevalonate, between the formation of acetate and mevalonate, and downregulating cellular expression of, but not directly inhibiting, HMG-CoA reductase. It also lowers LDL by enhancing the binding, uptake, and degradation of LDL-C in the endoplasmic reticulum.

Nevertheless, scientific knowledge of the exact mechanisms of policosanol's lipid-lowering activity remains incomplete and uncertain. High doses of policosanol can alter prostaglandin synthesis, lower platelet aggregation induced by arachidonic acid (AA), and inhibit proaggregatory thromboxane A_2 (TXA$_2$) generation induced by collagen; it does not inhibit and may increase levels of the antiaggregatory prostaglandin prostacyclin. Policosanol supports healthy endothelial function by preventing intimal thickening and smooth muscle cell proliferation while also preventing and possibly reversing atherosclerotic lesions and thrombosis. Policosanol may be active as an effective antioxidant in the cardiovascular system, particularly in preventing LDL oxidation, most likely by limiting microsomal lipid peroxidation.

NUTRIENT IN CLINICAL PRACTICE

Known or Potential Therapeutic Uses

Policosanol has primarily been proposed as part of a comprehensive approach to treating dyslipidemia. Some research suggests that it may be specifically effective in reducing elevated LDL-C and total cholesterol levels, particularly in type II hypercholesterolemia, including the IIa subtype (characterized by elevated total serum cholesterol and LDL-C levels), the IIb subtype (mixed hypercholesterolemia characterized by elevated total serum cholesterol, LDL-C, and triglyceride levels), and diabetes-related hypercholesterolemia. It also appears to increase levels of high-density lipoprotein cholesterol (HDL-C). Efficacy in the treatment of intermittent claudication is consistent with its known effects on platelet aggregation and endothelial function.

Historical/Ethnomedicine Precedent

Policosanol has not been used historically as an isolated nutrient.

Historical Note: Policosanol was largely developed in Cuba during the embargo that prevented access to many Western pharmaceuticals, and the initial laboratory and clinical research was done by Cuban scientists and physicians. Subsequent researchers and commentators, particularly after less successful trials, have suggested that politics may have played a role in earlier published findings of therapeutic efficacy.

Possible Uses

Dyslipidemia, hypercholesterolemia (type II), intermittent claudication, platelet aggregation.

Deficiency Symptoms

Not applicable.

Dietary Sources

Not applicable.

Dosage Forms Available

Capsule, tablet.

Source of Materials for Nutrient Preparations

Isolated constituents from sugarcane *(Saccharum officinarum)* wax; beeswax, rice bran.

Dosage Range
Adult
Dietary: Not applicable.
Supplemental/Maintenance: Not applicable.
Pharmacological/Therapeutic: 5 to 20 mg per day. A 6-month double-blind clinical trial found that daily dosages greater than 20 mg produce no significant additional cholesterol-lowering efficacy.[1] Many practitioners experienced in nutritional therapeutics advise patients to take their once-daily dose of policosanol in the evening because hepatic synthesis of cholesterol usually occurs primarily during the night.
Toxic: None reported, even at equivalent of approximately 620 times higher than the maximal recommended therapeutic dose (20 mg/day).[2]

SAFETY PROFILE
Overview

Clinical trials of policosanol lasting up to 3 years indicate that it is well tolerated and safe for most individuals at usual dosage levels.[3] Policosanol has not been associated with increases in hepatic enzymes or creatine kinase.

Nutrient Adverse Effects
General Adverse Effects
Quantifiable adverse effects include weight loss (1.8% of patients), polyuria (0.7%), and headache (0.6%). Other reported adverse effects include insomnia, somnolence, nervousness, dizziness, excitability, hypotension, hypertension, polyphagia, nausea, epigastric pain, diarrhea, constipation, erythema, pruritus, skin rash, and bleeding from the nose and gums.[4] These symptoms have been recorded in people taking policosanol; causality linking policosanol and these symptoms has not been established.

Research with Swiss mice shows no evidence of policosanol-induced carcinogenicity.[5]

Several animal studies, including rat model using doses up to 500 mg/kg, showed no evidence of significant reproductive or mutagenic toxicity.[2,6-9]

Adverse Effects Among Specific Populations
No dosage reduction is necessary in individuals with compromised hepatic function. No studies have been conducted involving individuals with compromised renal function.[4]

Pregnancy and Nursing
As of this writing, no reported adverse effects have been related to fetal development during pregnancy or to breast-fed infants. However, use during pregnancy is generally contraindicated because cholesterol and associated metabolic products are required for healthy fetal development. Likewise, administration during lactation should be discontinued because little is known about whether the product or some active metabolite is excreted in breast milk.

Infants and Children
Adequate long-term research is lacking, but no adverse effects have been reported in relation to policosanol use by children.

Contraindications
Pregnancy, breastfeeding.

Precautions and Warnings
Although potentially beneficial, concurrent use of policosanol and HMG-CoA reductase inhibitors may be inappropriate given the current lack of knowledge of policosanol's mechanism of action.

INTERACTIONS REVIEW
Strategic Considerations

Data from long-term formal studies of drug interactions, additive toxicity, or integrative therapeutics involving policosanol in humans are generally lacking. Pharmacokinetic research suggests that policosanol does not interact with drug-metabolizing processes involving the cytochrome P450 microsomal system.[2] Consequently, drug-to-drug interactions between policosanol and drugs metabolized through the cytochrome P450 hepatic system are not probable, although adverse pharmacodynamic drug-to-drug interactions cannot be excluded. Furthermore, the consistent lack of toxicity associated with sustained policosanol therapy and its proposed ability to shift lipid parameters positively and inhibit platelet aggregation significantly, without elevating liver enzymes or affecting coagulation parameters, suggest that therapeutic synergy is more likely to characterize potential interactions than is enhanced risk. Adjunctive therapies with a strong safety profile are much in demand given the wide range of uses emerging for statin medications and the widespread use of beta blockers, despite their known toxicities and risks. Thus, policosanol presents significant promise as a therapeutic agent in concert with statins, beta blockers, or other nutritional and botanical agents to treat dyslipidiemia and support lipid homeostasis and healthy cardiovascular function.

Even though largely undertaken by a relatively small number of researchers, mostly by a single research institute in Cuba, the initial positive evidence available on policosanol provides a substantial foundation for further large, well-designed clinical trials into its efficacy and interaction patterns. In contrast to data indicating that policosanol at 5 to 40 mg per day exerts lipoprotein-lowering effects comparable to statins, Berthold et al.[10] (2006) arrived at much less convincing findings. These investigators conducted a multicenter, randomized, double-blind, placebo-controlled, parallel-group trial in Germany involving 143 patients with "hypercholesterolemia or combined hyperlipidemia having baseline low-density lipoprotein cholesterol (LDL-C) levels of at least 150 mg/dL ... and either no or one cardiovascular risk factor other than known coronary heart disease, or baseline LDL-C levels of between 150 and 189 mg/dL ... and two or more risk factors." After a 6-week initial open-label placebo and diet run-in phase, they randomized subjects into five groups receiving sugarcane-derived policosanol (10, 20, 40, or 80 mg daily) or placebo for a double-blind 12-week treatment phase. None of the subjects in the five treatment groups exhibited decreases in LDL-C levels more than 10% from baseline, and "no statistically significant difference between policosanol and placebo was observed." Furthermore, after this relatively short treatment period, none of the secondary outcome measures—total cholesterol, HDL-C, very-low-density lipoprotein cholesterol (VLDL-C), triglycerides, lipoprotein(a), and ratio of total or LDL-C to HDL-C, exhibited any significant effects of policosanol.[10]

In an 8-week, double-blind, randomized controlled trial, Dulin et al.[11] reported that policosanol (20 mg/day) is "ineffective" in the treatment of "mild hypercholesterolemia."

These conflicting findings indicate that long-term, well-designed studies of adequate size are warranted to determine the therapeutic efficacy of policosanol monotherapy and suggest whether its role as a component of a more comprehensive protocol may be more effective. It should be noted that Berthold's study[10] of 143 patients randomized into five groups is very small (< 30 per group), particularly in comparison to statin trials, which typically involve many thousands of patients. Also, the experience with fish oil (omega-3 fatty acids) has shown more dramatic survival benefit than with statins in several trials, despite very modest changes in lipoprotein profiles. Given the earlier research with policosanol suggesting many mechanisms of action, it would seem premature to halt research with this agent after several small, negative clinical trials.

NUTRIENT-DRUG INTERACTIONS

Acetylsalicylic Acid (Aspirin) and Other Antiplatelet Medications

Antiplatelet Thromboprophylactics: Acetylsalicylic acid (acetosal, acetyl salicylic acid, ASA, salicylsalicylic acid; Arthritis Foundation Pain Reliever, Ascriptin, Aspergum, Asprimox, Bayer Aspirin, Bayer Buffered Aspirin, Bayer Low Adult Strength, Bufferin, Buffex, Cama Arthritis Pain Reliever, Easprin, Ecotrin, Ecotrin Low Adult Strength, Empirin, Extra Strength Adprin-B, Extra Strength Bayer Enteric 500 Aspirin, Extra Strength Bayer Plus, Halfprin 81, Heartline, Regular Strength Bayer Enteric 500 Aspirin, St. Joseph Adult Chewable Aspirin, ZORprin); combination drugs: ASA and caffeine (Anacin); ASA, caffeine, and propoxyphene (Darvon

Compound); ASA and carisoprodol (Soma Compound); ASA, codeine, and carisoprodol (Soma Compound with Codeine); ASA and codeine (Empirin with Codeine); ASA, codeine, butalbital, and caffeine (Fiorinal); cilostazol (Pletal), clopidogrel (Plavix), dipyridamole (Permole, Persantine), ticlopidine (Ticlid); combination drug: ASA and extended-release dipyridamole (Aggrenox, Asasantin).

Monoclonal Antibody Antiplatelet Agents: Abciximab (ReoPro), eptifibatide (Integrelin), tirofiban (Aggrastat).

Blood Viscosity Reducer Agent: Pentoxifylline (Pentoxil, Trental).

Interaction Type and Significance

✗✗   **Minimal to Mild Adverse Interaction—Vigilance Necessary**

⊕✗   **Bimodal or Variable Interaction, with Professional Management**

⊕⊕   **Beneficial or Supportive Interaction, with Professional Management**

Probability:
5. Improbable

Evidence Base:
◉ **Emerging**

Effect and Mechanism of Action

In high doses, policosanol can alter prostaglandin synthesis, lower platelet aggregation induced by AA, and inhibit proaggregatory TXA_2 generation induced by collagen.[12-14] Concomitant use of policosanol and antiplatelet medications such as aspirin may produce an additive interaction that, if clinically significant, could be beneficial or potentially detrimental, depending on the clinical circumstances (i.e., whether there is risk of clotting or bleeding).

Research

Arruzazabala et al.[15] conducted a randomized, double-blind, placebo-controlled study involving 43 healthy volunteers to compare the effects of policosanol, aspirin, and combination therapy on platelet aggregation. They found that policosanol alone significantly reduced platelet aggregation induced by adenosine diphosphate (ADP) (37.3%), epinephrine (32.6%), and collagen (40.5%), whereas aspirin alone significantly reduced platelet aggregation induced by collagen (61.4%) and epinephrine (21.9%) but not ADP-induced aggregation. Combined administration of the two agents significantly inhibited aggregation induced by all the agonists, reaching the highest reductions of platelet aggregation induced by collagen (71.3%) and epinephrine (57.5%). Coagulation time did not change significantly in any group. The researchers concluded that policosanol (20 mg/day) is as effective as aspirin (100 mg/day) on platelet aggregation and that combination therapy provided further activity compared with the respective monotherapies.

In a 2-week, randomized, double-blind, placebo-controlled trial involving healthy volunteers, Carbajal et al.[14] observed significant reductions of AA and collagen-induced platelet aggregation in vitro. Furthermore, policosanol also inhibited thromboxane, but not prostacyclin, generation induced by collagen. Likewise, clinical trials investigating the therapeutic effects of policosanol in the treatment of intermittent claudication have consistently demonstrated the agent's antiplatelet activity, with statistically significant improvement in walking distance before onset of pain.[16] In subsequent research involving healthy volunteers and hypercholesterolemic patients, Arruzazabala et al.[17] found that antiplatelet effects resulting from 40 mg/day policosanol versus 20 mg/day policosanol were similar after 30 days.

Nutritional Therapeutics, Clinical Concerns, and Adaptations

The effects of policosanol on platelet aggregation may alter the effects of aspirin and other antiplatelet medications when used concomitantly; modification of therapeutic dose may be necessary. Further research into these potential interactions, their clinical significance, occurrence, and management is warranted. Caution regarding coadministration is advised pending the emergence of such knowledge. Regular monitoring and appropriate titration is recommended. As with aspirin and other agents that inhibit platelet function, patients taking policosanol should be counseled to discontinue it 1 week before elective surgery. In emergency surgery with uncontrolled bleeding where pressure cannot be applied, such as intraspinal or intracranial bleeding, platelet transfusions should be considered in patients who have been taking antiplatelet agents, which may include policosanol.

Anticoagulant Medications

Oral Vitamin K Antagonist Anticoagulants: Anisindione (Miradon), dicumarol, ethyl biscoumacetate (Tromexan), nicoumalone (acenocoumarol; Acitrom, Sintrom), phenindione (Dindevan), phenprocoumon (Jarsin, Marcumar), warfarin (Coumadin, Marevan, Warfilone).
Heparin, Unfractionated (UFH): Heparin (Calciparine, Hepalean, Heparin Leo, Minihep Calcium, Minihep, Monoparin Calcium, Monoparin, Multiparin, Pump-Hep, Unihep, Uniparin Calcium, Uniparin Forte).
Heparinoids: Danaparoid (Orgaran), fondaparinux (Arixtra).
Low-Molecular-Weight (LMW) Heparin: Ardeparin (Normiflo), certoparin (Mono-Embolex), dalteparin (Fragmin), enoxaparin (Clexane, Lovenox), nadroparin (Fraxiparine), tinzaparin (Innohep).
Direct Thrombin Inhibitors: Argatroban, bivalirudin (Angiomax), dabigatran etexilate (Rendix; investigational), desirudin (Iprivask, Revasc), hirudin, lepirudin (Refludan).

Interaction Type and Significance

✗✗ **Minimal to Mild Adverse Interaction—Vigilance Necessary**

⊕✗ **Bimodal or Variable Interaction, with Professional Management**

⊕ **Potential or Theoretical Beneficial or Supportive Interaction, with Professional Management**

Probability:
5. Improbable

Evidence Base:
◉ **Emerging**

Effect and Mechanism of Action

In high doses, policosanol can alter prostaglandin synthesis, lower platelet aggregation induced by AA, and inhibit proaggregatory TXA_2 generation induced by collagen.[12-14] Some speculate whether the concurrent use of anticoagulant medications and policosanol might result in an additive effect. In the event that such interaction unintentionally produced unforeseen synergy or were not properly monitored and managed, excessive anticoagulant activity might result in adverse effects, such as excessive hemorrhage or inappropriate blood thinning. Conversely, if clinically significant, intentional coadministration might be efficacious and advantageous.

Research

Several clinical trials have demonstrated that policosanol can significantly inhibit platelet aggregation in humans without

affecting coagulation parameters.[13,14,18] Carbajal et al.[19] specifically investigated the effect of concomitant administration of warfarin and single or repeated doses of orally administered policosanol on bleeding time and experimentally induced venous thrombosis in rats. Policosanol alone did not significantly affect fibrinolytic activity or change the bleeding time. Either policosanol or warfarin monotherapy produced a significant reduction of thrombus weight. However, although the combination of policosanol and warfarin induced a moderate but significant prolongation of the bleeding time, this addition of policosanol to warfarin therapy did not enhance the prolongation of the bleeding time induced by warfarin alone. Further, when the combination was used instead of either agent alone, no significant benefits were observed on the reduction of thrombus weight. These findings indicate that any interaction between policosanol and warfarin (or similar agents [e.g., heparin]) is unlikely to be clinically significant.

Nutritional Therapeutics, Clinical Concerns, and Adaptations

Caution and regular monitoring remain appropriate, even though available evidence strongly suggests that any potential interaction between policosanol and common anticoagulant medications is unlikely to produce clinically significant adverse effects. It should be noted, however, that any agent with antiplatelet effects, including drugs (e.g., aspirin, Plavix, Persantine), botanicals (e.g., ginkgo, ginger, garlic), or policosanol, can increase the risk of bleeding in anticoagulated patients because both the major hemostatic pathways (platelets and coagulation cascade) are inhibited to some degree. Continued research into policosanol's mechanisms of action and therapeutic effects, along with observation deriving from its wider use, will provide opportunities to assess further the clinical significance (adverse or beneficial) of any interactions between policosanol and warfarin, heparin, or related anticoagulant agents and the frequency of any such events.

Beta-1-Adrenoceptor Antagonists (Beta-1-Adrenergic Blocking Agents) and Related Antihypertensive Medications

Oral forms (systemic).
Evidence: Propranolol (Inderal).
Extrapolated, based on similar properties: Acebutolol (Sectral), atenolol (Tenormin); combination drugs: atenolol and chlortalidone (Co-Tendione, Tenoretic); atenolol and nifedipine (Beta-Adalat, Tenif); betaxolol (Kerlone), bisoprolol (Zebeta), carteolol (Cartrol), esmolol (Brevibloc), labetalol (Normodyne, Trandate), metoprolol (Lopressor, Toprol XL); combination drug: metoprolol and hydrochlorothiazide (Lopressor HCT); nadolol (Corgard), nebivolol (Nebilet), oxprenolol (Trasicor), penbutolol (Levatol), pindolol (Visken), propranolol (Betachron, Inderal LA, Innopran XL, Inderal); combination drug: propranolol and bendrofluazide (Inderex); sotalol (Betapace, Betapace AF, Sorine), timolol (Blocadren).

Interaction Type and Significance

✗✗ **Minimal to Mild Adverse Interaction—Vigilance Necessary**

⊕✗ **Bimodal or Variable Interaction, with Professional Management**

⊕⊕ **Beneficial or Supportive Interaction, with Professional Management**

Probability:
4. Plausible

Evidence Base:
○ **Preliminary**

Effect and Mechanism of Action

Preliminary research, involving animals but also consistent with known mechanisms of action of policosanol and its constituents, suggests that the effects of policosanol on blood pressure may create additive hypotensive effects when combined with antihypertension medications such as beta blockers.

Research

Molina Cuevas et al.[20] investigated the effect of policosanol on arterial blood pressure in rats and its pharmacological interaction with propranolol and nifedipine (a calcium channel blocker). First, they observed that single doses of policosanol, at various potencies, orally administered to spontaneously hypertensive rats did not significantly change arterial pressure. After administering high doses of policosanol (200 mg/kg) to the rats followed by both antihypertensive agents, they found that such pretreatment with policosanol significantly increased propranolol-induced hypotensive effects without modifying cardiac frequency. No alterations were observed in the effects of nifedipine.

In a 3-year randomized trial, Castano et al.[21] investigated the concomitant use of policosanol and beta blockers in 205 "older hypercholesterolemic patients taking beta-blockers." After a 5-week diet-only baseline period, subjects were randomized to policosanol (5 mg/day) or placebo. After 1 year, subjects receiving policosanol exhibited significantly reduced LDL-C (20.9%), total cholesterol (TC) (19.3%), and triglycerides (TG) (25.7%), along with increased HDL-C levels (4.1%); these beneficial "effects did not wear off" during the 3-year follow-up. After the 3-year trial period, the authors reported that policosanol lowered LDL-C (34.3%), TC (23.2%), and TG (21.2%) and elevated HDL-C (12.3%), and that "reductions in systolic and diastolic blood pressure were observed in policosanol patients compared with those in the placebo group." Notably, of the 31 patients (15.1%) who discontinued the study, 20 (16 in placebo group and 4 in policosanol group) withdrew because of adverse effects. "The frequency of serious adverse events (SAE), mostly vascular," in policosanol patients (3.1%) was lower than in the placebo group (14.0%), with the frequency of policosanol patients reporting mild or moderate adverse effects (18.4%) also lower than in the placebo group (28.0%). The investigators concluded that "policosanol was well tolerated in elderly patients taking beta-blockers," and that additional "reduction of blood pressure and a lower frequency of SAE were observed in policosanol patients compared with those taking placebo." They added that "cholesterol-lowering efficacy of policosanol" was as "expected" and recommended the coadministration of policosanol in "hypercholesterolemic elderly individuals taking beta-blockers could provide additional benefits in lowering blood pressure."[21]

Nutritional Therapeutics, Clinical Concerns, and Adaptations

The apparent synergistic interaction observed between policosanol and beta blockers could produce unintended and potentially adverse effects or may be therapeutically efficacious, depending on therapeutic strategy, monitoring, respective dosage titration, and the particular needs and characteristics of the individual patient. Further research involving well-designed clinical trials is warranted to elucidate the potential risks and benefits of this pattern of interaction and enable development of safe and effective guidelines for clinical management. Pending such conclusive research, any concomitant use of policosanol and beta blockers should be approached cautiously, and collaboration between health care professionals trained and experienced in both conventional pharmacology and nutritional therapeutics would be judicious and most likely to enhance outcomes.

HMG-CoA Reductase Inhibitors (Statins)

Atorvastatin (Lipitor), fluvastatin (Lescol, Lescol XL), lovastatin (Altocor, Altoprev, Mevacor); combination drug: lovastatin and niacin (Advicor); pravastatin (Pravachol), rosuvastatin (Crestor), simvastatin (Zocor); combination drug: simvastatin and extended-release nicotinic acid (Niaspan).

Interaction Type and Significance

✗   **Potential or Theoretical Adverse Interaction of Uncertain Severity**

⊕✗   **Bimodal or Variable Interaction, with Professional Management**

⊕⊕   **Beneficial or Supportive Interaction, with Professional Management**

Probability: Evidence Base:
2. **Probable**   ☐ **Inadequate**

Effect and Mechanism of Action

Given the similar therapeutic objectives and related, if not sequential or redundant, activity and mechanisms of action, an additive or synergistic effect from concomitant use of HMG-CoA reductase inhibitors and policosanol appears possible, but unproven.

Research

Although several studies have compared the therapeutic effects of policosanol and various statin drugs, research is only beginning to emerge investigating the potential for adverse or beneficial effects from coadministration of statin drugs and policosanol.

The authors of the first trial directly investigating such concomitant therapy, however, have expressed a harsh judgment on the effectiveness of such combined treatment and questioned the value of continued research, despite the low dosage, small size, and short duration of their study. In a randomized, parallel, double-blind, double-dummy, placebo-controlled design involving 99 patients with LDL-C levels from 140 to 189 mg/dL, Cubeddu et al.[22] randomized subjects to one of four groups to receive policosanol, atorvastatin, combination therapy, or (double) placebo for 12 weeks. Starting with baseline characteristics that were similar among all treatment groups, the investigators reported that policosanol (20 mg/day) "did not significantly change plasma total cholesterol, LDL-C, high-density lipoprotein cholesterol, or triglyceride levels when compared with baseline values or with values of placebo-treated patients." In contrast, they found that subjects administered atorvastatin (10 mg/day) exhibited "reduced total cholesterol by 27% and LDL-C by 35%." Thus, while noting that policosanol "was safe and did not affect liver enzyme or creatinine phosphokinase levels," they concluded that the addition of "policosanol did not reduce LDL-C or total cholesterol levels either alone or in combination with atorvastatin." Consequently, they recommended that "observation supports the need for systematic evaluation of available products containing policosanol to determine their clinical lipid-lowering efficacy under rigorous experimental conditions." Pending conclusive evidence, they added, "We propose that policosanol should be added to the list of nutritional supplements lacking scientific validity to support their use."[22]

Further research through long-term, well-designed, and adequately powered trials using varying doses and combinations of these agents is warranted.

Nutritional Therapeutics, Clinical Concerns, and Adaptations

Unmanaged concurrent use might produce excessive inhibition of cholesterol formation, but adverse events from this hypothetical effect appear improbable. Coordinated use might allow reducing the dosage of the statin and thus moderation of inherent adverse effects on normal liver function. Many nutritionally oriented health care providers already administer policosanol, usually in conjunction with synergistic agents, to phase out and replace statin agents in patients who prefer to avoid the risks known to accompany use of these drugs. Further research involving well-designed clinical trials is warranted to elucidate the potential risks and benefits of this pattern of interaction and enable development of safe and effective guidelines for clinical management.

Pending such conclusive research, any concomitant use of policosanol and statin therapy should be undertaken only under professional supervision and with regular monitoring of lipid levels and liver function. Experienced practitioners of nutritional therapeutics typically combine policosanol and a program of dietary changes and regular exercise with agents such as fish oil, inositol hexaniacinate or time-release niacin, pantethine, and garlic based on the individual patient's particular pattern of dyslipidemia, family history, genomic variables, and other risk factors. Collaboration between health care professionals trained and experienced in both conventional pharmacology and nutritional therapeutics would be judicious and most likely to enhance outcomes. Epidemiological investigations have shown an increased risk of hemorrhagic stroke in individuals with very low serum cholesterol levels (< 120 mg/dL).

THEORETICAL, SPECULATIVE, AND PRELIMINARY INTERACTIONS RESEARCH, INCLUDING OVERSTATED INTERACTIONS CLAIMS

Ezetimibe

Ezetimibe (Zetia).

Ezetimibe is a potent and highly specific inhibitor of an intestinal sterol permease. Doses as low as 10 mg/day can suppress intestinal absorption of cholesterol and decrease serum LDL-C by approximately 18%. McCarty[23] hypothesized that coadministration of policosanol and ezetimibe may produce an additive efficacy "that could reduce LDL cholesterol by about 40%, without side effects, and that could be recommended to virtually anyone whose LDL cholesterol levels were not already ideal." Research appears warranted based on trials with each agent individually.

Salicylates

Including: Aspirin, choline salicylate, magnesium salicylate, salsalate, diflunisal, sodium salicylate, sodium thiosalicylate.

Some preliminary research has been interpreted to indicate that effects of policosanol on clotting may alter the effects of salicylates. Even though research findings focusing on policosanol's effects on platelet aggregation and coagulation indicate that adverse effects or interactions are unlikely, any concomitant use of policosanol and salicylates should be undertaken only under close observation and with regular monitoring, until further research provides direct and conclusive evidence of a clinically significant interaction and enables development of guidelines for clinical management of such cases.

See also earlier section on Acetylsalicylic Acid (Aspirin) and Other Antiplatelet Medications.

The 23 citations for this monograph, as well as additional reference literature, are located under Policosanol on the CD at the back of the book.

Probiotics

Nutrient Names: Probiotic intestinal flora and prebiotics.
Synonyms: Healthy bacteria, intestinal microbiota, probiotic flora, symbiotic flora.

Summary

Drug/Class Interaction Type	Mechanism and Significance	Management
Antibiotics Antimicrobials ☼/⊕⊕⊕/◇	Antibiotic agents, particulary repeated courses or high-dose administration, will damage the intestinal flora that are indigenous and intrinsic to the gut ecology and play significant roles in immune, endocrine, detoxification, and other body systems. Repletion of such commensal bacteria and rebuilding of gut ecology through diverse and vigorous probiotic cultures can provide both short- and long-term strategic benefits for preventing or treating many conditions, with minimal risk of adverse effects. Mechanisms and effects established, but controversy exists regarding necessity. Research warranted and ongoing as to particulars and strategies, such as species, strains, dose, and duration.	Administer, especially after high-dose or extended antibiotic therapy; several months may be necessary. *Saccharomyces boulardii* (an antibiotic-resistant probiotic yeast) during or after antibiotic course may also be necessary to counter adverse effects, such as *C. difficile* overgrowth (antibiotic-associated colitis).
Lansoprazole- Amoxicillin- Metronidazole (LAM) triple therapy ⊕⊕	Coadministration of probiotic flora with triple (or quadruple) therapy can enchance efficacy in eradicating *Helicobacter pylori*. Preliminary supportive evidence; mechanisms partially understood.	Coadminister.

NUTRIENT DESCRIPTION

Chemistry and Forms

Probiotics

Bifidobacterium adolescentis, B. animalis, B. bifidus (bifidum), B. breve, B. infantis, B. lactis, B. longum, B. thermophilum; Lactobacillus acidophilus, L. brevis, L. bulgaricus, L. casei, L. cellobiosus, L. crispatus, L. curvatus, L. fermentum, L., Lactobacillus GG (L. rhamnosus or *L. casei* subsp. *rhamnosus), L. johnsonii, L. plantarum, L. salivarus; Saccharomyces boulardii, S. cerevisiae.*

    Lactobacillus bulgaricus and *Streptococcus thermophilus* are the "yogurt species." *Lactococcus lactis* and *L. lactis* subspecies *cremoris (Streptococcus cremoris)* are also part of milk souring and are used as probiotics.

    Enterococcus faecium (also in the streptococcal family) has also been used in the management of diarrheal illness.

Prebiotics

The most common prebiotics are *inulin*, a long-chain oligosaccharide (2-60 sugars), and *fructooligosaccharide* (FOS), a short-chain oligosaccharide (2-7 sugars). Almost all fibers function as prebiotics to some extent, as do many of the sugar alcohols (e.g., lactitol, maltitol, xylitol).

Related Substances

Probiotics: Live-culture foods; kefir, yogurt.

Prebiotics: Artichokes, onions, chicory, garlic, leeks; foods known to contain low-molecular-weight carbohydrates classified as FOS.

Physiology and Function

Probiotics are known by many names, including "live foods," yogurt, lactobacilli, acidophilus, and "cultured" dairy products. The human gastrointestinal (GI) tract is home to more than a trillion live bacteria from about 400 species. The average adult body contains about 20 times more bacteria than it does somatic cells.[1] In the natural environment, a delicate symbiosis evolves between these endogenous bacteria and their host. These live organisms act beneficially by affecting the host animal, improving its intestinal microbial balance. The vital contribution of natural flora to normal intestinal development is underscored by studies of animals raised in a germ-free environment. These animals have hypoplastic intestinal epithelia, reduced gut immunity, and impaired peristalsis, all of which improve only when normal gut flora are introduced.[2] Scientific discoveries continue to highlight the multifaceted functions of intestinal microflora within multiple body systems. For example, emerging research regarding the vermiform appendix suggests that its major physiologic function may be to harbor and protect the commensal colonic flora, so that they are preserved and available to repopulate the colon after severe diarrheal illnesses such as cholera or other types of severe infectious gastroenteritis.[2a]

Probiotics change the metabolic activities or composition of microbiota and modulate immune system reactivity in ways that benefit healthy function. Exogenous probiotics are administered therapeutically to individuals in whom this naturally beneficial symbiosis has been disturbed, in an attempt to restore normal flora. A 2004 Cochrane review reports that probiotic therapy is effective in reducing diarrhea.[3] A 2005 report summarizing 185 studies found that probiotics successfully treated 68 different conditions in diverse populations.[4]

Lactobacillus and *Bifidobacterium* each represent a genus of probiotics most often used therapeutically. Some species and strains are derived from the intestinal microbiota of healthy humans. Some bifidobacteria that have been perpetuated as probiotics for babies have been derived from human milk. Other species are nonhuman probiotics used in the fermentation of dairy products. Species from other bacterial genera, such as *Streptococcus, Bacillus,* and *Enterococcus* have also been used as probiotics, but concerns surround the safety of such probiotics because these genera also contain pathogenic species, particularly *Enterococcus.*[5-9] Nonbacterial microorganisms such as yeasts from the genus *Saccharomyces,* most notably *S. boulardii,* have also been used as probiotics for many years.

Probiotics, as implied by their collective name, are a class of bacteria and yeast that are essentially life supporting in their action within human physiology. Historically, they have always been part of the human digestive tract ecology, with breast-feeding establishing the initial colonization process before the immune system has fully developed the distinction between self and other. Thus, in an immune sense, probiotics are within the boundaries of self in a presumably lifelong symbiotic relationship.

Microflora of the large intestine complete digestion through fermentation, playing a key role in the endogenous synthesis of vitamins (e.g., niacin, folic acid, biotin, K, B_{12}, B_6), short-chain fatty acids, amino acids (e.g., L-arginine, L-cysteine, L-glutamine), and other "gut" nutrients. Microflora protect against overgrowth of opportunistic bacteria and fungi. These layers of tissue facilitate detoxification and stimulate the development of the immune system. For example, the metabolism of food by *Lactobacillus acidophilus* results in the production of lactic acid, hydrogen peroxide, and other beneficial byproducts that support changes in the gut environment hostile to unwanted organisms. Many of these bacteria are able to tolerate environments with a pH of 3 and 2% to 8% concentrations of bile acid. Probiotics in the diet can modify the composition and some metabolic activities of the intestinal microflora.

Certain probiotics are found as the live microorganisms in foods, such as active yogurt culture. Acidophilus organisms can act as a source of lactase. The microorganisms can survive passage through the gut and temporarily bring the benefits of normal gut flora. Bifidobacteria are anaerobic pleomorphic rods or club-shaped organisms that normally have an important role in breaking down dietary carbohydrate and interact directly with the host metabolism. Bifidobacteria also excrete water-soluble vitamins, but species and strains are considerably different. The healthy human gut, without pharmacological disruption, contains a wide range of bacterial species, and once established, variable strains normally grow in number and diversity. Fructooligosaccharides are naturally occurring carbohydrates that support the growth of bifidobacteria and cannot be digested or absorbed by humans.

Pharmacokinetic data suggest that human intestinal flora are essential for hydrolysis of the glycoside forms of the anthocyanin and proanthocyanin moities, as well as the glycoside forms of isoflavones and phytoestrogens.[10-12] These data suggest that iatrogenic reduction in microflora induced by antibiotics may reduce the bioavailability of at least some plant food polyphenols, although clinical evidence is not available.

The ideal probiotic should remain viable at the level of the large intestine and should adhere to the intestinal epithelium to confer a significant health benefit. Viable bacteria have greater immunological effects than nonviable bacteria and killed bacteria have been associated with adverse effects in some cases.[13,14] Some of the best-characterized probiotics have been shown to adhere strongly to intestinal epithelium through in vivo and in vitro studies.[15] Probiotics must also be resistant to gastric acid digestion and to bile salts to reach the intestinal tract intact, and they should be nonpathogenic.[16]

NUTRIENT IN CLINICAL PRACTICE
Known or Potential Therapeutic Uses

Probiotics have been clinically used to protect against intestinal permeability resulting from intestinal inflammation induced by nonsteroidal anti-inflammatory drugs (NSAIDs). Probiotics are also used to help reduce the adverse side effect of antibiotic-induced diarrhea. The concern about overuse of antibiotics

has recently been noted because of the more frequent overgrowth of antibiotic-resistant bacteria such as *Clostridium difficile*, which causes a severe form of colitis due to antibiotic therapy. Probiotic yeast such as *Saccharomyces boulardii* have been used as specific therapy for *C. difficile* colitis. Probiotics are used to enhance immune system factors to aid in the sequelae of asthma, allergies, upper respiratory infections, eczema, and other autoimmune disorders. Probiotics help replenish the intestinal flora when it is depleted by the factors surrounding infectious diarrhea, irritable bowel syndrome, and other intestinal disorders partly created by a depletion of healthy gut flora.

Historical/Ethnomedicine Precedent

Probiotics in the form of *Streptococcus thermophilus* and *Lactobacillus bulgaricus* in fermented milk have been ingested by humans for thousands of years in the belief they have health benefits. Fermented dairy products such as yogurt have been prepared and consumed since the third millennium BCE, with the earliest uses most likely deriving from experiences of ingesting materials created through spontaneous fermentation by naturally occurring bacteria living on the goatskin bags used by the Bulgars (or Hunno-Bulgars). The development of food derived from fermentation of soy represents a parallel culinary evolution in East Asia. Likewise, in Biblical history, it was written that Abraham owed his fertility and longevity to the regular ingestion of yogurt. In the early twentieth century, the Russian immunologist Elie Metchnikoff proposed that lactic acid bacilli may have beneficial health effects and attributed his own longevity to regular probiotic ingestion.

Possible Uses

Allergic airway disease, allergic reactions (risk reduction and treatment), antibiotic-induced diarrhea, arthritis, atopy (particularly in infants), bone mineralization, calcium absorption, cancer, candidiasis, carcinogenic compound reduction in GI tract, cholesterol, constipation, Crohn's disease, diarrhea, digestive problems, dysbiosis, eczema, enteritis, food intolerances/sensitivities, food poisoning, glutamate synthase, *Helicobacter pylori* infection, hypercholesterolemia, immune enhancement/support, immune system development, intestinal permeability from NSAID-induced intestinal inflammation, irritable bowel disorder, irritable bowel syndrome, lactose intolerance, malnutrition, obesity, oral thrush, osteoporosis, pollen allergy, pouchitis, pseudomembranous colitis, seasonal allergies, sinusitis, surgery recovery, traveler's diarrhea, ulcerative colitis, vaginal infections, vulvovaginitis, workplace wellness (decreased sick leave), yeast infections.

Deficiency Symptoms

The absence of healthy live bacteria in the intestines have led to hypoplastic intestinal epithelia, reduced gut immunity, and impaired peristalsis.[2] The depletion of such organisms tend to increase gut permeability, leaky gut syndrome, dysbiosis, abdominal distention, bloating, abdominal cramping, loose stools, fatigue, constipation, and acute/chronic diarrhea.

Dietary Sources

A wide variety of foods have live bacteria that contain mixtures of lactobacilli and bifidobacteria. These foods include yogurt, kefir, fermented foods such as sauerkraut and kimchi, probiotic foods, and prebiotic foods; most yogurt preparations are usually mixtures of lactobacilli and bifidobacteria, sometimes with

Streptococcus thermophilus. Some "soil organisms" are primarily derived from soil, rather than mammals.

Nutrient Preparations Available

Bifidobacteria, acidophilus, lactobacillus, yogurt, yeasts, fermented foods. Probiotic *Escherichia coli* are available in Germany. The most common prebiotics are inulin and fructooligosaccharides (see Chemistry and Forms).

Dosage Forms Available

Capsule, enema, liquid (oral), liquid (topical), powder.

Most commercially available forms of probiotic supplements are refrigerated until consumption because culture viability remains an important issue in achieving therapeutic effects. Some manufacturers market probiotic products that they claim do not require refrigeration to maintain stability due to freeze-drying or other processes. Nevertheless, shelf life viability of all preparations is somewhat shorter at room temperature than under refrigeration.

Source Material for Nutrient Preparations

Cow's milk, goat milk, human milk; carrots, corn; soil.

Dosage Range

Dosage is represented as number of organisms per dose/serving (often noted as "CFU" for "colony-forming units").

Adult

Dietary: None established.
Supplemental/Maintenance: One capsule or teaspoon per day orally, typically providing 1 to 2 billion CFU.
Pharmacological/Therapeutic: Dosage in clinical trials has ranged from 1 to 20 billion microflora. A typical therapeutic dose of probiotic bacteria is 2 to 4 billion CFU, two to four times daily, and that of *Saccharomyces boulardii* yeast is 500 mg, standardized to provide 3 billion CFU per gram, twice daily. *S. boulardii* is usually administered concurrently with antibiotic therapy, and bacterial probiotics are given after completion of a course of antibiotics, for 1 to 6 months.
Toxic: No toxicity has been established.

Pediatric (< 18 Years)

Dietary: None established.
Supplemental/Maintenance: One capsule or teaspoon per day orally, typically providing 1 to 2 billion CFU.
Pharmacological/Therapeutic: See Adult.
Toxic: None established.

Laboratory Values

Select laboratories have tests for presence, number, types, and characteristics of bacteria, as well as presence of pathogenic microorganisms and excessive gut permeability.

SAFETY PROFILE

Overview

Generally, medical literature reports probiotics as safe for human consumption. Potential benefits must be considered against possible harm, knowing that the data will never be absolute. Relevant data can be divided into two categories: population surveys, both retrospective and prospective, and anecdotal case reports that retrospectively try to establish some connection to prior ingestion of probiotics. Neither category provides a definitive scientific evidence–based overview of the safety of probiotics. Some clinical scientists assert that there will never be definitive clinical data.[17]

Based on Finnish estimates that 0.02% of blood cultures test positive for lactobacilli, more than 166,000 patients would need to be studied prospectively to detect a 10% increase in bacteremia caused by *Lactobacillus*. Even with this estimate, given that blood was cultured in the Finnish study only for clinical indications, the expected yield would likely be lower if blood from healthy patients who ingested probiotics prophylactically were routinely cultured.

Although immunocompromised patients are especially vulnerable to infection, prospective studies have shown that probiotics are safe in immunocompromised adults and children with human immunodeficiency virus (HIV).[18,19]

In preterm neonates, probiotics reduce the incidence and severity of necrotizing enterocolitis, with no secondary probiotic infections seen to date.[20,21]

Sepsis from *Lactobacillus* has not been reported in prospective randomized studies of probiotics. The risk of sepsis from *Lactobacillus* should be weighed against risk of sepsis with more pathological species of bacteria and against risk of the disease that probiotic therapy was meant to prevent.[17] Many *Lactobacillus* species are intrinsically vancomycin resistant but have had a long history of safe use as probiotics. There is no indication thus far that vancomycin-resistant lactobacilli could transfer the resistance to other bacteria by plasmids or other means.[22] Although rare, reports indicating the presence of probiotic bacteria in samples isolated from infected tissues have raised concerns about their intrinsic properties as well as their potential pathogenicity.[23,24] Improperly stored probiotic products may cause nausea and minor GI distress resulting from degradation.

In a paper reviewing safety issues, Hammerman et al.[17] presented anecdotal adverse reports that clinical *Lactobacillus* infections do exist, most often in elderly patients. The most often cited case is a well-qualified report of a 74-year-old woman who developed a liver abscess after ingesting *Lactobacillus rhamnosus* for 4 months. After direct "gram-staining of a hepatic abscess aspirate demonstrated an abundance of polymorphonuclear leukocytes and gram-positive coccobacilli," the authors observed that the "fermentation pattern and enzymatic reactions of this isolate were compatible with a probiotic strain *L. rhamnosus* GG used in dairy products in Finland since 1990."[7] However, they also noted that the "incidence of severe infections caused by lactobacilli is very low." Notably, the case report does not disclose the comedications used by the woman, diagnosed as an adult-onset diabetic, which might reveal the impact of potential adverse effects of any pharmacodynamic interaction occurring with her liver. Another concern would be medications or conditions that might lead to intestinal ulceration, thus providing a portal of entry to the bloodstream for ingested probiotic bacteria. In other case reports, a 67-year-old man with mitral valve regurgitation developed *Lactobacillus* endocarditis and sepsis after a tooth extraction,[8] and a 6-week-old infant developed *Lactobacillus* sepsis, although the child had severe underlying medical problems.[25]

Nutrient Adverse Effects

General Adverse Effects

Mild to moderate flulike symptoms, flatulence, abdominal bloating, nausea, and loose stools, resulting from "die-off" of pathogenic yeast and bacteria in the gut, are common in the first week of dosing with probiotics, a phenomenon also known as Jarisch-Herxheimer reaction. Temporary dose reduction or temporary cessation and titration of dose and administration interval typically alleviates the discomfort.

Adverse Effects Among Specific Populations
None confirmed.

Pregnancy and Nursing
None established.

Infants and Children
None established. There have been numerous studies illustrating the safety and effectiveness of probiotics with infants.[26-32]

Effect and Mechanism of Action

Probiotics change the metabolic activities or composition of microbiota and modulate immune system reactivity that benefits health. Exogenous probiotics are given therapeutically to individuals in whom this naturally beneficial symbiosis has been disturbed, in an attempt to restore normal flora.

Contraindications

Probiotic agents are potentially contraindicated in immunosuppressed individuals, particularly those with or at risk for ulcerations of the GI tract. Although administration of probiotics is often a core tactic within integrative nutritional therapeutic strategies for immunocompromised patients, a single unqualified case report described an immunosuppressed patient who developed a *Lactobacillus* infection after eating yogurt.[33]

INTERACTIONS REVIEW
Strategic Considerations

Probiotics have been advocated for the prevention and treatment of a wide range of diseases, and strong evidence exists for their efficacy in some clinical scenarios. Probiotics are now widely used in many countries by both consumers and in clinical practice. Given the increasingly widespread use of probiotics, a thorough understanding of their risks and benefits is imperative.

Dietary modulation of gut microbiota with prebiotics and probiotics is an important function in nutritional sciences. In addition, some nutritional approaches use other nutraceuticals and botanicals, such as a modified butyric acid, as well as Chinese herbal formulae and the essential oil of oregano as sequential or symbiotic therapies. *Prebiotics* are defined as a functional food that has nondigestible food ingredients that beneficially affects the host by selectively stimulating the growth and activity of one or a limited number of symbiotic bacteria in the colon. Prebiotics can be nondigestible oligosaccharides and fibers, but also may be poorly absorbed sugars (e.g., D-tagatose) or sugar alcohols (e.g., lactitol, xylitol), which promote the growth of symbiotic colonic microflora. Among the oligosaccharides, inulin and oligofructose have been shown to inhibit growth of pathogens and to display clear bifidogenic properties.[34]

The status of human intestinal ecology radically changed in the past 60 years in a direction far removed from anything comparable to millennia of evolutionary experience. Up until the middle of the twentieth century, the GI tract of adult humans, in both industrialized and undeveloped cultures, was populated by trillions of diverse organisms that might compose 6 to 8 pounds of living mass.[35] However, the status of bacterial microbiota playing their symbiotic role in digestive, immune, and other functions has been significantly altered by the decline of breastfeeding, the introduction of chlorine in water supplies, declining levels of biological activity in agricultural soil, and the massive upsurge in the medical and animal husbandry use of antimicrobial agents, particularly broad-spectrum antibiotics. Subsequently, recognition has grown steadily as to the profound and widespread systemic implications of the depletion of this intimate natural resource within the human ecology and economy. Health care professionals have long recognized the immediate and long-term impact of antibiotic therapy on the intestinal flora, but the pervasive and cumulative, local and systemic sequelae of overgrowth of pathogenic yeast and anaerobic bacteria, with the attendant loss of metabolic activities and buffering presence for the gut mucosa of the symbiotic bacteria, have been more subtle.

Nevertheless, research into the particulars of such adverse effects has been absent or negligible. Scientific experiments and well-designed clinical trials are needed to investigate critical issues such as the variable susceptibilities within patient populations based on perinatal and infant nutrition, the divergent impact of antibiotics versus other medications as well as specific versus broad-spectrum antibiotics, and the differential effects of short-term versus chronic medication regimens and isolated versus repeated antibiotic administration. In addition, high-quality studies are needed regarding the efficacy of intake of cultured foods such as yogurt versus probiotic products on symbiont repletion, and on the effectiveness of various therapeutic repletion tactics, such as flora constituents (e.g., species, strains), methods of gut preparation and role of prebiotics in reestablishing a dynamic symbiotic microbiota, necessary numbers of organisms, combinations and duration of intake, methods of preparation, and methods of stabilization and delivery of probiotic organisms. In many respects, these concerns include the inherently related and increasingly critical issue of antibiotic-resistant pathogens. Moreover, critical investigation is required to determine the degree to which botanical and nutritional agents might also decimate and disrupt, or support and enhance, healthy flora and gut ecology.

Probiotic repletion and rejuvenation of the gut mucosa have long played a central role in the therapeutic strategies of experienced practitioners within nutritional, naturopathic, and integrative medicine. Given the patient population and their typical medical histories, it is often assumed that healthy flora are lacking and that degradation of the gut integrity and ecology has ensued to such a degree as to participate in a general decline in health and an increase in susceptibility because of decreased function and increased toxic load. Thus, in so many cases, whether labeled with such vaguely defined syndromes as "fibromyalgia," "chronic fatigue," or "food sensitivities," or more conventionally as asthma and atopy, irritable bowel, or constipation, the initial stages of treating a patient with chronic conditions centers around improving dietary habits and reconstructing the gut ecology. However, as in so many areas of integrative medicine's maturation, it is necessary to move past naive assumptions that naturally occurring substances are inherently benign and universally beneficial. Such an approach must give way to a scientifically based and clinically efficacious approach employing all agents, regardless of origins, as potential tools in evolving and multidisciplinary strategies personalized to optimal intervention, given individual pharmacogenomic and biochemical variability and responses to therapeutic interventions.

A cursory review of the scientific literature over the past 20 years reveals a rapidly ascending curve representing the numbers of scientific studies and published papers focusing on the physiology and therapeutics of probiotics, prebiotics, and related topics. For example, there is clinical evidence to show that probiotics may help children with food sensitivities, whereas there was no effect in those without food sensitivities.[36]

Probiotic therapy has been applied for decades, if not millennia, in many clinical circumstances, from treating asthma and irritable bowel syndrome to preventing thrush or constipation. Research into the safety, applicability, and efficacy of probiotics needs to keep pace with their rapidly expanding popularity in the consumer market and their continued expansion within professional medical contexts.

NUTRIENT-DRUG INTERACTIONS

Antibiotics/Antimicrobial Agents (Systemic)

Aminoglycoside Antibiotics: Amikacin (Amikin), gentamicin (G-mycin, Garamycin, Jenamicin), kanamycin (Kantrex), neomycin (Mycifradin, Myciguent, Neo-Fradin, NeoTab, Nivemycin), netilmicin (Netromycin), paromomycin (monomycin; Humatin), streptomycin, tobramycin (AKTob, Nebcin, TOBI, TOBI Solution, TobraDex, Tobrex).

Beta-Lactam Antibiotics: Methicillin (Staphcillin); aztreonam (Azactam injection); carbapenem antibiotics: meropenem (Merrem I.V.); combination drug: imipenem and cilastatin (Primaxin I.M., Primaxin I.V.); penicillin antibiotics: amoxicillin (Amoxicot, Amoxil, Moxilin, Trimox, Wymox); combination drug: amoxicillin and clavulanic acid (Augmentin, Augmentin XR, Clavulin); ampicillin (Amficot, Omnipen, Principen, Totacillin); combination drug: ampicillin and sulbactam (Unisyn); bacampicillin (Spectrobid), carbenicillin (Geocillin), cloxacillin (Cloxapen), dicloxacillin (Dynapen, Dycill), mezlocillin (Mezlin), nafcillin (Unipen), oxacillin (Bactocill), penicillin G (Bicillin C-R, Bicillin L-A, Pfizerpen, Truxcillin), penicillin V (Beepen-VK, Betapen-VK, Ledercillin VK, Pen-Vee K, Robicillin VK, Suspen, Truxcillin VK, V-Cillin K, Veetids), piperacillin (Pipracil); combination drug: piperacillin and tazobactam (Zosyn); ticarcillin (Ticar); combination drug: ticarcillin and clavulanate (Timentin).

Cephalosporin Antibiotics: Cefaclor (Ceclor), cefadroxil (Duricef), cefamandole (Mandol), cefazolin (Ancef, Kefzol), cefdinir (Omnicef), cefepime (Maxipime), cefixime (Suprax), cefoperazone (Cefobid), cefotaxime (Claforan), cefotetan (Cefotan), cefoxitin (Mefoxin), cefpodoxime (Vantin), cefprozil (Cefzil), ceftazidime (Ceptaz, Fortaz, Tazicef, Tazidime), ceftibuten (Cedax), ceftizoxime (Cefizox), ceftriaxone (Rocephin), cefuroxime (Ceftin, Kefurox, Zinacef), cephalexin (Keflex, Keftab), cephapirin (Cefadyl), cephradine (Anspor, Velocef); imipenem combination drug: imipenem and cilastatin (Primaxin I.M., Primaxin I.V.); loracarbef (Lorabid), meropenem (Merrem I.V.).

Fluoroquinolone (4-Quinolone) Antibiotics: Cinoxacin (Cinobac, Pulvules), ciprofloxacin (Ciloxan, Cipro), enoxacin (Penetrex), gatifloxacin (Tequin), levofloxacin (Levaquin), lomefloxacin (Maxaquin), moxifloxacin (Avelox), nalidixic acid (Neggram), norfloxacin (Noroxin), ofloxacin (Floxin, Ocuflox), sparfloxacin (Zagam), trovafloxacin (alatrofloxacin; Trovan).

Macrolide Antibiotics: Azithromycin (Zithromax), clarithromycin (Biaxin), dirithromycin (Dynabac), erythromycin, oral (EES, EryPed, Ery-Tab, PCE Dispertab, Pediazole), troleandomycin (Tao).

Sulfonamide Antibiotics: Sodium sulfacetamide (AK-Sulf, Bleph-10, Sodium Sulamyd), sulfamethoxazole (Gantanol), sulfanilamide (AVC), sulfasalazine (salazosulfapyridine, salicylazosulfapyridine, suphasalazine; Apo-Sulfasalazine, Azulfidine, Azulfidine EN-Tabs, PMS-Sulfasalazine, Salazopyrin, Salazopyrin EN-Tabs, SAS), sulfisoxazole (Gantrisin); combination drug: sulfamethoxazole and trimethoprim (cotrimoxazole, co-trimoxazole, SXT, TMP-SMX, TMP-sulfa; Bactrim, Bactrim DS, Cotrim, Septra, Septra DS, Sulfatrim, Uroplus); triple sulfa (Sultrin Triple Sulfa).

Chemotherapy, Cytotoxic Antibiotics: Bleomycin (Blenoxane), dactinomycin (Actinomycin D, Cosmegen, Cosmegen Lyovac), mitomycin (Mutamycin), plicamycin (Mithracin).

Miscellaneous Antibiotics/Antimicrobials: Bacitracin (Caci-IM), chloramphenicol (Chloromycetin), chlorhexidine (Peridex), clindamycin, oral (Cleocin), colistimethate (Coly-Mycin M), dapsone (DDS, diaminodiphenylsulphone; Aczone Gel, Avlosulfon), furazolidone (Furoxone), lincomycin (Lincocin), linezolid (Zyvox), nitrofurantoin (Macrobid, Macrodantin), trimethoprim (Proloprim, Trimpex), vancomycin (Vancocin).

Interaction Type and Significance

☼ **Prevention or Reduction of Drug Adverse Effect**

⊕⊕⊕ **Beneficial or Supportive Interaction, Not Requiring Professional Management**

◇ **Adverse Drug Effect on Nutritional Therapeutics, Strategic Concern**

Nutrient Depletion
Probability:
2. Probable or
1. Certain

Evidence Base:
○ **Preliminary** or
◉ **Emerging**

Coadministration Benefit
Probability:
4. Plausible or
2. Probable

Evidence Base:
○ **Preliminary,**
◉ **Emerging,** or
● **Consensus** (varies with topic)

Effect and Mechanism of Action

Probiotics play a critical role in normal functions of the digestive, immune, endocrine, and other body systems but also inhibit growth of potential pathogenic organisms. The potential pathogens produce indole, skatol, putricine, cadaverine, endo-, exo-, and enterotoxins as well as other pathogenic materials; notably, both pathogenic and probiotic bacteria are capable of producing lactic acid and bacteriocins. The inhibition caused by probiotics is antagonistic to pathogen growth. Probiotics provide a competitive environment that does not favor the growth of enteric pathogens. Probiotics trigger cytokine synthesis from enterocytes by attaching to their surfaces. Probiotics restore the normal intestinal flora after antibiotic therapy and produce metabolites, such as hydrogen peroxide and bacteriocins, that are toxic to many pathogenic bacteria. Probiotics also produce butyric and other short-chain fatty acids that both nourish and increase the turnover of enterocytes. Probiotics are also capable of neutralizing many dietary carcinogens.

Research

Antibiotic resistance of pathogens is at the forefront of medical challenges in both the clinical and the public health arena.

Bacteria have mutated over the last 60 years to become resistant to many antibiotic therapies. Even though antibiotics are an effective tool in the treatment of many serious infections, the spread of resistance genes and resistant bacteria impedes the effectiveness of antibiotics as a clinical tool.[37] The risks potentially associated with antibiotic therapy, as a general rule, are multifaceted. The selection of resistant forms can occur during or after microbial treatment. Antibiotic residues can be found for long periods after treatment. Stuart Levy[37] notes that "there is a mounting use of other agents aimed at destroying bacteria, namely the surface antibacterials now available in many household products." The term "multidrug resistance" (MDR) initially described resistant mammalian tumor cells and later strains of *Mycobacterium tuberculosis;* MDR now describes multidrug resistance in any organism—bacterium, fungus, or parasite.[38-44]

Diarrhea is a common adverse effect of antimicrobial therapy, largely from the elimination of beneficial bacteria normally found in the colon. Controlled studies have shown that coadministration of probiotic microorganisms such as *Lactobacillus casei*, *L. acidophilus*, *Bifidobacterium longum*, or *Saccharomyces boulardii* can prevent or resolve antibiotic-induced diarrhea.[45] The diarrhea experienced by many patients after antibiotic therapy is sometimes caused by an overgrowth of the anaerobic bacterium *Clostridium difficile*, which causes a disease known as pseudomembranous colitis. Controlled studies have shown that coadministration of probiotic yeast, specifically *S. boulardii* or *Saccharomyces cerevisiae*, helps prevent recurrence of this infection. In one study, administration of 500 mg *S. boulardii* twice daily enhanced the effectiveness of vancomycin in preventing recurrent *Clostridium* infection.[45,46]

The general literature suggests that two categories define the interactions between uses of probiotics and antibiotics. First, the antibiotics may deplete or interfere with the absorption, viability, or function of the probiotics; theoretically, ingesting these organisms may help replenish them. Second, the probiotic may reduce the likelihood or severity of the potential adverse effects of the antibiotics.

Probiotic therapies can offset the loss of GI flora associated with antibiotic therapy.[47] Probiotic therapy can be fundamental to strategic case management for a wide range of chronic conditions, particularly digestive and immune conditions, within the diverse disciplines of natural medicine, nutritional therapeutics, and integrative care. In persons with suspected or diagnosed yeast/fungal intestinal overgrowth, probiotics are typically administered in conjunction with or following antifungal agents, along with nutrients intended to reduce gut permeability and reestablish integrity and normal function of mucous membranes of the GI tract.

The strongest evidence for the use of probiotics is in the management of diarrheal diseases.[16] A meta-analysis of randomized controlled trials demonstrated that many probiotics are effective in preventing antibiotic-associated diarrhea.[48] The agents cited in this meta-analysis included the yeast strain *Saccharomyces boulardii,* as well as the bacterium *Lactobacillus acidophilus* in combination with *L. bulgaricus*, *L. rhamnosus* strain GG [American Type Culture Collection (ATCC) 53103;LGG], and *Enterococcus faecium* strain SF68. Separate meta-analysis of randomized controlled trials showed a variety of probiotics, including *Lactobacillus* species, *Enterococcus* species, and *S. boulardii*, to be efficacious with infective diarrhea in both children and adults.[16] Probiotics were found to reduce the duration of diarrhea by more than 30 hours. Efficacy in

this setting is also supported by a randomized clinical trial of a probiotics mix. The mix included 3×10^{11} CFU *L. bulgaricus, L. casei, L. plantarum, L. acidophilus, Bifidobacterium longum, B. breve, B. infantis*, and *Streptococcus thermophilus.*

A different probiotic mix, *Bifidobacterium lactis* Bb12 and *Lactobacillus reuteri* (ATCC55730) at 1×10^7 CFU, has been shown to be useful in preventing flares of chronic pouchitis in patients with inflammatory bowel disease and diarrheal illness in infants attending child care.[49,50] (*Pouchitis* refers to inflammation of the rectal stump in patients who are status/post–colectomy with ileostomy.) The use of probiotic species, including *B. longum, L. acidophilus, L. casei, S. boulardii,* and *Saccharomyces cerevisiae,* provide a reduction and prevention of the potential adverse effect of diarrhea with antibiotics.[3,45,46,51-55]

The scientific literature provides only minimal evidence from laboratory experiments and clinical trials investigating the differential impact of various antibiotic agents and classes on particular native species and strains of gut flora or the preventive or therapeutic application of probiotics in conjunction with or after particular antibiotics. However, the primary focus of scientific research and clinical administration of probiotic therapy continues to center on *Bifidobacterium longum, Lactobacillus acidophilus, Lactobacillus casei, Saccharomyces boulardii,* and *Saccharomyces cerevisiae,* which can prevent or reduce the severity of diarrhea, a significant and often serious potential adverse effect.[3,45,46,51-54] *S. boulardii* provides a supportive interaction that may support and enhance the therapeutic activity of the concomitant antibiotic.[55,56] In addition, *L. acidophilus* GG enables the recolonization of human colonic mucosa and enhances the therapeutic efficacy of the antibiotic agent.[15,57-59]

Important examples of clinical applications for probiotic therapy are discussed next.

Antibiotic-Induced Diarrhea. Many studies have examined probiotic therapy in the prevention of antibiotic-associated diarrhea. A study of patients receiving extensive antibiotic treatment indicates that 2 years of probiotic therapy (at 2×10^{10} CFU daily) provided a protective strategy for reestablishing healthy flora in these patients.[55]

Atopic Dermatitis and Food Sensitivity. The use of probiotic therapy as part of treatment for atopic dermatitis is well documented and is often considered most efficacious in treating patients with food sensitivities who are also affected by atopic dermatitis.[36]

Clostridium difficile *Pseudomembranous Colitis.* The higher risk of serious GI diseases caused by antibiotic therapy makes probiotics a unique protective and therapeutic agent. *Clostridium difficile* infection is usually curable but can be very debilitating, especially in elderly or seriously ill patients. It also recurs repeatedly in some patients and occasionally causes life-threatening inflammation of the colon. This strain presents a growing challenge across North America and Europe. A virulent, once-rare strain has driven a string of recent outbreaks and is suspected to be responsible for much of the overall increase in the disease. New resistance to widely used antibiotics seems to have made the microbe more likely to cause diarrhea in sick and elderly people. At the same time, researchers are concerned about scattered cases of *C. difficile* among people not normally susceptible to the organism. In the United States, "the rate of C-diff in hospital patients doubled between 2000 and 2003," reports McDonald et al.[60] of the Centers for Disease Control and Prevention (CDC) in Atlanta. *Saccharomyces boulardii* has been successfully used in treatment of *C. difficile* colitis, usually after failure of metronidazole and oral vancomycin.[45] Anecdotal clinical experience suggests that prophylactic use of 9 to 10 billion CFU daily of *S. boulardii* concomitantly with broad-spectrum antibiotics may prevent overgrowth of *C. difficile*. Adequately powered, randomized clinical trials of this strategy would appear justified in view of this growing problem among hospitalized patients.

Enteric Colonization of Candida in Neonatal Patients. Oral coadministration of *Lactobacillus casei* subspecies *rhamnosus* (LGG) reduces the incidence and intensity of enteric colonization by *Candida* species in very-low-birth-weight neonates. The ability of LGG to prevent colonization by fungi might translate into a similar ability to prevent fungal infections. In a randomized trial involving 80 preterm neonates, Manzoni et al.[61] administered LGG (6×10^9 CFU/day), delivered in human milk and compared to human milk alone, for 6 weeks until discharge from the neonatal intensive care unit. They observed that the incidence of fungal enteric colonization was significantly lower in the LGG group than in the control group (23.1% vs. 48.8%). Furthermore, the number of fungal isolates obta-ined from each neonate and each colonized neonate was also significantly lower in the LGG group. Overall, the reduction in GI colonization reached significance in neonates with a birth weight of 1001 to 1500 g, but was not significant in those with a lower birth weight. LGG was not isolated from blood cultures or other specimens, and there were no adverse effects.

Inflammatory Bowel Disease. Probiotics, prebiotics, and antibiotics can provide significant benefit to patients with inflammatory bowel disease (IBD). Probiotics and prebiotics are the type of therapy that appeals to most patients with IBD. Probiotics have no significant adverse effects, except possibly a transient increase in abdominal gas with prebiotics, and thus far appear to be entirely safe. More than a dozen studies using probiotics in IBD indicate clear benefit in pouchitis and possibly in Crohn's disease. Further clinical trials are warranted investigating treatment of ulcerative colitis. The use of oligosaccharide and other prebiotics within conventional therapy for IBD is in its infancy, although significant effects on both the luminal and the mucosa-associated flora have been demonstrated in healthy subjects. Probiotics and prebiotics could play a central role in standard treatment of patients with IBD, although these therapies carry an uncertain risk of potential adverse effects. Their efficacy in clinical studies varies, with Crohn's disease and pouchitis reporting more benefit than ulcerative colitis. However, the ideal combination of conventional interventions, probiotics, and prebiotics and criteria for their application has not been determined.[62]

Nutritional Therapeutics, Clinical Concerns, and Adaptations

Physicians can prevent and treat a wide range of disorders and support restoration of healthy physiological function by instituting a strategy built around probiotic repletion. Survey data and anecdotal experience strongly indicate that probiotics, usually in combination with prebiotics and other supportive measures, are often self-prescribed by individuals during or after antibiotic therapy.

Common therapeutic applications of probiotics include improving general gut health; improving the body's natural defenses; reversing patterns of fungal overgrowth, deteriorated intestinal function, and immune compromise; and reducing blood cholesterol levels. The American College of Nutrition recommends, in its nutrition specialist certification review materials, that 6 months of probiotic therapy, with at least 10 billion probiotic organisms daily, is usually indicated to reverse the effects of antibiotic therapy and reestablish healthy gut microbiota.

Helicobacter pylori Triple Therapy (LAM)/Quadruple Therapy

Lansoprazole-amoxicillin-metronidazole (LAM) triple-therapy regimen: Lansoprazole (Prevacid), amoxicillin (Amoxil, Polymox, Trimox, Wymox; Augmentin), metronidazole (Flagyl, Protostat).
Related: HeliMet (Wyeth; discontinued August 2005 in United Kingdom): Lansoprazole (Zoton), clarithromycin (Klaricid), metronidazole.

Interaction Type and Significance
⊕⊕ **Beneficial or Supportive Interaction, with Professional Management**

Probability:	Evidence Base:
2. Probable	◉ **Emerging**

Effect and Mechanism of Action
Probiotics can be incorporated into a triple-therapy (or quadruple-therapy) methodology using a proton pump inhibitor (PPI) and two antibiotics.[47,63] Higher eradication rates are found with the coadministration of probiotic agents and pharmaceutical agents.

Research
In a trial involving 138 patients in whom triple therapy failed, Sheu et al.[47] found that a 4-week pretreatment with *Lactobacillus*- and *Bifidobacterium*-containing yogurt (AB-yogurt) "can decrease *H. pylori* loads despite antimicrobial resistance, thus improving the efficacy of quadruple therapy in eradicating residual *H. pylori*."

Nutritional Therapeutics, Clinical Concerns, and Adaptations
Physicians prescribing triple (or quadruple) therapy for recalcitrant *Helicobacter pylori* infection are advised to consider coadministration of probiotic flora during and after such eradication therapy.

THEORETICAL, SPECULATIVE, AND PRELIMINARY INTERACTIONS RESEARCH, INCLUDING OVERSTATED INTERACTIONS CLAIMS

Sulfasalazine

Sulfazalzine (Salazosulfapyridine, salicylazosulfapyridine, suphasalazine; Apo-Sulfasalazine, Azulfidine, Azulfidine EN-Tabs, PMS-Sulfasalazine, Salazopyrin, Salazopyrin EN-Tabs, SAS).

Findings from an in vitro experiment suggest that *Lactobacillus acidophilus* may accelerate metabolism of sulfasalazine. The occurrence of this pharmacodynamic phenomenon has not been established in humans, nor has any pattern of clinical significance emerged. The authors studied bacterial metabolism of three drugs (sulfasalazine, phthalylsulfathiazole, and chloramphenicol palmitate) and two dyes (tartrazine and methyl red) using a resting culture technique. The strains used were isolated intestinal lactobacilli, *E. coli*, and mixed cultures of feces of mice. One strain of *L. acidophilus* exhibited degradation of sulfasalazine as high as 94.3%. In contrast, the highest degradation of phthalylsulfathiazole and chloramphenicol palmitate was found to be 17.6% and 8%, respectively. The authors also discussed toxicological aspects of degradation products in relation to the use of lactobacilli as dietary supplement or therapeutic aid.[64] Although highly preliminary, these data suggest that although probiotics may potentially have beneficial effects in inflammatory bowel disease, at least certain strains might increase the metabolism of sulfasalazine with coadministration. If unexpected relapse of symptoms were to occur in IBD patients taking both sulfasalzine and probiotics, consideration should be given to discontinuing probiotics and/or increasing the dose of sulfasalazine.

NUTRIENT-NUTRIENT INTERACTIONS

Oligosaccharides and Other Prebiotics

Health care professionals trained and experienced in nutritional therapeutics and integrative care strategies often use prebiotic therapy to "fertilize" the gut before probiotic therapy and thereby enhance its effectiveness. For example, using a murine influenza vaccination model examining a specific prebiotic-oligosaccharide mixture, with stimulation of delayed-type hypersensitivity, Vos et al.[65] suggest that application use of galactooligosaccharides (GOS) and fructooligosaccharides (FOS) in dietary products might provide an opportunity to stimulate the adaptive immune response in a direction favoring T-helper cell type 1 (Th1) immunity and subsequently inhibit infections and T-helper 2 (Th2)–related immune disorders (e.g., allergic/atopic disease) in humans.[65]

Oligosaccharides in breast milk or added to infant formula modulate postnatal immune development by altering bowel flora and have a potential role in primary allergy prevention during infancy. Infant formulas enhanced with prebiotic oligosaccharides were found to modify intestinal bacteria and more than halve the risk of atopic dermatitis among high-risk babies. In a 6-month, double-blind, randomized, placebo-controlled trial of 259 infants at risk for atopy, only 10 of 102 infants given prebiotics in their formula developed atopic dermatitis, according to an online report in the July 2006 *Archives of Disease in Childhood*. By contrast, 24 of 104 controls given formula without probiotics developed the disorder.[66]

The effect of oligofructose (OF, prebiotic) on microflora in infants is being increasingly studied. A double-blind placebo-controlled trial assessed the effect of daily OF administration on the intestinal microflora, intestinal tolerance, and well-being of healthy infants age 7 to 19 months, with 8 days of observation, 21 days of administration, and 15 days of post-treatment. Exclusion criteria included antibiotic use and intake of another prebiotic or probiotic any time after enrollment. Fecal flora were analyzed by culture methods, and health information was recorded daily. Bifidobacteria tended to increase slightly with OF administration, but not with placebo. Simultaneously, a decrease in potential pathogens, significant for clostridia but not for staphylococci, was observed in the OF group. These modifications did not persist during the post-treatment period. OF intake was accompanied by less flatulence, diarrhea, vomiting, and fever events.[34]

Administration of probiotics and prebiotics can reduce incidence of eczema in infants. Eczema, also known as atopic dermatitis (AD), is one of the first signs of allergy during the early days of life and is believed to result from delayed development of the immune system. According to the American Academy of Dermatologists, eczema affects 10% to 20% of all infants, but almost half will "grow out" of eczema between ages 5 and 15. The research adds to a 2003 study from Finland that reported children exposed to the *Lactobacillus rhamnosus* GG (LGG) bacteria around birth were 40% less likely to develop AD at 4 years of age compared with children in a placebo group. In the new study (2006), Kukkonen et al.[67] from the University

of Helsinki built on these earlier results by examining the effects of a probiotic and prebiotic combination on allergy prevention in a much larger population of allergy-prone infants than previously studied. The researchers randomized 1223 pregnant women to receive either placebo or daily probiotic formulation containing four probiotic strains: *Lactobacillus rhamnosus* GG, *L. rhamnosus* LC705, *Bifidobacterium breve* Bb99, and *Propionibacterium freudenreichii* ssp. *shermanii* JS. The women were treated for the 2 to 4 weeks before delivery. The newborns then received either the same probiotics in combination with GOS (461 babies) or placebo (464 babies) for 6 months. Researchers have found that breast milk naturally contains prebiotic oligosaccharides, believed to stimulate bifidobacteria that facilitate the release of energy and nutrients from the diet. No significant differences were observed between the treated and placebo groups with regard to allergic disease overall, but the researchers reported that administration of the probiotic/prebiotic mixture was associated with a 26% reduction in eczema and a 34% reduction in atopic eczema specifically. Fecal samples revealed that the probiotic/prebiotic group had significantly higher lactobacilli, propionibacteria, and bifidobacteria populations. This result indicated "successful intervention and good adherence." According to the researchers:

> Our prospective study indicates, for the first time to our knowledge, an inverse association between the prevalence of eczema and the abundance of certain species of the indigenous gut microbiota, thus supporting the important role of commensal bacteria in the pathogenesis of eczema.... Gut microbiota contact directly with extensions of dendritic cells, which orchestrate the mucosal immune homeostasis. Commensal bacteria stimulate the innate immune system and contribute to the generation of regulatory lymphocytes, which, through IL-10 and TGF-beta, establish and maintain mucosal immune tolerance.[67]

The results show that probiotics and prebiotics offer an "easily accessible, inexpensive, and safe" way of reducing eczema in infants, particularly high-risk infants. The researchers said that continued follow-up on these same infants will show if this effect is maintained later in life, and if any impact on airway allergies such as asthma is observed.[67]

Milk formulas containing prebiotics help floral inoculation with beneficial bacteria. Antibiotics exert deleterious effects on the intestinal microbiota, favoring the emergence of opportunistic bacteria, pathogenic yeasts, other fungi, and diarrhea. Prebiotics are nondigestible food components that stimulate the growth of bifidobacteria and other symbionts. To study the effects of probiotic administration after antibiotic treatment, Brunser et al.[68] conducted a randomized, double-blind, controlled clinical trial involving 140 infants 1 to 2 years of age distributed into two groups after being treated for acute bronchitis with a 1-week course of amoxicillin (50 mg/kg/day). For 3 weeks the children received greater than 500 mL/day of a prebiotic formula (4.5 g/L) or placebo. Fecal samples obtained at the beginning of the antibiotic treatment ("day seven"), at the end of the treatment and before formula administration ("day zero"), and during formula administration ("days seven and twenty-one") were evaluated for *Bifidobacterium, Lactobacillus-Enterococcus, Clostridium lituseburiense* cluster, *Clostridium histolyticum* cluster, *Escherichia coli*, and *Bacteroides-Prevotella*. The authors reported that amoxicillin decreased total fecal bacteria and increased *E. coli*, whereas the prebiotic group exhibited significantly increased bifidobacteria, from 8.17 ± 1.46 on day zero to 8.54 ± 1.20 on day seven, compared with the control 8.22 ± 1.24 on day zero versus 7.95 ± 1.54 on day seven. The *Lactobacillus* population showed a similar tendency, but the other bacteria were unaffected. Adverse GI symptoms were absent during the prebiotic administration. The authors concluded that prebiotics "in a milk formula increase fecal bifidobacteria early after amoxicillin treatment without inducing gastrointestinal symptoms."[68] Continued research is warranted to investigate further the synergistic use of prebiotics and probiotics directly after antibiotic therapy or in response to long-term sequelae associated with, or aggravated by, the adverse effects of antibiotic therapy.

Prebiotics and calcium exhibit a synergistic relationship in the process of bone mineralization. In a randomized, placebo-controlled trial, Abrams et al.[69] found that a combination of prebiotic short-chain and long-chain inulin-type fructans enhances calcium absorption and long-term bone mineralization in young adolescents. The investigators randomly assigned pubertal adolescents to receive 8 g/day of a mixed short and long degree of polymerization, inulin-type fructan product (fructan group) or maltodextrin placebo (as control). At baseline and after 1 year, they measured bone mineral content, bone mineral density, and calcium absorption; they also determined polymorphisms of the Fok1 vitamin D receptor gene. Subsequently, they observed that after both 8 weeks and 1 year, calcium absorption was significantly greater in the fructan group than in the control group. Notably, an "interaction with Fok1 genotype was present such that subjects with an ff genotype had the least initial response to fructan." After 1 year, the "fructan group had a greater increment in both whole-body bone mineral content ... and whole-body bone mineral density ... than did the control group." The authors concluded that daily "consumption of a combination of prebiotic short- and long-chain inulin-type fructans significantly increases calcium absorption and enhances bone mineralization during pubertal growth." They also added that effects of "dietary factors on calcium absorption may be modulated by genetic factors, including specific vitamin D receptor gene polymorphisms."[69]

These findings indicate that further research investigating this synergistic intervention is warranted (preferably with calcium, vitamin D, and magnesium administration controlled), especially given the critical importance of establishing maximal bone density during adolescence and early adulthood. Similar study of the potential impact of prebiotic nutritional support in adults of different age groups, particularly perimenopausal and postmenopausal women, also appears highly relevant.

HERB-NUTRIENT INTERACTIONS

Numerous botanical agents from European, American, and Asian traditions of herbal medicine appear to require the action of intestinal bacteria to attain their biologically active form (e.g., see Licorice monograph). Research is lacking on the effect of loss of gut bacteria on clinical efficacy of these traditional therapeutic interventions, but the implications could be profound not only for the indigenous populations employing these classical methods of healing in their native context, but also for researchers attempting to validate their effects in an average "Western" (i.e., modern) patient population who have presumably been treated with numerous courses

of antibiotics, but not with subsequent, thorough probiotic repletion.

Echinacea

Echinacea *(Echinacea angustifolia, Echinacea purpurea)*.

In a 10-day randomized trial involving 15 healthy adults, Hill, Foote, et al.[70] observed potentially problematic changes in intestinal microbiota after *Echinacea* administration. The investigators reported that standardized *E. purpurea* (1000 mg daily) stimulated the growth of certain *Bacteroides* species of intestinal bacteria, which may act as pathogens, particularly when the gut ecology has been disrupted. In stool samples they found *Echinacea* use associated with increased counts for three groups of organisms: the total group of aerobic bacteria, the anaerobic *Bacteroides* in general, and *Bacteroides fragilis* in particular. The authors concluded that the "health consequences associated with this change are unknown." Notably, reports of potentially related adverse events associated with echinacea use, such as irritable bowel syndrome or other pathological responses that might be predicted to result from such unfavorable alterations, are lacking.

Although similar findings for echinacea or other herbs (e.g., goldenseal, isatis) often used as antimicrobial/immunostimulant agents are generally absent in the scientific literature, such effects from chronic unsupervised use at high doses would not necessarily be unexpected. Further research and judicious pharmacovigilance are appropriate and necessary as the use of botanical medicine grows within the consumer self-care market and professional therapeutic application.

Ginseng, Chinese/Korean

Chinese/Korean ginseg *(Panax ginseng)*.

Ginseng interacts as a proactive factor with intestinal bacteria. It is activated in the body by intestinal bacterial deglycosylation. Orally ingested ginsenoside passes through the stomach and small intestine, without decomposition by either gastric juice or liver enzymes, into the large intestine, where ginsenoside is deglycosylated by colonic bacteria, followed by transit to the circulation. Colonic bacteria cleave the oligosaccharide connected to the aglycone stepwise from the terminal sugar to afford the major metabolites, 20S-protopanaxadiol 20-O-beta-D-glucopyranoside (M1) and 20S-protopanaxatriol (M4). These metabolites are further esterified with fatty acids, and the resultant fatty acid conjugates are sustained in their active state in the body longer than parental metabolites. Growing evidence indicates that ginsenoside is a prodrug that is activated in the human body by intestinal bacterial deglycosylation and fatty acid esterification.[71] Research investigating the potential decreased efficacy of treatment with ginseng preparation in individuals with diminished intestinal flora, and possible enhancement of effect with restoration of gut ecology through probiotic repletion, represents a promising direction for creative endeavor in integrative medical approaches.

The 72 citations for this monograph, as well as additional reference literature, are located under Probiotics on the CD at the back of the book.

S-Adenosylmethionine (SAMe)

Nutrient Name: S-adenosylmethionine (SAMe).
Synonyms: S-adenosyl-L-methionine, S-adenosyl methionine, ademetionine; AdoMet.

Summary

Drug/Class Interaction Type	Mechanism and Significance	Management
Acetaminophen ☼	SAMe reduces acetaminophen hepatotoxicity. Further research warranted to confirm efficacy and establish dosage and treatment guidelines.	May be effective with or in place of NAC as an antidote in treatment of acetaminophen toxicity.
Imipramine Tricyclic antidepressants (TCAs) ⊕⊕/⊕✗/✗✗	SAMe can accelerate onset of action of imipramine. Concomitant administration could be therapeutic with proper management. Additive or synergistic effect may theoretically result from concomitant use of SAMe and TCAs because of their potentially similar influences on CNS.	Coadministration may be beneficial. May need to modify drug dosage. Monitor and titrate.
Levodopa Antiparkinsonian medications ✗/◇◇/◇◇/⊕✗/⊕	SAMe tends to be low in Parkinson's disease and levodopa therapy depletes the body of SAMe. However, SAMe may contribute to Parkinson-like motor impairments and interfere with action of L-dopa by promoting methylation. Concomitant administration of L-dopa and SAMe might potentially amplify, distort, or harmonize endogenous L-dopa and SAMe equilibrium. Research lacking to provide conclusive advice.	Concomitant use could aggravate symptoms or interfere with drug action. If clinically appropriate, may need to modify drug dosage. Monitor closely and titrate.
Oral contraceptives (OCs) ☼	By enhancing liver detoxification, glutathione production, and related metabolic processes, SAMe may protect against tendency of OCs to raise cholesterol saturation of bile by increasing biliary cholesterol secretion. Clinical trials warranted to follow and validate findings from supportive indirect research.	Coadministration may be beneficial in patients at risk of hepatobiliary dysfunction.
Ursodeoxycholic acid (UDCA) Chenodeoxycholic acid (CDCA) ⊕⊕	Both UDCA and SAMe can be efficacious in treatment of conditions related to hepatobiliary dysfunction and disease, including pruritus and intrahepatic cholestasis of pregnancy (ICP). UDCA was more effective than SAMe in controlling some symptoms, but research indicates that coadministration can increase efficacy and reduce potential fetal toxicity of UDCA.	Coadministration may be beneficial in patients at risk of hepatobiliary dysfunction, particularly ICP.
Venlafaxine Selective serotonin reuptake inhibitor and serotonin-norepinephrine reuptake inhibitor (SSRI and SNRI) Antidepressants ⊕⊕	Coadministration of SAMe with SSRIs, including venlafaxine, may augment therapeutic effect, particularly in individuals with partial or resistant responses to standard antidepressant pharmacotherapy. Mechanisms of action not fully elucidated, but preliminary evidence suggests minimal adverse effects.	Coadministration may be beneficial. May need to modify drug dosage. Monitor and titrate.

NAC, N-acetylcysteine; CNS, central nervous system.

NUTRIENT DESCRIPTION

Chemistry and Forms

Sulfuradenosylmethionine, S-adenosyl-L-methionine; S-adenosyl-methionine butanedisulfonate, S-adenosylmethionine tosylate.

Physiology and Function

S-Adenosylmethionine (SAMe) is a naturally occurring compound functioning in a multitude of biochemical reactions and biosynthetic processes throughout the central nervous system (CNS), liver, connective tissue, and detoxification systems and within cellular metabolic activities. Dietary methionine is primarily metabolized in the liver, where it is combined with adenosine triphosphate (ATP) to form SAMe in a reaction catalyzed by methionine adenosyltransferase I/III (MAT I/III), the product of the MAT1A gene, which is exclusively expressed in the liver. SAMe serves as a precursor molecule to three main metabolic pathways within all cells: methylation, transulfuration, and aminopropylation.

S-Adenosylmethionine is the body's main biological methyl donor. After donating a methyl group in the synthesis of nucleic acids (DNA and RNA), choline, creatine, carnitine, proteins, phospholipids, catecholamines, epinephrine, and various neurotransmitters, SAMe is converted to S-adenosylhomocysteine (SAH). Subsequent trans-sulfuration reactions enable and regulate formation of sulfur-containing amino acids such as cysteine, glutathione, and taurine. After donating sulfur in this way, SAH gives up adenosine and is rapidly metabolized to homocysteine. Through the pathway known as aminopropylation, SAMe is metabolized to decarboxylated SAMe and functions as a cofactor in the synthesis of polyamines, including spermidine, puescine, and spermine, which are essential for cellular growth and differentiation, gene expression, DNA repair, protein phosphorylation, and neuron myelination and regeneration. As a key facilitator of phosphatidylcholine synthesis, SAMe plays a role in promoting flexible and responsive cellular membranes and supports healthy bile production and flow. SAMe influences levels of 5-hydroxyindoleacetic acid (5-HIAA), a serotonin metabolite, and homovanillic acid, a dopamine metabolite, in the cerebrospinal fluid (CSF) and appears to cross the blood-brain barrier via carrier-mediated transport.

NUTRIENT IN CLINICAL PRACTICE

Known or Potential Therapeutic Uses

Human clinical trials investigating SAMe have reported positive outcomes in the treatment of a range of conditions, reflecting the broad and diverse functions of this substance in human physiology. In particular, researchers have focused on depression, osteoarthritis, and liver disorders. Although a number of studies have shown clinical benefit, most have been limited by small numbers, brief duration, and preliminary or flawed design. Further, the research findings from human trials cannot be extrapolated readily to self-prescribed use or typical clinical practice, since oral dosages in European clinical trials have usually been significantly higher than those typically used by many individuals, and many studies have used intravenous (IV) or intramuscular (IM) modes of administration.

Historical/Ethnomedicine Precedent

S-Adenosylmethionine has not been used historically as an isolated nutrient.

Possible Uses

Alzheimer's disease, attention deficit–hyperactivity disorder (ADHD), cardiovascular disease, cirrhosis, dementia, depression, fibromyalgia, Gilbert's syndrome, infertility (male), insomnia, intrahepatic cholestasis of pregnancy, migraine, osteoarthritis, rheumatoid arthritis, Sjögren's syndrome, vacuolar myelopathy.

Dietary Sources

Methionine, from which SAMe is formed, can be obtained from a variety of dietary sources, but SAMe itself is not available through foods in any significant amounts. Dietary deficiencies in methionine, folate, or vitamin B_{12} can reduce SAMe levels.

Nutrient Preparations Available

S-Adenosylmethionine butanedisulfonate, S-adenosylmethionine tosylate.

In Europe, pharmaceutical preparations of SAMe are available mainly as IV, IM, and oral forms. In the United States, SAMe is primarily available in an over-the-counter (OTC) nutraceutical oral form as a capsule or tablet. SAMe is extremely hygroscopic and highly unstable; enteric-coated tablets packaged in foil or foil blister packs are considered the most stable form to avoid degradation.

Dosage Forms Available

Enteric-coated tablets. Parenteral preparations are available in Europe.

Source Materials for Nutrient Preparations

Biofermentation or synthesis from adenosine and methionine, generally complexed with a stabilizing salt, such as tosylate, disulfate tosylate, disulfate ditosylate, or 1,4-butanedisulfonate.

Dosage Range

Adult

Dietary: Not applicable.
  Estimated safe and adequate daily dietary intake: Not applicable.
  Average U.S. daily intake: Not applicable.
  Recommended dietary allowance (RDA): None established.

Supplemental/Maintenance: Not applicable.
Pharmacological/Therapeutic: 400 mg three or four times daily, based on clinical trials.
Oral: 200 to 1600 mg daily.

Adequate dose-escalation studies using the oral formulation of SAMe have yet to be performed to demonstrate the most effective oral dose of SAMe.

The most common dosage is 400 mg daily, even though this level is significantly below the efficacy threshold indicated by research and clinical experience. Its relatively high cost has often been considered a limiting factor in the effective use of SAMe as a nutraceutical, especially when self-prescribed.

Toxic: No dietary reference intake (DRI) has been set for S-adenosylmethionine.

Pediatric (< 18 Years)

No guidelines have been established for therapeutic or toxic dosage levels of SAMe for infants or children. Use within such populations is not usually recommended as appropriate.

Laboratory Values

Plasma levels of SAMe. Levels of L-methionine S-adenosyltransferase activity in erythrocytes, SAMe concentrations in CSF, and concentrations of SAMe and S-adenosylhomocysteine (SAH) in whole blood have also been used in clinical trials.

SAFETY PROFILE
Overview

In clinical trials and reported clinical use, SAMe has generally been well tolerated and considered safe.

Nutrient Adverse Effects

No toxic effects have been reported in research or clinical experience involving SAMe. Dry mouth, nausea, restlessness, and skin rashes are among the several minor adverse effects occasionally associated with SAMe intake and generally reported at higher doses. One case report of "serotonin syndrome" involving concomitant use of IM SAMe (100 mg/day) and clomipramine (75 mg/day) represents the most severe adverse event known.[1-4]

Adults

Mutagenicity: Research thus far indicates that SAMe is nonmutagenic in vitro and in vivo, even using high doses.

Adverse Effects Among Specific Populations
S-Adenosylmethionine use may trigger a manic episode in individuals with bipolar disorder.[5-7]

Pregnancy and Nursing
The safety of SAMe use in pregnant or breast-feeding women has not been established. However, several studies investigating SAMe in the treatment of intrahepatic cholestasis of pregnancy (ICP) have reported the agent as apparently safe during pregnancy.

Infants and Children
The safety of SAMe administration in infants and children has not been established.

Contraindications

Bipolar disorder, migraines, Parkinson's disease; individuals with active bleeding.

Precautions and Warnings

Given that SAMe is a precursor to homocysteine and that methionine may elevate homocysteine, it would be prudent to assess homocysteine levels before treating with SAMe in individuals with a significant family history of coronary heart disease.

INTERACTIONS REVIEW

Strategic Considerations

S-Adenosylmethionine's central role in several critical metabolic pathways indicates that both excessive intake and drug-induced depletion are likely to produce significant consequences. Well-designed studies will be required to clarify and articulate the particulars of these patterns in a systematic manner. Likewise, further research is needed to determine therapeutic approaches to synergistic use of SAMe as part of integrative therapeutics employing the nutraceutical in conjunction with various conventional therapies for treatment of the conditions for which SAMe shows promise.

The issue of SAMe use by individuals diagnosed with bipolar disorder continues to be controversial; well-designed research is needed to assess its efficacy as a therapeutic agent, alone or in conjunction with conventional pharmacological treatments.

The scientific understanding of the physiology and pharmacology of SAMe is generally in a preliminary state, particularly with regard to genetic variability and its pharmacogenomic implications. In particular, the critical roles of SAMe in the areas of DNA methylation, neurotransmitter self-regulatory processes, and hepatic conjugation of pharmaceutical agents all deserve continued research and will undoubtedly reveal significant implications for SAMe's therapeutic application and interactions with other medications. Recent clinical trial data suggest that SAMe appears to augment the antidepressant effect of SSRI and SSRI/SNRI agents. Large, randomized, placebo-controlled trials addressing the difficult clinical problem of antidepressant-refractory depression are warranted.

NUTRIENT-DRUG INTERACTIONS

Acetaminophen

Acetaminophen (APAP, paracetamol; Tylenol); combination drugs: acetaminophen and codeine (Capital and Codeine; Phenaphen with Codeine; Tylenol with Codeine); acetaminophen and hydrocodone (Anexsia, Anodynos-DHC, Co-Gesic, Dolacet, DuoCet, Hydrocet, Hydrogesic, Hy-Phen, Lorcet 10/650, Lorcet-HD, Lorcet Plus, Lortab, Margesic H, Medipain 5, Norco, Stagesic, T-Gesic, Vicodin, Vicodin ES, Vicodin HP, Zydone); acetaminophen and oxycodone (Endocet, Percocet 2.5/325, Percocet 5/325, Percocet 7.5/500, Percocet 10/650, Roxicet 5/500, Roxilox, Tylox); acetaminophen and pentazocine (Talacen); acetaminophen and propoxyphene (Darvocet-N, Darvocet-N 100, Pronap-100, Propacet 100, Propoxacet-N, Wygesic), acetaminophen, butalbital, and caffeine (Fioricet).

Interaction Type and Significance

☼ **Prevention or Reduction of Drug Adverse Effect**

Probability:	Evidence Base:
2. Probable	○ Preliminary

Effect and Mechanism of Action

S-Adenosylmethionine reduces acetaminophen hepatotoxicity and lethality by metabolism of the active moiety to glutathione.

Research

In mouse models, SAMe (intraperitoneal administration, 1 g/kg or 2.5 mmol/kg) within 1 to 5 hours reduced depletion of plasma and liver glutathione, liver damage, and release of aspartate transaminase (AST) after acetaminophen administration.[8,9] Other researchers concluded that SAMe presented a therapeutic alternative to *N*-acetylcysteine (NAC) as an antidote for poisoning with acetaminophen.[10]

Nutritional Therapeutics, Clinical Concerns, and Adaptations

Further research is indicated to confirm the efficacy and determine most effective dosage levels for use of SAMe, in place of or in conjunction with NAC, as an antidote in the treatment of acetaminophen poisoning.

Imipramine and Other Tricyclic Antidepressants

Evidence: Imipramine (Janimine, Tofranil).
Extrapolated, based on similar properties: Clomipramine (Anafranil)
Similar properties but evidence lacking for extrapolation: Amitriptyline (Elavil); combination drug: amitriptyline and perphenazine (Etrafon, Triavil, Triptazine); amoxapine (Asendin), desipramine (Norpramin, Pertofrane), doxepin (Adapin, Sinequan), nortriptyline (Aventyl, Pamelor), protriptyline (Vivactil), trimipramine (Surmontil).

Interaction Type and Significance

⊕⊕ **Beneficial or Supportive Interaction, with Professional Management**
⊕✗ **Bimodal or Variable Interaction, with Professional Management**
✗✗ **Minimal to Mild Adverse Interaction—Vigilance Necessary**

Probability:	Evidence Base:
2. Probable	◉ Emerging

Effect and Mechanism of Action

S-Adenosylmethionine accelerates the onset of action of imipramine. Experiments using rats demonstrated that SAMe prevents the 5-HT(1A) receptor upregulation induced by acute imipramine in the frontal cortex.[11] SAMe and tricyclic antidepressants (TCAs) exert potentially similar influences on the CNS and together can generate an additive or synergistic effect.

Research

Numerous clinical trials have investigated the efficacy of SAMe in the treatment of various degrees of depression, often in comparison to TCAs, particularly imipramine. TCAs and SAMe have both been used successfully in treatment of depression; double-blind clinical studies show approximately equivalent efficacy, both superior to placebo, with TCAs associated with more frequent adverse events and SAMe being better tolerated. Pancheri et al.[12] estimated IM 400 mg/day SAMe to be comparable to oral 150 mg/day imipramine in terms of antidepressive efficacy. Although many clinical trials of SAMe have involved IM, parenteral, or other modes of administering SAMe, oral administration of SAMe has demonstrated antidepressant activity, independent of its combination with imipramine or other antidepressants.[13]

Preliminary research has focused on the concomitant administration of these two agents with promising implications. In a double-blind clinical trial with 40 subjects receiving oral imipramine (150 mg/day initially and then according to symptoms), half also received IM 200 mg/day SAMe, and the other half also received placebo. The patients receiving the SAMe-imipramine combination reported a more rapid decrease in depressive symptoms than did those in the placebo-imipramine group.[14]

Report
In 1993, Iruela et al.[15] published a case report describing an episode of "serotonin syndrome" in a woman after combining IM 100 mg SAMe daily, with 75 mg/day clomipramine.

Nutritional Therapeutics, Clinical Concerns, and Adaptations
Physicians prescribing imipramine or other TCAs may consider use of SAMe within an integrative strategy combining the two agents and using SAMe as a support during weaning from TCA therapy. However, the potential for therapeutic synergy also invokes the risk of excessive pharmacological response. A clear need exists for well-designed clinical studies with larger numbers of subjects and a variety of combination therapies to determine conclusively which patients will benefit from conventional antidepressants, SAMe, or some combination and to establish appropriate dosage levels and therapeutic protocols. Pending such evidence, individuals should be dissuaded from unsupervised concomitant use of SAMe and TCAs or other antidepressant medications.

Significant potential exists for safe and effective therapy using coadministration within the context of integrative care, providing close supervision and regular monitoring by health care professionals trained and experienced in both conventional pharmacology and nutritional therapeutics. Clinical trials investigating the use of SAMe for treatment of depression suggests that an effective dose could be anywhere in the range of 800 to 1600 mg daily. Any concomitant use of SAMe and a TCA such as imipramine would need to be determined on the basis of the relative dose of the antidepressant and the particular needs of the individual being treated.

Levodopa and Related Antiparkinsonian Medications

Levodopa (L-dopa; Dopar, Larodopa); combination drugs: levodopa and benserazide (co-beneldopa; Madopar); levodopa and carbidopa (Atamet, Parcopa, Sinemet, Sinemet CR); levodopa, carbidopa and entacapone (Stalevo).

Related antiparkinsonian medications: Carbidopa (Lodosyn), selegiline (deprenyl, L-deprenil, L-deprenyl; Atapryl, Carbex, Eldepryl, Jumex, Movergan, Selpak).

Interaction Type and Significance
✗   **Potential or Theoretical Adverse Interaction of Uncertain Severity**
◇◇   **Drug-Induced Effect on Nutrient Function, Supplementation Contraindicated, Professional Management Appropriate**
⊕✗   **Bimodal or Variable Interaction, with Professional Management**

⊕   **Potential or Theoretical Beneficial or Supportive Interaction with Professional Management**

Probability: Evidence Base:
2. Probable   ◉ **Emerging**

Effect and Mechanism of Action
S-Adenosylmethionine levels tend to be low in individuals with Parkinson's disease, and levodopa therapy depletes the body of SAMe. However, SAMe may contribute to Parkinson-like motor impairments and interfere with the action of L-dopa. Thus, the dynamic equilibrium between endogenous L-dopa and SAMe can potentially be amplified, distorted, or harmonized by the introduction of exogenous L-dopa and SAMe.

SAMe promotes methylation and, as suggested by both rodent and human studies, excessive methylation can cause depletion of dopamine, is associated with Parkinson's disease, and can interfere with the effects of L-dopa. SAMe is the rate-limiting endogenous methyl donor, and its biochemical roles include the metabolism of dopamine and the synthesis of acetylcholine. Thus, SAMe may produce effects that resemble the changes that occur in Parkinson's disease, such as hypokinesia, tremor, rigidity, and abnormal posture. Therefore, SAMe may play a role in Parkinson-like motor impairments, particularly under conditions of excessive SAMe-dependent methylation.[16-18]

Levodopa is administered with dopa decarboxylase inhibitors (DDIs) to prevent its peripheral degradation. This increases conversion of levodopa to 3-O-methyldopa (3-OMD) by catechol-O-methyltransferase (COMT). SAMe serves as methyl donor for this O-metabolization of levodopa, with resulting conversion of SAMe to total homocysteine (tHcy) via S-adenosylhomocysteine (SAH).[19]

Research
Studies of the interaction between L-dopa and SAMe, both endogenous and exogenous, reveal several significant trends, but no conclusive patterns of substantive evidence have confirmed a safe and effective approach to clinical management. Whereas some evidence suggests that individuals with Parkinson's disease may benefit from SAMe therapy, other research indicates that SAMe may deplete dopamine, aggravate motor symptoms, and possibly block the intended therapeutic action of L-dopa.

In two early studies, Charlton et al.[16] and Crowell et al.[20] found that exogenous SAMe intake was associated with Parkinson-like symptoms in rats, specifically decreases in motor activity. Subsequent research with human subjects undergoing treatment of Parkinson's disease with L-dopa showed that L-dopa reacts avidly with SAMe to produce 3-OMD.[21]

Levodopa has been shown to deplete the concentration of SAMe in the brain and increase tHcy levels.[19,22] This depletion pattern may contribute to the depression often experienced by individuals with Parkinson's disease and may constitute a significant factor in the adverse effects associated with levodopa therapy.[22,23] General evidence regarding the function of SAMe and preliminary research both suggest that SAMe administration could benefit individuals with Parkinson's disease through positive effects on the depression and impaired cognitive function typically associated with the condition.[23] A double-blind, crossover study published by Carrieri et al.[24] in 1990 demonstrated beneficial effects of SAMe (400 mg orally, twice daily, plus 200 mg daily intramuscularly), versus placebo, against depression in 21 patients with Parkinson's disease. Parkinsonian symptoms appeared to be unchanged, adverse effects were moderate and of brief duration, and there was no indication that the effectiveness of levodopa had been reduced. Likewise, in a more recent (2000) open-label pilot study involving 13 subjects with Parkinson's disease and comorbid depression, Di Rocco et al.[24a] found that 10 of the 11 patients who completed the clinical trial demonstrated at least a 50% improvement on the 17-point Hamilton Depression Scale (HDS) after 800 to 3600 mg SAMe daily for 10 weeks.

Nutritional Therapeutics, Clinical Concerns, and Adaptations

The emerging pattern of evidence reflects the delicate interplay and dynamic equilibrium between L-dopa and SAMe. On the one hand, individuals with Parkinson's disease tend to be deficient in SAMe, inclined to depression, and subject to the depleting effects of levodopa therapy. On the other hand, SAMe could in theory contribute to excessive methylation, which appears to exacerbate motor impairments similar to parkinsonism, and concomitant SAMe may interfere with the therapeutic action of levodopa. Furthermore, the significant adverse effects associated with L-dopa (or carbidopa/levodopa) therapy cannot be easily overlooked, whereas SAMe is generally considered to produce minor adverse effects. Well-designed clinical trials with substantial numbers of human subjects will be required to clarify the diverse and paradoxical findings of the available preliminary research.

The possibility of enhanced synergistic benefits from combined therapy needs to be considered in light of the reasonable risk of serious exacerbation of symptoms. Given the weight of the evidence and the significant risk probability, it would be prudent to consider unsupervised and unmonitored use of SAMe during levodopa therapy as contraindicated. SAMe may benefit the person with Parkinson's disease as a whole while aggravating the pathophysiology.

The question of SAMe administration, particularly in conjunction with levodopa therapy, may be a matter of determining the individual (and dynamic) balance of SAMe depletion and excessive methylation effects or attendant risk. At this time, the balance of the evidence available warrants a cautionary avoidance of SAMe intake by individuals with Parkinson's disease, pending more conclusive research confirming safety and efficacy. In cases where SAMe administration is indicated by determination of a deficiency or depletion pattern and the broader clinical picture, any such use should only be undertaken within the context of close supervision and regular monitoring by health care professionals trained and experienced in both conventional pharmacology and nutritional therapeutics. In some of these individuals, levodopa dosage might need to be increased to compensate for any potential interference caused by SAMe coadministration. Given the lack of a comprehensive understanding of the pathophysiological processes involved and the complete implications of either of the therapeutic interventions, no dosage ranges for SAMe (or concomitant levodopa) can reasonably be suggested without reference to the particular individual being treated, his or her peculiar characteristics and needs, and clinical response. An integrative approach to personalized care will generally emphasize respecting and enabling, rather than imposing on or obstructing, the normal feedback cycles and self-regulatory processes involved in these neurotransmitters, their complex interrelationships, and pervasive influences.

Oral Contraceptives: Monophasic, Biphasic, and Triphasic Estrogen Preparations (Synthetic Estrogen and Progesterone Analogs)

Ethinyl estradiol and desogestrel (Desogen, Ortho-TriCyclen). Ethinyl estradiol and ethynodiol (Demulen 1/35, Demulen 1/50, Nelulen 1/25, Nelulen 1/50, Zovia).

Ethinyl estradiol and levonorgestrel (Alesse, Levlen, Levlite, Levora 0.15/30, Nordette, Tri-Levlen, Triphasil. Trivora). Ethinyl estradiol and norethindrone/norethisterone (Brevicon, Estrostep, Genora 1/35, GenCep. 1/35, Jenest-28, Loestrin 1.5/30, Loestrin1/20, Modicon, Necon 1/25, Necon 10/11, Necon 0.5/30, Necon 1/50, Nelova 1/35, Nelova 10/11, Norinyl 1/35, Norlestin 1/50, Ortho Novum 1/35, Ortho Novum 10/11, Ortho Novum 7/7/7, Ovcon-35, Ovcon-50, Tri-Norinyl, Trinovum). Ethinyl estradiol and norgestrel (Lo/Ovral, Ovral). Mestranol and norethindrone (Genora 1/50, Nelova 1/50, Norethin 1/50, Ortho-Novum 1/50). Related, internal application: Etonogestrel/ethinyl estradiol vaginal ring (Nuvaring).

Interaction Type and Significance

☼   **Prevention or Reduction of Drug Adverse Effect**

Probability:	Evidence Base:
4. Plausible	○ **Preliminary**

Effect and Mechanism of Action

Oral contraceptives (OCs) raise the cholesterol saturation of bile by increasing biliary cholesterol secretion.[25] SAMe enables liver detoxification and related metabolic processes, including glutathione production.

Research

Some women experience adverse reactions to the synthetic estrogens in OCs, including dysfunctional liver bile production, especially bile cholesterol supersaturation.[26] In particular, women with past histories of intrahepatic cholestasis of pregnancy (ICP), a relatively rare condition, exhibit an exaggerated genetic sensitivity to estrogens, which may express as abnormal hepatic reactivity to OC intake and increased risk of developing gallbladder disease. Studies have provided findings supporting the efficacy of SAMe in the treatment of ICP.[27,28] In a 1984 preliminary report of a controlled randomized trial, Di Padova[29] and a group of Italian researchers found that SAMe antagonizes OC-induced bile cholesterol supersaturation in healthy women. In a related small study published in 1988, Frezza et al.[30] found that oral SAMe (800 mg daily for 2 weeks) protects women with previous ICP from ethinyl estradiol–induced liver toxicity and normalizes bile cholesterol saturation index (CSI) in women who secrete lithogenic bile. These researchers concluded that SAMe acts as a physiological antidote against estrogen hepatobiliary toxicity caused by OCs in susceptible women.

Nutritional Therapeutics, Clinical Concerns, and Adaptations

Weight gain in women using OCs has been debated for decades, and concern remains over estrogen's role in contributing to liver dysfunction and increased susceptibility to weight gain and gallbladder disease among women entering their fourth decade. Although ICP is a relatively uncommon condition, the research into its pathophysiology suggests that SAMe administration might counter the adverse effects on hepatobiliary function and fat metabolism experienced by some women in relation to estrogen metabolism, particularly under the potential stress of OCs. In this situation the emerging tools of pharmacogenomics may provide effective means for assessing relative risk among women in relation to estrogen stress and exogenous hormones in particular. Further, the trend toward decreasing the estrogen dosage in OCs has undoubtedly reduced the frequency and degree of bile cholesterol supersaturation and other, more subtle manifestations of hepatobiliary dysfunction among susceptible women.

Clinicians might consider concomitant SAMe as a supportive adjunctive therapy, with minimal attendant risk, for female patients prescribed OCs (or in other cases involving potential liver and/or gallbladder reactivity to estrogen, including hormone replacement therapy) who have a history of or now exhibit changes in bile function, fat metabolism, or other indication of estrogenic distress. A dosage in the range of 200 to 400 mg per day, in divided doses, would be a reasonable starting point, subject to individual patient characteristics and needs and tailored to clinical response.

Ursodeoxycholic Acid and Chenodeoxycholic Acid

Evidence: Ursodeoxycholic acid (UDCA, ursodiol; Actigall, Destolit, Urdox, Urso, Ursofalk, Ursogal).
Extrapolated, based on similar properties: Chenodeoxycholic acid (CDCA, chenodiol; Chenix).

Interaction Type and Significance
⊕⊕   **Beneficial or Supportive Interaction, with Professional Management**

Probability: Evidence Base:
2. Probable   ◉ Emerging

Effect and Mechanism of Action
Ursodeoxycholic acid (UDCA) is used in the treatment of several hepatobiliary conditions to reduce pruritus, treat cholelithiasis, and improve biochemical parameters, particularly bile constituents. The medical use of bear gallbladder *(Xiongdan)* in Chinese medicine was first recorded in the *Yao Xing Lun* ("Treatise on the Nature of Medicinal Herbs"), a now-lost text from the Song Dynasty that originated in the early Tang Dynasty (ca. 600 CE). Currently, the material is produced synthetically or extracted from byproducts of slaughterhouses. In many respects, UDCA inhabits the intermediary zone where traditional "herbal" medicine and pharmaceuticals overlap. Within conventional practice, UDCA is considered the only therapeutic modality whose effectiveness in the treatment of ICP is supported by evidence from controlled trials.[28,31] Similarly, UDCA is used for symptomatic relief of itching in the treatment of primary sclerosing cholangitis. UDCA is also used in the treatment of primary biliary cirrhosis to improve liver biochemistry, increase survival, and delay liver transplantation. Recent research on the use of UDCA in the treatment of Huntington's disease is considered promising.

S-Adenosylmethionine exerts numerous metabolic effects within the liver that can assist detoxification functions and alter bile formation in ways that may provide an additive effect with, or alternative to, UDCA as a therapeutic agent.

Research
In a randomized clinical trial published in 1996 involving 20 women with ICP in the last trimester of pregnancy, Floreani et al.[32] compared the effects of SAMe (1000 mg/day intramuscularly) and UDCA (450 mg/day). The treatment was continued until delivery, at least 15 days, in all women. They found that UDCA was more effective than SAMe in controlling pruritus and total bile acids. Subsequently Nicastri et al.[27] conducted a randomized placebo-controlled study involving 32 women exhibiting ICP who were divided into four groups. These researchers determined that, after treatment for 20 days, a "combination of ursodeoxycholic acid and

S-adenosylmethionine is more effective than placebo and than either drug alone." Roncaglia et al.[33] conducted a randomized controlled trial of oral UDCA (300 mg twice daily) and oral S-adenosyl-L-methionine (500 mg twice daily) in the treatment of severe gestational cholestasis. They found that women receiving UDCA demonstrated a significantly greater improvement in tests of liver function (i.e., concentration of serum bile acids, aspartate transaminase [AST], alanine transaminase [ALT], and bilirubin) compared with those receiving SAMe. Duration of therapy was significantly greater in women receiving UDCA compared with SAMe.

Nutritional Therapeutics, Clinical Concerns, and Adaptations
A relatively rare disorder, ICP appears to be related to an exaggerated genetic sensitivity to estrogens and manifests during pregnancy with pruritus and icterus as the chief complaints. Although ICP is generally considered as carrying minimal medical risk to the mother, it is regarded as presenting significant risk of perinatal mortality to the fetus, preterm delivery, fetal distress, and meconium staining. Elevated alkaline phosphatase and serum bilirubin levels are characteristic, as are other increased values of parameters indicating altered liver function and bile composition. The trend in clinical trials reveals a pattern of research focusing on the relative efficacy of UDCA and SAMe in the treatment of ICP. There is general agreement that UDCA represents a therapeutic agent supported by both clinical experience and research evidence. The available studies, although all small in size, suggest that a combination therapy provides synergistic, or at least additive, therapeutic efficacy. Given the consensus and evidence that both substances are safe during pregnancy, for both mother and fetus, such approaches deserve further research and empirical investigation. The utility of SAMe in the treatment of other conditions for which UDCA has shown efficacy has yet to be investigated in well-designed clinical trials of adequate size.

Venlafaxine and Related Selective Serotonin Reuptake Inhibitor and Serotonin-Norepinephrine Reuptake Inhibitor (SSRI and SNRI) Antidepressants

Evidence: Venlafaxine (Effexor).
Extrapolated, based on similar properties:
SSRI: Citalopram (Celexa), duloxetine (Cymbalta), escitalopram (S-citalopram; Lexapro), fluoxetine (Prozac, Sarafem), fluvoxamine (Faurin, Luvox), paroxetine (Aropax, Deroxat, Paxil, Seroxat), sertraline (Zoloft).
SSRI/SNRI: Duloxetine (Cymbalta).

Interaction Type and Significance
⊕⊕   **Beneficial or Supportive Interaction, with Professional Management**

Probability: Evidence Base:
2. Probable   ○ Preliminary

Effect and Mechanism of Action
S-Adenosylmethionine and selective serotonin reuptake inhibitors (SSRIs) are both known to benefit individuals with depression. However, research data are as yet inadequate to elucidate fully the mechanisms of action involved and whether the effect is additive or synergistic.

Research
Alpert et al.[34] conducted an open clinical trial to evaluate the safety, tolerability, and efficacy of oral SAMe as an antidepressant adjunct among partial responders and nonresponders to

serotonin reuptake inhibitors or venlafaxine, a dual selective serotonin reuptake inhibitor and serotonin-norepinephrine reuptake inhibitor (SSRI/SNRI). They administered S-adenosyl-L-methionine tosylate (800-1600 mg) to 30 antidepressant-treated adult outpatients with persisting major depressive disorder. At the end of the 6-week treatment period, these researchers observed a response rate of 50% and a remission rate of 43% after augmentation of SSRI or venlafaxine with SAMe and reported minor gastrointestinal distress and headaches as the primary adverse effects.[34] These findings indicate that further research in the form of a well-designed, adequately powered placebo-controlled clinical trial is warranted to further determine the efficacy, assess safety parameters, and refine clinical management guidelines for the integrative treatment of depression using SAMe and venlafaxine or SSRI antidepressants.

Nutritional Therapeutics, Clinical Concerns, and Adaptations

A review of clinical practice and preliminary evidence suggests an emerging, but not yet coherent or articulate, proposition suggesting that SAMe, in graduated dosages in the range of 400 to 800 mg twice daily, can be used adjunctively with SSRI medications to enhance the clinical effectiveness of treatment for depression and other appropriate conditions. The variable mechanisms of action among different SSRIs, along with individual pharmacogenomic variability, life stage, and gender factors and other metabolic influences, may account for differing therapeutic responses and occurrences of adverse effects.

Such an integrative therapeutic strategy warrants close supervision and regular monitoring within the context of coordinated care by health care providers trained and experienced in both clinical nutrition and conventional pharmacology. The concomitant use of SAMe and SSRI medications and/or SSRI/SNRI agents such as venlafaxine should not be used outside of such context of active clinical management. Even though preliminary findings indicate a minimal level of adverse effects, unsupervised coadministration of SSRI drugs with SAMe must still be treated as a potential risk for higher incidence of serotonin-associated unintended effects and adverse events, pending more conclusive evidence. A rapid onset of symptoms indicating an adverse response, particularly CNS toxicity, is highly probable in the unlikely event that a serotonin syndrome or other adverse event does develop.

THEORETICAL, SPECULATIVE, AND PRELIMINARY INTERACTIONS RESEARCH, INCLUDING OVERSTATED INTERACTIONS CLAIMS

Anticoagulant and Antiplatelet Medications

Anticoagulant and Antiplatelet Medications

Limited in vitro studies of SAMe's effect on platelet activation, particularly platelet thromboxane and vascular prostacyclin, suggest that use by individuals with active bleeding disorders or undergoing anticoagulant therapy may be contraindicated, at a level of risk perhaps comparable to aspirin. The range of cautions and contraindications will be extensive in the event that such concerns are confirmed by high-quality clinical trials or a consistent pattern of well-documented case reports. Toward clarifying such potentially significant issues, physicians treating susceptible individuals or prescribing potentially interacting medications are advised to be cognizant of the plausibility of such concerns and document and report suspicious events in a thorough and systematic manner.[35,36]

Monoamine Oxidase (MAO) Inhibitors

MAO-A inhibitors: Isocarboxazid (Marplan), moclobemide (Aurorix, Manerix), phenelzine (Nardil), procarbazine (Matulane), tranylcypromine (Parnate).
MAO-B inhibitors: Selegiline (deprenyl, L-deprenil, L-deprenyl; Atapryl, Carbex, Eldepryl, Jumex, Movergan, Selpak); pargyline (Eutonyl); rasagiline (Azilect).

Concerns have been raised that unmanaged exogenous SAMe could produce an undesirable additive effect if taken in conjunction with MAO inhibitors or SSRI antidepressants. Although such interactions might be plausible, no readily available published evidence from animal studies or human trials supports the hypothesis that such an interaction actually occurs or describes its character and implications in human subjects. In the event that such a pattern of interaction should come to light, the example of TCAs suggests that synergistic coadministration might be efficacious within the context of integrative case management and personalized therapeutic adaptations. Although classic MAO inhibitors are no longer widely used, the potentially catastrophic nature of their interactions would dictate extreme caution in combining a neurotransmitter modulator such as SAMe with MAO inhibitors in the absence of any clinical trial or published anecdotal experience with the combination.

Vidarabine

Evidence: Vidarabine (Ara-A, arabinoside; Vira-A).
Potential: Ribaviran (Copegus, Rebetol, Ribasphere, Vilona, Virazole).

The most common use of vidarabine is as an ophthalmic preparation for the treatment of herpes simplex virus types 1 and 2 (HSV-1 and HSV-2) in acute keratoconjunctivitis and recurrent superficial keratitis. The therapeutic action of vidarabine is achieved by interfering with viral DNA synthesis, specifically inhibition of S-adenosylhomocysteine hydrolase (SAH), methionine synthesis, and SAMe-dependent DNA methylation. Vidarabine cannot be given orally because it is metabolized in the gut, so it is usually administered intravenously or topically.[37-39]

The action of vidarabine indicates a potential risk for interfering with methionine function in humans and potentially inducing a depletion of methionine with extended use. Any such depleting effect on methionine status is likely to be gradual and cumulative, but evidence from human trials is lacking. Concomitant administration of SAMe (or methionine) could theoretically interfere with the therapeutic activity of vidarabine or related antiviral medications.

Although the mechanism of interaction between vidarabine and SAMe is obvious and incontrovertible, the recognition of this interaction and its potential adverse effects has not been acknowledged or addressed in published scientific research. Human studies are lacking to determine whether vidarabine might induce clinically significant methionine depletion and whether methionine administration might interfere with the medication's antiviral activity. Further research is warranted.

Physicians prescribing vidarabine for an extended period may want to present a patient with options for countering the potential adverse effects of this drug. Some nutritionally oriented health care professionals have found value in monitoring serum methionine in their patients taking vidarabine. Coadministration of methionine could be used to counter this adverse effect of vidarabine. Concomitant use of SAMe has not been studied in this regard but may be appropriate. However, due consideration is appropriate, and future research could help clarify whether any such SAMe intake might be contraindicated as interfering with the intended therapeutic action of the medication.

NUTRIENT-NUTRIENT INTERACTIONS

5-Hydroxytryptophan (5-HTP)

The concomitant administration of SAMe with 5-HTP or other supplements or herbs thought to exert an antidepressant effect should be approached with caution and subject to close supervision and regular monitoring. Such therapeutic synergies are common in clinical practice and have a presumed history of empirical efficacy. However, the safety and effectiveness of such prescribing practices have yet to be studied in any well-designed and systematic clinical trials and must always be considered within the context of an evolving and personalized therapeutic plan managed by health care professionals trained and experienced in both conventional pharmacology and the appropriate herbal or nutritional disciplines.

Selenium

The toxicity of selenium at high dosages, especially in its inorganic forms, is largely attributable to its depletion of SAMe reserves. SAMe is the body's principal methyl donor, and the metabolism of inorganic selenium requires both extra methyl donors and higher levels of antioxidants on its way to becoming methylselenol.

The 40 citations for this monograph, as well as additional reference literature, are located under S-Adenosylmethionine on the CD at the back of the book.

Nutrient-Drug Interactions and Drug-Induced Nutrient Depletions

5-Alpha (5α)-Reductase Inhibitors: Black Cohosh, Saw Palmetto

5-Hydroxytryptamine Receptor Agonists (Triptans): 5-HTP, Feverfew

Alpha-1-Adrenoceptor Antagonists: Saw Palmetto, Vitamin B_3

Alpha-Glucosidase Inhibitors: Chromium, Vitamin B_3

Aminoglycoside Antibiotics: Alpha-Lipoic Acid, Calcium, Eleuthero, Ginger, Ginkgo, Horse Chestnut, Licorice, Magnesium, Potassium, Probiotic Intestinal Flora, Vitamin B_1, Vitamin B_6, Vitamin B_{12}, Vitamin K

Aminosalicylates: Vitamin B_{12}

Amphetamines: 5-HTP, Magnesium, Omega-3 Fatty Acids, Vitamin B_6, Zinc

Anabolic Steroids: Echinacea

Androgens: DHEA, Zinc

Anesthesia, General: Alpha-Lipoic Acid, Ephedra, Ginger, Ginkgo, Milk Thistle, St. John's Wort, Valerian

Angiotensin II Receptor Antagonists: Alpha-Lipoic Acid, Potassium

Angiotensin-Converting Enzyme (ACE) Inhibitors: Arginine, Cayenne, Iron, Omega-3 Fatty Acids, Potassium, Vitamin E, Zinc

Antacids (Generally): Calcium, Cayenne, Chromium, Copper, Folic Acid, Iron, Vitamin A, Vitamin B_1, Vitamin D, Zinc

Antacids, Calcium-Based Antacids: Zinc

Antacids, Magnesium-Containing Antacids: Magnesium

Anthelmintic Drugs: Beta-Carotene, Vitamin A

Antiarrhythmic Drugs: Cascara, Magnesium, Potassium

Antibiotic Combination Drugs: Licorice, Probiotic Intestinal Flora, Vitamin K, Zinc

Antibiotics, Systemic: Echinacea, Inositol, Licorice, Probiotic Intestinal Flora, Vitamin A, Vitamin B_1, Vitamin B_2, Vitamin B_{12}, Vitamin K, Zinc

Antibiotics, Topical: Zinc

Anticoagulants (Generally): Cayenne, Melatonin, S-Adenosylmethionine (SAMe), Turmeric (Curcumin)

Anticoagulants, Heparin, Unfractionated: Cayenne, Chondroitin Sulfate, DHEA, Policosanol, Vitamin C, Vitamin D

Anticoagulants, Heparinoids: Cayenne, Chondroitin Sulfate, DHEA, Policosanol

Anticoagulants, Low-Molecular-Weight Heparins: Cayenne, Chondroitin Sulfate, DHEA, Policosanol, Vitamin C

Anticoagulants, Oral Vitamin K Antagonist Anticoagulants: Bilberry, Cayenne, Chondroitin Sulfate, Coenzyme Q10, Dang Gui, Devil's Claw, DHEA, Feverfew, Garlic, Ginger, Ginkgo, Ginseng, Green Tea, Horse Chestnut, Kava, Licorice, Magnesium, Omega-3 Fatty Acids, Policosanol, Red Clover, Reishi, Saw Palmetto, St. John's Wort, Vitamin A, Vitamin B_3, Vitamin C, Vitamin E, Vitamin K, Zinc

Anticoagulants, Thrombin Inhibitors, Hirudins: Cayenne, DHEA, Policosanol

Anticonvulsant Medications (Antiepileptic Drugs): Calcium, Copper, DHEA, Folic Acid, Ginkgo, Inositol, Kava, Milk Thistle, Omega-3 Fatty Acids, Valerian, Vitamin A, Vitamin B_1, Vitamin B_2, Vitamin B_3, Vitamin B_6, Vitamin B_{12}, Vitamin C, Vitamin D, Vitamin E, Vitamin K, Vitex, Zinc

Antifungal Agents (Generally): Echinacea

Antihypertensive Medications (Generally): Omega-3 Fatty Acids, Vitamin C

Antimalarial Drugs: Vitamin B_2

Antimicrobials/Antibiotics, Miscellaneous: Licorice, Probiotic Intestinal Flora, Vitamin K, Zinc

Antiparkinsonian Medications: Folic Acid, Iron, S-Adenosylmethionine (SAMe), Vitamin B_6, Vitex

Antiplatelet Thromboprophylactics: Bilberry, Cayenne, Feverfew, Garlic, Ginger, Ginkgo, Omega-3 Fatty Acids, Policosanol, S-Adenosylmethionine (SAMe)

Antiplatelets, Monoclonal Antibody Antiplatelet Agents: Cayenne, Ginger, Policosanol, S-Adenosylmethionine (SAMe)

Antipsychotics (Neuroleptic Agents): Chromium, Ginkgo, Kava, Melatonin, Vitamin B_6, Vitamin C

Antiretroviral Agents, Reverse-Transcriptase Inhibitors (Nonnucleoside; NNRTIs): St. John's Wort, Vitamin B_2

Antiretroviral Agents, Reverse-Transcriptase Inhibitors (Nucleoside; NRTIs): Aloe, Carnitine, Coenzyme Q10, DHEA, Reishi, Vitamin B_1, Vitamin B_2, Vitamin B_{12}, Zinc

Antitubercular Agents: Folic Acid, Milk Thistle, Vitamin B_6, Vitamin C

Arachidonic Acid Cascade Inhibitors: Vitamin A

Atypical Antipsychotics: 5-HTP, Chromium, Echinacea, Ginkgo, Melatonin, Omega-3 Fatty Acids, Vitamin B_3, Vitamin B_6, Vitamin C

Barbiturates: DHEA, Gotu Kola, Valerian, Vitamin B_2

Benzodiazepines: DHEA, Gotu Kola, Melatonin, Valerian, Vitamin B_3

Beta-1-Adrenoceptor Agonists (Beta-1-Adrenergic Blocking Agents; Systemic): Calcium, Carnitine, Chromium, Coenzyme Q10, Folic Acid, Magnesium, Melatonin, Potassium, Vitamin B_2, Vitamin B_3, Vitamin B_6, Vitamin C

Beta-2-Adrenoceptor Agonists (Beta-2-Adrenergic Blocking Agents): Calcium, Magnesium, Potassium

Beta-Lactam Antibiotics: Ginseng, Licorice, Probiotic Intestinal Flora, Vitamin B_1, Vitamin K, Zinc

Biguanides: Alpha-Lipoic Acid, Astragalus, Bilberry, Calcium, Chromium, DHEA, Ephedra, Folic Acid, Garlic, Ginkgo, Ginseng, Glucosamine Sulfate, Gotu Kola, Horse Chestnut, Magnesium, Omega-3 Fatty Acids, Reishi, Turmeric (Curcumin), Vitamin B_3, Vitamin B_{12}

Bile Acid Sequestrants: Beta-Carotene, Calcium, Folic Acid, Iron, Omega-3 Fatty Acids, Vitamin A, Vitamin B_2, Vitamin B_3, Vitamin D, Vitamin E, Vitamin K, Zinc

Biological Response Modifiers (TNF-α Antagonists): Echinacea

Bisphosphonates: Calcium, Iron, Magnesium, Vitamin D, Zinc

Blood Viscosity–Reducing Agents: Cayenne, Policosanol

Butyrophenone Neuroleptics: Milk Thistle, Phenylalanine

Calcium Channel Blockers: Calcium, Carnitine, Folic Acid, Magnesium, St. John's Wort, Vitamin B_6, Vitamin D

Carbonic Anhydrase Inhibitors: Potassium

Cardiac Glycosides: Calcium, Cascara, Dang Gui, Eleuthero, Ephedra, Hawthorn, Licorice

Cephalosporin Antibiotics: Ginseng, Green Tea, Iron, Licorice, Probiotic Intestinal Flora, Reishi, Vitamin B$_1$, Vitamin K, Zinc

Chemotherapy (Various Cytotoxic Agents): Aloe, Eleuthero, Ginseng, Licorice, Omega-3 Fatty Acids, Vitamin A, Vitamin C, Vitamin E

Chemotherapy and Radiotherapy (Generally): Aloe, Ginseng, Melatonin, PABA, Reishi, Vitamin C, Vitamin E

Chemotherapy, Alkylating Agents: Astragalus, Carnitine, Echinacea, Eleuthero, Selenium

Chemotherapy, Anthracyclines: Alpha-Lipoic Acid, Carnitine, Coenzyme Q10, Garlic, Ginkgo, Green Tea, Hawthorn, Milk Thistle, Reishi, Selenium, Turmeric (Curcumin), Vitamin B$_2$, Vitamin E

Chemotherapy, Antimetabolites: Echinacea, Eleuthero, Folic Acid, Vitamin B$_1$

Chemotherapy, Aromatase Inhibitor Hormonal Anticancer Therapies: Green Tea

Chemotherapy, Cytotoxic Antibiotics: Echinacea, Eleuthero, Ginseng, Licorice, Probiotic Intestinal Flora, Vitamin B$_1$, Vitamin K

Chemotherapy, Estrogens: Black Cohosh

Chemotherapy, GnRH Antagonists/LHRH Antagonists: Black Cohosh

Chemotherapy, LHRH Agonists: Black Cohosh, Vitamin D

Chemotherapy, Mitotic Inhibitors: Echinacea, Eleuthero, St. John's Wort

Chemotherapy, Topoisomerase II Inhibitors: St. John's Wort

Corticosteroids, Oral: Calcium, Cayenne, Chromium, DHEA, Echinacea, Ephedra, Folic Acid, Horse Chestnut, Licorice, Magnesium, Melatonin, Omega-3 Fatty Acids, Potassium, Selenium, Vitamin A, Vitamin B$_6$, Vitamin C, Vitamin D, Vitamin K, Zinc

Corticosteroids, Topical: Aloe, Green Tea, Licorice, Vitamin C

COX-1 Inhibitors (NSAIDs): Calcium, Cayenne, Chondroitin Sulfate, Chromium, Copper, Devil's Claw, Feverfew, Folic Acid, Ginger, Glucosamine Sulfate, Gotu Kola, Iron, Licorice, Melatonin, Omega-3 Fatty Acids, Potassium, Turmeric (Curcumin), Vitamin B$_3$, Vitamin B$_6$, Vitamin C, Zinc

COX-2 Inhibitors (NSAIDs): Calcium, Cayenne, Chondroitin Sulfate, Chromium, Copper, Devil's Claw, Feverfew, Folic Acid, Ginger, Glucosamine Sulfate, Gotu Kola, Iron, Licorice, Melatonin, Omega-3 Fatty Acids, Potassium, Turmeric (Curcumin), Vitamin B$_3$, Vitamin C, Zinc

Cytochrome P450 1A2 Isoenzyme Substrates: Echinacea, Melatonin

Cytochrome P450 2C9 Isoenzyme Substrates: Melatonin

Cytochrome P450 3A4 Isoenzyme Substrates: Echinacea, Vitamin E

Diuretics, Combination Drugs: Glucosamine Sulfate, Hawthorn, Licorice, Magnesium, Potassium, Vitamin D, Zinc

Erythropoiesis-Stimulating Agents: Dang Gui, Iron, Vitamin B$_6$, Vitamin C

Estrogen-Containing and Synthetic Estrogen Analog Medications: Arginine, Black Cohosh, Boron, Calcium, Copper, Dang Gui, DHEA, Magnesium, Melatonin, Milk Thistle, St. John's Wort, Vitamin B$_6$, Vitamin D, Vitamin E, Vitex, Zinc

Fibrates: Coenzyme Q10, Copper, Folic Acid, Gotu Kola, Omega-3 Fatty Acids, Vitamin B$_3$, Vitamin B$_6$, Vitamin B$_{12}$, Zinc

Fluoroquinolone (4-Quinolone) Antibiotics: Calcium, Green Tea, Iron, Licorice, Magnesium, Potassium, Probiotic Intestinal Flora, Vitamin B$_1$, Vitamin K, Zinc

GABA Analogs: Vitamin B$_3$

Ganglionic Blocking Agents: Vitamin B$_3$

Glucocorticoids, Systemic: See *Corticosteroids, Oral.*

Halogenated Inhalational Anesthetic Agents: Alpha-Lipoic Acid, Ephedra, Milk Thistle, St. John's Wort, Valerian

Histamine (H$_2$) Receptor Antagonists: Calcium, Chromium, Copper, Folic Acid, Iron, Licorice, Magnesium, Vitamin B$_{12}$, Vitamin C, Zinc

HMG-CoA Reductase Inhibitors (Statins): Beta-Carotene, Carnitine, Coenzyme Q10, Garlic, Gotu Kola, Omega-3 Fatty Acids, Policosanol, Reishi, Selenium, St. John's Wort, Vitamin A, Vitamin B$_3$, Vitamin C, Vitamin E

Hormone Replacement Therapy, Estrogen/Progestin Combinations: Arginine, Black Cohosh, Boron, Calcium, Copper, Dang Gui, DHEA, Magnesium, Melatonin, Milk Thistle, St. John's Wort, Vitamin B$_6$, Vitamin D, Vitamin E, Vitex, Zinc

Hormone Replacement Therapy, Estrogen/Testosterone Combinations: Black Cohosh, Boron, Calcium, Copper, Dang Gui, DHEA, Magnesium, Melatonin, Milk Thistle, St. John's Wort, Vitamin B$_6$, Vitamin D, Vitamin E, Vitex, Zinc

Hormone Replacement Therapy, Estrogens: Arginine, Black Cohosh, Boron, Calcium, Copper, Dang Gui, DHEA, Magnesium, Melatonin, Milk Thistle, St. John's Wort, Vitamin B$_6$, Vitamin D, Vitamin E, Vitex, Zinc

Hormone Replacement Therapy, Progesterone: Vitamin D

Hormone Replacement Therapy, Progestins: Vitamin D

Imidazole Antibiotics: Probiotic Intestinal Flora, Vitamin B$_2$

Immunosuppressants (Generally): Echinacea

Laxatives (Generally): Licorice

Laxatives, Bulk-Forming Laxative Agents: Potassium, Vitamin B$_2$

Laxatives, Fast-Acting Laxative Agents: Potassium

Laxatives, Prescription Laxative Agents: Potassium

Laxatives, Stimulant: Calcium

Loop Diuretics: Calcium, Folic Acid, Ginseng, Glucosamine Sulfate, Licorice, Magnesium, Potassium, Vitamin B$_1$, Vitamin B$_6$, Vitamin C, Zinc

Macrolide Antibiotics: Calcium, Green Tea, Magnesium, Probiotic Intestinal Flora, Vitamin B$_1$, Vitamin B$_6$, Vitamin K, Zinc

Meglitinide Analog Oral Hypoglycemics: Chromium, Vitamin B$_3$

Mixed Alpha-1/Beta- Adrenoceptor Antagonists: Potassium

Monoamine Oxidase A (MAO-A) Inhibitors: 5-HTP, Cayenne, Chromium, Eleuthero, Ephedra, Ginkgo, Ginseng, Licorice, Phenylalanine, S-Adenosylmethionine (SAMe), St. John's Wort, Tryptophan, Tyrosine, Vitamin B$_6$

Monoamine Oxidase B (MAO-B) Inhibitors: 5-HTP, Cayenne, Chromium, Eleuthero, Ephedra, Ginkgo, Kava, Licorice, Phenylalanine, S-Adenosylmethionine (SAMe), St. John's Wort, Tryptophan, Tyrosine

Narcotic Analgesics (Opioids): Ephedra, Ginseng, Gotu Kola, Phenylalanine, Tyrosine

Neuromuscular Blocking Agents: Magnesium

Nitrates: Arginine, Carnitine, Folic Acid, Vitamin C

Nitrofuran Antibiotics: Licorice

Nitroimidazole Antiprotozoals: Milk Thistle

Nonsteroidal Anti-Inflammatory Drugs (NSAIDs): See *COX-1 Inhibitors (NSAIDs)* or *COX-2 Inhibitors (NSAIDs).*

Nucleic Acid Synthesis Inhibitors, Antiviral: *S*-Adenosylmethionine (SAMe)

Oral Contraceptives (Synthetic Estrogen and Progesterone Analogues): Arginine, Calcium, Copper, Dang Gui, DHEA, Folic Acid, Iron, Licorice, Magnesium, Melatonin, Milk Thistle, *S*-Adenosylmethionine (SAMe), Selenium, St. John's Wort, Tyrosine, Vitamin A, Vitamin B_1, Vitamin B_2, Vitamin B_3, Vitamin B_6, Vitamin B_{12}, Vitamin C, Vitamin E, Vitex, Zinc

Oral Hypoglycemic Agents, Combination Drugs: DHEA, Ginkgo, Glucosamine Sulfate, Omega-3 Fatty Acids

Oral Hypoglycemic Agents: Aloe, Alpha-Lipoic Acid, Astragalus, Bilberry, Chromium, Coenzyme Q10, DHEA, Ephedra, Garlic, Ginkgo, Ginseng, Glucosamine Sulfate, Gotu Kola, Horse Chestnut, Magnesium, Omega-3 Fatty Acids, Reishi, Turmeric (Curcumin), Vitamin B_3

Penicillin Antibiotics: Ginseng, Green Tea

Peripheral Adrenergic Blocking Agents: Ephedra

Phenothiazines: Coenzyme Q10, Milk Thistle, Vitamin B_2, Vitamin B_3, Vitamin C

Phosphodiesterase-5 Inhibitors: Arginine

Photosensitizing Agents: St. John's Wort

Pivalate Prodrugs: Carnitine

Potassium-Sparing Diuretics: Arginine, Calcium, Folic Acid, Glucosamine Sulfate, Magnesium, Zinc

Progestin Oral Contraceptives, Implants, and Postcoital Contraceptives: Magnesium, St. John's Wort

Progestin-Estrogen Injectable Contraceptives: Magnesium

Progestins/Progesterone Analogs: Vitex; see Hormone Replacement Therapy, Estrogen/Progestin Combinations

Protease Inhibitors: Copper, Garlic, St. John's Wort, Vitamin C

Proton Pump Inhibitors: Beta-Carotene, Calcium, Chromium, Iron, Kava, St. John's Wort, Vitamin B_{12}, Zinc

Purine Nucleoside Analog Antivirals: Astragalus

Quinolone Antibiotics: See *Fluoroquinolone (4-Quinolone) Antibiotics.*

Retinoids: Beta-Carotene, Calcium, Carnitine, Vitamin A, Vitamin E

Salicylates: Calcium, Omega-3 Fatty Acids, Policosanol, Vitamin K

Secale Alkaloids: Ephedra

Sedative-Hypnotics: Gotu Kola, Melatonin, Valerian

Selective Estrogen Receptor Modulators (SERMs): Black Cohosh, Dang Gui, Green Tea

Selective Serotonin Reuptake Inhibitor (SSRI) Antidepressants: Chromium, Ginkgo, Inositol, Omega-3 Fatty Acids, *S*-Adenosylmethionine (SAMe), St. John's Wort, Tryptophan, Vitamin B_3, Vitamin B_6, Vitamin B_{12}, Vitamin C, Zinc

Selective Serotonin Reuptake Inhibitor/Serotonin-Norepinephrine Reuptake Inhibitor (SSRI/SNRI) Antidepressants: 5-HTP, Ginkgo, Omega-3 Fatty Acids, *S*-Adenosylmethionine (SAMe), St. John's Wort, Tryptophan, Vitamin B_3, Vitamin B_6, Vitamin B_{12}

Serotonin Agonists: 5-HTP, Tryptophan

Stimulant Medications: 5-HTP; Magnesium, Omega-3 Fatty Acids, Potassium, Reishi, Tyrosine, Vitamin B_6, Vitamin C, Zinc

Stool Softeners: Potassium

Sulfonamide Antibiotics: Calcium, Folic Acid, Licorice, Magnesium, PABA, Probiotic Intestinal Flora, Vitamin B_1, Vitamin B_6, Vitamin K, Zinc

Sulfonylurea Oral Hypoglycemics: Aloe, Alpha-Lipoic Acid, Astragalus, Bilberry, Chromium, Coenzyme Q10, DHEA, Ephedra, Garlic, Ginkgo, Ginseng, Glucosamine Sulfate, Gotu Kola, Horse Chestnut, Magnesium, Omega-3 Fatty Acids, Reishi, Turmeric (Curcumin), Vitamin B_3

Surgery (Generally): Garlic, Ginkgo, St. John's Wort

Tetracycline Antibiotics: Calcium, Folic Acid, Iron, Magnesium, Potassium, Vitamin A, Vitamin B_1, Vitamin B_2, Vitamin B_3, Vitamin B_6, Vitamin C, Zinc

Thiazide Diuretics: Calcium, Coenzyme Q10, Folic Acid, Ginkgo, Glucosamine Sulfate, Hawthorn, Licorice, Magnesium, Potassium, Vitamin B_2, Vitamin D, Zinc

Thiazide-like Diuretics: Glucosamine Sulfate, Potassium

Thiazolidinediones (Glitazones): Chromium, Vitamin B_3

Thrombolytic Agents: Astragalus

Thyroid Hormones: Alpha-Lipoic Acid, Calcium, Carnitine, Coenzyme Q10, DHEA, Iron, Tyrosine, Vitamin B_2

Triazolobenzodiazepines: Kava, St. John's Wort

Tricyclic Antidepressants: 5-HTP, Coenzyme Q10, Milk Thistle, *S*-Adenosylmethionine (SAMe), St. John's Wort, Tryptophan, Tyrosine, Vitamin B_1, Vitamin B_2, Vitamin B_3, Vitamin B_6, Vitamin B_{12}, Zinc

Urinary pH Modifiers: Ephedra

Vaccine Immunotherapies: Ginseng

Vitamin B_6–Depleting Drugs: Melatonin

13-*cis* Retinoic Acid (Isotretinoin): Beta-Carotene, Calcium, Carnitine, Vitamin A, Vitamin E

4-Aminosalicylic Acid (4-ASA) (Para-Aminosalicylic Acid): Vitamin B$_{12}$

5-Aminosalicylic Acid (5-ASA) (Mesalazine): Vitamin B$_{12}$

5-FU (Fluorouracil): Aloe, Beta-Carotene, Echinacea, Eleuthero, Folic Acid, Garlic, Ginkgo, Ginseng, Melatonin, Omega-3 Fatty Acids, Vitamin A, Vitamin B$_1$, Vitamin B$_3$, Vitamin B$_6$, Vitamin C, Vitamin E

6-Mercaptopurine (6-MP): Echinacea, Eleuthero, Folic Acid, Vitamin B$_1$, Vitamin B$_3$

6-Thioguanine (6-TG) (Thioguanine): Echinacea, Eleuthero, Folic Acid, Vitamin B$_1$, Vitamin B$_3$

Abacavir: Aloe, Carnitine, Coenzyme Q10, DHEA, Reishi, Vitamin B$_1$, Vitamin B$_2$, Vitamin B$_{12}$, Zinc

Abciximab: Cayenne, Ginger, Policosanol, *S*-Adenosylmethionine (SAMe)

Aberelix: Black Cohosh

Acarbose: Chromium, Vitamin B$_3$

Acebutolol: Calcium, Carnitine, Chromium, Coenzyme Q10, Folic Acid, Magnesium, Melatonin, Potassium, Vitamin B$_2$, Vitamin B$_3$, Vitamin B$_6$, Vitamin C

Acenocoumarol (Nicoumalone): Bilberry, Cayenne, Chondroitin Sulfate, Coenzyme Q10, DHEA, Dang Gui, Devil's Claw, Feverfew, Garlic, Ginger, Ginkgo, Ginseng, Green Tea, Horse Chestnut, Kava, Licorice, Magnesium, Omega-3 Fatty Acids, Policosanol, Red Clover, Reishi, Saw Palmetto, St. John's Wort, Vitamin A, Vitamin B$_3$, Vitamin C, Vitamin E, Vitamin K, Zinc

Acetaminophen: Dang Gui, Devil's Claw, Garlic, Gotu Kola, Licorice, Methionine, Milk Thistle, *S*-Adenosylmethionine (SAMe), Vitamin C

Acetaminophen + Butalbital + Caffeine: Calcium, DHEA, Ephedra, Garlic, Gotu Kola, Licorice, Methionine, Milk Thistle, *S*-Adenosylmethionine (SAMe), Valerian, Vitamin B$_2$, Vitamin C

Acetaminophen + Chlorpheniramine + Dextromethorphan + Pseudoephedrine: Garlic, Licorice, Methionine, Milk Thistle, *S*-Adenosylmethionine (SAMe), Vitamin C

Acetaminophen + Codeine: Garlic, Licorice, Methionine, Milk Thistle, *S*-Adenosylmethionine (SAMe), Vitamin C

Acetaminophen + Dextropropoxyphene: Garlic, Licorice, Methionine, Milk Thistle, *S*-Adenosylmethionine (SAMe), Vitamin C

Acetaminophen + Oxycodone: Ephedra, Garlic, Ginseng, Gotu Kola, Licorice, Milk Thistle, Phenylalanine, Tyrosine, Vitamin C

Acetaminophen + Pentazocine: Ephedra, Garlic, Ginseng, Gotu Kola, Licorice, Methionine, Milk Thistle, Phenylalanine, Tyrosine, Vitamin C

Acetaminophen + Propoxyphene: Ephedra, Garlic, Ginseng, Gotu Kola, Licorice, Milk Thistle, Phenylalanine, Tyrosine, Vitamin C

Acetazolamide: Coenzyme Q10, Ephedra, Potassium

Acetohexamide: Aloe, Alpha-Lipoic Acid, Astragalus, Bilberry, Chromium, Coenzyme Q10, DHEA, Ephedra, Garlic, Ginkgo, Ginseng, Glucosamine Sulfate, Gotu Kola, Horse Chestnut, Magnesium, Omega-3 Fatty Acids, Reishi, Turmeric/Curcumin, Vitamin B$_3$

Acetophenazine + Hydrocodone: Coenzyme Q10, Milk Thistle, Vitamin B$_2$, Vitamin B$_3$, Vitamin C

Acetylsalicylic Acid: Bilberry, Calcium, Cayenne, Devil's Claw, Feverfew, Folic acid, Garlic, Ginger, Ginkgo, Gotu Kola, Iron, Licorice, Melatonin, Milk Thistle, Omega-3 Fatty acids, Policosanol, Potassium, *S*-Adenosylmethionine (SAMe), Vitamin B$_2$, Vitamin B$_3$, Vitamin C, Vitamin E, Vitamin K, Zinc

Acetylsalicylic Acid + Caffeine: Calcium, Cayenne, Devil's Claw, Ephedra, Feverfew, Ginkgo, Gotu Kola, Iron, Licorice, Melatonin, Milk Thistle, Policosanol, Potassium, Vitamin B$_2$, Vitamin B$_3$, Vitamin C, Vitamin E, Vitamin K, Zinc

Acetylsalicylic Acid + Caffeine + Propoxyphene: Calcium, Cayenne, Devil's Claw, Ephedra, Feverfew, Folic Acid, Ginkgo, Ginseng, Gotu Kola, Iron, Licorice, Melatonin, Milk Thistle, Phenylalanine, Policosanol, Potassium, Tyrosine, Vitamin B$_2$, Vitamin B$_3$, Vitamin C, Vitamin E, Vitamin K, Zinc

Acetylsalicylic Acid + Codeine: Calcium, Cayenne, Devil's Claw, Ephedra, Feverfew, Folic Acid, Ginkgo, Ginseng, Gotu Kola, Iron, Licorice, Melatonin, Milk Thistle, Phenylalanine, Policosanol, Potassium, Tyrosine, Vitamin B$_2$, Vitamin B$_3$, Vitamin C, Vitamin E, Vitamin K

Acetylsalicylic Acid + Codeine + Butalbital + Caffeine: Calcium, Cayenne, Devil's Claw, Ephedra, Feverfew, Folic Acid, Ginkgo, Ginseng, Gotu Kola, Iron, Licorice, Melatonin, Milk Thistle, Phenylalanine, Policosanol, Potassium, Tyrosine, Vitamin B$_2$, Vitamin B$_3$, Vitamin C, Vitamin E, Vitamin K, Zinc

Acetylsalicylic Acid + Dipyridamole (Extended-Release): Bilberry, Calcium, Cayenne, Devil's Claw, Feverfew, Folic Acid, Garlic, Ginger, Ginkgo, Gotu Kola, Iron, Licorice, Melatonin, Milk Thistle, Omega-3 Fatty Acids, Policosanol, Potassium, *S*-Adenosylmethionine (SAMe), Vitamin B$_2$, Vitamin B$_3$, Vitamin C, Vitamin E, Vitamin K, Zinc

Acetylsalicylic Acid + Oxycodone: Calcium, Cayenne, Devil's Claw, Ephedra, Feverfew, Folic Acid, Ginkgo, Ginseng, Gotu Kola, Iron, Licorice, Melatonin, Milk Thistle, Phenylalanine, Policosanol, Potassium, Tyrosine, Vitamin B$_2$, Vitamin B$_3$, Vitamin C, Vitamin E, Vitamin K, Zinc

Acetylsalicylic Acid + Pentazocine: Calcium, Ephedra, Folic Acid, Ginseng, Gotu Kola, Iron, Licorice, Magnesium, Melatonin, Milk Thistle, Phenylalanine, Potassium, Tyrosine, Vitamin B$_2$, Vitamin B$_3$, Vitamin E

Acetylsalicylic Acid + Propoxyphene: Calcium, Cayenne, Devil's Claw, Ephedra, Feverfew, Folic Acid, Ginkgo, Ginseng, Gotu Kola, Iron, Licorice, Melatonin, Milk Thistle, Phenylalanine, Policosanol, Potassium, Tyrosine, Vitamin B$_2$, Vitamin B$_3$, Vitamin C, Vitamin E, Vitamin K, Zinc

Acitretin: Beta-Carotene, Calcium, Carnitine, Omega-3 Fatty Acids, Vitamin A, Vitamin E

Actidone (Cycloheximide): Dang Gui, Echinacea

Actinomycin D (Dactinomycin): Echinacea, Eleuthero, Ginseng, Licorice, Probiotic Flora, Vitamin B$_1$, Vitamin K

Acyclovir: Aloe, Astragalus, Folic Acid, Reishi

Adalimumab: Echinacea

Adefovir Dipivoxil: Carnitine

Adinazolam: Kava, St. John's Wort

Agalsidase Beta: Echinacea, Eleuthero, Folic Acid, Vitamin B_1

Albendazole: Beta-Carotene, Vitamin A

Albuterol: Calcium, Magnesium, Potassium

Albuterol + Ipratropium Bromide: Calcium, Magnesium, Potassium

Alclometasone: Aloe, Green Tea, Licorice, Vitamin C

Aldesleukin: Astragalus, Echinacea, Melatonin

Alendronate: Calcium, Iron, Magnesium, Vitamin D, Zinc

Alfacalcidol: Vitamin D

All-*trans* Retinoic Acid (Tretinoin): Beta-Carotene, Calcium, Carnitine, Vitamin A, Vitamin E

Allopurinol: Carnitine, Copper, Iron, Tryptophan, Vitamin D

Almotriptan: 5-HTP, Feverfew, Tryptophan

Alprazolam: DHEA, Gotu Kola, Kava, Melatonin, St. John's Wort, Valerian, Vitamin B_3

Alteplase, Recombinant, Parenteral: Astragalus

Altretamine: Vitamin B_6

Aluminum Carbonate Gel: Calcium, Cayenne, Chromium, Copper, Folic Acid, Iron, Vitamin A, Vitamin B_1, Vitamin C, Vitamin D, Zinc

Aluminum Hydroxide: Calcium, Cayenne, Chromium, Copper, Ephedra, Folic Acid, Iron, Vitamin A, Vitamin B_1, Vitamin C, Vitamin D, Zinc

Aluminum Hydroxide + Magnesium Hydroxide: Calcium, Cayenne, Chromium, Copper, Folic Acid, Iron, Magnesium, Vitamin A, Vitamin B_1, Vitamin C, Vitamin D, Vitex, Zinc

Aluminum Hydroxide + Magnesium Hydroxide + Calcium Carbonate + Simethicone: Calcium, Cayenne, Chromium, Copper, Folic Acid, Iron, Magnesium, Vitamin A, Vitamin B_1, Vitamin C, Vitamin D, Vitex, Zinc

Aluminum Hydroxide + Magnesium Hydroxide + Simethicone: Calcium, Cayenne, Chromium, Copper, Folic Acid, Iron, Magnesium, Vitamin A, Vitamin B_1, Vitamin C, Vitamin D, Vitex, Zinc

Aluminum Hydroxide + Magnesium Trisilicate: Calcium, Cayenne, Chromium, Copper, Folic Acid, Iron, Magnesium, Vitamin A, Vitamin B_1, Vitamin C, Vitamin D, Vitex, Zinc

Amcinonide: Aloe, Green Tea, Licorice, Vitamin C

Amikacin: Alpha-Lipoic Acid, Calcium, Eleuthero, Ginger, Ginkgo, Horse Chestnut, Licorice, Magnesium, Potassium, Probiotic Flora, Vitamin B_1, Vitamin B_6, Vitamin B_{12}, Vitamin K

Amiloride: Arginine, Calcium, Folic Acid, Glucosamine Sulfate, Magnesium, Potassium, Zinc

Amiloride + Hydrochlorothiazide: Arginine, Calcium, Coenzyme Q10, Folic Acid, Glucosamine Sulfate, Hawthorn, Licorice, Magnesium, Potassium, Vitamin D, Zinc

Aminosalicylic Acid (Para-Aminosalicylic Acid): Vitamin B_{12}

Amiodarone: Cascara, Echinacea, Magnesium, Potassium, Vitamin B_6, Vitamin E

Amitriptyline: 5-HTP, Coenzyme Q10, Echinacea, Milk Thistle, S-Adenosylmethionine (SAMe), St. John's Wort, Tryptophan, Tyrosine, Vitamin B_1, Vitamin B_2, Vitamin B_3, Vitamin B_6, Vitamin B_{12}, Zinc

Amitriptyline + Perphenazine: Coenzyme Q10, Echinacea, Milk Thistle, St. John's Wort, Vitamin B_{12}

Amlodipine: Calcium, Carnitine, DHEA, Folic Acid, Magnesium, St. John's Wort, Vitamin B_6, Vitamin D

Amlodipine + Benazepril: Arginine, Calcium, Cayenne, Coenzyme Q10, DHEA, Potassium, St. John's Wort

Ammonium Chloride: Ephedra

Amobarbital: DHEA, Gotu Kola, Valerian, Vitamin B_2

Amoxapine: 5-HTP, Coenzyme Q10, Milk Thistle, S-Adenosylmethionine (SAMe), St. John's Wort, Tryptophan, Tyrosine, Vitamin B_1, Vitamin B_2, Vitamin B_3, Vitamin B_6, Vitamin B_{12}, Zinc

Amoxicillin: Ginseng, Green Tea, Licorice, Probiotic Flora, Vitamin B_1, Vitamin K, Zinc

Amoxicillin + Clavulanic Acid: Ginseng, Green Tea, Licorice, Probiotic Flora, Vitamin B_1, Vitamin K, Zinc

Amphetamine: 5-HTP, Magnesium, Omega-3 Fatty Acids, Potassium, Reishi, Tyrosine, Vitamin B_6, Vitamin C, Zinc

Amphetamine + Dextroamphetamine: 5-HTP, Magnesium, Omega-3 Fatty Acids, Potassium, Reishi, Tyrosine, Vitamin B_6, Vitamin C, Zinc

Amphotericin B (AMB): Calcium, Echinacea, Magnesium, Potassium

Amphotericin, Liposomal: Echinacea

Ampicillin: Ginseng, Green Tea, Licorice, Probiotic Flora, Vitamin B_1, Vitamin C, Vitamin K, Zinc

Ampicillin + Sulbactam: Ginseng, Green Tea, Licorice, Probiotic Flora, Vitamin B_1, Vitamin K, Zinc

Amprenavir: Copper, Garlic, St. John's Wort, Vitamin C

Amyl Nitrate: Arginine, Carnitine, Folic Acid, Vitamin C

Anastrozole: Green Tea

Anesthesia, General: Alpha-Lipoic Acid, Ginger, Ginkgo, St. John's Wort

Anisindione: Bilberry, Cayenne, Chondroitin Sulfate, Coenzyme Q10, DHEA, Dang Gui, Devil's Claw, Feverfew, Garlic, Ginger, Ginkgo, Ginseng, Green Tea, Horse Chestnut, Kava, Licorice, Magnesium, Omega-3 Fatty Acids, Policosanol, Red Clover, Reishi, Saw Palmetto, St. John's Wort, Vitamin A, Vitamin B_3, Vitamin C, Vitamin E, Vitamin K, Zinc

Anistreplase: Astragalus

Anthralin: Vitamin E

Aprobarbital: DHEA, Gotu Kola, Valerian, Vitamin B_2

Ara-A (Vidarabine): Methionine, Reishi, S-Adenosylmethionine (SAMe)

Ara-C (Cytarabine): Echinacea, Eleuthero, Folic Acid, Ginseng, Vitamin B_1

Arabinoside (Vidarabine): Methionine, Reishi, S-Adenosylmethionine (SAMe)

Ardeparin: Cayenne, Chondroitin Sulfate, DHEA, Policosanol, Vitamin C

Argatroban: Cayenne, DHEA, Policosanol

Aripiprazole: 5-HTP, Chromium, Echinacea, Ginkgo, Melatonin, Omega-3 Fatty Acids, Vitamin B_3, Vitamin B_6, Vitamin C

ASA: See *Acetylsalicylic Acid*.

Asathioprine (Azathioprine): Echinacea, Folic Acid, Vitamin B_3

Aspirin and Related Compounds: See *Acetylsalicylic Acid*.

Atazanavir: Copper, Garlic, St. John's Wort, Vitamin C

Atenolol: Calcium, Carnitine, Chromium, Coenzyme Q10, Folic Acid, Magnesium, Melatonin, Potassium, Vitamin B_2, Vitamin B_3, Vitamin B_6, Vitamin C

Atenolol + Chlorthalidone: Arginine, Calcium, Coenzyme Q10, Policosanol, Potassium, Vitamin C

Atenolol + Nifedipine: Arginine, Calcium, Coenzyme Q10, Dang Gui, Magnesium, Policosanol, Potassium, St. John's Wort, Vitamin C

Atorvastatin: Beta-Carotene, Carnitine, Coenzyme Q10, Garlic, Gotu Kola, Omega-3 Fatty Acids, Policosanol,

Reishi, Selenium, St. John's Wort, Vitamin A, Vitamin B$_3$, Vitamin C, Vitamin E

Atovaquone + Proguanil: Vitamin B$_2$

ATRA (Tretinoin): Beta-Carotene, Calcium, Carnitine, Vitamin A, Vitamin E

Atracurium: Ginger, Magnesium

Azathioprine: Echinacea, Folic Acid, Vitamin B$_3$

Azidothymidine (AZT; Zidovudine): Aloe, Carnitine, Coenzyme Q10, Copper, DHEA, Folic Acid, Reishi, Vitamin B$_1$, Vitamin B$_2$, Vitamin B$_{12}$, Vitamin E, Zinc

Azithromycin: Calcium, Green Tea, Magnesium, Probiotic Flora, Vitamin B$_1$, Vitamin B$_6$, Vitamin K, Zinc

AZT (Zidovudine): Aloe, Carnitine, Coenzyme Q10, Copper, DHEA, Folic Acid, Reishi, Vitamin B$_1$, Vitamin B$_2$, Vitamin B$_{12}$, Vitamin E, Zinc

AZT + 3TC (Zidovudine + Lamivudine): Aloe, Carnitine, Coenzyme Q10, Copper, DHEA, Folic Acid, Reishi, Vitamin B$_1$, Vitamin B$_2$, Vitamin B$_{12}$, Vitamin E, Zinc

Aztreonam: Ginseng, Green Tea, Iron, Licorice, Probiotic Flora, Reishi, Vitamin B$_1$, Vitamin C, Vitamin K, Zinc

Bacampicillin: Ginseng, Green Tea

Bacitracin: Licorice, Probiotic Flora, Vitamin K, Zinc

Baclofen: Phenylalanine

Beclomethasone Inhalant: Calcium

Beclomethasone Topical: Aloe, Green Tea, Licorice, Vitamin C

Benazepril: Arginine, Cayenne, Iron, Omega-3 Fatty Acids, Potassium, Vitamin E, Zinc

Bendrofluazide (Bendroflumethiazide): Calcium, Coenzyme Q10, Folic Acid, Ginkgo, Glucosamine Sulfate, Hawthorn, Licorice, Magnesium, Potassium, Vitamin B$_2$, Vitamin D, Zinc

Bendrofluazide + Propranolol: Arginine, Coenzyme Q10, Ginkgo, Glucosamine Sulfate, Hawthorn, Licorice, Magnesium, Policosanol, Potassium, Vitamin D, Zinc

Benperidol: Milk Thistle, Phenylalanine

Benserazide: Folic Acid, Iron, S-Adenosylmethionine (SAMe), Vitamin B$_6$, Vitex

Benzthiazide: Calcium, Coenzyme Q10, Folic Acid, Ginkgo, Glucosamine Sulfate, Hawthorn, Licorice, Magnesium, Potassium, Vitamin B$_2$, Vitamin D, Zinc

Benztropine: Vitamin B$_3$

Benzyl + Procaine Penicillin: Vitamin C

Bepridil: Calcium, Carnitine, Folic Acid, Magnesium, St. John's Wort, Vitamin B$_6$, Vitamin D

Betamethasone: Aloe, Calcium, Cayenne, Chromium, DHEA, Echinacea, Ephedra, Folic Acid, Green Tea, Horse Chestnut, Licorice, Magnesium, Melatonin, Omega-3 Fatty Acids, Potassium, Selenium, Vitamin A, Vitamin B$_6$, Vitamin C, Vitamin D, Vitamin K, Zinc

Betamethasone Topical: Aloe, Green Tea, Licorice, Vitamin C

Betanidine: Ephedra

Betaxolol: Calcium, Carnitine, Chromium, Coenzyme Q10, Folic Acid, Magnesium, Melatonin, Potassium, Vitamin B$_2$, Vitamin B$_3$, Vitamin B$_6$, Vitamin C

Bexarotene: Beta-Carotene, Calcium, Carnitine, Vitamin A, Vitamin E

Bezafibrate: Coenzyme Q10, Copper, Folic Acid, Gotu Kola, Omega-3 Fatty Acids, Vitamin B$_3$, Vitamin B$_6$, Vitamin B$_{12}$, Zinc

Bicalutamide: Black Cohosh, Vitamin D

Bisacodyl Tablets: Potassium

Bismuth Subsalicylate + Metronidazole + Tetracycline: Calcium, Folic Acid, Iron, Magnesium, Potassium,

Vitamin A, Vitamin B$_1$, Vitamin B$_2$, Vitamin B$_3$, Vitamin B$_6$, Vitamin C, Zinc

Bisoprolol: Calcium, Carnitine, Chromium, Coenzyme Q10, Folic Acid, Magnesium, Melatonin, Potassium, Vitamin B$_2$, Vitamin B$_3$, Vitamin B$_6$, Vitamin C

Bivalirudin: Cayenne, DHEA, Policosanol

Bleomycin: Aloe, Echinacea, Eleuthero, Garlic, Ginseng, Licorice, Omega-3 Fatty Acids, Probiotic Flora, Selenium, Turmeric/Curcumin, Vitamin A, Vitamin B$_1$, Vitamin C, Vitamin E, Vitamin K

Boldenone: Echinacea

Borate: Vitamin B$_2$

Boric Acid: Vitamin B$_2$

Brecanavir (GW640385): Copper, Garlic, St. John's Wort, Vitamin C

Bretylium: Ephedra

Brinzolamide (Ophthalmic Suspension): Potassium

Bromazepam: DHEA, Gotu Kola, Melatonin, Valerian, Vitamin B$_3$

Brotizolam: Kava, St. John's Wort

Buformin: Alpha-Lipoic Acid, Astragalus, Bilberry, Calcium, Chromium, DHEA, Ephedra, Folic Acid, Garlic, Ginkgo, Ginseng, Glucosamine Sulfate, Gotu Kola, Horse Chestnut, Magnesium, Omega-3 Fatty Acids, Reishi, Turmeric/Curcumin, Vitamin B$_3$, Vitamin B$_{12}$

Bumetanide: Calcium, Folic Acid, Ginseng, Glucosamine Sulfate, Licorice, Magnesium, Potassium, Vitamin B$_1$, Vitamin B$_6$, Vitamin C, Zinc

Buprenorphine: Ephedra, Ginseng, Gotu Kola, Phenylalanine, Tyrosine

Buprenorphine + Naloxone: Ephedra, Ginseng, Gotu Kola, Phenylalanine, Tyrosine

Bupropion: Melatonin

Buspirone: 5-HTP, St. John's Wort, Tryptophan

Busulfan: Astragalus, Carnitine, Echinacea, Eleuthero, Selenium

Butabarbital: DHEA, Gotu Kola, Valerian, Vitamin B$_2$

Butalbital: DHEA, Gotu Kola, Valerian, Vitamin B$_2$

Butorphanol: Ephedra, Ginseng, Gotu Kola, Phenylalanine, Tyrosine

Butoxamine: Potassium

Caffeine: Calcium, Ephedra, Kava, Melatonin

Calcitonin: Calcium, Vitamin D

Calcitriol: Vitamin D

Calcium Acetate: Calcium

Calcium Carbonate: Calcium, Cayenne, Chromium, Copper, Folic Acid, Iron, Vitamin A, Vitamin B$_1$, Vitamin D, Zinc

Calcium Carbonate + Magnesium Hydroxide + Simethicone: Calcium, Cayenne, Chromium, Copper, Folic Acid, Iron, Magnesium, Vitamin A, Vitamin B$_1$, Vitamin D, Vitex, Zinc

Camptothecin-11 (Irinotecan): Aloe, Ginseng, Omega-3 Fatty Acids, Vitamin A, Vitamin C, Vitamin E

Candesartan: Alpha-Lipoic Acid, Potassium

Candesartan + Hydrochlorothiazide: Alpha-Lipoic Acid, Potassium

Capecitabine: Echinacea, Eleuthero, Folic Acid, Vitamin B$_1$

Captopril: Arginine, Cayenne, Iron, Magnesium, Omega-3 Fatty Acids, Potassium, Vitamin E, Zinc

Captopril + Hydrochlorothiazide: Arginine, Calcium, Cayenne, Coenzyme Q10, Glucosamine Sulfate, Hawthorn, Licorice, Magnesium, Potassium, Vitamin D, Zinc

Carbamazepine: Calcium, Carnitine, Copper, DHEA, Folic Acid, Ginkgo, Inositol, Kava, Milk Thistle, Omega-3 Fatty Acids, Valerian, Vitamin A, Vitamin B_1, Vitamin B_2, Vitamin B_3, Vitamin B_6, Vitamin B_{12}, Vitamin C, Vitamin D, Vitamin E, Vitamin K, Vitex, Zinc

Carbenicillin: Ginseng, Green Tea

Carbenoxolone: Potassium

Carbidopa: 5-HTP, Folic Acid, Iron, Kava, S-Adenosylmethionine (SAMe), Vitamin B_3, Vitamin B_6, Vitamin C, Vitex

Carboplatin: Alpha-Lipoic Acid, Astragalus, Carnitine, Cayenne, Chondroitin Sulfate, Echinacea, Eleuthero, Ginger, Ginkgo, Ginseng, Milk Thistle, Selenium, Turmeric/Curcumin

Carteolol: Calcium, Carnitine, Chromium, Coenzyme Q10, Folic Acid, Magnesium, Melatonin, Potassium, Vitamin B_2, Vitamin B_3, Vitamin B_6, Vitamin C

Carvedilol: Potassium

CDDP (Cisplatin): Aloe, Alpha-Lipoic Acid, Astragalus, Beta-Carotene, Calcium, Carnitine, Cayenne, Chondroitin Sulfate, Echinacea, Eleuthero, Feverfew, Ginger, Ginkgo, Ginseng, Magnesium, Melatonin, Milk Thistle, Omega-3 Fatty Acids, Potassium, Selenium, Turmeric/Curcumin, Vitamin A, Vitamin B_6, Vitamin C, Vitamin E, Zinc

Cedilanin-D (deslanoside): Calcium, Cascara, Dang Gui, Eleuthero, Ephedra, Hawthorn, Licorice, Magnesium, Potassium, St. John's Wort

Cefaclor: Ginseng, Green Tea, Iron, Licorice, Probiotic Flora, Reishi, Vitamin B_1, Vitamin K, Zinc

Cefadroxil: Ginseng, Green Tea, Iron, Licorice, Probiotic Flora, Reishi, Vitamin B_1, Vitamin K, Zinc

Cefamandole: Ginseng, Green Tea, Iron, Licorice, Probiotic Flora, Reishi, Vitamin B_1, Vitamin K, Zinc

Cefazolin: Ginseng, Green Tea, Iron, Licorice, Probiotic Flora, Reishi, Vitamin B_1, Vitamin K, Zinc

Cefcapene Pivoxil: Carnitine

Cefdinir: Ginseng, Green Tea, Iron, Licorice, Probiotic Flora, Reishi, Vitamin B_1, Vitamin K, Zinc

Cefditoren Pivoxil: Carnitine

Cefepime: Ginseng, Green Tea, Iron, Licorice, Probiotic Flora, Reishi, Vitamin B_1, Vitamin K, Zinc

Cefetamet Pivoxil: Carnitine

Cefixime: Ginseng, Green Tea, Iron, Licorice, Probiotic Flora, Reishi, Vitamin B_1, Vitamin K, Zinc

Cefoperazone: Ginseng, Green Tea, Iron, Licorice, Probiotic Flora, Reishi, Vitamin B_1, Vitamin K, Zinc

Cefotaxime: Ginseng, Green Tea, Iron, Licorice, Probiotic Flora, Reishi, Vitamin B_1, Vitamin C, Vitamin K, Zinc

Cefotetan: Ginseng, Green Tea, Iron, Licorice, Probiotic Flora, Reishi, Vitamin B_1, Vitamin K, Zinc

Cefoxitin: Ginseng, Green Tea, Iron, Licorice, Probiotic Flora, Reishi, Vitamin B_1, Vitamin K, Zinc

Cefpodoxime: Ginseng, Green Tea, Iron, Licorice, Probiotic Flora, Reishi, Vitamin B_1, Vitamin K, Zinc

Cefprozil: Ginseng, Green Tea, Iron, Licorice, Probiotic Flora, Reishi, Vitamin B_1, Vitamin K, Zinc

Ceftazidime: Ginseng, Green Tea, Iron, Licorice, Probiotic Flora, Reishi, Vitamin B_1, Vitamin K, Zinc

Ceftibuten: Ginseng, Green Tea, Iron, Licorice, Probiotic Flora, Reishi, Vitamin B_1, Vitamin K, Zinc

Ceftizoxime: Ginseng, Green Tea, Iron, Licorice, Probiotic Flora, Reishi, Vitamin B_1, Vitamin K, Zinc

Ceftriaxone: Ginseng, Green Tea, Iron, Licorice, Probiotic Flora, Reishi, Vitamin B_1, Vitamin K, Zinc

Cefuroxime: Ginseng, Green Tea, Iron, Licorice, Probiotic Flora, Reishi, Vitamin B_1, Vitamin K, Zinc

Celecoxib: Calcium, Cayenne, Chondroitin Sulfate, Chromium, Copper, Devil's Claw, Feverfew, Folic Acid, Ginger, Glucosamine Sulfate, Gotu Kola, Iron, Licorice, Melatonin, Omega-3 Fatty Acids, Potassium, Turmeric/Curcumin, Vitamin B_3, Vitamin C, Zinc

Celiprolol: Potassium

Cephalexin: Ginseng, Green Tea, Iron, Licorice, Probiotic Flora, Reishi, Vitamin B_1, Vitamin K, Zinc

Cephapirin: Ginseng, Green Tea, Iron, Licorice, Probiotic Flora, Reishi, Vitamin B_1, Vitamin K, Zinc

Cephradine: Ginseng, Green Tea, Iron, Licorice, Probiotic Flora, Reishi, Vitamin B_1, Vitamin K, Zinc

Cerivastatin: Beta-Carotene, Carnitine, Coenzyme Q10, Garlic, Gotu Kola, Omega-3 Fatty Acids, Policosanol, Reishi, Selenium, St. John's Wort, Vitamin A, Vitamin B_3, Vitamin C, Vitamin E

Certoparin: Cayenne, Chondroitin Sulfate, DHEA, Policosanol, Vitamin C

Chenodeoxycholic Acid (CDCA): S-Adenosylmethionine (SAMe), Vitamin B_3

Chlorambucil: Astragalus, Carnitine, Echinacea, Eleuthero, Selenium

Chloramphenicol: Folic Acid, Iron, Licorice, Probiotic Flora, Vitamin B_{12}, Vitamin K, Zinc

Chlordiazepoxide: DHEA, Gotu Kola, Melatonin, Valerian, Vitamin B_3

Chlorhexidine Mouthwash: Iron, Licorice, Probiotic Flora, Vitamin K, Zinc

Chlorhexidine + Nystatin + Hydrocortisone: Iron, Licorice, Probiotic Flora, Vitamin K

Chlorimipramine (Clomipramine): 5-HTP, Coenzyme Q10, Echinacea, Milk Thistle, S-Adenosylmethionine (SAMe), St. John's Wort, Tryptophan, Tyrosine, Vitamin B_1, Vitamin B_2, Vitamin B_3, Vitamin B_6, Vitamin B_{12}, Zinc

Chloroquine: Calcium, Magnesium, Vitamin B_2, Vitamin E

Chlorothiazide: Calcium, Coenzyme Q10, Folic Acid, Ginkgo, Glucosamine Sulfate, Hawthorn, Licorice, Magnesium, Potassium, Vitamin B_2, Vitamin D, Zinc

Chlorotrianisene: Arginine, Black Cohosh, Boron, Calcium, Copper, DHEA, Dang Gui, Magnesium, Melatonin, Milk Thistle, St. John's Wort, Vitamin B_6, Vitamin D, Vitamin E, Vitex, Zinc

Chlorpromazine: Chromium, Coenzyme Q10, Ginkgo, Kava, Melatonin, Milk Thistle, Reishi, Vitamin B_2, Vitamin B_3, Vitamin B_6, Vitamin C, Vitamin E

Chlorpropamide: Aloe, Alpha-Lipoic Acid, Astragalus, Bilberry, Chromium, Coenzyme Q10, DHEA, Ephedra, Garlic, Ginkgo, Ginseng, Glucosamine Sulfate, Gotu Kola, Horse Chestnut, Magnesium, Omega-3 Fatty Acids, Reishi, Turmeric/Curcumin, Vitamin B_3

Chlortetracycline: Calcium, Folic Acid, Iron, Magnesium, Potassium, Vitamin A, Vitamin B_1, Vitamin B_2, Vitamin B_3, Vitamin B_6, Vitamin C, Zinc

Chlortetracycline + Demeclocycline + Tetracycline: Calcium, Folic Acid, Iron, Magnesium, Potassium, Vitamin A, Vitamin B_1, Vitamin B_2, Vitamin B_3, Vitamin B_6, Vitamin C, Zinc

Chlorthalidone: Calcium, Coenzyme Q10, Folic Acid, Ginkgo, Glucosamine Sulfate, Hawthorn, Licorice, Magnesium, Potassium, Vitamin B_2, Vitamin D, Zinc

Chlorzoxazone: Garlic, St. John's Wort

Cholestyramine: Beta-Carotene, Calcium, Folic Acid, Iron, Magnesium, Omega-3 Fatty Acids, Vitamin A, Vitamin B_2, Vitamin B_3, Vitamin B_{12}, Vitamin D, Vitamin E, Vitamin K, Zinc

Choline Salicylate: Calcium, Omega-3 Fatty Acids, Policosanol, Vitamin K

Ciclosporin (Cyclosporine): Arginine, Echinacea, Ginkgo, Magnesium, Melatonin, Omega-3 Fatty Acids, Potassium, St. John's Wort, Turmeric/Curcumin, Vitamin C, Vitamin E, Zinc

Cilazapril: Alpha-Lipoic Acid, Arginine, Cayenne, Iron, Omega-3 Fatty Acids, Potassium, Vitamin E, Zinc

Cilostazol: Bilberry, Cayenne, Feverfew, Garlic, Ginger, Ginkgo, Omega-3 Fatty Acids, Policosanol, S-Adenosylmethionine (SAMe)

Cimetidine: Calcium, Chromium, Copper, Folic Acid, Iron, Licorice, Magnesium, Vitamin B_{12}, Vitamin C, Vitamin D, Zinc

Cinoxacin: Calcium, Green Tea, Iron, Licorice, Magnesium, Potassium, Probiotic Flora, Vitamin B_1, Vitamin K, Zinc

Ciprofibrate: Coenzyme Q10, Copper, Folic Acid, Gotu Kola, Omega-3 Fatty Acids, Vitamin B_3, Vitamin B_6, Vitamin B_{12}, Zinc

Ciprofloxacin: Calcium, Copper, Green Tea, Iron, Licorice, Magnesium, Potassium, Probiotic Flora, Vitamin B_1, Vitamin K, Zinc

Cisatracurium: Magnesium

Cisplatin: Aloe, Alpha-Lipoic Acid, Astragalus, Beta-Carotene, Calcium, Carnitine, Cayenne, Chondroitin Sulfate, Echinacea, Eleuthero, Feverfew, Ginger, Ginkgo, Ginseng, Magnesium, Melatonin, Milk Thistle, Omega-3 Fatty Acids, Potassium, Selenium, Turmeric/Curcumin, Vitamin A, Vitamin B_6, Vitamin C, Vitamin E, Zinc

Citalopram: 5-HTP, Chromium, Folic Acid, Ginkgo, Inositol, Omega-3 Fatty Acids, S-Adenosylmethionine (SAMe), St. John's Wort, Tryptophan, Vitamin B_3, Vitamin B_6, Vitamin B_{12}, Vitamin C, Zinc

Cladribine: Echinacea, Eleuthero, Folic Acid, Vitamin B_1

Clarithromycin: Calcium, Green Tea, Magnesium, Probiotic Flora, Vitamin B_1, Vitamin B_6, Vitamin K, Zinc

Clindamycin Oral: Licorice, Probiotic Flora, Vitamin K, Zinc

Clindamycin Topical: Zinc

Clobetasol: Aloe, Green Tea, Licorice, Vitamin C, Zinc

Clobetasol Topical (Clobetasol): Aloe, Green Tea, Licorice, Vitamin C, Zinc

Clobetasone: Aloe, Green Tea, Licorice, Vitamin C

Clocortolone: Aloe, Green Tea, Licorice, Vitamin C

Clocortolone Pivalate Topical (Clocortolone): Aloe, Green Tea, Licorice, Vitamin C

Clodronate: Calcium, Iron, Magnesium, Vitamin D, Zinc

Clofibrate: Coenzyme Q10, Copper, Folic Acid, Gotu Kola, Iron, Omega-3 Fatty Acids, Vitamin B_3, Vitamin B_6, Vitamin B_{12}, Vitamin E, Zinc

Clomipramine: 5-HTP, Coenzyme Q10, Echinacea, Milk Thistle, S-Adenosylmethionine (SAMe), St. John's Wort, Tryptophan, Tyrosine, Vitamin B_1, Vitamin B_2, Vitamin B_3, Vitamin B_6, Vitamin B_{12}, Zinc

Clonazepam: Calcium, Carnitine, Copper, DHEA, Folic Acid, Ginkgo, Gotu Kola, Inositol, Kava, Melatonin, Milk Thistle, Omega-3 Fatty Acids, Valerian, Vitamin A, Vitamin B_1, Vitamin B_2, Vitamin B_3, Vitamin B_6, Vitamin B_{12}, Vitamin C, Vitamin D, Vitamin E, Vitamin K, Vitex, Zinc

Clonidine: DHEA, Ephedra, Melatonin

Clonidine + Chlorthalidone: Arginine, Coenzyme Q10, DHEA, Ephedra, Melatonin, Potassium

Clopidogrel: Bilberry, Cayenne, Feverfew, Garlic, Ginger, Ginkgo, Omega-3 Fatty Acids, Policosanol, S-Adenosylmethionine (SAMe)

Clorazepate: Calcium, Carnitine, Copper, DHEA, Folic Acid, Ginkgo, Gotu Kola, Inositol, Kava, Melatonin, Milk Thistle, Omega-3 Fatty Acids, Tryptophan, Valerian, Vitamin A, Vitamin B_1, Vitamin B_2, Vitamin B_3, Vitamin B_6, Vitamin B_{12}, Vitamin C, Vitamin D, Vitamin E, Vitamin K, Vitex, Zinc

Clotrimazole: Probiotic Flora, Vitamin B_2

Cloxacillin: Ginseng, Green Tea, Licorice, Probiotic Flora, Vitamin B_1, Vitamin K, Zinc

Clozapine: 5-HTP, Chromium, Echinacea, Ginkgo, Melatonin, Omega-3 Fatty Acids, Selenium, Vitamin B_3, Vitamin B_6, Vitamin C

Co-Beneldopa (Levodopa + Benserazide): 5-HTP, Folic Acid, Iron, Kava, Methionine, Phenylalanine, S-Adenosylmethionine (SAMe), Tyrosine, Vitamin B_3, Vitamin B_6, Vitamin C, Vitex

Cocaine: Ginseng

Codeine: Ephedra, Ginseng, Gotu Kola, Phenylalanine, Tyrosine

Codeine + Acetaminophen: Ephedra, Ginseng, Gotu Kola, Phenylalanine, Tyrosine

Colchicine: Beta-Carotene, Calcium, Folic Acid, Magnesium, Potassium, Vitamin A, Vitamin B_{12}

Colesevelam: Beta-Carotene, Calcium, Folic Acid, Iron, Omega-3 Fatty Acids, Vitamin A, Vitamin B_2, Vitamin B_3, Vitamin B_{12}, Vitamin D, Vitamin E, Vitamin K, Zinc

Colestipol: Beta-Carotene, Calcium, Folic Acid, Iron, Omega-3 Fatty Acids, Vitamin A, Vitamin B_2, Vitamin B_3, Vitamin B_{12}, Vitamin D, Vitamin E, Vitamin K, Zinc

Colestyramine (Cholestyramine): Beta-Carotene, Calcium, Folic Acid, Iron, Magnesium, Omega-3 Fatty Acids, Vitamin A, Vitamin B_2, Vitamin B_3, Vitamin B_{12}, Vitamin D, Vitamin E, Vitamin K, Zinc

Colistimethate: Licorice, Probiotic Flora, Vitamin K, Zinc

Conjugated Equine Estrogens: Arginine, Black Cohosh, Boron, Calcium, Copper, DHEA, Dang Gui, Magnesium, Melatonin, Milk Thistle, St. John's Wort, Vitamin B_6, Vitamin D, Vitamin E, Vitex, Zinc

Conjugated Equine Estrogens + Norgestrel: Arginine, Black Cohosh, Boron, Calcium, Copper, DHEA, Dang Gui, Magnesium, Melatonin, Milk Thistle, St. John's Wort, Vitamin B_6, Vitamin D, Vitamin E, Vitex, Zinc

Cortisone: Calcium, Cayenne, Chromium, DHEA, Echinacea, Ephedra, Folic Acid, Horse Chestnut, Licorice, Magnesium, Melatonin, Omega-3 Fatty Acids, Potassium, Selenium, Vitamin A, Vitamin B_6, Vitamin C, Vitamin D, Vitamin K, Zinc

Cortisone Eyedrops: Aloe, Green Tea, Licorice, Vitamin C

CPT-11 (Irinotecan): Aloe, Ginseng, Omega-3 Fatty Acids, Vitamin A, Vitamin C, Vitamin E

Cyclobenzaprine: Echinacea

Cycloheximide: Dang Gui, Echinacea

Cyclopenthiazide: Calcium, Coenzyme Q10, Folic Acid, Ginkgo, Glucosamine Sulfate, Hawthorn, Licorice, Magnesium, Potassium, Vitamin B_2, Vitamin D, Zinc

Cyclopenthiazide + Oxprenolol: Glucosamine Sulfate, Hawthorn, Licorice, Magnesium, Potassium, Vitamin D, Zinc

Cyclophosphamide: Aloe, Alpha-Lipoic Acid, Astragalus, Beta-Carotene, Carnitine, Echinacea, Eleuthero, Ginger, Ginseng, Licorice, Melatonin, Omega-3 Fatty Acids, Reishi, Selenium, Turmeric/Curcumin, Vitamin A, Vitamin C, Vitamin E

Cycloserine (CsA): Calcium, Folic Acid, Magnesium, Milk Thistle, Vitamin B_6, Vitamin B_{12}, Vitamin C, Vitamin D

Cyclosporine: Arginine, Echinacea, Ginkgo, Magnesium, Melatonin, Omega-3 Fatty Acids, Potassium, St. John's Wort, Turmeric/Curcumin, Vitamin C, Vitamin E, Zinc

Cyproterone: Black Cohosh, Vitamin D

Cytarabine: Echinacea, Eleuthero, Folic Acid, Ginseng, Vitamin B_1

D-Amphetamine (Dextroamphetamine): 5-HTP, Magnesium, Omega-3 Fatty Acids, Potassium, Reishi, Tyrosine, Vitamin B_6, Vitamin C, Zinc

D4T (Stavudine): Aloe, Carnitine, Coenzyme Q10, DHEA, Reishi, Vitamin B_1, Vitamin B_2, Vitamin B_{12}, Zinc

D600 (Gallopamil): Calcium, Carnitine, Folic Acid, Magnesium, St. John's Wort, Vitamin B_6, Vitamin D

Dabigatran: Cayenne, DHEA, Policosanol

Dacarbazine (DTIC): Astragalus, Carnitine, Echinacea, Eleuthero, Selenium

Dactinomycin: Echinacea, Eleuthero, Ginseng, Licorice, Probiotic Flora, Vitamin B_1, Vitamin K

Dalteparin: Cayenne, Chondroitin Sulfate, DHEA, Policosanol, Vitamin C

Danaparoid: Cayenne, Chondroitin Sulfate, DHEA, Policosanol

Dapsone (DDS): Folic Acid, Licorice, PABA, Probiotic Flora, Vitamin E, Vitamin K, Zinc

Darbepoetin Alpha (Darbepoetin Alfa): Dang Gui, Iron, Vitamin B_6, Vitamin C

Darunavir: Copper, Garlic, St. John's Wort, Vitamin C

Daunorubicin: Alpha-Lipoic Acid, Carnitine, Coenzyme Q10, Feverfew, Garlic, Ginkgo, Ginseng, Green Tea, Hawthorn, Milk Thistle, Reishi, Selenium, St. John's Wort, Turmeric/Curcumin, Vitamin B_2, Vitamin E

Daunorubicin, Liposomal: Alpha-Lipoic Acid, Carnitine, Coenzyme Q10, Feverfew, Garlic, Ginkgo, Ginseng, Green Tea, Hawthorn, Milk Thistle, Reishi, Selenium, St. John's Wort, Turmeric/Curcumin, Vitamin B_2, Vitamin E

Debrisoquine: Ephedra

Deferasirox: Vitamin C

Delavirdine: St. John's Wort, Vitamin B_2

Delta-Aminolevulinic Acid (d-ALA): St. John's Wort

Demeclocycline: Calcium, Folic Acid, Iron, Magnesium, Potassium, Vitamin A, Vitamin B_1, Vitamin B_2, Vitamin B_3, Vitamin B_6, Vitamin C, Zinc

Deprenyl (Selegiline): 5-HTP, Cayenne, Chromium, Eleuthero, Ephedra, Folic Acid, Ginkgo, Iron, Kava, Licorice, Phenylalanine, S-Adenosylmethionine (SAMe), St. John's Wort, Tryptophan, Tyrosine, Vitamin B_2, Vitamin B_6, Vitex

Desferoxamine: Copper, Iron, Vitamin C

Desflurane: Alpha-Lipoic Acid, Ephedra, Milk Thistle, St. John's Wort, Valerian

Desiccated Thyroid (L-Thyroxine + L-Triiodothyronine): Alpha-Lipoic Acid, Calcium, Carnitine, Coenzyme Q10, DHEA, Iron, Tyrosine, Vitamin B_2

Desipramine: 5-HTP, Coenzyme Q10, Melatonin, Milk Thistle, S-Adenosylmethionine (SAMe), St. John's Wort, Tryptophan, Tyrosine, Vitamin B_1, Vitamin B_2, Vitamin B_3, Vitamin B_6, Vitamin B_{12}, Vitamin E, Zinc

Desirudin: Cayenne, DHEA, Policosanol

Deslanoside: Calcium, Cascara, Dang Gui, Eleuthero, Ephedra, Hawthorn, Licorice, Magnesium, Potassium, St. John's Wort

Desogestrel: Arginine, Calcium, Copper, DHEA, Dang Gui, Folic Acid, Iron, Licorice, Magnesium, Melatonin, Milk Thistle, S-Adenosylmethionine (SAMe), Selenium, St. John's Wort, Tyrosine, Vitamin A, Vitamin B_1, Vitamin B_2, Vitamin B_3, Vitamin B_6, Vitamin B_{12}, Vitamin C, Vitamin E, Vitex, Zinc

Desonide: Aloe, Green Tea, Licorice, Vitamin C

Desoximetasone: Aloe, Green Tea, Licorice, Vitamin C

Desoxymethasone: Aloe, Green Tea, Licorice, Vitamin C

Dexamethasone: Aloe, Calcium, Ephedra, Green Tea, Licorice, Vitamin C

Dexamethasone + Tobramycin: Alpha-Lipoic Acid, Calcium, Eleuthero, Ginger, Ginkgo, Horse Chestnut, Licorice, Magnesium, Potassium, Probiotic Flora, Vitamin B_1, Vitamin B_6, Vitamin B_{12}, Vitamin K

Dexamphetamine (Amphetamine + Dextroamphetamine): 5-HTP, Magnesium, Omega-3 Fatty Acids, Potassium, Reishi, Tyrosine, Vitamin B_6, Vitamin C, Zinc

Dextroamphetamine: 5-HTP, Magnesium, Omega-3 Fatty Acids, Potassium, Reishi, Tyrosine, Vitamin B6, Vitamin C, Zinc

Dextrothyroxine: Alpha-Lipoic Acid, Calcium, Carnitine, Coenzyme Q10, DHEA, Iron, Tyrosine, Vitamin B_2

Diaminodiphenylsulphone (Dapsone): Folic Acid, Licorice, PABA, Probiotic Flora, Vitamin E, Vitamin K, Zinc

Diazepam: Carnitine, DHEA, Gotu Kola, Melatonin, Valerian, Vitamin B_3

Dichlorphenamide: Potassium

Diclofenac (Diclofenac Potassium; Diclofenac Sodium): Calcium, Cayenne, Chondroitin Sulfate, Chromium, Copper, Devil's Claw, Feverfew, Folic Acid, Ginger, Glucosamine Sulfate, Gotu Kola, Iron, Licorice, Melatonin, Omega-3 Fatty Acids, Potassium, Turmeric/Curcumin, Vitamin B_3, Vitamin B_6, Vitamin C, Zinc

Diclofenac + Misoprostol: Calcium, Cayenne, Chondroitin Sulfate, Chromium, Copper, Devil's Claw, Feverfew, Folic Acid, Ginger, Glucosamine Sulfate, Gotu Kola, Iron, Licorice, Magnesium, Melatonin, Omega-3 Fatty Acids, Potassium, Turmeric/Curcumin, Vitamin B_3, Vitamin B_6, Vitamin C, Zinc

Diclofenamide: Potassium

Dicloxacillin: Ginseng, Green Tea, Licorice, Probiotic Flora, Vitamin B_1, Vitamin K, Zinc

Dicumarol: Bilberry, Cayenne, Chondroitin Sulfate, Coenzyme Q10, DHEA, Dang Gui, Devil's Claw, Feverfew, Garlic, Ginger, Ginkgo, Ginseng, Green Tea, Horse Chestnut, Kava, Licorice, Magnesium, Omega-3 Fatty Acids, Policosanol, Red Clover, Reishi, Saw Palmetto, St. John's Wort, Vitamin A, Vitamin B_3, Vitamin C, Vitamin E, Vitamin K, Zinc

Didanosine (ddI): Aloe, Carnitine, Coenzyme Q10, Copper, DHEA, Reishi, Vitamin B_1, Vitamin B_2, Vitamin B_{12}, Zinc

Dideoxycytidine (ddC): Aloe, Carnitine, Coenzyme Q10, Copper, DHEA, Reishi, Vitamin B_1, Vitamin B_2, Vitamin B_{12}, Zinc

Dideoxyinosine (Didanosine): Aloe, Carnitine, Coenzyme Q10, Copper, DHEA, Reishi, Vitamin B_1, Vitamin B_2, Vitamin B_{12}, Zinc

Dienestrol: Arginine, Black Cohosh, Boron, Calcium, Copper, DHEA, Dang Gui, Magnesium, Melatonin, Milk Thistle, St. John's Wort, Vitamin B_6, Vitamin D, Vitamin E, Vitex, Zinc

Diflorasone: Aloe, Green Tea, Licorice, Vitamin C

Diflucortolone: Aloe, Green Tea, Licorice, Vitamin C

Diflunisal: Calcium, Cayenne, Chondroitin Sulfate, Chromium, Copper, Devil's Claw, Feverfew, Folic Acid, Ginger, Glucosamine Sulfate, Gotu Kola, Iron, Licorice, Melatonin, Omega-3 Fatty Acids, Policosanol, Potassium, Turmeric/Curcumin, Vitamin B_3, Vitamin B_6, Vitamin C, Vitamin K, Zinc

Digitoxin: Calcium, Cascara, Dang Gui, Eleuthero, Ephedra, Hawthorn, Licorice, Magnesium, Potassium, St. John's Wort

Digoxin: Calcium, Cascara, Dang Gui, Eleuthero, Ephedra, Hawthorn, Licorice, Magnesium, Potassium, St. John's Wort, Vitamin D

Dihydroergotamine (DHE-45): 5-HTP, Tryptophan

Dihydrotachysterol: Vitamin D

Diltiazem: Calcium, Carnitine, Folic Acid, Magnesium, St. John's Wort, Vitamin B_6, Vitamin D

Dimercaprol: Iron

Diphenylhydantoin: Calcium, Carnitine, Copper, DHEA, Folic Acid, Ginkgo, Inositol, Kava, Milk Thistle, Omega-3 Fatty Acids, Valerian, Vitamin A, Vitamin B_1, Vitamin B_2, Vitamin B_3, Vitamin B_6, Vitamin B_{12}, Vitamin C, Vitamin D, Vitamin E, Vitamin K, Vitex, Zinc

Dipyridamole: Bilberry, Cayenne, Feverfew, Garlic, Ginger, Ginkgo, Iron, Omega-3 Fatty Acids, Policosanol, S-Adenosylmethionine (SAMe)

Dirithromycin: Calcium, Green Tea, Magnesium, Probiotic Flora, Vitamin B_1, Vitamin B_6, Vitamin K, Zinc

Disopyramide: Cascara, Magnesium, Potassium

Disulfiram: Vitamin C

Divalproex Semisodium/Sodium: Calcium, Carnitine, Copper, DHEA, Folic Acid, Ginkgo, Inositol, Kava, Milk Thistle, Omega-3 Fatty Acids, Selenium, Valerian, Vitamin A, Vitamin B_1, Vitamin B_2, Vitamin B_3, Vitamin B_6, Vitamin B_{12}, Vitamin C, Vitamin D, Vitamin E, Vitamin K, Vitex, Zinc

DMPS: Iron

DMSA: Iron

Dobutamine: Calcium

Docetaxel: Aloe, Beta-Carotene, Echinacea, Eleuthero, Feverfew, Ginseng, Melatonin, Omega-3 Fatty Acids, St. John's Wort, Turmeric/Curcumin, Vitamin A, Vitamin B_6, Vitamin C, Vitamin E

Docusate: Magnesium, Potassium

Dofetilide: Cascara, Magnesium, Potassium

Donepezil: Ginkgo

Dorzolamide: Potassium

Dorzolamide + Timolol: Potassium

Doxacurium: Magnesium

Doxazosin: Saw Palmetto, Vitamin B_3

Doxepin: 5-HTP, Coenzyme Q10, Echinacea, Milk Thistle, S-Adenosylmethionine (SAMe), St. John's Wort, Tryptophan, Tyrosine, Vitamin B_1, Vitamin B_2, Vitamin B_3, Vitamin B_6, Vitamin B_{12}, Zinc

Doxorubicin: Aloe, Alpha-Lipoic Acid, Carnitine, Coenzyme Q10, Feverfew, Garlic, Ginkgo, Ginseng, Green Tea, Hawthorn, Melatonin, Milk Thistle, Omega-3 Fatty Acids, Reishi, Selenium, St. John's Wort, Turmeric/Curcumin, Vitamin A, Vitamin B_2, Vitamin C, Vitamin D, Vitamin E

Doxorubicin, Pegylated Liposomal: Alpha-Lipoic Acid, Carnitine, Coenzyme Q10, Feverfew, Garlic, Ginkgo, Green Tea, Hawthorn, Milk Thistle, Reishi, Selenium, St. John's Wort, Turmeric/Curcumin, Vitamin B_2, Vitamin B_6, Vitamin E

Doxycycline: Calcium, Folic Acid, Iron, Magnesium, Potassium, Vitamin A, Vitamin B_1, Vitamin B_2, Vitamin B_3, Vitamin B_6, Vitamin C, Zinc

Doxylamine: Vitamin B_6

Doxylamine + Pyridoxine: Vitamin B_6

Droperidol: Milk Thistle, Phenylalanine

Duloxetine: 5-HTP, Folic Acid, Ginkgo, Omega-3 Fatty Acids, S-Adenosylmethionine (SAMe), St. John's Wort, Tryptophan, Vitamin B_3, Vitamin B_6, Vitamin B_{12}

Dutasteride: Black Cohosh, Saw Palmetto

Dydrogesterone: Vitamin D, Vitex

Dyphylline: Potassium

Econazole: Echinacea

EDTA: Calcium, Copper, Iron, Vitamin C, Zinc

Efavirenz: St. John's Wort, Vitamin B_2

Eletriptan: 5-HTP, Feverfew, Tryptophan

Enalapril: Arginine, Cayenne, Iron, Omega-3 Fatty Acids, Potassium, Vitamin E, Zinc

Enalapril + Felodipine: Arginine, Calcium, Cayenne, Coenzyme Q10, Potassium, St. John's Wort, Zinc

Enalapril + Hydrochlorothiazide: Arginine, Calcium, Cayenne, Coenzyme Q10, Glucosamine Sulfate, Hawthorn, Licorice, Magnesium, Potassium, Vitamin D, Zinc

Enflurane: Alpha-Lipoic Acid, Ephedra, Milk Thistle, St. John's Wort, Valerian

Enoxacin: Calcium, Green Tea, Iron, Licorice, Magnesium, Potassium, Probiotic Flora, Vitamin B_1, Vitamin K, Zinc

Enoxaparin: Cayenne, Chondroitin Sulfate, DHEA, Policosanol, Vitamin C

Entacapone: Folic Acid, Iron, S-Adenosylmethionine (SAMe), Vitamin B_6, Vitex

Ephedrine: Selenium

Ephedrine + Guaifenesin + Theophylline: Cayenne, Magnesium

Epinephrine: Magnesium, Potassium, Vitamin C

Epirubicin: Alpha-Lipoic Acid, Carnitine, Coenzyme Q10, Feverfew, Garlic, Ginkgo, Green Tea, Hawthorn, Milk Thistle, Reishi, Selenium, St. John's Wort, Turmeric/Curcumin, Vitamin B_2, Vitamin E

Epo (Epoetin Alpha): Dang Gui, Iron, Vitamin B_6, Vitamin C

Epoetin Alpha/Epoetin Alfa (Erythropoietin): Dang Gui, Iron, Vitamin B_6, Vitamin C

Epoetin Beta: Dang Gui, Iron, Vitamin B_6, Vitamin C

Eprosartan: Alpha-Lipoic Acid, Potassium

Eptifibatide: Cayenne, Ginger, Policosanol, S-Adenosylmethionine (SAMe)

Ergotamine: 5-HTP, Tryptophan

Erythromycin + Benzoyl Peroxide: Vitamin E, Zinc

Erythromycin Oral: Calcium, Green Tea, Magnesium, Probiotic Flora, Vitamin B_1, Vitamin B_6, Vitamin B_{12}, Vitamin K, Zinc

Erythromycin Topical: Calcium, Green Tea, Magnesium, Probiotic Flora, Vitamin B_1, Vitamin B_6, Vitamin K, Zinc

Escitalopram: Chromium, Folic Acid, Ginkgo, Inositol, Omega-3 Fatty Acids, S-Adenosylmethionine (SAMe), St. John's Wort, Tryptophan, Vitamin B_3, Vitamin B_6, Vitamin B_{12}, Vitamin C, Zinc

Esmolol: Calcium, Carnitine, Chromium, Coenzyme Q10, Folic Acid, Magnesium, Melatonin, Potassium, Vitamin B_2, Vitamin B_3, Vitamin B_6, Vitamin C

Esomeprazole: Beta-Carotene, Calcium, Chromium, Iron, Kava, St. John's Wort, Vitamin B_{12}, Zinc

Estazolam: DHEA, Gotu Kola, Kava, Melatonin, St. John's Wort, Valerian, Vitamin B_3

Esterified Estrogens: Arginine, Black Cohosh, Boron, Calcium, Copper, DHEA, Dang Gui, Magnesium, Melatonin, Milk Thistle, St. John's Wort, Vitamin B_6, Vitamin D, Vitamin E, Vitex, Zinc

Esterified Estrogens + Methyltestosterone: Beta-Carotene, Black Cohosh, Boron, Calcium, Copper, DHEA, Dang Gui, Magnesium, Melatonin, Milk Thistle, St. John's Wort, Vitamin A, Vitamin B_6, Vitamin D, Vitamin E, Vitex, Zinc

Estradiol: Arginine, Black Cohosh, Boron, Calcium, Copper, DHEA, Dang Gui, Magnesium, Melatonin, Milk Thistle, St. John's Wort, Vitamin B_6, Vitamin D, Vitamin E, Vitex, Zinc

Estradiol + Dydrogesterone: Arginine, Black Cohosh, Boron, Calcium, Copper, DHEA, Dang Gui, Magnesium, Melatonin, Milk Thistle, St. John's Wort, Vitamin B_6, Vitamin D, Vitamin E, Vitex, Zinc

Estradiol + Norethindrone (Oral): Arginine, Black Cohosh, Boron, Calcium, Copper, DHEA, Dang Gui, Magnesium, Melatonin, Milk Thistle, St. John's Wort, Vitamin B_6, Vitamin D, Vitamin E, Vitex, Zinc

Estradiol + Norethindrone Patch (Estradiol + Norethindrone Acetate): Arginine, Black Cohosh, Boron, Calcium, Copper, DHEA, Dang Gui, Magnesium, Melatonin, Milk Thistle, St. John's Wort, Vitamin B_6, Vitamin D, Vitamin E, Vitex, Zinc

Estradiol + Norgestimate: Arginine, Black Cohosh, Boron, Calcium, Copper, DHEA, Dang Gui, Magnesium, Melatonin, Milk Thistle, St. John's Wort, Vitamin B_6, Vitamin D, Vitamin E, Vitex, Zinc

Estradiol Cypionate: Arginine, Black Cohosh, Boron, Calcium, Copper, DHEA, Dang Gui, Magnesium, Melatonin, Milk Thistle, St. John's Wort, Vitamin B_6, Vitamin D, Vitamin E, Vitex, Zinc

Estradiol Cypionate + Medroxyprogesterone Acetate: Beta-Carotene, Folic Acid, Magnesium, Vitamin A, Vitamin B_3, Vitamin D

Estradiol Hemihydrate: Arginine, Black Cohosh, Boron, Calcium, Copper, DHEA, Dang Gui, Magnesium, Melatonin, Milk Thistle, St. John's Wort, Vitamin B_6, Vitamin D, Vitamin E, Vitex, Zinc

Estradiol Topical: Arginine, Black Cohosh, Boron, Calcium, Copper, DHEA, Dang Gui, Magnesium, Melatonin, Milk Thistle, St. John's Wort, Vitamin B_6, Vitamin D, Vitamin E, Vitex, Zinc

Estradiol Transdermal: Arginine, Black Cohosh, Boron, Calcium, Copper, DHEA, Dang Gui, Magnesium, Melatonin, Milk Thistle, St. John's Wort, Vitamin B_6, Vitamin D, Vitamin E, Vitex, Zinc

Estradiol Vaginal Ring: Arginine, Black Cohosh, Boron, Calcium, Copper, DHEA, Dang Gui, Magnesium, Melatonin, Milk Thistle, St. John's Wort, Vitamin B_6, Vitamin D, Vitamin E, Vitex, Zinc

Estradiol Valerate: Arginine, Black Cohosh, Boron, Calcium, Copper, DHEA, Dang Gui, Magnesium, Melatonin, Milk Thistle, St. John's Wort, Vitamin B_6, Vitamin D, Vitamin E, Vitex, Zinc

Estradiol Valerate + Cyproterone Acetate: Arginine, Black Cohosh, Boron, Calcium, Copper, DHEA, Dang Gui, Magnesium, Melatonin, Milk Thistle, St. John's Wort, Vitamin B_6, Vitamin D, Vitamin E, Vitex, Zinc

Estradiol Valerate + Norgestrel: Arginine, Black Cohosh, Boron, Calcium, Copper, DHEA, Dang Gui, Magnesium,

Estrone: Arginine, Black Cohosh, Boron, Calcium, Copper, DHEA, Dang Gui, Magnesium, Melatonin, Milk Thistle, St. John's Wort, Vitamin B_6, Vitamin D, Vitamin E, Vitex, Zinc

Estropipate: Arginine, Black Cohosh, Boron, Calcium, Copper, DHEA, Dang Gui, Magnesium, Melatonin, Milk Thistle, St. John's Wort, Vitamin B_6, Vitamin D, Vitamin E, Vitex, Zinc

Eszopiclone: 5-HTP, Gotu Kola, Melatonin, Valerian

Etanercept: Echinacea

Ethacrynic Acid: Calcium, Folic Acid, Ginseng, Glucosamine Sulfate, Licorice, Magnesium, Potassium, Vitamin B_1, Vitamin B_6, Vitamin C, Zinc

Ethambutol: Copper, Folic Acid, Milk Thistle, Vitamin B_3, Vitamin B_6, Vitamin C, Vitamin D, Zinc

Ethanol: Ginseng, Gotu Kola, Kava, Licorice, Milk Thistle, Turmeric/Curcumin

Ethinyl Estradiol: Arginine, Boron, Calcium, Copper, DHEA, Dang Gui, Folic Acid, Iron, Licorice, Magnesium, Melatonin, Milk Thistle, S-Adenosylmethionine (SAMe), Selenium, St. John's Wort, Tyrosine, Vitamin A, Vitamin B_1, Vitamin B_2, Vitamin B_3, Vitamin B_6, Vitamin B_{12}, Vitamin C, Vitamin E, Vitex, Zinc

Ethinyl Estradiol + Desogestrel: Arginine, Calcium, Copper, DHEA, Dang Gui, Folic Acid, Iron, Licorice, Magnesium, Melatonin, Milk Thistle, S-Adenosylmethionine (SAMe), Selenium, St. John's Wort, Tyrosine, Vitamin A, Vitamin B_1, Vitamin B_2, Vitamin B_3, Vitamin B_6, Vitamin B_{12}, Vitamin C, Vitamin E, Vitex, Zinc

Ethinyl Estradiol + Ethynodiol: Arginine, Calcium, Copper, DHEA, Dang Gui, Folic Acid, Iron, Licorice, Magnesium, Melatonin, Milk Thistle, S-Adenosylmethionine (SAMe), Selenium, St. John's Wort, Tyrosine, Vitamin A, Vitamin B_1, Vitamin B_2, Vitamin B_3, Vitamin B_6, Vitamin B_{12}, Vitamin C, Vitamin E, Vitex, Zinc

Ethinyl Estradiol + Levonorgestrel: Arginine, Calcium, Copper, DHEA, Dang Gui, Folic Acid, Iron, Licorice, Magnesium, Melatonin, Milk Thistle, S-Adenosylmethionine (SAMe), Selenium, St. John's Wort, Tyrosine, Vitamin A, Vitamin B_1, Vitamin B_2, Vitamin B_3, Vitamin B_6, Vitamin B_{12}, Vitamin C, Vitamin E, Vitex, Zinc

Ethinyl Estradiol + Norethindrone: Arginine, Calcium, Copper, DHEA, Dang Gui, Folic Acid, Iron, Licorice, Magnesium, Melatonin, Milk Thistle, S-Adenosylmethionine (SAMe), Selenium, St. John's Wort, Tyrosine, Vitamin A, Vitamin B_1, Vitamin B_2, Vitamin B_3, Vitamin B_6, Vitamin B_{12}, Vitamin C, Vitamin E, Vitex, Zinc

Ethinyl Estradiol + Norethisterone (Ethinyl Estradiol + Norethindrone): Arginine, Calcium, Copper, DHEA, Dang Gui, Folic Acid, Iron, Licorice, Magnesium, Melatonin, Milk Thistle, S-Adenosylmethionine (SAMe), Selenium, St. John's Wort, Tyrosine, Vitamin A, Vitamin B_1, Vitamin B_2, Vitamin B_3, Vitamin B_6, Vitamin B_{12}, Vitamin C, Vitamin E, Vitex, Zinc

Ethinyl Estradiol + Norgestrel: Arginine, Calcium, Copper, DHEA, Dang Gui, Folic Acid, Iron, Licorice, Magnesium, Melatonin, Milk Thistle, S-Adenosylmethionine (SAMe), Selenium, St. John's Wort, Tyrosine, Vitamin A, Vitamin B_1, Vitamin B_2, Vitamin B_3, Vitamin B_6, Vitamin B_{12}, Vitamin C, Vitamin E, Vitex, Zinc

Ethionamide: Folic Acid, Milk Thistle, Vitamin B_6, Vitamin C, Vitamin D

Ethosuximide: Calcium, Carnitine, Copper, DHEA, Folic Acid, Ginkgo, Inositol, Kava, Milk Thistle, Omega-3 Fatty Acids, Valerian, Vitamin A, Vitamin B_1, Vitamin B_2, Vitamin B_3, Vitamin B_6, Vitamin B_{12}, Vitamin C, Vitamin D, Vitamin E, Vitamin K, Vitex, Zinc

Ethotoin: Calcium, Carnitine, Copper, DHEA, Folic Acid, Ginkgo, Inositol, Kava, Milk Thistle, Omega-3 Fatty Acids, Valerian, Vitamin A, Vitamin B_1, Vitamin B_2, Vitamin B_3, Vitamin B_6, Vitamin B_{12}, Vitamin C, Vitamin D, Vitamin E, Vitamin K, Vitex, Zinc

Ethyl Biscoumacetate: Bilberry, Cayenne, Chondroitin Sulfate, Coenzyme Q10, DHEA, Dang Gui, Devil's Claw, Feverfew, Garlic, Ginger, Ginkgo, Ginseng, Green Tea, Horse Chestnut, Kava, Licorice, Magnesium, Omega-3 Fatty Acids, Policosanol, Red Clover, Reishi, Saw Palmetto, St. John's Wort, Vitamin A, Vitamin B_3, Vitamin C, Vitamin E, Vitamin K, Zinc

Ethylphenacemide (Pheneturide): Calcium, Copper, DHEA, Folic Acid, Ginkgo, Inositol, Kava, Milk Thistle, Omega-3 Fatty Acids, Valerian, Vitamin A, Vitamin B_1, Vitamin B_2, Vitamin B_3, Vitamin B_6, Vitamin B_{12}, Vitamin C, Vitamin D, Vitamin E, Vitamin K, Vitex, Zinc

Ethynodiol: Arginine, Calcium, Copper, DHEA, Dang Gui, Folic Acid, Iron, Licorice, Magnesium, Melatonin, Milk Thistle, S-Adenosylmethionine (SAMe), Selenium, St. John's Wort, Tyrosine, Vitamin A, Vitamin B_1, Vitamin B_2, Vitamin B_3, Vitamin B_6, Vitamin B_{12}, Vitamin C, Vitamin E, Vitex, Zinc

Etidronate: Calcium, Iron, Magnesium, Vitamin D, Zinc

Etodolac: Calcium, Cayenne, Chondroitin Sulfate, Chromium, Copper, Devil's Claw, Feverfew, Folic Acid, Ginger, Glucosamine Sulfate, Gotu Kola, Iron, Licorice, Melatonin, Omega-3 Fatty Acids, Potassium, Turmeric/Curcumin, Vitamin B_3, Vitamin B_6, Vitamin C, Zinc

Etonogestrel/Ethinyl Estradiol Vaginal Ring: Arginine, Copper, Dang Gui, Iron, Licorice, Magnesium, Selenium, St. John's Wort, Tyrosine, Vitamin A, Vitamin B_1, Vitamin B_2, Vitamin B_3, Vitamin B_6, Vitamin B_{12}, Vitamin C, Vitamin E, Zinc

Etoposide: Aloe, Feverfew, Ginseng, Melatonin, Omega-3 Fatty Acids, St. John's Wort

Etretinate: Beta-Carotene, Calcium, Carnitine, Omega-3 Fatty Acids, Vitamin A, Vitamin E

Etrorelix: Black Cohosh

Exemestane: Green Tea

Ezetimibe: Policosanol

Famciclovir: Astragalus

Famotidine: Calcium, Chromium, Copper, Folic Acid, Iron, Licorice, Magnesium, Vitamin B_{12}, Vitamin C, Zinc

Felbamate: Calcium, Carnitine, Copper, DHEA, Folic Acid, Ginkgo, Inositol, Kava, Milk Thistle, Omega-3 Fatty Acids, Valerian, Vitamin A, Vitamin B_1, Vitamin B_2, Vitamin B_3, Vitamin B_6, Vitamin B_{12}, Vitamin C, Vitamin D, Vitamin E, Vitamin K, Vitex, Zinc

Felodipine: Calcium, Carnitine, Folic Acid, Magnesium, St. John's Wort, Vitamin B_6, Vitamin D

Felodipine + Ramipril: Arginine, Calcium, Coenzyme Q10, Magnesium, Potassium, St. John's Wort

Fenofibrate: Coenzyme Q10, Copper, Folic Acid, Gotu Kola, Omega-3 Fatty Acids, Vitamin B_3, Vitamin B_6, Vitamin B_{12}, Vitamin C, Vitamin E, Zinc

Fenoprofen: Calcium, Cayenne, Chondroitin Sulfate, Chromium, Copper, Devil's Claw, Feverfew, Folic Acid, Ginger, Glucosamine Sulfate, Gotu Kola, Iron, Licorice, Melatonin, Omega-3 Fatty Acids, Potassium, Turmeric/Curcumin, Vitamin B_3, Vitamin B_6, Vitamin C, Zinc

Fenoterol: Calcium, Magnesium, Potassium

Fentanyl: Ephedra, Ginger, Ginseng, Gotu Kola, Magnesium, Phenylalanine, Tyrosine

Fexofenadine: St. John's Wort

Filgrastim: Echinacea

Finasteride: Black Cohosh, Saw Palmetto

Flecainide: Cascara, Magnesium, Potassium

Floxuridine: Echinacea, Eleuthero, Folic Acid, Vitamin B_1

Fluconazole: Echinacea, St. John's Wort

Fludarabine: Echinacea, Eleuthero, Folic Acid, Vitamin B_1

Fludestrin (Testolactone): Beta-Carotene, DHEA, Vitamin A, Zinc

Fludroxycortide: Aloe, Green Tea, Licorice, Vitamin C

Fluocinonide: Aloe, Green Tea, Licorice, Vitamin C

Fluocortolone: Aloe, Green Tea, Licorice, Vitamin C

Fluorouracil (5-FU): Aloe, Beta-Carotene, Echinacea, Eleuthero, Folic Acid, Garlic, Ginkgo, Ginseng, Melatonin, Omega-3 Fatty Acids, Vitamin A, Vitamin B_1, Vitamin B_3, Vitamin B_6, Vitamin C, Vitamin E

Fluoxetine: 5-HTP, Chromium, DHEA, Folic Acid, Ginkgo, Inositol, Melatonin, Omega-3 Fatty Acids, S-Adenosylmethionine (SAMe), St. John's Wort, Tryptophan, Vitamin B_3, Vitamin B_6, Vitamin B_{12}, Vitamin C, Zinc

Fluoxymesterone: DHEA, Echinacea, Zinc

Fluphenazine: Chromium, Coenzyme Q10, Ginkgo, Kava, Melatonin, Milk Thistle, Vitamin B_2, Vitamin B_3, Vitamin B_6, Vitamin C

Flurandrenolide: Aloe, Green Tea, Licorice, Vitamin C

Flurazepam: DHEA, Gotu Kola, Melatonin, Valerian, Vitamin B_3

Flurbiprofen: Vitamin D

Flutamide: Black Cohosh, Vitamin D

Fluticasone: Aloe, Green Tea, Licorice, Vitamin C

Fluvastatin: Beta-Carotene, Carnitine, Coenzyme Q10, Garlic, Gotu Kola, Omega-3 Fatty Acids, Policosanol, Reishi, Selenium, St. John's Wort, Vitamin A, Vitamin B_3, Vitamin C, Vitamin E

Fluvoxamine: 5-HTP, Chromium, Folic Acid, Ginkgo, Inositol, Melatonin, Omega-3 Fatty Acids, S-Adenosylmethionine (SAMe), St. John's Wort, Tryptophan, Vitamin B_3, Vitamin B_6, Vitamin B_{12}, Vitamin C, Zinc

Folic Acid: Zinc

Fondaparinux: Cayenne, Chondroitin Sulfate, DHEA, Policosanol

Formoterol: Calcium, Magnesium, Potassium

Fosamprenavir: Copper, Garlic, St. John's Wort, Vitamin C

Foscarnet: Magnesium

Fosinopril: Arginine, Cayenne, Iron, Omega-3 Fatty Acids, Potassium, Vitamin E, Zinc

Fosphenytoin: Calcium, Carnitine, Copper, DHEA, Folic Acid, Ginkgo, Inositol, Kava, Milk Thistle, Omega-3 Fatty Acids, Valerian, Vitamin A, Vitamin B_1, Vitamin B_2, Vitamin B_3, Vitamin B_6, Vitamin B_{12}, Vitamin C, Vitamin D, Vitamin E, Vitamin K, Vitex, Zinc

Frovatriptan: 5-HTP, Feverfew, Tryptophan

Fujimycin (Tacrolimus): Echinacea, St. John's Wort

Furaltadone: Licorice, Probiotic Flora, Vitamin K, Zinc

Furazolidone: Licorice, Probiotic Flora, Vitamin K, Zinc

Furbiprofen: Calcium, Cayenne, Chondroitin Sulfate, Chromium, Copper, Devil's Claw, Feverfew, Folic Acid, Ginger, Glucosamine Sulfate, Gotu Kola, Iron, Licorice, Melatonin, Omega-3 Fatty Acids, Potassium,

Turmeric/Curcumin, Vitamin B_3, Vitamin B_6, Vitamin C, Zinc

Furosemide: Calcium, Folic Acid, Ginseng, Glucosamine Sulfate, Licorice, Magnesium, Potassium, Vitamin B_1, Vitamin B_6, Vitamin C, Zinc

G-Strophanthin (Ouabain): Calcium, Cascara, Dang Gui, Eleuthero, Ephedra, Hawthorn, Licorice, Magnesium, Potassium, St. John's Wort

Gabapentin: Carnitine, Folic Acid, Vitamin B_3, Vitamin B_6, Vitamin D

Gallopamil: Calcium, Carnitine, Folic Acid, Magnesium, St. John's Wort, Vitamin B_6, Vitamin D

Ganciclovir: Astragalus

Ganirelix: Black Cohosh

Gatifloxacin: Calcium, Green Tea, Iron, Licorice, Magnesium, Potassium, Probiotic Flora, Vitamin B_1, Vitamin K, Zinc

GCSF: Echinacea

Gemcitabine: Aloe, Echinacea, Eleuthero, Folic Acid, Ginseng, Melatonin, Omega-3 Fatty Acids, Vitamin A, Vitamin B_1, Vitamin C, Vitamin E

Gemfibrozil: Coenzyme Q10, Copper, Folic Acid, Gotu Kola, Omega-3 Fatty Acids, Vitamin B_3, Vitamin B_6, Vitamin B_{12}, Vitamin E, Zinc

Gentamicin: Alpha-Lipoic Acid, Calcium, Carnitine, Eleuthero, Ginger, Ginkgo, Horse Chestnut, Licorice, Magnesium, Potassium, Probiotic Flora, Vitamin B_1, Vitamin B_6, Vitamin B_{12}, Vitamin C, Vitamin E, Vitamin K

Glibenclamide (Glyburide): Aloe, Alpha-Lipoic Acid, Astragalus, Bilberry, Chromium, Coenzyme Q10, DHEA, Ephedra, Garlic, Ginkgo, Ginseng, Glucosamine Sulfate, Gotu Kola, Horse Chestnut, Magnesium, Omega-3 Fatty Acids, Reishi, Turmeric/Curcumin, Vitamin B_3, Vitamin E

Glimepiride: Aloe, Alpha-Lipoic Acid, Astragalus, Bilberry, Chromium, Coenzyme Q10, DHEA, Ephedra, Garlic, Ginkgo, Ginseng, Glucosamine Sulfate, Gotu Kola, Horse Chestnut, Magnesium, Omega-3 Fatty Acids, Reishi, Turmeric/Curcumin, Vitamin B_3

Glipizide: Aloe, Alpha-Lipoic Acid, Astragalus, Bilberry, Chromium, Coenzyme Q10, DHEA, Ephedra, Garlic, Ginkgo, Ginseng, Glucosamine Sulfate, Gotu Kola, Horse Chestnut, Magnesium, Omega-3 Fatty Acids, Reishi, Turmeric/Curcumin, Vitamin B_3

Glipizide + Metformin: Aloe, Alpha-Lipoic Acid, Calcium, Chromium, Coenzyme Q10, DHEA, Ephedra, Folic Acid, Garlic, Ginkgo, Ginseng, Glucosamine Sulfate, Horse Chestnut, Magnesium, Omega-3 Fatty Acids, Reishi, Turmeric/Curcumin, Vitamin B_3, Vitamin B_{12}

Glyburide: Aloe, Alpha-Lipoic Acid, Astragalus, Bilberry, Chromium, Coenzyme Q10, DHEA, Ephedra, Garlic, Ginkgo, Ginseng, Glucosamine Sulfate, Gotu Kola, Horse Chestnut, Magnesium, Omega-3 Fatty Acids, Reishi, Turmeric/Curcumin, Vitamin B_3, Vitamin E

Glyburide + Metformin: Aloe, Alpha-Lipoic Acid, Calcium, Chromium, Coenzyme Q10, DHEA, Ephedra, Folic Acid, Garlic, Ginkgo, Ginseng, Glucosamine Sulfate, Horse Chestnut, Magnesium, Omega-3 Fatty Acids, Reishi, Turmeric/Curcumin, Vitamin B_3, Vitamin B_{12}

Glycerin-Containing Suppositories: Potassium

Glyceryl Trinitrate (Nitroglycerin): Arginine, Carnitine, Folic Acid, Vitamin C

GMCSF: Echinacea

Goserelin: Black Cohosh, Vitamin D

Griseofulvin: Echinacea, Vitamin B_3, Vitamin E

GTN (Nitroglycerin): Arginine, Carnitine, Folic Acid, Vitamin C

Guaifenesin + Phenylpropanolamine: Potassium, Tyrosine

Guanadrel: Ephedra

Guanethidine: Ephedra, Vitamin B_3

Halcinonide: Aloe, Green Tea, Licorice, Vitamin C

Halobetasol: Aloe, Green Tea, Licorice, Vitamin C

Haloperidol: Alpha-Lipoic Acid, Chromium, Ginkgo, Iron, Kava, Melatonin, Milk Thistle, Phenylalanine, Potassium, Vitamin B_3, Vitamin B_6, Vitamin C, Vitamin E

Halothane: Alpha-Lipoic Acid, Ephedra, Milk Thistle, St. John's Wort, Valerian

Heparin: Cayenne, Chondroitin Sulfate, DHEA, Policosanol, Vitamin C, Vitamin D

Heparin + Phosphatidylcholine + Aescin: Horse Chestnut

Heparin, Unfractionated: Calcium, Cayenne, Chondroitin Sulfate, DHEA, Omega-3 Fatty Acids, Policosanol, Potassium, Vitamin C, Vitamin D

Hirudin: Cayenne, DHEA, Policosanol

Hizaricin (Cycloheximide): Dang Gui, Echinacea

Hydralazine: Melatonin, Vitamin B_6, Zinc

Hydralazine + Hydrochlorothiazide: Arginine, Coenzyme Q10, Melatonin, Potassium, Vitamin B_6

Hydrochlorothiazide: Calcium, Coenzyme Q10, Folic Acid, Ginkgo, Glucosamine Sulfate, Hawthorn, Licorice, Magnesium, Potassium, Vitamin B_2, Vitamin D, Zinc

Hydrocodone: Ephedra, Ginseng, Gotu Kola, Phenylalanine, Tyrosine

Hydrocodone + Acetaminophen: Ephedra, Ginseng, Gotu Kola, Phenylalanine, Tyrosine

Hydrocodone + Acetylsalicylic Acid: Ephedra, Ginseng, Gotu Kola, Phenylalanine, Tyrosine

Hydrocodone + Ibuprofen: Calcium, Cayenne, Chondroitin Sulfate, Chromium, Copper, Devil's Claw, Feverfew, Folic Acid, Ginger, Ginseng, Glucosamine Sulfate, Gotu Kola, Iron, Licorice, Melatonin, Omega-3 Fatty Acids, Potassium, Turmeric/Curcumin, Vitamin B_3, Vitamin B_6, Vitamin C, Zinc

Hydrocortisone: Calcium, Cayenne, Chromium, DHEA, Echinacea, Ephedra, Folic Acid, Horse Chestnut, Licorice, Magnesium, Melatonin, Omega-3 Fatty Acids, Potassium, Selenium, Vitamin A, Vitamin B_6, Vitamin C, Vitamin D, Vitamin K, Zinc

Hydrocortisone 17-Butyrate/Acetate/Probutate/Valerate: Aloe, Green Tea, Licorice, Vitamin C

Hydroflumethiazide: Calcium, Coenzyme Q10, Folic Acid, Ginkgo, Glucosamine Sulfate, Hawthorn, Licorice, Magnesium, Potassium, Vitamin B_2, Vitamin D, Zinc

Hydrogel Dressings: Aloe

Hydromorphone: Ephedra, Ginseng, Gotu Kola, Phenylalanine, Tyrosine

Hydroxychloroquine: Calcium, Magnesium, Vitamin B_2, Vitamin B_6, Vitamin D

Hyoscine Hydrobromide: Ginger

Hyoscyamine: Iron

Ibandronate: Calcium, Iron, Magnesium, Vitamin D, Zinc

Ibuprofen: Calcium, Cayenne, Chondroitin Sulfate, Chromium, Copper, Devil's Claw, Feverfew, Folic Acid, Ginger, Glucosamine Sulfate, Gotu Kola, Iron, Licorice, Melatonin, Omega-3 Fatty Acids, Potassium, Turmeric/Curcumin, Vitamin B_3, Vitamin B_6, Vitamin C, Zinc

Ibuprofen + Hydrocodone: Ephedra, Ginseng, Gotu Kola, Phenylalanine, Tyrosine

Ibutilide: Cascara, Magnesium, Potassium

Idarubicin: Alpha-Lipoic Acid, Carnitine, Coenzyme Q10, Feverfew, Garlic, Ginkgo, Green Tea, Hawthorn, Milk Thistle, Reishi, Selenium, St. John's Wort, Turmeric/Curcumin, Vitamin B_2, Vitamin E

Ifosfamide: Astragalus, Carnitine, Echinacea, Eleuthero, Selenium

Imatinib: St. John's Wort

Imidazole Carboxamide (Dacarbazine): Astragalus, Carnitine, Echinacea, Eleuthero, Selenium

Imipenem: Ginseng, Licorice, Probiotic Flora, Vitamin B_1, Vitamin K, Zinc

Imipenem + Cilastatin: Ginseng, Green Tea, Iron, Licorice, Probiotic Flora, Reishi, Vitamin B_1, Vitamin K, Zinc

Imipramine: 5-HTP, Coenzyme Q10, Echinacea, Milk Thistle, S-Adenosylmethionine (SAMe), St. John's Wort, Tryptophan, Tyrosine, Vitamin B_1, Vitamin B_2, Vitamin B_3, Vitamin B_6, Vitamin B_{12}, Zinc

Indapamide: Calcium, Coenzyme Q10, Folic Acid, Ginkgo, Glucosamine Sulfate, Hawthorn, Licorice, Magnesium, Potassium, Vitamin B_2, Vitamin D, Zinc

Indinavir: Copper, Garlic, St. John's Wort, Vitamin C

Indomethacin: Calcium, Cayenne, Chondroitin Sulfate, Chromium, Copper, Devil's Claw, Feverfew, Folic Acid, Ginger, Glucosamine Sulfate, Gotu Kola, Iron, Licorice, Melatonin, Omega-3 Fatty Acids, Potassium, Turmeric/Curcumin, Vitamin A, Vitamin B_3, Vitamin B_6, Vitamin C, Zinc

Infliximab: Echinacea

Influenza Vaccine: Ginseng

Insulin: Alpha-Lipoic Acid, Bilberry, Chromium, DHEA, Ephedra, Garlic, Ginkgo, Ginseng, Glucosamine Sulfate, Horse Chestnut, Licorice, Magnesium, Milk Thistle, Omega-3 Fatty Acids, Potassium, Reishi, Turmeric/Curcumin, Vitamin B_3, Vitamin E

Interferon Alpha: Astragalus, Echinacea, Iron, Licorice, Zinc

Interferon Gamma-1b: Echinacea

Intrauterine L-Norgestrel System: Vitamin D

Ipecac: Potassium

Irbesartan: Alpha-Lipoic Acid, Potassium

Irbesartan + Hydrochlorothiazide: Alpha-Lipoic Acid, Potassium

Irinotecan: Aloe, Feverfew, Ginseng, Melatonin, Omega-3 Fatty Acids, St. John's Wort, Turmeric/Curcumin, Vitamin A, Vitamin C, Vitamin E

Iron Salts (Nonheme Iron): Green Tea

Isocarboxazid: 5-HTP, Cayenne, Chromium, Eleuthero, Ephedra, Ginkgo, Ginseng, Licorice, Phenylalanine, S-Adenosylmethionine (SAMe), St. John's Wort, Tryptophan, Tyrosine, Vitamin B_6

Isoetharine: Calcium, Magnesium, Potassium

Isoflurane: Alpha-Lipoic Acid, Ephedra, Milk Thistle, St. John's Wort, Valerian

Isoniazid (Isonicotinic Acid Hydrazide): Calcium, Copper, Folic Acid, Magnesium, Milk Thistle, Vitamin B_3, Vitamin B_6, Vitamin C, Vitamin D, Vitamin E

Isoniazid + Pyrazinamide + Rifampicin: Calcium, Copper, Folic Acid, Magnesium, Milk Thistle, Vitamin B_3, Vitamin B_6, Vitamin C, Vitamin D, Vitamin E

Isoniazid + Rifampicin: Calcium, Copper, Folic Acid, Magnesium, Milk Thistle, Vitamin B_3, Vitamin B_6, Vitamin C, Vitamin D, Vitamin E

Isoproterenol: Garlic

Isosorbide Dinitrate: Arginine, Carnitine, Folic Acid, Vitamin C

Isosorbide Dinitrate + Hydralazine: Arginine, Carnitine, Folic Acid, Melatonin, Vitamin B_6, Vitamin C

Isosorbide Mononitrate: Arginine, Carnitine, Folic Acid, Vitamin C

Isotretinoin (13-*cis* Retinoic Acid): Beta-Carotene, Calcium, Carnitine, Vitamin A, Vitamin E

Isradipine: Calcium, Carnitine, Folic Acid, Magnesium, St. John's Wort, Vitamin B_6, Vitamin D

Itraconazole: Echinacea, St. John's Wort

Kaken (Cycloheximide): Dang Gui, Echinacea

Kanamycin: Alpha-Lipoic Acid, Calcium, Eleuthero, Ginger, Ginkgo, Horse Chestnut, Licorice, Magnesium, Potassium, Probiotic Flora, Vitamin B_1, Vitamin B_6, Vitamin B_{12}, Vitamin K

Kaolin Clay: Ephedra

Ketoconazole: Black Cohosh, Echinacea, Green Tea, Vitamin D

Ketoprofen: Calcium, Cayenne, Chondroitin Sulfate, Chromium, Copper, Devil's Claw, Feverfew, Folic Acid, Ginger, Glucosamine Sulfate, Gotu Kola, Iron, Licorice, Melatonin, Omega-3 Fatty Acids, Potassium, Turmeric/Curcumin, Vitamin B_3, Vitamin B_6, Vitamin C, Zinc

Ketorolac: Calcium, Cayenne, Chondroitin Sulfate, Chromium, Copper, Devil's Claw, Feverfew, Folic Acid, Ginger, Glucosamine Sulfate, Gotu Kola, Iron, Licorice, Melatonin, Omega-3 Fatty Acids, Potassium, Turmeric/Curcumin, Vitamin B_3, Vitamin B_6, Vitamin C, Zinc

L-Deprenyl/L-Deprenil (Selegiline): 5-HTP, Cayenne, Chromium, Eleuthero, Ephedra, Folic Acid, Ginkgo, Iron, Kava, Licorice, Phenylalanine, S-Adenosylmethionine (SAMe), St. John's Wort, Tryptophan, Tyrosine, Vitamin B_2, Vitamin B_6, Vitex

L-Norgestrel (Norgestrel, Oral): Magnesium, St. John's Wort

L-Thyroxine + L-Triiodothyronine: Alpha-Lipoic Acid, Calcium, Carnitine, Coenzyme Q10, DHEA, Iron, Tyrosine, Vitamin B_2

L-Triiodothyronine: Alpha-Lipoic Acid, Calcium, Carnitine, Coenzyme Q10, DHEA, Iron, Tyrosine, Vitamin B_2

Labetalol: Potassium

Lactulose: Potassium

Lamivudine: Aloe, Carnitine, Coenzyme Q10, Copper, DHEA, Reishi, Vitamin B_1, Vitamin B_2, Vitamin B_{12}, Zinc

Lamivudine + Zidovudine: Aloe, Carnitine, Coenzyme Q10, Copper, DHEA, Folic Acid, Reishi, Vitamin B_1, Vitamin B_2, Vitamin B_{12}, Vitamin E, Zinc

Lansoprazole: Beta-Carotene, Calcium, Chromium, Iron, Kava, Probiotic Flora, St. John's Wort, Vitamin B_{12}, Zinc

Lansoprazole + Amoxicillin + Clarithromycin: Licorice, Probiotic Flora, Vitamin C, Vitamin K, Zinc

Lepirudin: Cayenne, DHEA, Policosanol

Lercanidipine: Calcium, Carnitine, Folic Acid, Magnesium, St. John's Wort, Vitamin B_6, Vitamin D

Letrozole: Green Tea

Leuprolide: Black Cohosh, Vitamin D

Leurocristine (Vincristine): Alpha-Lipoic Acid, Echinacea, Eleuthero, Feverfew, Ginseng, St. John's Wort, Turmeric/Curcumin

Levalbuterol: Calcium, Magnesium, Potassium

Levamisole: Beta-Carotene, Echinacea, Vitamin A

Levetiracetam: Calcium, Carnitine, Copper, DHEA, Folic Acid, Ginkgo, Inositol, Kava, Milk Thistle, Omega-3 Fatty Acids, Valerian, Vitamin A, Vitamin B_1, Vitamin B_2, Vitamin B_3, Vitamin B_6, Vitamin B_{12}, Vitamin C, Vitamin D, Vitamin E, Vitamin K, Vitex, Zinc

Levodopa: Folic Acid, Iron, Kava, Methionine, Phenylalanine, Tyrosine, Vitamin B$_3$, Vitamin B$_6$, Vitamin C

Levodopa + Benserazide: 5-HTP, Folic Acid, Iron, Kava, Methionine, Phenylalanine, *S*-Adenosylmethionine (SAMe), Tyrosine, Vitamin B$_3$, Vitamin B$_6$, Vitamin C, Vitex

Levodopa + Carbidopa: 5-HTP, Folic Acid, Iron, Kava, Methionine, Phenylalanine, *S*-Adenosylmethionine (SAMe), Tyrosine, Vitamin B$_3$, Vitamin B$_6$, Vitamin C, Vitex

Levodopa + Carbidopa + Entacapone: 5-HTP, Folic Acid, Iron, Kava, Methionine, Phenylalanine, *S*-Adenosylmethionine (SAMe), Tyrosine, Vitamin B$_6$, Vitamin C, Vitex

Levofloxacin: Calcium, Green Tea, Iron, Licorice, Magnesium, Potassium, Probiotic Flora, Vitamin B$_1$, Vitamin K, Zinc

Levomepromazine (Methotrimeprazine): Coenzyme Q10, Milk Thistle, Vitamin B$_2$, Vitamin B$_3$, Vitamin C

Levonorgestrel, Implant: Magnesium, St. John's Wort

Levonorgestrel, Oral Postcoital Contraceptive: Magnesium, St. John's Wort

Levorphanol: Ephedra, Ginseng, Gotu Kola, Phenylalanine, Tyrosine

Levothyroxine (Levoxin): Alpha-Lipoic Acid, Calcium, Carnitine, Coenzyme Q10, DHEA, Iron, Tyrosine, Vitamin B$_2$

Lincomycin: Licorice, Probiotic Flora, Vitamin K, Zinc

Lindane: Vitamin E

Linezolid: Licorice, Probiotic Flora, Vitamin K, Zinc

Liothyronine Sodium (L-Triiodothyronine): Alpha-Lipoic Acid, Calcium, Carnitine, Coenzyme Q10, DHEA, Iron, Tyrosine, Vitamin B$_2$

Liothyronine Sodium (Synthetic T$_3$) (L-Triiodothyronine): Alpha-Lipoic Acid, Calcium, Carnitine, Coenzyme Q10, DHEA, Iron, Tyrosine, Vitamin B$_2$

Liotrix (L-Thyroxine + L-Triiodothyronine [Synthetic]): Alpha-Lipoic Acid, Calcium, Carnitine, Coenzyme Q10, DHEA, Iron, Tyrosine, Vitamin B$_2$

Liquid Parafin (Mineral Oil): Beta-Carotene, Calcium, Potassium, Vitamin A, Vitamin D, Vitamin E, Vitamin K

Lisinopril: Arginine, Cayenne, Iron, Omega-3 Fatty Acids, Potassium, Vitamin E, Zinc

Lisinopril + Hydrochlorothiazide: Arginine, Calcium, Cayenne, Coenzyme Q10, Glucosamine Sulfate, Hawthorn, Licorice, Magnesium, Potassium, Vitamin D, Zinc

Lithium Carbonate: 5-HTP, Chromium, Folic Acid, Inositol, Magnesium, Tryptophan

Lomefloxacin: Calcium, Green Tea, Iron, Licorice, Magnesium, Potassium, Probiotic Flora, Vitamin B$_1$, Vitamin K, Zinc

Lometrexol (T64): Echinacea, Eleuthero, Folic Acid, Vitamin B$_1$

Loperamide: St. John's Wort

Lopinavir + Ritonavir: Copper, Garlic, St. John's Wort, Vitamin C

Loracarbef: Ginseng, Green Tea, Iron, Licorice, Probiotic Flora, Reishi, Vitamin B$_1$, Vitamin K, Zinc

Lorazepam: DHEA, Gotu Kola, Melatonin, Valerian, Vitamin B$_3$

Losartan: Alpha-Lipoic Acid, Potassium

Losartan + Hydrochlorothiazide: Alpha-Lipoic Acid, Arginine, Calcium, Coenzyme Q10, Glucosamine Sulfate, Hawthorn, Licorice, Magnesium, Potassium, Vitamin D, Zinc

Lovastatin: Beta-Carotene, Carnitine, Coenzyme Q10, Garlic, Gotu Kola, Omega-3 Fatty Acids, Policosanol, Reishi, Selenium, St. John's Wort, Vitamin A, Vitamin B$_3$, Vitamin C, Vitamin E

Lovastatin + Niacin: Beta-Carotene, Carnitine, Coenzyme Q10, Garlic, Gotu Kola, Omega-3 Fatty Acids, Policosanol, Reishi, Selenium, St. John's Wort, Vitamin A, Vitamin B$_3$, Vitamin C, Vitamin E

Magnesium Hydroxide: Calcium, Cayenne, Chromium, Copper, Folic Acid, Iron, Magnesium, Vitamin A, Vitamin B$_1$, Vitamin D, Vitex, Zinc

Magnesium Salicylate: Calcium, Omega-3 Fatty Acids, Policosanol, Vitamin K

Magnesium Trisilicate: Calcium, Cayenne, Chromium, Copper, Folic Acid, Iron, Magnesium, Vitamin A, Vitamin B$_1$, Vitamin D, Vitex, Zinc

Magnesium-containing Products: Potassium

Mecamylamine: Vitamin B$_3$

Mecamylamine Hydrochloride (Mecamylamine): Vitamin B$_3$

Mechlorethamine: Astragalus, Carnitine, Echinacea, Eleuthero, Ginger, Selenium, Turmeric/Curcumin

Meclofenamate: Calcium, Cayenne, Chondroitin Sulfate, Chromium, Copper, Devil's Claw, Feverfew, Folic Acid, Ginger, Glucosamine Sulfate, Gotu Kola, Iron, Licorice, Melatonin, Omega-3 Fatty Acids, Potassium, Turmeric/Curcumin, Vitamin B$_3$, Vitamin B$_6$, Vitamin C, Zinc

Medazepam: DHEA, Gotu Kola, Melatonin, Valerian, Vitamin B$_3$

Medroxyprogesterone: Vitamin D

Medroxyprogesterone + Conjugated Estrogens (Medroxyprogesterone Conjugated Equine Estrogens): Arginine, Beta-Carotene, Black Cohosh, Boron, Calcium, Copper, DHEA, Dang Gui, Folic Acid, Magnesium, Melatonin, Milk Thistle, St. John's Wort, Vitamin A, Vitamin B$_6$, Vitamin D, Vitamin E, Vitex, Zinc

Medroxyprogesterone, Injection: Beta-Carotene, Calcium, Folic Acid, Vitamin A, Vitamin B$_3$, Vitamin D

Medroxyprogesterone, Oral: Beta-Carotene, Calcium, Folic Acid, Magnesium, St. John's Wort, Vitamin A, Vitamin D

Mefenamic Acid: Calcium, Cayenne, Chondroitin Sulfate, Chromium, Copper, Devil's Claw, Feverfew, Folic Acid, Ginger, Glucosamine Sulfate, Gotu Kola, Iron, Licorice, Melatonin, Omega-3 Fatty Acids, Potassium, Turmeric/Curcumin, Vitamin B$_3$, Vitamin B$_6$, Vitamin C, Zinc

Meloxicam: Calcium, Cayenne, Chondroitin Sulfate, Chromium, Copper, Devil's Claw, Feverfew, Folic Acid, Ginger, Glucosamine Sulfate, Gotu Kola, Iron, Licorice, Melatonin, Omega-3 Fatty Acids, Potassium, Turmeric/Curcumin, Vitamin B$_3$, Vitamin B$_6$, Vitamin C, Zinc

Melperon: Milk Thistle, Phenylalanine

Melphalan: Astragalus, Carnitine, Echinacea, Eleuthero, Selenium

Meperidine: Chromium, Ephedra, Ginseng, Gotu Kola, Phenylalanine, Tyrosine

Mephenytoin: Calcium, Carnitine, Copper, DHEA, Folic Acid, Ginkgo, Inositol, Kava, Milk Thistle, Omega-3 Fatty Acids, Valerian, Vitamin A, Vitamin B$_1$, Vitamin B$_2$, Vitamin B$_3$, Vitamin B$_6$, Vitamin B$_{12}$, Vitamin C, Vitamin D, Vitamin E, Vitamin K, Vitex, Zinc

Mephobarbital: Calcium, Carnitine, Copper, DHEA, Folic Acid, Ginkgo, Gotu Kola, Inositol, Kava, Milk Thistle, Omega-3 Fatty Acids, Valerian, Vitamin A, Vitamin B$_1$, Vitamin B$_2$, Vitamin B$_3$, Vitamin B$_6$, Vitamin B$_{12}$, Vitamin C, Vitamin D, Vitamin E, Vitamin K, Vitex, Zinc

Mercaptopurine (6-MP): Echinacea, Eleuthero, Folic Acid, Vitamin B_1, Vitamin B_3

Meropenem: Ginseng, Green Tea, Iron, Licorice, Probiotic Flora, Reishi, Vitamin B_1, Vitamin K, Zinc

Mesalamine (Mesalazine): Vitamin B_{12}

Mesoridazine: Coenzyme Q10, Milk Thistle, Vitamin B_2, Vitamin B_3, Vitamin C

Mestranol + Norethindrone: Arginine, Calcium, Copper, DHEA, Dang Gui, Folic Acid, Iron, Licorice, Magnesium, Melatonin, Milk Thistle, S-Adenosylmethionine (SAMe), Selenium, St. John's Wort, Tyrosine, Vitamin A, Vitamin B_1, Vitamin B_2, Vitamin B_3, Vitamin B_6, Vitamin B_{12}, Vitamin C, Vitamin E, Vitex, Zinc

Metaproterenol: Calcium, Magnesium, Potassium

Metformin: Alpha-Lipoic Acid, Astragalus, Bilberry, Calcium, Chromium, Coenzyme Q10, DHEA, Ephedra, Folic Acid, Garlic, Ginkgo, Ginseng, Glucosamine Sulfate, Gotu Kola, Horse Chestnut, Magnesium, Omega-3 Fatty Acids, Reishi, Turmeric/Curcumin, Vitamin B_3, Vitamin B_{12}

Methadone: Ephedra, Ginseng, Gotu Kola, Phenylalanine, Tyrosine

Methamphetamine: Ginseng

Methandrostenolone (Methandienone): Echinacea, Milk Thistle

Methazolamide: Potassium

Methenolone Enanthate: Echinacea

Methicillin: Ginseng, Green Tea, Licorice, Probiotic Flora, Vitamin B_1, Vitamin K, Zinc

Methohexital: DHEA, Gotu Kola, Valerian, Vitamin B_2

Methotrexate (MTX): Aloe, Beta-Carotene, Echinacea, Eleuthero, Folic Acid, Garlic, Ginseng, Iron, Melatonin, Milk Thistle, Omega-3 Fatty Acids, PABA, Vitamin A, Vitamin B_1, Vitamin B_2, Vitamin B_6, Vitamin B_{12}, Vitamin C, Vitamin E

Methotrimeprazine: Coenzyme Q10, Milk Thistle, Vitamin B_2, Vitamin B_3, Vitamin C

Methoxamine: Melatonin

Methsuximide: Calcium, Carnitine, Copper, DHEA, Folic Acid, Ginkgo, Inositol, Kava, Milk Thistle, Omega-3 Fatty Acids, Valerian, Vitamin A, Vitamin B_1, Vitamin B_2, Vitamin B_3, Vitamin B_6, Vitamin B_{12}, Vitamin C, Vitamin D, Vitamin E, Vitamin K, Vitex, Zinc

Methyclothiazide: Calcium, Coenzyme Q10, Folic Acid, Ginkgo, Glucosamine Sulfate, Hawthorn, Licorice, Magnesium, Potassium, Vitamin B_2, Vitamin D, Zinc

Methylcellulose: Potassium, Vitamin B_2

Methyldopa: Ephedra, Iron, Vitamin B_{12}

Methyldopa + Chlorothiazide: Arginine, Coenzyme Q10, Ephedra, Potassium, Vitamin B_{12}

Methyldopa + Hydrochlorothiazide: Arginine, Coenzyme Q10, Ephedra, Potassium, Vitamin B_{12}

Methylphenidate: 5-HTP, Iron, Reishi, Tyrosine, Zinc

Methylprednisolone: Calcium, Cayenne, Chromium, DHEA, Echinacea, Ephedra, Folic Acid, Horse Chestnut, Licorice, Magnesium, Melatonin, Omega-3 Fatty Acids, Potassium, Selenium, Vitamin A, Vitamin B_6, Vitamin C, Vitamin D, Vitamin K, Zinc

Methyltestosterone: Beta-Carotene, DHEA, Vitamin A, Zinc

Metoclopramide: Vitamin B_2, Zinc

Metocurine Iodide: Magnesium

Metolazone: Calcium, Coenzyme Q10, Folic Acid, Ginkgo, Glucosamine Sulfate, Hawthorn, Licorice, Magnesium, Potassium, Vitamin B_2, Vitamin D, Zinc

Metoprolol: Calcium, Carnitine, Chromium, Coenzyme Q10, Folic Acid, Magnesium, Melatonin, Potassium, Vitamin B_2, Vitamin B_3, Vitamin B_6, Vitamin C

Metoprolol + Hydrochlorothiazide: Arginine, Calcium, Coenzyme Q10, Glucosamine Sulfate, Hawthorn, Licorice, Magnesium, Policosanol, Potassium, Vitamin C, Vitamin D, Zinc

Metronidazole (Systemic): Licorice, Milk Thistle, Probiotic Flora, Vitamin K, Zinc

Metronidazole (Vaginal): Zinc

Mexiletine: Cascara, Magnesium, Potassium, Vitamin C

Mezlocillin: Ginseng, Green Tea, Licorice, Probiotic Flora, Vitamin B_1, Vitamin K, Zinc

Midazolam: DHEA, Gotu Kola, Kava, Melatonin, St. John's Wort, Valerian, Vitamin B_3

Mineral Oil: Beta-Carotene, Calcium, Potassium, Vitamin A, Vitamin D, Vitamin E, Vitamin K

Minocycline: Calcium, Folic Acid, Iron, Magnesium, Potassium, Vitamin A, Vitamin B_1, Vitamin B_2, Vitamin B_3, Vitamin B_6, Vitamin C, Zinc

Mipobroman: Astragalus, Carnitine, Echinacea, Eleuthero, Selenium

Mirtazapine: Melatonin

Misoprostol: Magnesium

Mitomycin: Echinacea, Eleuthero, Ginseng, Licorice, Probiotic Flora, Vitamin B_1, Vitamin K

Mitoxantrone: Alpha-Lipoic Acid, Carnitine, Coenzyme Q10, Garlic, Ginkgo, Green Tea, Hawthorn, Milk Thistle, Reishi, Selenium, St. John's Wort, Turmeric/Curcumin, Vitamin B_2, Vitamin E

Mivacurium: Magnesium

Moclobemide: 5-HTP, Cayenne, Chromium, Eleuthero, Ephedra, Ginkgo, Ginseng, Licorice, Phenylalanine, S-Adenosylmethionine (SAMe), St. John's Wort, Tryptophan, Tyrosine, Vitamin B_6

Modafinil: Reishi, Tyrosine

Moexipril: Arginine, Cayenne, Iron, Omega-3 Fatty Acids, Potassium, Vitamin E, Zinc

Monobasic Sodium Phosphate Monohydrate + Dibasic Sodium Phosphate Heptahydrate: Potassium

Monomycin (Paromomycin): Alpha-Lipoic Acid, Calcium, Eleuthero, Ginger, Ginkgo, Horse Chestnut, Licorice, Magnesium, Potassium, Probiotic Flora, Vitamin B_1, Vitamin B_6, Vitamin B_{12}, Vitamin K

Morphine: Ephedra, Ginseng, Gotu Kola, Phenylalanine, Tyrosine

Morphine Hydrochloride + Codeine Hydrochloride + Papaverine Hydrochloride: Ephedra, Ginger, Ginseng, Gotu Kola, Phenylalanine, Tyrosine

Morphine Sulfate (Morphine): Ephedra, Ginseng, Gotu Kola, Phenylalanine, Tyrosine

Moxifloxacin: Calcium, Green Tea, Iron, Licorice, Magnesium, Potassium, Probiotic Flora, Vitamin B_1, Vitamin K, Zinc

Mycophenolate: Echinacea, Magnesium, Turmeric/Curcumin

Nabumetone: Calcium, Cayenne, Chondroitin Sulfate, Chromium, Copper, Devil's Claw, Feverfew, Folic Acid, Ginger, Glucosamine Sulfate, Gotu Kola, Iron, Licorice, Melatonin, Omega-3 Fatty Acids, Potassium, Turmeric/Curcumin, Vitamin B_3, Vitamin B_6, Vitamin C, Zinc

Nadolol: Calcium, Carnitine, Chromium, Coenzyme Q10, Folic Acid, Magnesium, Melatonin, Potassium, Vitamin B_2, Vitamin B_3, Vitamin B_6, Vitamin C

Nadroparin: Cayenne, Chondroitin Sulfate, DHEA, Policosanol, Vitamin C

Nafcillin: Ginseng, Green Tea, Licorice, Probiotic Flora, Vitamin B$_1$, Vitamin K, Zinc

Nalidixic Acid: Calcium, Green Tea, Iron, Licorice, Magnesium, Potassium, Probiotic Flora, Vitamin B$_1$, Vitamin K, Zinc

Naloxone: Phenylalanine

Nandrolone: Echinacea

Naproxen: Calcium, Cayenne, Chondroitin Sulfate, Chromium, Copper, Devil's Claw, Feverfew, Folic Acid, Ginger, Glucosamine Sulfate, Gotu Kola, Iron, Licorice, Melatonin, Omega-3 Fatty Acids, Potassium, Turmeric/Curcumin, Vitamin B$_3$, Vitamin B$_6$, Vitamin C, Zinc

Naramycin, Naramycin A (Cycloheximide): Dang Gui, Echinacea

Naratriptan: 5-HTP, Feverfew, Tryptophan

Nateglinide: Chromium, Vitamin B$_3$

Nebivolol: Calcium, Carnitine, Chromium, Coenzyme Q10, Folic Acid, Magnesium, Melatonin, Potassium, Vitamin B$_2$, Vitamin B$_3$, Vitamin B$_6$, Vitamin C

Nefazodone: St. John's Wort

Nelfinavir: Copper, Garlic, St. John's Wort, Vitamin C

Neocycloheximide (Cycloheximide): Dang Gui, Echinacea

Neomycin: Alpha-Lipoic Acid, Beta-Carotene, Calcium, Eleuthero, Folic Acid, Ginger, Ginkgo, Horse Chestnut, Iron, Licorice, Magnesium, Potassium, Probiotic Flora, Vitamin A, Vitamin B$_1$, Vitamin B$_3$, Vitamin B$_6$, Vitamin B$_{12}$, Vitamin D, Vitamin K

NET EN (Norethindrone, Injectable): Magnesium, St. John's Wort, Vitamin B$_3$

Netilmicin: Alpha-Lipoic Acid, Calcium, Eleuthero, Ginger, Ginkgo, Horse Chestnut, Licorice, Magnesium, Potassium, Probiotic Flora, Vitamin B$_1$, Vitamin B$_6$, Vitamin B$_{12}$, Vitamin K

Nevirapine: St. John's Wort, Vitamin B$_2$

Niacin: Chromium, Omega-3 Fatty Acids

Nicardipine: Calcium, Carnitine, Folic Acid, Magnesium, St. John's Wort, Vitamin B$_6$, Vitamin D

Nicotine Transdermal Patches: Vitamin B$_3$

Nicoumalone: Bilberry, Cayenne, Chondroitin Sulfate, Coenzyme Q10, DHEA, Dang Gui, Devil's Claw, Feverfew, Garlic, Ginger, Ginkgo, Ginseng, Green Tea, Horse Chestnut, Kava, Licorice, Magnesium, Omega-3 Fatty Acids, Policosanol, Red Clover, Reishi, Saw Palmetto, St. John's Wort, Vitamin A, Vitamin B$_3$, Vitamin C, Vitamin E, Vitamin K, Zinc

Nifedipine: Black Cohosh, Calcium, Dang Gui, Magnesium, Saw Palmetto

Nilutamide: Black Cohosh, Vitamin D

Nimodipine: Calcium, Carnitine, Folic Acid, Magnesium, St. John's Wort, Vitamin B$_6$, Vitamin D

Nisoldipine: Calcium, Carnitine, Folic Acid, Magnesium, St. John's Wort, Vitamin B$_6$, Vitamin D

Nitrendipine: Calcium, Carnitine, Folic Acid, Magnesium, St. John's Wort, Vitamin B$_6$, Vitamin D

Nitrofurantoin: Licorice, Magnesium, Probiotic Flora, Vitamin B$_6$, Vitamin K, Zinc

Nitrofurazone: Licorice, Probiotic Flora, Vitamin K, Zinc

Nitrogen Mustard (Mechlorethamine): Astragalus, Carnitine, Echinacea, Eleuthero, Ginger, Selenium, Turmeric/Curcumin

Nitroglycerin: Arginine, Carnitine, Folic Acid, Vitamin C

Nitrous Oxide: Folic Acid, Vitamin B$_{12}$

Nizatidine: Calcium, Chromium, Copper, Folic Acid, Iron, Licorice, Magnesium, Vitamin B$_{12}$, Vitamin C, Zinc

Nor-Testosterone (Nandrolone): Echinacea

Nordihydroguaiaretic Acid (NDGA): Vitamin A

Norethindrone: Vitamin D, Vitex

Norethindrone, Oral: Magnesium, St. John's Wort

Norethisterone: Magnesium, St. John's Wort, Vitamin D

Norethisterone Enanthate (Norethindrone, Injectable): Magnesium, St. John's Wort, Vitamin B$_3$, Vitex

Norethisterone Enanthate + Estradiol Valerate: Magnesium, Vitamin B$_3$

Norfloxacin: Calcium, Green Tea, Iron, Licorice, Magnesium, Potassium, Probiotic Flora, Vitamin B$_1$, Vitamin K, Zinc

Norgestrel, Oral: Magnesium, St. John's Wort

Nortriptyline: 5-HTP, Coenzyme Q10, Milk Thistle, S-Adenosylmethionine (SAMe), St. John's Wort, Tryptophan, Tyrosine, Vitamin B$_1$, Vitamin B$_2$, Vitamin B$_3$, Vitamin B$_6$, Vitamin B$_{12}$, Zinc

Nystatin: Echinacea, Zinc

Nystatin, Topical: Echinacea

Ofloxacin: Calcium, Green Tea, Iron, Licorice, Magnesium, Potassium, Probiotic Flora, Vitamin B$_1$, Vitamin K, Zinc

Olanzapine: 5-HTP, Chromium, Echinacea, Ginkgo, Melatonin, Omega-3 Fatty Acids, Vitamin B$_3$, Vitamin B$_6$, Vitamin C, Zinc

Olestra: Vitamin K

Olmesartan: Alpha-Lipoic Acid, Potassium

Omeprazole: Beta-Carotene, Calcium, Chromium, Iron, Kava, St. John's Wort, Vitamin B$_{12}$, Vitamin E, Zinc

Opium and Belladonna: Ephedra, Ginseng, Gotu Kola, Phenylalanine, Tyrosine

Opium Tincture: Ephedra, Ginseng, Gotu Kola, Phenylalanine, Tyrosine

Opium, Camphor, Anise, Benzoic Acid, and Glycerin (Paregoric): Ephedra, Ginseng, Gotu Kola, Phenylalanine, Tyrosine

Oprelevkin: Echinacea

Orfloxacin: Calcium, Green Tea, Iron, Licorice, Magnesium, Potassium, Probiotic Flora, Vitamin B$_1$, Vitamin K, Zinc

Orlistat: Beta-Carotene, Coenzyme Q10, Vitamin A, Vitamin D, Vitamin E, Vitamin K

Ornidazole: Milk Thistle

Ouabain: Calcium, Cascara, Dang Gui, Eleuthero, Ephedra, Hawthorn, Licorice, Magnesium, Potassium, St. John's Wort

Oxacillin: Ginseng, Green Tea, Licorice, Probiotic Flora, Vitamin B$_1$, Vitamin K, Zinc

Oxaliplatin: Alpha-Lipoic Acid, Astragalus, Carnitine, Cayenne, Chondroitin Sulfate, Echinacea, Eleuthero, Ginger, Ginkgo, Ginseng, Milk Thistle, Selenium, St. John's Wort, Vitamin E

Oxandrolone: Echinacea

Oxaprozin: Calcium, Cayenne, Chondroitin Sulfate, Chromium, Copper, Devil's Claw, Feverfew, Folic Acid, Ginger, Glucosamine Sulfate, Gotu Kola, Iron, Licorice, Melatonin, Omega-3 Fatty Acids, Potassium, Turmeric/Curcumin, Vitamin B$_3$, Vitamin B$_6$, Vitamin C, Zinc

Oxazepam: DHEA, Gotu Kola, Melatonin, Valerian, Vitamin B$_3$

Oxcarbazepine (Oxycarbamazepine): Calcium, Carnitine, Copper, DHEA, Folic Acid, Ginkgo, Inositol, Kava, Milk Thistle, Omega-3 Fatty Acids, Valerian, Vitamin A, Vitamin B$_1$, Vitamin B$_2$, Vitamin B$_3$, Vitamin B$_6$, Vitamin B$_{12}$, Vitamin C, Vitamin D, Vitamin E, Vitamin K, Vitex, Zinc

Oxprenolol: Calcium, Carnitine, Chromium, Coenzyme Q10, Folic Acid, Magnesium, Melatonin, Potassium, Vitamin B_2, Vitamin B_3, Vitamin B_6, Vitamin C

Oxprenolol + Cyclopenthiazide: Arginine, Calcium, Coenzyme Q10, Potassium

Oxtriphylline: Potassium

Oxycodone: Ephedra, Ginseng, Gotu Kola, Phenylalanine, Tyrosine

Oxycodone + Acetaminophen: Ephedra, Garlic, Ginseng, Gotu Kola, Licorice, Milk Thistle, Phenylalanine, Tyrosine, Vitamin C

Oxycodone + Acetylsalicylic Acid: Calcium, Cayenne, Devil's Claw, Ephedra, Feverfew, Folic Acid, Ginkgo, Ginseng, Gotu Kola, Iron, Licorice, Melatonin, Milk Thistle, Phenylalanine, Policosanol, Potassium, Tyrosine, Vitamin B_2, Vitamin B_3, Vitamin C, Vitamin E, Vitamin K, Zinc

Oxymetholone: Echinacea

Oxymorphone: Ephedra, Ginseng, Gotu Kola, Phenylalanine, Tyrosine

Oxytetracycline: Calcium, Folic Acid, Iron, Magnesium, Potassium, Vitamin A, Vitamin B_1, Vitamin B_2, Vitamin B_3, Vitamin B_6, Vitamin C, Zinc

Oxytocin: Ephedra

***p*-Aminosalicylic Acid (Para-Aminosalicylic Acid):** Vitamin B_{12}

Paclitaxel: Aloe, Beta-Carotene, Echinacea, Eleuthero, Feverfew, Ginseng, Melatonin, Omega-3 Fatty Acids, PABA, St. John's Wort, Turmeric/Curcumin, Vitamin A, Vitamin C, Vitamin E

Paclitaxel, Protein-Bound: Echinacea, Eleuthero, Feverfew, Ginseng, St. John's Wort, Turmeric/Curcumin

Pamidronate: Calcium, Iron, Magnesium, Vitamin D, Zinc

Pancreatic Enzymes (Pancreatin): Folic Acid

Pancuronium: Magnesium

Pantoprazole: Beta-Carotene, Calcium, Chromium, Iron, Kava, St. John's Wort, Vitamin B_{12}, Zinc

Para-Aminosalicylic Acid (4-Aminosalicylic Acid): Vitamin B_{12}

Paregoric: Ephedra, Ginseng, Gotu Kola, Phenylalanine, Tyrosine

Pargyline: 5-HTP, Cayenne, Chromium, Eleuthero, Ephedra, Ginkgo, Kava, Licorice, Phenylalanine, *S*-Adenosylmethionine (SAMe), St. John's Wort, Tryptophan, Tyrosine, Vitamin B_3

Paromomycin: Alpha-Lipoic Acid, Calcium, Eleuthero, Ginger, Ginkgo, Horse Chestnut, Licorice, Magnesium, Potassium, Probiotic Flora, Vitamin B_1, Vitamin B_6, Vitamin B_{12}, Vitamin K

Paroxetine: 5-HTP, Chromium, Folic Acid, Ginkgo, Inositol, Omega-3 Fatty Acids, *S*-Adenosylmethionine (SAMe), St. John's Wort, Tryptophan, Vitamin B_3, Vitamin B_6, Vitamin B_{12}, Vitamin C, Zinc

PAS (Para-Aminosalicylic Acid): Vitamin B_{12}

Pegfilgastin: Echinacea

Pegylated Interferon Alpha-2b: Echinacea

Pegylated Liposomal Doxorubicin (Doxorubicin, Pegylated Liposomal): Alpha-Lipoic Acid, Carnitine, Coenzyme Q10, Feverfew, Garlic, Ginkgo, Green Tea, Hawthorn, Milk Thistle, Reishi, Selenium, St. John's Wort, Turmeric/Curcumin, Vitamin B_2, Vitamin B_6, Vitamin E

Pemetrexed: Echinacea, Eleuthero, Folic Acid, Vitamin B_1, Vitamin B_{12}

Pemetrexed + Cisplatin: Vitamin B_{12}

Pemoline: Reishi, Tyrosine

Penbutolol: Calcium, Carnitine, Chromium, Coenzyme Q10, Folic Acid, Magnesium, Melatonin, Potassium, Vitamin B_2, Vitamin B_3, Vitamin B_6, Vitamin C

Penicillamine: Copper, Iron, Magnesium, Vitamin B_6, Zinc

Penicillin G (Benzathine Penicillin): Ginseng, Green Tea, Licorice, Probiotic Flora, Vitamin B_1, Vitamin K, Zinc

Penicillin V (Pen VK): Ginseng, Green Tea, Licorice, Probiotic Flora, Vitamin B_1, Vitamin K, Zinc

Pentamidine: Magnesium

Pentazocine: Ephedra, Ginseng, Gotu Kola, Phenylalanine, Tyrosine

Pentobarbital: Calcium, Copper, DHEA, Folic Acid, Ginkgo, Gotu Kola, Inositol, Kava, Milk Thistle, Omega-3 Fatty Acids, Valerian, Vitamin A, Vitamin B_1, Vitamin B_2, Vitamin B_3, Vitamin B_6, Vitamin B_{12}, Vitamin C, Vitamin D, Vitamin E, Vitamin K, Vitex, Zinc

Pentostatin: Echinacea, Eleuthero, Folic Acid, Vitamin B_1

Pentoxifylline: Arginine, Cayenne, Coenzyme Q10, Policosanol, Vitamin E

Pericyazine: Coenzyme Q10, Milk Thistle, Vitamin B_2, Vitamin B_3, Vitamin C

Perindopril: Arginine, Cayenne, Iron, Omega-3 Fatty Acids, Potassium, Vitamin E, Zinc

Perphenazine: Coenzyme Q10, Milk Thistle, Vitamin B_2, Vitamin B_3, Vitamin C

Phenelzine: 5-HTP, Cayenne, Chromium, Eleuthero, Ephedra, Ginkgo, Ginseng, Licorice, Phenylalanine, *S*-Adenosylmethionine (SAMe), St. John's Wort, Tryptophan, Tyrosine, Vitamin B_6

Pheneturide: Calcium, Copper, DHEA, Folic Acid, Ginkgo, Inositol, Kava, Milk Thistle, Omega-3 Fatty Acids, Valerian, Vitamin A, Vitamin B_1, Vitamin B_2, Vitamin B_3, Vitamin B_6, Vitamin B_{12}, Vitamin C, Vitamin D, Vitamin E, Vitamin K, Vitex, Zinc

Phenformin: Alpha-Lipoic Acid, Astragalus, Bilberry, Calcium, Chromium, Coenzyme Q10, DHEA, Ephedra, Folic Acid, Garlic, Ginkgo, Ginseng, Glucosamine Sulfate, Gotu Kola, Horse Chestnut, Magnesium, Omega-3 Fatty Acids, Reishi, Turmeric/Curcumin, Vitamin B_3, Vitamin B_{12}

Phenindione: Bilberry, Cayenne, Chondroitin Sulfate, Coenzyme Q10, DHEA, Dang Gui, Devil's Claw, Feverfew, Garlic, Ginger, Ginkgo, Ginseng, Green Tea, Horse Chestnut, Kava, Licorice, Magnesium, Omega-3 Fatty Acids, Policosanol, Red Clover, Reishi, Saw Palmetto, St. John's Wort, Vitamin A, Vitamin B3, Vitamin C, Vitamin E, Vitamin K, Zinc

Phenobarbital (Phenobarbitone): Calcium, Carnitine, Copper, DHEA, Folic Acid, Ginkgo, Gotu Kola, Inositol, Kava, Milk Thistle, Omega-3 Fatty Acids, Reishi, Valerian, Vitamin A, Vitamin B_1, Vitamin B_2, Vitamin B_3, Vitamin B_6, Vitamin B_{12}, Vitamin C, Vitamin D, Vitamin E, Vitamin K, Vitex, Zinc

Phenprocoumon: Bilberry, Cayenne, Chondroitin Sulfate, Coenzyme Q10, DHEA, Dang Gui, Devil's Claw, Feverfew, Garlic, Ginger, Ginkgo, Ginseng, Green Tea, Horse Chestnut, Kava, Licorice, Magnesium, Omega-3 Fatty Acids, Policosanol, Red Clover, Reishi, Saw Palmetto, St. John's Wort, Vitamin A, Vitamin B_3, Vitamin C, Vitamin E, Vitamin K, Zinc

Phensuximide: Calcium, Carnitine, Copper, DHEA, Folic Acid, Ginkgo, Inositol, Kava, Milk Thistle, Omega-3 Fatty Acids, Valerian, Vitamin A, Vitamin B_1, Vitamin B_2, Vitamin B_3, Vitamin B_6, Vitamin B_{12}, Vitamin C, Vitamin D, Vitamin E, Vitamin K, Vitex, Zinc

Phenylalanine Mustard: Astragalus, Carnitine, Echinacea, Eleuthero, Ginger, Selenium

Phenylethylamine: Phenylalanine

Phenylpropanolamine: Potassium, Tyrosine

Phenylpropanolamine + Guaifenesin: Potassium, Tryosine

Phenytoin: Calcium, Carnitine, Copper, DHEA, Folic Acid, Ginkgo, Inositol, Kava, Milk Thistle, Omega-3 Fatty Acids, Valerian, Vitamin A, Vitamin B_1, Vitamin B_2, Vitamin B_3, Vitamin B_6, Vitamin B_{12}, Vitamin C, Vitamin D, Vitamin E, Vitamin K, Vitex, Zinc

Pindolol: Calcium, Carnitine, Chromium, Coenzyme Q10, Folic Acid, Magnesium, Melatonin, Potassium, Vitamin B_2, Vitamin B_3, Vitamin B_6, Vitamin C

Pioglitazone: Chromium, Vitamin B_3

Pipecuronium: Magnesium

Piperacillin: Ginseng, Green Tea, Licorice, Probiotic Flora, Vitamin B_1, Vitamin K, Zinc

Piperacillin + Tazobactam: Ginseng, Green Tea, Licorice, Probiotic Flora, Vitamin B_1, Vitamin K, Zinc

Pipobroman: Astragalus, Carnitine, Echinacea, Eleuthero, Selenium

Piracetam: Calcium, Carnitine, Copper, DHEA, Folic Acid, Ginkgo, Inositol, Kava, Milk Thistle, Omega-3 Fatty Acids, Valerian, Vitamin A, Vitamin B_1, Vitamin B_2, Vitamin B_3, Vitamin B_6, Vitamin B_{12}, Vitamin C, Vitamin D, Vitamin E, Vitamin K, Vitex, Zinc

Pirbuterol: Calcium, Magnesium, Potassium

Piroxicam: Calcium, Cayenne, Chondroitin Sulfate, Chromium, Copper, Devil's Claw, Feverfew, Folic Acid, Ginger, Glucosamine Sulfate, Gotu Kola, Iron, Licorice, Melatonin, Omega-3 Fatty Acids, Potassium, Turmeric/Curcumin, Vitamin B_3, Vitamin B_6, Vitamin C, Zinc

Pivampicillin: Carnitine

Pivanex: Carnitine

Pivmecillinam: Carnitine

***Plantago isphagula/ovata/psyllium* (Psyllium):** Potassium, Vitamin B_2

***Plantago* Seed Mucilage (Psyllium):** Potassium, Vitamin B_2

Plicamycin: Ginseng

Polycarbophil: Potassium, Vitamin B_2

Polyethylene Glycol: Potassium

Polyethylene Glycol–Electrolyte Solution: Potassium

Polyethylene Oxide Sheet Dressing: Aloe

Polythiazide: Calcium, Coenzyme Q10, Folic Acid, Ginkgo, Glucosamine Sulfate, Hawthorn, Licorice, Magnesium, Potassium, Vitamin B_2, Vitamin D, Zinc

Posaconazole: Echinacea, St. John's Wort

Pravastatin: Beta-Carotene, Carnitine, Coenzyme Q10, Garlic, Gotu Kola, Omega-3 Fatty Acids, Policosanol, Reishi, Selenium, St. John's Wort, Vitamin A, Vitamin B_3, Vitamin C, Vitamin E

Prazepam: DHEA, Gotu Kola, Melatonin, Valerian, Vitamin B_3

Praziquantl: Beta-Carotene, Vitamin A

Prazosin: Saw Palmetto, Vitamin B_3

Prednisolone: Calcium, Cayenne, Chromium, DHEA, Echinacea, Ephedra, Folic Acid, Horse Chestnut, Licorice, Magnesium, Melatonin, Omega-3 Fatty Acids, Potassium, Selenium, Vitamin A, Vitamin B_6, Vitamin C, Vitamin D, Vitamin K, Zinc

Prednisone: Calcium, Cayenne, Chromium, DHEA, Echinacea, Ephedra, Folic Acid, Horse Chestnut, Licorice, Magnesium, Melatonin, Omega-3 Fatty Acids, Potassium, Selenium, Vitamin A, Vitamin B_6, Vitamin C, Vitamin D, Vitamin K, Zinc

Pregabalin: Vitamin B_3

Primidone: Calcium, Carnitine, Copper, DHEA, Folic Acid, Ginkgo, Inositol, Kava, Milk Thistle, Omega-3 Fatty Acids, Valerian, Vitamin A, Vitamin B_1, Vitamin B_2, Vitamin B_3, Vitamin B_6, Vitamin B_{12}, Vitamin C, Vitamin D, Vitamin E, Vitamin K, Vitex, Zinc

Probenecid: Vitamin B_2, Vitamin B_3, Vitamin C

Probucol: Beta-Carotene

Procainamide: Cascara, Magnesium, Potassium

Procarbazine: 5-HTP, Cayenne, Chromium, Eleuthero, Ephedra, Ginkgo, Ginseng, Licorice, Phenylalanine, *S*-Adenosylmethionine (SAMe), St. John's Wort, Tryptophan, Tyrosine, Vitamin B_6

Prochlorperazine: Coenzyme Q10, Milk Thistle, Vitamin B_2, Vitamin B_3, Vitamin B_6, Vitamin C

Progesterone, Micronized: Vitamin D

Progestin(s)/Progestogen(s): Beta-Carotene, Calcium, Folic Acid, Magnesium, St. John's Wort, Vitamin A, Vitamin D

Promethazine: Coenzyme Q10, Milk Thistle, Vitamin B_2, Vitamin B_3, Vitamin C

Propiomazine: Coenzyme Q10, Milk Thistle, Vitamin B_2, Vitamin B_3, Vitamin C

Propoxyphene: Ephedra, Ginseng, Gotu Kola, Phenylalanine, Tyrosine

Propoxyphene + Acetaminophen: Ephedra, Ginseng, Gotu Kola, Phenylalanine, Tyrosine

Propranolol: Calcium, Carnitine, Chromium, Coenzyme Q10, Folic Acid, Magnesium, Melatonin, Policosanol, Potassium, Vitamin B_2, Vitamin B_3, Vitamin B_6, Vitamin C, Vitamin E

Propranolol + Bendrofluazide: Arginine, Calcium, Coenzyme Q10, Policosanol, Potassium, Vitamin C

Proteolytic Enzymes: Folic Acid

Protriptyline: 5-HTP, Coenzyme Q10, Milk Thistle, *S*-Adenosylmethionine (SAMe), St. John's Wort, Tryptophan, Tyrosine, Vitamin B_1, Vitamin B_2, Vitamin B_3, Vitamin B_6, Vitamin B_{12}, Zinc

Pseudoephedrine: Potassium

Psyllium Husk (Psyllium): Potassium, Vitamin B_2

Purgoxin (Digoxin): Calcium, Cascara, Dang Gui, Eleuthero, Ephedra, Hawthorn, Licorice, Magnesium, Potassium, St. John's Wort, Vitamin D

Pyrazinamide (PZA): Folic Acid, Milk Thistle, Vitamin B_3, Vitamin B_6, Vitamin C, Vitamin D

Pyrimethamine: Folic Acid, Iron

PZA: See *Pyrazinamide.*

Quazepam: DHEA, Gotu Kola, Melatonin, Valerian, Vitamin B_3

Quetiapine: 5-HTP, Chromium, Echinacea, Ginkgo, Melatonin, Omega-3 Fatty Acids, Vitamin B_3, Vitamin B_6, Vitamin C

Quinacrine: Vitamin B_2

Quinapril: Arginine, Cayenne, Iron, Omega-3 Fatty Acids, Potassium, Vitamin E, Zinc

Quinethazone: Calcium, Coenzyme Q10, Folic Acid, Ginkgo, Glucosamine Sulfate, Hawthorn, Licorice, Magnesium, Potassium, Vitamin B_2, Vitamin D, Zinc

Quinidine: Beta-Carotene, Cascara, Magnesium, Potassium

Rabeprazole: Beta-Carotene, Calcium, Chromium, Iron, Kava, St. John's Wort, Vitamin B_{12}, Zinc

Radiotherapy: Coenzyme Q10, Eleuthero, Ginseng, Melatonin, Vitamin B_3, Zinc; see also *Chemotherapy and Radiotherapy* in Drug Class Cross-Index.

Raloxifene: Black Cohosh, Dang Gui, Green Tea, Vitamin D

Raltitrexed (ZD-1694): Echinacea, Eleuthero, Folic Acid, Vitamin B_1

Ramipril: Arginine, Cayenne, Iron, Omega-3 Fatty Acids, Potassium, Vitamin E, Zinc

Ranitidine: Calcium, Chromium, Copper, Folic Acid, Iron, Licorice, Magnesium, Vitamin B_{12}, Vitamin C, Zinc

Ranitidine + Bismuth + Citrate: Calcium, Chromium, Copper, Folic Acid, Iron, Licorice, Magnesium, Vitamin B_{12}, Vitamin C, Zinc

Rasagiline: 5-HTP, Cayenne, Chromium, Eleuthero, Ephedra, Ginkgo, Kava, Licorice, Phenylalanine, S-Adenosylmethionine (SAMe), St. John's Wort, Tryptophan, Tyrosine

Recombinant Erythropoietin (Epoetin Alpha): Dang Gui, Iron, Vitamin B_6, Vitamin C

Repaglinide: Chromium, Vitamin B_3

Reserpine: Ephedra, Reishi

Reteplase, Recombinant: Astragalus

Ribavirin: S-Adenosylmethionine (SAMe)

Ribavirin + Interferon Alpha-2b: Iron, Licorice, Zinc

Rifampicin: Folic Acid, Milk Thistle, Vitamin B_3, Vitamin B_6, Vitamin C, Vitamin D, Vitamin E

Rimiterol: Calcium, Magnesium, Potassium

Risedronate: Calcium, Iron, Magnesium, Vitamin D, Zinc

Risperidone: 5-HTP, Chromium, Echinacea, Ginkgo, Melatonin, Omega-3 Fatty Acids, Vitamin B_3, Vitamin B_6, Vitamin C, Vitamin E

Ritonavir: Copper, Garlic, St. John's Wort, Vitamin C

Rizatriptan: 5-HTP, Feverfew, Tryptophan

Rocuronium: Magnesium

Rofecoxib: Calcium, Cayenne, Chondroitin Sulfate, Chromium, Copper, Devil's Claw, Feverfew, Folic Acid, Ginger, Glucosamine Sulfate, Gotu Kola, Iron, Licorice, Melatonin, Omega-3 Fatty Acids, Potassium, Turmeric/Curcumin, Vitamin B_3, Vitamin C, Zinc

Rosiglitazone: Chromium, Vitamin B_3

Rosuvastatin: Beta-Carotene, Carnitine, Coenzyme Q10, Garlic, Gotu Kola, Omega-3 Fatty Acids, Policosanol, Reishi, Selenium, St. John's Wort, Vitamin A, Vitamin B_3, Vitamin C, Vitamin E

Salazosulfapyridine (Sulfasalazine): Calcium, Folic Acid, Iron, Licorice, Magnesium, Omega-3 Fatty Acids, PABA, Probiotic Flora, Vitamin B_1, Vitamin B_6, Vitamin K, Zinc

Salbutamol: Calcium, Magnesium, Potassium

Salicylazosulfapyridine (Sulfasalazine): Calcium, Folic Acid, Iron, Licorice, Magnesium, Omega-3 Fatty Acids, PABA, Probiotic Flora, Vitamin B_1, Vitamin B_6, Vitamin K, Zinc

Salicylic Acid (Salsalate): Calcium, Folic Acid, Omega-3 Fatty Acids, Policosanol, Vitamin C, Vitamin K, Zinc

Salicylsalicylic Acid (Acetylsalicylic Acid): Bilberry, Calcium, Cayenne, Devil's Claw, Feverfew, Folic Acid, Garlic, Ginger, Ginkgo, Gotu Kola, Iron, Licorice, Melatonin, Milk Thistle, Omega-3 Fatty Acids, Policosanol, Potassium, S-Adenosylmethionine (SAMe), Vitamin B_2, Vitamin B_3, Vitamin C, Vitamin E, Vitamin K, Zinc

Salmeterol: Calcium, Magnesium, Potassium

Salsalate: Calcium, Cayenne, Chondroitin Sulfate, Chromium, Copper, Devil's Claw, Feverfew, Folic Acid, Ginger, Glucosamine Sulfate, Gotu Kola, Iron, Licorice, Melatonin, Omega-3 Fatty Acids, Policosanol, Potassium, Turmeric/Curcumin, Vitamin B_3, Vitamin B_6, Vitamin C, Vitamin K, Zinc

Saquinavir: Copper, Garlic, St. John's Wort, Vitamin C

Saquinavir + Ritonavir (SQV/RTV): Copper, Garlic, St. John's Wort, Vitamin C

Sargramostim: Echinacea

Scoline (Suxamethonium): Ginger, Magnesium

Scopolamine: Dang Gui, Vitamin B_1

Secale Alkaloids: Ephedra

Secnidazole: Milk Thistle

Secobarbital: DHEA, Gotu Kola, Valerian, Vitamin B_2

Selegiline: 5-HTP, Cayenne, Chromium, Ephedra, Folic Acid, Ginkgo, Iron, Kava, Licorice, Phenylalanine, S-Adenosylmethionine (SAMe), St. John's Wort, Tryptophan, Tyrosine, Vitamin B_2, Vitamin B_6, Vitex

Senna: Potassium

Sertraline: Chromium, Folic Acid, Ginkgo, Inositol, Omega-3 Fatty Acids, S-Adenosylmethionine (SAMe), St. John's Wort, Tryptophan, Vitamin B_3, Vitamin B_6, Vitamin B_{12}, Vitamin C, Zinc

Sevoflurane: Aloe, Alpha-Lipoic Acid, Ephedra, Milk Thistle, St. John's Wort, Valerian

Sibutramine: 5-HTP, Tryptophan

Sildenafil: Arginine

Silver Sulfadiazine: Calcium, Folic Acid, Licorice, Magnesium, PABA, Probiotic Flora, Vitamin B_1, Vitamin B_6, Vitamin K, Zinc

Simvastatin: Beta-Carotene, Carnitine, Coenzyme Q10, Garlic, Gotu Kola, Omega-3 Fatty Acids, Policosanol, Reishi, Selenium, St. John's Wort, Vitamin A, Vitamin B_3, Vitamin B_{12}, Vitamin C, Vitamin E

Simvastatin + Extended-Release Nicotinic Acid: Beta-Carotene, Carnitine, Coenzyme Q10, Garlic, Gotu Kola, Omega-3 Fatty Acids, Policosanol, Reishi, Selenium, St. John's Wort, Vitamin A, Vitamin B_3, Vitamin C, Vitamin E

Sodium Bicarbonate: Ephedra

Sodium Fluoride: Calcium, Vitamin D

Sodium Polystyrene Sulfonate: Magnesium

Sodium Salicylate: Calcium, Omega-3 Fatty Acids, Policosanol, Vitamin K

Sodium Sulfacetamide: Calcium, Folic Acid, Licorice, Magnesium, PABA, Probiotic Flora, Vitamin B_1, Vitamin B_6, Vitamin K, Zinc

Sodium Thiosalicylate: Calcium, Omega-3 Fatty Acids, Policosanol, Vitamin K

Sodium Valproate: Calcium, Carnitine, Copper, DHEA, Folic Acid, Ginkgo, Inositol, Kava, Milk Thistle, Omega-3 Fatty Acids, Valerian, Vitamin A, Vitamin B_1, Vitamin B_2, Vitamin B_3, Vitamin B_6, Vitamin B_{12}, Vitamin C, Vitamin D, Vitamin E, Vitamin K, Vitex, Zinc

Sotalol: Calcium, Carnitine, Cascara, Chromium, Coenzyme Q10, Folic Acid, Magnesium, Melatonin, Potassium, Vitamin B_2, Vitamin B_3, Vitamin B_6, Vitamin C

Sparfloxacin: Calcium, Green Tea, Iron, Licorice, Magnesium, Potassium, Probiotic Flora, Vitamin B_1, Vitamin K, Zinc

Spironolactone: Arginine, Calcium, Folic Acid, Glucosamine Sulfate, Licorice, Magnesium, Potassium, Zinc

Spironolactone + Hydrochlorothiazide: Arginine, Calcium, Coenzyme Q10, Folic Acid, Glucosamine Sulfate, Hawthorn, Licorice, Magnesium, Potassium, Vitamin D, Zinc

Stanozolol: Echinacea, Iron

Staphcillin (Methicillin): Ginseng, Green Tea, Licorice, Probiotic Flora, Vitamin B_1, Vitamin K, Zinc

Stavudine: Aloe, Carnitine, Coenzyme Q10, DHEA, Reishi, Vitamin B_1, Vitamin B_2, Vitamin B_{12}, Zinc

Streptokinase: Astragalus

Streptomycin: Alpha-Lipoic Acid, Calcium, Eleuthero, Ginger, Ginkgo, Horse Chestnut, Licorice, Magnesium, Potassium, Probiotic Flora, Vitamin B_1, Vitamin B_6, Vitamin B_{12}, Vitamin C, Vitamin K

Streptozocin: Astragalus, Carnitine, Echinacea, Eleuthero, Selenium

Succinylcholine (Suxamethonium): Ginger, Magnesium

Sucralfate: Calcium, Vitamin D

Sulfadoxine: Calcium, Folic Acid, Licorice, Magnesium, PABA, Probiotic Flora, Vitamin B_1, Vitamin B_6, Vitamin K, Zinc

Sulfadoxine + Pyrimethamine: Folic Acid, Iron, Vitamin B_2

Sulfaguanidine: Ginger

Sulfamethoxazole: Calcium, Folic Acid, Licorice, Magnesium, PABA, Potassium, Probiotic Flora, Vitamin B_1, Vitamin B_6, Vitamin K, Zinc

Sulfanilamide: Calcium, Folic Acid, Licorice, Magnesium, PABA, Probiotic Flora, Vitamin B_1, Vitamin B_6, Vitamin K, Zinc

Sulfasalazine (Sulphasalazine): Calcium, Folic Acid, Iron, Licorice, Magnesium, Omega-3 Fatty Acids, PABA, Probiotic Flora, Vitamin B_1, Vitamin B_6, Vitamin K, Zinc

Sulfinpyrazone: Vitamin B_2, Vitamin B_3

Sulfisoxazole: Calcium, Folic Acid, Licorice, Magnesium, PABA, Probiotic Flora, Vitamin B_1, Vitamin B_6, Vitamin K, Zinc

Sulindac: Calcium, Cayenne, Chondroitin Sulfate, Chromium, Copper, Devil's Claw, Feverfew, Folic Acid, Ginger, Glucosamine Sulfate, Gotu Kola, Iron, Licorice, Melatonin, Omega-3 Fatty Acids, Potassium, Turmeric/Curcumin, Vitamin B_3, Vitamin B_6, Vitamin C, Zinc

Sumatriptan: 5-HTP, Feverfew, Tryptophan

Surgery: Aloe, Garlic

Suxamethonium: Ginger, Magnesium

T_3 (L-Triiodothyronine): Alpha-Lipoic Acid, Calcium, Carnitine, Coenzyme Q10, DHEA, Iron, Tyrosine, Vitamin B_2

T_4 (Levothyroxine): Alpha-Lipoic Acid, Calcium, Carnitine, Coenzyme Q10, DHEA, Iron, Tyrosine, Vitamin B_2

T_4 + T_3 (L-Thyroxine + L-Triiodothyronine): Alpha-Lipoic Acid, Calcium, Carnitine, Coenzyme Q10, DHEA, Iron, Tyrosine, Vitamin B_2

Tacrine: Echinacea, Melatonin, Milk Thistle, Vitamin C

Tacrolimus (FK-506): Echinacea, St. John's Wort

Tadalafil: Arginine

Tamoxifen: Aloe, Black Cohosh, Calcium, Dang Gui, Feverfew, Ginseng, Green Tea, Melatonin, Omega-3 Fatty Acids, Vitamin A, Vitamin C, Vitamin E

Tamsulosin: Saw Palmetto, Vitamin B_3

Telmisartan: Alpha-Lipoic Acid, Potassium

Temazepam: DHEA, Gotu Kola, Melatonin, Valerian, Vitamin B_3

Temozolomide: Astragalus, Carnitine, Echinacea, Eleuthero, Selenium

Teniposide: St. John's Wort

Tenofovir: Aloe, Carnitine, Coenzyme Q10, DHEA, Reishi, Vitamin B_1, Vitamin B_2, Vitamin B_{12}, Zinc

Terazosin: Saw Palmetto, Vitamin B_3

Terbutaline: Potassium

Testolactone (Testolacton): Beta-Carotene, DHEA, Vitamin A, Zinc

Testosterone Cypionate (Methyltestosterone): Beta-Carotene, DHEA, Vitamin A, Zinc

Testosterone Undecanoate (Testosterone): Beta-Carotene, DHEA, Zinc

Tetracycline: Calcium, Folic Acid, Iron, Magnesium, Potassium, Vitamin A, Vitamin B_1, Vitamin B_2, Vitamin B_3, Vitamin B_6, Vitamin C, Zinc

Tetrathiomolybdate: Copper, Zinc

Theophylline: Arginine, Cayenne, Ephedra, Magnesium, Melatonin, Potassium, St. John's Wort, Vitamin B_6

Thiethylperazine: Milk Thistle

Thioguanine (6-TG): Echinacea, Eleuthero, Folic Acid, Vitamin B_1, Vitamin B_3

Thiopental: DHEA, Gotu Kola, Valerian, Vitamin B_2

Thiopentone: DHEA, Ginger, Gotu Kola, Valerian, Vitamin B_2

Thioproperazine: Coenzyme Q10, Milk Thistle, Vitamin B_2, Vitamin B_3, Vitamin C

Thioridazine: Coenzyme Q10, Milk Thistle, Potassium, Vitamin A, Vitamin B_2, Vitamin B_3, Vitamin C, Vitamin D

Thiotepa: Astragalus, Carnitine, Echinacea, Eleuthero, Selenium

Thyroxine (Levothyroxine): Alpha-Lipoic Acid, Calcium, Carnitine, Coenzyme Q10, DHEA, Iron, Tyrosine, Vitamin B_2

Tiagabine: Carnitine, Folic Acid, Vitamin B_3

Ticarcillin: Ginseng, Green Tea, Licorice, Probiotic Flora, Vitamin B_1, Vitamin K, Zinc

Ticarcillin + Clavulanic Acid: Ginseng, Green Tea, Licorice, Probiotic Flora, Vitamin B_1, Vitamin K, Zinc

Ticlopidine: Bilberry, Cayenne, Feverfew, Garlic, Ginger, Ginkgo, Omega-3 Fatty Acids, Policosanol, S-Adenosylmethionine (SAMe)

Tiludronate: Calcium, Iron, Magnesium, Vitamin D, Zinc

Timolol: Calcium, Carnitine, Chromium, Coenzyme Q10, Folic Acid, Magnesium, Melatonin, Potassium, Vitamin B_2, Vitamin B_3, Vitamin B_6, Vitamin C

Tinidazole: Milk Thistle

Tinzaparin: Cayenne, Chondroitin Sulfate, DHEA, Policosanol, Vitamin C

Tipranavir: Copper, Garlic, St. John's Wort, Vitamin C

Tirofiban: Cayenne, Ginger, Policosanol, S-Adenosylmethionine (SAMe)

TMC114 (Darunavir): Copper, Garlic, St. John's Wort, Vitamin C

Tobramycin: Alpha-Lipoic Acid, Calcium, Eleuthero, Ginger, Ginkgo, Horse Chestnut, Licorice, Magnesium, Potassium, Probiotic Flora, Vitamin B_1, Vitamin B_6, Vitamin B_{12}, Vitamin K

Tobramycin and Dexamethasone Ophthalmic Ointment (Dexamethasone + Tobramycin): Alpha-Lipoac Acid, Calcium, Eleuthero, Ginger, Ginkgo, Horse Chestnut, Licorice, Magnesium, Potassium, Probiotic Flora, Vitamin B_1, Vitamin B_6, Vitamin B_{12}, Vitamin K

Tolazamide: Aloe, Alpha-Lipoic Acid, Astragalus, Bilberry, Chromium, Coenzyme Q10, DHEA, Ephedra, Garlic, Ginkgo, Ginseng, Glucosamine Sulfate, Gotu Kola, Horse Chestnut, Magnesium, Omega-3 Fatty Acids, Reishi, Turmeric/Curcumin, Vitamin B_3

Tolbutamide: Aloe, Alpha-Lipoic Acid, Astragalus, Bilberry, Chromium, Coenzyme Q10, DHEA, Ephedra, Garlic, Ginkgo, Ginseng, Glucosamine Sulfate, Gotu Kola, Horse Chestnut, Magnesium, Omega-3 Fatty Acids, Reishi, Turmeric/Curcumin, Vitamin B_3

Tolmetin: Calcium, Cayenne, Chondroitin Sulfate, Chromium, Copper, Devil's Claw, Feverfew, Folic Acid, Ginger, Glucosamine Sulfate, Gotu Kola, Iron, Licorice, Melatonin, Omega-3 Fatty Acids, Potassium, Turmeric/Curcumin, Vitamin B_3, Vitamin B_6, Vitamin C, Zinc

Topiramate: Calcium, Carnitine, Copper, DHEA, Folic Acid, Ginkgo, Inositol, Kava, Milk Thistle, Omega-3 Fatty Acids, Potassium, Valerian, Vitamin A, Vitamin B_1, Vitamin B_2, Vitamin B_3, Vitamin B_6, Vitamin B_{12}, Vitamin C, Vitamin D, Vitamin E, Vitamin K, Vitex, Zinc

Topotecan: Feverfew

Toremifene: Black Cohosh, Dang Gui, Green Tea

Torsemide: Calcium, Folic Acid, Ginseng, Glucosamine Sulfate, Licorice, Magnesium, Potassium, Vitamin B_1, Vitamin B_6, Vitamin C, Zinc

Trandolapril: Arginine, Cayenne, Iron, Omega-3 Fatty Acids, Potassium, Vitamin E, Zinc

Trandolapril + Verapamil: Arginine, Calcium, Coenzyme Q10, Magnesium, Melatonin, Potassium, St. John's Wort, Vitamin E

Tranylcypromine: 5-HTP, Cayenne, Chromium, Eleuthero, Ephedra, Ginkgo, Ginseng, Licorice, Melatonin, Phenylalanine, S-Adenosylmethionine (SAMe), St. John's Wort, Tryptophan, Tyrosine, Vitamin B_6

Trastuzumab: Cascara, Green Tea

Trazodone: 5-HTP, Ginkgo, St. John's Wort

Trenbolone: Echinacea

Tretinoin: Beta-Carotene, Calcium, Carnitine, Vitamin A, Vitamin E

Triamcinolone + Nystatin: Licorice

Triamcinolone, Oral: Calcium, Cayenne, Chromium, DHEA, Echinacea, Ephedra, Folic Acid, Green Tea, Horse Chestnut, Licorice, Magnesium, Melatonin, Omega-3 Fatty Acids, Potassium, Selenium, Vitamin A, Vitamin B_6, Vitamin C, Vitamin D, Vitamin K, Zinc

Triamcinolone, Topical: Aloe, Calcium, Green Tea, Licorice, Vitamin C

Triamterene: Arginine, Calcium, Folic Acid, Glucosamine Sulfate, Magnesium, Potassium, Zinc

Triamterene + Hydrochlorothiazide: Arginine, Calcium, Coenzyme Q10, Folic Acid, Glucosamine Sulfate, Hawthorn, Licorice, Magnesium, Potassium, Vitamin D, Zinc

Triazolam: DHEA, Gotu Kola, Kava, Melatonin, St. John's Wort, Valerian, Vitamin B_3

Trichlormethiazide: Calcium, Coenzyme Q10, Folic Acid, Ginkgo, Glucosamine Sulfate, Hawthorn, Licorice, Magnesium, Potassium, Vitamin B_2, Vitamin D, Zinc

Trientine (Trien): Copper, Iron

Trienthylene Tetramine: Copper, Iron

Trifluoperazine: Coenzyme Q10, Milk Thistle, Vitamin B_2, Vitamin B_3, Vitamin C

Triflupromazine: Coenzyme Q10, Milk Thistle, Vitamin B_2, Vitamin B_3, Vitamin C

Trimethadione: Carnitine, Folic Acid

Trimethaphan: Vitamin B_3

Trimethoprim: Folic Acid, Licorice, Probiotic Flora, Vitamin B_2, Vitamin K, Zinc

Trimethoprim-Sulfamethoxazole: Calcium, Folic Acid, Licorice, Magnesium, PABA, Potassium, Probiotic Flora, Vitamin B_1, Vitamin B_2, Vitamin B_6, Vitamin C, Vitamin K, Zinc

Trimipramine: 5-HTP, Coenzyme Q10, Echinacea, Milk Thistle, Potassium, S-Adenosylmethionine (SAMe), St. John's Wort, Tryptophan, Tyrosine, Vitamin B_1, Vitamin B_2, Vitamin B_3, Vitamin B_6, Vitamin B_{12}, Zinc

Triperidol: Milk Thistle, Phenylalanine

Triple Sulfa: Calcium, Folic Acid, Licorice, Magnesium, PABA, Probiotic Flora, Vitamin B_1, Vitamin B_6, Vitamin K, Zinc

Triptorelin: Black Cohosh, Melatonin, Vitamin D

Troleandomycin: Calcium, Green Tea, Magnesium, Probiotic Flora, Vitamin B_1, Vitamin B_6, Vitamin K, Zinc

Trovafloxacin: Calcium, Green Tea, Iron, Licorice, Magnesium, Potassium, Probiotic Flora, Vitamin B_1, Vitamin K, Zinc

Tubocurarine: Magnesium

Tulobuterol: Calcium, Magnesium, Potassium

Tumor Necrosis Factor Alpha (TNF-α): Melatonin, Omega-3 Fatty Acids

UFH (Heparin, Unfractionated): Calcium, Cayenne, Chondroitin Sulfate, DHEA, Omega-3 Fatty Acids, Policosanol, Potassium, Vitamin C, Vitamin D

Uracil Mustard: Astragalus, Carnitine, Echinacea, Eleuthero, Ginger, Selenium

Uramustine (Uracil Mustard): Astragalus, Carnitine, Echinacea, Eleuthero, Ginger, Selenium

Urokinase: Astragalus

Ursodeoxycholic Acid (UDCA): S-Adenosylmethionine (SAMe), Vitamin B_3

Valciclovir: Astragalus

Valdecoxib: Calcium, Cayenne, Chondroitin Sulfate, Chromium, Copper, Devil's Claw, Feverfew, Folic Acid, Ginger, Glucosamine Sulfate, Gotu Kola, Iron, Licorice, Melatonin, Omega-3 Fatty Acids, Potassium, Turmeric/Curcumin, Vitamin B_3, Vitamin C, Zinc

Valproate Semisodium/Valproate Sodium: Calcium, Carnitine, Copper, DHEA, Folic Acid, Ginkgo, Inositol, Kava, Milk Thistle, Omega-3 Fatty Acids, Selenium, Valerian, Vitamin A, Vitamin B_1, Vitamin B_2, Vitamin B_3, Vitamin B_6, Vitamin B_{12}, Vitamin C, Vitamin D, Vitamin E, Vitamin K, Vitex, Zinc

Valproic Acid (Valproate): Calcium, Carnitine, Copper, DHEA, Folic Acid, Ginkgo, Inositol, Kava, Milk Thistle, Omega-3 Fatty Acids, Selenium, Valerian, Vitamin A, Vitamin B_1, Vitamin B_2, Vitamin B_3, Vitamin B_6, Vitamin B_{12}, Vitamin C, Vitamin D, Vitamin E, Vitamin K, Vitex, Zinc

Valsartan: Alpha-Lipoic Acid, Potassium

Valsartan + Hydrochlorothiazide: Alpha-Lipoic Acid, Potassium

Vancomycin: Licorice, Probiotic Flora, Vitamin K, Zinc

Vardenafil: Arginine

Vecuronium: Ginger, Magnesium

Venlafaxine: 5-HTP, Folic Acid, Ginkgo, Omega-3 Fatty Acids, S-Adenosylmethionine (SAMe), St. John's Wort, Tryptophan, Vitamin B_3, Vitamin B_6, Vitamin B_{12}

Verapamil: Calcium, Carnitine, Folic Acid, Magnesium, Melatonin, St. John's Wort, Vitamin B_6, Vitamin D, Vitamin E

Vidarabine: Methionine, Reishi, S-Adenosylmethionine (SAMe)

Vigabatrin: Calcium, Carnitine, Copper, DHEA, Folic Acid, Ginkgo, Inositol, Kava, Milk Thistle, Omega-3 Fatty Acids, Valerian, Vitamin A, Vitamin B_1, Vitamin B_2, Vitamin B_3, Vitamin B_6, Vitamin B_{12}, Vitamin C, Vitamin D, Vitamin E, Vitamin K, Vitex, Zinc

Vinblastine: Echinacea, Eleuthero, Feverfew, Ginseng, St. John's Wort, Turmeric/Curcumin

Vincristine: Alpha-Lipoic Acid, Echinacea, Eleuthero, Feverfew, Ginseng, St. John's Wort, Turmeric/Curcumin

Vincristine + Dactinomycin + Cyclophosphamide: Feverfew

Vinorelbine: Echinacea, Eleuthero, St. John's Wort

Voriconazole: Echinacea, St. John's Wort

Warfarin: Bilberry, Cayenne, Chondroitin Sulfate, Coenzyme Q10, DHEA, Dang Gui, Devil's Claw, Echinacea, Feverfew, Garlic, Ginger, Ginkgo, Ginseng, Green Tea, Horse Chestnut, Iron, Kava, Licorice, Magnesium, Omega-3 Fatty Acids, Policosanol, Red Clover, Reishi, Saw Palmetto, St. John's Wort, Vitamin A, Vitamin B_3, Vitamin C, Vitamin D, Vitamin E, Vitamin K, Zinc

Zafirlukast: Melatonin

Zalcitabine (Dideoxycytidine): Aloe, Carnitine, Coenzyme Q10, Copper, DHEA, Reishi, Vitamin B_1, Vitamin B_2, Vitamin B_{12}, Zinc

Zaleplon: Gotu Kola, Melatonin, Valerian

Zidovudine (AZT, ZDV): Aloe, Carnitine, Coenzyme Q10, Copper, DHEA, Folic Acid, Reishi, Vitamin B_1, Vitamin B_2, Vitamin B_{12}, Vitamin E, Zinc

Zidovudine + Lamivudine (AZT + 3TC): Aloe, Carnitine, Coenzyme Q10, Copper, DHEA, Folic Acid, Reishi, Vitamin B_1, Vitamin B_2, Vitamin B_{12}, Vitamin E, Zinc

Ziprasidone: 5-HTP, Chromium, Echinacea, Ginkgo, Melatonin, Omega-3 Fatty Acids, Vitamin B_3, Vitamin B_6, Vitamin C

Zoledronic Acid (Zoledronate): Calcium, Iron, Magnesium, Vitamin D, Zinc

Zolmitriptan: 5-HTP, Feverfew, Tryptophan

Zolpidem: 5-HTP, Gotu Kola, Melatonin, Valerian

Zonisamide: Calcium, Carnitine, Copper, DHEA, Folic Acid, Ginkgo, Inositol, Kava, Milk Thistle, Omega-3 Fatty Acids, Potassium, Valerian, Vitamin A, Vitamin B_1, Vitamin B_2, Vitamin B_3, Vitamin B_6, Vitamin B_{12}, Vitamin C, Vitamin D, Vitamin E, Vitamin K, Vitex, Zinc

3TC (lamivudine): Aloe, Carnitine, Coenzyme Q10, Copper, DHEA, Reishi, Vitamin B_1, Vitamin B_2, Vitamin B_{12}, Zinc

A-Spas S/L (hyoscyamine): Iron

A/T/S (erythromycin topical): Calcium, Green Tea, Magnesium, Probiotic Flora, Vitamin B_1, Vitamin B_6, Vitamin K, Zinc

Abbokinase (urokinase): Astragalus

Abbokinase Open-Cath (urokinase): Astragalus

Abilify (aripiprazole): 5-HTP, Chromium, Echinacea, Ginkgo, Melatonin, Omega-3 Fatty Acids, Vitamin B_3, Vitamin B_6, Vitamin C

Abilitat (aripiprazole): 5-HTP, Chromium, Echinacea, Ginkgo, Melatonin, Omega-3 Fatty Acids, Vitamin B_3, Vitamin B_6, Vitamin C

Abraxane (paclitaxel, protein-bound): Echinacea, Eleuthero, Feverfew, Ginseng, St. John's Wort, Turmeric/Curcumin

Accolate (zafirlukast): Melatonin

Accoleit (zafirlukast): Melatonin

Accupril (quinapril): Arginine, Cayenne, Iron, Omega-3 Fatty Acids, Potassium, Vitamin E, Zinc

Accutane (isotretinoin): Beta-Carotene, Calcium, Carnitine, Vitamin A, Vitamin E

Aceon (perindopril): Arginine, Cayenne, Iron, Omega-3 Fatty Acids, Potassium, Vitamin E, Zinc

Acezide (captopril + hydrochlorothiazide): Arginine, Calcium, Cayenne, Coenzyme Q10, Glucosamine Sulfate, Hawthorn, Licorice, Magnesium, Potassium, Vitamin D, Zinc

Achromycin (tetracycline): Calcium, Folic Acid, Iron, Magnesium, Potassium, Vitamin A, Vitamin B_1, Vitamin B_2, Vitamin B_3, Vitamin B_6, Vitamin C, Zinc

AcipHex (rabeprazole): Beta-Carotene, Calcium, Chromium, Iron, Kava, St. John's Wort, Vitamin B_{12}, Zinc

Acitrom (nicoumalone): Bilberry, Cayenne, Chondroitin Sulfate, Coenzyme Q10, DHEA, Dang Gui, Devil's Claw, Feverfew, Garlic, Ginger, Ginkgo, Ginseng, Green Tea, Horse Chestnut, Kava, Licorice, Magnesium, Omega-3 Fatty Acids, Policosanol, Red Clover, Reishi, Saw Palmetto, St. John's Wort, Vitamin A, Vitamin B_3, Vitamin C, Vitamin E, Vitamin K, Zinc

Aclovate (alclometasone): Aloe, Green Tea, Licorice, Vitamin C

Acti-Aid (cycloheximide): Dang Gui, Echinacea

Acticort 100 (hydrocortisone 17-butyrate/acetate/probutate/valerate): Aloe, Green Tea, Licorice, Vitamin C

ActiDione (cycloheximide): Dang Gui, Echinacea

Actigall (ursodeoxycholic acid): S-Adenosylmethionine (SAMe), Vitamin B_3

Actimmune (interferon gamma-1b): Echinacea

Actin-N (nitrofurazone): Licorice, Probiotic Flora, Vitamin K, Zinc

Actiq Oral Transmucosal (fentanyl): Ephedra, Ginger, Ginseng, Gotu Kola, Magnesium, Phenylalanine, Tyrosine

Actisite (tetracycline): Calcium, Folic Acid, Iron, Magnesium, Potassium, Vitamin A, Vitamin B_1, Vitamin B_2, Vitamin B_3, Vitamin B_6, Vitamin C, Zinc

Actispray (cycloheximide): Dang Gui, Echinacea

Activase (alteplase, recombinant, parenteral): Astragalus

Activella (estradiol + norethindrone [oral]): Arginine, Black Cohosh, Boron, Calcium, Copper, DHEA, Dang Gui, Magnesium, Melatonin, Milk Thistle, St. John's Wort, Vitamin B_6, Vitamin D, Vitamin E, Vitex, Zinc

Actonel (risedronate): Calcium, Iron, Magnesium, Vitamin D, Zinc

Actos (pioglitazone): Chromium, Vitamin B_3

Acular ophthalmic (ketorolac): Vitamin B_6

Acutrim (phenylpropanolamine): Potassium, Tyrosine

Aczone (dapsone): Folic Acid, Licorice, PABA, Probiotic Flora, Vitamin E, Vitamin K, Zinc

Adalat LA (nifedipine): Black Cohosh, Calcium, Dang Gui, Magnesium, Saw Palmetto

Adalat Retard (nifedipine): Black Cohosh, Calcium, Dang Gui, Magnesium, Saw Palmetto

Adalat (nifedipine): Black Cohosh, Calcium, Dang Gui, Magnesium, Saw Palmetto

Adapin (doxepin): 5-HTP, Coenzyme Q10, Echinacea, Milk Thistle, S-Adenosylmethionine (SAMe), St. John's Wort, Tryptophan, Tyrosine, Vitamin B_1, Vitamin B_2, Vitamin B_3, Vitamin B_6, Vitamin B_{12}, Zinc

Adcomag trisil (magnesium trisilicate): Calcium, Cayenne, Chromium, Copper, Folic Acid, Iron, Magnesium, Vitamin A, Vitamin B_1, Vitamin D, Vitex, Zinc

Adderall (amphetamine + dextroamphetamine): 5-HTP, Magnesium, Omega-3 Fatty Acids, Potassium, Reishi, Tyrosine, Vitamin B_6, Vitamin C, Zinc

Adipine MR (nifedipine): Black Cohosh, Calcium, Dang Gui, Magnesium, Saw Palmetto

Adrenalin (epinephrine): Magnesium, Potassium, Vitamin C

Adrenalin Chloride Solution, injectable (epinephrine): Magnesium, Potassium, Vitamin C

Adrenaline, Epi (epinephrine): Magnesium, Potassium, Vitamin C

Adriamycin (doxorubicin): Aloe, Alpha-Lipoic Acid, Carnitine, Coenzyme Q10, Feverfew, Garlic, Ginkgo, Ginseng, Green Tea, Hawthorn, Melatonin, Milk Thistle, Omega-3 Fatty Acids, Reishi, Selenium, St. John's Wort, Turmeric/Curcumin, Vitamin A, Vitamin B_2, Vitamin C, Vitamin D, Vitamin E

Adrucil (fluorouracil): Aloe, Beta-Carotene, Echinacea, Eleuthero, Folic Acid, Garlic, Ginkgo, Ginseng, Melatonin, Omega-3 Fatty Acids, Vitamin A, Vitamin B_1, Vitamin B_3, Vitamin B_6, Vitamin C, Vitamin E

Advanced Formula Di-Gel Tablets (calcium carbonate + magnesium hydroxide + simethicone): Calcium, Cayenne, Chromium, Copper, Folic Acid, Iron, Magnesium, Vitamin A, Vitamin B_1, Vitamin D, Vitex, Zinc

Advicor (lovastatin + niacin): Beta-Carotene, Carnitine, Coenzyme Q10, Garlic, Gotu Kola, Omega-3 Fatty Acids, Policosanol, Reishi, Selenium, St. John's Wort, Vitamin A, Vitamin B_3, Vitamin C, Vitamin E

Advil (ibuprofen): Calcium, Cayenne, Chondroitin Sulfate, Chromium, Copper, Devil's Claw, Feverfew, Folic Acid, Ginger, Glucosamine Sulfate, Gotu Kola, Iron, Licorice, Melatonin, Omega-3 Fatty Acids, Potassium, Turmeric/Curcumin, Vitamin B_3, Vitamin B_6, Vitamin C, Zinc

Aeroseb-Dex (dexamethasone): Aloe, Calcium, Ephedra, Green Tea, Licorice, Vitamin C

Aeroseb-HC (hydrocortisone 17-butyrate/acetate/probutate/valerate): Aloe, Green Tea, Licorice, Vitamin C

Afrinol (pseudoephedrine): Potassium

Agenerase (amprenavir): Copper, Garlic, St. John's Wort, Vitamin C

Aggrastat (tirofiban): Cayenne, Ginger, Policosanol, S-Adenosylmethionine (SAMe)

Aggrenox (acetylsalicylic acid + dipyridamole [extended-release]): Bilberry, Calcium, Cayenne, Devil's Claw, Feverfew, Folic Acid, Garlic, Ginger, Ginkgo, Gotu Kola, Iron, Licorice, Melatonin, Milk Thistle, Omega-3 Fatty Acids, Policosanol, Potassium, S-Adenosylmethionine (SAMe), Vitamin B_2, Vitamin B_3, Vitamin C, Vitamin E, Vitamin K, Zinc

Agoral (mineral oil): Beta-Carotene, Calcium, Potassium, Vitamin A, Vitamin D, Vitamin E, Vitamin K

Agrylin (anagrelide)

Airomir (salbutamol): Potassium

AK-Sulf (sodium sulfacetamide): Calcium, Folic Acid, Licorice, Magnesium, PABA, Probiotic Flora, Vitamin B_1, Vitamin B_6, Vitamin K, Zinc

Akne-Mycin (erythromycin topical): Calcium, Green Tea, Magnesium, Probiotic Flora, Vitamin B_1, Vitamin B_6, Vitamin K, Zinc

AKTob (tobramycin): Alpha-Lipoic Acid, Calcium, Eleuthero, Ginger, Ginkgo, Horse Chestnut, Licorice, Magnesium, Potassium, Probiotic Flora, Vitamin B_1, Vitamin B_6, Vitamin B_{12}, Vitamin K

Ala-Cort (hydrocortisone 17-butyrate/acetate/probutate/valerate): Aloe, Green Tea, Licorice, Vitamin C

Ala-Scalp HP (hydrocortisone 17-butyrate/acetate/probutate/valerate): Aloe, Green Tea, Licorice, Vitamin C

Albuterol Inhaled (albuterol): Calcium, Magnesium, Potassium

Aldactazide (spironolactone + hydrochlorothiazide): Arginine, Calcium, Coenzyme Q10, Folic Acid, Glucosamine Sulfate, Hawthorn, Licorice, Magnesium, Potassium, Vitamin D, Zinc

Aldactone (spironolactone): Arginine, Calcium, Folic Acid, Glucosamine Sulfate, Licorice, Magnesium, Potassium, Zinc

Aldoclor (methyldopa + chlorothiazide): Arginine, Coenzyme Q10, Ephedra, Potassium, Vitamin B_{12}

Aldomet (methyldopa): Ephedra, Iron, Vitamin B_{12}

Aldoril (methyldopa + hydrochlorothiazide): Arginine, Coenzyme Q10, Ephedra, Potassium, Vitamin B12

Alenic Alka (aluminum hydroxide + magnesium trisilicate): Calcium, Cayenne, Chromium, Copper, Folic Acid, Iron, Magnesium, Vitamin A, Vitamin B_1, Vitamin C, Vitamin D, Vitex, Zinc

Alesse (ethinyl estradiol + levonorgestrel): Arginine, Calcium, Copper, DHEA, Dang Gui, Folic Acid, Iron, Licorice, Magnesium, Melatonin, Milk Thistle, S-Adenosylmethionine (SAMe), Selenium, St. John's Wort, Tyrosine, Vitamin A, Vitamin B_1, Vitamin B_2, Vitamin B_3, Vitamin B_6, Vitamin B_{12}, Vitamin C, Vitamin E, Vitex, Zinc

Alferon N (interferon alpha): Astragalus, Echinacea, Iron, Licorice, Zinc

Alimta (pemetrexed): Echinacea, Eleuthero, Folic Acid, Vitamin B_1, Vitamin B_{12}

Alka-Seltzer (aspirin + citric acid + sodium bicarbonate): Calcium, Cayenne, Chromium, Copper, Folic Acid, Iron, Vitamin A, Vitamin B_1, Vitamin D, Zinc

Alkaban-AQ (vinblastine): Echinacea, Eleuthero, Feverfew, Ginseng, St. John's Wort, Turmeric/Curcumin

Alkeran (melphalan): Astragalus, Carnitine, Echinacea, Eleuthero, Selenium

Allegra (fexofenadine): St. John's Wort

Allercort (hydrocortisone 17-butyrate/acetate/probutate/valerate): Aloe, Green Tea, Licorice, Vitamin C

alli (orlistat): Beta-Carotene, Coenzyme Q10, Vitamin A, Vitamin D, Vitamin E, Vitamin K

Allohexal (allopurinol): Carnitine, Copper, Iron, Tryptophan, Vitamin D

Aloprim (allopurinol): Carnitine, Copper, Iron, Tryptophan, Vitamin D

Alora Transdermal (estradiol): Arginine, Black Cohosh, Boron, Calcium, Copper, DHEA, Dang Gui, Magnesium, Melatonin, Milk Thistle, St. John's Wort, Vitamin B_6, Vitamin D, Vitamin E, Vitex, Zinc

Alphaderm (hydrocortisone 17-butyrate/acetate/probutate/valerate): Aloe, Green Tea, Licorice, Vitamin C

Alphatrex (betamethasone dipropionate/valerate): Aloe, Green Tea, Licorice, Vitamin C

Altace (ramipril): Arginine, Cayenne, Iron, Omega-3 Fatty Acids, Potassium, Vitamin E, Zinc

Alternagel (aluminum hydroxide): Calcium, Cayenne, Chromium, Copper, Ephedra, Folic Acid, Iron, Vitamin A, Vitamin B_1, Vitamin C, Vitamin D, Zinc

Altocor (lovastatin): Beta-Carotene, Carnitine, Coenzyme Q10, Garlic, Gotu Kola, Omega-3 Fatty Acids, Policosanol, Reishi, Selenium, St. John's Wort, Vitamin A, Vitamin B_3, Vitamin C, Vitamin E

Altoprev (lovastatin): Beta-Carotene, Carnitine, Coenzyme Q10, Garlic, Gotu Kola, Omega-3 Fatty Acids, Policosanol, Reishi, Selenium, St. John's Wort, Vitamin A, Vitamin B_3, Vitamin C, Vitamin E

Alupent (metaproterenol): Calcium, Magnesium, Potassium

Alurate (aprobarbital): DHEA, Gotu Kola, Valerian, Vitamin B_2

Aluvia (lopinavir + ritonavir): Copper, Garlic, St. John's Wort, Vitamin C

Amaryl (glimepiride): Aloe, Alpha-Lipoic Acid, Astragalus, Bilberry, Chromium, Coenzyme Q10, DHEA, Ephedra, Garlic, Ginkgo, Ginseng, Glucosamine Sulfate, Gotu Kola, Horse Chestnut, Magnesium, Omega-3 Fatty Acids, Reishi, Turmeric/Curcumin, Vitamin B_3

Ambien (zolpidem): 5-HTP, Gotu Kola, Melatonin, Valerian

AmBisome (amphotericin, liposomal): Echinacea

Amerge (naratriptan): 5-HTP, Feverfew, Tryptophan

Amficot (ampicillin): Ginseng, Green Tea, Licorice, Probiotic Flora, Vitamin B_1, Vitamin C, Vitamin K, Zinc

Ami-Tex LA (guaifenesin + phenylpropanolamine): Potassium, Tryosine

Amigesic (salsalate): Calcium, Folic Acid, Omega-3 Fatty Acids, Policosanol, Vitamin C, Vitamin K, Zinc

Amikin (amikacin): Alpha-Lipoic Acid, Calcium, Eleuthero, Ginger, Ginkgo, Horse Chestnut, Licorice, Magnesium, Potassium, Probiotic Flora, Vitamin B_1, Vitamin B_6, Vitamin B_{12}, Vitamin K

Amoxicot (amoxicillin): Ginseng, Green Tea, Licorice, Probiotic Flora, Vitamin B_1, Vitamin K, Zinc

Amoxil (amoxicillin): Ginseng, Green Tea, Licorice, Probiotic Flora, Vitamin B_1, Vitamin K, Zinc

Amphojel (aluminum hydroxide): Calcium, Cayenne, Chromium, Copper, Ephedra, Folic Acid, Iron, Vitamin A, Vitamin B_1, Vitamin C, Vitamin D, Zinc

Amytal (amobarbital): DHEA, Gotu Kola, Valerian, Vitamin B_2

Ana-Gard (epinephrine): Magnesium, Potassium, Vitamin C

Anacin (acetylsalicylic acid): Bilberry, Calcium, Cayenne, Devil's Claw, Feverfew, Folic Acid, Garlic, Ginger, Ginkgo, Gotu Kola, Iron, Licorice, Melatonin, Milk Thistle, Omega-3 Fatty Acids, Policosanol, Potassium, S-adenosylmethionine (SAMe), Vitamin B_2, Vitamin B_3, Vitamin C, Vitamin E, Vitamin K, Zinc

Anadrol-50 (oxymetholone): Echinacea

Anafranil (clomipramine): 5-HTP, Coenzyme Q10, Echinacea, Milk Thistle, S-Adenosylmethionine (SAMe), St. John's Wort, Tryptophan, Tyrosine, Vitamin B_1, Vitamin B_2, Vitamin B_3, Vitamin B_6, Vitamin B_{12}, Zinc

Anandrone (nilutamide): Black Cohosh, Vitamin D

Anaprox (naproxen): Calcium, Cayenne, Chondroitin Sulfate, Chromium, Copper, Devil's Claw, Feverfew, Folic Acid, Ginger, Glucosamine Sulfate, Gotu Kola, Iron, Licorice, Melatonin, Omega-3 Fatty Acids, Potassium, Turmeric/Curcumin, Vitamin B_3, Vitamin B_6, Vitamin C, Zinc

Anaspaz (hyoscyamine): Iron

Anavar (oxandrolone): Echinacea

Ancef (cefazolin): Ginseng, Green Tea, Iron, Licorice, Probiotic Flora, Reishi, Vitamin B_1, Vitamin K, Zinc

Androcur (cyproterone): Black Cohosh, Vitamin D

Android (methyltestosterone): Beta-Carotene, DHEA, Vitamin A, Zinc

Andromaco Gliporal (buformin): Alpha-Lipoic Acid, Astragalus, Bilberry, Calcium, Chromium, DHEA, Ephedra, Folic Acid, Garlic, Ginkgo, Ginseng, Glucosamine Sulfate, Gotu Kola, Horse Chestnut, Magnesium, Omega-3 Fatty Acids, Reishi, Turmeric/Curcumin, Vitamin B_3, Vitamin B_{12}

Anectine (suxamethonium): Ginger, Magnesium

Anexsia (hydrocodone + acetaminophen): Ephedra, Ginseng, Gotu Kola, Phenylalanine, Tyrosine

Angiomax (bivalirudin): Cayenne, DHEA, Policosanol

Angiopine (nifedipine): Black Cohosh, Calcium, Dang Gui, Magnesium, Saw Palmetto

Angiopine LA (nifedipine): Black Cohosh, Calcium, Dang Gui, Magnesium, Saw Palmetto

Angiopine MR (nifedipine): Black Cohosh, Calcium, Dang Gui, Magnesium, Saw Palmetto

Anodynos-DHC (hydrocodone + acetaminophen): Ephedra, Ginseng, Gotu Kola, Phenylalanine, Tyrosine

Anquil (benperidol): Milk Thistle, Phenylalanine

Ansaid (furbiprofen): Calcium, Cayenne, Chondroitin Sulfate, Chromium, Copper, Devil's Claw, Feverfew, Folic Acid, Ginger, Glucosamine Sulfate, Gotu Kola, Iron, Licorice, Melatonin, Omega-3 Fatty Acids, Potassium, Turmeric/Curcumin, Vitamin B_3, Vitamin B_6, Vitamin C, Vitamin D, Zinc

Anspor (cephradine): Ginseng, Green Tea, Iron, Licorice, Probiotic Flora, Reishi, Vitamin B_1, Vitamin K, Zinc

Antabus (disulfiram): Vitamin C

Antabuse (disulfiram): Vitamin C

Antagon (ganirelix): Black Cohosh

Anthra-Derm (anthralin): Vitamin E

Anturane (sulfinpyrazone): Vitamin B_2, Vitamin B_3

Apexicon (diflorasone): Aloe, Green Tea, Licorice, Vitamin C

Apo-Clonidine (clonidine): DHEA, Ephedra, Melatonin

Apo-Gemfibrozil (gemfibrozil): Coenzyme Q10, Copper, Folic Acid, Gotu Kola, Omega-3 Fatty Acids, Vitamin B_3, Vitamin B_6, Vitamin B_{12}, Vitamin E, Zinc

Apo-Guanethidine (guanethidine): Ephedra, Vitamin B_3

Apo-Hydral (hydralazine): Melatonin, Vitamin B_6, Zinc

Apo-Hydralazine (hydralazine): Melatonin, Vitamin B_6, Zinc

Apo-Nifed (nifedipine): Black Cohosh, Calcium, Dang Gui, Magnesium, Saw Palmetto

Apo-Salvent (salbutamol): Potassium

Apo-Sulfasalazine (sulfasalazine): Calcium, Folic Acid, Iron, Licorice, Magnesium, Omega-3 Fatty Acids, PABA, Probiotic Flora, Vitamin B_1, Vitamin B_6, Vitamin K, Zinc

Apresazide (hydralazine + hydrochlorothiazide): Arginine, Coenzyme Q10, Melatonin, Potassium, Vitamin B_6

Apresoline (hydralazine): Melatonin, Vitamin B_6, Zinc

Apresoline Injection (hydralazine): Melatonin, Vitamin B_6, Zinc

Aprovel (irbesartan): Alpha-Lipoic Acid, Potassium

Aptivus (tipranavir): Copper, Garlic, St. John's Wort, Vitamin C

Aquazide (hydrochlorothiazide): Calcium, Coenzyme Q10, Folic Acid, Ginkgo, Glucosamine Sulfate, Hawthorn, ?>Licorice, Magnesium, Potassium, Vitamin B_2, Vitamin D, Zinc

Aquest (estrone): Arginine, Black Cohosh, Boron, Calcium, Copper, DHEA, Dang Gui, Magnesium, Melatonin, Milk Thistle, St. John's Wort, Vitamin B_6, Vitamin D, Vitamin E, Vitex, Zinc

Aralen (chloroquine): Calcium, Magnesium, Vitamin B_2, Vitamin E

Aralen HCl (chloroquine): Calcium, Magnesium, Vitamin B_2, Vitamin E

Aranesp (darbepoetin alpha): Dang Gui, Iron, Vitamin B_6, Vitamin C

Aredia (pamidronate): Calcium, Iron, Magnesium, Vitamin D, Zinc

Arfonad (trimethaphan): Vitamin B_3

Argatroban (argatroban): Cayenne, DHEA, Policosanol

Aricept (donepezil): Ginkgo

Arimidex (anastrozole): Green Tea

Aristocort (triamcinolone, oral): Calcium, Cayenne, Chromium, DHEA, Echinacea, Ephedra, Folic Acid, Horse Chestnut, Licorice, Magnesium, Melatonin, Omega-3 Fatty Acids, Potassium, Selenium, Vitamin A, Vitamin B_6, Vitamin C, Vitamin D, Vitamin K, Zinc

Arixtra (fondaparinux): Cayenne, Chondroitin Sulfate, DHEA, Policosanol

Arm-A-Med (isoetharine): Calcium, Magnesium, Potassium

Armour Thyroid (L-thyroxine + L-triiodothyronine): Alpha-Lipoic Acid, Calcium, Carnitine, Coenzyme Q10, DHEA, Iron, Tyrosine, Vitamin B_2

Aromasin (exemestane): Green Tea

Aropax (paroxetine): 5-HTP, Chromium, Folic Acid, Ginkgo, Inositol, Omega-3 Fatty Acids, S-Adenosylmethionine (SAMe), St. John's Wort, Tryptophan, Vitamin B_3, Vitamin B_6, Vitamin B_{12}, Vitamin C, Zinc

Arthritis Foundation Pain Reliever (acetylsalicylic acid): Bilberry, Calcium, Cayenne, Devil's Claw, Feverfew, Folic Acid, Garlic, Ginger, Ginkgo, Gotu Kola, Iron, Licorice, Melatonin, Milk Thistle, Omega-3 Fatty Acids, Policosanol, Potassium, S-Adenosylmethionine (SAMe), Vitamin B_2, Vitamin B_3, Vitamin C, Vitamin E, Vitamin K, Zinc

Arthrotec (diclofenac + misoprostol): Calcium, Cayenne, Chondroitin Sulfate, Chromium, Copper, Devil's Claw, Feverfew, Folic Acid, Ginger, Glucosamine Sulfate, Gotu Kola, Iron, Licorice, Magnesium, Melatonin, Omega-3 Fatty Acids, Potassium, Turmeric/Curcumin, Vitamin B_3, Vitamin B_6, Vitamin C, Zinc

Asacol (mesalazine): Vitamin B_{12}

Asasantin (acetylsalicylic acid + dipyridamole [extended-release]): Bilberry, Calcium, Cayenne, Devil's Claw, Feverfew, Folic Acid, Garlic, Ginger, Ginkgo, Gotu Kola, Iron, Licorice, Melatonin, Milk Thistle, Omega-3 Fatty Acids, Policosanol, Potassium, S-Adenosylmethionine (SAMe), Vitamin B$_2$, Vitamin B$_3$, Vitamin C, Vitamin E, Vitamin K, Zinc

Ascriptin (acetylsalicylic acid): Bilberry, Calcium, Cayenne, Devil's Claw, Feverfew, Folic Acid, Garlic, Ginger, Ginkgo, Gotu Kola, Iron, Licorice, Melatonin, Milk Thistle, Omega-3 Fatty Acids, Policosanol, Potassium, S-Adenosylmethionine (SAMe), Vitamin B$_2$, Vitamin B$_3$, Vitamin C, Vitamin E, Vitamin K, Zinc

Asendin (amoxapine): 5-HTP, Coenzyme Q10, Milk Thistle, S-Adenosylmethionine (SAMe), St. John's Wort, Tryptophan, Tyrosine, Vitamin B$_1$, Vitamin B$_2$, Vitamin B$_3$, Vitamin B$_6$, Vitamin B$_{12}$, Zinc

Aspergum (acetylsalicylic acid): Bilberry, Calcium, Cayenne, Devil's Claw, Feverfew, Folic Acid, Garlic, Ginger, Ginkgo, Gotu Kola, Iron, Licorice, Melatonin, Milk Thistle, Omega-3 Fatty Acids, Policosanol, Potassium, S-Adenosylmethionine (SAMe), Vitamin B$_2$, Vitamin B$_3$, Vitamin C, Vitamin E, Vitamin K, Zinc

Asprimox (acetylsalicylic acid): Bilberry, Calcium, Cayenne, Devil's Claw, Feverfew, Folic Acid, Garlic, Ginger, Ginkgo, Gotu Kola, Iron, Licorice, Melatonin, Milk Thistle, Omega-3 Fatty Acids, Policosanol, Potassium, S-Adenosylmethionine (SAMe), Vitamin B$_2$, Vitamin B$_3$, Vitamin C, Vitamin E, Vitamin K, Zinc

AsthmaHaler (epinephrine): Magnesium, Potassium, Vitamin C

AsthmaNefrin (epinephrine): Magnesium, Potassium, Vitamin C

Astramorph PF (morphine): Ginseng, Gotu Kola, Phenylalanine, Tyrosine

Atabrine (quinacrine): Vitamin B$_2$

Atacand (candesartan): Alpha-Lipoic Acid, Potassium

Atacand HCT (candesartan + hydrochlorothiazide): Alpha-Lipoic Acid, Potassium

Atamet (levodopa + carbidopa): 5-HTP, Folic Acid, Iron, Kava, Methionine, Phenylalanine, S-Adenosylmethionine (SAMe), Tyrosine, Vitamin B$_3$, Vitamin B$_6$, Vitamin C, Vitex

Atapryl (selegiline): 5-HTP, Cayenne, Chromium, Eleuthero, Ephedra, Folic Acid, Ginkgo, Iron, Kava, Licorice, Phenylalanine, S-Adenosylmethionine (SAMe), St. John's Wort, Tryptophan, Tyrosine, Vitamin B$_2$, Vitamin B$_6$, Vitex

Ativan (lorazepam): DHEA, Gotu Kola, Melatonin, Valerian, Vitamin B$_3$

Atragen (tretinoin): Beta-Carotene, Calcium, Carnitine, Vitamin A, Vitamin E

Atridox (doxycycline): Calcium, Folic Acid, Iron, Magnesium, Potassium, Vitamin A, Vitamin B$_1$, Vitamin B$_2$, Vitamin B$_3$, Vitamin B$_6$, Vitamin C, Zinc

Atromid-S (clofibrate): Coenzyme Q10, Copper, Folic Acid, Gotu Kola, Iron, Omega-3 Fatty Acids, Vitamin B$_3$, Vitamin B$_6$, Vitamin B$_{12}$, Vitamin E, Zinc

Augmentin (amoxicillin + clavulanic acid): Ginseng, Green Tea, Licorice, Probiotic Flora, Vitamin B$_1$, Vitamin K, Zinc

Augmentin XR (amoxicillin + clavulanic acid): Ginseng, Green Tea, Licorice, Probiotic Flora, Vitamin B$_1$, Vitamin K, Zinc

Aurorix (moclobemide): 5-HTP, Cayenne, Chromium, Eleuthero, Ephedra, Ginkgo, Ginseng, Licorice, Phenylalanine, S-Adenosylmethionine (SAMe), St. John's Wort, Tryptophan, Tyrosine, Vitamin B$_6$

Avalide (irbesartan + hydrochlorothiazide): Alpha-Lipoic Acid, Potassium

Avandia (rosiglitazone): Chromium, Vitamin B$_3$

Avapro (irbesartan): Alpha-Lipoic Acid, Potassium

AVC (sulfanilamide): Calcium, Folic Acid, Licorice, Magnesium, PABA, Probiotic Flora, Vitamin B$_1$, Vitamin B$_6$, Vitamin K, Zinc

Avelox (moxifloxacin): Calcium, Green Tea, Iron, Licorice, Magnesium, Potassium, Probiotic Flora, Vitamin B$_1$, Vitamin K, Zinc

Aventyl (nortriptyline): 5-HTP, Coenzyme Q10, Milk Thistle, S-Adenosylmethionine (SAMe), St. John's Wort, Tryptophan, Tyrosine, Vitamin B$_1$, Vitamin B$_2$, Vitamin B$_3$, Vitamin B$_6$, Vitamin B$_{12}$, Zinc

Avidart (dutasteride): Black Cohosh, Saw Palmetto

Avinza (morphine): Ginseng, Gotu Kola, Phenylalanine, Tyrosine

Avita (tretinoin): Beta-Carotene, Calcium, Carnitine, Vitamin A, Vitamin E

Avlosulfon (dapsone): Folic Acid, Licorice, PABA, Probiotic Flora, Vitamin E, Vitamin K, Zinc

Avodart (dutasteride): Black Cohosh, Saw Palmetto

Avolve (dutasteride): Black Cohosh, Saw Palmetto

Axert (almotriptan): 5-HTP, Feverfew, Tryptophan

Axid (nizatidine): Calcium, Chromium, Copper, Folic Acid, Iron, Licorice, Magnesium, Vitamin B$_{12}$, Vitamin C, Zinc

Axid AR (nizatidine): Calcium, Chromium, Copper, Folic Acid, Iron, Licorice, Magnesium, Vitamin B$_{12}$, Vitamin C, Zinc

Aygestin (norethindrone, oral): Magnesium, St. John's Wort

Azactam injection (aztreonam): Ginseng, Green Tea, Iron, Licorice, Probiotic Flora, Reishi, Vitamin B$_1$, Vitamin C, Vitamin K, Zinc

Azamun (azathioprine): Echinacea, Folic Acid, Vitamin B$_3$

Azilect (rasagiline): 5-HTP, Cayenne, Chromium, Eleuthero, Ephedra, Ginkgo, Kava, Licorice, Phenylalanine, S-Adenosylmethionine (SAMe), St. John's Wort, Tryptophan, Tyrosine

Azopt ophthalmic suspension (brinzolamide, ophthalmic suspension): Potassium

Azulfidine (sulfasalazine): Calcium, Folic Acid, Iron, Licorice, Magnesium, Omega-3 Fatty Acids, PABA, Probiotic Flora, Vitamin B$_1$, Vitamin B$_6$, Vitamin K, Zinc

Azulfidine EN-Tabs (sulfasalazine): Calcium, Folic Acid, Iron, Licorice, Magnesium, Omega-3 Fatty Acids, PABA, Probiotic Flora, Vitamin B$_1$, Vitamin B$_6$, Vitamin K, Zinc

B&O Supprettes (opium and belladonna): Ephedra, Ginseng, Gotu Kola, Phenylalanine, Tyrosine

Bactine (hydrocortisone 17-butyrate/acetate/probutate/valerate): Aloe, Green Tea, Licorice, Vitamin C

Bactocill (oxacillin): Ginseng, Green Tea, Licorice, Probiotic Flora, Vitamin B$_1$, Vitamin K, Zinc

Bactrim (trimethoprim + sulfamethoxazole): Calcium, Folic Acid, Licorice, Magnesium, PABA, Potassium, Probiotic Flora, Vitamin B$_1$, Vitamin B$_2$, Vitamin B$_6$, Vitamin C, Vitamin K, Zinc

Bapadin (bepridil): Calcium, Carnitine, Folic Acid, Magnesium, St. John's Wort, Vitamin B$_6$, Vitamin D

Basajel (aluminum carbonate gel): Calcium, Cayenne, Chromium, Copper, Folic Acid, Iron, Vitamin A, Vitamin B$_1$, Vitamin C, Vitamin D, Zinc

Baycol (cerivastatin): Beta-Carotene, Carnitine, Coenzyme Q10, Garlic, Gotu Kola, Omega-3 Fatty Acids,

Policosanol, Reishi, Selenium, St. John's Wort, Vitamin A, Vitamin B_3, Vitamin C, Vitamin E

Bayer Aspirin (acetylsalicylic acid): Bilberry, Calcium, Cayenne, Devil's Claw, Feverfew, Folic Acid, Garlic, Ginger, Ginkgo, Gotu Kola, Iron, Licorice, Melatonin, Milk Thistle, Omega-3 Fatty Acids, Policosanol, Potassium, S-Adenosylmethionine (SAMe), Vitamin B_2, Vitamin B_3, Vitamin C, Vitamin E, Vitamin K, Zinc

Bayer Buffered Aspirin (acetylsalicylic acid): Bilberry, Calcium, Cayenne, Devil's Claw, Feverfew, Folic Acid, Garlic, Ginger, Ginkgo, Gotu Kola, Iron, Licorice, Melatonin, Milk Thistle, Omega-3 Fatty Acids, Polico-sanol, Potassium, S-Adenosylmethionine (SAMe), Vitamin B_2, Vitamin B_3, Vitamin C, Vitamin E, Vitamin K, Zinc

Bayer Low Adult Strength (acetylsalicylic acid): Bilberry, Calcium, Cayenne, Devil's Claw, Feverfew, Folic Acid, Garlic, Ginger, Ginkgo, Gotu Kola, Iron, Licorice, Melatonin, Milk Thistle, Omega-3 Fatty Acids, Polico-sanol, Potassium, S-Adenosylmethionine (SAMe), Vitamin B_2, Vitamin B_3, Vitamin C, Vitamin E, Vitamin K, Zinc

Beclovent (beclomethasone inhalant): Calcium

Beconase (beclomethasone inhalant): Calcium

Beconase AQ (beclomethasone inhalant): Calcium

Beepen-VK (penicillin V): Ginseng, Green Tea, Licorice, Probiotic Flora, Vitamin B_1, Vitamin K, Zinc

Bendectin (doxylamine + pyridoxine): Vitamin B_6

Benemid (probenecid): Vitamin B_2, Vitamin B_3, Vitamin C

Benicar (olmesartan): Alpha-Lipoic Acid, Potassium

Benperidol-neuraxpharm (benperidol): Milk Thistle, Phenylalanine

Benzamycin (erythromycin + benzoyl peroxide): Vitamin E, Zinc

Berotec (fenoterol): Calcium, Magnesium, Potassium

Beta-Adalat (atenolol + nifedipine): Arginine, Calcium, Coenzyme Q10, Dang Gui, Magnesium, Policosanol, Potassium, St. John's Wort, Vitamin C

Beta-HC (hydrocortisone 17-butyrate/acetate/probutate/valerate): Aloe, Green Tea, Licorice, Vitamin C

Beta-Val (betamethasone dipropionate/valerate): Aloe, Green Tea, Licorice, Vitamin C

Betachron (propranolol): Calcium, Carnitine, Chromium, Coenzyme Q10, Folic Acid, Magnesium, Melatonin, Policosanol, Potassium, Vitamin B_2, Vitamin B_3, Vitamin B_6, Vitamin C, Vitamin E

Betaderm (betamethasone dipropionate/valerate): Aloe, Green Tea, Licorice, Vitamin C

Betanate (betamethasone dipropionate/valerate): Aloe, Green Tea, Licorice, Vitamin C

Betapace (sotalol): Calcium, Carnitine, Cascara, Chromium, Coenzyme Q10, Folic Acid, Magnesium, Melatonin, Potassium, Vitamin B_2, Vitamin B_3, Vitamin B_6, Vitamin C

Betapace AF (sotalol): Calcium, Carnitine, Cascara, Chromium, Coenzyme Q10, Folic Acid, Magnesium, Melatonin, Potassium, Vitamin B_2, Vitamin B_3, Vitamin B_6, Vitamin C

Betapen-VK (penicillin V): Ginseng, Green Tea, Licorice, Probiotic Flora, Vitamin B_1, Vitamin K, Zinc

Betatrex (betamethasone dipropionate/valerate): Aloe, Green Tea, Licorice, Vitamin C

Bexophene (acetylsalicylic acid + propoxyphene): Calcium, Cayenne, Devil's Claw, Ephedra, Feverfew, Folic Acid, Ginkgo, Ginseng, Gotu Kola, Iron, Licorice, Melatonin, Milk Thistle, Phenylalanine, Policosanol, Potassium, Tyrosine, Vitamin B_2, Vitamin B_3, Vitamin C, Vitamin E, Vitamin K, Zinc

Bextra (valdecoxib): Calcium, Cayenne, Chondroitin Sulfate, Chromium, Copper, Devil's Claw, Feverfew, Folic Acid, Ginger, Glucosamine Sulfate, Gotu Kola, Iron, Licorice, Melatonin, Omega-3 Fatty Acids, Potassium, Turmeric/Curcumin, Vitamin B_3, Vitamin C, Zinc

Bezalip (bezafibrate): Coenzyme Q10, Copper, Folic Acid, Gotu Kola, Omega-3 Fatty Acids, Vitamin B_3, Vitamin B_6, Vitamin B_{12}, Zinc

Biaxin (clarithromycin): Calcium, Green Tea, Magnesium, Probiotic Flora, Vitamin B_1, Vitamin B_6, Vitamin K, Zinc

Bicillin C-R (penicillin G): Ginseng, Green Tea, Licorice, Probiotic Flora, Vitamin B_1, Vitamin K, Zinc

Bicillin L-A (penicillin G): Ginseng, Green Tea, Licorice, Probiotic Flora, Vitamin B_1, Vitamin K, Zinc

BiDil (isosorbide dinitrate + hydralazine): Arginine, Carnitine, Folic Acid, Melatonin, Vitamin B_6, Vitamin C

Bifenabid (probucol): Beta-Carotene

Biltricide (praziquantl): Beta-Carotene, Vitamin A

Black-Draught (senna): Potassium

Blenoxane (bleomycin): Aloe, Echinacea, Eleuthero, Garlic, Ginseng, Licorice, Omega-3 Fatty Acids, Probiotic Flora, Selenium, Turmeric/Curcumin, Vitamin A, Vitamin B_1, Vitamin C, Vitamin E, Vitamin K

Bleph-10 (sodium sulfacetamide): Calcium, Folic Acid, Licorice, Magnesium, PABA, Probiotic Flora, Vitamin B_1, Vitamin B_6, Vitamin K, Zinc

Blocadren (timolol): Calcium, Carnitine, Chromium, Coenzyme Q10, Folic Acid, Magnesium, Melatonin, Potassium, Vitamin B_2, Vitamin B_3, Vitamin B_6, Vitamin C

Bondronat (ibandronate): Calcium, Iron, Magnesium, Vitamin D, Zinc

Bonefos (clodronate): Calcium, Iron, Magnesium, Vitamin D, Zinc

Boniva (ibandronate): Calcium, Iron, Magnesium, Vitamin D, Zinc

Brelomax (tulobuterol): Calcium, Magnesium, Potassium

Brethaire (terbutaline): Potassium

Brethine (terbutaline): Potassium

Brevibloc (esmolol): Calcium, Carnitine, Chromium, Coenzyme Q10, Folic Acid, Magnesium, Melatonin, Potassium, Vitamin B_2, Vitamin B_3, Vitamin B_6, Vitamin C

Brevicon (ethinyl estradiol + norethindrone): Arginine, Calcium, Copper, DHEA, Dang Gui, Folic Acid, Iron, Licorice, Magnesium, Melatonin, Milk Thistle, S-Adenosylmethionine (SAMe), Selenium, St. John's Wort, Tyrosine, Vitamin A, Vitamin B_1, Vitamin B_2, Vitamin B_3, Vitamin B_6, Vitamin B_{12}, Vitamin C, Vitamin E, Vitex, Zinc

Brevital (methohexital): DHEA, Gotu Kola, Valerian, Vitamin B_2

Bricanyl (terbutaline): Potassium

Bronchaid (epinephrine): Magnesium, Potassium, Vitamin C

Bronkaid Mist (epinephrine): Magnesium, Potassium, Vitamin C

Bronkometer (isoetharine): Calcium, Magnesium, Potassium

Bronkosol (isoetharine): Calcium, Magnesium, Potassium

Brontin Mist (epinephrine): Magnesium, Potassium, Vitamin C

Bufferin (acetylsalicylic acid): Bilberry, Calcium, Cayenne, Devil's Claw, Feverfew, Folic Acid, Garlic, Ginger, Ginkgo, Gotu Kola, Iron, Licorice, Melatonin, Milk Thistle, Omega-3 Fatty Acids, Policosanol, Potassium, S-Adenosylmethionine (SAMe), Vitamin B_2, Vitamin B_3, Vitamin C, Vitamin E, Vitamin K, Zinc

Buffex (acetylsalicylic acid): Bilberry, Calcium, Cayenne, Devil's Claw, Feverfew, Folic Acid, Garlic, Ginger, Ginkgo,

Gotu Kola, Iron, Licorice, Melatonin, Milk Thistle, Omega-3 Fatty Acids, Policosanol, Potassium, S-Adenosylmethionine (SAMe), Vitamin B_2, Vitamin B_3, Vitamin C, Vitamin E, Vitamin K, Zinc

Buformina (buformin): Alpha-Lipoic Acid, Astragalus, Bilberry, Calcium, Chromium, DHEA, Ephedra, Folic Acid, Garlic, Ginkgo, Ginseng, Glucosamine Sulfate, Gotu Kola, Horse Chestnut, Magnesium, Omega-3 Fatty Acids, Reishi, Turmeric/Curcumin, Vitamin B_3, Vitamin B_{12}

Bumex (bumetanide): Calcium, Folic Acid, Ginseng, Glucosamine ·Sulfate, Licorice, Magnesium, Potassium, Vitamin B_1, Vitamin B_6, Vitamin C, Zinc

Buprenex (buprenorphine): Ephedra, Ginseng, Gotu Kola, Phenylalanine, Tyrosine

Buronil (melperon): Milk Thistle, Phenylalanine

Buspar (buspirone): 5-HTP, St. John's Wort, Tryptophan

Butisol (butabarbital): DHEA, Gotu Kola, Valerian, Vitamin B_2

Caci-IM (bacitracin): Licorice, Probiotic Flora, Vitamin K, Zinc

Caelyx (doxorubicin, pegylated liposomal): Alpha-Lipoic Acid, Carnitine, Coenzyme Q10, Feverfew, Garlic, Ginkgo, Green Tea, Hawthorn, Milk Thistle, Reishi, Selenium, St. John's Wort, Turmeric/Curcumin, Vitamin B_2, Vitamin B_6, Vitamin E

Cafcit (caffeine): Calcium, Ephedra, Kava, Melatonin

Caffedrine (caffeine): Calcium, Ephedra, Kava, Melatonin

Calan (verapamil): Calcium, Carnitine, Folic Acid, Magnesium, Melatonin, St. John's Wort, Vitamin B_6, Vitamin D, Vitamin E

Calan SR (verapamil): Calcium, Carnitine, Folic Acid, Magnesium, Melatonin, St. John's Wort, Vitamin B_6, Vitamin D, Vitamin E

Calanif (nifedipine): Black Cohosh, Calcium, Dang Gui, Magnesium, Saw Palmetto

Calcimar (calcitonin): Calcium, Vitamin D

Calciparine (heparin): Calcium, Cayenne, Chondroitin Sulfate, DHEA, Omega-3 Fatty Acids, Policosanol, Potassium, Vitamin C, Vitamin D

Calcium Rich Rolaids (calcium carbonate): Calcium, Cayenne, Chromium, Copper, Folic Acid, Iron, Vitamin A, Vitamin B_1, Vitamin D, Zinc

Caldecort Anti-Itch (hydrocortisone 17-butyrate/acetate/probutate/valerate): Aloe, Green Tea, Licorice, Vitamin C

Cama Arthritis Pain Reliever (acetylsalicylic acid): Bilberry, Calcium, Cayenne, Devil's Claw, Feverfew, Folic Acid, Garlic, Ginger, Ginkgo, Gotu Kola, Iron, Licorice, Melatonin, Milk Thistle, Omega-3 Fatty Acids, Policosanol, Potassium, S-Adenosylmethionine (SAMe), Vitamin B_2, Vitamin B_3, Vitamin C, Vitamin E, Vitamin K, Zinc

Camcolit (lithium carbonate): 5-HTP, Chromium, Folic Acid, Inositol, Magnesium, Tryptophan

Camila (norethindrone, oral): Magnesium, St. John's Wort

Campto (irinotecan): Aloe, Feverfew, Ginseng, Melatonin, Omega-3 Fatty Acids, St. John's Wort, Turmeric/Curcumin, Vitamin A, Vitamin C, Vitamin E

Camptosar (irinotecan): Aloe, Feverfew, Ginseng, Melatonin, Omega-3 Fatty Acids, St. John's Wort, Turmeric/Curcumin, Vitamin A, Vitamin C, Vitamin E

Canasa (mesalazine): Vitamin B_{12}

Capital and Codeine (codeine + acetaminophen): Ephedra, Ginseng, Gotu Kola, Phenylalanine, Tyrosine

Capoten (captopril): Arginine, Cayenne, Iron, Magnesium, Omega-3 Fatty Acids, Potassium, Vitamin E, Zinc

Capto-Co (captopril + hydrochlorothiazide): Arginine, Calcium, Cayenne, Coenzyme Q10, Glucosamine Sulfate, Hawthorn, Licorice, Magnesium, Potassium, Vitamin D, Zinc

Captozide (captopril + hydrochlorothiazide): Arginine, Calcium, Cayenne, Coenzyme Q10, Glucosamine Sulfate, Hawthorn, Licorice, Magnesium, Potassium, Vitamin D, Zinc

Carafate (sucralfate): Calcium, Vitamin D

Carbatrol (carbamazepine): Calcium, Carnitine, Copper, DHEA, Folic Acid, Ginkgo, Inositol, Kava, Milk Thistle, Omega-3 Fatty Acids, Valerian, Vitamin A, Vitamin B_1, Vitamin B_2, Vitamin B_3, Vitamin B_6, Vitamin B_{12}, Vitamin C, Vitamin D, Vitamin E, Vitamin K, Vitex, Zinc

Carbex (selegiline): 5-HTP, Cayenne, Chromium, Eleuthero, Ephedra, Folic Acid, Ginkgo, Iron, Kava, Licorice, Phenylalanine, S-Adenosylmethionine (SAMe), St. John's Wort, Tryptophan, Tyrosine, Vitamin B_2, Vitamin B_6, Vitex

Carbolith (lithium carbonate): 5-HTP, Chromium, Folic Acid, Inositol, Magnesium, Tryptophan

Cardene (nicardipine): Calcium, Carnitine, Folic Acid, Magnesium, St. John's Wort, Vitamin B_6, Vitamin D

Cardene I.V. (nicardipine): Calcium, Carnitine, Folic Acid, Magnesium, St. John's Wort, Vitamin B_6, Vitamin D

Cardene SR (nicardipine): Calcium, Carnitine, Folic Acid, Magnesium, St. John's Wort, Vitamin B_6, Vitamin D

Cardif (nitrendipine): Calcium, Carnitine, Folic Acid, Magnesium, St. John's Wort, Vitamin B_6, Vitamin D

Cardilate MR (nifedipine): Black Cohosh, Calcium, Dang Gui, Magnesium, Saw Palmetto

Cardizem (diltiazem): Calcium, Carnitine, Folic Acid, Magnesium, St. John's Wort, Vitamin B_6, Vitamin D

Cardizem CD (diltiazem): Calcium, Carnitine, Folic Acid, Magnesium, St. John's Wort, Vitamin B_6, Vitamin D

Cardizem SR (diltiazem): Calcium, Carnitine, Folic Acid, Magnesium, St. John's Wort, Vitamin B_6, Vitamin D

Cardura (doxazosin): Saw Palmetto, Vitamin B_3

Cartia XT (diltiazem): Calcium, Carnitine, Folic Acid, Magnesium, St. John' Wort, Vitamin B_6, Vitamin D

Cartrol (carteolol): Calcium, Carnitine, Chromium, Coenzyme Q10, Folic Acid, Magnesium, Melatonin, Potassium, Vitamin B_2, Vitamin B_3, Vitamin B_6, Vitamin C

Casodex (bicalutamide): Black Cohosh, Vitamin D

Cataflam (diclofenac): Calcium, Cayenne, Chondroitin Sulfate, Chromium, Copper, Devil's Claw, Feverfew, Folic Acid, Ginger, Glucosamine Sulfate, Gotu Kola, Iron, Licorice, Melatonin, Omega-3 Fatty Acids, Potassium, Turmeric/Curcumin, Vitamin B_3, Vitamin B_6, Vitamin C, Zinc

Catapres Oral (clonidine): DHEA, Ephedra, Melatonin

Catapres-TTS Transdermal Dixarit (clonidine): DHEA, Ephedra, Melatonin

Ceclor (cefaclor): Ginseng, Green Tea, Iron, Licorice, Probiotic Flora, Reishi, Vitamin B_1, Vitamin K, Zinc

Cedax (ceftibuten): Ginseng, Green Tea, Iron, Licorice, Probiotic Flora, Reishi, Vitamin B_1, Vitamin K, Zinc

Cefadyl (cephapirin): Ginseng, Green Tea, Iron, Licorice, Probiotic Flora, Reishi, Vitamin B_1, Vitamin K, Zinc

Cefizox (ceftizoxime): Ginseng, Green Tea, Iron, Licorice, Probiotic Flora, Reishi, Vitamin B_1, Vitamin K, Zinc

Cefobid (cefoperazone): Ginseng, Green Tea, Iron, Licorice, Probiotic Flora, Reishi, Vitamin B_1, Vitamin K, Zinc

Cefotan (cefotetan): Ginseng, Green Tea, Iron, Licorice, Probiotic Flora, Reishi, Vitamin B_1, Vitamin K, Zinc

Ceftin (cefuroxime): Ginseng, Green Tea, Iron, Licorice, Probiotic Flora, Reishi, Vitamin B_1, Vitamin K, Zinc

Cross-Indexes

Cefzil (cefprozil): Ginseng, Green Tea, Iron, Licorice, Probiotic Flora, Reishi, Vitamin B_1, Vitamin K, Zinc

Celebrex (celecoxib): Calcium, Cayenne, Chondroitin Sulfate, Chromium, Copper, Devil's Claw, Feverfew, Folic Acid, Ginger, Glucosamine Sulfate, Gotu Kola, Iron, Licorice, Melatonin, Omega-3 Fatty Acids, Potassium, Turmeric/Curcumin, Vitamin B_3, Vitamin C, Zinc

Celestone (betamethasone): Calcium, Cayenne, Chromium, DHEA, Echinacea, Ephedra, Folic Acid, Horse Chestnut, Licorice, Magnesium, Melatonin, Omega-3 Fatty Acids, Potassium, Selenium, Vitamin A, Vitamin B_6, Vitamin C, Vitamin D, Vitamin K, Zinc

Celexa (citalopram): 5-HTP, Chromium, Folic Acid, Ginkgo, Inositol, Omega-3 Fatty Acids, S-Adenosylmethionine (SAMe), St. John's Wort, Tryptophan, Vitamin B_3, Vitamin B6, Vitamin B_{12}, Vitamin C, Zinc

CellCept (mycophenolate): Echinacea, Magnesium, Turmeric/Curcumin

Celontin (methsuximide): Calcium, Carnitine, Copper, DHEA, Folic Acid, Ginkgo, Inositol, Kava, Milk Thistle, Omega-3 Fatty Acids, Valerian, Vitamin A, Vitamin B_1, Vitamin B_2, Vitamin B_3, Vitamin B_6, Vitamin B_{12}, Vitamin C, Vitamin D, Vitamin E, Vitamin K, Vitex, Zinc

Cenafed (pseudoephedrine): Potassium

Cenestin (conjugated synthetic estrogens): Arginine, Black Cohosh, Boron, Calcium, Copper, DHEA, Dang Gui, Magnesium, Melatonin, Milk Thistle, St. John's Wort, Vitamin B_6, Vitamin D, Vitamin E, Vitex, Zinc

Centrax (prazepam): DHEA, Gotu Kola, Melatonin, Valerian, Vitamin B_3

Ceptaz (ceftazidime): Ginseng, Green Tea, Iron, Licorice, Probiotic Flora, Reishi, Vitamin B_1, Vitamin K, Zinc

Cerebyx (fosphenytoin): Calcium, Carnitine, Copper, DHEA, Folic Acid, Ginkgo, Inositol, Kava, Milk Thistle, Omega-3 Fatty Acids, Valerian, Vitamin A, Vitamin B_1, Vitamin B_2, Vitamin B_3, Vitamin B_6, Vitamin B_{12}, Vitamin C, Vitamin D, Vitamin E, Vitamin K, Vitex, Zinc

Cerubidine (daunorubicin): Alpha-Lipoic Acid, Carnitine, Coenzyme Q10, Feverfew, Garlic, Ginkgo, Ginseng, Green Tea, Hawthorn, Milk Thistle, Reishi, Selenium, St. John's Wort, Turmeric/Curcumin, Vitamin B_2, Vitamin E

Cetacort (hydrocortisone 17-butyrate/acetate/probutate/valerate): Aloe, Green Tea, Licorice, Vitamin C

Cetrotide (etrorelix): Black Cohosh

Chenix (chenodeoxycholic acid): S-Adenosylmethionine (SAMe), Vitamin B_3

Chimax (flutamide): Black Cohosh, Vitamin D

Chlor Trimeton (pseudoephedrine): Potassium

Chlorohex (chlorhexidine): Iron, Licorice, Probiotic Flora, Vitamin K, Zinc

Chloromycetin (chloramphenicol): Folic Acid, Iron, Licorice, Probiotic Flora, Vitamin B_{12}, Vitamin K, Zinc

Choledyl (oxtriphylline): Potassium

Choloxin (dextrothyroxine): Alpha-Lipoic Acid, Calcium, Carnitine, Coenzyme Q10, DHEA, Iron, Tyrosine, Vitamin B_2

Chronulac (lactulose): Potassium

Cialis (tadalafil): Arginine

Cibacalcin (calcitonin): Calcium, Vitamin D

Ciloxan (ciprofloxacin): Calcium, Copper, Green Tea, Iron, Licorice, Magnesium, Potassium, Probiotic Flora, Vitamin B_1, Vitamin K, Zinc

Cinobac (cinoxacin): Calcium, Green Tea, Iron, Licorice, Magnesium, Potassium, Probiotic Flora, Vitamin B_1, Vitamin K, Zinc

Cipro (ciprofloxacin): Calcium, Copper, Green Tea, Iron, Licorice, Magnesium, Potassium, Probiotic Flora, Vitamin B_1, Vitamin K, Zinc

Ciproterona (cyproterone): Black Cohosh, Vitamin D

Citrucel (methylcellulose): Potassium, Vitamin B_2

Claforan (cefotaxime): Ginseng, Green Tea, Iron, Licorice, Probiotic Flora, Reishi, Vitamin B_1, Vitamin C, Vitamin K, Zinc

Clavulin (amoxicillin + clavulanic acid): Ginseng, Green Tea, Licorice, Probiotic Flora, Vitamin B_1, Vitamin K, Zinc

Cleocin (clindamycin oral): Licorice, Probiotic Flora, Vitamin K, Zinc

Cleocin T (clindamycin topical): Zinc

Clexane (enoxaparin): Cayenne, Chondroitin Sulfate, DHEA, Policosanol, Vitamin C

Climagest (estradiol + norethindrone, oral): Arginine, Black Cohosh, Boron, Calcium, Copper, DHEA, Dang Gui, Magnesium, Melatonin, Milk Thistle, St. John's Wort, Vitamin B_6, Vitamin D, Vitamin E, Vitex, Zinc

Climara Transdermal (estradiol): Arginine, Black Cohosh, Boron, Calcium, Copper, DHEA, Dang Gui, Magnesium, Melatonin, Milk Thistle, St. John's Wort, Vitamin B_6, Vitamin D, Vitamin E, Vitex, Zinc

Climens (estradiol valerate + cyproterone acetate): Arginine, Black Cohosh, Boron, Calcium, Copper, DHEA, Dang Gui, Magnesium, Melatonin, Milk Thistle, St. John's Wort, Vitamin B_6, Vitamin D, Vitamin E, Vitex, Zinc

Climesse (estradiol + norethindrone, oral): Arginine, Black Cohosh, Boron, Calcium, Copper, DHEA, Dang Gui, Magnesium, Melatonin, Milk Thistle, St. John's Wort, Vitamin B_6, Vitamin D, Vitamin E, Vitex, Zinc

Clindaderm (clindamycin topical): Zinc

Clinoril (sulindac): Calcium, Cayenne, Chondroitin Sulfate, Chromium, Copper, Devil's Claw, Feverfew, Folic Acid, Ginger, Glucosamine Sulfate, Gotu Kola, Iron, Licorice, Melatonin, Omega-3 Fatty Acids, Potassium, Turmeric/Curcumin, Vitamin B_3, Vitamin B_6, Vitamin C, Zinc

Cloderm (clocortolone): Aloe, Green Tea, Licorice, Vitamin C

Cloxapen (cloxacillin): Ginseng, Green Tea, Licorice, Probiotic Flora, Vitamin B_1, Vitamin K, Zinc

Clozaril (clozapine): 5-HTP, Chromium, Echinacea, Ginkgo, Melatonin, Omega-3 Fatty Acids, Selenium, Vitamin B_3, Vitamin B_6, Vitamin C

Co-Gesic (hydrocodone + acetaminophen): Ephedra, Ginseng, Gotu Kola, Phenylalanine, Tyrosine

Co-Magaldrox (aluminum hydroxide + magnesium hydroxide + simethicone): Calcium, Cayenne, Chromium, Copper, Folic Acid, Iron, Magnesium, Vitamin A, Vitamin B_1, Vitamin C, Vitamin D, Vitex, Zinc

Co-Proxamol (acetaminophen + dextropropoxyphene): Garlic, Licorice, Methionine, Milk Thistle, S-Adenosylmethionine (SAMe), Vitamin C

Co-Tendione (atenolol + chlorthalidone): Arginine, Calcium, Coenzyme Q10, Policosanol, Potassium, Vitamin C

Co-Zidocapt (captopril + hydrochlorothiazide): Arginine, Calcium, Cayenne, Coenzyme Q10, Glucosamine Sulfate, Hawthorn, Licorice, Magnesium, Potassium, Vitamin D, Zinc

Cogentin (benztropine): Vitamin B_3

Cognex (tacrine): Echinacea, Melatonin, Milk Thistle, Vitamin C

Colace (docusate): Magnesium, Potassium

Colestid (colestipol): Beta-Carotene, Calcium, Folic Acid, Iron, Omega-3 Fatty Acids, Vitamin A, Vitamin B_2, Vitamin B_3, Vitamin B_{12}, Vitamin D, Vitamin E, Vitamin K, Zinc

ColyMycin M (colistimethate): Licorice, Probiotic Flora, Vitamin K, Zinc

CoLyte (polyethylene glycol–electrolyte solution): Potassium

CombiPatch (estradiol + norethindrone patch): Arginine, Black Cohosh, Boron, Calcium, Copper, DHEA, Dang Gui, Magnesium, Melatonin, Milk Thistle, St. John's Wort, Vitamin B_6, Vitamin D, Vitamin E, Vitex, Zinc

Combipres (clonidine + chlorthalidone): Arginine, Coenzyme Q10, DHEA, Ephedra, Melatonin, Potassium

Combivent (albuterol + ipratropium bromide): Calcium, Magnesium, Potassium

Combivir (zidovudine + lamivudine): Aloe, Carnitine, Coenzyme Q10, Copper, DHEA, Folic Acid, Reishi, Vitamin B_1, Vitamin B_2, Vitamin B_{12}, Vitamin E, Zinc

Compazine (prochlorperazine): Coenzyme Q10, Milk Thistle, Vitamin B_2, Vitamin B_3, Vitamin B_6, Vitamin C

Concerta (methylphenidate): 5-HTP, Iron, Reishi, Tyrosine, Zinc

Copegus (ribavirin): S-Adenosylmethionine (SAMe)

Coracten/SR/XL (nifedipine): Black Cohosh, Calcium, Dang Gui, Magnesium, Saw Palmetto

Cordarone (amiodarone): Cascara, Echinacea, Magnesium, Potassium, Vitamin B_6, Vitamin E

Cordran (flurandrenolide): Aloe, Green Tea, Licorice, Vitamin C

Corgard (nadolol): Calcium, Carnitine, Chromium, Coenzyme Q10, Folic Acid, Magnesium, Melatonin, Potassium, Vitamin B_2, Vitamin B_3, Vitamin B6, Vitamin C

Cormax (clobetasol): Aloe, Green Tea, Licorice, Vitamin C, Zinc

Coroday MR (nifedipine): Black Cohosh, Calcium, Dang Gui, Magnesium, Saw Palmetto

Corsodyl (chlorhexidine): Iron, Licorice, Probiotic Flora, Vitamin K, Zinc

Cort-Dome (hydrocortisone): Aloe, Green Tea, Licorice, Vitamin C

Cortaid (hydrocortisone): Aloe, Green Tea, Licorice, Vitamin C

Cortef (hydrocortisone): Aloe, Calcium, Cayenne, Chromium, DHEA, Echinacea, Ephedra, Folic Acid, Green Tea, Horse Chestnut, Licorice, Magnesium, Melatonin, Omega-3 Fatty Acids, Potassium, Selenium, Vitamin A, Vitamin B_6, Vitamin C, Vitamin D, Vitamin K, Zinc

Cortifair (hydrocortisone): Aloe, Green Tea, Licorice, Vitamin C

Cortizone (hydrocortisone): Aloe, Green Tea, Licorice, Vitamin C

Cortone (hydrocortisone): Aloe, Calcium, Cayenne, Chromium, DHEA, Echinacea, Ephedra, Folic Acid, Green Tea, Horse Chestnut, Licorice, Magnesium, Melatonin, Omega-3 Fatty Acids, Potassium, Selenium, Vitamin A, Vitamin B_6, Vitamin C, Vitamin D, Vitamin K, Zinc

Cortril (hydrocortisone): Aloe, Green Tea, Licorice, Vitamin C

Corvert (ibutilide): Cascara, Magnesium, Potassium

Cosmegen (dactinomycin): Echinacea, Eleuthero, Ginseng, Licorice, Probiotic Flora, Vitamin B_1, Vitamin K

Cosmegen Lyovac (dactinomycin): Echinacea, Eleuthero, Ginseng, Licorice, Probiotic Flora, Vitamin B_1, Vitamin K

Cosopt (dorzolamide + timolol): Potassium

Cotrim (trimethoprim + sulfamethoxazole): Calcium, Folic Acid, Licorice, Magnesium, PABA, Potassium, Probiotic Flora, Vitamin B_1, Vitamin B_2, Vitamin B_6, Vitamin C, Vitamin K, Zinc

Coumadin (warfarin): Bilberry, Cayenne, Chondroitin Sulfate, Coenzyme Q10, DHEA, Dang Gui, Devil's Claw, Echinacea, Feverfew, Garlic, Ginger, Ginkgo, Ginseng, Green Tea, Horse Chestnut, Iron, Kava, Licorice, Magnesium, Omega-3 Fatty Acids, Policosanol, Red Clover, Reishi, Saw Palmetto, St. John's Wort, Vitamin A, Vitamin B_3, Vitamin C, Vitamin D, Vitamin E, Vitamin K, Zinc

Covera-HS (verapamil): Calcium, Carnitine, Folic Acid, Magnesium, Melatonin, St. John's Wort, Vitamin B_6, Vitamin D, Vitamin E

Cozaar (losartan): Alpha-Lipoic Acid, Potassium

Creg (carvedilol): Potassium

Crestor (rosuvastatin): Beta-Carotene, Carnitine, Coenzyme Q10, Garlic, Gotu Kola, Omega-3 Fatty Acids, Policosanol, Reishi, Selenium, St. John's Wort, Vitamin A, Vitamin B_3, Vitamin C, Vitamin E

Crixivan (indinavir): Copper, Garlic, St. John's Wort, Vitamin C

Cuprimine (penicillamine): Copper, Iron, Magnesium, Vitamin B_6, Zinc

Cutivate (fluticasone): Aloe, Green Tea, Licorice, Vitamin C

Cyclocort (amcinonide): Aloe, Green Tea, Licorice, Vitamin C

Cyclofem (estradiol cypionate + medroxyprogesterone acetate): Beta-Carotene, Folic Acid, Magnesium, Vitamin A, Vitamin B_3, Vitamin D

Cycrin (medroxyprogesterone, oral): Beta-Carotene, Calcium, Folic Acid, Magnesium, St. John's Wort, Vitamin A, Vitamin D

Cylert (pemoline): Reishi, Tyrosine

Cymbalta (duloxetine): 5-HTP, Folic Acid, Ginkgo, Omega-3 Fatty Acids, S-Adenosylmethionine (SAMe), St. John's Wort, Tryptophan, Vitamin B_3, Vitamin B_6, Vitamin B_{12}

Cyprohexal (cyproterone): Black Cohosh, Vitamin D

Cyprone (cyproterone): Black Cohosh, Vitamin D

Cyprostat (cyproterone acetate): Black Cohosh, Vitamin D, Vitex

Cyproteron (cyproterone): Black Cohosh, Vitamin D

Cyproteronum (cyproterone): Black Cohosh, Vitamin D

Cystodigin (digitoxin): Calcium, Cascara, Dang Gui, Eleuthero, Ephedra, Hawthorn, Licorice, Magnesium, Potassium, St. John's Wort

Cystospaz (hyoscyamine): Iron

Cystospaz-M (hyoscyamine): Iron

Cytomel (L-triiodothyronine): Alpha-Lipoic Acid, Calcium, Carnitine, Coenzyme Q10, DHEA, Iron, Tyrosine, Vitamin B_2

Cytosar-U (cytarabine): Echinacea, Eleuthero, Folic Acid, Ginseng, Vitamin B_1

Cytotec (misoprostol): Magnesium

Cytovene (ganciclovir): Astragalus

Cytoxan (cyclophosphamide): Aloe, Alpha-Lipoic Acid, Astragalus, Beta-Carotene, Carnitine, Echinacea, Eleuthero, Ginger, Ginseng, Licorice, Melatonin, Omega-3 Fatty Acids, Reishi, Selenium, Turmeric/Curcumin, Vitamin A, Vitamin C, Vitamin E

Dalfon (fenoprofen): Calcium, Cayenne, Chondroitin Sulfate, Chromium, Copper, Devil's Claw, Feverfew, Folic Acid, Ginger, Glucosamine Sulfate, Gotu Kola, Iron, Licorice, Melatonin, Omega-3 Fatty Acids, Potassium, Turmeric/Curcumin, Vitamin B_3, Vitamin B_6, Vitamin C, Zinc

Dalmane (flurazepam): DHEA, Gotu Kola, Melatonin, Valerian, Vitamin B_3

Daranide (dichlorphenamide): Potassium

Daraprim (pyrimethamine): Folic Acid, Iron

Darvocet-N (acetaminophen + propoxyphene): Ephedra, Garlic, Ginseng, Gotu Kola, Licorice, Milk Thistle, Phenylalanine, Tyrosine, Vitamin C

Darvocet-N 100 (acetaminophen + propoxyphene): Ephedra, Garlic, Ginseng, Gotu Kola, Licorice, Milk Thistle, Phenylalanine, Tyrosine, Vitamin C

Darvon (propoxyphene): Ephedra, Ginseng, Gotu Kola, Phenylalanine, Tyrosine

Darvon Compound (acetylsalicylic acid + caffeine + propoxyphene): Calcium, Cayenne, Devil's Claw, Ephedra, Feverfew, Folic Acid, Ginkgo, Ginseng, Gotu Kola, Iron, Licorice, Melatonin, Milk Thistle, Phenylalanine, Policosanol, Potassium, Tyrosine, Vitamin B_2, Vitamin B_3, Vitamin C, Vitamin E, Vitamin K, Zinc

Darvon Compound-65 Pulvules (acetylsalicylic acid + propoxyphene): Calcium, Cayenne, Devil's Claw, Ephedra, Feverfew, Folic Acid, Ginkgo, Ginseng, Gotu Kola, Iron, Licorice, Melatonin, Milk Thistle, Phenylalanine, Policosanol, Potassium, Tyrosine, Vitamin B_2, Vitamin B_3, Vitamin C, Vitamin E, Vitamin K, Zinc

Darvon-N (propoxyphene): Ephedra, Ginseng, Gotu Kola, Phenylalanine, Tyrosine

DaunoXome (daunorubicin, liposomal): Alpha-Lipoic Acid, Carnitine, Coenzyme Q10, Feverfew, Garlic, Ginkgo, Ginseng, Green Tea, Hawthorn, Milk Thistle, Reishi, Selenium, St. John's Wort, Turmeric/Curcumin, Vitamin B_2, Vitamin E

Daypro (oxaprozin): Calcium, Cayenne, Chondroitin Sulfate, Chromium, Copper, Devil's Claw, Feverfew, Folic Acid, Ginger, Glucosamine Sulfate, Gotu Kola, Iron, Licorice, Melatonin, Omega-3 Fatty Acids, Potassium, Turmeric/Curcumin, Vitamin B_3, Vitamin B_6, Vitamin C, Zinc

De-capeptyl Trelstar (triptorelin): Black Cohosh, Melatonin, Vitamin D

Debeone (phenformin): Alpha-Lipoic Acid, Astragalus, Bilberry, Calcium, Chromium, Coenzyme Q10, DHEA, Ephedra, Folic Acid, Garlic, Ginkgo, Ginseng, Glucosamine Sulfate, Gotu Kola, Horse Chestnut, Magnesium, Omega-3 Fatty Acids, Reishi, Turmeric/Curcumin, Vitamin B_3, Vitamin B_{12}

Deca-durabolin (nandrolone): Echinacea

Decaderm (dexamethasone): Aloe, Calcium, Ephedra, Green Tea, Licorice, Vitamin C

Decadron (dexamethasone): Aloe, Calcium, Ephedra, Green Tea, Licorice, Vitamin C

Decapryn (doxylamine): Vitamin B_6

Decaspray (dexamethasone): Aloe, Calcium, Ephedra, Green Tea, Licorice, Vitamin C

Declomycin (demeclocycline): Calcium, Folic Acid, Iron, Magnesium, Potassium, Vitamin A, Vitamin B_1, Vitamin B_2, Vitamin B_3, Vitamin B_6, Vitamin C, Zinc

Decofed (pseudoephedrine): Potassium

Delacort (hydrocortisone 17-butyrate/acetate/probutate/valerate): Aloe, Green Tea, Licorice, Vitamin C

Delestrogen (estradiol valerate): Arginine, Black Cohosh, Boron, Calcium, Copper, DHEA, Dang Gui, Magnesium, Melatonin, Milk Thistle, St. John's Wort, Vitamin B_6, Vitamin D, Vitamin E, Vitex, Zinc

Delta-Cortef (prednisolone): Calcium, Cayenne, Chromium, DHEA, Echinacea, Ephedra, Folic Acid, Horse Chestnut, Licorice, Magnesium, Melatonin, Omega-3 Fatty Acids, Potassium, Selenium, Vitamin A, Vitamin B_6, Vitamin C, Vitamin D, Vitamin K, Zinc

Deltasone (prednisone): Calcium, Cayenne, Chromium, DHEA, Echinacea, Ephedra, Folic Acid, Horse Chestnut, Licorice, Magnesium, Melatonin, Omega-3 Fatty Acids, Potassium, Selenium, Vitamin A, Vitamin B_6, Vitamin C, Vitamin D, Vitamin K, Zinc

Demadex (torsemide): Calcium, Folic Acid, Ginseng, Glucosamine Sulfate, Licorice, Magnesium, Potassium, Vitamin B_1, Vitamin B_6, Vitamin C, Zinc

Demerol (meperidine): Chromium, Ephedra, Ginseng, Gotu Kola, Phenylalanine, Tyrosine

Demulen 1/35 (ethinyl estradiol + ethynodiol): Arginine, Calcium, Copper, DHEA, Dang Gui, Folic Acid, Iron, Licorice, Magnesium, Melatonin, Milk Thistle, S-Adenosylmethionine (SAMe), Selenium, St. John's Wort, Tyrosine, Vitamin A, Vitamin B_1, Vitamin B_2, Vitamin B_3, Vitamin B_6, Vitamin B_{12}, Vitamin C, Vitamin E, Vitex, Zinc

Demulen 1/50 (ethinyl estradiol + ethynodiol): Arginine, Calcium, Copper, DHEA, Dang Gui, Folic Acid, Iron, Licorice, Magnesium, Melatonin, Milk Thistle, S-Adenosylmethionine (SAMe), Selenium, St. John's Wort, Tyrosine, Vitamin A, Vitamin B_1, Vitamin B_2, Vitamin B_3, Vitamin B_6, Vitamin B_{12}, Vitamin C, Vitamin E, Vitex, Zinc

Dep-Gynogen (estradiol cypionate): Arginine, Black Cohosh, Boron, Calcium, Copper, DHEA, Dang Gui, Magnesium, Melatonin, Milk Thistle, St. John's Wort, Vitamin B_6, Vitamin D, Vitamin E, Vitex, Zinc

Depacon (sodium valproate): Calcium, Carnitine, Copper, DHEA, Folic Acid, Ginkgo, Inositol, Kava, Milk Thistle, Omega-3 Fatty Acids, Valerian, Vitamin A, Vitamin B_1, Vitamin B_2, Vitamin B_3, Vitamin B_6, Vitamin B_{12}, Vitamin C, Vitamin D, Vitamin E, Vitamin K, Vitex, Zinc

Depacon (valproate sodium): Calcium, Carnitine, Copper, DHEA, Folic Acid, Ginkgo, Inositol, Kava, Milk Thistle, Omega-3 Fatty Acids, Selenium, Valerian, Vitamin A, Vitamin B_1, Vitamin B_2, Vitamin B_3, Vitamin B_6, Vitamin B_{12}, Vitamin C, Vitamin D, Vitamin E, Vitamin K, Vitex, Zinc

Depakene (valproic acid): Calcium, Carnitine, Copper, DHEA, Folic Acid, Ginkgo, Inositol, Kava, Milk Thistle, Omega-3 Fatty Acids, Selenium, Valerian, Vitamin A, Vitamin B_1, Vitamin B_2, Vitamin B_3, Vitamin B_6, Vitamin B_{12}, Vitamin C, Vitamin D, Vitamin E, Vitamin K, Vitex, Zinc

Depakote Delayed Release (divalproex sodium): Calcium, Carnitine, Copper, DHEA, Folic Acid, Ginkgo, Inositol, Kava, Milk Thistle, Omega-3 Fatty Acids, Selenium, Valerian, Vitamin A, Vitamin B_1, Vitamin B_2, Vitamin B_3, Vitamin B_6, Vitamin B_{12}, Vitamin C, Vitamin D, Vitamin E, Vitamin K, Vitex, Zinc

Depakote ER (divalproex sodium): Calcium, Carnitine, Copper, DHEA, Folic Acid, Ginkgo, Inositol, Kava, Milk Thistle, Omega-3 Fatty Acids, Selenium, Valerian, Vitamin A, Vitamin B_1, Vitamin B_2, Vitamin B_3, Vitamin B_6, Vitamin B_{12}, Vitamin C, Vitamin D, Vitamin E, Vitamin K, Vitex, Zinc

Depen (penicillamine): Copper, Iron, Magnesium, Vitamin B_6, Zinc

Depo-Estradiol (estradiol cypionate): Arginine, Black Cohosh, Boron, Calcium, Copper, DHEA, Dang Gui, Magnesium, Melatonin, Milk Thistle, St. John's Wort, Vitamin B_6, Vitamin D, Vitamin E, Vitex, Zinc

Depo-Provera (medroxyprogesterone, injection): Beta-Carotene, Calcium, Folic Acid, Vitamin A, Vitamin B_3, Vitamin D

Depo-subQ Provera 104 (medroxyprogesterone, injection): Beta-Carotene, Calcium, Folic Acid, Vitamin A, Vitamin B_3, Vitamin D

DepoCyt (cytarabine): Echinacea, Eleuthero, Folic Acid, Ginseng, Vitamin B_1

Depogen (estradiol cypionate): Arginine, Black Cohosh, Boron, Calcium, Copper, DHEA, Dang Gui, Magnesium, Melatonin, Milk Thistle, St. John's Wort, Vitamin B_6, Vitamin D, Vitamin E, Vitex, Zinc

Deponit (nitroglycerin): Arginine, Carnitine, Folic Acid, Vitamin C

Deracyn (adinazolam): Kava, St. John's Wort

Derma-Smoothe/FS (fluocinolone): Aloe, Green Tea, Licorice, Vitamin C

Dermacort (hydrocortisone): Aloe, Green Tea, Licorice, Vitamin C

Dermarest (hydrocortisone): Aloe, Green Tea, Licorice, Vitamin C

DermiCort (hydrocortisone): Aloe, Green Tea, Licorice, Vitamin C

Dermotyl (clobetasol): Aloe, Green Tea, Licorice, Vitamin C, Zinc

Dermoval (clobetasol): Aloe, Green Tea, Licorice, Vitamin C, Zinc

Dermovate (clobetasol): Aloe, Green Tea, Licorice, Vitamin C, Zinc

Dermovate-NN (neomycin + nystatin + clobetasol): Aloe, Beta-Carotene, Green Tea, Licorice, Vitamin C, Zinc

Dermoxin (clobetasol): Aloe, Green Tea, Licorice, Vitamin C, Zinc

Dermtex HC (hydrocortisone 17-butyrate/acetate/probutate/valerate): Aloe, Green Tea, Licorice, Vitamin C

Deroxat (paroxetine): 5-HTP, Chromium, Folic Acid, Ginkgo, Inositol, Omega-3 Fatty Acids, S-Adenosylmethionine (SAMe), St. John's Wort, Tryptophan, Vitamin B_3, Vitamin B_6, Vitamin B_{12}, Vitamin C, Zinc

Desferal (desferoxamine): Copper, Iron, Vitamin C

Desogen (ethinyl estradiol + desogestrel): Arginine, Calcium, Copper, DHEA, Dang Gui, Folic Acid, Iron, Licorice, Magnesium, Melatonin, Milk Thistle, S-Adenosylmethionine (SAMe), Selenium, St. John's Wort, Tyrosine, Vitamin A, Vitamin B_1, Vitamin B_2, Vitamin B_3, Vitamin B_6, Vitamin B_{12}, Vitamin C, Vitamin E, Vitex, Zinc

DesOwen (desonide): Aloe, Green Tea, Licorice, Vitamin C

Destolit (ursodeoxycholic acid): S-Adenosylmethionine (SAMe), Vitamin B_3

Desyrel (trazodone): 5-HTP, Ginkgo, St. John's Wort

Deteclo (chlortetracycline + demeclocycline + tetracycline): Calcium, Folic Acid, Iron, Magnesium, Potassium, Vitamin A, Vitamin B_1, Vitamin B_2, Vitamin B_3, Vitamin B_6, Vitamin C, Zinc

Dex-A-Diet (phenylpropanolamine): Potassium, Tyrosine

Dexatrim (phenylpropanolamine): Potassium, Tyrosine

Dexedrine (dextroamphetamine): 5-HTP, Magnesium, Omega-3 Fatty Acids, Potassium, Reishi, Tyrosine, Vitamin B_6, Vitamin C, Zinc

Diabeta (glyburide): Aloe, Alpha-Lipoic Acid, Astragalus, Bilberry, Chromium, Coenzyme Q10, DHEA, Ephedra, Garlic, Ginkgo, Ginseng, Glucosamine Sulfate, Gotu Kola, Horse Chestnut, Magnesium, Omega-3 Fatty Acids, Reishi, Turmeric/Curcumin, Vitamin B_3, Vitamin E

Diabinese (chlorpropamide): Aloe, Alpha-Lipoic Acid, Astragalus, Bilberry, Chromium, Coenzyme Q10, DHEA, Ephedra, Garlic, Ginkgo, Ginseng, Glucosamine Sulfate,

Gotu Kola, Horse Chestnut, Magnesium, Omega-3 Fatty Acids, Reishi, Turmeric/Curcumin, Vitamin B_3

Diamox Sequels (acetazolamide): Coenzyme Q10, Ephedra, Potassium

Diamox (acetazolamide): Coenzyme Q10, Ephedra, Potassium

Dianabol (methandrostenolone): Echinacea, Milk Thistle

Dianben (metformin): Alpha-Lipoic Acid, Astragalus, Bilberry, Calcium, Chromium, Coenzyme Q10, DHEA, Ephedra, Folic Acid, Garlic, Ginkgo, Ginseng, Glucosamine Sulfate, Gotu Kola, Horse Chestnut, Magnesium, Omega-3 Fatty Acids, Reishi, Turmeric/Curcumin, Vitamin B_3, Vitamin B_{12}

Diastat (diazepam): Carnitine, DHEA, Gotu Kola, Melatonin, Valerian, Vitamin B_3

Diclectin (doxylamine + pyridoxine): Vitamin B_6

Didronel (etidronate): Calcium, Iron, Magnesium, Vitamin D, Zinc

Diflucan (fluconazole): Echinacea, St. John's Wort

Digitek (digoxin): Calcium, Cascara, Dang Gui, Eleuthero, Ephedra, Hawthorn, Licorice, Magnesium, Potassium, St. John's Wort, Vitamin D

Dilacor XR (diltiazem): Calcium, Carnitine, Folic Acid, Magnesium, St. John's Wort, Vitamin B_6, Vitamin D

Dilantin (phenytoin): Calcium, Carnitine, Copper, DHEA, Folic Acid, Ginkgo, Inositol, Kava, Milk Thistle, Omega-3 Fatty Acids, Valerian, Vitamin A, Vitamin B_1, Vitamin B_2, Vitamin B_3, Vitamin B_6, Vitamin B_{12}, Vitamin C, Vitamin D, Vitamin E, Vitamin K, Vitex, Zinc

Dilaudid-5 (hydromorphone): Ephedra, Ginseng, Gotu Kola, Phenylalanine, Tyrosine

Dilaudid-HP (hydromorphone): Ephedra, Ginseng, Gotu Kola, Phenylalanine, Tyrosine

Dilaudid (hydromorphone): Ephedra, Ginseng, Gotu Kola, Phenylalanine, Tyrosine

Dilor (dyphylline): Potassium

Diltia XT (diltiazem): Calcium, Carnitine, Folic Acid, Magnesium, St. John's Wort, Vitamin B_6, Vitamin D

Dimetapp Decongestant (pseudoephedrine): Potassium

Dindevan (phenindione): Bilberry, Cayenne, Chondroitin Sulfate, Coenzyme Q10, DHEA, Dang Gui, Devil's Claw, Feverfew, Garlic, Ginger, Ginkgo, Ginseng, Green Tea, Horse Chestnut, Kava, Licorice, Magnesium, Omega-3 Fatty Acids, Policosanol, Red Clover, Reishi, Saw Palmetto, St. John's Wort, Vitamin A, Vitamin B_3, Vitamin C, Vitamin E, Vitamin K, Zinc

Diovan (valsartan): Alpha-Lipoic Acid, Potassium

Diovan HCT (valsartan + hydrochlorothiazide): Alpha-Lipoic Acid, Potassium

Diprolene (betamethasone dipropionate/valerate): Aloe, Green Tea, Licorice, Vitamin C

Diprolene AF (betamethasone dipropionate/valerate): Aloe, Green Tea, Licorice, Vitamin C

Diprosone (betamethasone dipropionate/valerate): Aloe, Green Tea, Licorice, Vitamin C

Disalcid (salsalate): Calcium, Cayenne, Chondroitin Sulfate, Chromium, Copper, Devil's Claw, Feverfew, Folic Acid, Ginger, Glucosamine Sulfate, Gotu Kola, Iron, Licorice, Melatonin, Omega-3 Fatty Acids, Policosanol, Potassium, Turmeric/Curcumin, Vitamin B_3, Vitamin B_6, Vitamin C, Vitamin K, Zinc

Dithranol (anthralin): Vitamin E

Diucardin (hydroflumethiazide): Calcium, Coenzyme Q10, Folic Acid, Ginkgo, Glucosamine Sulfate, Hawthorn, Licorice, Magnesium, Potassium, Vitamin B_2, Vitamin D, Zinc

Diuril (chlorothiazide): Calcium, Coenzyme Q10, Folic Acid, Ginkgo, Glucosamine Sulfate, Hawthorn, Licorice, Magnesium, Potassium, Vitamin B_2, Vitamin D, Zinc

Dobutrex (dobutamine): Calcium

Dolacet (hydrocodone + acetaminophen): Ephedra, Ginseng, Gotu Kola, Phenylalanine, Tyrosine

Dolobid (diflunisal): Calcium, Cayenne, Chondroitin Sulfate, Chromium, Copper, Devil's Claw, Feverfew, Folic Acid, Ginger, Glucosamine Sulfate, Gotu Kola, Iron, Licorice, Melatonin, Omega-3 Fatty Acids, Policosanol, Potassium, Turmeric/Curcumin, Vitamin B_3, Vitamin B_6, Vitamin C, Vitamin K, Zinc

Dolophine (methadone): Ephedra, Ginseng, Gotu Kola, Phenylalanine, Tyrosine

Donnamar (hyoscyamine): Iron

Doral (quazepam): DHEA, Gotu Kola, Melatonin, Valerian, Vitamin B_3

Doryx (doxycycline): Calcium, Folic Acid, Iron, Magnesium, Potassium, Vitamin A, Vitamin B_1, Vitamin B_2, Vitamin B_3, Vitamin B_6, Vitamin C, Zinc

Doxil (doxorubicin, pegylated liposomal): Alpha-Lipoic Acid, Carnitine, Coenzyme Q10, Feverfew, Garlic, Ginkgo, Green Tea, Hawthorn, Milk Thistle, Reishi, Selenium, St. John's Wort, Turmeric/Curcumin, Vitamin B_2, Vitamin B_6, Vitamin E

Doxy (doxycycline): Calcium, Folic Acid, Iron, Magnesium, Potassium, Vitamin A, Vitamin B_1, Vitamin B_2, Vitamin B_3, Vitamin B_6, Vitamin C, Zinc

Drenison (flurandrenolide): Aloe, Green Tea, Licorice, Vitamin C

DriCort (hydrocortisone 17-butyrate/acetate/probutate/valerate): Aloe, Green Tea, Licorice, Vitamin C

Dridol (droperidol): Milk Thistle, Phenylalanine

Drithocreme (anthralin): Vitamin E

Drixoral (pseudoephedrine): Potassium

Drogenil (flutamide): Black Cohosh, Vitamin D

DTIC-Dome (dacarbazine): Astragalus, Carnitine, Echinacea, Eleuthero, Selenium

Duagen (dutasteride): Black Cohosh, Saw Palmetto

Dulcolax (bisacodyl tablets): Potassium

DuoCet (hydrocodone + acetaminophen): Ephedra, Ginseng, Gotu Kola, Phenylalanine, Tyrosine

Duofem (levonorgestrel, oral postcoital contraceptive): Magnesium, St. John's Wort

Duphaston (dydrogesterone): Vitamin D, Vitex

Duprost (dutasteride): Black Cohosh, Saw Palmetto

Dura-Estrin (estradiol cypionate): Arginine, Black Cohosh, Boron, Calcium, Copper, DHEA, Dang Gui, Magnesium, Melatonin, Milk Thistle, St. John's Wort, Vitamin B_6, Vitamin D, Vitamin E, Vitex, Zinc

Duraclon (clonidine): DHEA, Ephedra, Melatonin

Duragesic Transdermal (fentanyl): Ephedra, Ginger, Ginseng, Gotu Kola, Magnesium, Phenylalanine, Tyrosine

Duralith (lithium carbonate): 5-HTP, Chromium, Folic Acid, Inositol, Magnesium, Tryptophan

Duramorph (morphine): Ephedra, Ginseng, Gotu Kola, Phenylalanine, Tyrosine

Duricef (cefadroxil): Ginseng, Green Tea, Iron, Licorice, Probiotic Flora, Reishi, Vitamin B_1, Vitamin K, Zinc

Dutagen (dutasteride): Black Cohosh, Saw Palmetto

Dutas (dutasteride): Black Cohosh, Saw Palmetto

Dyazide (triamterene + hydrochlorothiazide): Arginine, Calcium, Coenzyme Q10, Folic Acid, Glucosamine Sulfate, Hawthorn, Licorice, Magnesium, Potassium, Vitamin D, Zinc

Dycill (dicloxacillin): Ginseng, Green Tea, Licorice, Probiotic Flora, Vitamin B_1, Vitamin K, Zinc

Dymelor (acetohexamide): Aloe, Alpha-Lipoic Acid, Astragalus, Bilberry, Chromium, Coenzyme Q10, DHEA, Ephedra, Garlic, Ginkgo, Ginseng, Glucosamine Sulfate, Gotu Kola, Horse Chestnut, Magnesium, Omega-3 Fatty Acids, Reishi, Turmeric/Curcumin, Vitamin B_3

Dynabac (dirithromycin): Calcium, Green Tea, Magnesium, Probiotic Flora, Vitamin B_1, Vitamin B_6, Vitamin K, Zinc

Dynacin (minocycline): Calcium, Folic Acid, Iron, Magnesium, Potassium, Vitamin A, Vitamin B_1, Vitamin B_2, Vitamin B_3, Vitamin B_6, Vitamin C, Zinc

DynaCirc (isradipine): Calcium, Carnitine, Folic Acid, Magnesium, St. John's Wort, Vitamin B_6, Vitamin D

DynaCirc CR (isradipine): Calcium, Carnitine, Folic Acid, Magnesium, St. John's Wort, Vitamin B_6, Vitamin D

DynaCirc I.V. (isradipine): Calcium, Carnitine, Folic Acid, Magnesium, St. John's Wort, Vitamin B_6, Vitamin D

Dynapen (dicloxacillin): Ginseng, Green Tea, Licorice, Probiotic Flora, Vitamin B_1, Vitamin K, Zinc

Dyrenium (triamterene): Arginine, Calcium, Folic Acid, Glucosamine Sulfate, Magnesium, Potassium, Zinc

Easprin (acetylsalicylic acid): Bilberry, Calcium, Cayenne, Devil's Claw, Feverfew, Folic Acid, Garlic, Ginger, Ginkgo, Gotu Kola, Iron, Licorice, Melatonin, Milk Thistle, Omega-3 Fatty Acids, Policosanol, Potassium, S-Adenosylmethionine (SAMe), Vitamin B_2, Vitamin B_3, Vitamin C, Vitamin E, Vitamin K, Zinc

Ecostatin (econazole): Echinacea

Ecotrin (acetylsalicylic acid): Bilberry, Calcium, Cayenne, Devil's Claw, Feverfew, Folic Acid, Garlic, Ginger, Ginkgo, Gotu Kola, Iron, Licorice, Melatonin, Milk Thistle, Omega-3 Fatty Acids, Policosanol, Potassium, S-Adenosylmethionine (SAMe), Vitamin B_2, Vitamin B_3, Vitamin C, Vitamin E, Vitamin K, Zinc

Ecotrin Low Adult Strength (acetylsalicylic acid): Bilberry, Calcium, Cayenne, Devil's Claw, Feverfew, Folic Acid, Garlic, Ginger, Ginkgo, Gotu Kola, Iron, Licorice, Melatonin, Milk Thistle, Omega-3 Fatty Acids, Policosanol, Potassium, S-Adenosylmethionine (SAMe), Vitamin B_2, Vitamin B_3, Vitamin C, Vitamin E, Vitamin K, Zinc

ED-SPAZ (hyoscyamine): Iron

Edecrin (ethacrynic acid): Calcium, Folic Acid, Ginseng, Glucosamine Sulfate, Licorice, Magnesium, Potassium, Vitamin B_1, Vitamin B_6, Vitamin C, Zinc

EES (erythromycin oral): Calcium, Green Tea, Magnesium, Probiotic Flora, Vitamin B_1, Vitamin B_6, Vitamin B_{12}, Vitamin K, Zinc

Effexor (venlafaxine): 5-HTP, Folic Acid, Ginkgo, Omega-3 Fatty Acids, S-Adenosylmethionine (SAMe), St. John's Wort, Tryptophan, Vitamin B_3, Vitamin B_6, Vitamin B_{12}

Efidac (pseudoephedrine): Potassium

Efudex (fluorouracil): Aloe, Beta-Carotene, Echinacea, Eleuthero, Folic Acid, Garlic, Ginkgo, Ginseng, Melatonin, Omega-3 Fatty Acids, Vitamin A, Vitamin B_1, Vitamin B_3, Vitamin B_6, Vitamin C, Vitamin E

Efudix (fluorouracil): Aloe, Beta-Carotene, Echinacea, Eleuthero, Folic Acid, Garlic, Ginkgo, Ginseng, Melatonin, Omega-3 Fatty Acids, Vitamin A, Vitamin B_1, Vitamin B_3, Vitamin B_6, Vitamin C, Vitamin E

Elavil (amitriptyline): 5-HTP, Coenzyme Q10, Echinacea, Milk Thistle, S-Adenosylmethionine (SAMe), St. John's Wort, Tryptophan, Tyrosine, Vitamin B_1, Vitamin B_2, Vitamin B_3, Vitamin B_6, Vitamin B_{12}, Zinc

Eldepryl (selegiline): 5-HTP, Cayenne, Chromium, Eleuthero, Ephedra, Folic Acid, Ginkgo, Iron, Kava, Licorice, Phenylalanine, S-Adenosylmethionine (SAMe), St. John's Wort, Tryptophan, Tyrosine, Vitamin B_2, Vitamin B_6, Vitex

Ellence (epirubicin): Alpha-Lipoic Acid, Carnitine, Coenzyme Q10, Feverfew, Garlic, Ginkgo, Green Tea, Hawthorn, Milk Thistle, Reishi, Selenium, St. John's Wort, Turmeric/Curcumin, Vitamin B_2, Vitamin E

Eloxatin (oxaliplatin): Alpha-Lipoic Acid, Astragalus, Carnitine, Cayenne, Chondroitin Sulfate, Echinacea, Eleuthero, Ginger, Ginkgo, Ginseng, Milk Thistle, Selenium, St. John's Wort, Vitamin E

Eltroxin (levothyroxine): Alpha-Lipoic Acid, Calcium, Carnitine, Coenzyme Q10, DHEA, Iron, Tyrosine, Vitamin B_2

Eludril (chlorhexidine): Iron, Licorice, Probiotic Flora, Vitamin K, Zinc

Eminase (anistreplase): Astragalus

Empirin (acetylsalicylic acid): Bilberry, Calcium, Cayenne, Devil's Claw, Feverfew, Folic Acid, Garlic, Ginger, Ginkgo, Gotu Kola, Iron, Licorice, Melatonin, Milk Thistle, Omega-3 Fatty Acids, Policosanol, Potassium, S-Adenosylmethionine (SAMe), Vitamin B_2, Vitamin B_3, Vitamin C, Vitamin E, Vitamin K, Zinc

Empirin with Codeine (acetylsalicylic acid + codeine): Calcium, Cayenne, Devil's Claw, Ephedra, Feverfew, Folic Acid, Ginkgo, Ginseng, Gotu Kola, Iron, Licorice, Melatonin, Milk Thistle, Phenylalanine, Policosanol, Potassium, Tyrosine, Vitamin B_2, Vitamin B_3, Vitamin C, Vitamin E, Vitamin K

Enbrel (etanercept): Echinacea

Endocet (acetaminophen + oxycodone): Ephedra, Garlic, Ginseng, Gotu Kola, Licorice, Milk Thistle, Phenylalanine, Tyrosine, Vitamin C

Endocodone (oxycodone): Ephedra, Ginseng, Gotu Kola, Phenylalanine, Tyrosine

Endodan (acetylsalicylic acid + oxycodone): Calcium, Cayenne, Devil's Claw, Ephedra, Feverfew, Folic Acid, Ginkgo, Ginseng, Gotu Kola, Iron, Licorice, Melatonin, Milk Thistle, Phenylalanine, Policosanol, Potassium, Tyrosine, Vitamin B_2, Vitamin B_3, Vitamin C, Vitamin E, Vitamin K, Zinc

Endoxana (cyclophosphamide): Aloe, Alpha-Lipoic Acid, Astragalus, Beta-Carotene, Carnitine, Echinacea, Eleuthero, Ginger, Ginseng, Licorice, Melatonin, Omega-3 Fatty Acids, Reishi, Selenium, Turmeric/Curcumin, Vitamin A, Vitamin C, Vitamin E

Enduron (methyclothiazide): Calcium, Coenzyme Q10, Folic Acid, Ginkgo, Glucosamine Sulfate, Hawthorn, Licorice, Magnesium, Potassium, Vitamin B_2, Vitamin D, Zinc

Enerjets (caffeine): Calcium, Ephedra, Kava, Melatonin

Entex LA (guaifenesin + phenylpropanolamine): Potassium, Tyrosine.

Epifin (epinephrine): Magnesium, Potassium, Vitamin C

Epifoam (hydrocortisone 17-butyrate/acetate/probutate/valerate): Aloe, Green Tea, Licorice, Vitamin C

Epinal (epinephrine): Magnesium, Potassium, Vitamin C

EpiPen (epinephrine): Magnesium, Potassium, Vitamin C

EpiPen Auto-Injector, injectable (epinephrine): Magnesium, Potassium, Vitamin C

Epitrate (epinephrine): Magnesium, Potassium, Vitamin C

Epivir (lamivudine): Aloe, Carnitine, Coenzyme Q10, Copper, DHEA, Reishi, Vitamin B_1, Vitamin B_2, Vitamin B_{12}, Zinc

Epogen (epoetin alpha): Dang Gui, Iron, Vitamin B_6, Vitamin C

Eposin (etoposide): Aloe, Feverfew, Ginseng, Melatonin, Omega-3 Fatty Acids, St. John's Wort

Eppy/N (epinephrine): Magnesium, Potassium, Vitamin C

Eprex (epoetin alpha): Dang Gui, Iron, Vitamin B_6, Vitamin C

Equipoise (boldenone): Echinacea

Ergamisol (levamisole): Beta-Carotene, Echinacea, Vitamin A

Errin (norethindrone, oral): Magnesium, St. John's Wort

Ery-Tab (erythromycin oral): Calcium, Green Tea, Magnesium, Probiotic Flora, Vitamin B_1, Vitamin B_6, Vitamin B_{12}, Vitamin K, Zinc

Erycette (erythromycin topical): Calcium, Green Tea, Magnesium, Probiotic Flora, Vitamin B_1, Vitamin B_6, Vitamin K, Zinc

Eryderm (erythromycin topical): Calcium, Green Tea, Magnesium, Probiotic Flora, Vitamin B_1, Vitamin B_6, Vitamin K, Zinc

Erygel (erythromycin topical): Calcium, Green Tea, Magnesium, Probiotic Flora, Vitamin B_1, Vitamin B_6, Vitamin K, Zinc

EryPed (erythromycin oral): Calcium, Green Tea, Magnesium, Probiotic Flora, Vitamin B_1, Vitamin B_6, Vitamin B_{12}, Vitamin K, Zinc

Esbatal (betanidine): Ephedra

Escapelle (levonorgestrel, oral postcoital contraceptive): Magnesium, St. John's Wort

Esidrix (hydrochlorothiazide): Calcium, Coenzyme Q10, Folic Acid, Ginkgo, Glucosamine Sulfate, Hawthorn, Licorice, Magnesium, Potassium, Vitamin B_2, Vitamin D, Zinc

Eskalith (lithium carbonate): 5-HTP, Chromium, Folic Acid, Inositol, Magnesium, Tryptophan

Essaven (topical) (heparin + phosphatidylcholine + Aescin): Horse Chestnut

Estinyl (ethinyl estradiol): Arginine, Boron, Calcium, Copper, DHEA, Dang Gui, Folic Acid, Iron, Licorice, Magnesium, Melatonin, Milk Thistle, S-Adenosylmethionine (SAMe), Selenium, St. John's Wort, Tyrosine, Vitamin A, Vitamin B_1, Vitamin B_2, Vitamin B_3, Vitamin B_6, Vitamin B_{12}, Vitamin C, Vitamin E, Vitex, Zinc

Estra-D (estradiol cypionate): Arginine, Black Cohosh, Boron, Calcium, Copper, DHEA, Dang Gui, Magnesium, Melatonin, Milk Thistle, St. John's Wort, Vitamin B_6, Vitamin D, Vitamin E, Vitex, Zinc

Estra-L 40 (estradiol valerate): Arginine, Black Cohosh, Boron, Calcium, Copper, DHEA, Dang Gui, Magnesium, Melatonin, Milk Thistle, St. John's Wort, Vitamin B_6, Vitamin D, Vitamin E, Vitex, Zinc

Estrace (estradiol): Arginine, Black Cohosh, Boron, Calcium, Copper, DHEA, Dang Gui, Magnesium, Melatonin, Milk Thistle, St. John's Wort, Vitamin B_6, Vitamin D, Vitamin E, Vitex, Zinc

Estradot (estradiol): Arginine, Black Cohosh, Boron, Calcium, Copper, DHEA, Dang Gui, Magnesium, Melatonin, Milk Thistle, St. John's Wort, Vitamin B_6, Vitamin D, Vitamin E, Vitex, Zinc

Estragyn 5 (estrone): Arginine, Black Cohosh, Boron, Calcium, Copper, DHEA, Dang Gui, Magnesium, Melatonin, Milk Thistle, St. John's Wort, Vitamin B_6, Vitamin D, Vitamin E, Vitex, Zinc

Estratab (esterified estrogens): Arginine, Black Cohosh, Boron, Calcium, Copper, DHEA, Dang Gui, Magnesium, Melatonin, Milk Thistle, St. John's Wort, Vitamin B_6, Vitamin D, Vitamin E, Vitex, Zinc

Estratest (esterified estrogens + methyltestosterone): Beta-Carotene, Black Cohosh, Boron, Calcium, Copper, DHEA,

Dang Gui, Magnesium, Melatonin, Milk Thistle, St. John's Wort, Vitamin A, Vitamin B_6, Vitamin D, Vitamin E, Vitex, Zinc

Estratest H.S. (esterified estrogens + methyltestosterone): Beta-Carotene, Black Cohosh, Boron, Calcium, Copper, DHEA, Dang Gui, Magnesium, Melatonin, Milk Thistle, St. John's Wort, Vitamin A, Vitamin B_6, Vitamin D, Vitamin E, Vitex, Zinc

Estreva (estradiol hemihydrate): Arginine, Black Cohosh, Boron, Calcium, Copper, DHEA, Dang Gui, Magnesium, Melatonin, Milk Thistle, St. John's Wort, Vitamin B_6, Vitamin D, Vitamin E, Vitex, Zinc

Estring (estradiol): Arginine, Black Cohosh, Boron, Calcium, Copper, DHEA, Dang Gui, Magnesium, Melatonin, Milk Thistle, St. John's Wort, Vitamin B_6, Vitamin D, Vitamin E, Vitex, Zinc

Estro-A (estrone): Arginine, Black Cohosh, Boron, Calcium, Copper, DHEA, Dang Gui, Magnesium, Melatonin, Milk Thistle, St. John's Wort, Vitamin B_6, Vitamin D, Vitamin E, Vitex, Zinc

Estro-Cyp (estradiol cypionate): Arginine, Black Cohosh, Boron, Calcium, Copper, DHEA, Dang Gui, Magnesium, Melatonin, Milk Thistle, St. John's Wort, Vitamin B_6, Vitamin D, Vitamin E, Vitex, Zinc

Estroject-LA (estradiol cypionate): Arginine, Black Cohosh, Boron, Calcium, Copper, DHEA, Dang Gui, Magnesium, Melatonin, Milk Thistle, St. John's Wort, Vitamin B_6, Vitamin D, Vitamin E, Vitex, Zinc

Estrone '5' (estrone): Arginine, Black Cohosh, Boron, Calcium, Copper, DHEA, Dang Gui, Magnesium, Melatonin, Milk Thistle, St. John's Wort, Vitamin B_6, Vitamin D, Vitamin E, Vitex, Zinc

Estronol-LA (estradiol cypionate): Arginine, Black Cohosh, Boron, Calcium, Copper, DHEA, Dang Gui, Magnesium, Melatonin, Milk Thistle, St. John's Wort, Vitamin B_6, Vitamin D, Vitamin E, Vitex, Zinc

Estrostep (ethinyl estradiol + norethindrone): Arginine, Calcium, Copper, DHEA, Dang Gui, Folic Acid, Iron, Licorice, Magnesium, Melatonin, Milk Thistle, S-Adenosylmethionine (SAMe), Selenium, St. John's Wort, Tyrosine, Vitamin A, Vitamin B_1, Vitamin B_2, Vitamin B_3, Vitamin B_6, Vitamin B_{12}, Vitamin C, Vitamin E, Vitex, Zinc

Ethide (ethionamide): Folic Acid, Milk Thistle, Vitamin B_6, Vitamin C, Vitamin D

Ethiocid (ethionamide): Folic Acid, Milk Thistle, Vitamin B_6, Vitamin C, Vitamin D

Ethomid (ethionamide): Folic Acid, Milk Thistle, Vitamin B_6, Vitamin C, Vitamin D

Ethrane (enflurane): Alpha-Lipoic Acid, Ephedra, Milk Thistle, St. John's Wort, Valerian

Etomide (ethionamide): Folic Acid, Milk Thistle, Vitamin B_6, Vitamin C, Vitamin D

Etopophos (etoposide): Aloe, Feverfew, Ginseng, Melatonin, Omega-3 Fatty Acids, St. John's Wort

Etrafon (amitriptyline + perphenazine): Coenzyme Q10, Echinacea, Milk Thistle, St. John's Wort, Vitamin B_{12}

Eulexin (flutamide): Black Cohosh, Vitamin D

Eumosone (clobetasol): Aloe, Green Tea, Licorice, Vitamin C, Zinc

Eumovate (clobetasone): Aloe, Green Tea, Licorice, Vitamin C

Euthroid (L-thyroxine + L-triiodothyronine [synthetic]): Alpha-Lipoic Acid, Calcium, Carnitine, Coenzyme Q10, DHEA, Iron, Tyrosine, Vitamin B_2

Euthyral (L-thyroxine + L-triiodothyronine [synthetic]): Alpha-Lipoic Acid, Calcium, Carnitine, Coenzyme Q10, DHEA, Iron, Tyrosine, Vitamin B_2

Eutonyl (pargyline): 5-HTP, Cayenne, Chromium, Eleuthero, Ephedra, Ginkgo, Kava, Licorice, Phenylalanine, S-Adenosylmethionine (SAMe), St. John's Wort, Tryptophan, Tyrosine, Vitamin B_3

Evista (raloxifene): Black Cohosh, Dang Gui, Green Tea, Vitamin D

Excedrin IB (ibuprofen): Calcium, Cayenne, Chondroitin Sulfate, Chromium, Copper, Devil's Claw, Feverfew, Folic Acid, Ginger, Glucosamine Sulfate, Gotu Kola, Iron, Licorice, Melatonin, Omega-3 Fatty Acids, Potassium, Turmeric/Curcumin, Vitamin B_3, Vitamin B_6, Vitamin C, Zinc

Exirel (pirbuterol): Calcium, Magnesium, Potassium

Exjade (deferasirox): Vitamin C

Exna (benzthiazide): Calcium, Coenzyme Q10, Folic Acid, Ginkgo, Glucosamine Sulfate, Hawthorn, Licorice, Magnesium, Potassium, Vitamin B_2, Vitamin D, Zinc

Extra Strength Adprin-B (acetylsalicylic acid): Bilberry, Calcium, Cayenne, Devil's Claw, Feverfew, Folic Acid, Garlic, Ginger, Ginkgo, Gotu Kola, Iron, Licorice, Melatonin, Milk Thistle, Omega-3 Fatty Acids, Policosanol, Potassium, S-Adenosylmethionine (SAMe), Vitamin B_2, Vitamin B_3, Vitamin C, Vitamin E, Vitamin K, Zinc

Extra Strength Bayer Enteric 500 Aspirin (acetylsalicylic acid): Bilberry, Calcium, Cayenne, Devil's Claw, Feverfew, Folic Acid, Garlic, Ginger, Ginkgo, Gotu Kola, Iron, Licorice, Melatonin, Milk Thistle, Omega-3 Fatty Acids, Policosanol, Potassium, S-Adenosylmethionine (SAMe), Vitamin B_2, Vitamin B_3, Vitamin C, Vitamin E, Vitamin K, Zinc

Extra Strength Bayer Plus (acetylsalicylic acid): Bilberry, Calcium, Cayenne, Devil's Claw, Feverfew, Folic Acid, Garlic, Ginger, Ginkgo, Gotu Kola, Iron, Licorice, Melatonin, Milk Thistle, Omega-3 Fatty Acids, Policosanol, Potassium, S-Adenosylmethionine (SAMe), Vitamin B_2, Vitamin B_3, Vitamin C, Vitamin E, Vitamin K, Zinc

Ezide (hydrochlorothiazide): Calcium, Coenzyme Q10, Folic Acid, Ginkgo, Glucosamine Sulfate, Hawthorn, Licorice, Magnesium, Potassium, Vitamin B_2, Vitamin D, Zinc

Fabrazyme (agalsidase beta): Echinacea, Eleuthero, Folic Acid, Vitamin B_1

Famvir (famciclovir): Astragalus

Fansidar (sulfadoxine + pyrimethamine): Folic Acid, Iron, Vitamin B_2

Fareston (toremifene): Black Cohosh, Dang Gui, Green Tea

Fasigyn (tinidazole): Milk Thistle

Faurin (fluvoxamine): 5-HTP, Chromium, Folic Acid, Ginkgo, Inositol, Melatonin, Omega-3 Fatty Acids, S-Adenosylmethionine (SAMe), St. John's Wort, Tryptophan, Vitamin B_3, Vitamin B_6, Vitamin B_{12}, Vitamin C, Zinc

Felbatol (felbamate): Calcium, Carnitine, Copper, DHEA, Folic Acid, Ginkgo, Inositol, Kava, Milk Thistle, Omega-3 Fatty Acids, Valerian, Vitamin A, Vitamin B_1, Vitamin B_2, Vitamin B_3, Vitamin B_6, Vitamin B_{12}, Vitamin C, Vitamin D, Vitamin E, Vitamin K, Vitex, Zinc

Feldene (piroxicam): Calcium, Cayenne, Chondroitin Sulfate, Chromium, Copper, Devil's Claw, Feverfew, Folic Acid, Ginger, Glucosamine Sulfate, Gotu Kola, Iron, Licorice, Melatonin, Omega-3 Fatty Acids, Potassium, Turmeric/Curcumin, Vitamin B_3, Vitamin B_6, Vitamin C, Zinc

Femara (letrozole): Green Tea

FemHRT (estradiol + norethindrone, oral): Arginine, Black Cohosh, Boron, Calcium, Copper, DHEA, Dang Gui, Magnesium, Melatonin, Milk Thistle, St. John's Wort, Vitamin B$_6$, Vitamin D, Vitamin E, Vitex, Zinc

Femoston (estradiol + dydrogesterone): Arginine, Black Cohosh, Boron, Calcium, Copper, DHEA, Dang Gui, Magnesium, Melatonin, Milk Thistle, St. John's Wort, Vitamin B$_6$, Vitamin D, Vitamin E, Vitex, Zinc

Fenformin (phenformin): Alpha-Lipoic Acid, Astragalus, Bilberry, Calcium, Chromium, Coenzyme Q10, DHEA, Ephedra, Folic Acid, Garlic, Ginkgo, Ginseng, Glucosamine Sulfate, Gotu Kola, Horse Chestnut, Magnesium, Omega-3 Fatty Acids, Reishi, Turmeric/Curcumin, Vitamin B$_3$, Vitamin B$_{12}$

Fentanyl Oralet (fentanyl): Ephedra, Ginger, Ginseng, Gotu Kola, Magnesium, Phenylalanine, Tyrosine

FiberCon (polycarbophil): Potassium, Vitamin B$_2$

Fina (trenbolone): Echinacea

Fioricet (paracetamol + butalbital + caffeine): Calcium, DHEA, Ephedra, Garlic, Gotu Kola, Licorice, Methionine, Milk Thistle, S-Adenosylmethionine (SAMe), Valerian, Vitamin B$_2$, Vitamin C

Fiorinal (acetylsalicylic acid + codeine + butalbital + caffeine): Calcium, Cayenne, Devil's Claw, Ephedra, Feverfew, Folic Acid, Ginkgo, Ginseng, Gotu Kola, Iron, Licorice, Melatonin, Milk Thistle, Phenylalanine, Policosanol, Potassium, Tyrosine, Vitamin B$_2$, Vitamin B$_3$, Vitamin C, Vitamin E, Vitamin K, Zinc

Flagyl (metronidazole, systemic): Licorice, Milk Thistle, Probiotic Flora, Vitamin K, Zinc

Fleet (Glycerin-containing Suppositories): Potassium

Fleet enema, Fleet Phospho-soda Oral Saline Laxative (monobasic sodium phosphate monohydrate + dibasic sodium phosphate heptahydrate): Potassium

Fletchers Castoria (senna): Potassium

Flexeril (cyclobenzaprine): Echinacea

Flomax (tamsulosin): Saw Palmetto, Vitamin B$_3$

Flomaxtra (tamsulosin): Saw Palmetto, Vitamin B$_3$

Florone (diflorasone): Aloe, Green Tea, Licorice, Vitamin C

Floxin (ofloxacin): Calcium, Green Tea, Iron, Licorice, Magnesium, Potassium, Probiotic Flora, Vitamin B$_1$, Vitamin K, Zinc

Fludara (fludarabine): Echinacea, Eleuthero, Folic Acid, Vitamin B$_1$

Fluonex (fluocinonide): Aloe, Green Tea, Licorice, Vitamin C

Fluonid (fluocinolone): Aloe, Green Tea, Licorice, Vitamin C

Fluorigard (sodium fluoride): Calcium, Vitamin D

Fluorinse (sodium fluoride): Calcium, Vitamin D

Fluoritab (sodium fluoride): Calcium, Vitamin D

Fluorodex (sodium fluoride): Calcium, Vitamin D

Fluoroplex (fluorouracil): Aloe, Beta-Carotene, Echinacea, Eleuthero, Folic Acid, Garlic, Ginkgo, Ginseng, Melatonin, Omega-3 Fatty Acids, Vitamin A, Vitamin B$_1$, Vitamin B$_3$, Vitamin B$_6$, Vitamin C, Vitamin E

Fluothane (halothane): Alpha-Lipoic Acid, Ephedra, Milk Thistle, St. John's Wort, Valerian

Flura-Drops (sodium fluoride): Calcium, Vitamin D

Flura-Tab (sodium fluoride): Calcium, Vitamin D

Flurandrenolone (fludroxycortide): Aloe, Green Tea, Licorice, Vitamin C

Foamicon (magnesium trisilicate): Calcium, Cayenne, Chromium, Copper, Folic Acid, Iron, Magnesium, Vitamin A, Vitamin B$_1$, Vitamin D, Vitex, Zinc

Folex (methotrexate): Aloe, Beta-Carotene, Echinacea, Eleuthero, Folic Acid, Garlic, Ginseng, Iron, Melatonin, Milk Thistle, Omega-3 Fatty Acids, PABA, Vitamin A, Vitamin B$_1$, Vitamin B$_2$, Vitamin B$_6$, Vitamin B$_{12}$, Vitamin C, Vitamin E

Foradil (formoterol): Calcium, Magnesium, Potassium

Forane (isoflurane): Alpha-Lipoic Acid, Ephedra, Milk Thistle, St. John's Wort, Valerian

Fortaz (ceftazidime): Ginseng, Green Tea, Iron, Licorice, Probiotic Flora, Reishi, Vitamin B1, Vitamin K, Zinc

Fortipine LA 40 (nifedipine): Black Cohosh, Calcium, Dang Gui, Magnesium, Saw Palmetto

Fortovase (saquinavir): Copper, Garlic, St. John's Wort, Vitamin C

Fosamax (alendronate): Calcium, Iron, Magnesium, Vitamin D, Zinc

Foscavir (foscarnet): Magnesium

Fragmin (dalteparin): Cayenne, Chondroitin Sulfate, DHEA, Policosanol, Vitamin C

Fraxiparine (nadroparin): Cayenne, Chondroitin Sulfate, DHEA, Policosanol, Vitamin C

Frenactil (benperidol): Milk Thistle, Phenylalanine

Frova (frovatriptan): 5-HTP, Feverfew, Tryptophan

FUDR (floxuridine): Echinacea, Eleuthero, Folic Acid, Vitamin B$_1$

Fulvicin (griseofulvin): Echinacea, Vitamin B$_3$, Vitamin E

Fungisome (amphotericin, liposomal): Echinacea

Fungizone (amphotericin B): Calcium, Echinacea, Magnesium, Potassium

Furacin (nitrofurazone): Licorice, Probiotic Flora, Vitamin K, Zinc

Furadantin (nitrofurantoin): Licorice, Magnesium, Probiotic Flora, Vitamin B$_6$, Vitamin K, Zinc

Furoxone (furazolidone): Licorice, Probiotic Flora, Vitamin K, Zinc

G-mycin (gentamicin): Alpha-Lipoic Acid, Calcium, Carnitine, Eleuthero, Ginger, Ginkgo, Horse Chestnut, Licorice, Magnesium, Potassium, Probiotic Flora, Vitamin B$_1$, Vitamin B$_6$, Vitamin B$_{12}$, Vitamin C, Vitamin E, Vitamin K

Gabitril (tiagabine): Carnitine, Folic Acid, Vitamin B$_3$

Gantanol (sulfamethoxazole): Calcium, Folic Acid, Licorice, Magnesium, PABA, Potassium, Probiotic Flora, Vitamin B$_1$, Vitamin B$_6$, Vitamin K, Zinc

Gantrisin (sulfisoxazole): Calcium, Folic Acid, Licorice, Magnesium, PABA, Probiotic Flora, Vitamin B$_1$, Vitamin B$_6$, Vitamin K, Zinc

Garamycin (gentamicin): Alpha-Lipoic Acid, Calcium, Carnitine, Eleuthero, Ginger, Ginkgo, Horse Chestnut, Licorice, Magnesium, Potassium, Probiotic Flora, Vitamin B$_1$, Vitamin B$_6$, Vitamin B$_{12}$, Vitamin C, Vitamin E, Vitamin K

Gastrosed (hyoscyamine): Iron

Gaviscon Chewable (aluminum hydroxide + magnesium trisilicate): Calcium, Cayenne, Chromium, Copper, Folic Acid, Iron, Magnesium, Vitamin A, Vitamin B$_1$, Vitamin C, Vitamin D, Vitex, Zinc

Gaviscon Regular Strength (magnesium trisilicate): Calcium, Cayenne, Chromium, Copper, Folic Acid, Iron, Magnesium, Vitamin A, Vitamin B$_1$, Vitamin D, Vitex, Zinc

Gemzar (gemcitabine): Aloe, Echinacea, Eleuthero, Folic Acid, Ginseng, Melatonin, Omega-3 Fatty Acids, Vitamin A, Vitamin B$_1$, Vitamin C, Vitamin E

Gen-Nifedipine (nifedipine): Black Cohosh, Calcium, Dang Gui, Magnesium, Saw Palmetto

Gen-Xene (clorazepate): Calcium, Carnitine, Copper, DHEA, Folic Acid, Ginkgo, Gotu Kola, Inositol, Kava, Melatonin, Milk Thistle, Omega-3 Fatty Acids, Tryptophan, Valerian,

Vitamin A, Vitamin B$_1$, Vitamin B$_2$, Vitamin B$_3$, Vitamin B$_6$, Vitamin B$_{12}$, Vitamin C, Vitamin D, Vitamin E, Vitamin K, Vitex, Zinc

Genaphed (pseudoephedrine): Potassium

GenCept 1/35 (ethinyl estradiol + norethindrone): Arginine, Calcium, Copper, DHEA, Dang Gui, Folic Acid, Iron, Licorice, Magnesium, Melatonin, Milk Thistle, S-Adenosylmethionine (SAMe), Selenium, St. John's Wort, Tyrosine, Vitamin A, Vitamin B$_1$, Vitamin B$_2$, Vitamin B$_3$, Vitamin B$_6$, Vitamin B$_{12}$, Vitamin C, Vitamin E, Vitex, Zinc

Genora 1/35 (ethinyl estradiol + norethindrone): Arginine, Calcium, Copper, DHEA, Dang Gui, Folic Acid, Iron, Licorice, Magnesium, Melatonin, Milk Thistle, S-Adenosyl-methionine (SAMe), Selenium, St. John's Wort, Tyrosine, Vitamin A, Vitamin B$_1$, Vitamin B$_2$, Vitamin B$_3$, Vitamin B$_6$, Vitamin B$_{12}$, Vitamin C, Vitamin E, Vitex, Zinc

Genora 1/50 (mestranol + norethindrone): Arginine, Calcium, Copper, DHEA, Dang Gui, Folic Acid, Iron, Licorice, Magnesium, Melatonin, Milk Thistle, S-Adenosylmethionine (SAMe), Selenium, St. John's Wort, Tyrosine, Vitamin A, Vitamin B$_1$, Vitamin B$_2$, Vitamin B$_3$, Vitamin B$_6$, Vitamin B$_{12}$, Vitamin C, Vitamin E, Vitex, Zinc

Gentlax (senna): Potassium

Geocillin (carbenicillin): Ginseng, Green Tea

Geodon (ziprasidone): 5-HTP, Chromium, Echinacea, Ginkgo, Melatonin, Omega-3 Fatty Acids, Vitamin B$_3$, Vitamin B$_6$, Vitamin C

Glauctabs (methazolamide): Potassium

Gleevec (imatinib): St. John's Wort

Glianimon (benperidol): Milk Thistle, Phenylalanine

Glivec (imatinib): St. John's Wort

Glucobay (acarbose): Chromium, Vitamin B$_3$

Glucophage (metformin): Alpha-Lipoic Acid, Astragalus, Bilberry, Calcium, Chromium, Coenzyme Q10, DHEA, Ephedra, Folic Acid, Garlic, Ginkgo, Ginseng, Glucosamine Sulfate, Gotu Kola, Horse Chestnut, Magnesium, Omega-3 Fatty Acids, Reishi, Turmeric/Curcumin, Vitamin B$_3$, Vitamin B$_{12}$

Glucophage XR (metformin): Alpha-Lipoic Acid, Astragalus, Bilberry, Calcium, Chromium, Coenzyme Q10, DHEA, Ephedra, Folic Acid, Garlic, Ginkgo, Ginseng, Glucosamine Sulfate, Gotu Kola, Horse Chestnut, Magnesium, Omega-3 Fatty Acids, Reishi, Turmeric/Curcumin, Vitamin B$_3$, Vitamin B$_{12}$

Glucotrol (glipizide): Aloe, Alpha-Lipoic Acid, Astragalus, Bilberry, Chromium, Coenzyme Q10, DHEA, Ephedra, Garlic, Ginkgo, Ginseng, Glucosamine Sulfate, Gotu Kola, Horse Chestnut, Magnesium, Omega-3 Fatty Acids, Reishi, Turmeric/Curcumin, Vitamin B$_3$

Glucotrol XL (glipizide): Aloe, Alpha-Lipoic Acid, Astragalus, Bilberry, Chromium, Coenzyme Q10, DHEA, Ephedra, Garlic, Ginkgo, Ginseng, Glucosamine Sulfate, Gotu Kola, Horse Chestnut, Magnesium, Omega-3 Fatty Acids, Reishi, Turmeric/Curcumin, Vitamin B$_3$

Glucovance (glyburide + metformin): Aloe, Alpha-Lipoic Acid, Calcium, Chromium, Coenzyme Q10, DHEA, Ephedra, Folic Acid, Garlic, Ginkgo, Ginseng, Glucosamine Sulfate, Horse Chestnut, Magnesium, Omega-3 Fatty Acids, Reishi, Turmeric/Curcumin, Vitamin B$_3$, Vitamin B$_{12}$

Gly-Cort (hydrocortisone 17-butyrate/acetate/probutate/valerate): Aloe, Green Tea, Licorice, Vitamin C

Glynase (glyburide): Aloe, Alpha-Lipoic Acid, Astragalus, Bilberry, Chromium, Coenzyme Q10, DHEA, Ephedra, Garlic, Ginkgo, Ginseng, Glucosamine Sulfate, Gotu Kola,

Horse Chestnut, Magnesium, Omega-3 Fatty Acids, Reishi, Turmeric/Curcumin, Vitamin B$_3$, Vitamin E

Glynase Prestab (glyburide): Aloe, Alpha-Lipoic Acid, Astragalus, Bilberry, Chromium, Coenzyme Q10, DHEA, Ephedra, Garlic, Ginkgo, Ginseng, Glucosamine Sulfate, Gotu Kola, Horse Chestnut, Magnesium, Omega-3 Fatty Acids, Reishi, Turmeric/Curcumin, Vitamin B$_3$, Vitamin E

GoLYTELY (polyethylene glycol–electrolyte solution): Potassium

Grifulvin (griseofulvin): Echinacea, Vitamin B$_3$, Vitamin E

Gris-PEG (griseofulvin): Echinacea, Vitamin B$_3$, Vitamin E

Grisactin (griseofulvin): Echinacea, Vitamin B$_3$, Vitamin E

Gristatin (griseofulvin): Echinacea, Vitamin B$_3$, Vitamin E

Gynodiol (ethinyl estradiol): Arginine, Boron, Calcium, Copper, DHEA, Dang Gui, Folic Acid, Iron, Licorice, Magnesium, Melatonin, Milk Thistle, S-Adenosylmethionine (SAMe), Selenium, St. John's Wort, Tyrosine, Vitamin A, Vitamin B$_1$, Vitamin B$_2$, Vitamin B$_3$, Vitamin B$_6$, Vitamin B$_{12}$, Vitamin C, Vitamin E, Vitex, Zinc

Gynogen L.A. 20 (estradiol valerate): Arginine, Black Cohosh, Boron, Calcium, Copper, DHEA, Dang Gui, Magnesium, Melatonin, Milk Thistle, St. John's Wort, Vitamin B$_6$, Vitamin D, Vitamin E, Vitex, Zinc

Habitrol (nicotine transdermal patches): Vitamin B$_3$

Halcion (triazolam): DHEA, Gotu Kola, Kava, Melatonin, St. John's Wort, Valerian, Vitamin B$_3$

Haldol (haloperidol): Alpha-Lipoic Acid, Chromium, Ginkgo, Iron, Kava, Melatonin, Milk Thistle, Phenylalanine, Potassium, Vitamin B$_3$, Vitamin B$_6$, Vitamin C, Vitamin E

Halfprin 81 (acetylsalicylic acid): Bilberry, Calcium, Cayenne, Devil's Claw, Feverfew, Folic Acid, Garlic, Ginger, Ginkgo, Gotu Kola, Iron, Licorice, Melatonin, Milk Thistle, Omega-3 Fatty Acids, Policosanol, Potassium, S-Adenosylmethionine (SAMe), Vitamin B$_2$, Vitamin B$_3$, Vitamin C, Vitamin E, Vitamin K, Zinc

Halog (halcinonide): Aloe, Green Tea, Licorice, Vitamin C

Halotestin (fluoxymesterone): DHEA, Echinacea, Zinc

Harmonyl (reserpine): Ephedra, Reishi

Heartline (acetylsalicylic acid): Bilberry, Calcium, Cayenne, Devil's Claw, Feverfew, Folic Acid, Garlic, Ginger, Ginkgo, Gotu Kola, Iron, Licorice, Melatonin, Milk Thistle, Omega-3 Fatty Acids, Policosanol, Potassium, S-Adenosylmethionine (SAMe), Vitamin B$_2$, Vitamin B$_3$, Vitamin C, Vitamin E, Vitamin K, Zinc

Helidac (bismuth subsalicylate + metronidazole + tetracycline): Calcium, Folic Acid, Iron, Magnesium, Potassium, Vitamin A, Vitamin B$_1$, Vitamin B$_2$, Vitamin B$_3$, Vitamin B$_6$, Vitamin C, Zinc

HeliMet (lansoprazole + metronidazole + clarithromycin): Probiotic Flora

Hepalean (heparin): Calcium, Cayenne, Chondroitin Sulfate, DHEA, Omega-3 Fatty Acids, Policosanol, Potassium, Vitamin C, Vitamin D

Heparin Leo (heparin): Calcium, Cayenne, Chondroitin Sulfate, DHEA, Omega-3 Fatty Acids, Policosanol, Potassium, Vitamin C, Vitamin D

Herceptin (trastuzumab): Cascara, Green Tea

Hexalen (altretamine): Vitamin B$_6$

Hi-Cor (hydrocortisone): Aloe, Green Tea, Licorice, Vitamin C

Hivid (dideoxycytidine): Aloe, Carnitine, Coenzyme Q10, Copper, DHEA, Reishi, Vitamin B$_1$, Vitamin B$_2$, Vitamin B$_{12}$, Zinc

Humanlog (insulin): Alpha-Lipoic Acid, Bilberry, Chromium, DHEA, Ephedra, Garlic, Ginkgo, Ginseng,

Glucosamine Sulfate, Horse Chestnut, Licorice, Magnesium, Milk Thistle, Omega-3 Fatty Acids, Potassium, Reishi, Turmeric/Curcumin, Vitamin B$_3$, Vitamin E

Humatin (paromomycin): Alpha-Lipoic Acid, Calcium, Eleuthero, Ginger, Ginkgo, Horse Chestnut, Licorice, Magnesium, Potassium, Probiotic Flora, Vitamin B$_1$, Vitamin B$_6$, Vitamin B$_{12}$, Vitamin K

Humira (adalimumab): Echinacea

Humulin (insulin): Alpha-Lipoic Acid, Bilberry, Chromium, DHEA, Ephedra, Garlic, Ginkgo, Ginseng, Glucosamine Sulfate, Horse Chestnut, Licorice, Magnesium, Milk Thistle, Omega-3 Fatty Acids, Potassium, Reishi, Turmeric/Curcumin, Vitamin B$_3$, Vitamin E

Hy-Phen (hydrocodone + acetaminophen): Ephedra, Ginseng, Gotu Kola, Phenylalanine, Tyrosine

Hycamtin (topotecan): Feverfew

Hydro-Tex (hydrocortisone): Aloe, Green Tea, Licorice, Vitamin C

Hydrocet (hydrocodone + acetaminophen): Ephedra, Ginseng, Gotu Kola, Phenylalanine, Tyrosine

Hydrocot (hydrochlorothiazide): Calcium, Coenzyme Q10, Folic Acid, Ginkgo, Glucosamine Sulfate, Hawthorn, Licorice, Magnesium, Potassium, Vitamin B$_2$, Vitamin D, Zinc

HydroDiuril (hydrochlorothiazide): Calcium, Coenzyme Q10, Folic Acid, Ginkgo, Glucosamine Sulfate, Hawthorn, Licorice, Magnesium, Potassium, Vitamin B$_2$, Vitamin D, Zinc

Hydrogesic (hydrocodone + acetaminophen): Ephedra, Ginseng, Gotu Kola, Phenylalanine, Tyrosine

Hydromox (quinethazone): Calcium, Coenzyme Q10, Folic Acid, Ginkgo, Glucosamine Sulfate, Hawthorn, Licorice, Magnesium, Potassium, Vitamin B$_2$, Vitamin D, Zinc

Hygroton (chlorthalidone): Calcium, Coenzyme Q10, Folic Acid, Ginkgo, Glucosamine Sulfate, Hawthorn, Licorice, Magnesium, Potassium, Vitamin B$_2$, Vitamin D, Zinc

Hylorel (guanadrel): Ephedra

Hypnovel (midazolam): DHEA, Gotu Kola, Kava, Melatonin, St. John's Wort, Valerian, Vitamin B$_3$

Hypolar Retard 20 (nifedipine): Black Cohosh, Calcium, Dang Gui, Magnesium, Saw Palmetto

Hytone (hydrocortisone): Aloe, Green Tea, Licorice, Vitamin C

Hytrin (terazosin): Saw Palmetto, Vitamin B$_3$

Hyzaar (losartan + hydrochlorothiazide): Alpha-Lipoic Acid, Arginine, Calcium, Coenzyme Q10, Glucosamine Sulfate, Hawthorn, Licorice, Magnesium, Potassium, Vitamin D, Zinc

Idamycin (idarubicin): Alpha-Lipoic Acid, Carnitine, Coenzyme Q10, Feverfew, Garlic, Ginkgo, Green Tea, Hawthorn, Milk Thistle, Reishi, Selenium, St. John's Wort, Turmeric/Curcumin, Vitamin B$_2$, Vitamin E

Ifex (ifosfamide): Astragalus, Carnitine, Echinacea, Eleuthero, Selenium

Iletin (insulin): Alpha-Lipoic Acid, Bilberry, Chromium, DHEA, Ephedra, Garlic, Ginkgo, Ginseng, Glucosamine Sulfate, Horse Chestnut, Licorice, Magnesium, Milk Thistle, Omega-3 Fatty Acids, Potassium, Reishi, Turmeric/Curcumin, Vitamin B$_3$, Vitamin E

Imdur (isosorbide mononitrate): Arginine, Carnitine, Folic Acid, Vitamin C

Imitrex (sumatriptan): 5-HTP, Feverfew, Tryptophan

Imodium A-D (loperamide): St. John's Wort

Imodium A-D Caplets (loperamide): St. John's Wort

Imuran (azathioprine): Echinacea, Folic Acid, Vitamin B$_3$

Inapsine (droperidol): Milk Thistle, Phenylalanine

Inderal (propranolol): Calcium, Carnitine, Chromium, Coenzyme Q10, Folic Acid, Magnesium, Melatonin, Policosanol, Potassium, Vitamin B$_2$, Vitamin B$_3$, Vitamin B6, Vitamin C, Vitamin E

Inderal LA (propranolol): Calcium, Carnitine, Chromium, Coenzyme Q10, Folic Acid, Magnesium, Melatonin, Policosanol, Potassium, Vitamin B$_2$, Vitamin B$_3$, Vitamin B$_6$, Vitamin C, Vitamin E

Inderex (propranolol + bendrofluazide): Arginine, Calcium, Coenzyme Q10, Glucosamine Sulfate, Hawthorn, Licorice, Magnesium, Policosanol, Potassium, Vitamin C, Vitamin D, Zinc

Indocin (indomethacin): Calcium, Cayenne, Chondroitin Sulfate, Chromium, Copper, Devil's Claw, Feverfew, Folic Acid, Ginger, Glucosamine Sulfate, Gotu Kola, Iron, Licorice, Melatonin, Omega-3 Fatty Acids, Potassium, Turmeric/Curcumin, Vitamin A, Vitamin B$_3$, Vitamin B$_6$, Vitamin C, Zinc

Indocin-SR (indomethacin): Calcium, Cayenne, Chondroitin Sulfate, Chromium, Copper, Devil's Claw, Feverfew, Folic Acid, Ginger, Glucosamine Sulfate, Gotu Kola, Iron, Licorice, Melatonin, Omega-3 Fatty Acids, Potassium, Turmeric/Curcumin, Vitamin A, Vitamin B$_3$, Vitamin B$_6$, Vitamin C, Zinc

Infumorph (morphine): Ephedra, Ginseng, Gotu Kola, Phenylalanine, Tyrosine

INH (isoniazid): Calcium, Copper, Folic Acid, Magnesium, Milk Thistle, Vitamin B$_3$, Vitamin B$_6$, Vitamin C, Vitamin D, Vitamin E

Inhibace (cilazapril): Alpha-Lipoic Acid, Arginine, Cayenne, Iron, Omega-3 Fatty Acids, Potassium, Vitamin E, Zinc

Innohep (tinzaparin): Cayenne, Chondroitin Sulfate, DHEA, Policosanol, Vitamin C

Innopran XL (propranolol): Calcium, Carnitine, Chromium, Coenzyme Q10, Folic Acid, Magnesium, Melatonin, Policosanol, Potassium, Vitamin B$_2$, Vitamin B$_3$, Vitamin B$_6$, Vitamin C, Vitamin E

Integrelin (eptifibatide): Cayenne, Ginger, Policosanol, S-Adenosylmethionine (SAMe)

Intron A (interferon alpha): Astragalus, Echinacea, Iron, Licorice, Zinc

Inversine (mecamylamine): Vitamin B$_3$

Invirase (saquinavir): Copper, Garlic, St. John's Wort, Vitamin C

Ipocal (mesalazine): Vitamin B$_{12}$

Iprivask (desirudin): Cayenne, DHEA, Policosanol

ISDN (isosorbide dinitrate): Arginine, Carnitine, Folic Acid, Vitamin C

Ismelin (guanethidine): Ephedra, Vitamin B$_3$

ISMN (isosorbide mononitrate): Arginine, Carnitine, Folic Acid, Vitamin C

ISMO (isosorbide mononitrate): Arginine, Carnitine, Folic Acid, Vitamin C

Isoptin/SR/XL (verapamil): Calcium, Carnitine, Folic Acid, Magnesium, Melatonin, St. John's Wort, Vitamin B$_6$, Vitamin D, Vitamin E

Isopto Hyoscine Ophthalmic (scopolamine): Dang Gui, Vitamin B$_1$

Isordil (isosorbide dinitrate): Arginine, Carnitine, Folic Acid, Vitamin C

Isotrate (isosorbide mononitrate): Arginine, Carnitine, Folic Acid, Vitamin C

Isuprel (isoproterenol): Garlic

Jadelle (levonorgestrel, implant): Magnesium, St. John's Wort

Janimine (imipramine): 5-HTP, Coenzyme Q10, Echinacea, Milk Thistle, *S*-Adenosylmethionine (SAMe), St. John's Wort, Tryptophan, Tyrosine, Vitamin B_1, Vitamin B_2, Vitamin B_3, Vitamin B_6, Vitamin B_{12}, Zinc

Jarsin (phenprocoumon): Bilberry, Cayenne, Chondroitin Sulfate, Coenzyme Q10, DHEA, Dang Gui, Devil's Claw, Feverfew, Garlic, Ginger, Ginkgo, Ginseng, Green Tea, Horse Chestnut, Kava, Licorice, Magnesium, Omega-3 Fatty Acids, Policosanol, Red Clover, Reishi, Saw Palmetto, St. John's Wort, Vitamin A, Vitamin B_3, Vitamin C, Vitamin E, Vitamin K, Zinc

Jenamicin (gentamicin): Alpha-Lipoic Acid, Calcium, Carnitine, Eleuthero, Ginger, Ginkgo, Horse Chestnut, Licorice, Magnesium, Potassium, Probiotic Flora, Vitamin B_1, Vitamin B_6, Vitamin B_{12}, Vitamin C, Vitamin E, Vitamin K

Jenest-28 (ethinyl estradiol + norethindrone): Arginine, Calcium, Copper, DHEA, Dang Gui, Folic Acid, Iron, Licorice, Magnesium, Melatonin, Milk Thistle, *S*-Adenosylmethionine (SAMe), Selenium, St. John's Wort, Tyrosine, Vitamin A, Vitamin B_1, Vitamin B_2, Vitamin B_3, Vitamin B_6, Vitamin B_{12}, Vitamin C, Vitamin E, Vitex, Zinc

Jolivette (norethindrone, oral): Magnesium, St. John's Wort

Jumex (selegiline): 5-HTP, Cayenne, Chromium, Eleuthero, Ephedra, Folic Acid, Ginkgo, Iron, Kava, Licorice, Phenylalanine, S-Adenosylmethionine (SAMe), St. John's Wort, Tryptophan, Tyrosine, Vitamin B_2, Vitamin B_6, Vitex

Kadian (morphine): Ephedra, Ginseng, Gotu Kola, Phenylalanine, Tyrosine

Kaletra (lopinavir + ritonavir): Copper, Garlic, St. John's Wort, Vitamin C

Kantrex (kanamycin): Alpha-Lipoic Acid, Calcium, Eleuthero, Ginger, Ginkgo, Horse Chestnut, Licorice, Magnesium, Potassium, Probiotic Flora, Vitamin B_1, Vitamin B_6, Vitamin B_{12}, Vitamin K

Kaopectate 1-D (loperamide): St. John's Wort

Karidium (sodium fluoride): Calcium, Vitamin D

Karvea (irbesartan): Alpha-Lipoic Acid, Potassium

Keflex (cephalexin): Ginseng, Green Tea, Iron, Licorice, Probiotic Flora, Reishi, Vitamin B_1, Vitamin K, Zinc

Keftab (cephalexin): Ginseng, Green Tea, Iron, Licorice, Probiotic Flora, Reishi, Vitamin B_1, Vitamin K, Zinc

Kefurox (cefuroxime): Ginseng, Green Tea, Iron, Licorice, Probiotic Flora, Reishi, Vitamin B_1, Vitamin K, Zinc

Kefzol (cefazolin): Ginseng, Green Tea, Iron, Licorice, Probiotic Flora, Reishi, Vitamin B_1, Vitamin K, Zinc

Kemstro (baclofen): Phenylalanine

Keppra (levetiracetam): Calcium, Carnitine, Copper, DHEA, Folic Acid, Ginkgo, Inositol, Kava, Milk Thistle, Omega-3 Fatty Acids, Valerian, Vitamin A, Vitamin B_1, Vitamin B_2, Vitamin B_3, Vitamin B_6, Vitamin B_{12}, Vitamin C, Vitamin D, Vitamin E, Vitamin K, Vitex, Zinc

Kerlone (betaxolol): Calcium, Carnitine, Chromium, Coenzyme Q10, Folic Acid, Magnesium, Melatonin, Potassium, Vitamin B_2, Vitamin B_3, Vitamin B_6, Vitamin C

Kestrone-5 (estrone): Arginine, Black Cohosh, Boron, Calcium, Copper, DHEA, Dang Gui, Magnesium, Melatonin, Milk Thistle, St. John's Wort, Vitamin B_6, Vitamin D, Vitamin E, Vitex, Zinc

Klonopin (clonazepam): Calcium, Carnitine, Copper, DHEA, Folic Acid, Ginkgo, Gotu Kola, Inositol, Kava, Melatonin, Milk Thistle, Omega-3 Fatty Acids, Valerian, Vitamin A, Vitamin B_1, Vitamin B_2, Vitamin B_3, Vitamin B_6, Vitamin B_{12}, Vitamin C, Vitamin D, Vitamin E, Vitamin K, Vitex, Zinc

Kondremul Plain (mineral oil): Beta-Carotene, Calcium, Potassium, Vitamin A, Vitamin D, Vitamin E, Vitamin K

Konsyl-D (psyllium): Potassium, Vitamin B_2

Kwell Shampoo (lindane): Vitamin E

LactiCare-HC (hydrocortisone 17-butyrate/acetate/probutate/valerate): Aloe, Green Tea, Licorice, Vitamin C

Lanacort (hydrocortisone 17-butyrate/acetate/probutate/valerate): Aloe, Green Tea, Licorice, Vitamin C

Laniazid (isoniazid): Calcium, Copper, Folic Acid, Magnesium, Milk Thistle, Vitamin B_3, Vitamin B_6, Vitamin C, Vitamin D, Vitamin E

Lanoxicaps (digoxin): Calcium, Cascara, Dang Gui, Eleuthero, Ephedra, Hawthorn, Licorice, Magnesium, Potassium, St. John's Wort, Vitamin D

Lanoxin (digoxin): Calcium, Cascara, Dang Gui, Eleuthero, Ephedra, Hawthorn, Licorice, Magnesium, Potassium, St. John's Wort, Vitamin D

Lanvis (thioguanine): Echinacea, Eleuthero, Folic Acid, Vitamin B_1, Vitamin B_3

Largactil (chlorpromazine): Chromium, Coenzyme Q10, Ginkgo, Kava, Melatonin, Milk Thistle, Reishi, Vitamin B_2, Vitamin B_3, Vitamin B_6, Vitamin C, Vitamin E

Largon (propiomazine): Coenzyme Q10, Milk Thistle, Vitamin B_2, Vitamin B_3, Vitamin C

Lasix (furosemide): Calcium, Folic Acid, Ginseng, Glucosamine Sulfate, Licorice, Magnesium, Potassium, Vitamin B_1, Vitamin B_6, Vitamin C, Zinc

Ledercillin VK (penicillin V): Ginseng, Green Tea, Licorice, Probiotic Flora, Vitamin B_1, Vitamin K, Zinc

Lemoderm (hydrocortisone 17-butyrate/acetate/probutate/valerate): Aloe, Green Tea, Licorice, Vitamin C

Lendormin (brotizolam): Kava, St. John's Wort

Lescol (fluvastatin): Beta-Carotene, Carnitine, Coenzyme Q10, Garlic, Gotu Kola, Omega-3 Fatty Acids, Policosanol, Reishi, Selenium, St. John's Wort, Vitamin A, Vitamin B_3, Vitamin C, Vitamin E

Lescol XL (fluvastatin): Beta-Carotene, Carnitine, Coenzyme Q10, Garlic, Gotu Kola, Omega-3 Fatty Acids, Policosanol, Reishi, Selenium, St. John's Wort, Vitamin A, Vitamin B_3, Vitamin C, Vitamin E

Lesterol (probucol): Beta-Carotene

Leukeran (chlorambucil): Astragalus, Carnitine, Echinacea, Eleuthero, Selenium

Leukine (GMCSF): Echinacea

Leustatin (cladribine): Echinacea, Eleuthero, Folic Acid, Vitamin B_1

Levaquin (levofloxacin): Calcium, Green Tea, Iron, Licorice, Magnesium, Potassium, Probiotic Flora, Vitamin B_1, Vitamin K, Zinc

Levatol (penbutolol): Calcium, Carnitine, Chromium, Coenzyme Q10, Folic Acid, Magnesium, Melatonin, Potassium, Vitamin B_2, Vitamin B_3, Vitamin B_6, Vitamin C

Levbid (hyoscyamine): Iron

Levitra (vardenafil): Arginine

Levlen (ethinyl estradiol + levonorgestrel): Arginine, Calcium, Copper, DHEA, Dang Gui, Folic Acid, Iron, Licorice, Magnesium, Melatonin, Milk Thistle, *S*-Adenosylmethionine (SAMe), Selenium, St. John's Wort, Tyrosine, Vitamin A, Vitamin B_1, Vitamin B_2, Vitamin B_3, Vitamin B_6, Vitamin B_{12}, Vitamin C, Vitamin E, Vitex, Zinc

Levlite (ethinyl estradiol + levonorgestrel): Arginine, Calcium, Copper, DHEA, Dang Gui, Folic Acid, Iron, Licorice, Magnesium, Melatonin, Milk Thistle, *S*-Adenosylmethionine (SAMe), Selenium, St. John's

Wort, Tyrosine, Vitamin A, Vitamin B_1, Vitamin B_2, Vitamin B_3, Vitamin B_6, Vitamin B_{12}, Vitamin C, Vitamin E, Vitex, Zinc

Levo-Dromoran (levorphanol): Ephedra, Ginseng, Gotu Kola, Phenylalanine, Tyrosine

Levo-T (levothyroxine): Alpha-Lipoic Acid, Calcium, Carnitine, Coenzyme Q10, DHEA, Iron, Tyrosine, Vitamin B_2

Levonelle (levonorgestrel, oral postcoital contraceptive): Magnesium, St. John's Wort

Levonelle-2 (levonorgestrel, oral postcoital contraceptive): Magnesium, St. John's Wort

Levora 0.15/30 (ethinyl estradiol + levonorgestrel): Arginine, Calcium, Copper, DHEA, Dang Gui, Folic Acid, Iron, Licorice, Magnesium, Melatonin, Milk Thistle, S-Adenosylmethionine (SAMe), Selenium, St. John's Wort, Tyrosine, Vitamin A, Vitamin B_1, Vitamin B_2, Vitamin B_3, Vitamin B_6, Vitamin B_{12}, Vitamin C, Vitamin E, Vitex, Zinc

Levothroid (levothyroxine): Alpha-Lipoic Acid, Calcium, Carnitine, Coenzyme Q10, DHEA, Iron, Tyrosine, Vitamin B_2

Levoxyl (levothyroxine): Alpha-Lipoic Acid, Calcium, Carnitine, Coenzyme Q10, DHEA, Iron, Tyrosine, Vitamin B_2

Levsin (hyoscyamine): Iron

Levsin/SL (hyoscyamine): Iron

Levsinex (hyoscyamine): Iron

Lexapro (escitalopram): Chromium, Folic Acid, Ginkgo, Inositol, Omega-3 Fatty Acids, S-Adenosylmethionine (SAMe), St. John's Wort, Tryptophan, Vitamin B_3, Vitamin B_6, Vitamin B_{12}, Vitamin C, Zinc

Lexiva (fosamprenavir): Copper, Garlic, St. John's Wort, Vitamin C

Lexotan (bromazepam): DHEA, Gotu Kola, Melatonin, Valerian, Vitamin B_3

Lexxel (enalapril + felodipine): Arginine, Calcium, Cayenne, Coenzyme Q10, Iron, Potassium, St. John's Wort, Zinc

Li-Liquid (lithium carbonate): 5-HTP, Chromium, Folic Acid, Inositol, Magnesium, Tryptophan

Libritabs (chlordiazepoxide): DHEA, Gotu Kola, Melatonin, Valerian, Vitamin B_3

Librium (chlordiazepoxide): DHEA, Gotu Kola, Melatonin, Valerian, Vitamin B_3

Lidex-E (fluocinonide): Aloe, Green Tea, Licorice, Vitamin C

Lidex (fluocinonide): Aloe, Green Tea, Licorice, Vitamin C

Lincocin (lincomycin): Licorice, Probiotic Flora, Vitamin K, Zinc

Lioresal (baclofen): Phenylalanine

Lipitor (atorvastatin): Beta-Carotene, Carnitine, Coenzyme Q10, Garlic, Gotu Kola, Omega-3 Fatty Acids, Policosanol, Reishi, Selenium, St. John's Wort, Vitamin A, Vitamin B_3, Vitamin C, Vitamin E

Liquid Pred (prednisone): Calcium, Cayenne, Chromium, DHEA, Echinacea, Ephedra, Folic Acid, Horse Chestnut, Licorice, Magnesium, Melatonin, Omega-3 Fatty Acids, Potassium, Selenium, Vitamin A, Vitamin B_6, Vitamin C, Vitamin D, Vitamin K, Zinc

Liskonum (lithium carbonate): 5-HTP, Chromium, Folic Acid, Inositol, Magnesium, Tryptophan

Litarex (lithium carbonate): 5-HTP, Chromium, Folic Acid, Inositol, Magnesium, Tryptophan

Lithane (lithium carbonate): 5-HTP, Chromium, Folic Acid, Inositol, Magnesium, Tryptophan

Lithobid (lithium carbonate): 5-HTP, Chromium, Folic Acid, Inositol, Magnesium, Tryptophan

Lithonate (lithium carbonate): 5-HTP, Chromium, Folic Acid, Inositol, Magnesium, Tryptophan

Lithotabs (lithium carbonate): 5-HTP, Chromium, Folic Acid, Inositol, Magnesium, Tryptophan

Lo/Ovral (ethinyl estradiol + norgestrel): Arginine, Calcium, Copper, DHEA, Dang Gui, Folic Acid, Iron, Licorice, Magnesium, Melatonin, Milk Thistle, S-Adenosylmethionine (SAMe), Selenium, St. John's Wort, Tyrosine, Vitamin A, Vitamin B_1, Vitamin B_2, Vitamin B_3, Vitamin B_6, Vitamin B_{12}, Vitamin C, Vitamin E, Vitex, Zinc

Lobate (clobetasol): Aloe, Green Tea, Licorice, Vitamin C, Zinc

Locholest (cholestyramine): Beta-Carotene, Calcium, Folic Acid, Iron, Magnesium, Omega-3 Fatty Acids, Vitamin A, Vitamin B_2, Vitamin B_3, Vitamin B_{12}, Vitamin D, Vitamin E, Vitamin K, Zinc

Locoid (hydrocortisone 17-butyrate/acetate/probutate/valerate): Aloe, Green Tea, Licorice, Vitamin C

Lodine (etodolac): Calcium, Cayenne, Chondroitin Sulfate, Chromium, Copper, Devil's Claw, Feverfew, Folic Acid, Ginger, Glucosamine Sulfate, Gotu Kola, Iron, Licorice, Melatonin, Omega-3 Fatty Acids, Potassium, Turmeric/Curcumin, Vitamin B_3, Vitamin B_6, Vitamin C, Zinc

Lodosyn (carbidopa): 5-HTP, Folic Acid, Iron, Kava, S-Adenosylmethionine (SAMe), Vitamin B_3, Vitamin B_6, Vitamin C, Vitex

Loestrin (ethinyl estradiol + norethindrone): Arginine, Calcium, Copper, DHEA, Dang Gui, Folic Acid, Iron, Licorice, Magnesium, Melatonin, Milk Thistle, S-Adenosylmethionine (SAMe), Selenium, St. John's Wort, Tyrosine, Vitamin A, Vitamin B_1, Vitamin B_2, Vitamin B_3, Vitamin B_6, Vitamin B_{12}, Vitamin C, Vitamin E, Vitex, Zinc

Lofibra (fenofibrate): Coenzyme Q10, Copper, Folic Acid, Gotu Kola, Omega-3 Fatty Acids, Vitamin B_3, Vitamin B_6, Vitamin B_{12}, Vitamin C, Vitamin E, Zinc

Lonide (fluocinonide): Aloe, Green Tea, Licorice, Vitamin C

Lopid (gemfibrozil): Coenzyme Q10, Copper, Folic Acid, Gotu Kola, Omega-3 Fatty Acids, Vitamin B_3, Vitamin B_6, Vitamin B_{12}, Vitamin E, Zinc

Lopressor (metoprolol): Calcium, Carnitine, Chromium, Coenzyme Q10, Folic Acid, Magnesium, Melatonin, Potassium, Vitamin B_2, Vitamin B_3, Vitamin B_6, Vitamin C

Lopressor HCT (metoprolol + hydrochlorothiazide): Arginine, Calcium, Coenzyme Q10, Glucosamine Sulfate, Hawthorn, Licorice, Magnesium, Policosanol, Potassium, Vitamin C, Vitamin D, Zinc

Lopurin (allopurinol): Carnitine, Copper, Iron, Tryptophan, Vitamin D

Lorabid (loracarbef): Ginseng, Green Tea, Iron, Licorice, Probiotic Flora, Reishi, Vitamin B_1, Vitamin K, Zinc

Lorcet 10/650 (hydrocodone + acetaminophen): Ephedra, Ginseng, Gotu Kola, Phenylalanine, Tyrosine

Lorcet Plus (hydrocodone + acetaminophen): Ephedra, Ginseng, Gotu Kola, Phenylalanine, Tyrosine

Lorcet-HD (hydrocodone + acetaminophen): Ephedra, Ginseng, Gotu Kola, Phenylalanine, Tyrosine

Lorelco (probucol): Beta-Carotene

Lortab (hydrocodone + acetaminophen): Ephedra, Ginseng, Gotu Kola, Phenylalanine, Tyrosine

Lortab ASA (hydrocodone + acetylsalicylic acid): Ephedra, Ginseng, Gotu Kola, Phenylalanine, Tyrosine

Losec (omeprazole): Beta-Carotene, Calcium, Chromium, Iron, Kava, St. John's Wort, Vitamin B_{12}, Vitamin E, Zinc

Lotensin (benazepril): Arginine, Cayenne, Iron, Omega-3 Fatty Acids, Potassium, Vitamin E, Zinc

Lotrel (amlodipine + benazepril): Arginine, Calcium, Cayenne, Coenzyme Q10, DHEA, Potassium, St. John's Wort

Lovenox (enoxaparin): Cayenne, Chondroitin Sulfate, DHEA, Policosanol, Vitamin C

Lozol (indapamide): Calcium, Coenzyme Q10, Folic Acid, Ginkgo, Glucosamine Sulfate, Hawthorn, Licorice, Magnesium, Potassium, Vitamin B_2, Vitamin D, Zinc

Lufyllin (dyphylline): Potassium

Luminol (phenobarbital): Calcium, Carnitine, Copper, DHEA, Folic Acid, Ginkgo, Gotu Kola, Inositol, Kava, Milk Thistle, Omega-3 Fatty Acids, Reishi, Valerian, Vitamin A, Vitamin B_1, Vitamin B_2, Vitamin B_3, Vitamin B_6, Vitamin B_{12}, Vitamin C, Vitamin D, Vitamin E, Vitamin K, Vitex, Zinc

Lunelle (estradiol cypionate + medroxyprogesterone acetate): Beta-Carotene, Folic Acid, Magnesium, Vitamin A, Vitamin B_3, Vitamin D

Lunesta (eszopiclone): 5-HTP, Gotu Kola, Melatonin, Valerian

Lupron (leuprolide): Black Cohosh, Vitamin D

Luride (sodium fluoride): Calcium, Vitamin D

Lurselle (probucol): Beta-Carotene

Luvox (fluvoxamine): 5-HTP, Chromium, Folic Acid, Ginkgo, Inositol, Melatonin, Omega-3 Fatty Acids, S-Adenosylmethionine (SAMe), St. John's Wort, Tryptophan, Vitamin B_3, Vitamin B_6, Vitamin B_{12}, Vitamin C, Zinc

Luxiq (betamethasone): Aloe, Green Tea, Licorice, Vitamin C

Lynoral (ethinyl estradiol): Arginine, Boron, Calcium, Copper, DHEA, Dang Gui, Folic Acid, Iron, Licorice, Magnesium, Melatonin, Milk Thistle, S-Adenosylmethionine (SAMe), Selenium, St. John's Wort, Tyrosine, Vitamin A, Vitamin B_1, Vitamin B_2, Vitamin B_3, Vitamin B_6, Vitamin B_{12}, Vitamin C, Vitamin E, Vitex, Zinc

Lyrica (pregabalin): Vitamin B_3

Maalox (aluminum hydroxide + magnesium hydroxide + simethicone): Calcium, Cayenne, Chromium, Copper, Folic Acid, Iron, Magnesium, Vitamin A, Vitamin B_1, Vitamin C, Vitamin D, Vitex, Zinc

Maalox Anti-Diarrheal (loperamide): St. John's Wort

Macrobid (nitrofurantoin): Licorice, Magnesium, Probiotic Flora, Vitamin B_6, Vitamin K, Zinc

Macrodantin (nitrofurantoin): Licorice, Magnesium, Probiotic Flora, Vitamin B_6, Vitamin K, Zinc

Madopar (levodopa + benserazide): 5-HTP, Folic Acid, Iron, Kava, Methionine, Phenylalanine, S-Adenosylmethionine (SAMe), Tyrosine, Vitamin B_3, Vitamin B_6, Vitamin C, Vitex

Majeptil (thioproperazine): Coenzyme Q10, Milk Thistle, Vitamin B_2, Vitamin B_3, Vitamin C

Malarone (atovaquone + proguanil): Vitamin B_2

Mandol (cefamandole): Ginseng, Green Tea, Iron, Licorice, Probiotic Flora, Reishi, Vitamin B_1, Vitamin K, Zinc

Manerix (moclobemide): 5-HTP, Cayenne, Chromium, Eleuthero, Ephedra, Ginkgo, Ginseng, Licorice, Phenylalanine, S-Adenosylmethionine (SAMe), St. John's Wort, Tryptophan, Tyrosine, Vitamin B_6

Marcumar (phenprocoumon): Bilberry, Cayenne, Chondroitin Sulfate, Coenzyme Q10, DHEA, Dang Gui, Devil's Claw, Feverfew, Garlic, Ginger, Ginkgo, Ginseng, Green Tea, Horse Chestnut, Kava, Licorice, Magnesium, Omega-3 Fatty Acids, Policosanol, Red Clover, Reishi, Saw Palmetto, St. John's Wort, Vitamin A, Vitamin B_3, Vitamin C, Vitamin E, Vitamin K, Zinc

Marevan (warfarin): Bilberry, Cayenne, Chondroitin Sulfate, Coenzyme Q10, DHEA, Dang Gui, Devil's Claw, Echinacea, Feverfew, Garlic, Ginger, Ginkgo, Ginseng, Green Tea, Horse Chestnut, Iron, Kava, Licorice, Magnesium, Omega-3 Fatty Acids, Policosanol, Red Clover, Reishi, Saw Palmetto, St. John's Wort, Vitamin A, Vitamin B_3, Vitamin C, Vitamin D, Vitamin E, Vitamin K, Zinc

Margesic H (hydrocodone + acetaminophen): Ephedra, Ginseng, Gotu Kola, Phenylalanine, Tyrosine

Marplan (isocarboxazid): 5-HTP, Cayenne, Chromium, Eleuthero, Ephedra, Ginkgo, Ginseng, Licorice, Phenylalanine, S-Adenosylmethionine (SAMe), St. John's Wort, Tryptophan, Tyrosine, Vitamin B_6

Marthritic (salsalate): Calcium, Folic Acid, Omega-3 Fatty Acids, Policosanol, Vitamin C, Vitamin K, Zinc

Matulane (procarbazine): 5-HTP, Cayenne, Chromium, Eleuthero, Ephedra, Ginkgo, Ginseng, Licorice, Phenylalanine, S-Adenosylmethionine (SAMe), St. John's Wort, Tryptophan, Tyrosine, Vitamin B_6

Mavik (trandolapril): Arginine, Cayenne, Iron, Omega-3 Fatty Acids, Potassium, Vitamin E, Zinc

Maxalt (rizatriptan): 5-HTP, Feverfew, Tryptophan

Maxaquin (lomefloxacin): Calcium, Green Tea, Iron, Licorice, Magnesium, Potassium, Probiotic Flora, Vitamin B_1, Vitamin K, Zinc

Maxiflor (diflorasone): Aloe, Green Tea, Licorice, Vitamin C

Maxipime (cefepime): Ginseng, Green Tea, Iron, Licorice, Probiotic Flora, Reishi, Vitamin B_1, Vitamin K, Zinc

Maxivate (betamethasone dipropionate/valerate): Aloe, Green Tea, Licorice, Vitamin C

Maxtrex (methotrexate): Aloe, Beta-Carotene, Echinacea, Eleuthero, Folic Acid, Garlic, Ginseng, Iron, Melatonin, Milk Thistle, Omega-3 Fatty Acids, PABA, Vitamin A, Vitamin B_1, Vitamin B_2, Vitamin B_6, Vitamin B_{12}, Vitamin C, Vitamin E

Maxzide (triamterene + hydrochlorothiazide): Arginine, Calcium, Coenzyme Q10, Folic Acid, Glucosamine Sulfate, Hawthorn, Licorice, Magnesium, Potassium, Vitamin D, Zinc

Mebaral (mephobarbital): Calcium, Carnitine, Copper, DHEA, Folic Acid, Ginkgo, Gotu Kola, Inositol, Kava, Milk Thistle, Omega-3 Fatty Acids, Valerian, Vitamin A, Vitamin B_1, Vitamin B_2, Vitamin B_3, Vitamin B_6, Vitamin B_{12}, Vitamin C, Vitamin D, Vitamin E, Vitamin K, Vitex, Zinc

Meclomen (meclofenamate): Calcium, Cayenne, Chondroitin Sulfate, Chromium, Copper, Devil's Claw, Feverfew, Folic Acid, Ginger, Glucosamine Sulfate, Gotu Kola, Iron, Licorice, Melatonin, Omega-3 Fatty Acids, Potassium, Turmeric/Curcumin, Vitamin B_3, Vitamin B_6, Vitamin C, Zinc

Medihaler-Epi (epinephrine): Magnesium, Potassium, Vitamin C

Medihaler-Iso (isoproterenol): Garlic

Medipain 5 (hydrocodone + acetaminophen): Ephedra, Ginseng, Gotu Kola, Phenylalanine, Tyrosine

Medrol (methylprednisolone): Calcium, Cayenne, Chromium, DHEA, Echinacea, Ephedra, Folic Acid, Horse Chestnut, Licorice, Magnesium, Melatonin, Omega-3 Fatty Acids, Potassium, Selenium, Vitamin A, Vitamin B_6, Vitamin C, Vitamin D, Vitamin K, Zinc

Mefoxin (cefoxitin): Ginseng, Green Tea, Iron, Licorice, Probiotic Flora, Reishi, Vitamin B_1, Vitamin K, Zinc

Mellaril (thioridazine): Coenzyme Q10, Milk Thistle, Potassium, Vitamin A, Vitamin B_2, Vitamin B_3, Vitamin C, Vitamin D

Melphalan (phenylalanine mustard): Astragalus, Carnitine, Echinacea, Eleuthero, Ginger, Selenium

Menest (esterified estrogens): Arginine, Black Cohosh, Boron, Calcium, Copper, DHEA, Dang Gui, Magnesium, Melatonin, Milk Thistle, St. John's Wort, Vitamin B_6, Vitamin D, Vitamin E, Vitex, Zinc

Mepacrine (quinacrine): Vitamin B_2

Meridia (sibutramine): 5-HTP, Tryptophan

Merrem I.V. (meropenem): Ginseng, Green Tea, Iron, Licorice, Probiotic Flora, Reishi, Vitamin B_1, Vitamin K, Zinc

Mesantoin (fosphentoin): Calcium, Carnitine, Copper, DHEA, Folic Acid, Ginkgo, Inositol, Kava, Milk Thistle, Omega-3 Fatty Acids, Valerian, Vitamin A, Vitamin B_1, Vitamin B_2, Vitamin B_3, Vitamin B_6, Vitamin B_{12}, Vitamin C, Vitamin D, Vitamin E, Vitamin K, Vitex, Zinc

Mesigyna (norethisterone enanthate + estradiol valerate): Magnesium, Vitamin B_3

Metadate (methylphenidate): 5-HTP, Iron, Reishi, Tyrosine, Zinc

Metaglip (glipizide + metformin): Aloe, Alpha-Lipoic Acid, Calcium, Chromium, Coenzyme Q10, DHEA, Ephedra, Folic Acid, Garlic, Ginkgo, Ginseng, Glucosamine Sulfate, Horse Chestnut, Magnesium, Omega-3 Fatty Acids, Reishi, Turmeric/Curcumin, Vitamin B_3, Vitamin B_{12}

Metamucil (psyllium): Potassium, Vitamin B_2

Methadose (methadone): Ephedra, Ginseng, Gotu Kola, Phenylalanine, Tyrosine

Methitest (methyltestosterone): Beta-Carotene, DHEA, Vitamin A, Zinc

Methylin (methylphenidate): 5-HTP, Iron, Reishi, Tyrosine, Zinc

Meticorten (prednisone): Calcium, Cayenne, Chromium, DHEA, Echinacea, Ephedra, Folic Acid, Horse Chestnut, Licorice, Magnesium, Melatonin, Omega-3 Fatty Acids, Potassium, Selenium, Vitamin A, Vitamin B_6, Vitamin C, Vitamin D, Vitamin K, Zinc

MetroGel Vaginal (metronidazole, vaginal): Zinc

Mevacor (lovastatin): Beta-Carotene, Carnitine, Coenzyme Q10, Garlic, Gotu Kola, Omega-3 Fatty Acids, Policosanol, Reishi, Selenium, St. John's Wort, Vitamin A, Vitamin B_3, Vitamin C, Vitamin E

Mexitil (mexiletine): Cascara, Magnesium, Potassium, Vitamin C

Mezlin (mezlocillin): Ginseng, Green Tea, Licorice, Probiotic Flora, Vitamin B_1, Vitamin K, Zinc

Miacalcin Nasal (calcitonin): Calcium, Vitamin D

Micanol Cream (anthralin): Vitamin E

Micardis (telmisartan): Alpha-Lipoic Acid, Potassium

Microlut (levonorgestrel, oral postcoital contraceptive): Magnesium, St. John's Wort

Micronase (glyburide): Aloe, Alpha-Lipoic Acid, Astragalus, Bilberry, Chromium, Coenzyme Q10, DHEA, Ephedra, Garlic, Ginkgo, Ginseng, Glucosamine Sulfate, Gotu Kola, Horse Chestnut, Omega-3 Fatty Acids, Reishi, Turmeric/Curcumin, Vitamin B_3, Vitamin E

Micronor (norethindrone, oral): Magnesium, St. John's Wort, Vitamin D

Microval (levonorgestrel, oral postcoital contraceptive): Magnesium, St. John's Wort

Microzide (hydrochlorothiazide): Calcium, Coenzyme Q10, Folic Acid, Ginkgo, Glucosamine Sulfate, Hawthorn, Licorice, Magnesium, Potassium, Vitamin B_2, Vitamin D, Zinc

Midamor (amiloride): Arginine, Calcium, Folic Acid, Glucosamine Sulfate, Magnesium, Potassium, Zinc

Milkinol (mineral oil): Beta-Carotene, Calcium, Potassium, Vitamin A, Vitamin D, Vitamin E, Vitamin K

Milontin (phensuximide): Calcium, Carnitine, Copper, DHEA, Folic Acid, Ginkgo, Inositol, Kava, Milk Thistle, Omega-3 Fatty Acids, Valerian, Vitamin A, Vitamin B_1, Vitamin B_2, Vitamin B_3, Vitamin B_6, Vitamin B_{12}, Vitamin C, Vitamin D, Vitamin E, Vitamin K, Vitex, Zinc

Minihep (heparin): Calcium, Cayenne, Chondroitin Sulfate, DHEA, Omega-3 Fatty Acids, Policosanol, Potassium, Vitamin C, Vitamin D

Minihep Calcium (heparin): Calcium, Cayenne, Chondroitin Sulfate, DHEA, Omega-3 Fatty Acids, Policosanol, Potassium, Vitamin C, Vitamin D

Minipress (prazosin): Saw Palmetto, Vitamin B_3

Minitran (nitroglycerin): Arginine, Carnitine, Folic Acid, Vitamin C

Minocin (minocycline): Calcium, Folic Acid, Iron, Magnesium, Potassium, Vitamin A, Vitamin B_1, Vitamin B_2, Vitamin B_3, Vitamin B_6, Vitamin C, Zinc

Miradon (anisindione): Bilberry, Cayenne, Chondroitin Sulfate, Coenzyme Q10, DHEA, Dang Gui, Devil's Claw, Feverfew, Garlic, Ginger, Ginkgo, Ginseng, Green Tea, Horse Chestnut, Kava, Licorice, Magnesium, Omega-3 Fatty Acids, Policosanol, Red Clover, Reishi, Saw Palmetto, St. John's Wort, Vitamin A, Vitamin B_3, Vitamin C, Vitamin E, Vitamin K, Zinc

Miralax (polyethylene glycol): Potassium

Mirena (intrauterine L-norgestrel system): Vitamin D

Mithracin (plicamycin): Ginseng

Mitoxana (ifosfamide): Astragalus, Carnitine, Echinacea, Eleuthero, Selenium

Mivacron (mivacurium): Magnesium

Mobic (meloxicam): Calcium, Cayenne, Chondroitin Sulfate, Chromium, Copper, Devil's Claw, Feverfew, Folic Acid, Ginger, Glucosamine Sulfate, Gotu Kola, Iron, Licorice, Melatonin, Omega-3 Fatty Acids, Potassium, Turmeric/Curcumin, Vitamin B_3, Vitamin B_6, Vitamin C, Zinc

Modalim (ciprofibrate): Coenzyme Q10, Copper, Folic Acid, Gotu Kola, Omega-3 Fatty Acids, Vitamin B_3, Vitamin B_6, Vitamin B_{12}, Zinc

Modecate (fluphenazine): Coenzyme Q10, Milk Thistle, Vitamin B_2, Vitamin B_3, Vitamin C

Modicon (ethinyl estradiol + norethindrone): Arginine, Calcium, Copper, DHEA, Dang Gui, Folic Acid, Iron, Licorice, Magnesium, Melatonin, Milk Thistle, S-Adenosylmethionine (SAMe), Selenium, St. John's Wort, Tyrosine, Vitamin A, Vitamin B_1, Vitamin B_2, Vitamin B_3, Vitamin B_6, Vitamin B_{12}, Vitamin C, Vitamin E, Vitex, Zinc

Modrasone (alclometasone): Aloe, Green Tea, Licorice, Vitamin C

Moduretic (amiloride + hydrochlorothiazide): Arginine, Calcium, Coenzyme Q10, Folic Acid, Ginkgo, Glucosamine Sulfate, Hawthorn, Licorice, Magnesium, Potassium, Vitamin D, Zinc

Mono Gesic (salsalate): Calcium, Folic Acid, Omega-3 Fatty Acids, Policosanol, Vitamin C, Vitamin K, Zinc

Mono-Embolex (certoparin): Cayenne, Chondroitin Sulfate, DHEA, Policosanol, Vitamin C

Monodox (doxycycline): Calcium, Folic Acid, Iron, Magnesium, Potassium, Vitamin A, Vitamin B_1, Vitamin B_2, Vitamin B_3, Vitamin B_6, Vitamin C, Zinc

Monoket (isosorbide mononitrate): Arginine, Carnitine, Folic Acid, Vitamin C

Monoparin (heparin): Calcium, Cayenne, Chondroitin Sulfate, DHEA, Omega-3 Fatty Acids, Policosanol, Potassium, Vitamin C, Vitamin D

Monoparin Calcium (heparin): Calcium, Cayenne, Chondroitin Sulfate, DHEA, Omega-3 Fatty Acids, Policosanol, Potassium, Vitamin C, Vitamin D

Monopril (fosinopril): Arginine, Cayenne, Iron, Omega-3 Fatty Acids, Potassium, Vitamin E, Zinc

Motrin (ibuprofen): Calcium, Cayenne, Chondroitin Sulfate, Chromium, Copper, Devil's Claw, Feverfew, Folic Acid, Ginger, Glucosamine Sulfate, Gotu Kola, Iron, Licorice, Melatonin, Omega-3 Fatty Acids, Potassium, Turmeric/Curcumin, Vitamin B_3, Vitamin B_6, Vitamin C, Zinc

Motrin IB (ibuprofen): Calcium, Cayenne, Chondroitin Sulfate, Chromium, Copper, Devil's Claw, Feverfew, Folic Acid, Ginger, Glucosamine Sulfate, Gotu Kola, Iron, Licorice, Melatonin, Omega-3 Fatty Acids, Potassium, Turmeric/Curcumin, Vitamin B_3, Vitamin B_6, Vitamin C, Zinc

Movergan (selegiline): 5-HTP, Cayenne, Chromium, Eleuthero, Ephedra, Folic Acid, Ginkgo, Iron, Kava, Licorice, Phenylalanine, S-Adenosylmethionine (SAMe), St. John's Wort, Tryptophan, Tyrosine, Vitamin B_2, Vitamin B_6, Vitex

Moxilin (amoxicillin): Ginseng, Green Tea, Licorice, Probiotic Flora, Vitamin B_1, Vitamin K, Zinc

MS Contin (morphine): Ephedra, Ginseng, Gotu Kola, Phenylalanine, Tyrosine

MSIR (morphine): Ephedra, Ginseng, Gotu Kola, Phenylalanine, Tyrosine

Multiparin (heparin): Calcium, Cayenne, Chondroitin Sulfate, DHEA, Omega-3 Fatty Acids, Policosanol, Potassium, Vitamin C, Vitamin D

Mustargen (mechlorethamine): Astragalus, Carnitine, Echinacea, Eleuthero, Ginger, Selenium, Turmeric/Curcumin

Mutamycin (mitomycin): Echinacea, Eleuthero, Ginseng, Licorice, Probiotic Flora, Vitamin B_1, Vitamin K

Myambutol (ethambutol): Copper, Folic Acid, Milk Thistle, Vitamin B_3, Vitamin B_6, Vitamin C, Vitamin D, Zinc

Mycelex (clotrimazole): Probiotic Flora, Vitamin B_2

Mycifradin (neomycin): Alpha-Lipoic Acid, Beta-Carotene, Calcium, Eleuthero, Folic Acid, Ginger, Ginkgo, Horse Chestnut, Iron, Licorice, Magnesium, Potassium, Probiotic Flora, Vitamin A, Vitamin B_1, Vitamin B_3, Vitamin B_6, Vitamin B_{12}, Vitamin D, Vitamin K

Myciguent (neomycin): Alpha-Lipoic Acid, Beta-Carotene, Calcium, Eleuthero, Folic Acid, Ginger, Ginkgo, Horse Chestnut, Iron, Licorice, Magnesium, Potassium, Probiotic Flora, Vitamin A, Vitamin B_1, Vitamin B_3, Vitamin B_6, Vitamin B_{12}, Vitamin D, Vitamin K

Mycolog II (triamcinolone + nystatin): Licorice

MyCort (hydrocortisone 17-butyrate/acetate/probutate/valerate): Aloe, Green Tea, Licorice, Vitamin C

Mycostatin (nystatin): Echinacea, Zinc

Mycostatin (topical) (nystatin, topical): Echinacea

Mycotuf (ethionamide): Folic Acid, Milk Thistle, Vitamin B_6, Vitamin C, Vitamin D

Mykrox (metolazone): Calcium, Coenzyme Q10, Folic Acid, Ginkgo, Glucosamine Sulfate, Hawthorn, Licorice, Magnesium, Potassium, Vitamin B_2, Vitamin D, Zinc

Mylanta (aluminum hydroxide + magnesium hydroxide + simethicone): Calcium, Cayenne, Chromium, Copper, Folic Acid, Iron, Magnesium, Vitamin A, Vitamin B_1, Vitamin C, Vitamin D, Vitex, Zinc

Myleran (busulfan): Astragalus, Carnitine, Echinacea, Eleuthero, Selenium

Myobid (ethionamide): Folic Acid, Milk Thistle, Vitamin B_6, Vitamin C, Vitamin D

Myocet (doxorubicin, pegylated liposomal): Alpha-Lipoic Acid, Carnitine, Coenzyme Q10, Feverfew, Garlic, Ginkgo, Green Tea, Hawthorn, Milk Thistle, Reishi, Selenium, St. John's Wort, Turmeric/Curcumin, Vitamin B_2, Vitamin B_6, Vitamin E

Mysoline (primidone): Calcium, Carnitine, Copper, DHEA, Folic Acid, Ginkgo, Inositol, Kava, Milk Thistle, Omega-3 Fatty Acids, Valerian, Vitamin A, Vitamin B_1, Vitamin B_2, Vitamin B_3, Vitamin B_6, Vitamin B_{12}, Vitamin C, Vitamin D, Vitamin E, Vitamin K, Vitex, Zinc

Naprosyn (naproxen): Calcium, Cayenne, Chondroitin Sulfate, Chromium, Copper, Devil's Claw, Feverfew, Folic Acid, Ginger, Glucosamine Sulfate, Gotu Kola, Iron, Licorice, Melatonin, Omega-3 Fatty Acids, Potassium, Turmeric/Curcumin, Vitamin B_3, Vitamin B_6, Vitamin C, Zinc

Naqua (trichlormethiazide): Calcium, Coenzyme Q10, Folic Acid, Ginkgo, Glucosamine Sulfate, Hawthorn, Licorice, Magnesium, Potassium, Vitamin B_2, Vitamin D, Zinc

Narcan (naloxone): Phenylalanine

Nardil (phenelzine): 5-HTP, Cayenne, Chromium, Eleuthero, Ephedra, Ginkgo, Ginseng, Licorice, Phenylalanine, S-Adenosylmethionine (SAMe), St. John's Wort, Tryptophan, Tyrosine, Vitamin B_6

Naturetin (bendroflumethiazide): Calcium, Coenzyme Q10, Folic Acid, Ginkgo, Glucosamine Sulfate, Hawthorn, Licorice, Magnesium, Potassium, Vitamin B_2, Vitamin D, Zinc

Navelbine (vinorelbine): Echinacea, Eleuthero, St. John's Wort

Navidrex (cyclopenthiazide): Calcium, Coenzyme Q10, Folic Acid, Ginkgo, Glucosamine Sulfate, Hawthorn, Licorice, Magnesium, Potassium, Vitamin B_2, Vitamin D, Zinc

Nebcin (tobramycin): Alpha-Lipoic Acid, Calcium, Eleuthero, Ginger, Ginkgo, Horse Chestnut, Licorice, Magnesium, Potassium, Probiotic Flora, Vitamin B_1, Vitamin B_6, Vitamin B_{12}, Vitamin K

Nebilet (nebivolol): Calcium, Carnitine, Chromium, Coenzyme Q10, Folic Acid, Magnesium, Melatonin, Potassium, Vitamin B_2, Vitamin B_3, Vitamin B_6, Vitamin C

NebuPent (pentamidine): Magnesium

Necon 0.5/30 (ethinyl estradiol + norethindrone): Arginine, Calcium, Copper, DHEA, Dang Gui, Folic Acid, Iron, Licorice, Magnesium, Melatonin, Milk Thistle, S-Adenosylmethionine (SAMe), Selenium, St. John's Wort, Tyrosine, Vitamin A, Vitamin B_1, Vitamin B_2, Vitamin B_3, Vitamin B_6, Vitamin B_{12}, Vitamin C, Vitamin E, Vitex, Zinc

Necon 1/25 (ethinyl estradiol + norethindrone): Arginine, Calcium, Copper, DHEA, Dang Gui, Folic Acid, Iron, Licorice, Magnesium, Melatonin, Milk Thistle, S-Adenosylmethionine (SAMe), Selenium, St. John's Wort, Tyrosine, Vitamin A, Vitamin B_1, Vitamin B_2, Vitamin B_3, Vitamin B_6, Vitamin B_{12}, Vitamin C, Vitamin E, Vitex, Zinc

Necon 1/50 (ethinyl estradiol + norethindrone): Arginine, Calcium, Copper, DHEA, Dang Gui, Folic Acid, Iron, Licorice, Magnesium, Melatonin, Milk Thistle, S-Adenosylmethionine (SAMe), Selenium, St. John's Wort, Tyrosine, Vitamin A, Vitamin B_1, Vitamin B_2, Vitamin B_3, Vitamin B_6, Vitamin B_{12}, Vitamin C, Vitamin E, Vitex, Zinc

Necon 10/11 (ethinyl estradiol + norethindrone): Arginine, Calcium, Copper, DHEA, Dang Gui, Folic Acid, Iron, Licorice, Magnesium, Melatonin, Milk Thistle,

S-Adenosylmethionine (SAMe), Selenium, St. John's Wort, Tyrosine, Vitamin A, Vitamin B$_1$, Vitamin B$_2$, Vitamin B$_3$, Vitamin B$_6$, Vitamin B$_{12}$, Vitamin C, Vitamin E, Vitex, Zinc

Neggram (nalidixic acid): Calcium, Green Tea, Iron, Licorice, Magnesium, Potassium, Probiotic Flora, Vitamin B$_1$, Vitamin K, Zinc

Nelova 1/35 (ethinyl estradiol + norethindrone): Arginine, Calcium, Copper, DHEA, Dang Gui, Folic Acid, Iron, Licorice, Magnesium, Melatonin, Milk Thistle, *S*-Adenosyl-methionine (SAMe), Selenium, St. John's Wort, Tyrosine, Vitamin A, Vitamin B$_1$, Vitamin B$_2$, Vitamin B$_3$, Vitamin B$_6$, Vitamin B$_{12}$, Vitamin C, Vitamin E, Vitex, Zinc

Nelova 1/50 (mestranol + norethindrone): Arginine, Calcium, Copper, DHEA, Dang Gui, Folic Acid, Iron, Licorice, Magnesium, Melatonin, Milk Thistle, *S*-Adenosyl-methionine (SAMe), Selenium, St. John's Wort, Tyrosine, Vitamin A, Vitamin B$_1$, Vitamin B$_2$, Vitamin B$_3$, Vitamin B$_6$, Vitamin B$_{12}$, Vitamin C, Vitamin E, Vitex, Zinc

Nelova 10/11 (ethinyl estradiol + norethindrone): Arginine, Calcium, Copper, DHEA, Dang Gui, Folic Acid, Iron, Licorice, Magnesium, Melatonin, Milk Thistle, S-Adenosyl-methionine (SAMe), Selenium, St. John's Wort, Tyrosine, Vitamin A, Vitamin B$_1$, Vitamin B$_2$, Vitamin B$_3$, Vitamin B$_6$, Vitamin B$_{12}$, Vitamin C, Vitamin E, Vitex, Zinc

Nelulen 1/25 (ethinyl estradiol + ethynodiol): Arginine, Calcium, Copper, DHEA, Dang Gui, Folic Acid, Iron, Licorice, Magnesium, Melatonin, Milk Thistle, *S*-Adenosylmethionine (SAMe), Selenium, St. John's Wort, Tyrosine, Vitamin A, Vitamin B$_1$, Vitamin B$_2$, Vitamin B$_3$, Vitamin B$_6$, Vitamin B$_{12}$, Vitamin C, Vitamin E, Vitex, Zinc

Nelulen 1/50 (ethinyl estradiol + ethynodiol): Arginine, Calcium, Copper, DHEA, Dang Gui, Folic Acid, Iron, Licorice, Magnesium, Melatonin, Milk Thistle, *S*-Adenosylmethionine (SAMe), Selenium, St. John's Wort, Tyrosine, Vitamin A, Vitamin B$_1$, Vitamin B$_2$, Vitamin B$_3$, Vitamin B$_6$, Vitamin B$_{12}$, Vitamin C, Vitamin E, Vitex, Zinc

Nembutal (pentobarbital): Calcium, Copper, DHEA, Folic Acid, Ginkgo, Gotu Kola, Inositol, Kava, Milk Thistle, Omega-3 Fatty Acids, Valerian, Vitamin A, Vitamin B$_1$, Vitamin B$_2$, Vitamin B$_3$, Vitamin B$_6$, Vitamin B$_{12}$, Vitamin C, Vitamin D, Vitamin E, Vitamin K, Vitex, Zinc

Neo-Cultol (mineral oil): Beta-Carotene, Calcium, Potassium, Vitamin A, Vitamin D, Vitamin E, Vitamin K

Neo-Estrone (esterified estrogens): Arginine, Black Cohosh, Boron, Calcium, Copper, DHEA, Dang Gui, Magnesium, Melatonin, Milk Thistle, St. John's Wort, Vitamin B$_6$, Vitamin D, Vitamin E, Vitex, Zinc

Neo-Fradin (neomycin): Alpha-Lipoic Acid, Beta-Carotene, Calcium, Eleuthero, Folic Acid, Ginger, Ginkgo, Horse Chestnut, Iron, Licorice, Magnesium, Potassium, Probiotic Flora, Vitamin A, Vitamin B$_1$, Vitamin B$_3$, Vitamin B$_6$, Vitamin B$_{12}$, Vitamin D, Vitamin K

Neoproxil (cyproterone): Black Cohosh, Vitamin D

Neoral (cyclosporine): Arginine, Echinacea, Ginkgo, Magnesium, Melatonin, Omega-3 Fatty Acids, Potassium, St. John's Wort, Turmeric/Curcumin, Vitamin C, Vitamin E, Zinc

NeoRecormon (epoetin beta): Dang Gui, Iron, Vitamin B$_6$, Vitamin C

Neosar (cyclophosphamide): Aloe, Alpha-Lipoic Acid, Astragalus, Beta-Carotene, Carnitine, Echinacea, Eleuthero, Ginger, Ginseng, Licorice, Melatonin, Omega-3 Fatty Acids, Reishi, Selenium, Turmeric/Curcumin, Vitamin A, Vitamin C, Vitamin E

NeoTab (neomycin): Alpha-Lipoic Acid, Beta-Carotene, Calcium, Eleuthero, Folic Acid, Ginger, Ginkgo, Horse

Chestnut, Iron, Licorice, Magnesium, Potassium, Probiotic Flora, Vitamin A, Vitamin B$_1$, Vitamin B$_3$, Vitamin B$_6$, Vitamin B$_{12}$, Vitamin D, Vitamin K

Neptazane (methazolamide): Potassium

Nerisona (diflucortolone): Aloe, Green Tea, Licorice, Vitamin C

Nerisone (diflucortolone): Aloe, Green Tea, Licorice, Vitamin C

Netromycin (netilmicin): Alpha-Lipoic Acid, Calcium, Eleuthero, Ginger, Ginkgo, Horse Chestnut, Licorice, Magnesium, Potassium, Probiotic Flora, Vitamin B$_1$, Vitamin B$_6$, Vitamin B$_{12}$, Vitamin K

Neulasts: Echinacea

Neuleptil (pericyazine): Coenzyme Q10, Milk Thistle, Vitamin B$_2$, Vitamin B$_3$, Vitamin C

Neumega: Echinacea

Neupogen: Echinacea

Neurontin (gabapentin): Carnitine, Folic Acid, Vitamin B$_3$, Vitamin B$_6$, Vitamin D

Nexium (esomeprazole): Beta-Carotene, Calcium, Chromium, Iron, Kava, St. John's Wort, Vitamin B$_{12}$, Zinc

Niaspan (simvastatin + extended-release nicotinic acid): Beta-Carotene, Carnitine, Coenzyme Q10, Garlic, Gotu Kola, Omega-3 Fatty Acids, Policosanol, Reishi, Selenium, St. John's Wort, Vitamin A, Vitamin B$_3$, Vitamin C, Vitamin E

NicoDerm CQ (nicotine transdermal patches): Vitamin B$_3$

Nicotrol (nicotine transdermal patches): Vitamin B$_3$

Nifedipress MR (nifedipine): Black Cohosh, Calcium, Dang Gui, Magnesium, Saw Palmetto

Nifedotard 20 MR (nifedipine): Black Cohosh, Calcium, Dang Gui, Magnesium, Saw Palmetto

Nifelease (nifedipine): Black Cohosh, Calcium, Dang Gui, Magnesium, Saw Palmetto

Nifopress Retard (nifedipine): Black Cohosh, Calcium, Dang Gui, Magnesium, Saw Palmetto

Nighttime Sleep Aid (doxylamine): Vitamin B$_6$

Nilandron (nilutamide): Black Cohosh, Vitamin D

Nilstat (nystatin): Echinacea, Zinc

Nilstat (topical) (nystatin, topical): Echinacea

Nimbex (cisatracurium): Magnesium

Nimodrel MR (nifedipine): Black Cohosh, Calcium, Dang Gui, Magnesium, Saw Palmetto

Nimotop (nimodipine): Calcium, Carnitine, Folic Acid, Magnesium, St. John's Wort, Vitamin B$_6$, Vitamin D

Nipent (pentostatin): Echinacea, Eleuthero, Folic Acid, Vitamin B$_1$

Nitrek (nitroglycerin): Arginine, Carnitine, Folic Acid, Vitamin C

Nitrepin (nitrendipine): Calcium, Carnitine, Folic Acid, Magnesium, St. John's Wort, Vitamin B$_6$, Vitamin D

Nitro-Bid (nitroglycerin): Arginine, Carnitine, Folic Acid, Vitamin C

Nitro-Dur (nitroglycerin): Arginine, Carnitine, Folic Acid, Vitamin C

Nitro-Time (nitroglycerin): Arginine, Carnitine, Folic Acid, Vitamin C

Nitrodisc (nitroglycerin): Arginine, Carnitine, Folic Acid, Vitamin C

Nitrogard (nitroglycerin): Arginine, Carnitine, Folic Acid, Vitamin C

Nitroglyn (nitroglycerin): Arginine, Carnitine, Folic Acid, Vitamin C

Nitrol (nitroglycerin): Arginine, Carnitine, Folic Acid, Vitamin C

Nitrolingual (nitroglycerin): Arginine, Carnitine, Folic Acid, Vitamin C

Nitrostat (nitroglycerin): Arginine, Carnitine, Folic Acid, Vitamin C

Nivaten Retard (nifedipine): Black Cohosh, Calcium, Dang Gui, Magnesium, Saw Palmetto

Nivemycin (neomycin): Alpha-Lipoic Acid, Beta-Carotene, Calcium, Eleuthero, Folic Acid, Ginger, Ginkgo, Horse Chestnut, Iron, Licorice, Magnesium, Potassium, Probiotic Flora, Vitamin A, Vitamin B_1, Vitamin B_3, Vitamin B_6, Vitamin B_{12}, Vitamin D, Vitamin K

Nizoral (ketoconazole): Black Cohosh, Echinacea, Green Tea, Vitamin D

Nobrium (medazepam): DHEA, Gotu Kola, Melatonin, Valerian, Vitamin B_3

NoDoz (caffeine): Calcium, Ephedra, Kava, Melatonin

Nolvadex (tamoxifen): Black Cohosh, Calcium, Dang Gui, Feverfew, Ginseng, Green Tea, Melatonin, Omega-3 Fatty Acids, Vitamin A, Vitamin C, Vitamin E

Nootropyl (piracetam): Calcium, Carnitine, Copper, DHEA, Folic Acid, Ginkgo, Inositol, Kava, Milk Thistle, Omega-3 Fatty Acids, Valerian, Vitamin A, Vitamin B_1, Vitamin B_2, Vitamin B_3, Vitamin B_6, Vitamin B_{12}, Vitamin C, Vitamin D, Vitamin E, Vitamin K, Vitex, Zinc

Nor-QD (norethindrone, oral): Magnesium, St. John's Wort

Norco (hydrocodone + acetaminophen): Ephedra, Ginseng, Gotu Kola, Phenylalanine, Tyrosine

Norcuron (vecuronium): Ginger, Magnesium

Nordette (ethinyl estradiol + levonorgestrel): Arginine, Calcium, Copper, DHEA, Dang Gui, Folic Acid, Iron, Licorice, Magnesium, Melatonin, Milk Thistle, S-Adenosylmethionine (SAMe), Selenium, St. John's Wort, Tyrosine, Vitamin A, Vitamin B_1, Vitamin B_2, Vitamin B_3, Vitamin B_6, Vitamin B_{12}, Vitamin C, Vitamin E, Vitex, Zinc

Norethin 1/50 (mestranol + norethindrone): Arginine, Calcium, Copper, DHEA, Dang Gui, Folic Acid, Iron, Licorice, Magnesium, Melatonin, Milk Thistle, S-Adenosylmethionine (SAMe), Selenium, St. John's Wort, Tyrosine, Vitamin A, Vitamin B_1, Vitamin B_2, Vitamin B_3, Vitamin B_6, Vitamin B_{12}, Vitamin C, Vitamin E, Vitex, Zinc

Norgeston (levonorgestrel, oral postcoital contraceptive): Magnesium, St. John's Wort

Norinyl 1/35 (ethinyl estradiol + norethindrone): Arginine, Calcium, Copper, DHEA, Dang Gui, Folic Acid, Iron, Licorice, Magnesium, Melatonin, Milk Thistle, S-Adenosylmethionine (SAMe), Selenium, St. John's Wort, Tyrosine, Vitamin A, Vitamin B_1, Vitamin B_2, Vitamin B_3, Vitamin B_6, Vitamin B_{12}, Vitamin C, Vitamin E, Vitex, Zinc

Noristerat (norethindrone, injectable): Magnesium, St. John's Wort, Vitamin B_3

Norlestin 1/50 (ethinyl estradiol + norethindrone): Arginine, Calcium, Copper, DHEA, Dang Gui, Folic Acid, Iron, Licorice, Magnesium, Melatonin, Milk Thistle, S-Adenosylmethionine (SAMe), Selenium, St. John's Wort, Tyrosine, Vitamin A, Vitamin B_1, Vitamin B_2, Vitamin B_3, Vitamin B_6, Vitamin B_{12}, Vitamin C, Vitamin E, Vitex, Zinc

NorLevo (levonorgestrel, oral post-coital contraceptive): Magnesium, St. John's Wort

Normiflo (ardeparin): Cayenne, Chondroitin Sulfate, DHEA, Policosanol, Vitamin C

Normodyne (labetalol): Potassium

Noroxin (norfloxacin): Calcium, Green Tea, Iron, Licorice, Magnesium, Potassium, Probiotic Flora, Vitamin B_1, Vitamin K, Zinc

Norpace (disopyramide): Cascara, Magnesium, Potassium

Norplant-2 (levonorgestrel, implant): Magnesium, St. John's Wort

Norplant (levonorgestrel, implant): Magnesium, St. John's Wort

Norpramin (desipramine): 5-HTP, Coenzyme Q10, Melatonin, Milk Thistle, S-Adenosylmethionine (SAMe), St. John's Wort, Tryptophan, Tyrosine, Vitamin B_1, Vitamin B_2, Vitamin B_3, Vitamin B_6, Vitamin B_{12}, Vitamin E, Zinc

Norvasc (amlodipine): Calcium, Carnitine, DHEA, Folic Acid, Magnesium, St. John's Wort, Vitamin B_6, Vitamin D

Norvir (ritonavir): Copper, Garlic, St. John's Wort, Vitamin C

Novantrone (mitoxantrone): Alpha-Lipoic Acid, Carnitine, Coenzyme Q10, Garlic, Ginkgo, Green Tea, Hawthorn, Milk Thistle, Reishi, Selenium, St. John's Wort, Turmeric/Curcumin, Vitamin B_2, Vitamin E

Novo-Clonidine (clonidine): DHEA, Ephedra, Melatonin

Novo-Gemfibrozil (gemfibrozil): Coenzyme Q10, Copper, Folic Acid, Gotu Kola, Omega-3 Fatty Acids, Vitamin B_3, Vitamin B_6, Vitamin B_{12}, Vitamin E, Zinc

Novo-Hylazin (hydralazine): Melatonin, Vitamin B_6, Zinc

Novo-Nifedin (nifedipine): Black Cohosh, Calcium, Dang Gui, Magnesium, Saw Palmetto

Novolin (insulin): Alpha-Lipoic Acid, Bilberry, Chromium, DHEA, Ephedra, Garlic, Ginkgo, Ginseng, Glucosamine Sulfate, Horse Chestnut, Licorice, Magnesium, Milk Thistle, Omega-3 Fatty Acids, Potassium, Reishi, Turmeric/Curcumin, Vitamin B_3, Vitamin E

NovoRapid (insulin): Alpha-Lipoic Acid, Bilberry, Chromium, DHEA, Ephedra, Garlic, Ginkgo, Ginseng, Glucosamine Sulfate, Horse Chestnut, Licorice, Magnesium, Milk Thistle, Omega-3 Fatty Acids, Potassium, Reishi, Turmeric/Curcumin, Vitamin B_3, Vitamin E

Noxafil (posaconazole): Echinacea, St. John's Wort

Nozinan (methotrimeprazine): Coenzyme Q10, Milk Thistle, Vitamin B_2, Vitamin B_3, Vitamin C

Nu-Clonidine (clonidine): DHEA, Ephedra, Melatonin

Nu-Nifed (nifedipine): Black Cohosh, Calcium, Dang Gui, Magnesium, Saw Palmetto

Nu-Nifedipine-PA (nifedipine): Black Cohosh, Calcium, Dang Gui, Magnesium, Saw Palmetto

Nuclav (amoxicillin + clavulanic acid): Ginseng, Green Tea, Licorice, Probiotic Flora, Vitamin B_1, Vitamin K, Zinc

NuLytely (polyethylene glycol-electrolyte solution): Potassium

Numorphan (oxymorphone): Ephedra, Ginseng, Gotu Kola, Phenylalanine, Tyrosine

Nuprin (ibuprofen): Calcium, Cayenne, Chondroitin Sulfate, Chromium, Copper, Devil's Claw, Feverfew, Folic Acid, Ginger, Glucosamine Sulfate, Gotu Kola, Iron, Licorice, Melatonin, Omega-3 Fatty Acids, Potassium, Turmeric/Curcumin, Vitamin B_3, Vitamin B_6, Vitamin C, Zinc

Nutracort (hydrocortisone): Aloe, Green Tea, Licorice, Vitamin C

Nuvaring (etonogestrel/ethinyl estradiol vaginal ring): Arginine, Copper, Dang Gui, Iron, Licorice, Magnesium, Selenium, St. John's Wort, Tyrosine, Vitamin A, Vitamin B_1, Vitamin B_2, Vitamin B_3, Vitamin B_6, Vitamin B_{12}, Vitamin C, Vitamin E, Zinc

Nydrazid (isoniazid): Calcium, Copper, Folic Acid, Magnesium, Milk Thistle, Vitamin B_3, Vitamin B_6, Vitamin C, Vitamin D, Vitamin E

Nyquil (acetaminophen + chlorpheniramine + dextromethorphan + pseudoephedrine + alcohol): Garlic, Licorice,

Methionine, Milk Thistle, *S*-Adenosylmethionine (SAMe), Vitamin C

Nystex (nystatin): Echinacea, Zinc

Nystex Ointment (nystatin, topical): Echinacea

Nystop (nystatin, topical): Echinacea

Ocuflox (ofloxacin): Calcium, Green Tea, Iron, Licorice, Magnesium, Potassium, Probiotic Flora, Vitamin B_1, Vitamin K, Zinc

Ogen (estropipate): Arginine, Black Cohosh, Boron, Calcium, Copper, DHEA, Dang Gui, Magnesium, Melatonin, Milk Thistle, St. John's Wort, Vitamin B_6, Vitamin D, Vitamin E, Vitex, Zinc

Olean (olestra): Vitamin K

Olux (clobetasol): Aloe, Green Tea, Licorice, Vitamin C, Zinc

Omnicef (cefdinir): Ginseng, Green Tea, Iron, Licorice, Probiotic Flora, Reishi, Vitamin B_1, Vitamin K, Zinc

Omnipen (ampicillin): Ginseng, Green Tea, Licorice, Probiotic Flora, Vitamin B_1, Vitamin C, Vitamin K, Zinc

Oncovin (vincristine): Alpha-Lipoic Acid, Echinacea, Eleuthero, Feverfew, Ginseng, St. John's Wort, Turmeric/Curcumin

Onkotrone (mitoxantrone): Alpha-Lipoic Acid, Carnitine, Coenzyme Q10, Garlic, Ginkgo, Green Tea, Hawthorn, Milk Thistle, Reishi, Selenium, St. John's Wort, Turmeric/Curcumin, Vitamin B_2, Vitamin E

Oralin (insulin): Alpha-Lipoic Acid, Bilberry, Chromium, DHEA, Ephedra, Garlic, Ginkgo, Ginseng, Glucosamine Sulfate, Horse Chestnut, Licorice, Magnesium, Milk Thistle, Omega-3 Fatty Acids, Potassium, Reishi, Turmeric/Curcumin, Vitamin B_3, Vitamin E

Oramorph SR (morphine): Ephedra, Ginseng, Gotu Kola, Phenylalanine, Tyrosine

Orapred (prednisolone): Calcium, Cayenne, Chromium, DHEA, Echinacea, Ephedra, Folic Acid, Horse Chestnut, Licorice, Magnesium, Melatonin, Omega-3 Fatty Acids, Potassium, Selenium, Vitamin A, Vitamin B_6, Vitamin C, Vitamin D, Vitamin K, Zinc

Orasone (prednisone): Calcium, Cayenne, Chromium, DHEA, Echinacea, Ephedra, Folic Acid, Horse Chestnut, Licorice, Magnesium, Melatonin, Omega-3 Fatty Acids, Potassium, Selenium, Vitamin A, Vitamin B_6, Vitamin C, Vitamin D, Vitamin K, Zinc

Oretic (hydrochlorothiazide): Calcium, Coenzyme Q10, Folic Acid, Ginkgo, Glucosamine Sulfate, Hawthorn, Licorice, Magnesium, Potassium, Vitamin B_2, Vitamin D, Zinc

Orgaran (danaparoid): Cayenne, Chondroitin Sulfate, DHEA, Policosanol

Orinase (tolbutamide): Aloe, Alpha-Lipoic Acid, Astragalus, Bilberry, Chromium, Coenzyme Q10, DHEA, Ephedra, Garlic, Ginkgo, Ginseng, Glucosamine Sulfate, Gotu Kola, Horse Chestnut, Magnesium, Omega-3 Fatty Acids, Reishi, Turmeric/Curcumin, Vitamin B_3

Oro-Clense (chlorhexidine): Iron, Licorice, Probiotic Flora, Vitamin K, Zinc

Ortho Dienestrol (dienestrol): Arginine, Black Cohosh, Boron, Calcium, Copper, DHEA, Dang Gui, Magnesium, Melatonin, Milk Thistle, St. John's Wort, Vitamin B_6, Vitamin D, Vitamin E, Vitex, Zinc

Ortho Novum 1/35 (ethinyl estradiol + norethindrone): Arginine, Calcium, Copper, DHEA, Dang Gui, Folic Acid, Iron, Licorice, Magnesium, Melatonin, Milk Thistle, *S*-Adenosylmethionine (SAMe), Selenium, St. John's Wort, Tyrosine, Vitamin A, Vitamin B_1, Vitamin B_2, Vitamin B_3, Vitamin B_6, Vitamin B_{12}, Vitamin C, Vitamin E, Vitex, Zinc

Ortho Novum 10/11 (ethinyl estradiol + norethindrone): Arginine, Calcium, Copper, DHEA, Dang Gui, Folic Acid, Iron, Licorice, Magnesium, Melatonin, Milk Thistle, *S*-Adenosylmethionine (SAMe), Selenium, St. John's Wort, Tyrosine, Vitamin A, Vitamin B_1, Vitamin B_2, Vitamin B_3, Vitamin B_6, Vitamin B_{12}, Vitamin C, Vitamin E, Vitex, Zinc

Ortho Novum 7/7/7 (ethinyl estradiol + norethindrone): Arginine, Calcium, Copper, DHEA, Dang Gui, Folic Acid, Iron, Licorice, Magnesium, Melatonin, Milk Thistle, *S*-Adenosylmethionine (SAMe), Selenium, St. John's Wort, Tyrosine, Vitamin A, Vitamin B_1, Vitamin B_2, Vitamin B_3, Vitamin B_6, Vitamin B_{12}, Vitamin C, Vitamin E, Vitex, Zinc

Ortho-Est (estropipate): Arginine, Black Cohosh, Boron, Calcium, Copper, DHEA, Dang Gui, Magnesium, Melatonin, Milk Thistle, St. John's Wort, Vitamin B_6, Vitamin D, Vitamin E, Vitex, Zinc

Ortho-Micronor (norethindrone, oral): Magnesium, St. John's Wort

Ortho-Novum 1/50 (mestranol + norethindrone): Arginine, Calcium, Copper, DHEA, Dang Gui, Folic Acid, Iron, Licorice, Magnesium, Melatonin, Milk Thistle, *S*-Adenosylmethionine (SAMe), Selenium, St. John's Wort, Tyrosine, Vitamin A, Vitamin B_1, Vitamin B_2, Vitamin B_3, Vitamin B_6, Vitamin B_{12}, Vitamin C, Vitamin E, Vitex, Zinc

Ortho-Prefest (estradiol + norgestimate): Arginine, Black Cohosh, Boron, Calcium, Copper, DHEA, Dang Gui, Magnesium, Melatonin, Milk Thistle, St. John's Wort, Vitamin B_6, Vitamin D, Vitamin E, Vitex, Zinc

Ortho-TriCyclen (ethinyl estradiol + desogestrel): Arginine, Calcium, Copper, DHEA, Dang Gui, Folic Acid, Iron, Licorice, Magnesium, Melatonin, Milk Thistle, *S*-Adenosylmethionine (SAMe), Selenium, St. John's Wort, Tyrosine, Vitamin A, Vitamin B_1, Vitamin B_2, Vitamin B_3, Vitamin B_6, Vitamin B_{12}, Vitamin C, Vitamin E, Vitex, Zinc

Orudis (ketoprofen): Calcium, Cayenne, Chondroitin Sulfate, Chromium, Copper, Devil's Claw, Feverfew, Folic Acid, Ginger, Glucosamine Sulfate, Gotu Kola, Iron, Licorice, Melatonin, Omega-3 Fatty Acids, Potassium, Turmeric/Curcumin, Vitamin B_3, Vitamin B_6, Vitamin C, Zinc

Oruvail (ketoprofen): Calcium, Cayenne, Chondroitin Sulfate, Chromium, Copper, Devil's Claw, Feverfew, Folic Acid, Ginger, Glucosamine Sulfate, Gotu Kola, Iron, Licorice, Melatonin, Omega-3 Fatty Acids, Potassium, Turmeric/Curcumin, Vitamin B_3, Vitamin B_6, Vitamin C, Zinc

Ostac (clodronate): Calcium, Iron, Magnesium, Vitamin D, Zinc

Ovcon-35 (ethinyl estradiol + norethindrone): Arginine, Calcium, Copper, DHEA, Dang Gui, Folic Acid, Iron, Licorice, Magnesium, Melatonin, Milk Thistle, *S*-Adenosylmethionine (SAMe), Selenium, St. John's Wort, Tyrosine, Vitamin A, Vitamin B_1, Vitamin B_2, Vitamin B_3, Vitamin B_6, Vitamin B_{12}, Vitamin C, Vitamin E, Vitex, Zinc

Ovcon-50 (ethinyl estradiol + norethindrone): Arginine, Calcium, Copper, DHEA, Dang Gui, Folic Acid, Iron, Licorice, Magnesium, Melatonin, Milk Thistle, *S*-Adenosylmethionine (SAMe), Selenium, St. John's Wort, Tyrosine, Vitamin A, Vitamin B_1, Vitamin B_2, Vitamin B_3, Vitamin B_6, Vitamin B_{12}, Vitamin C, Vitamin E, Vitex, Zinc

Ovral (ethinyl estradiol + norgestrel): Arginine, Calcium, Copper, DHEA, Dang Gui, Folic Acid, Iron, Licorice, Magnesium, Melatonin, Milk Thistle, *S*-Adenosylmethionine (SAMe), Selenium, St. John's Wort, Tyrosine, Vitamin A, Vitamin B_1, Vitamin B_2, Vitamin B_3, Vitamin B_6, Vitamin B_{12}, Vitamin C, Vitamin E, Vitex, Zinc

Ovrette (norgestrel, oral): Magnesium, St. John's Wort

OxyContin (oxycodone): Ephedra, Ginseng, Gotu Kola, Phenylalanine, Tyrosine

OxyIR (oxycodone): Ephedra, Ginseng, Gotu Kola, Phenylalanine, Tyrosine

Pamelor (nortriptyline): 5-HTP, Coenzyme Q10, Milk Thistle, S-Adenosylmethionine (SAMe), St. John's Wort, Tryptophan, Tyrosine, Vitamin B_1, Vitamin B_2, Vitamin B_3, Vitamin B_6, Vitamin B_{12}, Zinc

Pandel (hydrocortisone 17-butyrate/acetate/probutate/valerate): Aloe, Green Tea, Licorice, Vitamin C

Panesclerina (probucol): Beta-Carotene

Papaveretum (morphine hydrochloride + codeine hydrochloride + papaverine hydrochloride): Ephedra, Ginger, Ginseng, Gotu Kola, Phenylalanine, Tyrosine

Paraflex (chlorzoxazone): Garlic, St. John's Wort

Parafon Forte (chlorzoxazone): Garlic, St. John's Wort

Paraplatin (carboplatin): Alpha-Lipoic Acid, Astragalus, Carnitine, Cayenne, Chondroitin Sulfate, Echinacea, Eleuthero, Ginger, Ginkgo, Ginseng, Milk Thistle, Selenium, Turmeric/Curcumin

Parbenem (probenecid): Vitamin B_2, Vitamin B_3, Vitamin C

Parcopa (levodopa + carbidopa): 5-HTP, Folic Acid, Iron, Kava, Methionine, Phenylalanine, S-Adenosylmethionine (SAMe), Tyrosine, Vitamin B_3, Vitamin B_6, Vitamin C, Vitex

Pariet (rabeprazole): Beta-Carotene, Calcium, Chromium, Iron, Kava, St. John's Wort, Vitamin B_{12}, Zinc

Parnate (tranylcypromine): 5-HTP, Cayenne, Chromium, Eleuthero, Ephedra, Ginkgo, Ginseng, Licorice, Melatonin, Phenylalanine, S-Adenosylmethionine (SAMe), St. John's Wort, Tryptophan, Tyrosine, Vitamin B_6

Paser (para-aminosalicylic acid): Vitamin B_{12}

Pavulon (pancuronium): Magnesium

Paxene (paclitaxel): Aloe, Beta-Carotene, Echinacea, Eleuthero, Feverfew, Ginseng, Melatonin, Omega-3 Fatty Acids, PABA, St. John's Wort, Turmeric/Curcumin, Vitamin A, Vitamin C, Vitamin E

Paxil (paroxetine): 5-HTP, Chromium, Folic Acid, Ginkgo, Inositol, Omega-3 Fatty Acids, S-Adenosylmethionine (SAMe), St. John's Wort, Tryptophan, Vitamin B_3, Vitamin B_6, Vitamin B_{12}, Vitamin C, Zinc

PC-Cap (acetylsalicylic acid + propoxyphene): Calcium, Cayenne, Devil's Claw, Ephedra, Feverfew, Folic Acid, Ginkgo, Ginseng, Gotu Kola, Iron, Licorice, Melatonin, Milk Thistle, Phenylalanine, Policosanol, Potassium, Tyrosine, Vitamin B_2, Vitamin B_3, Vitamin C, Vitamin E, Vitamin K, Zinc

PCE Dispertab (erythromycin oral): Calcium, Green Tea, Magnesium, Probiotic Flora, Vitamin B_1, Vitamin B_6, Vitamin B_{12}, Vitamin K, Zinc

Pedi Dri Topical Powder (nystatin, topical): Echinacea

PediaCare Fever Drops (ibuprofen): Calcium, Cayenne, Chondroitin Sulfate, Chromium, Copper, Devil's Claw, Feverfew, Folic Acid, Ginger, Glucosamine Sulfate, Gotu Kola, Iron, Licorice, Melatonin, Omega-3 Fatty Acids, Potassium, Turmeric/Curcumin, Vitamin B_3, Vitamin B_6, Vitamin C, Zinc

PediaCare Infant Drops (pseudoephedrine): Potassium

Pediaflor (sodium fluoride): Calcium, Vitamin D

Pediapred (prednisolone): Calcium, Cayenne, Chromium, DHEA, Echinacea, Ephedra, Folic Acid, Horse Chestnut, Licorice, Magnesium, Melatonin, Omega-3 Fatty Acids, Potassium, Selenium, Vitamin A, Vitamin B_6, Vitamin C, Vitamin D, Vitamin K, Zinc

Pediazole (erythromycin oral): Calcium, Green Tea, Magnesium, Probiotic Flora, Vitamin B_1, Vitamin B_6, Vitamin B_{12}, Vitamin K, Zinc

Peg-Intron: Enchinacea

Peganone (ethotoin): Calcium, Carnitine, Copper, DHEA, Folic Acid, Ginkgo, Inositol, Kava, Milk Thistle, Omega-3 Fatty Acids, Valerian, Vitamin A, Vitamin B_1, Vitamin B_2, Vitamin B_3, Vitamin B_6, Vitamin B_{12}, Vitamin C, Vitamin D, Vitamin E, Vitamin K, Vitex, Zinc

Pen-Vee K (penicillin V): Ginseng, Green Tea, Licorice, Probiotic Flora, Vitamin B_1, Vitamin K, Zinc

Penecort (hydrocortisone): Aloe, Green Tea, Licorice, Vitamin C

Penetrex (enoxacin): Calcium, Green Tea, Iron, Licorice, Magnesium, Potassium, Probiotic Flora, Vitamin B_1, Vitamin K, Zinc

Pentacarinat (pentamidine): Magnesium

Pentacort (hydrocortisone): Aloe, Green Tea, Licorice, Vitamin C

Pentam 300 (pentamidine): Magnesium

Pentasa (mesalazine): Vitamin B_{12}

Pentothal (thiopental): DHEA, Gotu Kola, Valerian, Vitamin B_2

Pentoxil (pentoxifylline): Arginine, Cayenne, Coenzyme Q10, Policosanol, Vitamin E

Pepcid RPD (famotidine): Calcium, Chromium, Copper, Folic Acid, Iron, Licorice, Magnesium, Vitamin B_{12}, Vitamin C, Zinc

Pepcid (famotidine): Calcium, Chromium, Copper, Folic Acid, Iron, Licorice, Magnesium, Vitamin B_{12}, Vitamin C, Zinc

Pepcid AC (famotidine): Calcium, Chromium, Copper, Folic Acid, Iron, Licorice, Magnesium, Vitamin B_{12}, Vitamin C, Zinc

Pepto Diarrhea Control (loperamide): St. John's Wort

Percocet 10/650 (acetaminophen + oxycodone): Ephedra, Garlic, Ginseng, Gotu Kola, Licorice, Milk Thistle, Phenylalanine, Tyrosine, Vitamin C

Percocet 2.5/325 (acetaminophen + oxycodone): Ephedra, Garlic, Ginseng, Gotu Kola, Licorice, Milk Thistle, Phenylalanine, Tyrosine, Vitamin C

Percocet 5/325 (acetaminophen + oxycodone): Ephedra, Garlic, Ginseng, Gotu Kola, Licorice, Milk Thistle, Phenylalanine, Tyrosine, Vitamin C

Percocet 7.5/500 (acetaminophen + oxycodone): Ephedra, Garlic, Ginseng, Gotu Kola, Licorice, Milk Thistle, Phenylalanine, Tyrosine, Vitamin C

Percodan (acetylsalicylic acid + oxycodone): Calcium, Cayenne, Devil's Claw, Ephedra, Feverfew, Folic Acid, Ginkgo, Ginseng, Gotu Kola, Iron, Licorice, Melatonin, Milk Thistle, Phenylalanine, Policosanol, Potassium, Tyrosine, Vitamin B_2, Vitamin B_3, Vitamin C, Vitamin E, Vitamin K, Zinc

Percodan-Demi (acetylsalicylic acid + oxycodone): Calcium, Cayenne, Devil's Claw, Ephedra, Feverfew, Folic Acid, Ginkgo, Ginseng, Gotu Kola, Iron, Licorice, Melatonin, Milk Thistle, Phenylalanine, Policosanol, Potassium, Tyrosine, Vitamin B_2, Vitamin B_3, Vitamin C, Vitamin E, Vitamin K, Zinc

Percolone (oxycodone): Ephedra, Ginseng, Gotu Kola, Phenylalanine, Tyrosine

Peridex (chlorhexidine): Iron, Licorice, Probiotic Flora, Vitamin K, Zinc

Periochip (chlorhexidine): Iron, Licorice, Probiotic Flora, Vitamin K, Zinc

Periogard Oral Rinse (chlorhexidine): Iron, Licorice, Probiotic Flora, Vitamin K, Zinc

Periostat (doxycycline): Calcium, Folic Acid, Iron, Magnesium, Potassium, Vitamin A, Vitamin B$_1$, Vitamin B$_2$, Vitamin B$_3$, Vitamin B$_6$, Vitamin C, Zinc

Permitil (fluphenazine): Coenzyme Q10, Milk Thistle, Vitamin B$_2$, Vitamin B$_3$, Vitamin C

Permole (dipyridamole): Bilberry, Cayenne, Feverfew, Garlic, Ginger, Ginkgo, Iron, Omega-3 Fatty Acids, Policosanol, S-Adenosylmethionine (SAMe)

Persantine (dipyridamole): Bilberry, Cayenne, Feverfew, Garlic, Ginger, Ginkgo, Iron, Omega-3 Fatty Acids, Policosanol, S-Adenosylmethionine (SAMe)

Pertofrane (desipramine): 5-HTP, Coenzyme Q10, Melatonin, Milk Thistle, S-Adenosylmethionine (SAMe), St. John's Wort, Tryptophan, Tyrosine, Vitamin B$_1$, Vitamin B$_2$, Vitamin B$_3$, Vitamin B$_6$, Vitamin B$_{12}$, Vitamin E, Zinc

Petrogalar Plain (mineral oil): Beta-Carotene, Calcium, Potassium, Vitamin A, Vitamin D, Vitamin E, Vitamin K

Pfizerpen (penicillin G): Ginseng, Green Tea, Licorice, Probiotic Flora, Vitamin B$_1$, Vitamin K, Zinc

Pharmorubicin (epirubicin): Alpha-Lipoic Acid, Carnitine, Coenzyme Q10, Feverfew, Garlic, Ginkgo, Green Tea, Hawthorn, Milk Thistle, Reishi, Selenium, St. John's Wort, Turmeric/Curcumin, Vitamin B$_2$, Vitamin E

Phenaphen with Codeine (codeine + acetaminophen): Ephedra, Ginseng, Gotu Kola, Phenylalanine, Tyrosine

Phenergan (promethazine): Coenzyme Q10, Milk Thistle, Vitamin B$_2$, Vitamin B$_3$, Vitamin C

Phenidone (1-Phenyl-3-Pyrazolidone): Vitamin A

Phenldrine (phenylpropanolamine): Potassium, Tyrosine

Phenoxine (phenylpropanolamine): Potassium, Tyrosine

Phenytek (phenytoin): Calcium, Carnitine, Copper, DHEA, Folic Acid, Ginkgo, Inositol, Kava, Milk Thistle, Omega-3 Fatty Acids, Valerian, Vitamin A, Vitamin B$_1$, Vitamin B$_2$, Vitamin B$_3$, Vitamin B$_6$, Vitamin B$_{12}$, Vitamin C, Vitamin D, Vitamin E, Vitamin K, Vitex, Zinc

Phillips Milk of Magnesia Magnesium Citrate Solution (magnesium-containing products): Potassium

Phillips' Milk of Magnesia MOM (magnesium hydroxide): Calcium, Cayenne, Chromium, Copper, Folic Acid, Iron, Magnesium, Vitamin A, Vitamin B$_1$, Vitamin D, Vitex, Zinc

PhosLo (calcium acetate): Calcium

Phyllocontin (theophylline): Arginine, Cayenne, Ephedra, Magnesium, Melatonin, Potassium, St. John's Wort, Vitamin B$_6$

Pipracil (piperacillin): Ginseng, Green Tea, Licorice, Probiotic Flora, Vitamin B$_1$, Vitamin K, Zinc

Pitocin (oxytocin): Ephedra

Plan B (levonorgestrel, oral postcoital contraceptive): Magnesium, St. John's Wort

Plaquenil (hydroxychloroquine): Calcium, Magnesium, Vitamin B$_2$, Vitamin B$_6$, Vitamin D

Platinol-AQ (cisplatin): Aloe, Alpha-Lipoic Acid, Astragalus, Beta-Carotene, Calcium, Carnitine, Cayenne, Chondroitin Sulfate, Echinacea, Eleuthero, Feverfew, Ginger, Ginkgo, Ginseng, Magnesium, Melatonin, Milk Thistle, Omega-3 Fatty Acids, Potassium, Selenium, Turmeric/Curcumin, Vitamin A, Vitamin B$_6$, Vitamin C, Vitamin E, Zinc

Platinol (cisplatin): Aloe, Alpha-Lipoic Acid, Astragalus, Beta-Carotene, Calcium, Carnitine, Cayenne, Chondroitin Sulfate, Echinacea, Eleuthero, Feverfew, Ginger, Ginkgo, Ginseng, Magnesium, Melatonin, Milk Thistle, Omega-3 Fatty Acids, Potassium, Selenium, Turmeric/Curcumin, Vitamin A, Vitamin B$_6$, Vitamin C, Vitamin E, Zinc

Plavix (clopidogrel): Bilberry, Cayenne, Feverfew, Garlic, Ginger, Ginkgo, Omega-3 Fatty Acids, Policosanol, S-Adenosylmethionine (SAMe)

Plendil (felodipine): Calcium, Carnitine, Folic Acid, Magnesium, St. John's Wort, Vitamin B$_6$, Vitamin D

Pletal (cilostazol): Bilberry, Cayenne, Feverfew, Garlic, Ginger, Ginkgo, Omega-3 Fatty Acids, Policosanol, S-Adenosylmethionine (SAMe)

PMS-Lithium (lithium carbonate): 5-HTP, Chromium, Folic Acid, Inositol, Magnesium, Tryptophan

PMS-Nifedipine (nifedipine): Black Cohosh, Calcium, Dang Gui, Magnesium, Saw Palmetto

PMS-Sulfasalazine (sulfasalazine): Calcium, Folic Acid, Iron, Licorice, Magnesium, Omega-3 Fatty Acids, PABA, Probiotic Flora, Vitamin B$_1$, Vitamin B$_6$, Vitamin K, Zinc

Pneumopent (pentamidine): Magnesium

Pondocillin (pivampicillin): Carnitine

Ponstel (mefenamic acid): Calcium, Cayenne, Chondroitin Sulfate, Chromium, Copper, Devil's Claw, Feverfew, Folic Acid, Ginger, Glucosamine Sulfate, Gotu Kola, Iron, Licorice, Melatonin, Omega-3 Fatty Acids, Potassium, Turmeric/Curcumin, Vitamin B3, Vitamin B6, Vitamin C, Zinc

Postinor-2 (levonorgestrel, oral postcoital contraceptive): Magnesium, St. John's Wort

Prandin (repaglinide): Chromium, Vitamin B$_3$

Pravachol (pravastatin): Beta-Carotene, Carnitine, Coenzyme Q10, Garlic, Gotu Kola, Omega-3 Fatty Acids, Policosanol, Reishi, Selenium, St. John's Wort, Vitamin A, Vitamin B$_3$, Vitamin C, Vitamin E

Precose (acarbose): Chromium, Vitamin B3

Prelone (prednisolone): Calcium, Cayenne, Chromium, DHEA, Echinacea, Ephedra, Folic Acid, Horse Chestnut, Licorice, Magnesium, Melatonin, Omega-3 Fatty Acids, Potassium, Selenium, Vitamin A, Vitamin B$_6$, Vitamin C, Vitamin D, Vitamin K, Zinc

Premarin (conjugated equine estrogens): Arginine, Black Cohosh, Boron, Calcium, Copper, DHEA, Dang Gui, Magnesium, Melatonin, Milk Thistle, St. John's Wort, Vitamin B$_6$, Vitamin D, Vitamin E, Vitex, Zinc

Premelle cycle 5 (medroxyprogesterone + conjugated equine estrogens): Arginine, Beta-Carotene, Black Cohosh, Boron, Calcium, Copper, DHEA, Dang Gui, Folic Acid, Magnesium, Melatonin, Milk Thistle, St. John's Wort, Vitamin A, Vitamin B$_6$, Vitamin D, Vitamin E, Vitex, Zinc

Prempak-C (conjugated equine estrogens + norgestrel): Arginine, Black Cohosh, Boron, Calcium, Copper, DHEA, Dang Gui, Magnesium, Melatonin, Milk Thistle, St. John's Wort, Vitamin B$_6$, Vitamin D, Vitamin E, Vitex, Zinc

Prempro (medroxyprogesterone + conjugated equine estrogens): Arginine, Beta-Carotene, Black Cohosh, Boron, Calcium, Copper, DHEA, Dang Gui, Folic Acid, Magnesium, Melatonin, Milk Thistle, St. John's Wort, Vitamin A, Vitamin B$_6$, Vitamin D, Vitamin E, Vitex, Zinc

Pres Tab (glyburide): Aloe, Alpha-Lipoic Acid, Astragalus, Bilberry, Chromium, Coenzyme Q10, DHEA, Ephedra, Garlic, Ginkgo, Ginseng, Glucosamine Sulfate, Gotu Kola, Horse Chestnut, Magnesium, Omega-3 Fatty Acids, Reishi, Turmeric/Curcumin, Vitamin B$_3$, Vitamin E

Prevacid (lansoprazole): Beta-Carotene, Calcium, Chromium, Iron, Kava, Probiotic Flora, St. John's Wort, Vitamin B$_{12}$, Zinc

Prevalite (cholestyramine): Beta-Carotene, Calcium, Folic Acid, Iron, Magnesium, Omega-3 Fatty Acids, Vitamin A, Vitamin B$_2$, Vitamin B$_3$, Vitamin B$_{12}$, Vitamin D, Vitamin E, Vitamin K, Zinc

PreviDent (sodium fluoride): Calcium, Vitamin D

Prevpac (lansoprazole + amoxicillin + clarithromycin): Licorice, Probiotic Flora, Vitamin C, Vitamin K, Zinc

Prezista (darunavir): Copper, Garlic, St. John's Wort, Vitamin C

Priadel (lithium carbonate): 5-HTP, Chromium, Folic Acid, Inositol, Magnesium, Tryptophan

Prilosec (omeprazole): Beta-Carotene, Calcium, Chromium, Iron, Kava, St. John's Wort, Vitamin B_{12}, Vitamin E, Zinc

Primatene Dual Action (ephedrine + guaifenesin + theophylline): Cayenne, Magnesium

Primatene Mist (epinephrine): Magnesium, Potassium, Vitamin C

Primaxin I.M. (imipenem + cilastatin): Ginseng, Green Tea, Iron, Licorice, Probiotic Flora, Reishi, Vitamin B_1, Vitamin K, Zinc

Primaxin I.V. (imipenem + cilastatin): Ginseng, Green Tea, Iron, Licorice, Probiotic Flora, Reishi, Vitamin B1, Vitamin K, Zinc

Primobolan (methenolone enanthate): Echinacea

Principen (ampicillin): Ginseng, Green Tea, Licorice, Probiotic Flora, Vitamin B_1, Vitamin C, Vitamin K, Zinc

Prinivil (lisinopril): Arginine, Cayenne, Iron, Omega-3 Fatty Acids, Potassium, Vitamin E, Zinc

Prinzide (lisinopril + hydrochlorothiazide): Arginine, Calcium, Cayenne, Coenzyme Q10, Glucosamine Sulfate, Hawthorn, Licorice, Magnesium, Potassium, Vitamin D, Zinc

Pro-Banthine (propantheline bromide): Vitamin B_2

Probalan (probenecid): Vitamin B_2, Vitamin B_3, Vitamin C

Procan-SR (procainamide): Cascara, Magnesium, Potassium

Procardia (nifedipine): Black Cohosh, Calcium, Dang Gui, Magnesium, Saw Palmetto

Procrit (epoetin alpha): Dang Gui, Iron, Vitamin B_6, Vitamin C

Proctocort (hydrocortisone): Aloe, Green Tea, Licorice, Vitamin C

Procur (cyproterone): Black Cohosh, Vitamin D

Procytox (cyclophosphamide): Aloe, Alpha-Lipoic Acid, Astragalus, Beta-Carotene, Carnitine, Echinacea, Eleuthero, Ginger, Ginseng, Licorice, Melatonin, Omega-3 Fatty Acids, Reishi, Selenium, Turmeric/Curcumin, Vitamin A, Vitamin C, Vitamin E

Progout (allopurinol): Carnitine, Copper, Iron, Tryptophan, Vitamin D

Prograf (tacrolimus): Echinacea, St. John's Wort

Progyluton (estradiol valerate + norgestrel): Arginine, Black Cohosh, Boron, Calcium, Copper, DHEA, Dang Gui, Magnesium, Melatonin, Milk Thistle, St. John's Wort, Vitamin B_6, Vitamin D, Vitamin E, Vitex, Zinc

Progynova (estradiol valerate): Arginine, Black Cohosh, Boron, Calcium, Copper, DHEA, Dang Gui, Magnesium, Melatonin, Milk Thistle, St. John's Wort, Vitamin B_6, Vitamin D, Vitamin E, Vitex, Zinc

Prokine (GMCSF): Echinacea

Proleukin (aldesleukin): Astragalus, Echinacea, Melatonin

Prolixin (fluphenazine): Chromium, Coenzyme Q10, Ginkgo, Kava, Melatonin, Milk Thistle, Vitamin B_2, Vitamin B_3, Vitamin B_6, Vitamin C

Prolixin Decanoate (fluphenazine): Coenzyme Q10, Milk Thistle, Vitamin B_2, Vitamin B_3, Vitamin C

Prolixin Enanthate (fluphenazine): Coenzyme Q10, Milk Thistle, Vitamin B_2, Vitamin B_3, Vitamin C

Proloprim (trimethoprim): Folic Acid, Licorice, Probiotic Flora, Vitamin B_2, Vitamin K, Zinc

Promacot (promethazine): Coenzyme Q10, Milk Thistle, Vitamin B_2, Vitamin B_3, Vitamin C

Promethegan (promethazine): Coenzyme Q10, Milk Thistle, Vitamin B_2, Vitamin B_3, Vitamin C

Prometrium (progesterone, micronized): Vitamin D

Pronap-100 (acetaminophen + propoxyphene): Ephedra, Garlic, Ginseng, Gotu Kola, Licorice, Milk Thistle, Phenylalanine, Tyrosine, Vitamin C

Pronestyl (procainamide): Cascara, Magnesium, Potassium

Pronil (secnidazole): Milk Thistle

Propacet 100 (acetaminophen + propoxyphene): Ephedra, Garlic, Ginseng, Gotu Kola, Licorice, Milk Thistle, Phenylalanine, Tyrosine, Vitamin C

Propagest (phenylpropanolamine): Potassium, Tyrosine

Propecia (finasteride): Black Cohosh, Saw Palmetto

Propoxacet-N (acetaminophen + propoxyphene): Ephedra, Garlic, Ginseng, Gotu Kola, Licorice, Milk Thistle, Phenylalanine, Tyrosine, Vitamin C

Proscar (finasteride): Black Cohosh, Saw Palmetto

ProSom (estazolam): DHEA, Gotu Kola, Kava, Melatonin, St. John's Wort, Valerian, Vitamin B_3

Protium (pantoprazole): Beta-Carotene, Calcium, Chromium, Iron, Kava, St. John's Wort, Vitamin B_{12}, Zinc

Protonix (pantoprazole): Beta-Carotene, Calcium, Chromium, Iron, Kava, St. John's Wort, Vitamin B_{12}, Zinc

Protostat (metronidazole, systemic): Licorice, Milk Thistle, Probiotic Flora, Vitamin K, Zinc

Provel (ibuprofen): Calcium, Cayenne, Chondroitin Sulfate, Chromium, Copper, Devil's Claw, Feverfew, Folic Acid, Ginger, Glucosamine Sulfate, Gotu Kola, Iron, Licorice, Melatonin, Omega-3 Fatty Acids, Potassium, Turmeric/Curcumin, Vitamin B_3, Vitamin B_6, Vitamin C, Zinc

Proventil (albuterol): Calcium, Magnesium, Potassium

Provera (medroxyprogesterone, oral): Beta-Carotene, Calcium, Folic Acid, Magnesium, St. John's Wort, Vitamin A, Vitamin D

Provigil (modafinil): Reishi, Tyrosine

Prozac (fluoxetine): 5-HTP, Chromium, DHEA, Folic Acid, Ginkgo, Inositol, Melatonin, Omega-3 Fatty Acids, S-Adenosylmethionine (SAMe), St. John's Wort, Tryptophan, Vitamin B_3, Vitamin B_6, Vitamin B_{12}, Vitamin C, Zinc

Psorcon (diflorasone): Aloe, Green Tea, Licorice, Vitamin C

Pulmadil (rimiterol): Calcium, Magnesium, Potassium

Pulvules (cinoxacin): Calcium, Green Tea, Iron, Licorice, Magnesium, Potassium, Probiotic Flora, Vitamin B_1, Vitamin K, Zinc

Pump-Hep (heparin): Calcium, Cayenne, Chondroitin Sulfate, DHEA, Omega-3 Fatty Acids, Policosanol, Potassium, Vitamin C, Vitamin D

Purinethol (mercaptopurine): Echinacea, Eleuthero, Folic Acid, Vitamin B_1, Vitamin B_3

Questran (cholestyramine): Beta-Carotene, Calcium, Folic Acid, Iron, Magnesium, Omega-3 Fatty Acids, Vitamin A, Vitamin B_2, Vitamin B_3, Vitamin B_{12}, Vitamin D, Vitamin E, Vitamin K, Zinc

Quick Pep (caffeine): Calcium, Ephedra, Kava, Melatonin

Quilonum SR (lithium carbonate): 5-HTP, Chromium, Folic Acid, Inositol, Magnesium, Tryptophan

Quinaglute (quinidine): Beta-Carotene, Cascara, Magnesium, Potassium

Quinidex (quinidine): Beta-Carotene, Cascara, Magnesium, Potassium

Quinora (quinidine): Beta-Carotene, Cascara, Magnesium, Potassium

QVAR (beclomethasone inhalant): Calcium

Rebetol (ribavirin): S-Adenosylmethionine (SAMe)

Rebetron (ribavirin + interferon alpha-2b): Iron, Licorice, Zinc

Rederm (hydrocortisone 17-butyrate/acetate/probutate/valerate): Aloe, Green Tea, Licorice, Vitamin C

Reductil (sibutramine): 5-HTP, Tryptophan

Refludan (lepirudin): Cayenne, DHEA, Policosanol

Reglan (metoclopramide): Vitamin B_2, Zinc

Regular Strength Bayer Enteric 500 Aspirin (acetylsalicylic acid): Bilberry, Calcium, Cayenne, Devil's Claw, Feverfew, Folic Acid, Garlic, Ginger, Ginkgo, Gotu Kola, Iron, Licorice, Melatonin, Milk Thistle, Omega-3 Fatty Acids, Policosanol, Potassium, S-Adenosylmethionine (SAMe), Vitamin B_2, Vitamin B_3, Vitamin C, Vitamin E, Vitamin K, Zinc

Regulin (betanidine): Ephedra

Relafen (nabumetone): Calcium, Cayenne, Chondroitin Sulfate, Chromium, Copper, Devil's Claw, Feverfew, Folic Acid, Ginger, Glucosamine Sulfate, Gotu Kola, Iron, Licorice, Melatonin, Omega-3 Fatty Acids, Potassium, Turmeric/Curcumin, Vitamin B_3, Vitamin B_6, Vitamin C, Zinc

Relaxazone (chlorzoxazone): Garlic, St. John's Wort

Relpax (eletriptan): 5-HTP, Feverfew, Tryptophan

Remeron (mirtazapine): Melatonin

Remicade (infliximab): Echinacea

Remular-S (chlorzoxazone): Garlic, St. John's Wort

Rendix (dabigatran): Cayenne, DHEA, Policosanol

Renese (polythiazide): Calcium, Coenzyme Q10, Folic Acid, Ginkgo, Glucosamine Sulfate, Hawthorn, Licorice, Magnesium, Potassium, Vitamin B_2, Vitamin D, Zinc

Renova (tretinoin): Beta-Carotene, Calcium, Carnitine, Vitamin A, Vitamin E

ReoPro (abciximab): Cayenne, Ginger, Policosanol, S-Adenosylmethionine (SAMe)

Reprexain (hydrocodone + ibuprofen): Calcium, Cayenne, Chondroitin Sulfate, Chromium, Copper, Devil's Claw, Feverfew, Folic Acid, Ginger, Ginseng, Glucosamine Sulfate, Gotu Kola, Iron, Licorice, Melatonin, Omega-3 Fatty Acids, Potassium, Turmeric/Curcumin, Vitamin B_3, Vitamin B_6, Vitamin C, Zinc

Reprexain (ibuprofen + hydrocodone): Ephedra, Ginseng, Gotu Kola, Phenylalanine, Tyrosine

Rescriptor (delavirdine): St. John's Wort, Vitamin B_2

Restoril (temazepam): DHEA, Gotu Kola, Melatonin, Valerian, Vitamin B_3

Retavase (reteplase, recombinant): Astragalus

Retin-A (tretinoin): Beta-Carotene, Calcium, Carnitine, Vitamin A, Vitamin E

Retrovir (zidovudine): Aloe, Carnitine, Coenzyme Q10, Copper, DHEA, Folic Acid, Reishi, Vitamin B_1, Vitamin B_2, Vitamin B_{12}, Vitamin E, Zinc

Revasc (desirudin): Cayenne, DHEA, Policosanol

Reyataz (atazanavir): Copper, Garlic, St. John's Wort, Vitamin C

Rheumatrex (methotrexate): Aloe, Beta-Carotene, Echinacea, Eleuthero, Folic Acid, Garlic, Ginseng, Iron, Melatonin, Milk Thistle, Omega-3 Fatty Acids, PABA, Vitamin A, Vitamin B_1, Vitamin B_2, Vitamin B_6, Vitamin B_{12}, Vitamin C, Vitamin E

Rhindecon (phenylpropanolamine): Potassium, Tyrosine

Ribasphere (ribavirin): S-Adenosylmethionine (SAMe)

Ridafed (pseudoephedrine): Potassium

Rifadin (rifampicin): Folic Acid, Milk Thistle, Vitamin B_3, Vitamin B_6, Vitamin C, Vitamin D, Vitamin E

Rifadin IV (rifampicin): Folic Acid, Milk Thistle, Vitamin B_3, Vitamin B_6, Vitamin C, Vitamin D, Vitamin E

Rifamate (isoniazid + rifampicin): Calcium, Copper, Folic Acid, Magnesium, Milk Thistle, Vitamin B_3, Vitamin B_6, Vitamin C, Vitamin D, Vitamin E

Rifater (isoniazid + pyrazinamide + rifampicin): Calcium, Copper, Folic Acid, Magnesium, Milk Thistle, Vitamin B_3, Vitamin B_6, Vitamin C, Vitamin D, Vitamin E

Rimactane (isoniazid + rifampicin): Calcium, Copper, Folic Acid, Magnesium, Milk Thistle, Vitamin B_3, Vitamin B_6, Vitamin C, Vitamin D, Vitamin E

Risperdal (risperidone): 5-HTP, Chromium, Echinacea, Ginkgo, Melatonin, Omega-3 Fatty Acids, Vitamin B_3, Vitamin B6, Vitamin C, Vitamin E

Ritalin (methylphenidate): 5-HTP, Iron, Reishi, Tyrosine, Zinc

Ritalin-SR (methylphenidate): 5-HTP, Iron, Reishi, Tyrosine, Zinc

Rivotril (clonazepam): Calcium, Carnitine, Copper, DHEA, Folic Acid, Ginkgo, Gotu Kola, Inositol, Kava, Melatonin, Milk Thistle, Omega-3 Fatty Acids, Valerian, Vitamin A, Vitamin B_1, Vitamin B_2, Vitamin B_3, Vitamin B_6, Vitamin B_{12}, Vitamin C, Vitamin D, Vitamin E, Vitamin K, Vitex, Zinc

RMS (morphine): Ephedra, Ginseng, Gotu Kola, Phenylalanine, Tyrosine

Robicillin VK (penicillin V): Ginseng, Green Tea, Licorice, Probiotic Flora, Vitamin B_1, Vitamin K, Zinc

Rocephin (ceftriaxone): Ginseng, Green Tea, Iron, Licorice, Probiotic Flora, Reishi, Vitamin B_1, Vitamin K, Zinc

Roferon-A (interferon alpha): Astragalus, Echinacea, Iron, Licorice, Zinc

Rowasa (mesalazine): Vitamin B_{12}

Roxanol (morphine): Ephedra, Ginseng, Gotu Kola, Phenylalanine, Tyrosine

Roxanol Rescudose (morphine): Ephedra, Ginseng, Gotu Kola, Phenylalanine, Tyrosine

Roxanol T (morphine): Ephedra, Ginseng, Gotu Kola, Phenylalanine, Tyrosine

Roxicet 5/500 (acetaminophen + oxycodone): Ephedra, Garlic, Ginseng, Gotu Kola, Licorice, Milk Thistle, Phenylalanine, Tyrosine, Vitamin C

Roxicodone (oxycodone): Ephedra, Ginseng, Gotu Kola, Phenylalanine, Tyrosine

Roxilox (acetaminophen + oxycodone): Ephedra, Garlic, Ginseng, Gotu Kola, Licorice, Milk Thistle, Phenylalanine, Tyrosine, Vitamin C

Rubex (doxorubicin): Aloe, Alpha-Lipoic Acid, Carnitine, Coenzyme Q10, Feverfew, Garlic, Ginkgo, Ginseng, Green Tea, Hawthorn, Melatonin, Milk Thistle, Omega-3 Fatty Acids, Reishi, Selenium, St. John's Wort, Turmeric/Curcumin, Vitamin A, Vitamin B_2, Vitamin C, Vitamin D, Vitamin E

Rufen (ibuprofen): Calcium, Cayenne, Chondroitin Sulfate, Chromium, Copper, Devil's Claw, Feverfew, Folic Acid, Ginger, Glucosamine Sulfate, Gotu Kola, Iron, Licorice, Melatonin, Omega-3 Fatty Acids, Potassium, Turmeric/Curcumin, Vitamin B_3, Vitamin B_6, Vitamin C, Zinc

S-2 (epinephrine): Magnesium, Potassium, Vitamin C

S-T Cort (hydrocortisone 17-butyrate/acetate/probutate/valerate): Aloe, Green Tea, Licorice, Vitamin C

Sabril (vigabatrin): Calcium, Carnitine, Copper, DHEA, Folic Acid, Ginkgo, Inositol, Kava, Milk Thistle, Omega-3 Fatty Acids, Valerian, Vitamin A, Vitamin B_1, Vitamin B_2, Vitamin B_3, Vitamin B_6, Vitamin B_{12}, Vitamin C, Vitamin D, Vitamin E, Vitamin K, Vitex, Zinc

Salazopyrin (sulfasalazine): Calcium, Folic Acid, Iron, Licorice, Magnesium, Omega-3 Fatty Acids, PABA, Probiotic Flora, Vitamin B_1, Vitamin B_6, Vitamin K, Zinc

Salazopyrin EN-Tabs (sulfasalazine): Calcium, Folic Acid, Iron, Licorice, Magnesium, Omega-3 Fatty Acids, PABA, Probiotic Flora, Vitamin B_1, Vitamin B_6, Vitamin K, Zinc

Salflex (salsalate): Calcium, Cayenne, Chondroitin Sulfate, Chromium, Copper, Devil's Claw, Feverfew, Folic Acid, Ginger, Glucosamine Sulfate, Gotu Kola, Iron, Licorice, Melatonin, Omega-3 Fatty Acids, Policosanol, Potassium, Turmeric/Curcumin, Vitamin B_3, Vitamin B_6, Vitamin C, Vitamin K, Zinc

Salofalk (mesalazine): Vitamin B_{12}

Salsitab (salsalate): Calcium, Folic Acid, Omega-3 Fatty Acids, Policosanol, Vitamin C, Vitamin K, Zinc

Sandimmune (cyclosporine): Arginine, Echinacea, Ginkgo, Magnesium, Melatonin, Omega-3 Fatty Acids, Potassium, St. John's Wort, Turmeric/Curcumin, Vitamin C, Vitamin E, Zinc

SangCya (cyclosporine): Arginine, Echinacea, Ginkgo, Magnesium, Melatonin, Omega-3 Fatty Acids, Potassium, St. John's Wort, Turmeric/Curcumin, Vitamin C, Vitamin E, Zinc

Sarafem (fluoxetine): 5-HTP, Chromium, DHEA, Folic Acid, Ginkgo, Inositol, Melatonin, Omega-3 Fatty Acids, S-Adenosylmethionine (SAMe), St. John's Wort, Tryptophan, Vitamin B_3, Vitamin B_6, Vitamin B_{12}, Vitamin C, Zinc

SAS (sulfasalazine): Calcium, Folic Acid, Iron, Licorice, Magnesium, Omega-3 Fatty Acids, PABA, Probiotic Flora, Vitamin B_1, Vitamin B_6, Vitamin K, Zinc

Scopace Tablet (scopolamine): Dang Gui, Vitamin B_1

Seclopen (benzyl + procaine penicillin): Vitamin C

Seconal (secobarbital): DHEA, Gotu Kola, Valerian, Vitamin B_2

Sectral (acebutolol): Calcium, Carnitine, Chromium, Coenzyme Q10, Folic Acid, Magnesium, Melatonin, Potassium, Vitamin B_2, Vitamin B_3, Vitamin B_6, Vitamin C

Selexid (pivmecillinam): Carnitine

Selpak (selegiline): 5-HTP, Cayenne, Chromium, Eleuthero, Ephedra, Folic Acid, Ginkgo, Iron, Kava, Licorice, Phenylalanine, S-Adenosylmethionine (SAMe), St. John's Wort, Tryptophan, Tyrosine, Vitamin B_2, Vitamin B_6, Vitex

Senexon (senna): Potassium

Senna-Gen (senna): Potassium

Senokot (senna): Potassium

Senolax (senna): Potassium

Septra (trimethoprim + sulfamethoxazole): Calcium, Folic Acid, Licorice, Magnesium, PABA, Potassium, Probiotic Flora, Vitamin B_1, Vitamin B_2, Vitamin B_6, Vitamin C, Vitamin K, Zinc

Serax (oxazepam): DHEA, Gotu Kola, Melatonin, Valerian, Vitamin B_3

Serentil (mesoridazine): Coenzyme Q10, Milk Thistle, Vitamin B_2, Vitamin B_3, Vitamin C

Serevent (salmeterol): Calcium, Magnesium, Potassium

Seromycin (cycloserine): Calcium, Folic Acid, Magnesium, Milk Thistle, Vitamin B_6, Vitamin B_{12}, Vitamin C, Vitamin D

Seroquel (quetiapine): 5-HTP, Chromium, Echinacea, Ginkgo, Melatonin, Omega-3 Fatty Acids, Vitamin B_3, Vitamin B_6, Vitamin C

Seroxat (paroxetine): 5-HTP, Chromium, Folic Acid, Ginkgo, Inositol, Omega-3 Fatty Acids, S-Adenosylmethionine (SAMe), St. John's Wort, Tryptophan, Vitamin B_3, Vitamin B_6, Vitamin B_{12}, Vitamin C, Zinc

Serzone (nefazodone): St. John's Wort

Sevorane (sevoflurane): Aloe, Alpha-Lipoic Acid, Ephedra, Milk Thistle, St. John's Wort, Valerian

Silvadene (silver sulfadiazine): Calcium, Folic Acid, Licorice, Magnesium, PABA, Probiotic Flora, Vitamin B_1, Vitamin B_6, Vitamin K, Zinc

Sinemet (levodopa + carbidopa): 5-HTP, Folic Acid, Iron, Kava, Methionine, Phenylalanine, S-Adenosylmethionine (SAMe), Tyrosine, Vitamin B_3, Vitamin B_6, Vitamin C, Vitex

Sinemet CR (levodopa + carbidopa): 5-HTP, Folic Acid, Iron, Kava, Methionine, Phenylalanine, S-Adenosylmethionine (SAMe), Tyrosine, Vitamin B_3, Vitamin B_6, Vitamin C, Vitex

Sinequan (doxepin): 5-HTP, Coenzyme Q10, Echinacea, Milk Thistle, S-Adenosylmethionine (SAMe), St. John's Wort, Tryptophan, Tyrosine, Vitamin B_1, Vitamin B_2, Vitamin B_3, Vitamin B_6, Vitamin B_{12}, Zinc

Sintrom (nicoumalone): Bilberry, Cayenne, Chondroitin Sulfate, Coenzyme Q10, DHEA, Dang Gui, Devil's Claw, Feverfew, Garlic, Ginger, Ginkgo, Ginseng, Green Tea, Horse Chestnut, Kava, Licorice, Magnesium, Omega-3 Fatty Acids, Policosanol, Red Clover, Reishi, Saw Palmetto, St. John's Wort, Vitamin A, Vitamin B_3, Vitamin C, Vitamin E, Vitamin K, Zinc

Siterone (cyproterone): Black Cohosh, Vitamin D

Skelid (tiludronate): Calcium, Iron, Magnesium, Vitamin D, Zinc

Sleep Aid (doxylamine): Vitamin B_6

Slo-Bid (theophylline): Arginine, Cayenne, Ephedra, Magnesium, Melatonin, Potassium, St. John's Wort, Vitamin B_6

Slo-Phyllin (theophylline): Arginine, Cayenne, Ephedra, Magnesium, Melatonin, Potassium, St. John's Wort, Vitamin B_6

Slofedipine XL (nifedipine): Black Cohosh, Calcium, Dang Gui, Magnesium, Saw Palmetto

Snap Back (caffeine): Calcium, Ephedra, Kava, Melatonin

Sodium Sulamyd (sodium sulfacetamide): Calcium, Folic Acid, Licorice, Magnesium, PABA, Probiotic Flora, Vitamin B_1, Vitamin B_6, Vitamin K, Zinc

Solfoton (phenobarbital): Calcium, Carnitine, Copper, DHEA, Folic Acid, Ginkgo, Gotu Kola, Inositol, Kava, Milk Thistle, Omega-3 Fatty Acids, Reishi, Valerian, Vitamin A, Vitamin B_1, Vitamin B_2, Vitamin B_3, Vitamin B_6, Vitamin B_{12}, Vitamin C, Vitamin D, Vitamin E, Vitamin K, Vitex, Zinc

Soma Compound (ASA + carisoprodol): Bilberry, Calcium, Cayenne, Devil's Claw, Feverfew, Folic Acid, Garlic, Ginger, Ginkgo, Gotu Kola, Iron, Licorice, Melatonin, Milk, Thistle, Omega-3 Fatty Acids, Policosanol, Potassium, S-Adenosylmethionine (SAMe), Vitamin B_2 Vitamin B_3, Vitamin C, Vitamin E, Vitamin K, Zinc

Somac (pantoprazole): Beta-Carotene, Calcium, Chromium, Iron, Kava, St. John's Wort, Vitamin B_{12}, Zinc

Sonata (zaleplon): Gotu Kola, Melatonin, Valerian

Sorbitrate (isosorbide dinitrate): Arginine, Carnitine, Folic Acid, Vitamin C

Soriatane (acitretin): Beta-Carotene, Calcium, Carnitine, Omega-3 Fatty Acids, Vitamin A, Vitamin E

Sorine (sotalol): Calcium, Carnitine, Cascara, Chromium, Coenzyme Q10, Folic Acid, Magnesium, Melatonin, Potassium, Vitamin B_2, Vitamin B_3, Vitamin B_6, Vitamin C

Spectazole (econazole): Echinacea

Spectracef (cefditoren pivoxil): Carnitine

Spectrobid (bacampicillin): Ginseng, Green Tea

Sporanox (itraconazole): Echinacea, St. John's Wort

SSD (silver sulfadiazine): Calcium, Folic Acid, Licorice, Magnesium, PABA, Probiotic Flora, Vitamin B_1, Vitamin B_6, Vitamin K, Zinc

St Joseph Adult Chewable Aspirin (acetylsalicylic acid): Bilberry, Calcium, Cayenne, Devil's Claw, Feverfew, Folic Acid, Garlic, Ginger, Ginkgo, Gotu Kola, Iron, Licorice, Melatonin, Milk Thistle, Omega-3 Fatty Acids, Policosanol, Potassium, S-Adenosylmethionine (SAMe), Vitamin B_2, Vitamin B_3, Vitamin C, Vitamin E, Vitamin K, Zinc

Stadol (butorphanol): Ephedra, Ginseng, Gotu Kola, Phenylalanine, Tyrosine

Stadol NS (butorphanol): Ephedra, Ginseng, Gotu Kola, Phenylalanine, Tyrosine

Stagesic (hydrocodone + acetaminophen): Ephedra, Ginseng, Gotu Kola, Phenylalanine, Tyrosine

Stalevo (levodopa + carbidopa + entacapone): 5-HTP, Folic Acid, Iron, Kava, Methionine, Phenylalanine, S-Adenosylmethionine (SAMe), Tyrosine, Vitamin B_6, Vitamin C, Vitex

Starlix (nateglinide): Chromium, Vitamin B_3

Stay Alert (caffeine): Calcium, Ephedra, Kava, Melatonin

Stelazine (trifluoperazine): Coenzyme Q10, Milk Thistle, Vitamin B_2, Vitamin B_3, Vitamin C

Stemetil (prochlorperazine): Coenzyme Q10, Milk Thistle, Vitamin B_2, Vitamin B_3, Vitamin B_6, Vitamin C

Stilnoct (zolpidem): 5-HTP, Gotu Kola, Melatonin, Valerian

Stilphostrol (diethylstilbestrol): Black Cohosh

Streptase (streptokinase): Astragalus

Sublimaze Injection (fentanyl): Ephedra, Ginger, Ginseng, Gotu Kola, Magnesium, Phenylalanine, Tyrosine

Suboxone (buprenorphine + naloxone): Ephedra, Ginseng, Gotu Kola, Phenylalanine, Tyrosine

Subutex (buprenorphine): Ephedra, Ginseng, Gotu Kola, Phenylalanine, Tyrosine

Sudafed (pseudoephedrine): Potassium

Sudrine (pseudoephedrine): Potassium

Sular (nisoldipine): Calcium, Carnitine, Folic Acid, Magnesium, St. John's Wort, Vitamin B_6, Vitamin D

Sulfatrim Pediatric (trimethoprim + sulfamethoxazole): Calcium, Folic Acid, Licorice, Magnesium, PABA, Potassium, Probiotic Flora, Vitamin B_1, Vitamin B_2, Vitamin B_6, Vitamin C, Vitamin K, Zinc

Sultrin Triple Sulfa (triple sulfa): Calcium, Folic Acid, Licorice, Magnesium, PABA, Probiotic Flora, Vitamin B_1, Vitamin B_6, Vitamin K, Zinc

Sumycin (tetracycline): Calcium, Folic Acid, Iron, Magnesium, Potassium, Vitamin A, Vitamin B_1, Vitamin B_2, Vitamin B_3, Vitamin B_6, Vitamin C, Zinc

Superlipid (probucol): Beta-Carotene

Suphedrin (pseudoephedrine): Potassium

Suprane (desflurane): Alpha-Lipoic Acid, Ephedra, Milk Thistle, St. John's Wort, Valerian

Suprax (cefixime): Ginseng, Green Tea, Iron, Licorice, Probiotic Flora, Reishi, Vitamin B_1, Vitamin K, Zinc

Surfak (docusate): Magnesium, Potassium

Surmontil (trimipramine): 5-HTP, Coenzyme Q10, Echinacea, Milk Thistle, Potassium, S-Adenosylmethionine (SAMe), St. John's Wort, Tryptophan, Tyrosine, Vitamin B_1, Vitamin B_2, Vitamin B_3, Vitamin B_6, Vitamin B_{12}, Zinc

Sus-Phrine (epinephrine): Magnesium, Potassium, Vitamin C

Suspen (penicillin V potassium): Ginseng, Green Tea, Licorice, Probiotic Flora, Vitamin B_1, Vitamin K, Zinc

Sustiva (efavirenz): St. John's Wort, Vitamin B_2

Symbyax (olanzapine): 5-HTP, Chromium, Echinacea, Ginkgo, Melatonin, Omega-3 Fatty Acids, Vitamin B_3, Vitamin B_6, Vitamin C, Zinc

Synacort (hydrocortisone 17-butyrate/acetate/probutate/valerate): Aloe, Green Tea, Licorice, Vitamin C

Synelar (fluocinolone): Aloe, Green Tea, Licorice, Vitamin C

Synemol (fluocinolone): Aloe, Green Tea, Licorice, Vitamin C

Synthroid (levothyroxine): Alpha-Lipoic Acid, Calcium, Carnitine, Coenzyme Q10, DHEA, Iron, Tyrosine, Vitamin B_2

Syntocinon (oxytocin): Ephedra

Syprine (trientine): Copper, Iron

T-Gesic (hydrocodone + acetaminophen): Ephedra, Ginseng, Gotu Kola, Phenylalanine, Tyrosine

Tabloid (thioguanine): Echinacea, Eleuthero, Folic Acid, Vitamin B_1, Vitamin B_3

Tace (chlorotrianisene): Arginine, Black Cohosh, Boron, Calcium, Copper, DHEA, Dang Gui, Magnesium, Melatonin, Milk Thistle, St. John's Wort, Vitamin B_6, Vitamin D, Vitamin E, Vitex, Zinc

Tagamet (cimetidine): Calcium, Chromium, Copper, Folic Acid, Iron, Licorice, Magnesium, Vitamin B_{12}, Vitamin C, Vitamin D, Zinc

Tagamet HB (cimetidine): Calcium, Chromium, Copper, Folic Acid, Iron, Licorice, Magnesium, Vitamin B_{12}, Vitamin C, Vitamin D, Zinc

Talacen (acetaminophen + pentazocine): Ephedra, Garlic, Ginseng, Gotu Kola, Licorice, Methionine, Milk Thistle, Phenylalanine, Tyrosine, Vitamin C

Talwin (pentazocine): Ephedra, Ginseng, Gotu Kola, Phenylalanine, Tyrosine

Talwin Compound (acetylsalicylic acid + pentazocine): Calcium, Ephedra, Folic Acid, Ginseng, Gotu Kola, Iron, Licorice, Magnesium, Melatonin, Milk Thistle, Phenylalanine, Potassium, Tyrosine, Vitamin B_2, Vitamin B_3, Vitamin E

Talwin NX (pentazocine): Ephedra, Ginseng, Gotu Kola, Phenylalanine, Tyrosine

Tambocor (flecainide): Cascara, Magnesium, Potassium

Tao (troleandomycin): Calcium, Green Tea, Magnesium, Probiotic Flora, Vitamin B_1, Vitamin B_6, Vitamin K, Zinc

Tarabine PFS (cytarabine): Echinacea, Eleuthero, Folic Acid, Ginseng, Vitamin B_1

Targretin (bexarotene): Beta-Carotene, Calcium, Carnitine, Vitamin A, Vitamin E

Tarka (trandolapril + verapamil): Arginine, Calcium, Coenzyme Q10, Magnesium, Melatonin, Potassium, St. John's Wort, Vitamin E

Taxol (paclitaxel): Aloe, Beta-Carotene, Echinacea, Eleuthero, Feverfew, Ginseng, Melatonin, Omega-3 Fatty Acids, PABA, St. John's Wort, Turmeric/Curcumin, Vitamin A, Vitamin C, Vitamin E

Taxotere (docetaxel): Aloe, Beta-Carotene, Echinacea, Eleuthero, Feverfew, Ginseng, Melatonin, Omega-3 Fatty Acids, St. John's Wort, Turmeric/Curcumin, Vitamin A, Vitamin B_6, Vitamin C, Vitamin E

Tazicef (ceftazidime): Ginseng, Green Tea, Iron, Licorice, Probiotic Flora, Reishi, Vitamin B_1, Vitamin K, Zinc

Tazidime (ceftazidime): Ginseng, Green Tea, Iron, Licorice, Probiotic Flora, Reishi, Vitamin B_1, Vitamin K, Zinc

Tebrazid (pyrazinamide): Folic Acid, Milk Thistle, Vitamin B_3, Vitamin B_6, Vitamin C, Vitamin D

Tegison (etretinate): Beta-Carotene, Calcium, Carnitine, Omega-3 Fatty Acids, Vitamin A, Vitamin E

Tegretol (carbamazepine): Calcium, Carnitine, Copper, DHEA, Folic Acid, Ginkgo, Inositol, Kava, Milk Thistle, Omega-3 Fatty Acids, Valerian, Vitamin A, Vitamin B_1, Vitamin B_2, Vitamin B_3, Vitamin B_6, Vitamin B_{12}, Vitamin C, Vitamin D, Vitamin E, Vitamin K, Vitex, Zinc

Teladar (betamethasone dipropionate/valerate): Aloe, Green Tea, Licorice, Vitamin C

Temodar (temozolomide): Astragalus, Carnitine, Echinacea, Eleuthero, Selenium

Temovate (clobetasol): Aloe, Green Tea, Licorice, Vitamin C, Zinc

Tempo Tablets (aluminum hydroxide + magnesium hydroxide + calcium carbonate + simethicone): Calcium, Cayenne, Chromium, Copper, Folic Acid, Iron, Magnesium, Vitamin A, Vitamin B_1, Vitamin C, Vitamin D, Vitex, Zinc

Tenif (atenolol + nifedipine): Arginine, Calcium, Coenzyme Q10, Dang Gui, Magnesium, Policosanol, Potassium, St. John's Wort, Vitamin C

Tenoretic (atenolol + chlorthalidone): Arginine, Calcium, Coenzyme Q10, Policosanol, Potassium, Vitamin C

Tenormin (atenolol): Calcium, Carnitine, Chromium, Coenzyme Q10, Folic Acid, Magnesium, Melatonin, Potassium, Vitamin B_2, Vitamin B_3, Vitamin B_6, Vitamin C

Tensipine MR (nifedipine): Black Cohosh, Calcium, Dang Gui, Magnesium, Saw Palmetto

Teolit (testolactone): Beta-Carotene, DHEA, Vitamin A, Zinc

Tequin (gatifloxacin): Calcium, Green Tea, Iron, Licorice, Magnesium, Potassium, Probiotic Flora, Vitamin B_1, Vitamin K, Zinc

Terramycin (oxytetracycline): Calcium, Folic Acid, Iron, Magnesium, Potassium, Vitamin A, Vitamin B_1, Vitamin B_2, Vitamin B_3, Vitamin B_6, Vitamin C, Zinc

Teslac (testolactone): Beta-Carotene, DHEA, Vitamin A, Zinc

Teslak (testolactone): Beta-Carotene, DHEA, Vitamin A, Zinc

Testred (methyltestosterone): Beta-Carotene, DHEA, Vitamin A, Zinc

Tetracyn (tetracycline): Calcium, Folic Acid, Iron, Magnesium, Potassium, Vitamin A, Vitamin B_1, Vitamin B_2, Vitamin B_3, Vitamin B_6, Vitamin C, Zinc

Tetrathiomolybdate (tetrathiomolybdate): Copper, Zinc

Teveten (eprosartan): Alpha-Lipoic Acid, Potassium

Texacort (hydrocortisone 17-butyrate/acetate/probutate/valerate): Aloe, Green Tea, Licorice, Vitamin C

Theo-24 (theophylline): Arginine, Cayenne, Ephedra, Magnesium, Melatonin, Potassium, St. John's Wort, Vitamin B_6

Theo-Bid (theophylline): Arginine, Cayenne, Ephedra, Magnesium, Melatonin, Potassium, St. John's Wort, Vitamin B_6

Theo-Dur (theophylline): Arginine, Cayenne, Ephedra, Magnesium, Melatonin, Potassium, St. John's Wort, Vitamin B_6

Theocron (theophylline): Arginine, Cayenne, Ephedra, Magnesium, Melatonin, Potassium, St. John's Wort, Vitamin B_6

Theolair (theophylline): Arginine, Cayenne, Ephedra, Magnesium, Melatonin, Potassium, St. John's Wort, Vitamin B_6

Thiopental (thiopentone): DHEA, Ginger, Gotu Kola, Valerian, Vitamin B_2

Thioplex (thiotepa): Astragalus, Carnitine, Echinacea, Eleuthero, Selenium

Thioprine (azathioprine): Echinacea, Folic Acid, Vitamin B_3

Thorazine (chlorpromazine): Chromium, Coenzyme Q10, Ginkgo, Kava, Melatonin, Milk Thistle, Reishi, Vitamin B_2, Vitamin B_3, Vitamin B_6, Vitamin C, Vitamin E

Thyar (L-thyroxine + L-triiodothyronine, synthetic): Alpha-Lipoic Acid, Calcium, Carnitine, Coenzyme Q10, DHEA, Iron, Tyrosine, Vitamin B_2

Thyrolar (L-thyroxine + L-triiodothyronine, synthetic): Alpha-Lipoic Acid, Calcium, Carnitine, Coenzyme Q10, DHEA, Iron, Tyrosine, Vitamin B_2

Tiamate (diltiazem): Calcium, Carnitine, Folic Acid, Magnesium, St. John's Wort, Vitamin B_6, Vitamin D

Tiazac (diltiazem): Calcium, Carnitine, Folic Acid, Magnesium, St. John's Wort, Vitamin B_6, Vitamin D

Tiberal (ornidazole): Milk Thistle

Ticar (ticarcillin): Ginseng, Green Tea, Licorice, Probiotic Flora, Vitamin B_1, Vitamin K, Zinc

Ticlid (ticlopidine): Bilberry, Cayenne, Feverfew, Garlic, Ginger, Ginkgo, Omega-3 Fatty Acids, Policosanol, S-Adenosylmethionine (SAMe)

Tikosyn (dofetilide): Cascara, Magnesium, Potassium

Timentin (ticarcillin + clavulanic acid): Ginseng, Green Tea, Licorice, Probiotic Flora, Vitamin B_1, Vitamin K, Zinc

Tindamax (tinidazole): Milk Thistle

Titralac (calcium carbonate): Calcium, Cayenne, Chromium, Copper, Folic Acid, Iron, Vitamin A, Vitamin B_1, Vitamin D, Zinc

TOBI (tobramycin): Alpha-Lipoic Acid, Calcium, Eleuthero, Ginger, Ginkgo, Horse Chestnut, Licorice, Magnesium, Potassium, Probiotic Flora, Vitamin B_1, Vitamin B_6, Vitamin B_{12}, Vitamin K

TOBI Solution (tobramycin): Alpha-Lipoic Acid, Calcium, Eleuthero, Ginger, Ginkgo, Horse Chestnut, Licorice, Magnesium, Potassium, Probiotic Flora, Vitamin B_1, Vitamin B_6, Vitamin B_{12}, Vitamin K

Tobradex (dexamethasone + tobramycin): Alpha-Lipoic Acid, Calcium, Eleuthero, Ginger, Ginkgo, Horse Chestnut, Licorice, Magnesium, Potassium, Probiotic Flora, Vitamin B_1, Vitamin B_6, Vitamin B_{12}, Vitamin K

Tobrex (tobramycin): Alpha-Lipoic Acid, Calcium, Eleuthero, Ginger, Ginkgo, Horse Chestnut, Licorice, Magnesium, Potassium, Probiotic Flora, Vitamin B_1, Vitamin B_6, Vitamin B_{12}, Vitamin K

Tofranil (imipramine): 5-HTP, Coenzyme Q10, Echinacea, Milk Thistle, S-Adenosylmethionine (SAMe), St. John's Wort, Tryptophan, Tyrosine, Vitamin B_1, Vitamin B_2, Vitamin B_3, Vitamin B_6, Vitamin B_{12}, Zinc

Tol-Tab (tolbutamide): Aloe, Alpha-Lipoic Acid, Astragalus, Bilberry, Chromium, Coenzyme Q10, DHEA, Ephedra, Garlic, Ginkgo, Ginseng, Glucosamine Sulfate, Gotu Kola, Horse Chestnut, Magnesium, Omega-3 Fatty Acids, Reishi, Turmeric/Curcumin, Vitamin B_3

Tolectin (tolmetin): Calcium, Cayenne, Chondroitin Sulfate, Chromium, Copper, Devil's Claw, Feverfew, Folic Acid, Ginger, Glucosamine Sulfate, Gotu Kola, Iron, Licorice, Melatonin, Omega-3 Fatty Acids, Potassium, Turmeric/Curcumin, Vitamin B_3, Vitamin B_6, Vitamin C, Zinc

Tolinase (tolazamide): Aloe, Alpha-Lipoic Acid, Astragalus, Bilberry, Chromium, Coenzyme Q10, DHEA, Ephedra, Garlic, Ginkgo, Ginseng, Glucosamine Sulfate, Gotu Kola, Horse Chestnut, Magnesium, Omega-3 Fatty Acids, Reishi, Turmeric/Curcumin, Vitamin B3

Tomudex (raltitrexed): Echinacea, Eleuthero, Folic Acid, Vitamin B_1

Topamax (topiramate): Calcium, Carnitine, Copper, DHEA, Folic Acid, Ginkgo, Inositol, Kava, Milk Thistle, Omega-3 Fatty Acids, Potassium, Valerian, Vitamin A, Vitamin B_1, Vitamin B_2, Vitamin B_3, Vitamin B_6, Vitamin B_{12}, Vitamin C, Vitamin D, Vitamin E, Vitamin K, Vitex, Zinc

Topicort (desoximetasone): Aloe, Green Tea, Licorice, Vitamin C

Topicort LP (desoximetasone): Aloe, Green Tea, Licorice, Vitamin C

Topifort (clobetasol): Aloe, Green Tea, Licorice, Vitamin C, Zinc

Toradol (ketorolac): Calcium, Cayenne, Chondroitin Sulfate, Chromium, Copper, Devil's Claw, Feverfew, Folic Acid, Ginger, Glucosamine Sulfate, Gotu Kola, Iron, Licorice, Melatonin, Omega-3 Fatty Acids, Potassium, Turmeric/Curcumin, Vitamin B_3, Vitamin B_6, Vitamin C, Zinc

Torecan (thiethylperazine): Milk Thistle

Totacillin (ampicillin): Ginseng, Green Tea, Licorice, Probiotic Flora, Vitamin B_1, Vitamin C, Vitamin K, Zinc

Tracrium (atracurium): Ginger, Magnesium

Tramake (tramadol): 5-HTP

Trandate (labetalol): Potassium

Transderm Scop Patch (scopolamine): Dang Gui, Vitamin B_1

Transderm-Nitro (nitroglycerin): Arginine, Carnitine, Folic Acid, Vitamin C

Tranxene (clorazepate): Calcium, Carnitine, Copper, DHEA, Folic Acid, Ginkgo, Gotu Kola, Inositol, Kava, Melatonin, Milk Thistle, Omega-3 Fatty Acids, Tryptophan, Valerian, Vitamin A, Vitamin B_1, Vitamin B_2, Vitamin B_3, Vitamin B_6, Vitamin B_{12}, Vitamin C, Vitamin D, Vitamin E, Vitamin K, Vitex, Zinc

Trasicor (oxprenolol): Calcium, Carnitine, Chromium, Coenzyme Q10, Folic Acid, Magnesium, Melatonin, Potassium, Vitamin B_2, Vitamin B_3, Vitamin B_6, Vitamin C

Trasidrex (oxprenolol + cyclopenthiazide): Arginine, Calcium, Coenzyme Q10, Ginkgo, Glucosamine Sulfate, Hawthorn, Licorice, Magnesium, Potassium, Vitamin D, Zinc

Trecator SC (ethionamide): Folic Acid, Milk Thistle, Vitamin B_6, Vitamin C, Vitamin D

Trelstar LA (triptorelin): Black Cohosh, Melatonin, Vitamin D

Trental (pentoxifylline): Arginine, Cayenne, Coenzyme Q10, Policosanol, Vitamin E

Tri-Levlen (ethinyl estradiol + levonorgestrel): Arginine, Calcium, Copper, DHEA, Dang Gui, Folic Acid, Iron, Licorice, Magnesium, Melatonin, Milk Thistle, S-Adenosylmethionine (SAMe), Selenium, St. John's Wort, Tyrosine, Vitamin A, Vitamin B_1, Vitamin B_2, Vitamin B_3, Vitamin B_6, Vitamin B_{12}, Vitamin C, Vitamin E, Vitex, Zinc

Tri-Norinyl (ethinyl estradiol + norethindrone): Arginine, Calcium, Copper, DHEA, Dang Gui, Folic Acid, Iron, Licorice, Magnesium, Melatonin, Milk Thistle, S-Adenosylmethionine (SAMe), Selenium, St. John's Wort, Tyrosine, Vitamin A, Vitamin B_1, Vitamin B_2, Vitamin B_3, Vitamin B_6, Vitamin B_{12}, Vitamin C, Vitamin E, Vitex, Zinc

Triaminic A.M. (pseudoephedrine): Potassium

Triapin (felodipine + ramipril): Arginine, Calcium, Coenzyme Q10, Magnesium, Potassium, St. John's Wort

Triavil (amitriptyline + perphenazine): Coenzyme Q10, Echinacea, Milk Thistle, St. John's Wort, Vitamin B_{12}

Tricor (fenofibrate): Coenzyme Q10, Copper, Folic Acid, Gotu Kola, Omega-3 Fatty Acids, Vitamin B_3, Vitamin B_6, Vitamin B_{12}, Vitamin C, Vitamin E, Zinc

Tridesilon (desonide): Aloe, Green Tea, Licorice, Vitamin C

Tridil (nitroglycerin): Arginine, Carnitine, Folic Acid, Vitamin C

Tridione (trimethadione): Carnitine, Folic Acid

Trifluperidol (triperidol): Milk Thistle, Phenylalanine

Triglide (fenofibrate): Coenzyme Q10, Copper, Folic Acid, Gotu Kola, Omega-3 Fatty Acids, Vitamin B_3, Vitamin B_6, Vitamin B_{12}, Vitamin C, Vitamin E, Zinc

Trilafon (perphenazine): Coenzyme Q10, Milk Thistle, Vitamin B_2, Vitamin B_3, Vitamin C

Trileptal (oxcarbazepine): Calcium, Carnitine, Copper, DHEA, Folic Acid, Ginkgo, Inositol, Kava, Milk Thistle, Omega-3 Fatty Acids, Valerian, Vitamin A, Vitamin B_1, Vitamin B_2, Vitamin B_3, Vitamin B_6, Vitamin B_{12}, Vitamin C, Vitamin D, Vitamin E, Vitamin K, Vitex, Zinc

Trimovate (neomycin + nystatin + clobetasone): Aloe, Beta-Carotene, Green Tea, Licorice, Vitamin C, Zinc

Trimox (amoxicillin): Ginseng, Green Tea, Licorice, Probiotic Flora, Vitamin B_1, Vitamin K, Zinc

Trimpex (trimethoprim): Folic Acid, Licorice, Probiotic Flora, Vitamin B_2, Vitamin K, Zinc

Trinovum (ethinyl estradiol + norethindrone): Arginine, Calcium, Copper, DHEA, Dang Gui, Folic Acid, Iron, Licorice, Magnesium, Melatonin, Milk Thistle, S-Adenosylmethionine (SAMe), Selenium, St. John's Wort, Tyrosine, Vitamin A, Vitamin B_1, Vitamin B_2, Vitamin B_3, Vitamin B_6, Vitamin B_{12}, Vitamin C, Vitamin E, Vitex, Zinc

Triostat (injection) (L-triiodothyronine): Alpha-Lipoic Acid, Calcium, Carnitine, Coenzyme Q10, DHEA, Iron, Tyrosine, Vitamin B_2

Triphasil (ethinyl estradiol + levonorgestrel): Arginine, Calcium, Copper, DHEA, Dang Gui, Folic Acid, Iron, Licorice, Magnesium, Melatonin, Milk Thistle, S-Adenosylmethionine (SAMe), Selenium, St. John's Wort, Tyrosine, Vitamin A, Vitamin B_1, Vitamin B_2, Vitamin B_3, Vitamin B_6, Vitamin B_{12}, Vitamin C, Vitamin E, Vitex, Zinc

Triptazine (amitriptyline + perphenazine): Coenzyme Q10, Echinacea, Milk Thistle, St. John's Wort, Vitamin B_{12}

Trisequens (estradiol + norethindrone, oral): Arginine, Black Cohosh, Boron, Calcium, Copper, DHEA, Dang Gui, Magnesium, Melatonin, Milk Thistle, St. John's Wort, Vitamin B_6, Vitamin D, Vitamin E, Vitex, Zinc

Tritec (ranitidine + bismuth + citrate): Calcium, Chromium, Copper, Folic Acid, Iron, Licorice, Magnesium, Vitamin B_{12}, Vitamin C, Zinc

Trivora (ethinyl estradiol + levonorgestrel): Arginine, Calcium, Copper, DHEA, Dang Gui, Folic Acid, Iron, Licorice, Magnesium, Melatonin, Milk Thistle, S-Adenosylmethionine (SAMe), Selenium, St. John's Wort, Tyrosine, Vitamin A, Vitamin B_1, Vitamin B_2, Vitamin B_3, Vitamin B_6, Vitamin B_{12}, Vitamin C, Vitamin E, Vitex, Zinc

Trizivir (abacavir + lamivudine + zidovudine): Aloe, Carnitine, Coenzyme Q10, Copper, DHEA, Folic Acid, Reishi, Vitamin B_1, Vitamin B_2, Vitamin B_{12}, Vitamin E, Zinc

Tromexan (ethyl biscoumacetate): Bilberry, Cayenne, Chondroitin Sulfate, Coenzyme Q10, DHEA, Dang Gui, Devil's Claw, Feverfew, Garlic, Ginger, Ginkgo, Ginseng, Green Tea, Horse Chestnut, Kava, Licorice, Magnesium, Omega-3 Fatty Acids, Policosanol, Red Clover, Reishi, Saw Palmetto, St. John's Wort, Vitamin A, Vitamin B_3, Vitamin C, Vitamin E, Vitamin K, Zinc

Trovan (trovafloxacin): Calcium, Green Tea, Iron, Licorice, Magnesium, Potassium, Probiotic Flora, Vitamin B_1, Vitamin K, Zinc

Truphylline (theophylline): Arginine, Cayenne, Ephedra, Magnesium, Melatonin, Potassium, St. John's Wort, Vitamin B_6

Trusopt (dorzolamide): Potassium

Truxcillin (penicillin V potassium): Ginseng, Green Tea, Licorice, Probiotic Flora, Vitamin B_1, Vitamin K, Zinc

Truxcillin VK (penicillin V): Ginseng, Green Tea, Licorice, Probiotic Flora, Vitamin B_1, Vitamin K, Zinc

Tums (calcium carbonate): Calcium, Cayenne, Chromium, Copper, Folic Acid, Iron, Vitamin A, Vitamin B_1, Vitamin D, Zinc

Tylenol (acetaminophen): Dang Gui, Devil's Claw, Garlic, Gotu Kola, Licorice, Methionine, Milk Thistle, S-Adenosylmethionine (SAMe), Vitamin C

Tylenol Cold (acetaminophen + chlorpheniramine + dextromethorphan + pseudoephedrine): Garlic, Licorice, Methionine, Milk Thistle, S-Adenosylmethionine (SAMe), Vitamin C

Tylenol with Codeine (acetaminophen + codeine): Ephedra, Garlic, Ginseng, Gotu Kola, Licorice, Methionine, Milk Thistle, Phenylalanine, S-Adenosylmethionine (SAMe), Tyrosine, Vitamin C

Tylox (acetaminophen + oxycodone): Ephedra, Garlic, Ginseng, Gotu Kola, Licorice, Milk Thistle, Phenylalanine, Tyrosine, Vitamin C

Ultane (sevoflurane): Aloe, Alpha-Lipoic Acid, Ephedra, Milk Thistle, St. John's Wort, Valerian

Ultralan (fluocortolone): Aloe, Green Tea, Licorice, Vitamin C

Ultram (tramadol): 5-HTP

Ultravate (halobetasol): Aloe, Green Tea, Licorice, Vitamin C

Uni-Dur (theophylline): Arginine, Cayenne, Ephedra, Magnesium, Melatonin, Potassium, St. John's Wort, Vitamin B_6

Unihep (heparin): Calcium, Cayenne, Chondroitin Sulfate, DHEA, Omega-3 Fatty Acids, Policosanol, Potassium, Vitamin C, Vitamin D

Uniparin Calcium (heparin): Calcium, Cayenne, Chondroitin Sulfate, DHEA, Omega-3 Fatty Acids, Policosanol, Potassium, Vitamin C, Vitamin D

Uniparin Forte (heparin): Calcium, Cayenne, Chondroitin Sulfate, DHEA, Omega-3 Fatty Acids, Policosanol, Potassium, Vitamin C, Vitamin D

Unipen (nafcillin): Ginseng, Green Tea, Licorice, Probiotic Flora, Vitamin B_1, Vitamin K, Zinc

Uniphyl (theophylline): Arginine, Cayenne, Ephedra, Magnesium, Melatonin, Potassium, St. John's Wort, Vitamin B_6

Unipine XL (nifedipine): Black Cohosh, Calcium, Dang Gui, Magnesium, Saw Palmetto

Unisom (doxylamine): Vitamin B_6

Unisyn (ampicillin + sulbactam): Ginseng, Green Tea, Licorice, Probiotic Flora, Vitamin B_1, Vitamin K, Zinc

Unithroid (levothyroxine): Alpha-Lipoic Acid, Calcium, Carnitine, Coenzyme Q10, DHEA, Iron, Tyrosine, Vitamin B_2

Unitrol (phenylpropanolamine): Potassium, Tyrosine

Univasc (moexipril): Arginine, Cayenne, Iron, Omega-3 Fatty Acids, Potassium, Vitamin E, Zinc

Urdox (ursodeoxycholic acid): S-Adenosylmethionine (SAMe), Vitamin B_3

Urso (ursodeoxycholic acid): S-Adenosylmethionine (SAMe), Vitamin B_3

Ursofalk (ursodeoxycholic acid): S-Adenosylmethionine (SAMe), Vitamin B_3

Ursogal (ursodeoxycholic acid): S-Adenosylmethionine (SAMe), Vitamin B_3

Uticort (betamethasone dipropionate/valerate): Aloe, Green Tea, Licorice, Vitamin C

Utrogestan (progesterone, micronized): Vitamin D

V-Cillin K (penicillin V): Ginseng, Green Tea, Licorice, Probiotic Flora, Vitamin B_1, Vitamin K, Zinc

Vagifem (estradiol hemihydrate): Arginine, Black Cohosh, Boron, Calcium, Copper, DHEA, Dang Gui, Magnesium, Melatonin, Milk Thistle, St. John's Wort, Vitamin B_6, Vitamin D, Vitamin E, Vitex, Zinc

Valergen 20 (estradiol valerate): Arginine, Black Cohosh, Boron, Calcium, Copper, DHEA, Dang Gui, Magnesium, Melatonin, Milk Thistle, St. John's Wort, Vitamin B_6, Vitamin D, Vitamin E, Vitex, Zinc

Valisone (betamethasone dipropionate/valerate): Aloe, Green Tea, Licorice, Vitamin C

Valium (diazepam): Carnitine, DHEA, Gotu Kola, Melatonin, Valerian, Vitamin B_3

Vancenase (beclomethasone inhalant): Calcium

Vancenase AQ (beclomethasone inhalant): Calcium

Vanceril (beclomethasone inhalant): Calcium

Vancocin (vancomycin): Licorice, Probiotic Flora, Vitamin K, Zinc

Vanos (fluocinonide): Aloe, Green Tea, Licorice, Vitamin C

Vanticon (zafirlukast): Melatonin

Vantin (cefpodoxime): Ginseng, Green Tea, Iron, Licorice, Probiotic Flora, Reishi, Vitamin B_1, Vitamin K, Zinc

Vascor (bepridil): Calcium, Carnitine, Folic Acid, Magnesium, St. John's Wort, Vitamin B_6, Vitamin D

Vaseretic (enalapril + hydrochlorothiazide): Arginine, Calcium, Cayenne, Coenzyme Q10, Glucosamine Sulfate, Hawthorn, Licorice, Magnesium, Potassium, Vitamin D, Zinc

Vasotec (enalapril): Arginine, Cayenne, Iron, Omega-3 Fatty Acids, Potassium, Vitamin E, Zinc

Vasoxyl (methoxamine): Melatonin

Vectrin (minocycline): Calcium, Folic Acid, Iron, Magnesium, Potassium, Vitamin A, Vitamin B_1, Vitamin B_2, Vitamin B_3, Vitamin B_6, Vitamin C, Zinc

Veetids (penicillin V potassium): Ginseng, Green Tea, Licorice, Probiotic Flora, Vitamin B_1, Vitamin K, Zinc

Velban (vinblastine): Echinacea, Eleuthero, Feverfew, Ginseng, St. John's Wort, Turmeric/Curcumin

Velocef (cephradine): Ginseng, Green Tea, Iron, Licorice, Probiotic Flora, Reishi, Vitamin B_1, Vitamin K, Zinc

Velsar (vinblastine): Echinacea, Eleuthero, Feverfew, Ginseng, St. John's Wort, Turmeric/Curcumin

Ventolin (albuterol): Calcium, Magnesium, Potassium

Vepesid (etoposide): Aloe, Feverfew, Ginseng, Melatonin, Omega-3 Fatty Acids, St. John's Wort

Vercyte (pipobroman): Astragalus, Carnitine, Echinacea, Eleuthero, Selenium

Verelan (verapamil): Calcium, Carnitine, Folic Acid, Magnesium, Melatonin, St. John's Wort, Vitamin B_6, Vitamin D, Vitamin E

Verelan PM (verapamil): Calcium, Carnitine, Folic Acid, Magnesium, Melatonin, St. John's Wort, Vitamin B_6, Vitamin D, Vitamin E

Versed (midazolam): DHEA, Gotu Kola, Kava, Melatonin, St. John's Wort, Valerian, Vitamin B_3

Vesanoid (tretinoin): Beta-Carotene, Calcium, Carnitine, Vitamin A, Vitamin E

Vesprin (triflupromazine): Coenzyme Q10, Milk Thistle, Vitamin B_2, Vitamin B_3, Vitamin C

Vfend (voriconazole): Echinacea, St. John's Wort

Viagra (sildenafil): Arginine

Vibra-Tabs (doxycycline): Calcium, Folic Acid, Iron, Magnesium, Potassium, Vitamin A, Vitamin B_1, Vitamin B_2, Vitamin B_3, Vitamin B_6, Vitamin C, Zinc

Vibramycin (doxycycline): Calcium, Folic Acid, Iron, Magnesium, Potassium, Vitamin A, Vitamin B_1, Vitamin B_2, Vitamin B_3, Vitamin B_6, Vitamin C, Zinc

Vicodin (hydrocodone + acetaminophen): Ephedra, Ginseng, Gotu Kola, Phenylalanine, Tyrosine

Vicodin ES (hydrocodone + acetaminophen): Ephedra, Ginseng, Gotu Kola, Phenylalanine, Tyrosine

Vicodin HP (hydrocodone + acetaminophen): Ephedra, Ginseng, Gotu Kola, Phenylalanine, Tyrosine

Vicoprofen (ibuprofen + hydrocodone): Calcium, Cayenne, Chondroitin Sulfate, Chromium, Copper, Devil's Claw,

Cross-Indexes

Ephedra, Feverfew, Folic Acid, Ginger, Ginseng, Glucosamine Sulfate, Gotu Kola, Iron, Licorice, Melatonin, Omega-3 Fatty Acids, Phenylalanine, Potassium, Turmeric/Curcumin, Tyrosine, Vitamin B$_3$, Vitamin B$_6$, Vitamin C, Zinc

Videx (didanosine): Aloe, Carnitine, Coenzyme Q10, Copper, DHEA, Reishi, Vitamin B$_1$, Vitamin B$_2$, Vitamin B$_{12}$, Zinc

Vigilon (polyethylene oxide sheet dressing): Aloe

Vika (levonorgestrel, oral postcoital contraceptive): Magnesium, St. John's Wort

Vikela (levonorgestrel, oral postcoital contraceptive): Magnesium, St. John's Wort

Vilona (ribavirin): S-Adenosylmethionine (SAMe)

Vincasar PFS (vincristine): Alpha-Lipoic Acid, Echinacea, Eleuthero, Feverfew, Ginseng, St. John's Wort, Turmeric/Curcumin

Vioxx (rofecoxib): Calcium, Cayenne, Chondroitin Sulfate, Chromium, Copper, Devil's Claw, Feverfew, Folic Acid, Ginger, Glucosamine Sulfate, Gotu Kola, Iron, Licorice, Melatonin, Omega-3 Fatty Acids, Potassium, Turmeric/Curcumin, Vitamin B$_3$, Vitamin C, Zinc

Vira-A (vidarabine): Methionine, Reishi, S-Adenosylmethionine (SAMe)

Viracept (nelfinavir): Copper, Garlic, St. John's Wort, Vitamin C

Viramune (nevirapine): St. John's Wort, Vitamin B$_2$

Virazole (ribavirin): S-Adenosylmethionine (SAMe)

Viread (tenofovir): Aloe, Carnitine, Coenzyme Q10, DHEA, Reishi, Vitamin B$_1$, Vitamin B$_2$, Vitamin B$_{12}$, Zinc

Virilon (methyltestosterone): Beta-Carotene, DHEA, Vitamin A, Zinc

Visken (pindolol): Calcium, Carnitine, Chromium, Coenzyme Q10, Folic Acid, Magnesium, Melatonin, Potassium, Vitamin B$_2$, Vitamin B$_3$, Vitamin B$_6$, Vitamin C

Vitinoin (tretinoin): Beta-Carotene, Calcium, Carnitine, Vitamin A, Vitamin E

Vivactil (protriptyline): 5-HTP, Coenzyme Q10, Milk Thistle, S-Adenosylmethionine (SAMe), St. John's Wort, Tryptophan, Tyrosine, Vitamin B$_1$, Vitamin B$_2$, Vitamin B$_3$, Vitamin B$_6$, Vitamin B$_{12}$, Zinc

Vivarin (caffeine): Calcium, Ephedra, Kava, Melatonin

Vivelle-Dot (estradiol): Arginine, Black Cohosh, Boron, Calcium, Copper, DHEA, Dang Gui, Magnesium, Melatonin, Milk Thistle, St. John's Wort, Vitamin B$_6$, Vitamin D, Vitamin E, Vitex, Zinc

Vivelle Transdermal (estradiol): Arginine, Black Cohosh, Boron, Calcium, Copper, DHEA, Dang Gui, Magnesium, Melatonin, Milk Thistle, St. John's Wort, Vitamin B$_6$, Vitamin D, Vitamin E, Vitex, Zinc

Voltaren (diclofenac): Calcium, Cayenne, Chondroitin Sulfate, Chromium, Copper, Devil's Claw, Feverfew, Folic Acid, Ginger, Glucosamine Sulfate, Gotu Kola, Iron, Licorice, Melatonin, Omega-3 Fatty Acids, Potassium, Turmeric/Curcumin, Vitamin B$_3$, Vitamin B$_6$, Vitamin C, Zinc

VP-16 (etoposide): Aloe, Feverfew, Ginseng, Melatonin, Omega-3 Fatty Acids, St. John's Wort

Vumon (teniposide): St. John's Wort

Warfilone (warfarin): Bilberry, Cayenne, Chondroitin Sulfate, Coenzyme Q10, DHEA, Dang Gui, Devil's Claw, Echinacea, Feverfew, Garlic, Ginger, Ginkgo, Ginseng, Green Tea, Horse Chestnut, Iron, Kava, Licorice, Magnesium, Omega-3 Fatty Acids, Policosanol, Red Clover, Reishi, Saw Palmetto, St. John's Wort, Vitamin A, Vitamin B$_3$, Vitamin C, Vitamin D, Vitamin E, Vitamin K, Zinc

WelChol (colesevelam): Beta-Carotene, Calcium, Folic Acid, Iron, Omega-3 Fatty Acids, Vitamin A, Vitamin B$_2$, Vitamin B$_3$, Vitamin B$_{12}$, Vitamin D, Vitamin E, Vitamin K, Zinc

Wellbutrin (bupropion): Melatonin

Westcort (hydrocortisone 17-butyrate/acetate/probutate/valerate): Aloe, Green Tea, Licorice, Vitamin C

Westhroid (L-thyroxine + L-triiodothyronine): Alpha-Lipoic Acid, Calcium, Carnitine, Coenzyme Q10, DHEA, Iron, Tyrosine, Vitamin B$_2$

Winstrol (stanozolol): Echinacea, Iron

Wygesic (acetaminophen + propoxyphene): Ephedra, Garlic, Ginseng, Gotu Kola, Licorice, Milk Thistle, Phenylalanine, Tyrosine, Vitamin C

Wymox (amoxicillin): Ginseng, Green Tea, Licorice, Probiotic Flora, Vitamin B$_1$, Vitamin K, Zinc

Xanax (alprazolam): DHEA, Gotu Kola, Kava, Melatonin, St. John's Wort, Valerian, Vitamin B$_3$

Xeloda (capecitabine): Echinacea, Eleuthero, Folic Acid, Vitamin B$_1$

Xenical (orlistat): Beta-Carotene, Coenzyme Q10, Vitamin A, Vitamin D, Vitamin E, Vitamin K

Xopenex (levalbuterol): Calcium, Magnesium, Potassium

Zagam (sparfloxacin): Calcium, Green Tea, Iron, Licorice, Magnesium, Potassium, Probiotic Flora, Vitamin B$_1$, Vitamin K, Zinc

Zamadol (tramadol): 5-HTP

Zanidip (lercanidipine): Calcium, Carnitine, Folic Acid, Magnesium, St. John's Wort, Vitamin B$_6$, Vitamin D

Zanosar (streptozocin): Astragalus, Carnitine, Echinacea, Eleuthero, Selenium

Zantac (ranitidine): Calcium, Chromium, Copper, Folic Acid, Iron, Licorice, Magnesium, Vitamin B$_{12}$, Vitamin C, Zinc

Zarontin (ethosuximide): Calcium, Carnitine, Copper, DHEA, Folic Acid, Ginkgo, Inositol, Kava, Milk Thistle, Omega-3 Fatty Acids, Valerian, Vitamin A, Vitamin B$_1$, Vitamin B$_2$, Vitamin B$_3$, Vitamin B$_6$, Vitamin B$_{12}$, Vitamin C, Vitamin D, Vitamin E, Vitamin K, Vitex, Zinc

Zaroxolyn (metolazone): Calcium, Coenzyme Q10, Folic Acid, Ginkgo, Glucosamine Sulfate, Hawthorn, Licorice, Magnesium, Potassium, Vitamin B$_2$, Vitamin D, Zinc

Zavedos (idarubicin): Alpha-Lipoic Acid, Carnitine, Coenzyme Q10, Feverfew, Garlic, Ginkgo, Green Tea, Hawthorn, Milk Thistle, Reishi, Selenium, St. John's Wort, Turmeric/Curcumin, Vitamin B$_2$, Vitamin E

Zebeta (bisoprolol): Calcium, Carnitine, Chromium, Coenzyme Q10, Folic Acid, Magnesium, Melatonin, Potassium, Vitamin B$_2$, Vitamin B$_3$, Vitamin B$_6$, Vitamin C

Zentel (albendazole): Beta-Carotene, Vitamin A

Zerit (stavudine): Aloe, Carnitine, Coenzyme Q10, DHEA, Reishi, Vitamin B$_1$, Vitamin B$_2$, Vitamin B$_{12}$, Zinc

Zestoretic (lisinopril + hydrochlorothiazide): Arginine, Calcium, Cayenne, Coenzyme Q10, Glucosamine Sulfate, Hawthorn, Licorice, Magnesium, Potassium, Vitamin D, Zinc

Zestril (lisinopril): Arginine, Cayenne, Iron, Omega-3 Fatty Acids, Potassium, Vitamin E, Zinc

Zetia (ezetimibe): Policosanol

Ziagen (abacavir): Aloe, Carnitine, Coenzyme Q10, DHEA, Reishi, Vitamin B$_1$, Vitamin B$_2$, Vitamin B$_{12}$, Zinc

Zinacef (cefuroxime): Ginseng, Green Tea, Iron, Licorice, Probiotic Flora, Reishi, Vitamin B$_1$, Vitamin K, Zinc

Zithromax (azithromycin): Calcium, Green Tea, Magnesium, Probiotic Flora, Vitamin B$_1$, Vitamin B$_6$, Vitamin K, Zinc

Zocor (simvastatin): Beta-Carotene, Carnitine, Coenzyme Q10, Garlic, Gotu Kola, Omega-3 Fatty Acids, Policosanol, Reishi, Selenium, St. John's Wort, Vitamin A, Vitamin B$_3$, Vitamin B$_{12}$, Vitamin C, Vitamin E

Zoladex (goserelin): Black Cohosh, Vitamin D

Zoloft (sertraline): Chromium, Folic Acid, Ginkgo, Inositol, Omega-3 Fatty Acids, S-Adenosylmethionine (SAMe), St. John's Wort, Tryptophan, Vitamin B$_3$, Vitamin B$_6$, Vitamin B$_{12}$, Vitamin C, Zinc

Zometa (zoledronic acid): Calcium, Iron, Magnesium, Vitamin D, Zinc

Zomig (zolmitriptan): 5-HTP, Feverfew, Tryptophan

Zonegran (zonisamide): Calcium, Carnitine, Copper, DHEA, Folic Acid, Ginkgo, Inositol, Kava, Milk Thistle, Omega-3 Fatty Acids, Potassium, Valerian, Vitamin A, Vitamin B$_1$, Vitamin B$_2$, Vitamin B$_3$, Vitamin B$_6$, Vitamin B$_{12}$, Vitamin C, Vitamin D, Vitamin E, Vitamin K, Vitex, Zinc

ZORprin (acetylsalicylic acid): Bilberry, Calcium, Cayenne, Devil's Claw, Feverfew, Folic Acid, Garlic, Ginger, Ginkgo, Gotu Kola, Iron, Licorice, Melatonin, Milk Thistle, Omega-3 Fatty Acids, Policosanol, Potassium, S-Adenosyl-methionine (SAMe), Vitamin B$_2$, Vitamin B$_3$, Vitamin C, Vitamin E, Vitamin K, Zinc

Zosyn (piperacillin + tazobactam): Ginseng, Green Tea, Licorice, Probiotic Flora, Vitamin B$_1$, Vitamin K, Zinc

Zoton (lansoprazole): Beta-Carotene, Calcium, Chromium, Iron, Kava, Probiotic Flora, St. John's Wort, Vitamin B$_{12}$, Zinc

Zovia (ethinyl estradiol + ethynodiol): Arginine, Calcium, Copper, DHEA, Dang Gui, Folic Acid, Iron, Licorice, Magnesium, Melatonin, Milk Thistle, S-Adenosylmethionine (SAMe), Selenium, St. John's Wort, Tyrosine, Vitamin A, Vitamin B$_1$, Vitamin B$_2$, Vitamin B$_3$, Vitamin B$_6$, Vitamin B$_{12}$, Vitamin C, Vitamin E, Vitex, Zinc

Zovirax (acyclovir): Aloe, Astragalus, Folic Acid, Reishi

Zydol (tramadol): 5-HTP

Zydone (hydrocodone + acetaminophen): Ephedra, Ginseng, Gotu Kola, Phenylalanine, Tyrosine

Zyloprim (allopurinol): Carnitine, Copper, Iron, Tryptophan, Vitamin D

Zyprexa (olanzapine): 5-HTP, Chromium, Echinacea, Ginkgo, Melatonin, Omega-3 Fatty Acids, Vitamin B$_3$, Vitamin B$_6$, Vitamin C, Zinc

Zyvox (linezolid): Licorice, Probiotic Flora, Vitamin K, Zinc

Quick Guide to Interactions Evaluation System

Interaction Probability Guide

I. PROBABILITY OF CLINICALLY SIGNIFICANT INTERACTION:

1. Certain
2. Probable
3. Possible
4. Plausible
5. Improbable
6. Unknown

II. TYPE AND CLINICAL SIGNIFICANCE OF INTERACTION:

✗   Potential or Theoretical Adverse Interaction of Uncertain Severity

✗✗   Minimal to Mild Adverse Interaction—Vigilance Necessary

✗✗✗   Potentially Harmful or Serious Adverse Interaction—Avoid

◇   Impaired Drug Absorption and Bioavailability, Negligible Effect

◇◇   Impaired Drug Absorption and Bioavailability, Precautions Appropriate

◇◇◇   Impaired Drug Absorption and Bioavailability, Avoidance Appropriate

◇   Adverse Drug Effect on Herbal Therapeutics, Strategic Concern

◇   Adverse Drug Effect on Nutrient Therapeutics, Strategic Concern

◇≈≈   Drug-Induced Adverse Effect on Nutrient Function, Coadministration Therapeutic, with Professional Management

◇≈≈   Drug-Induced Adverse Effect on Nutrient Function, Supplementation Therapeutic, Not Requiring Professional Management

◇◇   Drug-Induced Effect on Nutrient Function, Supplementation Contraindicated, Professional Management Appropriate

⊕✗   Bimodal or Variable Interaction, with Professional Management

⊕   Potential or Theoretical Beneficial or Supportive Interaction, with Professional Management

⊕⊕   Beneficial or Supportive Interaction, with Professional Management

⊕⊕⊕   Beneficial or Supportive Interaction, Not Requiring Professional Management

≈≈   Drug-Induced Nutrient Depletion, Supplementation Therapeutic, with Professional Management

≈≈≈   Drug-Induced Nutrient Depletion, Supplementation Therapeutic, Not Requiring Professional Management

≈◇◇   Drug-Induced Nutrient Depletion, Supplementation Contraindicated, Professional Management Appropriate

☼   Prevention or Reduction of Drug Adverse Effect

☼   Prevention or Reduction of Herb or Nutrient Adverse Effect

?   Interaction Possible but Uncertain Occurrence and Unclear Implications

III. STRENGTH AND QUALITY OF SOURCE EVIDENCE:

● Consensus
◉ Emerging
○ Preliminary
▽ Mixed
☐ Inadequate

Index

Printed and bound by CPI Group (UK) Ltd, Croydon, CR0 4YY

03/10/2024

01040364-0011